PATHOPHYSIOLOGY

The Biologic Basis for Disease in Adults and Children

PATHOPHYSIOLOGY

The Biologic Basis for Disease in Adults and Children

SECOND EDITION

Kathryn L. McCance, RN, PhD

Professor, College of Nursing,
University of Utah, Salt Lake City, Utah

Sue E. Huether, RN, PhD

Associate Professor, College of Nursing,
University of Utah, Salt Lake City, Utah

with 1030 *illustrations*

St. Louis Baltimore Boston Chicago London Madrid Philadelphia Sydney Toronto

Dedicated to Publishing Excellence

Editor: Sally Schrefer
Developmental Editor: Penny Rudolph
Project Manager: Karen Edwards
Production Editor: Gail Brower
Designer: Elizabeth Fett
Manufacturing Supervisor: Karen Lewis

SECOND EDITION

Printed in the United States of America
Composition by The Clarinda Company
Printing/binding by Von Hoffmann Press, Inc.

Mosby–Year Book, Inc.
11830 Westline Industrial Drive
St. Louis, Missouri 63146

Library of Congress Cataloging in Publication Data

McCance, Kathryn L.
    Pathophysiology: the biologic basis for diseases in adults and
children / Kathryn L. McCance, Sue E. Huether. —2nd ed.
      p.   cm.
    Includes bibliographical references and index.
    ISBN 0-8016-6902-2
    1. Physiology, Pathological. 2. Nursing. I. Huether, Sue E.
II. Title.
    [DNLM: 1. Disease—nurses' instruction. 2. Pathology—nurses'
instruction. 3. Physiology—nurses' instruction. QZ 4 M478p 1993]
RB113.M35 1993
616.07—dc20
DNLM/DLC
for Library of Congress
                             93-31475
                              CIP

94 95 96 97 98   9 8 7 6 5 4 3 2 1

Contributors

Margaret M. Andrews, RN, PhD
Chair, Department of Nursing,
Nazareth College of Rochester,
Rochester, New York

Barbara J. Boss, PhD, RN
Professor of Nursing,
School of Nursing,
University of Mississippi Medical Center,
Jackson, Mississippi

Margorie Cengiz Budd, RN, MS
Clinical Associate Professor,
College of Nursing,
University of Utah,
Salt Lake City, Utah

Pamela F. Cipriano, PhD, RN, FAAN
Medical University of South Carolina,
Hollings Oncology Center,
Charleston, South Carolina

Gale D. Danek, RN, MSN
Clinical Nurse Specialist, Children's Health,
Shands Hospital at the University of Florida,
Gainesville, Florida

Sheryl S. Davey, RN, MS
Clinical Assistant Professor,
College of Nursing,
University of Utah,
Salt Lake City, Utah

Katherine M. Donohoe, RN, MS
Doctoral Candidate, School of Nursing,
Clinician, Department of Neurology,
University of Rochester,
Rochester, New York

Judith A. Farley, MSN, RN, CNRN
Clinical Nurse Specialist,
Pediatric Neuroscience,
Children's Hospital,
Boston, Massachusetts

Rosemary B. Field, RN, MS, OCN
Oncology/Bone Marrow Transplant Clinical Nurse
  Specialist,
Assistant Professor, Clinical,
University Hospital,
College of Nursing,
University of Utah Health Sciences Center,
Salt Lake City, Utah

Cyrena M. Gilman, RN, MN, CNN
Unit Director, Pediatric Dialysis,
Riley Hospital for Children,
Indiana University Medical Center,
Indianpolis, Indiana

D. Patricia Gray, RN, PhD
Associate Professor of Adult Health Nursing,
Georgia State University,
Atlanta, Georgia

Deborah L. Greener, CNM, PhD
Assistant Professor,
Johns Hopkins,
Department of Obstetrics and Gynecology,
Baltimore, Maryland

Sandra W. Haak, MS, PhD
Associate Professor, Clinical,
College of Nursing,
University of Utah,
Salt Lake City, Utah

Joleen Heath, RN, MS
Neurological Clinical Specialist,
Veteran's Administration Medical Center,
Salt Lake City, Utah

Katherine Hoare, RN, DNSC
Assistant Director of Nursing,
Nursing Systems,
Quality Assurance and Research,
Santa Clara Valley Medical Center,
San Jose, California

Lynn B. Jorde, PhD
Associate Professor,
Department of Human Genetics,
University of Utah School of Medicine,
Salt Lake City, Utah

Melva Kravitz, RN, PhD, CCRN
Associate Chief, Nursing Service/Research,
Veterans Administration Medical Center,
Albuquerque, New Mexico

Patti Ludwig-Beymer, PhD, RN
Nursing Research and Affiliation Coordinator,
Lutheran General Hospital,
Park Ridge, Illinois

Thom J. Mansen, RN, PhD
Assistant Professor,
College of Nursing,
University of Utah,
Salt Lake City, Utah

Frances Lynn McCullough, MNSc, RNP, ONC
Orthopaedic Nurse Specialist,
Arkansas Spine Center,
Little Rock, Arkansas

Kathleen Hardin Mooney, RN, PhD, FAAN
Professor,
College of Nursing,
University of Utah,
Salt Lake City, Utah

Leona A. Mourad, MS, RN, ONC
Associate Professor, Emeritus,
Ohio State University;
Nursing Consultant,
Mourad Consultant Associates,
Columbus, Ohio

Noreen Heer Nicol, MS, RN, FNP
Dermatology Clinical Specialist/Nurse Practitioner,
National Jewish Center for Immunology and Respiratory
  Medicine;
Clinical Senior Instructor,
University of Colorado Health Sciences Center, School of
  Nursing,
Denver, Colorado

Pamela D. Parker-Cohen, MD, RN, MS, FNPc
Thomas Jefferson Medical College,
Philadelphia, Pennsylvania

Stephanie J. Richardson, RN, PhD(c), MS
Instructor and Doctoral Student,
College of Nursing,
University of Utah,
Salt Lake City, Utah

Lee K. Roberts, PhD
Associate Research Fellow,
Advanced Product Research,
Schering/Phough HealthCare Products,
Memphis, Tennessee

Kristynia M. Robinson, PhD(c), RN, FNPc
Family Nurse Practitioner/Associate Professor of
  Nursing,
St. Mark's–Westminster School of Nursing,
Westminster College,
Salt Lake City, Utah

Neal S. Rote, PhD
Professor and Chair, Microbiology and Immunology,
Professor, Obstetrics and Gynecology,
Wright State University School of Medicine,
Dayton, Ohio

Mary Schoessler, RN, MS
Assistant Director, Education,
Providence Medical Center,
Portland, Oregon

Jane Shelby, BS, MS, PhD
Research Associate,
Department of Surgery,
College of Medicine,
University of Utah,
Salt Lake City, Utah

Sharon L. Sims, RN, PhD
Assistant Professor,
Indiana University School of Nursing,
Indianapolis, Indiana

Peter M. Sunderland, PhD, RN
Assistant Professor,
Director of Clinical Research,
Department of Neurosurgery,
University of Utah,
Salt Lake City, Utah

Mary Suzanne Tarmina, RN, PhD
Associate Clinical Professor,
College of Nursing,
University of Utah,
Salt Lake City, Utah

Roger R. Williams, MD
Professor of Medicine,
Director, Cardiovascular Genetics Research Clinic,
University of Utah,
Salt Lake City, Utah

Reviewers

Sr. Rose Terese Bahr, RN, PhD, FAAN*
Professor of Nursing and Chair,
Division of Community Health Nursing,
School of Nursing,
Catholic University of America,
Washington, DC

Jane Ball, RN, CPNP, DrPH*
Trauma Services,
Children's Hospital National Medical Center,
Washington, DC

Beverly Bartlett, RN, PhD*
Assistant Professor,
College of Nursing,
University of Rhode Island,
Kingston, Rhode Island

Carroll Conner Bouman, RN, MS*
Clinical Nurse Specialist in Cardiopulmonary Nursing;
Faculty Member and Doctoral Candidate,
School of Nursing,
University of Rochester,
Rochester, New York

John Carey, MD, MPH*
Associate Professor,
Chief, Division of Medical Genetics,
School of Medicine,
University of Utah,
Salt Lake City, Utah

*First edition reviewer.

Miguel da Cunha, PhD*
Associate Professor,
University of Texas Health Sciences Center at Houston,
Houston, Texas

Joyce Dains, RN, DrPH*
Assistant Professor,
School of Nursing,
University of Texas Health Sciences Center at Houston,
Houston, Texas

Carol DeMoss, RN, MN, CS*
Clinical Nurse Specialist,
Visiting Nurse Association of Allegheny County,
Pittsburgh, Pennsylvania

Dennis M. DePace, PhD
Department of Anatomy,
Hahnemann University,
Philadelphia, Pennsylvania

Dorothy Doughty, RN, MN, CETN*
Program Director,
Emory University,
Enterostomal Therapy Nursing Education Program,
Atlanta, Georgia

Harmon J. Eyre, MD*
Professor of Medicine,
Division of Hematology/Oncology,
School of Medicine,
University of Utah,
Salt Lake City, Utah

Nancy Gibson, RN, FNP
Salt Lake City, Utah

Mikel Gray, PhD, PNP, CURN*
Clinical Urodynamics,
Henrietta Egleston Hospital for Children,
Scottish Rite Children's Hospital,
Shepherd Spinal Center;
Adjunct Professor,
Georgia State University School of Nursing,
Atlanta, Georgia

Judith Hall, RN, PhD*
Assistant Professor,
School of Nursing,
University of Texas at Arlington,
Arlington, Texas

Laurel Halloran, RN, MSN*
Assistant Professor;
Clinical Nurse Specialist, Doctoral Candidate,
Department of Nursing,
Western Connecticut State University,
Danbury, Connecticut

K.C. Hayes, DVM, PhD*
Director, Foster Biomedical Research Center;
Professor and Chairman, Biology Department,
Brandeis University,
Waltham, Massachusetts

Mary Beth Hayward, RN, MSN*
Associate Professor,
School of Nursing,
Medical College of Ohio,
Toledo, Ohio

Ruthellyn Hinton, RN, MS, MN*
Associate Professor,
Department of Nursing,
Pittsburg State University,
Pittsburg, Kansas

Marilyn Humphrey, RN, MA
Coordinator, Nursing Program,
Chabot College,
Hayward, California

Linda Jones, RN, MS, CS, OCN*
Assistant to the Associate Director for Nursing Oncology,
University of Rochester Cancer Center;
Assistant Professor of Clinical Nursing,
University of Rochester School of Nursing,
Rochester, New York

Sr. Joan Klemballa, RN, MA*
Associate Professor,
Division of Nursing Education,
University of District of Columbia,
Washington, DC

Helene J. Krouse, RN, C, PhD*
Assistant Professor,
School of Nursing,
Boston College,
Chestnut Hill, Massachusetts

Renee Leasure, PhD, RN, CCRN
Assistant Professor,
University of Oklahoma,
College of Nursing,
Oklahoma City, Oklahoma

Mary Lentz, RN, PhD*
Assistant Professor,
School of Nursing,
University of Pittsburgh,
Pittsburgh, Pennsylvania

Stacey Levine, RN, PhD*
Associate Professor,
University of Alberta,
Clinical Sciences Department,
Edmonton, Alberta, Canada

Leslie Marshall, PhD, RN
Associate Professor,
University of Iowa College of Nursing,
Iowa City, Iowa

Patricia Maybee, RN, MS, CCRN*
College of Nursing,
Clemson University,
Department of Instruction,
Clemson, South Carolina

Mary Beth McDowell, RN, MN*
Assistant Professor,
College of Allied Health and Nursing,
Eastern Kentucky University,
Richmond, Kentucky

Mary Ellen McMorrow, RN, EdD, CCRN*
College of Staten Island,
School of Nursing,
Staten Island, New York

Diane Melancon, RN, MSN*
Associate Professor of Nursing Education,
San Antonio College,
San Antonio, Texas

Kenneth Morgan, PhD*
Associate Professor,
Department of Epidemiology and Biostatistics,
McGill University,
Montreal, Canada

Leona Mourad, RN, MS*
Associate Professor Emeritus,
College of Nursing,
Ohio State University,
Columbus, Ohio

Christine Mudge-Grout, RN, MS*
Clinical Nurse Specialist, Nephrology/Transplant,
Department of Nursing,
University of California at San Francisco,
San Francisco, California

*First edition reviewer.

Virginia J. Neelon, RN, PhD*
Associate Professor,
School of Nursing,
University of North Carolina at Chapel Hill,
Chapel Hill, North Carolina

Donna Patterson, RN, MSN*
Assistant Professor,
Villanova University,
College of Nursing,
Villanova, Pennsylvania

Ann Peterson, RN, BS, BSN*
Endocrine Clinical Nurse Specialist,
Nursing Department,
National Institutes of Health,
Bethesda, Maryland

Karen A. Pfeifer, MSN, RN, CNA, ONC
Director of Nursing Resources,
Zale Lipshy University Hospital,
Dallas, Texas

Nancy Redeker, RN, C, MSN, PhD*
Instructor,
Rutgers University,
College of Nursing,
Newark, New Jersey

Gayle Reiber, RN, PhD*
Associate Professor,
School of Public Health,
University of Washington
Seattle, Washington

Linda L. Robertson, RN, PhD*
Assistant Professor,
School of Nursing,
University of Pittsburgh,
Pittsburgh, Pennsylvania

Connie Robinson, RN, MN*
Assistant Professor,
School of Nursing,
University of California at San Francisco,
San Francisco, California

David B. Roll, PhD*
Professor of Medicinal Chemistry,
College of Pharmacy,
University of Utah,
Salt Lake City, Utah

Amy Perrin Ross, RN, MSN, CNRN*
Neuroscience Clinical Nurse Specialist,
Loyola University Medical Center,
Maywood, Illinois;
Triton College,
Continuing Education Center for Health Professionals,
River Grove, Illinois

Phyllis Russo, RN, EdD*
Chairperson, Undergraduate Nursing,
College of Nursing,
Seton Hall University,
South Orange, New Jersey

*First edition reviewer.

Ann Sedore, RN, PhD*
Associate Professor,
College of Nursing,
Syracuse University,
Syracuse, New York

Janice Selekman, RN, DNSc*
Associate Professor,
Generic Baccalaureate Program Director,
Department of Nursing,
Thomas Jefferson University,
Philadelphia, Pennsylvania

Mary Ann Siefert, RN, MS*
Primary Childrens Hospital,
Salt Lake City, Utah

Barbara Peterson Sinclair, RN, MN*
Director, OB/GYN Nurse Practitioner Program,
School of Nursing,
California State University,
Los Angeles, California

Patricia A. Stuckey, MSN, RN, OCN
Assistant Professor, Medical-Surgical Nursing,
Virginia Commonwealth University,
Medical College of Virginia School of Nursing,
Richmond, Virginia

Lydia DeCastro-Svetich, RN, MS*
Associate Professor,
Orvis School of Nursing,
University of Nevada, Reno,
Reno, Nevada

Patricia J. Thompson, PhD, RN
Associate Professor,
University of Arkansas for Medical Sciences,
College of Nursing,
Little Rock, Arkansas

Arthur Vander, PhD*
Department of Physiology,
University of Michigan,
Ann Arbor, Michigan

Filomena Varvaro, RN, PhD*
Assistant Professor,
School of Nursing,
University of Pittsburgh,
Pittsburgh, Pennsylvania

Sharon Wahl, RN, MSN, EdDc*
Assistant Professor,
Department of Nursing,
San Jose State University,
San Jose, California

Eleanor A. Walker, BSN, MS*
Assistant Professor,
School of Nursing,
Catholic University of America,
Washington, DC

Connie A. Walleck, RN, MS, FCCM
Senior Associate Director of Nursing,
University Hospital,
SUNY Health Science Center,
Syracuse, New York

Lin C. Weeks, RN, MS, CNAA*
Administrative Director,
Hospital Education,
Hermann Hospital,
Houston, Texas

Pamela B. Weilitz, RN, MSN
Pulmonary Clinical Nurse Specialist,
Barnes Hospital,
St. Louis, Missouri

Raymond L. White, PhD*
Professor and Co-Chairman, Human Genetics Department,
Investigator of Howard Hughes Medical Institute,
School of Medicine,
University of Utah,
Salt Lake City, Utah

*First edition reviewer.

Gail M. Wilkes, RN, MS, OCN*
Clinical Nurse Specialist in Oncology,
Boston City Hospital,
Boston, Massachusetts

Elizabeth Hahn Winslow, PhD, RN, FAAN
Associate Professor,
School of Nursing,
University of Texas at Arlington,
Arlington, Texas

Maxwell Wintrobe, MD, BSc (Med), PhD, DSc (Hon. Manitoba), DSc (Hon. Utah), DSc (Hon. Wisc.), MACP, MD (Hon. Athens)*
Late Distinguished Professor of Internal Medicine,
School of Medicine,
University of Utah,
Salt Lake City, Utah

To Kallie, Margot, and their parents,
Beth and Greg,
their aunt and uncles,
Anne, Eric, and Mark,
and their grandfather,
Papa John
. . . all Wolfers
*"Here's lookin at **all** the kids!"*

KLM

To the many wonderful
teachers and students who have
taught me through the years.

SEH

Preface

Spectacular advances in modern biology are revolutionizing our understanding of pathophysiology. Although the knowledge explosion—so overwhelming—is comprehensive and progressing rapidly, we have made every effort to stay current. Each chapter has been updated and in several instances revised extensively. Yet, we have retained our initial three broad objectives in offering this second edition:

- We have continued to provide comprehensive presentations of underlying principles common to all disease processes.
- We have retained, updated, and consistently revised coverage of disease processes in all age groups.
- We have paid scrupulous attention to making this edition an even more effective learning tool.

Specifically, we have added new two-color illustrations and updated and revised first edition illustrations appropriately. Algorithms have been added, and many have been revised to facilitate ease of learning.

ORGANIZATION OF THE BOOK

The basic organization has not changed from the first edition. The book is divided into two parts: *Part One, Central Concepts of Pathophysiology: Cells and Tissues,* and *Part Two, Pathophysiologic Alterations: Organs and Systems.*

Part One: Central Concepts of Pathophysiology: Cells and Tissues

> **PART ONE: CENTRAL CONCEPTS OF PATHOPHYSIOLOGY: CELLS AND TISSUES**
>
> The Cell
> Genes and Gene-Environment Interaction
> Mechanisms of Self-Defense
> Cellular Proliferation—Cancer

As before, Part One begins with an indepth study of the cell, its workings, and other processes related to cells, but now has the addition of new areas of study:

- Completely revised chapters on cancer
- Cell signaling and cell communication processes
- Cytokines and their biologic activities
- Updated information on the identification of the genome and gene therapy
- Gender and life expectancy and cellular aging
- Mechanisms of immune defense

- Significantly revised content on AIDS and psychoneuroimmunologic regulation
- Concepts of stress, coping, and illness

Part One lays the foundation for organ system diseases and disorders that are presented in Part Two. Physical laws and principles, for example, fluid movement, energy expenditures, and electrical conductances, are emphasized to increase student awareness of how these laws and principles can be applied to understanding mechanisms and complications of disease. Cells of the immune system and inflammatory responses are activated with every type of trauma or disease. Understanding these mechanisms of protection and healing provides a powerful source of knowledge that can be generalized to disorders of many organ systems. Once the normal responses are understood, students can more easily comprehend the consequences of both immune deficiencies or hyperactive responses.

Knowledge of the rapidly expanding information on the genetic basis of disease and gene-environment interaction is critical to understanding developmental alterations, cancer, cardiovascular disease, diabetes, cystic fibrosis, degenerative neural diseases, and other common disorders. Therefore both cellular and population genetics have been updated to provide the student the necessary knowledge base for appreciating the importance of risk factors, diagnostic procedures, and treatments that are influenced by genetics.

Part Two: Pathophysiologic Alterations: Organs and Systems

PART TWO: PATHOPHYSIOLOGIC ALTERATIONS: ORGANS AND SYSTEMS

The Neurologic System
The Endocrine System
The Reproductive System
The Hematologic System
The Cardiovascular and Lymphatic Systems
The Pulmonary System
The Renal and Urologic Systems
The Digestive System
The Musculoskeletal System
The Integumentary System

Part Two is still a survey of specific diseases from the traditional systems organization but adds new information and some strategic changes in pedagogy. Because student and faculty response to the format of this text has been overwhelmingly enthusiastic, each system unit still begins with a chapter on the normal anatomy and physiology of the system. We have paid scrupulous attention to updating these chapters, knowing that normal function *directly* informs the discussion of the specific diseases that follow. These chapters have been extensively edited to include new diagnostic tests and updated information on the normal aging process unique to each system.

Throughout Part Two updated or new content has been added, including:

- Reorganization of the alterations of neurologic function chapter to include new information on head trauma and diffuse axonal injury
- Neurologic complications of AIDS and a new section on HIV infection in children
- Expansion of content on sexual dysfunction and cancer of the reproductive organs
- New information on tuberculosis and lung cancer
- New algorithms on conditions such as multiple organ system dysfunction, septic shock, disseminated intravascular coagulation, asthma, adult respiratory distress syndrome, and glomerulonephritis
- More tables to increase clarity of content on topics such as croup syndromes, glomerulonephritis, pneumonia in children, cancer of the GI tract, and hepatitis
- Application of cytokine function from Part One to pathophysiologic processes in Part Two, including the role of colony-stimulating factor (CSF) in hematopoiesis, leukemia, and leukopenia
- Pathologic effects of interleukins and tumor necrosis factor
- Cellular mechanisms of atherosclerosis leading to myocardial infarction and Kawasaki disease in children

Many features of the first edition have been retained for most of the disorders, including:

- Epidemiology and risk factors
- Pathogenesis and clinical manifestations
- Evaluation and treatment
- Clinical commentaries (listed on p. xvii)
- Use of physical laws to aid students in understanding pathophysiologic alterations
- Extensive integration of cancer research data

New features that enhance the second edition include revised historical openers with new art, new two-color illustrations, figure titles in boldface type, updated and easily retrieved content on aging, detailed chapter outlines with page numbers, updated and revised key terms, and complete updated summary reviews. The reference lists have been divided into cited references and references for additional reading to aid further study.

Although major emphasis is devoted to pathophysiology and clinical manifestations, significant attention is also paid to epidemiology and risk factors. Throughout the book, we have continued to extensively cross-reference to fully integrate the two parts of the book. Rather than delete controversial material, for example the role of estrogens in breast cancer, we have summarized theoretical positions and identified gaps in current understanding. Sensitivity to gender differences in the development and manifestations of various diseases and disorders has been included as appropriate.

LIFESPAN CONTENT
Aging Content

Beginning in Chapter 2, theories of aging are presented. Reference is made to this content throughout Part Two as the normal changes associated with aging are presented in the normal anatomy and physiology chapter of each system unit. The pathophysiology of diseases associated with advanced age is discussed in the alterations chapters. In this way, we attempt to make it clear to students that there are physiologic changes related to aging that are normal and healthy, and that old age should not be considered synonymous with sickness and death.

Pediatric Content

In the same fashion, content related to alterations in children is firmly rooted in Part One of the book, and frequent reference is made to cellular content during the discussion of specific diseases of childhood presented in the systems units in Part Two. Material in Part One includes considerations related to childhood, such as congenital immune deficiencies, genetic disorders, familial diseases, and cancer in children. We take the opportunity in the systems chapters on children in Part Two to summarize, when appropriate, the differences between diseases in adults and children, such as differences in tumors.

ADDITIONAL LEARNING AIDS
Study Guide and Workbook

A most exciting addition to the second edition is a new Study Guide and Workbook for students written by Dr. Clayton Parkinson. Dr. Parkinson has designed the study guide to help students learn pathophysiology by reinforcing key concepts and integrating workbook-like exercises. To this end, he has designed the anatomy and physiology chapters to have review objectives keyed to the text and keyed to practice examinations with answers. The pathophysiology chapters have prerequisite objectives with review assignments referenced to the text. The pathophysiology objectives are in boldface type and are keyed to study assignments and have an abbreviated outline narrative with summary charts. A practice examination with answers and a case study follow the narrative for application of concepts.

Instructor's Resource Manual and Test Bank

The instructor's manual has been significantly revised and updated. The revisions include updated chapter objectives; new sections on difficult concepts, with suggested teaching and learning approaches; and integrative content questions (i.e., critical thinking exercises). The integrative questions are designed to reinforce the application of physical laws and principles for problem solving. For example, students are asked to apply the concepts of osmotic gradient to the clinical problem of dehydration and to Starling's forces for understanding edema formation in an individual with hypertension.

A 1200-item test bank is available in the instructor's manual. Questions include multiple choice, true/false, matching, and short answer. Answers and page references to the text are provided.

Transparency Acetates

A new package of transparency acetates is available. This includes 150 transparencies, primarily of disorders. A legend booklet is included, and the acetates have been 3-hole punched so they can be stored in a binder.

■   ■   ■   ■

With the revisions, updated material, and new student learning aids, we believe this new edition offers a *state of the art and science* approach to learning pathophysiology.

Kathryn L. McCance
Sue E. Huether

Acknowledgments

Many people worked on this book! Most significant was Sue Meeks, who generated the manuscript. Sue's astute and scrupulous approach kept us consistently on target. Thanks again, Sue, for your energy and remarkable attention to detail.

Again, we thank our colleagues and friends at the University of Utah College of Nursing. Special thanks to Debbie Bachan and Molly Berigan-Spira for their critical assistance with many details related to the revision and transmittal of the manuscript. Thanks to Mary Youngkin and Jeanne La Ber for their generous and skilled attention as reference librarians in Eccles Health Sciences Library. In addition, retrieving and securing hundreds of references was facilitated by Cheryl Mansen. Thank you, Cheryl. We acknowledge the librarians at the National Library of Medicine for their very helpful assistance in retrieving illustrations for the historical unit openers.

To our outstanding editors—thank you. Sally Schrefer, our editor, inherited us part way through revision. Sally got us focused and kept us on track and managed the entire project with "grit and grace." To Sally, thank you, and we'll have you in cowboy boots yet!

Penny Rudolph was our developmental editor. Penny is quick, thorough, and gently persistent. Thank you, Penny, for managing such detail completely and confidently. To Brian Dennison, thanks for all the administrative help and kindness, especially when we lost or forgot things.

Gail Brower was our chief production editor. Gail's ability to orchestrate thousands of details easily and accurately was astonishing. Thank you, Gail.

Again, we had the great fortune of having two extremely talented artists—Donald O'Connor and George Wassilchenko. Thanks, not only from us, but from many faculty and students who have written to tell us how the art program made the book!

Reviewers for this edition included faculty, students, clinicians, and investigators. Many comments and suggestions were essential and notably consistent—saving us invaluable time and energy. To all of the reviewers, thank you.

Contents

PART TWO   Pathophysiologic Alterations: Organs and Systems

Detailed Contents

UNIT IV Cellular Proliferation: Cancer

PART TWO   Pathophysiologic Alterations: Organs and Systems

UNIT VII   The Reproductive System

19   Structure and Function of the Reproductive Systems, 711

Kristynia M. Robinson
Sue E. Huether

20   Alterations of the Reproductive System, 745

Kristynia M. Robinson
Kathryn L. McCance

21 Sexually Transmitted Diseases, 800

Thom J. Mansen

UNIT VIII   The Hematologic System

22 Structure and Function of the Hematologic System, 830

Kathryn L. McCance
Pamela F. Cipriano

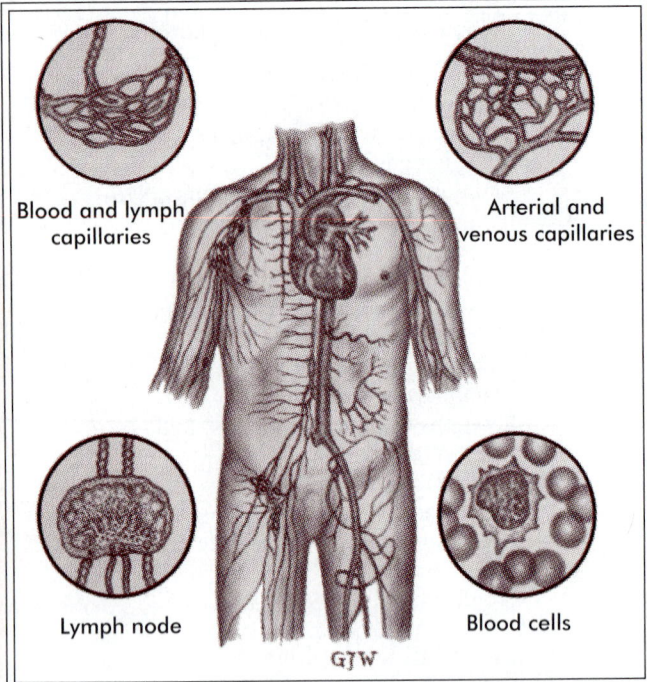

Blood and lymph capillaries

Arterial and venous capillaries

Lymph node

Blood cells

GJW

UNIT IX   **The Cardiovascular and Lymphatic Systems**

26   **Structure and Function of the Cardiovascular and Lymphatic Systems, 943**

Kathryn L. McCance
Stephanie J. Richardson

UNIT XI   The Renal and Urologic Systems

37 Alterations of Digestive Function in Children, 1376

Gale D. Danek
Sue E. Huether

UNIT XIII   The Musculoskeletal System

38 Structure and Function of the Musculoskeletal System, 1404

Leona A. Mourad

CLINICAL COMMENTARIES

AGING CONTENT

PEDIATRIC CONTENT

PART ONE

Central Concepts of Pathophysiology
Cells and Tissues

UNIT I

The Cell

THE STUDY OF CELLULAR BIOLOGY really began in the seventeenth century, primarily from the discoveries of Englishman Robert Hooke (1635-1723) and Dutchman Anthony van Leeuwenhoek (1632-1723). Hooke was the first to use the term *cell* in biology. He describes in a collection of essays, *Micrographia*, a honeycomb of chambers in cork, which he called "cells." He thought the cells were similar to the veins and arteries of animals, although his microscope did not permit the observation of any intracellular structures.

After improving the microscope lens, Van Leeuwenhoek described a variety of single-celled life forms, including bacteria, in 1683. This was an incredible feat because the dimensions of bacteria are typically about 1 or 2 μm.

In 1824, with improved microscopy, R. J. H. Dutrochet noted that all animal and plant tissues are aggregates of cells of various kinds. Although he observed that growth results from an increase in either the size or the number of cells, or both, he did not realize that each cell is capable of reproduction.

Matthias Schleiden and Theodor Schwann, in 1838 and 1839, were the first to argue convincingly that each cell is capable of its own growth and development. Rudolf Virchow (1821-1902), often called the "Pope of Medicine," extended the findings of Schleiden and Schwann by attributing every cell's existence to that of a preexisting cell (*omnis cellula e cellula*— every cell from a cell). The ideas of Schleiden, Schwann, and Virchow became

The human immunodeficiency virus.
(Courtesy National Library of Medicine.)

embryology, histology, cytology, genetics, anatomy, physiology, pathophysiology, and the applied clinical sciences. Approaches to learning the molecular events in cell function have also changed significantly. Traditionally, students studied prokaryotic cells (cells lacking a distinct nucleus), especially descriptions of bacterial and viral experiments, as core subjects of molecular biology. Today, emphasis is on the eukaryotic cell. General principles of eukaryotic cell structure and function, and the proteins responsible for this structure and function, have no counterparts in bacterial cells. In addition, there are many differences between the eukaryotic and prokaryotic cells in the organization and expression of their genes.

known as the cell theory, or cell doctrine, which states that (1) all living things are composed of one or more compartments called cells, (2) each cell is capable of maintaining its own unique vitality, and (3) cells can arise only from other cells. The cell theory radically changed the understanding of disease, which could now be studied with respect to alterations in cellular structure and function. Virchow was not a strong supporter of the bacterial theory of disease, but his view that the reactions of the body's cells to invading microorganisms can have more deleterious effects than the invading organism itself is still an essential tenet in the study of disease.

Modern biology is molecular biology. The determination for understanding cell function in molecular terms is spectacular. The molecular approach to biology has already affected

Before the birth of molecular biology, biological sciences grew independently of each other, including biochemistry and genetics. The first event in which a relation was discovered between a genetic trait and a biochemical abnormality occurred in the study of human disease. Archibald Garrod realized by 1909 that the disease *alkaptonuria* was caused by a rare inherited recessive mutation characterized by a deficiency of the enzyme homogentisic acid oxidase. He identified the nature of the genetic defect in his treatise on "Inborn Errors of Metabolism." It was too early, however, in the history of genetics or biochemistry to understand that genes do, in fact, control the structure of enzymes.

In 1931, Barbara McClintock (1902-1992) associated visible rearrangements of gene segments within and between chromosomes with the distribution of specific genetic traits in strains of corn. Because of her classical studies, genes were no longer "theoretical" objects but accepted as physical entities and determinants of biological specificity. Her work was recognized a number of years later in 1983 with the Nobel Prize in Physiology and Medicine. The merging of biochemistry and genetics, between 1930 and 1950, enabled the discovery of the chemical nature of the gene in the 1950s (see Chapter 4 historical overview).

The birth of molecular biology, which has been mainly concerned with how genes govern cell activity, began in 1953, when James D. Watson (1928-) and Francis H. C. Crick (1916-) identified the double-helical structure of DNA. During the 1930s and early 1940s, while geneticists and biochemists were engaged in identifying the gene and finding enzymes, little attention was paid to other structures within the cell. When the electron microscope became available, new structures emerged before a spellbound audience. A new, striking fact also emerged: all eukaryotic cells have certain cell structures in common. Much of the early electron-microscopic identification of cell structures and biochemical analysis of cell functions was the work of Albert Claude (1899-1983), George Palade (1912-), and Keith Porter (1912-).

Thus, by the end of the 1950s, the fundamental observations made independently by geneticists, biochemists, and structural cell biologists were ready to be woven together into a pattern that would become the design for molecular cell biology. Three important discoveries were made in the 1960s: (1) messenger RNA carries the information from DNA to the endoplasmic reticulum, (2) the genetic code, and (3) proteins are translated by transfer RNA and ribosomes. By 1975, new technology allowed segments of DNA to be isolated and purified and allowed the sequencing and synthesis of DNA and peptides.

Research that began in the 1980s, and still continues, has produced an overwhelming amount of information. Gradually, essential principles of molecular cell biology are emerging, including the identity of the genome, recognition of cell movement, cell adhesion, cell communication, mechanisms of cell transport, and mechanisms of cellular defense. New techniques of molecular analysis are revealing an astonishing account of cell activity and a unity in the principles that govern cell function.

CHAPTER 1

Cellular Biology

Kathryn L. McCance

A*n understanding of cellular biology is increasingly necessary for an understanding of disease. An overwhelming amount of information is revealing how cells behave as a multicellular "social" organism. At the heart of it all is cellular communication—how messages originate, are transmitted, re-*ceived, interpreted, and used by the cell, "cell talk." When the cell talk is not understood, is blocked, or is abruptly interrupted, disease within itself occurs. Streamlined conversation between, among, and within cells maintains social acceptance. Cells must demonstrate a "chemical fondness" for other cells to*

5

maintain the integrity of the entire organism. When they no longer tolerate this fondness, the conversation breaks down, and cells either adapt (sometimes altering function) or become vulnerable to isolation, injury, or disease.

PROKARYOTES AND EUKARYOTES

Living cells are generally divided into two major classes, the eukaryotes and prokaryotes. The cells of higher animals and plants are eukaryotes, as are the single-celled organisms fungi, protozoa, and most algae. Prokaryotes include cyanobacteria (blue-green algae), bacteria, and rickettsiae. Prokaryotes traditionally were studied as core subjects of molecular biology. Today emphasis is on the eukaryotic cell; much of its structure and function has no counterpart in bacterial cells.

Eukaryotes (*eu* = good; *karyon* = nucleus) are larger and have more extensive intracellular anatomy and organization than prokaryotes. Eukaryotic cells have a characteristic set of membrane-bounded intracellular compartments, called organelles, that includes a well-defined nucleus. The **prokaryotes** contain no organelles, and their nuclear material is not encased by a nuclear membrane. Prokaryotic cells are characterized by lack of a distinct nucleus.

Besides having structural differences, prokaryotic and eukaryotic cells differ in chemical composition and biochemical activity. The *nuclei* of prokaryotic cells carry genetic information in a single circular chromosome, and they lack a class of proteins called histones, which in eukaryotic cells bind with deoxyribonucleic acid (DNA) and are involved in the supercoiling of DNA. Eukaryotic cells have several or many chromosomes. Protein production, or synthesis, in the two classes of cells also differs because of major structural differences in ribonucleic acid (RNA) protein complexes. Other distinctions include differences in mechanisms of transport across the outer cellular membrane and in enzyme content.

CELLULAR FUNCTIONS

Cells become specialized through the process of differentiation, or maturation, so that some cells eventually perform one kind of function and other cells perform other functions. Highly developed functions, such as movement, are often associated with the absence of some other property, such as hormone production, which is more highly developed in some other type of specialized cell.

The seven chief cellular functions are the following:

1. *Movement.* Muscle cells can generate forces that produce motion. Muscles that are attached to bones produce limb movements, whereas those that enclose hollow tubes or cavities move or empty contents when they contract. For example, the contraction of smooth muscle cells surrounding blood vessels changes the diameter of the vessels; the contraction of muscles in walls of the urinary bladder expels urine.

2. *Conductivity.* Conduction as a response to a stimulus is manifested by a wave of excitation, an electrical potential, that passes along the surface of the cell to reach its other parts. Conductivity is the chief function of nerve cells.

3. *Metabolic absorption.* All cells can take in and use nutrients and other substances from their surroundings. Cells of the intestine and the kidney are specialized to carry out absorption. Cells of the kidney tubules reabsorb fluids and synthesize proteins. Intestinal epithelial cells reabsorb fluids and synthesize protein enzymes.

4. *Secretion.* Certain cells, such as mucous gland cells, can synthesize new substances from substances they absorb and secrete the new substances to serve as needed elsewhere. Cells of the adrenal gland, testis, and ovary can secrete hormonal steroids.

5. *Excretion.* All cells can rid themselves of waste products resulting from the metabolic breakdown of nutrients. Membrane-bounded sacs (lysosomes) within cells contain enzymes that break down, or digest, large molecules, turning them into waste products that are released from the cell.

6. *Respiration.* Cells absorb oxygen, which is used to transform nutrients into energy in the form of adenosine triphosphate (ATP). Cellular respiration, or oxidation, occurs in organelles called mitochondria.

7. *Reproduction.* Tissue growth occurs as cells enlarge and reproduce themselves. Even without growth, tissue maintenance requires that new cells be produced to replace cells that are lost normally through cellular death. Not all cells are capable of continuous division, and some cells, such as nerve cells, cannot reproduce.

STRUCTURE AND FUNCTION OF CELLULAR COMPONENTS

A "typical" eukaryotic cell is shown in Fig. 1-1. It consists of three components: an outer membrane called the **plasma membrane,** or **plasmalemma;** a fluid "filling,"

FIG. 1-1 **Typical components of a eukaryotic cell. A,** Diagram. **B,** Electron micrograph of a eukaryotic cell (×40,500). (From Raven & Johnson, 1992.)

called **cytoplasm;** and the "organs" of the cell—the membrane-bounded intracellular **organelles,** among them the nucleus.

Nucleus

The **nucleus,** which is surrounded by the cytoplasm and is generally located in the center of the cell, is the largest membrane-bounded organelle. Two membranes compose the **nuclear envelope** (Fig. 1-2, *A*). The outer membrane is continuous with membranes of the endoplasmic reticulum. The nucleus contains the **nucleolus,** most of the cellular DNA, and the DNA-binding proteins, the histones, that regulate its activity. The length of DNA in eukaryotic cells is so great that the risk of

breakage is high. Therefore, the histones that bind to DNA cause the folding of DNA into chromosomes (Fig. 1-2, *C*). The wrapping of DNA into tight packages of chromosomes is essential for cell division in eukaryotes.

The primary functions of the nucleus are cell division and control of genetic information. Other functions include the replication and repair of DNA and the transcription of the information stored in DNA. Genetic information is transcribed into RNA, which can be processed into messenger, transport, and ribosomal RNA and introduced into the cytoplasm, where it directs cellular activities. Most of the processing of RNA occurs in the nucleolus. (The role of DNA and RNA in protein synthesis is discussed in Chapter 4.)

FIG. 1-2 The nucleus. The nucleus is composed of a double membrane, called a nuclear envelope, that encloses the fluid-filled interior, called nucleoplasm. The chromosomes are suspended in the nucleoplasm (here shown much larger than real size to show the tightly packed DNA strands). Swelling at one or more points of the chromosome, shown in **A,** occurs at a nucleolus where genes are being copied into RNA. The nuclear envelope is studded with pores. **B,** The pores are visible as dimples in this freeze etch of a nuclear envelope. **C,** Histone-folding DNA in chromosomes. (From Raven & Johnson, 1992.)

Cytoplasmic Organelles

Cytoplasm is an aqueous solution (cytosol) that fills the intracellular compartment known as the **cytoplasmic matrix**—the space between the nuclear envelope and the plasma membrane. The cytosol represents about half the volume of a eukaryotic cell. It contains thousands of enzymes involved in intermediate metabolism and is crowded with ribosomes making proteins. Newly synthesized proteins remain in the cytosol if they lack a signal for transport to a cell organelle (Alberts et al., 1989). The organelles suspended in the cytoplasm are enclosed in biologic membranes, which enables them simultaneously to carry out functions that require different biochemical environments. These functions, many of which are directed by coded messages carried from the nucleus by RNA, include synthesis of proteins and hormones and their transport out of the cell, isolation and elimination of waste products from the cell, metabolic processes, breakdown and disposal of cellular debris and foreign proteins (antigens), and maintenance of cellular structure and motility.

Ribosomes

Ribosomes are RNA-protein complexes (nucleoproteins) that are synthesized in the nucleolus and secreted into the cytoplasm, possibly through pores in the nuclear envelope. These tiny organelles may float free in the cytoplasm or attach themselves to the outer membranes of the endoplasmic reticulum (see Fig. 1-1). Their chief function is to provide sites for cellular protein synthesis.

Endoplasmic Reticulum

The **endoplasmic reticulum** (*endo* = within; *plasm* = cytoplasm; *reticulum* = network) is a membrane factory that specializes in the synthesis and transport of the protein and lipid components of most of the cell's organelles. It consists of a network of tubular or saclike channels (cisternae) that extend throughout the cytoplasm and are continuous with the outer nuclear membrane (see Fig. 1-1). The folded membranes that form the cisternae of the endoplasmic reticulum may be rough (granular) or smooth (agranular). The rough endoplasmic reticulum is "rough" because ribosomes and ribonucleoprotein particles are attached to it (Fig. 1-3). Some of the proteins synthesized by these ribosomes remain in the endoplasmic reticulum, and others are used to construct membranes of other organelles (the Golgi complex, lysosomes, peroxisomes, nucleus) and of the cell itself.

Smooth endoplasmic reticulum does not contain ribosomes or ribonucleoprotein particles (see Fig. 1-1).

FIG. 1-3 Electron micrograph of rough endoplasmic reticulum. (From Raven & Johnson, 1992.)

Rather, membranous surfaces of the smooth endoplasmic reticulum contain enzymes involved in the synthesis of steroid hormones and are responsible for a variety of reactions required to remove toxic substances from the cell. The endoplasmic reticulum communicates with the Golgi complex and interacts with other organelles, particularly lysosomes and peroxisomes.

Golgi Complex

The **Golgi complex** (or **Golgi apparatus**) is a network of flattened, smooth membranes and vesicles frequently located near the nucleus of the cell (Fig. 1-4). Proteins from the endoplasmic reticulum are processed and packaged into small, membrane-bounded vesicles called **secretory vesicles** or **secretory granules,** which break off from the Golgi complex and migrate to a variety of intracellular and extracellular destinations, including the plasma membrane. The vesicles fuse with the plasma membrane, and their contents are released from the cell. Many molecules, including lipids, proteins, glycoproteins, and enzymes of lysosomes, pass through the Golgi complex at some stage in their maturation.

The biochemical changes that take place in the Golgi complex are not clearly understood, but the Golgi complex is probably the director of macromolecular traffic (e.g., protein, polynucleotide, and polysaccharide molecules) in the cell (Alberts et al., 1989).

Lysosomes

Lysosomes (*lyso* = dissolution; *soma* = body) are sac-like structures that originate from the Golgi complex (Fig. 1-5; see also Fig. 1-1). They contain over 40 digestive enzymes called hydrolases, which catalyze the hydrolytic cleavage of carbon-oxygen, carbon-nitrogen,

carbon-sulfur, and oxygen-phosphorus bonds in proteins, lipids, nucleic acids, and carbohydrates. Lysosomes function as the intracellular digestive system. Lysosomal enzymes are capable of digesting most cellular constituents down to their basic forms, such as amino acids, fatty acids, and sugars.

The lysosomal membrane acts as a protective shield between the powerful digestive enzymes within the lysosome and the cytoplasm, preventing their leakage into the cytoplasmic matrix. Disruption of the membrane by various treatments or cellular injury leads to a release of the lysosomal enzymes, which can then react with their specific substrates, causing cellular self-digestion. Lysosomal abnormalities are involved in a number of conditions that involve cellular injury and death.

Lysosomal storage diseases may be due to a genetic defect or lack of one or more lysosomal enzymes. For example, the lack of lysosomal alpha-1,4-glucosidase leads to an accumulation of glycogen in lysosomes known as Pompe's disease. Tay-Sachs disease is characterized by an accumulation of GM_2 ganglioside (a lipid) in lysosomes as a result of the deficiency or absence of lysosomal hexosaminidase A. In gout, undigested uric acid accumulates within lysosomes, damaging the lysosomal membrane. Subsequent enzyme leakage results in cell death and tissue injury.

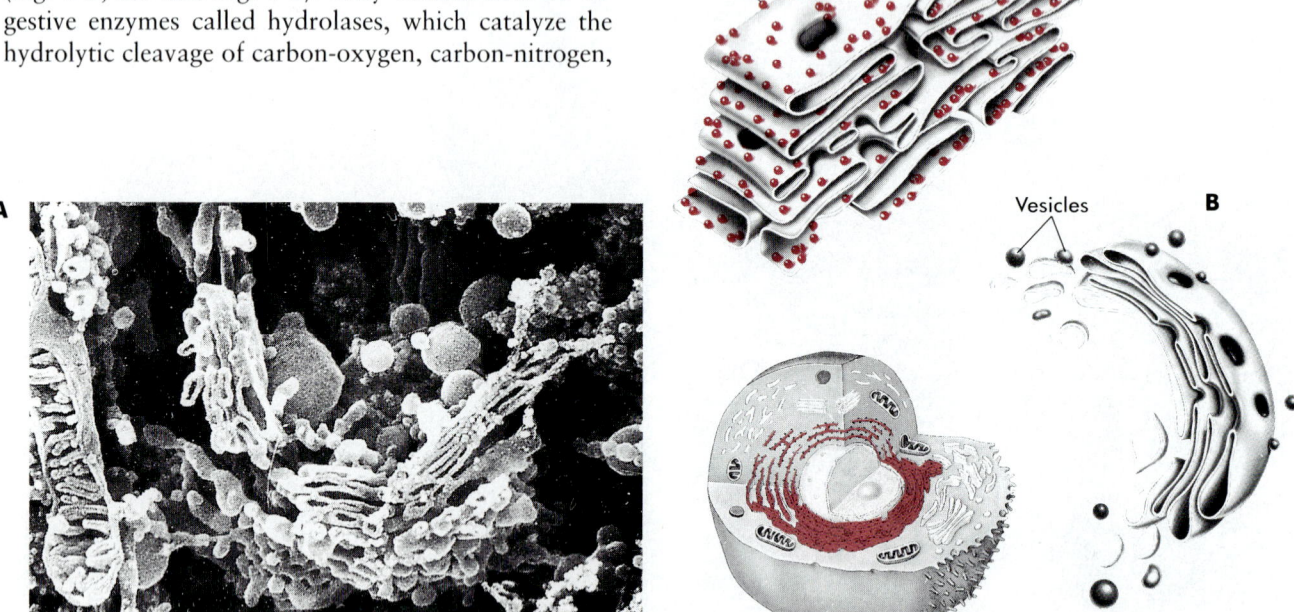

FIG. 1-4 Golgi complex. A, Electron micrograph (×6300). **B,** Diagram—proteins synthesized from ribosomes are processed by the Golgi complex. (**A,** From Erlandsen & Magney, 1992; **B,** from Raven & Johnson, 1992.)

Lysosomes are necessary for normal digestion of cellular nutrients, intracellular debris, and potentially harmful extracellular substances that must be removed from the body. Extracellular substances are taken into the cell and encapsulated in a membrane-bounded vesicle. Lysosomes merge with the vesicle to form a digestive vacuole. Merging releases lysosomal enzymes into the vacuole, and the foreign substance is digested and converted to products that can enter the cytoplasm and be used by the cell. **Primary lysosomes** are lysosomes that have not merged with encapsulated foreign substances and whose enzymes are not as yet involved in the digestive process. **Secondary lysosomes** (digestive vacuoles) are those in which digestion is under way.

As cells complete their life span and die, lysosomes digest the resultant cellular debris. Lysosomes involved in this process, which is called **autodigestion,** are called **autolysosomes.** In living cells, cellular debris is encapsulated within a vesicle that reacts with a lysosome to complete its degradation. This process is called **autophagy.** Autophagy also occurs during starvation, enabling the cell to use a part of its own substance for fuel without doing itself irreparable harm.

Products of autophagy (and of phagocytosis, the ingestion of harmful foreign substances, see Chapter 7)

pass out of the lysosome and are reused by the cell. Indigestible material is stored in vesicles called **residual bodies,** whose contents are actively expelled from the cell (see Fig. 1-23). High concentrations of lipids may accumulate within the residual bodies and remain there for a long time. The lipids are eventually oxidized, and a pigmented substance containing polyunsaturated fatty acids and proteins accumulates in the cell. This pigmented substance, termed *lipofuscin,* is often called "age pigment" and is noted in older individuals (see Chapter 2).

Peroxisomes

Peroxisomes (**microbodies**) are similar to lysosomes in microscopic appearance, but they are larger and oval or irregular in shape. Peroxisomes contain several enzymes that either produce or use hydrogen peroxide, for example, the enzyme catalase, which accelerates, or catalyzes, the conversion of two hydrogen peroxides to water and oxygen. Hydrogen peroxide is produced in the peroxisomes by enzymes that oxidize D-amino acids, uric acid, and various 1-hydroxy acids. Beyond their participation in metabolic oxidations involving hydrogen peroxide, the function of peroxisomes is little understood.

FIG. 1-5 Lysosomes in a white blood cell. A, Electron micrograph (×82,000) and **B,** diagram. (**A,** From Erlandsen & Magney, 1992; **B,** from Raven & Johnson, 1992.)

Mitochondria

Mitochondria (*mito* = thread; *chondros* = granule) are of much interest because of their role in cellular energy metabolism (see p. 21). These cytoplasmic organelles appear as spheres, rods, or filamentous bodies that are bounded by a double membrane (Fig. 1-6). The outer membrane is smooth and surrounds the mitochondrion itself; the inner membrane is convoluted in the mitochondrial matrix to form partitions called cristae. The inner membrane contains the enzymes of the respiratory chain—the name given to the electron transport chain. These enzymes are essential to the process of oxidative phosphorylation that generates most of the cell's ATP. Metabolic pathways involved in the metabolism of carbohydrates, lipids, and amino acids and special pathways involving urea and heme synthesis are located in the mitochondrial matrix.

The outer membrane is permeable (passable) to many substances, but the inner membrane is highly selective and contains many transmembranous transport systems. The inner membrane contains a transporter to move electrically charged calcium (calcium ions) (Devlin, 1992). (Membrane transport is discussed on p. 23.)

Cytoskeleton

All eukaryotic cells contain elaborate and specialized internal structures that provide the "bones and muscles" of the cell—the **cytoskeleton.** The cytoskeleton maintains the cell's shape and internal organization, and it permits movement of substances within the cell and movement of external projections (cilia or microvilli) outside the plasma membrane. The internal skeleton is composed of a network of protein filaments; two of the most important are microtubules and actin filaments, or microfilaments.

Microtubules are small, hollow, cylindrical, unbranched tubules made of protein. When found together, microtubules exhibit rigidity, unlike the rest of the cytoplasm. Microtubules thus add strength to the cell's structure (Fig. 1-7, *A*). Within the cell, microtubules support and move organelles from one part of the cytoplasm to another, facilitate transport of impulses along nerve cells, and have roles in the inflammatory and immune responses and hormone secretion. Microtubules are also involved in external movement, or motility, of some cells.

Microtubules are arranged in the thickened base, or basal body, of a protrusion from the cell's plasma membrane. This arrangement occurs in the basal bodies of sperm flagella and the cilia of certain other cells. The long, whiplike flagella enable sperm cells to move. Cilia usually move substances past the cell, which remains stationary. For example, cilia on cells lining the respiratory tract move together to "beat" mucus toward the throat so it can be removed by coughing.

While the cell is not in the process of division, only a few microtubules are assembled; cellular division (mitosis) or defense (phagocytosis) does, however, induce a cycle of rapid assembly and disassembly. Microtubules involved in cellular division are arranged as shown in Fig. 1-7, *B*. This arrangement is called a **centriole.** Centrioles always consist of nine bundles containing three microtubules each. During division, the pairs of centrioles split and migrate to opposite poles of the cell (see p. 34).

A

Outer membrane
Inner membrane
Matrix
Crista
Outer compartment

B

FIG. 1-6 Mitochondrion. A, Electron micrograph (×34,000) and **B,** diagram. (**A,** From Erlandsen & Magney, 1992; **B,** from Raven & Johnson, 1992.)

FIG. 1-7 Cytoskeletal organelles. A, Network of mitochondria, ribosomes, and endoplasmic reticulum supported by a network of filaments, through which pass microtubules. **B,** The centriole is composed of nine triplets of microtubules. **C,** Cytoskeleton showing several actin filaments (×52,500). (**A** and **B,** From Raven & Johnson, 1992; **C,** from Erlandsen & Magney, 1992.)

Alterations of microtubular function are implicated in disease processes. For example, defective protein synthesis has been related to a decreased number of microtubules as a result of increased cellular levels of acetaldehyde (a product of alcohol metabolism) found in chronic alcoholism.

Actin filaments (microfilaments) are smaller fibrils that generally occur in bundles rather than singly (Fig. 1-7, C). Like microtubules, actin filaments are associated with cellular locomotion and maintenance of cell and tissue shape. Cellular locomotion depends on contractile properties that involve both microtubules and actin filaments. Anesthetic drugs can affect both structures, disrupting intracellular movement and cellular motility.

Plasma Membranes

Whether they surround the cell or enclose an intracellular organelle, membranes are exceedingly important to normal physiologic function because they control the composition of the space, or compartment, they enclose. Membranes can include or exclude a variety of molecules, and because of selective transport systems, they can move molecules into or out of the space. By controlling the movement of substances from one compartment to another, membranes exert a powerful influence on metabolic pathways. In addition to these functions,

the plasma membrane has an important role in cell-to-cell recognition. For example, protein receptors for hormones and for other chemical signals are associated with the membrane and act as markers that identify a cell to its neighbors. Other functions of the plasma membrane include cellular mobility and the maintenance of cellular shape (Table 1-1).

Plasma membranes are usually thicker than the membranes of intracellular organelles. The outer surfaces of plasma membranes in many cells are not smooth but are studded with cilia or even smaller cylindrical projections called microvilli. Both are capable of movement.

Membrane Composition

The major chemical components of all membranes are lipids and proteins, but the percentage of each varies among different membranes. Lipid molecules are the most abundant, but the protein molecules are so large that in total mass these two constituents are roughly equal. The structure of a plasma membrane is shown in Fig. 1-8. Intracellular membranes have a higher percentage of proteins than plasma membranes, presumably because most enzymatic activity occurs within organelles. Carbohydrates are mainly associated with plasma membranes, where they are combined chemically with lipids, forming glycolipids, and with proteins, forming glycoproteins.

TABLE 1-1

Plasma Membrane Functions

Cellular mechanism	Membrane functions
Structure	Containment of cellular organelles
	Maintenance of relationship with cytoskeleton, endoplasmic reticulum, and other organelles
	Maintenance of fluid and electrolyte balance
Protection	Barrier to toxic molecules and macromolecules (proteins, nucleic acid, polysaccharides)
	Barrier to foreign organisms and cells
Activation of cell	Hormones (regulation of cellular activity)
	Mitogens (cellular division, see Chapter 4)
	Antigens (antibody synthesis, see Chapter 8)
	Growth factors (proliferation and differentiation, see Chapter 10)
Transport	Diffusion and exchange diffusion
	Endocytosis (pinocytosis and phagocytosis)
	Exocytosis (secretion)
	Active transport
Cell-to-cell interaction	Communication and attachment at junctional complexes
	Symbiotic nutritive relationships
	Release of enzymes and antibodies to extracellular environment
	Relationships with extracellular matrix

Modified from King, D.W., Fenoglio, C.M., & Lefkowitch, J.H. (1983). *General pathology: Principles and dynamics.* Philadelphia: Lea & Febiger.

Lipids

The basic component of the plasma membrane is a bilayer of lipid molecules—phospholipids, glycolipids, and cholesterol (respective ratios 70:5:25). The lipids are responsible for the structural integrity of the membrane. Each lipid molecule is said to be polar, or amphipathic. An **amphipathic molecule** is one in which one part is hydrophobic (uncharged, or "water hating") and another part is hydrophilic (charged, or "water loving") (Fig. 1-9).

The membrane spontaneously organizes itself into a bilayer because of these two incompatible solubilities. The hydrophobic region (hydrophobic tail) of each lipid molecule is protected from water, whereas the hydrophilic region (hydrophilic head) is immersed in it. The bilayer's structure accounts for one of the essential functions of the plasma membrane: it is impermeable to most water-soluble molecules (molecules that dissolve in water) because they are insoluble in the oily core region. The bilayer serves as a barrier to the diffusion of water and hydrophilic substances, while allowing lipid-soluble molecules, such as oxygen (O_2) and carbon dioxide (CO_2), to diffuse through it readily. Because the bilayer is fluid at temperatures above freezing, components of the cellular environment move slowly and selectively across the membrane all the time. (Components of the cellular environment are discussed in Chapter 3.)

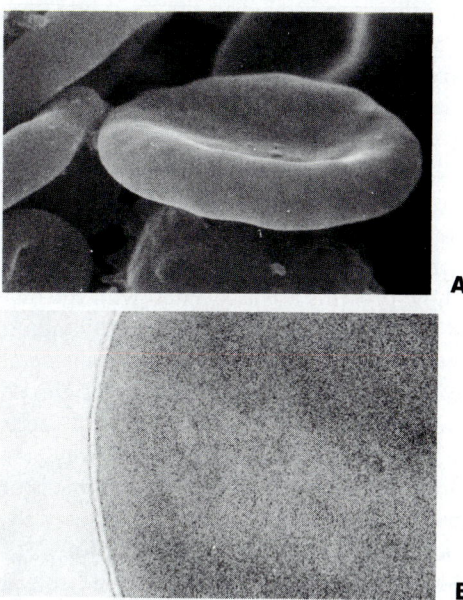

FIG. 1-8 Human red blood cell. A, Electron micrograph of a human red blood cell. **B,** The membrane bilayer that encases the cell is clearly visible in the micrograph. (From Raven & Johnson, 1992.)

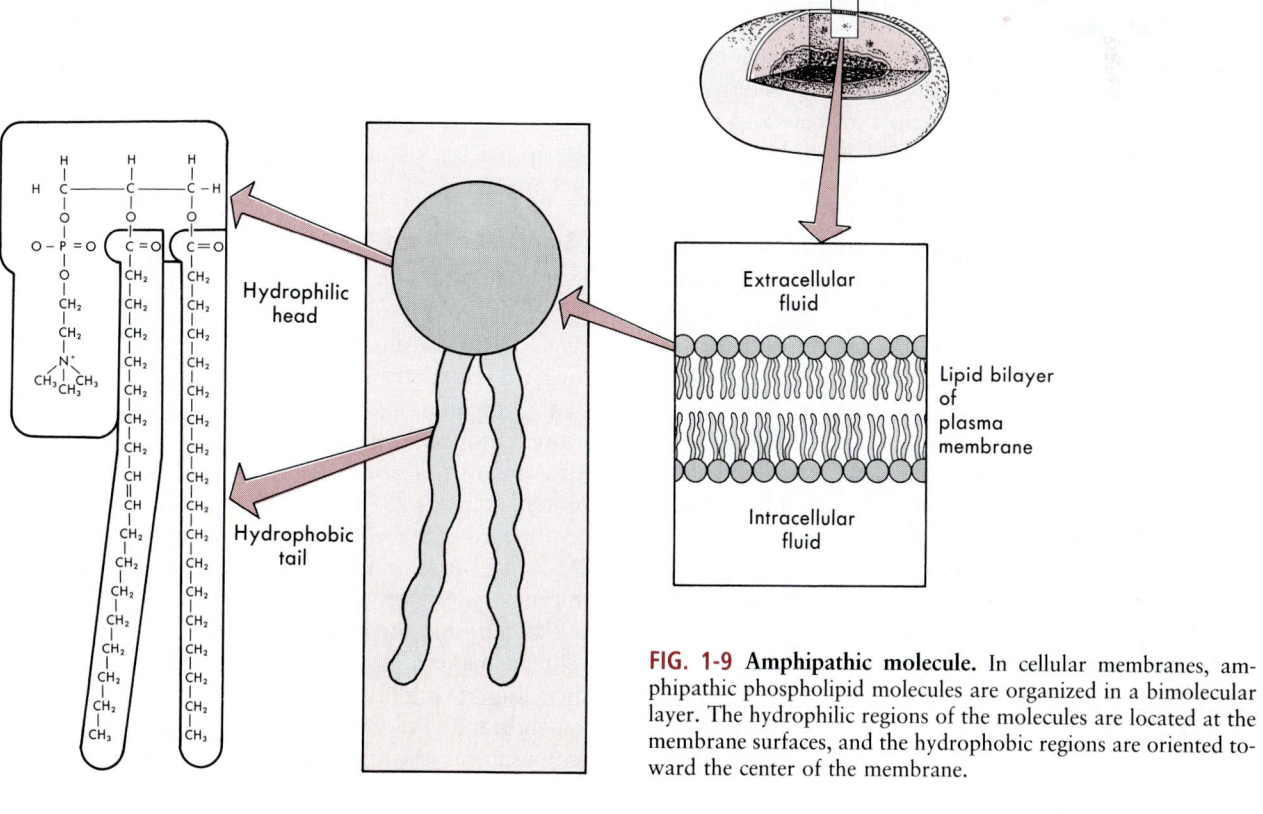

FIG. 1-9 Amphipathic molecule. In cellular membranes, amphipathic phospholipid molecules are organized in a bimolecular layer. The hydrophilic regions of the molecules are located at the membrane surfaces, and the hydrophobic regions are oriented toward the center of the membrane.

Proteins

Recent research suggests two ways to classify membrane proteins. One way is classification as peripheral or integral proteins (see Fig. 1-12). **Integral membrane proteins** are those embedded in the lipid bilayer linked to either *phosphatidylinositol*, a minor phospholipid, or a fatty acid chain. The integral proteins can be removed from the membrane only by detergents that solubilize (dissolve) the lipid. **Peripheral membrane proteins** are not embedded in the bilayer but reside at one surface or the other, bound to an integral protein.

Although the classification of membrane proteins as peripheral or integral is commonly used, it does not describe how proteins are associated with the bilayer. The second mode of classification does so by taking into account the membrane-spanning, or transmembranous, nature of membrane proteins (Alberts et al., 1989) (Fig. 1-10). According to this classification, proteins are associated with the lipid bilayer in four ways:

1. Some proteins, called **transmembrane proteins,** extend across the bilayer and are exposed to an aqueous environment on both sides of it.
2. Some intracellular proteins extend their polypeptide chain partway through the bilayer by means of a fatty acid chain.
3. Some cell-surface proteins are attached to the bilayer by a covalent linkage (i.e., a specific oligosaccharide).
4. Some proteins do not extend even partway through the bilayer but are bound to the membrane by noncovalent linkages with other membrane proteins.

Proteins exist in densely folded molecular configurations rather than straight chains, so an excess of hydrophilic units is at the surface of the molecule and an excess of hydrophobic units is inside. Although membrane structure is determined by the lipid bilayer, membrane functions are determined largely by proteins. For example, proteins facilitate transport across membranes by serving as receptors, enzymes, or transporters. Proteins act as (1) recognition and binding units (receptors) for substances moving in and out of the cell, (2) pores or channels for various electrically charged particles called ions or electrolytes, (3) specific carriers for amino acids and monosaccharides, and (4) specific enzymes that drive active pumps that promote concentration of certain ions, particularly potassium (K^+), within the cell, while keeping concentrations of other ions, for example, sodium (Na^+), below concentrations found in the extracellular environment. (Membrane transport is discussed on p. 23.)

The interaction of plasma membrane proteins with lipids is complex and is currently the subject of much research. The role of proteins in the onset and progression of disease is important because of their enzymatic,

FIG. 1-10 Four ways in which proteins in the lipid bilayer can be associated with the bilayer. (1) Transmembrane proteins extend across the bilayer; (2) some intracellular proteins extend their polypeptide chain partway through the bilayer by means of a fatty acid chain; (3) some cell surface proteins are attached to the bilayer by a covalent linkage; and (4) some proteins are not embedded in the lipid bilayer at all, but are bound by noncovalent linkages with other membrane proteins.

transport, and recognition-receptor functions in cellular physiology.

Carbohydrates

A significant amount of carbohydrate is contained within the plasma membrane in the form of glycoprotein. Intercellular recognition, which is required for tissue formation, is an important function of membrane glycoproteins.

Membrane Fluidity: The Fluid Mosaic Model

In the 1960s, G. L. Nicholson and S. J. Singer proposed the popular **fluid mosaic model** for biologic membranes (Fig. 1-11). The model, which is continually being modified, presents integral proteins as pieces of a mosaic that float singly or as aggregates in the fluid lipid bilayer. The protein molecules serve to (1) transport other molecules into and out of the cell, (2) facilitate (catalyze) membrane reactions, (3) receive messages, thus acting as receptors for extracellular and intracellular signals, and (4) create structural linkages between the external and internal cellular environments.

The fluid mosaic model accounts for the flexibility of cellular membranes, their self-sealing properties, and their impermeability to many substances. The degree of a membrane's fluidity depends on temperature. At lower temperatures, the lipids are in a gel crystalline state, and

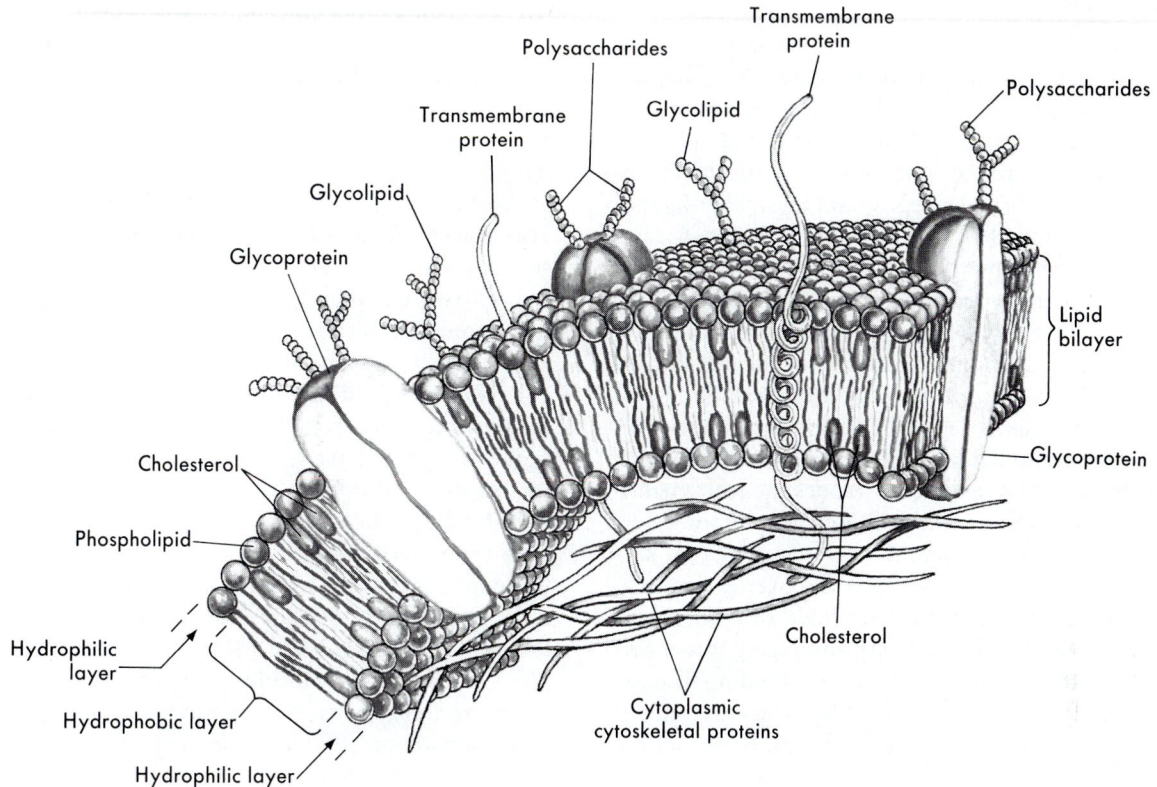

FIG. 1-11 Fluid mosaic model. Schematic, three-dimensional view of the fluid mosaic model of membrane structure. The lipid bilayer provides the basic structure and serves as a relatively impermeable barrier to most water-soluble molecules.

at higher temperatures they become highly fluid. These properties are critical for cellular growth, division, and receptor function. Because *some* proteins are free to move within the plasma membranes (like floating icebergs), certain foreign proteins (antigens) may become buried in the bilayer, emerging at the surface only after injury and then attracting antibodies (proteins produced by the immune system), which attack host cells. Antigens and antibodies, which are the cause and effect of the immune response, are discussed in Chapter 6. The burial and reemergence of antigens may be one cause of autoimmune disease, described in Chapter 8.

In the fluid mosaic model, cellular membranes are dynamic. Not only do some lipids and proteins move laterally on the membrane, but ions and other molecules also move through it. Cells, however, do have ways of immobilizing specific membrane proteins in a specific region of the membrane. Confinement may be necessary for certain functions to occur, for example, the proteins that form intercellular junctions. The fluid mosaic model is logical in that it describes the membrane as existing in a state of change and modulation, which allows the cell to protect itself actively against injurious agents. Hormones, bacteria, viruses, drugs, antibodies,

chemicals that transmit nerve impulses (neurotransmitters), and other substances attach to the plasma membrane by means of receptor molecules on its outer layer. The number of receptors present may vary at different times, and the cell is capable of modulating the effects of injurious agents by altering receptor number and pattern (Catt et al., 1979). This aspect of the fluid mosaic model has drastically modified previously held concepts concerning the onset of disease.

The concentration of cholesterol in the plasma membrane affects membrane fluidity. Increased concentration results in less fluidity on the membrane's hydrophilic outer surface and more fluidity at its hydrophobic core. Cholesterol content changes are factors in some diseases. In cirrhosis of the liver, for example, the cholesterol content of the red blood cell's plasma membrane increases. This causes an overall decrease in membrane fluidity that seriously affects the cell's ability to transport oxygen. The implications of changes in membrane integrity and their role in subsequent disease states are largely unknown. As measurement techniques for studying membrane physiology improve, the pathologic manifestations of many diseases may be explained according to changes in membrane structure and function.

Cellular Receptors

Cellular receptors are protein molecules on the plasma membrane, in the cytoplasm, or in the nucleus that are capable of recognizing and binding with specific smaller molecules called **ligands.** Hormones, for example, are ligands. Recognition and binding depend on the chemical configuration of the receptor and its smaller ligand, which must fit together somewhat like pieces of a jigsaw puzzle (see Chapter 17).

Plasma membrane receptors are particularly important for cellular uptake of ligands. They protrude from or are exposed at the external surface of the membrane, often attached to integral proteins (Fig. 1-12). Some of these recognition units have all the mobile properties related to membrane fluidity. The ligands that bind with membrane receptors include hormones, neurotransmitters, antigens, complement components, lipoproteins, infectious agents, drugs, and metabolites. The past several years have brought many new discoveries concerning the specific interactions of cellular receptors with their respective ligands. In many instances, this information has provided a basis for understanding disease.

Although the chemical nature of both ligands and the receptors to which they bind is different, receptors are classified on the basis of their location and function (see Cell-to-Cell Communication). Cellular type determines overall cellular function, but plasma membrane receptors determine which ligands a cell will bind with and how the cell will respond to binding with each. For example, the ability of a hormone or a neurotransmitter to stimulate a cell is regulated by the specificity and number of receptors present on the plasma membrane. Specific processes also control intracellular mechanisms. Hormone binding, for example, depends on special messenger molecules that regulate protein synthesis within the cell (see Chapter 17). Neurotransmitters (discussed in Chapter 12) also operate by causing special messengers to react with specific receptors.

Receptors for different drugs are found on the plasma membrane, in the cytoplasm, and in the nucleus. Membrane receptors have been found for certain anesthetics, opiates, endorphins, enkephalins, antibiotics, cancer chemotherapeutic agents, digitalis, and other drugs. Membrane receptors for endorphins, which are opiate-like peptides isolated from the pituitary gland, are found in large quantities in pain pathways of the nervous system (see Chapters 12 and 13). With binding, the endorphins (or drugs like morphine) change the cell's permeability to ions, increase the concentration of molecules that regulate intracellular protein synthesis, and initiate molecular events that modulate pain perception.

Receptors for infectious microorganisms, or antigen

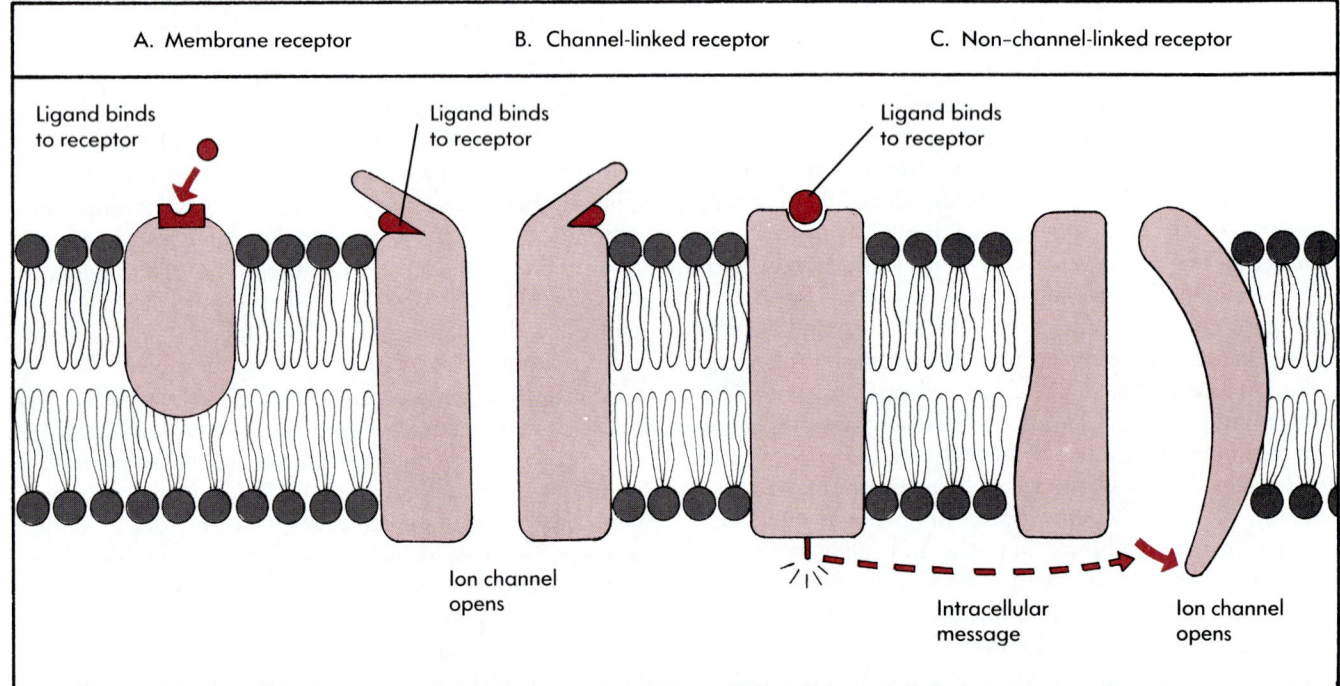

FIG. 1-12 Cellular receptors. A, Plasma membrane receptor for a ligand (here, a hormone molecule) on the surface of an integral protein. **B** and **C,** A neurotransmitter can exert its effect on a postsynaptic cell by means of two fundamentally different types of receptor proteins: channel-linked receptors and non–channel–linked receptors. Channel-linked receptors are also known as ligand-gated channels. (**B** and **C,** Modified from Alberts et al., 1989.)

receptors, bind bacteria, viruses, and parasites. Antigen receptors on white blood cells (lymphocytes, monocytes, macrophages, and granulocytes) recognize and bind with antigenic microorganisms and activate the immune and inflammatory responses (see Chapters 6 and 7).

CELL-TO-CELL COMMUNICATION

Cells need to communicate with each other to regulate their growth and division, their development and organization into tissues, and to coordinate their functions. Cells communicate in three ways: (1) they form protein channels (gap junctions) that directly coordinate the activities of adjacent cells; (2) they display plasma-membrane–bound signaling molecules (receptors) that affect the cell itself and other cells in direct physical contact; and (3) they secrete chemicals that signal to cells some distance away (Fig. 1-13). Alterations in cellular communication affect disease onset and progression. In fact, if a cell is unable to perform gap junctional intercellular communication, it is hypothesized that normal growth control and cell differentia-

tion would not be possible, thereby favoring cancerous tumor development (see Chapter 10). (Communication through gap junctions is discussed on p. 36 and contact signaling by plasma-membrane–bound molecules is discussed on pp. 20 and 31.) Secreted chemical signals involve communication at a distance. Three primary modes of chemical signaling include endocrine, paracrine, and synaptic (Fig. 1-14).

Endocrine signaling involves specialized endocrine cells that secrete hormone chemicals released by one set of cells and travel through the tissue through the bloodstream to produce a response in other sets of cells (see Chapter 17). In **paracrine signaling**, cells secrete local chemical mediators that are quickly taken up, destroyed, or immobilized. The mediators act only on nearby cells. In **synaptic signaling**, cells secrete chemicals, or **neurotransmitters**, at specialized junctions called **chemical synapses**; the neurotransmitter diffuses across the synaptic cleft and acts on the postsynaptic target cell (see Fig. 1-14). In each type of chemical signaling, the target cell receives the signal by first attaching to its receptors. Many of the same signaling molecules are receptors used in endocrine, paracrine, and synaptic sig-

FIG. 1-13 **Cellular communication.** Three ways in which cells communicate with one another. (Modified from Alberts et al., 1989.)

FIG. 1-14 **Primary modes of chemical signaling.** Three forms of signaling mediated by secreted molecules. Not all neurotransmitters act in the strictly synaptic mode shown; some act in a paracrine mode as local chemical mediators that influence multiple target cells in the area. (Modified from Alberts et al., 1989.)

Cell surface receptors

Signaling molecule

G-protein

Enzyme

cAMP

Target protein

Signaling molecule

G-protein

Enzyme

Ca++

Target protein

cAMP pathway   Ca++ pathway

FIG. 1-15 **Intracellular messengers.** Two major pathways by which G-protein–linked cell-surface receptors generate intracellular messengers. In both cases the binding of an extracellular ligand alters the conformation of the cytoplasmic domain of the receptor so that it binds to a G-protein, which in turn activates (or inactivates) a plasma membrane enzyme. In other cases the G-protein binds to an ion channel rather than to an enzyme. In the cyclic AMP pathway, the enzyme produces cyclic AMP. In the Ca++ pathway, the enzyme produces a soluble mediator that releases Ca++ from an intracellular storage site. Both cyclic AMP and Ca++ bind to other specific proteins in the cell, thereby altering their activity. (Redrawn from Alberts et al., 1989.)

TABLE 1-2

Cellular Responses Mediated by the Inositol-Phospholipid Signaling Pathway

Target tissue	Signaling molecule	Physiologic function
Liver	Antidiuretic hormone	Glycogen breakdown
Pancreas	Acetylcholine	Amylase secretion
Smooth muscle	Acetylcholine	Contraction
Pancreatic B cells	Acetylcholine	Insulin secretion
Mast cells	Antigen	Histamine secretion
Blood platelets	Thrombin	Serotonin and platelet-derived growth factor secretion

Modified from Alberts et al., 1989.

naling. The important differences lie in the speed and selectivity with which the signals are delivered to their targets (Alberts et al., 1989).

Plasma membrane receptors belong to one of three classes that are defined by the signaling (transduction) mechanism used. **Channel-linked receptors,** or ligand-gated channels, involve rapid synaptic signaling between electrically excitable cells (see Fig. 1-12, *B*). The gated ion channels open or close briefly in response to neurotransmitters changing the ion permeability of the plasma membrane of the postsynaptic cell.

Catalytic receptors, once activated by ligands, function directly as enzymes. These receptors are transmembrane proteins that intracellularly function as a tyrosine-specific protein kinase.

G-protein–linked receptors indirectly activate or inactivate a plasma membrane enzyme or ion channel. The interaction between the receptor and the enzyme or ion channel is mediated by a different protein called a **GTP-binding regulatory protein (G-protein).** Activation of the G-protein–linked receptors activates a chain of reactions that alters the concentration of intracellular messengers or signaling molecules. These intracellular messengers alter the behavior of other target proteins in the cell, including cyclic adenosine monophosphate (AMP) and calcium (Ca++) (Fig. 1-15). Other G-protein–linked receptors interact with the inositol phospholipids found in small quantities in the plasma membrane. The inositol phospholipids are significant in cell signaling, and the molecules involved are called the **inositol-phospholipid transduction pathway.** A G-protein–linked receptor activates the enzyme phosphoinositide-specific phospholipase that in turn generates two intracellular messengers: (1) inositol triphosphate (InsP$_3$) releases Ca++, increasing the intracellular concentration of Ca++; and (2) diacylglycerol remains in the plasma membrane and activates protein kinase C. Protein kinase C further activates various cell proteins. Several different plasma membrane receptors have been shown to use the inositol phospholipid transduction pathway (Table 1-2) (Alberts et al., 1989). Breakdown of the signal transduction pathways can cause pathophysiologic alterations because of disturbances between the signaling molecule and the corresponding target tissue response (see Table 1-2).

CELLULAR METABOLISM

All of the chemical tasks of maintaining essential cellular functions are referred to as **cellular metabolism.** The energy-using process of metabolism is called **anabolism** (*ana* = upward), and the energy-releasing process is known as **catabolism** (*kata* = downward). Metabolism provides the cell with the energy it needs to synthesize (produce) cellular structures.

Dietary proteins, fats, and starches are hydrolyzed in the intestinal tract into amino acids, fatty acids, and glucose. These constituents are then absorbed, circulated, and taken up by the cell where they may be used for various vital cellular processes including the production of adenosine triphosphate (ATP). The process by which ATP is produced is one example of a series of reactions called a **metabolic pathway**. A metabolic pathway involves several intermediate steps whose end products are not always detectable. A key feature of cellular metabolism is the directing of biochemical reactions by protein catalysts, or enzymes. Most biochemical reactions in a pathway are catalyzed by a specific enzyme. Each enzyme has a high affinity for a **substrate**—a specific substance that is converted to a product of the reaction.

Role of Adenosine Triphosphate

For a cell to function, the cell must be able to extract and use the chemical energy contained within the structure of organic molecules. When a mole of glucose is metabolically broken down in the presence of oxygen into carbon dioxide and water, 686 kilocalories (kcal) of energy is released. In a test tube, this energy is released as heat. Because a cell cannot transform heat into work, chemical energy, rather than heat, is created by metabolism. The chemical energy lost by one molecule is transferred to the chemical structure of another molecule by an energy-carrying or transferring molecule, such as ATP. The energy stored in ATP can be used in a variety of energy-requiring reactions and in the process is generally converted to adenosine diphosphate (ADP) and inorganic phosphate (Pi). The energy available as a result of this reaction is about 7 kcal/mol of ATP. In addition to its use in synthesis (anabolism) of organic molecules, ATP is used by the cell for muscle contraction and active transport of molecules across cellular membranes. The function of ATP is not only to *store* energy but also to *transfer* it from one molecule to another. Energy is stored by molecules of carbohydrate, lipid, and protein, which, when catabolized, transfer energy to ATP.

Food and Production of Cellular Energy

The process of catabolism of the proteins, lipids, and polysaccharides found in food can be divided into three phases (Fig. 1-16). In phase 1, large molecules are broken down into their smaller subunits—proteins into amino acids, polysaccharides into simple sugars, and fats into fatty acids and glycerol. These processes are called **digestion** and occur outside of the cell by the action of secreted enzymes.

In phase 2, the small molecules enter cells and are further broken down in the cytoplasm. Most of the sugars are converted into pyruvate. Pyruvate then enters mitochondria and is converted to the acetyl groups of acetyl coenzyme A (acetyl CoA). Acetyl CoA, like ATP, releases energy when it is hydrolyzed. The most important part of phase 2 is the lysis (splitting) of glucose, known as **glycolysis** (Fig. 1-17). Glycolysis produces a net of two molecules of ATP per glucose molecule through the process of **oxidation,** or the removal and transfer of a pair of electrons. This process, often called **oxidative cellular metabolism,** involves nine biochemical reactions. In reactions 1 to 4, glucose is converted to the three-carbon aldehyde (glyceraldehyde 3-phosphate), which requires energy in the form of ATP. In reactions 5 and 6, the aldehyde group of the glyceraldehyde 3-phosphate is oxidized (loses electrons) to carboxylic acid, and the energy from this reaction creates a new high-energy phosphate (ATP) for each molecule of aldehyde. In reactions 7, 8, and 9, a net profit of two molecules of ATP per glucose molecule is produced.

Phase 3 occurs when the acetyl group of acetyl CoA is completely degraded to carbon dioxide (CO_2) and water (H_2O). It is in this final phase that most of the ATP is generated. Phase 3 begins with the **citric acid cycle** (also called the **Krebs cycle,** or the **tricarboxylic acid cycle**) and ends with oxidative phosphorylation. The citric acid cycle accounts for approximately two thirds of the total oxidation of carbon compounds in most cells. Its major end products are CO_2 and two dinucleotides, NADH and $FADH_2$. NADH and $FADH_2$ transfer their electrons into the electron-transport chain.

Oxidative Phosphorylation

Oxidative phosphorylation occurs in the mitochondria and is the mechanism by which the energy produced from carbohydrates, fats, and proteins is transferred to ATP. During the breakdown (catabolism) of foods, many of the reactions involve the removal of electrons from various intermediates. These reactions generally require a coenzyme (a nonprotein carrier molecule), such as nicotinamide adenine dinucleotide (NAD), to transfer the electrons and thus are called **transfer reactions.**

In oxidative phosphorylation, molecules of NAD and flavin adenine nucleotide (FAD) transfer electrons they have gained from the oxidation of substrates to molecular oxygen, O_2. The electrons from reduced NAD and FAD, NADH and $FADH_2$, are transferred to a series of carrier molecules (the **electron-transport chain**), on the inner surfaces of the mitochondria with the release of hydrogen ions. Some of the carrier molecules are a group of brightly colored iron-containing proteins

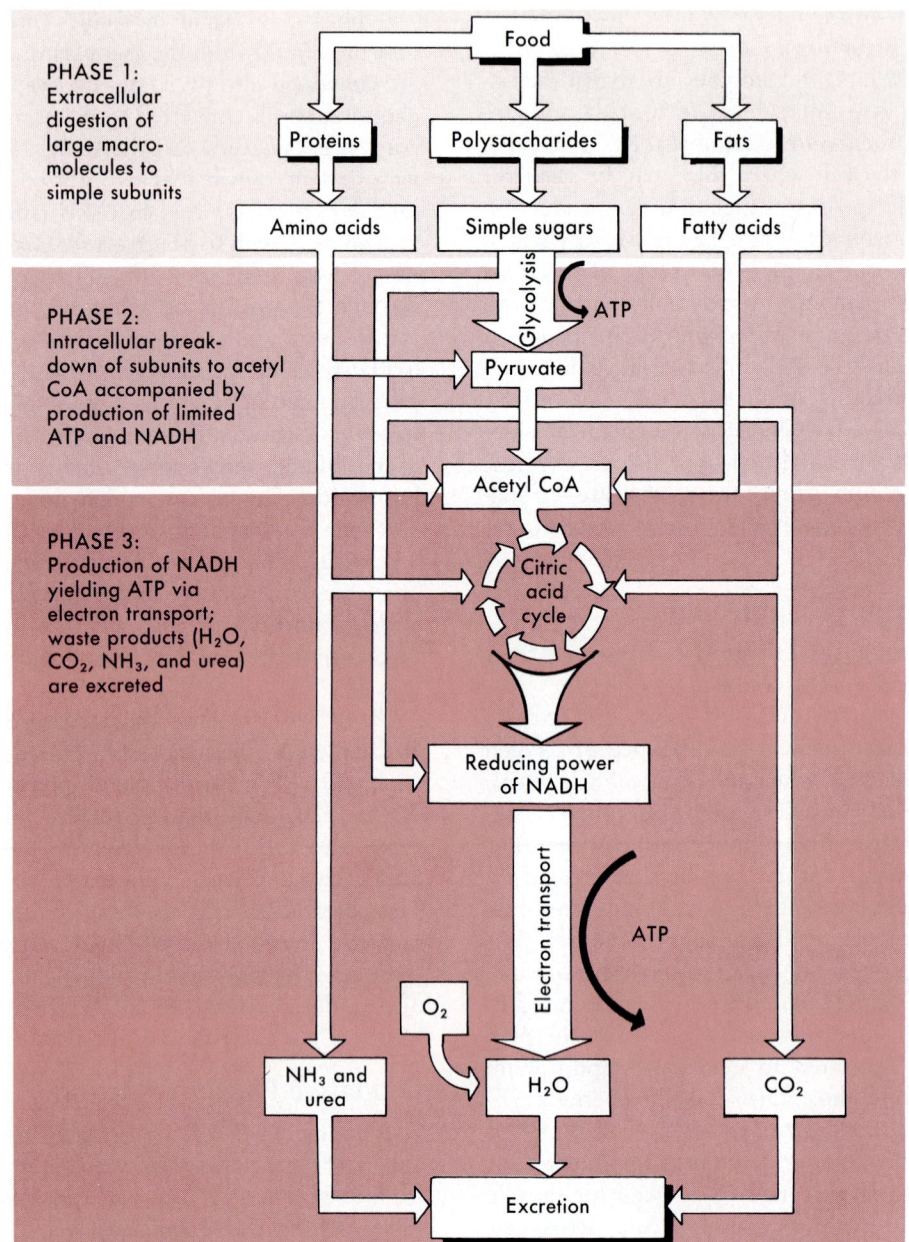

FIG. 1-16 Three phases of catabolism, which leads from food to waste products. These reactions produce ATP, which is used to drive other processes in the cell. (Modified from Alberts et al., 1989.)

known as cytochromes that accept a pair of electrons. After passing through a sequence of different cytochromes, these electrons are eventually combined with molecular oxygen. If oxygen is not available to the electron-transport chain, ATP will not be formed by the mitochondria. Instead, an anaerobic (without oxygen) metabolic pathway synthesizes ATP. This process, called **substrate phosphorylation,** or **anaerobic glycolysis,** does not take place in the mitochondria and is linked

to the breakdown (glycolysis) of carbohydrate as shown in Fig. 1-17.

Since glycolysis occurs in the cytoplasm of the cell, it provides energy for cells that lack mitochondria. However, as noted above, glycolysis also provides energy to the cell when oxygen delivery is insufficient or delayed. The reactions in anaerobic glycolysis involve the conversion of glucose to pyruvic acid (pyruvate) with the simultaneous production of ATP. With the glycolysis of

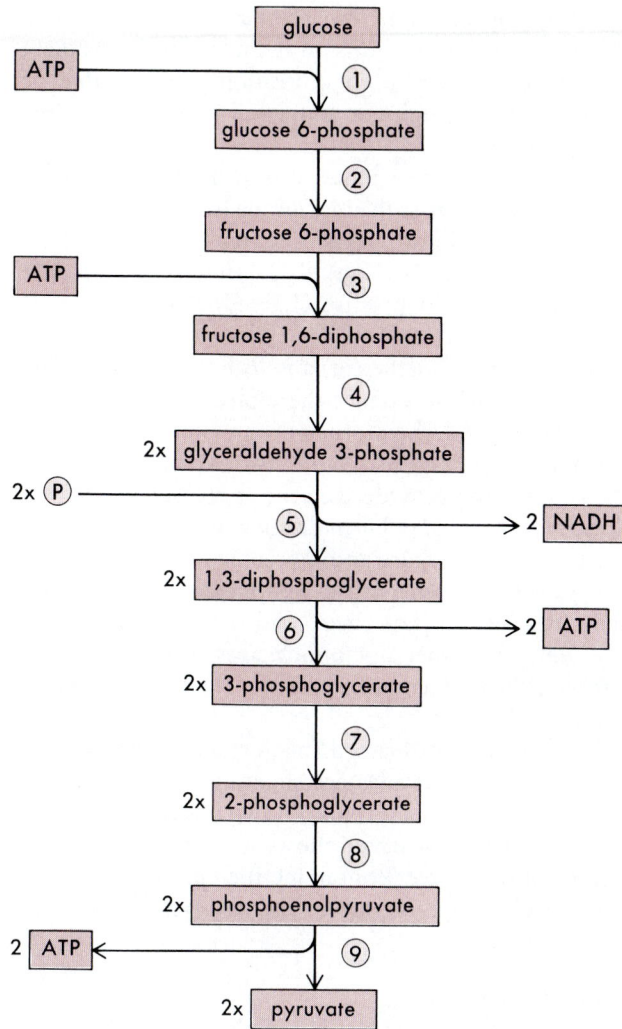

FIG. 1-17 Glycolysis. Each of the numbered reactions is catalyzed by a different enzyme. At step 4, a six-carbon sugar is broken down to give two three-carbon sugars, so that the number of molecules at every step after this is doubled. Reactions 5 and 6 are the reactions responsible for the net synthesis of ATP and NADH molecules. (Modified from Alberts et al., 1989.)

one molecule of glucose, two ATP molecules and two molecules of pyruvate are liberated. If oxygen is present, the two molecules of pyruvate move into the mitochondria, where they enter the citric acid cycle. If oxygen is absent, pyruvate is converted to lactic acid and released into the extracellular fluid. The conversion of pyruvic acid to lactic acid is reversible; therefore, once oxygen is restored, lactic acid is quickly converted back to either pyruvic acid or glucose. The anaerobic generation of ATP from glucose, through the reactions of glycolysis, is not as efficient as aerobic generation of ATP. The addition of an oxygen-requiring stage to the catabolic process (stage 3) provides cells with a much more powerful method for extracting energy from food molecules.

PROCESSES OF CELLULAR INTAKE AND OUTPUT

Cells continually take in nutrients, fluids, and chemical messengers from the extracellular environment and expel metabolites or the products of metabolism and end products of lysosomal digestion. Intake and output, or transport, occurs by different mechanisms, depending on the characteristics of the substance to be transported. Water and small, electrically uncharged molecules move easily through pores in the plasma membrane's lipid bilayer. This process, called **passive transport,** will occur naturally through any semipermeable barrier. It is driven by osmosis, hydrostatic pressure, and diffusion, all of which depend on the laws of physics and do not require life. The process is passive in that it does not require any expenditure of energy by the cell.

Other molecules cannot be driven across the plasma membrane solely by forces of diffusion, hydrostatic pressure, or osmosis because they are too large or are ligands that have bound with receptors on the cell's plasma membrane. Some of these molecules are moved into the cell by mechanisms of **active transport,** which requires life, biologic activity, and the expenditure of metabolic energy by the cell. Unlike passive transport, which can be duplicated across any semipermeable barrier in a laboratory, active transport occurs only across living membranes that (1) use energy generated by cellular metabolism and (2) have receptors that are capable of recognizing and binding with the substance to be transported. Large molecules (macromolecules), along with fluids, are transported by means of endocytosis (taking in) and exocytosis (expelling). Water and electrically charged molecules are transported by protein channels embedded in the plasma membrane. Ligands enter the cell by means of receptor-mediated endocytosis.

Movement of Water and Solutes

Cellular membranes are semipermeable and generally allow passage of water and small particles of dissolved substances called **solutes.** The movement of solute molecules through membranes is related to their size, solubility, electrical properties, and concentration on either side of the membrane. Small, lipid-soluble particles, such as oxygen, carbon dioxide, and urea, can readily pass the lipid bilayers of the plasma membrane. Larger, water-soluble particles may pass through pores in the membranes. Although large protein molecules, such as albumin and globulin, pass through membranes by endocytosis, they influence the movement of water by exerting an osmotic effect (see p. 25).

Body fluids are composed of two types of solutes: **electrolytes,** which are electrically charged and dissociate into constituent **ions** when placed in solution, and nonelectrolytes, such as glucose, urea, and creatinine, which do not dissociate. Electrolytes account for approximately 95% of the solute molecules in body water. Electrolytes exhibit **polarity** by orienting themselves toward the positive or negative pole. Ions with a positive charge are known as **cations** and migrate toward the negative pole, or cathode, if an electrical current is passed through the electrolyte solution. **Anions** carry a negative charge and migrate toward the positive pole, or anode, in the presence of electrical current. Anions and cations are located in both the intracellular fluid (ICF) and extracellular fluid (ECF) compartments, although concentration of particular ions varies depending on their location. (Fluid and electrolyte balance between body compartments is discussed in Chapter 3.) For example, sodium (Na^+) is the predominant extracellular cation, and potassium (K^+) is the principal intracellular cation. The difference in ICF and ECF concentrations of these ions is important to the transmission of electrical impulses across the plasma membranes of nerve and muscle cells.

Electrolytes are measured in milliequivalents per liter (mEq/L) or milligrams per deciliter (mg/dl). Milliequivalents per liter indicate the number of electrical charges per unit volume of fluid. The term *milliequivalent* thus indicates the chemical-combining activity of an ion, which depends on the electrical charge, or **valence**, of its ions. In abbreviations, valence is indicated by the *number* of plus or minus signs. Monovalent ions, or ions with one charge, include sodium (Na^+), chlorine (Cl^-), and potassium (K^+). Divalent ions, which have two charges, include calcium (Ca^{++}) and magnesium (Mg^{++}). One milliequivalent of any cation can combine chemically with 1 mEq of any anion: one monovalent anion will combine with one monovalent cation. Divalent ions combine more strongly than monovalent ions. To maintain electrochemical balance, one divalent ion will combine with two monovalent ions (e.g., $Ca^{++} + 2Cl^- = CaCl_2$).

Passive Transport

Diffusion

Diffusion is the movement of a solute molecule from an area of greater solute concentration to an area of lesser solute concentration. This difference in concentration is known as a **concentration gradient.** Particles in a solution move randomly in any direction. If the concentration of particles in one part of the solution is greater than in another part, the particles distribute themselves evenly throughout the solution. According to the same principle, if the concentration of particles is greater on one side of a permeable membrane than on the other side, the particles diffuse spontaneously from the area of greater concentration to the area of lesser concentration until equilibrium is reached. The higher the con-

centration on one side, the greater the diffusion rate. The overall effect of diffusion is the passive movement of particles "down" a concentration gradient, that is, from an area of high concentration to an area of low concentration.

The diffusion rate is influenced by differences of electrical potential across the membrane (see p. 32.) Because the pores in the lipid bilayer are often lined with Ca^{++}, other cations (e.g., Na^+ and K^+) diffuse slowly because they are repelled by positive charges in the pores.

The rate of diffusion of a substance depends also on its size (diffusion coefficient) and its lipid solubility (Fig. 1-18). Usually, the smaller the molecule and the more soluble it is in oil, the more hydrophobic or nonpolar it is, and the more rapidly it will diffuse across the bilayer. Oxygen, carbon dioxide, and the steroid hormones are all examples of nonpolar molecules. Water-soluble substances, such as sugars and inorganic ions, diffuse very slowly, whereas uncharged lipophilic ("lipid-loving") molecules, such as fatty acids and steroids, diffuse rapidly. Ions and other polar molecules generally diffuse across cellular membranes more slowly than lipid-soluble substances.

Water readily diffuses through biologic membranes because water molecules are small and uncharged. Although the mechanism is not known with certainty, the dipolar structure of water allows it to cross rapidly the regions of the bilayer containing the lipid head groups. Lipid head groups constitute the two outer regions of the lipid bilayer.

Hydrostatic pressure

Hydrostatic pressure is the mechanical force of water pushing against cellular membranes. In the vascular system, hydrostatic pressure is the blood pressure generated in vessels by the contraction of the heart. Blood reaching the capillary bed has a hydrostatic pressure of 25 to 30 mm Hg, which is sufficient force to push water across the thin capillary membranes into the interstitial space, a process known as *filtration*. Hydrostatic pressure is partially balanced by osmotic pressure: there is a net movement of water out of the capillary partially balanced by osmotic forces that tend to pull water into the capillaries. Water that is not osmotically attracted back into the capillaries moves into the lymph system (see Starling's forces in Chapter 3).

Osmosis

Osmosis is the movement of *water* "down" a concentration gradient; that is, across a semipermeable membrane from a region of higher water concentration to a region of lower water concentration. For osmosis to occur, the membrane must be more permeable to water than to solutes, and there must be a greater concentration of solutes so that water moves more easily. Osmo-

FIG. 1-18 **Passive diffusion of solute molecules across the plasma membrane.** Oxygen, nitrogen, water, urea, glycerol, and carbon dioxide can diffuse readily down the concentration gradient. Macromolecules are too large to diffuse through pores in the plasma membrane. Ions may be repelled if the pores contain substances with identical charges. If the pores are lined with cations, for example, other cations will have difficulty diffusing because the positive charges will repel one another. Diffusion can still occur, but it occurs more slowly.

sis is directly related to both hydrostatic pressure and solute concentration, but *not* to particle size or weight. For example, particles of the plasma protein albumin are small but more concentrated in body fluids than the larger and heavier particles of globulin. Therefore albumin exerts a greater osmotic force than globulin.

Osmolality controls distribution and movement of water between body compartments. The terms osmolality and osmolarity are often used interchangeably in reference to osmotic activity, but they define different measurements. **Osmolality** is a measure of the number of milliosmoles per kilogram of water, or the concentration of molecules per *weight* of water. **Osmolarity** is a measure of the number of milliosmoles per liter of solution, or the concentration of molecules per *volume* of solution. When solute is added to water, the volume is expanded and includes the original liter of water plus the volume occupied by the solute particles. In measuring osmolarity, the volume of water is therefore reduced by an amount equal to the volume of added solute.

In solutions that contain only dissociable substances, such as sodium and chloride, the difference between the two measurements is negligible. In considering all the different solutes in plasma (proteins, glucose, lipids, etc.), however, the difference between osmolality and osmolarity becomes more significant. In plasma, less of the plasma weight is water, and the overall concentration of particles is therefore greater. The osmolality will be greater than the osmolarity because of the smaller proportion of water. Osmolality is thus the preferred measure of osmotic activity in clinical assessment of individuals.

The normal osmolality of body fluids is 280 to 294 mOsm/kg. The osmolality of intracellular and extracellular fluid tends to equalize and so provides a measure of body fluid concentration and thus the body's hydration status. Hydration is also affected by hydrostatic pressure, since the movement of water by osmosis can be opposed by an equal amount of hydrostatic pressure. The amount of hydrostatic pressure required to oppose the osmotic movement of water is called the **osmotic pressure** of the solution. Factors that determine osmotic pressure are the type and thickness of the plasma membrane, the size of the molecules, the concentration of molecules or the concentration gradient, and the solubility of molecules within the membrane. Examples of the movement of water in relation to hydrostatic and osmotic forces occur in the glomerulus in the kidney (see Chapter 32) and in the capillaries of the microcirculation (see Chapter 26).

Effective osmolality is sustained osmotic activity and depends on the concentration of solutes remaining on one side of a permeable membrane. If the solutes penetrate the membrane and equilibrate with the solution on the other side of the membrane, the osmotic effect will be diminished or lost. For example, urea is a small solute that readily diffuses across cellular membranes. Solutions containing urea rapidly lose their effective osmolality because they rapidly equilibrate. Solutes too large to pass through the membrane thus sustain an effective osmolality, meaning that they enhance osmotic activity. Plasma proteins are examples of molecules that provide effective osmolality because they normally do not cross cellular membranes.

Plasma proteins also influence osmolality because they have a negative charge. The principle by which the plasma protein charge influences osmolality is known as Gibbs-Donnan equilibrium, and it affects the distribution of ions across cellular membranes. Gibbs-Donnan equilibrium occurs when fluid in one compartment contains small diffusible ions such as Na^+ and Cl^-, together with large, nondiffusible charged particles, such as plasma proteins. Because the body tends to maintain an electrical equilibrium, the nondiffusible protein molecules cause asymmetry in the distribution of small ions. Anions such as Cl^- are thus driven out of the cell or plasma, and cations like Na^+ are attracted. The protein-containing compartment will maintain a state of electroneutrality, but the osmolality will be higher. The overall osmotic effect of colloids, such as plasma proteins, is called the **oncotic pressure,** or **colloid osmotic pressure.**

Tonicity describes the effective osmolality of a solution. (The terms *osmolality* and *tonicity* may be used interchangeably.) Solutions, then, have relative degrees of tonicity. An **isotonic solution** (or iso-osmotic solution) has the same osmolality or concentration of particles (285 mOsm) as the ICF or ECF. Examples of isotonic solutions include 5% dextrose in water and normal (0.9%) saline solution. A **hypotonic solution** has a lower concentration and is thus more dilute than body fluids. Water is a hypotonic solution. Consequently, water is osmotically pulled into the cells, causing them to swell or burst. A **hypertonic solution** has a concentration greater than 285 to 294 mOsm/kg. An example of hypertonic solution is 3% saline solution. Water can be pulled out of the cells by a hypertonic solution, so that the cells shrink. The concept of tonicity is important when correcting water and solute imbalances by administering different types of replacement solutions.

Mediated and Active Transport
Mediated transport

Mediated transport (passive and active) involves integral or transmembrane proteins with receptors having a high degree of specificity for the substance being transported. Inorganic anions and cations (e.g., Na^+, K^+, Ca^{++}, Cl^-, and HCO_3^-) and charged and uncharged organic compounds (e.g., amino acids and sugars) require specific transport systems to facilitate movement through different cellular membranes. Rates at which substances are moved by mediated transport mechanisms have often been measured, yet the specific membrane proteins involved have not been identified. Mediated transport is much faster than simple diffusion.

A **transport protein** *(carrier protein)* is a transmembrane or integral protein that binds with and transfers a specific solute molecule across the lipid bilayer. Each transport protein, or **transporter,** has receptors for a specific solute. When the transporter is saturated—that is, when all receptor sites are occupied by solute molecules—the rate of transport is maximal. Solute binding can be blocked by **competitive inhibitors** that compete for the same receptor site and may or may not be transported by the transport protein. Noncompetitive inhibitors bind elsewhere but can alter the structure of the transporter.

The transporter protein is a multipass, transmembrane protein; that is, their polypeptide chain crosses the lipid bilayer multiple times. This chain forms a continuous pathway enabling solutes to pass across the membrane without coming into direct contact with the hydrophobic interior of the lipid bilayer (Alberts et al., 1989) (Fig. 1-19). (Transmembrane proteins are illustrated in Figs. 1-10 and 1-11.)

Another mechanism of mediated transport is the channel protein. The protein transporter creates a water-filled pore or channel across the bilayer through which specific ions can diffuse. These channels are sometimes called ion channels, and because they are permeable mainly to K^+, they are also called K^+ leak channels (Fig. 1-20). The channel is controlled by a gate mechanism that determines which receptor-bound solutes can move into the channel that is created after receptor-solute contact. Binding stimulates conformational changes in the protein transporter that move the solute through the channel short distances at a time until it reaches the other side of the membrane. Ion channels are responsible for the electrical excitability of nerve and muscle cells and play a critical role in the membrane potential (Devlin, 1992).

Mediated transport systems can move solute molecules singly or two at a time. Two molecules can be moved simultaneously in one direction (a process called **symport**) or in opposite directions (called **antiport**), or a single molecule can be moved in one direction (called **uniport**) (Fig. 1-21).

In **passive mediated transport,** also called **facilitated diffusion,** the protein transporter moves solute molecules through cellular membranes without expending

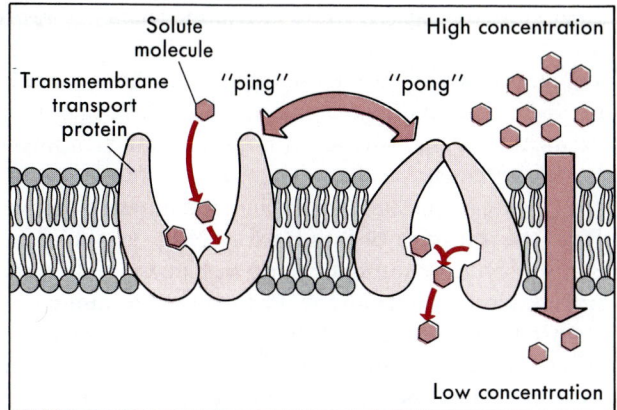

FIG. 1-19 Conformational-change model of mediated transport (facilitated diffusion). The transporter protein has two states, "ping" and "pong." In the ping state, sites for molecules of a specific solute are exposed on the outside of the bilayer. In the pong state, the sites are exposed to the inner side of the bilayer.

FIG. 1-20 Channel mode of mediated transport (facilitated diffusion). A channel protein forms a water-filled pore across the bilayer through which specific ions can diffuse. (Redrawn from Alberts et al., 1989.)

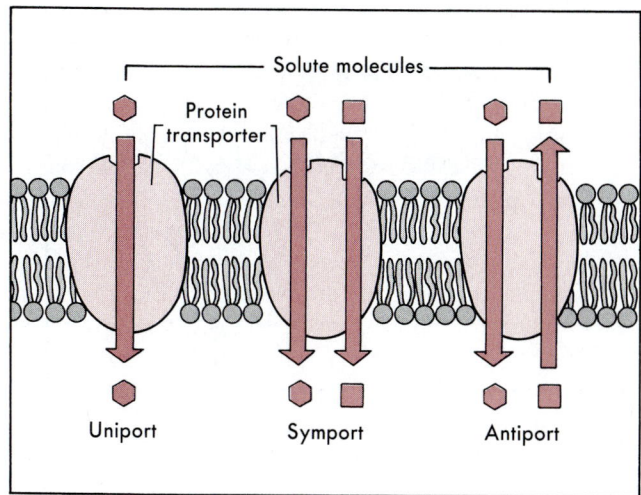

FIG. 1-21 Mediated transport. Simultaneous movement of a single solute molecule in one direction (uniport), of two different solute molecules in one direction (symport), and of two different solute molecules in opposite directions (antiport).

metabolic energy. The direction of movement is the same as in simple diffusion—down the concentration gradient. Perhaps the most widely referred to passive transport system is that for glucose in erythrocytes (red blood cells). Glucose is transported by a uniport mechanism and demonstrates saturation kinetics; that is, the transport system is saturated when all the glucose-specific receptors on the membrane are occupied and operating at their maximal capacity.

The anions Cl^- and HCO_3^- also undergo passive mediated transport in the erythrocyte. This antiport mechanism allows Cl^- movement in one direction and simultaneous HCO_3^- movement in the opposite direction. The directions of movement depend on the concentration gradients of the ions across the membrane.

In **active mediated transport,** also called active transport, the protein transporter moves molecules against, or up, the concentration gradient. Unlike passive mediated transport, active mediated transport requires the expenditure of energy. Many active mediated transport systems, or pumps, have ATP as their primary energy source, but not all. Some use the electrochemical gradient of Na^+ across the membrane (Fig. 1-22). Energy in the form of ATP, however, is required for activation of the Na^+ gradient.

A "carrier" mechanism in the plasma membrane mediates the transport of ions, such as Na^+, K^+, H^+, Cl^-, HCO_3^-, and of nutrients, such as glucose and amino acids. Energy supplied by ATP is required to pump ions against a concentration gradient. The best-known pump is the $Na^+ + K^+$-dependent ATPase pump. It continuously regulates the cells' volume by controlling leaks through pores or protein channels and maintains the ionic concentration gradients necessary for cellular excitation and membrane conductivity (see p. 32). The maintenance of intracellular K^+ concentrations is also required for enzyme activity, including that of enzymes involved in protein synthesis.

FIG. 1-22 Active mediated transport. Metabolic energy (ATP; P) controls the active transport of many substances, including Na^+. ATP is necessary for active mediated transport. (Redrawn from Alberts et al., 1989.)

Active transport of Na⁺ and K⁺

Active transport of Na^+ and K^+

The active transport system for Na^+ and K^+ is found in virtually all mammalian cells. The Na^+, K^+ antiport system, Na^+ moving out of and K^+ moving into the cell, uses the direct energy of ATP to move these cations. The transporter protein is an enzyme, ATPase. ATPase has a requirement for Na^+, K^+, and Mg^{++} ions. The concentration of ATPase in plasma membranes is directly related to Na^+, K^+ transport activity. Approximately 60% to 70% of the ATP synthesized by cells, especially muscle and nerve cells, is used to maintain the Na^+, K^+ transport system. Excitable tissues (e.g., muscle and nerve tissues) have a high concentration of Na^+, K^+ ATPase, as do other tissues that transport significant amounts of Na^+, for example, kidneys and salivary glands. For every ATP molecule hydrolyzed, three molecules of Na^+ are transported out of the cell, whereas only two molecules of K^+ move into the cell. The process leads to an electrical potential and is called *electrogenic,* with the inside of the cell more negative than the outside. The exact mechanism for transport of Na^+ and K^+ across the membrane is uncertain. One proposal is that ATPase induces the transporter protein to undergo several conformational changes, causing Na^+ and K^+ to move short distances (see Fig. 1-22). The conformational change creates a lowering of affinity for Na^+ and K^+ to the ATPase transporter, resulting in the release of the cations after transport.

The sarcoplasmic reticulum of heart muscle and skeletal muscle has an ATP-dependent Ca^{++} active transport system that regulates the Ca^{++} levels in the cell's cytoplasm, which in turn regulates muscle contraction and relaxation cycles (see Chapter 26). The Ca^{++} transport system depends on ATPase activity and is similar to that of Na^+, K^+ ATPase.

The transport of sugars and amino acids across the

TABLE 1-3

Major Transport Systems in Mammalian Cells

Substance transported	Mechanism of transport	Tissues
Sugars		
Glucose	Passive protein channel	Most tissues
	Active: symport with Na^+	Small intestines and renal tubular cells
Fructose	Passive	Intestines and liver
Amino acids	Coupled channels	
Amino acid specific transporters	Active: symport with Na^+	Intestines, kidney, and liver
All amino acids except proline	Active: group translocation	Liver
Specific amino acids	Passive	Small intestine
Other organic molecules		
Cholic acid, deoxycholic acid, and taurocholic acid	Active: symport with Na^+	Intestines
Organic anions, e.g., malate, α-ketoglutarate, glutamate	Antiport with counter-organic anion	Mitochondria of liver cells
ATP-ADP	Antiport transport of nucleotides; can be active	Mitochondria of liver cells
Inorganic ions		
Na^+	Passive	Distal renal tubular cells
Na^+/H^+	Active antiport, proton pump	Proximal renal tubular cells and small intestines
Na^+/K^+	Active: ATP driven, protein channel	Plasma membrane of most cells
Ca^{++}	Active: ATP driven, antiport with Na^+	All cells, antiporter in red cells
H^+/K^+	Active	Parietal cells of gastric cells secreting H^+
Cl^-/HCO_3^- (perhaps other anions)	Mediated: antiport	Erythrocytes and many other cells

From Devlin, 1992; Raven & Johnson, 1992.

NOTE: The known transport systems are listed here; others have been proposed. Most transport systems have been studied in only a few tissues and their sites of activity may be more limited than indicated.

plasma membrane depends on the simultaneous movement (symport) of Na^+ or Na^+-dependent transport (see Fig. 1-21). Na^+-dependent symport occurs primarily in the plasma membrane of epithelial cells of the kidney tubules and intestines. The transport of glucose is not directly dependent on the hydrolysis of ATP; however, the Na^+ gradient is ATP dependent, and thus ATP is indirectly involved in glucose transport.

The epithelial cells that line the intestines depend on Na^+ to transport various amino acids. Similarly, the uptake of Cl^- by the small intestine depends on Na^+ symport and antiport mechanisms for the secretion of Ca^{++} from the cell.

Table 1-3 summarizes the major mechanisms of transport through pores and protein transporters in the plasma membranes. Many disease states are caused and/or manifested by loss of these membrane transport systems.

Transport by Vesicle Formation
Endocytosis and Exocytosis

Pores and protein transporters cannot move large proteins, polynucleotides, or polysaccharides (macromolecules) across the plasma membrane, yet most cells are able to take in and eject these macromolecules. The active transport mechanisms by which the cells do this are very different from those that mediate small solute and ion transport. Transport of macromolecules involves the sequential formation and fusion of membrane-bounded vesicles.

In **endocytosis,** a section of the plasma membrane enfolds substances from outside the cell, invaginates (folds inward), and separates from the plasma membrane, forming a vesicle that moves into the inside of the cell (Fig. 1-23, *A*). Two types of endocytosis are designated based on the size of the vesicle formed. **Pinocytosis** (cell drinking) involves the ingestion of fluids and solute mol-

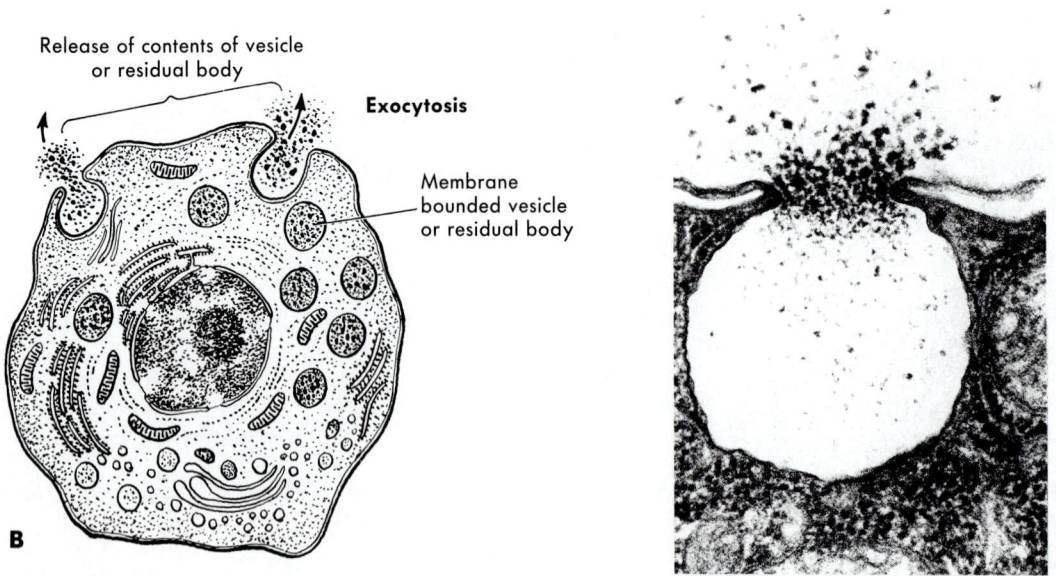

FIG. 1-23 Endocytosis and exocytosis. A, Endocytosis and fusion with lysosome. **B,** Exocytosis. **C,** Electron micrograph of exocytosis. (From Raven & Johnson, 1992.)

ecules through formation of small vesicles, and **phago-cytosis** (cell eating) involves the ingestion of large particles, such as bacteria, through formation of large vesicles (also called vacuoles).

Since most kinds of cells are continually ingesting fluid and solutes by pinocytosis, the terms *pinocytosis* and *endocytosis* are often used interchangeably. In pinocytosis the vesicle containing fluids, solutes, or both fuses with a lysosome, and lysosomal enzymes digest them for use by the cell. In phagocytosis the large molecular substances are engulfed by the plasma membrane and enter the cell so that they can be isolated and destroyed by lysosomal enzymes (see Chapter 7). Substances that are not degraded by lysosomes are isolated in residual bodies and released by the cell by exocytosis. Both pinocytosis and phagocytosis require metabolic energy and often involve binding of the substance with plasma membrane receptors before membrane invagination and fusion with lysosomes in the cell.

In eukaryotic cells, secretion of macromolecules almost always occurs by **exocytosis** (Fig. 1-23, *B* and *C*).

For example, to secrete macromolecules of insulin across plasma membranes, insulin-producing cells store and package insulin molecules in intracellular vesicles, which fuse with the plasma membrane and open to the extracellular space, or matrix, releasing the insulin. Not all secreted substances are secreted into the extracellular matrix. Some adhere to the plasma membrane and are thought to replace segments of the membrane lost through endocytosis or diffuse into the blood to nourish or signal other cells. Exocytosis has two main functions: (1) replacement of portions of the plasma membrane that have been removed by endocytosis, and (2) release of molecules synthesized by the cells into the extracellular matrix.

Receptor-Mediated Endocytosis

Ligand binding to *some* plasma membrane receptors leads to clustering, aggregation, and immobilization of the receptors in specialized areas of the membrane called **coated pits** (Fig. 1-24). The pits, which are coated with bristlelike structures (clathrin), deepen and enfold (in-

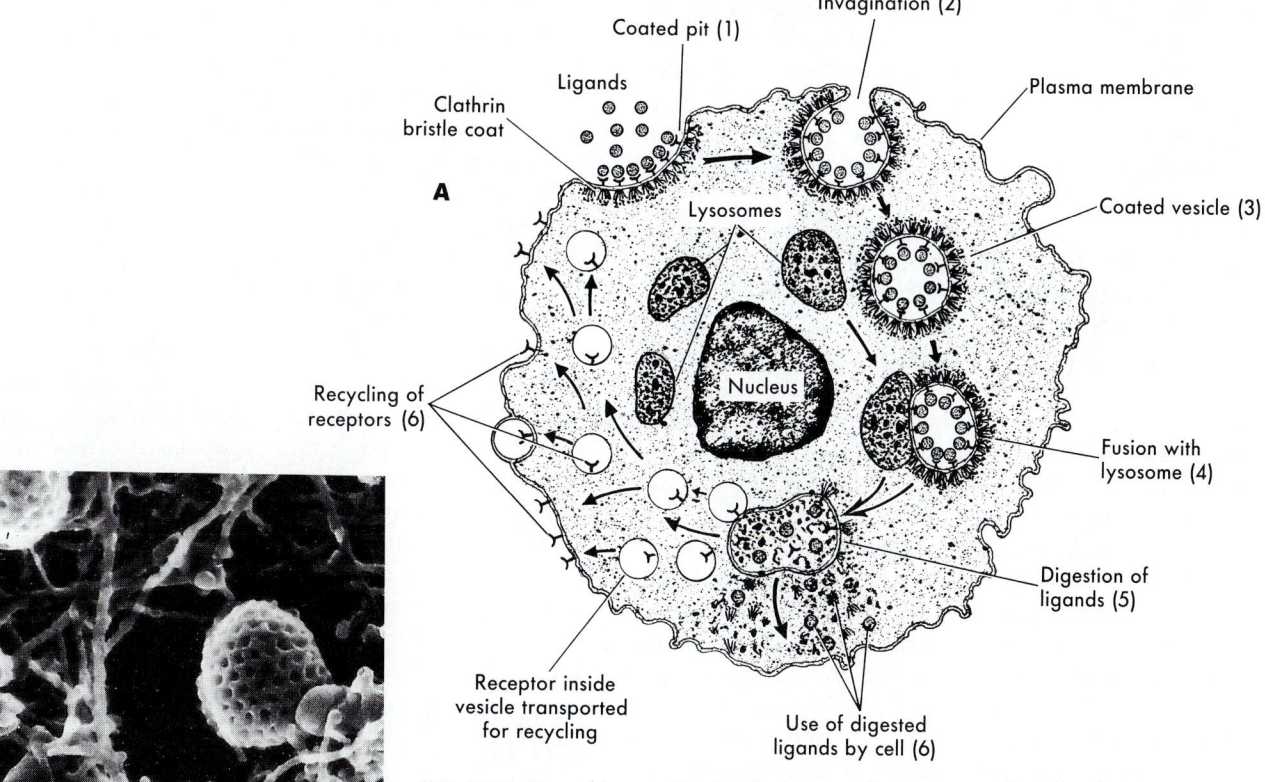

FIG. 1-24 **Ligand internalization by means of receptor-mediated endocytosis. A,** The ligand attaches to its surface receptor (through the bristle coat or clathrin coat) and, through receptor-mediated endocytosis, enters the cell. The ingested material fuses with a lysosome and is processed by hydrolytic lysosomal enzymes. Processed molecules can then be transferred to other cellular components. **B,** Electron micrograph of a coated pit showing different sizes of filaments of the cytoskeleton (×82,000). (**B,** From Erlandsen & Magney, 1992.)

vaginate), internalizing ligand-receptor complexes and forming a coated vesicle. The clathrin coat or bristles are thought to be responsible for trapping membrane receptors in coated pits. This internalization process, called **receptor-mediated endocytosis** (**ligand internalization**), is rapid and enables the cell to ingest large amounts of specific ligands without ingesting large volumes of extracellular fluid. Inside the cell, the ingested material is processed by lysosomal enzymes.

The cellular uptake of cholesterol, for example, depends on receptor-mediated endocytosis. Cholesterol (a ligand) is primarily carried in blood plasma attached to an acceptor protein. This cholesterol-protein complex is called low-density lipoprotein (LDL). LDL receptors, which bind LDL to the plasma membrane, control the rate at which cholesterol is transferred into the cell (see Chapter 27).

Movement of Electrical Impulses: Membrane Potentials

All body cells are electrically polarized, with the inside of the cell more negatively charged than the outside. The difference in electrical charge, or voltage, is known as the **resting membrane potential** and is about -70 to -85 millivolts. The difference in voltage across the plasma membrane is a result of the differences in ionic composition of ICF and ECF. Sodium ions have a greater concentration in the ECF, and potassium ions have a greater concentration in the ICF. The concentration difference is maintained by the active transport of Na^+ and K^+ (the sodium-potassium pump), which transports sodium outward and potassium inward (Fig. 1-25). Because the resting plasma membrane is more permeable to K^+ than to Na^+, K^+ can diffuse easily from its area of higher concentration in the ICF to its area of lower concentration in the ECF. Because sodium and potassium are both cations, the net result is an excess of anions inside the cell, resulting in the resting membrane potential.

Nerve and muscle cells are excitable and can change their resting membrane potential in response to electrochemical stimuli. Changes in resting membrane potential convey messages from cell to cell. When a nerve or muscle cell receives a stimulus that exceeds the membrane threshold value, there is a rapid change in the resting membrane potential known as the **action potential**. The action potential carries signals along the nerve or muscle cell and conveys information from one cell to another. (Nerve impulses are described in Chapter 12.) When a resting cell is stimulated through voltage-regulated channels, the cell membranes become more permeable to sodium. There is a net movement of sodium into the cell, and the membrane potential decreases, or "moves forward," from a negative value (in millivolts) to zero. This decrease is known as **depolar-**

ization. The depolarized cell is more positively charged, and its polarity is neutralized.

To generate an action potential and the resulting depolarization, a critical value known as the **threshold potential** must be reached. Generally this occurs when the cell has depolarized by 15 to 20 millivolts. When the threshold is reached, the cell will continue to depolarize with no further stimulation. The sodium gates open and sodium rushes into the cell, causing the membrane potential to reduce to zero and then become positive (depolarization). The rapid reversal in polarity results in the action potential.

During **repolarization** the negative polarity of the resting membrane potential is reestablished. As the voltage-gated sodium channels begin to close, voltage-gated potassium channels open. Membrane permeability to sodium decreases, and potassium permeability increases, with an outward movement of potassium ions. The sodium gates close, and with the outward movement of potassium, the membrane potential becomes more negative. The Na^+, K^+ pump then returns the membrane to the resting potential by pumping potassium back into the cell and sodium out of the cell.

During most of the action potential, the plasma membrane is unable to respond to an additional stimulus. This time is known as the **absolute refractory period** and is related to changes in permeability to sodium. During the latter phase of the action potential, when permeability to potassium increases, a stronger-than-normal stimulus can evoke an action potential known as the **relative refractory period.**

When the membrane potential is more negative than normal, the cell is in a hyperpolarized (less excitable) state. A larger-than-normal stimulus is then required to reach the threshold potential and generate an action potential. When the membrane potential is more positive than normal, the cell is in a hypopolarized (more excitable than normal) state, and a smaller-than-normal stimulus is required to reach the threshold potential. Changes in the intracellular and extracellular concentration of ions or a change in membrane permeability can cause these alterations in membrane excitability.

CELLULAR REPRODUCTION: THE CELL CYCLE

Cells of the human body are subject to wear and tear, and most do not last for the lifetime of the individual. In almost all tissues, new cells are created as fast as old cells die. Cellular reproduction is therefore necessary for the maintenance of life. Reproduction of gametes (sperm and egg cells) occurs through a process called meiosis, described in Chapter 4. The reproduction, or division, of other body cells (somatic cells) involves two

FIG. 1-25 Sodium-potassium and propagation of an action potential. A, Concentration difference of Na⁺ and K⁺ intracellularly and extracellularly. The direction of active transport by the sodium-potassium pump is also shown. **B,** Top diagram represents the polarized state of a neuronal membrane when at rest. The lower diagrams represent changes in sodium and potassium membrane permeabilities with the generation and propagation of an action potential. (**B,** From Anthony, C. P., & Thibodeau, G. A. [1979]. *Textbook of anatomy and physiology* [10th ed.]. St. Louis: Mosby–Year Book.)

sequential phases: **mitosis,** or nuclear division, and **cytokinesis,** or cytoplasmic division. These two phases occur in close succession, with cytokinesis beginning toward the end of mitosis. Before a cell can divide, however, it must double its mass and duplicate all of its contents. Most of the work of preparing for division occurs during the growth phase, called **interphase.** The alternation between mitosis and interphase in all tissues with cellular turnover is known as the **cell cycle.**

Most of the early work on the cell cycle was limited to microscopic observation of mitosis and cytokinesis. Interphase was considered the "resting stage" of the cell. With recent technologic advances, a considerable amount has been learned about the interphase part of the cell cycle. During interphase many important processes are taking place as the cell produces DNA, RNA, protein, lipids, and other substances, and each pair of **chromosomes** (paired organelles that carry genetic information) also make exact copies of themselves.

There are four designated phases of the cell cycle (Fig. 1-26). They are (1) the S phase (S = synthesis), in which DNA is synthesized in the cell nucleus; (2) the G_2 phase (G = gap), in which RNA and protein synthesis occurs, the period between the completion of DNA synthesis and the next phase (M); (3) the M phase (M = mitosis), which includes both nuclear and cytoplasmic division; and (4) the G_1 phase, which is the period between the M phase and the start of DNA synthesis.

Phases of Mitosis and Cytokinesis

Interphase (the G_1, S, and G_2 phases) is the longest phase of the cell cycle. During interphase, chromosomes are not visible under a light microscope. An electron microscope shows that during interphase the chromatin consists of very long, slender rods that are jumbled together in the nucleus. Late in interphase, strands of **chromatin** (the substance that gives the nucleus its granular appearance) begin to coil, causing them to shorten and thicken. This allows the strands to absorb more staining material, so that they become visible as chromosomes under a light microscope.

The M phase of the cell cycle, mitosis and cytokinesis, begins with **prophase,** the first appearance of chromosomes. As the phase proceeds, each chromosome is seen as two identical halves called **chromatids,** which lie together and are attached at some point by a spindle attachment site called a **centromere.** (The two chromatids of each chromosome, which are genetically identical, are sometimes called sister chromatids.) The nuclear membrane, which surrounds the nucleus, disappears. **Spindle fibers** are microtubules formed in the cytoplasm. Spindle fibers radiate from two centrioles located at opposite poles of the cell. The role of the spindle fibers is to pull the chromosomes to opposite sides of the cell.

During **metaphase,** the next phase of mitosis and cytokinesis, the spindle fibers begin to pull the centromeres of the chromosomes. The centromeres become aligned

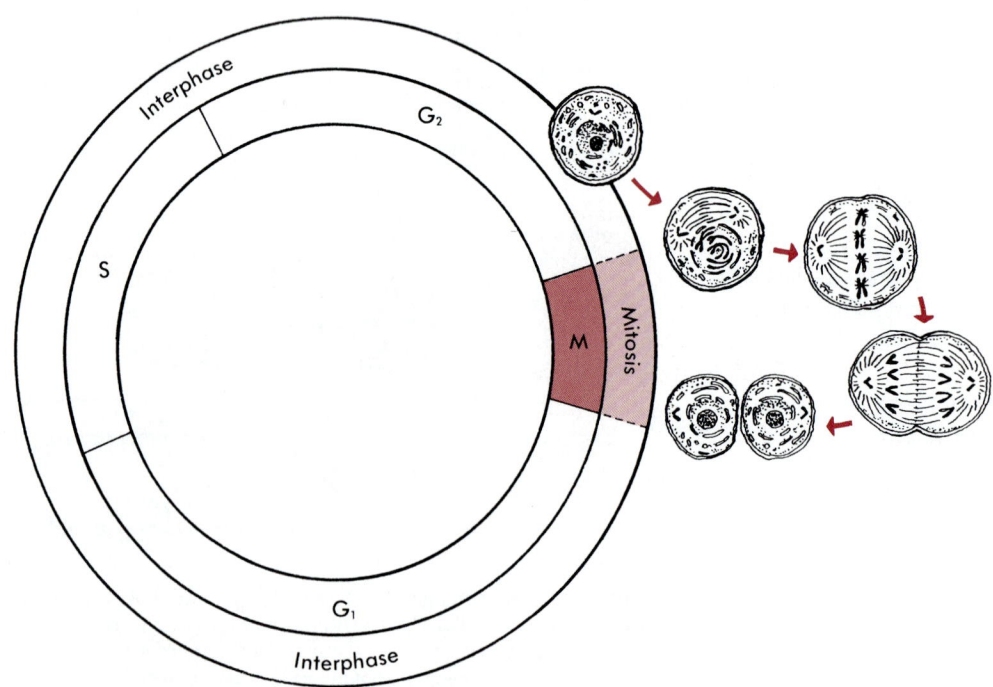

FIG. 1-26 Interphase and the phases of mitosis.

in the middle of the spindle, which is called the **equatorial plate** (or **metaphase plate**) of the cell. This is the stage in which chromosomes are easiest to observe microscopically, since they are highly condensed and arranged in a relatively organized fashion in the two-dimensional equatorial plate.

Anaphase begins when the centromeres split and the sister chromatids are pulled apart. The spindle fibers shorten, causing the sister chromatids to be pulled, centromere first, toward opposite sides of the cell. When the sister chromatids are separated, each is considered to be a chromosome. Thus the cell has 92 chromosomes during this stage. By the end of anaphase, there are 46 chromosomes lying at each side of the cell. Barring mitotic errors, each of the two groups of 46 chromosomes is identical to the original 46 chromosomes present at the start of the cell cycle.

Telophase is the final stage. During telophase, a new nuclear membrane is formed around each group of 46 chromosomes, the spindle fibers disappear, and the chromosomes begin to uncoil. Cytokinesis causes the cytoplasm to divide into roughly equal parts during this phase. At the end of telophase, two identical diploid cells, called **daughter cells,** have been formed from the original cell.

Rates of Cellular Division

Although the complete cell cycle lasts from 12 to 24 hours, about 1 hour is generally required for the four stages of mitosis and cytokinesis: prophase, metaphase, anaphase, and telophase. All types of cells undergo mitosis during formation of the embryo, but in many adult cells, such as nerve cells, lens cells of the eye, and muscle cells, they lose their ability to replicate and divide. The cells of other tissues, particularly epithelial cells (e.g., of the intestine, lung, and skin), divide continuously and rapidly, completing the entire cell cycle in less than 10 hours.

The difference between cells that divide slowly and cells that divide rapidly is the length of time spent in the G_1 phase of the cell cycle. Some cells that divide very slowly remain in the G_1 phase for days or even years. Once the S phase begins, however, progression through mitosis takes a relatively constant amount of time. Once a cell has progressed out of the G_1 phase, there is no turning back, it is committed to completing the S, G_2, and M phases. Times associated with the four successive phases differ.

The mechanisms that control cell division depend on "social control genes" and protein growth factors. Individual cells are members of a complex cellular society in which survival of the entire organism is key and not survival or proliferation of just the individual cells. When a need arises for new cells, as in repair of injured cells, previously nondividing cells must be rapidly triggered to reenter the cell cycle. With continual wear and tear, the cell birth rate and the cell death rate must be kept in balance. Therefore, there must be cell-division controls that govern this balance. Protein growth factors governing the proliferation of different cell types and genes involved in the social control on cell division have recently been identified and are called "social control genes" (Alberts et al., 1989).

The best model for understanding disruption of cell division and study of these so-called social control genes

TABLE 1-4

Examples of Growth Factors and Their Actions

Growth factor	Physiologic actions
Platelet-derived growth factor (PDGF)	Stimulates proliferation of connective tissue cells and neuroglial cells
Epidermal growth factor (EGF)	Stimulates proliferation of epidermal cells and other cell types
Insulin-like growth factor I (IGF-I)	Collaborates with PDGF and EGF; stimulates proliferation of fat cells and connective tissue cells
Insulin-like growth factor II (IGF-II)	Collaborates with PDGF and EGF; stimulates proliferation of fat cells and connective tissue cells
Transforming growth factor B (TGF-B)	Stimulates or inhibits response of most cells to other growth factors; regulates differentiation of some cell types (e.g., cartilage)
Fibroblast growth factor (FGF)	Stimulates proliferation of fibroblasts, endothelial cells, myoblasts, and other cell types
Interleukin-2 (IL-2)	Stimulates proliferation of T-lymphocytes (see p. 228)
Nerve growth factor (NGF)	Promotes axon growth and survival of sympathetic and some sensory and CNS neurons
Hemopoietic cell growth factors (IL-3, GM-CSF, M-CSF, G-CSF, erythropoietin)	See Fig. 22-6 and specific functions

is tumor biology. Current emphasis in locating and identifying these genes is to study tumor cells that have presumably originated because of mutations to these genes, or proto-oncogenes. Proto-oncogenes are thought to encode key components of the normal system of social controls of cell division (Alberts et al., 1989). Some proto-oncogenes code for growth factors, some for growth factor receptors, some for intracellular regulatory proteins that are involved in cell adhesion, and some for proteins that help relay signals for cell division to the cell nucleus (Alberts et al., 1989). Although more than 50 proto-oncogenes have been identified, many more are yet to be discovered (see Chapter 10).

Growth Factors

Cells require highly specific proteins that stimulate cell division called **growth factors**. Different types of cells require different growth factors that are present in the serum in very low concentrations. For example, **platelet-derived growth factor** (**PDGF**) stimulates the production of connective tissue cells. Table 1-4 summarizes the most significant growth factors. Cells that respond to a particular growth factor have specific receptors for the growth factor in their plasma membrane. Recent evidence shows that some growth factors are also regulators of other cell processes, like cellular differentiation. In addition to growth factors that stimulate cellular processes, there are factors that inhibit functions; these factors are not well understood. Cells that are starved of growth factors come to a halt after mitosis and enter the arrested, or G_0, state of the cell cycle (see p. 34 for cell cycle) (Alberts et al., 1989). Growth factors are also discussed in Chapters 10 and 22.

TISSUES

The cells of the body are organized hierarchically: cells of one or more types are organized into tissues, and different types of tissues compose organs. Finally, organs are integrated to perform complex functions as tracts or systems.

All cells are in contact with a network of extracellular macromolecules known as the **extracellular matrix.** The extracellular matrix not only holds cells and tissues together but also provides an organized latticework within which cells can migrate and interact with one another.

Tissue Formation

To form tissues, cells must exhibit intercellular recognition and adhesion. Specialized cells are thought to form a tissue in one of two different ways. First and simplest is mitosis of one or more **founder cells** (the most basic precursor cell). Founder cells are prevented from "wan-

dering away" by macromolecules in the extracellular matrix and by adherence to one another at specialized junctions on their plasma membranes. Mitosis of founder cells forms, for example, epithelial cell sheets (Fig. 1-27).

The second way in which specialized cells form tissues involves their migration to and subsequent assembly at the site of tissue formation. During embryonic development, for example, cells from the neural crest migrate to several different regions, where they differentiate and assemble into a variety of tissues, including those of the peripheral nervous system. Migrant cells are thought to arrive at the site of tissue formation through chemotaxis or contact guidance. **Chemotaxis** is movement along a chemical gradient caused by chemical attraction (see Chapter 7). Cells at the migrant cells' destination secrete a chemical, called chemotactic factor, that attracts specific migrant cells. **Contact guidance** is movement along a pathway, or "pavement," in the extracellular matrix (Alberts et al., 1989).

Tissues are not randomly arranged into organs. No matter how tissue is formed, staying together in groups means that cells must recognize each other and remain distinct from the cells of surrounding tissues. Little is known about the mechanisms involved in these processes.

Intercellular Communication

Cells in direct physical contact with neighboring cells are often linked together at specialized regions of their plasma membranes called **cell junctions**. Cell junctions have two main functions: (1) to hold cells together and (2) to allow small molecules to pass from cell to cell, allowing coordination of the activities of cells that form tissues. There are three main types of cell junctions: (1) desmosomes (macula adherens), (2) tight junctions (zonula occludens), and (3) gap junctions (Fig. 1-28). Together they form the **junctional complex. Desmosomes** hold cells together by forming either continuous bands or belts of epithelial sheets or buttonlike points of contact. Desmosomes also act as a system of braces to maintain structural stability. **Tight junctions** serve as a barrier to diffusion, prevent the movement of substances through transport proteins in the plasma membrane, and prevent the leakage of small molecules between the plasma membranes of adjacent cells. **Gap junctions** are clusters of protein channels that allow small ions and molecules to pass directly from the inside of one cell to the inside of another. Cells connected by gap junctions are considered ionically (electrically) and metabolically coupled. Gap junctions coordinate the activities of adjacent cells. They are important, for example, in synchronizing contractions of heart muscle cells through ionic coupling and in permitting action potentials to spread rapidly from cell to cell in neural tis-

FIG. 1-27 Tissue formation by mitosis and migration. **A,** Tissue formation by mitosis. Founder cells are kept in place by extracellular matrix and recognition and adherence at cell junctions. **B,** Tissue formation by migration. Specialized cells are attracted to the site of tissue formation by chemotaxis or contact guidance; then they aggregate and differentiate into organized tissue.

sues. The reason that gap junctions occur in tissues that are not electrically active is unknown. Although most gap junctions are associated with junctional complexes, they sometimes exist as independent structures.

The junctional complex is a very permeable part of the plasma membrane. Its permeability is controlled by a process called **gating,** which depends on concentrations of calcium ions in the cytoplasm. Increased cytoplasmic calcium causes decreased permeability at the junctional complex. Gating is an important cellular defense mechanism because it enables uninjured cells to "seal themselves off" from injured neighbors. As damaged cells release calcium, it travels through the junctional complex and increases calcium levels in neighboring cells. (The damaging effects of calcium influx are described in Chapter 2.) This decreases the permeability of the junctional complexes of the neighboring cells, which form a relatively impermeable wall around the injured area.

Types of Tissues

There are four basic types of tissues: epithelial, muscle, nerve, and connective tissues. The structure and func-

tion of these four types underlie the structure and function of each organ system.

Epithelial Tissue

Epithelial tissue covers most internal and external surfaces of the body. Epithelial cells are closely joined and are attached to a **basement membrane (basement lamina),** which provides a supporting layer and separates the epithelium from underlying connective tissue (see Fig. 1-27, A). Because of its variety of locations, epithelial tissue has several diverse functions, including protection, absorption, secretion, and excretion. For example, the epidermis provides a protective barrier between the host and the outside environment, whereas the linings of the internal body organs help absorb substances into the body, excrete waste products, and secrete substances into body cavities.

Epithelial cell surfaces differ according to their location and function. Epithelial cells that line body cavities and blood vessels are smooth, whereas other epithelial cells have tiny cytoplasmic projections called **microvilli** on their free surfaces. Microvilli considerably increase the cell's surface area and are found on cells

Epithelial cells

Belt
desmosome →

Spot
Desmosomes

Hemidesmosomes

Cell
viewed from
above

Belt desmosome

Junctional complex

Tight junction
(zonula occludens)

Belt desmosome
(zonula adherens)

Filamentous
material in
intercellular
space

Spot desmosome
(macula adherens)

Intercellular filaments

Gap
junction

Intercellular channel

Intercellular units
forming channels for
extracellular transport

A

B

FIG. 1-28 **Junctional complex. A,** Schematic drawing of a belt desmosome between epithelial cells. This junction, also called zonula adherens, encircles each of the interacting cells. The spot desmosomes and hemidesmosomes, like the belt desmosomes, are adhering junctions. This tight junction is an impermeable junction that holds cells together but seals them in such a way that molecules cannot leak between them. The gap junction, as a communicating junction, mediates the passage of small molecules from one interacting cell to the other. **B,** Electron micrograph of desmosomes. (From Raven & Johnson, 1992.)

whose main functions are absorption and secretion, such as the epithelial cells lining the digestive tract. **Cilia,** which are hairlike projections that propel mucus, pus, and dust particles out of the body, are characteristic of cells lining the respiratory passages.

Epithelial tissue is classified in two ways: (1) according to the number and arrangement of cell layers and (2) according to cell shape. Epithelium that is formed by a single layer of cells, all of which are in contact with the basement membrane, is called **simple epithelium.** **Stratified epithelium** has two or more layers of cells, and only the deepest layer is in contact with the basement membrane. Tissue that appears to consist of several cellular layers, but is actually a single layer with all cells contacting the basement membrane, is called **pseudostratified epithelium.**

Three basic cell shapes are found in epithelium: squamous, cuboidal, and columnar. **Squamous cells** are flat and thin; **cuboidal cells** are as high as they are wide and thus appear square in vertical sections; and **columnar cells** are taller than they are wide and appear rectangular in vertical sections. Overall classifications of epithelial tissue, which take into account both the number of cell layers and cell shape, are summarized in Table 1-5.

TABLE 1-5

Characteristics of Epithelial Tissues

Type of epithelium	Structure	Location	Function
Simple squamous epithelium (Fig. 1-29)	Single layer of cells	Lining of blood vessels	Diffusion and filtration Separation of blood from fluids in tissues
		Lining of pulmonary alveoli (air sacs)	Separation of air from fluids in tissues
		Bowman's capsule (kidney)	Filtration of substances from blood, forming urine

Nucleus   Epithelial cell membrane

FIG. 1-29 **Simple squamous epithelial cell.** A, Diagram. B, Photomicrograph of simple squamous epithelial cell in parietal wall of Bowman's capsule in kidney. *Pointer* is touching a typical flattened squamous epithelial cell. (×140.) (From Thibodeau, G. A. [1987]. *Anatomy and physiology.* St. Louis: Mosby–Year Book.)

Type of epithelium	Structure	Location	Function
Stratified squamous epithelium (Fig. 1-30)	Two or more layers, depending on location, with cells closest to basement membrane tending to be cuboidal	Epidermis of skin Linings of mouth, pharynx, esophagus, anus, vagina	Protection and secretion

Cornified layer

Basement membrane   Basal cells   Dermis

FIG. 1-30 **Cornified stratified squamous epithelium.** A, Diagram. B, Photomicrograph of stratified squamous epithelium of the skin. (×140.) (From Thibodeau & Patton, 1993.)

Continued.

TABLE 1-5

Characteristics of Epithelial Tissues—cont'd

Type of epithelium	Structure	Location	Function
Transitional epithelium (Fig. 1-31)	Vary in shape from cuboidal to squamous depending on whether basal cells of the bladder are columnar and comprise many layers; when the bladder is full and stretched, the cells flatten and stretch like squamous cells	Linings of urinary bladder and other hollow structures	Stretching that permits expansion of hollow organs

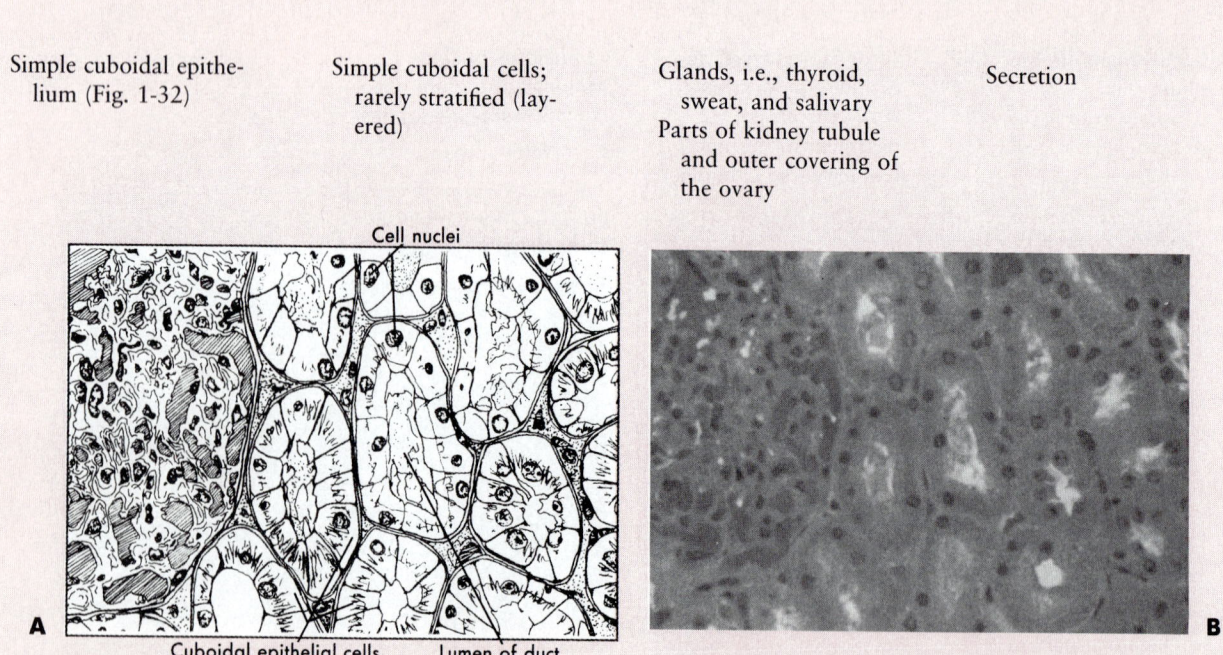

FIG. 1-31 **Stratified squamous transitional epithelium. A,** Diagram. **B,** Photomicrograph of stratified squamous transitional epithelium of the vagina. (×140.) (From Thibodeau & Patton, 1993.)

Simple cuboidal epithelium (Fig. 1-32)	Simple cuboidal cells; rarely stratified (layered)	Glands, i.e., thyroid, sweat, and salivary Parts of kidney tubule and outer covering of the ovary	Secretion

FIG. 1-32 **Simple cuboidal epithelium. A,** Diagram. **B,** Photomicrograph of simple cuboidal epithelium of the distal convoluted tubule of the kidney. (×140.) (From Thibodeau & Patton, 1993.)

TABLE 1-5

Characteristics of Epithelial Tissues—cont'd

Type of epithelium	Structure	Location	Function
Simple columnar epithelium (Fig. 1-33)	Large amounts of cytoplasm and cellular organelles	Lining of digestive tube from stomach to anus Ducts of many glands	Secretion and absorption

FIG. 1-33 **Simple columnar epithelium. A,** Diagram. **B,** Photomicrograph of simple columnar epithelium of the colon. (×140.) (From Thibodeau, G. A. ([1987]. *Anatomy and physiology.* St. Louis: Mosby–Year Book.)

Type of epithelium	Structure	Location	Function
Ciliated simple columnar epithelium	Same as that of simple columnar epithelium, but ciliated	Linings of bronchi of the lungs, nasal cavity, and oviducts	Secretion, absorption, and propulsion of fluids and particles
Stratified columnar epithelium (Fig. 1-34)	Small and rounded basement membrane (columnar cells do not touch basement membrane)	Linings of epiglottis, part of pharynx, anus, and male urethra	Protection

FIG. 1-34 **Stratified columnar epithelium. A,** Diagram. **B,** Photomicrograph of stratified columnar epithelium of a large duct in the sublingual gland. (×280.) (**A,** From Thibodeau, G. A. [1987]. *Anatomy and physiology.* St. Louis: Mosby–Year Book; **B,** courtesy Richard Ash, University of Utah.)

Continued.

TABLE 1-5

Characteristics of Epithelial Tissues—cont'd

Type of epithelium	Structure	Location	Function
Pseudostratified ciliated columnar epithelium (Fig. 1-35)	All cells in contact with basement membrane Nuclei found at different levels within the cell, giving stratified appearance Free surface often ciliated	Linings of large ducts of some glands (parotid, salivary), male urethra, respiratory passages, and eustachian tubes of ears	Transport of substances

FIG. 1-35 **Pseudostratified ciliated columnar epithelium.** A, Diagram. B, Photomicrograph of pseudostratified ciliated columnar epithelium of the trachea. (×280.) (From Thibodeau & Patton, 1993.)

Connective Tissue

Connective tissue varies considerably in structure and function but is most common as the framework on which epithelial cells cluster to form organs. Other functions include binding various tissues and organs together, supporting them in their locations, and serving as storage sites for excess nutrients.

In contrast to epithelial tissue, connective tissue is characterized by an abundant extracellular matrix that surrounds few cells. The extracellular matrix is composed of ground substance and fibers. **Ground substance** is a homogeneous mass that varies in consistency from fluid to semisolid gel. Fibers are produced by connective tissue cells (fibroblasts) found within the ground substance. There are three types of fibers: collagenous (white), elastic (yellow), and reticular. **Collagenous fibers** are formed of bundles of smaller fibrils appearing as wavy bands under the microscope. These fibers are composed of the protein collagen and are strong and inelastic. (Collagen synthesis by fibroblasts is described

with respect to tissue repair in Chapter 7.) **Elastic fibers** are long, branching fibers composed of a protein called elastin that enables the fibers to return to their original length after stretching. Elastin occurs not only as fibers but also as membranes, particularly the membranes of blood vessels. **Reticular fibers** are thin, short, branching fibers that form an inelastic network made from a collagen-like protein called reticulum. Reticular fibers form the internal framework (stroma) to which the epithelial cells of glands are attached. They are found in loose connective tissue, generally in bone marrow and in the **parenchyma** (i.e., the essential substance of an organ rather than its framework) of the liver, spleen, and lymph nodes.

Connective tissues are classified according to the consistency (e.g., as loose or dense) of the ground substance and the type and organization of the fibers within it. Table 1-6 summarizes the characteristics of connective tissues.

TABLE 1-6

Connective Tissues

Classification	Structure	Function and location
Loose or areolar tissue (Fig. 1-36)	Unorganized; spaces between fibers Most fibers collagenous, some elastic and reticular Includes many types of cells (fibroblasts and macrophages most common) and large amount of intercellular fluid	Attaches skin to underlying tissue, holds organs in place by filling the spaces between them, supports blood vessels Intercellular fluid transports nutrients and waste products Fluid accumulation causes swelling (edema)

FIG. 1-36 Loose areolar connective tissue.

Classification	Structure	Function and location
Dense, irregular tissue (Fig. 1-37)	Dense, compact, and areolar tissue, with fewer cells and more, closely woven collagenous fibers than in loose tissue	Acts as protective barrier; dermis layer of the skin

FIG. 1-37 Dense, irregular connective tissue.

Continued.

TABLE 1-6

Connective Tissues—cont'd

Classification	Structure	Function and location
Dense, regular (white fibrous) tissue (Fig. 1-38)	Collagenous fibers and some elastic fibers, tightly packed into parallel bundles, with only fibroblast cells	Forms strong tendons of muscle, ligaments of joints, some fibrous membranes, and fascia that surrounds the organs and muscles

FIG. 1-38 Dense regular (white fibrous) connective tissue.

Elastic tissue (Fig. 1-39)	Elastic fibers, some collagenous fibers, fibroblasts	Lends strength and elasticity to walls of arteries, trachea, vocal chords, and other structures

FIG. 1-39 Elastic connective tissue.

TABLE 1-6

Connective Tissues—cont'd

Classification	Structure	Function and location
Adipose tissue (Fig. 1-40)	Fat cells dispersed in loose tissues; each cell containing a large droplet of fat flattens nucleus and forces cytoplasm into a ring around cell's periphery	Stores fat, which provides padding and protection

Venule

Fat droplets
(adipose cell)

Loose
connective
tissue

Artery

Capillaries

Nucleus of
adipose cell

FIG. 1-40 Adipose tissue.

Cartilage (hyaline, elastic, and fibrocartilage) (Fig. 1-41)	Collagenous fibers embedded in a firm matrix (chondrin); no blood supply	Gives form, support, and flexibility to joints, trachea, nose, ear, vertebral disks, embryonic skeleton, and many internal structures

Matrix

Nucleus of
chondrocyte

Elastic
fibers

Perichondrium

Lacuna

Chondrocytes
(cartilage cells)

A   Lacuna   Chondrocytes
(cartilage cells)

B   Chondrocytes
(cartilage cells)

Collagenous
fibers

C   Nuclei of
chondrocytes

FIG. 1-41 Cartilage. A, Hyaline cartilage. B, Elastic cartilage. C, Fibrous cartilage.

Continued.

TABLE 1-6

Connective Tissues—cont'd

Classification	Structure	Function and location
Bone (Fig. 1-42)	Collagenous fibers and inorganic salts called osteoblasts Well supplied by blood vessels (see Chapter 38)	Lends skeleton rigidity and strength

FIG. 1-42 Bone.

Special connective tissues 　Plasma 　Macrophages in tissue, reticuloendothelia, or macrophage system	Fluid Scattered macrophages (phagocytes) called Kupffer's cells (in liver), alveolar macrophages (in lungs), microglia (in central nervous system)	Serves as matrix for blood cells Facilitate inflammatory response and carry out phagocytosis in loose connective, lymphatic, digestive, medullary (bone marrow), splenic, adrenal, and pituitary tissues

Muscle Tissue

Muscle tissue is composed of long, thin, cells or fibers called myocytes. Myocytes are highly contractile. Three different types of muscle tissue are skeletal, cardiac, and smooth (Table 1-7). (Muscles are discussed in detail in Chapter 38.)

Neural Tissue

Neural tissue is composed of highly specialized cells called neurons that receive and transmit electrical impulses very rapidly across junctions called synapses. Synapses are points of functional contact between neurons. At synapses, impulses pass from neuron to neuron or from a neuron to a muscle cell as chemical messengers called neurotransmitters are released (see Chapter 12). The total number of neurons is fixed at birth, and replacement is impossible thereafter.

Different types of neurons have special characteristics that depend on their distribution and function within the nervous system. All neurons, however, are composed of the following parts: (1) a cell body, (2) a single axon, and (3) one or more dendrites (see Fig. 1-46). The cell body contains special cytoplasmic structures, as well as microtubules, actin filaments, Golgi complex, lysosomes, and lipofuscin. The axons and dendrites can be very long. Generally, the axon conducts nerve impulses away from the cell body; dendrites conduct nerve impulses toward the cell body. (Neuronal transmission is discussed in Chapter 12.)

TABLE 1-7

Muscle Tissues

Type of muscle	Structural characteristics of cells	Function	Location
Skeletal (striated) muscle (Fig. 1-43)	Long, cylindrical cells that extend throughout length of muscles Striated myofibrils (proteins) Many nuclei on periphery	Voluntary movement of skeleton; maintenance of posture	Attached to bones directly or by tendons

FIG. 1-43 Skeletal (striated) muscle.

Cardiac muscle (Fig. 1-44)	Branching networks throughout muscle tissue Striated myofibrils	Involuntary pumping action of heart	Cells attached end-to-end at intercalated disks; tissue forms walls of heart (myocardium)

FIG. 1-44 Cardiac muscle.

Continued.

TABLE 1-7

Muscle Tissues—cont'd

Type of muscle	Structural characteristics of cells	Function	Location
Smooth (visceral) muscle (Fig. 1-45)	Long spindles that taper to a point Absence of striated myofibrils	Voluntary and involuntary contractions that move substances through hollow structures	Walls of hollow internal structures, such as digestive tract and blood vessels (viscera)

Nucleus of smooth muscle cell

Smooth muscle cell

Smooth muscle cell fibers (transverse)

Venule

FIG. 1-45 Smooth (visceral) muscle.

Dendrites   Nucleus

FIG. 1-46 Typical neuron. The axon conducts electrical signals away from the cell body. Signals are produced by a flux of ions across the neuron's plasma membrane. At the synapse, the neuron forms a specialized junction with another neuron (or with a muscle cell) across which electrochemical signals (neurotransmitters) pass. (From Raven & Johnson, 1992.)

Cell body

Axon

Myelin sheath

Node of Ranvier

Schwann cell

Terminal branches of axon

SUMMARY REVIEW

Cellular Functions

1 Cells become specialized through the process of differentiation or maturation.

2 There are seven specialized cellular functions: movement, conductivity, metabolic absorption, secretion, excretion, respiration, and reproduction.

3 The eukaryotic cell consists of three general components: the plasma membrane, the cytoplasm, and the intracellular organelles.

4 The nucleus is the largest membrane-bounded organelle and is usually found in the cell's center. The chief function of the nucleus is cell division and control of genetic information.

5 Cytoplasm, or the cytoplasmic matrix, is an aqueous solution (cytosol) that fills the space between the nucleus and the plasma membrane.

6 The organelles are suspended in the cytoplasm and are enclosed in biologic membranes.

7 The endoplasmic reticulum is a network of tubular channels (cisternae) that extend throughout the outer nuclear membrane. It specializes in the synthesis and transport of protein and lipid components of most of the organelles.

8 The Golgi complex is a network of smooth membranes and vesicles located near the nucleus. The Golgi complex is responsible for processing and packaging proteins into secretory vesicles that break away from the Golgi complex and migrate to a variety of intracellular and extracellular destinations, including the plasma membrane.

9 Lysosomes are saclike structures that originate from the Golgi complex and contain digestive enzymes. These enzymes are responsible for digesting most cellular substances down to their basic form, such as amino acids, fatty acids, and sugars.

10 Cellular injury leads to a release of the lysosomal enzymes causing cellular self-digestion.

11 Peroxisomes are similar to lysosomes, but contain several enzymes that either produce or use hydrogen peroxide.

12 Mitochondria contain the metabolic machinery necessary for cellular energy metabolism. The enzymes of the respiratory chain (electron transport chain), found in the inner membrane of the mitochondria, generate most of the cell's ATP.

13 The cytoskeleton is the "bone and muscle" of the cell. The internal skeleton is composed of a network of protein filaments including microtubules and actin filaments (microfilaments)

14 The plasma membrane encloses the cell and, by controlling the movement of substances across it, exerts a powerful influence on metabolic pathways.

15 Protein receptors (recognition units) on the plasma membrane enable the cell to interact with other cells and with extracellular substances.

16 The plasma membrane is a bilayer of lipids (phospholipids and glycolipids) and cholesterol, which gives the membrane its structural integrity.

17 Membrane functions are determined largely by proteins. These functions include recognition by protein receptors and transport of substances into and out of the cell.

18 The fluid mosaic model accounts for the fluidity of the lipid bilayer and the flexibility, self-sealing properties, and selective impermeability of the plasma membrane.

19 Cellular receptors are protein molecules on the plasma membrane, in the cytoplasm, or in the nucleus, capable of recognizing and binding smaller molecules, called ligands.

20 The dynamic nature of the fluid plasma membrane enables it to vary the number of receptors on its surface. The cell is, therefore, capable of "hiding" from injurious agents by altering receptor number and pattern.

21 The ligand-receptor complex initiates a series of protein interactions, causing adenylate cyclase to catalyze the transformation of cellular ATP to messenger molecules that stimulate specific responses within the cell.

Cell-to-Cell Communication

1 Cells communicate in three ways: (1) they form protein channels (gap junctions), (2) they display receptors that affect intracellular processes or other cells in direct physical contact, and (3) they secrete signals for long distance communication.

2 Three modes of chemical signaling include endocrine, paracrine, and synaptic.

Cellular Metabolism

1 The chemical tasks of maintaining essential cellular functions are referred to as cellular metabolism. Anabolism is the energy-using process of metabolism, whereas catabolism is the energy-releasing process.

2 Adenosine triphosphate (ATP) functions as an energy-transferring molecule. Energy is stored by molecules of carbohydrate, lipid, and protein, which, when catabolized, transfer energy to ATP.

3 Oxidative phosphorylation occurs in the mitochondria and is the mechanism by which the energy produced from carbohydrates, fats, and proteins is transferred to ATP.

Processes of Cellular Intake and Output

1 Water and small, electrically uncharged molecules move through pores in the plasma membrane's lipid bilayer in the process called passive transport.

2 Passive transport does not require the expenditure of energy; rather it is driven by the physical effects of osmosis, hydrostatic pressure, and diffusion.

3 Larger molecules and molecular complexes (e.g., ligand-receptor complexes) are moved into the cell by active transport, which requires expenditure of energy (by means of ATP) by the cell.

4 The largest molecules (macromolecules) and fluids are transported by the processes of endocytosis (ingestion) and exocytosis (expulsion).

5 Two types of solutes exist in body fluids: (1) electrolytes and (2) nonelectrolytes. Electrolytes are electrically charged and dissociate into constituent ions when placed in solution. Nonelectrolytes do not dissociate when placed in solution.

6 Diffusion is the passive movement of a solute from an area of higher solute concentration to an area of lower solute concentration.

7 Hydrostatic pressure is the mechanical force of water pushing against cellular membranes.

8 Osmosis is the movement of water across a semipermeable membrane from a region of lower solute concentration to a region of higher solute concentration.

9 The amount of hydrostatic pressure required to oppose the osmotic movement of water is called the osmotic pressure of the solution.

10 The overall osmotic effect of colloids, such as plasma proteins, is called the oncotic pressure or colloid osmotic pressure.

11 Mediated transport can be passive or active. Mediated transport includes the movement of two molecules simultaneously in one direction (symport) or in opposite directions (antiport), or the movement of a single molecule in one direction (uniport).

12 Passive mediated transport is also called facilitated diffusion. It does not require the expenditure of metabolic energy.

13 Active mediated transport requires metabolic energy (ATP) to move molecules against the concentration gradient.

14 Active transport also occurs by endocytosis, or vesicle formation, in which the substance to be transported is engulfed by a segment of the plasma membrane, forming a vesicle that moves into the cell.

15 Pinocytosis is a type of endocytosis in which fluids and solute molecules are ingested through formation of small vesicles.

16 Phagocytosis is a type of endocytosis in which large particles, such as bacteria, are ingested through formation of large vesicles, called vacuoles.

17 In receptor-mediated endocytosis, the plasma membrane receptors are clustered, along with bristlelike structures, in specialized areas called coated pits.

18 Endocytosis occurs when coated pits invaginate, internalizing ligand-receptor complexes in coated vesicles.

19 Inside the cell, material ingested by endocytosis is processed and digested by lysosomal enzymes.

20 All body cells are electrically polarized, with the inside of the cell more negatively charged than the outside. The difference in voltage across the plasma membrane is the resting membrane potential.

21 When an excitable (nerve or muscle) cell receives an electrochemical stimulus, cations enter the cell, causing a rapid change in the resting membrane potential known as the action potential. The action potential "moves" along the cell's plasma membrane and is transmitted to an adjacent cell. This is how electrochemical signals convey information from cell to cell.

Cellular Reproduction: The Cell Cycle

1 Cellular reproduction in body tissues involves mitosis (nuclear division) and cytokinesis (cytoplasmic division).

2 Only mature cells are capable of division. Maturation occurs during a stage of cellular life called interphase (growth phase).

3 The cell cycle is the reproductive process that begins after interphase in all tissues with cellular turnover. There are four phases of the cell cycle: (1) the S phase, during which DNA synthesis takes place in the cell nucleus; (2) the G_2 phase, the period between the completion of DNA synthesis and the next phase (M); (3) the M phase, which involves both nuclear (mitotic) and cytoplasmic (cytokinetic) division; and (4) the G phase (growth phase, or interphase), after which the cycle begins again.

4 The M phase (mitosis) involves four stages: prophase, metaphase, anaphase, and telophase.

5 The mechanisms that control cell division depend on "social control genes" and protein growth factors.

Tissues

1 Cells of one or more types are organized into tissues, and different types of tissues compose organs. Organs are organized so as to function as tracts or systems.

2 Specialized cells are thought to form tissue by (1) mitosis of one or more founder cells or (2) migration of founder cells and their subsequent assembly at the site of tissue formation.

3 Tissue cells are linked at cell junctions, which are specialized regions on their plasma membranes called desmosomes, tight junctions, and gap junctions. Cell junctions attach adjacent cells and allow small molecules to pass between them.

4 The four basic types of tissues are epithelial, muscle, nerve, and connective tissues.
5 Epithelial tissue covers most internal and external surfaces of the body. The functions of epithelial tissue include protection, absorption, secretion, and excretion.
6 Connective tissue binds various tissues and organs together, supporting them in their locations and serving as storage sites for excess nutrients.

7 Muscle tissue is composed of long, thin, highly contractile cells or fibers called myocytes. Muscle tissue that is attached to bones enables voluntary movement. Muscle tissue in internal organs enables involuntary movement, such as the heartbeat.
8 Neural tissue is composed of highly specialized cells called neurons that receive and transmit electrical impulses very rapidly across junctions called synapses.

KEY TERMS

Absolute refractory period, 32
Actin filament (microfilament), 14
Action potential, 32
Active mediated transport, 28
Active transport, 23
Amphipathic molecule, 15
Anabolism, 20
Anaerobic glycolysis, 22
Anaphase, 35
Anion, 24
Antiport, 26
Autodigestion, 11
Autolysosome, 11
Autophagy, 11
Basement membrane (basement lamina), 37
Catabolism, 20
Catalytic receptor, 20
Cation, 24
Cell cycle, 34
Cell junction, 36
Cellular metabolism, 20
Cellular receptor, 18
Centriole, 12
Centromere, 34
Channel-linked receptor, 20
Chemical synapse, 19
Chemotaxis, 36
Chromatid, 34
Chromatin, 34
Chromosome, 34
Cilium, 38
Citric acid cycle (Krebs cycle, tricarboxylic acid cycle), 21
Coated pit, 31
Collagenous fiber, 42
Columnar cell, 38
Competitive inhibitor, 26
Concentration gradient, 24
Contact guidance, 36
Cuboidal cell, 38
Cytokinesis, 34

Cytoplasm, 7
Cytoplasmic matrix, 9
Cytoskeleton, 12
Daughter cell, 35
Depolarization, 32
Desmosome, 36
Diffusion, 24
Digestion, 21
Effective osmolality, 26
Elastic fiber, 42
Electrolyte, 23
Electron-transport chain, 21
Endocrine signaling, 19
Endocytosis, 30
Endoplasmic reticulum, 9
Equatorial plate (metaphase plate), 35
Eukaryote, 6
Exocytosis, 31
Extracellular matrix, 36
Fluid mosaic model, 16
Founder cell, 36
Gap junction, 36
Gating, 37
Glycolysis, 21
Golgi complex (Golgi apparatus), 10
G-protein–linked receptor, 20
Ground substance, 42
Growth factor, 36
GTP-binding regulatory protein (G-protein), 20
Hydrostatic pressure, 24
Hypertonic solution, 26
Hypotonic solution, 26
Inositol-phospholipid transduction pathway, 20
Integral membrane protein, 16
Interphase, 34
Ion, 23
Isotonic solution, 26
Junctional complex, 36
Ligand, 18
Lysosome, 10

Mediated transport, 26
Metabolic pathway, 21
Metaphase, 34
Microtubule, 12
Microvillus, 37
Mitochondrion, 12
Mitosis, 34
Neurotransmitter, 19
Nuclear envelope, 7
Nucleolus, 7
Nucleus, 7
Oncotic pressure (colloid osmotic pressure), 26
Organelle, 7
Osmolality, 25
Osmolarity, 25
Osmosis, 24
Osmotic pressure, 25
Oxidation, 21
Oxidative cellular metabolism (oxidation), 21
Oxidative phosphorylation, 21
Paracrine signaling, 19
Parenchyma, 42
Passive mediated transport (facilitated diffusion), 26
Passive transport, 23
Peripheral membrane protein, 16
Peroxisome (microbody), 11
Phagocytosis, 31
Pinocytosis, 30
Plasma membrane (plasmalemma), 6
Plasma membrane receptor, 18
Platelet-derived growth factor (PDGF), 36
Polarity, 24
Primary lysosome, 11
Prokaryote, 6
Prophase, 34
Pseudostratified epithelium, 38
Receptor-mediated endocytosis (ligand internalization), 32

Relative refractory period, 32
Repolarization, 32
Residual body, 11
Resting membrane potential, 32
Reticular fiber, 42
Ribosome, 9
Secondary lysosome, 11
Secretory vesicle (secretory granule), 10

Simple epithelium, 38
Solute, 23
Spindle fiber, 34
Squamous cell, 38
Stratified epithelium, 38
Substrate, 21
Substrate phosphorylation, 22
Symport, 26
Synaptic signaling, 19

Telophase, 35
Threshold potential, 32
Tight junction, 36
Tonicity, 26
Transfer reaction, 21
Transmembrane protein, 16
Transport protein (transporter), 26
Uniport, 26
Valence, 24

REFERENCES

Alberts, B., Bray, D., Lewis, J., Raff, M., Roberts, K., & Watson, J. D. (1989). *Molecular biology of the cell* (2nd ed.). New York: Garland.

Anthony, C. P., & Thibodeau G. A. (1979). *Textbook of anatomy and physiology* (10th ed.). St. Louis: Mosby–Year Book.

Catt, K. J., Harwood, J. P., Aguilera, G., & Dufau, M. L. (1979). Hormonal regulation of peptide receptors and target cell responses. *Nature, 280,* 109-116.

Devlin, T. M. (Ed.). (1992). *Textbook of biochemistry: With clinical correlations* (3rd ed.). New York: Wiley.

Erlandsen, S. L., & Magney, J. E. (1992). *Color atlas of histology.* St. Louis: Mosby–Year Book.

King, D. W., Fenoglio, C. M., & Lefkowitch, J. H. (1983). *General pathology: Principles and dynamics.* Philadelphia: Lea & Febiger.

Kissane, J. M. (Ed.). (1990). *Anderson's pathology* (9th ed.). St. Louis: Mosby–Year Book.

Raven, P. H., & Johnson, G. B. (1992). *Biology.* St. Louis: Mosby–Year Book.

Thibodeau, G. A., & Patton, K. I. (1993). *Anatomy & physiology* (2nd ed.). St. Louis: Mosby–Year Book.

SUGGESTED READINGS

Berne, R. M., & Levy, M. N. (Eds.). (1993). *Physiology.* (3rd ed.). St. Louis: Mosby–Year Book.

Berridge, M. J. (1985, October). The molecular basis of communication within the cell. *Scientific American, 253*(4), 142.

Hasler, C. M., Bennick, M. R., Troskp, J. E. (1991). Inhibition of gap junction-mediated intercellular communication by α-linolenate. *Amerian Journal of Physiology, 261*(1), C161-C168.

Hobbs, A. S., & Albers, R. W. (1980). The structure of proteins involved in active membrane transport. *Annual Review of Biophysics and Bioengineering, 9,* 259-291.

Research News. (1991). The cell cycle: Spinning farther afield. *Science, 252*(5012), 1490-1492.

Singer, S. J. (1977). Thermodynamics: The structure of integral membrane proteins and transport. *Journal of Supramolecular Structure, 6,* 313-323.

Singer, S. J., & Nicolson, G. L. (1972). The fluid mosaic model of the structure of cell membranes. *Science, 175,* 720-731.

Trosko, J. E., Chang, C. C., & Mudhukar, B. V. (1990). Symposium: Cell communication in normal and uncontrolled growth. *Modulation of Intercellular Communication During Radiation and Chemical Carcinogenesis, 123*(3), 241-251.

CHAPTER 2

Altered Cellular and Tissue Biology

Kathryn L. McCance

K nowledge of the structural and functional reactions of cells and tissues to injurious agents, including genetic defects, is key for the understanding of disease processes. Currently diseases are defined and interpreted in molecular terms and not just in general descriptions of altered structure. Altered cellular and tissue biology can be the result of adaptation, injury, neoplasia, aging, or death. (Neoplasia is discussed in Chapters 10 and 11.) Adaptation occurs in response to both normal, or physiologic, conditions and adverse, or pathologic, conditions. For example, the uterus adapts to pregnancy—a normal

53

physiologic state—by enlarging. Enlargement occurs because of an increase in the size and number of uterine cells. In an adverse condition, such as high blood pressure, myocardial cells are stimulated to enlarge by the increased work of pumping. Like most of the body's adaptive mechanisms, however, cellular adaptations to adverse conditions are usually only temporarily successful. Severe or long-term stressors overwhelm adaptive processes, and cellular injury or death ensues.

Cellular injury can be caused by any factor that disrupts cellular structures or deprives the cell of oxygen and nutrients required for survival. Injury may be reversible (sublethal) or irreversible (lethal) and is classified broadly as chemical, hypoxic (lack of sufficient oxygen), or infectious. Cellular injuries from various causes have different clinical and pathophysiologic manifestations.

Cellular death is confirmed by structural changes seen when cells are stained and examined under a microscope. No biochemical indicators of cellular death are universally applicable because we still do not know precisely what biochemical functions must be compromised before a cell dies (Orrenius, McConkey, & Nicotera, 1991; Scarpelli & Iannaccone, 1990).

Cellular aging causes structural and functional changes that eventually may lead to cellular death or a decreased capacity to recover from injury. Mechanisms explaining how and why cells age are not known, and distinguishing between pathologic changes and physiologic changes that occur with aging is often difficult. Aging clearly causes alterations in cellular structure and function, yet senescence is both inevitable and normal.

CELLULAR ADAPTATION

Cells adapt to their environment to escape and protect themselves from injury. An adapted cell is neither normal nor injured—its condition lies somewhere between these two states. Cellular adaptations, however, are a common and central part of many disease states. In the early stages of a successful adaptive response, cells may have enhanced function; thus, it is hard to know what is a pathologic response versus an extreme adaptation to an excessive functional demand (Kissane, 1990). The most significant adaptive changes in cells include atrophy (decrease in cell size), hypertrophy (increase in cell size), hyperplasia (increase in cell number), and metaplasia (reversible replacement of one mature cell type by another, less mature cell type). Dysplasia (deranged cellular growth) is not considered a true cellular adapta-

FIG. 2-1 Adaptive and dysplastic alterations in simple cuboidal epithelial cells.

tion, but rather an atypical hyperplasia. These changes are shown in Fig. 2-1.

Atrophy

Atrophy is a decrease or shrinkage in cellular size. If atrophy occurs in a sufficient number of an organ's cells, the entire organ shrinks or becomes atrophic. Atrophy can affect any organ, but it is most common in skeletal muscle, the heart, secondary sex organs, and the brain. The causes of atrophy include decreases in work load, use, blood supply, nutrition, hormonal stimulation, and nervous stimulation. Individuals immobilized in bed for a prolonged time exhibit a type of skeletal muscle atrophy called disuse atrophy. Aging causes brain cells to become atrophic (presumably as arteriosclerosis obstructs the brain's blood supply) and endocrine-dependent organs, such as the gonads, to shrink as hormonal stimulation decreases. Brain atrophy occurs in a large percentage of individuals infected with the human immunodeficiency virus (HIV) (Pedersen, Thomsen, Arlein-Soberg et al., 1991). Whether atrophy is caused by normal physiologic conditions or by pathologic conditions, atrophic cells exhibit the same basic changes.

The atrophic muscle cell contains less endoplasmic reticulum and fewer mitochondria and myofilaments (part of the muscle fiber that controls contraction) than does the normal cell. In muscular atrophy caused by nerve loss, there is an immediate reduction in oxygen consumption and amino acid uptake. The biochemical changes of atrophy are not well understood, but mechanisms probably include decreased protein synthesis, increased protein catabolism, or both (Scarpelli & Iannaccone, 1990).

Atrophy, as a result of chronic malnutrition, is often accompanied by an increase in the number of **autophagic vacuoles,** which are membrane-bound vesicles within the cell that contain cellular debris—small fragments of mitochondria and endoplasmic reticulum—and hydrolytic enzymes. Atrophic change causes a rapid increase in hydrolytic enzymes, which are isolated in autophagic vacuoles to prevent uncontrolled cellular destruction. Thus, the vacuoles proliferate as needed to protect the uninjured organelles from the injured organelles and are eventually taken up and destroyed by lysosomes (a process described in Chapter 1). Certain contents of the autophagic vacuole may resist destruction by lysosomal enzymes and persist in membrane-bound residual bodies. An example of such content is granules that contain **lipofuscin,** the yellow-brown age pigment. Lipofuscin accumulates primarily in liver cells, myocardial cells, and atrophic cells.

Hypertrophy

Hypertrophy is an increase in the size of cells and consequently in the size of the affected organ. The cells of the heart and kidneys are particularly responsive to enlargement. The increase in cellular size is associated with an increased accumulation of protein in the cellular components (plasma membrane, endoplasmic reticulum, myofilaments, and mitochondria), and *not* with an increase in cellular fluid. The exact physiologic mechanism of hypertrophy in various cells remains uncertain. Muscular hypertrophy might involve an increase in the rate of protein synthesis, a decrease in the rate of protein degradation, or both. If protein degradation decreases and the rate of protein synthesis is normal or slightly increased, the net effect is an accumulation of cellular protein. In myocardial hypertrophy, initial enlargement is caused by dilation of the cardiac chambers, but this is short-lived and is followed by increased synthesis of cardiac muscle proteins, allowing muscle fibers to do more work. The nucleus is also hypertrophic with increased synthesis of DNA (Kissane, 1990). Although fully matured (e.g., terminally differentiated), muscle cells are unable to undergo further mitosis; they are, however, capable of increased DNA synthesis. Why cardiac muscle cells are unable to progress through the cell cycle to mitosis is unclear; it may be because of a block that prevents them from entering G_2 of the cell cycle (Scarpelli & Iannaccone, 1990) (Fig. 2-2). The cell cycle is discussed in Chapters 1 and 10. Eventually, however, advanced hypertrophy can lead to myocardial failure (see Chapter 27). Muscular hypertrophy tends to diminish if the excessive work load diminishes.

After removal of one kidney, the other kidney adapts to increased demand for work with an increase in both the size and the number of cells. The major contribution to renal enlargement is hypertrophy. An example of normal or physiologic hypertrophy is the increased growth of the uterus and mammary glands in response to pregnancy.

FIG. 2-2 Cell cycle and possible sites of block.

Hyperplasia

Hyperplasia is an increase in the number of cells resulting from an increased rate of cellular division. Hyperplasia, as a response to injury, occurs when the injury has been severe and prolonged enough to have caused cell death (Kissane, 1990). Loss of epithelial cells and cells of the liver and kidney triggers DNA synthesis and mitotic division. Increased cell growth is a multistep process involving the production of growth factors, which stimulate the remaining cells to synthesize new cell components and, ultimately, to divide. Hyperplasia and hypertrophy often occur together, although the specific mechanism is unknown. Hyperplasia and hypertrophy both take place if the cells are capable of synthesizing DNA, which enables mitotic division to occur.

Two types of normal, or physiologic, hyperplasia are (1) compensatory hyperplasia and (2) hormonal hyperplasia. **Compensatory hyperplasia** is an adaptive mechanism that enables certain organs to regenerate. For example, removal of part of the liver leads to hyperplasia of the remaining liver cells (hepatocytes) to compensate for the loss. Even with removal of 70% of the liver, regeneration is complete in about 2 weeks. The remarkable regenerating capacity of the liver was even noted by the ancient Greeks. According to the story, Prometheus was chained to a mountain, and his liver was eaten daily by a vulture, only to regenerate every night. A recently identified new protein, **hepatocyte growth factor** (HGF), is thought to be a mediator of liver regeneration (Bottaro et al., 1991).

Not all types of mature cells have the same capacity for compensatory hyperplastic growth. Some cells, such as nerve, skeletal muscle, and myocardial cells and the lens cells of the eye, do not regenerate. Significant compensatory hyperplasia occurs in epidermal and intestinal epithelia, hepatocytes, bone marrow cells, and fibroblasts, and some hyperplasia is noted in bone, cartilage, and smooth muscle cells. An example of compensatory hyperplasia is a callus, or thickening, of the skin as a result of hyperplasia of epidermal cells in response to a mechanical stimulus (Fig. 2-3).

Hormonal hyperplasia occurs chiefly in estrogen-dependent organs, such as the uterus and breast. After ovulation, for example, estrogen stimulates the endometrium to grow and thicken for reception of the fertilized ovum. If pregnancy occurs, hormonal hyperplasia, as well as hypertrophy, enables the uterus to enlarge. (Hormone function is described in Chapters 17 and 19.)

Pathologic hyperplasia is the abnormal proliferation of normal cells, usually in response to excessive hormonal stimulation. The most common example is pathologic hyperplasia of the endometrium (which is caused by an imbalance between estrogen and progesterone secretion, with oversecretion of estrogen (see Chapter 20). Pathologic endometrial hyperplasia, which causes excessive menstrual bleeding, is under the influence of regu-

FIG. 2-3 Callus formation and hyperkeratosis or thickening of the skin. (From Thibodeau, G. A. [1987]. *Anatomy and physiology.* St. Louis: Mosby–Year Book.)

lar growth-inhibition controls. If these controls fail, hyperplastic endometrial cells can undergo malignant transformation. (Malignant cell transformation is discussed in Chapter 10.)

Dysplasia

Dysplasia refers to abnormal changes in the size, shape, and organization of mature cells. Dysplasia, although not considered a true "adaptive process," is related to hyperplasia and is often called **atypical hyperplasia.** Dysplastic changes frequently are encountered in epithelial tissue of the cervix and respiratory tract, where they are strongly associated with common neoplastic growths and often are found adjacent to cancerous cells. Recent data indicate that atypical hyperplasia is a strong predictor of breast cancer development (London, Connolly, Schnitt, & Colditz, 1992). Neoplasia is a term associated with malignant tumors. If the inciting stimulus is removed, dysplastic changes are often reversible.

Metaplasia

Metaplasia is the reversible replacement of one mature cell type by another, sometimes less differentiated, cell type. The best example of metaplasia is replacement of normal columnar ciliated epithelial cells of the bronchial

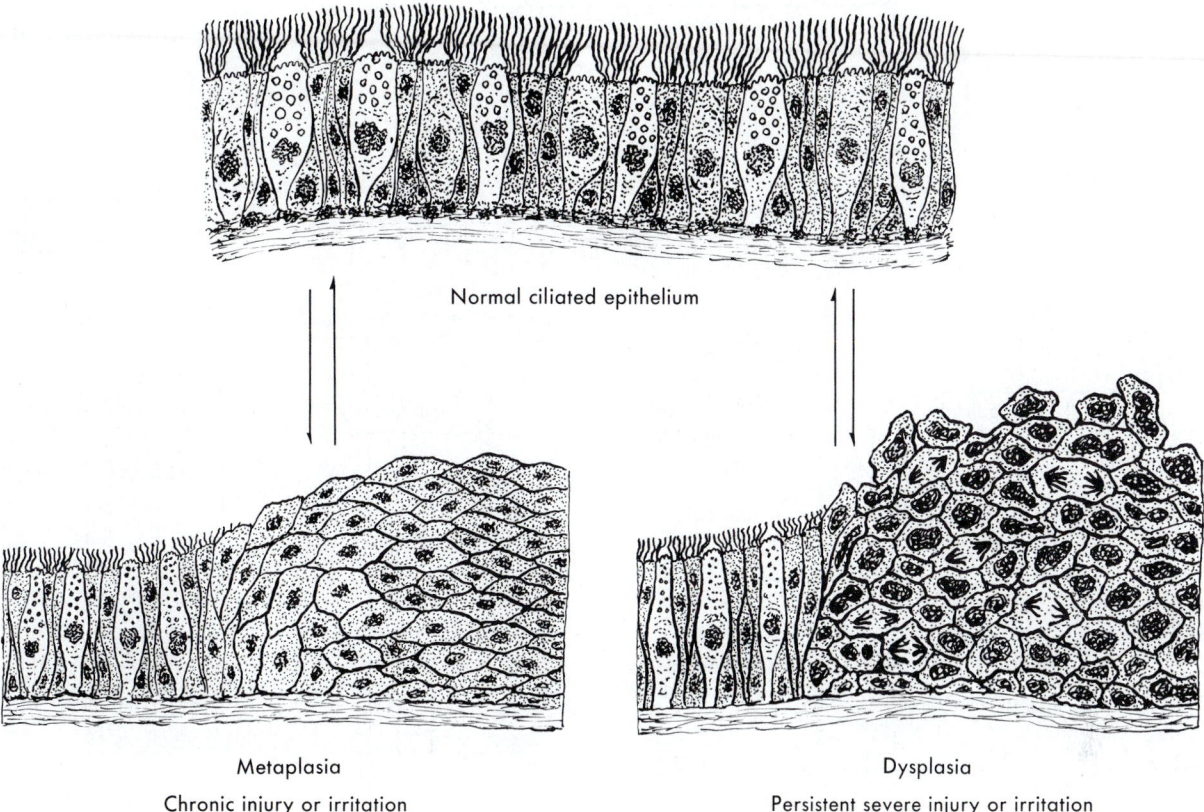

Normal ciliated epithelium

Metaplasia

Chronic injury or irritation

Dysplasia

Persistent severe injury or irritation

FIG. 2-4 Reversible changes in cells lining the bronchi.

(airway) lining by stratified squamous epithelial cells (Fig. 2-4). The newly formed squamous epithelial cells do not secrete mucus or have cilia, causing loss of a vital protective mechanism. (Protective mechanisms of the respiratory tract are described in Chapter 29.)

Bronchial metaplasia can be reversed if the inducing stimulus, usually cigarette smoking, is removed. With prolonged exposure to the inducing stimulus, however, cancerous transformation can occur.

CELLULAR INJURY

The precise biologic processes responsible for cellular injury are complex, interdependent, and in many cases unknown. In general, cellular injury occurs if the cell is unable to maintain homeostasis—a normal or adaptive steady state—in the face of injurious stimuli. Injurious stimuli include chemical agents, lack of sufficient oxygen (hypoxia), infectious agents, physical and mechanical factors, immunologic reactions, genetic factors, and nutritional imbalances.

The mechanisms causing chemical and hypoxic injury are perhaps the best understood. Both of these mechanisms can lead to disruption of selective permeability (i.e., transport mechanisms) of the plasma membrane;

reduction or cessation of cellular metabolism; lack of protein synthesis; damage to lysosomal membranes, with leakage of destructive enzymes into the cytoplasm; enzymatic destruction of cellular organelles; cellular death (exhibited by nuclear changes); and phagocytosis of the dead cell by cellular components of the acute inflammatory response (see Chapter 7). The extent of cellular injury depends on the type, state (including level of cell differentiation and increased susceptibility to fully differentiated cells), and adaptive processes of the cell, as well as the type, severity, and duration of the injurious stimulus. Two individuals exposed to an identical stimulus may incur varying degrees of cellular injury. Modifying factors, such as nutritional status, can profoundly influence the extent of injury. The precise "point of no return" that leads to cellular death is a biochemical puzzle, and the exact mechanisms responsible for the transition from reversible to irreversible cellular damage are currently debated.

Hypoxic Injury

Hypoxia, or lack of sufficient oxygen, is the single most common cause of cellular injury (Fig. 2-5). Hypoxia can result from a decreased amount of oxygen in the air, loss of hemoglobin or hemoglobin function, decreased production of red blood cells, diseases of the respira-

FIG. 2-5 Hypoxic injury induced by ischemia.

tory and cardiovascular systems, and poisoning of the oxidative enzymes (cytochromes) within the cells. The most common cause of hypoxia is **ischemia** (reduced blood supply).

Ischemic injury is often caused by gradual narrowing of arteries (arteriosclerosis) and complete blockage by blood clots (thrombosis). Progressive hypoxia caused by gradual arterial obstruction is better tolerated than the sudden acute **anoxia** (total lack of oxygen) caused by a sudden obstruction, such as can occur with an embolus (a blood clot or other plug in the circulation). An acute obstruction in a coronary artery can cause myocardial cell death (infarction) within minutes if the blood supply is not restored, whereas gradual onset of ischemia usually results in myocardial adaptation. The most common causes of death in the United States, myocardial infarction and stroke, generally result from atherosclerosis (a type of arteriosclerosis) and consequent ischemic

injury. (Vascular obstruction is discussed in Chapter 27.)

Cellular responses to hypoxic injury caused by ischemia have been demonstrated in studies of the heart muscle (Jennings & Reimer, 1981; Vlessis, Muller, Bartos, & Trunkey, 1991). Within a minute of interruption of blood supply to the myocardium, the heart becomes pale and has difficulty contracting normally. Within 3 to 5 minutes, the ischemic portion of the myocardium ceases to contract. The abrupt lack of contraction is caused by a rapid decrease in mitochondrial phosphorylation, which results in insufficient adenosine triphosphate (ATP) production. Lack of ATP leads to an increase in anaerobic metabolism, which generates ATP from glycogen when there is insufficient oxygen. When glycogen stores are depleted, even anaerobic metabolism ceases. (Aerobic and anaerobic cellular metabolism are described in Chapter 1.)

A reduction in ATP levels causes the plasma membrane's sodium-potassium pump and sodium-calcium exchange to fail, which leads to an intracellular accumulation of sodium and calcium and diffusion of potassium out of the cell. (The sodium-potassium pump is discussed in Chapter 1.) Sodium and water then can enter the cell freely, and cellular swelling results. The movement of water and ions into the cell causes early dilation of the endoplasmic reticulum. Dilation causes the ribosomes to detach from the rough endoplasmic reticulum, resulting in reduced protein synthesis. With continued hypoxia, the entire cell becomes markedly swollen, with increased concentrations of sodium, water, and chloride and decreased concentrations of potassium. These disruptions are reversible if oxygen is restored. If oxygen is not restored, however, there is vacuolation (formation of vacuoles) within the cytoplasm and marked swelling of the mitochondria resulting from mitochondrial membrane damage. Structurally, this stage is associated with irreversible cell injury. With plasma membrane damage, extracellular calcium moves into the cell and accumulates in the mitochondria.

All cells in the body are bathed in a fluid rich in calcium ions. In muscle cells, calcium is necessary for the activation of the contractile proteins, actin and myosin. If the plasma membrane's barrier to calcium ions is eliminated or damaged, calcium readily enters and accumulates in the mitochondria, resulting in mitochondrial swelling and rapid death of the cell (Farber, 1981). Death is caused by calcium accumulation compromising ATP production by the mitochondria. In hypoxic injury caused by atherosclerosis, failure of ATP production further deprives the myocardium of the energy needed for contraction.

Chemical Injury
Mechanisms of Chemical Injury

Chemical injury begins with a biochemical interaction between a toxic substance and the cell's plasma membrane, which is ultimately damaged, leading to increased permeability. Not all of the mechanisms causing chemically induced membrane destruction are known.

Because it has been investigated extensively, carbon tetrachloride (CCl_4) injury is a useful example of chemical injury. Carbon tetrachloride, an agent formerly used in dry cleaning, is injurious to cells because an enzyme system in the smooth endoplasmic reticulum of liver cells converts it into CCl_3 (chloromethyl), a highly toxic free radical. A **free radical** is an electrically uncharged atom or group of atoms having an unpaired electron that is capable of injurious chemical bond formation. Free radicals are highly reactive, are difficult to control, and induce chain reactions. The formation of free radicals in biologic materials requires an extreme energy source, such as ionizing radiation (e.g., x-rays) or interactions with other molecules, such as CCl_4 or oxygen. Free radicals can damage cellular membranes by **lipid peroxidation,** which is the destruction of polyunsaturated lipids (the same process by which fats become rancid). Peroxidation involves the reaction of oxygen-derived free radicals, such as free hydroxyl groups (OH), and lipids to form free-radical intermediates and moderately stable peroxides (Scarpelli & Iannaccone, 1990). These actions can lead to chain reactions, causing auto-oxidation of the fatty-acid content of lipids in cellular membranes. The formation of free radicals also occurs during phagocytosis as a way of killing bacteria (See Chapter 7.).

In CCl_4 injury, newly formed CCl_3 rapidly destroys the endoplasmic reticulum of the liver cell by breaking down the reticulum's lipid component. The next event in CCl_3 injury is an accumulation of lipid molecules within the cytoplasm, starting within cisternae of the endoplasmic reticulum (Fig. 2-6). Fatty liver develops because CCl_4 poisoning blocks the synthesis of **lipid-acceptor proteins (apoproteins)** that normally bind with triglycerides to form lipoproteins, which are transported out of the cell. Blockage of triglyceride (lipoprotein) secretion begins 10 to 15 minutes after CCl_4 exposure. Fat droplets that accumulate in cisternae of the endoplasmic reticulum combine to form larger droplets and fill vacuoles that, in turn, fill the entire cytoplasm (Fig. 2-7). Approximately 10 to 12 hours later, the liver appears grossly enlarged and pale because of the accumulation of fat. (Accumulation of fat is discussed further on p. 72.)

In the meantime, cellular swelling progresses because of alterations in the selective permeability of the plasma membrane. Cellular swelling becomes severe when the plasma membrane loses its ability to prevent the passive inward diffusion of sodium ions and water. The most serious consequence of plasma membrane damage is, as in hypoxic injury, to the mitochondria. An influx of calcium ions from the extracellular compartment and their accumulation in the mitochondria cause the mitochondria to swell, an occurrence that is associated with irreversible cellular injury. The injured mitochondria can no longer generate ATP, but they do continue to accumulate calcium ions. The influx of calcium into the mitochondria interferes with oxidative metabolism (by uncoupling oxidative phosphorylation). Like hypoxic injury, chemical injury causes reduction in ATP, causing failure of the sodium-potassium pump, which results in intracellular accumulation of sodium and diffusion of potassium out of the cell. Sodium and water freely enter the cell and cellular swelling results. As ATP generation fails, the cell loses its capacity for active transport of ions and oxidization of fatty acids, which lowers pH and may lead to further lipid accumulation.

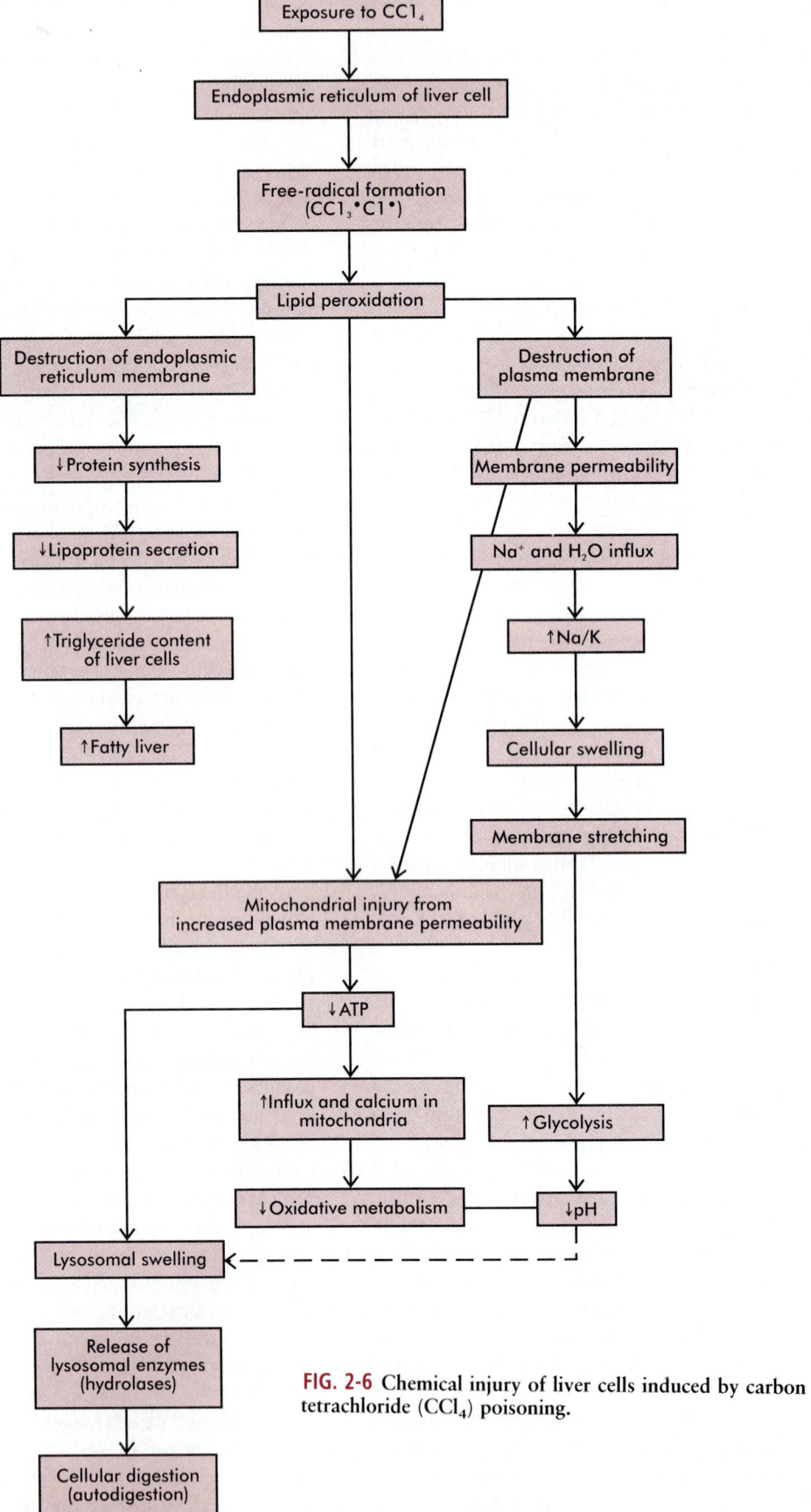

FIG. 2-6 Chemical injury of liver cells induced by carbon tetrachloride (CCl_4) poisoning.

FIG. 2-7 **Electron micrograph of liver cells 8 hours after administration of CCl$_4$.** Hepatocytes are large and edematous with a finely granular cytoplasm; clear vacuoles probably represent infiltration of triglycerides. Nuclei appear normal. (From Kissane, 1990.)

Decreasing cellular pH (caused by the loss of oxidative phosphorylation and ATP-stimulating glycolysis), together with fluid and electrolyte imbalances (increased sodium and water and decreased potassium), lead to lysosomal membrane injury, causing a leakage of lysosomal enzymes into the cytoplasm. Enzymatic digestion of cellular organelles, including the nucleus and nucleolus, ensues, halting synthesis of deoxyribonucleic acid (DNA) and ribonucleic acid (RNA). The leakage of lysosomal enzymes apparently occurs late in chemical injury, well after irreversible lipid accumulation, mitochondrial swelling, and ATP loss. The lysosomal phase of chemical injury is probably similar to that which occurs in hypoxic injury.

Chemical Agents

A number of chemical agents, too numerous to list, cause cellular injury. Highly toxic substances are known as poisons. Minute amounts of some, such as arsenic and cyanide, can rapidly destroy enough cells to cause somatic death (death of the individual). Chronic exposure to air pollutants, insecticides, and herbicides can cause cellular injury. Carbon monoxide, carbon tetrachloride, and social drugs, such as alcohol, can significantly alter cellular function and injure cellular structures. Over-the-counter and prescribed drugs also may cause cellular injury, sometimes leading to death. Accidental or suicidal poisonings by chemical agents cause numerous deaths. The injurious effects of some of these agents—lead, carbon monoxide, and ethyl alcohol—exemplify common cellular injuries.

Lead

Heavy metals, such as lead, cause a significant number of childhood poisonings. Lead-based paint, which has a sweet taste, is often ingested by children. Other sources of lead include dust and soil in inner-city urban areas, debris from household renovations, and formula mixed with lead-contaminated tap water (Shannon & Graef, 1992). Children are particularly vulnerable to lead toxicity because, compared with adults, they absorb lead more readily through the intestines. If nutrition is compromised, especially if dietary intake of iron, calcium, and vitamin D is insufficient, lead's toxic effects are enhanced (Hazardous Substances and Public Health, 1991).

The organ systems primarily affected by lead include the nervous system, the hematopoietic system (tissues that produce blood cells), and the kidneys. A suggested mechanism by which lead acts on the central nervous system is interference with neurotransmitters, which may cause hyperactive behavior and proliferation of capillaries of the white matter and intercerebral arteries (Kissane, 1990). Lead inhibits several enzymes involved in hemoglobin synthesis. A significant manifestation of lead toxicity is anemia caused by lysis of red blood cells (hemolysis). Manifestations of brain involvement include convulsions and delirium and, with peripheral nerve involvement, wrist, finger, and sometimes foot paralysis. Renal lesions can cause tubular dysfunction resulting in glycosuria (glucose in the urine), aminoaciduria (amino acids in the urine), and hyperphosphaturia (excess phosphate in the urine). Gastrointestinal symptoms are less severe and include nausea, loss of appetite, weight loss, and abdominal cramping.

Carbon monoxide

Gaseous substances can be classified according to their ability to asphyxiate (interrupt respiration) or irritate. Toxic asphyxiants, such as carbon monoxide, hydrogen cyanide, and hydrogen sulfide, directly interfere with cellular respiration. Carbon monoxide is widely available.

Carbon monoxide is odorless, colorless, and undetectable unless it is mixed with a visible or odorous pollutant. It is produced by the incomplete combustion of such fuels as gasoline. Although carbon monoxide is a chemical agent, the ultimate injury it produces is a hypoxic injury, namely, oxygen deprivation. Normally, oxygen molecules are carried to tissues bound to hemoglobin in red blood cells (see Chapter 29). Because carbon monoxide's affinity for hemoglobin is 300 times greater than that of oxygen, it quickly binds with the hemoglobin, preventing oxygen molecules from doing so. Minute amounts of carbon monoxide can produce significant percentages of carboxyhemoglobin (carbon monoxide bound with hemoglobin).

Symptoms related to carbon monoxide poisoning include headache, giddiness, tinnitus (ringing in the ears), nausea, weakness, and vomiting. At risk for carbon monoxide exposure are those who (1) breathe air polluted by gasoline engines or defective furnaces, (2) work in such occupations as coal mining, fire fighting, or engine repair, and (3) smoke cigarettes, cigars, or pipes. The fetus is especially at risk from the effects of carbon monoxide because fetal carboxyhemoglobin levels are likely to be 10% to 15% greater than maternal levels (Holbrook, 1983).

Ethanol

Alcohol (ethanol) is the number one favorite mood-altering drug in the United States (Lieber, 1991). Because alcohol is not only a psychoactive drug but also a food, it is considered part of the basic food supply in many societies. A large intake of alcohol has enormous effects on nutritional status. Liver and nutritional disorders are the most serious consequences of alcohol abuse. New understandings of the mechanisms of ethanol-induced liver injury have emerged through the clarification of a new pathway for ethanol oxidation, the microsomal P-450 oxidase pathway.

The major effects of acute alcoholism involve the central nervous system. After ingestion, it is absorbed, un-altered, in the stomach and small intestine. Fatty foods and milk slow absorption (Cotran, Kumar, & Robbins, 1989). Alcohol then is distributed to all tissues and fluids of the body in direct proportion to the blood concentration.

Most of the alcohol in the blood is metabolized in the liver through one major and two accessory pathways. The major pathway involves hepatic alcohol dehydrogenase (ADH), an enzyme of the cytosol that catalyzes the conversion of ethanol to acetaldehyde (Fig. 2-8).

The microsomal ethanol oxidizing system (MEOS) is dependent on cytochrome P-450, an enzyme necessary for cellular oxidation (Lieber, 1991). Activation of MEOS requires a high ethanol concentration and, thus, is thought to be important in the accelerated ethanol metabolism (i.e., tolerance) noted in chronic alcoholics (Lieber, 1991).

Individuals differ in their capability to metabolize alcohol. Genetic differences in metabolism of liver alcohol, including aldehyde dehydrogenases, have been identified (Lieber, 1988). Chronic alcoholics develop certain levels of tolerance because of enzyme induction, leading to an increased rate of metabolism (e.g., P-450).

Acute alcoholism exerts its effects mainly on the central nervous system (CNS), but it also may induce hepatic and gastric changes that are reversible in the absence of continued alcohol intake (Cotran et al., 1989). The hepatic changes, initiated from acetaldehyde, include deposition in fat, enlargement of the liver, interruption of microtubular transport of proteins and their secretion, increase in intracellular water, depression of fatty acid oxidation in the mitochondria, increased membrane rigidity, and acute liver cell necrosis (see Chapter 36). In the CNS, alcohol is, itself, a depressant, initially affecting subcortical structures (probably the brainstem reticular formation) (Cotran et al., 1989). Consequently, motor and intellectual activity becomes disoriented. Acute alcoholism contributes significantly to over 50% of motor vehicle fatalities (Cotran et al., 1989). At higher blood levels, medullary centers become depressed, affecting respiration. Much investigation is under way on the relationship of alcohol and snoring and obstructive sleep apnea (cessation of breathing) (Stradling & Crosby, 1991).

Chronic alcoholism is responsible for structural alterations in practically all organs and tissues in the body, especially the liver and stomach. The precise mechanisms for these widespread effects is controversial. Acetaldehyde, because of its reactive nature, is proposed as the mediator of the widespread tissue and organ damage (Lieber, 1991). Chronic alcoholism is related to several disorders, including increased tendency to hypertension, a higher incidence of acute and chronic pancreatitis, and regressive changes in skeletal muscle (see Chapter 36). The deleterious effects of prenatal alcohol

FIG. 2-8 Major pathway of metabolism of alcohol in the liver through ADH. (Modified from Cotran, Kumar, & Robbins, 1989.)

exposure (e.g., fetal alcohol syndrome) are the subject of numerous research studies.

Whatever the cause, chronic alcoholics have a significantly shortened lifespan related mainly to damage to the liver, stomach, brain, and heart. Alcohol is a well-known cause of hepatic injury, terminating in cirrhosis (p. 1356). Although still controversial, moderate amounts of alcohol may decrease the incidence of coronary heart disease (see Chapter 27).

Infectious Injury

The pathogenicity (virulence) of microorganisms lies in their ability to survive and proliferate in the human body, where they injure cells and tissues. The disease-producing potential of a microorganism depends on its ability to (1) invade and destroy cells, (2) produce toxins, and (3) produce damaging hypersensitivity reactions.

Bacteria

Bacterial survival and growth depend on the effectiveness of the body's defense mechanisms and on the bacterium's ability to resist these defenses (see Chapter 7). One mode of resistance is a coating that protects the bacterium from ingestion and destruction by specialized cells called phagocytes. Such coatings include the thick polysaccharide covering of the pneumococcus, the waxy capsule surrounding the tubercle bacillus, and the M protein cell wall of the streptococcus. Not all virulent extracellular pathogens are encapsulated types. For example, *Mycobacterium tuberculosis* can survive within and be transported by phagocytes.

Bacteria that survive and proliferate in the body produce substances that injure cells and tissues. Some bacteria produce destructive enzymes. For example, a variety of clostridia, *Clostridum perfringens,* produces both collagenases and lecithinases—powerful lytic enzymes that destroy connective tissues and cellular membranes.

Toxins are produced by many microorganisms. Gram-positive bacteria, such as *Corynebacterium diphtheriae, Clostridium tetani,* and *Clostridium botulinum,* produce powerful exotoxins. The term **exotoxin** seems to be a misnomer because exotoxins are toxins contained *within* the bacterium. They are called exotoxins because their toxic effects are produced on their release as metabolic products during bacterial growth.

Exotoxins are proteins and have highly specific effects. For example, the diphtheria toxin produces its effects by inactivating enzymes critical to protein synthesis. *C. tetani* produces a neurotoxin that acts on the central and sympathetic nervous systems by blocking motor inhibition, chiefly in the motor anterior horn cells of the spinal cord. This exotoxin also acts on the respiratory center of the brain, causing spasm or depression of the respiratory muscles, resulting in asphyxia and death. *C. botulinum* produces an exotoxin that causes severe food poisoning. The exotoxin is resistant to gastric digestion and is absorbed into the blood. It interferes with the motor end plates of skeletal muscles and causes paralysis, mainly of the eye orbit, pharynx, larynx, and respiratory muscles.

Bacteria that produce endotoxins are also called pyrogenic bacteria because they activate the inflammatory process and produce fever. (The physiology of fever is discussed in Chapter 13; the inflammatory response is discussed in Chapter 7.) **Endotoxins** are contained in the cell walls of gram-negative bacteria and are released as phospholipids and polysaccharides of cell walls during lysis, or destruction, of the bacteria. Thus the endotoxin is also called **lipopolysaccharide** (LPS). Endotoxin can be released from the membrane of the bacteria, either during bacterial growth or during treatment with antibiotics, which therefore cannot prevent the toxic effects of endotoxin (Calandra, Baumgartner, & Glauser, 1991). The innermost part of the LPS, the *lipid A*, made of fatty acids, is the structure responsible for the toxic effects of LPS.

Over the last decades, the incidence of gram-negative infections has increased significantly in major medical centers (Calandra et al., 1991). One of the most key and disappointing observations is that the survival of gram-negative bacteria remains in the range of 10% to 40% (Calandra et al., 1991). In individuals developing gram-negative toxic manifestations (e.g., septic shock), fatality rates may be 50% or more (Calandra et al., 1991; Veterans Administration Systemic Sepsis Cooperative Study Group, 1987).

A major achievement in the understanding of the pathophysiology of gram-negative infections has been the recent recognition of the role played by tumor necrosis factor/cachectin (TNF) in the pathogenesis of endotoxic shock (Calandra et al., 1991; Sherry & Cerami, 1988). Tumor necrosis factor is a cytokine (mediator) produced by activated macrophages (e.g., large phagocytic cells) on exposure to endotoxin. Tumor necrosis factor is sometimes called cachectin because of its role in promoting a group of symptoms in the individual with cancer called cachexia. (Cachexia is discussed in Chapter 11; cytokines are discussed in Chapter 6.)

Fever is caused by the release of endogenous pyrogens from macrophages or circulating white blood cells (interleukin-1 and tumor necrosis factor-α) attracted to the site of injury. Fever is caused also by the release of biochemicals (certain prostaglandins) during the inflammatory response. Endogenous pyrogens are proteins that act on the thermoregulatory centers of the hypothalamus. Mechanisms by which prostaglandins (PGE_1 and PGE_2) cause fever are not well defined (see Chapter 13).

Inflammation is the body's response to the presence of the bacteria. The inflammatory response increases capillary permeability, allowing substances involved in bacterial destruction to migrate from the capillaries to the site of infection. Endotoxins increase capillary permeability further through activation of a plasma protein system, the complement cascade (see Chapter 7). Capillary permeability may increase sufficiently to permit escape of large quantities of blood, contributing to the syndrome of disseminated (or diffuse) intravascular coagulation or, in severe cases, cardiovascular shock (see Chapter 27).

The ability to produce hypersensitivity reactions is an important pathogenic mechanism of bacterial toxins. Tissue lesions of many chronic infections are related to the induction of hypersensitivity to the toxin. For example, *M. tuberculosis* causes inflammatory lesions known as granulomas. The inflammatory response to bacterial toxins causes a destructive, or "granulomatous," reaction. Some bacteria alter host tissues so that the tissues evoke self-destructive (autoimmune) reactions. Other bacteria produce substances that "look like" host proteins and cause the body to produce substances (antibodies) that later "recognize" and react with the look-alike host proteins in normal tissues. (Hypersensitivity reactions and autoimmune disease are described in Chapter 8.)

Bacteremia, or **septicemia,** is the proliferation of microorganisms in the blood. Bacteremia is caused by a failure of the body's defense mechanisms. The most frequent cause of bacteremia is proliferation of gram-negative bacteria, although a few gram-positive bacteria and fungi are sometimes the cause. (The gram-negative bacteria include *Escherichia coli, Serratia marcescens, Proteus mirabilis, Enterobacter aerogenes, Pseudomonas aeruginosa,* and *Bacteroides* species.) Symptoms of bacteremia are produced by the endotoxins that are released from the cell walls of the bacteria. Once in the blood, endotoxins cause the release of vasoactive peptides that affect blood vessels. One vascular effect is vasodilation that reduces blood pressure, which in turn causes decreased oxygen delivery and subsequent cardiovascular shock (see Chapter 27). Lymphangitis, or inflamed lymphatic vessels, is a manifestation of bacteremia that causes red streaks under the skin of an arm or leg radiating from the infection site.

Viruses

Viruses are intracellular parasites that take over the metabolic machinery of host cells and use it for their own survival and replication. This results in decreased synthesis of macromolecules vital to the host. Viral diseases are the most common afflictions of humans. The common cold affects most people annually. The ubiquitous role of viruses ranges from the "cold sore" of herpes simplex to the causation of cancer (discussed in detail in Chapter 10).

Viruses do not produce exotoxins or endotoxins. The protein coat (capsid) that encapsulates most viruses enables them to resist phagocytosis but evokes a very strong immune response. Viruses, however, can rapidly produce irreversible and lethal injury in highly susceptible cells in an immunosuppressed host. If a symbiotic relationship is maintained between the host cell and the virus, however, persistent unapparent infection may result. Cell injury does not occur, and the virus persists until it is activated to replicate (e.g., fever blister). (The role of foreign proteins in stimulating the creation of immunity is described in Chapter 6.) Immunity may protect the individual from an acute exacerbation only or may be sufficiently strong to prevent disease.

Viral replication

Virions, or **viral particles,** do not possess any of the metabolic organelles that are contained within either procaryotes (e.g., bacteria) or eucaryotes (e.g., human cells) (Fig. 2-9). Thus viruses have no metabolism. Unlike bacteria, viruses are incapable of independent reproduction. Their replication is totally dependent on their ability to infect a **permissive host cell**—a cell that cannot resist viral invasion and replication. The replication cycle of most viruses can be divided into two distinct phases, infection and integration. Infection begins when a virion binds to receptors on the plasma membrane of a host cell (Fig. 2-10). Specificity of these receptors dictates the range of host cells with which a particular virus can bind. For example, one known receptor is the CD4 pro-

tein of helper lymphocytes for the human immunodeficiency virus (HIV). Once bound, the virion *penetrates* the plasma membrane by receptor-mediated endocytosis, by envelope fusion with the plasma membrane, or by directly crossing the plasma membrane.

Viruses contain either DNA or RNA and thus are known as DNA or RNA viruses. After *uncoating,* the viral DNA enters the cell's nucleus, where it becomes incorporated into the host cell's chromosomal DNA. This is the *integration* phase, during which the viral genome (a complete set of hereditary factors) essentially regulates the metabolic activities of the host cell by directing its own *replication.* New virions then are released from the cell for transmission of the viral infection to other host cells. The replication of RNA viruses is essentially the same as for DNA viruses, except that different mechanisms of messenger RNA (mRNA) formation occur among different groups of RNA viruses. In all cases, RNA replication is facilitated by specific RNA-dependent RNA polymerase enzymes (replicases) encoded by the viral RNA chromosome. Viral DNA not only replicates in the host cell but also becomes integrated with host DNA and transmitted to the host's daughter cells during host cell mitosis. By this process, viral genes can become part of the vertically transmitted (inherited) genetic information of the host cell and its progeny. (The process by which DNA transmits genetic information is discussed in Chapter 4.)

FIG. 2-9 **Electron micrograph of virion inclusion in the nucleus of a glial cell.** The individual was diagnosed with progressive multifocal leukocephalopathy. (From Kissane, 1990.)

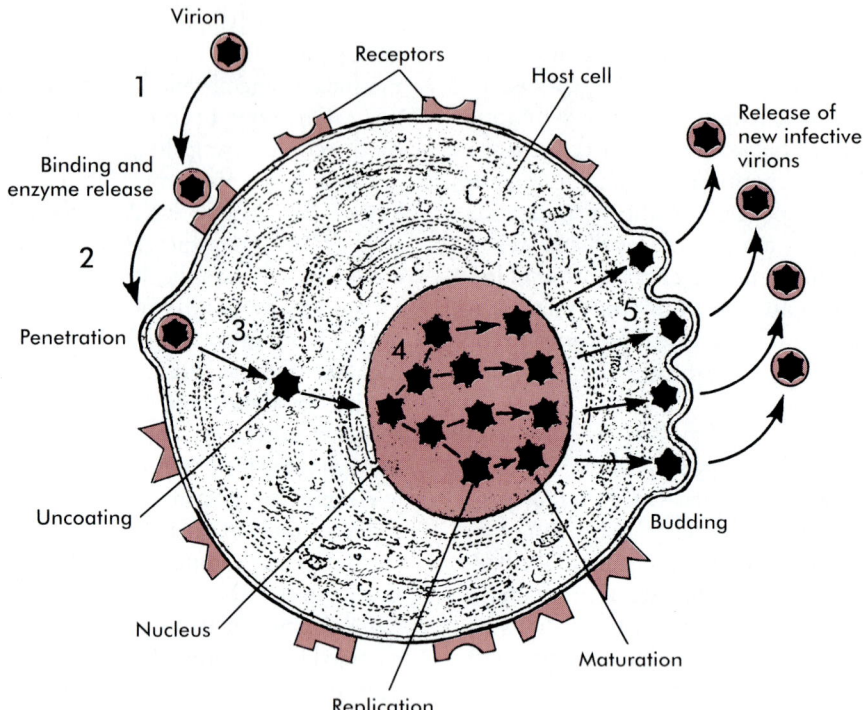

FIG. 2-10 Stages of viral infection of a host cell. The virion (1) becomes attached to receptors on the cell's plasma membrane; (2) releases enzymes that weaken the membrane and allow it to penetrate the cell; (3) uncoats itself; (4) replicates; and (5) matures and escapes from the cell by budding from the plasma membrane. The infection then can spread to other host cells.

Cellular effects of viruses

Besides taking over the host cell's metabolic machinery, viral infection can injure cellular structures. In some viral infections, cellular destruction results from plasma membrane damage that occurs when a virion binds with receptors on the host cell and releases enzymes that change the configuration of the membrane's fatty acids, altering the lipid bilayer (see Fig. 2-10). Alteration of the plasma membrane can incite an immune response with injury of the host's cells (e.g., hepatitis B virus). (The lipid bilayer is described and illustrated in Chapter 1.)

Once inside the host cell, virions have many cytopathic effects, including the following:

1. The cessation of protein synthesis. Herpes simplex, for example, stops cell division.
2. Disruption of lysosomal membranes, resulting in release of lysosomal enzymes that can kill the cell (see Chapter 1).
3. Formation of **inclusion bodies** (sites where synthesis of viral nucleic acids or proteins is occurring or has occurred). Some viral infections (e.g., smallpox) are associated with cytoplasmic inclusions.
4. Fusion of host cells, producing multinucleated giant cells. Fusion is seen with measles, influenza, and herpes simplex infections.
5. Alteration of the antigenic properties, or "identity" of the host cell, causing the host's immune system to attack the cell as if it were a foreign protein. (Antigenic properties and autoimmune disease are discussed in Unit III.)
6. Transformation of host cells into cancerous cells, resulting in uninhibited and unregulated growth. The Epstein-Barr virus, for example, is implicated in Burkitt lymphoma.

Human diseases caused by specific viruses are listed in Table 2-1.

Immunologic and Inflammatory Injury

Cellular membranes are injured by direct contact with cellular and chemical components of the immune and inflammatory responses, such as phagocytic cells (lymphocytes and macrophages) and such substances as histamine, antibodies, lymphokines, complement, and proteases (see Chapter 7). Complement is responsible for many of the membrane alterations that occur during immunologic injury.

Membrane alterations are associated with rapid leak-

TABLE 2-1

Characteristics and Pathophysiologic Effects of Viruses

Virus	Pathophysiologic effects
Papovaviruses (DNA) (papilloma)	Small viruses that induce tumors and cancers in animals, warts (papilloma) in humans
Adenoviruses (DNA)	Medium-sized viruses that cause various respiratory infections in humans; some cause tumors in animals
Herpesviruses (DNA) (herpes simplex, herpes zoster)	Medium-sized viruses that cause various diseases in humans, such as fever blisters, chickenpox, shingles, and infectious mononucleosis; implicated in a type of human cancer called Burkitt lymphoma
Poxvirus (DNA) (variola, cowpox, vaccinia)	Very large, complex, brick-shaped viruses that cause diseases such as smallpox (variola), molluscum contagiosum (wartlike skin lesions), cowpox, and vaccinia; vaccinia virus gives immunity to smallpox
Hepatitis B (DNA)	Widespread throughout the world; blood and blood products are the best-documented routes for transmission
Picornaviruses (RNA) (poliovirus, rhinovirus)	Smallest RNA-containing viruses; at least 70 human enteroviruses are known, including the polio-, coxsackie-, and echoviruses; more than 100 rhinoviruses exist and are the most common cause of colds
Myxoviruses (RNA) (influenza A, B, C)	Medium-sized viruses with a spiked envelope; have the ability to agglutinate red blood cells; cause influenza
Paramyxoviruses (RNA) (measles, mumps)	Structurally similar to myxoviruses, but generally larger; cause parainfluenza, measles, mumps
Coronaviruses (RNA)	Associated with upper respiratory tract infections and the common cold
Retroviruses (RNA)	Tumor-associated viruses; cause leukemia and tumors in animals; some members produce "slow" viral infections, cause of AIDS
Arenaviruses (RNA) (lassa)	Possess RNA-containing granules; some members produce "slow" viral infections in humans
Reoviruses (RNA)	Relation to human disease not clear; may be involved in mild respiratory infections and infantile gastroenteritis
Hepatitis A (RNA)	Isolated from chimpanzees; is known to be transmitted by humans by close person-to-person contact

Modified from Tortora, Funke, & Case, 1989.

age of K^+ out of the cell and rapid influx of water. Antibodies can interfere with membrane function by binding to and occupying receptor molecules on the plasma membrane. This type of injury is found in certain forms of diabetes mellitus and in myasthenia gravis. Antibodies also can block or destroy cellular junctions, interfering with intercellular communication. (See Chapter 6 for a discussion of antibody binding and Chapter 1 for a description of intercellular junctions and communication.)

Injurious Genetic Factors

Genetic disorders may be the result of genetic factors that alter the cell's nucleus and the plasma membrane's structure, shape, receptors, or transport mechanisms. For example, enzymatic genetic defects can lead to abnormalities in membrane transport. Genetic disorders that cause structural alterations of the red blood cell include sickle cell anemia, Huntington's disease, muscular dystrophy, and abetalipoproteinemia. (Mechanisms causing genetic abnormalities are discussed in Unit II.)

Injurious Nutritional Imbalances

Cells require adequate amounts of essential nutrients—proteins, carbohydrates, lipids (fats), vitamins, and minerals—to function normally. If these nutrients are not consumed in the diet and transported to the body's cells, or if excessive amounts of nutrients are consumed and transported, pathophysiologic cellular effects develop.

Proteins, which consist of chains of amino acids, are the major structural units of the cell and participate in many enzymatic and hormonal functions. Protein deficiency causes a decrease in the intestinal mucosal mass, decreasing the absorptive function. The integrity of the pancreas is also affected, resulting in diminished exocrine secretion. With starvation or malnutrition, the lowered plasma proteins, particularly albumin, cause fluid to move into the interstitium (edema). Protein-calorie malnutrition (PCM) is the predominant world-wide type of malnutrition. Children suffering from malnutrition are very susceptible and often die of infectious diseases. Even with adequate protein intake, cellular injury can occur if amino acid transport mechanisms fail or are defective. In Fanconi syndrome, for example, renal tubular cells may contain accumulated protein droplets that have been absorbed but cannot be transported. (Alterations of renal function are the subject of Chapter 33.)

Glucose is the major carbohydrate obtained from the breakdown of starch (see Chapter 1). Hyperglycemia (excessive glucose in the blood) caused by excessive carbohydrate intake may lead to obesity. Deficiencies of glucose result from starvation or from lack of use, as in diabetes. In both of these conditions, the body compensates by metabolizing fat (lipids). (For details on diabetes, see Chapter 18.)

In lipid deficiency, or **hypolipidemia**, the body compensates by mobilizing fatty acids from adipose tissue. This causes an increase in the production and circulation of ketone bodies, which are acidic by-products of lipid metabolism. The excretion of ketone bodies results in loss of water and electrolytes and causes dehydration and thirst. Severe increases in ketone bodies cause ketoacidosis, coma, and death. **Hyperlipidemia,** or an increase in lipoproteins in the blood, results in deposits of fat in the heart, liver, and muscle.

Vitamins are not sources of energy but are necessary for maintaining normal cellular function. Adequate vitamin intake is necessary because most vitamins are not synthesized by the body. Vitamins are classified as water-soluble (thiamine, pyridoxal, cobalamin, ascorbic acid, riboflavin, nicotinic acid, and folic acid) or fat-soluble (A, D, E, and K). They are involved in many reactions, including metabolism of visual pigments (vitamin A), calcium and phosphate metabolism (vitamin D), prothrombin synthesis (vitamin K), and antioxidation reactions (vitamin E). Pyridoxal (vitamin B_6) affects amino acid transfer reactions; flavin adenine dinucleotide (FAD), flavin mononucleotide (FMN), and nicotinamide-adenine dinucleotide (NAD) help the reaction transfer of electrons (see Chapter 1). Deficiencies in vitamin C result in poor wound healing and scurvy. Vitamin D deficiency causes rickets and problems with healing of fractures. Folate deficiency is associated with plasma and membrane changes of the red blood cell and is particularly a problem in individuals with severe liver dysfunction. Vitamin deficiencies are associated with several other disease states, including cancer (see Chapter 10).

Alterations in plasma membrane functions can be induced by certain nutritional substances. For example,

increases in vitamin A consumption can cause lysis of the plasma membrane, releasing hydrolases that damage lysosomal membranes. With insulin deficiency, glucose cannot cross the plasma membrane to enter the cell, causing energy deficits. Nutritional deficiencies also are associated with abnormalities of the chromosomes, nucleus, and DNA synthesis.

Injurious Physical Agents

Injurious physical agents include temperature extremes, changes in atmospheric pressure, radiation, illumination, mechanical factors, noise, and prolonged vibration. Physical injury can result from excessive exposure to many environmental agents, as well as to agents used for the diagnosis and treatment of illness.

Temperature Extremes

Chilling or freezing of cells causes **hypothermic injury** directly by creating high intracellular sodium concentrations, which result from the formation and dissolution of ice crystals. Indirect forms of injury occur because of changes in small blood vessels (the microcirculation). Slow chilling can cause vasoconstriction followed by paralysis of vasomotor control, resulting in vasodilation and increased membrane permeability. This causes cellular and tissue swelling. With an abrupt drop in temperature, vasoconstriction and increased viscosity of the blood cause ischemic injury—infarction and necrosis (cellular death) in affected tissues. With continued exposure to freezing temperatures, vasodilation produces severe swelling that causes degenerative changes in the myelin sheath that surrounds peripheral nerves, resulting in sensory and motor disturbances. Thrombosis also can occur and may lead to gangrene of the affected part. (Gangrene is discussed on p. 78.) These conditions often are called *frostbite.*

Hyperthermic injury (injury caused by excessive heat) varies depending on the nature, intensity, and extent of the injury. A full-thickness burn is an open wound involving skin layers—epidermis, dermis, and subcutaneous layers—and causing extensive loss of fluids and plasma proteins. Cellular regeneration is not possible, so that skin from a donor or from the host must be grafted to the site. Partial-thickness burns result in reddening of the area as a result of dilation of small blood vessels and increased permeability of cellular membranes, with loss of protein-rich fluid, resulting in the typical "burn blister." In surface epithelial cells, membrane permeability increases, causing both cytoplasmic and nuclear swelling. Temperature-sensitive enzymes within certain cells respond to heat by increasing cellular metabolism, with detrimental effects. Intense heat also damages the vascular endothelium and causes coagulation of the blood vessels. (Burns are discussed further in Chapter 41.)

Epidemiologic investigators have recently reported a relationship between overheating in infants, that is, overdressing infants in the winter, and sudden infant deaths (Ponsonby et al., 1992). Increased deaths were significantly related to more thermal insulation. Further studies are being done. (Other conditions related to temperature changes are discussed in Chapter 13.)

Changes in Atmospheric Pressure

Sudden increases or decreases in atmospheric pressure cause **blast injury,** which can be transmitted by either air (air blast) or water (immersion blast). With sudden increases in pressure, such as in air blast or explosive injuries, tissue injury is caused by compressive waves of air impinging on the body, followed by a sudden wave of decreased pressure. The pressure changes may collapse the thorax, rupture internal solid organs, and cause widespread hemorrhage (Cotran et al., 1989). In increased pressure caused by immersion blast, water pressure is applied suddenly to all sides of the body, forcing the body up out of water. The positive pressure compresses the abdomen and ruptures hollow internal organs, such as the spleen, kidneys, and liver.

With sudden decreases in pressure, carbon dioxide and nitrogen that are normally dissolved in the blood come out of solution and form tiny bubbles called gas emboli. At low atmospheric pressure, such as occurs at altitudes above 15,000 feet, there is a significant decrease in available oxygen. This causes hypoxic injury, and compensatory vasoconstriction shunts blood from the peripheral circulation (in the extremities) to the visceral organs, including the lungs. The combination of increases in pulmonary blood flow and systemic hypoxia causes "high-altitude pulmonary edema" (Roy et al., 1969). (Pulmonary edema is described in Chapter 30.)

Deep sea divers and underwater construction workers who return to the surface too quickly develop a form of gas embolism called **decompression sickness** or **caisson disease** ("the bends"). If water pressure is reduced too rapidly, the gases dissolved in blood bubble out of solution, forming emboli. Oxygen is quickly redissolved, but nitrogen bubbles may persist and obstruct blood vessels. Ischemia resulting from gas emboli causes cellular hypoxia, particularly in the muscles, joints, and tendons, which are especially susceptible to changes in oxygen supply. Emboli and interstitial gas accumulate around the joints and skeletal muscles, causing the individual to double up in pain. Tissues of the heart and brain also may be affected by emboli, causing necrosis. The gases can be promptly redissolved in blood by raising the atmospheric pressure. This is accomplished by placing the individual in a decompression chamber. First, pressure is increased until it approximates pressure at the depth to which the diver had descended. This

redissolves the gas bubbles in the blood. Then the pressure in the chamber is decreased gradually until it equals pressure at the surface of the water. The slow decrease in pressure slows the gases from bubbling out of solution.

Ionizing Radiation

Ionizing radiation is any form of radiation capable of removing orbital electrons from atoms. Ionizing radiation is emitted by x-rays, gamma rays, alpha- and beta-particles (which are emitted from atomic nuclei in the process of radioactive decay), and from neutrons, deuterons, protons, and pions (all of which are emitted from cobalt or linear accelerators). Occupational exposure to ionizing radiation is mostly limited to alpha- and beta-particle exposure and exposure to x-rays, gamma rays, and neutrons. Radiant energy from sunlight (solar radiation) also can injure cells.

The most abundant source of exposure to ionizing radiation is the environment. This source includes emissions from radioactive material inside the body, cosmic rays from outer space, and radiation emitted from such substances as soil and building materials. Environmental radioactivity is primarily emitted by uranium, thorium, and potassium. Other sources are x-rays used for medical diagnosis and treatment, uranium and thorium mines, nuclear weapons, and nuclear reactors that generate electricity. Table 2-2 includes types of ionizing radiation and their magnitude of tissue penetration.

The mechanism by which ionizing radiation damages cells is shown in Fig. 2-11. DNA is the most vulnerable target of radiation, particularly the bonds within the DNA molecule. All phases of the cell cycle can be affected by ionizing radiation. Sensitivity of the cell appears to be greatest in G_2, that gap of the cell just before mitosis; irradiation during this phase retards the onset of cell division. Irradiation during mitosis induces

---

TABLE 2-2

Types of Ionizing Radiation and Their Tissue Penetration

Type	Tissue penetration
X-rays	High
Gamma (γ) rays	High
Beta (β) particles	Low
Alpha (α) particles	Very low
Protons	Intermediate between α and β
Neutrons	High

Modified from Kissane, 1990.

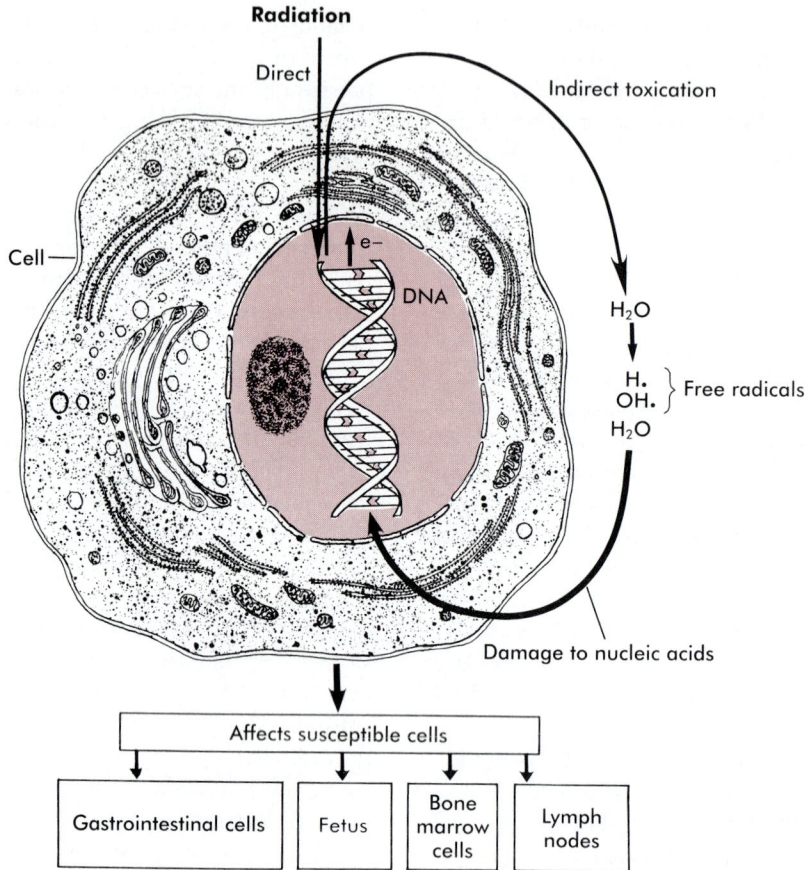

FIG. 2-11 Cellular damage caused by ionizing radiation. Radiation can damage macromolecules in two ways: (1) directly, where the micromolecules are ionized; and (2) indirectly, where water is ionized and produces free radicals that in turn damage macromolecules. Cells that are particularly susceptible to damage are those of the gastrointestinal tract, bone marrow, lymph nodes, fetus, and ovarian follicles. (Modified from King et al., 1983.)

chromosome aberrations. Chromosomal aberrations include breaks, deletions, translocations, and many other structural abnormalities. Membrane molecules and enzymes also are damaged by radiation. The intensity, duration, and cumulative effects of exposure to ionizing radiation determine the extent of injury.

Not all cells and tissues have the same sensitivity to radiation, although all cells can be affected. Radiosensitivity depends on rate of mitosis and cellular maturity. Because fetal cells are both immature and undergoing rapid cycling, the fetus is at great risk for injury caused by ionizing radiation. Particularly vulnerable are embryonic germ cells, which are precursors of ova and sperm. Throughout life, cells of the bone marrow, intestinal mucosa, testicular seminiferous epithelium, and ovarian follicles are susceptible to injury because they are always undergoing mitosis, which ensures the presence of vulnerable, immature daughter cells.

The effects of ionizing radiation may be acute or delayed. Acute effects of high doses, such as skin redness, skin damage, or chromosomal aberrations, occur within hours, days, or months. The delayed effects of low doses may not be evident for years. Effects are usually (1) somatic (involving the exposed individual's entire body), for example, leukemia and other cancers; (2) genetic, involving offspring of the exposed individual; or (3) fetal, involving fetuses that are exposed in utero (McGuigan, 1992). (The carcinogenic effects of radiation are discussed in Chapter 11, and radiation-induced cancers of the thyroid gland, breast, liver, and bone are discussed in Chapters 18, 20, 32, and 39, respectively.)

Illumination

Most discussions about the effects of light and illumination have been limited to questions of occupational safety and efficiency. Researchers have found, however, that illumination has biologic effects related to health (Weston, 1948; Wilkins & Wilkinson, 1991; Ziegman, Sutliff, & Rounds, 1991).

The harmful effects of fluorescent lighting include

eyestrain, obscured vision, and possibly cataract formation (Wilkins & Wilkinson, 1991). The rapid modulation of light from fluorescent lamps is responsible for eyestrain and headaches (Wilkins & Wilkinson, 1991). The modulation can be reduced by wearing tinted glasses. The shorter wavelengths in radiant energy in environmental lighting influence the absorption, scattering, and fluorescence, thus obscuring vision (Ziegman et al., 1991).

Recent studies have demonstrated the in vitro toxicity of halogen lamps (DeFlora & D'Agostini, 1992). A pilot study of 12 mice illuminated with varying intensities and durations of halogen exposure resulted in benign forms of skin cancer (papillomas), as well as malignant tumor growth. Emission of far-ultraviolet radiation from halogen lamps is thought to be in the range of wavelength responsible for inducing melanoma (DeFlora & D'Agostini, 1992). Fortunately, prevention is simple, whereby commercial models should be available with glass or plastic covers.

Mechanical Stresses

Mechanical injury is caused by physical impact or irritation. The response of tissue to mechanical stress is the major focus of occupational biomechanics. A major focus of occupational biomechanics is the prevention of overexertion disorders of the low back and upper extremities. Many mechanical stresses can cause *overt* injuries (e.g., a head injury when a worker is struck in the head with a dropped object). Most stresses, however, are subtle and can cause *accumulative* injuries and disorders (Keyserling & Armstrong, 1992). Table 2-3 summarizes common types of occupational mechanical stresses and associated types of injury.

Noise

Noise is sound that has the potential for inflicting bodily harm. The most common pathophysiologic effect of noise is hearing impairment. Noise trauma can be caused by acute loud noise, as well as by the cumulative effects of various intensities, frequencies, and durations of noise.

Two types of hearing loss are associated with noise: (1) acoustic trauma, or instantaneous damage caused by a single sharply rising wave of sound (e.g., gunfire), and (2) noise-induced hearing loss, the more common type, which is the result of prolonged exposure to intense sound (e.g., work place and leisure-time activities). Acoustic trauma can rupture the eardrum, displace the ossicles of the middle ear, and damage the organ of Corti in the inner ear.

If noise has not been too loud or the exposure too long, hearing will return to its original level, a type of hearing loss called a temporary threshold shift (TTS). If the noise is louder than a certain value or the exposure

TABLE 2-3

Common Types of Occupational Mechanical Stresses and Associated Types of Injury

Mechanical stresses	Type of injury
Forceful exertions (e.g., lifting, pushing, pulling of heavy loads)	Low back pain
Awkward trunk postures (e.g., flexion, lateral bending, axial twisting, prolonged sitting)	Low back pain
Whole body vibration (e.g., vibrating seat or platform)	Low back pain; bone deformities; alteration nerve conduction (carpal tunnel syndrome)
Repetitive or prolonged exposure (e.g., to any of the above)	Low back pain
Extreme reaching	Trauma disorders of the
Low temperatures (e.g., exposure to cold air, tools, materials)	upper arms (synovitis, Raynaud phenomenon, bursitis, tendinitis)
Vibration (segmental and whole)	
Forceful exertions (e.g., friction, balance, posture, pace, use of heavy objects)	
Ulnar deviation of the wrist	
Repetitive functions (e.g., walking, climbing stairs, carrying, shoveling, pushing, lifting objects)	Localized and/or whole body fatigue (shortness of breath, general weakness, hypoxic injury)

time is long, then the hearing threshold never returns to its original value, causing a permanent threshold shift (PTS). Structural changes associated with TTS, although not fully established, include intracellular changes in the sensory cells (hair cells) and swelling of the auditory nerve endings (Consensus Conference, 1990). With PTS, cochlear blood flow may be impaired and hair cells are damaged with each exposure. Noise-induced hearing loss is gradual and painless. Symptoms of noise-induced hearing loss include loudness recruitment and tinnitus. In loudness recruitment, soft sounds are not heard, but loud sounds are heard normally. Tinnitus is a constant, high-pitched ringing that annoys the individual and contributes to loss of sleep.

MANIFESTATIONS OF CELLULAR INJURY

Cellular Manifestations: Accumulations

Cellular accumulations, also known as *infiltrations,* not only occur when injury is sublethal and sustained in injured cells, but also can occur in normal cells. Common accumulations consist of substances that are normally present, such as fluids and electrolytes, triglycerides (lipids), glycogen, calcium, uric acid, proteins, melanin, and bilirubin. Abnormal accumulations of these substances can occur in the cytoplasm (frequently in the lysosomes) or in the nucleus if (1) the normal, endogenous substance is produced in excess or at an increased rate; (2) an endogenous substance (normal or abnormal) is not effectively catabolized, usually because of lack of a vital lysosomal enzyme; or (3) harmful exogenous materials, such as heavy metals, mineral dusts, or microorganisms, accumulate because of inhalation, ingestion, or infection.

In all the storage diseases, the cells attempt to digest, or catabolize, the "stored" substances. As a result, excessive amounts of metabolites (products of catabolism) accumulate in the cells and are expelled into the extracellular matrix, where they are taken up by phagocytic cells called macrophages (see Chapter 7). Some of these scavenger cells circulate throughout the body, whereas others remain fixed in certain tissues, such as the liver or spleen. As more and more macrophages and other phagocytes migrate to tissues that are producing excessive metabolites, the affected tissues begin to swell. This is the mechanism that causes enlargement of the liver (hepatomegaly) or the spleen (splenomegaly). Enlargement of one of these organs is a clinical manifestation of many of the storage diseases.

Water

Cellular swelling, the most common degenerative change, is caused by the shift of extracellular water into the cells. In hypoxic injury, movement of fluid and ions into the cell is associated with acute failure of metabolism and loss of ATP production. Normally, the pump that transports sodium ions out of the cell is maintained by the presence of ATP and ATPase, the active-transport enzyme. In metabolic failure caused by hypoxia, reduced ATP and ATPase permit sodium to accumulate in the cell, whereas potassium diffuses outward. The increase of intracellular sodium increases osmotic pressure, which draws more water into the cell (transport mechanisms are described in Chapter 1). The cisternae of the endoplasmic reticulum become distended, rupture, and coalesce to form large vacuoles that isolate the water from the cytoplasm. This process is called **vacuolation.** Progressive vacuolation results in a more seri-

ous condition called **hydropic degeneration** (Fig. 2-12). If cellular swelling affects all of the cells in an organ, the organ increases in weight and becomes distended and pale.

Cellular swelling is reversible and is considered to be sublethal. It is, in fact, an early manifestation of almost all types of cellular injury, including severe or lethal cell injury. It is also associated with high fever, hypokalemia (abnormally low concentrations of potassium in the blood; see Chapter 3), and certain infections.

Lipids and Carbohydrates

Certain metabolic disorders result in the abnormal intracellular accumulation of carbohydrates and lipids. These substances may accumulate throughout the body, but are found primarily in cells of the spleen, liver, and central nervous system. Accumulations in cells of the central nervous system can cause neurologic dysfunction and severe mental retardation. Lipids accumulate in Tay-Sachs, Neimann-Pick, and Gaucher's disease, whereas in the diseases known as mucopolysaccharidoses, the excess is of carbohydrates. The mucopolysaccharidoses are progressive disorders that usually involve multiple organs, including liver, spleen, heart, and blood vessels. The accumulated mucopolysaccharides are found in reticuloendothelial cells, endothelial cells, inti-

FIG. 2-12 **The process of hydropic degeneration.**

mal smooth muscle cells, and fibroblasts throughout the body. These carbohydrate accumulations can cause clouding of the cornea, joint stiffness, and mental retardation (Kissane, 1990).

Although lipids sometimes accumulate in heart and kidney cells, the most common site of intracellular lipid accumulation, or **fatty change**, is in liver cells. Because hepatic metabolism and secretion of lipids are crucial to proper body function, imbalances and deficiencies in these processes lead to major pathologic changes. Lipid accumulation in liver cells causes an organic condition known as fatty liver, or fatty change (Fig. 2-13). As lipids fill the cells, vacuolation pushes the nucleus and other organelles aside. Grossly, the liver looks yellowish and greasy.

Lipid accumulation in liver cells occurs after cellular injury sets one or more of the following mechanisms in motion:

1. Increased movement of free fatty acids into the liver. (Starvation, for example, increases breakdown of triglycerides in adipose tissue, releasing fatty acids that subsequently enter liver cells.)
2. Failure of the metabolic process that converts fatty acids to phospholipids, resulting in the preferential conversion of the fatty acids to triglycerides.
3. Increased synthesis of triglycerides from fatty acids. (Increases in an enzyme, alpha-glycerophosphatase, can accelerate triglyceride synthesis.)
4. Decreased synthesis of apoproteins (lipid-acceptor proteins).
5. Failure of lipids to bind with apoproteins and form lipoproteins.
6. Failure of mechanisms that transport lipoproteins out of the cell.

Alcohol abuse is one of the most common causes of fatty liver. (See Chapter 36 for a discussion of liver abnormalities.) Although the exact mechanism by which alcohol causes fatty change is uncertain, the following defects are implicated: (1) increased movement of free fatty acids into the liver, (2) alternative synthesis of triglycerides, (3) decreased triglyceride use, (4) problems with apoprotein synthesis or lipoprotein transport, and (5) direct damage to the endoplasmic reticulum by free radicals released by alcohol's toxic effects (Lieber, 1991).

Fatty change caused by alcohol can lead to a form of liver fibrosis called cirrhosis. If alcohol intake ceases, the cirrhotic liver can return to a normal size and function. Fatty change from other causes, notably carbon tetrachloride poisoning, is often irreversible.

Glycogen

Intracellular accumulations of glycogen are seen in genetic disorders called glycogen storage diseases and in disorders of glucose and glycogen metabolism. Like water and lipid accumulation, glycogen accumulation results in excessive vacuolation of the cytoplasm.

The most common cause of glycogen accumulation is the disorder of glucose metabolism, diabetes mellitus (see Chapter 18). In diabetes mellitus, glycogen accumulates in the epithelial cells of the proximal convoluted renal tubules, the loop of Henle, liver cells, myocardial cells, and the beta cells of the islets of Langerhans. With the decrease in insulin, glucose concentrations increase in the blood (hyperglycemia) and in the urine (glycosuria) as blood glucose levels rise above the renal threshold. The renal tubular cells reabsorb the excess quantities of glucose and store it as glycogen. With the administration of insulin, glycogen accumulation is reversed, as long as no renal tubular dysfunction is present.

Proteins

Proteins provide cellular structure and constitute most of the cell's dry weight. They are synthesized on ribosomes in the cytoplasm from the essential amino acids lysine, threonine, leucine, isoleucine, methionine, tryptophan, valine, phenylalanine, and histidine. Protein accumulation probably damages cells in two ways. First, metabolites, produced when the cell attempts to digest some proteins, are enzymes that, when released from ly-

FIG. 2-13 Fatty liver of an alcoholic. The liver is enlarged, swollen, greasy, and yellow. (From Kissane, 1990.)

sosomes, can damage cellular organelles. Second, excessive amounts of protein in the cytoplasm push against cellular organelles, disrupting organelle function and intracellular communication.

Protein excess accumulates primarily in the epithelial cells of the renal convoluted tubule and in the antibody-forming plasma cells (B lymphocytes) of the immune system. (The immune system is described in Chapter 6.) Several types of renal disorders cause excessive excretion of protein molecules in the urine (proteinuria) (see Chapter 33). Normally, little or no protein is present in the urine, and its presence in significant amounts indicates cellular injury and altered cellular function. For example, certain renal disorders can cause glomerular damage, which allows proteins to leak across the glomerular membrane and into the glomerular filtrate. The protein then moves into the proximal tubule and is resorbed by the epithelial cells through the process of pinocytosis ("cell drinking"), which is discussed in Chapter 1. The protein-containing pinocytotic vesicles fuse with lysosomes, after which the protein is released into the cytoplasm as a product of lysosomal digestion. Protein accumulations in the cytoplasm of renal tubular cells do not cause direct cellular dysfunction, but they do signify a pathologic process.

Accumulations of protein in B lymphocytes can occur during active synthesis of antibodies during the immune response. The excess aggregates of protein are called Russell bodies (see Chapter 6). Russell bodies have been identified in multiple myeloma (plasma cell tumor). (See Chapters 24 and 39.)

Pigments

Pigment accumulations may be normal or abnormal, endogenous (produced within the body) or exogenous (produced outside the body). Endogenous pigments are derived, for example, from amino acids (e.g., tyrosine, tryptophan). They include melanin and the blood proteins—porphyrins, hemoglobin, and hemosiderin (ferritin). Lipid-rich pigments such as lipofuscin (the aging pigment) give a yellow-brown color to cells undergoing slow, regressive, and often atrophic changes. Exogenous pigments include mineral dusts containing silica and iron particles, lead, silver salts, and dyes for tattoos.

Melanin

Melanin accumulates in epithelial cells (keratinocytes) of the skin and retina. It is an extremely important pigment because it protects the skin against long exposure to sunlight and is considered an essential factor in the prevention of skin cancer (see Chapters 11 and 41). Ultraviolet light (e.g., sunlight) stimulates the synthesis of melanin, which probably absorbs ultraviolet rays during subsequent exposure. Melanin also may protect the skin by trapping the injurious free radicals produced by the action of ultraviolet light on skin.

Melanin is a brown-black pigment derived from the amino acid tryptosine. It is synthesized by epidermal cells called melanocytes, and is stored in membrane-bounded cytoplasmic vesicles called melanosomes. Melanosomes are particularly abundant in projections of melanocytic cytoplasm, called dendrites, from which they are transmitted to neighboring keratinocytes, where melanin accumulation occurs (Cotran et al., 1989). (Keratinocytes, which constitute 95% of epidermal cells, are discussed with other skin components in Chapter 41.) The dendritic melanocytes form bridges between neighboring keratinocytes and inject melanosomes into the keratinocytes by an unknown mechanism.

Melanin also can accumulate in melanophores (melanin-containing pigment cells), macrophages, or other phagocytic cells in the dermis. Presumably these cells acquire the melanin from nearby melanocytes or from pigment that has been extruded from dying epidermal cells. This is the mechanism that causes freckles.

Although rare, melanin accumulation occurs in the skin of individuals with Addison's disease (adrenocortical insufficiency resulting from disorders of the adrenal cortex; see Chapter 18). The increased melaninogenesis (melanin production) seen in Addison's disease is caused by the loss of feedback control of adrenocorticotropic hormone (ACTH). Decreased hormonal secretion from the adrenal gland causes increased release of ACTH from the pituitary gland. In Addison's disease, the increase in melanin occurs presumably because a segment of the ACTH molecule contains the melanin-stimulating hormone (MSH).

An increase in melanin also occurs in the benign form of "pigmented moles" called nevi (See Chapter 41.). Malignant melanoma is a cancerous skin tumor that contains melanin and invades normal tissue early and widely and often leads to death.

A decrease in melanin production occurs in the inherited disorder of melanin metabolism called albinism. Albinism is often diffuse, involving all the skin, the eyes, and the hair. Albinism is also related to phenylalanine metabolism. In classic types, the albino is unable to convert tyrosine to DOPA (3,4-dihydroxyphenylalanine), an intermediate in melanin biosynthesis. Melanin-producing cells are present in normal numbers, but they are unable to make melanin. Individuals with albinism are very sensitive to sunlight and quickly become sunburned. They are also at high risk for skin cancer.

Hemoproteins

Hemoproteins are among the most essential of the normal endogenous pigments. They include hemoglobin and the oxidative enzymes, the cytochromes. Central to an understanding of disorders involving these pigments is knowledge of iron uptake, metabolism, excretion, and storage (see Chapter 22). Hemoprotein accumulations in cells are caused by excessive storage of iron, which is transferred to the cells from the bloodstream. Iron enters the blood from three primary sources: (1) tissue stores, (2) the intestinal mucosa, and (3) macrophages that remove and destroy dead or defective red blood cells. The amount of iron in blood plasma also depends on the metabolism of the major iron-transport protein, transferrin.

Iron is stored in tissue cells in two forms: as ferritin and, when greater levels of iron are present, as hemosiderin. **Hemosiderin** is a yellow-brown pigment derived from hemoglobin. With pathologic states, excesses of iron cause hemosiderin to accumulate within cells. Accumulation of hemosiderin often occurs in areas of bruising and hemorrhage and in the lungs and spleen after congestion caused by heart failure. With a local hemorrhage, the skin first appears red-blue, then lysis of the escaped red blood cell occurs, causing the hemoglobin to be transformed to hemosiderin. The color changes noted in bruising reflect this transformation.

Hemosiderosis is a condition in which excess iron is stored as hemosiderin in the cells of many organs and tissues. This condition is common in individuals who have received repeated blood transfusions or prolonged parenteral administration of iron. Hemosiderosis is also associated with increased absorption of dietary iron, conditions in which iron storage and transport are impaired, and hemolytic anemia. Excessive alcohol (wine) ingestion also can lead to hemosiderosis. Normally, absorption of excessive dietary iron is prevented by an iron-absorption process in the intestines. Failure of this process can lead to total-body iron accumulations in the range of 60 to 80 g, compared with normal iron stores of 4.5 to 5 g (Kissane, 1990). Excessive accumulations of iron, such as occurs in hemochromatosis (a genetic disorder of iron metabolism and the most severe example of iron overload) are associated with liver and pancreatic cell damage.

It is debatable whether iron accumulation itself causes cellular injury or whether injury is the result of the basic defect that leads to iron storage. The finding that the extent of liver injury (cirrhosis) is related to the extent of iron accumulation (Powell & Kerr, 1975) suggests that excessive iron accumulation does injure cells.

Bilirubin is a normal, yellow-to-green pigment of bile derived from the porphyrin structure of hemoglobin. Excesses of bilirubin within cells and tissues cause jaundice (icterus), or yellowing of the skin. Jaundice occurs when the bilirubin level exceeds 1.5 to 2 mg/dl of plasma, compared with the normal values of 0.4 to 1 mg/dl. Hyperbilirubinemia occurs with (1) destruction of red blood cells (erythrocytes), such as in hemolytic jaundice; (2) diseases affecting the metabolism and excretion of bilirubin in the liver; and (3) diseases that cause obstruction of the common bile duct, such as gall-stones or pancreatic tumors. (For a detailed description of these diseases, see Chapter 36.) Certain drugs can cause the obstruction of normal bile flow through the liver. They are chlorpromazine and other phenothiazine derivatives; estrogenic hormones; and halothane, an anesthetic.

Because unconjugated bilirubin is lipid soluble, it can injure the lipid components of the plasma membrane, but the exact mechanism or mechanisms that produce injury are not clearly known. Albumin, a plasma protein, provides significant protection by binding unconjugated bilirubin in plasma. Albumin-coupled bilirubin has been experimentally shown to be nontoxic to tissue-culture cells (Cowger, 1971). Cowger's experiments demonstrated that unconjugated bilirubin causes two cellular effects: uncoupling of oxidative phosphorylation and a loss of cellular proteins. These two effects could cause structural injury to the various membranes of the cell.

Calcium

Calcium salts accumulate in both injured and dead tissues. An important mechanism of cellular calcification is the influx of extracellular calcium in injured mitochondria (see pp. 58 and 59). Another mechanism that causes calcium accumulation in alveoli (gas-exchange airways of the lungs), gastric epithelium, and renal tubules is the excretion of acid at these sites, leading to the local production of hydroxyl ions. Hydroxyl ions result in precipitation of calcium hydroxide ($Ca[OH]_2$) and hydroxyapatite ($3Ca_3[PO_4]_2Ca[OH]_2$), a mixed salt. Damage occurs when calcium salts clump and harden, interfering with normal cellular structure and function.

Pathologic calcification can be dystrophic or metastatic. **Dystrophic calcification** is the calcification of dying and dead tissues. This type of calcification occurs in chronic tuberculosis of the lungs and lymph nodes, in arteries with advanced atherosclerosis (narrowing as a result of plaque accumulation), and often in injured heart valves (Fig. 2-14). Calcification of the heart valves interferes with opening and closing of the valves, causing heart murmurs (see Chapter 27). Calcification of the coronary arteries predisposes them to severe narrowing and thrombosis, which can lead to myocardial infarction. Another site of dystrophic calcification is the center of tumors. Over time the center is deprived of oxygen supply, dies, and becomes calcified. The calcium salts appear as gritty, clumped granules that can become hard as stone. When several layers clump together, they resemble grains of sand and are called **psammoma bodies.**

The exact pathogenic mechanisms responsible for dystrophic calcification are unknown. A popular hypothesis is that with progressive deterioration of dead cells, the exposed denatured (changed) proteins prefer-

FIG. 2-14 Aortic valve calcification. This aortic valve was unable to close because of calcification caused by rheumatic heart disease. (From Kissane, 1990.)

entially bind with phosphate ions. The phosphate ions then react with calcium ions to form deposits of phosphate carbonate precipitates and, sometimes, crystalline formations of calcium phosphate. Dystrophic calcification develops slowly and is an explicit marker for the site of dead cells.

Metastatic calcification consists of mineral deposits that occur in undamaged normal tissues as the result of hypercalcemia (an excess of calcium in the blood; see Chapter 3). Conditions that cause hypercalcemia include hyperparathyroidism, toxic levels of vitamin D, hyperthyroidism, idiopathic hypercalcemia of infancy, Addison's disease (adrenal cortical insufficiency), systemic sarcoidosis, milk-alkali syndrome, and the increased bone demineralization that results from bone tumors, leukemia, and disseminated cancers. Hypercalcemia also can occur in some instances of advanced renal failure with phosphate retention, resulting in hyperparathyroidism (Kissane, 1990).

Urate

In humans, uric acid (**urate**) is the major end-product of purine catabolism because of the absence of the enzyme urate oxidase. Serum urate concentration is, in general, stable; approximately 5 mg/dl in postpubertal males and 4.1 mg/dl in postpubertal females. Balance among the production of purine-nucleotides occurs from catabolism of purine-containing compounds to produce free purine, oxidation of purine to uric acid by xanthine oxidase, tubular reabsorption of urate, and finally, tubular secretion of urate. Disturbances of this balance result in hyperuricemia and deposition of sodium urate crystals in the tissues, leading to painful disorders collectively called gout. These disorders include acute arthritis, chronic gouty arthritis, tophus (firm modular subcutaneous deposits of urate crystals surrounded by fibrosis), and nephritis (inflammation of the nephron).

Chronic hyperuricemia results in the deposition of urate in tissues, cell injury, and inflammation. Because urate crystals are not degraded by lysosomal enzymes, they persist in dead cells.

Systemic Manifestations

Systemic manifestations of cellular injury include a general sense of fatigue and malaise, a loss of well-being, and altered appetite. Fever is frequently present because of biochemicals produced during the inflammatory response (see Chapters 2 and 7). Table 2-4 summarizes the most significant systemic manifestations of cellular injury.

CELLULAR DEATH

Necrosis

Cellular death eventually leads to the process of cellular dissolution, or **necrosis**. Necrosis is the sum of cellular changes after local cell death and the process of cellular self-digestion known as autodigestion, or **autolysis** (Fig. 2-15). The structural signs that indicate irreversible injury and progression to necrosis are the dense clumping and progressive disruption of genetic material and disruption of the plasma and organelle membranes. In later stages of necrosis, most organelles are disrupted, and **karyolysis** (nuclear dissolution from the action of hydrolytic enzymes) is under way. In some cells, the nucleus shrinks and becomes a small, dense mass of genetic material—a process called nuclear **pyknosis**. The pyknotic nucleus eventually dissolves (by karyolysis) as a result of the action of hydrolytic lysosomal enzymes on DNA.

Different types of necrosis tend to occur in different organs or tissues and sometimes can indicate the mechanism or cause of cellular injury. There are four major types of necrosis: coagulative, liquefactive, caseous, and fatty. Another type, gangrenous necrosis, is *not* a distinctive type of cell death but refers to larger areas of tissue death.

Coagulative necrosis, which occurs primarily in the kidneys, heart, and adrenal glands, commonly results from hypoxia caused by severe ischemia. Another mechanism is hypoxia caused by chemical injury, particularly

TABLE 2-4

Systemic Manifestations of Cellular Injury

Manifestation	Cause
Fever	Release of endogenous pyrogens (interleukin-1, tumor necrosis factor alpha, and prostaglandins) from bacteria or macrophages; acute inflammatory response
Increased heart rate	Increase in oxidative metabolic processes resulting from fever
Increase in leukocytes (leukocytosis)	Increase in total number of white blood cells because of infection; normal is 5000-9000/mm^3 (increase is directly related to the severity of the infection)
Pain	Various mechanisms, such as release of bradykinins, obstruction, pressure
Presence of cellular enzymes in extracellular fluid	Release of enzymes from cells of tissue*
Lactate dehydrogenase (LDH) (LDH isoenzymes)	Release from red blood cells, liver, kidney, skeletal muscle
Creatine kinase (CK) (CK isoenzymes)	Release from skeletal muscle, brain, heart
Aspartate aminotransferase (AST/SGOT)	Release from heart, liver, skeletal muscle, kidney, pancreas
Alanine aminotransferase (ALT/SGPT)	Release from liver, kidney, heart
Alkaline phosphatase (ALP)	Release from liver, bone
Amylase	Release from pancreas
Aldolase	Release from skeletal muscle, heart

*The rapidity of enzyme transfer is a function of the weight of the enzyme and the concentration gradient across the cellular membrane. The specific metabolic and excretory rates of the enzymes determine how long levels of enzymes remain elevated.

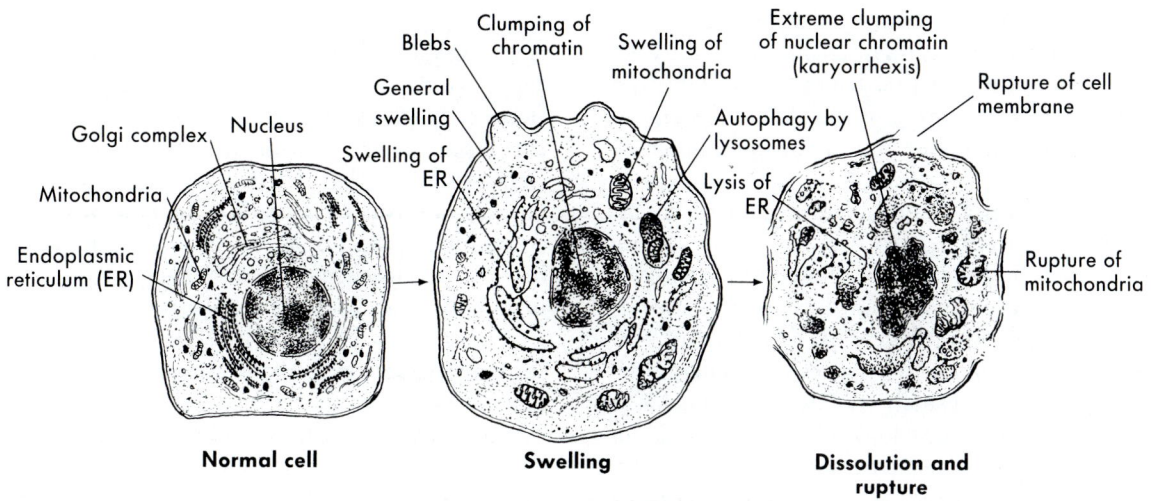

FIG. 2-15 Stages of necrosis.

the ingestion of mercuric chloride. Coagulation is caused by protein denaturation, which causes the protein albumin to change from a gelatinous, transparent state to a firm, opaque state, similar to that of a cooked egg white. The necrotic tissues appear firm and slightly swollen. Recent evidence indicates that an abnormality in intracellular levels of Ca^{++} (e.g., increased) may be a critical event in coagulation necrosis (Scarpelli & Iannaccone, 1990).

Liquefactive necrosis commonly results from ischemic injury to neurons and glial cells in the brain. Dead brain tissue is readily affected by liquefaction necrosis because brain cells are rich in the digestive hydrolytic enzymes and lipids, and the brain contains little connective tissue. As the cells are digested by their own hydrolases, the tissue becomes soft, liquefies, and is walled off from healthy tissue, forming cysts. (Cyst formation is described in Chapter 7.)

Liquefactive necrosis can result also from bacterial infection, particularly by staphylococci, streptococci, and *E. coli*. In this case, the hydrolases are released from the lysosomes of neutrophils, which are phagocytes attracted to the infected area to kill the bacteria. (This action is part of the acute inflammatory response, which is discussed in Chapter 7.) Liquefaction of bacterial cells and neighboring tissue cells by neutrophilic hydrolases results in the accumulation of pus.

Caseous necrosis, which commonly results from tuberculous pulmonary infection, particularly by *M. tuberculosis,* is a combination of coagulative and liquefactive necrosis. The dead cells disintegrate, but the debris is not digested completely by hydrolases. Tissues appear soft and granular and resemble clumped cheese, which gives this type of necrosis its name. A granulomatous inflammatory wall encloses areas of caseous necrosis.

Fat necrosis, which occurs in the breast, pancreas, and other abdominal structures, is a specific type of cellular dissolution caused by powerful enzymes called lipases. Lipases break down triglycerides, releasing free fatty acids, which then combine with calcium, magnesium, and sodium ions, creating soaps (a process known as saponification). The necrotic tissue appears opaque and chalk white.

Gangrenous necrosis, a term commonly used in surgical clinical practice, refers to death of tissue and results from severe hypoxic injury, commonly occurring because of arteriosclerosis, or blockage, of major arteries, especially in the lower leg. With hypoxia and subsequent bacterial invasion, the tissues can undergo necrosis. **Dry gangrene** is usually the result of coagulative necrosis. **Wet gangrene** develops when neutrophils invade the site, causing liquefactive necrosis. In dry gangrene, the skin becomes very dry and shrinks, resulting

FIG. 2-16 **Foot of an individual with gangrene caused by small vessel disease.** (From Levin M. E., & O'Neal, L. W. [1988]. *The diabetic foot* [4th ed.]. St. Louis: Mosby–Year Book.)

in wrinkles, and its color changes to dark brown or black (Fig. 2-16).

In wet gangrene, which usually occurs in internal organs, the site is cold, swollen, and black. A foul odor produced by the accumulation of pus is usually present. If systemic symptoms become severe, death can ensue.

Gas gangrene, a special type of gangrene, is due to infection of injured tissue by one of many species of *Clostridium.* These anaerobic bacteria produce hydrolytic enzymes and toxins that destroy connective tissue and cellular membranes, and cause bubbles of gas to form in muscle cells. Gas gangrene can be fatal if enzymes lyse the membranes of red blood cells, destroying their oxygen-carrying capacity. Death is due to shock. The condition is treated with antitoxins and supplemental oxygen delivered in a hyperbaric (pressurized) chamber.

Apoptosis

Apoptosis (Greek for "dropping off") is a name recently suggested for an important, distinct type of cell death (Kerr & Searle, 1980) that differs from necrosis in several respects. Apoptosis is an active process of cellular self-destruction that is implicated in both normal and pathologic tissue changes. It is the type of cell death responsible for local deletion of cells during normal embryonic development, neurons dying during synaptogenesis, lymphocytes dying during receptor repertoire selection, and so on (Raff, 1992). Recent results have shown that apoptosis plays a major role in endocrine-dependent tissues that are undergoing atrophic change (Sandford, Searle, & Kerr, 1984; Tomei & Cope, 1991). Apoptosis is known to occur spontaneously in malignant tumors and in normal, rapidly proliferating cells treated with cancer chemotherapeutic agents and ionizing radiation (Wyllie, Kerr, & Currie, 1980). Its significance in aging is unknown. Necrosis and apoptosis affect tissues differently. Unlike necrosis, apoptosis affects scattered, single cells. Apoptosis is nuclear and cytoplasmic shrinkage of a cell (i.e., unlike necrosis, in which cells swell and lyse) followed by fragmentation into membrane-bound fragments and subsequent phagocytosis by neighboring, healthy cells (Cotran et al., 1989).

Normal cell death has recently gained new attention (Raff, 1992). Although the molecular mechanisms are unknown, it is thought that the normal cells that die might kill themselves by activating a "suicide programme" (Raff, 1992; Tomei & Cope, 1991). The survival of many developing vertebrate neurons depends on neurohormonal factors that are secreted by the target cells they innervate; those that fail to get enough die, apparently by active suicide because their death can be prevented for days by drugs that inhibit RNA or protein synthesis (Raff, 1992). Among nonneural tissues, it is not only endocrine-dependent cells that require specific signaling molecules to survive. In culture at least, blood cell precursor cells require one or more colony-stimulating factors, T lymphoblasts (immature lymphocytes) require interleukin-2, and endothelial cells require growth factors, such as fibroblast growth factor; in all of these examples, cells deprived of survival signals die by programmed (normal) cell death. Although much more molecular research needs to be done to determine how normal cell death occurs in higher animals, it seems reasonable that dependence on specific survival signals provides a simple way to eliminate misplaced cells for regulating cell numbers and, perhaps, for selecting the fittest cells (Raff, 1992).

AGING

Aging is usually defined as a normal physiologic process. Fundamental to the definition of aging is its universal and inevitable nature. To understand the basic mechanisms of aging, one must be able to identify the irreversible and universal processes at the cellular and molecular level—a very difficult task. It is difficult because it requires the separation of irreversible processes from potentially reversible mechanisms (i.e., those that result from disease or age-related debilities).

Aging traditionally has been excluded from the domain of disease because it is "normal"; disease is usually considered "abnormal." Conceptually, this distinction seems clear until the concept of "injury" is introduced; disease has been defined by some pathologists as the result of injury. Aging has been defined as the time-dependent loss of structure and function that proceeds very slowly and in such small increments that it appears to be the result of the accumulation of small, impercep-

FIG. 2-17 **Microinsults.** (Redrawn from Johnson, 1985.)

tible injuries—a gradual result of "wear and tear."

Injuries may result from unavoidable and universal microinsults caused by continuous bombardment by ultraviolet light, countless mechanical insults, and reactions to metabolites (Johnson, 1985) (Fig. 2-17). In this context, the distinction between aging and disease is unclear. For example, some degree of atrophy of the brain is considered "normal" in old age until it proceeds far enough to cause clinically significant disability and is called "disease." Likewise, most human beings have atherosclerosis, and the plaques progress with age, but at what point in this progression is it considered abnormal? These conceptual distinctions have given rise to two general categories of theories of aging. The first category proposes that aging is the result of the accumulation of random injuries and events. The second category proposes that aging is the result of a genetically controlled developmental program, or built-in self-destructive processes.

Normal Life Span

The **maximal life span** of humans is between 80 and 100 years and does not vary among populations significantly. Few individuals, however, in primitive societies reach the maximal life span; most die in infancy and the early years (Ory & Warner, 1990). In societies with improvements in sanitation, housing, nutrition, and health care, many persons attain the maximal life span. Although the maximal life span has not changed significantly over time, the average life span, or **life expect-**

ancy, has increased. In recent years, the death rate for people 65 years of age and older has declined significantly. This decline has been largely due to decreases in cardiovascular disease (Cassel, Riesenberg, Sorensen, & Walsh, 1990). In each successive age group from 65 and older, women outnumber men; thus women have a greater life expectancy than men. Increases in life expectancy have resulted in a large elderly population with inherent problems of disability, disease, and socioeconomic hardship.

Life Expectancy and Gender Differences

In all developed countries, life expectancy for females exceeds that for males (the gender gap): The female advantage is 7 years in North America and 4 to 8 years in other developed countries (Ory & Warner, 1990). These figures reflect a widening of gender mortality over the course of the twentieth century. Race has a key impact on the gender mortality differences in the United States (Fig. 2-18). Between 1920 and 1970, the gender gap increased among whites by a factor of 6, and by a factor

of 8 among blacks. Since 1970, however, the size of the gap has narrowed sharply among whites and has begun to decline among blacks (Nathanson, 1990).

Factors responsible for these differences in the gender gap in the United States include: (1) more rapid *improvement* in female compared with male death rates and (2) an *increasing* male disadvantage in death rates from the chronic conditions that are the leading causes of death in developed countries (Nathanson, 1990). The narrowing of the gender gap between 1970 and 1986 in the United States was due to two factors: (1) A *decline* in the rate of increase in female life expectancy and (2) a sharp *increase* in life expectancy by males (Nathanson, 1990). Today the gender gap is a 7-year difference in longevity—between 71 for men and 78 for women (Riley, 1990).

Causes of the gender gap have been divided into three very broad areas: biologic, behavioral, and sociocultural. Current biologic hypotheses include genetic predispositions, hormonal and immunologic differences, and greater in utero mortality (Table 2-5).

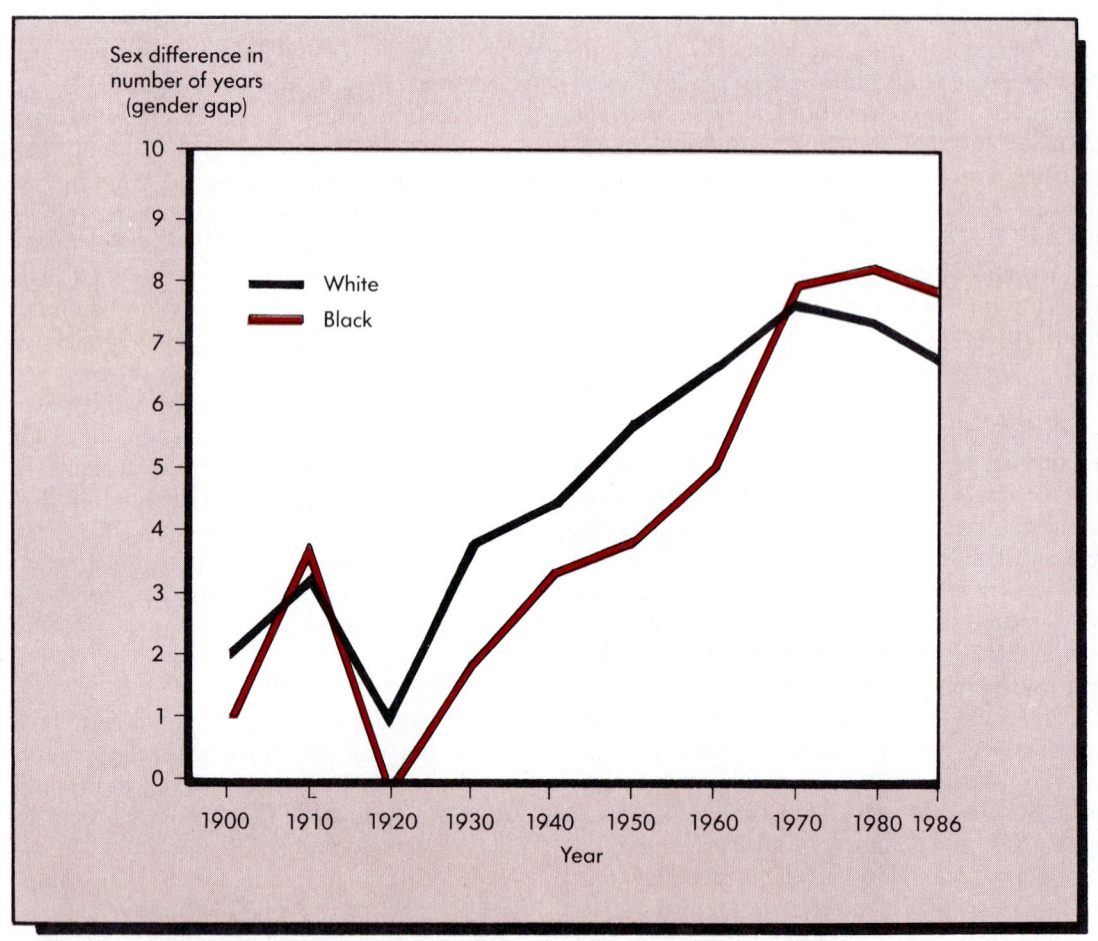

FIG. 2-18 Gender gap difference in life expectancy at birth by race: United States, 1900-1986. (Redrawn from Ory & Warner, 1990.)

TABLE 2-5

Causes of the Current Longevity and Health Differences Between Men and Women

Biologic hypotheses	Comments
Genetic	
Female genotype (XX) compared to male genotype (XY)	Little is known about the Y chromosome compared to the X chromosome, especially the significance of the X chromosome to longevity; however, certain genes on the X chromosome are involved in vital functions including blood clotting, muscle function, protection against oxidative damage, DNA synthesis, nucleotide synthesis, and immune response; thus the question raised is, To what extent are these genes critical to longevity?
Increased male mortality during the prenatal period	The incidence in excess male mortality or early die-off during the prenatal period may be attributed to homozygosity of the genes of the X chromosome (one allele instead of two alleles for each gene)
Characteristics of the Y chromosome	The Y chromosome is about one third of the size of the X chromosome; few recognized genes are mapped to the Y chromosome
Genetic and/or hormonal	
Sex hormones	The levels and balance of the cholesterol-carrying lipoproteins by sex hormones are major factors in the gender gap; sex hormones result in a *healthier* pattern of lipoproteins in women than in men; exogenous estrogens raise protective lipoproteins (high density lipoproteins [HDL]) and lower nonprotective lipoproteins (low density lipoproteins [LDL]); male androgens have the opposite effect (see Chapter 27); the pattern in women undergoes a disadvantageous change after menopause; however, the increased death rate for women from cardiovascular disease lags behind that of men by several years
Neuroendocrine effects, hormones, and the immune system	Sex hormones regulate longevity through their effects on behavior and through the immune system; these effects are interrelated and the central nervous system is at the center of these relationships; behaviorally, sex hormones affect aggressiveness, territoriality, mate selection, and mating behavior; how these behaviors affect longevity is incompletely understood; reproductive senescence, although life-threatening, can contribute to increasing "wear and tear" and includes cell depletion, cell death, and organ involution; the central nervous system affects the immune system through neuroendocrine mechanisms; sex hormones also affect the immune system; an important question is, How do men and women differ in their perception, handling, and physiologic consequences of stress, and how do these differences relate to the gender gap?
Immune function	The immune system in female mice does appear to be more robust than that in males; it is not clear whether this is related to the antibody genes that map to the X chromosome (Smith & Warner, 1990)
Social roles	
Multiple roles held by middle-aged women	Differing social roles of men and women are often cited as major causes of the gender gap; the key question is, To what extent do the different roles become sources of stress and thus differentially effect longevity?; data from women 45-55 years old reveal that the majority of these women are performing multiple roles; although these roles are sources of stress, surprisingly the reported stresses are not translated into negative health outcomes (Ory & Warner, 1990); working may play a protective role by alleviating the stress of nurturing roles and thereby prevent morbidity
Blue collar vs. white collar occupations and social class	There continues to be an increase in the relative mortality disadvantage of manual relative to nonmanual workers (for many causes of death) for both men and women; from 1957 to 1983, there was a decline in age-adjusted incidence of myocardial infarction in both white and blue collar male workers; however, the decline in white collar workers was double that of blue collar workers (Nathanson, 1990); no consistent trends in myocardial infarction were observed in women
Risky behavior and social class	Social class differences in smoking behavior (most documented risky behavior) do correspond to observed gender–social class mortality relationships; men with lower levels of education are substantially more likely to smoke than either better educated men or women (Nathanson, 1990); however, as the prevalence of smoking among men has declined more rapidly than among women, gender differences in smoking within the blue collar group, although still present, have become less marked

Continued.

TABLE 2-5

Causes of the Current Longevity and Health Differences Between Men and Women—cont'd

Biologic hypotheses	Comments
Social roles—*cont'd*	
Health service use and morbidity differences	Although women report greater use of physician services (particularly preventive services) than men, elderly men have higher hospitalization rates than women; with fewer work obligations, women are more likely to curtail activities and get more bed rest when ill; a more flexible daily schedule made possible by a lower employment rate is a key reason why women make more doctor visits for chronic problems (Verbrugge, 1990); overall, however, women have higher rates of morbidity and therapeutic care than men; women more frequently have short-term illnesses, with higher rates of daily symptoms and higher incidence rates for acute illnesses; thus women have a higher prevalence of many nonfatal chronic conditions, such as arthritis, chronic sinusitis, and digestive conditions; by contrast, men have higher prevalence rates of heart disease, atherosclerosis, emphysema, and other fatal conditions
Other social, psychologic, and emotional issues	Women's excess morbidity in contemporary life is driven by social factors, risks from less satisfying employment, keenly "felt" stress and unhappiness, stronger feelings of illness vulnerability, fewer formal time constraints, and less physically strenuous leisure activities

Theories and Mechanisms of Aging

The theories of aging are multiple and diverse because there is relatively little "indisputable" knowledge on the subject. Table 2-6 presents the historical development of aging research. Many of the theories proposed to explain aging have focused on a single mechanism—the so-called magic bullet approach to arrest aging. It is doubtful that a single theory will explain all the mechanisms of aging. As stated earlier, there are two general categories of theories of aging: (1) that aging is due to the accumulation of injurious events, sometimes called damage-accumulation theories; or (2) that biologic changes of aging are due to a genetically controlled developmental program. In the first category, random accumulation of errors in protein structure, mutations in somatic cells, the accumulation of metabolic waste products, and free-radical mediated damage (from highly reactive intermediates produced in the normal course of metabolism, such as hydroperoxides, aldehydes, and ketones) decrease the ability to maintain a physiologic steady state. The accumulation of these insults or injuries increases one's susceptibility to disease. The second category, the developmentally programmed theories of aging, focuses on the possibility that aging is the result of certain genes that program senescence and cell death. Supporters of this theory claim that because maximal life span is genetically determined, the aging process is also.

There is evidence both for and against any particular theory of aging. Three major areas of the mechanisms of aging have retained their appeal or have been extensively tested, however: (1) cellular changes produced by genetic and environmental factors; (2) changes in cellular regulatory, or control mechanisms, especially in cells of the neuroendocrine, immune, and central nervous systems; and (3) degenerative extracellular and vascular alterations (Norwood, 1990; Warner, Butler, Sprott, & Schneider, 1987).

Genetic and Environmental Factors

Cellular aging may be the consequence of "wear and tear" that causes functional changes and eventual cellular death. Many investigators propose that cellular damage may occur during replication as a result of factors within the cell, such as DNA and protein mechanisms, or factors outside the cell, such as ionizing radiation. They further propose that cells are already programmed at birth or are injured during life so as to cause errors in mitotic division and in the replication of genetic material that eventually lead to either cellular atrophy or death. Atrophy is common in the thymus, testis, ovary, uterus, and breast of aged individuals, although these organs age differently. For example, the ovary begins to lose function at an average age of 45, whereas the thymus gland begins to atrophy before adolescence.

One of the genetic mechanisms of aging is programmed aging. Regardless of damaging environmental factors, some investigators think that each normal cell may have a finite life span during which it is capable of replication. A classic experiment done by Hayflick (1965) demonstrated that fibroblasts are limited to a finite number of generations (40 to 60 doublings). This phenomenon has not been demonstrated for epithelial cells. Although this theory proposes that human cells have a finite number of replications, its proponents do not propose that aging is the result of cells losing their ability to divide. Rather, they believe that an intrinsic program within the human genome progressively slows or shuts down certain physiologic mechanisms, including mitosis (Russell, 1987).

Another genetic mechanism of aging suggests that mutations in somatic cells cause aging. The **somatic mutation hypothesis** is designed to evaluate DNA damage and efficiency of repair, and integrity of DNA synthesis. Most experimental evidence thus far does not support the hypothesis that aging is due to somatic mutation. With more sensitive laboratory methods, however, the future of DNA repair studies appears to be full of promise (Norwood, 1990; Warner et al., 1987).

The **catastrophic** or **error-prone theory,** initially proposed by Orgel in 1963, stated that the presence of errors in those enzymes involved in transcription and translation, and thus their own synthesis, leads to an increase in errors and eventually to the death of the cell. The theory was later modified by Orgel in 1970, with the possibility that nongrowing cells may not be subject to error catastrophe if the rate of error production did not increase significantly during protein synthesis. Abnormal forms of some, but not all, cellular proteins do appear during senescence but not as a result of errors in protein synthesis as originally predicted (Dice & Goff, 1987). Rather, the abnormal proteins appear to reflect several types of posttranslational modifications (Dice & Goff, 1987). The error-catastrophe theory has attracted a great deal of interest. Most of the evidence, however, argues against this theory as originally formulated. The accumulation of altered proteins in aging may result from an increased production or decreased ability of aged cells to degrade their cellular proteins, or both.

Alterations of Cellular Control Mechanisms

Many investigators suggest that the overall effects of aging are due to changes in certain cell populations that exert regulatory or control functions, such as cells of the central nervous system, neuroendocrine system, and immune system (Bliznakov, Wan, Chang, & Folkers, 1978; Denckla, 1981; Everitt & Burgess, 1976; Greenberg & Yunis, 1978; Walford, 1980). The **neuroendocrine theory** of aging purports that a genetic program

TABLE 2-6

Theories of Aging

Theory	Year	Proponent
Waste product theory	1923	Carrell & Ebeling
Wear-and-tear theory	1924	Pearl
Rate of living theory[a]	1928	Pearl
Endocrine theory	1947	Korenchevsky & Jones
Free-radical theory	1955	Harman
Collagen theory[b]	1957	Verzar
Metabolic theory[a]	1957; 1961	Carlson et al; Johnson et al.
Somatic mutation theory	1959	Sziliard
Error-catastrophe theory	1963; 1970	Orgel
Cross-linking theory[b]	1968	Bjorksten
Programmed senescence theory	1969	Hayflick
Immunologic theory	1969	Walform

From Schneider, E.L. (1987). Theories of aging: A perspective. In H.R. Warner, R.N. Butler, R.L. Sprott, & E.L. Schneider (Eds.) *Modern biological theories of aging.* New York: Raven Press.
NOTE: Theories with the same superscript may represent the same theory.

for aging is encoded in the brain and is controlled and relayed to peripheral tissues through hormonal and neural agents. Controversy exists as to what neuroendocrine mechanisms are responsible for aging. Possible mechanisms include (1) increased hormonal degradation, (2) decreased rate of hormonal synthesis and secretion, and (3) decreased target-organ sensitivity related to the number of cellular receptors for hormonal ligands, ligand–receptor binding, or ligand internalization (see Chapter 1). (The neuroendocrine theory of aging is discussed further in Chapter 17.)

Proponents of immune theories of aging believe that the immune system is implicated in aging because (1) immune function declines with age; (2) the decline in immune function is related to certain diseases, such as cancer, and to many other secondary effects; and (3) the number of autoantibodies (antibodies that attack body tissues) increases with age. (Changes in the immune system with age are discussed in Chapter 6.)

Degenerative Extracellular Changes

Extracellular factors that affect the aging process include the binding of collagen; the increase in free radicals' effects on cells; the structural alterations of fascia, tendons, ligaments, bones, and joints; and peripheral vascular disease, particularly arteriosclerosis (King, Fenoglio, & Lefkowich, 1983; Norwood, 1990). (See Chapter 27.)

Aging affects the extracellular matrix with increased cross-linking (e.g., aging collagen becomes more insoluble, chemically stable but rigid, resulting in a decrease of cell permeability), decreased synthesis, and increased degradation of collagen. These changes, together with the disappearance of elastin and changes in proteoglycans and plasma proteins, cause disorders of the ground substance that result in dehydration and wrinkling of the skin (see Chapter 41). Other age-related defects in the extracellular matrix include skeletal muscle alterations (e.g., atrophy, decreased tone, and loss of contractility), cataracts, diverticula, hernias, and rupture of intervertebral disks.

Free radicals of oxygen that result from oxidative cellular metabolism (e.g., respiratory chain, phagocytosis, prostaglandin synthesis) are thought to damage tissues during the aging process. The oxygen radicals produced include singlet oxygen, superoxide radical, hydroxyl radical, and hydrogen peroxide. (Free radicals are discussed in Chapter 1.) These oxygen products are extremely reactive and can damage nucleic acids, destroy polysaccharides, oxidize proteins, peroxide unsaturated fatty acids, and kill and lyse cells. Oxidant effects on target cells can give rise to malignant transformation through DNA damage (Cochrane, 1991). Investigators have proposed that progressive and cumulative damage from oxygen radicals leads to harmful alterations in cellular function consistent with those of aging (Harman, 1955, 1985). This hypothesis has its foundation from an older theory, the "wear-and-tear" theory of aging, which states that damages accumulate with time, decreasing the organism's ability to maintain a steady state. The hypothesis is controversial because there is no evidence that free radicals increase with aging, nor have higher levels been found in animals with short life spans than in animals with long life spans (Kanugo, 1980; Pryor, 1987).

Of much interest is the relationship between aging and the disappearance or alteration of extracellular substances important for vessel integrity. With aging, lipid, calcium, and plasma proteins are deposited in the walls of vessels. These depositions cause serious basement membrane thickening and alterations in smooth muscle functioning, resulting in arteriosclerosis. Arteriosclerosis is a progressive disease that causes serious problems in the aged individual, including stroke, myocardial infarction, renal disease, and peripheral vascular disease.

Cellular Aging

Cellular changes characteristic of aging include atrophy, decreased function, and loss of cells, possibly caused by apoptosis. Loss of cellular function from any of these causes initiates the compensatory mechanisms of hypertrophy and hyperplasia of remaining cells, which can lead to metaplasia, dysplasia, and neoplasia. All these changes can alter receptor placement and function, nutrient pathways, secretion of cellular products, and neuroendocrine control mechanisms. In the aged cell, DNA, RNA, cellular proteins, and membranes are most susceptible to injurious stimuli. DNA is particularly vulnerable to such injuries as breaks, deletions, and additions. Although DNA generally repairs itself with time, the aged cell's capacity for DNA repair is decreased (King et al., 1983; Norwood, 1990; Setlow, 1987). (The processes of DNA replication and repair are discussed in Chapter 4.) Lack of DNA repair increases the cell's susceptibility to mutations that may be lethal or may promote the development of neoplasia (see Chapter 10).

Tissue and Systemic Aging

It is probably safe to say that every physiologic process can be shown to function less efficiently with increasing age. The most characteristic tissue change with age is a progressive stiffness or rigidity (Cassel et al., 1990). The rigidity changes affect many systems, including the arterial, pulmonary, and musculoskeletal systems. A consequence of blood vessel and organ stiffness is a progressive increase in peripheral resistance to blood flow. The movement of intracellular and extracellular substances is also usually decreased with age. The diffusion capacity of the lung decreases with advancing age (Morris, 1990). Blood flow through organs decreases; for example, renal plasma flow decreases as a function of age.

Changes in the endocrine and immune systems occur with aging. The thymus atrophies at puberty, causing a decreased immune response to T-dependent antigens (foreign proteins). Later in life, an increase in autoantibodies and immune complexes (antibodies that are bound to antigens) and an overall decrease of immunologic tolerance for the host's own cells further diminish the effectiveness of the immune system. In women, the reproductive system loses ova, and in men spermatogenesis is decreased. Responsiveness to hormones decreases in the breast and endometrium.

The stomach is affected by a decreased rate of emptying and decreased secretion of hormones and hydrochloric acid. Muscular atrophy diminishes mobility by decreasing motor tone and contractility. The skin of the aged individual is affected by atrophy and wrinkling of the epidermis and alterations in underlying dermis, fat, and muscle.

Total-body changes include a decrease in height; a reduction in circumference of the neck, thighs, and arms; widening of the pelvis; and lengthening of the nose and ears. Several of these changes are due to tissue atrophy and to decreased bone mass caused by osteoporosis and osteoarthritis. Changes in body weight are mostly related to body fat. Men usually gain weight until approximately age 50, whereas women gain until approximately age 70 before losing. As fat increases, total body water decreases. Total body potassium also decreases because of decreased cellular mass. An increased sodium/potassium ratio suggests that the decreased cellular mass is accompanied by an increased extracellular compartment.

Although some of these alterations are probably inherent in aging, others represent consequences of aging. Advanced age increases susceptibility to disease, and death occurs after an injury or insult because of diminished cellular, tissue, and organic function. To determine that an individual "died of old age" would truly be a monumental task if not an impossible one.

SOMATIC DEATH

Somatic death is death of the entire organism. Unlike the changes that follow cellular death in a live body, **postmortem change** is diffuse and does not involve components of the inflammatory response. Within minutes of death, manifestations of postmortem change appear, eliminating any difficulty in determining that death has occurred. The most notable manifestations are complete cessation of respiration and circulation. The surface of the skin usually becomes pale and yellowish; however, the lifelike color of the cheeks and lips may persist after death of causes such as carbon monoxide poisoning, drowning, and chloroform poisoning (Shennan, 1935).

Body temperature falls gradually immediately after death, then more rapidly (approximately 1.0° to 1.5° F/hr) until, after 24 hours, body temperature equals that of the environment (Minckler, Anstall, & Minckler, 1971). After death caused by certain infective diseases, body temperature may continue to rise for a short time. Postmortem reduction of body temperature is called **algor mortis.**

Blood pressure within the retinal vessels decreases, causing muscle tension to decrease and the pupils to become dilated. The face, nose, and chin become "sharp-" or "peaked-looking" as blood and fluids drain away (Shennan, 1935). Gravity causes blood to settle in the most dependent, or lowest tissues, which develop a purple discoloration called **livor mortis.** Incisions at this time usually fail to cause bleeding. The skin loses its elasticity and transparency.

Within 6 hours after death, acidic compounds accumulate within the muscles because of the breakdown of carbohydrate and depletion of ATP. This interferes with ATP-dependent detachment of myosin from actin (contractile proteins), and muscle stiffening, or **rigor mortis,** sets in. The smaller muscles are usually affected first, particularly the muscles of the jaw. Within 12 to 14 hours, rigor mortis usually affects the entire body.

Signs of putrefaction are generally obvious about 24 to 48 hours after death. Rigor mortis gradually diminishes, and the body becomes flaccid in 12 to 14 hours. Putrefactive changes vary depending on the temperature of the environment. The most visible is greenish discoloration of the skin, particularly on the abdomen. The discoloration is thought to be related to the diffusion of hemolyzed blood into the tissues and the production of sulfhemoglobin (Minckler et al., 1971). Slippage or loosening of the skin from underlying tissues occurs at the same time. After this, swelling or bloating of the body and liquefactive changes occur, sometimes causing opening of the body cavities. At a microscopic level, putrefactive changes are associated with the release of enzymes and lytic dissolution called **postmortem autolysis.**

CLINICAL COMMENTARY
CRITERIA FOR SOMATIC DEATH

Issues involving death and dying are among the most difficult in clinical practice. Contrary to what some law books state as the criterion for death, arrest of the heart is not proof that life has ended, because the heart can sometimes be restored to action. If cardiac arrest is not reversed, hypoxic injury to other vital organs ensues. Because of its high oxygen demands, the brain is usually the first such organ to be destroyed. This phenomenon, along with the advent of transplantation procedures requiring viable organs from a donor, has led to the development of criteria for determining "brain death" as proof of somatic death. These criteria are as follows:

1. Coma with cerebral unresponsiveness, including cessation of all brainstem reflexes (pupillary reactions, ocular movement, blinking, and swallowing)
2. Cessation of breathing (no respiratory movement after removal from the respirator for 1 to 2 minutes)
3. Isoelectric ("flat") electroencephalogram (EEG).

SUMMARY REVIEW

Cellular Adaptation

1 Cellular adaptation is an alteration that enables the cell to maintain a steady state despite adverse conditions.

2 Atrophy is a decrease in cellular size caused by aging, disuse, or lack of blood supply, hormonal stimulation, or neural stimulation. Amounts of endoplasmic reticulum, mitochondria, and microfilaments are decreased.

3 Hypertrophy is an increase in the size of cells caused by increased work demands or hormonal stimulation. Amounts of protein in the plasma membrane, endoplasmic reticulum, microfilaments, and mitochondria are increased.

4 Hyperplasia is an increase in the number of cells caused by an increased rate of cellular division. Normal hyperplasia is stimulated by hormones or the need to replace lost tissues.

5 Dysplasia, or atypical hyperplasia, is an abnormal change in the size, shape, and organization of mature tissue cells.

6 Metaplasia is the reversible replacement of one mature cell type by another, less mature cell type.

Cellular Injury

1 Cellular injury is caused by lack of oxygen (hypoxia), caustic or toxic chemicals, infectious agents, inflammatory and immune responses, genetic factors, insufficient nutrients, or physical trauma from many causes.

2 Sublethal injury, which does not kill the cell, may result in cellular adaptation. Lethal injury, which does kill the cell, always involves disruption of cellular metabolism.

3 Metabolism cannot occur if the cell's oxygen supply is cut off or if damage to the plasma membrane causes the cell to "drown" in an influx of extracellular fluids and charged solutes. Both insults disable ATP production, which is essential for both metabolism and maintenance of active transport processes that prevent fluid and solute influx.

4 The sequence of events leading to cell death is commonly decreased ATP production, failure of active transport mechanisms (the sodium-potassium pump), cellular swelling, detachment of ribosomes from the endoplasmic reticulum, cessation of protein synthesis, mitochondrial swelling as a result of calcium accumulation, vacuolation, leakage of digestive enzymes from lysosomes, autodigestion of intracellular structures, lysis of the plasma membrane, and death.

5 The initial insult in hypoxic injury is usually ischemia, the cessation of blood flow into vessels that supply the cell with oxygen and nutrients.

6 The initial insult in chemical injury is damage or destruction of the plasma membrane. Examples of chemical agents that cause cellular injury include carbon tetrachloride, lead, carbon monoxide, and ethyl alcohol.

7 Bacteria injure cells by producing destructive enzymes, exotoxins, or endotoxins. Enzymes can damage the plasma membranes of host cells, exotoxins can inactivate enzymes critical to protein synthesis, and endotoxins activate the inflammatory response and produce fever.

8 Bacteremia, or septicemia, is the proliferation of bacteria in the blood. Endotoxins released by bloodborne bacteria cause the release of vasoactive enzymes that increase the permeability of blood vessels. Leakage from vessels causes hypotension that can result in septic shock.

9 Viruses enter host cells and use the metabolic processes of host cells to proliferate.

10 Viruses that have invaded host cells decrease protein synthesis, disrupt lysosomal membranes, form inclusion bodies where synthesis of viral nucleic acids is occurring, fuse with host cells to produce giant cells, alter antigenic properties of the host cell, and transform host cells into cancerous cells.

11 Activation of inflammation and immunity, which occurs after cellular injury or infection, involves powerful biochemicals and proteins capable of damaging normal (uninjured and uninfected) cells.

12 Genetic disorders injure cells by altering the nucleus and the plasma membrane's structure, shape, receptors, or transport mechanisms.

13 Deprivation of essential nutrients (proteins, carbohydrates, lipids, and vitamins) can cause cellular injury by altering cellular structure and function, particularly of transport mechanisms, chromosomes, the nucleus, and DNA.

14 Injurious physical agents include temperature extremes, changes in atmospheric pressure, ionizing radiation, illumination, mechanical stresses (such as repetitive body movements), and noise.

Manifestations of Cellular Injury

1 Cellular manifestations of cellular injury include accumulations of water, lipids, carbohydrates, glycogen, proteins, pigments, hemosiderin, bilirubin, calcium, and urate.

2 Accumulations harm cells by "crowding" the organelles and by causing excessive (and sometimes harmful) metabolites to be produced during their catabolism. The metabolites are released into the cytoplasm or expelled into the extracellular matrix.

3 Cellular swelling, the accumulation of excessive water in the cell, is due to the failure of transport mechanisms and is a sign of many types of cellular injury.

4 Accumulations of organic substances—lipids, carbohydrates, glycogen, proteins, and pigments—are due to disorders in which (a) cellular uptake of the substance exceeds the cell's capacity to catabolize (digest) or use it or (b) cellular anabolism (synthesis) of the substance exceeds the cell's capacity to use or secrete it.

5 Dystrophic calcification (accumulation of calcium salts) is always a sign of pathologic change because it only occurs in injured or dead cells. Metastatic calcification, however, can occur in uninjured cells in individuals with hypercalcemia.

6 Disturbances in urate metabolism can result in hyperuricemia and deposition of sodium urate crystals in tissue—leading to painful disorders called gout.

7 Systemic manifestations of cellular injury include fever, leukocytosis, increased heart rate, pain, and serum elevations of enzymes in the plasma.

Cellular Death

1 Cellular death is manifested as cellular dissolution, or necrosis. Necrosis is the sum of the changes after local cell death and includes the process of autolysis, or cellular self-destruction.

2 There are four major types of necrosis: coagulative, liquefactive, caseous, and fat necrosis. Different types of necrosis occur in different tissues.

3 Structural signs that indicate irreversible injury and progression to necrosis are the dense clumping and disruption of genetic material and the disruption of the plasma and organelle membranes.

4 Apoptosis, a distinct type of cellular death, is a process of selective cellular self-destruction that occurs in both normal and pathologic tissue changes.

5 Gangrenous necrosis, or gangrene, is tissue necrosis due to hypoxia and subsequent bacterial invasion.

Aging

1 It is difficult to determine the physiologic (normal) from the pathologic changes of aging.

2 Humans have an inherent maximal life span (80 to 100 years) that is dictated by currently unknown intrinsic mechanisms.

3 Although the maximal life span has not changed significantly over time, the average life span, or life expectancy, has increased. Life expectancy for men is about 71 years and women 78 years.

4 The physiologic mechanisms of aging are apparently associated with (a) cellular changes produced by genetic and environmental factors, (b) changes in cellular regulatory or control mechanisms, and (c) degenerative extracellular and vascular alterations.

Somatic Death

1 Somatic death is death of the entire organism. Postmortem change is diffuse and does not involve the inflammatory response.

2 Manifestations of somatic death include cessation of respiration and circulation, gradual lowering of body temperature, pupil dilation, loss of elasticity and transparency in the skin, muscle stiffening (rigor mortis), and skin discoloration (livor mortis). Signs of putrefaction are obvious about 24 to 48 hours after death.

KEY TERMS

Algor mortis, 85
Anoxia, 58
Apoptosis, 78
Atrophy, 54
Autolysis, 76
Autophagic vacuole, 55
Bacteremia (septicemia), 64
Bilirubin, 75
Blast injury, 69
Caseous necrosis, 78
Catastrophic (error-prone) theory, 83
Cellular accumulation (infiltration), 72
Cellular swelling, 72
Coagulative necrosis, 76
Compensatory hyperplasia, 56
Decompression sickness (caisson disease), 69
Dry gangrene, 78
Dysplasia (atypical hyperplasia), 56
Dystrophic calcification, 75
Endotoxin, 64
Exotoxin, 63
Fat necrosis, 78
Fatty change, 73

Free radical, 59
Gangrenous necrosis, 78
Gas gangrene, 78
Hemoprotein, 74
Hemosiderin, 75
Hemosiderosis, 75
Hepatocyte growth factor, 56
Hormonal hyperplasia, 56
Hydropic degeneration, 72
Hyperlipidemia, 68
Hyperplasia, 56
Hyperthermic injury, 68
Hypertrophy, 55
Hypolipidemia, 68
Hypothermic injury, 68
Hypoxia, 57
Inclusion body, 66
Ionizing radiation, 69
Ischemia, 58
Karyolysis, 76
Life expectancy, 79
Lipid-acceptor protein (apoprotein), 59
Lipid peroxidation, 59

Lipofuscin, 55
Lipopolysaccharide, 64
Liquefactive necrosis, 78
Livor mortis, 85
Maximal life span, 79
Melanin, 74
Metaplasia, 56
Metastatic calcification, 76
Necrosis, 76
Neuroendocrine theory, 83
Noise, 71
Pathologic hyperplasia, 56
Permissive host cell, 65
Postmortem autolysis, 85
Postmortem change, 85
Psammoma body, 75
Pyknosis, 76
Rigor mortis, 85
Somatic death, 85
Somatic mutation hypothesis, 83
Urate, 76
Vacuolation, 72
Virion (viral particle), 65
Wet gangrene, 78

REFERENCES

Bliznakov, E. G., Wan, Y. P., Chang, D., & Folkers, K. (1978). Partial reaction of impaired immune competence in aged mice by synthetic thymus factors. *Biochemistry/Biophysics Research Communication, 80*, 631-636.

Bottaro, D. P., Rubin, J. S., Faletto, D. L. M.-L., Chan, A., Kmiecik, T. E., Vande Woude, G. F., & Aaroson, S. A. (1991). Identification of the hepatocyte growth factor receptor as the c-met proto-oncogene product. *Science, 251*(4995), 802-805.

Calandra, T., Baumgartner, J., & Glauser, M. P. (1991). Anti-lipopolysaccharide and anti-tumor necrosis factor/cachectin antibodies for the treatment of gram-negative bacteremia and septic shock. *Proceedings of Clinical Biological Research, 367*, 141-159.

Cassel, C. K., Risenberg, D. E., Sorensen, L. B., & Walsh, J. R. (Eds.). (1990). *Geriatric medicine* (2nd ed.). New York: Springer-Verlag.

Cochrane, C. G. (1991). Cellular injury by oxidants. *American Journal of Medicine, 91*(3C), 235-305.

Consensus Conference. (1990). Noise and hearing loss. *Journal of the American Medical Association, 263*(23), 3185-3190.

Cotran, R. S., Kumar, V., & Robbins, S. L. (1989). *Robbins pathologic basis of disease* (4th ed.). Philadelphia: W. B. Saunders.

Cowger, M. L. (1971). Mechanisms of bilirubin toxicity on tissue culture cells: Factors that affect toxicity reversibility by albumin, and comparison with other respiratory poisons by albumin, and comparison with other respiratory poisons and surfactants. *Biochemical Medicine, 5*, 1-16.

DeFlora, S., & D'Agostini, F. (1992). Halogen lamp carcinogenicity. *Nature, 356*(6370), 569.

Denckla, W. D. (1981). Aging, dying, and the pituitary. In R. T. Schimke (Ed.). *Biological mechanisms in aging* (NIH Publication No. 81-2 194.). Bethesda, MD: National Institutes on Aging.

Dice J. F., & Goff, S. A. (1987). Molecular determinants of protein half life. *Eucara FASEBJ, Nov 1*(5), 349-357.

Everitt, A. V., & Burgess, J. A. (1976). *Hypothalamus, pituitary, and aging.* Springfield, IL: Charles C Thomas.

Farber, J. L. (1981). Minireview: The role of calcium in cell death. *Life Sciences, 29*, 1289.

Greenberg, L. K., & Yunis, E. J. (1978). Histocompatibility determinants, immune responsiveness, and aging in man. *Federal Proceedings, 37*, 1258.

Harman, D. (1955). Aging: A theory based on free radical and radiation chemistry. *University of California Radiology Lab Report,* 3078.

Harman, D. (1985). Role of free radicals in aging and disease. In H. A. Johnson (Ed.), *Aging: Relations between normal aging and disease* (vol. 28). New York: Raven Press.

Hayflick, L. (1965). The limited in vitro lifetime of human diploid cell strains. *Experimental Cell Research, 37*, 614.

Hazardous Substances and Public Health. (1991). *Death of toddler holds message for primary care providers, 89*, 87-90.

Holbrook, J. (1983). Cigarette smoking. In W. H. Rom (Ed.). *Environmental and occupational medicine.* Boston: Little, Brown.

Jennings, R. B. & Reimer, K. A. (1981). Lethal myocardial ischemic injury. *American Journal of Pathology, 102*, 241.

Johnson, H. A. (Ed.). (1985). Is aging physiological or pathological? In *Relations between normal aging and disease.* New York: Raven Press.

Kanugo, M. S. (1980). *Biochemistry of aging* (pp. 182-192). New York & London: Academic Press.

Kerr, J. F. R., & Searle, J. (1980). Apoptosis: Its nature and kinetic role. In R. E. Meyn & H. R. Withers (Eds.), *Radiation biology in cancer research* (pp. 367-384). New York: Raven Press.

Keyserling, W. M., & Armstrong, T. J. (1992). Ergonomics. In J. M. Last & R. B. Wallace (Eds.), *Maxey-Roseneau-Last: Public health and preventive medicine* (13th ed.). Norwalk, CT: Appleton & Lange.

King, D. W., Fenoglio, C. M., & Lefkowich, J. H. (1983). *General pathology principles & dynamics*. Philadelphia: Lea & Febiger.

Kissane, J. M. (Ed.). (1990). *Anderson's pathology* (9th ed.). St. Louis: Mosby—Year Book.

Levin, M. E., & O'Neal, L. W. (1992). *The diabetic foot* (5th ed.). St. Louis: Mosby—Year Book.

Leiber, C. S. (1988). Metabolic effects of ethanol and its interaction with other drugs, hepatoxic agents, vitamins, and carcinogens: A 1988 update. *Seminars in Liver Disease 8* (1), 47-68.

Lieber, C. S. (1991). Hepatic, metabolic, and toxic effects of ethanol: 1991 update. *Alcohol, Clinical Experimental Research, 15*(4), 574-592.

London, S. J., Connolly, J. L., Schnitt, S. J., & Colditz, G. A. (1992). A prospective study of benign breast disease and the risk of breast cancer. *Journal of the American Medical Association, 267*(7), 941-944.

McGuigan, M. A. (1992). Teratogenesis and reproductive toxicology. In J. B. Sullivan & G. R. Krieger (Eds.), *Hazardous materials toxicology clinical principles of environmental health*. Baltimore: Williams & Wilkins.

Minckler, J., Anstall, H. B., & Minckler, T. M. (1971). *Pathobiology: An introduction*. St. Louis: Mosby—Year Book.

Morris, J. F. (1990). Pulmonary diseases. In C.K. Cassel, D.E. Risenberg, L. B. Sorensen, & J. R. Walsh (Eds.), *Geriatric medicine* (2nd ed.). New York: Springer-Verlag.

Nathanson, C. A. (1990). The gender-mortality differential in developed countries: Demographic and sociocultural dimensions. In M. G. Ory & H. R. Warner (Eds.), *Gender, health, and longevity: Multidisciplinary perspectives*. New York: Springer Publishing Co.

Norwood, T. H. (1990). Cellular aging. In C. K. Cassel, D. E. Risenberg, L. B. Sorensen, & J. R. Walsh (Eds.), *Geriatric medicine* (2nd ed.). New York: Springer-Verlag.

Orrenius, S., McConkey, D. J., & Nicotera, P. (1991). Role of calcium in toxic and programmed cell death. *Advances in Experimental Medical Biology, 283*, 419-425.

Ory, M. G., & Warner, H. R. (Eds.). (1990). *Gender, health, and longevity: Multidisciplinary perspectives*. New York: Springer Publishing Co.

Pedersen, C., Thomsen, C., Arlien-Soborg, P., Praestholm, J., Kjaer, L., Boesen, F., Hansen, H. S., & Nielsen, J. O. (1991). Central nervous system involvement in human immunodeficiency virus disease: A prospective study including neurological examination, computerized tomography, and magnetic resonance imaging. *Danish Medical Bulletin, 38*(4), 374-379.

Ponsonby, A. L., Dwyer, T., Gibbons, L. E., Cochrane, J. A., Jones, M. E., & McCall, M. J. (1992). Thermal environment and sudden infant death syndrome: Case-control study. *British Medical Journal, 304*, 277-282.

Powell, L. W., & Kerr, J. F. R. (1975). Pathology of the liver in hemochromatosis. *Pathobiological Annual, 5*, 317.

Pryor, W. A. (1987). The free-radical theory of aging revisited: A critique and a suggested disease-specific theory. In H. R. Warner (Ed.), *Biological theories of aging*. New York: Raven Press.

Raff, M. C. (1992). Social controls on cell survival and cell death. *Nature, 356*, 397-401.

Riley, M. W. (1990). Foreword: The gender paradox. In M. G. Ory & H. R. Warner (Eds.), *Gender, health, and longevity: Multidisciplinary perspectives*. New York: Springer Publishing Co.

Roy, S. B., Gulena, J. S., Khanna, P. K., Manchanda, S. C., Pande, J. N., & Subba, P. S. (1969). Haemodynamic studies in high altitude pulmonary edema. *British Heart Journal, 31*, 52.

Russell, R. L. (1987). Evidence for and against the theory of developmentally programmed aging. In H. R. Warner, R. N. Butler, R. L. Sprott, & E. L. Schneider (Eds.), *Modern biological theories of aging*. New York: Raven Press.

Sandford, N. L., Searle, J. W., & Kerr, J. F. R. (1984). Successive waves of apoptosis in the rat prostate after repeated withdrawal of testosterone stimulation. *Pathology, 16*(4), 406-410.

Scarpelli, D. G., & Iannaccone, P. M. (1990). Cell injury and errors of metabolism. In J. M. Kissane (Ed.), *Anderson's pathology* (9th ed.). St. Louis: Mosby—Year Book.

Setlow, R. B. (1987). Theory presentation and background summary. In H. R. Warner, R. N. Butler, R. L. Sprott, & E. L. Schneider (Eds.). *Modern biological theories of aging*. New York: Raven Press.

Shannon, M. W., & Graef, J. W. (1992). Lead intoxication in infancy. *Pediatrics, 89*(1), 87-90.

Shennan, T. (1935). *Postmortems and morbid anatomy* (3rd ed.). Baltimore: William Wood.

Sherry, B., & Cerami, A. (1988). Cachectin/tumor necrosis factor exerts endocrine, paracrine, and autocrine control of inflammatory responses. *Journal of Cellular Biology, 107*, 1269-1277.

Smith, D. W. E., & Warner, H. R. (1990). Overview of biomedical perspectives: Possible relationships between genes on the sex chromosomes and longevity. In M. G. Ory & H. R. Warner (Eds.), *Gender, health, and longevity: Multidisciplinary perspectives*. New York: Springer Publishing Co.

Stradling, J. R., & Crosby, J. H. (1991). Predictors and prevalence of obstructive sleep apnea and snoring in 1001 middle-aged men. *Thorax, 46*(2), 85-90.

Thibodeau, G. A. & Patton, K. T. (1993). *Anatomy and physiology*. St. Louis: Mosby—Year Book.

Tomei, L. D., & Cope, F. O. (Eds.). (1991). *Apoptosis: The molecular basis of cell death*. New York: Cold Spring Harbor Laboratory Press.

Tortora, G. J., Funke, B. R., & Case, C. L. (1989). *Microbiology: An introduction* (3rd ed.). Menlo Park, CA: Benjamin Cummings.

Verbrugge, L. M. (1990). The twain meet: Empirical explanations of sex differences in health and mortality. In M. G. Ory & H. R. Warner (Eds.), *Gender, health, and longevity: Multidisciplinary perspectives*. New York: Springer Publishing.

Veterans Administration Systemic Sepsis Cooperative Study Group. (1987). Effect of high-dose glucocorticoid therapy on mortality in patients with clinical signs of systemic sepsis. *New England Journal of Medicine, 317*, 659-665.

Vlessis, A. A., Muller, P., Bartos, D., & Trunkey, D. (1991). Mechanisms of peroxide-induced cellular injury in cultured adult myocytes. *FASEB J, 5*(11), 2600-2605.

Walford, T. L. (1980). Immunology and aging. *American Journal of Clinical Pathology, 74*, 247.

Warner, H. R., Butler, R. N., Sprott, R. L., & Schneider, E. L. (1987). *Modern biological theories of aging*. New York: Raven Press.

Weston, H. C. (1948). The effects of age and illumination upon visual performance with clore sights. *British Journal of Ophthalmology, 32*, 645.

Wilkins, A. J., & Wilkinson, P. (1991). A tint to reduce eye-strain from fluorescent lighting? *Ophthalmic Physiology, 11*(2), 172-175.

Wyllie, A. H., Kerr, J. F. R., & Currie, A. R. (1980). Cell death: The significance of apoptosis. In G. H. Bourne & J. F. Danielli (Eds.), *International Review of Cytology, 68*, 251-306.

Ziegman, S., Sutliff, G., & Rounds, M. (1991). Relationships between human cataracts and environmental radiant energy: Cataract formation, light scattering, and fluorescence. *Lens Eye Toxic Research, 8*(23), 259-280.

SUGGESTED READINGS

Brody, J. A., & Brock, D. W. (1985). Epidemiologic and statistical characteristics of the United States elderly population. In C. E. Finch & E. L. Schneider (Eds.), *Handbook of the biology of aging* (2nd ed.). New York: Van Nostrand Reinhold.

Hayflick, L. (1980). The biology of human aging. *Advances in Pathobiology, 7*, 80.

Leaf, A., (1982). Long-lived populations: Extreme old age. *Journal of the American Geriatric Association, 30*, 485-487.

Monti, D., Grassilli, E., Troiano, L., Cossarizza, A., Salvioli, S., Barbieri, D., Agnesini, C., Bettuzzi, S., Ingletti, M. C., Corti, A., et al. (1992). Senescence, immortalization, and apoptosis: An intriguing relationship. *Annals of New York Academy of Science, 673,* 70-82.

Orgel, L. E. (1970). The maintenance of the accuracy of protein synthesis and its relevance to aging: A correction. *Proceedings of the National Academy of Sciences, 67,* 1476.

Schneider, E. L. (1987). Theories of aging: A perspective. In H. R. Warner, R. N. Butler, R. L. Sprott, & E. L. Schneider (Eds.). *Modern biological theories of aging.* New York: Raven Press.

Searle, J., Kerr, J. F. R., & Bishop, C. (1982). Necrosis and apoptosis: Distinct modes of cell death with fundamentally different significance. *Pathology Annual, 17* (2), 244.

U. S. Department of Health and Human Services (USDHHS) (1991). Special issue on lead toxicity. *ATSDR, 2*(1), 1-8.

CHAPTER 3

The Cellular Environment: Fluids and Electrolytes, Acids and Bases

Sue E. Huether

Chapter Outline

The cells of the body live in a fluid environment that requires an electrolyte concentration and pH value that is maintained within a very narrow range. Changes in the composition of electrolytes affect electrical potentials of excitatory cells and cause shifts of fluid from one compartment to another. Alterations in pH disrupt the cellular function of enzyme systems. Fluid fluctuations affect blood volume and cellular function. Disturbances in these functions are common and can be life-threatening. Understanding how alterations occur and the body's ability to compensate or correct the disturbance is important to understanding many pathophysiologic conditions.

DISTRIBUTION OF BODY FLUIDS

The fluids of the body are distributed among functional compartments, or spaces, and provide a transport medium for cellular and tissue function. The **intracellular fluid (ICF)** comprises all of the fluid contained within cells. The **extracellular fluid (ECF)** is all of the fluid outside the cells and is divided into smaller compartments. The two main ECF compartments are the **interstitial fluid**, or the space between cells and outside the blood vessels (i.e., connective tissue, cartilage, and bone), and the **intravascular fluid**, which is the blood plasma. Other ECF compartments include the lymph and the transcellular fluids such as the synovial, intestinal, and cerebrospinal fluid; sweat; urine; and pleural, synovial, peritoneal, pericardial, and intraocular fluids.

The sum of fluids within all compartments constitutes the **total body water (TBW)** (Table 3-1). The volume of TBW is usually expressed as a percentage of body weight in kilograms. The standard value for TBW is 60% of a 70-kg adult male, which is equivalent to 42 L of fluid (Table 3-2). The rest of the body weight is made up of fat and fat-free solids, particularly bone.

Although the amount of fluid within the various compartments is relatively constant, there is exchange of solutes and water between compartments to maintain their unique compositions. Fluid volume is usually measured in liters (L), or milliliters (1 ml = $\frac{1}{1000}$ of a liter). The percentage of TBW varies with the amount of body fat and age. Because fat is water-repelling (hydrophobic), very little water is contained in adipose cells. Individuals with more body fat have proportionately less TBW and tend to be more susceptible to fluid imbalances that cause dehydration.

☐ AGING and Distribution of Body Fluids

The distribution and amount of TBW change with age (see Table 3-2). In newborn infants, TBW is about 75% to 80% of body weight. The percentage of TBW decreases to about 67% of body weight during the first year of life. In the immediate postnatal period there is a physiologic loss of body water amounting to 5% of body weight as the infant adjusts to a new environment. Infants are particularly susceptible to significant changes in TBW, because of their high metabolic rate. The turnover of body fluids in infants is caused by their greater body surface area and by their high metabolic rate. The turnover of body fluid, therefore, is much faster. Loss of fluids from diarrhea can represent a significant proportion of body weight. Renal mechanisms of fluid and electrolyte conservation also may not be mature enough to counter the losses so that dehydration may develop rapidly.

During childhood, TBW slowly decreases to 60% to 65% of body weight. At adolescence, the percentage of TBW approaches adult proportions, and sex differences begin to appear. Males eventually have a greater percentage of body water as a function of increasing muscle mass. Females have more body fat and less muscle as a function of estrogens and therefore have less water.

In the elderly, there is a further decline in the percentage of TBW. The decrease is due in part to an increased amount of fat and a decreased amount of muscle and to a reduced ability to regulate sodium and water balance. With age, the kidney becomes less efficient in pro-

TABLE 3-2

Total Body Water in Relation to Body Weight

Body build	TBW (%) Adult male	TBW (%) Adult female	TBW (%) Infant
Normal	60	50	70
Lean	70	60	80
Obese	50	42	60

NOTE TBW (total body water) is a percentage of body weight.

TABLE 3-1

Distribution of Body Water

	Percentage of body weight	Volume (L)
Intracellular fluid (ICF)	40	28
Extracellular fluid (ECF)	20	14
Interstitial	(15)	(11)
Intravascular	(5)	(3)
Total body water (TBW)	60	42

TABLE 3-3

Normal Water Gains and Losses (70-kg man)

	Daily intake (ml)		Daily output (ml)
Drinking	1400-1800	Urine	1400-1800
Water in food	700-1000	Stool	100
Water of oxidation	300-400	Skin	300-500
		Lungs	600-800
TOTAL	2400-3200		2400-3200

ducing concentrated urine, and the responses for conserving sodium become sluggish. The normal reduction of TBW in the elderly becomes clinically important with stress, such as fever or dehydration from any cause; loss of body fluids at such times can be severe and life-threatening.

Although daily fluid intake may fluctuate widely, the body regulates water volume within a relatively narrow range. The primary sources of body water are drinking, ingestion of water in food, and water derived from oxidative metabolism. Normally, the largest amounts of water are lost through renal excretion. Lesser amounts are eliminated through the stool and through vaporization from the skin and lungs (this is insensible water loss) (Table 3-3).

Water Movement between ICF and ECF

The movement of water between ICF and ECF compartments is primarily a function of osmotic forces. (Osmosis and other mechanisms of passive transport are discussed in Chapter 1.) Water moves freely across cell membranes, so that the osmolality of TBW is normally at equilibrium. Sodium is the most abundant ECF ion and is responsible for the osmotic balance of the ECF space. Potassium maintains the osmotic balance of the ICF space. The osmotic force of ICF proteins and other

nondiffusible substances is balanced by the active transport of ions out of the cell. Normally, the ICF is not subject to rapid changes in osmolality, but when there are changes in ECF osmolality, a net transfer of water from one compartment to another occurs until osmotic equilibrium is reestablished. A model of the maintenance of osmotic equilibrium is illustrated in Fig. 3-1.

Water Movement between Plasma and Interstitial Fluid

The distribution of water and the movement of nutrients and waste products among the capillary, plasma, and the interstitial spaces occurs as a result of changes in hydrostatic pressure and osmotic forces at the arterial and venous ends of the capillary. Because water, sodium, and glucose readily move across the capillary membrane, the plasma proteins maintain the effective osmolality by generating plasma oncotic pressure. Osmotic forces within the capillary are balanced by the hydrostatic pressure, which arises from cardiac contraction. The movement of fluid back and forth across the capillary wall is called **net filtration** and is best described by **Starling's hypothesis:**

$$\text{Net filtration} = (\text{force favoring filtration}) - (\text{forces opposing filtration})$$

A Normal osmotic equilibrium

B Addition of solute to ECF osmotic disequilibrium

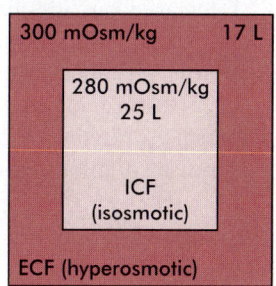

C Reestablishment of osmotic equilibrium

Water moves from ICF to ECF according to osmotic gradient. Osmotic equilibrium is reestablished with smaller ICF compartment.

D Addition of free water to ECF osmotic disequilibrium

E Reestablishment of osmotic equilibrium

Water moves from ECF to ICF according to osmotic gradient. Osmotic equilibrium is reestablished with larger ICF and ECF compartments.

FIG. 3-1 Model of osmotic equilibrium.

The forces favoring filtration, or movement of water out of the capillary and into the interstitial space, include the capillary hydrostatic pressure and the interstitial oncotic pressure. The forces opposing filtration are the plasma oncotic pressure and the interstitial hydrostatic pressure. Normally, the interstitial forces are negligible, because only a very small percentage of plasma proteins cross the capillary membrane, and interstitial fluid moves into cells or is drawn back into the plasma. Thus the major forces for filtration are within the capillary.

As the plasma flows from the arterial to the venous end of the capillary, changes in the force of hydrostatic pressure facilitate the movement of water across the capillary membrane. Oncotic pressure remains fairly constant because plasma proteins normally do not cross the capillary membrane. At the arterial end of the capillary, hydrostatic pressure is greater than capillary oncotic pressure and water filters into the interstitial space. Because of oncotic forces, there is some movement of water back into the capillary, but the net effect is loss of water from the capillary. The movement of water from the plasma causes the hydrostatic pressure within the capillary to decrease. Thus at the venous end of the capillary, oncotic pressure exceeds hydrostatic pressure. Fluids then are attracted back into the circulation, balancing the movement of fluids between the plasma and the interstitial space. The overall effect is filtration at the arterial end and reabsorption at the venous end (Fig. 3-2).

An important factor in capillary filtration of fluid is the integrity of the capillary membrane. Changes in membrane permeability may permit the escape of plasma proteins into the interstitial space. The normal relationship defined by Starling's hypothesis is altered with the osmotic movement of water into the interstitial space, causing tissue edema.

ALTERATIONS IN WATER MOVEMENT
Edema

Edema is the accumulation of fluid within the interstitial spaces. It is a problem of fluid distribution and does not necessarily indicate a fluid excess. In some conditions, sequestered fluids can cause both edema and dehydration. The pathophysiologic process is related to an increase in the forces favoring fluid filtration from the capillaries or lymphatic channels into the tissues. The most common mechanisms include increased hydrostatic pressure, decreased plasma oncotic pressure, increased capillary membrane permeability, and lymphatic obstruction (Fig. 3-3).

Pathophysiology

An increase in hydrostatic pressure can result from venous obstruction or salt and water retention. Venous obstruction can cause the hydrostatic pressure of fluid within the capillaries to become great enough to cause fluid to escape into the interstitial spaces. Thrombophlebitis, hepatic obstruction, tight clothing around the extremities, and prolonged standing are common causes of venous obstruction. Congestive heart failure and renal failure are both conditions associated with salt and water retention, which in turn cause volume overload and edema. Additionally, renal failure may be associated with loss of plasma proteins that contributes to the edema of nephrosis.

Losses or diminished production of plasma albumin contributes to a decrease in plasma oncotic pressure. Decreased oncotic attraction of fluid within the capillary causes fluid to move into the interstitial space. Decreased production of plasma protein may occur with liver disease or protein malnutrition. The escape of plasma proteins from the serum into the interstitial space also enhances the movement of water from the

FIG. 3-2 Capillary net filtration forces.

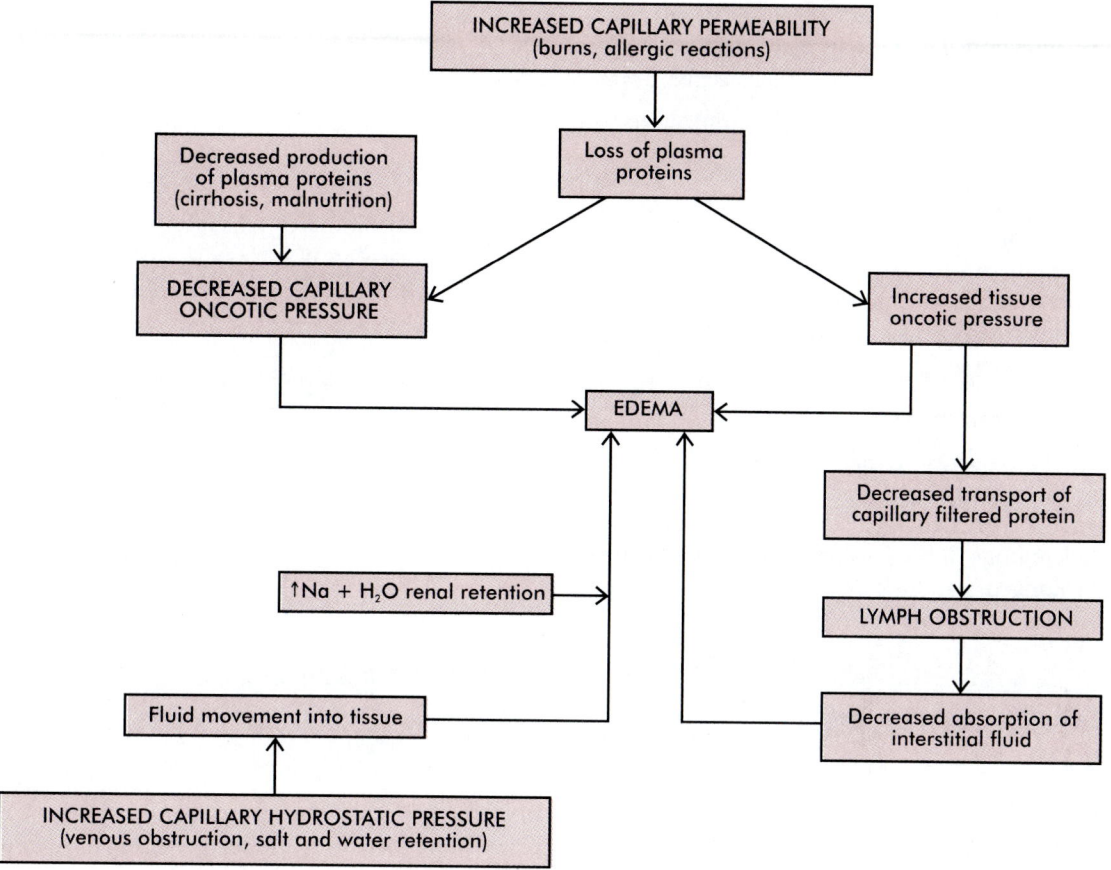

FIG. 3-3 Mechanisms of edema formation.

plasma into the tissues. Losses of plasma proteins occur with glomerular diseases of the kidney, serous drainage from open wounds, hemorrhage, burns, and cirrhosis of the liver.

Increases in capillary permeability are usually associated with inflammation and the immune response. (Immunity is discussed in Chapter 6; inflammation is discussed in Chapter 7.) These responses are often the result of trauma such as burns or crushing injuries, neoplastic disease, and allergic reactions. Proteins then escape from the vascular bed and produce edema through a loss of capillary oncotic pressure and a gain in interstitial fluid proteins.

The lymphatic system normally absorbs interstitial fluid and the small amount of proteins that normally pass across the capillary membrane. When the lymphatic channels are blocked (because of infection) or are surgically removed, proteins and fluid accumulate in the interstitial space. For example, lymphedema of the arm or leg will occur after surgical removal of axillary and femoral lymph nodes for treatment of carcinoma. Inflammation or tumors may be a cause of lymphatic obstruction leading to edema.

Clinical Manifestations

Edema may be localized or generalized. Some localized edema is limited to the site of trauma, as in a sprained finger. Another kind of localized edema is the accumulation of fluid within particular organ systems. This includes cerebral edema, pulmonary edema, pleural effusion, pericardial effusion, and ascites (accumulation of fluid in the peritoneal space). Dependent edema, in which fluid accumulates in gravity-dependent areas of the body, might be a sign of more generalized edema. Dependent edema might appear in the feet and legs when standing and in the sacrum and buttocks when lying down. Dependent edema can be identified by using the fingers to press away edematous fluid in tissues overlying bony prominences. A pit will be left in the skin; hence the term *pitting edema.*

Edema is usually associated with weight gain, swelling and puffiness, tight-fitting clothes and shoes, limited movement of the affected area, and symptoms associated with the underlying pathologic condition. The accumulation of fluid increases the distance required for nutrients and waste to move between capillaries and tissues. Increased tissue pressure may diminish capillary blood flow. Therefore, wounds heal more slowly, and the risks of infection and formation of pressure sores increase. Edema of specific organs, such as the brain, lung, or larynx, can be life-threatening.

Although the accumulation of fluid is excessive, it is trapped in a "third space" and is not available for metabolic processes. Therefore a state of dehydration can develop as a result of the sequestering of the edematous fluid. An example of such sequestration occurs with severe burns, in which large amounts of vascular fluid are lost to the interstitial spaces, reducing plasma volume and causing shock (see Chapter 27).

Evaluation and Treatment

Specific conditions causing edema require diagnosis. Edema may be treated symptomatically until the underlying disorder is corrected. Correction measures include elevating edematous limbs, using support stockings, avoiding prolonged standing, restricting salt intake, or taking diuretics.

SODIUM, CHLORIDE, AND WATER BALANCE

Because water follows the osmotic gradients established by changes in salt concentration, sodium and water balance are intimately related. Water balance is primarily regulated by antidiuretic hormone (ADH; also known as vasopressin); sodium is regulated by aldosterone.

Water Balance

Secretion of ADH and perception of thirst are primary factors in the regulation of water balance. Thirst is a sensation that stimulates water-drinking behavior. Thirst is experienced when water loss equals 2% of an individual's body weight or when there is an increase in osmolality. Dry mouth, hyperosmolality, and plasma volume depletion activate **osmoreceptors** (neurons located in the hypothalamus that are stimulated by increased osmolality). The action of the osmoreceptors then causes thirst. Drinking water restores plasma volume and dilutes the ECF osmolality.

The secretion of ADH is initiated by an increase in plasma osmolality or a decrease in circulating blood volume and a lowered blood pressure. An increase in plasma osmolality occurs with a deficit of water or an excess of sodium in relation to water. The increased osmolality results in decreased extracellular and interstitial fluid volume and stimulates hypothalamic osmoreceptors. In addition to causing thirst, the stimulated osmoreceptors increase the release of ADH from the posterior pituitary gland. The action of ADH is to increase the permeability of renal tubular cells to water, and water is then reabsorbed into the plasma from the distal

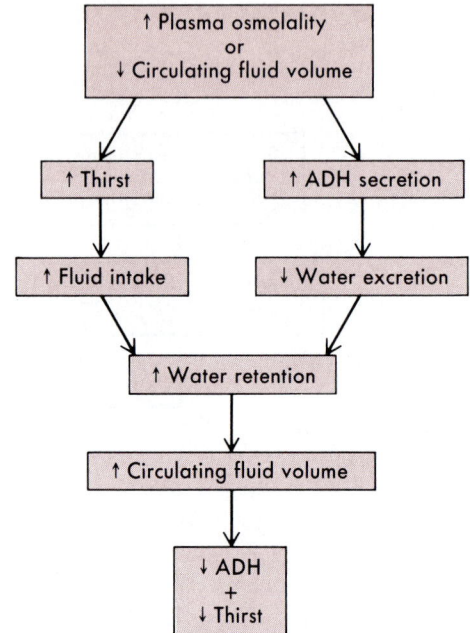

FIG. 3-4 Regulation of thirst and ADH secretion.

tubules and collecting ducts of the kidney. Urine concentration increases, and the reabsorbed water decreases plasma osmolality, returning it toward normal. Like most hormones, ADH is regulated by a feedback mechanism, as illustrated in Fig. 3-4.

With volume depletion, such as dehydration from vomiting, diarrhea, or excessive sweating, **volume-sensitive receptors** and **baroreceptors** (nerve endings that are sensitive to changes in volume and pressure) stimulate release of ADH from the pituitary gland. The volume receptors are located in the right and left atrium and thoracic vessels; baroreceptors are in the aorta and pulmonary arteries, and carotid sinus. Secretion of ADH is caused also by a decrease in atrial pressure, as occurs with decreased blood volume. The reabsorption of water mediated by ADH then promotes the restoration of plasma volume.

Sodium and Chloride Balance

Sodium accounts for 90% of the ECF cations (positively charged ions) and is the most powerful cation in the ECF. (The distribution of electrolytes in body compartments is summarized in Table 3-4.) As the most abundant ECF cation, along with its constituent anions (negatively charged ions) chloride and bicarbonate, sodium regulates osmotic forces and therefore regulates water balance. Sodium has many important body functions, including regulation of osmolality (interstitial and intravascular fluid volume), working with potassium and calcium to maintain neuromuscular irritability for conduction of nerve impulses, regulation of acid-base balance (through sodium bicarbonate and sodium phosphate), participation in cellular chemical reactions, and membrane transport.

Chloride is the major anion in the extracellular fluid. It provides electroneutrality, particularly in relation to sodium. The transport of chloride is generally passive and follows the active transport of sodium, so that increases or decreases in chloride are proportional to changes in sodium. Because bicarbonate is the other major anion in the ECF, the concentration of chloride tends to vary inversely with changes in bicarbonate concentration.

The concentration of sodium is maintained within a narrow range (136 to 145 mEq/L) primarily by the kidney in conjunction with neural and hormonal mediators. The average dietary intake of sodium ranges from 5 to 6 g/day; the minimal daily requirement of sodium is 500 mg. Sweating depletes sodium and water volume and increases the body's sodium requirement.

The kidney regulates sodium primarily through renal tubular reabsorption. Under normal rates of sodium intake, the tubules of the kidney function to reabsorb sodium. With an excess or deficit of sodium in relation to water, a combination of hormonal, neural, and renal mechanisms acts synergistically to control sodium balance.

The hormonal regulation of sodium balance is mediated by **aldosterone**, a mineralocorticoid synthesized and secreted from the adrenal cortex (see Chapter 17). The secretion of aldosterone is influenced by both circulating blood volume and plasma concentrations of Na^+ and K^+ (i.e., aldosterone is secreted when sodium levels are depressed or potassium levels are increased). The action of aldosterone is to increase the reabsorption of sodium and secretion of potassium by the distal tubule of the kidney. As a result, sodium concentration of the ECF is enhanced, and potassium is excreted with the urine.

When circulating blood volume is reduced, **renin**, an enzyme secreted by the juxtaglomerular cells of the kidney, is released in response to sympathetic nerve stimulation and decreased perfusion of the renal vasculature. Renin stimulates the formation of **angiotensin I**, an inactive polypeptide, which is then converted into **angiotensin II**, which acts as a hormone. Angiotensin II has two major functions. It stimulates the secretion of aldosterone, and it causes vasoconstriction. The aldosterone then promotes sodium and water reabsorption. The vasoconstriction elevates the systemic blood pressure and restores renal perfusion. The restoration of sodium levels, fluid volume, and renal perfusion then inhibits the further release of renin. This mechanism of sodium and water regulation is known as the **renin-angiotensin system** (see Chapter 32).

TABLE 3-4

Distribution of Electrolytes in Body Compartments

	Extracellular fluid (mEq/L)	Intracellular fluid (mEq/L)
Cations		
Sodium	142	10
Potassium	5	156
Calcium	5	4
Magnesium	2	26
TOTALS	154	196
Anions		
Bicarbonate	24	12
Chloride	104	4
Phosphate	2	40-95
Proteins	16	54
Other anions	8	31-86
TOTALS	154	196

In addition to sodium regulation by aldosterone, a **natriuretic hormone** (a hormone that promotes urinary excretion of sodium) decreases tubular reabsorption of sodium and causes loss of salt and water. Atrial natriuretic factor is a hormone produced by the atrial muscle of the heart, and one of its functions is renal elimination of sodium for control of sodium and water balance. (It also increases glomerular filtration rate and inhibits aldosterone production and secretion [Rosenzweig & Seidman, 1991]). Natriuretic hormone is sometimes called the "third factor" in sodium regulation. (Increased glomerular filtration rate is thus the "first factor" and aldosterone the "second factor.") The effect of a "third factor" is apparent when there is prolonged elevation of aldosterone from chronic retention of fluid or excessive secretion from an adrenal tumor. In such cases, the sodium-retaining action of aldosterone is overcome, and salt is excreted followed by a water diuresis.

ALTERATIONS IN SODIUM, CHLORIDE, AND WATER BALANCE

Alterations in sodium and water balance are closely related. Water imbalances may develop because of changes in osmotic gradients caused by gain or loss of salt. Likewise, sodium imbalances occur with alterations in body water volume. Generally, the alterations can be classified as changes in tonicity, the change in concen-

TABLE 3-5

Water and Solute Imbalances

Tonicity	Mechanism
Isotonic (isosmolar) imbalance	Gain or loss of ECF resulting in a concentration equivalent to a 0.9% sodium chloride (salt) solution (normal saline); no shrinking or swelling of cells
Hypertonic (hyperosmolar) imbalance	Imbalances that result in an ECF concentration greater than 0.9% salt solution, i.e., water loss or solute gain; cells shrink in a hypertonic fluid
Hypotonic (hypoosmolar) imbalance	Imbalance that results in an ECF less than 0.9% salt solution, i.e., water gain or solute loss; cells swell in a hypotonic fluid

tration of particles in relation to water (see Chapter 1). Alterations can therefore be classified as isotonic, hypertonic, or hypotonic (Table 3-5).

Isotonic Alterations

Isotonic alterations occur when changes in TBW are accompanied by proportional changes in electrolytes. For example, if an individual loses pure plasma or ECF, fluid volume is depleted, but the number and type of electrolytes and the osmolality remain in a normal range. Excessive amounts of isotonic body fluids can result from excessive administration of intravenous normal saline or oversecretion of aldosterone with renal retention of both sodium and water. Losses of isotonic body fluids include hemorrhage, severe wound drainage, and excessive diaphoresis.

Isotonic volume depletion (isotonic dehydration) causes contraction of the ECF volume with weight loss, dryness of skin and mucous membranes, decreased urine output, and symptoms of hypovolemia. Indicators of hypovolemia include a rapid heart rate, flattened neck veins, and normal or decreased blood pressure. In severe states, hypovolemic shock can occur (see Chapter 27).

Isotonic volume excesses are most commonly the result of excessive administration of intravenous fluids, hypersecretion of aldosterone, or the effects of drugs

such as cortisone. As the plasma volume expands, symptoms of hypervolemia develop. There will be weight gain and a decrease in hematocrit and plasma proteins caused by the diluting effect of excess plasma volume. The neck veins may distend, and the blood pressure increases. Increased capillary hydrostatic pressure leads to edema formation. If the plasma volume is great enough, pulmonary edema and heart failure develop.

Hypertonic Alterations

Hypertonic fluid alterations develop when the osmolality of the ECF is elevated above normal. The most common causes are an increased concentration of ECF sodium (hypernatremia) or a deficit of ECF water. In both instances, the hypertonicity of the ECF attracts water from the intracellular space, causing ICF dehydration. A primary increase in ECF sodium causes an osmotic attraction of water and symptoms of hypervolemia. In contrast, a hypertonic state caused primarily by water loss leads to hypovolemia (Table 3-6).

Hypernatremia
Pathophysiology

Hypernatremia occurs when serum sodium levels exceed 147 mEq/L. Excessive serum sodium may be caused by an acute gain in sodium or a loss of water. Sodium gains cause intracellular dehydration; the movement of water to the ECF may cause hypervolemia. With an accompanying water loss, both ICF and ECF dehydration occur. Hyperosmolality is a common result of hypernatremia.

High amounts of dietary sodium rarely cause hypernatremia. More commonly, high sodium levels occur with inappropriate administration of hypertonic saline solution (e.g., as sodium bicarbonate for treatment of acidosis during cardiac arrest), or sodium levels are high because of oversecretion of aldosterone, as in primary hyperaldosteronism, or Cushing syndrome caused by excess secretion of adrenocorticotropic hormone (ACTH), which also causes increased secretion of aldosterone.

Increased sodium in relation to water loss is associated with fever or respiratory infections, which increase the respiratory rate and enhance water loss from the lungs. Diabetes insipidus, diabetes mellitus, polyuria, profuse sweating, and also diarrhea cause water loss in relation to sodium. Infants with severe diarrhea are particularly vulnerable. Insufficient water intake also can cause hypernatremia, particularly in individuals who are comatose, confused, or immobilized.

Clinical Manifestations

Water is redistributed to the extracellular space, and intracellular dehydration ensues. Convulsions and pulmonary edema are the most serious symptoms. Thirst, fe-

TABLE 3-6

Causes and Consequences of Hypertonic Imbalances

Cause	Elevated sodium (hypernatremia)	Water deficit	Other factors
Contributing factors	**Excessive administration of hypertonic salt solutions** Intravenous hypertonic sodium Saline-induced abortions Selected infant formulas Near saltwater drownings **Hyperaldosteronism** **Cushing's syndrome**	**Water deprivation** Confusion or coma Inability to communicate Loss of thirst **Water loss** Watery diarrhea Diabetes insipidus Excessive diuresis Excessive diaphoresis	Hyperglycemia
ECF effects	**Hypervolemia** Weight gain Bounding pulse Increased blood pressure Edema Venous distention **Neuromuscular symptoms** Muscle weakness Seizures	**Hypovolemia** Weight loss Weak pulses Postural hypotension Tachycardia	Initial dilutional hyponatremia Poluria Polydipsia Weight loss Hypovolemia Late hypernatremia
ICF effects	Intracellular dehydration	Intracellular dehydration Thirst Fever Decreased urine output Shrinkage of brain cells: Confusion Coma Cerebral hemorrhage	Intracellular dehydration

ver, dry mucous membranes, and restlessness are associated with hypernatremia as a result of water loss.

Evaluation and Treatment

The serum sodium level is usually above 147 mEq/L. If there is water loss, urine specific gravity will be greater than 1.030, and hematocrit and plasma proteins will be elevated. The treatment of hypernatremia is to give an isotonic salt-free fluid (i.e., 5% dextrose in water) until the serum sodium level returns to normal. Hypervolemia and edema require treatment of the underlying clinical condition.

Water Deficit
Pathophysiology

Dehydration is an appropriate term to describe water deficit, but dehydration is also commonly used to indicate both sodium loss and water loss (isotonic or isoosmolar dehydration). Pure **water deficits** (hyperosmolar or hypertonic dehydration) are rare because most people have access to water. Individuals who are comatose or paralyzed will continue insensible water losses through the skin and lungs with a minimal obligatory formation of urine. Hyperventilation caused by fever also may precipitate water deficit. The most frequent cause of water loss is increased renal clearance of free water as a result of impaired tubular function or inability to concentrate the urine, as with diabetes insipidus (see Chapter 18).

Clinical Manifestations

Marked water deficit is manifested by symptoms of dehydration: thirst, dry skin and mucous membranes, elevated temperature, weight loss, and concentrated urine (with the exception of diabetes insipidus). Skin turgor may be normal or decreased. Symptoms of hypovolemia, including tachycardia, weak pulses, and postural hypotension, may be present.

Evaluation and Treatment

An elevated hematocrit and serum sodium concentration are associated with moderate water loss in addition to clinical signs and symptoms.

Treatment is to give water. When intravenous replacement is required, 5% dextrose in water should be used because pure water lyses red blood cells.

Hyperchloremia

Hyperchloremia occurs clinically when there is an excess of sodium or a deficit of bicarbonate. Greater than normal amounts of chloride can be expected with hypernatremia or metabolic acidosis (See p. 000). Ingestion of excessive chloride infrequently accompanies the use of an ammonium chloride diuretic. There are no specific symptoms associated with chloride deficit.

Alterations in chloride levels are usually secondary to their pathophysiologic processes. Treatment therefore is usually related to management of the underlying disorder.

Hypotonic Alterations

Hypotonic fluid imbalances occur when the osmolality of the ECF is less than normal. The most common causes are sodium deficit (**hyponatremia**) or water excess. Either of these causes leads to an intracellular overhydration (edema). When there is a sodium deficit, the osmotic pressure of the ECF decreases, and water moves into the cell, where the osmotic pressure is greater. The plasma volume then decreases, leading to symptoms of hypovolemia. With a water excess, both the ICF and ECF volume increase, causing symptoms of hypervolemia (Table 3-7).

TABLE 3-7

Causes and Consequences of Hypotonic Imbalances

Cause	Decreased sodium (hyponatremia)	Water excess	Other factors
Contributing factors	Inadequate intake, hypoaldosteronism, excessive diuretic therapy	Excessive pure water intake	Isotonic dehydration treated with intravenous D5W
		Excessive administration of hypotonic intravenous solutions	(Glucose in the D5W solution is metabolized to water, contributing to hyponatremia)
	Furosemide	Drinking water to replace isotonic fluid losses	Nephrotic syndrome
	Ethacrinic acid		Cirrhosis
	Thiazides	Tap water enemas	Cardiac failure
		Psychogenic polydipsia	
		Renal water retention	
		Syndrome of inappropriate antidiuretic hormone (SIADH)	
ECF effects	Hypovolemia (May not be present if there is water excess)	Hypervolemia (May not be present if fluid trapped in intracellular space)	
ICF effects	Edema	Edema	Edema
		Brain cell swelling: irritability, depression, confusion	
		Seizures	
		Coma	
		Systemic cellular edema: weakness, anorexia, nausea, diarrhea	

Hyponatremia
Pathophysiology

Hyponatremia develops when the serum sodium concentration decreases to below 135 mEq/L. Sodium deficits usually cause hypoosmolality with movement of water into cells. Several clinical syndromes may cause hyponatremia. These may be caused by sodium loss, inadequate sodium intake, or dilution of the body's sodium level.

Pure sodium deficits usually are caused by extrarenal losses such as vomiting, diarrhea, gastrointestinal suctioning, or burns. **Inadequate intake** of dietary sodium is rare but can occur in individuals on low-sodium diets, particularly among those taking diuretics. **Dilutional hyponatremias** occur when there is an excess of TBW in relation to total body sodium. Replacement of fluid loss with intravenous 5% dextrose in water also can cause a dilutional hyponatremia once the glucose is metabolized, leaving a hypotonic solution with a diluting effect. Excessive sweating also may stimulate thirst and intake of large amounts of water, which dilute sodium. Hyponatremia also may be hypoosmolar or hypertonic. During acute oliguric renal failure, severe congestive heart failure, or cirrhosis, renal excretion of water is impaired. Both TBW and sodium levels are increased, but TBW exceeds the increase in sodium, producing a **hypoosmolar hyponatremia**. **Hypertonic hyponatremia** develops with hyperlipidemia, hyperproteinemia, and hyperglycemia. Increases in plasma lipids and proteins displace water volume and decrease sodium concentration. Hyperglycemia increases ECF osmolality and attracts water from the ICF compartment. The osmotic fluid shift to the ECF in turn dilutes the concentration of sodium and other electrolytes.

Clinical Manifestations

Deficits of sodium alter the ability of cells to depolarize and repolarize normally (see Chapter 1). Behavioral and neurologic changes characteristic of hyponatremia include lethargy, confusion, apprehension, seizures, and coma. Pure sodium losses may be accompanied by loss of ECF causing an isotonic **hypovolemia** with symptoms of hypotension, tachycardia, and decreased urine output. Weight gain, edema, ascites, and jugular vein distention are characteristic of dilutional hyponatremias.

Evaluation and Treatment

In hyponatremic states, serum sodium concentration falls below 135 mEq/L. With pure sodium deficits, the hematocrit and plasma protein levels may be elevated. Urine specific gravity is less than 1.010 when renal function is normal because sodium is maximally conserved.

Treatment of hyponatremia is related to the contributing disorder. Losses of sodium and water volume are calculated from the clinical evaluation, and appropriate solutions then are selected for replacement. Restriction of water intake is required in most cases of dilutional hyponatremia because body sodium levels may be normal or increased even though serum levels are low. Hypertonic saline solutions are used cautiously with such severe symptoms as seizures.

Water Excess
Pathophysiology

When the body is functioning normally, it is almost impossible to produce an excess of TBW. Some individuals with psychogenic disorders develop water intoxication from **compulsive water drinking**. Acute renal failure, severe congestive heart failure, and cirrhosis are clinical conditions that can precipitate water excess during intravenous infusion of 5% dextrose in water. **Decreased urine formation** from intrinsic renal disease or decreased renal blood flow contributes to water excess. The overall effect is dilution of the ECF with the movement of water to the intracellular space by osmosis. Water excess produces a hypotonic or hypoosmolar water imbalance.

The **syndrome of inappropriate secretion of ADH (SIADH)** is another circumstance contributing to excess water. The syndrome occurs when factors other than hyperosmolality or hypovolemia stimulate the secretion of ADH. Several clinical conditions associated with stress result in SIADH. These include fear, pain, acute infection, brain trauma, surgery, and drugs such as analgesics and anesthetics. The most common cause is bronchogenic cancer. Syndrome of inappropriate secretion of ADH is not caused by excess water intake but by decreased renal excretion of water. Therefore, the presence of SIADH increases the risk of water excess if intravenous fluids are being administered. Serum sodium and osmolality are reduced. The kidney continues to excrete sodium and urine specific gravity is elevated, but urine volume is decreased.

Clinical Manifestations

The symptoms of water excess are related to the rate at which water loading has occurred. Acute excesses cause confusion and convulsions. Weakness, nausea, muscle twitching, headache, and weight gain are common symptoms of chronic water accumulation.

Evaluation and Treatment

Serum sodium concentration can be decreased, but this also can occur with a pure sodium deficit. Serum osmolality is decreased because water will be in excess of sodium. The hematocrit therefore is reduced from the dilutional effect of water excess.

Withholding fluid for 24 hours is effective treatment

if there are no convulsions. Small amounts of intravenous hypertonic sodium chloride can be given when symptoms are severe.

Hypochloremia

Loss of chloride, **hypochloremia**, is usually the result of hyponatremia or elevated bicarbonate concentration, as in metabolic alkalosis (see p. 116). Hypochloremia develops with vomiting and loss of hydrochloric acid. Sodium deficit related to restricted intake or use of diuretics is accompanied by chloride deficiency. Cystic fibrosis, for example, is also characterized by hypochloremia. As with hyperchloremia, treatment of the underlying condition is required.

ALTERATIONS IN POTASSIUM, CALCIUM, PHOSPHATE, AND MAGNESIUM BALANCE

Potassium

Potassium is the major intracellular electrolyte and contributes to many important cellular functions. Total body potassium content is about 4000 mEq, with most of it located in the cells. Daily dietary intake of potassium is 40 to 150 mEq/day, with an average of 1.5 mEq/kg body weight. The ICF concentration of K^+ is 150 to 160 mEq/L; the ECF concentration is 3.5 to 4.5 mEq/L.

The difference in the concentration is maintained by a sodium-potassium active transport system (Na^+, K^+ ATPase pump). The ratio of ECF K^+ to ICF K^+ is the major determinant of the resting membrane potential, which is necessary for the transmission of nerve impulses. (Membrane transport and membrane potentials are discussed in Chapter 1.) Changes in the ratio of ICF to ECF potassium are responsible for many of the symptoms associated with potassium imbalance.

Potassium is necessary for a variety of metabolic functions. As the predominant ICF ion, it exerts a major influence in the regulation of ICF osmolality and provides the balance for intracellular electrical neutrality in relation to H^+ and Na^+. Potassium is required for glycogen deposition in liver and skeletal muscle cells. The significant role of potassium in maintaining the resting membrane potential is reflected in transmission and conduction of nerve impulses, maintenance of normal cardiac rhythms, and skeletal and smooth muscle contraction.

Generally, the amount of K^+ excreted varies in proportion to the dietary intake (40 to 120 mEq/day). Although potassium is found in most body fluids (Table 3-8), the kidney provides the most efficient regulation of potassium balance. Potassium is freely filtered by the renal glomerulus, and 90% is reabsorbed by the proximal tubule and loop of Henle. The distal tubule secretes potassium and determines the amount of K^+ excreted from the body. The transport is passive, so that principles of passive transport govern K^+ excretion. Unlike sodium, however, the renal mechanism for conserving K^+ is weak, even when total body potassium stores are depleted.

Several factors related to passive transport and aldosterone contribute to renal regulation of potassium. These factors include the concentration gradients for potassium at the distal tubule and collecting duct, changes in pH (causing acidosis or alkalosis), changes in electrical potential differences across the distal tubule, and aldosterone levels. (Renal mechanisms are described in more detail in Chapter 32.)

The concentration of potassium in the distal tubular cell is primarily determined by the plasma concentration in the peritubular capillaries. When plasma K^+ concentration increases from increased dietary intake or shifts of K^+ from the ICF occur, potassium is secreted into the urine by the distal tubules. Decreases in plasma potassium result in decreased distal tubular secretion, although approximately 5 to 15 mEq of K^+/day will continue to be lost. Changes in the rate of filtrate flow through the distal tubule also influence the concentration gradient for K^+ secretion. When the flow rate is high, as occurs with the administration of diuretics, the concentration of potassium in the distal tubular urine will be lower, favoring the secretion of potassium.

TABLE 3-8

Approximate Concentration of Electrolytes in Body Fluids

Fluid	Na^+ (mEq/L)	K^+ (mEq/L)	Cl^- (mEq/L)	HCO_3^- (mEq/L)
Saliva	33	20	34	0
Gastric juice*	60	9	84	0
Bile	149	5	101	45
Pancreatic juice	141	5	77	92
Ileal fluid	129	11	116	29
Cecal fluid	80	21	48	22
Cerebrospinal fluid	141	3	127	23
Sweat	45	5	58	0

From Smith, L.H., & Thier, S.O. (1981). *Pathophysiology: The biological principles of disease.* Philadelphia: W.B. Saunders. Adapted from Arieff, A. In Maxwell, M.H., & Kleeman, C.R. (Eds.). (1972). *Clinical disorders of fluid and electrolyte metabolism* (2nd ed.). New York: McGraw-Hill.
*The Cl concentration exceeds the Na^+, K^+ concentration by 15 mEq/L in gastric juice. This largely represents the secretion of H^+ by the parietal cells.

Changes in pH and thus in hydrogen ion concentration also can affect K^+ balance. Hydrogen ions accumulate in the ICF during states of acidosis. Intracellular fluid levels of hydrogen are diminished during states of alkalosis. During acidosis, potassium shifts out of the cell to the ECF to maintain a balance of cations across the cell membrane. The decreased ICF K^+ results in decreased secretion of K^+ by the distal tubular cells, contributing to hyperkalemia. In contrast, alkalosis causes potassium to shift into the cell, so that the distal tubular cells increase their secretion of K^+, contributing to hypokalemia.

Besides acting to conserve sodium, aldosterone is a major factor in potassium regulation. When potassium concentration is increased, aldosterone is released, stimulating secretion of potassium into the urine by the distal tubules of the kidney. Aldosterone also increases the secretion of K^+ from the sweat glands.

Insulin contributes to the regulation of plasma potassium levels by promoting the movement of potassium into liver and muscle cells. Insulin therefore can be used to treat hyperkalemia, and dangerously low levels of plasma potassium can result from the administration of insulin when potassium levels are depressed. Potassium balance is especially significant in the treatment of conditions requiring insulin administration, such as insulin-dependent diabetes.

An interesting aspect of K^+ regulation is the ability of the body to adapt to increased levels of potassium intake over time. A sudden increase in potassium may be fatal, but if the intake of potassium is slowly increased by amounts greater than 120 mEq/day, the kidney is able to increase the urinary excretion of potassium and maintain potassium balance. This tolerance to increasing amounts of potassium is known as **potassium adaptation**.

Hypokalemia
Pathophysiology

Potassium deficiency, or **hypokalemia**, develops when the serum potassium concentration decreases to below 3.5 mEq/L. Because cellular and total body stores of potassium are difficult to measure, changes in potassium balance are described by the plasma concentration, although changes in total body potassium are not always reflected in the plasma potassium concentration. Generally, the lowered serum potassium indicates a loss of total body potassium. Because potassium is lost from the ECF, the change in the concentration gradient favors movement of K^+ from the cell to the ECF. The ICF/ECF concentration ratio is maintained, but total body K^+ is depleted.

Extracellular fluid hypokalemia can, however, develop without losses of total body potassium. For example, potassium shifts into the cell during states of re-

spiratory or metabolic alkalosis or after administration of insulin. In the event of alkalosis, K^+ shifts into the cell in exchange for H^+ to maintain plasma acid-base balance. Insulin also promotes cellular uptake of K^+, causing a deficit in ECF potassium.

Plasma K^+ levels may be normal or elevated when total body potassium is depleted. In such instances, potassium shifts from the ICF to the ECF. One of the common causes of this problem is diabetic ketoacidosis in which the increased hydrogen ion concentration in the ECF causes H^+ to shift into the cell in exchange for potassium. A normal level of potassium is maintained in the plasma, but potassium continues to be lost in the urine, causing a deficit in total body potassium. Severe, even fatal, hypokalemia may occur if insulin is administered without also providing potassium supplements. Thus total body potassium depletion becomes evident when insulin treatment is initiated.

Potassium loss also occurs through normal body functions without causing hypokalemia. Average daily losses of potassium are as follows:

Location	Daily loss (mEq/L)
Stool	5-10
Sweat	0-20
Kidney	40-120

Factors contributing to the development of hypokalemia include reduced intake of potassium, increased entry of potassium into cells, and increased losses of body potassium. Dietary deficiency of potassium is a rare cause of hypokalemia. It may occur in elderly individuals with both low protein intake and inadequate intake of fruits and vegetables and in those with alcoholism or anorexia nervosa. Generally, reduced potassium intake becomes a problem when combined with other causes of potassium depletion.

Shifts of potassium from the extracellular to intracellular space cause apparent deficits in total body potassium. Alkalosis, particularly respiratory alkalosis, is the most common clinical problem. Extracellular fluid potassium will exchange with ICF hydrogen and correct the alkalosis by increasing the pH of the ECF. Treatment of pernicious anemia with vitamin B_{12} or folate also may precipitate hypokalemia if the formation of new red blood cells causes enough potassium uptake to cause an extracellular decrease in potassium. Familial hypokalemic periodic paralysis is a rare genetically transmitted disease that also causes potassium to shift into the intracellular space.

Losses of potassium from body stores are most commonly caused by gastrointestinal and renal disorders. Diarrhea (from any cause), intestinal drainage tubes or fistulae, and laxative abuse also may result in hypokalemia. Normally, only 5 to 10 mEq of potassium and 100 to 150 ml of water are excreted in the stool each day. With diarrhea, fluid and electrolyte losses can be voluminous, with several liters of fluid and 100 to 200 mEq of potassium lost per day. Vomiting or continuous nasogastric suction frequently is associated with potassium depletion, partly because of the potassium lost from the gastric fluid, but principally because of renal compensation for volume depletion and the metabolic alkalosis (elevated bicarbonate levels) that occurs from sodium, chloride, and hydrogen ion losses. The loss of fluid and sodium stimulates the secretion of aldosterone, which in turn causes renal losses of potassium. The elevated flow of bicarbonate at the distal tubule contributes to renal excretion of potassium because of increased tubular lumen electronegativity.

Renal losses of potassium are related to increased secretion of potassium by the distal tubule. Use of diuretics, excessive aldosterone secretion, increased distal tubular flow rate, and low plasma magnesium concentration all may contribute to urinary losses of potassium. Many diuretics, including thiazides, furosemide, ethacrynic acid, and osmotic diuretics, inhibit the reabsorption of sodium chloride, causing the diuretic effect. The distal tubular flow rate then increases, promoting potassium secretion. If sodium loss is severe, the compensating aldosterone secretion (which causes secondary hyperaldosteronism) may further deplete potassium stores. Primary hyperaldosteronism with excessive secretion of aldosterone from an adrenal adenoma also causes potassium wasting. Many kidney diseases result in a reduced ability to conserve sodium. The disordered sodium reabsorption produces a diuretic effect, and the increased distal tubule flow rate favors the secretion of potassium. Magnesium deficits stimulate renin release and hyperaldosteronism causing hypokalemia. Several antibiotics, including amphotericin B, gentamicin, and carbenicillin, are known to cause hypokalemia.

Clinical Manifestations

A wide range of metabolic dysfunctions may result from potassium deficiency. Carbohydrate metabolism is affected because hypokalemia depresses insulin secretion and alters hepatic and skeletal muscle glycogen synthesis. Renal function is impaired, with a decreased ability to concentrate urine. Polyuria (increased urine) and polydipsia (increased thirst) are associated with decreased responsiveness to ADH. Chronic potassium deficits lasting more than 1 month may damage renal tissue, with interstitial fibrosis and tubular atrophy.

Neuromuscular and cardiac effects of hypokalemia produce the most common symptoms. Neuromuscular excitability is decreased, causing skeletal muscle weakness, smooth muscle atony, and cardiac dysrhythmias. As Chapter 1 describes, the resting membrane potential (E_m) is determined by the *ratio* of extracellular to intracellular potassium ion concentration. Because the concentration of potassium in the ECF is small, only small changes in ECF potassium are required to influence the resting membrane potential and affect neuromuscular excitability. When extracellular potassium levels decrease rapidly and intracellular potassium concentration does not change, the resting membrane potential becomes more negative, and the cell membrane is **hyperpolarized**. If the threshold potential (E_t) remains stable, the difference between resting membrane potential and threshold potential increases, requiring a stronger stimulus to initiate an action potential (Fig. 3-5).

Factors such as calcium concentration and pH also contribute to the changes in neuromuscular excitability associated with hypokalemia. Increases in ECF calcium concentration tend to make the threshold potential less negative and decrease membrane excitability, potentiating the neuromuscular effects of hypokalemia.

The onset of symptoms is related to the rate of potassium depletion. Because the body can accommodate slow losses of potassium, the decrease in ECF concentration may be slow enough to allow potassium to shift from the intracellular space. The extracellular to intracellular potassium concentration gradient then is restored toward normal, with less severe neuromuscular changes. With acute losses of potassium, changes in neuromuscular excitability are more profound. Skeletal muscle weakness initially occurs in the larger muscles of the legs and arms and ultimately affects the diaphragm and depresses ventilation. Paralysis and respiratory arrest then can occur. Loss of smooth muscle tone is manifested by constipation, intestinal distention, anorexia, nausea, vomiting, and paralytic ileus.

The cardiac effects of hypokalemia are related also to changes in membrane excitability (see Fig. 3-5). Because potassium contributes to the repolarization phase of the action potential, hypokalemia delays ventricular repolarization. A variety of dysrhythmias may occur, including sinus bradycardia, atrioventricular block, and paroxysmal atrial tachycardia. The characteristic changes in the electrocardiogram reflect delayed repolarization. For instance, the amplitude of the T wave is decreased; the amplitude of the U wave is increased; and the S-T segment is depressed (Fig. 3-6). In severe states of hypokalemia, there is peaking of the P waves and prolonging of the QRS complex. Hypokalemia also increases the risk of digitalis toxicity.

Evaluation and Treatment

The diagnosis of hypokalemia is significantly related to the medical history and the identification of disorders associated with potassium loss. Treatment involves an estimation of total body potassium losses and correction of acid-base imbalances. Further losses of potassium should be prevented, and the individual should be encouraged to eat foods rich in potassium. The maxi-

FIG. 3-5 Effects of potassium and calcium on membrane excitability. (Modified from Leaf & Cotran, 1985.)

mal rate of oral replacement is 40 to 80 mEq/day if renal function is normal. A maximal safe rate of intravenous replacement is 20 mEq/hour. Because potassium is irritating to blood vessels, a maximal concentration of 40 mEq/L should be used. Serum potassium values can be monitored until normokalemia is achieved.

Hyperkalemia
Pathophysiology

An elevation of ECF potassium *above 5.5 mEq/L* constitutes **hyperkalemia**. Because of efficient renal excretion, increases in total body potassium are relatively rare. Acute increases in serum potassium are handled quickly through an increase in cellular uptake and renal excretion of body potassium excesses. Excretion is partially mediated by the secretion of aldosterone, because it facilitates losses of potassium in the urine.

Excesses of potassium may be caused by increased intake, a shift of potassium from cells to the ECF, or decreased renal excretion. If renal function is normal, slow, chronic increases in potassium intake are usually well tolerated through potassium adaptation, although acute potassium loading can exceed renal excretion rates. Use of stored whole blood and intravenous boluses of penicillin G or replacement potassium can precipitate hyperkalemia, particularly if renal function is impaired. Dietary excesses of potassium are uncommon, but accidental ingestion of potassium salt substitutes can cause toxicity.

Movement of potassium from the ICF to ECF occurs with cell trauma or change in cell membrane permeability, acidosis, insulin deficiency, or cell hypoxia. Burns,

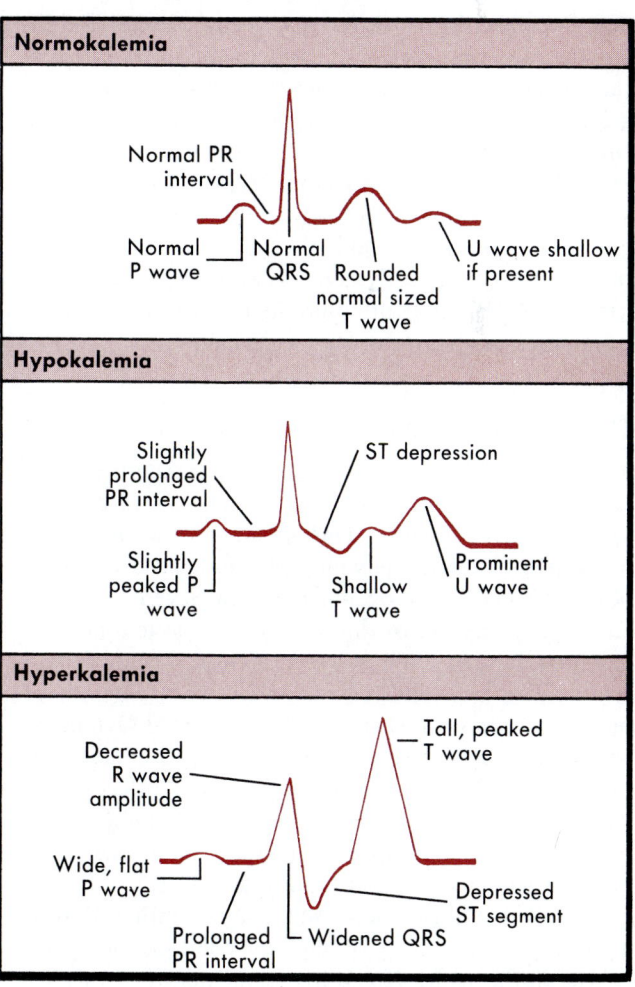

FIG. 3-6 ECG changes with potassium imbalance.

massive crushing injuries, and extensive surgeries can cause loss of potassium to the ECF. If renal function is sustained, potassium will be excreted. As cell repair begins, hypokalemia develops without an adequate intake of potassium.

In states of acidosis, hydrogen ions shift into the cells in exchange for ICF potassium and sodium; hyperkalemia and acidosis therefore often occur together. Because insulin promotes cellular entry of potassium, insulin deficits, which occur with such conditions as diabetic ketoacidosis, are accompanied by hyperkalemia. Hypoxia can lead to hyperkalemia by diminishing the efficiency of cell membrane active transport, resulting in the escape of potassium to the ECF. Digitalis overdose may cause hyperkalemia by inhibiting the sodium-potassium ATPase pump, which maintains high intracellular potassium and high extracellular sodium (see Chapter 1).

Decreased renal excretion of potassium is commonly associated with hyperkalemia. Renal failure that results in oliguria (urine output less than 30 ml/hr) is accompanied by elevations of serum potassium. The severity of hyperkalemia is related to the amount of potassium intake, the degree of acidosis, and the rate of cell damage. Decreases in the secretion or renal effects of aldosterone also can cause decreases in the urinary excretion of potassium. For example, Addison's disease results in decreased production and secretion of aldosterone and thus contributes to hyperkalemia. Potassium-sparing diuretics (such as spironolactone, which inhibits sodium reabsorption) and potassium and hydrogen secretion by the distal tubule also may contribute to hyperkalemia. (Frequently, however, these diuretics are used in combination with diuretics that cause potassium wasting in an attempt to balance renal potassium gains and losses.)

Clinical Manifestations

Symptoms of hyperkalemia vary, but common characteristics are muscle weakness or paralysis and changes in the electrocardiogram. During mild attacks, increased neuromuscular irritability may be manifested as restlessness, intestinal cramping, and diarrhea. Severe hyperkalemia causes muscle weakness, loss of muscle tone, and paralysis. In mild states of hyperkalemia, the more rapid repolarization is reflected in the electrocardiogram as narrow and taller T waves with a shortened Q-T interval. Severe hyperkalemia depresses the S-T segment, prolongs the P-R interval, and widens the QRS complex (see Fig. 3-6). Bradyarrhythmias are common in hyperkalemia with alterations in cardiac conduction causing ventricular fibrillation or cardiac arrest.

As with hypokalemia, changes in the ratio of intracellular to extracellular potassium concentration contribute to the symptoms of hyperkalemia. If extracellular potassium concentration increases without a significant change in intracellular potassium, the resting membrane potential decreases, and the cell membrane is **hypopolarized** (the inside of the cell becomes less negative or partially depolarized). (Electrical properties of cells are discussed in Chapter 1.) With relatively mild elevations in extracellular potassium, the cell more rapidly repolarizes and becomes more irritable. An action potential then is initiated more rapidly because the distance between the resting membrane potential and the threshold potential has been shortened. With more severe hyperkalemia, the resting membrane potential approaches or exceeds the threshold potential. In this case, the cell is not able to repolarize and therefore does not respond to excitation stimuli. The most serious consequence is cardiac standstill.

Like the effects of hypokalemia, the neuromuscular effects of hyperkalemia are related to the rate of increase in the ECF potassium concentration and the presence of other contributing factors such as acidosis and calcium balance. Chronic increases in ECF potassium concentration result in shifts of potassium into the cell, because the tendency is to maintain a normal ratio of intracellular/extracellular potassium concentrations. Acute elevations of extracellular potassium affect neuromuscular irritability as this ratio is disrupted.

Because calcium influences the threshold potential, changes in extracellular fluid calcium concentration can augment or override the effects of hyperkalemia. With hypocalcemia, the threshold potential becomes more negative, enhancing the neuromuscular effects of hyperkalemia. Hypercalcemia causes the threshold potential to become less negative, counteracting the effects of hyperkalemia (see Fig. 3-5).

Evaluation and Treatment

Hyperkalemia should be investigated when there is a history of renal disease, massive trauma, insulin deficiency, Addison's disease, use of potassium salt substitutes, or metabolic acidosis. The acuity of the onset of symptoms may be related to the underlying cause.

Management of hyperkalemia is related to treating the contributing causes and correcting the potassium excess. Normalizing the extracellular potassium concentration can be achieved with a variety of methods; the treatment chosen is related to the cause and severity of the problem. Calcium gluconate can be administered to restore normal neuromuscular irritability when serum potassium levels are dangerously high. Administration of insulin and glucose facilitates cellular entry of potassium, and sodium bicarbonate corrects metabolic acidosis and lowers serum potassium. Oral or rectal administration of cation exchange resins, which exchange sodium for potassium in the intestine, can be effective. Dialysis effectively removes potassium when there is renal failure.

Calcium and Phosphate

The total body content of calcium is about 1200 g. Most calcium (99%) is located in bone as hydroxyapatite (an inorganic compound that contributes to bone rigidity), and the remainder is in the plasma and body cells. Of the calcium in the plasma, 50% is bound to plasma proteins (2.5 mEq/L); about 40% is in the free or ionized form (2.4 mEq/L). The total fraction of calcium circulating in the blood is small (4.5 to 5.5 mEq/L, 8.6 to 10.5 mg/dl). Ionized calcium has the most important physiologic functions.

Calcium is a necessary ion for many fundamental metabolic processes. It is the major cation for the structure of bone and teeth. It serves as an enzymatic cofactor for blood clotting and is required for hormone secretion and the function of cell receptors. Plasma membrane stability and permeability are directly related to calcium ions, as is the transmission of nerve impulses and the contraction of muscles.

Phosphate is found primarily in bone, with smaller amounts within the intracellular and extracellular spaces. In the serum, phosphate exists in phospholipids and phosphate esters and as inorganic phosphate, which is the ionized form. The normal serum levels of inorganic phosphate range from 2.5 to 4.5 mg/dl and may be as high as 6.0 to 7.0 mg/dl in infants and young children. Intracellular phosphate has many metabolic forms, including the high-energy structures, creatine phosphate, and adenosine triphosphate (ATP). Phosphate acts as an intracellular and extracellular anion buffer in the regulation of acid-base balance; in the form of ATP it provides energy for muscle contraction.

Calcium and phosphate concentrations are rigidly controlled. They are related by the product of calcium and phosphate, which is a constant ($Ca^{++} \times HPO_4^{=} = K$). Thus, if the concentration of one ion increases, that of the other decreases.

Calcium and phosphate balance is mediated by the interaction among three hormones: parathyroid hormone (PTH), vitamin D, and calcitonin. Acting together, these substances determine the amount of dietary calcium and phosphate absorbed from the intestine, the deposition and absorption of calcium and phosphate from the bone, and the renal reabsorption and excretion of calcium and phosphate by the kidney.

The parathyroid glands are sensitive to changes in serum calcium concentrations. The parathyroid glands secrete PTH in response to low serum calcium. Parathyroid hormone initiates renal activation of vitamin D. (The specific actions of PTH in relation to calcium and phosphorus are described in Chapter 17.)

The renal regulation of calcium and phosphate balance requires PTH. As PTH secretion is stimulated by low levels of serum calcium, there is increased reabsorption of calcium along the distal part of the nephron and inhibition of phosphate resorption by the proximal segment of the nephron. The net result is an increase in serum calcium and urinary excretion of phosphate. Fig. 3-7 summarizes hormonal regulation of calcium.

Another hormone important to calcium and phosphate regulation is vitamin D. Vitamin D (cholecalciferol) is a fat-soluble steroid ingested in food or synthesized in the skin in the presence of ultraviolet light. Several steps of activation are required before vitamin D can act at target tissues. The first step occurs in the liver; final activation is in the kidney. The renal activation of vitamin D begins when the serum calcium level decreases and stimulates secretion of PTH. Parathyroid hormone then acts to increase calcium reabsorption and enhance renal excretion of phosphate, producing decreased phosphate levels. The combination of low calcium, PTH secretion, and low phosphate thus causes the renal activation of vitamin D. The activated vitamin D then circulates in the plasma and acts to increase ab-

FIG. 3-7 Hormonal regulation of calcium balance.

sorption of calcium in the small intestine. When there is renal failure, vitamin D will not be activated; serum calcium levels will decrease; and phosphate levels increase.

The exchange of calcium and phosphate between serum and bone is regulated also by hormones. When serum calcium levels are low, PTH and vitamin D stimulate the osteoclasts in bone to resorb bone and release calcium and phosphate into the plasma. As calcium levels increase above 12 mg/dl, the thyroid hormone calcitonin opposes the action of PTH and lowers the serum calcium level by stimulating osteoblasts to deposit calcium and form new bone. When calcium levels are low, the secretion of calcitonin is suppressed.

The fractions of serum calcium that are freely ionized or bound to plasma proteins are influenced by pH. In states of acidosis, there is an increase in levels of ionized calcium. When alkalosis develops, with an increase in pH, there is an increase in protein-bound calcium and a decrease in the physiologically active, ionized calcium. The decreased concentration of ionized calcium may be great enough to cause symptoms of hypocalcemia, such as tetany.

Hypocalcemia
Pathophysiology

Hypocalcemia occurs when serum calcium concentrations are lower than 8.5 mg/dl. Deficits in calcium are related to inadequate intestinal absorption, deposition of ionized calcium into bone or soft tissue, blood administration, or decreases in PTH and vitamin D.

Nutritional deficiencies of calcium can occur with inadequate sources of dairy products or green leafy vegetables. Excessive amounts of dietary phosphorus also bind with calcium, so that neither mineral is absorbed. Blood transfusions are also a common cause of hypocalcemia because the citrate solution used in storing whole blood binds with calcium. Pancreatitis causes release of lipases into soft tissue spaces, so that the free fatty acids that are formed bind calcium, causing decrease in ionized calcium. Neoplastic bone metastases tend to inhibit bone resorption and increase calcium deposition into bone, thereby decreasing serum calcium levels.

Vitamin D deficiency, which can result from inadequate intake or avoidance of sunlight, causes decreased intestinal absorption of calcium. Malabsorption of fat, including fat-soluble vitamin D, may also contribute to calcium deficiency. Removal of the parathyroid glands with the resulting loss of PTH also causes hypocalcemia. Metabolic or respiratory alkalosis causes symptoms of hypocalcemia because the change in pH enhances protein binding of ionized calcium.

Clinical Manifestations

The clinical manifestations of hypocalcemia are primarily caused by an increase in neuromuscular excitability.

Calcium deficits cause partial depolarization of nerves and muscle from a decrease in the threshold potential to a level close to resting membrane potential (see Fig. 3-5). Therefore, a smaller stimulus is required for initiating the action potential. The symptoms include confusion, paresthesias around the mouth and in the digits, carpopedal spasm (muscle spasms in the hands and feet), and hyperreflexia.

Two clinical signs are Chvostek's sign and Trousseau's sign. Chvostek's sign is elicited by tapping on the facial nerve just below the temple. A positive sign is a twitch of the nose or lip. Trousseau's sign is contraction of the hand and fingers when the arterial blood flow in the arm is occluded for 5 minutes.

Severe symptoms include convulsions and tetany, a continuous severe muscle spasm that can interfere with breathing and cause death. The characteristic electrocardiographic (ECG) change is a prolonged Q-T interval, indicating prolonged ventricular depolarization. Intestinal cramping and hyperactive bowel sounds also may be present because hypocalcemia affects the smooth muscles of the gastrointestinal tract.

Evaluation and Treatment

The health history may signify underlying pathologic conditions that require further evaluation and treatment. Severe symptoms of hypocalcemia require emergency treatment with intravenous 10% calcium gluconate. Oral calcium replacement should be initiated, and serum calcium levels should be monitored. Decreasing phosphate intake facilitates long-term management of hypocalcemia.

Hypercalcemia
Pathophysiology

Hypercalcemia with serum calcium concentrations exceeding 12 mg/dl can be caused by a number of diseases. The most common among these are hyperparathyroidism; bone metastases with calcium resorption from breast, prostate, and cervical cancer; sarcoidosis; and excess vitamin D. Many tumors produce PTH and elevate the serum calcium levels. Sarcoidosis appears to increase vitamin D levels.

Clinical Manifestations

Many of the symptoms of hypercalcemia are nonspecific. Because serum calcium levels are increased, a greater amount of calcium is also contained inside the cells. The threshold potential becomes more positive, and the cell membrane becomes refractory to depolarization. Thus many of the symptoms are related to loss of cell membrane excitability. (Membrane potentials and membrane excitability are discussed in Chapter 1.) Fatigue, weakness, lethargy, anorexia, nausea, and constipation are common. Impaired renal function frequently develops, and kidney stones form as precipitates of calcium salts. A shortened Q-T segment and depressed T waves also may be observed on the ECG.

Evaluation and Treatment

With elevated serum calcium levels, there is often a reciprocal decrease in serum phosphate values. Specific diagnostic procedures to identify the contributing pathologic condition are required.

Treatment is related to severity of symptoms and the underlying disease. When renal function is normal, oral phosphate administration is effective. When there is acute illness and high calcium levels, intravenous administration of large amounts of normal saline will enhance renal excretion of calcium. Corticosteroids and the cytotoxic drug mithramycin also are used to treat hypercalcemia. Ultimately, the underlying pathologic condition must be treated.

Hypophosphatemia
Pathophysiology

Hypophosphatemia is a serum phosphate level lower than 2.0 mg/dl and is usually an indication of phosphate deficiency. In some conditions, total body phosphate is normal, but serum volumes are low. The most common causes are intestinal malabsorption and increased renal excretion of phosphate. Inadequate absorption is associated with vitamin D deficiency, use of magnesium- and aluminum-containing antacids (which bind with phosphorus), chronic alcohol abuse, and malabsorption syndromes. Respiratory alkalosis can cause severe hypophosphatemia because of cellular use of phosphorus for an accelerated glucose metabolism. Increased renal excretion of phosphorus is associated with hyperparathyroidism.

Clinical Manifestations

The consequences of phosphate deficiency are related to reduced capacity for oxygen transport by red blood cells and to disturbed energy metabolism. Transport and release of oxygen are associated with 2,3-diphosphoglycerate (2,3-DPG) and ATP. When phosphate is depleted, 2,3-DPG and ATP levels become low and diminish release of oxygen to the tissues. The oxyhemoglobin curve shifts to the left (see Chapter 29), and hypoxia can occur.

Leukocyte and platelet dysfunction are also associated with hypophosphatemia. There is greater risk of infection and blood-clotting impairment, with potential for hemorrhage. Nerve and muscle function can be affected with derangement in energy metabolism. Irritability, confusion, numbness, coma, and convulsions develop with severe phosphate losses. Muscle weakness may become serious enough to cause respiratory failure, and cardiomyopathies also can develop. In response to low phosphate levels, bone resorption occurs and may lead to rickets or osteomalacia.

Evaluation and Treatment

To correct the condition, the underlying cause must be identified and treated. Although serum phosphate levels are below normal, the administration of phosphate salts is dangerous, and low phosphate levels are usually not considered life-threatening.

Hyperphosphatemia
Pathophysiology

Hyperphosphatemia, or an elevated serum phosphate level above 4.5 mg/dl, develops with acute or chronic renal failure with significant loss of glomerular filtration. Because most phosphate is located in cells, the cell destruction associated with treatment of metastatic tumors with chemotherapy can release large amounts of phosphate into the serum. Chronic use of phosphate-containing enemas or laxatives also may lead to hyperphosphatemia. Hyperparathyroidism can cause elevated phosphate by increasing renal tubular reabsorption of phosphate.

High levels of serum phosphate also lower serum calcium levels, and increased amounts of phosphate and calcium are deposited in bone and soft tissues. Serum calcium levels may become low enough to cause symptoms of hypocalcemia, including tetany.

Clinical Manifestations

Symptoms of hyperphosphatemia are primarily related to low serum calcium levels and thus are comparable to symptoms of hypocalcemia. With prolonged hyperphosphatemia, calcification of soft tissues occurs in the lungs, kidneys, and joints.

Evaluation and Treatment

To correct the condition, the underlying pathologic condition must be identified and treated. Aluminum hydroxide may be administered because it binds phosphate in the gastrointestinal tract and is eliminated. Dialysis is required for management of renal failure.

Magnesium

Magnesium (Mg^{++}) is a major intracellular cation. About 40% to 60% is stored in muscle and bone. Plasma concentration is 1.8 to 2.4 mEq/L with about one third bound to plasma proteins. Regulation of magnesium metabolism is not well understood. Low serum magnesium appears to have a direct effect on the kidney to cause conservation of magnesium. Magnesium is a cofactor in intracellular enzymatic reactions and is a cause of neuromuscular excitability. Calcium and magnesium often interact in reactions at the cellular level.

Hypomagnesemia, a rare condition in which serum magnesium concentration is less than 1.5 mEq/L, increases neuromuscular excitability and can be a cause of tetany. Malnutrition, malabsorption syndromes, alcoholism, renal tubular dysfunction, and thiazide diuretics can cause magnesium losses. Symptoms of hypomagnesemia are similar to those of hypocalcemia. Behavioral changes, irritability, increased reflexes, muscle weakness, ataxia, nystagmus, tetany, and convulsions may be observed. Treatment is intramuscular or intravenous administration of magnesium sulfate.

Hypermagnesemia, in which concentration is greater than 2.5 mEq/L, is rare and usually is caused by renal failure. Magnesium-containing antacids (e.g., Gaviscon, Gelusil) can potentiate excess magnesium. Excess magnesium depresses skeletal muscle contraction and nerve function. Symptoms include nausea and vomiting, muscle weakness, hypotension, bradycardia, and respiratory depression (Kokko & Tanner, 1990). Treatment is avoidance of magnesium-containing substances and removal by dialysis.

ACID-BASE BALANCE

Hydrogen ion concentration must be regulated within a narrow range for the body to function normally. Slight changes in amounts of hydrogen can significantly alter biologic processes in cells and tissues. Hydrogen ion is necessary to maintain membrane integrity and the speed of enzymatic reactions. Most pathologic conditions disturb acid-base balance, and the degree of severity may be more harmful than the disease process.

Hydrogen Ion and pH

The hydrogen ion concentration $[H^+]$ is commonly expressed as the pH, the negative logarithm of hydrogen ions in solution. The logarithmic value means that as the pH changes one unit (e.g., 7.0 to 6.0), the $[H^+]$ changes tenfold. The relationship is commonly expressed as follows:

$$pH = \log \frac{1}{[H^+]}$$

or

$$pH = -\log[H^+]$$

As the $[H^+]$ increases, the pH decreases; likewise, as the $[H^+]$ decreases, the pH increases. The greater the $[H^+]$, the more acidic the solution and the lower the pH. The lower the $[H^+]$, the more basic the solution and the higher the pH. In biologic fluids, a pH of less than 7.4 is defined as acidic and a pH greater than 7.4 is defined as basic.

Different body fluids have different pH values as follows:

Body Fluid	pH
Gastric juices	1.0-3.0
Urine	5.0-6.0
Arterial blood	7.38-7.42
Venous blood	7.37
Cerebrospinal fluid	7.32
Pancreatic fluid	7.8-8.0

Body acids are formed as end products of cellular metabolism. The average person generates 50 to 100 mEq acid/day from the metabolism of protein, carbohydrates, and fats, and from loss of base in the stools. To maintain a normal pH, an equal amount of acid therefore must be neutralized or excreted. The lungs, kidneys, and bone are the major organs involved in the regulation of acid-base balance. The systems are interrelated and work together to regulate acute or chronic changes in acid-base status. Body acids exist in two forms: **volatile** (can be eliminated as CO_2 gas) and **nonvolatile.** The volatile acid is carbonic acid (H_2CO_3), which is formed from the hydration of carbon dioxide:

$$CO_2 + H_2O \rightleftarrows H_2CO_3$$
(carbonic anhydrase)

Carbonic acid is a weak acid, and, in the presence of carbonic anhydrase, it readily dissociates into carbon dioxide. Approximately 12,000 to 15,000 millimoles of CO_2 are produced per day (Rose, 1989). The carbon dioxide is then eliminated by pulmonary ventilation. Sulfuric, phosphoric, and other organic acids are nonvolatile strong acids produced from the metabolism of proteins, carbohydrates, and fats. (Strong acids are those that readily give up their hydrogen; weak acids do not.) Nonvolatile acids are eliminated by the renal tubules. Thus the lungs and kidneys, with the help of body buffer systems, are the prime regulators of acid-base balance.

Buffer Systems

Buffering is a process that occurs in response to changes in acid-base status. **Buffers** are substances that can absorb excessive H^+ (acid) or OH^- (base) without a significant change in pH. Although acids are normally added to the body daily, buffers are available to maintain pH within the normal range (7.35 to 7.45). The buffer systems are located in both the ICF and ECF compartments, and they function at different rates. Buffer systems exist as buffer pairs, consisting of a weak acid and its conjugate base (Table 3-9). The most important plasma buffer systems are carbonic acid–bicarbonate and hemoglobin. Phosphate and protein are the most important intracellular buffers.

An important factor for effective buffering is a func-

TABLE 3-9

TABLE 3-9

Buffer Systems

Buffer pairs	Buffer system	pK values	Reaction	Rate
HCO_3^-/H_2CO_3	Bicarbonate	6.1	$H^+ + HCO_3^- \gtrless H_2O + CO_2$	Instantaneous
Hb^-/HHb	Hemoglobin	7.3	$HHb \rightleftharpoons H^+ + Hb^-$	Instantaneous
$HPO_4^-/H_2PO_4^-$	Phosphate	6.8	$H_2PO_4 \rightleftharpoons H^+ + HPO_4^-$	Instantaneous
Pr^-/HPr	Plasma proteins	6.7	$HPr \rightleftharpoons H^+ + Pr^-$	Instantaneous

Organs	Mechanism	Rate
Lungs	Regulates retention or elimination of CO_2 and therefore H_2CO_3 concentration	Minutes-hours
Ionic shifts	Exchange of intracellular potassium and sodium for hydrogen	2-4 hours
Kidneys	Bicarbonate reabsorption and regeneration, ammonia formation, phosphate buffering	Hours-days
Bone	Exchanges of calcium, phosphate, and release of carbonate	Hours-days

tion known as the *pK value*, which represents the pH at which a buffer pair is half dissociated. Buffer pairs can associate and dissociate (see Table 3-9).

The pK provides a rate constant for the chemical reaction. A buffer system is most effective when the pK for the buffer is close to the pH of the fluid in which the buffer is acting. For the bicarbonate–carbonic acid buffer system, the pK is 6:1. This value is not as high as the pK for other buffer systems (see Table 3-9), but this buffer system is still very effective because carbon dioxide is rapidly removed from the blood by the lungs.

The pK value is also a term in the equation used to determine pH. The relationships among pH, pK, and the ratio of bicarbonate/carbonic acid can be expressed as follows by the *Henderson-Hasselbalch equation*:

$$pH = pK + \log \frac{[HCO_3^-]}{[H_2CO_3]}$$

The pH then can be determined when specific values are included in the equation:

$$
\begin{aligned}
pH &= 6.1 + \log \frac{[HCO_3^-]}{[H_2CO_3]} \\
&= 6.1 + \log \frac{24}{1.2} \\
&= 6.1 + \log \frac{20}{1} \\
&= 6.1 + 1.3 \\
&= 7.40
\end{aligned}
$$

Carbonic Acid–Bicarbonate Buffering

The major buffering system is the carbonic acid–bicarbonate buffer pair, which operates in both the lung and the kidney. The volatile feature of this buffer pair is significant because the amount of carbonic acid formed is a function of the partial pressure of carbon dioxide (Pco_2). The greater the Pco_2, the more carbonic acid is formed. The relationship that exists between carbonic acid (H_2CO_3) and carbon dioxide (Pco_2) can be expressed as follows:

$$H_2CO_3 = 0.03 \times Pco_2 \text{ (mm Hg)}$$

The 0.03 represents the solubility coefficient for carbon dioxide. The Pco_2 of arterial blood is normally about 40 mm Hg. Therefore the amount of H_2CO_3 is equal to about 1.2 mmol/L (0.03×40). As the amount of carbon dioxide increases or decreases, the amount of H_2CO_3 changes in the same direction.

The relationship between bicarbonate and carbonic acid is usually expressed as a ratio. When the pH is 7.40, this ratio is 20:1 (bicarbonate/carbonic acid). The ratio is defined by the amount of bicarbonate and carbon dioxide (carbonic acid) in the arterial blood. Bicarbonate concentration (HCO_3^-) is normally about 24 mEq/L. Therefore the 20:1 ratio can be developed as follows:

$$\frac{[HCO_3] = 24 \text{ mEq/L}}{[H_2CO_3] = (0.03 \times 40 \text{ mm Hg})} = \frac{24}{1.2} = \frac{20}{1}$$

or

$$\frac{[HCO_3] = 24 \text{ mEq/L}}{[H_2CO_3] = 1.2 \text{ mmol/L}} = \frac{24}{1.2} = \frac{20}{1}$$

The significance of the ratio is that the values for HCO_3^- and P_{CO_2} (H_2CO_3) can increase or decrease proportionately, but the 20:1 ratio is maintained.

Another important component of the bicarbonate–carbonic acid buffer system is the renal regulation of bicarbonate. The lungs can decrease the amount of carbonic acid by blowing off CO_2 and leaving water. The kidneys can reabsorb bicarbonate or regenerate new bicarbonate from CO_2 and water. The renal mechanism does not act as rapidly as the lungs, but the two systems are very effective together because acid concentration can be rapidly adjusted by the lungs and bicarbonate is easily reabsorbed or regenerated by the kidneys. Because the lungs and kidneys function at different rates and regulate different components of the bicarbonate–carbonic acid buffer system, the pH equation can be symbolically expressed as:

$$pH = \frac{\text{Renal regulation (slow)}}{\text{Pulmonary regulation (fast)}}$$

or

$$pH = \frac{\text{Base}}{\text{Acid}}$$

or

$$pH = \frac{\text{Metabolic acid} - \text{base function}}{\text{Respiratory acid} - \text{base function}}$$

Changes in either the numerator or the denominator will change the pH. For example, if the amount of bicarbonate is decreased, the pH also decreases, causing a state of acidosis. The pH can be returned to a normal range if the value of the denominator or the amount of carbonic acid also decreases.

This type of adjustment in pH is known as **compensation**. With compensation, a 20:1 ratio may be achieved, but the actual values for HCO_3^- and H_2CO_3 are not normal. The respiratory system thus compensates for changes in pH by increasing or decreasing ventilation. The renal system compensates by producing more acidic or more alkaline urine. For example, the respiratory system compensates for metabolic acidosis (Fig. 3-8).

Correction, a process distinctly different from compensation, occurs when the values for both components of the buffer pair are returned to normal. In this example, pH would be corrected when the bicarbonate and carbonic acid return to their normal concentrations.

Protein Buffering

Both intracellular and extracellular proteins have negative charges and can serve as buffers for H^+, but because most proteins are inside cells, they are primarily an intracellular buffer system. Hemoglobin (Hb) is an excellent intracellular buffer because of its ability to bind with H^+ (forming HHb) and carbon dioxide ($HHbCO_2$). Hemoglobin bound to H^+ becomes a weak acid. Unsaturated hemoglobin (venous blood) is a better buffer than hemoglobin saturated with oxygen (arterial blood). The hemoglobin buffer system is illustrated in Fig. 3-9.

Renal Buffering

The distal tubule of the kidney regulates acid-base balance by secreting hydrogen into the urine and reabsorbing bicarbonate. The maximal acidity that can be achieved in the distal tubular fluid of the kidney is a pH of about 4.4 to 4.7. Buffers in the tubular fluid combine with hydrogen ions, allowing more H^+ to be secreted before the limiting pH value is reached. Dibasic phosphate ($HPO_4^=$) and ammonia (NH_3) are two important renal buffers. Dibasic phosphate is filtered at the glomerulus. About 75% is reabsorbed and the remainder is available for buffering H^+. Secreted H^+ combines with $HPO_4^=$ to form monobasic phosphate ($H_2PO_4^-$). The remaining negative charge on the molecule makes it lipid insoluble, and it cannot diffuse back across the tubular cell and into the blood. Thus it is excreted in the urine (Fig. 3-10).

Ammonia (NH_3) is an important renal buffer. The major source of ammonia is derived from the synthesis and enzymatic conversion of glutamine by the renal tubular cells. Ammonia is not ionized (does not carry a charge), and therefore it is lipid soluble and can cross

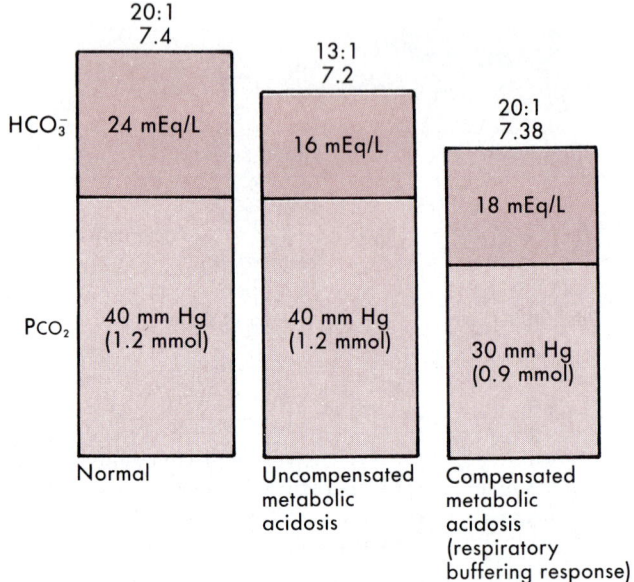

FIG. 3-8 Maintenance of HCO_3^-:P_{CO_2} (H_2CO_3) ratio in metabolic acidosis.

FIG. 3-9 **Buffering of hydrogen with hemoglobin and CO_2 transport.** CO_2 is produced in tissue cells and diffuses to the plasma, where it is transported as dissolved CO_2, or it combines with water to form carbonic acid (H_2CO_3), or it combines with protein from which hydrogen has been released. Most of the CO_2 diffuses into the red blood cell and combines with water to form H_2CO_3. The H_2CO_3 dissociates to form hydrogen (H^+) and bicarbonate (HCO_3^-). The HCO_3^- shifts into the plasma and chloride (Cl^-) shifts into the red blood cell to maintain electroneutrality. Hydrogen combines with hemoglobin that has released its oxygen to form HHb, which buffers the hydrogen and makes venous blood slightly more acidic than arterial blood. *CA, Carbonic anhydrase.*

the cell membrane. The presence of NH_3 in the cell creates a concentration gradient and it diffuses into the renal tubular fluid, where it combines with hydrogen to form ammonium ion (NH_4^+), which is eliminated in the urine (see Fig. 3-10). The renal buffering of hydrogen ions requires the use of CO_2 to form H_2CO_3. The enzyme carbonic anhydrase catalyzes the formation of H^+ + HCO_3^-. The hydrogen is secreted from the tubular cell and buffered in the lumen by phosphate and ammonia. The bicarbonate is reabsorbed. The end effect is the addition of new bicarbonate, which contributes to the alkalinity of the plasma, because the hydrogen ion is excreted from the body (see Fig. 3-10).

Other Buffers

A cellular ion exchange mechanism is also an important buffering system. The best example is the shift of po-

tassium in exchange for hydrogen during states of acidosis or alkalosis. During acidosis, potassium tends to leave the intracellular space in exchange for hydrogen. The reverse occurs during alkalosis. Although the ionic shifts facilitate buffering, the changes in intracellular or extracellular potassium concentrations may have serious consequences.

Acid-Base Imbalances

Pathophysiologic changes in the concentration of hydrogen ion in the blood lead to acid-base imbalances. **Acidemia** is a state in which the pH of arterial blood is less than 7.35. A systemic increase in hydrogen ion concentration is termed **acidosis**. **Alkalemia** is a state in which the pH of arterial blood is greater than 7.45. A systemic decrease in hydrogen ion concentration is termed **alkalosis**.

EPITHELIAL
FILTRATE   CELL   CAPILLARY

FIG. 3-10 Renal excretion of acid. *1,* Conservation of filtered bicarbonate. Filtered bicarbonate combines with secreted hydrogen in the presence of carbon anhydrase (CA) to form carbonic acid (H_2CO_3), which then dissociates to water (H_2O) and carbon dioxide (CO_2); both diffuse into the epithelial cell. The CO_2 and H_2O combine to form H_2CO_3 in the presence of CA, and the resulting HCO_3^- is converted by reabsorption into the capillary. *2,* Formation of titratable acid. Hydrogen ion is secreted and combines with dibasic phosphate ($HPO_4^=$) to form monobasic phosphate (H_2P^{4-}). The secreted hydrogen is formed from the dissociation of H_2CO_3, and the remaining HCO_3^- is reabsorbed into the capillary. *3,* Formation of ammonium. Ammonia (NH_3) is produced from glutamine in the epithelial cell and diffused to the tubular lumen, where it combines with H^+ to form ammonium (NH_4). Once NH_4^+ has been formed, it cannot return to the epithelial cell (diffusional trapping), and the bicarbonate remaining in the epithelial cell is reabsorbed into the capillary. (From Berne & Levy, 1993.)

An abnormal decrease in bicarbonate concentration or an increase in hydrogen ion concentration is called **metabolic acidosis.** Conversely, an increase in bicarbonate concentration or a decrease in hydrogen ion concentration is known as **metabolic alkalosis.** Changes in the rate of alveolar ventilation produce changes in the Pco_2.

TABLE 3-10

Primary and Compensatory Acid-Base Changes

	Primary disturbance			Compensations		
	pH	Pco_2	HCO_3-	pH	Pco_2	HCO_3-
Metabolic acidosis	↓	N	↓	↑-N	↓	↓
Metabolic alkalosis	↑	N	↑	↓-N	↑	↑
Respiratory acidosis	↓	↑	N	↑-N	↑	↑
Respiratory alkalosis	↑	↓	N	↓-N	↓	↓

NOTE: ↑-N, Increase toward normal; ↓-N, decrease toward normal.

When less CO_2 is removed in relation to the amount of CO_2 generated, the Pco_2 increases. The resulting condition is known as **respiratory acidosis** because carbonic acid increases. When more CO_2 is removed in relation to the amount of CO_2 generated, the Pco_2 decreases. The resulting condition is known as **respiratory alkalosis.** Table 3-10 summarizes changes occurring in pH, Pco_2, and HCO_3^- with respiratory or metabolic acid-base disorders. Fig. 3-11 summarizes the relationships between pH, Pco_2, and bicarbonate during different acid-base alterations.

Metabolic Acidosis
Pathophysiology

Metabolic acidosis can be caused from an increase in noncarbonic acids or loss of bicarbonate from the extracellular fluid (Table 3-11). The development of metabolic acidosis can occur quickly, as in lactic acidosis from poor perfusion, or more slowly, as in renal failure or diabetic ketoacidosis.

The buffer systems compensate for the excess acid and attempt to maintain the arterial pH within a normal range. Buffering by bicarbonate lowers the serum value of this ion. The respiratory system compensates for a metabolic acidosis as the reduced pH stimulates hyperventilation, lowering the $PaCO_2$ and the amount of H_2CO_3 circulating in the blood. The kidneys excrete the excess acid as (NH_4^+) and titratable acid. When the acidosis is severe, the buffers are unable to compensate for the increasing H^+ load, and the pH continues to decrease. The result is a decrease in the 20:1 ratio of bicarbonate to carbonic acid (Fig. 3-12).

The evaluation of the **anion gap** can be useful for distinguishing different types of metabolic acidosis. Nor-

TABLE 3-11

Causes of Metabolic Acidosis

Increased noncarbonic acids (elevated anion gap)	Bicarbonate loss (normal anion gap)
Increased H⁺ load	Diarrhea
Ketoacidosis (e.g., diabetes mellitus, starvation)	Ureterosigmoidoscopy
	Renal failure
Lactic acidosis (e.g., shock)	Proximal renal tubule acidosis
Ingestions (e.g., ammonium chloride, ethylene glycol, methanol, salicylates, paraldehyde)	
Decreased H⁺ excretion	
Uremia	
Distal renal tubule acidosis	

FIG. 3-11 Graph of pH, Pco₂, and bicarbonate relationships. *Solid black lines* represent different Pco₂ values. *Vertical axis* represents bicarbonate concentration, and *horizontal axis* represents pH values. Thus for any indicated Pco₂, there is a corresponding pH and bicarbonate concentration. Any point on the graph predicts the required Pco₂, pH, and bicarbonate values. *Dashed horizontal line* shows behavior of bicarbonate as a pure buffer at 24 mEq/L. The normal blood buffer line represents values that would be obtained if blood were equilibrated at different CO₂ values. Point N represents normal values. A represents **metabolic alkalosis,** indicated by a normal Pco₂ of 40 and pH greater than 7.4. Respiratory compensation is achieved by hypoventilation, which raises the Pco₂ to point B and decreases the pH. **Respiratory alkalosis** is represented by point C and reflects hypocapnia (decreased Pco₂). Renal compensation for respiratory alkalosis is increased renal excretion of bicarbonate to normalize the pH at point D. **Metabolic acidosis** at point E represents normal Pco₂ and a decrease in bicarbonate and pH. Respiratory compensation by hyperventilation is indicated by point F. **Respiratory acidosis** at point G indicates high Pco₂ and low pH values. Renal compensation for chronic high Pco₂ values is indicated by point H. (Modified from Berne & Levy, 1993.)

$$Anion\ gap =$$
$$[Na^+(140) + K^+(4.0)] -$$
$$[HCO_3^-(24) + Cl^-(110)]$$
$$= 10 - 12\ mEq/L$$

In metabolic acidosis a normal anion gap is characteristic of conditions related to bicarbonate loss with retention of chloride to maintain an ionic balance. This is called **hyperchloremic metabolic acidosis.** An elevated anion gap is characteristic of acidosis associated with accumulation of anions other than chloride (e.g., lactate and ketoacids) (see Table 3-11).

Clinical Manifestations

Metabolic acidosis is manifested by changes in the neurologic, respiratory, gastrointestinal, and cardiovascular systems. Headache and lethargy are early symptoms, which progress to coma with severe acidosis. Deep, rapid respirations (Kussmaul's respirations) are indicative of respiratory compensation. Anorexia, nausea, vomiting, diarrhea, and abdominal discomfort are common. Severe acidosis can compromise ventricular contraction and produce life-threatening dysrhythmias.

Evaluation and Treatment

The diagnosis of metabolic acidosis is established from the health history, clinical symptoms, and laboratory findings. Arterial blood pH is below 7.35, and bicarbonate concentration is less than 24 mEq/L. The underlying condition must be diagnosed to establish effective

mally, the concentrations of cations and anions in the plasma are equivalent. Some anions, such as protein, sulfates, phosphates, and organic acids, however, are not measured in the common laboratory evaluations of the blood. Therefore, the **normal anion gap** represents the difference between the sum of Na⁺ and K⁺ and the sum of HCO₃⁻ and Cl⁻, or about 10 to 12 mEq.

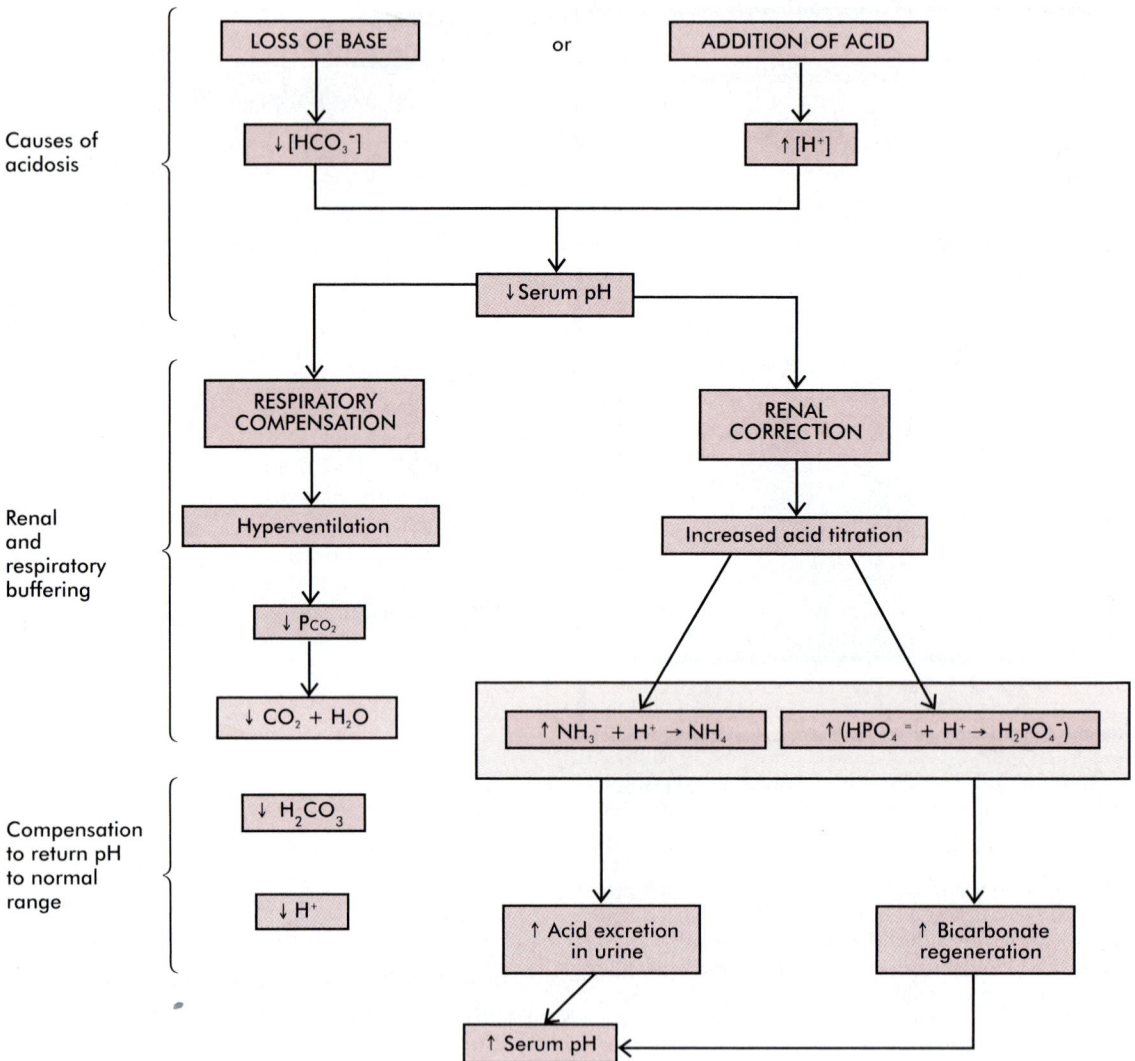

FIG. 3-12 Metabolic acidosis with compensation and correction.

treatment. During severe acidosis (pH ≤ 7.1), sodium bicarbonate administration is required to elevate the pH to a safe level.

Metabolic Alkalosis
Pathophysiology

Metabolic alkalosis occurs when there is an increase in bicarbonate, usually caused by excessive loss of metabolic acids. Among the conditions that can result in metabolic alkalosis are prolonged vomiting, gastrointestinal suctioning, excessive bicarbonate intake, hyperaldosteronism, and diuretic therapy.

When acid loss is caused by vomiting with depletion of ECF and chloride (**hypochloremic metabolic alkalosis**), renal compensation is not very effective because the volume depletion and loss of electrolytes (Na$^+$, K$^+$, H$^+$, and Cl$^-$) stimulate a paradoxical response by the kid-

neys. The kidneys increase sodium and bicarbonate reabsorption with excretion of hydrogen. Bicarbonate is reabsorbed because the ECF chloride concentration is decreased. When the potassium concentration is depleted, hydrogen is excreted to maintain an electrochemical balance. The urine is acidic, and the reabsorbed bicarbonate prevents correction of the alkalosis (Fig. 3-13). Correction is achieved when the ECF is expanded with a solution of sodium chloride and potassium. The volume replacement decreases the renal stimulus to reabsorb Na$^+$ and chloride as an anion is replaced. Bicarbonate then can be lost in the urine and hydrogen ion excretion decreases, correcting the pH.

Hyperaldosteronism has a pathophysiologic process different from the volume depletion that leads to hypochloremic alkalosis. With hyperaldosteronism, the excess aldosterone causes sodium retention and loss of hy-

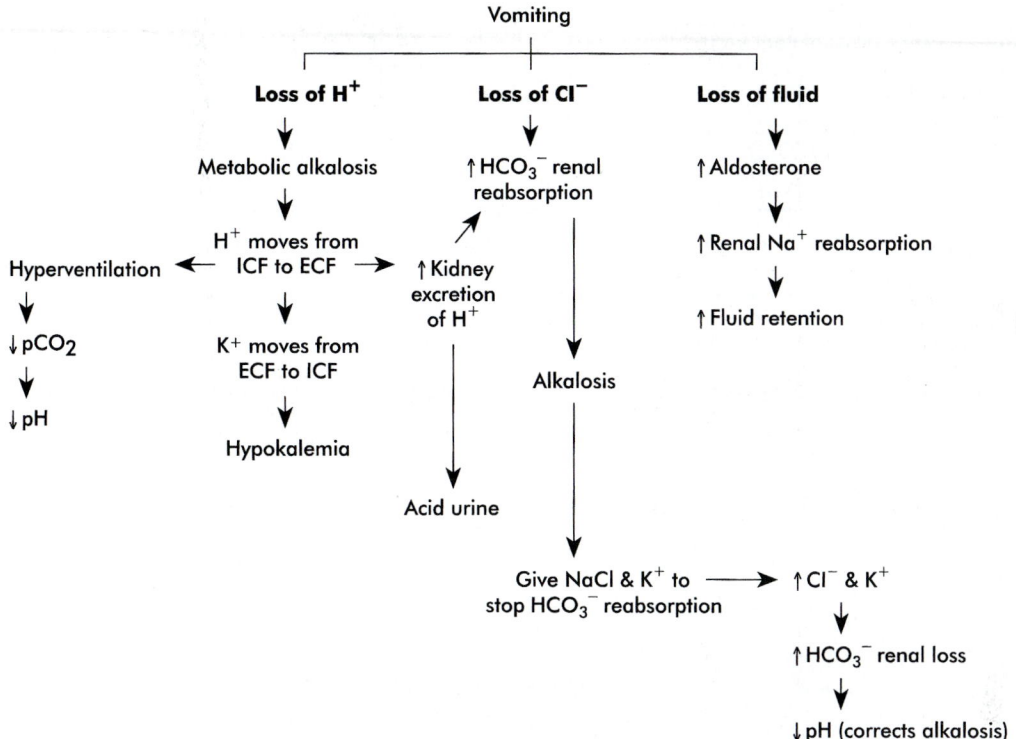

FIG. 3-13 Hypochloremic metabolic alkalosis.

drogen and potassium. Mild volume expansion ensues, and bicarbonate is retained with the sodium, causing alkalosis.

Diuretics such as thiazides, ethacrynic acid, and furosemide produce mild alkalosis by enhancing sodium, potassium, and chloride excretion more than bicarbonate excretion.

Respiratory compensation for metabolic alkalosis occurs when the elevated pH inhibits the respiratory center. The rate and depth of ventilation are decreased, causing retention of carbon dioxide. The ratio of HCO_3^- to H_2CO_3 is reduced toward normal. Respiratory compensation is not very efficient, however, and chronic or severe metabolic alkalosis requires therapeutic intervention (Fig. 3-14).

Clinical Manifestations

Because of the many causes of metabolic alkalosis, the symptoms are varied. Some common symptoms, such as weakness, muscle cramps, and hyperactive reflexes, are related to volume depletion and electrolyte losses. Because alkalosis causes a decrease in ionized calcium, tetany may develop.

Respirations are slow and shallow to increase carbon dioxide content. Confusions and convulsions occur with severe alkalosis. Atrial tachycardia is a potential problem. The oxyhemoglobin curve is shifted to the left (see Chapter 29), decreasing the dissociation of oxyhemoglobin and increasing the risk of dysrhythmias.

Evaluation and Treatment

The health history provides significant clues to the diagnosis of metabolic alkalosis. The arterial pH is above 7.45, and bicarbonate levels exceed 26 mEq/L. With respiratory compensation, the P_{CO_2} rises above 40 mm Hg. With hypochloremic alkalosis, serum chloride values are below normal. Potassium levels are usually depleted because hydrogen is released from the cells in exchange for potassium to help regulate the pH level. The K^+ is then secreted from the distal tubule or kidney cells into the urine.

With hypochloremic alkalosis or contraction alkalosis with volume depletion, a sodium chloride solution is required for correction. The renal stimulus to increase ECF volume by retaining Na^+ is diminished, and HCO_3^- can be excreted as $NaHCO_3$ in the urine. The administration of potassium corrects alkalosis caused by hyperaldosteronism or hypokalemia. The potassium causes hydrogen to move back into the ECF and decreases loss of hydrogen from the distal tubule.

Respiratory Acidosis
Pathophysiology

Respiratory disorders of acid-base balance are due to increases or decreases of alveolar ventilation in relation to the metabolic production of carbon dioxide. Respiratory acidosis occurs when there is depression of ventilation. Carbon dioxide is retained, increasing $[H^+]$ (as H_2CO_3) and producing acidosis. Carbon dioxide excess

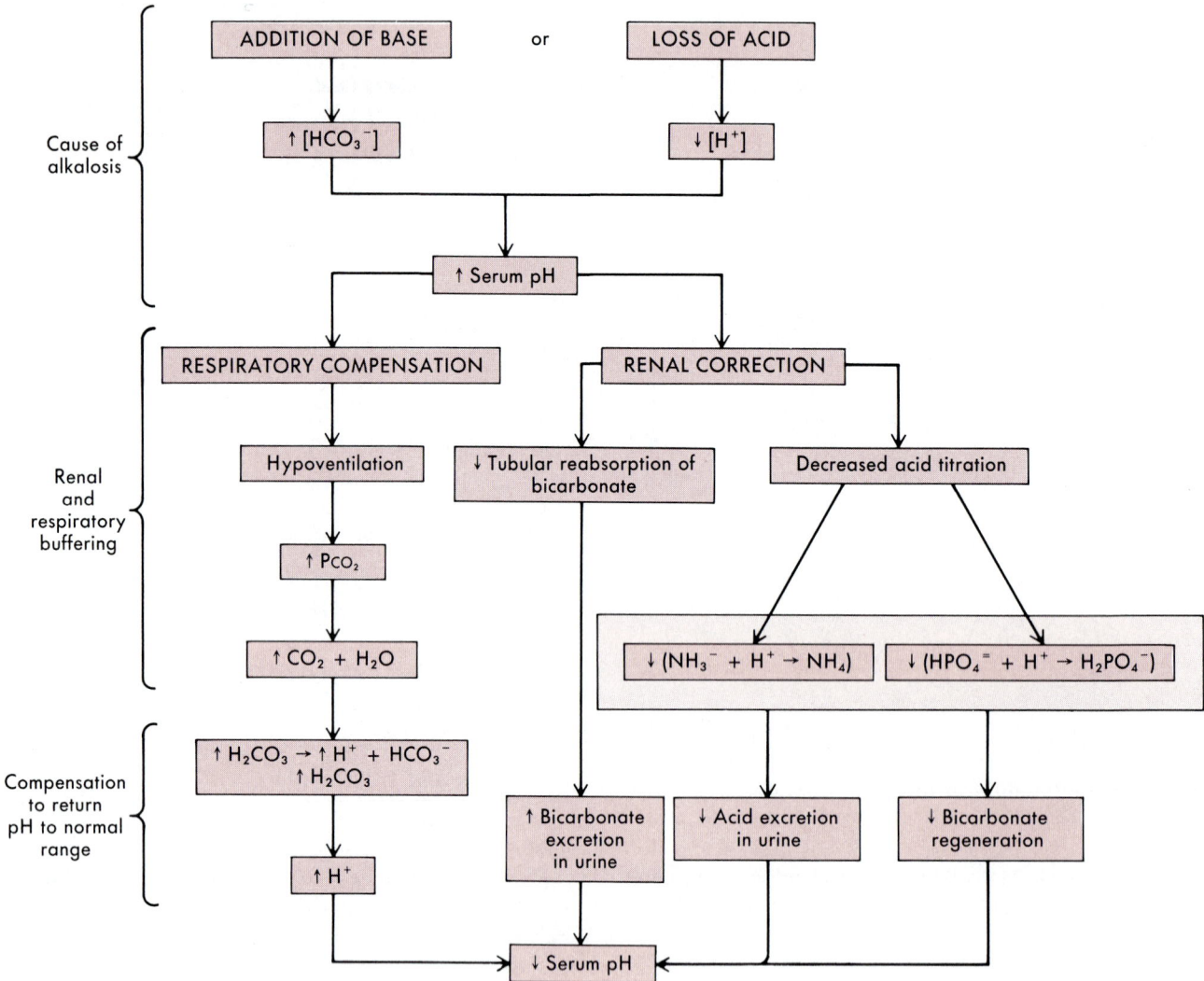

FIG. 3-14 Metabolic alkalosis with compensation and correction.

is called **hypercapnia.** The common causes include depression of the respiratory center (brainstem trauma and oversedation), respiratory muscle paralysis, disorders of the chest wall (kyphoscoliosis, Pickwickian syndrome, and flail chest), and disorders of the lung parenchyma (pneumonia, pulmonary edema, emphysema, asthma, and bronchitis).

Respiratory acidosis may be acute or chronic. Airway obstruction is the most common cause of acute respiratory acidosis. Compensation for respiratory acidosis is not effective because the renal buffer mechanism takes time to function. Furthermore, the protein buffers provide marginal compensation, and HCO_3^- is not a good buffer for CO_2. Acute uncompensated respiratory acidosis is characterized by a decreased pH, elevated PCO_2, and normal or slightly increased bicarbonate level.

Chronic respiratory acidosis is commonly associated with chronic obstructive pulmonary disease and defor-

mities of the chest wall. Renal compensation is effective and is established over several days. The acidosis produced from CO_2 retention stimulates the kidney to secrete hydrogen ion and regenerate bicarbonate. Serum bicarbonate and arterial PCO_2 are elevated, and pH will be restored toward normal (Fig. 3-15).

Clinical Manifestations

The symptoms of respiratory acidosis are related to acuity of onset and severity of PCO_2 retention. Initial symptoms include restlessness and apprehension followed by lethargy, muscle twitching, tremors, convulsions, and coma. Neurologic symptoms are due to a decrease in the pH of cerebrospinal fluid and vasodilation because CO_2 readily crosses the blood-brain barrier. The respiratory rate is rapid at first and gradually becomes depressed because, over time, the respiratory center adapts to increasing levels of CO_2. Cyanosis does not occur un-

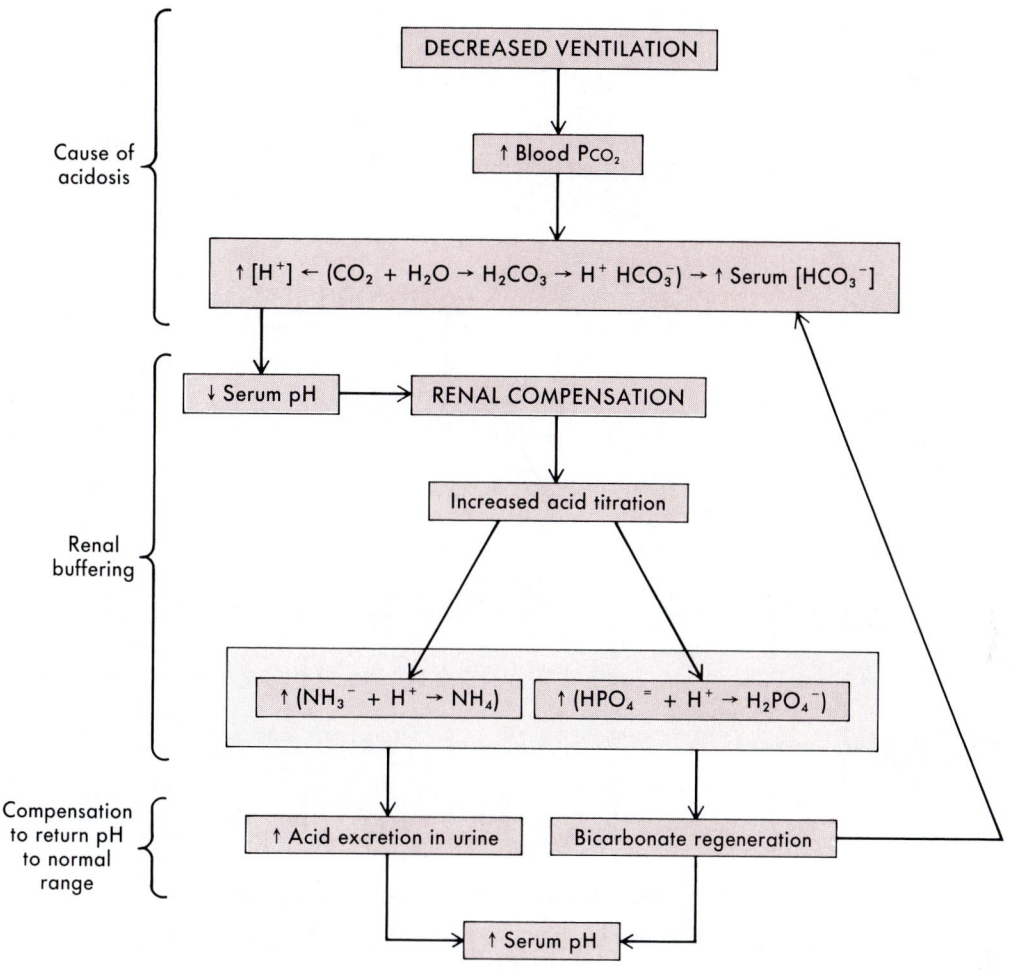

FIG. 3-15 Respiratory acidosis with compensation and correction.

less there is an accompanying hypoxemia, and the skin may instead be pink from vasodilation caused by the acidosis.

Evaluation and Treatment

The primary diagnostic indicators are an arterial pH less than 7.35 and hypercapnia. Acute respiratory acidosis must be distinguished from chronic acidosis; the health history and clinical laboratory data are therefore helpful. With renal compensation, bicarbonate levels are elevated, and the pH is restored toward normal.

The restoration of adequate alveolar ventilation removes excess CO_2. If alveolar ventilation cannot be maintained spontaneously because of drug overdose or neuromuscular disorders, mechanical ventilation is required. The arterial pH, PCO_2, PO_2, and HCO_3^- must be carefully monitored. Rapid reduction of PCO_2 can cause respiratory alkalosis with seizures and death.

Renal buffering is usually effective in compensating for uncomplicated chronic respiratory acidosis. The underlying diseases are treated to achieve maximal ventilation. In the presence of hypoxemia and hypercapnia, oxygen can function as a respiratory depressant when the respiratory center is no longer stimulated by the lower pH and elevated PCO_2. Therefore, oxygen should be given cautiously.

Respiratory Alkalosis
Pathophysiology

Respiratory alkalosis occurs when there is alveolar hyperventilation and excessive reduction of carbon dioxide (termed **hypocapnia**). Stimulation of ventilation is precipitated by hypoxemia, which may be caused by pulmonary disease, congestive heart failure, or high altitudes; hypermetabolic states such as fever, anemia, and thyrotoxicosis; early salicylate intoxication; hyste-

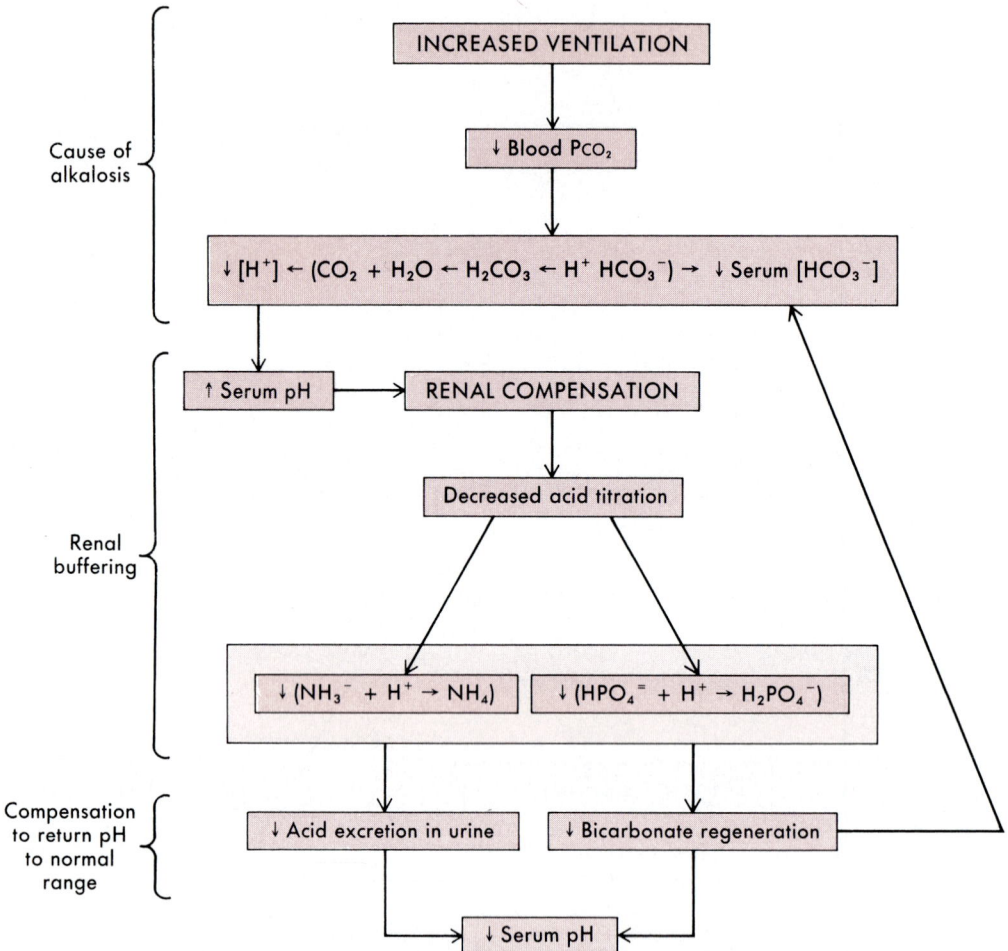

FIG. 3-16 Respiratory alkalosis with compensation and correction.

ria; cirrhosis; and gram-negative sepsis. Improper use of mechanical ventilators can cause iatrogenic respiratory alkalosis. Secondary respiratory alkalosis may develop from hyperventilation stimulated by metabolic or respiratory acidosis.

The onset of respiratory alkalosis occurs within minutes of hyperventilation. Cellular buffers provide immediate compensation with shifts of H^+ from ICF to ECF. The H^+ shifts are not very effective, however, if there is a significant decrease in P_{CO_2}. When there is chronic respiratory alkalosis, renal compensation restores pH toward normal by decreasing H^+ excretion and bicarbonate absorption (Fig. 3-16).

Clinical Manifestations

Respiratory alkalosis, like metabolic alkalosis, is irritating to the central and peripheral nervous system. Symptoms include dizziness, confusion, tingling of extremities (paresthesias), convulsions, and coma. Carpopedal

spasm and other symptoms of hypocalcemia are similar to those of metabolic alkalosis. Deep and rapid respirations (tachypnea) are primary symptoms that cause respiratory alkalosis.

Evaluation and Treatment

The underlying disturbance must be identified. The arterial pH is above 7.45, and the P_{CO_2} is less than 38 mm Hg. In acute states, bicarbonate levels are normal. With chronic respiratory alkalosis, there is a compensatory decrease in the bicarbonate level and the pH is closer to normal.

Treating the underlying disturbance is the most effective treatment. Hypoxemia must be corrected and hypermetabolic states reversed. Symptoms from hysterical hyperventilation can be corrected by rebreathing from a paper bag, which increases the concentration of inspired carbon dioxide and reverses the respiratory alkalosis.

SUMMARY REVIEW

Distribution of Body Fluids

1 Body fluids are distributed among functional compartments and are classified as intracellular fluid (ICF) and extracellular fluid (ECF).
2 The sum of all fluids is the total body water (TBW), which varies with age and amount of body fat.
3 Water moves between the ICF and ECF compartments principally by osmosis.
4 Water moves between the plasma and interstitial fluid by osmosis and hydrostatic pressure, which occur across the capillary membrane.
5 Movement across the capillary wall is called net filtration and is described according to Starling's law.

Alterations in Water Movement

1 Edema is a problem of fluid distribution that results in accumulation of fluid within the interstitial spaces.
2 The pathophysiologic process that leads to edema is related to an increase in forces favoring fluid filtration from the capillaries or lymphatic channels into the tissues.
3 Edema is caused by arterial dilation, venous or lymphatic obstruction, and increased vascular volume.
4 Edema may be localized or generalized and is usually associated with weight gain, swelling and puffiness, tighter-fitting clothes and shoes, and limited movement of the affected area.

Sodium, Chloride, and Water Balance

1 Sodium and water balance are intimately related; chloride levels are generally proportional to changes in sodium levels.
2 Water balance is regulated by the sensation of thirst and by antidiuretic hormone, which is initiated by an increase in plasma osmolality or a decrease in circulating blood volume.
3 Sodium balance is regulated by aldosterone, which increases reabsorption of sodium by the distal tubule of the kidney.
4 Renin and angiotensin are enzymes that promote or inhibit secretion of aldosterone and thus regulate sodium and water balance.
5 Atrial natriuretic hormone is also involved in decreasing tubular resorption and promoting urinary excretion of sodium.

Alterations in Sodium, Chloride, and Water Balance

1 Alterations in water balance may be classified as isotonic, hypertonic, or hypotonic.
2 Isotonic alterations occur when changes in TBW are accompanied by proportional changes in electrolytes.

3 Hypertonic alterations develop when the osmolality of the ECF is elevated above normal, usually because of an increased concentration of ECF sodium or a deficit of ECF water.
4 Hypernatremia (sodium levels greater than 147 mEq/L) may be caused by an acute increase in sodium or a loss of water.
5 Water deficit, or hypertonic dehydration, is rare but can be caused by lack of access to water, pure water losses, hyperventilation, arid climates, and increased renal clearance.
6 Hyperchloremia is caused by an excess of sodium or a deficit of bicarbonate.
7 Hypotonic alterations occur when the osmolality of the ECF is less than normal.
8 Hyponatremia (serum sodium concentration less than 135 mEq/L) usually causes movement of water into cells.
9 Hyponatremia may be caused by sodium loss, inadequate sodium intake, or dilution of the body's sodium level.
10 Water excess is rare but can be caused by compulsive water drinking, decreased urine formation, or syndrome of inappropriate secretion of ADH.
11 Hypochloremia is usually the result of hyponatremia or elevated bicarbonate concentrations.

Alterations in Potassium, Calcium, Phosphate, and Magnesium

1 Potassium is the predominant ICF ion; it functions to regulate ICF osmolality, maintain the resting membrane potential, and deposit glycogen in liver and skeletal muscle cells.
2 Potassium balance is regulated by the kidney, by aldosterone and insulin secretion, and by changes in pH.
3 A mechanism known as potassium adaptation allows the body to accommodate slowly increased levels of potassium intake.
4 Hypokalemia (serum potassium concentration less than 3.5 mEq/L) indicates loss of total body potassium, although ECF hypokalemia can develop without losses of total body potassium and plasma K^+ levels may be normal or elevated when total body potassium is depleted.
5 Hypokalemia may be caused by reduced potassium intake, increased ICF-to-ECF potassium concentration, loss of potassium from body stores, increased aldosterone secretion (e.g., caused by hypernatremia), and increased renal excretion.

6 Hyperkalemia (potassium levels that are greater than 5.5 mEq/L) may be caused by increased potassium intake, a shift from ICF to ECF potassium, or decreased renal excretion.

7 Calcium is a necessary ion in the structure of bones and teeth, in blood clotting, in hormone secretion and the function of cell receptors, and in membrane stability.

8 Phosphate acts as a buffer in acid-base regulation and provides energy for muscle contraction.

9 Calcium and phosphate concentrations are rigidly controlled by parathyroid hormone (PTH), vitamin D, and calcitonin.

10 Hypocalcemia (serum calcium concentration less than 8.5 mg/dl) is related to inadequate intestinal absorption, deposition of ionized calcium into bone or soft tissue, blood administration, or decreased PTH and vitamin D levels.

11 Hypercalcemia (serum calcium concentration greater than 12 mg/dl) can be caused by a number of diseases, including hyperparathyroidism, bone metastases, sarcoidosis, and excess vitamin D.

12 Hypophosphatemia is usually caused by intestinal malabsorption and increased renal excretion of phosphate.

13 Hyperphosphatemia develops with acute or chronic renal failure with significant loss of glomerular filtration.

14 Magnesium is a major intracellular cation and is principally regulated by PTH.

15 Magnesium functions in enzymatic reactions and often interacts with calcium at the cellular level.

16 Hypomagnesemia (serum magnesium concentrations less than 1.5 mEq/L) may be caused by malabsorption syndromes.

17 Hypermagnesemia (serum magnesium concentrations greater than 2.5 mEq/L) is rare and is usually due to renal failure.

Acid-Base Balance

1 Hydrogen ions, which maintain membrane integrity and the speed of enzymatic reactions, must be concentrated within a narrow range if the body is to function normally.

2 Hydrogen ion concentration is expressed as pH, which represents the negative logarithm of hydrogen ions in solution.

3 Different body fluids have different pH values.

4 The renal and respiratory systems, together with the body's buffer systems, are the principal regulators of acid-base balance.

5 Buffers are substances that can absorb excessive acid or base without a significant change in pH.

6 Buffers exist as acid-base pairs; the principal plasma buffers are carbonic acid—bicarbonate, protein (hemoglobin), and phosphate.

7 Buffer pairs can associate and dissociate; the pK value is the pH at which a buffer pair is half dissociated.

8 The lungs and kidneys act to compensate for changes in pH by increasing or decreasing ventilation and by producing more acidic or more alkaline urine.

9 Correction is a process different from compensation; correction occurs when the values for both components of the buffer pair are returned to normal.

10 Acid-base imbalances are caused by changes in the concentration of H^+ in the blood; an increase causes acidosis, and a decrease causes alkalosis.

11 An abnormal increase or decrease in bicarbonate concentration causes metabolic acidosis or metabolic alkalosis; changes in the rate of alveolar ventilation produce respiratory acidosis or respiratory alkalosis.

12 Metabolic acidosis is caused by an increase in noncarbonic acids or loss of bicarbonate from the extracellular fluid.

13 Metabolic alkalosis occurs with an increase in bicarbonate usually caused by loss of metabolic acids from conditions such as vomiting, gastrointestinal suctioning, excessive bicarbonate intake, hyperaldosteronism, and diuretic therapy.

14 Respiratory acidosis occurs with a decrease of alveolar ventilation and increase in levels of carbon dioxide, which in turn causes hypercapnia.

15 Respiratory alkalosis occurs with alveolar hyperventilation and excessive reduction of carbon dioxide, or hypocapnia.

KEY TERMS

REFERENCES

Berne, R. M., & Levy, M. N. (Eds.). (1993). *Physiology,* (3rd ed.). St. Louis: Mosby–Year Book.
Kokko, J. P., & Tanner, R. L. (1990). *Fluids and electrolytes* (2nd ed.). Philadelphia: W. B. Saunders.
Leaf, A., & Cotran, R. (1985). *Renal pathology* (3rd ed., p. 127). New York: Oxford University Press.
Rose, D. B. (1989). *Clinical physiology of acid-base and electrolyte disorders* (3rd ed.). New York: McGraw-Hill.
Rosenzweig, A., & Seidman, E. (1991). Atrial natriuretic factor and related peptide hormones. *Annual Review of Biochemistry, 60,* 229-255.

SUGGESTED READINGS

Brenner, M., & Williver, J. (1990). Pulmonary and acid-base assessment. *Nursing Clinics of North America, 25*(4), 761-777.
Carroll, H. J. (1992). Whole body acid-base balance. *Contributors to Nephrology 100,* 89-104.
Catehpole, M. (1982, October). Electrolytes, their physiological action and interaction: A review. *Journal of the American Association of Nurse Anesthetists,* 476-481.
Cogan, M. (1991). *Fluid and electrolytes: Physiology and pathophysiology.* Norwalk: Appleton-Lange.
D'Addesio, J. (1992). Metabolic and respiratory acidosis. *Topics in Emergency Medicine, 14*(1), 51-55.
DuBose, T. D. (1992). Acid-base emergencies. *Patient Care, 26*(3), 214-220, 223-231.

Halperin, M. L., Vasuvattakul, S., & Bayoumi, A. (1992). A modified classification of metabolic acidosis: A pathophysiologic approach. *Nephron, 60,* 129-133.
Kovacs, L., & Robertson, G. L. (1992). Syndrome of inappropriate diuresis. *Endocrinology and Metabolism Clinics of North America 21* (4), 859-875.
Lane, G., & Poirce, A. G. (1982, January). When persistence pays off: Resolving the mystery of unexplained electrolyte imbalance. *Nursing 82, 12*(1).
Levy, I. J. (1977, June). Clinical problems in acid-base balance. *Journal of the American Association of Nurse Anesthetists,* 279-289.
Maxwell, M. H., & Kleeman, C. (1980). *Clinical disorders of fluid and electrolyte metabolism.* New York: McGraw-Hill.
McBroom, M. J. (1977, February). Fundamentals of acid-base balance. *Journal of the American Association of Nurse Anesthetists,* 23-36.
Quinlan, M. (1984, April). Edema: What really causes it, how to control it. *RN,* 55-59.
Schrier, R. (1992). *Renal and electrolyte disorders* (4th ed.). Boston: Little, Brown, & Co.
Terry, J. (1991). The other electrolytes: Magnesium, calcium, and phosphorus. *Journal of Intravenous Nursing, 14*(3), 167-176.
Toto, R. D. (1991). Acid-base balance in the CCU patient. *Hospital Medicine, 27*(8), 103-105.
Williams, A. V. (1992). Hyperkalemia: Mechanisms, etiology, and treatment. *Journal of South Carolina Medical Association 88* (12), 561-565.

UNIT II

Genes and Gene-Environment Interaction

GREGOR MENDEL, an Austrian monk who lived in the nineteenth century, is usually credited as the father of genetics. The ancient Hebrews and Greeks and later scholars of the Middle Ages also observed many important genetic phenomena and proposed theories to account for them, but many of their theories were incorrect. Mendel's great contribution was to formulate several important principles of heredity through careful experimentation with living organisms. His laws of segregation and independent assortment form the foundation of modern genetics. Mendel's findings were published in 1865 in an obscure journal. They remained unnoticed until 1900, when they were simultaneously rediscovered by three scientists working independently in three different countries. One of the great ironies of biologic science is that Charles Darwin, the nineteenth-century founder of the theory of evolution, formulated his theories in complete ignorance of Mendel's discoveries.

The first decade after 1900 saw many important advances in genetics. Landsteiner discovered the ABO blood group in 1900. In 1902 Garrod reported on alkaptonuria, the first recognized "inborn error of metabolism." In 1907 Johannsen coined the term *gene* to denote the basic unit of inheritance.

The next four decades were a time of considerable theoretical work and experimentation. The fruit fly, *Drosophila*, became a main-

GENETIC BASIS OF HUMAN DISEASE

Molecular mechanisms and strategies for therapy (1988). (Courtesy National Library of Medicine.)

temporary molecular genetics. Only in 1956, however, was the correct number of human chromosomes (46) identified by cytologists. Until then, it was thought that humans had 48 chromosomes. Three years later, Down syndrome was found to be caused by an extra twenty-first chromosome.

Since 1960 technologic developments in the form of computers and vastly improved laboratory facilities have spurred revolutionary progress in genetics. Laboratory analysis of proteins has demonstrated much more genetic variation in organisms than scientists once thought existed. Analysis of biochemical pathways involved in genetic diseases has pinpointed much more closely the specific defects responsible for the diseases. Increasing refinement of cytogenetic techniques has enabled researchers to uncover many new types of chromosomal abnormalities. Through the use of elaborate statistical techniques, much has been learned about inheritance patterns of complex genetic diseases and about the interactions of genes and environment (see Chapter 5).

stay of genetics laboratories and was also used by H. J. Muller to demonstrate the genetic effects of ionizing radiation. Many fundamental concepts of evolutionary genetics were developed by Ronald Fisher, Sewall Wright, and J. B. S. Haldane. The eugenics movement, which sought to "improve" the genetic quality of the human species through differential breeding, gained popularity in the 1920s and 1930s and then rapidly lost favor after the Nazi atrocities. The inheritance patterns of many important hereditary diseases, such as phenylketonuria, cystic fibrosis, and Huntington disease, were elucidated during this period.

The most significant development in genetics during the 1950s was the specification of the physical structure of deoxyribonucleic acid (DNA) by James Watson and Francis Crick (1953). Their work formed the basis for con-

Perhaps the most rapidly progressing area of genetics is molecular genetics. The precise molecular defects involved in several genetic diseases have been discovered, greatly improving prospects for treating, and perhaps curing, those diseases. In addition, new molecular techniques have allowed scientists to identify the locations of many individual genes on each chromosome. This progress will greatly enhance the already important role of genetics in preventive health care.

Genes and Genetic Diseases

Lynn B. Jorde

In the nineteenth century, microscopic studies of cells led scientists to suspect that the nucleus of the cell contained the important mechanisms of inheritance. Scientists found that chromatin, the substance that gives the nucleus a granular appearance, is observable in nondividing cells. Just before the cell divides, the chromatin condenses to form discrete, dark-staining organelles, which are called chromo-

somes. (Cell division is discussed in Chapter 1.) With the rediscovery of Mendel's important breeding experiments at the turn of the twentieth century, it soon became apparent that the chromosomes contained **genes**, the basic units of inheritance. Chromosomes were the subject of much study, but because of poorly developed laboratory techniques, progress was slow. Since the mid-1950s, however, technologic advances *have permitted a rapid increase in scientific knowledge of the form, composition, and function of chromosomes.*

The primary constituent of the chromatin is **deoxyribonucleic acid (DNA).** *Genes are composed of sequences of DNA. By serving as the blueprints of proteins in the body, genes ultimately influence all aspects of body structure and function.* **Structural genes** *dictate the makeup of proteins. Estimates suggest that there are approximately 50,000 to 100,000 structural genes. An error in one of these genes often leads to a recognizable genetic disease.*

To date, nearly 5000 genetic conditions have been identified and cataloged (McKusick, 1992). As infectious diseases come under increasingly effective control, the proportion of beds of pediatric hospitals occupied by children with genetic diseases has risen to one third (Hall, Powers, McIlvaine, & Ean, 1978). In addition, many common diseases that primarily affect adults, such as hypertension, coronary heart disease, diabetes, and cancer, are now known to have important genetic components. (These diseases are also affected by environmental factors. The interaction between genetic and environmental components is discussed in Chapter 5.)

Great progress is being made in the diagnosis of genetic diseases and the understanding of genetic mechanisms underlying them. With the huge strides being made in molecular genetics, "gene therapy"— the replacement of disease genes with normal ones— has begun. Genetics is now one of the most rapidly advancing fields of medicine.

DNA, RNA, AND PROTEINS: HEREDITY AT THE MOLECULAR LEVEL

DNA

Composition and Structure of DNA

Genes are composed of DNA, which has three basic components: the pentose sugar molecule, deoxyribose; a phosphate molecule; and four types of nitrogenous bases. Two of the bases, **cytosine** and **thymine,** are single carbon-nitrogen rings called **pyrimidines.** The other two bases, **adenine** and **guanine,** are double carbon-nitrogen rings called **purines.** The four bases are commonly represented by their first letters: *A, C, T,* and *G.*

One of Watson and Crick's contributions was to demonstrate how these molecules are physically assembled together as DNA. They proposed the now-famous **double-helix** model, in which DNA can be envisioned as a twisted ladder with chemical bonds as its rungs (Fig. 4-1). The two sides of the ladder are composed of the sugar and phosphate molecules, held together by strong

phosphodiester bonds. Projecting from each side of the ladder, at regular intervals, are the nitrogenous bases. The base projecting from one side is bound to the base projecting from the other by a weak hydrogen bond. Therefore, the nitrogenous bases form the rungs of the ladder; adenine pairs with thymine, and guanine pairs with cytosine. Each DNA subunit—consisting of one deoxyribose molecule, one phosphate group, and one base—is called a **nucleotide.**

DNA as the Genetic Code

To serve as the basis of genetic inheritance, DNA must be able to direct the synthesis of all the body's proteins. Proteins are composed of one or more **polypeptides** (intermediate protein compounds), which are in turn composed of sequences of **amino acids** (organic acids containing NH_2). The body contains 20 different types of amino acids, and the amino acid sequences that make up polypeptides must in some way be specified by the DNA molecule.

Because there are 20 possible amino acids and only 4 possible bases, each single nucleotide cannot specify an

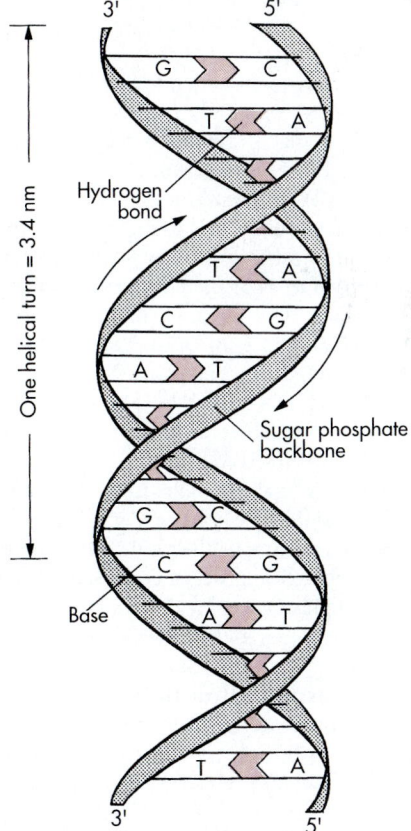

FIG. 4-1 Structure of the double helix that forms the DNA molecule. Sugar-phosphate bonds are the backbones of the two polynucleotide chains. The nitrogenous bases are in the center of the molecule and correspond to the "rungs" in the usual schematic representation of DNA.

Terms such as *cloning, genetic engineering,* and *recombinant DNA* have received a great deal of exposure in the popular press during the past several years as the news media have recognized the potential importance of these techniques. Indeed they are part of the scientific revolution sometimes known as the "new genetics."

Recombinant DNA

Genetic engineering refers to laboratory alteration of genes. Most alterations are accomplished by using recombinant DNA techniques, which involve combining the DNA of two or more different organisms. A number of sophisticated methods have been invented to alter genes. A common approach that is similar in principle to most other approaches is described here.

Among the key components of recombinant DNA research are bacterial plasmids, small circular pieces of self-replicating DNA that reside in many bacteria but often are not essential to the growth or survival of the bacteria. Plasmids can therefore be extracted from or inserted into bacteria without seriously disrupting bacterial growth or reproduction. Once they have been extracted from their bacterial hosts, the plasmids are exposed to restriction endonucleases, which are enzymes that cleave, or cut, the plasmid DNA at a specific nucleotide sequence, called a restriction site.

Different restriction endonucleases have different restriction sites. A commonly used restriction endonuclease is called *Eco*RI (from the bacteria that produce it, *Escherichia coli*). *Eco*RI cleaves DNA only when the sequence GAATTC is found on one DNA strand and the complementary sequence is found on the other strand. The DNA of another organism, such as a human, can also be exposed to *Eco*RI and can be cleaved at the same restriction sites. The resulting human restriction fragments, which are pieces of DNA, have exposed ends that have base sequences complementary to those of the cleaved plasmid DNA. The human DNA and plasmid DNA, if mixed together, undergo complementary base pairing (that is, they recombine).

The result is that the human DNA is incorporated within the plasmid. The plasmids, which now contain human genes in addition to their own, are allowed to reenter bacteria. Selection processes can be applied to extract the bacteria that contain the desired human genes. These bacteria are cultured and allowed to form clones (or genetically identical copies) through normal cell division. Through continued cell division, millions of bacterial clones are formed, all containing the same human gene. Like any other gene, the human gene directs protein synthesis in the bacteria, resulting in the production of human proteins by bacteria.

Because bacteria multiply rapidly, large amounts of a given human protein can be manufactured by using this procedure. It has already been used successfully to produce human insulin in mass quantities. Because the insulin produced this way is actually human insulin, it causes fewer allergic reactions than the insulin taken from animal pancreases. Interferon, a substance that may help the body to fight cancer and viral infections, has also been produced this way, as has human growth hormone, a substance that can be used to cure pituitary dwarfism.

In trying to isolate a particular gene, it is often more convenient to begin work with the messenger RNA (mRNA) that codes for the gene product. The mRNA can be purified from body cells, and then an enzyme called reverse transcriptase can be used to generate the DNA sequence that is complementary to the mRNA. This complementary DNA (cDNA) can be inserted into plasmids and cloned by using the same recombinant techniques, so that virtually unlimited quantities of the desired gene product can be manufactured.

Recombinant DNA methods have been applied toward the understanding of the single-gene disorder phenylketonuria (PKU), which is the result of a lack of the enzyme phenylalanine hydroxylase. First, mRNA coding for this enzyme was purified from rat liver cells. After attachment of a radioactive "label" to cDNA produced from this mRNA, the cDNA was used as a probe. The probe was exposed to a series of cells that had been manipulated in the laboratory so that each cell line contained only one or a few chromosomes. When the probe hybridized consistently with only the cells containing chromosome 12, it proved that the gene that produces phenylalanine hydroxylase and thus causes PKU is located on this chromosome. Knowing the chromosome location of a gene is a very important step in the diagnosis and understanding of a genetic disease. Ultimately, therapeutic techniques might be developed to correct such disorders by replacing or repairing the abnormal gene.

The use of recombinant DNA techniques to clone DNA sequences has been, and continues to be, of great importance in genetics. However, the cloning process can take a great deal of time, even for well-studied genes. When genetic diagnosis is done, it is often necessary to obtain results very quickly. A newer technique, the polymerase chain reaction (PCR), provides a very rapid means of making millions of copies of a DNA sequence in only a few hours (as opposed to a week or longer when cloning techniques are used). PCR basically involves the artificial replication of a DNA sequence, achieved by exposing the DNA strand to alterations in temperature in the presence of free DNA bases. At lower temperatures the DNA undergoes complementary base pairing. At higher temperatures the DNA strands separate to form new templates for another cycle of replication when the temperature is again lowered. By repeating this temperature cycling again and again, DNA copies can be produced rapidly (Erlich, Gelfand, & Sninsky, 1991). This technique is very useful for diagnostic purposes because it requires only a very small sample of blood or other tissue and because many copies can be made in a very short time. In theory, even a single DNA molecule can be copied millions of times by using PCR. PCR is also used extensively in forensic medicine (e.g., in identifying the DNA of criminal suspects by using blood, semen, or hair samples left at the scene of a crime).

Process by which DNA is recombined.

A

Plasmid

E. coli — Bacterial chromosome

tet^r

GAATTC
CTTAAG
Cleavage site

B Plasmid

EcoRI

tet^r

G
AATTC
Sticky ends

CTTAAG

Anneal

tet^r

GAATTC
CTTAA

D Recombinant DNA

Insert into E. coli
E

Replicate

Replicate
F

AATTC
G
Sticky ends
CTTAA

C Human DNA

GAATTC   GAATTC
CTTAAG   CTTAAG

The advent of this technology has led to fears that organisms that could pose grave threats to the human species might be created. In 1974 a group of molecular geneticists themselves called a moratorium on recombinant DNA research when its implications began to be realized. However, after much study and the introduction of rules regarding laboratory containment, research was resumed. Because of the elaborate precautions taken to prevent inadvertent creation of harmful organisms and because of the very low probability that such organisms could survive outside the laboratory, the possibility of such an occurrence is now considered to be extremely remote.

Gene therapy

An area in which recombinant DNA techniques have generated a great deal of interest is gene therapy, which essentially involves the insertion of normal genes. For example, by recombinant DNA methods, a normal gene might be inserted into a human chromosome to counteract the effects of an abnormal or missing gene.

Gene therapy can be applied in two ways. The less controversial approach is somatic cell therapy, which consists of inserting normal genes into the cells of an individual who has a genetic disease. In this way a particular tissue, such as bone marrow cells that produce abnormal erythrocytes, would be treated. More controversial is the application of gene therapy very early in embryonic development. By inserting genes into the embryos, all body cells could be altered, including the germ cells. Thus not only would the genetic constitution of the embryo and resulting individual be changed, but all the descendants of that individual also would have altered genetic constitutions. This procedure is sometimes referred to as germ cell therapy.

Somatic cell therapy has been initiated for several human genetic diseases, including a form of severe combined immune deficiency caused by adenosine deaminase deficiency (Anderson, 1992). The procedure has been quite successful in individuals with such diseases, and no serious side effects have been encountered. It is likely that many additional genetic diseases will be treated through somatic cell therapy in the near future (Miller, 1992). Because of several important technical and ethical considerations, germ line therapy will not be attempted in humans in the foreseeable future.

amino acid. Similarly, the amino acids cannot be specified by couplets of bases (e.g., adenine-guanine, thymine-guanine, guanine-cytosine) because there are only 4 times 4, or 16, possible couplets. If series of three bases are translated into amino acids, however, there are 4 times 4 times 4, or 64, possible combinations—more than enough to specify each different amino acid. By manufacturing synthetic nucleotide sequences and allowing them to direct the formation of amino acids in the laboratory, it was proved that amino acids were specified by these triplets of bases, or **codons.**

Of the 64 possible codons, 3 signal the end of a gene and are known as **termination** or **nonsense codons.** The remaining 61 *all* specify amino acids, which means that most amino acids can be specified by more than 1 codon. The genetic code is thus said to be redundant, although each codon can specify only one amino acid.

Another significant feature of the genetic code is that it is universal: *all* living organisms use precisely the same DNA codes to specify proteins. The one known exception to this rule occurs in mitochondria, cytoplasmic organelles that are the sites of cellular respiration (see Chapter 1). The mitochondria have their own extranuclear DNA. Several codons of mitochondrial DNA code for different amino acids than do the same nuclear DNA codons.

Replication of DNA

In addition to having the ability to specify amino acid sequences, DNA must be able to replicate itself accurately during cell division if it is to serve as the basic genetic material. DNA replication consists of the breaking of the weak hydrogen bonds between the bases, leaving a single strand with each base unpaired. The consistent pairing of adenine with thymine and of guanine with cytosine, known as **complementary base pairing,** is the key to accurate replication. The principle of complementary base pairing dictates that the unpaired base will attract a free nucleotide only if the nucleotide has the proper complementary base. Thus a portion of a single strand with a sequence of bases labeled ATTGCT will bond with a series of free nucleotides with the bases TAACGA. When replication is complete, a new double-stranded molecule identical to the original is formed (Fig. 4-2). The single strand is said to be a **template,** or molecule on which a complementary molecule is built, and is the basis for synthesizing the new double strand.

Several different proteins are involved in DNA replication. One protein unwinds the double helix, one holds the strands apart, and others perform different distinct functions. The most important of these proteins is an enzyme known as **DNA polymerase.** This enzyme travels along the single DNA strand, adding the correct nucleotides to the free end of the new strand. Besides adding the new nucleotides, the DNA polymerase performs

FIG. 4-2 Replication of DNA. The two chains of the double helix separate, and each chain serves as the template for a new complementary chain.

a proofreading procedure. After the new nucleotide has been added to the chain, the DNA polymerase checks to make sure that its base is actually complementary to the template base. If it is not, the incorrect nucleotide is excised and replaced with a correct one. This procedure, one of the mechanisms of DNA repair, substantially enhances the accuracy of DNA replication.

Mutation

A **mutation** is any inherited alteration of genetic material. Chromosome aberrations that cause congenital defects are examples of mutations. Other mutations are subtle and are not observable as chromosome aberrations. One such mutation is the **base pair substitution,** in which one base pair is replaced by another. This substitution sometimes results in a change in amino acid sequence, but because of the redundancy of the genetic code, it may have no consequence. Such mutations are often called **silent substitutions.** Profound consequences can result, however, when an amino acid sequence is altered by a base pair substitution. (Many of the serious genetic diseases discussed later are the result of base pair substitutions.)

The second major type of mutation is the **frameshift mutation.** This alteration involves the insertion or deletion of one or more base pairs to the DNA molecule. As Fig. 4-3 shows, these mutations can change the entire "reading frame" of the DNA sequence because codons consist of groups of three base pairs. A frameshift mutation thus can greatly alter the resulting amino acid sequence.

A large number of agents are known to increase the frequency of mutations. These agents are known collectively as **mutagens.** Radiation, such as that produced by x-rays and nuclear fallout, is an important mutagen and is known to cause cell damage (see Chapter 2). Radiation forms electrically charged ions that can produce chemical reactions that in turn change DNA bases. A variety of chemicals can also induce mutations, often because they are chemically similar to DNA bases. Other chemicals mimic the effects of ionizing radiation, and still others interfere with the process of base pairing. Hundreds of chemicals are now known to be mutagenic in humans and/or laboratory animals. Among these are nitrogen mustard, vinyl chloride, alkylating agents, formaldehyde, sodium nitrite, and saccharin. Some of these chemicals, however, are much more potent mutagens than others. Nitrogen mustard, for example, is extremely mutagenic, whereas saccharin is a relatively weak mutagen.

Measurement of the mutation rate in humans is difficult, in part because mutations are very rare events. Current estimates are that the rate of **spontaneous mutation** (a mutation that occurs in the absence of exposure to known mutagens) in humans is about 10^{-4} to 10^{-7} per gene per generation. This rate appears to vary from one gene to another. Certain areas of some chromosomes have particularly high mutation rates and are known as **mutational hot spots.** In particular, sequences consisting of a cytosine base followed by a guanine base (CG) are highly susceptible to mutation and are known to account for a disproportionately large percentage of disease-causing mutations (Cooper & Youssoufian, 1988).

From Genes to Proteins

Whereas DNA is formed and replicated in the cell nucleus, protein synthesis takes place in the cytoplasm. The transport of the DNA code from nucleus to cytoplasm and subsequent protein formation involves two basic processes, **transcription** and translation. Both of

FIG. 4-3 Different kinds of mutations.

these processes are mediated by **ribonucleic acid (RNA),** a type of nucleic acid that is chemically very similar to DNA. RNA is also composed of sugar molecules, phosphate groups, and nitrogenous bases. RNA differs from DNA in that the sugar molecule is ribose rather than deoxyribose and in that uracil rather than thymine is one of the four bases. The other bases of RNA, as in DNA, are adenine, cytosine, and guanine. Uracil is structurally very similar to thymine, so it also can pair with adenine. The final difference between RNA and DNA is that, whereas DNA usually occurs as a double strand, RNA usually occurs as a single strand.

Transcription

Transcription is the process by which RNA is synthesized from a DNA template. The result is the formation of **messenger RNA (mRNA)** from the base sequence specified by the DNA molecule. An enzyme called DNA-dependent RNA polymerase, or **RNA polymerase,** binds to a **promoter** site on the DNA. A promoter site is a sequence of DNA that specifies the beginning of a gene. The RNA polymerase then pulls a portion of the DNA strands apart from one another, allowing unattached DNA bases to be exposed. One of the DNA strands then provides the template for the sequence of mRNA nucleotides.

The sequence of bases in the mRNA is thus complementary to that of the template strand, and with the exception of the presence of uracil instead of thymine, the mRNA sequence is identical to that of the other DNA strand. Transcription continues until a DNA sequence called a **termination sequence** is reached. Then the RNA polymerase detaches from the DNA, and the transcribed mRNA is freed to move out of the nucleus and into the cytoplasm. The process of transcription is summarized in Fig. 4-4.

Gene Splicing

After the mRNA first has been transcribed from the DNA template, it reflects exactly the base sequence of the DNA. The RNA in this state is sometimes called **heterogeneous nuclear RNA (hnRNA).** In eukaryotes an important step takes place before this RNA leaves the nucleus. Many of the RNA sequences are removed by nuclear enzymes, and the remaining sequences are spliced together to form the functional mRNA that will migrate to the cytoplasm.

The excised sequences are called **introns,** and the sequences that are left to code for proteins are called **exons.** The function, if any, of introns is not yet understood.

Translation

Translation is the process by which RNA directs the synthesis of a polypeptide. However, mRNA cannot code directly for amino acids. Instead, it interacts with **transfer RNA (tRNA),** a cloverleaf-shaped strand of about 80 nucleotides. As Fig. 4-5 illustrates, the tRNA molecule has a site for the attachment of an amino acid. At the opposite side of the cloverleaf is a sequence of three nucleotides called the **anticodon.** The anticodon undergoes complementary base pairing with an appropriate codon in the mRNA. The mRNA thus specifies the sequence of amino acids by acting through the tRNA.

The site of actual protein synthesis is the **ribosome,** which consists of roughly equal parts of protein and **ribosomal RNA (rRNA).** During translation, depicted in Fig. 4-6, the ribosome first binds to an initiation site on the mRNA sequence. The ribosome then binds the tRNA to its surface so that base pairing can occur between tRNA and mRNA. The ribosome then moves along the mRNA sequence, codon by codon. As each codon is processed, an amino acid is translated by the interaction of mRNA and tRNA.

DNA chains   RNA chains

☐ Cytosine
☐ Adenine
☐ Guanine
▨ Uracil
◖ Thymine

RNA polymerase

RNA nucleotide

FIG. 4-4 General scheme of RNA transcription (see text for explanation).

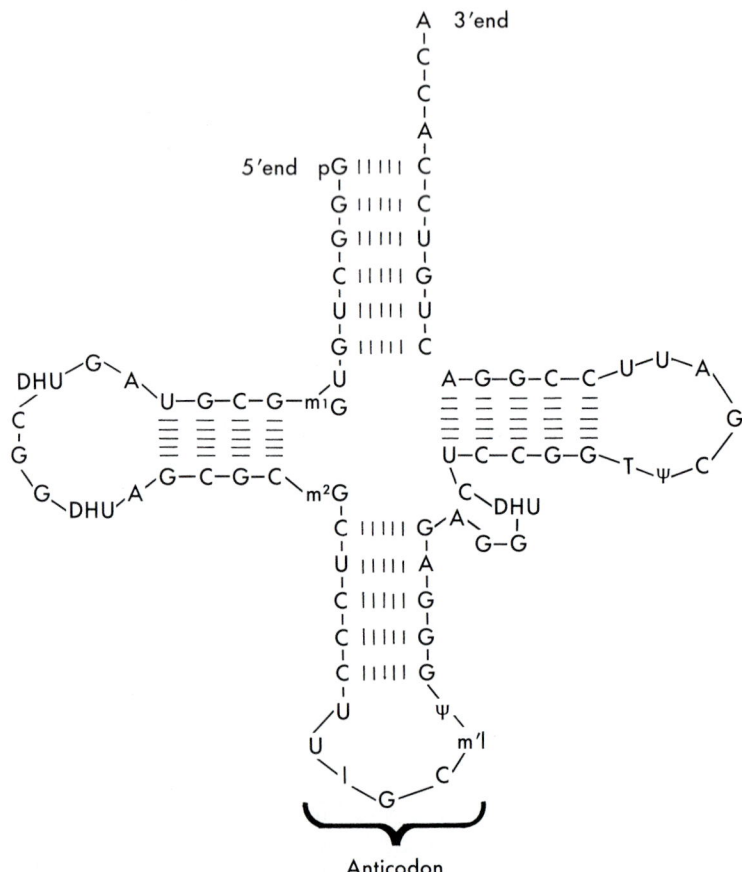

FIG. 4-5 Cloverleaf structure of transfer RNA.

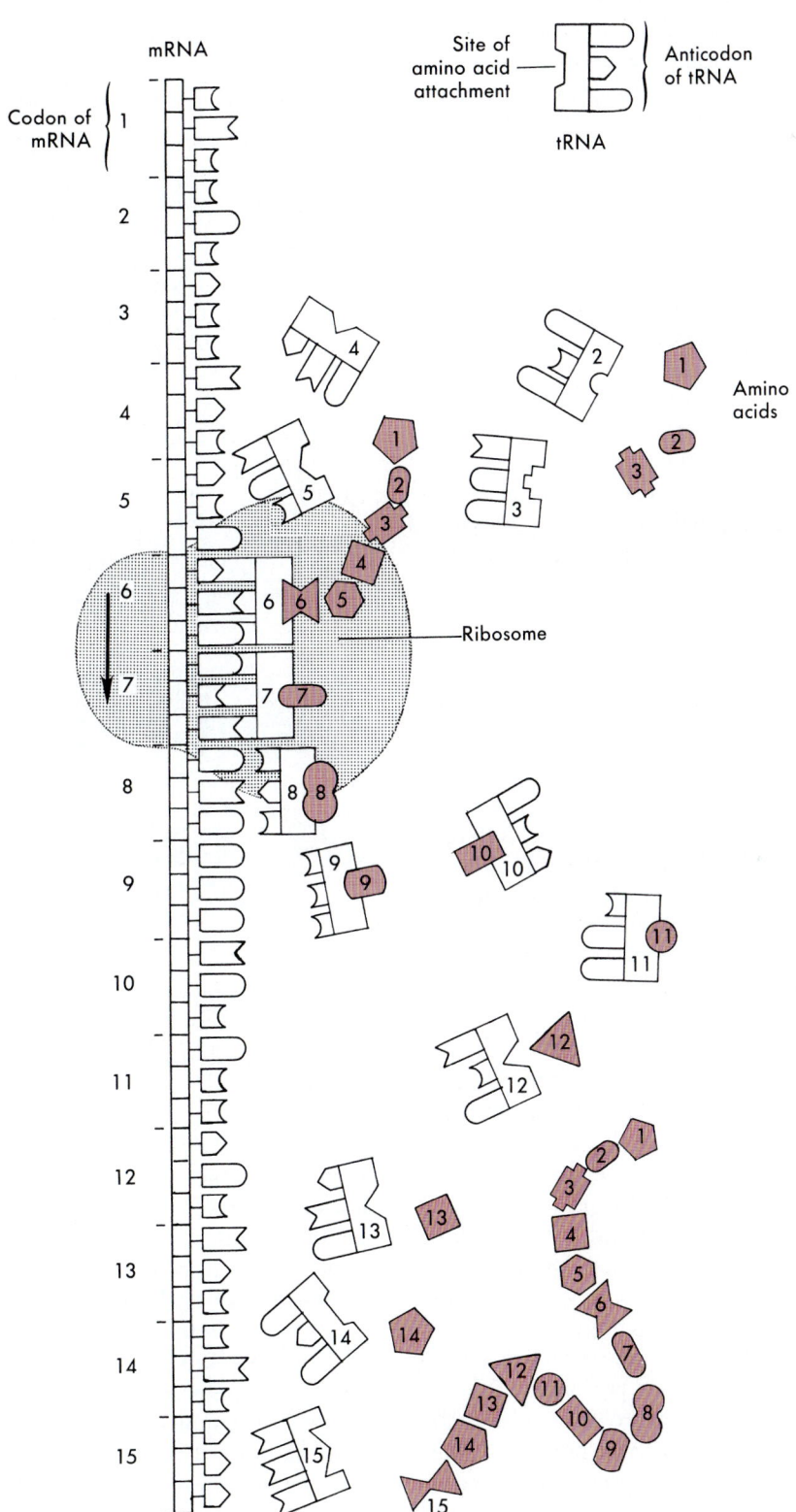

FIG. 4-6 A ribosome "reading" the code of mRNA and assembling a polypeptide chain.

In this process the ribosome provides an enzyme that catalyzes the formation of covalent peptide bonds between the adjacent amino acids, resulting in a growing polypeptide. When the ribosome arrives at a termination signal on the mRNA sequence, translation and polypeptide formation cease. The mRNA, ribosome, and polypeptide separate from one another, and the polypeptide is released into the cytoplasm to perform its required function.

CHROMOSOMES

Human cells can be categorized into two types: the **gametes** (sperm and egg cells) and the **somatic cells,** which include all cells other than gametes. Each somatic cell has 46 chromosomes in its nucleus. These are **diploid cells,** meaning that the chromosomes occur in pairs. Thus each cell actually contains 23 pairs of chromosomes. One member of each pair comes from the individual's mother, and one comes from the father. New somatic cells are formed through mitosis and cytokinesis, through which the cell nucleus and cytoplasm are replicated. (The division process that creates new copies of somatic cells is described in Chapter 1.) Gametes are **haploid cells:** they have only one member of each chromosome pair, giving them a total of 23 chromosomes. The process by which these haploid cells are formed from diploid cells is called **meiosis** and is illustrated in Fig. 4-7.

In 22 of the 23 chromosome pairs, the two members of each pair are virtually identical in microscopic appearance and are thus said to be **homologous** to one another. These 22 chromosome pairs are homologous in both males and females and are termed **autosomes.** The remaining pair of chromosomes, the **sex chromosomes,** consist of two homologous X chromosomes in females and a nonhomologous pair, X and Y, in males.

Fig. 4-8, *A,* illustrates a **metaphase spread,** which is a photograph of the chromosomes as they appear in the nucleus of a somatic cell during metaphase. (Chromosomes are easiest to visualize during this stage of mitosis.) A **karyotype** is an ordered display of chromosomes. In Fig. 4-8, *B,* the chromosomes in this photograph are cut out and arranged according to size, with the **homologous chromosomes** paired together. The 22 autosomes are numbered according to length, with chromosome number 1 as the longest and chromosome 22 as the shortest. Some natural variation in relative chromosome length can be expected from person to person, however, so it is not always possible to distinguish each chromosome by its length. Therefore the position of the centromere is also used to classify the chromosomes (Fig. 4-9).

The chromosomes shown in Fig. 4-8 were stained

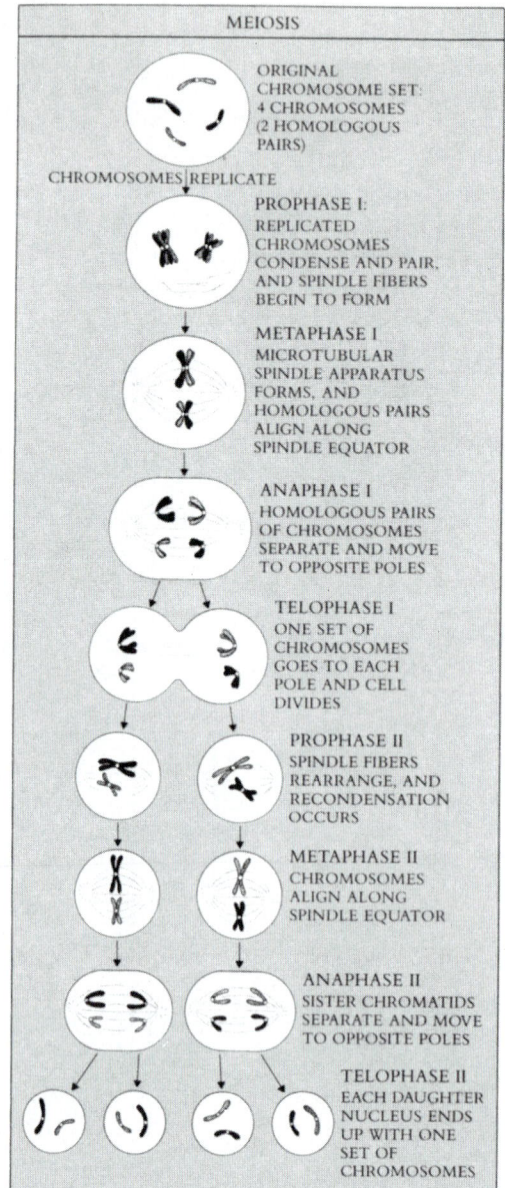

FIG. 4-7 Phases of meiosis. (From Raven & Johnson, 1992.)

with a substance that penetrates all areas of the chromosome (a "solid stain"). In the late 1960s and early 1970s several staining materials were found to bind preferentially to certain areas of chromosomes. The resulting distinctive **chromosome bands** are evident in various patterns in the different chromosomes so that each chromosome can be distinguished easily. One of the most commonly used stains is **Giemsa stain.** By using banding techniques, chromosomes can be unambiguously numbered, and individual variation in chromosome composition can be studied. Missing or duplicated portions of chromosomes, which often result in serious diseases, can also be readily identified.

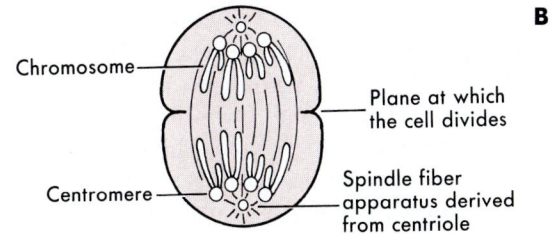

FIG. 4-8 Karyotype of chromosomes. A, Chromosomes of normal male (×2000). **B,** Karyotype of chromosomes seen in **A.** Chromosomes were obtained from a leukocyte, or white blood cell, taken from the blood of a male donor. (From Thibodeau, G. A. [1987]. *Anatomy and physiology.* St. Louis: Mosby–Year Book.)

FIG. 4-9 Structure of chromosomes. A, Human chromosomes 1, 5, and 13. Each is replicated and consists of two chromatids. Chromosome 1 is a metacentric chromosome because the centromere is close to the middle; chromosome 5 is submetacentric because the centromere is set off from the middle; chromosome 13 is acrocentric because the centromere is at or very near the end. **B,** During mitosis the centromere divides, and the chromosomes move to opposite poles of the cell. At the time of centromere division, the chromatids are designated chromosomes.

Chromosome Aberrations and Associated Diseases

Chromosome abnormalities are the leading known cause of mental retardation and miscarriage. Estimates indicate that a major chromosome aberration occurs in at least 1 in 12 conceptions. Most of these fetuses do not survive to term; in fact, about 50% of all recovered spontaneous abortuses have major chromosome aberrations (Hassold, 1986). The number of live births affected by these abnormalities is not, however, insignificant; about 1 in 150 has a major diagnosable chromosome abnormality (de Grouchy & Turleau, 1990).

Polyploidy

Cells that have a multiple of the normal number of chromosomes are said to be **euploid cells** (Greek *eu* = good or true). Because normal gametes are haploid and most normal somatic cells are diploid, they are both euploid forms. When a euploid cell has more than the diploid number of chromosomes, it is said to be a **polyploid cell.** Several types of body tissues, including some liver, bronchial, and epithelial tissues, are normally polyploid. A zygote having three copies of each chromosome, rather than the usual two, has a form of polyploidy called **triploidy. Tetraploidy,** a condition in which euploid cells have 92 chromosomes, has also been observed. Both of these conditions are incompatible with postnatal survival. Nearly all triploid fetuses are spontaneously aborted or stillborn. A few have survived to term but have died shortly after birth. Tetraploidy has been found primarily in early abortuses, although occasionally affected infants have been born alive. Like triploid infants, however, they do not survive. Triploidy and tetraploidy are relatively common conditions, accounting for approximately 10% of all known miscarriages (Hassold, 1986).

Aneuploidy

A somatic cell that does not contain a multiple of 23 chromosomes is an **aneuploid cell.** A cell containing three copies of one chromosome is said to be trisomic (a condition termed **trisomy**) and is aneuploid. **Monosomy,** the presence of only one copy of a given chromosome in a diploid cell, is the other common form of aneuploidy. Among the autosomes, monosomy of any chromosome is lethal, but newborns with trisomy of some chromosomes can survive. This difference illustrates an important principle: *in general, loss of chromosome material has more serious consequences than duplication of chromosome material.*

Aneuploidy of the sex chromosomes is less serious than that of the autosomes. For the Y chromosome, this is true because very little genetic material seems to be located on this chromosome. For the X chromosome, inactivation of extra chromosomes largely diminishes their effect. A zygote bearing *no* X chromosome, however, will not survive.

Aneuploidy is usually the result of **nondisjunction,** an error in which homologous chromosomes or sister chromatids fail to separate normally during meiosis or mitosis (Fig. 4-10). Nondisjunction during either stage of meiosis produces some gametes that have two copies of a given chromosome and others that have no copies of the chromosome. When such gametes unite with normal haploid gametes, the resulting zygote is monosomic or trisomic for that chromosome. Occasionally, a cell can be monosomic or trisomic for more than one chromosome.

Autosomal aneuploidy

Trisomy can occur for any chromosome, but the only forms seen with an appreciable frequency in live births are trisomies of the thirteenth, eighteenth, or twenty-first chromosomes. Fetuses with most other chromosomal trisomies *do not* survive to term. Trisomy 16, for example, is the most commonly known trisomy among abortuses, but it is not seen in live births (Hassold & Jacobs, 1984).

Partial trisomy, in which only an extra portion of a chromosome is present in each cell, can also occur. As one would expect, the consequences of partial trisomies are not as severe as those of complete trisomies. Trisomies may also occur in only some cells of the body. Individuals thus affected are said to be **chromosomal mosaics,** meaning that the body has two or more different cell lines, each of which has a different karyotype. Mosaics are usually formed by early mitotic nondisjunction occurring in one embryo cell but not in others.

The best-known example of aneuploidy in an autosome is trisomy of the twenty-first chromosome, which causes **Down syndrome** (named after J. Langdon Down, who first described the disease in 1866). This disease was formerly called "mongolism," but because of its racist connotations, this term is no longer used. Down syndrome is seen in 1 in 800 live births (Hassold & Jacobs, 1984). Individuals with this disease are mentally retarded, with intelligence quotients (IQs) usually ranging from 25 to 50. The facial appearance is distinctive (Fig. 4-11), with a low nasal bridge, epicanthal folds (which produce the superficially Oriental appearance), protruding tongue, and flat, low-set ears. Poor muscle tone (hypotonia) and short stature are both characteristic. Congenital heart defects affect about one third to one half of live-born children with Down syndrome; a reduced ability to fight respiratory infections and an increased susceptibility to leukemia also contribute to reduced survival rate. By age 40, individuals with Down syndrome virtually always develop symptoms that are nearly identical to those of Alzheimer disease. About three fourths of fetuses known to have Down syndrome

CLINICAL COMMENTARY   PRENATAL DIAGNOSIS OF CHROMOSOME ABNORMALITIES

All the chromosome abnormalities discussed here can be detected prenatally, using a procedure called *amniocentesis*. At about the sixteenth week of gestation, a sufficient amount of amniotic fluid is available to enable the withdrawal of a small amount of fluid (2 to 20 ml). This fluid contains live skin cells (fibroblasts) shed by the fetus. These cells can be cultured and karyotyped, and chromosome abnormalities can be detected.

Other disorders can be detected with this procedure. These include most neural tube defects, which cause an elevation of α-fetoprotein in the amniotic fluid, and more than 100 diseases caused by mutations of single genes. The procedure involves a risk of losing the fetus, estimated to be about 0.5%. Thus amniocentesis is recommended only for pregnancies known to have an elevated risk for a genetic disease. These include pregnancies of women older than 35, in which the risk for Down syndrome and other aneuploidies is elevated, and pregnancies in which parents are known to carry translocations or certain disease genes.

One of the problems with prenatal diagnosis by amniocentesis is that by the time the sixteenth week of gestation is reached and another 2 or 3 weeks to culture the fibroblasts and test for genetic disease elapse, the mother is near the twentieth week of pregnancy. Pregnancy termination involving an affected fetus at this stage can present serious emotional and personal dilemmas as well as some medical risks. For many parents, abortion would be more acceptable for a fetus at an earlier gestational age. A newer technique, *chorionic villus sampling*, consists of extracting a small amount of villous tissue directly from the chorion. This procedure can be performed at about 10 weeks' gestation and does not require in vitro culturing of cells because sufficient numbers are directly available in the extracted tissue. Thus the procedure allows prenatal diagnosis at about 2 months' gestation rather than at nearly 5 months' gestation. Chorionic villus sampling involves a slightly higher fetal loss rate than does amniocentesis, with most estimates ranging from 1% to 2%.

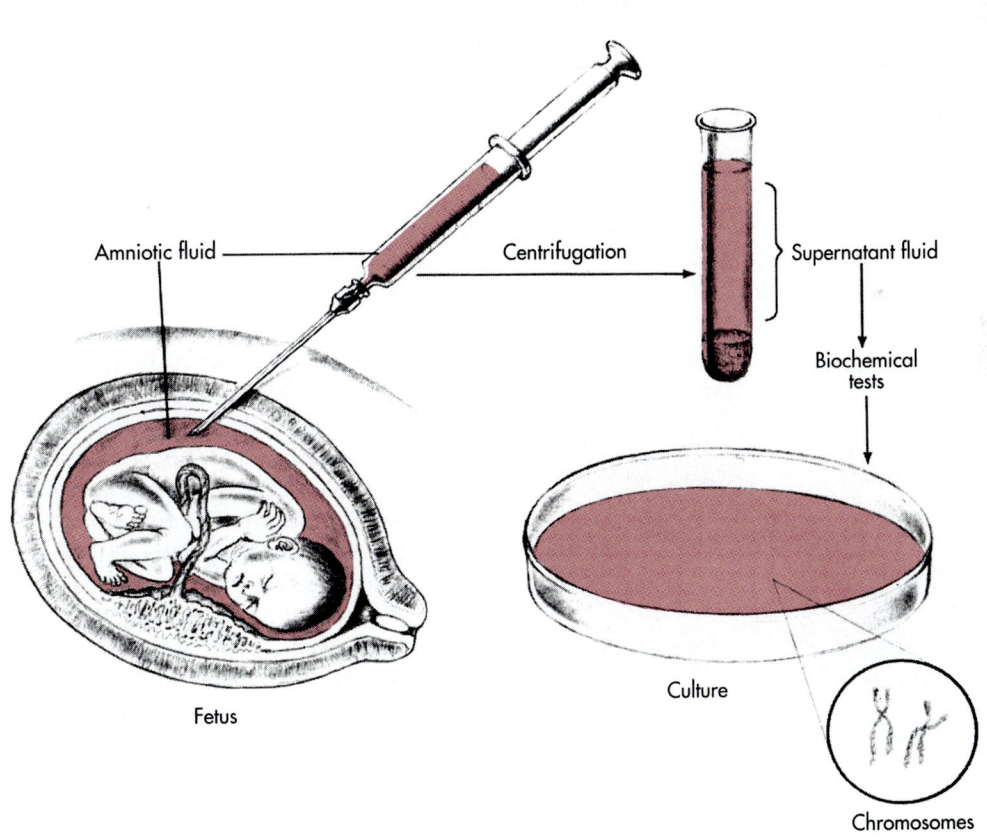

Amniotic fluid   Centrifugation   Supernatant fluid

Biochemical tests

Fetus   Culture   Chromosomes

Amniocentesis, a technique for prenatal diagnosis.

	Metaphase I	Anaphase I	Telophase I	Metaphase II	Anaphase II	Telophase II
a Normal mitosis	X / Y		XY XY			
b Normal meiosis	X Y		X Y			XX / YY
c Mitotic nondisjunction	X / Y		XXY YO			
d Nondisjunction in meiosis II	X Y		X Y			XX / YY
e Nondisjunction in meiosis I	X Y		XY			XY / XY

FIG. 4-10 **Nondisjunction.** Causes aneuploidy when chromosomes or sister chromatids fail to divide properly.

FIG. 4-11 **Down syndrome (trisomy 21).** (From Whaley & Wong, 1991.)

are spontaneously aborted or stillborn. About 20% of infants born with Down syndrome die during their first 10 years of life. For those who survive beyond age 10, average life expectancy is now about 60 years.

About 97% of Down syndrome cases are caused by nondisjunction during the formation of one of the parent's gametes or during early embryonic development. The remaining 3% result from translocations (discussed later). In approximately 90% to 95% of cases, the nondisjunction occurs in the formation of the mother's egg cell. Paternal nondisjunction is responsible for the remaining cases. Among individuals with Down syndrome, about 1% are known to be mosaics. Because mosaics have a large number of normal cells, the effects of the trisomic cells are attenuated and symptoms are generally less severe.

The risk of having a child with Down syndrome increases greatly with maternal age. As Fig. 4-12 demonstrates, women under the age of 30 have a risk ranging from about 1 in 1000 births to 1 in 2000 births. The risk begins to rise substantially after age 35, and it

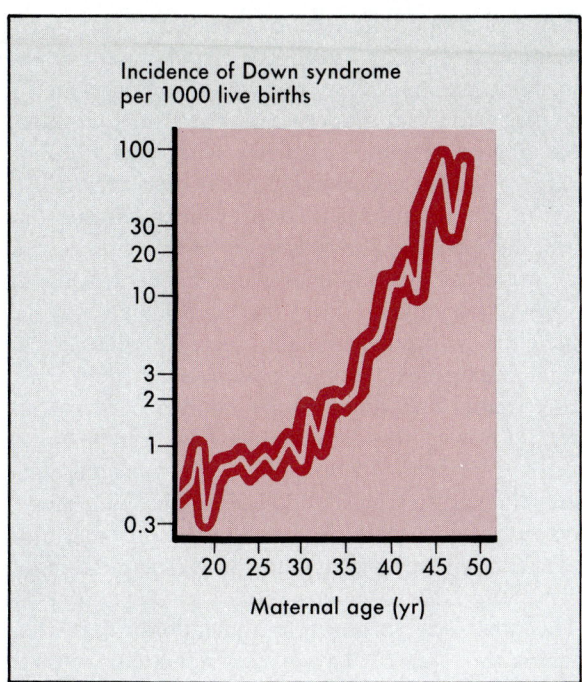

FIG. 4-12 Down syndrome increases with maternal age. Rate is per 1000 live births related to maternal age.

FIG. 4-13 Turner syndrome. A sex chromosome is missing and the person's chromosomes are 45,X. Characteristic signs are short stature, female genitalia, webbed neck, shieldlike chest with underdeveloped breasts and widely spaced nipples, and imperfectly developed ovaries. (From Goodman & Gorlin, 1977.)

reaches 3% to 5% for women over the age of 45. This dramatic increase in risk may be caused by the age of maternal egg cells, which are held in an arrested state of prophase I from the time they are formed in the female embryo until they are shed in ovulation. Thus an egg cell formed by a 45-year-old woman is itself 45 years old. This long suspended state may allow for the accumulation of errors leading to nondisjunction. The risk of Down syndrome, as well as other trisomies, does not increase with paternal age (Martin & Rademaker, 1987).

Sex chromosome aneuploidy

The incidence of sex chromosome aneuploidies is fairly high. Among live births, about 1 in 500 males and 1 in 900 females has a form of sex chromosome aneuploidy (Thompson, McInnes, & Willard, 1991). Because these conditions are generally less severe than autosomal aneuploidies, all forms except complete absence of an X chromosome allow at least some individuals to survive.

One of the most common sex chromosome aneuploidies, affecting about 1 in 1000 newborn females, is trisomy X. Instead of two X chromosomes, these females have three X chromosomes in each cell. Most of them have no overt physical abnormalities, although sterility, menstrual irregularity, or mental retardation is sometimes seen. Some females have four X chromosomes, and they are more often mentally retarded. Those with

five or more X chromosomes generally have more severe mental retardation and various physical defects.

A condition that leads to somewhat more serious problems is the presence of a single X chromosome and no homologous X or Y chromosome, so that the individual has a total of 45 chromosomes. The karyotype is usually designated 45,X, and it causes a set of symptoms known as **Turner syndrome** (Fig. 4-13). Because they have no Y chromosomes, people with Turner syndrome are females. They are usually sterile, however, and have gonadal streaks rather than ovaries. These streaks of connective tissue are susceptible to cancer. Other features of the disorder include short stature, characteristic webbing of the neck, widely spaced nipples, coarctation (narrowing) of the aorta, edema of the feet in newborns, reduced carrying angle at the elbow (cubitus valgus), and sparse body hair. They are not considered retarded, although there is evidence for some impairment of spatial and mathematical reasoning ability. About three fourths of recognized 45,X conceptions inherit their X chromosome from the mother. Thus most cases are caused by a **meiotic error** in the father.

The frequency of Turner syndrome is low compared to that of other sex chromosome aneuploidies: only about 1 in 3000 newborn females is affected (de la Chapelle, 1990). About one half of individuals with Turner syndrome have simple monosomy of the X chromosome; others have one of several more complex X chromosome abnormalities. The 45,X karyotype is extremely common among conceptions, however, and about 15% to 20% of spontaneous abortions with chromosome abnormalities have this karyotype, making it one of the most common single-chromosome aberrations. Thus the condition is highly lethal during gestation: only about 0.5% of 45,X conceptions survive to term. The condition may be relatively benign among live-born females because many or most of these individuals are mosaics. Combinations of 45,X cells with XX, XXX, or XY cells are common among those with Turner syndrome.

Individuals with at least two X chromosomes and a Y chromosome in each cell (47,XXY karyotype) have a disorder known as **Klinefelter syndrome** (Fig. 4-14). Because of the presence of a Y chromosome, these individuals have a male appearance, but they are usually sterile, and about half develop femalelike breasts (a condition called gynecomastia). The testicles are small and firm, body hair is sparse, the voice is often somewhat high pitched, and a moderate degree of mental impairment may be present. Klinefelter syndrome is found in about 1 in 1000 male births. About two thirds of the cases are due to nondisjunction of the X chromosomes in the mother, and the frequency of the disorder rises with maternal age. Individuals with the XXXY and XXXXY karyotypes are also considered to have Klinefelter syndrome, and the degree of physical and mental impairment increases with each additional X chromosome. Regardless of the number of X chromosomes, however, these individuals have a male appearance. The presence of a single Y chromosome, which causes the undifferentiated gonads to become testes, always produces a male. As in Turner syndrome, mosaicism is fairly common; the most prevalent combination is XXY and XY cells.

The other sex chromosome aneuploidy that affects males is the 47,XYY karyotype. Individuals with this karyotype tend to be taller than average, and they have a 10- to 15-point reduction in average IQ. This condition, which causes few serious physical problems, achieved great notoriety when it was found that its incidence in prison populations was about 1 in 30 (compared with 1 in 1000 in the general male population). This discovery led to the suggestion that this chromosome might predispose affected individuals to violent, criminal behavior. Several dozen studies have addressed this issue, and they have shown that XYY males are not inclined to commit violent crimes. However, even after adjusting for the effects of decreased IQ, there is some evidence for an increased propensity to commit minor, nonviolent crimes.

Abnormalities of Chromosome Structure

In addition to the loss or gain of whole chromosomes, parts of chromosomes can be lost or duplicated as gametes are formed, and the arrangement of genes on chromosomes can be altered. Unlike aneuploidy and polyploidy, these changes sometimes do not have serious consequences for an individual's health. Some of them can even go entirely unnoticed, especially when very small pieces of chromosomes are involved. Nevertheless, abnormalities of chromosome structure can also produce serious disease in individuals or their offspring.

During meiosis and mitosis, chromosomes usually maintain their structural integrity very well, but **chromosome breakage** does occasionally occur. Mechanisms exist to "heal" these breaks, and generally the break is repaired perfectly with no damage resulting to the daughter cell. Sometimes, however, the breaks remain, or they heal in a fashion that alters the structure of the chromosome. The extent of chromosome breakage is in-

FIG. 4-14 Klinefelter syndrome. The affected person carries an extra sex chromosome and is XXY. Characteristic signs are normal male genitalia but with small testicles, sparse body hair, some female breast development, and a rather female body shape. (From Whaley & Wong, 1991.)

creased in the presence of certain harmful agents, called **clastogens.** Identified clastogens include ionizing radiation, some viral infections, and certain chemicals.

Deletions

Broken chromosomes and loss of DNA cause **deletions** (Fig. 4-15). Usually, a gamete with a deletion unites with a normal gamete to form a zygote. The zygote thus has one chromosome with the normal complement of genes and one with some missing genes. Because a fairly large number of genes can be lost in a deletion, serious consequences can result even though one chromosome is normal. The most often cited example of a disease caused by a chromosomal deletion is the **cri du chat syndrome** (Fig. 4-16). The term, which literally means "cry of the cat," describes the characteristic cry of the affected child. Other symptoms include low birth weight, severe mental retardation, microcephaly

(smaller than normal head size), heart defects, and the typical facial appearance shown in Fig. 4-16. The disease is caused by a deletion of part of the short arm of chromosome 5.

Duplications

Duplications of chromosome material are, like deletions, a form of chromosome aberration. Because a deficiency of genetic material is more harmful than an excess, duplications usually have less serious consequences than deletions. For example, a deletion of a region of chromosome 5 causes cri du chat syndrome, but a duplication of the same region causes mental retardation but physical traits that are nearly normal.

Inversions

An **inversion** is the occurrence of two breaks on a chromosome, followed by the reinsertion of the missing frag-

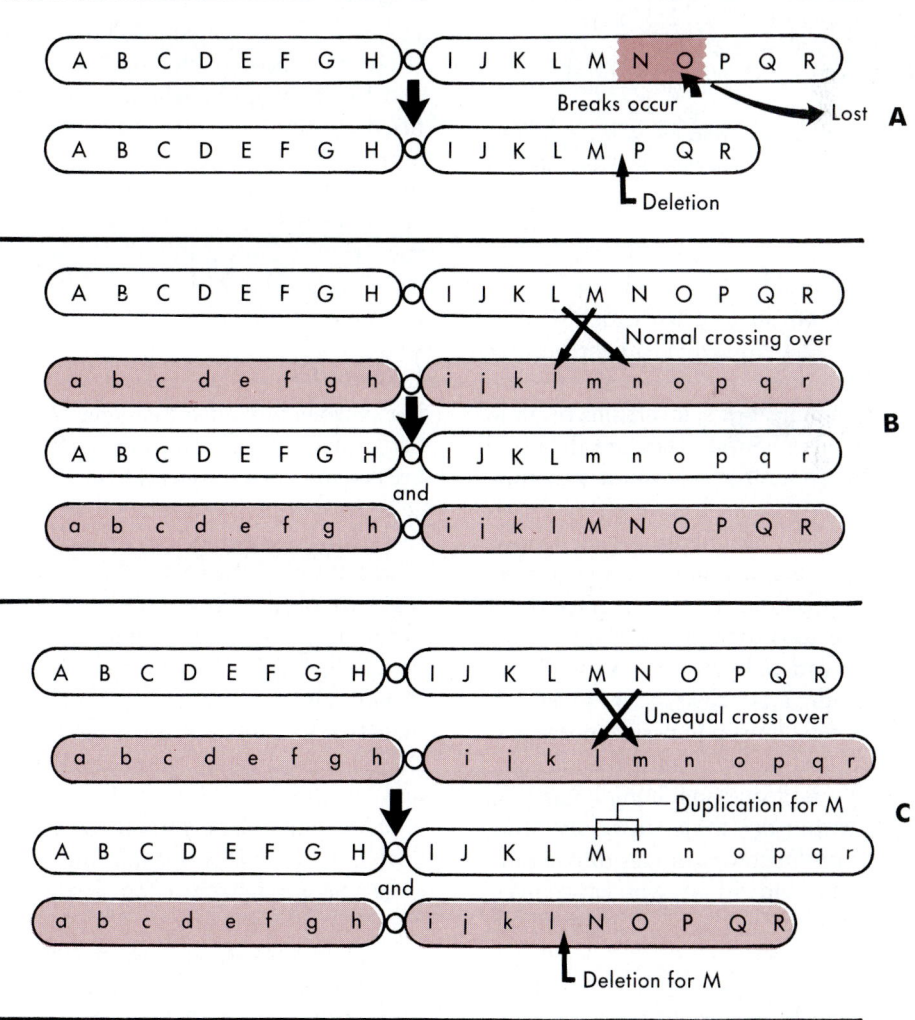

FIG. 4-15 **Abnormalities of chromosome structure. A,** Deletion occurs when a chromosome segment is lost. **B,** Normal crossing-over. **C,** The generation of duplication and deletion through unequal crossing-over.

FIG. 4-16 Infant with cri du chat syndrome. Caused by deletion of part of the short arm of chromosome 5. (From Thompson et al., 1991.)

ment at its original site but in inverted order. Thus a chromosome symbolized as ABCDEFG might become ABEDCFG after an inversion.

Unlike deletions and duplications, inversions result in no loss or gain of genetic material. They are thus said to be a "balanced" alteration of chromosome structure, and they often have no apparent physical effect. Genes are sometimes influenced by neighboring genes, however, and this **position effect,** a change in a gene's expression caused by its position, does sometimes result in physical defects in persons with inversions.

The serious problems caused by inversions usually occur in the offspring of individuals carrying the inversion. Because chromosomes must line up in perfect order during prophase I, a chromosome with an inversion must form a loop to line up with its normal homologue (Fig. 4-17). Crossing-over within this loop can result in duplications or deletions in the chromosomes of daughter cells. Thus the offspring of individuals who carry inversions often have chromosome deletions or duplications.

Translocations

The interchanging of genetic material between nonhomologous chromosomes is called **translocation.** A reciprocal translocation occurs when breaks take place in two different chromosomes and the material is ex-

changed (Fig. 4-18, *A*). As with inversions, the carrier of a reciprocal translocation is usually normal because the individual has a normal complement of genetic material. As Fig. 4-18, *B*, illustrates, however, the carrier's gametes can be normal, can carry the translocation, or can have duplications and deletions.

A second, and clinically more important, type of translocation is termed a **Robertsonian translocation.** In this type of translocation, the long arms of two nonhomologous chromosomes fuse at the centromere, forming a single chromosome. Robertsonian translocations are confined to chromosomes 13 through 15, 21, and 22 since the short arms of these chromosomes are very small and contain no essential genetic material. When a Robertsonian translocation takes place, the short arms are usually lost during subsequent cell divisions. Since the carriers of Robertsonian translocations lose no important genetic material, they are normal, although they have only 45 chromosomes in each cell. Their offspring, however, may have serious deletions or duplications. For example, a common Robertsonian translocation involves the fusion of the long arms of chromosomes 21 and 14. An offspring who inherits a gamete carrying the fused chromosome receives an extra copy of the long arm of chromosome 21 and thus develops Down syndrome. Robertsonian translocations are responsible for approximately 3% to 5% of Down syndrome cases. Parents who carry a Robertsonian translocation involving chromosome 21 have an increased risk for producing multiple offspring with Down syndrome.

Fragile sites

For reasons not yet fully understood, there are a number of areas on chromosomes that develop distinctive breaks and gaps (observable microscopically) when the cells are cultured in a folate-deficient medium. Most of these **fragile sites** have no apparent relationship to disease. However, one particular fragile site, located on the long arm of the X chromosome, is associated with a disorder of considerable importance, both clinically and genetically. This disorder is known as the *fragile X syndrome.* The most important feature of this syndrome is mental retardation. With a relatively high population prevalence (affecting approximately 1 in 1500 males and 1 in 3000 to 5000 females), the fragile X syndrome is the second most common genetic cause of mental retardation (after Down syndrome).

Fragile X syndrome involves a puzzling pattern of inheritance. In particular, males who inherit the mutation do not necessarily express the disease condition, but they can pass it on to descendants who do express it. Ordinarily, a male who inherits a disease gene on the X chromosome expresses the condition since he has only one X chromosome. Another uncommon feature of this disease is that about one third of carrier females are af-

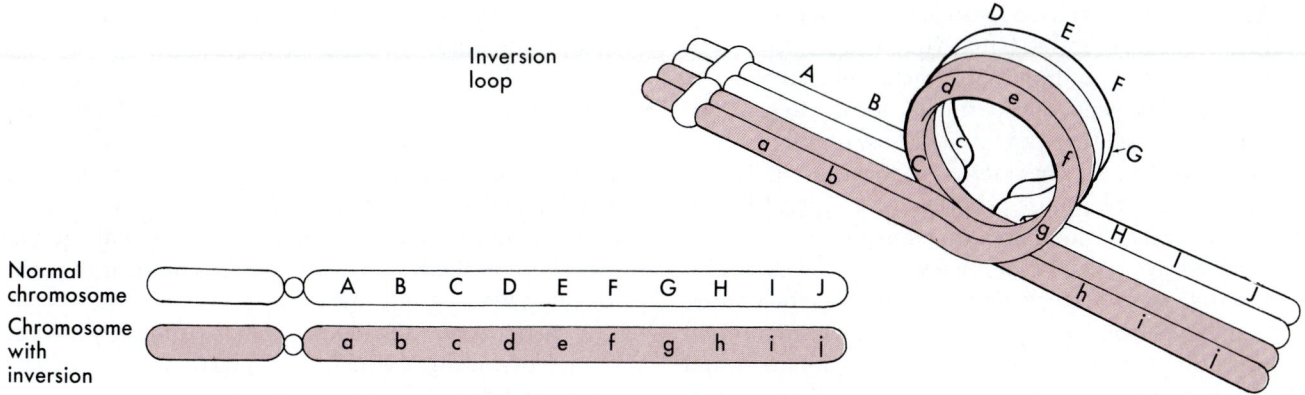

FIG. 4-17   Inversion loop. The loop forms when a chromosome carrying an inversion pairs with a normal (noninverted) homologue.

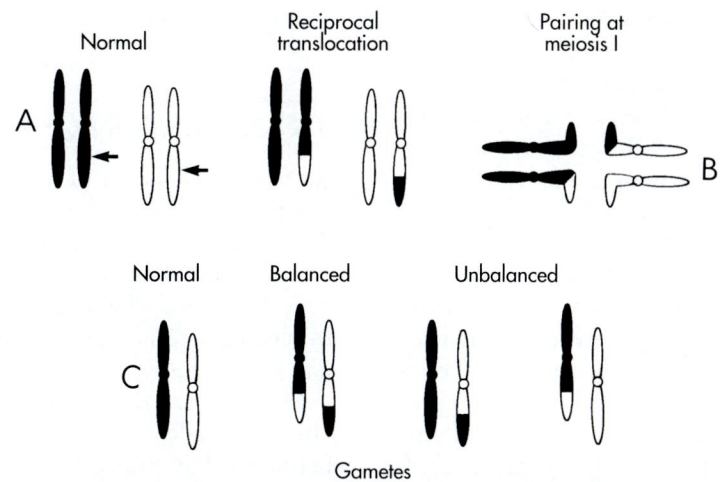

FIG. 4-18   Normal and chromosome translocation. A, Normal chromosomes and reciprocal translocation. **B,** Pairing at meiosis. **C,** Consequences of translocation in gametes; unbalanced gametes result in zygotes that are partially trisomic and partially monosomic and consequently develop abnormally. (From Thompson et al., 1991.)

fected, although less severely than males. Many mechanisms have been proposed to account for the complex mode of inheritance of the fragile X syndrome. Recently, it has been shown that unaffected transmitting males have an elevated number (more than about 50) of repeated DNA sequences in the first exon of the fragile X gene. These "repeats" consist of CGG sequences that are duplicated again and again. Affected males have a much larger number of these repeats, often 100 or more (Fu et al., 1991). It appears that an increase in the number of these repeated sequences in successive generations can lead to expression of the fragile X syndrome. Several other genetic diseases also appear to be caused by this mechanism (Caskey, Pizzuti, Fu, Fenwick, & Nelson, 1992).

ELEMENTS OF FORMAL GENETICS

The mechanisms by which an individual's set of paired chromosomes produces traits are the principles of genetic inheritance. Mendel's work with garden peas first defined these principles. Later geneticists have refined Mendel's work to explain patterns of inheritance for traits and diseases that appear in families.

Analysis of traits that occur with defined, predictable patterns has helped geneticists link the pieces of the human gene map. Current research focuses on assigning genes to specific locations on chromosomes. Eventually, diseases and defects caused by single genes can be traced, and therapies to prevent and treat such diseases can be developed.

Many traits are caused by single genes and are often called mendelian traits (after Gregor Mendel). Each gene occupies a position along a chromosome known as a **locus**. The genes at a particular locus can take different forms (i.e., they can be composed of different nucleotide sequences). These different forms are called **alleles.** For example, most people have a type of hemoglobin known as hemoglobin A, whose protein sequence is dictated by a single gene. A few individuals have an alternative form of hemoglobin, termed hemoglobin S, which differs from hemoglobin A by a single amino acid substitution. The genes coding for hemoglobins A and S are thus two different alleles at a locus. A locus that has two or more alleles that occur with an appreciable frequency in a population is said to be **polymorphic** or a **polymorphism.**

Because humans are diploid organisms, each chromosome is represented twice, with one member of the chromosome pair contributed by the father and one by the mother. At a given locus, an individual has one gene whose origin is paternal and one whose origin is maternal. When the two genes are identical, the individual is **homozygous** at that locus. When the genes are not identical, the individual is **heterozygous** at the locus.

Phenotype and Genotype

The composition of genes at a given locus is known as the **genotype.** The outward appearance of an individual, which is the result of both genotype and environment, is the **phenotype.** For example, an infant who is born with an inability to metabolize the amino acid phenylalanine has the single-gene disorder known as phenylketonuria (PKU) and thus has the PKU genotype. If the condition is left untreated, abnormal metabolites of phenylalanine will begin to accumulate in the infant's brain, and irreversible mental retardation will occur. Mental retardation is thus one aspect of the PKU phenotype. By imposing dietary restrictions to exclude food containing phenylalanine, however, retardation can be prevented. Although the child still has the PKU genotype, a modification of the environment (in this case the child's diet) produces an outwardly normal phenotype.

Dominance and Recessiveness

In many loci, the effects of one allele mask those of another when the two are found together in a **heterozygote.** The allele whose effects are observable is said to be **dominant.** The allele whose effects are hidden is said to be **recessive** (from the Latin root for "hiding"). Traditionally, for loci having two alleles, the dominant allele is denoted by an uppercase letter, and the recessive allele is denoted by a lowercase letter. When one allele is dominant over another, the heterozygote genotype, Aa, has the same phenotype as the dominant homozy-

gote, AA. For the recessive allele to be expressed, it must exist in the **homozygote** form, aa.

When the heterozygote is distinguishable from both homozygotes, the locus is said to exhibit **codominance.** For example, in the MN blood group, both alleles, M and N, of the heterozygote are detectable and therefore codominant. Another example is the ABO blood group, in which heterozygotes having the A and B alleles express both of them as A and B antigens on their red cells (forming blood group AB).

A **carrier** is an individual who has a disease gene but is phenotypically normal. The great majority of the genes for a recessive disease occur in heterozygotes who carry one copy of the gene but do not express the disease. Because many recessive genes are lethal in the homozygous state, they are eliminated from the population when they occur in homozygotes. By "hiding" in carriers, however, most recessive genes for diseases survive to be passed on to the next generation.

TRANSMISSION OF GENETIC DISEASES

An important aspect of a genetic disease is the pattern in which it is inherited through the generations of a family, or its **mode of inheritance.** Once the mode of inheritance is known, much can be learned about the disease gene itself, and reliable genetic counseling can be given to members of families in which the disease is present (see Chapter 5).

Modes of inheritance were systematically studied by Gregor Mendel, who formulated two basic laws of inheritance. His **principle of segregation** states that homologous genes separate from one another during reproduction and that each reproductive cell carries only one of the homologous genes. Mendel's second law, the **principle of independent assortment,** states that the hereditary transmission of one gene has no effect on the transmission of another. Mendel discovered these laws in the mid–nineteenth century by performing breeding experiments with garden peas. He had no knowledge of chromosomes. Early in the twentieth century geneticists found that the behavior of chromosomes does essentially correspond to Mendel's laws, which now form the basis for the **chromosome theory of inheritance.**

The known single-gene diseases can be classified into four major modes of inheritance: autosomal dominant, autosomal recessive, X-linked dominant, and X-linked recessive. The first two types involve genes known to occur on the 22 pairs of autosomes. The last two types occur on the X chromosome; there is no good documentation of disease genes occurring on the Y chromosome. The number of diseases assigned to each category is growing rapidly. Current catalogs of single-gene traits, which include disease-producing and nonclinical traits (such as attached earlobes), list 2470 known autosomal dominant traits, 647 autosomal recessive traits, and 190 X-linked traits (McKusick, 1992). In addition, there are 2403 traits whose modes of inheritance are tentatively defined.

An important tool in the analysis of modes of inheritance is the **pedigree** chart. This pedigree chart summarizes family relationships and shows which members of a family are affected by a genetic disease (Fig. 4-19). Generally, the pedigree begins with one individual in the family, the **proband,** also termed the **propositus** (male) or **proposita** (female). This individual is usually the first person in the family diagnosed or seen in a clinic.

Autosomal Dominant Inheritance
Characteristics of Pedigrees

Diseases caused by autosomal dominant genes are rare in populations. The most common occur in fewer than 1 in 500 individuals, so that it is uncommon for two individuals both affected by the same autosomal dominant disease to produce offspring together. Fig. 4-20, *A,* illustrates this unusual pattern. More often, affected offspring are produced by the union of a normal parent with an affected heterozygous parent. The diagram (Punnett square) in Fig. 4-20 illustrates this mating. The affected parent can pass either a disease gene or a normal gene to his or her children. Each event has a probability of .5; thus, on the average, half of the children will be heterozygous and will express the disease, and half will be normal.

Fig. 4-21, *A,* is a typical pedigree showing the transmission of an autosomal dominant gene. The gene shown here causes achondroplasia (Fig. 4-21, *B*). Several important characteristics of this pedigree support the conclusion that the trait is caused by an autosomal dominant gene:

1. The two sexes exhibit the trait in approximately equal proportions, and males and females are equally likely to transmit the trait to their offspring.
2. There is no skipping of generations. If an individual has achondroplasia, one parent must also have it. If neither parent has the trait, none of the children has it (with the exception of new mutations, as discussed later).
3. Affected heterozygous individuals transmit the trait to approximately half of their children, but because gamete transmission is subject to chance fluctuations, it is possible that all or none of the children of an affected parent may have the trait. When large numbers of matings of this type are studied, however, the proportion of affected children will closely approach one half.

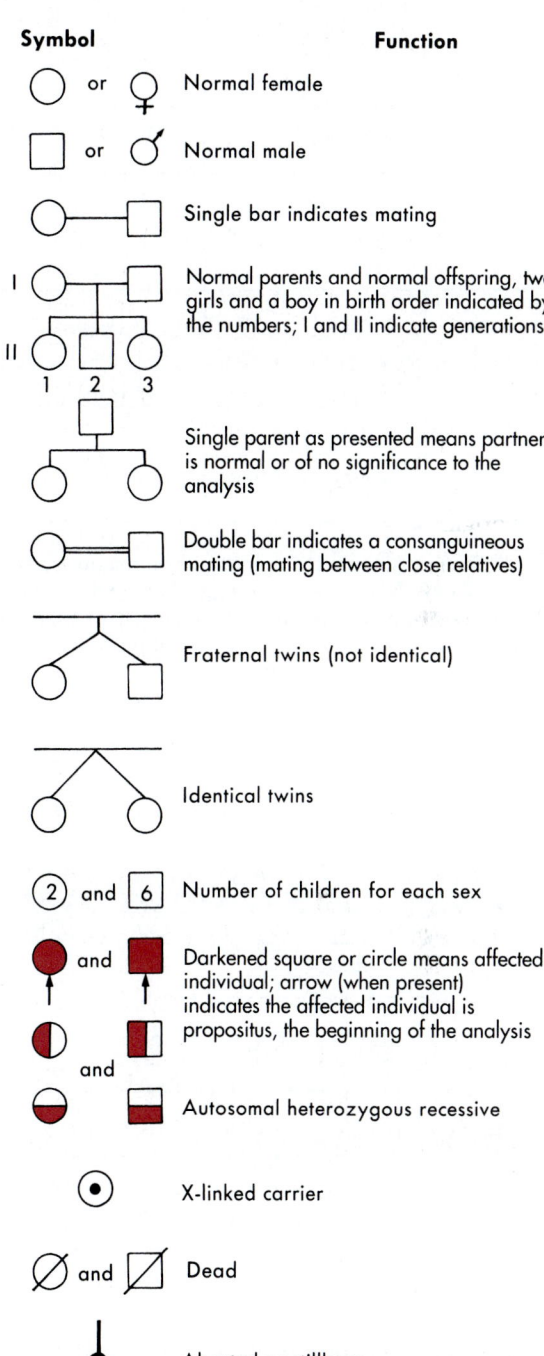

FIG. 4-19 Symbols commonly used in pedigrees.

A

	Affected parent	
	D	**d**
D	DD Homozygous affected (usually rare)	Dd Heterozygous affected
d	Dd Heterozygous affected	dd Homozygous normal

Affected parent

B

	Normal parent	
	d	**d**
D	Dd Heterozygous affected	Dd Heterozygous affected
d	dd Homozygous normal	dd Homozygous normal

Affected parent

FIG. 4-20 Punnett square and autosomal dominant traits. A, Punnett square for the mating of two individuals with an autosomal dominant gene. Here both parents are affected by the trait. **B,** Punnett square for the mating of a normal individual with a carrier for an autosomal dominant gene.

Recurrence Risks

Parents at risk for producing children with a genetic disease nearly always ask the question, What is the *chance* that our child will have this disease? When one child has already been born with a genetic disease, the parents can be given a **recurrence risk,** which is the probability that subsequent children will also have the disease. If the parents have not yet had children, but are known to be at risk for having children with a genetic disease, an **occurrence risk** (the probability that a child will have a specific disease) can be given. When one parent is affected by an autosomal dominant disease (and is a heterozygote) and the other is normal, the occurrence and recurrence risks for each child are one half.

An important principle is that each birth is an independent event, much like a coin toss. Thus, even though parents may have already had a child with the disease, their recurrence risk remains one half. Even if they have had several children, all affected (or all unaffected) by the disease, the law of independence dictates that the probability that their next child will have the disease is still one half. Parents' misunderstanding of this principle is a common problem encountered in genetic counseling.

If a child has been born with an autosomal dominant disease and there is no history of the disease in the family, the child is probably the product of a new muta-

A

FIG. 4-21 Pedigree for achondroplasia. A, Pedigree showing the transmission of an autosomal dominant disease. **B,** Achondroplasia, an autosomal dominant disorder. (**B,** From McKusick, 1990.)

tion. The gene transmitted by one of the parents has thus undergone a mutation from a normal to a disease-causing allele. The genes at this locus in most of the parent's other germ cells would still be normal. In this situation the recurrence risk for the parent's subsequent offspring is not greater than that of the general population. The offspring of the affected child, however, will have an occurrence risk of one half. Because these diseases often reduce the potential for reproduction, a large proportion of the observed cases of many autosomal dominant diseases are the result of new mutations. For example, approximately seven eighths of all cases of achondroplasia are caused by new mutations.

Occasionally, two or more offspring will present symptoms of an autosomal dominant disease when there is no family history of the disease. Since mutation is a rare event, it is unlikely that this disease would be a result of multiple mutations in the same family. The mechanism most likely to be responsible is termed **germ-line mosaicism.** During the embryonic development of one of the parents, a mutation occurred that affected all or part of the germline but few or none of the somatic cells of the embryo. Thus the parent carries the mutation in his or her germline but does not actually express the disease. As a result, the unaffected parent can transmit the mutation to multiple offspring. This phenomenon, although relatively rare, can have significant effects on recurrence risks (Hall, 1988).

Delayed Age of Onset

One of the most well-known autosomal dominant diseases is Huntington disease, a neurologic disorder whose main features are progressive dementia and increasingly uncontrollable movements of the limbs (discussed further in Chapter 15). The latter is known as chorea (Greek *khoreia* = dance), and the disease was formerly called Huntington chorea.

One of the key features of this disease is its **delayed age of onset:** symptoms are not usually seen until age 40 or later. Thus those who develop the disease have often had children before they are aware that they have the gene. If the disease were present at birth, nearly all affected persons would die before reaching reproductive age, and the occurrence of the gene in the population would be much lower. From the gene's "point of view," a delayed age of onset is quite advantageous. An individual whose parent has the disease has a 50% chance of developing it during middle age. He or she is thus confronted with a torturous question: Should I have children, knowing that there is a 50:50 chance that I may have this disease gene and pass it to half of my children?

Penetrance and Expressivity

Another important variation seen in some autosomal dominant diseases is incomplete penetrance. The **penetrance** of a trait is the percentage of individuals with a specific genotype who also exhibit the expected phenotype. Incomplete penetrance means that individuals who have the gene for a disease may not exhibit the disease phenotype at all, even though the gene and the associated disease may be transmitted to the next generation. A pedigree illustrating the transmission of an autosomal dominant gene with incomplete penetrance is given in Fig. 4-22. Retinoblastoma, the most common malignant eye tumor affecting children, is one disease that typically exhibits incomplete penetrance. About 10% of the individuals who are **obligate carriers** of the gene (i.e., those who have an affected parent and affected children and therefore must themselves carry the gene) do not have the disease. The penetrance of the gene is then said to be 90%.

The gene responsible for retinoblastoma has been mapped to the long arm of chromosome 13, and its DNA sequence has been studied extensively. This gene is known as a **tumor-suppressor gene:** the normal function of its protein product is to regulate the cell cycle so that cells do not grow uncontrollably. When the protein is altered, its tumor-suppressing capacity is lost, and a tumor can form (see Weinberg [1991] for a review of tumor-suppressor genes) (see also Chapters 10 and 16).

A similar complication is variable expressivity. **Expressivity** is the extent of variation in phenotype associated with a particular genotype. If expressivity of a disease is variable, the penetrance may be complete but the severity of the disease can vary greatly. The best-known example of variable expressivity in an autosomal dominant disease is type 1 neurofibromatosis, or von Recklinghausen disease. The gene that causes neurofibromatosis has been mapped to the long arm of chromosome 17, and studies of its DNA sequence indi-

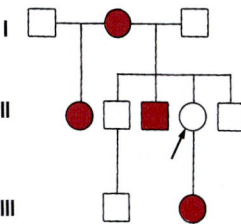

FIG. 4-22 Pedigree for retinoblastoma showing incomplete penetrance. Female with marked arrow in line II must be heterozygous, but she does not express the trait.

FIG. 4-23 Neurofibromatosis. Patient is severely affected with neurofibromatosis. (Courtesy National Library of Medicine.)

cate that it, like the retinoblastoma gene, is probably a tumor-suppressor gene (White & O'Connell, 1991). This disease is sometimes called the "elephant man's disease." However, Joseph Merrick, the man to whom this term was originally applied, probably had a rare disorder called Proteus syndrome. The expression of this gene can vary from a few harmless *café-au-lait* spots ("coffee with milk," describing the light-brown color) on the skin to numerous malignant neurofibromas, scoliosis, seizures, gliomas, neuromas, hypertension, and mental retardation (Fig. 4-23).

A parent with mild expression of the disease—so mild that he or she is not aware of it—can transmit the gene to a child, who can then exhibit severe expression of the disease. As with delayed age of onset and incomplete penetrance, variable expressivity provides a mechanism by which autosomal dominant genes can be maintained at higher prevalence rates in populations.

Several different factors can cause variation in expressivity. Genes at other loci can sometimes modify the expression of a disease gene (these are termed modifier genes). Environmental factors can also influence the expression of a disease gene. Finally, different types of mutations at a locus can cause variation in severity. For example, a base substitution resulting in a single amino acid change usually produces a mild form of the clotting disorder hemophilia A (see box, p. 153). A base substitution resulting in a "stop" codon (and thus pre-mature termination of translation) usually produces a more severe form of hemophilia A.

Genomic Imprinting

Mendel's experimental work with garden peas established that the phenotype is the same whether a given allele is inherited from the mother or the father. Indeed, this principle has been part of the central dogma of genetics. Recently, however, it has become increasingly apparent that this principle does not always hold. For example, the average age of onset of Huntington disease is substantially earlier if the gene is inherited from the father rather than from the mother (33 years vs. 42 years). Even more striking are the results of a deletion on the long arm of chromosome 15 (15q11-q13). When the deleted chromosome is inherited from the father, the offspring manifest a disease known as Prader-Willi syndrome. This disease phenotype includes short stature, obesity, and hypogonadism. When the deleted chromosome is inherited from the mother, the offspring develop Angelman syndrome, which is characterized by mental retardation, seizures, and an ataxic gait. The deletions inherited from the father and the mother are cytogenetically indistinguishable.

What could cause these differences? It appears that they involve the phenomenon of **genomic imprinting** (Hall, 1990). The allele inherited from the mother has a different "imprint" from the allele inherited from the father. The imprint alters the activity level of the allele, causing the differences described. The precise way in which genomic imprinting works is not yet understood. However, research with transgenic mice (mice that have had a single foreign gene placed in their genome through recombinant DNA techniques) indicates that the expression level of these transgenes is influenced by the parental origin of the gene (imprinting) *and* that the activity level is associated with the degree of methylation of the gene. Genes that are more highly methylated tend to be transcriptionally less active (i.e., less of the gene is transcribed into messenger RNA). The attachment of methyl groups to DNA may inhibit the binding of proteins that promote transcription. Methylation, which can vary in degree depending on which parent transmits the gene, thus may represent the imprint itself. At this point, however, only an *association* between methylation and imprinting has been established. It is not at all clear whether methylation is the actual *mechanism* of genomic imprinting.

Autosomal Recessive Inheritance
Characteristics of Pedigrees

Like autosomal dominant diseases, diseases caused by autosomal recessive genes are rare in populations, although the number of carriers for recessive diseases can be high. The most common lethal recessive disease in

Caucasian children, cystic fibrosis, occurs in about 1 in 2000 births. Approximately 1 in 23 Caucasians carries one copy of the gene for cystic fibrosis (see Chapter 31). Because an individual must be homozygous for a recessive gene to express the disease, the carriers are phenotypically normal. Because most genes for recessive diseases are maintained in normal carriers, they are able to survive in the population from one generation to the next. As with some autosomal dominant diseases, some autosomal recessive diseases are characterized by delayed age of onset, incomplete penetrance, and variable expressivity.

Fig. 4-24 shows a pedigree for cystic fibrosis. The cystic fibrosis gene, which has been mapped to the long arm of chromosome 7, encodes a protein product that is involved in the transport of chloride ions across epithelial cell membranes (Collins, 1992). In fact, the gene product may be the chloride ion channel itself. Defective transport of chloride ions leads to a salt imbalance that results in secretions of abnormally thick, dehydrated mucus. Some of the digestive organs, particularly the pancreas, become obstructed with mucus, causing malnutrition, and the lungs become clogged with mucus, making them highly susceptible to bacterial infections (especially *Pseudomonas*). Death from lung disease or heart failure usually occurs before age 30. In the pedigree shown here, the two affected individuals are the offspring of the marriage of two first cousins. Marriage between related individuals, termed **consanguinity** (from the Latin root meaning "common blood"), is often a factor in producing children with recessive diseases because related individuals are more likely to share the same recessive genes. Consanguinity is seen most often in rare recessive diseases, since carriers of common recessive diseases have a fairly high probability of encountering one another just by chance.

The important criteria for discerning autosomal recessive inheritance include the following:
1. Males and females are affected in equal proportions.
2. Consanguinity is often present.
3. The disease is seen in siblings but usually not in their parents.
4. On the average, one fourth of the offspring of carrier parents will be affected.

Recurrence Risks

In most cases of recessive disease, the parents of affected individuals are both heterozygous carriers. On the average, one fourth of their offspring will be normal homozygotes, one half will be phenotypically normal carrier heterozygotes, and one fourth will be homozygotes with the disease (Fig. 4-25). Thus the recurrence risk for the offspring of carrier parents is 25%. As before, these are the *average* figures. In any given family, there will

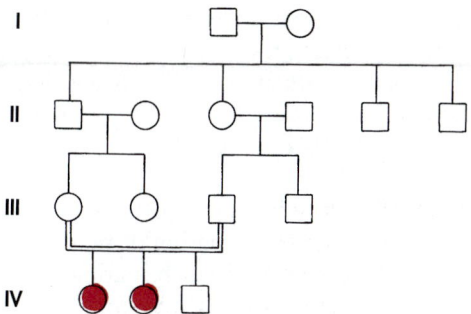

FIG. 4-24 Pedigree for cystic fibrosis.

	D	d
D	DD Homozygous normal	Dd Heterozygous carrier
d	Dd Heterozygous carrier	dd Homozygous affected

FIG. 4-25 Punnett square for the mating of heterozygous carriers typical of most cases of recessive disease.

likely be chance fluctuations, but a study of a large number of families would yield figures close to these proportions.

If two parents have a recessive disease, they each must be homozygous for the disease. Therefore, when two parents are affected by a recessive disease, all their children must also be affected. This observation helps to distinguish recessive from dominant inheritance because two parents both affected by a dominant gene are nearly always both heterozygotes, and thus one fourth of their children will be unaffected.

Because carrier parents usually are unaware that they both carry the same recessive gene, they often produce an affected child before knowing of their condition. Increasingly, **carrier detection tests** that can identify heterozygotes by measuring the reduced amount of a critical enzyme are becoming available. The critical enzyme would be totally lacking in a homozygous recessive individual, but an essentially normal phenotype is seen when it is present in a reduced quantity in the carrier. Often carriers can also be detected by direct examination of the disease locus for a mutation. Such testing is especially valuable for siblings of known carriers, who may themselves be carriers. Some recessive diseases for which carrier detection tests are now available are PKU, sickle cell disease, cystic fibrosis, Tay-Sachs disease, and galactosemia.

Consanguinity

Consanguinity and **inbreeding** are related concepts. *Consanguinity* refers to the mating of two related individuals, and the offspring of such matings are said to be *inbred*. Consanguinity is often an important characteristic of pedigrees for recessive diseases because relatives share a certain proportion of genes received from a common ancestor. The proportion of shared genes depends on the closeness of their biologic relationship. For example, siblings share one half of their genes on average. With each decreasing degree of relationship, this proportion is reduced by one half. Uncles share one fourth of their genes with nephews and nieces, first cousins share one eighth; first cousins once removed* share one sixteenth; second cousins share one thirty-second, and so on. With consanguineous matings there is a significant increase in recessive disorders. Most empirical studies show that the proportion of offspring of marriages of first cousins who are affected by genetic diseases is approximately double that of the general population (Jorde, 1991). Marriages between first cousins are prohibited in most states of the United States. Marriages between closer relatives (except between double first cousins†) are prohibited throughout the United States.

X-Linked Inheritance

Not all genetic diseases are caused by genes located on the 22 autosomes. Some conditions are instead caused by genes located on the sex chromosomes, and that mode of inheritance is **sex-linked.** Because the Y chromosome is not yet known to carry any disease-causing genes, the terms **X-linked** and *sex-linked* are sometimes equated. The former, however, is a more specific term. Only a few diseases are known to be inherited as X-linked dominant traits. Because these diseases are so seldom encountered, only the much more common X-linked recessive diseases are discussed here.

Because females receive two X chromosomes, one from the father and one from the mother, they can be homozygous for a disease allele at a given locus, homozygous for the normal allele at the locus, or heterozygous. Males, having only one X chromosome, are said to be **hemizygous** for genes on this chromosome. If a

male inherits a recessive disease gene on the X chromosome, he will be affected by the disease because the Y chromosome does not carry a normal allele to counteract the effects of the disease gene. Males are always more frequently affected by X-linked recessive diseases, with the difference becoming more pronounced as the disease becomes rarer.

X Inactivation

In the late 1950s Mary Lyon proposed that one X chromosome in the somatic cells of females is permanently inactivated, a process termed X inactivation (Lyon, 1962). This proposal, known as the Lyon hypothesis, explains why most gene products coded by the X chromosome are present in equal amounts in males and females, even though males have only one X chromosome and females have two X chromosomes. This phenomenon is called **dosage compensation.** The inactivated X chromosomes are observable in many interphase cells as highly condensed intranuclear chromatin bodies, termed **Barr bodies** (after Barr and Bertram, who discovered them in the late 1940s). Normal females have one Barr body in each somatic cell, whereas normal males have no Barr bodies.

The actual process of inactivation occurs very early in embryonic development, approximately 7 to 14 days after fertilization. In each somatic cell one of the two X chromosomes is inactivated. In some cells, the X chromosome contributed by the father is inactivated; in others, the maternal X chromosome is inactivated. Because the inactivation process is random, the maternal X chromosome is inactivated in approximately half of the cells, and the paternal X chromosome is inactivated in approximately half of the cells. Once the X chromosome has been inactivated in a cell, all the descendants of that cell have the same chromosome inactivated. Thus inactivation is said to be *random* but *fixed*.

Some individuals do not have the normal number of X chromosomes in their somatic cells. For example, males with Klinefelter syndrome typically have two X chromosomes and one Y chromosome. These males *do* have one Barr body in each cell. Females whose cell nuclei have three X chromosomes have two Barr bodies in each cell, and females whose cell nuclei have four X chromosomes have three Barr bodies in each cell. Females with Turner syndrome have only one X chromosome and no Barr bodies. Thus the number of Barr bodies is always one less than the number of X chromosomes in the cell. All but one X chromosome is always inactivated.

Persons with abnormal numbers of X chromosomes, such as those with Turner syndrome or Klinefelter syndrome, are not physically normal. This situation presents a puzzle because they presumably have only one active X chromosome, just as individuals with normal

---

*First cousins once removed are the offspring of one's own first cousins.

†Double first cousins share both sets of grandparents; ordinary first cousins share just one set of grandparents.

numbers of chromosomes do. One hypothesis is that the abnormal number of chromosomes exerts some influence very early in embryogenesis, before inactivation occurs. Furthermore, the distal part of the short arm of the X chromosome, as well as several other regions on the chromosome arm, is not inactivated. Thus X inactivation is also known to be *incomplete.*

The actual mechanism underlying X inactivation is still not well understood, although the gene responsible for initiating X inactivation has recently been located (Brown et al., 1991). **Methylation** of X chromosome DNA, a process in which DNA is inactivated when cytosine bases are enzymatically converted to 5-methylcytosine, appears to be involved. Inactive X chromosomes can be at least partially reactivated in vitro by administering 5-azacytidine, a demethylating agent.

Sex Determination

The process of sexual differentiation, in which the embryonic gonads become either testes or ovaries, begins during the sixth week of gestation. A key principle of sex determination in the human is that one copy of the Y chromosome is sufficient to initiate the process of gonadal differentiation that produces a male fetus. The number of X chromosomes does not alter this process. For example, an individual with two X chromosomes and one Y chromosome in each cell is still phenotypically a male. Thus it is logical that the Y chromosome must contain a gene that begins the process of male gonadal development.

This gene, termed *SRY* (for "sex-determining region on the Y"), has been located on the short arm of the Y chromosome (Sinclair et al., 1990). The SRY gene lies immediately proximal to the distal tip of the Y chromosome, known as the **pseudoautosomal** region (Fig. 4-26). This portion of the Y chromosome is so named because it pairs with the distal tip of the short arm of the X chromosome during meiosis and exchanges genetic material with it (crossover), just as autosomes do. The DNA sequences of these regions on the X and Y chromosomes are highly similar. The remainder of the X and Y chromosomes, however, do not exchange material and are not similar in DNA sequence. An important piece of evidence that supports SRY as the male-determining gene is that female mouse embryos injected with this gene develop as phenotypic males (Koopman, Gubbay, Vivian, Goodfellow, & Lovell-Badge, 1991).

Although the SRY gene is located on the Y chromosome, the other genes that contribute to male differentiation are located on other chromosomes. Thus SRY appears to act as a trigger that initiates the action of genes on other chromosomes (e.g., those that control Sertoli cell differentiation, or secretion of Müllerian-inhibiting substance, and so forth). This concept is sup-

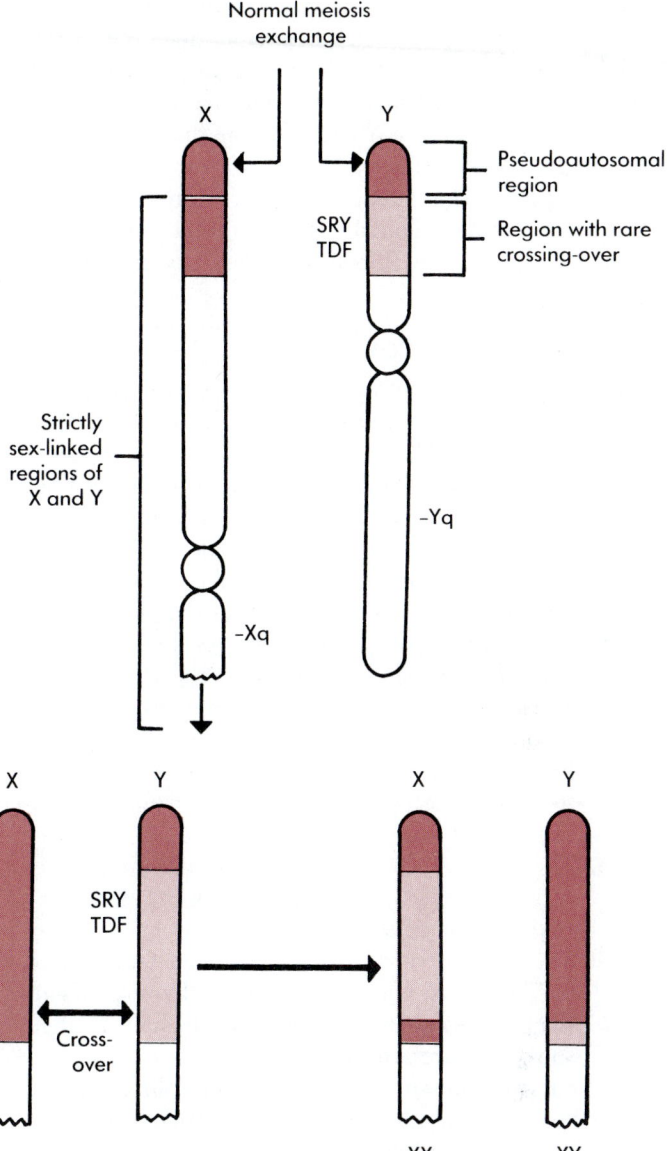

FIG. 4-26 Etiology of XX male phenotype by aberrant exchange between X- and Y-linked sequences. X and Y chromosomes normally recombine within the pseudoautosomal segment in male meiosis. If recombination occurs below the pseudoautosomal boundary, between the X-specific and Y-specific portions of the chromosomes, sequences responsible for male sexual differentiation may be translocated from the Y to the X chromosome. Fertilization by a sperm containing such an X chromosome leads to an XX male. (Modified from Thompson et al., 1991.)

ported by the fact that the SRY gene is similar in sequence to other genes that are known to regulate the transcription of DNA (i.e., they turn other genes on and off).

Occasionally, the crossover between X and Y occurs closer to the centromere than it should, placing the SRY gene on the X chromosome after crossover. This variation can result in offspring with an apparently normal XX karyotype but a male phenotype. Such XX males are seen in about 1 in 20,000 live births and closely resemble males with Klinefelter syndrome. Conversely, it is possible to inherit a Y chromosome that has lost the SRY gene (due to either a crossover error or a deletion of the gene). This situation produces an XY female. Such females have gonadal streaks rather than ovaries and have poorly developed secondary sex characteristics.

Characteristics of Pedigrees

X-linked pedigrees show distinctive modes of inheritance. The most striking characteristic is that females are seldom affected. To express an X-linked recessive trait, a female must be homozygous: either both of her parents are affected or her father is affected and her mother is a carrier. Such matings are rare.

An important example of an X-linked recessive disease is hemophilia A. The pedigree in the accompanying clinical commentary demonstrates the following principles of X-linked recessive inheritance:

1. The trait is seen much more frequently in males than in females.
2. Because a father can give a son only a Y chromosome, the trait is never transmitted from father to son.
3. The gene can be transmitted through a series of carrier females, causing the appearance of a "skipped generation."
4. The gene is passed from an affected father to all his daughters, who, as phenotypically normal carriers, transmit it to approximately half of their sons, who are affected.

The most common and severe of all X-linked recessive disorders is Duchenne muscular dystrophy (DMD), which affects approximately 1 in 3500 males. As its name suggests, this disorder is characterized by progressive muscle degeneration. Affected individuals are usually unable to walk by age 10 or 12 years. The disease affects the heart and respiratory muscles, and death caused by respiratory or cardiac failure usually occurs before age 20. Until recently, the underlying pathologic origin of this disorder was a mystery. However, mapping and cloning of the disease gene (on the short arm of the X chromosome) have greatly increased our understanding of the disorder (Chamberlain, 1991). The DMD gene is the largest gene ever found in the human, spanning over 2 million DNA bases. It encodes a previously undiscovered muscle protein, termed **dystrophin**. Extensive study of dystrophin indicates that it plays an essential role in maintaining the structural integrity of muscle cells: it may also help to regulate the activity of membrane proteins. When dystrophin is absent, as in individuals with DMD, the cell cannot survive, and muscle deterioration ensues.

Most cases of Duchenne muscular dystrophy are due to deletions of portions of the DMD gene. They generally involve frameshift deletions in which all the amino acids following the deletion are altered. It is interesting that an "in frame" deletion (in which a multiple of three bases is deleted, and the amino acids following the deletion are *not* altered) produces a milder form of muscular dystrophy, the Becker type. These two types of dystrophy are examples of a disease in which different types of mutations at the same locus produce variable expression of the disease.

Recurrence Risks

The most common mating type involving X-linked recessive genes is the combination of a carrier female and a normal male. On the average, the carrier mother will transmit the disease gene to half of her sons and half of her daughters. As Fig. 4-27, *A*, shows, half of the daughters in such a mating will be carriers, whereas half will be normal. Half of the sons will be normal, whereas half will have the disease. These are probabilities that indicate what risks can be expected on the *average*.

The other common mating type is an affected father and a normal mother (Fig. 4-27, *B*). In this situation all the sons must be normal because the father can transmit only his Y chromosome to them. Because all the daughters must receive the father's X chromosome, they will all be heterozygous carriers. Because the sons *must* receive the Y chromosome and the daughters *must* receive the X with the disease gene, these are predictions and not probabilities. None of the children will inherit the disease.

The final mating pattern, less common than the other two, involves an affected father and a carrier mother (Fig. 4-27, *C*). With this pattern, on average, half of the daughters will be heterozygous carriers, and half will be homozygous for the disease gene and thus affected. Half of the sons will be normal, and half will be affected. Some X-linked recessive diseases, such as DMD, are fatal or incapacitating before the affected individual reaches reproductive age, and therefore affected fathers are rare or nonexistent.

Sex-Limited and Sex-Influenced Traits

Confusion sometimes exists between traits that are sex-linked and those that are sex-limited or sex-influenced. A **sex-limited trait** is one that can occur in only one of the sexes, often because of anatomic differences. Inherited uterine and testicular defects are two obvious examples.

A **sex-influenced trait** is one that occurs much more frequently in one sex than in the other. A good exam-

CLINICAL COMMENTARY   HEMOPHILIA A AND THE RUSSIAN REVOLUTION

The figure (partial pedigree for descendants of Queen Victoria) is one of the best-known disease pedigrees in existence. It shows the transmission of hemophilia A in the European royal families. This disease, often called a "bleeder syndrome," is caused by a defect in one of the blood-clotting factors, factor VIII, and can cause severe hemorrhages. In this pedigree Queen Victoria of England was the first known carrier of the disease, and several of her male descendants were affected by it. One of the most historically significant consequences of this pedigree involves the hemophiliac Czarevich Alexis, son of Czar Nicholas II of Russia. Grigori Rasputin, the "mad monk," was reputedly the only person able to prevent the young boy's bleeding episodes and was thus able to gain considerable power over the royal family. Rasputin's destabilizing influence is thought to have hastened the 1917 Bolshevik revolution.

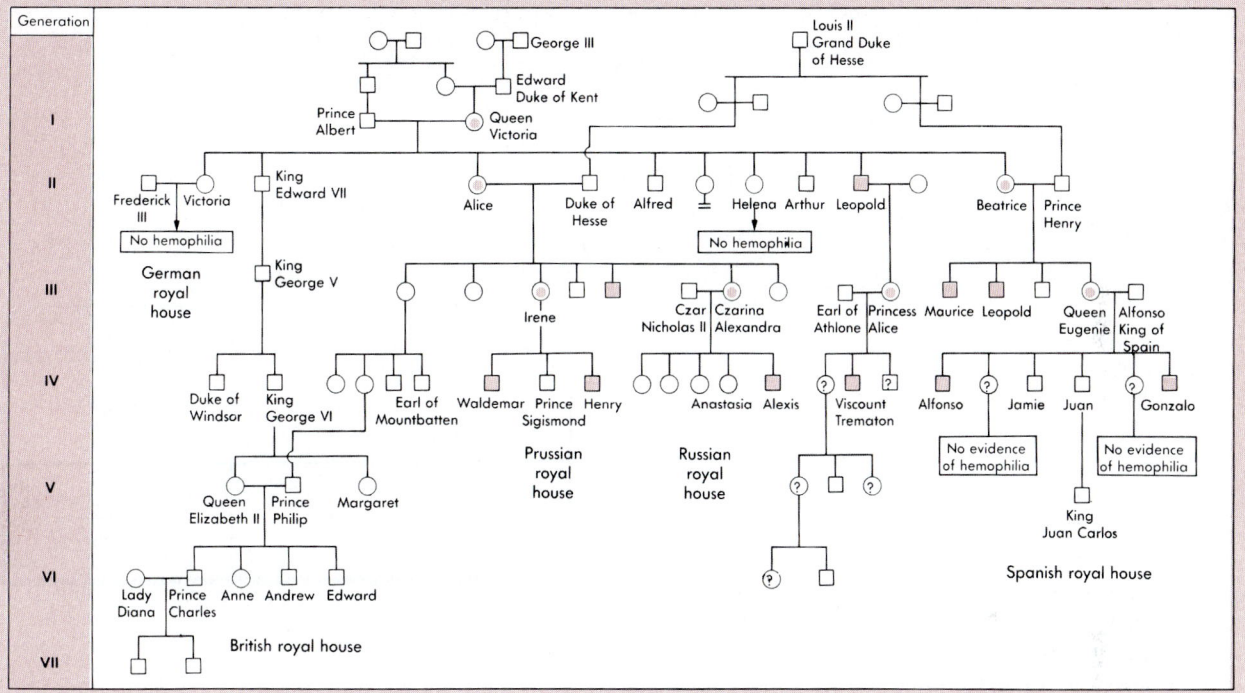

Partial pedigree for descendants of Queen Victoria showing the appearance of hemophilia A in one of her sons, in the descendants of that son, and in the descendants of her daughters and granddaughters. The royal families of Prussia, Hesse, Battenberg (Mountbatten), Russia, and Spain were thus affected with the disease. The present royal family of England, however, is free of the disease, in spite of inbreeding. (Modified from Raven & Johnson, 1992.)

FIG. 4-27 **Punnett square and X-linked recessive traits. A,** Punnett square for the mating of a normal male ($X_H Y$) and a female carrier of an X-linked recessive gene ($X_H X_h$). **B,** Punnett square for the mating of a normal female ($X_H X_H$) with a male affected by an X-linked recessive disease ($X_h Y$). **C,** Punnett square for the mating of a female who carries an X-linked recessive gene ($X_H X_h$) with a male who is affected with the disease caused by the gene ($X_h Y$).

ple of a sex-influenced trait is male-pattern baldness, which occurs in both males and females but is much more common in males. In males it is inherited as a dominant trait, whereas in females it is inherited as a recessive trait. Because of their hormonal constitution, females need two copies of the gene to express male-pattern baldness.

Evaluation of Pedigrees

With complications such as incomplete penetrance, variable expressivity, delayed age of onset, and sex-influenced traits, it is not always possible simply to look at a disease pedigree and determine the mode of inheritance. A sophisticated statistical methodologic approach has evolved to deal with such complications. Incorporated into computer programs, these statistical techniques assess the probability of observing a certain pedigree if a particular mode of inheritance (e.g., autosomal dominant with incomplete penetrance) is in effect.

LINKAGE ANALYSIS AND GENE MAPPING

Locating genes on chromosomes and on specific areas of chromosomes is one of the most important endeavors in human genetics. The location of a gene can tell much about the function of the gene, its interaction with other genes, and the likelihood that certain individuals will develop a genetic disease.

Classic Pedigree Analysis

Mendel's second law, the principle of independent assortment, states that an individual's genes will be transmitted to the next generation independently of one another. This law is only partly true, however, because genes located close together on the same chromosome *do* tend to be transmitted together to the offspring. Thus Mendel's principle of independent assortment holds true for most pairs of genes but not those that occupy the

Homologous chromosomes   Meiosis gametes

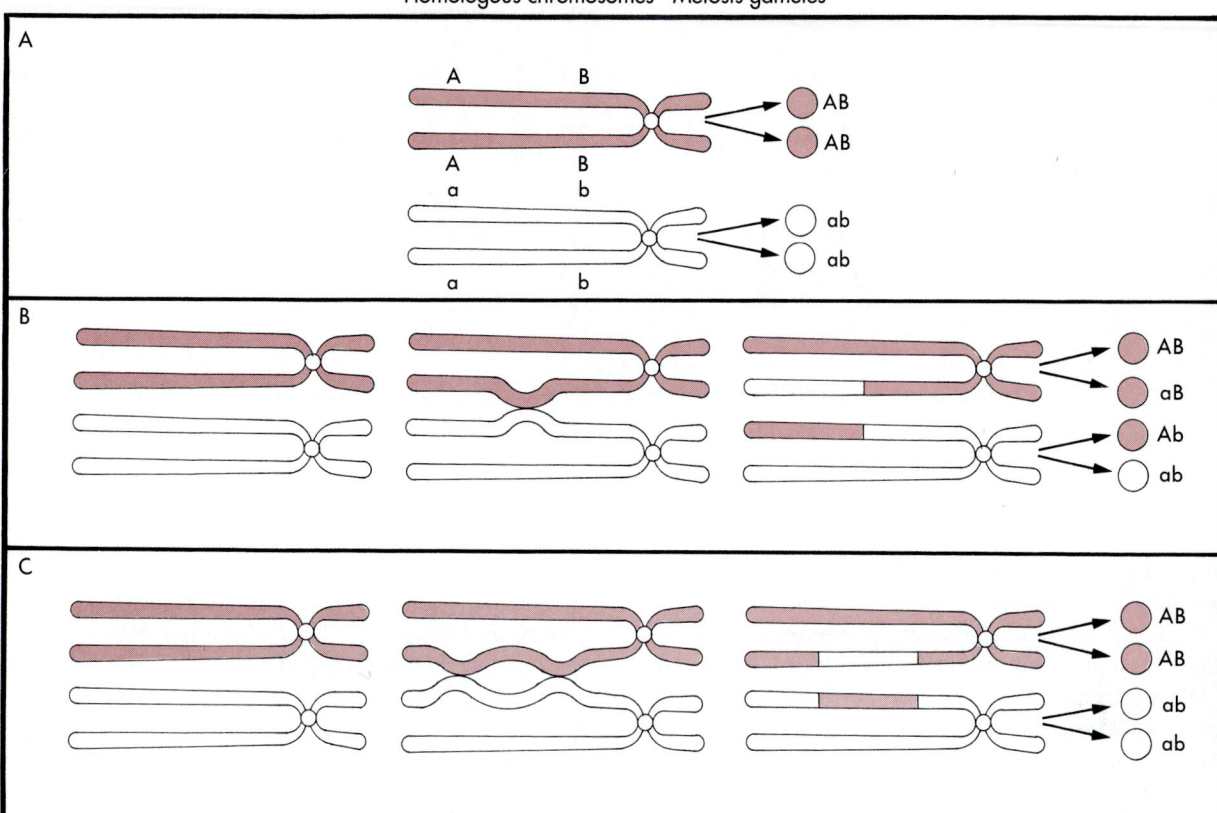

FIG. 4-28 **The genetic results of crossing-over. A,** No crossing-over. **B,** Crossing-over with recombination. **C,** Double crossing-over resulting in no recombination.

same region of a chromosome. Such loci demonstrate **linkage** and are said to be linked.

During the first meiotic stage, the arms of homologous chromosome pairs intertwine and sometimes exchange portions of their DNA (Fig. 4-28) in a process known as **crossing-over.** During crossing-over new combinations of alleles can be formed. For example, two loci on a chromosome have alleles A and a and alleles B and b. Alleles A and B are located together on one chromosome arm, and alleles a and b are located on the other arm. The genotype of this individual is denoted as AB/ab.

As Fig. 4-28, *A,* shows, the allele pairs AB and ab would be transmitted together when no crossing-over occurs. However, when crossing-over occurs (Fig. 4-28, *B*), all four possible pairs of alleles can be transmitted to the offspring: AB, aB, Ab, and ab. The process of forming such new arrangements of alleles is called **recombination.** Crossing-over does not necessarily lead to

recombination, however, because double crossing-over between two loci can result in no actual recombination of the alleles at the loci (Fig. 4-28, *C*).

The rate of crossing-over can be used to infer the distance between two loci on a chromosome because the probability of crossovers occurring between two loci increases as the loci become more distant. For example, if an individual with genotype AB/ab produces recombinant offspring gametes (composition of Ab and aB) 2% of the time, it is said that the two loci are two map units apart. One **map unit** equals a 1% recombination rate between two loci. When loci on the same chromosome are 50 or more map units apart, they are considered unlinked because their recombination frequency is just as great as it would be if they were on different chromosomes (where the probability of being transmitted together must equal one half). Because they are on the same chromosome, they are said to be unlinked but **syntenic loci.** Recombination frequencies provide a

FIG. 4-29 **The ABO nail-patella linkage in three generations of a family.** Letters below symbols indicate ABO blood groups. Individual III-6 shows recombination.

good estimate of actual physical distance between loci at smaller distances, but because of double crossovers, they tend to yield underestimates at larger distances. On average, each map unit is equal to approximately 1 million DNA base pairs.

Pedigrees can be used to determine recombination rates between loci. Fig. 4-29 shows a pedigree in which the rare disease nail-patella syndrome (an autosomal dominant disease consisting of malformed patellae and nails) is being transmitted. The individuals in this pedigree have also been typed for the ABO blood group, whose locus is also located on chromosome 9. Examination of generations one and two shows that the nail-patella gene must be on the same chromosome arm as the gene for blood type A because the mother, whose blood type was B, was unaffected with the disease. The daughter's genotype would then be AN/Bn, where N indicates the disease allele and n indicates the normal allele. The daughter's husband (individual II-1) must have the genotype On/On. If the loci for nail-patella syndrome and the ABO blood group are linked, the children of this union who are affected with nail-patella syndrome should have blood type A; those who are unaffected should have blood type B. In six of seven cases we find this to be true. In one case a recombination occurred (individual III-6), indicating a recombination rate of 1 in 7, or 14%. The two loci are therefore 14 map units apart.

In practice, a much larger sample of families would be used to ensure against statistical artifacts. Also, as with the determination of mode of inheritance, the situation is not always as clear as in Fig. 4-29. Elaborate statistical procedures have been devised to evaluate the probabilities that two loci are linked at a given map distance.

Once a close linkage has been established between a disease locus and a "marker" locus (such as a blood group) and once the alleles of the two loci that are inherited together within a family have been determined, reliable predictions of whether a member of a family will develop the disease can be made. If, for example, the recombination rate between a disease locus and a "marker" locus, such as the ABO blood group, is less than 1%, family members can simply have their ABO blood type assayed to find out, with 99% or greater certainty, whether each member carries the disease gene.

This capability is especially important for diseases with delayed age of onset. Linkage has been established between several DNA polymorphisms and the gene for Huntington disease. Determining this kind of linkage means that it will be possible for offspring of an individual with Huntington disease to know whether they also carry the gene and thus could pass it on to their own children. The difficult decision of whether to have children will be made easier for these individuals, although, of course, some individuals may prefer to remain uninformed of their genotypes. Other delayed-onset diseases for which linked markers have been found include adult polycystic kidney disease, familial Alzheimer disease, and an autosomal dominant form of breast cancer (about 5% of breast cancer cases are caused by an autosomal dominant gene).

For some genetic diseases, prophylactic treatment is available if the condition can be diagnosed in time. An example of this is hemochromatosis, a recessive genetic disease in which excess iron is retained, causing degeneration of the heart, liver, brain, and other vital organs. Diagnosis is usually made at about 40 years of age in males, after which most individuals survive only a few years. If earlier tests could determine whether an individual had the disease, preventive treatment, consisting of phlebotomies to remove blood and thus excess iron, could be administered before degeneration began. This has been made easier by establishing that the gene for hemochromatosis is closely linked to the human leukocyte antigen (HLA) (see Chapter 6) complex on chromosome 6. Individuals at risk for developing the disease can be determined by assaying their HLA type, and preventive therapy can be given, ensuring an ordinary life span. This example is one instance in which genetics contributes to preventive medicine in its best sense.

Complete Human Gene Map: Prospects and Benefits

Rapid progress is currently being made in assigning genes to their chromosomal locations. A number of important genetic diseases have been located on specific areas of individual chromosomes: these include Huntington disease, retinoblastoma, DMD, hemophilia A, cystic fibrosis, PKU, neurofibromatosis, and familial Alzheimer disease (Williamson et al., 1991). Table 4-1 contains a partial list of mapped diseases. The development of thousands of new DNA markers is especially helpful in this effort. Geneticists now talk about a "complete" map of the human genome as a goal achievable within one or two decades. Achievement of this goal will serve several purposes:

1. Marker genes will be available to establish close linkages for many genetic diseases. The biggest single drawback to linkage studies now is the lack of markers distributed throughout the genome. As this drawback is overcome, accurate prediction can be made for the inheritance of many (or even most) genetic diseases.
2. Knowing the location of genes often yields valuable information about the way genes function and interact with one another. A number of genes with similar functions (e.g., some of the globin genes) are located close to one another on the same chromosome. This characteristic can have important implications for the diseases caused by these genes.
3. Mapping a disease gene is an important step toward isolating and **cloning** the gene (clones are identical copies of genes). Once a gene can be cloned, its DNA sequence can be studied to determine the nature and function of the protein encoded by the gene. Cloning the genes that cause diseases such as cystic fibrosis and DMD has contributed immensely to our understanding of the pathophysiologic aspect of these disorders. In addition, the ability to clone a gene opens up the possibility of gene therapy for the disorder.

TABLE 4-1

Some Important Genetic Diseases That Have Been Mapped to Specific Chromosome Locations

Disease	Chromosome location	Gene cloned*
Huntington disease	4p16	Yes
Cystic fibrosis	7q31	Yes
Hemophilia A	Xq28	Yes
Marfan syndrome	15q15-21	Yes
Sickle cell anemia	11p15	Yes
β-Thalassemia	11p15	Yes
α-Thalassemia	16pter-p12	Yes
Familial breast cancer	17q21	No
Fragile X syndrome	Xq27	Yes
Phenylketonuria	12q21-qter	Yes
Duchenne muscular dystrophy	Xp21	Yes
Becker muscular dystrophy†	Xp21	Yes
Retinoblastoma	13q14	Yes
Hemochromatosis	6p21	No
Familial hypercholesterolemia (LDL receptor defect)	19p13	Yes
Polycystic kidney disease	16p	No
α-1-antitrypsin deficiency	14q31-32	Yes
Familial Alzheimer disease‡	21q11-q21	No
Cleft palate	Xq13-21	No
Tay-Sachs disease	15q22-q25	Yes
Neurofibromatosis (classical)	17q11	Yes
Neurofibromatosis (bilateral acoustic form)	22q11-13	No
Familial polyposis coli	5q21-22	Yes

*Cloning may be partial or complete.
†Becker muscular dystrophy is an allelic form of Duchenne muscular dystrophy.
‡Familial Alzheimer disease is a complex, heterogeneous disease. The single gene now located for this disease is associated with only *some* of the known cases.

CLINICAL COMMENTARY   ASSIGNING LOCI TO SPECIFIC CHROMOSOMES

Gene markers

Morphologic variations can occasionally be seen microscopically on a chromosome. A good example of such variation is the "uncoiled" appearance of the long arm of chromosome 1, a rare feature that is transmitted in families. Donahue, Bias, Renwick, and McKusick (1968) first assigned a gene to a specific autosome by studying this variation. Families in which this variant is inherited were typed for a number of blood groups and serum proteins, and it was found that the Duffy blood group locus was closely linked (within 2.5 map units) to the uncoiler locus. Other types of gene markers, such as distinct banding patterns, can also be used in this way.

Gene dosage analysis

The amount or dosage of an enzyme associated with a specific gene can sometimes be measured. When a specific portion of a chromosome is deleted, it is sometimes possible to show that only half of the level of an enzyme is present in the organism. If the gene coding for this enzyme is known, the gene can then be associated with the specific area of the chromosome that has been deleted. For example, this method has been used to map the enzymes acid phosphatase (to chromosome 2) and adenylate kinase (to chromosome 9). Assigning loci to chromosomes by analyzing deletions is called deletion mapping.

The same method can be applied when a portion of a chromosome is duplicated or when an individual has a partial or complete trisomy. When a 150% level of enzyme activity (caused by three alleles instead of two) is shown, the amount of enzyme may indicate that a gene coding for the enzyme is located on the duplicated region of the chromosome. For example, superoxide dismutase-1 (SOD-1) has been assigned to the long arm of chromosome 21 in this way. Because individuals with Down syndrome have an additional long arm of this chromosome (trisomy 21), one speculation is that SOD-1 may play a causal role in this disease. Assigning loci to chromosomes by analyzing duplications is called duplication mapping.

Somatic cell hybridization

One of the more surprising biologic discoveries in recent years is that somatic cells from different species, when grown in the same culture, occasionally fuse together to form hybrid cells. This fusion has been done with cells from humans and mice. The resulting hybrid cells contain 86 chromosomes: the 46 human chromosomes together with the 40 mouse chromosomes. The percentage of successful cell fusions can be greatly increased by exposing the cells to certain agents, such as Sendai virus or polyethylene glycol. The cells are then exposed to selective media such as hypoxanthine, aminopterin, and thymidine (HAT) medium to weed out those that do not fuse. The hybrid cells are then cloned, and all clones of a cell necessarily have identical karyotypes.

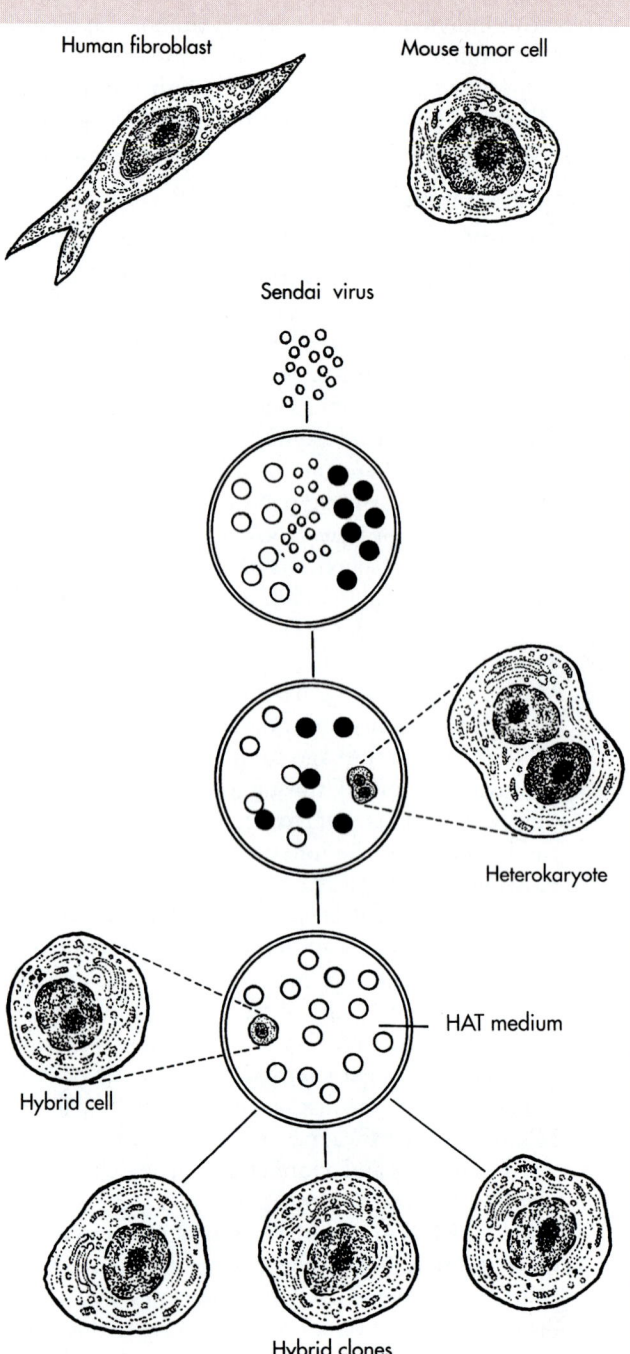

Somatic cell hybridization. Human fibroblasts are fused to mouse tumor cells that lack either HGPRT or TK enzymes. Sendai viruses promote the fusion. Some of the cells first fuse to produce cells with two nuclei (heterokaryons) and then form true hybrids. The hybrid cells are grown in a selective medium (HAT), where the hybrids thrive at the expense of the nonfused cells. As the hybrid cells divide, they lose human chromosomes randomly, then stabilize into different clones containing different human chromosomes.

Because the hybrid cells are unstable, they begin to lose the chromosomes of one of the species as they undergo cell divisions. Eventually cells are left having a full set of mouse chromosomes but only one or a few human chromosomes. The cells are karyotyped to determine which chromosomes remain. These sets of cells can then be studied to determine which enzymes they produce. The mouse and human enzymes are sufficiently different that they can be distinguished from one another. By looking at different cell lines with different groups of human chromosomes, it is possible to establish that a certain chromosome must always be present when a certain enzyme is detected. Thus the gene coding for that enzyme must be located on that chromosome.

Sometimes a gene can be assigned to a specific *segment* of a chromosome by using somatic cell hybridization. Translocations in which only part of a single human chromosome is attached to one of the mouse chromosomes occur infrequently. If a human enzyme is still detectable, the gene coding for this enzyme must be located on the translocated segment of the human chromosome.

In situ hybridization

In situ hybridization involves hybridizing a specific piece of radioactively labeled DNA or RNA (a probe) to fixed metaphase chromosomes that have been denatured so that their DNA is single-stranded. If the radioactive probe matches the DNA of a chromosome segment, it hybridizes and remains at a particular position on the chromosome (hence the term *in situ*). Its position can then be located by autoradiography, a procedure in which the radioactive emissions from the hybridized probe mark its location when exposed to x-ray film.

In situ hybridization is often combined with somatic cell hybridization to locate genes on chromosomes. Once the cell lines with different combinations of human chromosomes are created by somatic cell hybridization, they can be exposed to radioactively labeled probes. Consistent hybridization of a probe with cell lines containing a certain chromosome demonstrates that the gene corresponding to the probe is located on that chromosome. In some ways this approach is superior to the enzyme assay technique described previously since it does not require the in vitro expression of a phenotype (the enzyme).

Uncoiled chromosome   **Normal** chromosome   Normal pair

Two pairs of chromosomes. *Left,* From an individual who is heterozygous for the variant "uncoiler" chromosome. *Right,* From a related person who does not carry the variant. (From Donohue, R. P., Bias, W. B., Renwick, J. H., & McKusick, V. A. [1968]. *Proceedings of the National Academy of Sciences, 61.*)

MULTIFACTORIAL INHERITANCE

Not all traits are produced by single genes; some traits are the result of several genes acting together. These are usually referred to as **polygenic traits**. When environmental factors are also known to influence the expression of the trait (as is usually the case), the term **multifactorial inheritance** is used. Many multifactorial and polygenic traits tend to follow a normal distribution in populations (the familiar "bell-shaped curve"). Fig. 4-30 shows how three loci acting together can cause grain color in wheat to vary in a gradual way from white to red, exemplifying multifactorial inheritance. If both the alleles at each of the three loci are "white" alleles, the color is pure white. If most alleles are white but a few are red, the color is somewhat darker; if all are red, then the color is dark red.

Other examples of multifactorial traits include height and IQ. Although both height and IQ are determined in part by genes, they are also strongly influenced by

environment. For example, the average height of many human populations has increased by 5 to 10 cm since the turn of the century because of improvements in nutrition and health care. Also, IQ scores can be improved by exposing individuals (especially children) to enriched learning environments. Thus both genes *and* environment contribute to variation in these traits.

A number of diseases do not follow the bell-shaped distribution. Instead they appear to be either present in or absent from an individual. Yet they do not follow the patterns expected of single-gene diseases. Many of these are probably polygenic or multifactorial, but a certain **threshold of liability** must be crossed before the disease is expressed. Below the threshold the individual appears normal; above it the individual is affected by the disease (Fig. 4-31).

One of the best-known examples of such a threshold trait is pyloric stenosis, a disorder characterized by a narrowing or obstruction of the pylorus, the area between the stomach and intestine. Chronic vomiting, constipation, weight loss, and electrolyte imbalance can result from the condition, but it is easily corrected by surgery. The prevalence of pyloric stenosis is about 3 in 1000 live births in Caucasians. This disorder is much more common in males than females, affecting 1 in 200 males and 1 in 1000 females. The reason for this difference is that the threshold of liability is much lower in males than females, as shown in Fig. 4-31. Thus fewer defective alleles are required to generate the disorder in males. This situation also means that the offspring of affected females are more likely to have pyloric stenosis because affected females necessarily carry more disease-causing alleles than do most affected males. Table 4-2 gives the occurrence risks for offspring of males and females with pyloric stenosis, showing a varying threshold of liability.

A number of other common diseases are thought to correspond to this model. They include cleft lip and/or cleft palate, neural tube defects (anencephaly and spina bifida), clubfoot (talipes), and some forms of congenital heart disease.

Although recurrence risks can be given with confidence for single-gene diseases (50% for autosomal dominants, 25% for autosomal recessives, etc.), it is considerably more difficult to do so for multifactorial diseases. The number of genes contributing to the disease is not known, the precise allelic constitution of the parents is not known, and the extent of environmental effects can vary from one population to another. For most multifactorial diseases, **empiric risks** (i.e., those based on direct observation) have been derived. To determine empiric risks, a large population of families in which one child has developed the disease is examined. Then the siblings of each child are surveyed to calculate what percentage of them also develop the disease. For example, in Great Britain about 5% of the siblings of children

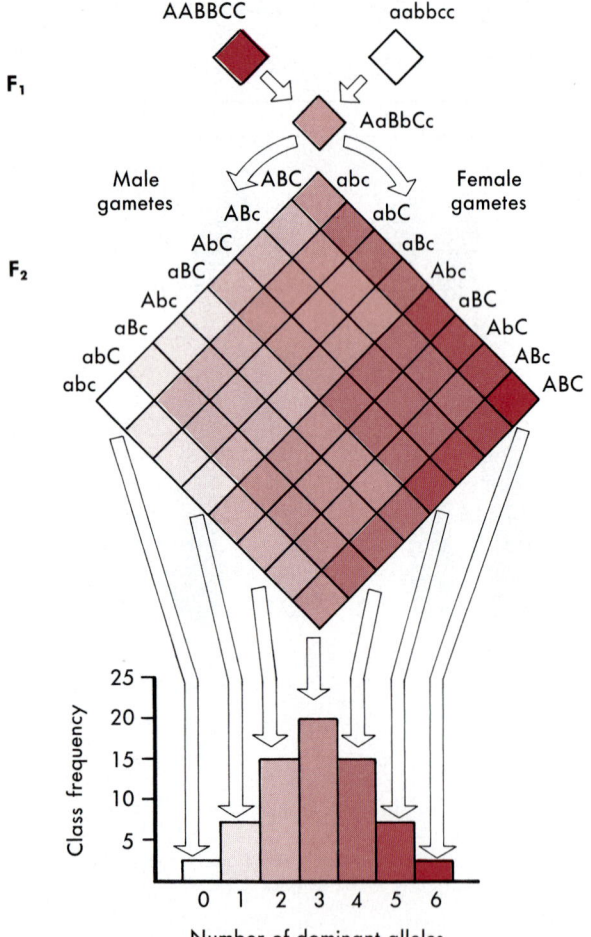

FIG. 4-30 Multifactorial inheritance. Analysis of mode of inheritance for grain color in wheat. The trait is controlled by three independently assorting gene loci.

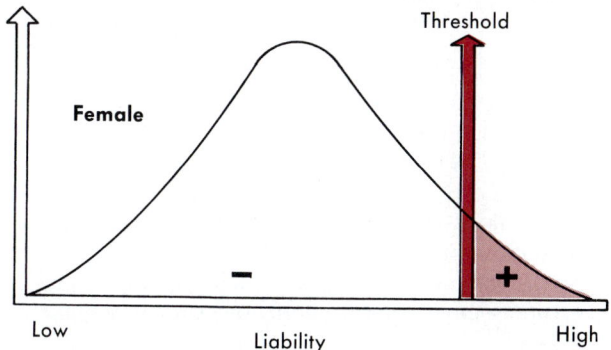

FIG. 4-31 Threshold of liability for pyloric stenosis in males and in females.

Threshold
Male
−   +

TABLE 4-2

The Incidence of Pyloric Stenosis in Offspring of Affected Persons as Compared with the Incidence of the General Population

Relatives	Risk
Sons of male patients	1 in 18
Daughters of male patients	1 in 42
Sons of female patients	1 in 5
Daughters of female patients	1 in 14

having neural tube defects also have neural tube defects. Thus the recurrence risk for parents who have had one child with a neural tube defect is 5%. Unlike risks for single-gene diseases, those for multifactorial diseases can change from one population to another. The empiric risk for neural tube defects in North America is about 2% to 3%, only half that of the British population.

Another difficulty is distinguishing polygenic or multifactorial diseases from single-gene diseases that have incomplete penetrance or variable expressivity. Large data sets and good epidemiologic data are often necessary to make the distinction. The box on the right lists criteria that are usually used to define multifactorial diseases.

Pinpointing the individual genes that contribute to the causation of multifactorial disorders is a formidable challenge. However, by using extensive gene maps created in humans and other organisms, it has been possible to identify genes that underlie complex multifactorial disorders such as hypertension (Hilbert et al., 1991) and insulin-dependent diabetes mellitus (Todd et al., 1991).

The genetics of common disorders such as hypertension, heart disease, and diabetes is complex and often confusing. Nevertheless, the public health impact of these diseases, together with the evidence for hereditary factors in their etiology, demands that genetic studies be pursued. The next decade will undoubtedly witness substantial advancements in our understanding of these disorders.

CRITERIA USED TO DEFINE MULTIFACTORIAL DISEASES

1. The recurrence risk becomes higher if more than one family member is affected. For example, the recurrence risk for neural tube defects in a British family increases to 10% if two siblings have been born with the disease. By contrast, the recurrence risk for single-gene diseases remains the same regardless of the number of siblings affected.

2. If the expression of the disease is more severe, the recurrence risk is higher. This is consistent with the liability model; a more severe expression indicates that the individual is at the extreme end of the liability distribution. Relatives of the affected individual are thus at a higher risk for inheriting disease genes. Cleft lip and/or cleft palate is a disease in which this has been shown to be true.

3. Relatives of probands of the less commonly affected sex are more likely to develop the disease. As with pyloric stenosis, this occurs because an affected individual of the less susceptible sex is usually at a more extreme position on the liability distribution.

4. Generally, if the population frequency of the disease is f, the risk for offspring and siblings of probands is approximately $\sqrt{f}$. This does not usually hold true for single-gene traits.

5. The recurrence risk for the disease decreases rapidly in more remotely related relatives. Although the recurrence risk for single-gene diseases decreases by 50% with each degree of relationship (e.g., an autosomal dominant disease has a 50% recurrence risk for siblings, 25% for uncle-nephew relationship, 12.5% for first cousins), the risk for multifactorial inheritance decreases much more quickly.

SUMMARY REVIEW

DNA, RNA, and Proteins: Heredity at the Molecular Level

1 Genes, the basic units of inheritance, are composed of deoxyribonucleic acid (DNA) and are located on the chromosomes.

2 DNA is composed of deoxyribose, a phosphate molecule, and four types of nitrogenous bases. The physical structure of DNA is a double helix.

3 The DNA bases code for amino acids, which in turn make up proteins. The amino acids are specified by triplet codons of nitrogenous bases.

4 DNA replication is based on complementary base pairing, in which a single strand of DNA serves as the template for attracting bases that form a new strand of DNA.

5 DNA polymerase is the primary enzyme involved in replication. It adds bases to the new DNA strand and performs "proofreading" functions.

6 A mutation is an inherited alteration of genetic material (i.e., DNA).

7 Substances that cause mutations are called mutagens.

8 The mutation rate in humans varies from locus to locus and ranges from 10^{-4} to 10^{-7} per gene per generation.

9 Transcription and translation, the two basic processes in which proteins are specified by DNA, both involve ribonucleic acid (RNA). RNA is chemically similar to DNA, but it is single-stranded, has a ribose sugar molecule, and has uracil rather than thymine as one of its four nitrogenous bases.

10 Transcription is the process by which DNA specifies a sequence of messenger RNA (mRNA).

11 Much of the RNA sequence is spliced from the mRNA before the mRNA leaves the nucleus. The excised sequences are called introns, and those that remain to code for proteins are called exons.

12 Translation is the process by which RNA directs the synthesis of polypeptides. This process takes place in the ribosomes, which consist of proteins and ribosomal RNA (rRNA).

13 During translation mRNA interacts with transfer RNA (tRNA), a molecule that has an attachment site for a specific amino acid.

Chromosomes

1 Human cells consist of diploid somatic cells (body cells) and haploid gametes (sperm and egg cells).

2 Humans have 23 pairs of chromosomes. Twenty-two of these pairs are autosomes. The remaining pair consists of the sex chromosomes. Females have two homologous X chromosomes as their sex chromosomes; males have an X and a Y chromosome.

3 A karyotype is an ordered display of chromosomes arranged according to length and the location of the centromere.

4 Various types of stains can be used to make chromosome bands more visible.

5 About 1 in 150 live births has a major diagnosable chromosome abnormality. Chromosome abnormalities are the leading known cause of mental retardation and miscarriage.

6 Polyploidy is a condition in which a euploid cell has some multiple of the normal number of chromosomes. Humans have been observed to have triploidy (three copies of each chromosome) and tetraploidy (four copies of each chromosome); both conditions are lethal.

7 Somatic cells that do not have a multiple of 23 chromosomes are aneuploid. Aneuploidy is usually the result of nondisjunction.

8 Trisomy is a type of aneuploidy in which one chromosome is present in three copies in somatic cells. A partial trisomy is one in which only part of a chromosome is present in three copies.

9 Monosomy is a type of aneuploidy in which one chromosome is present in only one copy in somatic cells.

10 In general, monosomies cause more severe physical defects than do trisomies, illustrating the principle that the loss of chromosome material has more severe consequences than the duplication of chromosome material.

11 Down syndrome, a trisomy of chromosome 21, is the best-known disease caused by a chromosome aberration. It affects 1 in 800 live births and is much more likely to occur in women over age 35.

12 Most aneuploidies of the sex chromosomes have less severe consequences than those of the autosomes.

13 The most commonly observed sex chromosome aneuploidies are the 47,XXX karyotype, 45,X karyotype (Turner syndrome), 47,XXY karyotype (Klinefelter syndrome), and 47,XYY karyotype.

14 Abnormalities of chromosome structure include deletions, duplications, inversions, and translocations.

Elements of Formal Genetics

1 Mendelian traits are caused by single genes, each of which occupies a position, or locus, on a chromosome.

2 Alleles are different forms of genes located at the same locus on the chromosome.

3 At any given locus in a somatic cell, an individual has two genes, one from each parent. An individual may be homozygous or heterozygous for a locus.

4 An individual's genotype is his or her genetic makeup, and the phenotype reflects the interaction of genotype and environment.

5 At a heterozygous locus, a dominant gene's effects mask those of a recessive gene. The recessive gene is expressed only when it is present in two copies.

Transmission of Genetic Diseases

1 Genetic diseases caused by single genes usually follow autosomal dominant, autosomal recessive, or X-linked recessive modes of inheritance.

2 Pedigree charts are an important tool in the analysis of modes of inheritance.

3 Recurrence risks specify the probability that future offspring will inherit a genetic disease. For single-gene diseases, recurrence risks remain the same for each offspring, regardless of the number of affected or unaffected offspring.

4 The recurrence risk for autosomal dominant diseases is usually 50%.

5 Germ-line mosaicism can alter recurrence risks for genetic diseases since unaffected parents can produce multiple affected offspring. This situation occurs because the germ line of one parent is affected by a mutation but the parent's somatic cells are unaffected.

6 Skipped generations are not seen in classic autosomal dominant pedigrees.

7 Males and females are equally likely to exhibit autosomal dominant diseases and to pass them on to their offspring.

8 Many genetic diseases have a delayed age of onset.

9 A gene that is not always expressed phenotypically is said to have incomplete penetrance.

10 Variable expressivity is a characteristic of many genetic diseases.

11 Genomic imprinting, which may involve methylation, results in differing expressions of a disease gene, depending on which parent transmitted the gene.

12 Most commonly, parents of children with autosomal recessive diseases are both heterozygous carriers of the disease gene.

13 The recurrence risk for autosomal recessive diseases is 25%.

14 Males and females are equally likely to be affected by autosomal recessive diseases.

15 Consanguinity is often present in families with autosomal recessive diseases, and it becomes more prevalent with rarer recessive diseases.

16 Carrier detection tests for an increasing number of autosomal recessive diseases are available.

17 The frequency of genetic diseases approximately doubles in the offspring of first-cousin matings.

18 In each normal female somatic cell, one of the two X chromosomes is inactivated early in embryogenesis.

19 X inactivation is random, fixed, and incomplete (i.e., only part of the chromosome is actually inactivated). It may involve methylation.

20 Gender is determined embryonically by the presence of the SRY gene on the Y chromosome. Embryos that have a Y chromosome (and thus the SRY gene) become males, whereas those lacking the Y chromosome become females. When the Y chromosome lacks the SRY gene, an XY female can be produced. Similarly, an X chromosome that contains the SRY gene can produce an XX male.

21 X-linked genes are those that are located on the X chromosome. Nearly all known X-linked diseases are caused by X-linked recessive genes.

22 Males are hemizygous for genes on the X chromosome.

23 X-linked recessive diseases are seen much more frequently in males than in females because males need only one copy of the gene to express the disease.

24 Fathers cannot pass X-linked genes to their sons.

25 Skipped generations are often seen in X-linked recessive disease pedigrees because the gene can be transmitted through carrier females.

26 Recurrence risks for X-linked recessive diseases depend on the carrier and affected status of the mother and father.

27 A sex-limited trait is one that occurs only in one of the sexes.

28 A sex-influenced trait is one that occurs more frequently in one sex than in the other.

Linkage Analysis and Gene Mapping

1 During meiosis I, crossing-over occurs and can cause recombinations of alleles located on the same chromosome.

2 The frequency of recombinations can be used to infer the map distance between loci on the same chromosome.

3 Loci that are on the same chromosome are syntenic.

4 A marker locus, when closely linked to a disease-gene locus, can be used to predict whether an individual will develop a genetic disease.

5 A more complete gene map will facilitate marker studies, studies of gene function and interaction, and gene therapy.

Multifactorial Inheritance

1 Traits that result from the combined effects of several loci are polygenic. When environmental factors also influence the trait, they are multifactorial.

2 Many multifactorial traits have a threshold of liability. Once the threshold of liability has been crossed, the disease may be expressed.

3 Empiric risks, based on direct observation of large numbers of families, are used to estimate recurrence risks for multifactorial diseases.

4 Recurrence risks for multifactorial diseases become higher if more than one family member is affected and/or if the expression of the disease in the proband is more severe.

5 If the population frequency of a multifactorial disease is f, the recurrence risk in offspring and siblings is approximately $\sqrt{f}$.

6 Recurrence risks for multifactorial diseases decrease rapidly for more remote relatives.

KEY TERMS

Adenine, 127
Allele, 144
Amino acid, 127
Aneuploid cell, 136
Anticodon, 132
Autosome, 134
Barr body, 150
Base pair substitution, 130
Carrier, 144
Carrier detection test, 149
Chromosomal mosaic, 136
Chromosome band, 134
Chromosome breakage, 140
Chromosome theory of inheritance, 144
Clastogen, 141
Cloning, 128
Codominance, 144
Codons, 130
Complementary base pairing, 130
Consanguinity, 149
Cri du chat syndrome, 141
Crossing-over, 155
Cytosine, 127
Delayed age of onset, 147
Deletion, 141
Deoxyribonucleic acid (DNA), 127
Diploid cell, 134
DNA polymerase, 130
Dominant, 144
Dosage compensation, 150
Double helix, 127
Down syndrome, 136
Duplication, 141
Dystrophin, 152
Empiric risk, 160
Euploid cell, 136
Exon, 132
Expressivity, 147
Fragile site, 142
Frameshift mutation, 131
Gamete, 134
Gene, 126
Genomic imprinting, 148

Genotype, 144
Germ line mosaicism, 147
Giemsa stain, 134
Guanine, 127
Haploid cell, 134
Hemizygous, 150
Heterogeneous nuclear RNA (hnRNA), 132
Heterozygote, 144
Heterozygous, 144
Homologous, 134
Homologous chromosome, 134
Homozygote, 144
Homozygous, 144
Inbreeding, 150
Intron, 132
Inversion, 141
Karyotype, 134
Klinefelter syndrome, 140
Linkage, 155
Locus, 144
Map unit, 155
Meiosis, 134
Meiotic error, 140
Messenger RNA (mRNA), 131
Metaphase spread, 134
Methylation, 151
Mode of inheritance, 144
Monosomy, 136
Multifactorial inheritance, 160
Mutagen, 131
Mutation, 130
Mutational hot spot, 131
Nondisjunction, 136
Nucleotide, 127
Obligate carrier, 147
Occurrence risk, 146
Partial trisomy, 136
Pedigree, 145
Penetrance, 147
Phenotype, 144
Polygenic trait, 160
Polymorphic (polymorphism), 144
Polypeptide, 127

Polyploid cell, 136
Position effect, 142
Principle of independent assortment, 144
Principle of segregation, 144
Proband (propositus/proposita), 145
Promoter site, 131
Pseudoautosomal, 151
Purine, 127
Pyrimidine, 127
Recessive, 144
Reciprocal translocation, 142
Recombination, 155
Recurrence risk, 146
Ribonucleic acid (RNA), 131
Ribosomal RNA (rRNA), 132
Ribosome, 132
RNA polymerase, 131
Robertsonian translocation, 142
Sex chromosome, 134
Sex-influenced trait, 152
Sex-limited trait, 152
Sex-linked (inheritance), 150
Silent substitution, 131
Somatic cell, 134
Spontaneous mutation, 131
Structural gene, 127
Syntenic loci, 155
Template, 130
Termination or nonsense codon, 130
Termination sequence, 131
Tetraploidy, 136
Threshold of liability, 160
Thymine, 127
Transcription, 131
Transfer RNA (tRNA), 132
Translation, 132
Translocation, 142
Triploidy, 136
Trisomy, 136
Tumor-suppressor gene, 147
Turner syndrome, 139
X-linked (inheritance), 150

REFERENCES

Anderson, W. F. (1992). Human gene therapy. *Science, 256,* 808-813.

Brown, C. J., Lafraniere, R. G., Powers, V. E., Sebastio, G., Ballabio, A., Pettigrew, A. L., Ledbetter, D. H., Levy, E., Craig, I. W., & Willard, H. F. (1991). Localization of the X inactivation center on the human X chromosome in Xq13. *Nature, 349,* 82-84.

Caskey, C. T., Pizzuti, A., Fu, Y–H., Fenwick, R. G., & Nelson, D. L. (1992). Triplet repeat mutations in human disease. *Science, 256,* 784-789.

Chamberlain, J. S. (1991). Duchenne muscular dystrophy. *Current Opinion in Genetics and Development, 1,* 11-14.

Collins, F. S. (1992). Cystic fibrosis: Molecular biology and therapeutic implications. *Science, 256,* 774-779.

Cooper, D. N., & Youssoufian, H. (1988). The CpG dinucleotide and human genetic disease. *Human Genetics, 78,* 151-155.

de Grouchy, J., & Turleau, C. (1990). Autosomal disorders. In A. E. H. Emery & D. L. Rimoin (Eds.), *Principles and practice of medical genetics* (Vol. 1, pp. 247-271). Edinburgh: Churchill Livingstone.

de la Chapelle, A. (1990). Sex chromosome abnormalities. In A. E. H. Emery & D. L. Rimoin (Eds.), *Principles and practice of medical genetics* (Vol. 1, pp. 273-299). Edinburgh: Churchill Livingstone.

Donahue, R. P., Bias, W. B., Renwick, J. H., & McKusick, V. A. (1968). Probable assignment of the Duffy blood-group locus to chromosome 1 in man. *Proceedings of the National Academy of Science, 61*, 949.

Erlich, H. A., Gelfand, D., & Sninsky, J. J. (1991). Recent advances in the polymerase chain reaction. *Science, 252*, 1643-1651.

Fu, Y., Kuhl, D. P. A., Pizzuti, A., Pieretti, M., Sutcliffe, J. S., Richards, S., Verkerk, A. J. M. H., Holden, J. J. A., Fenwick, R. G., Warren, S. T., Oostra, B. A., Nelson, D. L., & Caskey, C. T. (1991). Variation of the CGG repeat at the fragile X site results in genetic instability: Resolution of the Sherman paradox. *Cell, 67*, 1047-1058.

Goodman, R. M. & Gorlin, R. J. (1977). *Atlas of the face in genetic disorders* (2nd ed.). St. Louis: Mosby–Year Book.

Hall, J. G. (1988). Review and hypotheses: Somatic mosaicism: Observations related to clinical genetics. *American Journal of Human Genetics, 43*, 355-363.

Hall, J. G. (1990). Genomic imprinting: Review and relevance to human diseases. *American Journal of Human Genetics, 46*, 857-873.

Hall, J. G., Powers, E. K., McIlvaine, R. T., & Ean, V. H. (1978). The frequency and financial burden of genetic disease in a pediatric hospital. *American Journal of Medical Genetics, 1*, 417.

Hassold, T. J. (1986). Chromosome abnormalities in human reproductive wastage. *Trends in Genetics, 2*, 105-110.

Hassold, T. J., & Jacobs, P. A. (1984). Trisomy in man. *Annual Review of Genetics, 18*, 69.

Hilbert, P., Lindpainter, K., Beckmann, J. S., Serikawa, T., Soubrier, F., Dubay, C., Cartwright, P., De Gouyon, B., Julier, C., Takahasi, S., Vincent, M., Ganten, D., Georges, M., & Lathrop, G. M. (1991). Chromosomal mapping of two genetic loci associated with blood-pressure regulation in hereditary hypertensive rats. *Nature, 353*, 521-529.

Jorde, L. B. (1991). Inbreeding in human populations. In R. Dulbecco (Ed.), *Encyclopedia of human biology* (Vol. 4, pp. 431-441). New York: Academic Press.

Koopman, P., Gubbay, J., Vivian, N., Goodfellow, P. N., & Lovell-Badge, R. (1991). Male development of chromosomally female mice transgenic for SRY. *Nature, 351*, 117-121.

Lyon, M. F. (1962). Sex chromatin and gene action in the mammalian X-chromosome. *American Journal of Human Genetics, 14*, 135.

Martin, R. H., & Rademaker, A. W. (1987). The effect of age on the frequency of sperm chromosomal abnormalities in normal men. *American Journal of Human Genetics, 41*, 484-492.

McKusick, V. A. (1992). *Mendelian inheritance in man* (10th ed.). Baltimore: Johns Hopkins University Press.

Miller, A. D. (1992). Human gene therapy comes of age. *Nature, 357*, 455-460.

Raven, P. H., & Johnson, G. B. (1992). *Biology* (3rd ed.). St. Louis: Mosby–Year Book.

Sinclair, A. H., Berta, P., Palmer, M. S., Hawkins, J. R., Griffiths, B. L., Smith, M. J., Foster, J. W., Frischauf, A., Lovell-Badge, R., & Goodfellow, P. N. (1990). A gene from the human sex-determining region encodes a protein with homology to a conserved DNA-binding motif. *Nature, 346*, 240-244.

Thibodeau, G. A. (1987). *Anatomy and physiology*. St. Louis: Mosby–Year Book.

Thompson, M. W., McInnes, R. R., & Willard, H. F. (1991). *Genetics in medicine* (5th ed.). Philadelphia: W. B. Saunders.

Todd, J. A., Aitman, T. J., Cornall, R. J., Ghosh, S., Hall, J. R. S., Hearne, C. M., Knight, A. M., Love, J. M., McAleer, M. A., Prins, J., Rodrigues, N., Lathrop, M., Pressey, A., DeLarato, N. H., Peterson, L. B., & Wicker, L. S. (1991). Genetic analysis of autoimmune type 1 diabetes mellitus in mice. *Nature, 351*, 542-547.

Watson, J. D., & Crick, F. H. C. (1953). Molecular structure of nucleic acids—A structure for deoxyribonucleic acid. *Nature, 171*, 737.

Weinberg, R. A. (1991). Tumor suppressor genes. *Science, 254*, 1138-1146.

Whaley, L. F. & Wong, D. L. (1991). *Nursing care of infants and children* (4th ed.). St. Louis: Mosby–Year Book.

White, R., & O'Connell, P. (1991). Identification and characterization of the gene for neurofibromatosis type 1. *Current Opinion in Genetics and Development, 1*, 15-19.

Williamson, R., Bowcock, A., Kidd, K., Pearson, P., Schmidtke, J., Ceverha, P., Chipperfield, M., Cooper, D. N., Coutelle, C., Hewitt, J., Klinger, K., Langley, K., Beckmann, J., Tolley, M., & Maidak, B. (1991). Report of the DNA committee and catalogues of cloned and mapped genes, markers formatted for PCR and DNA polymorphisms. *Cytogenetics and Cell Genetics, 58* (3-4), 1190-1832.

SUGGESTED READINGS

Biggs, R. (1990). Defects in coagulation. In A. E. H. Emery & D. L. Rimoin (Eds.), *Principles and practice of medical genetics* (2nd ed., Vol. 2.). Edinburgh: Churchill Livingstone.

Cooper, D. N., & Schmidtke, J. (1989). Diagnosis of genetic disease using recombinant DNA: Second edition. *Human Genetics, 83*, 307-334.

de Grouchy, J., & Turleau, C. (1984). *Clinical atlas of human chromosomes* (2nd ed.). New York: John Wiley & Sons.

Emery, A. E. H., & Rimoin, D. L. (Eds.). (1990). *Principles and practice of medical genetics* (2nd ed., 2 vols.). Edinburgh: Churchill Livingstone.

Harper, P. S. (1988). *Practical genetic counselling* (3rd ed.). London: Wright.

Jenkins, J. B. (1990). *Human genetics* (2nd ed.). Menlo Park, CA: Benjamin/Cummings.

Mange, A. P., & Mange, E. J. (1990). *Genetics: Human aspects* (2nd ed.). Sunderland, MA: Sinauer.

McKusick, V. A. (1988). The new genetics and clinical medicine: A summing up. *Hospital Practice* (July 15), 177-191.

Rhoads, G. G., Jackson, L. G., Schlesselman, S., de la Cruz, F. F., Desnick, R. J., Golbus, M. S., Ledbetter, D. H., Lubs, H. A., Mahoney, M. J., Pergament, E., Simpson, J. L., Carpenter, R. J., Elias, S., Ginsberg, N. A., Goldberg, J. D., Hobbins, J. C., Lynch, L., Shiono, P. H., Wapner, R. J., & Zachary, J. M. (1989). The safety and efficacy of chorionic villus sampling for early prenatal diagnosis of cytogenetic abnormalities. *New England Journal of Medicine, 320*, 609-617.

Vogel, F., & Motulsky, A. G. (1986). *Human genetics: Problems and approaches* (2nd ed.). Berlin: Springer-Verlag.

Watson, J. D., Hopkins, N. H., Roberts, J. W., Steitz, J. A., & Weiner, A. M. (1987). *Molecular biology of the gene* (4th ed.). Menlo Park, CA: Benjamin/Cummings.

Weatherall, D. J. (1991). *The new genetics and clinical practice* (3rd ed.). Oxford: Oxford University Press.

White, R. L., & Lalouel, J. M. (1987). Investigation of genetic linkage in human families. *Advances in Human Genetics, 16*, 121.

Genes and Environmental Interaction: Familial Diseases

Roger R. Williams

Chapter Outline

E*pidemiology is the study of factors governing the occurrence and distribution of disease and disorders in a population. The most significant goal of epidemiology is to acquire the necessary knowledge of causal mechanisms in order to formulate and implement preventive measures against diseases. Almost 2400 years ago, Hippocrates suspected a connection between disease and environment (Hippocrates, republished, 1938). He states, "One should consider attentively the waters which inhabitants use . . . the mode in which the inhabitants live—whether*

they are fond of drinking and eating to excess or are fond of exercise and labor." Despite this recorded suspicion, virtually no disease-causing characteristics of the environment were discovered in the subsequent 2000 years.

In 1662 John Grant published the first quantitative examination of mortality and birth rates and noted the major impact of the bubonic plague in a defined population. Only after an additional 200 years had passed did similar observations lead to the beginning of a sustained interest in epidemiology. In

166

1839 the distribution of cholera was tabulated for England and Wales by William Farr.

In 1855 John Snow published a classic epidemiologic study demonstrating that cholera was caused by water distributed by the Southwark and Vauxhall Water Company in London, which was drawing drinking water from the Thames River at a location heavily polluted by sewage. Two competing water companies supplied water to two different parts of town, causing marked differences in cholera rates and leading to the initial suspicion. Conclusive evidence was found by studying a large portion of London in which the two companies were supplying water to neighboring houses. In this manner individuals could be matched for socioeconomic status and other characteristics, although they had different water supplies. The death rate from cholera was eight times higher among the individuals supplied by the company with polluted water, providing evidence for Snow's hypothesis and eventually leading to a considerable amount of disease prevention.

The studies of Grant, Farr, and Snow were all observational studies. A careful record of disease occurrence in an existing population was correlated with other recorded factors in an effort to determine the cause of a disease. Another test for epidemiologic hypotheses required intervention to observe whether or not a predicted outcome was associated with a change in a particular environmental factor. Two classic examples include Lind's attempt at using fresh fruit to prevent scurvy in 1753 and Jenner's trying cowpox vaccination to prevent smallpox in 1798.

More current epidemiologic methods have also emphasized common chronic diseases, particularly infectious diseases. The term epidemic once meant an outbreak of an infectious disease. It is now often used by the public and professionals to indicate any disease that seems to have an excessive occurrence. Comparisons between different populations or comparisons of frequencies in different time periods can document changes in disease occurrence. For example, in the United States coronary atherosclerosis accounts for nearly one third of all deaths, although in some areas of the world it occurs relatively infrequently. Lung cancer is now over 30 times more common in the United States than it was 50 years ago. Both of these diseases are considered epidemic. Because the rates of occurrence for these diseases have grown relatively slowly, the magnitude of the problem is often not appreciated by the general public. To an American man, the risk of dying of coronary heart disease, for example, equals the risk of major infectious epidemics in past centuries. Current epidemiology also concentrates on unusually low disease fre-quencies, which may provide other clues to what causes and what may prevent disease.

Over the last several decades, epidemiology has rapidly grown into a well-developed discipline. Large observational studies of cardiovascular disease and cancer have involved thousands of investigators, millions of people, and hundreds of millions of dollars. However, even the sophistication of large multicenter, randomized, clinical trials using state-of-the-art biostatistics, laboratory methods, and clinical protocols has left many important questions unanswered.

Evidence currently indicates that many common chronic diseases occur because of a mismatch between genetic and environmental factors. Some inherited traits have helped human beings survive in hostile environments, but these traits now increase susceptibility to chronic disease and early death. For example, genes for an efficient metabolism probably helped women survive pregnancy and lactation during food shortages common throughout history. For women with access to enough food, however, the same genes can lead to obesity, diabetes, hypertension, and stroke. Clearly, environmental factors affect the expression of inherited traits. Scientists of the past generally studied epidemiology and genetics separately. Only within the last two decades have scientific efforts increasingly included both of these disciplines in the study of the causes of disease. Today the goal is to identify the exact genetic and environmental influences that lead to major diseases. This approach allows individuals with specific susceptibilities to modify environmental factors and avoid tragic consequences. Knowledge of environmental factors should lead to dramatic public health efforts involving screening, identification of high-risk individuals, and effective risk-reduction programs designed to prevent disease.

WHAT FACTORS CAUSE DISEASE?

Factors causing disease can be simplistically classified as genetic or environmental (Table 5-1). Age and gender play important roles in the development of most diseases. Age often represents the accumulated effects of genetic and environmental factors over time. Sex differences may represent either environmental or genetic factors. Thus diseases with rates of occurrence that differ between men and women may reflect life-style or environmental differences or anatomic and hormonal differences.

When little is known about the cause of a disease, its occurrence often appears to be a chance or random

TABLE 5-1

Environmental Factors Affecting the Occurrence of Disease

Type	Examples
Microorganisms and immunologic exposures	Bacteria Viruses Fungi Protozoa Vectors (e.g., insects and animals) Allergens
Personal habits and life-style	Smoking Physical exercise Dietary intake
Chemical substances	Toxins Pollutants Medications Solvents, fumes Contaminants
Physical environment	Climate Radiation Physical trauma Geographic location (e.g., sun exposure, altitude) Community (e.g., water and food supplies)
Psychosocial milieu	Family status (e.g., bereavement, loss, status, change) Stress Coping skills Social isolation Ethnic and racial customs Religious customs

event. As scientific research identifies more genetic and environmental causes and pathophysiologic mechanisms, however, the number of diseases that seem to occur at random diminishes. Theoretically, causal factors could be identified for all diseases and therefore no disease occurrence could be considered truly random. Furthermore, subtle initiating events, such as mutations or uncommon exposures, might eventually lead researchers to classify all causal factors as either genetic or environmental.

In some cases, of course, the difficulty lies in distinguishing between the effects of shared environmental factors and the effects of a genetic background common to a population. Groups of individuals are often reported to have distinctively higher or lower disease rates, either because of shared environmental factors or because of a common gene pool (Carmelli, Williams, &

Rissanen, 1982). For example, dietary customs are shared by ethnic groups; genes for some traits are shared by particular racial groups; climate is common to those in shared geographic locations; and health codes may be shared by religious groups (Table 5-2). Often notable contrasts in disease occurrences are first observed within different populations, leading to the subsequent investigation of possible underlying environmental factors.

Finding and understanding environmental factors that affect the penetrance of specific genes is the single most important approach in preventing chronic familial diseases (see p. 147). For many common chronic diseases, studies suggest that genetic makeup predisposes an individual to the disease but that environmental factors then cause the disease to develop. For example, one hypothesis suggests that genetic predisposition to arterial hypertension is brought out by high salt intake (Williams & Hopkins, 1979). If this theory is true, most of the United States population is exposed to sufficient levels of the environmental factor (high dietary intake of sodium chloride) to allow "salt-sensitive hypertension genes" to be expressed in those who carry them. Many inherited traits, including some disease states, probably represent the blending of effects of many different genes in which none predominate. As Chapter 4 explains, these reflect polygenic inheritance; they are therefore termed **polygenic traits.** Environmental influences may then enhance an individual's predisposition to disease, producing a truly multifactorial set of causal factors for any given disease occurrence or observed trait.

Although geneticists often model theories of polygenic traits on the assumption of an infinite number of genes, the wide diversity of genotypes resulting from even three or four loci with two alleles probably approaches a range of expression similar to the classic polygenic models. Even with only two alleles, two loci produce 9 different genotypes, three loci produce 27 genotypes, and four loci produce 81 genotypes. Even a single locus with three, four, or five alleles will respectively produce 6, 10, or 15 different genotypes. Once environmental influences cause variations in the phenotype for each of these genotypes, a blended spectrum of phenotypes becomes a **multifactorial trait.**

Height is a classic example of a multifactorial trait resulting from many genes with superimposed environmental influences. Heights of individuals in the general population vary across the spectrum from short to tall, although the most common expression of the trait is near the middle of the spectrum. Children reach their adult height when they are approximately halfway between the height of both parents, after adjustment for the fact that females are commonly somewhat shorter than males. Because of improved nutrition, recent generations are also somewhat taller.

TABLE 5-2

Populations with Shared Disease Tendencies (due to shared environmental factors, common gene pool, or both)

Disease	Populations	Suggested environmental factors	Shared gene pool
Early coronary heart disease	Very high in Finland (very low in Japan)	Animal fat intake	Genes for high blood cholesterol
Colon cancer	Low in developing countries (e.g., Africa); high in "westernized" countries (USA, Europe)	Dietary fiber and fat intake	
Thalassemia (type of anemia)	High in persons of Mediterranean descent; low in other areas		Major dominant gene for thalassemia
Malaria (many other infectious diseases)	High in some parts of Africa and Asia; low in USA and Europe	Trypanosomes, mosquitoes, disease control measures	
Early non-insulin dependent diabetes and obesity	Native Americans	Change from scarce food supply to plenty	Apparent shared gene pool among various Indian tribes
Lung cancer	Low rates in Mormons and Seventh Day Adventists	Health code against use of tobacco	
Skin cancers	Higher rates among whites than among blacks; higher rates in "sun belt" than in other locations	Ultraviolet light	Inherited level of skin pigmentation

The notion of a threshold of liability (defined in Chapter 4) suggests that some disease states may depend on a similar multifactorially determined continuous risk level. A set of multifactorial traits may lead to a varying degree of liability for a disease, but actual expression of the disease occurs only after the liability surpasses some discrete threshold (Cavalli-Storza & Bodner, 1971). For example, serum cholesterol level is a multifactorial trait that is expressed on a continuum. Coronary heart attacks are rarely seen in men with serum cholesterol levels below a threshold of 160 mg/dl but are often seen in men with levels above 300 mg/dl.

Even when genetic factors are a primary cause of a condition, other factors also might be present. With serum cholesterol levels, for example, a major gene may produce strikingly high levels of cholesterol in some individuals, but polygenic inheritance and environmental factors can then cause considerable variation in cholesterol levels among those with this genotype. Many physiologic traits—such as serum cholesterol levels, blood pressure levels, and height—are probably multifactorial

traits that result from both polygenic inheritance and environmental factors. The effects of a single gene are observable only when a disease entity emerges, as in the case of striking elevations of cholesterol, high blood pressure, or retarded stature.

Types of genetic factors affecting disease occurrence are described in Table 5-3. Single genes are often expressed as relatively discrete, noticeable phenotypes or as observable genetic defects. The frequency of genetic disease in the general population depends on the gene frequency and the penetrance of a genetic trait (these concepts are defined in Chapter 4). Statistically, dominant genes are more penetrant than recessive genes, but, even with genetic predisposition to a specific disorder, individuals with a single dominant gene or with two copies of a recessive gene might not express the genetic disorder. Penetrance can depend on the person's age, gender, environmental factors, and other genes. The effects of these other factors on a particular gene's penetrance are called **interactions** (gene-environment interactions or gene-gene interactions).

TABLE 5-3

Genetic Factors Affecting the Occurrence of Disease

Mode of transmission	Considerations	Example

Single genes	Dominant, recessive, or additive?
	Gene frequencies high or low?
	Autosomal or X-linked?
	Totally or partially penetrant?
	Factors affecting penetrance?
	    (e.g., age, gender, environment,
	        other genes, chance)
		Rh blood type

Polygenic	Blending of effects of several genes (of- ten combined with environmental factors to produce multifactorial in- heritance)	Height

Multifactorial	Noticeable effect of single major gene
	    in addition to background variation
	    in phenotype due to polygenes
	Major gene effects determine the "ball-
	    park location" for a trait value,
	    whereas polygenes and environmen-
	    tal factors can affect which "base"
	    within that major gene phenotype or
	    "ballpark"
		Serum cholesterol

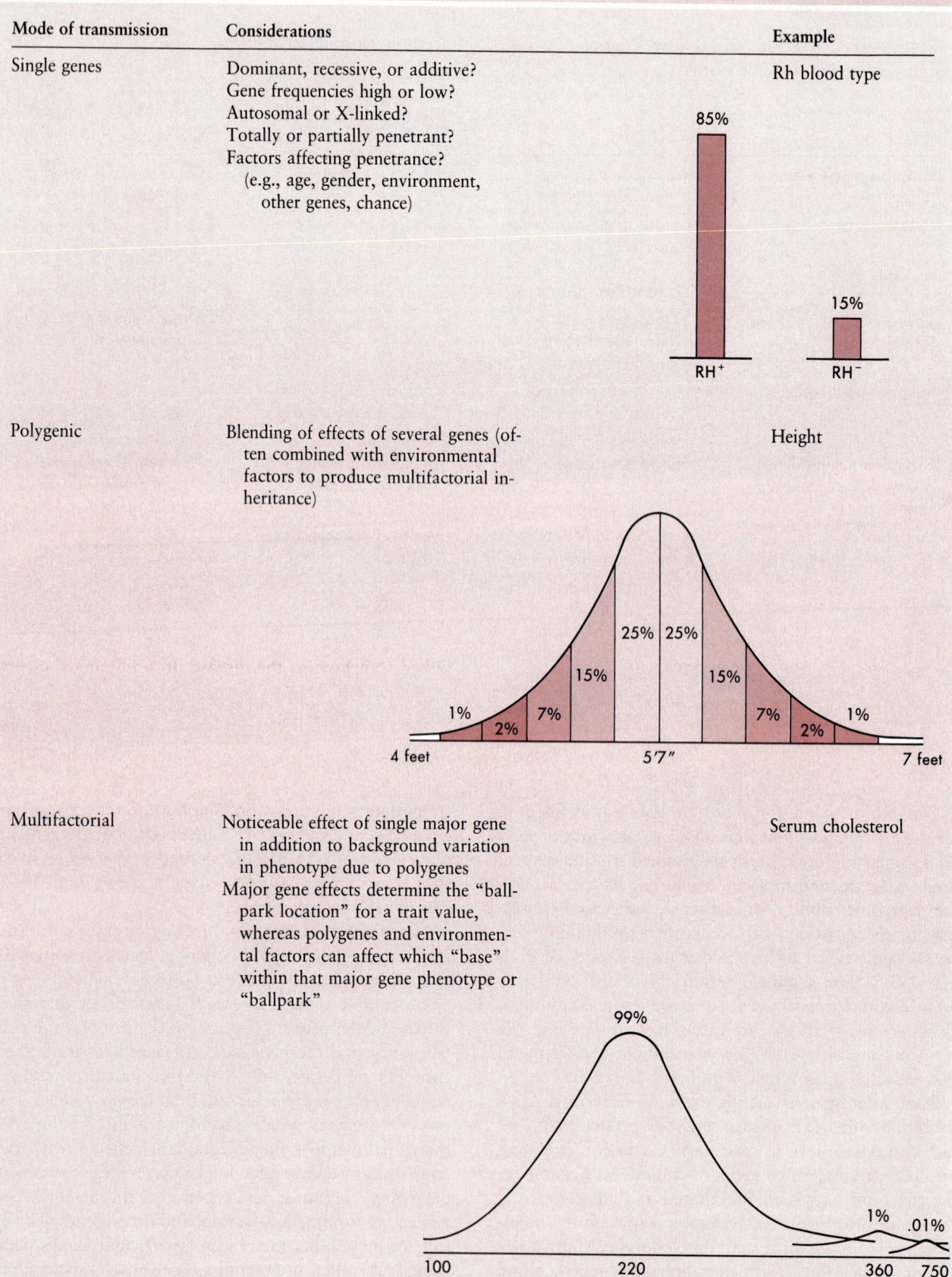

GENETICS AND EPIDEMIOLOGY: NEW APPLICATIONS FOR CLINICAL PRACTICE

An ultimate understanding of the causes of disease, individual susceptibility, and methods of prevention encompasses the disciplines of genetics and epidemiology together. It also draws on the knowledge of many different disciplines, including pathology, biostatistics, physiology, and numerous subdivisions within each of these disciplines. Epidemiologists identify specific chemicals in the environment that are thought to induce cancer or cardiovascular disease. Biochemists and molecular physiologists identify cell receptors, the keys to the cellular processes affected by molecules that have been absorbed or manufactured from environmental substances. Biochemists determine the amino acid sequences of cell receptors or enzymes controlling biochemical processes. Population geneticists and clinicians identify specific high-risk families with disorders suspected to involve newly identified biochemical mechanisms, and they obtain ordinary blood samples and important pertinent information about disease occurrence and environmental exposure. Molecular geneticists use this information to develop genetic "probes," extracting DNA from the chromosomes in the nuclei of white blood cells. Like keys in a lock, such probes help to find those individuals in whom a "good fit" indicates an inherited predisposition or a specific environmental factor leading to disease.

Although this approach may sound like science fiction, it is an accurate description of a rapidly evolving technology. Such scientific advances will ultimately lead to the identification and chromosomal location of many genes that cause either susceptibility or resistance to specific diseases. Markers for genetic susceptibility will be developed in conjunction with the identification of the appropriate modifiable environmental variables that work in conjunction with inherited predispositions to cause important chronic disease. Because this field is growing rapidly, a basic understanding of the principles needed to understand these applications will be important for health professionals in future decades.

ANALYZING DISEASE RISK

Disease Rates

The concepts and terminology used by epidemiologists who assess disease risk provide a foundation for understanding the causes of disease. Several basic rates help to describe the occurrence of disease. All these rates require accurate surveillance and reporting of disease and a census count of the base population. The **incidence rate** is the number of new cases detected during a given interval (usually 1 year) per number of persons in the population surveyed. The **prevalence rate** refers to the number of persons *living* with the disease (accumulated new and old cases) per number of persons in the population. Thus the prevalence rate is determined by the incidence rate and length of survival for persons with the disease. The **mortality rate** is the number of persons who have died from the disease during a given period (often 1 year) per number of persons in the surveyed population. In 1970 coronary heart disease in American men aged 50 to 64 years showed a prevalence rate of 9.7%, an annual incidence rate of 2.2%, and an annual mortality rate of 0.92% of the base population.

Disease rates can be determined separately in populations with and without exposure to suspected causal factors. If the disease rate is significantly higher in the exposed population, it suggests that the exposure is linked somehow to the disease. In preliminary investigations most data can only indicate an association or statistical connection between a particular factor and a particular disease. Years of research and a large body of experimental data are often required to determine which disease-associated factors also played a causal role. For example, initial studies showed that lung cancer was most common among cigarette smokers and among men, suggesting that men might have a greater predisposition for developing the disease. Subsequent data, however, showed that the association of male sex with lung cancer is easily explained by the increased level of smoking exhibited by men. Prospective population studies and experimental laboratory investigations have since provided convincing evidence that cigarette smoking causes lung cancer.

Risk Factor Analysis

Risk factors are indicators of a person's predisposition to developing a disease. A particular risk factor or set of risk factors predicts increased disease rates in a group of individuals (e.g., smokers more commonly develop lung cancer than nonsmokers do). Risk factors cannot precisely predict whether a specific person will contract or avoid a disease (many smokers do not develop lung cancer). As with the example of male sex and lung cancer, risk factors do not always suggest a cause for a dis-

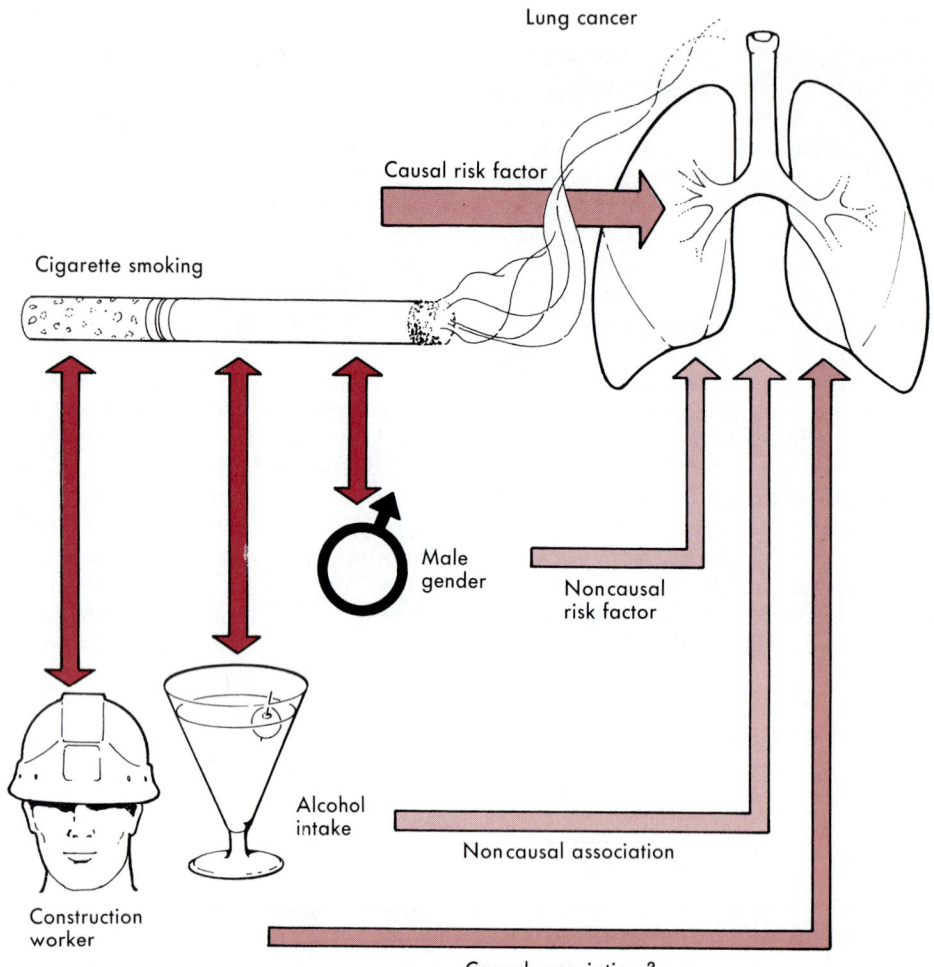

FIG. 5-1 Causal and noncausal risk factors associated with lung cancer. Smoking is a causal risk factor for lung cancer. Men and alcohol drinkers have a higher than average incidence rate for lung cancer because they are also more often smokers. Although construction workers also smoke more, they have more lung cancer even if they are nonsmokers, probably because of exposure to fumes and dust.

ease, but identifying them often provides clues toward identifying the cause of a particular disease.

Sets of risk factors have been developed for many common chronic diseases. Although scientists suspect a causal role for some of these risk factors, solid evidence establishing a causal relationship is lacking for many. The distinction between causal and noncausal risk factors is illustrated in Fig. 5-1. **Causal risk factors** are those that, when removed or eliminated, will result in the delay or prevention of the disease. **Noncausal risk factors** are helpful in predicting a person's chances of developing the disease, but they have no direct effect on the underlying cause of the disease.

Cigarette smoking, for example, is a proven causal risk factor leading to lung cancer. Since men and alcohol drinkers are more often smokers, they are also more

likely to develop lung cancer. Nonsmoking men and alcohol drinkers do not, however, have an increased risk for lung cancer. Therefore male gender and alcohol intake are noncausal risk factors for lung cancer. As Fig. 5-1 also shows, the greater incidence of lung cancer among construction workers also suggests a causal association. This incidence may, however, be a result of the dust and fumes associated with construction work (Williams & Horn, 1977; Williams, Stegens, & Goldsmith, 1977).

Analysis with Contingency Tables

The correlation between cigarette smoking and lung cancer also illustrates genetic susceptibility precipitated by environmental exposure. If, as studies indicate, cigarette smoking induces lung cancer more often among

TABLE 5-4

Statistical Measures Used to Calculate Risk

	Application	Calculation
Contingency table	Lists number of persons according to disease and exposure status	
Disease rate (incidence, prevalence, or mortality)	Measures occurrence rate of the disease	$$\dfrac{\text{Number of cases, new cases, or deaths}}{\text{Number of persons in the population}}$$
Relative risk	Measures the degree of increased disease rate in the exposed population compared to the unexposed population	$$\dfrac{\text{Number of exposed cases} \div \text{Number of exposed persons}}{\text{Number of unexposed cases} \div \text{Number of unexposed persons}}$$
Population attributable risk (%)*	Measures the percentage of disease cases in a specific population attributable to a specific risk factor	$$\dfrac{\left(\begin{array}{c}\text{Number of observed cases}\\\text{in the exposed}\\\text{population}\end{array}\right) - \left(\begin{array}{c}\text{Number of expected cases}\\\text{in the exposed}\\\text{population}\end{array}\right)}{\text{Total number of cases}} \times 10$$
Preventive efficiency	Measures the percentage of exposed persons in a defined population in whom a disease would be prevented if all avoided the causal exposure	$$\left(\begin{array}{c}\text{Population-}\\\text{attributable}\\\text{risk}\end{array}\right) \times \left(\dfrac{\text{Disease rate}}{\text{Proportion exposed}}\right)$$

*Another formula to get same result:

$$\begin{array}{c}\text{Population}\\\text{attributable}\\\text{risk}\end{array} = \dfrac{\left(\begin{array}{c}\text{Disease rate}\\\text{in total}\\\text{population}\end{array}\right) - \left(\begin{array}{c}\text{Disease rate}\\\text{in unexposed}\\\text{population}\end{array}\right)}{(\text{Disease rate in total population})} \times 100$$

The contingency table in the Calculation column:

Disease

Exposure	Yes	No	Totals:
Yes	a	b	m_1 Exposed persons
No	c	d	m_2 Nonexposed persons
	n_1	n_2	
	Disease cases	Healthy controls	Grand total

individuals who are genetically susceptible (Tokuhata, 1965), the effects of both genetics and environment can be analyzed using **contingency tables.**

The association of a disease with a particular risk factor is often evaluated by using 2-by-2 contingency tables, which are illustrated in Table 5-4. The contingency table lists the number of individuals who respectively do or do not have the disease and have or have not experienced exposure to a risk factor. The data that compose the contingency table are then used to calculate various statistical measures.

The **relative risk** of developing the disease is expressed as the ratio of the disease rate among the exposed population to the disease rate in the unexposed population. For lung cancer and cigarette smoking, a relative risk of 13.3 implies a lung cancer rate among smokers that is 13.3 times higher than the rate among nonsmokers. The **population-attributable risk** indicates the percentage of disease cases in the general population that are attributable to a causal risk factor. Although the relative risks and population-attributable risks may be similar measures in susceptible and resistant persons, pre-

TABLE 5-5

Chronic Disease Rates and Relative Risks from Exposure to Risk Factors

Risk factor	Possible mechanisms
Genetic predisposition or resistance	Number of different loci promoting or preventing the disease
	Gene frequency of each locus in the population
	Mode of transmission (dominant, polygenic, etc.) of each locus
	Factors increasing or decreasing each gene's survival and effects over generations
	Death or illness during reproductive years (insulin-dependent diabetes in past)
	Heterozygote advantage (e.g., sickle-cell erythrocytes resist malaria)
	New treatment that improves survival (advances in insulin-dependent diabetes)
	Changing environment (e.g., mismatch or "thrifty gene" in Indian tribes surviving for centuries with meager food supply develop obesity and non-insulin-dependent diabetes with oversupply of food?)
	Penetrance (sometimes variable depending on interactions with other genes and environmental factors)
Environmental and life-style factors that promote or protect	Number and type of exposures or protective factors (e.g., lung cancer and cigarette smoking, and uranium and hydrocarbon fumes)
	Level of exposure (e.g., packs smoked per day)
	Duration of exposure (e.g., years of smoking)
	Potency of exposure (e.g., filtered and nonfiltered cigarettes)
	Proportion of the general population exposed
Age	Cumulative effects of genes and environment over time
	Biologic "alarm clock" synchronized to changing metabolism
Gender	X-linked transmission on X chromosome (e.g., hemophilia)
	Sex-limited expression from hormonal or anatomic differences (e.g., breast cancer)
	Environmental differences (e.g., men smoke more and have more lung cancer)
	Combinations (e.g., coronary heart disease and smoking combined with high-density lipoproteins)
Interactions	Combined risk factors (likely present for many familial chronic diseases)

ventive measures help a higher proportion of people within the genetically susceptible subgroup. This difference is noted by comparing the genetically susceptible persons to genetically resistant persons with respect to the **preventive efficiency,** which is the percentage of exposed persons who would be saved from the disease if they all avoided the causal exposure. A higher preventive efficiency is seen in genetically susceptible persons.

In general, relative risks show how strongly exposures are linked to specific diseases. Population-attributable risks show which exposures account for the greatest amount of a given disease. Preventive efficiency indicates the cost-effectiveness of prevention programs in specifically defined populations. **High-risk persons** are those exposed to sufficient levels of causal risk factors to increase their disease risk significantly. If they are both genetically susceptible and exposed to the risk factor, they are at a very high risk of disease. Such individuals are good targets for disease-prevention programs. Factors affecting disease rates and relative risks are summarized in Table 5-5.

Prevention programs must also take into account the difference between cumulative effects leading to disease and acute effects. For example, the accumulated cancer-causing chemicals from cigarette smoking do lead to lung cancer, but the effects require time to develop. Preventing lung cancer thus requires years of smoking avoidance. In contrast, the risk of coronary death seems to be related more to the acute effects of carbon monoxide in cigarette smoke. Even after 20 years of smoking, the risk of coronary death drops to levels similar to those for nonsmokers within 2 years, according to some studies (Feinleib & Williams, 1976).

Analysis with Correlation Coefficients

Sometimes disease characteristics and risk factors can be assessed quantitatively as continuous traits rather than as purely dichotomous (absence or presence) outcomes. In an analysis of disease, **continuous traits** are those that are expressed across a range of severity. Obesity and blood pressure elevation, for example, are related conditions that appear with various degrees of severity. An-

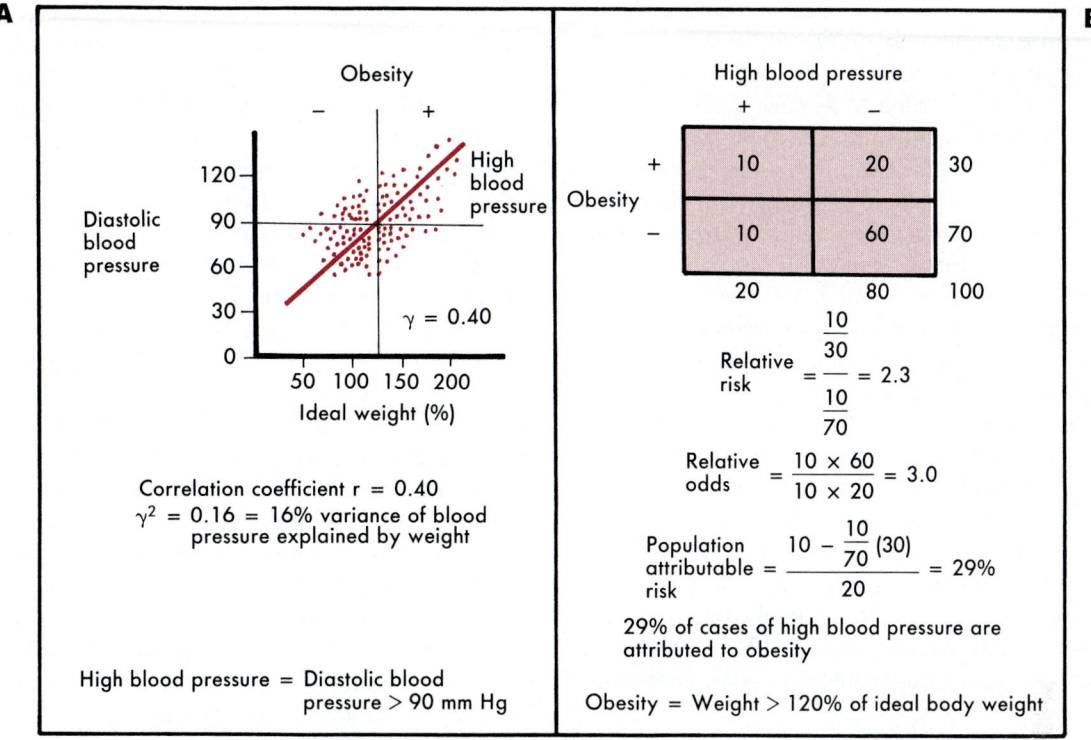

FIG. 5-2 Two methods used to test for an association between specific diseases and causal risk factors for that disease. **A,** Plots and correlation coefficients are used for continuous traits. **B,** A contingency table is used to analyze risk exposure with the presence or absence of disease. The horizontal line at 90 mm Hg diastolic blood pressure arbitrarily separates points into observations that would be considered to be hypertensive and normotensive individuals. A vertical line at 120% of ideal weight separates individuals arbitrarily into obese and nonobese individuals. These lines thus divide the plotted points into four sections that correspond to the number of observations tabulated in the contingency table.

alyzing obesity as a risk factor in a contingency table requires the choice of numerical dividing lines to obtain simple definition of what constitutes a dichotomous (opposites) classification of subjects into two single groups. Subjects must be either obese or nonobese, hypertensive or normotensive. In such cases quantitative methods may provide greater statistical power for detecting associations between risk factors and disease.

The statistic commonly used to quantify the degree of association between two continuous traits is called the **correlation coefficient** (γ). Fig. 5-2 illustrates both a contingency table and a correlation coefficient as methods of analysis applied to simulated data of blood pressure and ideal weight. As Fig. 5-2 shows, each point in the plotted data indicates the blood pressure level and percentage of ideal weight of a single individual. Summarizing the data for many individuals shows graphically a general, but not perfect, correlation between blood pressure values and weight levels. If the correlation between two characteristics were perfect, then all plotted points would fall along a single line, and the cor-

relation coefficient would be 1.00 (this is a positive number for direct relationships and negative for inverse relationships). If there were no correlation, there would be a correlation coefficient of 0.00, and plotted points would show a randomly scattered distribution. The square of the correlation coefficient is also a useful statistic because it indicates the percentage of variation of the dependent variable (in this case diastolic blood pressure) that is explained by the independent test variable (here the percentage of ideal weight).

The same set of data could be analyzed by means of a contingency table by setting a defined point to separate quantitative values for individuals considered obese or nonobese and hypertensive or normotensive. As shown in Fig. 5-2, a contingency table would thus produce a relative risk and a population-attributable risk.

Some statistics can be calculated only when the data are available from the entire general population. For example, disease rates in the exposed and unexposed populations are required for calculations of relative risk and population-attributable risk. To obtain accurate disease rates, surveillance or screening data must be collected from an entire population of mostly healthy people. Large community examination projects such as the Framingham Study (Gordon & Kannel, 1971) or tumor surveillance efforts such as the Third National Cancer Survey (Williams, Stegens et al., 1977) are examples of such extensive but informative studies. In large-scale studies a small percentage of subjects are generally found to have the disease of interest.

Initial studies of diseases and risk factors are usually carried out in more cost-efficient, case-control settings. Considerable cost savings result from examining a collection of disease cases and a matched number of healthy controls to see whether the exposure to suspected causal risk factors is more common among disease cases. Although epidemiologists cannot calculate relative risk, studies have shown that for case-control studies, the **relative odds** (or cross-products ratio determined from the data in the contingency table and illustrated in Fig. 5-2) are a reasonable approximation of the relative risk that would be obtained if cross-sectional or population data were available (MacMahon & Pugh, 1970).

For rare diseases and uncommon environmental exposures, the relative odds will be almost identical to the value of the relative risk. When either the disease or the exposure variable becomes common, the relative odds will be inflated, as compared to the relative risk (as it is in the simulated example of two relatively common disorders in Fig. 5-2).

ENVIRONMENTAL RISK FACTORS
Biologic and Immunologic Exposures

Several major types of environmental risk factors known to affect disease occurrence are categorized in Table 5-1. Some of these are environmental pathogens that cause such infectious diseases as pneumonia, tuberculosis, smallpox, poliomyelitis, and malaria. Immunologic reactions triggered by microbes and other environmental stimuli also play a prominent role in causing such diseases as asthma, rheumatic heart disease, and probably also type I diabetes and multiple sclerosis. (Immune mechanisms are discussed in Chapter 6.)

Life-Style

Personal habits and life-style factors have been found to be associated with some of the most common chronic diseases, including cancer and atherosclerosis. The frequency of this kind of environmental exposure in the general population is often the single most important factor in determining changing disease rates over time. For example, a dramatic increase in the frequency of cig-

arette smoking from the beginning of the century until the end of World War II was associated with parallel increases in lung cancer and coronary heart disease. Several decades after it became common for men to smoke, greater numbers of women began to increase their cigarette consumption, and similar increases in disease rates were ultimately seen in women. The effects of exposure to smoke can reflect varying degrees of exposure (e.g., packs of cigarettes smoked) or different kinds of environmental exposure, some of which are more potent than others. (For example, cigarette smoking is usually more hazardous than industrial smog.)

Physical and Chemical Substances

Chemical substances introduced into the environment have been associated with diseases ranging from liver damage to rare cancers and cardiac dysrhythmias. Among these exposures are medications, such as the chemotherapeutic agents used to treat cancer. These agents often produce beneficial effects, but they sometimes cause adverse effects greater than the ailments they were designed to eliminate (cancer treatment is discussed in Chapter 11). Toxins, pollutants, solvents, fumes, and contaminants in food, air, and water are other examples of disease-causing chemical exposures (see Chapter 2).

Some environmental exposures are identified indirectly. For example, population data show that Mormons develop less lung cancer and myocardial infarction than the general population. The association between disease and this group shows that these individuals share some characteristics, one of which is that they avoid cigarette use. Presumably, this is one of the causal risk factors linked to these diseases (Lyon, Klauber et al., 1977; Lyon, Wetzler et al., 1978).

Different components of the physical environment also promote diseases. Climate, for example, is associated with the occurrence of malaria, other infectious diseases, and multiple sclerosis. Different types of radiation exposure lead to disorders ranging from sunburn and heat exhaustion to radiation-induced skin cancer and leukemia (see Chapters 24 and 41). A nuclear holocaust with associated physical trauma, burns, and radiation sickness is the most serious possible environmental exposure, but ordinary burns and lacerations are other illnesses stemming from the physical environment.

Psychologic and Social Factors

Emotional disorders are often associated with other major diseases, either as a contributing cause or as a result of physical illness. Social and psychologic factors have been difficult to define accurately and are challenging to treat. The ill effects of these factors, however, consume a large portion of medical attention.

Increased total mortality and incidence rates of some

major cardiovascular diseases and/or cancer have been suggested in studies of several social factors, including (1) "type A" hard-driving personality, (2) decreased social supporting networks (friends, relatives, churches), (3) being unmarried (divorced, widowed, or never married), (4) stressful life events (death of a spouse, divorce, bankruptcy), (5) anger, (6) hostility, (7) low self-esteem, and (8) lower socioeconomic status. Investigators suggest a significant role for psychologic stress (see Chapter 9), anxiety, and depression in the development and progression of cancers, hypertension, coronary artery disease, and many other chronic illnesses.

COMBINED EFFECTS AND INTERACTION AMONG RISK FACTORS

Unraveling the pathophysiology of many common diseases requires understanding complex combinations and interactions of variables that may be difficult to define. Some risk factors are known and measurable, but other undefined genetic and environmental risk factors also contribute to the disease. When one or more risk factors interact, the individual effects of risk factors may be greatly magnified in a multiplicative or exponential manner, as illustrated in Fig. 5-3. Some factors alone may present little or no risk for disease, but in the presence of another factor, the risk increases substantially. For example, the combined effects of cigarette smoking and oral contraceptives increase the chance of myocardial infarction by approximately eighteenfold in young women (Jick et al., 1978). Either oral contraceptives or cigarette smoking alone has far less effect on coronary disease than do both factors combined.

One of the major goals of current research is to define the **heterogeneity,** or variety of causal factors, of common chronic diseases. When a disease is initially studied in a general population, several different types

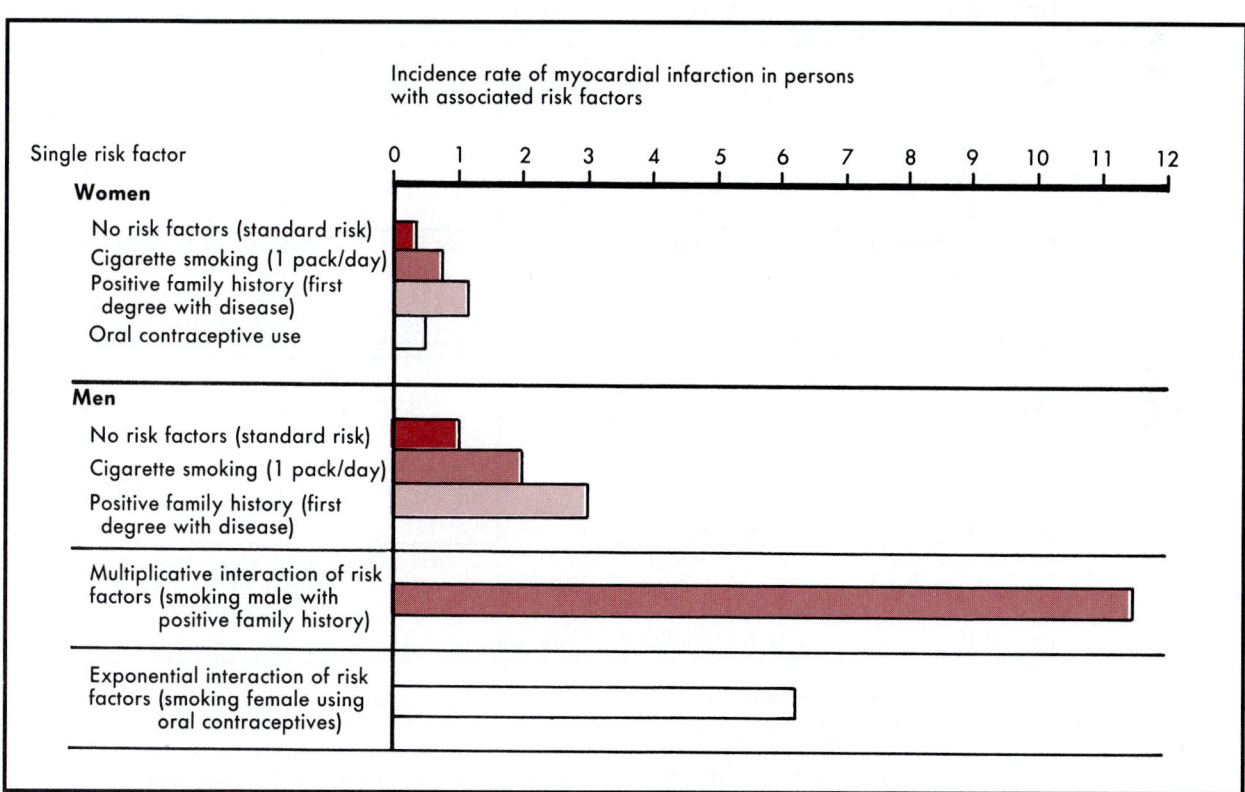

FIG. 5-3 Magnified risks from interactions among risk factors. The rate of myocardial infarction is indicated for 35- to 45-year-old adults in nine different risk settings. Beginning with males and females with standard myocardial infarction (MI) risk, the risk of MI is increased 2 to 3 times each by male gender, smoking, and a positive family history as isolated risk factors. A multiplicative interaction of smoking with a positive family history magnifies the risk well beyond the additive effects of each risk factor alone. Oral contraceptive pill users have little or no increased risk of MI unless they smoke cigarettes too. Their risk is then increased exponentially from that for other women. These data suggest a dramatic reduction in MI risk for high-risk persons who avoid smoking. The data presented are approximations extrapolated from several different reports of actual data (Feinleib & Williams, 1976; Hopkins, Williams, & Hunt, 1984; Jink, 1976).

of the disease with different causes may be combined in a single population of subjects. Careful definition of environmental risk factors, biochemical and genetic markers, and disease characteristics can often lead to the separation of cases into distinctive categories or syndromes with differing pathophysiologic mechanisms. This separation, in turn, suggests differing strategies for treatment and prevention. For example, chronic diseases with defined or suspected multiple causes include coronary atherosclerosis, diabetes, essential hypertension, and cancers of the breast and colon. All involve several environmental risk factors and also show familial predispositions in a substantial proportion of cases.

Familial Disease Tendency

Initial assessments of aggregation of disease in families can be made by collecting observations about sets of relatives such as siblings, parents with offspring, spouse

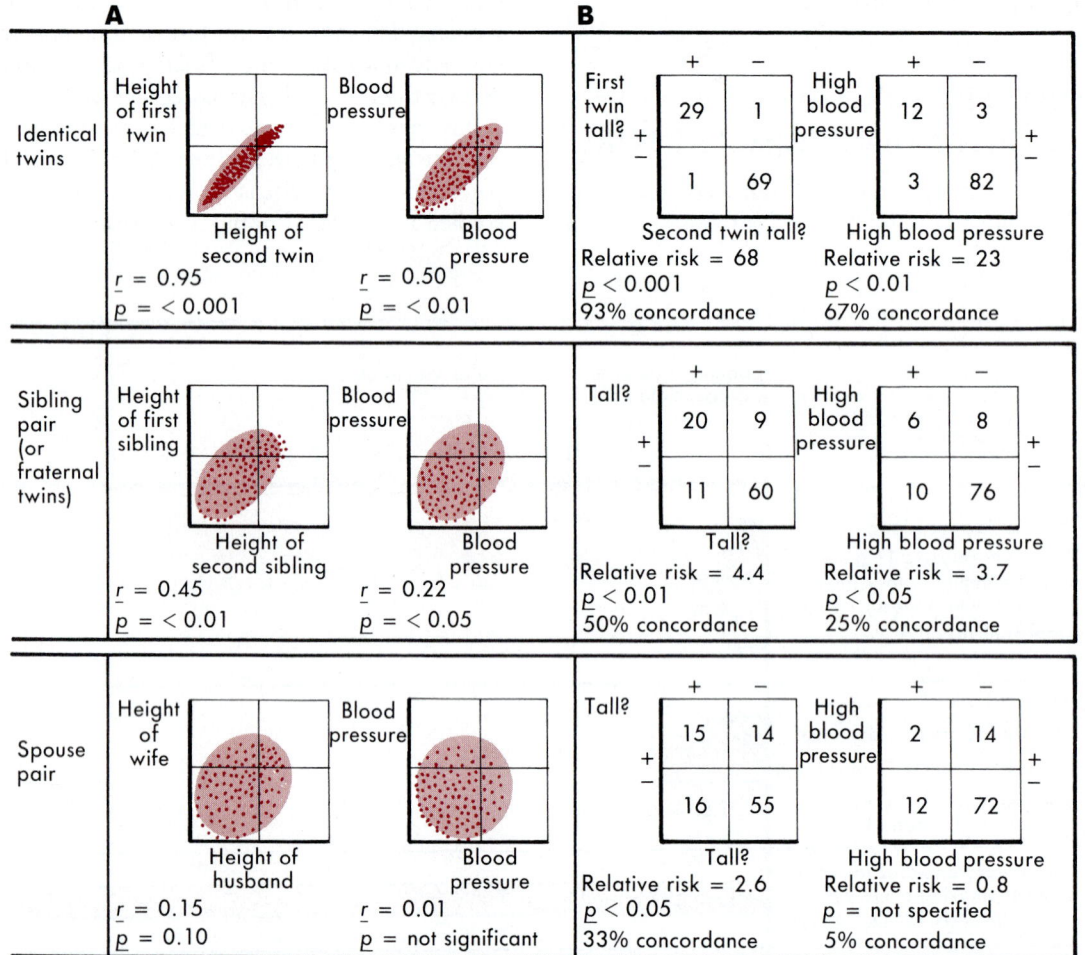

r = Correlation of coefficient; p = probability of occurrence (0.05 or less is considered significant);
Concordance rate = percentage of pairs that share a given trait.

Thirty percent of the general population is defined as tall; 15% of the general population has high blood pressure.

FIG. 5-4 Analysis of familial aggregation of traits and diseases with correlation coefficients and contingency tables. A, Horizontal and vertical lines within the correlation plots separate the individual points into four groups corresponding to the number of individuals listed in the four cells of the contingency table to test for familial aggregation or correlation of specific traits or diseases. Each point in the correlation plot represents a pair of relatives. For example, in the top left-hand plot, one point represents the height of the first twin along the vertical axis and the height of the second twin along the horizontal axis. The horizontal and vertical lines arbitrarily divide these twin pairs into individuals who would be considered tall or not tall. **B,** The corresponding contingency table indicates that 29 of these twin pairs were both considered to be tall and 69 were both considered to be not tall, whereas in 2 pairs of twins one individual was considered to be tall and the other considered to be not tall.

CLINICAL COMMENTARY   HYPERCHOLESTEROLEMIA AND CORONARY HEART DISEASE

The gene for hypercholesterolemia is totally penetrant in the last two generations, as illustrated in the pedigree. Four individuals born before 1880 found to be definitely heterozygous for this problem survived, respectively, to ages 62, 68, 71, and 81, unlike their grandsons and great-grandsons, who died in their thirties, forties, and fifties because of the same autosomal dominant gene.

The pedigree shows 361 persons in six generations of a pedigree. Dark symbols indicate 40 individuals who carried a gene for early coronary death mediated by very high serum cholesterol levels. Half of the children of affected adults have very high cholesterol levels, and none of them had been screened before their involvement in this study. The founder survived to age 81, but great-grandsons from two different wives show coronary disease usually with onset by age 45. Two of the sons from his first wife and another son from his second wife also had normal life expectancies. Pedigree analysis confirms that they carried this dominant gene that led to early coronary death in their grandsons (Williams, Hasstedt et al., 1986). This gene has been linked in a DNA marker for low density lipoprotein (LDL) receptors on chromosome 19 (Leppert et al., 1986).

Furthermore, variable expression of this gene can be observed in a woman and her two sons in the third and fourth generations of the pedigree. All three were known to have very high serum cholesterol values consistent with heterozygous familial hypercholesterolemia. One of the men was a smoker and died of coronary disease at age 32; his nonsmoking brother died of coronary disease at age 45. This information suggests approximately 13 years' difference in longevity potentially attributable to smoking in these high-risk men. This factor is in contrast to approximately 2 years' difference in the longevity of smokers and nonsmokers in the general population and approximately 7 years' difference in longevity between smokers and nonsmokers who die of coronary disease. The mother of these two men was examined at age 67, was found to have a cholesterol level of 365, and yet still was free of any manifestations of coronary disease by history, physical examination, and electrocardiogram.

A six-generation pedigree showing patterns of coronary death and high levels of cholesterol.

pairs, and twin sets. Statistical tests of those observations determine whether pairs of relatives both have a specific disease (or similar test results for continuous traits) more often than two randomly selected individuals from the general population (Hunt, Hasstedt, & Williams, 1986).

Analyses often involve the simple comparison of the outcome of pairs of individuals with a defined relationship. The same statistical methods—correlation coefficients and contingency tables—are used to assess the familial aggregation of the disease, as illustrated in Fig. 5-4. In the first column, height is shown to correlate very highly between identical twin pairs and quite strongly among sibling pairs, suggesting a strong genetic determination. Some detectable correlation at a lower level among spouse pairs might suggest selective mating (i.e., persons tend to marry individuals of similar height).

In the correlation plots in Fig. 5-4, even the two twins who are considered tall and not tall are very close to the boundaries used to separate tall and not tall, indicating a very high degree of correlation and concordance for this trait. In contrast, the lack of similarity of blood pressure in spouse pairs is indicated by plotted points that seem to have a randomly scattered distribution. Significant familial correlations are indicated for blood pressure values in pairs of twins and siblings.

If a point of separation is defined for these continuous traits, the data can be analyzed by using contingency tables. Here relative risks and associated levels of statistical significance are objective measures of familial aggregation of diseases. The concordance rate is a useful descriptive statistic reflecting the degree of familial disease aggregation. It defines the percentage of pairs in which both individuals are affected as a proportion of all pairs in which at least one person is affected.

Familial correlations and contingency table analyses can identify familial aggregation of risk factors, which may be either genetic or shared environmental factors. Contrasting identical and nonidentical twin pairs and related individuals and nonrelated persons living together (such as spouses or adopted children) provide initial impressions of whether or not genetic or environmental factors are responsible for familial disease aggregation.

Definitive understanding of genetic and environmental familial disease aggregations requires sophisticated analyses of many nuclear families or large pedigrees to define gene frequencies, modes of genetic transmission, effects of shared environment, and the factors affecting the penetrance of genetic predispositions. Definitive results often require large and expensive studies with large sample sizes, sophisticated data collection (including DNA markers), and complex mathematical analysis. Unfortunately, few such analyses are currently available for common chronic diseases. Many will likely become available in the future.

❏ AGING

Age is a risk factor for many diseases and may be compared to a clock ticking relentlessly until the alarm goes off and the disease is expressed (Table 5-6). Heart attacks, strokes, cancers, high blood pressure, diabetes, obesity, arthritis, and emotional illness are all more

TABLE 5-6

Age-related Disorders

Age	Disorders correlated with age range
Birth-14 years	Congenital disorders Allergy Infection Cancer (leukemia, Wilms tumor, medulloblastoma, retinoblastoma) Accidents Diabetes (early onset)
15-30 years	Allergy (asthma) Endocrine Accidents (suicide) Venereal disease
30-40 years	Ulcer Hypertension Breast cancer Homicide Suicide Complications of pregnancy Alcoholism
40-60 years	Heart disease (hypertension, rheumatic, infarction) Kidney disease (glomerular nephritis) Liver disease (cirrhosis) Cancer (lung, colon, breast, ovary)
60-80 years	Cardiovascular Cancer (lung, colon, prostate)
80-100 years	Cancer (leukemia, lymphoma, prostate) Dementia (Alzheimer, Parkinson) Osteoporosis Infection Cardiovascular Accidents (fracture)

Modified from King, D.W., Fenoglio, C.M., & Lefkowitch, J.H. (1983). *General pathology: Principles and dynamics.* Philadelphia: Lea & Febiger.

common with increasing age. Because age is accurately determined and is a strong predictor of disease risk, epidemiologists usually test and adjust for the effects of age in their search for the causes of diseases.

Age is not, however, only a confounder and an unmodifiable risk factor. In many cases age probably represents the cumulative effects of environmental exposures and inherited biochemical processes. Understanding both genetic and environmental causes of disease may eventually lead to "stopping the clock" for some diseases or at least "slowing down the ticking" and delaying the age of disease expression. (Theories of aging are discussed in Chapter 2.)

The general degeneration that accompanies aging can also result from deterioration of genetic templates (i.e., malfunction in RNA repair) and loss of immunologic defenses (i.e., against cancer or infection). Tissue integrity is also compromised through changes in elastin, bone matrix, or collagen or through loss of neurons. (The systemic effects of aging are discussed in appropriate units in Part Two.)

FAMILIAL DISEASES AND ASSOCIATED RISK FACTORS

"You can't change your genes, so inherited diseases cannot be prevented, right?" Wrong! Unfortunately, some clinicians and many persons in high-risk families have this misconception and take no steps to avoid the serious consequences of disorders such as early coronary heart disease or breast and colon cancer. A **familial tendency,** the increased possibility for genetically related family members to develop a disease, can combine with environmental risk factors to cause many diseases. An understanding of the genetic and environmental components in the pathophysiologic chain of events leading to a particular disease therefore can provide a solid rationale for more effective prevention, earlier detection, and more specific and more effective treatment of these diseases (Williams, 1984c; Williams, 1988).

Table 5-7 lists some of the known familial diseases and some suggested environmental factors that might play important roles in causing and eventually preventing disease. Table 5-8 lists some chronic diseases caused by single-gene defects mapped to specific chromosomal locations using genetic linkage or mutation detection. Research in this area is progressing so rapidly that these data cannot be comprehensive. What is significant is the variety of diseases that are apparently familial and the wide variety of potential interacting environmental factors. The promise of more definitive data suggests tremendous opportunities for future detection and prevention of familial disorders.

Recurrence risks for some multifactorial **congenital defects** (birth defects) are estimates based on empiric ob-

servations of the frequency of multiple cases seen in families (Emery & Rimoin, 1983). Some genetic disorders follow well-defined genetic patterns of expression, but even in those disorders that are present at birth, a wide range of expression is evident in relatives sharing the same gene. For example, a proband (the subject or individual being studied) having a neural tube defect expressed as marked deformities of the spinal cord (i.e., spina bifida) might have first-degree relatives with minor defects found on spinal x-ray films but causing no symptoms (a disorder termed spina bifida occulta). Congenital heart defects can be severe or minor in members of the same family. Furthermore, not all congenital disorders are genetically transmitted. Environmental factors such as drugs, radiation, alcohol, and cigarette smoke probably take their toll on the fetus early in pregnancy, perhaps with greater effect among genetically susceptible fetuses.

Factors used in estimating risks for these multifactorial traits include presence of the disease in parents, siblings, or other relatives; severity of the disorder in those already affected; sex-specific predominance for some disorders (e.g., pyloric stenosis occurs five times more often in males than in females); and any environmental factors known. Consanguinity of parents has little effect on the risk of most of these multifactorial disorders. Genetic evaluation and counseling for these birth defects (see Chapter 4) are often quite different from counseling provided for the common chronic diseases that show a familial predisposition.

Immunologic Disorders

Several immunologic diseases seem to have strong familial tendencies (Emery & Rimoin, 1983; Goodman, 1970; Stobo, 1982). Recent developments in identifying cellular markers, such as antigens, have considerably aided the investigation of these disorders (see Chapter 6). These include rheumatoid arthritis, systemic lupus erythematosus, idiopathic Addison disease, thyroid disorders (e.g., autoimmune thyroiditis and Graves disease), and possibly idiopathic thrombocytopenic purpura (ITP). For example, researchers propose that in the case of rheumatoid arthritis, genetically susceptible individuals become sensitive to collagen (Stobo, 1982).

Allergies and asthma also tend to run very strongly in some families (Emery & Rimoin, 1983; Goodman, 1970), and, again, interaction with environmental factors is evident. Early exposure to foods in infants and exposure to animal fur, dust, and other pollutants in young children prone to asthma are thought to aid in the progression of allergic diseases. Preventive measures include identifying allergy-prone children and having them avoid exposure to environmental allergens.

Many infectious diseases, such as rheumatic fever, may also involve immunologic susceptibility to severe effects. Furthermore, certain rare and well-defined im-

TABLE 5-7

Chronic Diseases Thought to Have Genetic Predisposition

Disease	Associated pathophysiology or hypothesis	Genetic factors	Environmental factors
Coronary heart disease (especially early disease) (several different syndromes)	Familial hypercholesterol-emia	Dominant	Dietary fat, saturated fat, polyunsaturated fat, total fat intake
	LDL receptor defects	Dominant	
	Other high cholesterol?	Unknown	Exercise, alcohol, diet
	Low HDL	Dominant	Smoking
	Endothelial factors?	Unknown	
	Platelet factors?	Unknown	
	Apolipoproteins, etc.?	(Apo B dominant?)	
		(Apo A-I recessive)	
		(Lipoprotein [a] codominant)	
	Diabetes	Unknown	
	Hypertension (especially early onset)	Unknown	
		Unknown	
	Multiplicative interactions of history and risk factors		
Stroke	Hypertension and diabetes	Unknown	
Hypertension	Heterogenous?	Polygenic?	Salt, stress, obesity
	Age at onset?	Major gene?	Polyunsaturated fat, calcium, exercise
	Severity? Etiology?	Quite penetrant?	
Insulin-dependent diabetes	Islet cell destruction	Recessive?	Viral infection
	Immunologic cause	<50% penetrant	Seasonal variation
		HLA linkage and association with chromosome 6	Complications a function of blood sugar control for years
Non-insulin-dependent diabetes	Insulin resistance or decreased production	80%-100% penetrant	Obesity
		Rare dominant form mapped to chromosome 7p	Dietary sugar and fiber
			Exercise protective
			Complications a function of blood sugar control and function
Breast cancer	Possibly estrogen and progesterone related	Linkage with chromosome 17	Age at first birth
			Obesity?
	Certain benign tumor precursors	50%-90% penetrant in some families	Dietary fat?
			Alcohol?
			Female hormones
Colon cancer	Several different types of syndromes	Gene for familial polyposis mapped to chromosomes	Fiber intake
	Often benign polyps are precursors		Dietary fat? (converted by bacteria to carcinogens)
Lung cancer	Chemical carcinogens from environment encounter enzymatically susceptible subjects	Known familial aggregation ± smoking	Cigarette smoke
			Environmental pollutants
			Radiation exposure
Rheumatic heart disease	Immunologic cross-reactivity to bacteria and heart valves	Familial aggregation	Group A β-strep bacterial infection
			Penicillin prevents
Asthma and other allergies	Immunologically reactive	Familial aggregation	Many possible allergens—fur, dust, pollen, mold, etc.
			Avoidance to prevent

TABLE 5-7

Chronic Diseases Thought to Have Genetic Predisposition—cont'd

Disease	Associated pathophysiology or hypothesis	Genetic factors	Environmental factors
Autoimmune disorders: rheumatic arthritis, Hashimoto thyroiditis and Graves disease, Addison disease, idiopathic thrombocytopenic purpura (ITP), IDDM, systemic lupus erythematosus	Autoantibodies to thyroid, adrenal, synovium, platelets	HLA linked on chromosome 6	Viral infections trigger immune responses
Psychiatric disorders: manic-depressive, depression, schizophrenia	Neurochemical disorders in brain tissue	Strongly familial and likely genetic in twin, adoption, and family studies	Uncertain influence Dramatic success with drug treatment for first two
Kidney stones	Mineral—acid-base imbalance	Very familial	Milk? Soda pop? Other fluids?
Gallstones	Fat, cholesterol, bilirubin balance	Quite familial	Dietary fat Obesity?
Obesity (probably very heterogenous)	Less energy wasted? Decreased thermogenesis in brown fat? Other basic energy differences like ATPase pumps? "Thrifty gene?"	Major genes in animals Clusters in families Assortative mating MZ* twins > DZ† twins Racial group (American Indians and Polynesians)	Dietary fat, sugar, and total calories Stress, etc., affecting appetite Exercise level Cultural perceptions, attractive to be fat or thin
Gout	Several different enzyme defects found	Several autosomal major genes	Dietary intake of meat, etc.
Multiple sclerosis	Autoimmune demyelination of nerve fibers	HLA association Poorly penetrant MZ twins often discordant	Slow virus? Climate dependent
Peptic ulcer disease	Excess acid production and/or decreased mucosal resistance	Biochemical markers of affected Variable penetrance	Stress Diet Dramatic drug Rx
Hemolytic anemia	G6PD deficiency Red cell hemolysis precipitated by exposure to drugs or infections	X-linked recessive	Aspirin Antibiotics Infections
Lactose intolerance	Deficiency of lactase enzyme in intestinal mucosa	Very common in blacks	Milk products
Alcoholism	Possible neurochemical origin? Associated with other psychiatric disorders	Quite familial (due to genes and/or family environment?)	Ethyl alcohol intake Social factors
Hemochromatosis	Increased iron absorption	Linked to HLA on chromosome 6 Recessive Quite penetrant	Treat with phlebotomy and prevent organ damage from iron loading

*Monozygotic.
†Dizygotic.

TABLE 5-8

Treatable Chronic Diseases from Single Gene Loci

Treatable disorder	Consequences without treatment	Transmission	Gene location
LDL receptor defect	Early coronary death	Dominant	19p
Defective apolipoprotein B	Early coronary death	Dominant	2p
Type III hyperlipidemia	Early coronary death	Recessive	19g
High lipoprotein [a]	Early coronary death	Dominant	6g
Heterozygous LDL deficiency	↑ Triglyceride, ↓ HDL	Dominant	8p
Hypertrophic cardiomyopathy	Heart failure and death	Dominant	14g
Prolonged QT syndrome	Sudden cardiac death	Dominant	11p
Hemochromatosis	Heart and liver failure	Recessive	6p
Myotonic dystrophy	Heart and muscle dysfunction	Dominant	19g
Abdominal aortic aneurysm	Ruptured aneurysm	Dominant	2g
Marfan syndrome	Ruptured aneurysm	Dominant	15g
Glucocorticoid remediable aldosteronism	Early hypertension and stroke	Dominant	8g
Cystic fibrosis	Chronic lung infection and death	Recessive	7g
Alpha-antitrypsin deficiency	Chronic lung disease	Dominant	14g
Antithrombin 3 deficiency	Venous and arterial thrombosis	Dominant	1g
Protein C deficiency	General thrombosis	Dominant	2g
Thalassemia	Severe anemia	Dominant	16p
Sickle cell anemia	Severe anemia	Dominant	11p
Spherocytosis	Severe anemia	Dominant	8p
G6PD deficiency	Hemolysis after certain medications	X-recessive	Xg
Hemophilia A and B	Hemorrhage with minor trauma	X-recessive	Xg
Von Willebrand disease	Fragile capillaries and hemorrhage	Dominant	12p

From Cooper & Schmidtke, 1992; Lifton et al., 1992; Keating et al., 1991.

munodeficiency syndromes are inherited, and more subtle susceptibilities to viral and bacterial diseases may also run in families, accounting for more common and less severe infectious problems. General susceptibility to cancer may, in some cases, be associated with an inherited decrease in immunologic defenses.

Cancer

Some cancers tend to be familial. Breast, colon, lung, and prostate are the most common sites of cancers with familial aggregation. Ovarian, uterine, and colon cancer in combination also occur in some families. If certain forms of cancer are identified in a family, increased surveillance and special screening procedures can be instituted to help detect cancers at an early and curable stage. (Theories of cancer development are discussed in Chapter 11.)

Perhaps the most preventable familial cancer is lung cancer. As Fig. 5-5 shows, the incidence of lung cancer is strikingly elevated among individuals who have positive family histories and are also cigarette smokers (Tokuhata, 1965). Because of their elevated risk of lung cancer, members of such families should be strongly encouraged to avoid smoking.

Breast Cancer

Breast cancer ranks along with lung cancer as one of the most common cancers in women. Breast cancer aggregates strongly in families. If a woman has one affected first-degree relative (e.g., sister, daughter, or mother), her risk of developing breast cancer doubles. This risk increases if the age of onset of the affected relative is early and if the cancer occurs in both breasts.

Known risk factors for breast cancer include late age at first delivery, early menarche, late menopause, obesity, atypia, hyperplasia, and positive family history of breast cancer. Other possible risk factors include alcohol intake, estrogen level, and estrogen replacement medications.

Identified risk factors suggest that gene-environment interactions are sometimes a cause of breast cancer. For example, a late age of first pregnancy is one of the greatest risk factors for breast cancer. As Fig. 5-6 shows, this factor enhances the risk for women already at risk, as indicated by pedigrees comparing them to women without positive family histories of breast cancer (Hunt, 1980). Other studies have suggested that the use of oral contraceptives ordinarily does not increase the risk for breast cancer in the general population but might in-

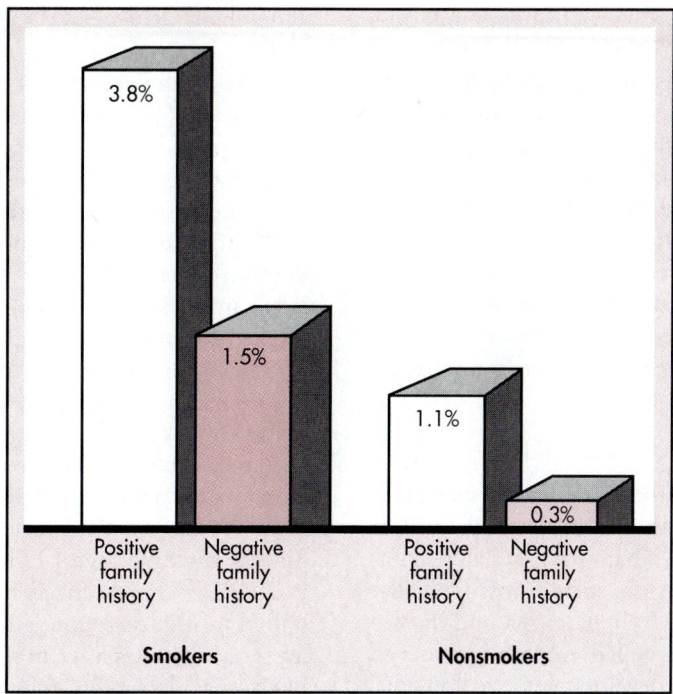

FIG. 5-5 **Smokers, nonsmokers, and rates of lung cancer.** Actual data from a case control study show that the highest rate of lung cancer occurs in smokers with familial predisposition. A familial predisposition was defined as one parent or sibling with lung cancer.

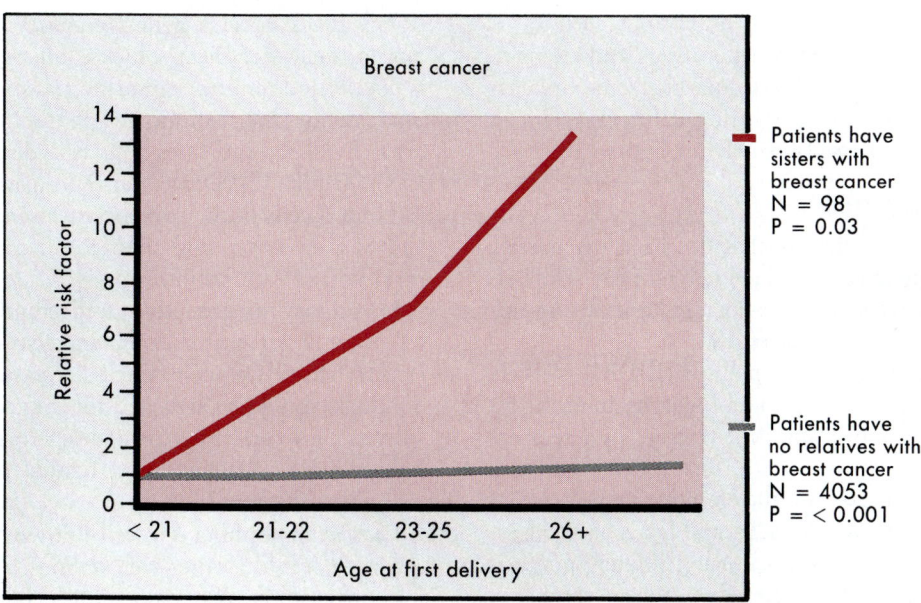

FIG. 5-6 **Relative risks of breast cancer.** Relative risk of breast cancer according to age of first delivery for women who have no relatives with breast cancer and for women who have a sister with breast cancer.

crease the risk among women with positive family histories of the disease (Brinton et al., 1979).

Many well-developed programs are available to help detect breast cancer at a curable stage. Breast self-examination is a procedure that should be taught to all women. Clinical screening and mammography should also be applied conscientiously for all women, especially those at high risk. Identification of the breast cancer susceptibility gene will offer potential of early diagnosis for women in affected families. When the gene is cloned, it should yield valuable evidence on the cause of breast cancer (Hall et al., 1992). (Breast cancer is discussed further in Chapter 20.)

Colorectal Cancer

Colorectal cancer is one of the most common cancers in both men and women and shows a strong familial tendency in some pedigrees. Familial tendency combined with environmental factors such as low-fiber diet and high fat intake may lead to hyperplasia and the development of benign polyps, which eventually undergo malignant degeneration and development of colon cancer. The risk of colorectal cancer in individuals with one affected first-degree relative is 2 to 3 times higher than that of the gneral population.

A small proportion of colorectal cancers are inherited in an autosomal dominant fashion. Familial polyposis coli occurs in approximately 1 in 8000 Americans. The gene responsible for familial polyposis coli was mapped to chromosome 5 several years ago, and recently, the gene was cloned (Groden et al., 1991; Kinzler et al., 1991). In addition to the study of familial polyposis coli, investigators are studying the role of genes on common colon cancer (Solomon, 1990; Stanbridge, 1990). A complex interaction of genetic alterations and environmental factors, such as high-fat, low-fiber diet, appears to play an etiologic role in causing colorectal cancer. (Colon cancer is discussed further in Chapter 36.)

Endocrine Disorders

Diabetes mellitus is a disease that has been extensively studied by both geneticists and epidemiologists. The heterogeneity of diabetes and its associated underlying disorders are described in Chapter 18.

Insulin-dependent diabetes mellitus (IDDM) is likely to occur as a result of an immunologic mechanism. Inherited factors probably "cock the trigger," whereas environmental factors (e.g., a viral insult) seem to "pull the trigger" and initiate an autoimmune response that destroys the pancreatic islet cells and leads to total insulin deficiency. Recent studies using linkage analysis have revealed two susceptible loci. One "candidate gene" is thought to be on chromosome 17 and the other on chromosome 1 or 4 (Todd, Aitman, & Cornall, 1991). Twin studies show that identical twins of IDDM

individuals have risks ranging from 30% to 50%. IDDM, however, is not 100% concordant among identical twins, indicating that genetic factors are not solely responsible for the disorder.

For individuals with a positive family history of diabetes mellitus, the best response at present is reassurance and support. If future advances can help not only to identify individuals who carry the trait but also to develop schemes for preventing the immunologic reaction, immunizations or other preventive techniques might be developed to prevent this disorder altogether.

Non-insulin-dependent diabetes mellitus (NIDDM) accounts for about 75% of all diabetes cases in the United States. Studies of identical twins show high concordance rates of 90% or more. NIDDM typically occurs among people over age 40, although a rare autosomal dominant form recently mapped to chromosone 7p has an early age of onset (Froguel et al., 1992). NIDDM is characterized by insulin resistance and impaired insulin secretion. Although the insulin and insulin receptor genes have both been cloned, it appears unlikely that defects in either gene are responsible for a large portion of NIDDM. The two most significant risk factors for NIDDM are positive family history and obesity (the latter contributes to insulin resistance).

Hematologic Disorders

Several hematologic disorders are genetically determined and interact with environmental factors (McKusick, 1992). Probably one of the best examples is drug-induced hemolytic anemia associated with glucose-6-phosphate dehydrogenase (G6PD) deficiency. This disorder is found chiefly, but not entirely, among members of the black race; a gene frequency of 11% is found among male American blacks. This enzyme deficiency is also found among Sephardic Jews and other individuals tracing their ethnic origin to the Mediterranean area. Evidence indicates that this disorder is inherited as an X-linked recessive trait and leads to hemolysis of red blood cells in the presence of uremia, diabetic ketoacidosis, infection, and a variety of drugs (including aspirin and certain antibiotics).

Hereditary spherocytosis and elliptocytosis are both uncommon autosomal dominant disorders that can also lead to hemolytic anemia. Close relatives of affected individuals should be screened for these disorders because splenectomy can be performed to prevent further hemolytic anemia. (Anemias and related disorders are discussed in Chapter 23.)

Classic hemophilia is a well-known X-linked recessive disorder, but like other well-defined bleeding disorders, it is uncommon. A person with bleeding problems and a positive family history of bleeding disorders should receive screening tests available to distinguish among different types of genetic bleeding disorders. Although classic hemophilia is relatively easy to recognize clinically because of the episodes of bleeding into the joints, subtle forms of the disease may be less easy to recognize. For example, women who are heterozygous carriers may have variable levels of clotting factors because of the phenomenon of X inactivation (see Chapter 4).

Hematochromatosis is a defect that leads to iron collection in tissues and has been identified as a single-gene defect carried on chromosome 6 (linked to HLA haplotypes [Edwards et al., 1977]). (HLA linkage is discussed in Chapter 6.) Hematochromatosis is apparently more common than previously thought. If untreated, it causes liver disease, heart disease, and diabetes.

Cardiovascular Disorders

Some forms of cardiovascular disease also show strong familial tendencies (Goodman, 1970). Rheumatic valvular heart disease seems to run strongly in some families. Although this tendency, in part, might result from transmission of the streptococcal organism among family members, research suggests that some individuals have an immunologic predisposition to the rheumatic complications of streptococcal infections.

Recently, investigators mapped the gene for the autosomal dominant disorder *long QT syndrome* on chromosome 11p (diagnosed by an abnormal electrocardiogram) (Keating et al., 1991). This disorder is associated with severe ventricular fibrillations and sudden death. Because prolonged QT segment is difficult to diagnose accurately, the reported close linkage will allow more accurate diagnoses of affected family members. Several myocardiopathies, including obstructive cardiomyopathy (idiopathic hypertrophic subaortic stenosis), also appear to be caused by a single gene in some pedigrees.

Probably one of the most common heart abnormalities is mitral valve prolapse. The exact frequency of occurrence and associated functional problems remain to be defined, but at least some individuals with the disease have symptomatic or even life-threatening arrhythmias. Mitral valve prolapse also tends to run in some families and may be associated with familial connective tissue disorders. Several forms of congenital heart disease, including atrial and ventricular septal defects, seem to be genetically transmitted, at least in some cases.

As a clearer understanding of the exact causal mechanisms for these diseases emerges, better detection and more effective screening procedures will help to prevent some of the associated problems. For example, in cases of rheumatic fever, prophylactic penicillin therapy is effective and should be considered for anyone with frequent streptococcal infections and a family history of rheumatic complications. (Cardiovascular diseases are discussed further in Chapter 27.)

Coronary Heart Disease

Early **coronary heart disease** (CHD) is one of the most common serious chronic diseases with a strong familial tendency. Fig. 5-7 summarizes the major risk factors. Several risk factors are usually associated with early coronary heart disease. Numerous studies have examined the role of family history in CHD. Findings from these studies show that an individual with a positive family history is 2 to 7 times more likely to suffer from heart disease than is an individual with no family history. The risk for CHD increase if (1) there are more affected relatives; (2) the affected relative is female (less commonly affected sex) rather than male; and (3) age of onset in the affected individual is early (before age 55).

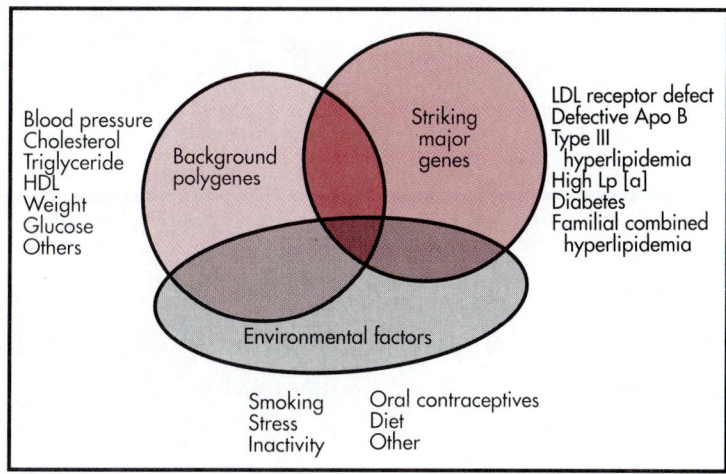

FIG. 5-7 Schematic for model of gene-environment interaction. Interacting effects of major genes, background polygenes, and environmental factors produce the unique coronary risk in given individuals.

Studies also suggest that several different genetic factors lead to early coronary diseases including familial hypercholesterolemia (McKusick, 1992), early severe hypertension (Hilbert et al., 1991), low levels of high-density lipoprotein cholesterol (HDL-cholesterol) (Hasstedt, Ash, & Williams, 1986), low serum apolipoprotein A-I (a protein that attaches to LDL-cholesterol) (Moll et al., 1986), high apolipoprotein B (attaches to LDL-cholesterol) (Hasstedt, Wu, & Williams, 1987), and congenital variations in coronary arteries (Neufeld & Goldbourt, 1983). Platelet factors and susceptibility to the adverse effects of cigarette smoking may also be inherited mechanisms leading to early familial coronary heart disease.

Recent evidence indicates a substantial interaction of genetic predisposition to early coronary disease with environmental risk factors, as illustrated in Fig. 5-7 (Williams, 1984a).

One of the most striking and penetrant examples of familial patterns of coronary disease occurs in males who are heterozygous for familial hypercholesterolemia. Data from one study have shown a distinctive time trend (mid-1800s to present) toward decreasing age at coronary death for affected males, as summarized in Fig. 5-8 (Williams, 1984a). This change in the degree of pene-

trance suggests that environmental factors also affect expression of the trait. Therefore, changes in environmental factors have increased the level of penetrance of this particular gene from being essentially unexpressed in the mid-1800s to the occurrence of severe early coronary death in current generations of at least one pedigree.

Population data suggest that many of the risk factors are multiplicative. Therefore, in any individual at high risk for coronary disease, careful screening and prompt treatment of all risk factors are important. For example, the magnified effects of smoking may be part of the decreasing age at death evident in an analysis of coronary disease. Additional factors such as dietary intake and exercise level (with its known effects on HDL levels) might also be playing a role. Until menopause, female hormones may help protect women against the effects of hypercholesterolemia.

Current theories of atherogenesis indicate that 10 to 20 years or more of exposure to certain risk factors at high enough levels is required for significant coronary artery disease to develop. This cumulative effect suggests that the most effective preventive measures should be instituted by the late teens or the early adult years of life. Exploratory studies and analyses further indicate

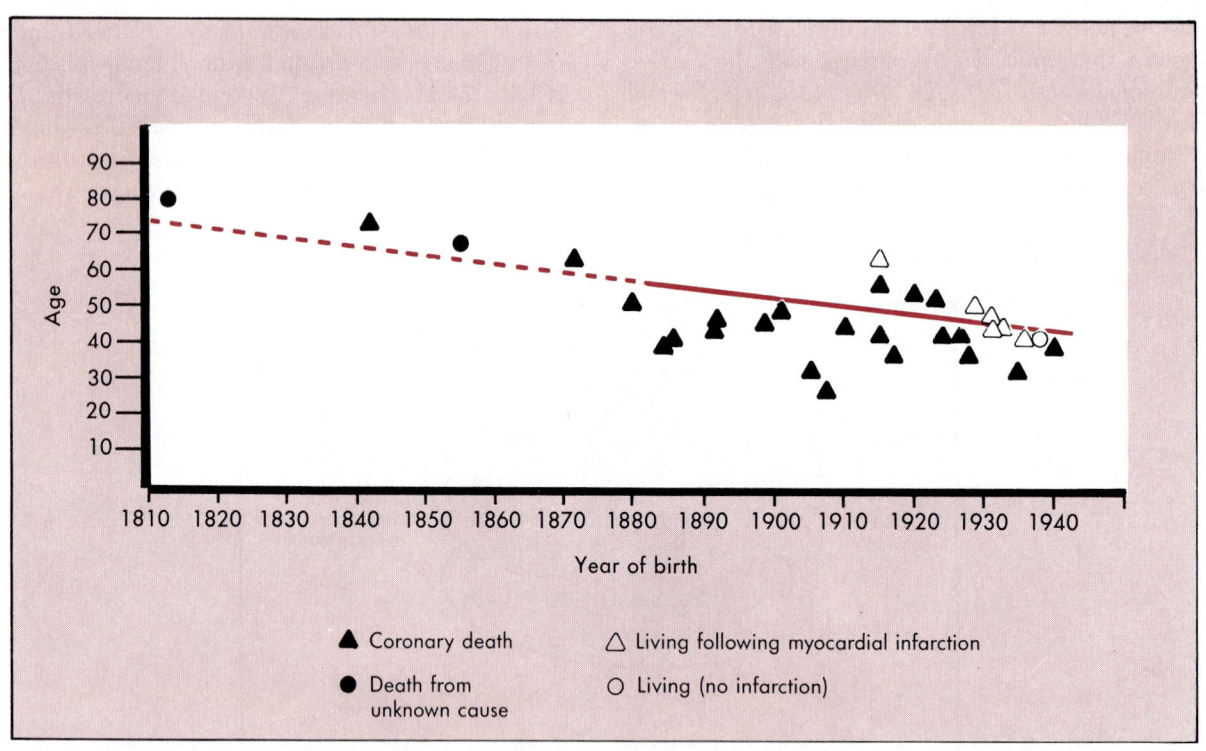

FIG. 5-8 Age and status of men heterozygous for familial hypercholesterolemia. Graph shows generally early onset of coronary death in current generations with considerable variation and normal life span for four males born before 1880. These data suggest that environmental factors changing over time markedly affect the expression of this potentially lethal gene.

that lowering serum cholesterol levels for those under age 35 may prevent up to 40% of cases of coronary artery disease, whereas delaying treatment until after age 55 might prevent only 5% of such cases (Whyte, 1975). Even severe genetic risk, such as heterozygous familial hypercholesterolemia (FH), can be managed with proper therapy. In a 3-year drug treatment study of 72 persons with heterozygous FH, coronary angiograms performed before and after the treatment showed significant regression of coronary atherosclerosis (Kane, Malloy, Ports et al., 1990). (Coronary heart disease is discussed further in Chapter 27.)

Hypertension and Stroke

Hypertension and stroke are both strongly familial cardiovascular diseases. Hypertension appears to be the most prominent risk factor for strokes (Kannel & Gordon, 1974). The continual improvement in detection and treatment of hypertension is probably responsible for the dramatic decline in the mortality rate from strokes over the last three decades in the United States

(Ward, 1990). Diabetes is also a significant risk factor for stroke, with a lesser level of possible contribution from hyperlipidemia and smoking (Kannel & Gordon, 1974). Some reported pedigrees have a striking aggregation of stroke and high blood pressure (Williams et al., 1984; Ward, 1990). As Fig. 5-9 indicates, hypertension, coronary disease, and stroke tend to aggregate in some families. Careful detection and treatment of hypertension, therefore, may prevent both strokes and coronary disease in high-risk families (Hopkins et al., 1984; Joint National Committee, 1984).

"Essential hypertension" is one of the most common forms of familial disease. Studies of twins and families consistently indicate approximately 50% heritability for blood pressure as a continuous trait and show significant coaggregation of hypertension. Essential hypertension demonstrates 85% to 100% concordance in identical twins and approximately 50% concordance in siblings (Feinleib et al., 1975; Hunt, Williams, & Barlow, 1986; Vander Molen et al., 1970; Williams, 1979; Williams, Dadone, Hunt, & Kuida, 1984). International

FIG. 5-9 Example of a pedigree in which early strokes, high blood pressure, and early coronary disease occur together. Hypertension is apparently the major underlying risk factor.

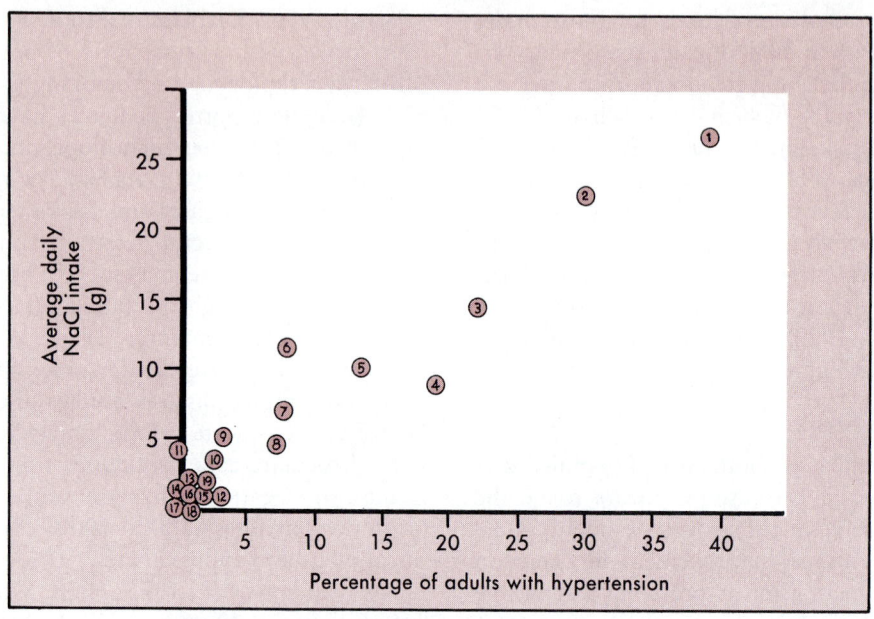

FIG. 5-10 Salt intake versus hypertension in nineteen populations. *r* = 0.96; *p* <0.001; *1*, Japanese, Northern Japan; *2*, Bahama natives, Bahama Islands; *3*, Japanese, Southern Japan; *4*, Rorotongans, Cook Islands; *5*, Americans, United States; *6*, Lau tribesmen, Solomon Islands; *7*, Marshall Islanders, Pacific; *8*, Chimbu Highlanders, New Guinea; *9*, Hasioi and Nagovisis, Solomon Islands; *10*, Pukapukans, Cook Islands; *11*, Eskimos, Alaska; *12*, Tukisenta natives, New Guinea Highlands; *13*, Aita and Baegu tribesmen, Solomon Islands; *14*, Cuna Indians, Amazon Forest, Brazil; *15*, Kwaio tribesmen, Solomon Islands; *16*, Yanomamo Indians, Brazil; *17*, Carajas Indians, Brazil; *18*, Murapins, New Guinea; *19*, Kung Bushmen, Botswana. (Williams, 1979.)

studies have shown a strong correlation between dietary sodium intake and prevalence of hypertension (Fig. 5-10). Studies have also confirmed a strong relationship between obesity and both blood pressure and hypertension (Kannel & Gordon, 1974; Williams et al., 1984). The role of environmental stress, however, has still been poorly defined in the etiology of chronic hypertension. Blacks have repeatedly demonstrated a prevalence of hypertension that is approximately twice that noted in other populations (Cassel, 1972; Blaustein & Grim, 1991).

A popular theory of inherited susceptibility to salt-induced hypertension suggests that hypertension can result from high salt intake and an inherited inability of the kidneys to excrete sodium efficiently without raising arterial blood pressure (Williams, 1979; Williams et al., 1984; Williams, Hunt, Dadone, Smith, Ash, & Kuida, 1984). Initially, either low salt intake or absent gene(s) for high blood pressure could prevent hypertension. In some susceptible persons, salt-initiated hypertension may be perpetuated by other mechanisms (such as reset baroreceptors or nephrosclerosis), even with low salt intake.

This long-held theory is currently being modified to account for developing evidence regarding the important role of other factors, including potassium, calcium, magnesium, chloride, and dietary fat intake and metabolism (Kesteloot, 1985; McCarron, 1983; Puska et al., 1983; Smith-Barbaro & Pucak, 1983; Whitescarver et al., 1984). Evidence for this theory is as follows:

1. Blood pressure is estimated to be 50% to 80% heritable in studies of twins, with the strong genetic role also supported by family and adoption studies.

2. High blood pressure is practically unknown in countries with diet containing less than 1 g salt daily, and high blood pressure prevalence correlates closely with salt intake in different countries.

3. High blood pressure is often lowered by diuretics, which enhance sodium excretion, or by a low-sodium diet.

4. Individual sodium intake correlates with blood pressure level in normotensive persons with a family history of high blood pressure but not in persons without hypertensive relatives (some differences between studies).

5. Sodium and potassium flux tested on human erythrocytes suggests altered sodium membrane transport for persons with essential high blood pressure and some of their relatives, compared to rapid sodium transport for normotensive persons without a family history of high blood pressure.

6. Certain rat strains are either susceptible or resistant to salt-induced high blood pressure. The inherited susceptibility to high blood pressure can be transplanted with kidneys.

Some biochemical correlates of hypertension related to sodium have been found to be highly heritable, including intraerythrocytic sodium (Dadone, 1987) and sodium-lithium countertransport (Dadone, 1985). These biochemical variables and hypertension also correlate with obesity and plasma lipids (Hunt, Williams, Smith, & Ash, 1986).

Studies of early familial coronary disease have consistently shown that hypertension seems to account for approximately the same magnitude of early coronary disease as hyperlipidemia (Glover et al., 1982; Hopkins & Williams, 1981; Hopkins et al., 1984; Rissanen, 1979; Williams, 1979). A more accurate definition of hypertensive syndromes and their expected outcomes should be helpful in allowing clinicians to pinpoint more precisely those individuals who need specific levels of treatment. Ongoing studies attempting to characterize different hypertension syndromes indicate that certain new tests may help to distinguish among different types of hypertension (Falkner et al., 1979; Perloff, Sokolow, & Cowan, 1983; Wilson & Meyer, 1981; Wood et al., 1984).

Renal Disorders

Several renal disorders are familial and can be managed quite effectively. For example, gout has been shown to occur with several different types of single-gene enzyme defects (Emery & Rimoin, 1983; Goodman, 1970; McKusick, 1992). Trauma to joints, dietary changes, and other factors are thought to precipitate symptoms by dislodging uric acid crystals (physically or chemically) from the synovial lining of asymptomatic carriers. Medications are available to prevent the accumulation of uric acid crystals in the kidneys and joints of persons with symptoms. Asymptomatic persons with high blood uric acid are at risk for the disorder and can be advised to avoid these precipitating factors and to recognize early symptoms.

Kidney stones commonly occur in some families and recur often in some individuals. Intake of certain dietary fluids, such as milk or carbonated beverages, is thought to be a precipitating environmental factor. Some common dietary recommendations therefore are believed to help prevent kidney stones. (The pathophysiology of kidney stones is discussed in Chapter 33.)

Gastrointestinal Disorders
Malabsorption Disorders

Several relatively common disorders of the digestive system are known or suspected to illustrate underlying interactions of environmental and genetic factors. For example, persons with gluten-sensitive enteropathy (celiac sprue) cannot tolerate gluten contained in wheat. Damage to the lining of the small bowel leads to malabsorption and diarrhea. If symptoms are prolonged and appropriate action is not taken, malnutrition and associated medical problems can result. Strict avoidance of wheat and wheat-containing foods produces dramatic improvement. This condition is thought to be inherited as a dominant gene with incomplete penetrance, although the reasons for variable penetrance are not yet understood (Goodman, 1970; McKusick, 1992).

Deficiencies of intestinal disaccharidases have been thought to be genetically transmitted. One example is lactase deficiency (lactose intolerance). A lactose tolerance test has been applied to different populations, indicating that 73% of the adult black population may have decreased intestinal lactase levels, in contrast to approximately 5% of the adult white population with the same deficiency (Goodman, 1970). Persons who are symptomatic for the disorder experience abdominal pain and diarrhea after milk consumption; symptoms usually diminish when milk is withdrawn from the diet. Similar symptoms sometimes occur secondarily after other diseases have damaged the intestinal mucosa.

Common inflammatory bowel diseases, including ulcerative colitis and Crohn disease, are thought to be caused, in part, by a genetic predisposition. Markedly increased rates of the disease occur in certain ethnic groups, especially Ashkenazic Jews, as compared to other races and to Sephardic Jews (Goodman, 1970). (Problems in absorption and digestion are discussed further in Chapter 36.)

Peptic Ulcers

Peptic ulcers occur in 5% to 10% of studied general populations and have been established to occur on a familial basis in studies of twins, families, and blood groups. Either duodenal or gastric ulcers can predominate within given families. Further evidence of genetic subtypes shows that approximately one half of individuals with a duodenal ulcer have hyperpepsinogenemia I, as do 50% of the offspring of persons with an ulcer and elevated levels of pepsinogen. This biochemical marker is thought to reflect an inherited increase in the mass of acid-secreting cells in the wall of the stomach (Rotter et al., 1979).

Both psychologic stress and cigarette smoking, through their effects on the nervous system and acid secretion, have long been recognized as precipitating or aggravating environmental factors. Cimetidine and other similar drugs that inhibit acid secretion have revolutionized both the treatment and the prevention of serious problems from peptic ulcer disease. (Peptic ulcers are discussed further in Chapter 36.)

Gallstones

Gallstones are eventually found in approximately 30% of all women and 15% of all men during their lifetimes. Cholecystectomy is one of the most common operations performed in North America. Multiple cases occurring among relatives suggest a familial predisposition, although genetic and environmental determinants of gallstones and associated complications remain to be defined in most cases. Some underlying genetic and environmental factors may be shared with obesity, which is commonly associated with gallstones.

Obesity

Perhaps one of the most challenging metabolic disorders is **obesity.** It is associated with hypertension, diabetes, elevated blood lipid levels, and cardiovascular disease (Kannel & Gordon, 1974). Obesity is probably a highly heterogeneous group of disorders with multiple etiologic factors. Significant familial aggregation of obesity has been found in many different kinds of studies, including twin and adoption studies. Single-gene mechanisms have been identified in animal studies, but in humans shared environmental factors and polygenic determinants probably play important roles in a large proportion of obesity cases.

A growing body of supportive data suggests the possibility that single genes are causal risk factors for such extreme cases as morbid obesity (defined as an excess weight of 100 pounds or weight approximately twice an individual's ideal weight [Williams, 1984b]). This severe form of obesity occurs in less than 1% of the general population but is found quite commonly among relatives of approximately half of morbidly obese individuals. One hypothesis is that basic cell membrane transport mechanisms might be different in these persons, although the condition is still influenced significantly by dietary caloric intake (Ash et al., 1983). (Metabolic regulation is discussed further in Chapter 35.)

Some interesting biochemical and metabolic studies of obesity indicate that, for some individuals who remain thin throughout their lives despite relatively high caloric intake, factors such as conversion of chemical energy directly into heat energy in brown adipose tissue may buffer excess sugar and fat calories. In one experimental study, volunteer prisoners who were thin and had relatives who were thin were able to consume approximately twice their normal caloric intake for several months without any significant weight gain (Sims et al., 1973). At the other end of the spectrum are morbidly obese individuals who lose weight very slowly, even when placed on vitamins and intravenous fluids with little or no caloric intake.

For example, after gastric surgery (stapling) for mor-bid obesity, individuals lose approximately 100 to 150 pounds over a 12-month period on approximately 600 calories of daily intake. This stringent restriction is aided, of course, by the staple bypass operation, which physically limits the passage of food and consequently helps enforce restricted caloric intake. After approximately 1 year, individuals who have undergone such surgery are able to consume approximately 1000 calories per day and seem to maintain a relatively stable weight on this diet, which would result in considerable weight loss by other persons.

Apparently, some people are endowed with a metabolism that can waste consumed energy as heat and thus prevent obesity from developing, whereas others are endowed with an efficient metabolism that may have been an advantage in time of famine but is a considerable detriment in a society saturated with excess calories. Whole-body calorimeter studies have indicated that some slender individuals can burn approximately 25% of excess fat and sugar calories within 1 hour of a meal; very obese individuals show little or no heat production, indicating they are storing excess calories rather than burning them (Beers & Bassett, 1981; Cioffi, James, & VanItallie, 1981). (Theories concerning the pathophysiology of obesity are discussed in Chapter 36.)

Although proven and established methods for preventing obesity are not yet available, some of the data regarding metabolic factors in obesity suggest several possibilities. Studies of both animals and humans seem to indicate that refined carbohydrates and fat calories contribute to the problem of obesity in individuals and therefore should be avoided (Beers & Bassett, 1981; Cioffi et al., 1981). Some suggest that increased physical activity not only consumes calories during the exercise but also has beneficial effects in influencing metabolic processes. In some families with patterns of obesity, an early age of onset seems to be prominent, so that dietary changes and increased activity levels could be promoted among youngsters in obesity-prone families, with the aim of preventing future obesity. Of course, shared environmental factors, such as common family dietary habits, must also contribute to a significant proportion of cases of obesity. Whether the etiologic basis is genetic or environmental, healthful dietary factors and increased physical activity levels remain worthwhile recommendations.

Current studies provide evidence for several different types of obesity syndromes. A more accurate characterization of these syndromes should lead to a better understanding of the underlying pathophysiology of each type. For example, complications such as diabetes may be much more common in some types, such as central obesity (as opposed to peripheral obesity).

CLINICAL COMMENTARY   A HYPOTHETICAL MODEL: GENES + ENVIRONMENT = DISEASE

Research suggests that genetic and environmental factors could combine to produce obesity (Williams, 1984b). To illustrate how this situation could happen, consider a hypothetical example that two autosomal genes might help to control a person's likelihood of developing obesity. Let us call the first gene the "BAT gene" (BAT signifying brown adipose tissue). The homozygous form of this gene (bb) is assumed to be associated with a marked defect in metabolic pathways that normally buffer excess caloric intake. The expression of this gene could be seen by sampling observations at various points in a chain of events leading from the genotype to the expression in obesity.

Obesity could be considered to be a phenotype of this gene, but the condition is at the end of a continuum that is preceded by several intermediate steps. Along the continuum are opportunities for other genes and environmental factors to modify the gene's expression. Obesity might, therefore, be considered as a "confounded ex-

pression" of this gene because it reflects the genetic effect only partially and also reflects the effect of other undetermined factors.

For this model, the "BAT gene" has a very strong effect, and the only other factors affecting obesity include environmental sugar and caloric intake and another well-defined hypothetical gene we shall call the "tooth gene." The "tooth gene" is manifested by a craving for sugar with its associated tendency toward obesity. Its effects are modified by the environmental availability of dietary sugar. The "tooth gene" has a mild effect on obesity.

Obesity can be entirely the result of environmental factors, but a higher level of obesity results from a combined effect of environmental factors and the "tooth gene." A striking level of obesity is found to occur when these two factors interact with the "BAT gene." Thus different levels of obesity depend on the combination of these three variables.

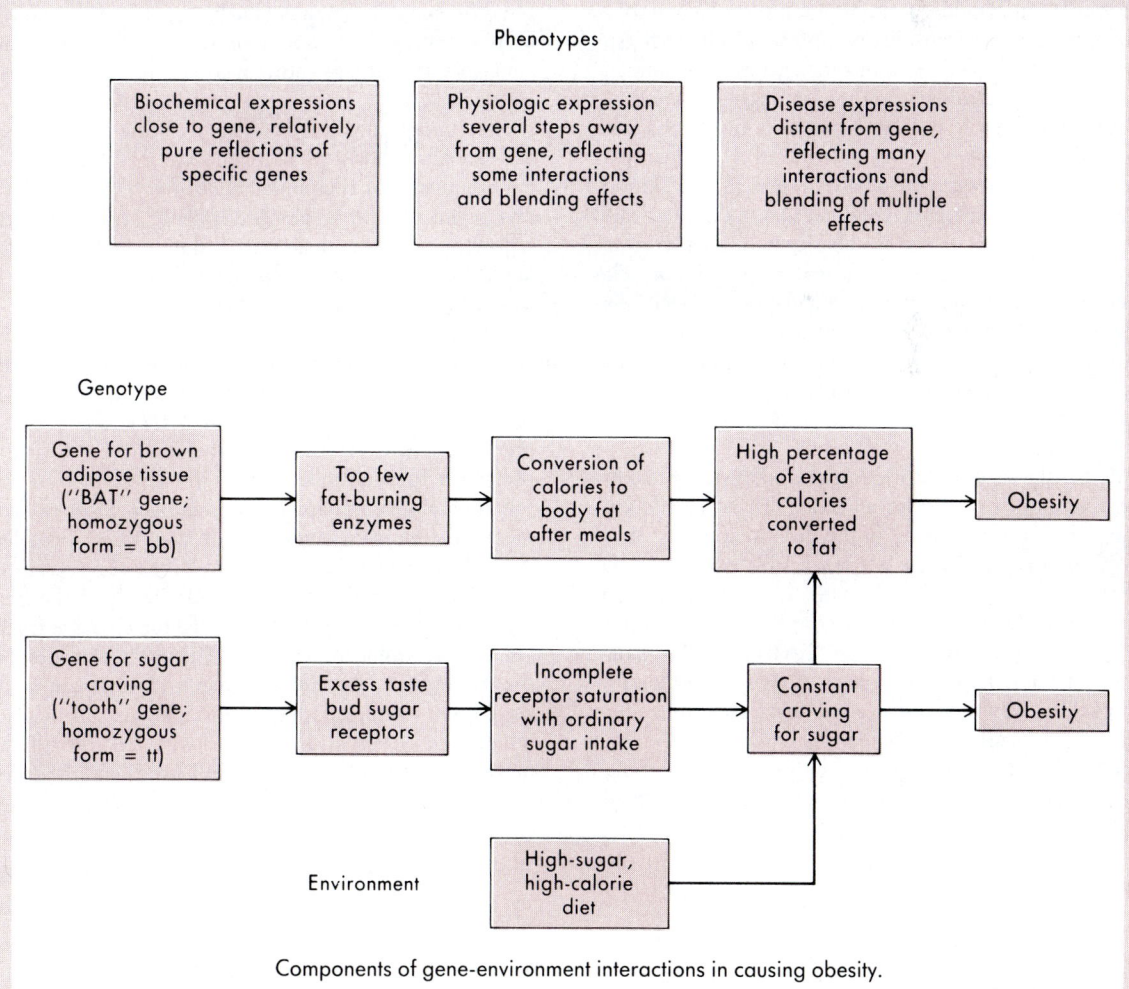

Components of gene-environment interactions in causing obesity.

Continued.

A HYPOTHETICAL MODEL:
GENES + ENVIRONMENT = DISEASE — cont'd

The phenotype frequency distribution illustrates the principal effect of each of these two genes and the effects of their interaction with each other and with the environment. In part *A*, the distribution of persons in the population by weight as a percentage of ideal weight is represented for individuals who have each of the three possible genotypes with respect to the BAT locus: BB (normal), Bb (heterozygous for the abnormal BAT allele), and bb (homozygous for the abnormal BAT allele). Means for individuals with each of these three genotypes are, respectively, 110%, 140%, and 195% of ideal weight. This spread demonstrates the dramatic effect of the homozygous state of this "BAT gene," leading to morbid obesity with a much milder form of obesity seen in heterozygous individuals. A considerable spread within each genotype reflects the influence of other genes, environmental factors, and random variation among individuals.

The considerable overlap between homozygous normal and heterozygous individuals shows the difficulty in distinguishing between the two in the general population. The homozygous affected individuals have a dramatically displaced outcome of morbid obesity with little overlap, making them easier to find in the general population. The single dotted curve in part *A* represents the frequency distribution of all individuals without identification of genotype. The expression of a major gene appears in the form of a "bimodal distribution" (two peaks, one for normal individuals and the other for those who have the major gene defect).

Part *B* shows the distribution of weight status for different genotypes of the "tooth gene." There is little separation between the means of the three genotypes (98%, 116%, 126%), and there is considerable overlap in the weight status of individuals with all three genotypes. Both the large spread and the overlap are caused primarily by the strong influence of the "BAT gene." The same general phenotype distribution in the entire population is represented by the upper dotted line. Part *B* thus illustrates the difficulty of detecting the mild effects of minor genes when they are confounded by strong effects of major genes or other factors that have not yet been defined.

Part *C* characterizes all subjects according to the genotype of both genes. Nine distinct genotypes are represented by all possible combinations of the two genes. The predominant separation is still attributable to the "BAT gene," but within genotypes for the "BAT gene" is an additional separation according to genotypes for the "tooth gene." Of course, the most striking obesity (220%) is observed in the individuals who are homozygously affected by both genes.

Part *D* illustrates the important role of age. The accumulation of extra calories stored as adipose tissue over time is less prevalent in children than in adults. Less separation in weight status is thus evident in children with the different genotypes. At birth they may show no separation, young children may show a mild separation, and teenagers and adults show a clear separation, as illustrated in Part *C*.

The important roles of dietary calorie and sugar intake are also evident in the phenotype distribution. In an environment that is completely devoid of excess calories and sugar, there may be no difference in weight status, regardless of genotype, as part *E* shows. An environment abundant with calories and sugar, however, is likely to cause genetic expression of obesity.

An actual understanding of the pathophysiologic basis of obesity requires a more complicated model, and major effects need to be carefully defined before less prominent factors can be detected. Whenever possible, phenotypes close to the genotype should be studied in preference to distant phenotypes influenced by other factors. In a more complex model, other genetic or environmental determinants may include such factors as television advertisements or the absence of taste bud receptors.

Any phenotype that corresponds closely to the genotype can serve as a genetic marker for classifying individuals according to genotype. Then, within genotypes, the different effects of environmental factors can be observed. For example, a high-calorie, high-sugar diet may not lead to obesity in individuals who are normally homozygous with respect to the "BAT gene" and the "tooth gene."

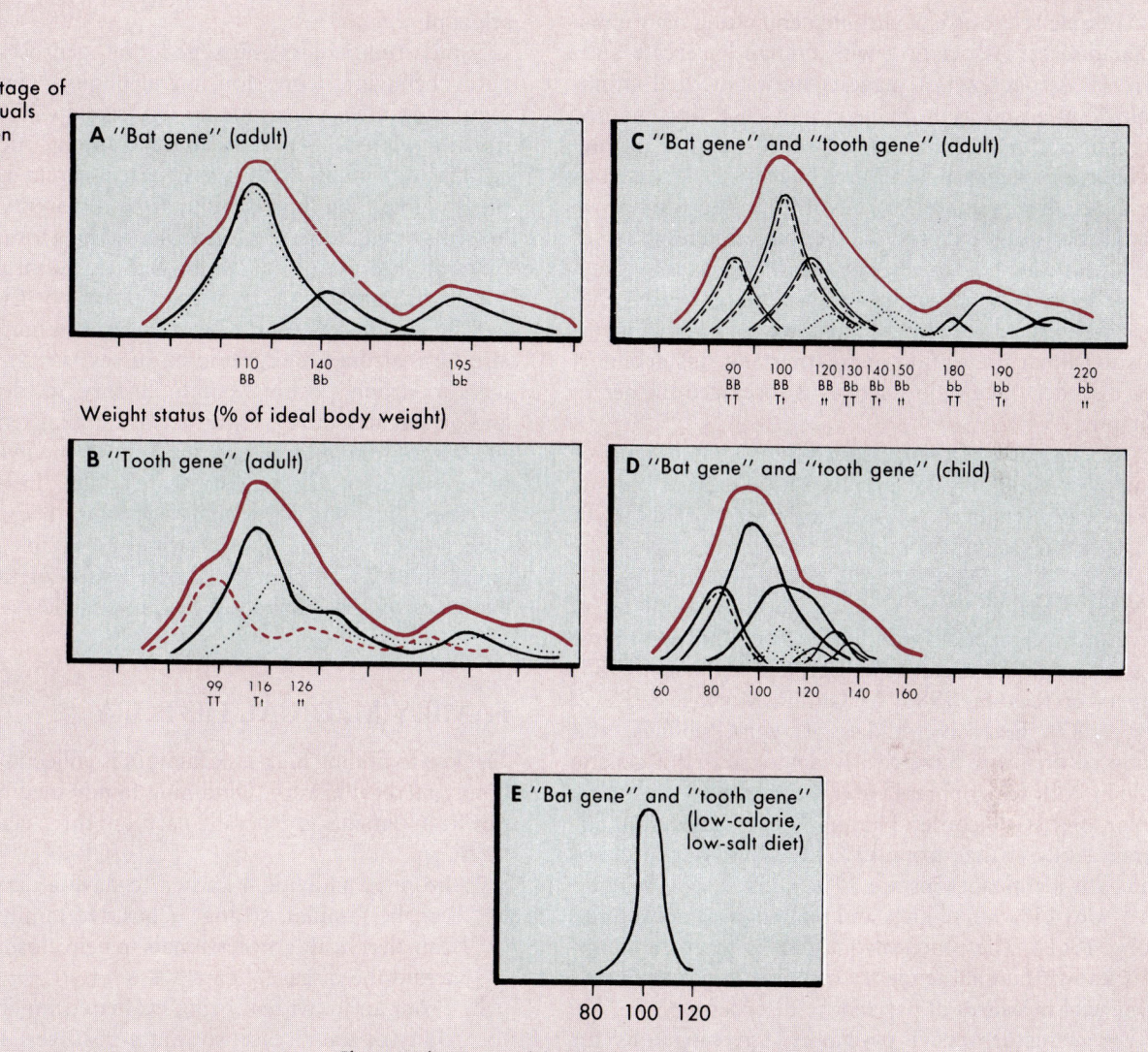

Phenotype frequency and distribution by genotype.

Neuromuscular Disorders

A variety of neuromuscular disorders are known or suspected to have genetic determinants (Emery & Rimoin, 1983; Goodman, 1970; McKusick, 1992). Disorders such as Huntington disease and muscular dystrophy are known to be genetically determined; however, they are not preventable and are currently managed with symptomatic treatment (see Chapter 15).

Multiple sclerosis is a chronic debilitating neuromuscular disease. Association with human leukocyte antigen (HLA) phenotypes suggests some inherited immunologic predisposition (Haile et al., 1981; Spielman & Nathanson, 1982) (see Chapter 6). The disease appears to have low penetrance. Viruses have been suspected to be the environmental factor involved in the pathophysiologic basis of the disease. Lower disease rates in lower latitudes (e.g., Los Angeles vs. Seattle) suggest protective climate factors. Further studies are required to define the exact pathophysiologic steps and better methods for either prevention or treatment of this debilitating disorder. (Multiple sclerosis is discussed further in Chapter 15.)

Alzheimer disease is a relatively common type of tragic dementia. Genetic predisposition in at least some of the cases has been suggested by the reported link to a DNA marker on chromosome 21.

Psychiatric Disorders

Several psychiatric disorders have been shown to have a strong familial occurrence (Egeland & Sussex, 1985; Emery & Rimoin, 1983; McGuffin, Murray, & Reveley, 1987). Extensive studies of twins, siblings, and adopted offspring have clearly demonstrated a genetic role in both schizophrenia and manic-depressive, or bipolar affective, disorder. Heritability estimates from different studies range from 40% to 100%. Concordance rates for identical twins are 50% to 80%, as compared to 5% to 15% for siblings and nonidentical twins (Gregory, 1968). The practical question is whether or not this known familial tendency can lead to preventive or beneficial measures in psychiatric disorders.

For manic-depressive psychoses, screening tests for detecting the disease in early stages are available. Early reports suggest linkage of bipolar affective disorder on chromosome 11; however, recent reports refute this association. New evidence exists for an X-linked dominant form of bipolar affective disorder (the gene is closely linked to the colorblindness loci on the X chromosome). Thus far this report has not been contraindicated.

Schizophrenia appears to be caused by inherited defects in neurochemistry, brain trauma, or both (Murray & Lewis, 1985). The recurrence risk for schizophrenia among the offspring of one affected parent is about 10%, which is about 10 times higher than the risk in the general population (McGuffin et al., 1987). Differ-ences in levels of monoamine oxidase or its metabolites have been observed in platelets or cerebrospinal fluid of schizophrenics whose disease shows familial tendencies. Birth trauma, prematurity, soft neurologic signs, abnormal electroencephalograms, or abnormal brain CT scans are found in up to one third of all schizophrenics. Evidence indicates that inherited susceptibility and environmental insult combine to produce some cases of schizophrenia.

Some studies have suggested that neuroses, sociopathic behavior, depression, and alcoholism may also be familial and may sometimes be associated with more serious psychoses. The risk of developing alcoholism among individuals with one affected parent is 3 to 5 times higher than those with unaffected parents. Studies of twins have shown the concordance rates for dizygotic twins are less than 30%, whereas the rates for monozygotic twins are greater than 60% (Devor & Cloninger, 1989). Suicide and depression can occur in families that also have alcoholics (Egeland & Sussex, 1985). Persons with a strong positive family history of depression and/or suicide could be warned of familial tendencies. Their spouses could be educated about the availability of effective antidepressant medications. Information about medications is especially important because most clinicians consider depression to be a treatable disorder and because, when untreated, the effects of the disorder are profound enough to lead to suicide.

FAMILY MEDICAL HISTORY

The key to finding high-risk families is collecting a good family medical history. Obtaining family medical histories from patients is generally useful in three clinical settings:

1. From an individual known to have a disease that can be familial, so that a positive family history can alert health professionals to help close relatives avoid the disease
2. From an individual being evaluated for the possibility of the disease, so that a positive family history will increase clinical suspicion and may help to justify further diagnostic tests
3. From a healthy individual, so that a general screening tool will identify a person with a positive family history that needs further attention

The most efficient use of a family medical history is to chart the history of a proband who has familial disease. For example, approximately one half of men with early coronary disease will have a strong positive family history of the disease. This type of family history indicates a familial tendency that can often be addressed by appropriately informed and motivated close relatives (see box on p. 197).

FAMILY MEDICAL HISTORY

When?

1. *Individual with disease* that is often familial (e.g., male coronary at age 36)
2. Individual *might* have disease but has nondiagnostic symptoms (e.g., 36-year-old man with vague chest discomfort)
3. General screening tool (broad family history overview during new patient workup)

How? (What data should be collected)

1. *Sex, age, vital status for all target relatives and spouse*
   First-degree relatives: parents, siblings, and offspring
   Second-degree relatives: grandparents, aunts, and uncles
2. *Disease and cause of death*
   Age at diagnosis?
   Prescriptions given?
3. *Risk factors*
   Year of exposure?
   Modification and outcome?

Why?

1. *Identify high-risk families:* If the family history is strongly positive, it will help indentify close relatives who can be helped to avoid the same problem
2. *Use like a diagnostic test:* Positive family history increases suspicion; special tests or monitoring may be justified
3. *Use to focus future attention:* Be alert to family tendencies; plan future procedures for screening and prevention

What can be learned?

1. Is the disease familial?
2. How strong is the tendency?
3. Does it affect males and females alike?
4. Is onset at the usual age?
5. Which risk factors are invloved?
6. What is the pathphysiology?
7. Which relatives need help?
8. At what age should screening start?
9. What is the best way to prevent, screen for, or treat the disease?

SUMMARY REVIEW

What Factors Cause Disease?

1 Factors causing disease can be fundamentally classified as genetic or environmental.
2 Finding and understanding environmental factors that affect the penetrance of specific genes is an important approach in preventing chronic familial diseases.
3 A polygenic trait is an inherited trait caused by the blending of effects of many different genes.
4 A multifactorial trait is produced by the blending of multiple genetic and environmental influences.
5 The penetrance of a single gene or number of genes can depend on the person's age, gender, genetic makeup, and environmental factors.
6 The effects of other factors on a single gene's penetrance are called interactions. They may be gene-gene or gene-environment interactions.
7 Environmental factors that can lead to disease in susceptible individuals include personal habits and life-styles; exposure to chemicals, toxins, pollutants, and medications; psychologic status; and microorganisms or other immunologic stimuli.

Analyzing Disease Risk

1 Statistical measurements important in determining disease risk are the incidence rate, the prevalence rate, and the mortality rate.
2 Risk factors are indicators of a person's predisposition to developing a disease; risk factors may be either causal or noncausal.
3 Risk factors may be statistically measured by using either contingency tables or correlation coefficients.
4 Measurement of the relative risk, population-attributable risk, and preventive efficiency for a particular population indicates the degree of familiality and efficiency of targeted intervention among high-risk persons who may be able to avoid disease with appropriate preventive measures.
5 Continuous traits (e.g., obesity) are traits expressed across a range of severity. Such traits can be analyzed with either correlation coefficients or contingency tables, using a threshold that defines an affected person.

Environmental Risk Factors

1 Environmental pathogens are associated with a variety of infectious diseases, including some that involve immunologic reactions triggered by microbes.
2 Personal habits have been associated with some of the most common chronic diseases.
3 Physical and chemical substances can be both causal factors and protective mechanisms in the development of some diseases.
4 Psychologic and social factors may be direct causes of contributing factors in the development of disease.

Combined Effects and Interaction among Risk Factors

1 Interactions and combined effects of causal risk factors are involved in many disease processes.
2 A goal of current research is to define the heterogeneity, or variety of factors that lead to common chronic diseases.
3 Analyzing disease tendencies in families involves collecting data about sets of relatives and identifying patterns of disease and exposure to risk factors.
4 Age is a risk factor for many diseases. It often represents the effects of exposure to various risk factors and inherited physiologic processes that cause human beings to age.

Familial Diseases and Associated Risks

1 A great variety of diseases are known to show a familial tendency, often in combination with some environmental interactions.
2 For many inherited disorders, expression of the trait depends on environmental exposures.
3 Immunologic disorders that show some familial tendency include rheumatoid arthritis, systemic lupus erythematosus, idiopathic Addison disease, autoimmune thyroiditis, Graves disease, and idiopathic thrombocytopenic purpura (ITP).
4 Allergies and asthma also show familial patterns, and susceptibility to certain infections may be an inherited trait.
5 Cancers that show some familial predisposition include cancer of the breast, colon, lung, ovary, uterus, and prostate.

6 Both types of diabetes mellitus (IDDM and NIDDM) show an inherited tendency that is probably expressed because of other causal risk factors.
7 Hematologic disorders that are inherited and expressed because of environmental risk factors include hemolytic anemia, glucose-6-phosphate dehydrogenase (G6PD) deficiency, hereditary spherocytosis and elliptocytosis, hemophilia, and hemochromatosis.
8 Cardiovascular disorders that show a familial tendency include rheumatic valvular heart disease, a prolonged QT segment (on electrocardiogram), myocardiopathies, mitral valve prolapse, septal defects, coronary heart disease, hypertension, and stroke.
9 Renal disorders that show a familial tendency include gout and kidney stones.
10 Gastrointestinal disorders that show an inherited susceptibility include malabsorptive syndrome (gluten-sensitive enteropathy, lactase deficiency), ulcerative colitis, Crohn disease, peptic ulcers, and obesity.
11 Neuromuscular disorders that have inherited determinants include Huntington disease, muscular dystrophy, and multiple sclerosis.
12 Psychiatric disorders with some familial tendency include schizophrenia and bipolar affective disorder.

Family Medical History

1 The family medical history is useful in screening susceptible individuals, indicating the need for more diagnostic evaluation, and identifying those at risk for certain diseases.
2 Patterns of familial diseases in particular families allow health professionals to begin risk-reduction efforts to prevent a disease occurrence or to minimize its severity.
3 Methods for collecting data for a family history include brief screening during routine health assessment, self-administered questionnaires, detailed interviews, verification of data about relatives, and screening and examination of selected relatives.

KEY TERMS

REFERENCES

Ash, K. O., Smith, J. B., Kemp, J. W., Lynch, M. B., Moody, F. G., Raymond, J. L., McKnight, M. R., & Williams, R. R. (1983). The effect of diet on ouabain binding to erythrocytes from obese subjects. *Clinical Physiology and Biochemistry, 1,* 293-299.

Beers, R. F., & Bassett, E. G. (1981). *Nutritional factors: Modulating effects on metabolic processes.* (p. 568). New York: Raven Press.

Blaustein, M. P., & Grim, C. E. (1991). The pathogenesis of hypertension: Black-white differences. *Cardiovascular Clinics, 21* (3), 97-114.

Brinton, L. A., Williams, R. R., Hoover, R. N., Stegens, N. L., Feinleib, M., & Fraumeni, J. F. (1979). Breast cancer risk factors among screening program participants. *Journal of the National Cancer Institute, 62,* 37-44.

Carmelli, D., Williams, R. R., & Rissanen, A. (1982). Contrasting patterns of familiality for cholesterol and triglyceride in Finland according to type of coronary manifestations and locations. *American Journal of Epidemiology, 116,* 617-621.

Cassel, J. C. (1972). Evans County cardiovascular and cerebrovascular epidemiologic study. *Archives of Internal Medicine, 128,* 883-895.

Cavalli-Storza, L. L., & Bodner, W. F. (1971). *The genetics of human populations.* San Francisco: W. H. Freeman.

Cioffi, L. A., James, W. P. T., & VanItallie, T. B. (1981). *The body weight regulatory system: Normal and disturbed mechanisms* (p. 380). New York: Raven Press.

Cooper, D. N., & Schmidtke, J. (1992). Molecular genetic approaches: Overview. *Annals of Medicine, 24,* 29-42.

Dadone, M. M. (1987). Preliminary evidence for genetic determination of intraerythrocytic sodium concentration in Utah pedigrees. *American Journal of Medical Genetics, 27*(1), 39-44.

Devor, E. J., & Cloninger, C. R. (1989). Genetics of alcoholism. *Annual Review of Genetics, 23,* 19-36.

Edwards, C. Q., Carroll, M., Bray, P. F., & Cartwright, G. E. (1977). Hereditary hemochromatosis: Diagnosis in siblings and children. *New England Journal of Medicine, 279,* 7-13.

Egeland, J. A., & Sussex, J. N. (1985, August). Suicide and family loading for affective disorders. *Journal of the American Medical Association, 254*(7), 915-918.

Emery, A. E. H., & Rimoin, D. L. (1983). *Principles and practice of medical genetics* (p. 1502). New York: Churchill Livingstone.

Falkner, B., Onesti, G., Angelakos, E. T., Fernandes, M., & Langman, C. (1979). Cardiovascular response to mental stress in normal adolescents with hypertensive parents. *Hypertension, 1,* 23-30.

Feinleib, M., Garrison, M. D., Barhani, N., Rosenman, R., & Christian, J. (1975). Studies of hypertension in twins. In O. Paul (Ed.), *Epidemiology and control of hypertension.* New York: Stratton.

Feinleib, M., & Williams, R. R. (1976). Relative risks of myocardial infarction, cardiovascular disease, and peripheral vascular disease by type of smoking. *Proceedings of Third World Conference on Smoking and Health.* In E. L. Wynder, D. Hoffman, & G. B. Gori (Eds.), *Smoking and health. I. Modifying the risk for the smoker.* Washington, DC: U. S. Government Printing Office.

Froguel, P., Vaxillaire, M., Sun, F., Velho, G., Zoualil, H., Butel, M. L., Lesage, S., Bionnet, N., Clement, K., Fougerousse, F., et al. (1992). Close linkage of glucokinase locus on chromosome 7p to early-onset non–insulin-dependent diabetes mellitus. *Nature, 356,* 162-164.

Glover, M. U., Kuber, M. T., Warren, S. E., & Vieweg, W. V. R. (1982). Myocardial infarction before age 36: Risk factor and arteriographic analysis. *American Journal of Cardiology, 49,* 1600-1603.

Goodman, R. M. (1970). *Genetic disorders of man* (p. 995). Boston: Little, Brown.

Gordon, T., & Kannel, W. B. (1971). Section 1: Introduction and general background. *The Framingham Study: An epidemiological investigation of cardiovascular disease.* Washington, DC: U.S. Public Health Service.

Gregory, I. (1968). *Fundamentals of psychiatry* (p. 647). Philadelphia: W. B. Saunders.

Groden, J., Thliveris, A., Samowitz, W., Carlson, M., Gelbert, L., Albertsen, H., Joslyn, G., Stevens, J., Spirio, L., Robertson, M., et al. (1991). Identification and characterization of the familial adenomatous polyposis coli gene. *Cell, 66,* 589-600.

Haile, R. W., Iselius, L., Hodge, S. E., Morton, N. E., & Detels, R. (1981). Segregation and linkage analysis of 40 multiplex multiple sclerosis families. *Human Heredity, 31,* 252-258.

Hall, J. M., Friedman, L., Guenther, C., Lee, M. K., Weber, J. L., Black, D. M., & King, M. C. (1992). Closing in on a breast cancer gene on chromosome 17q. *American Journal of Human Genetics, 15* (6), 1235-1242.

Hall, J. M., Lee, M. K., Newman, B., Morrow, J. E., Andersen, L. A., Huey, B., & King, M. C. (1990). Linkage of early-onset familial breast cancer to chromosome 17q21. *Science, 250* (4988), 1684-1689.

Hasstedt, S. J., Ash, K. O., & Williams, R. R. (1986). A re-examination of major locus hypotheses for high-density lipoprotein cholesterol level using 2170 persons screened in 55 Utah pedigrees. *American Journal of Medical Genetics, 24,* 57-67.

Hasstedt, S. J., Wu, L. L., & Williams, R. R. (1987). Major locus inheritance of apolipoprotein B in Utah pedigrees. *Genetic Epidemiology, 4*(2), 67-76.

Hilbert, P., Lindpainter, K., Beckmann, J. S., Serikawa, T., Soubrier, F., Dubay, C., Cartwright, P., De-Gouyon, B., Julier, C., Takahase, S., et al. (1991). Chromosomal mapping of two genetic loci associated with blood-pressure regulation in hereditary hypertensive rats. *Nature, 353,* 521-529.

Hippocrates (1938). On airs, waters, and places. Translated and republished in *Medical Classics, 3,* 19-42.

Hopkins, P. N., & Williams, R. R. (1981). A review of 246 suggested coronary risk factors. *Atherosclerosis, 40,* 1-52.

Hopkins, P. N., Williams, R. R., & Hunt, S. C. (1984). Magnified risks from cigarette smoking for coronary prone families in Utah. *Western Journal of Medicine, 141,* 196-202.

Hunt, S. C. (1980). The epidemiology of reproductive factors associated with breast cancer. Doctoral dissertation. University of Utah, Salt Lake City, Utah.

Hunt, S. C., Hasstedt, S. J., & Williams, R. R. (1986). Testing for familial aggregation of dichotomous trait. *Genetic Epidemiology, 3,* 299-312.

Hunt, S. C., Williams, R. R., & Barlow, G. K. (1986). A comparison of positive family history definitions for defining risk of future disease. *Journal of Chronic Disease, 39,* 809-821.

Hunt, S. C., Williams, R. R., Smith, J. B., & Ash, K. O. (1986). Association of three erythrocyte cation transport systems with plasma lipids in Utah subjects. *Hypertension, 8,* 30-36.

Jick, N., Dinan, B., Herman, R., & Rothman, K. J. (1978). Myocardial infarction and other vascular diseases in young women. *Journal of the American Medical Association, 240,* 2548-2552.

Jink, H. K. (1976). Cigarette smoking, use of oral contraceptives, and myocardial infarction. *American Journal of Obstetrics and Gynecology, 126,* 301-307.

Joint National Committee on Detection, Evaluation, & Treatment of High Blood Pressure. (1984). The 1984 report. *Archives of Internal Medicine, 144,* 1045-1057.

Kane, J. P., Malloy, M. J., Ports, T. A., Phillips, N. R., Diehl, J. C., & Havel, R. J. (1990). Regression of coronary atherosclerosis during treatment of familial hypercholesterolemia with combined drug regimens. *Journal of the American Medical Association, 265,* 3007-3012.

Kannel, W. B., & Gordon, T. (1974). *The Framingham Study. An epidemiological investigation of cardiovascular disease* (Section 30, Eighteen Year Follow-up). Washington, DC: U.S. Government Printing Office [DHEW Publication No. NIH 74-599].

Keating, M., Atkinson, D., Dunn, C., Timothy, K., Vincent, G. M., & Leppert, M. (1991). Linkage of a cardiac arrhythmia, the long QT syndrome, and the Harvey ras-1 gene. *Science, 252,* 704-706.

Kesteloot, H. (1985). Epidemiological studies on the relationship between sodium, potassium, and magnesium and arterial blood pressure. *Journal of Cardiovascular Pharmacology, 6,* S192-S196.

Kinzler, K. W., Nilbert, M. C., Su, L., Vogelstein, B., Bryan, T. M., Levy, D. B., Smith, K. J., Preisinger, A. C., Hedge, P., McKechnie, et al. (1991). Identification of FAP locus genes from chromosome 5q21. *Science, 253,* 661-665.

Leppert, M. F., Hasstedt, S. J., Holm, J., O'Connell, P., Wu, L., Ash, O., Williams, R. R., & White, R. (1986). A DNA probe for the LDL receptor gene is tightly linked to hypercholesterolemia in a pedigree with early coronary disease. *American Journal of Human Genetics, 39,* 300-306.

Lyon, J. L., Klauber, M. R., Gardner, J. W., & Smart, C. R. (1977). Cancer incidence in Mormons and non-Mormons in Utah, 1966-1970. *New England Journal of Medicine, 294,* 129-133.

Lyon, J. L., Wetzler, J. P., Klauber, M. R., & Williams, R. R. (1978). Cardiovascular mortality in Mormons and non-Mormons in Utah, 1969-1971. *American Journal of Epidemiology, 108,* 357-366.

MacMahon, B., & Pugh, T. F. (1970). *Epidemiology, principles and methods* (p. 375). Boston: Little, Brown.

McCarron, D. A. (1983). Calcium and magnesium nutrition in human hypertension. *Annals of Internal Medicine, 98,* 800-805.

McGuffin, P., Murray, R. M., & Reveley, A. M. (1987). Genetic influence on the psychoses. *British Medical Bulletin, 43,* 531-536.

McKusick, V. A. (1992). *Mendelian inheritance in man* (10th ed.). Baltimore: Johns Hopkins Press.

Moll, P. P., Sing, C. F., Williams, R. R., Mao, S. J. T., & Kottke, B. A. (1986). The genetic determinant of plasma apolipoprotein A-I levels measured by radioimmunoassay: A study of high-risk pedigrees. *American Journal of Human Genetics, 38*(3), 361-372.

Murray, R. M., & Lewis, S. W. (1985, May). Towards an etiological classification of schizophrenia. *The Lancet,* 1023-1026.

Neufeld, H. N., & Goldbourt, M. A. (1983). Coronary heart disease: Genetic aspects. *Circulation, 67*(5), 943-954.

Perloff, D., Sokolow, M., & Cowan, M. (1983). The prognostic value of ambulatory blood pressures. *Journal of the American Medical Association, 3,* 236-240.

Puska, P., Iacono, J. M., Nissinen, A., Korhanen, H. J., Vartiainen, E., Pietinen, P., Dougherty, R., Leino, U., Mutanen, M., Moisio, S., & Huttunen, J. (1983). Controlled randomized trial of the effect of dietary fat on blood pressure. *Lancet, 1,* 1-5.

Rissanen, A. M. (1979). Familial occurrence of coronary heart disease—Effect of age at diagnosis. *American Journal of Cardiology, 44,* 60-66.

Rotter, J. I., Sones, J. Q., Samloff, I. M., Richardson, C. T., Gurski, J. T., Walsh, J. H., & Rimoin, D. L. (1979). Duodenal ulcer disease associated with elevated serum pepsinogen I, an inherited autosomal dominant disorder. *New England Journal of Medicine, 300,* 63-66.

Sims, E. A. H., Danforth, E., Horton, E. S., Bray, G. A., Glennon, J. A., & Salans, L. B. (1973). Endocrine and metabolic defects of experimental obesity in man. *Recent Progress in Hormonal Research, 29,* 457-496.

Smith-Barbaro, P. A., & Pucak, G. J. (1983). Dietary fat and blood pressure. *Annals of Internal Medicine, 98,* 828-831.

Solomon, E. (1990). Colorectal cancer genes. *Nature, 343,* 412-414.

Spielman, R. S., & Nathanson, N. (1982). The genetics of susceptibilty to multiple sclerosis. *Epidemiologic Review, 4,* 45-65.

Stanbridge, E. (1990). Identifying tumor suppressor genes in human colorectal cancer. *Science, 247,* 12-13.

Stobo, J. D. (1982). Rheumatoid arthritis—From Rubens to restriction maps. *Western Journal of Medicine, 137,* 109-115.

Todd, J. A., Aitman, T. J., Cornall, R. J., Ghosh, S., Hall, J. R., Hearne, C. M., Knight, A. M., Love, J. M., McAleer, M. A., Prins, J., Rodriques, N., Lathrop, M., Pressey, A., DeLarato, N. H., Peterson, L. B., & Wicker, L. S. (1991). Genetic analysis of autoimmune type I diabetes mellitus in mice. *Nature, 351,* 542-547.

Tokuhata, G. K. (1965). Familial factors in lung cancer and smoking. In J. V. Neal, M. W. Shaw, & W. J. Schull (Eds.), *Genetics and the epidemiology of chronic diseases* (pp. 339-353). Washington, DC: Public Health Service Publication No. 1163.

Vander Molen, R., Brewer, G., Honeyman, M. S., Morrison, J., & Hoobler, S. W. (1970). A study of hypertension in twins. *American Heart Journal, 79,* 454-457.

Ward, R. (1990). Familial aggregation and genetic epidemiology of blood pressure. In J. H. Laragh & B. M. Brenner (Eds.), *Hypertension: Pathophysiology, diagnosis, and management* (pp. 81-100). New York: Raven Press.

Whitescarver, S. A., Cobern, E. O., Jackson, E. A., Gutherie, G. P., & Kotchen, T. A. (1984). Salt-sensitive hypertension: Contribution of chloride. *Science, 233,* 1430-1432.

Whyte, H. M. (1975). Potential effects of coronary heart disease morbidity of lowering the blood cholesterol. *Lancet, 1,* 906.

Williams, R. R. (1979). The role of genes in coronary atherosclerosis. In J. W. Hurst (Ed.), *Update IV: The heart.* (pp. 89-118). New York: McGraw-Hill.

Williams, R. R. (1984a). Population-based perspectives of the genetic epidemiology of *early* coronary disease in Framingham and Utah. In D. C. Rao, R. C. Elston, L. H. Kuller, M. Feinleib, C. Carter, & R. Havlik (Eds.), *Genetic epidemiology of coronary heart disease: Past, present, and future* (pp. 89-91). New York: Alan R. Liss, Inc.

Williams, R. R. (1984b). The role of genetic analysis in characterizing obesity. *International Journal of Obesity, 8,* 551-559.

Williams, R. R. (1984c). Understanding genetic and environmental risk factors in susceptible persons. *Western Journal of Medicine, 141,* 799-806.

Williams, R. R. (1988). Nature, nurture, and family predisposition. *New England Journal of Medicine, 318*(12), 767-771.

Williams, R. R., Dadone, M., Hunt, S. C., & Kuida, H. (1984). The genetic epidemiology of hypertension: A review of past studies and current results in 948 persons in 48 Utah pedigrees. In D. C. Rao, R. C. Elston, L. H. Kuller, M. Feinleib, C. Carter, & R. Havli, (Eds.), *Genetic epidemiology of coronary heart disease: Past, present, and future* (pp. 420-444). New York: Alan R. Liss, Inc.

Williams, R. R., Hasstedt, S. J., Wilson, D. E., Ash, K. O., Yanowitz, F. G., Reiber, G. E., & Kuida, H. (1986). Evidence that man with familial hypercholesterolemia can avoid early coronary heart disease: An analysis of 77 gene carriers in four Utah pedigrees. *Journal of the American Medical Association, 255,* 219-224.

Williams, R. R., & Hopkins, P. N. (1979). Salt, hypertension, and genetic-environmental interaction. In C. F. Sing & M. Skolnick (Eds.), *The genetic analysis of common diseases* (pp. 183-194). New York: Alan R. Liss, Inc.

Williams, R. R., & Horn, J. W. (1977). Association of cancer sites with tobacco and alcohol consumption and socioeconomic status: Patient interview study from the third national cancer survey. *Journal of the National Cancer Institute, 58,* 525-546.

Williams, R. R., Hunt, S. C., Dadone, M. M., Smith, J. B., Ash, K. O. & Kuida, H. (1984). Cation flux and other possible biological markers of genetically predisposed hypertension. In L. J. Filer & R. M. Lauder (Eds.), *Children's blood pressure, report of the eighty-eighth Ross Conference on Pediatric Research.* (pp. 100-123). Columbus, Ohio: Ross Laboratories.

Williams, R. R., Stegens, N. L., & Goldsmith, J. R. (1977). Industries and occupations associated with cancer sites from the TNCS interview study. *Journal of the National Cancer Institute, 59,* 1147-1185.

Wilson, N. V., & Meyer, B. M. (1981). Early prediction of hypertension using exercise blood pressure. *Preventive Medicine, 10,* 62-68.

Wood, D. L., Sheps, S. G., Elveback, L. R., & Schirger, A. (1984). Cold pressor test as a predictor of hypertension. *Hypertension, 6,* 301-306.

SUGGESTED READINGS

Botstein, D., White, R. L., Skolnick, M., & Davis, R. W. (1980). Construction of a genetic linkage map in man using restriction fragment length polymorphism. *American Journal of Human Genetics, 32,* 314-331.

Clover, J. (1993). Genetic susceptibility to multiple sclerosis linked to mylen basic protein gene [letter]. *Lancet, 341*(8836), 56.

Jenkins, C. D. (1971). Psychologic and social precursors of coronary disease. *New England Journal of Medicine, 284,* 244-255, 307-317.

Shapiro, L. J. (1993). Human genome project. *Western Journal of Medicine, 158*(2), 181.

Snow, J. (1855). *On the mode of communication of cholera* (2nd ed.). London: Churchill. Reprinted in 1936, in *Snow on cholera,* New York: Commonwealth Fund; reprinted in 1965, New York: Hafner.

Yamori, Y., Nara, Y., Mizushima, S., Murakami, S., Ikeda, K., Sawamura, M., Nabika, T., & Horrie, R. (1992). Gene-environment interaction in hypertension, stroke, and atherosclerosis in experimental models and supportive findings from a world-wide cross-sectional epidemiological survey: A WHO cardiac study. *Clinical and Experimental Pharmacological and Physiological Supplement, 20,* 43-52.

UNIT III

Mechanisms of Self-Defense

IMMUNOLOGY IS A RELATIVELY NEW SCIENCE, yet anecdotal evidence shows that people in ancient times were aware of mysterious phenomena that are recognized today as basic concepts of immunology. The ancient Egyptians drew hieroglyphics that represented inflammation. The Greeks, even as far back as the fifth century BC, recognized that individuals who survived a disease seldom contracted the disease a second time. These observations of immune and inflammatory processes were made before the discovery that infectious agents, such as bacteria and viruses, even existed.

The accidental and serendipitous application of immunologic principles ended in the late eighteenth century, when the investigative study of immunology began with the work of an English physician, Edward Jenner. Jenner performed the first experiment in the science that was to become immunology (Jenner, 1798). There are many stories about Jenner's experiment, many fanciful. It is known that Jenner recognized that milkmaids were protected from smallpox if they had developed cowpox, a bovine equivalent of smallpox that causes only mild disease in humans. Jenner took material from a cowpox pustule on the hand of an infected milkmaid (reputed to be named Sarah Nelmes in some stories) and injected it into the arm of James Phipps, an 8-year-old boy. After the boy's initial inflammatory reaction to the injection subsided, Jenner injected him with material from a small-

MECHANISMS OF SELF-DEFENSE

*A physician is inoculating a young child held in the arms of its mother (1827).
(Courtesy National Library of Medicine.)*

pox pustule. Fortunately the experiment was a success, because Jenner is reported to have re-injected smallpox bacteria into the boy at least 20 times. In 1798 Jenner used the term *vaccination* (*vacca* = cow) to describe his technique.

Further advancement of our knowledge about immunity has resulted from carefully planned, well-executed, and well-interpreted experiments, as well as serendipity and chance.

The earliest debates among researchers raged around the relative importance of serum (humoral) factors and cellular factors in immune function. It took years to identify the role of humoral factors—*antibodies*—in the development of immunity. In 1890 Emile von Behring and Shibasaburo Kitasato injected animals with diphtheria toxin, causing the animals to produce antitoxin that could be identified in

sera withdrawn for examination (von Behring & Kitasato, 1890). Rodolf Kraus later demonstrated that the antitoxin, which he called a precipitin, could cause diphtheria toxin to precipitate out of solution in vitro (Kraus, 1897). Other workers showed that the contents of sera from immunized animals could also lyse (dissolve) bacteria (the bacteriolysins) (Pfeiffer, 1894) and agglutinate (clump) bacteria (the agglutinins) (von Gruber & Durham, 1896). In the 1930s researchers finally learned that each of these functions could be attributed to antibody.

The role of cells in immune function was also investigated for the first time late in the nineteenth century. In the 1880s the Russian zoologist Elie Metchnikoff studied large, ameboid white blood cells (macrophages) in starfish and concluded that their function was to accumulate at a site of inflammation and ingest invaders (Metchnikoff, 1883). Later proponents of the cellular theory of immunity proposed that the role of antibody was to prepare (opsonize) the invader for ingestion by the macrophages. The role of other white blood cells (lymphocytes) was suggested in the 1890s by Robert Koch, during his study of tuberculosis. Koch was the first to describe the tuberculin reaction (Koch phenomenon) in which lymphocytes interact with the tuberculin bacillus (Koch, 1891).

In the 1950s extensive research by many scientists led to the realization that antibody and lymphocytes are both effectors of the same immune response. One of the most important breakthroughs was the recognition that discrete lymphoid organs are responsible for the development of these two effectors. Bruce Glick identified the lymphoid organ responsible for the development of antibody-producing cells (Glick, Chang, & Jaap, 1956). He observed that when the bursa of Fabricius (an organ that opens into the terminal portion of the digestive tract of chickens) was removed, the birds lost the ability to produce antibody in response to injected microorganisms. It was later observed that these birds retained cell-mediated immunity. When Glick and his co-workers attempted to publish a paper reporting their findings, it was reportedly rejected by editors of prestigious medical journals and was finally published in *Poultry Science.*

The lymphoid tissue responsible for the development of cellular, or cell-mediated, immunity—the thymus—was identified in the 1960s by Jacques Miller (1961) and Robert Good and colleagues (1962). They observed that experimental animals that had the thymus removed at birth could not elicit a cell-mediated immune response; that is, their non-antibody-producing lymphocytes did not react to the introduction of infectious agents. They could, however, produce fairly good antibody responses. As a result of the work of these and many other researchers, the study of immunology has risen from a fledgling science in the nineteenth century to what is perhaps the most exciting, diverse, and rapidly advancing discipline in biology today.

Immunity

Neal S. Rote

Chapter Outline

T he body's first lines of defense are anatomic barriers: the skin and mucous membranes lining the respiratory, gastrointestinal, and genitourinary tracts. These surfaces are biochemical barriers as well. Sebaceous glands in the skin secrete antibacterial and antifungal fatty acids and lactic acid. Perspiration, tears, and saliva contain an enzyme (lysozyme) that attacks the cell walls of gram-positive bacteria. As a result of these glandular secretions, the surface of the skin is acidic (pH 3 to 5), making it inhospitable to most bacteria.

If an injurious chemical, foreign body, or microorganism penetrates these defenses, the body attempts to eliminate it by mechanical clearance. It may be sloughed off with skin, caught in respiratory mucus and coughed up, vomited from the stomach, or flushed from the urinary tract by urine. Auxiliary defenses are present in the form of the body's normal *population of bacteria, or flora, which produce chemicals that inhibit the growth of some invading bacteria. All of these defenses are both external and nonspecific; that is, they protect the host as needed against any and all invaders.*

Once external barriers have been compromised, permitting harmful chemicals, foreign bodies, or microorganisms to penetrate cells and tissues, the **inflammatory response**, *or* **inflammation**, *occurs. This response, which begins within seconds of injury or invasion, is also nonspecific. It begins with the immediate marshaling of resources by vascular structures at the site of invasion. The affected tissues are soon surrounded by cells and fluids that are equipped to isolate, destroy, and remove the invaders, and thereby to promote healing.*

The third and last line of defense is the **immune response**, *or* **immunity**. *It occurs much more slowly than the inflammatory response and is specific in that it can confer permanent or long-term protection against specific microorganisms. It can also be induced by vaccination or inoculation. Unlike inflammation, which involves many different plasma systems and cell types, immunity is effected by one type*

of serum protein (immunoglobulin, or **antibody***) and one type of blood cell (lymphocyte). The many defenses against microorganisms are summarized in Table 6-1.*

The inflammatory and immune responses complement one another and interact in complex ways. Because many inflammatory processes are triggered or affected by simultaneous immune processes, an understanding of the immune response is necessary for an understanding of many aspects of inflammation. Therefore, the chapters in this unit will be presented in the sequence of immunity, inflammation, and diseases of immunity and inflammation. Chapter 6 will discuss normal immunity, including the role of antibodies and lymphocytes in protection against infectious organisms. Chapter 7 will discuss normal inflammation, including the interactions of the immune and inflammatory responses. Chapter 8 will discuss medically relevant aberrations in immunity and inflammation, including allergies, diseases that involve unwanted immunologic destruction of healthy tissue, and diseases that are caused by a deficiency in the normal immune or inflammatory responses.

TABLE 6-1

Defenses Against Infection

Type of defense	Specific mechanism
Surface defenses	Physical barriers: skin, conjunctivae, mucous membranes Mechanical removal: desquamation of skin, tears, mucus, ciliary action, coughing, salivation, swallowing, urination, defecation Normal bacterial flora: antibacterial factors Chemical inhibitors: gastric acid, lactic acid, fatty acids, spermine, lactoperoxidase, bile salts Antimicrobial substances: lysozyme, secretory IgA
Nonspecific resistance factors	Fever, interferons, complement, lysozyme, C-reactive protein (reacts with bacterial surface polysaccharides and activates complement), lactoferrin (binds and removes iron as a bacterial nutrient), α-1-antitrypsin (inhibits bacterial enzymes)

Inflammation	Soluble factors
	  Clotting system: Hageman factor (factor XII)
	  Complement system: chemotactic factors, anaphylatoxins
	  Kinin system: bradykinin
	Phagocytes
	  Circulating neutrophils, eosinophils, monocytes, macrophages
	  Fixed cells (of mononuclear phagocyte system) in alveoli, spleen, liver, bone marrow

Immune response	Humoral immune response: B cells, plasma cells, immunoglobulins Cell-mediated immune response: T cells, lymphokines

CHARACTERISTICS OF THE IMMUNE RESPONSE

The immune system of the normal adult is continually challenged by a spectrum of chemical substances that it recognizes as foreign, or "nonself." These substances are called **antigens.** Some antigens are on infectious agents, such as viruses, bacteria, fungi, or parasites; some are on noninfectious substances from the environment, such as pollens, foods, and bee venoms; and others are on drugs, vaccines, transfusions, and transplanted tissues.

The body's reaction to antigenic challenges is the immune response, in which physiologic and biochemical interactions cause the maturation and activation of two types of **immunocytes,** or **immunocompetent cells** (Fig. 6-1). The two types of immunocytes, B lymphocytes (B cells) and T lymphocytes (T cells), act in different ways to recognize and destroy specific antigens. They differ from the cells involved in inflammation in two ways. First, they have specificity, so that each individual B or T cell only recognizes one specific antigen. The B cells produce antibodies, which incapacitate the antigen, whereas the T cells attack the antigen directly. Second, once the B cells and T cells have been exposed to a particular antigen, some of them, called memory cells, become capable of "remembering" the antigen and of acting even faster if it invades the host again. Thus the immune system possesses memory and specificity and creates long-lasting protection against specific antigens. This process is termed **immunity.**

The immune response can be amplified or suppressed by both exogenous (external) and endogenous (internal) modulators. Some exogenous factors, such as trauma, disease, pollutants, radiation, ultraviolet light, and drugs, have profound effects on the capacity of an individual's immune system to respond to an antigenic challenge. The immune system is also modulated by certain endogenous factors, such as the individual's age, sex, nutritional status, genetic background, and reproductive status. The quality and intensity of the immune response are therefore a sum of the effects of all these factors: antigenic challenge, exogenous modulators, and endogenous factors.

Sometimes the normal immune response does not function in the best interests of the host and must be suppressed. For example, transplanted organs from donors are in danger of rejection as a result of the immune response. One means of lessening the likelihood of rejection is to match host tissues and donor tissues for antigenic compatibility, or histocompatibility. The other means is pharmacologic suppression of the immune response.

Another example of a functioning but detrimental immune response is an allergic reaction. Allergies are det-

FIG. 6-1 Scanning electron micrograph shows a mixed population of B and T lymphocytes (*L*). *Arrows* designate red blood cells. (From King, Fenoglio, & Lefkowitch, 1983.)

rimental immune responses in which the host's immune system "overreacts," or is hypersensitive, to the antigenic properties of certain substances, such as house dust, animal danders, and certain foods. (Immune deficiency diseases, autoimmune diseases, and allergic hypersensitivity are the subject of Chapter 8.)

Natural versus Acquired Immunity

Natural immunity, also called native or innate resistance, is not produced by the immune response. One type of natural immunity, which is present at birth, is species-dependent. Human beings are naturally immune to some of the infectious agents that cause illness in other species. For example, humans do not contract canine distemper or, as Jenner observed, serious cases of cowpox. The other type of natural immunity is host-dependent and involves the individual's characteristics that play some role in the development of specific diseases. (Analysis of risk factors, as described in Chapter 5, has identified some of these characteristics.)

Acquired immunity is gained after birth as a result of the immune response. Acquired immunity can be either active or passive, depending on whether the components of the immune response have been produced by the host or by a donor. **Active acquired immunity** is produced by the host after either natural exposure to an antigen or immunization. **Passive acquired immunity** does not involve the host's immune response. Rather, preformed antibodies or T lymphocytes are transferred to the recipient. This can occur naturally, as in the passage of maternal antibodies to the fetus, or artificially as in a clinical treatment. Clinically preformed antibodies from a donor (human or animal) are administered in the form of immune serum, which is antibody-containing blood from which the clotting factors and cells have been removed. Passive immunity is temporary and is used in the treatment of such clinical emergencies as rabies exposure, tetanus, and snakebite.

Primary and Secondary Immune Responses

The immune response to antigenic challenge has classically been divided into two phases, the primary and secondary responses. These phases can be demonstrated by serologic tests that measure plasma concentrations of antibody over time (Fig. 6-2). The initial administration of (or exposure to) most antigens is followed by a latent period during which mature B cells (called plasma cells) produce no detectable antibodies (immunoglobulin [Ig]). After approximately 5 days, one class of antibody (IgM) can be detected in the circulation. This marks the beginning of the initial or **primary immune response,** which is usually dominated by IgM, with lesser amounts of IgG (another class of immunoglobulin). With no further exposure to the antigen, the circulating antibody is catabolized (broken down) and measurable quantities fall. The individual's immune system,

however, has been primed. A second challenge by the same antigen results in the **secondary (or anamnestic) immune response,** which is characterized by the more rapid production of a larger amount of antibody than the primary response. The rapidity of the secondary immune response is the result of the presence of memory cells. The quantity of IgM produced in the secondary response is about the same as that produced in the primary response. IgG is the predominant antibody class of the secondary response and is frequently present in concentrations several times those of IgM. The greatest differences between the primary and secondary responses are in the amount of IgG that is produced and the rapidity with which antibody appears after antigen challenge.

The primary and secondary responses confer active acquired immunity. When an antigen, such as that on varicella (chickenpox) virus, enters the host for the first time, the primary immune response is activated. Antibody levels are not high, and the host becomes ill but recovers. If the host is exposed to varicella later in life, the secondary response occurs: antibody levels rise immediately, and the virus is neutralized before it can cause active infection.

The same thing happens as a result of immunization, except that the antigen is made less infectious (attenuated) or otherwise altered before administration so that it is strong enough to elicit the primary immune re-

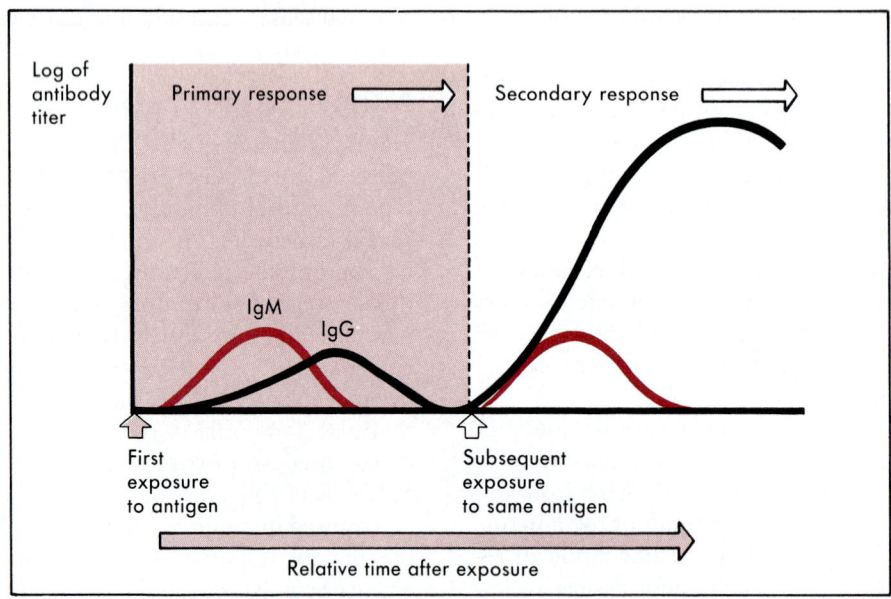

FIG. 6-2 Primary and secondary immune responses. The introduction of antigen induces a response dominated by two classes of immunoglobulins, IgM and IgG. IgM predominates in the primary response, with some IgG appearing later. After the host's immune system is primed, another challenge with the same antigen induces the secondary response, in which some IgM and large amounts of IgG are produced.

FIG. 6-3 Scanning electron micrograph of lymphocytes and macrophages. The lymphocytes are small and spherical; the macrophages are larger and more irregular in shape. (From Raven & Johnson, 1992.)

sponse but not strong enough to cause illness. Later exposure to the same antigen elicits the secondary immune response, preventing illness. In Jenner's experiment the antigens on cowpox and smallpox viruses were sufficiently similar that the cowpox antigen functioned as an altered, or attenuated, smallpox antigen. The antibodies and lymphocytes sensitized to recognize and destroy cowpox were also able to recognize the smallpox virus, thereby protecting the immunized child against smallpox.

Humoral versus Cell-Mediated Immunity

The primary immunocyte of the immune response is the lymphocyte (Fig. 6-3). The mature **lymphocyte** is a small, round, white blood cell approximately 6 to 10 micrometers (μm) in diameter.

Lymphocytes originate in the liver and spleen of the fetus and the bone marrow of the child or adult as lym-

FIG. 6-4 Lymphoid tissues: sites of B cell and T cell differentiation. Immature lymphocytes migrate through central lymphoid tissues: the bone marrow (probable central lymphoid tissue for B lymphocytes) and the thymus (central lymphoid tissue for T lymphocytes). Mature lymphocytes later reside in the T and B lymphocyte–rich areas of the peripheral lymphoid tissues.

phocyte precursors or stem cells. (Lymphocyte precursors are described in Unit IX.) They are not capable of implementing the immune response. To become immunocompetent, they must migrate through the lymphatics and blood vessels, then through lymphoid tissues in various parts of the body (Fig. 6-4). While passing through these tissues, they mature and undergo changes that commit them to one of two cellular lineages. The lymphocytes that migrate through one set of lymphoid tissues become **B lymphocytes, or B cells.** When B cells encounter antigens, they are stimulated to mature into plasma cells that produce antibodies. B cells are ultimately responsible for **humoral immunity** (see p. 214).

The lymphocytes that migrate through the thymus gland become **T lymphocytes, or T cells.** T cells are capable of becoming sensitized to and recognizing specific antigens, which they then attack directly. They are responsible for **cell-mediated immunity** (see p. 224).

The success of the immune response depends on the interaction between the humoral and cell-mediated responses, which share some components and processes. Differentiation (maturation) of T cells and B cells is shown in Fig. 6-5.

INDUCTION OF THE IMMUNE RESPONSE

Antigens and Immunogens

Although the terms *antigen* and *immunogen* are commonly used as synonyms, some technical differences between them are significant. An **antigen** is a molecule or molecular complex that reacts with preformed components of the immune system, such as lymphocytes and antibodies. Antigenicity is the molecule's innate capacity *to react with* those preformed components and is determined by the chemical structure of the antigen molecule. An **immunogen** is an antigen that can also *induce the formation of* components of the immune system (i.e., maturation of T and B lymphocytes and production of antibodies). Therefore, a substance may be antigenic—able to react with existing antibodies and mature lymphocytes—yet not immunogenic, that is, not able to induce the immune response.

A molecule is not antigenic unless at least a portion of its chemical structure can be recognized by and bound to specific (matching) receptors on a lymphocyte

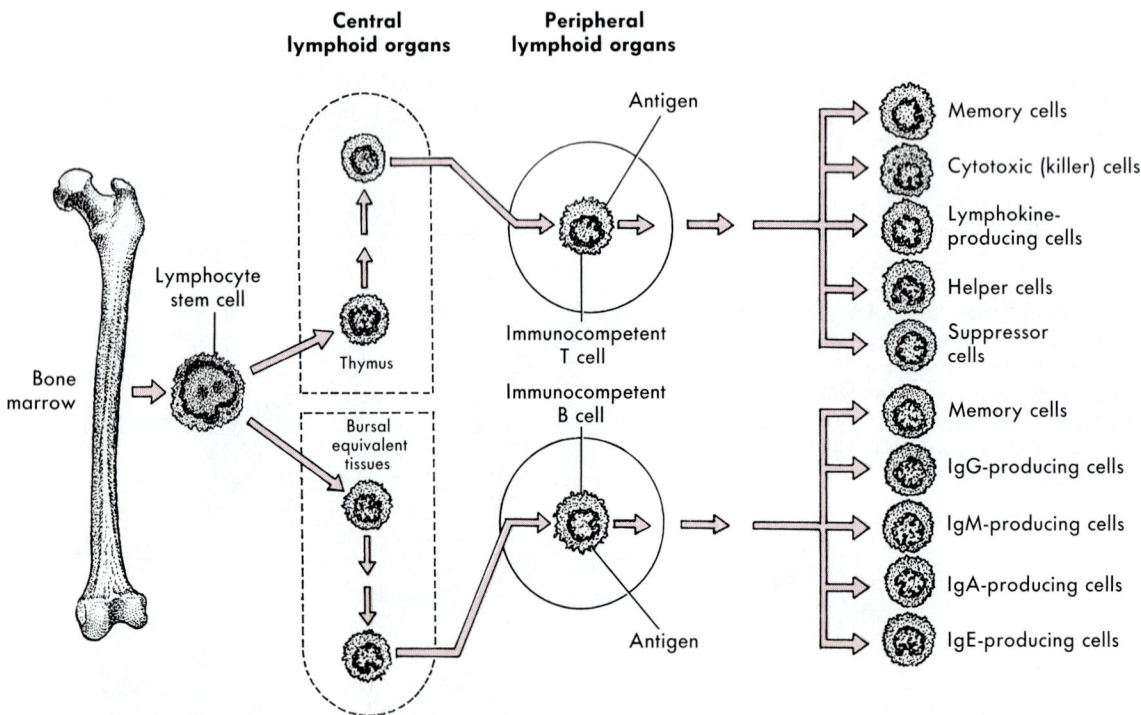

FIG. 6-5 Outcome of T (thymus-derived) and B (bursal-derived) pathways of lymphocyte maturation. Mature cells of the T cell lineage that have different functions usually develop from separate immature T cells. Mature B cells, on the other hand, may directly progress through the production of different classes of antibody against the same antigen. IgD is not shown because it does not circulate in the blood.

or antibody molecule. (Receptor function is described in Chapter 1.) The portion of the antigen molecule that is configured for recognition and binding is called an **antigenic determinant,** or **epitope.** The matching portion of the receptor on the lymphocyte or antibody is sometimes referred to as an antigen-binding, or antigen-combining, site, or **paratope.**

To be immunogenic, the antigenic molecule also must be (1) sufficiently foreign to the host, (2) sufficiently large, (3) sufficiently complex, and (4) present in sufficient amounts. In addition, the antigenic determinant sites must be accessible. Even if an antigen fulfills all these criteria, its ability to act as an immunogen may be affected by its route of entry into the host and by the host's endogenous characteristics, particularly genetic makeup.

Foremost among the criteria for immunogenicity is the antigen's foreignness. The immune system has the exquisite ability to distinguish self (**self-antigens**) from nonself (foreign antigens). Under normal conditions the immune system does not recognize self-antigens. This is the reason that the immune system is normally tolerant of the host's tissues but is able to reject foreign tissues and destroy infectious agents. **Tolerance,** once thought to be a state of nonresponsiveness in which the immune system passively allowed self-antigens to persist, is now known to be part of the active immune response. Rather than merely tolerating self-antigens, the immune system prevents their recognition by lymphocytes and antibodies. The response to self-antigens is active suppression of the immune system by specialized T lymphocytes called **suppressor T cells,** abbreviated **Ts** (see Fig. 6-5), and by specialized antibody called **anti-idiotypic antibody,** abbreviated **anti-ID.** Therefore, an antigen that fulfills the criteria of foreignness, size, complexity, and quantity will be immunogenic, whereas a self-antigen, which fulfills all the criteria *except* foreignness, will be **tolergenic.**

Molecular size also contributes to an antigen's immunogenicity. In general, large molecules (those greater than 10,000 daltons), such as proteins, polysaccharides, and nucleic acids, are most immunogenic. Low−molecular weight molecules, such as amino acids, monosaccharides, fatty acids, and the purine and pyrimidine bases, tend to be unable to induce the immune response. Many molecules in this size range can function as **haptens:** antigens that are too small to be immunogens by themselves but become immunogenic in combination with larger molecules.

The route and vehicle of entry or administration to the host are critical to the immunogenicity of some antigens. This has important clinical implications. The most common routes for clinical administration of antigen are the intravenous, intraperitoneal, subcutaneous, intranasal, and oral routes. Each route preferentially stimulates a different set of lymphocyte-containing (lymphoid) tissues (see Fig. 6-4), inducing different types of cell-mediated or humoral immune responses. Immunogenicity may also be altered by adjuvants (substances that stimulate the immune response) or by other agents that alter the processing of and the response to an antigen.

The genetic makeup of the host plays a critical role in the immune system's ability to respond to many antigens. The genes that affect the immune response are located on chromosome 6 and control the quality and quantity of the host's immune response. (Chromosomes and genetic inheritance are described in Chapter 4.)

Histocompatibility Antigens

How does the body actually recognize that a substance is foreign? The "code" that brings about this recognition consists of the major **histocompatibility antigens** (also called **HLA antigens** or **HLA determinants**), which are proteins found on the surface of nearly every cell in the body. HLA antigens play a role not only in defending the body against infection, but also in distinguishing each individual's tissue from the tissues of others.

HLA Complex

The major group of genes producing the HLA antigens is known as the **HLA complex,** or the **major histocompatibility complex (MHC).** This complex consists of four closely linked loci located on the short arm of chromosome 6. They are labeled A, B, C, and D complex. The antigens produced by the A, B, and C loci (class I antigens) are found on the surfaces of virtually all cells except erythrocytes (red blood cells), and they are involved in the rejection of foreign tissue. The D complex (class II antigens), on the other hand, consists of three separate and independent loci (DR, DP, and DQ) and are confined mostly to B lymphocytes, macrophages, some epithelial cells, and transiently to subpopulations of stimulated T lymphocytes.

Each HLA locus has many alleles: at least 20 at A, 40 at B, 10 at C, 14 at DR, 7 at DQ, and 6 at DP. With so many alleles at each HLA locus, many possible allele combinations exist, making it unlikely that two unrelated individuals will have the same HLA composition.

The specific alleles at the six HLA loci on one chromosome are termed the *haplotype.* Each individual has two HLA haplotypes, one for each chromosome. Because the loci are closely linked, the haplotypes are not usually disrupted by recombination and are thus transmitted intact to the offspring. Each parent passes one HLA haplotype to his or her offspring. The offspring then share one haplotype with each parent, and on the average, they share one haplotype with one half of their siblings, both haplotypes with one fourth of their siblings, and no haplotypes with one fourth of their siblings. Monozygotic twins, of course, have identical HLA haplotypes. This coexpression of both maternal and paternal alleles and the tremendous polymorphism make the HLA antigen system useful in determining paternity.

The HLA complex is particularly important, following discussion in determining the success of tissue grafts and organ transplants. The more similar two individuals are in their HLA makeup, the more likely the success of a transplant from one to the other (they must also have the same ABO blood type). Even when two people have the same HLA makeup, however, grafts sometimes are rejected because a number of other loci also determine tissue compatibility, although their effects are weaker than those of the HLA system. Thus it is always preferable to obtain a graft or transplant from a closely related individual, such as a sibling, because of a greater chance that a sibling will have the same histocompatibility antigens other than HLA.

Role of HLA Antigens

Although a certain degree of HLA matching is necessary for survival of grafted tissue in recipients, the function of the gene products of the major histocompatibility complex remains a partial puzzle. Obviously, these products have not evolved in order to confound transplanters of kidneys or hearts.

One function of class I and II antigens appears to be distinguishing of self from nonself. Many of the cellular interactions of the immune system require the recognition of foreign antigens in the context of self-antigens, either class I or II antigenic determinants.

Genetic loci within the HLA complex also control the quality and quantity of an immune response. These are referred to as **immune response genes,** or **Ir genes.**

Blood Group Antigens

The HLA antigens are not found on the surfaces of erythrocytes, but a number of other antigens that determine compatibility are found there. These are known collectively as the **blood group antigens.** More than 80 different red cell antigens are grouped into several dozen blood group systems, each determined by a different locus or set of loci. The most important of these, because they provoke the strongest humoral immune response, are the ABO and Rh systems.

Rh System

The **Rh blood group** (named after the rhesus monkey, the animal in which it was first discovered), with its high degree of polymorphism, is an antigen system second in complexity only to the HLA system. At least five major antigens and a large number of rare variants have been identified and are expressed only on erythrocytes (Rote, 1982). It appears to consist of three very tightly linked

genetic loci, labeled C, D, and E. Each locus has two alleles labeled C and c, D and d, or E and e. Distinct antigens are expressed by C, c, E, e, and D, whereas no distinct antigen has been observed for d. Therefore, d is considered a lack of D. The locus of greatest interest is the D locus, more commonly expressed as $Rh_o(D)$, because it is responsible for Rh maternal-fetal incompatibility and the resulting hemolytic disease of the newborn (see Chapter 25). Persons who have the DD or Dd genotype have the Rh antigen on their erythrocytes and are called Rh-positive. The recessive homozygotes, with genotype dd, are Rh-negative and do not have the Rh antigen. About 85% of North Americans are Rh-positive and about 15% are Rh-negative.

ABO System

Human blood transfusions were carried out as early as 1818, but they were often unsuccessful. Sometimes after a transfusion, the recipient's red blood cells would clump together, thereby blocking the capillaries, and cause death in some instances. In 1901 Karl Landsteiner reported that this reaction was caused by the ABO antigens located on the erythrocyte plasma membranes.

The **ABO blood group** consists of two major antigens, labeled A and B (Fig. 6-6). These appear to be codominant, so individuals can have one of four blood types. Individuals with blood type A carry the A antigen on their erythrocytes; individuals with blood type B carry the B antigen; those with blood type AB carry both A and B; those with type O carry neither antigen. A person with "type A blood" also has anti-B antibodies in the blood. If this person receives blood containing B antigens (i.e., blood from a type AB or B individual), a severe antibody reaction occurs. Similarly, a type B individual (whose blood contains anti-A antibodies) cannot receive blood from a type A or AB donor. Type O individuals, who have neither antigen but have both anti-A and anti-B antibodies, cannot accept blood from any of the other three types. These naturally occurring antibodies are immunoglobulins of the IgM class and are called **isohemagglutinins.**

Because individuals with type O blood lack both types of antigens, they can be "universal donors" and anyone can accept small volumes of their blood. Similarly, type AB individuals are "universal recipients," because they lack both anti-A and anti-B antibodies. When large volumes of *whole* blood are transfused, however, the donor's antibodies can bind to antigenic determinants on the recipient's erythrocytes. This reaction causes clumping of erythrocytes in the blood. Clumping (agglutination) and lysis are the causes of harmful transfusion reactions, which can be prevented only by complete and careful ABO matching between donor and recipient.

CLINICAL COMMENTARY   DETECTION OF HLA ANTIGENS

Different methods are used to detect classes I and II antigens. Class I antigens are identified by using an antibody-mediated, complement-dependent cytotoxicity assay devised by Terasaki and McClelland (1964). Lymphocytes are used as target cells because they are rich in HLA determinants and are easily obtained. The typing sera used are human sera obtained from either recipients of blood transfusions who have begun to produce antibodies against the leukocytes or multiparous women who have begun to produce antibodies against the HLA antigens of their mates.

Class II antigens have been detected by two different techniques. Originally, differences were determined by the mixed lymphocyte reaction (MLR). In the MLR, lymphocytes from two individuals are mixed under tissue-culture conditions. HLA-D antigens expressed on the surface of B lymphocytes from one donor (stimulator cells)

stimulate T lymphocytes from the other donor (responder cells). Lymphocyte stimulation is usually measured by incorporating a radioactive precursor, tritiated thymidine, into newly forming DNA. Other measures of proliferation, including increased cell number and formation of new RNA or protein, could also be used. In a two-way MLR, both donors' lymphocytes are allowed to respond, and proliferation is measured as the sum of both responses. More commonly, one-way MLRs, in which the lymphocytes of one donor are prevented from responding by preincubation with metabolic inhibitors, such as mitomycin C, or by preirradiation, are performed.

Panels of sera that identify molecules that appear to be identical with or very closely associated with the D antigens are now available. These serologically determined markers are termed HLA-DR, DP, and DQ.

Mixed lymphocyte reaction (MLR). The MLR measures the proliferation of responding T lymphocytes to HLA-D antigenic differences expressed on stimulator cells. Stimulator cells are initially inactivated by irradiation or by incubation with metabolic inhibitors to prevent their uptake of tritiated thymidine.

FIG. 6-6 Blood types. The relationship of antigens and antibodies involved in the ABO blood group system.

HUMORAL IMMUNE RESPONSE

B Lymphocytes

In birds, an organ called the bursa of Fabricius is responsible for the maturation of B lymphocytes (Glick, Chang, & Japp, 1956). Humans have no discrete bursa but do have tissues (probably the bone marrow) that make up the so-called **human bursal equivalent** (see Fig. 6-4). Lymphocytes destined to become B cells circulate through the bursal equivalent, where they undergo hormonally directed proliferation that gives them the capacity to react with antigen and generate diverse antibodies that protect the host against infection (see Fig. 6-5). B cell precursors cannot react with antigen, whereas postbursal B cells produce plasma membrane-bound antibodies of the IgM class, which can bind antigen.

It has been suggested that as many as 10^8 different antigenic determinants may be recognized by the immature B cells. Several theories have been generated to explain how such recognition occurs (Burnet, 1959; Jerne, 1955). The one most commonly held as correct is that of **clonal selection.** According to this concept, a large number of B cells with plasma membrane receptors for all potential antigenic determinants are spontaneously generated during fetal life, independent of the presence of antigen (Fig. 6-7). Each B cell, however, responds to only one specific antigen. When the immunocompetent B cells encounter an antigen for the first time, those with specific membrane receptors complementary to that antigen's determinant sites are stimulated to proliferate. B cells that have undergone this process are called **plasma cells** and can be found in the blood, secondary lymphoid organs (primarily spleen and lymph nodes), and some inflammatory sites. Thus two proliferative steps take place before antibody production can occur. The first, the generation of clonal diversity, probably takes place in the bursal-equivalent tissues, is hormonally driven and antigen-independent, and results in the generation of immature but immunocompetent B cells with plasma membrane receptors that can recognize virtually any antigenic molecule. The second, clonal selection, occurs in the peripheral lymphoid organs, is antigen-specific and antigen-driven, and results in the proliferation and maturation of antibody-secreting plasma cells. At about the eighth week of gestation in humans, antigen-driven differentiation may begin, although generation of clonal diversity probably continues in the bone marrow throughout most of adult life.

The immune response is initiated when an antigen

FIG. 6-7 Antibody production: generation of clones of antigen-specific B lymphocytes (B cells).
Under the control of hormones and without antigen, B lymphocyte precursors undergo cellular division
in the central lymphoid organs (bursal-equivalent tissues, probably bone marrow) and generate receptors against all possible antigens that may be encountered in the host's adult life. Later, primarily in the
peripheral lymphoid organs (spleen and lymph nodes), antigen presented by macrophages (phagocytic
cells of inflammation) reacts with the clones of B cells having appropriate receptors on their surfaces,
causing those cells to proliferate and produce antibody.

Physicochemical Properties of the Immunoglobulins

Class	Subclass	Heavy chain	Molecular weight (daltons)	Adult serum levels (mg/dl)
IgG	IgG1	γ_1	146,000	800-900
	IgG2	γ_2	146,000	280-300
	IgG3	γ_3	165,000	90-100
	IgG4	γ_4	146,000	50
IgM	IgM	μ	970,000	120-150
IgA	IgA1	α_1	160,000	280-300
	IgA2	α_2		50
	sIgA	α_1, α_2	385,000	5
IgD	IgD	δ	184,000	3
IgE	IgE	ϵ	190,000	0.03

binds and interacts with receptors on the surface of the immature B cell, triggering it into a sequence of proliferation and differentiation that results in the production of (1) immunoglobulin-secreting plasma cells and (2) a set of long-lived **memory cells** (see Figs. 6-5 and 6-7). The immunoglobulin-secreting plasma cells are active during the primary immune response. The memory cells are responsible for the secondary response that occurs on future exposure to the antigen (see Fig. 6-2). In other words, the memory cells are responsible for long-term immunity.

Immunoglobulins

Antibodies, or immunoglobulins, are serum glycoproteins produced by plasma cells in response to a challenge by an immunogen. The term **immunoglobulin** is used to denote all molecules of this type. **Antibodies,** on the other hand, are immunoglobulins known to have specificity for a particular antigen. The five molecular classes of immunoglobulins are IgG, IgA, IgM, IgE, and IgD. These classes are characterized by antigenic, structural, and functional differences (Table 6-2). Within the classes are several distinct subclasses, including four subclasses of IgG and two subclasses of IgA.

Structure of Immunoglobulin Molecules

Structural analysis of the immunoglobulins began with Porter's early studies on the effects of the enzyme papain on IgG (Porter, 1959). Limited papain digestion cleaved IgG into three fragments, two of which were identical (Fig. 6-8). The two identical fragments were found to retain the antigen-binding activity of the molecule and were termed **antigen-binding fragments (Fab).**

The third piece crystallized when separated from the Fab portions and was termed the **crystalline fragment (Fc).**

The Fab portions contain the recognition sites (receptors) for antigenic determinants and confer specificity. The Fc portion is responsible for most of the biologic functions of the molecule, including interactions with the nonspecific effector systems of inflammation, such as the complement cascade (see p. 240), for transport of maternal antibody to the fetus, and for binding to the surface of the effector cells of inflammation (polymorphonuclear neutrophils, macrophages, lymphocytes, mast cells, and platelets).

The antibody molecule consists of four polypeptide chains, two identical light (L) chains and two identical heavy (H) chains. Both light and heavy chains are divided into variable (V) and constant (C) regions. Among different antibodies the variable region is characterized by a large number of amino acid differences. The light chains of an antibody molecule are of either the kappa or lambda type and also consist of a variable (VL) and a constant (CL) region. Within the same molecule, the two heavy chains and two light chains are identical. Each class of antibody has a unique type of heavy chain: gamma (IgG), mu (IgM), alpha (IgA), epsilon (IgE), or delta (IgD) (Fig. 6-9). The light and heavy chains are held together by two major forces: noncovalent bonds and disulfide linkages.

The interaction of the variable region's amino acid sequences on both the heavy and light chains determines the conformation of the antigen-combining site and therefore the antigenic specificity of the immunoglobulin molecule (Fig. 6-10). In some cases the substitution of a single critical amino acid may have a significant effect on the shape of the combining site and specificity of the antibody molecule. The antigen fits into this binding site like a key into a lock and is held there by noncovalent chemical interactions.

Function of Antibodies

The chief functions of antibodies are to protect the host by (1) neutralizing bacterial toxins, (2) neutralizing viruses, (3) opsonizing bacteria (i.e., promoting phagocytosis [see p. 248]), and (4) activating components of the inflammatory response (Fig. 6-11 and Table 6-3).

Normally an antibody circulates in the blood or is suspended in body secretions until it encounters and binds to its appropriate antigen. At that time the antibody may play two roles: (1) it may have a direct effect on the antigen and (2) it may have an indirect effect on other mechanisms of self-defense. Directly, the antibody may produce **agglutination** (cause to clump together), **precipitation** (cause to fall out of solution), or **neutralization** (inactivate) of the antigen. Which of these occurs is determined by the class of antibody and the char-

FIG. 6-8 Molecular structure of an antibody. A, The molecule consists of four chains, two light *(L)* and two heavy *(H)*, held together by intra- and interchain disulfide linkages. The molecule can be divided into regions with variable *(V)* and relatively constant *(C)* amino acid structures (CH$_1$, CH$_2$, and CH$_3$ on the heavy chain). Between the CH$_1$ and CH$_2$ regions is the flexible hinge region *(Hi)*. **B,** Experimental fragmentation of IgG into its functional components by limited papain digestion.

FIG. 6-9 Structure of different immunoglobulins. Secretory IgA, IgD, IgE, IgG, and IgM.

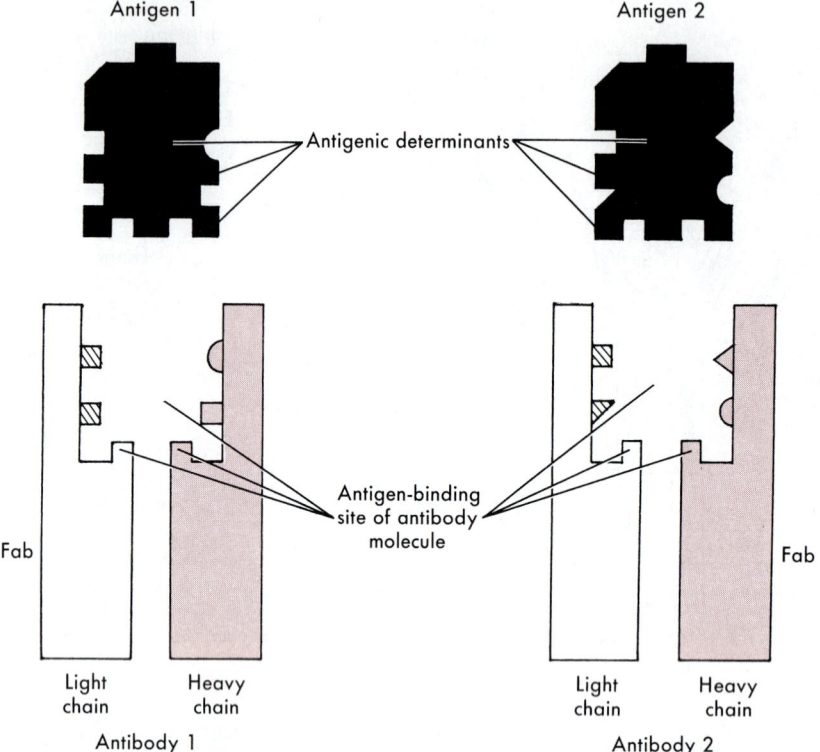

FIG. 6-10 Antigen-antibody binding. The specificity required for antibody binding with an antigen is determined by the shape of the combining site on the antibody.

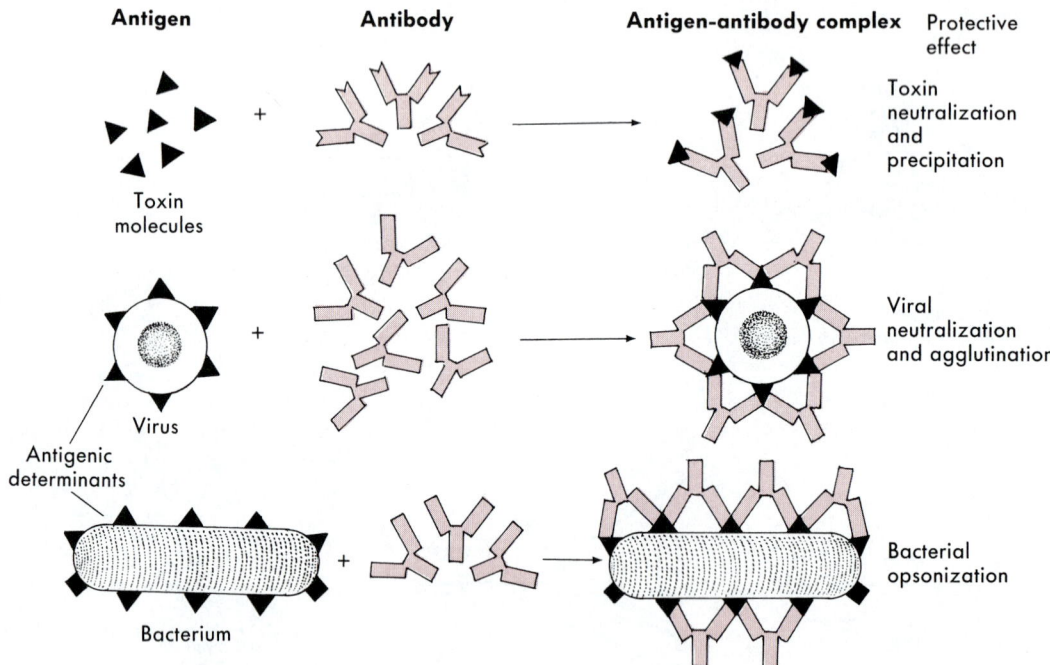

FIG. 6-11 Functions of antibody. Protective activities of antibodies include neutralization of bacterial exotoxins, neutralization of viruses and prevention of their interactions with cellular membranes, and opsonization of bacteria. All of these mechanisms are followed by removal of the antigen by phagocytosis, drainage along with body fluid, or both.

TABLE 6-3

Biologic Properties of the Immunoglobulins

Subclass	Complement activation		Binding to Fc receptors on				Placental transfer	Presence in secretions	Induction of agglutination
	Classical	Alternate	Macrophages	PMNs	Mast cells	Platelets			
IgG1	++	−	+	+	−	+	+++	±	+
IgG2	+	−	−	−	−	+	+	±	+
IgG3	+++	−	+	+	−	+	+++	±	+
IgG4	−	−	−	±	+	+	++	±	+
IgM	++++	−	−	−	−	−	−	+	+++
IgA1	−	+	−	±	−	−	−	+	−
IgA2	−	+	−	±	−	−	−	+	−
sIgA	−	−	−	−	−	−	−	++++	−
IgD	−	±	−	−	−	−	−	−	−
IgE	−	±	?	−	+++	−	−	+	−

NOTE: Minus sign = lack of activity; plus sign = relative degree of activity; PMN = polymorphonuclear neutrophil. (Complement activation and the function of monocytes, PMNs, mast cells, and platelets are described in the section on inflammation, beginning on p. 235.)

acteristics of the antigen. Protection always begins with antigen-antibody binding. The antibody molecule's Fab portions bind with antigenic determinant sites on the antigen. Binding results in **antigen-antibody complexes,** also called **immune complexes.** Antigen-antibody binding may directly affect the antigen by occupying its antigenic determinant sites, rendering them unable to bind with receptors on host cells. For example, viruses that are neutralized in this way are unable to infect cells because the first step in penetrating a host cell is binding with receptors on the cell's plasma membrane.

The indirect effects of antibodies also involve the binding of antigen into antigen-antibody complexes. Once bound, however, it is the Fc portion of the antibody molecule that confers indirect protection. Indirect protection consists of (1) enhancement of phagocytosis and (2) activation of plasma proteins that are capable of destroying the antigen. Both of these activities involve components of the inflammatory response: phagocytes (see p. 248) and proteins of the complement cascade (see p. 240).

Neutralization of bacterial toxins

Many bacteria produce toxins that enhance their pathogenic effects and harm the host in a variety of ways. (The injurious effects of bacterial toxins are described in Chapter 2.) Fortunately for the host, bacterial toxins are immunogens and are capable of initiating the humoral immune response. One of the principal roles of the antibodies subsequently produced is to function as antitoxins that neutralize bacterial toxins.

The mechanism of neutralization is the formation of antigen-antibody complexes (in this case, toxin-antitoxin complexes), which is the result of antigen-antibody binding (see Figs. 6-10 and 6-11). Simply stated, the antibodies "capture" the toxin molecules by occupying their antigenic determinant sites. This prevents the toxins from binding to tissue cells and exerting their harmful effects. Once the antigen-antibody complexes are formed, they may precipitate out of solution in body fluids or be removed from the body by **phagocytosis** (ingestion by phagocytic cells; see p. 248 for a discussion of phagocytosis).

Detection of the presence of specific antitoxins can aid in the diagnosis of diseases. For example, laboratory tests that detect antistreptolysin O or anti-DNAse B measure antibodies produced against those toxins and can be very useful in the diagnosis of group A streptococcal infections.

Actively induced immunity against many pathogens can be achieved by immunization (vaccination) with their toxins. To prevent harming the recipient, the toxins are chemically inactivated, resulting in a toxoid that has few toxic properties but retains immunogenicity. Vaccines against such diseases as diphtheria and tetanus are toxoids.

Neutralization of viruses

Antibodies protect the host against some viral infections by preventing the attachment and entrance of viruses into host cells. The mechanism of viral neutralization is shown schematically in Fig. 6-11. Neutralized viral particles may agglutinate or be ingested and removed by phagocytes.

Many viruses (e.g., measles, herpes) are usually inaccessible to antibody because they do not circulate in the bloodstream. Instead they remain in extravascular tissue cells and tend to spread by direct cell-to-cell contact. Antibodies against these viruses are most effective in preventing the initial infection but usually play only a minor role in recovery from a primary (initial) infection or in preventing recurrent infection. Other viruses, such as polio and influenza, spread from cell to cell through the blood and are more susceptible to the effects of circulating antibodies. These viruses can be controlled by antibodies even after the initial infection.

Protection against many viral infections, such as rubella, can be elicited effectively by vaccination with inactivated viruses. Levels of circulating IgG are usually a good indication of the degree of protection. Because antibody protects against reinfection, some vaccines have been designed to induce antibody production at the site of viral entrance into the body. For example, both oral and injected polio vaccines prevent systemic infection in the recipient, but only the oral preparation readily protects against the carrier state by inducing a secretory IgA response at the usual site of viral entry, which is the gastrointestinal tract.

Opsonization of bacteria

An **opsonin** is a substance that renders bacteria susceptible to phagocytosis. Antibodies themselves are opsonins; antibodies also induce opsonization by complement component C3b (see p. 248). **Opsonization,** the process of opsonin-enhanced phagocytosis, is necessary because many bacteria have an outer capsule that resists phagocytosis unless antibody is produced against it.

Activation of inflammatory processes

One function of an antibody is essentially translation: it acts as a bridge that lends specificity to the inflammatory response. One end of the immunoglobulin molecule, Fab, specifically binds to antigens, and the other end, Fc, informs the nonspecific amplifiers of the inflammatory response, both molecular and cellular, that an unwanted substance has invaded the body, either from the outside (e.g., infectious agents) or from within the body (e.g., a malignancy). Antigens are usually complex and bind several antibodies so that when an antigen reacts with the Fab regions of antibody, the Fc portions are held in close proximity to other Fc regions. The clustering of Fc regions results in (1) the binding to and activation of the complement cascade (see p. 248) and (2) the recognition of and binding to receptors (Fc receptors) on the surfaces of inflammatory cells.

Classes of Immunoglobulins

Fig. 6-9 illustrates the structure of the immunoglobulins. IgG constitutes 80% to 85% of the circulating immunoglobulins. The biologic activities attributed to the IgG subclasses are summarized in Table 6-3. IgG is the major class of immunoglobulin in the immune response and is responsible for most of the antibody functions, such as precipitation, agglutination, and complement activation. As a result of selective transport across the placenta, maternal IgG is also the major antibody found in fetal blood.

IgA has two subclasses, IgA1 and IgA2. The predominant antibody in normal body secretions is secretory IgA, which is predominantly IgA2. IgA in the blood is predominantly IgA1. The secretory piece is attached to IgA dimers in the mucosal cells and may protect the molecule against degradative enzymes in secretions. (The biologic role of IgA is discussed on p. 222.)

IgM is the largest immunoglobulin and has 10 theoretical antigenic binding sites, although only 5 are functional. It is the first antibody produced during the initial, or primary, response to antigen (see Fig. 6-2). IgM is synthesized early in neonatal life, and its synthesis may be increased as a response to infection in utero. The trophoblast cells that cover the surface of the placenta lack Fc receptors for IgM; therefore, the molecule does not cross the placenta under normal conditions.

Information on the role of IgD is very limited. It is found in very low concentrations in the blood and is primarily located on the surfaces of developing B lymphocytes.

IgE is the least concentrated of any of the immunoglobulins in the circulation (see Table 6-3). It is also the principal antibody in the allergic response (see Chapter 8) and in the prevention of parasitic infections.

Antibodies as Antigens

Because antibodies are proteins, they can also serve as strong antigens and immunogens. For instance, if human IgG is injected into a rabbit, the animal will recognize the human antibody as foreign and begin producing an immune response. That response will be characterized by the production of rabbit antibody that is reactive with the immunogen, the human IgG. Antibody molecules usually contain antigenic determinants that can be classified into one of three groups: isotypic, allotypic, and idiotypic (Fig. 6-12).

Isotypic antigens are species-specific, so the antigen differs between species of animals but is the same within the species. These determinants are usually found within the constant regions and are used to differentiate between kappa and lambda light chains and among the different subclasses of heavy chains. For instance, the

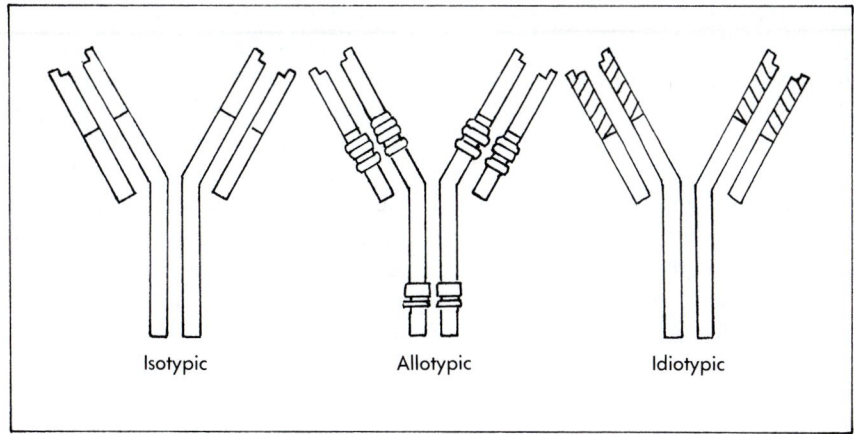

FIG. 6-12 Antibodies as antigens. Antibodies contain three types of antigenic determinants: isotypic, allotypic, and idiotypic.

human gamma heavy chain in IgG1 has an antigenic determinant that is found on IgG1 antibodies in all humans and differs from determinants found on any other class or subclass of human antibody and from those found on IgG1 antibodies from other species of animals. All members of the species will express in their blood a mixture of all isotypes representative of that species. Antibodies against isotypic determinants are commonly used in research and clinical laboratories to differentiate between classes of antibody and between antibodies from different species.

Allotypic antigens are those that are alleles expressed within a species. Antibodies from some members of a species would have a particular antigenic determinant that would differ from the same class and subclass of antibody from another member of the species. Allotypic determinants are also generally found in the constant region of both heavy and light chains, although they differ from the isotypic determinants found in the same general region. Each class and subclass of heavy or light chain has its own set of allelic determinants. For instance, the gamma heavy chain has a region called Gm that is allotypic, of which there are at least 25 known allotypes. Kappa chain has an allotypic region called Km, of which there are at least three known allotypes: Km(1), Km(2), and Km(3). Some members of the same species may have kappa chains that bear the Km(1) determinant and other members of the species will have the Km(2) or Km(3) determinant. If IgG from a Km(1)-bearing individual were injected into a person who possessed only the Km(2) allotype, an antiallotypic antibody against the Km(1) antigenic determinant would be produced.

Idiotypic antigenic determinants are found in the variable regions of heavy and light chains. Commonly an idiotypic determinant will consist of amino acids contributed by each variable region. Because of their location, many idiotypic antigens are found in the combining site on antibody and are characteristic of the antigenic specificity of that molecule. For instance, IgG3 produced against an antigen on the mumps virus will have a characteristic variable region that allows it to bind specifically to that antigen. IgG3 produced in the same individual but against a different antigen, such as tetanus toxoid, will have a different variable region that determines its specificity. Each IgG3 will have a unique set of amino acids in the variable region that will determine the antibody's specificity but will also be recognized as unique idiotypic antigenic determinants. Thus the IgG3 molecules produced in the same individual against mumps and tetanus toxoid will have different idiotypic determinants, although the isotypic and allotypic determinants may be identical. Antibodies produced against idiotypic determinants are called **antiidiotypic antibodies** and may be normally involved in controlling an individual's immune response against a specific antigen.

Monoclonal Antibodies

Most humoral immune responses are polyclonal; that is, a mixture of antibodies is produced from multiple clones of B lymphocytes (see Fig. 6-7). This occurs because most immunogens have multiple antigenic determinants and may stimulate a spectrum of B lymphocytes to proliferate. Each clone secretes antibody that differs slightly from that secreted by other clones, even though all the B cells were stimulated to proliferate by the same immunogen. The antibodies are heterogeneous in immunoglobulin class, amino acid sequence, specificity, and function, and some react more strongly with the antigen than others.

In 1975 César Milstein and Georges Kohler produced an antibody, called a **monoclonal antibody,** that would (1) act against a single specific antigen and (2) be produced by a single clone of B cells that could be maintained indefinitely in the laboratory. Monoclonal antibody was produced by hybridizing B cells from the spleens of mice that had been injected with a specific antigen and "immortal" plasma cells (B cells) from a plasma cell tumor (malignant myeloma). The result was a **hybridoma:** a B cell clone that was both antigenspecific and capable of indefinite proliferation. The hybridoma produced monoclonal antibodies. The advantages of monoclonal antibodies over conventional antisera (antibody-containing sera) are that (1) a single antibody of known antigenic specificity is generated rather than a mixture of different antibodies; (2) monoclonal antibodies have a single, constant binding affinity; (3) monoclonal antibodies can be diluted to a constant titer (concentration in fluid) because the actual antibody concentration is known; and (4) the antibody can be easily purified to homogeneity.

The generation of monoclonal antibodies is creating new therapeutic and diagnostic possibilities, particularly in the treatment of cancer and early detection of viral infections. Detection of viral infections thus far has been limited to verification that a particular virus is the cause of disease because diagnosis is generally performed by measuring the specific antibody response against the virus and any antibody that is produced immediately reacts with circulating antigen and therefore cannot be detected by routine serologic tests. Diagnosis is made after viral antigen has been removed from the blood, and the patient is recovering. Monoclonal antisera, on the other hand, can be selected against specific antigenic determinants of the virus, produced in large quantities, and used in tests for elevations in circulating viral antigen that appears early in the disease. Over the next 10 years and as a result of hybridoma technology, the clinician will be able to order tests for viral antigens that are specific and diagnostic and detect the disease early in its course.

Secretory Immune System

The immune system within the body is called the **systemic immune system.** A distinct set of lymphoid tissues make up another, partially independent, immune system at the external surfaces of the body, the **secretory (mucosal) immune system.** Most humoral immune responses occur when antibodies or B cells encounter antigens in the blood, but sometimes this encounter occurs in other body fluids. Some antibodies are present in secretions such as tears, sweat, saliva, mucus, and breast milk, where they can protect the body (or the neonate) against antigens that have not yet penetrated the skin or mucous membranes.

Although antibodies in both blood and secretions are produced by B cells that have matured into plasma cells, antibodies in blood are produced by cells of the systemic immune system, whereas antibodies in secretions are produced by cells of the secretory (mucosal) immune system. The B cells of these two systems follow a different pattern of migration once they leave the bone marrow and enter the lymphatics. Lymphocytes of the systemic immune system travel through the spleen and most lymph nodes (see Fig. 6-4). Lymphocytes of the secretory immune system travel through a different group of lymphoid tissues (Fig. 6-13): the lacrimal (tearproducing) and salivary glands, and lymphoid tissues in the breast, bronchi, intestines, and genitourinary tract. Immunoglobulins that are secreted at these sites are called secretory immunoglobulins (hence secretory IgA) and act locally rather than systemically.

Local protection is necessary to combat antigens (chiefly infectious microorganisms) that are inhaled, are swallowed, or otherwise come in contact with external body surfaces. Once they have taken up residence in the external layers of the body, harmful microorganisms can multiply, and the host becomes a carrier. These microorganisms may (1) cause local disease (e.g., cholera); (2) penetrate the skin or mucosa and cause systemic disease (e.g., gram-negative bacterial infection of the blood—septicemia—if the integrity of the gut is disturbed); (3) not cause disease in the carrier (because of effective systemic immunity) but be spread to other individuals; or (4) pass out of the body without any ill effects (e.g., in feces). The major function of the secretory immune system is to halt viral and bacterial invasion before local or systemic disease develops. When secretory immunoglobulins bind and react with microorganisms, they are unable to attach to and invade mucosal tissue.

IgA is the dominant secretory immunoglobulin, although IgM and IgG are also present in secretions. The primary role of IgA is to prevent the attachment and invasion of pathogens through mucosal membranes, such as those of the gastrointestinal, pulmonary, and genitourinary tracts. To induce protective immunity against some pathogens that enter through these routes, providing local immunization seems to be preferable to inducing only systemic immunity. The Sabin vaccine against polio is administered orally as an attenuated live virus. This route causes a transient, limited infection and induces effective systemic immunity and secretory immunity, preventing both the disease and the establishment of a carrier state. The Salk vaccine, on the other

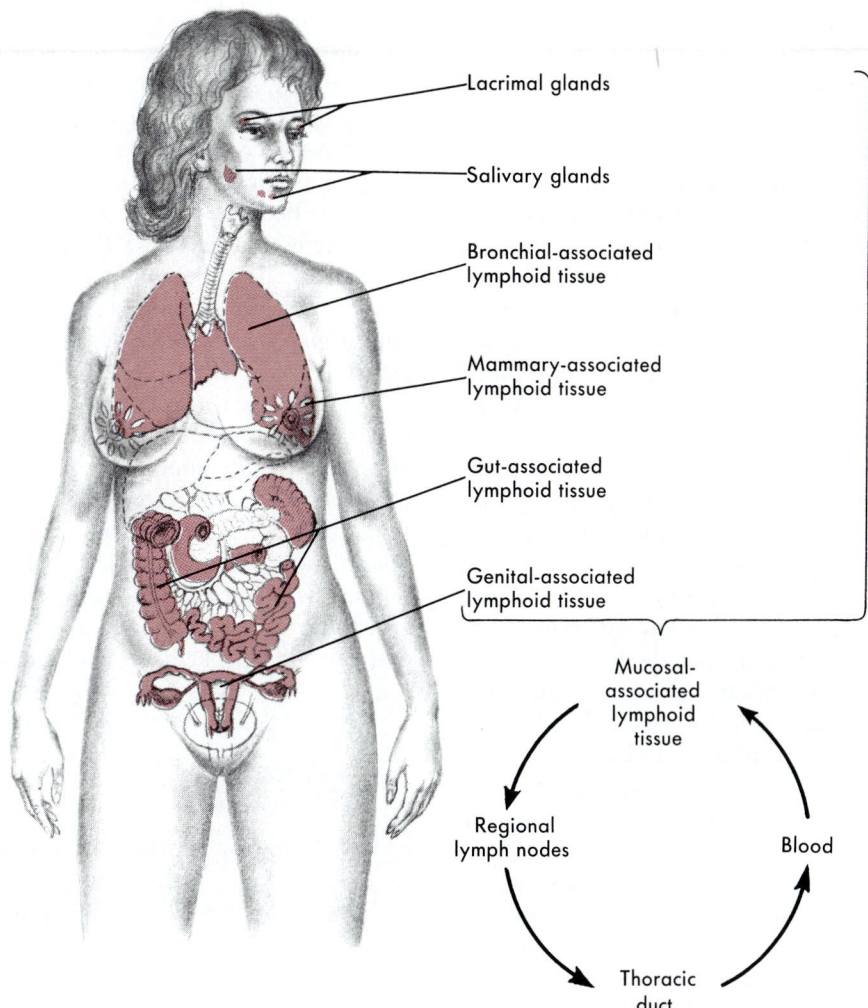

- Lacrimal glands
- Salivary glands
- Bronchial-associated lymphoid tissue
- Mammary-associated lymphoid tissue
- Gut-associated lymphoid tissue
- Genital-associated lymphoid tissue

Mucosal-associated lymphoid tissue

Regional lymph nodes

Blood

Thoracic duct

FIG. 6-13 **Mucosal-associated lymphoid tissues of the secretory immune system.** Lymphocytes from the mucosal-associated lymphoid tissues circulate throughout the body in a pattern separate from other lymphocytes. For example, lymphocytes from the gut-associated lymphoid tissue circulate through the regional lymph nodes, the thoracic duct, and the blood and return to other mucosal-associated lymphoid tissues rather than to lymphoid tissue of the systemic immune system.

hand, consists of killed viruses that are administered intradermally. It induces adequate systemic protection but does not generally prevent an intestinal carrier state.

The breast-associated lymphoid tissue is in the trafficking pattern of cells of the secretory immune system, so most antigens to which the mother has been exposed gastrointestinally induce sensitized lymphocytes that migrate to the breast and secrete IgA, IgM, and IgG into the milk. Antibodies against infectious disease agents are found in the milk and may provide protection to the newborn against those pathogens, such as polio, that invade through the gut. Colostral antibodies do not cross the newborn's gut after the first 24 hours of life and do not have a role in the newborn's systemic immunity.

The mechanisms of antigen-antibody binding are the same in the secretory and systemic immune systems; that is, binding neutralizes or opsonizes the antigen, preventing it from harming the host. The major differences between the two systems are that:

1. Their lymphocytes follow different paths of migration and pass through different lymphoid tissues.
2. The secretory immune response is one of the body's first lines of defense, whereas the systemic response is the body's final defense.
3. The secretory response occurs locally and externally (in body secretions), whereas the systemic response occurs systemically and internally (in blood and tissues).

CELL-MEDIATED IMMUNE RESPONSE

Some lymphocytes are destined to develop into T lymphocytes (T cells), which are responsible for cell-mediated immunity. They are called *T cells* because they are processed through the thymus gland. There are five types of mature T cells, each with a different immune function. Memory cells induce the secondary immune response; **lymphokine-producing cells** transfer delayed hypersensitivity (Td) and secrete proteins (lymphokines) that activate other cells such as **macrophages** (see Chapter 8); **cytotoxic (Tc) cells** attack antigens directly and destroy cells that bear foreign antigens, and **helper T (Th)** and **suppressor T (Ts) cells** control both cell-mediated and humoral processes. (The maturation of T cells is shown in Fig. 6-5.) The Td cell phenotype is probably a subset of Th cells that produces the appropriate lymphokines for activating macrophages but does not provide any other helper function.

The process of T cell proliferation and differentiation shown in Fig. 6-14 is similar to that shown in Fig. 6-7 for B cells. The chief difference is that the generation of clonal diversity takes place in the thymus for T cells and in the human bursal equivalent for B cells.

The role of the thymus in the maturation of the immune system did not become apparent until relatively recently (Miller, 1961; Mitchell & Miller, 1968). Lymphocytes destined to become T cells journey through the thymus, where, under the pressure and guidance of the thymic hormones and without the presence of antigen, they are driven to proliferate and simultaneously generate the capacity to recognize the diversity of antigens that the host will encounter throughout life. They exit the thymus as immature (i.e., inactive) but antigenically committed (immunocompetent) T cells. Immature T cells produce plasma membrane receptors that are not antibody but are related molecules with similar specificity for antigens. The **thymus**, which atrophies at puberty and practically disappears in adulthood, consists of a cortex and a medulla interspersed with connective tissue. Prethymic lymphocytes from the fetal liver, spleen, and bone marrow circulate through the bloodstream and seed the thymus during embryonic life. In the postcapillary venules of the thymic medulla, prethymic lymphocytes interact with thymic endothelial cells and enter the body of the thymus. Entrance into the thymus appears to be highly restricted to lymphocytes and also to be unidirectional. The lymphocytes distribute themselves in the thymic meshwork, where they rapidly proliferate in the cortex of the organ and probably migrate inward to the medulla as they mature into T cells capable of recognizing many different antigens.

During maturation in the thymus, T cells begin producing new proteins that are differentiation related and inserted into the plasma membrane of the cell. These proteins have been identified using monoclonal antibodies and are classified as "cluster of differentiation" or CD antigens. At least 80 different antigens comprise the CD system. The functional roles of many of these proteins have been determined, and several important CD antigens participate in the development of the immune response. Because of their association with different immune activities, several CD antigens are markers for particular cells of the immune system. The most important of these are listed in Table 6-4, and their order of appearance in thymocyte development is listed in Table 6-5.

The thymic epithelium produces several hormones involved in the maturation of T cells. These include forms of thymosin, thymopoietin, ubiquitin, thymostimulin, and several other hormones. The biologic roles of many thymic hormones are known. Thymic peptide hormones not only are involved in T cell differentiation within the thymus itself but also may diffuse into the bloodstream and influence uncommitted lymphocytes in the bone marrow and peripheral lymphoid tissues to travel to the

TABLE 6-4

CD Antigenic Markers of T Cell Development

CD no.	Cell type
1	Early thymocytes
2	Early thymocytes, receptor for sheep RBCs
3	T cells, interacts with T cell receptor
4	Th cells, adhesion molecule for class II HLA binding
5	T cells
7	Early thymocytes
8	Tc and Ts cells, adhesion molecule for class I HLA binding

TABLE 6-5

Order of CD Marker Appearance in Thymocyte Development

Earliest thymocyte	CD2,7+
	CD1,2,7+
	CD1,2,3,5,7+
	CD1,2,3,5,7,TCR+
	CD1,2,3,5,7,TCR,4,8+
Most mature thymocyte	CD1,2,3,5,7,TCR,4+ or CD1,2,3,5,7,TCR,8+

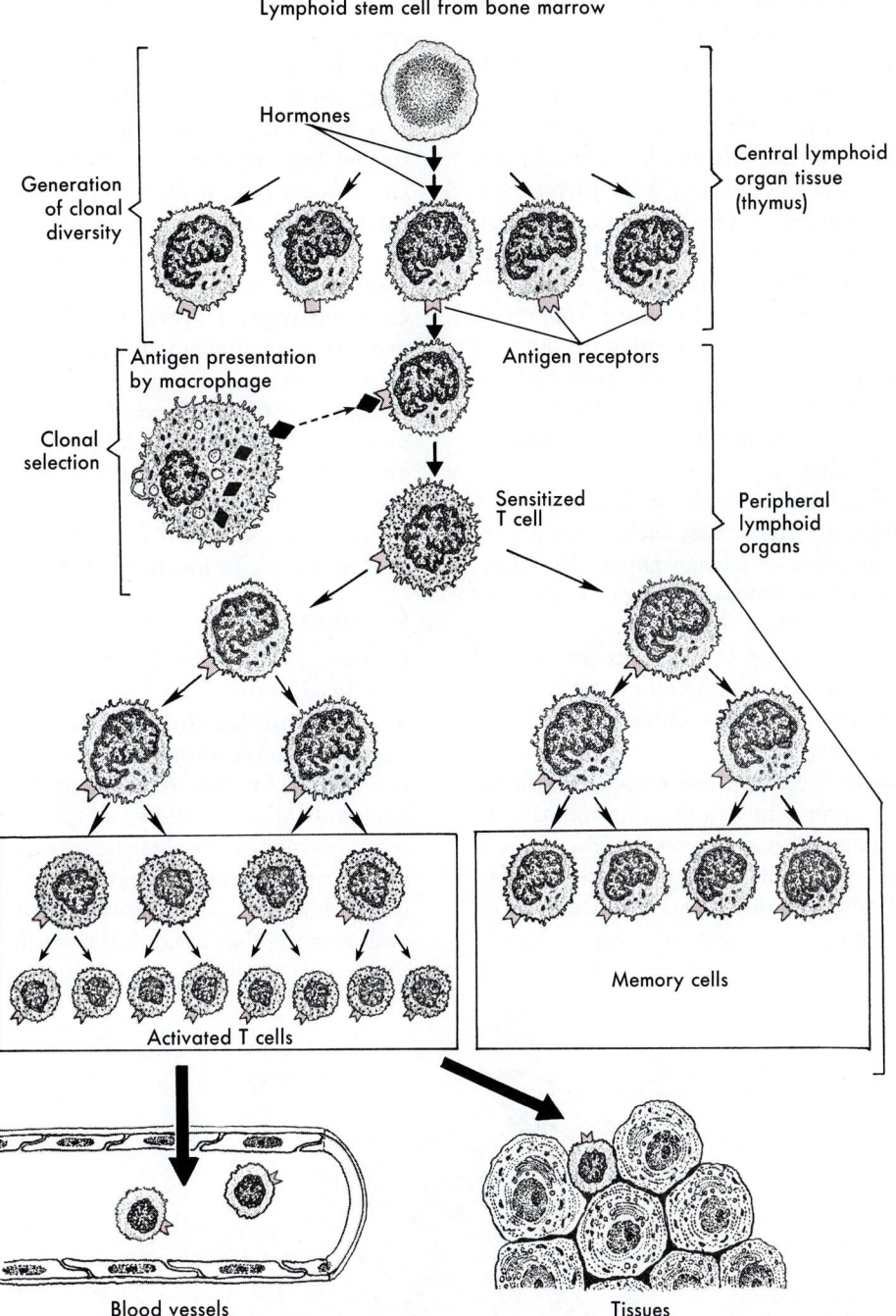

FIG. 6-14 T cell production: generation of clones of antigen-reactive T lymphocytes. Under the control of hormones and without antigen, T lymphocyte precursors undergo cellular division in the central lymphoid organ (the thymus) and generate receptors against all possible antigens that may be encountered in the host's adult life. Later, antigen encountered in the peripheral lymphoid organs reacts with the clones of cells expressing appropriate receptors on their surfaces, causing those cells to proliferate and produce functional T lymphocytes. (Modified from Tortora, Funke, & Case, 1986.)

thymus. In other words, immature precursor lymphocytes may become irreversibly committed to thymic maturation even before entering the thymus.

Antigenically committed but immature T cells exit the thymus through the blood vessels and lymphatics. When immature T cells encounter an antigen they are capable of binding with, they are stimulated to proliferate. This step is different from the proliferation that occurred in the thymus in that (1) all the cells produced are capable of recognizing the same antigen; (2) proliferation is driven by antigen and not dependent on thymic hormones; and (3) subpopulations of the immature T cells produce mature T cells having different functions (cytotoxicity, memory, helper functions, or suppressor functions). Therefore, the end product of antigen-driven proliferation is a large number of T cells capable of acting against the same antigen in a variety of ways.

The major effects of the cell-mediated immune response are the following:

1. *Cytotoxicity*: Cytotoxic T cells mediate the direct, cellular killing of target cells, such as virally infected cells, tumors, or foreign grafts. This function requires cellular contact, binding, and release of toxic substances from the Tc cell.
2. *Delayed hypersensitivity*: The Td cells are involved in the inflammatory response and produce soluble mediators (lymphokines) that influence other cells, such as macrophages.
3. *Memory*: Memory cells are also responsible for the accelerated response to a second antigenic challenge (the secondary immune response).
4. *Control*: Helper T cells facilitate and suppressor T cells inhibit both humoral and cell-mediated immune responses.

CELLULAR INTERACTIONS IN THE IMMUNE RESPONSE

Very few antigens can act alone as immunogens. For example, very few can directly induce immature B lymphocytes to become antibody-producing plasma cells. Antigens that do have this capacity are likely to have repeating antigenic determinants (multiple identical antigenic determinant sites). Because these antigens can stimulate B cells without the help of T cells, they are called T-independent antigens (Fig. 6-15). The repeating antigenic determinants interact with the B cell's membrane receptors at multiple sites, inducing the cross-linking of receptors and the activation of antibody production. Antigens that cannot induce the immune response independently must first interact with several populations of cells, including T helper (Th) cells and **antigen-presenting cells (APC)**. Antigen-presenting cells are usually macrophage or macrophage-like cells in tissue (i.e., Langerhans cell in the skin, B cells, and endothelial cells; see Figs. 6-7 and 6-14), with the participation of soluble products of these cells (cytokines).

Cytokines

Cytokines were originally characterized as small molecular weight proteins or glycoproteins (proteins containing carbohydrate) that are secreted by cells participating in the immune response. They function as "messengers" of the immune response in that cytokines provide communication among macrophages and various subsets of lymphocytes. During an immune response one of the participants may produce a cytokine that is released, binds to a specific receptor on a neighboring cell, and instructs that target cell to respond in a genetically

FIG. 6-15 Activation of a B cell by a T cell independent antigen. Repeating and identical antigenic determinants interact with several receptors on the surface of the B cell and mainly induce the production of IgM.

programmed fashion. Cytokines produced by lymphocytes are referred to as **lymphokines**, and those produced by monocytes/macrophages are called **monokines**. Because of their role in intercellular communication, cytokines have been called "hormones" of the immune response. The effects of these hormones may be on neighboring cells (paracrine), or they may bind to and affect the same cell that produced them (autocrine). (Paracrine, autocrine, and endocrine forms of cellular communication are discussed in Chapters 1 and 10.)

After cytokine stimulation a target cell may respond in many ways. One of the most common responses is increased production of proteins that are inserted in the plasma membrane and function as receptors. Many of these receptors are specific for various cytokines, but others are necessary for protection against infectious agents, such as receptors for complement component C3b or receptors for the Fc portion of antibody. Most cytokines will also cause the target cell to initiate proliferation and differentiation. Because this effect is common among cytokines, there is a great deal of redundancy in that different cytokines will have similar effects on the same target. The participation of cytokines is absolutely essential to the development of an adequate immune response.

Cytokines are produced by a wide variety of cells and guide many other cellular activities beyond the immune response. Many are growth factors that induce the proliferation and differentiation of cells other than lymphocytes, for example, other hemopoietic blood cells (see Chapter 22). In addition, the development and growth of the placenta during pregnancy are dependent on a variety of cytokines produced by both the mother and the child.

Antigen Processing, Presentation, and Recognition

When an antigen enters the host, it first equilibrates throughout body fluids. Antigen circulates through the spleen if it enters intraperitoneally or intravenously and to the regional draining lymph nodes if it enters by the subcutaneous or gastrointestinal routes. Antigen entering by the bloodstream is usually filtered through the red pulp of the spleen, where it encounters splenic lymphocytes. Antigen entering through the interstitial spaces is usually drained by the afferent lymphatics to the regional lymph nodes, where it enters the sinusoids. These spaces in the lymph node architecture are lined with phagocytic cells that ingest antigen. (Lymph nodes and lymphatic vessels are described in Chapter 26.)

At this point a process known as **antigen processing** occurs (Fig. 6-16). After its ingestion by a macrophage in the lymph node, the antigen is degraded. A portion of the degraded antigen is reexposed, or expressed, on the plasma membrane of the phagocyte, which "pre-

FIG. 6-16 Antigen processing and presentation. Circulating antigen is phagocytosed by macrophages. Remnants of the digested antigen are expressed on the membrane of the phagocyte and, in conjunction with HLA determinants, are presented to lymphocytes to initiate the immune response. The macrophage produces interleukin-1 (IL-1) that helps the T cell respond to antigen.

sents" it to T or B cells (see Figs. 6-7 and 6-14). Antigen processing and presentation are necessary for an immune response to occur. Antigen processing can also occur at many other sites including other lymphoid organs, the skin, and mucous membranes.

For presentation to occur effectively, the antigen must be in a complex with molecules of class I HLA antigens or class II HLA antigens. The particular HLA class that bears the antigen helps to determine which cell will respond to the presentation of that antigen. For Th cells to respond, the antigen must be presented in a complex with class II HLA antigens, those of the HLA-D/DR series. For Tc cells and Ts cells to respond, the antigen must be presented in a complex with class I HLA antigens of the HLA-A and B series. Th cell recognition of antigen, therefore, is referred to as "class II restricted," whereas Tc and Ts cell recognition of antigen is referred to as "class I restricted."

The T cell "sees" the presented antigen through a set of receptors found on the surface of the cell. At least two sets of receptors participate in this interaction; one is antigen specific (the T cell receptor), and the other is independent of the presented antigen (CD4 or CD8). The T cell receptor (TCR) is similar to the Fab portion of an antibody in that it consists of two protein chains and contains a combining site that specifically recognizes antigen. The two chains are referred to as alpha and beta chains, each of which has a variable region and a constant region. The TCR is inserted into the membrane in association with another set of proteins that make up the complex referred to as CD3. The combined effects of antigen binding to the TCR, the interaction with CD3, and the activation of other molecules in the lymphocyte membrane result in a signal being communicated to the cell as one of the signals for differentiation to begin.

A recently recognized group of antigens has the property of binding to certain groups of TCRs at sites away from the normal antigen-specific combining site. Because the antigen is not limited to reacting with only a few T cells that bear the appropriate antigen-specific TCR, many more T cells will be given an activation signal and initiate differentiation. The resultant increase in the immune response has led to these antigens being referred to as "super-antigens."

Before differentiation can proceed, however, a second signal is necessary. That signal is provided through CD4 for Th cells or CD8 for Tc and Ts cells. CD4 and CD8 are also proteins that are exposed on the lymphocyte surface. Neither will recognize the presented antigen directly. Each will bind specifically to regions of the HLA molecule that are away from the site where antigen is being presented. CD4 recognizes a particular amino acid sequence found on class II HLA molecules, and CD8 recognizes a sequence found on class I HLA molecules.

The interaction of these molecules contributes to the physical association of T cells and antigen-presenting cells and provides a second signal to initiate T cell differentiation.

The macrophage also produces a hormone, interleukin-1 (IL-1), that helps the T cell respond. During antigen presentation, IL-1 is released by the macrophage and binds to specific IL-1 receptors on the surface of the Th cell. One of the first steps in Th cell differentiation in response to these multiple signals is the production of another cytokine, IL-2. Without IL-2 production, the Th cell cannot efficiently mature into a functional helper cell. IL-2 has an autocrine effect in that it binds to specific IL-2 receptors on the surface of the same cell that is producing it. The results of the interaction of IL-2 and its receptor are an increased production of both IL-2 and IL-2 receptor, further differentiation of the Th cell, proliferation of the Th cell, and the production of other cytokines, such as IL-4 and IL-6.

T Cell and B Cell Differentiation
T Cell Differentiation

The development of cytotoxic T cells (Tc), which are responsible for the cell-mediated destruction of such targets as tumor cells or virally infected cells, requires the presentation of foreign antigen in association with class I antigens of the major histocompatibility complex. Tc cells can see antigen on the surface of antigen-presenting cells or other target cells. For instance, some viruses that infect cells will produce viral-specific antigens that complex with class I HLA antigens on the surface of the infected cell. The Tc cell binds presented antigen with a TCR identical with that found on Th cells. The interaction of CD8 with a portion of the class I molecule provides another differentiation signal. As with Th-antigen–presenting cell interactions, a cytokine must also interact with the Tc cell to induce complete maturation and development of cytotoxic activity. IL-2 from the Th cell fulfills this role.

B Cell Differentiation

B lymphocytes can also recognize antigen, either on the surface of antigen-presenting cells or in soluble form, although the particular antigenic determinant recognized may differ from that recognized by the Th cell. This recognition is apparent from studies using carriers and haptens. Haptens are not normally immunogenic. When haptens are covalently bound to high–molecular weight proteins (carriers) and injected into an animal, however, the B lymphocytes frequently recognize the hapten, and the Th cell recognizes the carrier portion. The result is the production of antibody against the hapten.

The antibody response of the B lymphocyte is under the control of hormones (interleukin-2 and other interleukins) secreted by the activated Th cell. Some of these hormones probably mimic the effects of antigens with repeating determinants by directly activating the B lymphocytes. Interleukins are not antigen-specific, so the Th cell activated by one antigen (i.e., the carrier) can produce a factor that facilitates the production of antibody against another antigen (i.e., the hapten).

B cell differentiation proceeds through multiple stages, each of which is under the control of cytokines. After interaction with antigen, B cells will proliferate, undergo class switch during which the class of antibody produced by the cell may change, and differentiate into plasma cells that are antibody "factors" with no further capacity to undergo cell division. IL-1, IL-2, and IL-4 most likely provide some of the signal to begin differentiation and proliferation. Class switch appears to be under the control of a variety of interleukins. For instance, IL-4 induces class switch to IgG1 and IgE, TGF-B (transforming growth factor-beta) helps class

switch to IgA, and IL-6 induces differentiation into IgG- and IgM-secreting plasma cells. The production of pentameric IgM is enhanced by IL-2, which controls J chain expression. Most of these cytokines are produced by Th cells, and each cytokine binds to its target through specific cell membrane receptors.

Control of B and T Cell Development

Like most systems of the body that are activated by outside influences, the immune system is conserved by being activated only during time of need and then completely or partially turned off after the threat to the individual has been repelled. Concurrently, the immune system is normally prevented from recognizing and rejecting its own tissue.

Several types of suppressor cells, including Ts cells and some monocytes and macrophages, control both the humoral and cell-mediated activities of the immune sys-

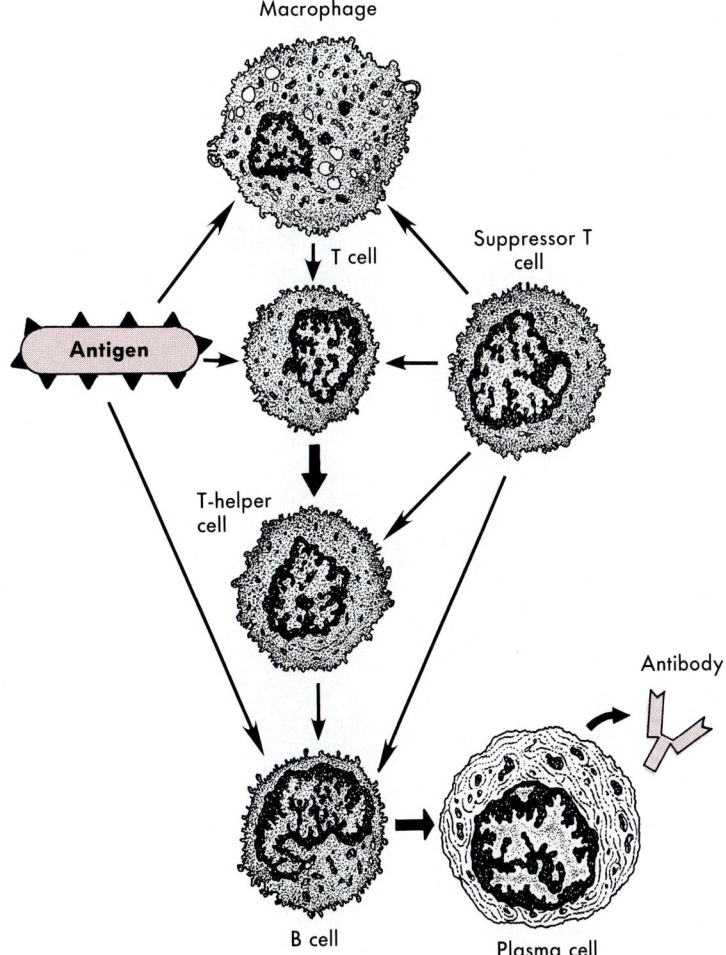

FIG. 6-17 Possible sites of suppressor T lymphocyte (Ts) effects on the production of antibody. The effect of one cell on another *(thin arrows)* and the maturation of one cell type into another *(thick arrows)* are represented. The effect of Ts cells appears to be on the early induction or proliferation phases of the immune response. The principal target of soluble suppressor factors is probably the Th cell, although other interactions have not been ruled out.

tem. Suppressor cells appear to vary in specificity, some being antigen-specific and others relatively nonspecific for a particular antigen or specific for only one class of antibody or effector cell (Fig. 6-17). Some suppressor cells affect the recognition of antigen and others suppress the proliferative steps that follow antigen recognition. Tolerance of self-antigens is apparently another suppressor cell function. Although the role of suppressor cells is currently under intense investigation, the degree of their heterogeneity of derivation, function, and specificity is far from determined.

FETAL AND NEONATAL IMMUNE FUNCTION

The normal human infant is immunologically immature at birth. Although cell-mediated immunologic capabilities begin developing early in gestation and are probably completely functional at birth, antibody production, phagocytic activity, and complement activity are clearly deficient. In the last trimester, the fetus appears capable of producing a primary immune response (almost entirely IgM) to antigenic challenge in utero and to infections such as cytomegalovirus, rubella virus, and *Toxoplasma gondii*. The fetus is unable to produce a significant IgG response, however. The capacity to produce IgA is underdeveloped, although some IgA can be detected.

To protect the child against infectious agents in utero and during the first few postnatal months, a system of active transport facilitates the passage of maternal antibodies into the fetal circulation (Fig. 6-18). In the placenta, maternal and fetal blood is separated by a layer of specialized cells termed *trophoblasts*. Immunoglobulins are too large to diffuse across the trophoblastic layer. The trophoblastic cells actively transport immunoglobulins from the maternal to the fetal circulation. Active transport of maternal IgG is mediated by surface receptors that are specific for the Fc portion of free IgG, but not for IgM, IgE, or IgA. Active transport sometimes results in higher antibody titers in umbilical cord blood than in maternal blood. (Active transport mechanisms are discussed in Chapter 1.)

At birth total IgG levels in the umbilical cord are near adult levels. When the source of maternal antibodies is severed at birth, antibody titers in the newborn begin to drop as maternal antibody is catabolized (Fig. 6-19). Thus antibody titers drop rapidly even though the neonate's production of IgG is beginning to rise. This occurs because the rate of catabolism is more rapid than the rate of production. Total immunoglobulin levels

Maternal circulation

IgG

Fetal circulation

FIG. 6-18 Transport of IgG across the trophoblast. The transport of maternal IgG across the trophoblast and into the fetal circulation is an active process. Maternal IgG binds to Fc receptors on the surface of the trophoblast and is enclosed in vacuoles by the process of endocytosis. Receptors on the trophoblast are specific for the Fc portion of IgG and do not bind other classes of immunoglobulins. The interaction of IgG with the receptors protects the antibody from digestion during transport of the vacuole across the cell. On the fetal side, IgG is released into the fetal circulation by exocytosis (see Chapter 1).

reach a minimum at 5 to 6 months in the normal child, occasionally causing transient hypogammaglobulinemia (insufficient quantities of circulating immunoglobulins). Many normal infants experience recurrent respiratory tract infections at this time.

AGING and Immune Function in the Elderly

Immune function decreases in old age. T cell function and specific antibody responses to antigenic challenge diminish, yet there is an increase in levels of circulating autoantibodies (antibodies against self-antigens) and immune complexes. In addition, there is an increased incidence of spontaneous monoclonal antibody production without concurrent B cell malignancy (myeloma).

The central lymphoid organ for T cell development, the thymus, reaches maximum size at sexual maturity and then begins involuting until it is a vestigial remnant by middle age. By age 45 to 50, thymic size is only 15% of its maximum. The level of thymic hormone production and the capacity of the thymus to mediate T cell differentiation decrease with thymic atrophy. Numbers of circulating T cells do not decrease with age, but T cell function may deteriorate. Individuals over 60 years of age generally exhibit decreased delayed hypersensitivity response (as demonstrated by milder positive reactions in tuberculin skin tests), decreased T cell–mediated responses to infections, and decreased T cell activity (as demonstrated by laboratory assays of T cell function).

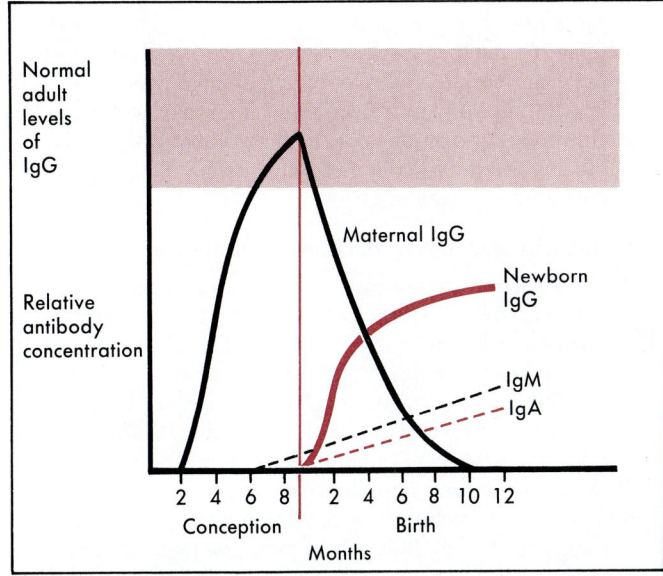

FIG. 6-19 Antibody levels in the umbilical cord blood and neonatal circulation. Early in gestation, maternal IgG crosses the placenta and enters the fetal circulation. At the time of birth, the fetal circulation contains nearly adult levels of IgG, which is almost exclusively maternal, and small amounts of fetal IgM and IgA. After the delivery of the infant, maternal IgG is rapidly catabolized while neonatal IgG production increases.

SUMMARY REVIEW

Characteristics of the Immune System

1 Immunity is a state of protection, primarily against infectious agents, characterized by memory and specificity.
2 Antigens are chemical substances that react with preformed components of the immune response. Immunogens are antigens that can also induce an immune response. Haptens are antigens that cannot be immunogenic unless they are bound to larger molecules called carriers.
3 Self-antigens are antigens on host cells. Self-antigens are normally not recognized as immunogenic by the host's immune system, a condition known as tolerance.

Induction of the Immune Response

1 The immune response is characterized by the activation of two types of immunocytes: B lymphocytes (B cells) and T lymphocytes (T cells). The activities of B cells compose the humoral immune response, those of T cells the cell-mediated immune response.

2 A B cell develops from a stem cell that matures under hormonal control in bursal-equivalent tissues and develops into a mature plasma cell capable of producing antibody against a specific antigen.
3 Antibodies are plasma glycoproteins that can be classified by chemical structure and biologic activity as IgG, IgM, IgA, IgE, or IgD.
4 Antibodies may protect the host from harmful antigens by recognizing and binding with the antigen's antigenic determinant sites. Occupied antigenic determinants on viruses and bacterial toxins are unable to bind with receptors on host cells and are, therefore, unable to have injurious effects.
5 The protective effects of antibodies vary with the identity of the antigen. Antibodies opsonize bacteria, neutralize toxins and viruses, and activate inflammatory processes.
6 Antibodies of the systemic immune system function internally, in the bloodstream and tissues. Antibodies of the secretory, or mucosal, immune system function externally, in the secretions of mucous membranes.

7 A T cell develops from a stem cell that matures under hormonal control in the thymus and develops into a cytotoxic T cell, which can kill target cells directly; a delayed hypersensitivity T cell, which produces lymphokines that affect other cells (especially macrophages); a helper T cell, which induces B cells to produce antibody; or a suppressor T cell, which suppresses antibody production and immune function.

8 Antibody production is the final stage of a process requiring the interaction of B cells, helper T cells, and antigen-presenting cells.

Cellular Interactions in the Immune Response

1 Antigens that cannot induce the immune response independently must first interact with several populations of cells, including T-helper cells, macrophages (as antigen-presenting cells), and cytokines.

2 Cytokines are proteins or glycoproteins secreted by cells participating in the immune response. They function as "messengers" enabling communication among macrophages and lymphocytes.

3 When an antigen enters a host, it first equilibrates throughout body fluids. Eventually, antigen encounters macrophages, for example, by circulating through interstitial spaces in the lymph node. At this point, antigen processing occurs.

4 For antigen presentation to lymphocytes to occur, it must be in a complex with molecules of class I HLA antigens or class II HLA antigens. For Th cells to respond, the antigen must be presented in a complex with class II HLA antigens (HLA-D/DR). For Tc cells and Ts cells to respond, the antigen must be presented in a complex with class I HLA antigens. During antigen presentation, interleukin-1 (IL-1) is released by the macrophage and binds to receptors of the Th cell. The Th cell then responds by producing IL-2. IL-1 and IL-2 most likely provide a signal to begin differentiation and proliferation of B lymphocytes or antibody production.

Fetal and Neonatal Immune Function

1 Mechanisms of self-defense are naturally somewhat deficient in the fetus, the neonate, and the elderly.

2 The primary immune response is adequate in the fetus and neonate, but the secondary immune response does not develop fully until about 6 months of age. Maternal antibodies protect the neonate for the first 6 months, after which they are catabolized.

Aging and Immune Function in the Elderly

1 T cell function and antibody production in response to specific antigenic challenge are somewhat deficient in the elderly. The elderly also tend to have increased levels of circulating autoantibodies (antibodies against self-antigens).

KEY TERMS

ABO blood group, 212
Acquired immunity, 207
Active acquired immunity, 207
Agglutination, 216
Allotypic antigen, 221
Antibody, 206, 216
Antigen, 207, 210
Antigen-antibody complex, 219
Antigen-binding fragment (Fab), 216
Antigenic determinant, 211
Antigen presenting cell, 226
Antigen processing, 227
Anti-idiotypic antibody (anti-ID), 211, 221
Blood group antigen, 212
B lymphocyte (B cell), 210
Cell-mediated immunity, 210
Clonal selection, 214
Crystalline fragment (Fc), 216
Cytokine, 226
Cytotoxic cell (Tc), 224
Epitope, 211
Hapten, 211
Helper T cell (Th), 224
Histocompatibility antigen (HLA antigen, HLA determinant), 211

HLA complex, 211
Human bursal equivalent, 214
Humoral immunity, 210
Hybridoma, 222
Idiotypic antigenic determinant, 221
Immune complex, 219
Immune response (immunity), 206
Immune response gene (Ir gene), 212
Immunity, 207
Immunocyte (immunocompetent cell), 207
Immunogen, 210
Immunoglobulin, 216
Inflammatory response (inflammation), 206
Interleukin-1 (IL-1), 228
Isohemagglutinin, 212
Isotypic antigen, 220
Lymphocyte, 209
Lymphokine, 227
Lymphokine-producing cell, 224
Macrophage, 224
Major histocompatibility complex (MHC), 211
Memory cell, 216

Monoclonal antibody, 222
Monokine, 227
Natural immunity, 207
Neutralization, 216
Opsonin, 220
Opsonization, 220
Paratope, 211
Passive acquired immunity, 207
Phagocytosis, 219
Plasma cell, 214
Precipitation, 216
Primary immune response, 208
Rh blood group, 212
Secondary immune response (anamnestic response), 208
Secretory (mucosal) immune system, 222
Self-antigen, 211
Suppressor T cell (Ts), 211, 224
Systemic immune system, 222
T cell receptor (TCR), 228
Thymus, 224
T lymphocyte (T cell), 210
Tolerance, 211
Tolergenic antigen, 211

REFERENCES

Burnet, F. M. (1959). *The clonal selection theory of acquired immunity*. London: Cambridge University Press.

Glick, B., Chang, T. S., & Jaap, R. G. (1956). The bursa of Fabricius and antibody production. *Poultry Science, 35,* 224-225.

Good, R. A., Dalmasso, A. O., Martinez, C., Archer, O. D., Pierce, J. C., & Papermaster, B. W. (1962). The role of the thymus in development of immunologic capacity in rabbits and mice. *Journal of Experimental Medicine, 116,* 773-796.

Jenner, E. (1798). *An inquiry into the causes and effects of the variolae vaccinae: A disease discovered in some of the western counties of England, particularly Gloucestershire, and known by the name of the cow pox*. London: Sampson Low.

Jerne, N. K. (1955). The natural-selection theory of antibody formation. *Proceedings of the National Academy of Sciences, 41,* 849.

King, D. W., Fenoglio, C. M., & Lefkowitch, J. H. (1983). *General pathology: Principles and dynamics*. Philadelphia: Lea & Febiger.

Koch, R. (1891). Fortsetzung der Mitteilungen über ein Heilmittel Gegen Tuberkulose. *Deutsche Medizinische Wochenschrift, 9,* 101-102.

Kraus, R. (1897). Über spezifische Reaktionen in Keimfreien Flitraten aus Cholera, Typhus, and Pestbouillonculturen, erzeugt durch Homologes Serum. *Weiner Klinische Wochenschrift, 10,* 736-738.

Landsteiner, K. (1901). Uber Aggluanohn-Verschenungen Normaten Menschlichen Blutes. *Weiner Klinische Wochenschrift, 14,* 1132-1134.

Metchnikoff, E. (1883). Untersuchungen über die Intracelluláre Verdauung bei Wirbellosen Tieren. *Arb Zool Inst Wein und Zool Station Triest, 5,* 141-168.

Miller, J. F. A. P. (1961). Immunological function of the thymus. *Lancet, 2,* 748-749.

Mitchell, G. F., & Miller, J. F. A. P. (1968). Immunological activity of thymus and thoracic duct lymphocytes. *Proceedings of the National Academy of Sciences, 59,* 296.

Pfeiffer, R. (1894). Weitere Untersuchungen über das wesen der Choleraimmunität und über specifische Baktericide Prozesse. *Z Hyg Infekt Krankh, 18,* 1-16.

Porter, R. R. (1959). The hydrolysis of rabbit gammaglobulin and antibodies with crystalline papain. *Biochemistry Journal, 73,* 119.

Raven, P. H., & Johnson, G. B. (1992). *Biology*. St. Louis: Mosby—Year Book.

Rote, N. S. (1982). Pathophysiology of Rh isoimmunization. *Clinical Obstetrics and Gynecology, 25,* 243-254.

Terasaki, P. I., & McClelland, J. D. (1964). Microdroplet assay of human serum cytotoxins. *Nature, 204,* 998.

Tortora, G. J., Funke, B. R., & Case, C. L. (1986.) *Microbiology: An introduction* (2nd ed.). (p. 450). Menlo Park, CA: Benjamin/Cummings.

von Behring, E., & Kitasato, S. (1890). Úber das Zustandekommen der Diphtherie-immunität und der Tetanus-immunität bei Thieren. *Deutsche Medizinische Wochenschrift, 16,* 1113-1114.

von Gruber, M., & Durham, H. E. (1896). Eine neue Methode zur raschen Erkennung des Choleravibrio und des Typhusbacillus. *Muenchener Medizinische Wochenschrift, 43,* 285-286.

SUGGESTED READINGS

Ballanti, J. (1985). *Immunology III*. Philadelphia: W. B. Saunders.

Bordet, J. (1895). Les leucocytes et les proprietes actives du serum chez les vaccines. *Annals of the Institute of Pasteur, 9,* 462-509.

Dausset, J. (1981). The major histocompatibility complex in man. *Science, 213,* 1469.

Ehrlich, P. (1877). Beitage zur Kenntnis der Anilinfarbungen und Ihrer Verwendung in der Mikroskopischen technik. *Arch Mikr Anat, 13,* 263-277.

Hildemann, W. H., Clark, E. A., & Raison, R. L. (1981). *Comprehensive immunogenetics*. New York: Elsevier.

Klein, J. (1990). *Immunology*. New York: Blackwell Scientific.

Kohler, G., & Milstein, C. (1975). Continuous cultures of fused cells secreting antibody of predefined specificity. *Nature, 256,* 495.

Kuby, J. (1992). *Immunology*. New York: Freeman.

Milanese, C., Richardson, N. E., & Reinherez, E. L. (1986). Identification of a T helper cell-derived lymphokine that activates resting T lymphocytes. *Science, 231,* 1118-1122.

Nossal, G. J. V. (1987). Current concepts—immunology: The basic components of the immune system. *New England Journal of Medicine, 316,* 1320-1325.

Rosenbaum, J. T., & Engleman, E. G. (1982). Histocompatibility antigens and disease susceptibility. In J. J. Twomey (Ed.), *The pathophysiology of human immunologic disorders* (p. 51). Baltimore: Urban & Schwarzenberg.

Scott, J. R., & Rote, N. S. (1985). *Immunology in obstetrics and gynecology*. Norwalk, CT: Appleton-Century-Crofts.

Stites, D. P., & Terr, A. I. (1991). *Basic and clinical immunology* (7th ed.). Los Altos, CA: Lange Medical.

Terasaki, P. I. (Ed.). (1980). *Histocompatibility testing*. Los Angeles: UCLA Tissue Typing Laboratory.

Inflammation

Neal S. Rote

Chapter Outline

I nflammation is a biochemical and cellular process that occurs in vascularized tissues. Most of the essential components of the inflammatory process are found in the circulation, and most of the early mediators (facilitators) of inflammation affect the vascular bed so as to increase the movement of plasma and blood cells from the circulation into the tissues surrounding the injury. These substances, known collectively as **exudate**, defend the host against infection and facilitate tissue repair and healing.

As described in antiquity, the superficial hallmarks of inflammation include redness (rubor), swelling (tumor), heat (calor), pain (dolor), and loss of function (functio laesa). The development of the microscope, however, enabled investigators to detect inflammatory changes at the cellular level. In the nineteenth century, Julius Cohnheim observed three characteristic changes in the microcirculation (arterioles, capillaries, and venules) near the site of an injury. He saw that (1) blood vessels were dilated, increasing blood flow to the area; (2) vascular permeability was increased, resulting in the outward leakage of plasma, which formed an inflammatory exudate; and (3) white blood cells adhered to the inner walls of vessels, then emigrated through vessel walls to the site of injury.

Inflammation and repair can be divided into several phases (Fig. 7-1). The characteristics of the early inflammatory response differ from those of the later response, and each phase involves different biochemical mediators and cells that function together to (1) destroy injurious agents and remove them from the inflammatory site; (2) wall off and confine these agents so as to limit their effects on the host; (3) stimulate and enhance the immune response; and (4) promote healing.

In contrast to the immune system, which is antigen-specific and has memory, the inflammatory response is nonspecific because it takes place in about the same way no matter what the stimulus and occurs in the same manner even on second exposure to the same stimulus. Unlike chronic inflammation, the acute response is self-limiting; that is, it continues only until the threat to the host is eliminated. This usually takes 8 to 10 days, from onset to healing. Inflammation is considered chronic if it persists longer than 2 weeks.

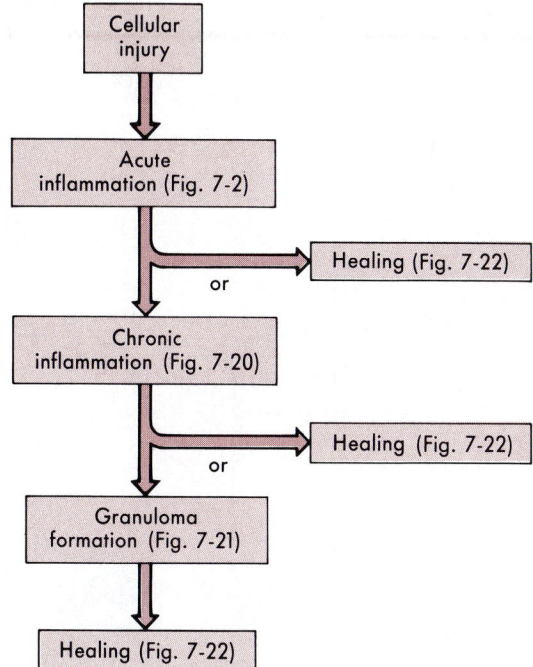

FIG. 7-1 The inflammatory process. Cellular injury leads to acute inflammation, which may result in resolution and healing of the injured site or progress into chronic inflammation. Chronic inflammation, in turn, may result either in healing or progress into the development of a granuloma. The final step of the process is usually healing and reconstruction of the damaged tissue. The figure numbers refer to those in which more detailed information may be found on that portion of the process.

THE ACUTE INFLAMMATORY RESPONSE

The acute inflammatory response begins after lethal or nonlethal cellular injury (Fig. 7-2). Cellular injury may be caused by trauma (mechanical forces), oxygen or nutrient deprivation, genetic or immune defects, chemical agents, microorganisms, temperature extremes, or ionizing radiation. (Mechanisms of cellular injury are described in Chapter 2.) Inflammation is also triggered by the presence of dead cells, which may be host cells, microorganisms, or cells of dead parasites.

Unlike the immune response, which takes days to develop, the vascular effects of inflammation are immediate, occurring in seconds. First, arterioles near the site of injury constrict briefly. Vasoconstriction is followed by vasodilation, which increases blood flow to the inflamed site. Arteriolar dilation increases pressure in the microcirculation, which may increase the exudation of plasma and blood cells into the tissues. Exudation causes edema and swelling. As plasma moves outward, blood remaining in the microcirculation flows more slowly and becomes more viscous (thick and sticky).

Leukocytes (white blood cells) migrate to vessel walls and adhere there. At the same time biochemical mediators stimulate the endothelial cells that line capillaries and venules to retract, creating spaces at junctions between the cells. (Intercellular junctions are described in Chapter 1.) The leukocytes, which otherwise could not penetrate vessel walls, are able to squeeze out through the spaces created by endothelial retraction (Fig. 7-3).

This state of vascular permeability continues throughout acute inflammation, permitting blood cells and plasma proteins to exude continuously into inflamed tissues. Once in the tissues, these cells and proteins act in concert to (1) stimulate and control subsequent inflammatory processes and (2) interact with components of the immune response.

Neutrophils are the first phagocytic leukocytes to arrive at the inflamed site. They phagocytose (ingest) bacteria, dead cells, and cellular debris, then die and are removed as pus through the epithelium or the lymphatic system. (The lymphatic system is described in Chapter 26.) The next phagocytes on the scene are monocytes and macrophages, which perform many of the same functions as neutrophils but for a longer time and later

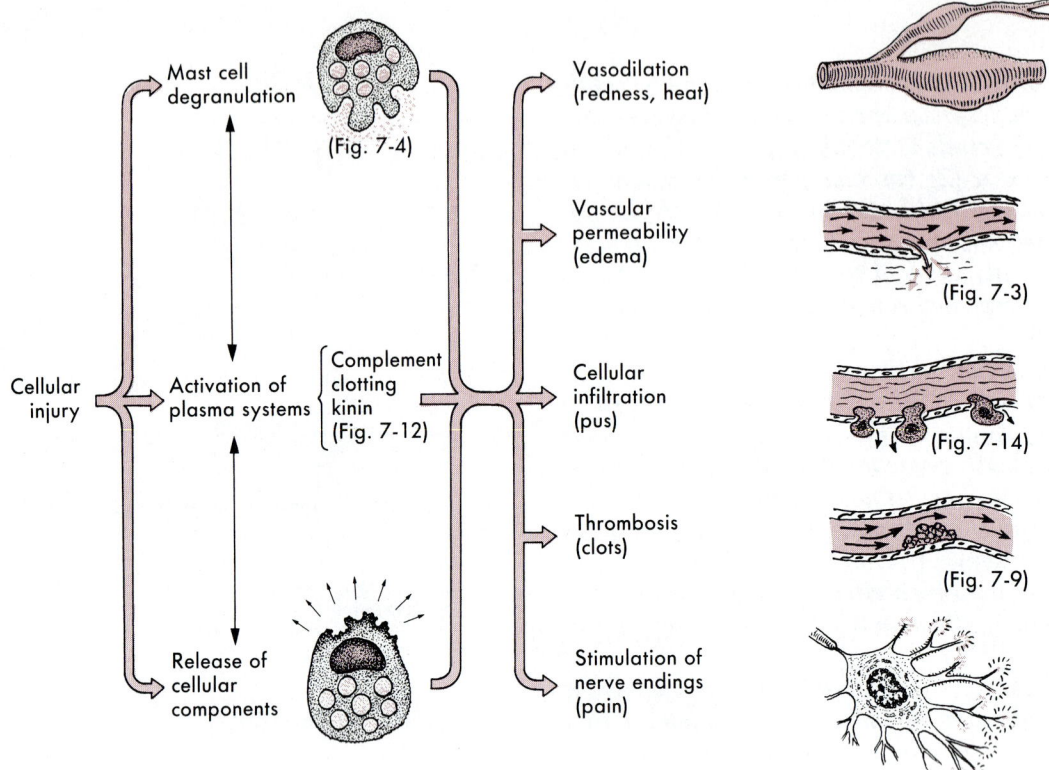

FIG. 7-2 **The acute inflammatory response.** Inflammation is usually initiated by cellular injury. Mast cell degranulation, the activation of three plasma systems, and the release of subcellular components from the damaged cells occur as a consequence of cellular injury. These systems are interdependent, so that induction of one (e.g., mast cell degranulation) can result in the induction of the other two. The end result is the development of microscopic changes in the inflamed site, as well as characteristic clinical manifestations. The figure numbers refer to those in which more detailed information may be found on that portion of the response.

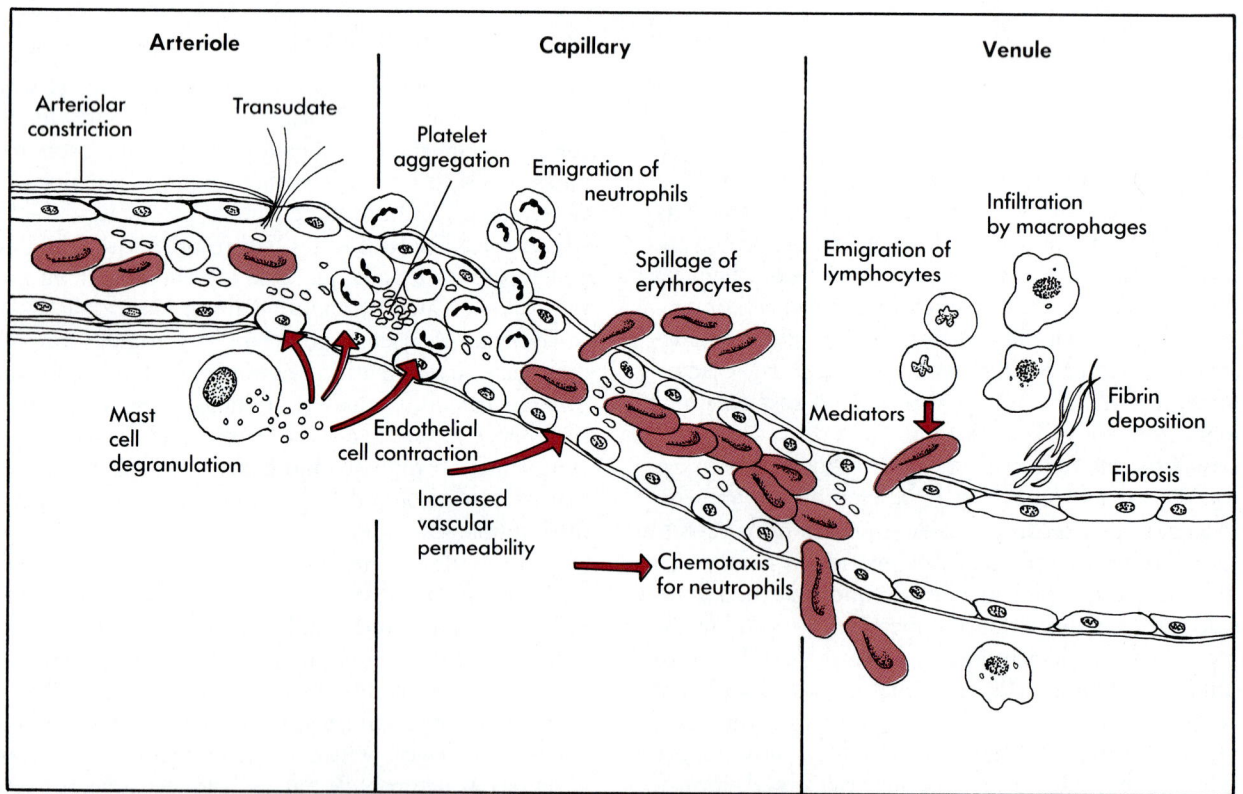

FIG. 7-3 **The sequence of events in the process of inflammation.** See text for details.

in the inflammatory response. Other cells found in inflamed tissues are eosinophils, which help to control the inflammatory response and act directly against parasites; basophils, which have a function similar to that of mast cells (described on p. 238); and **platelets,** which are cytoplasmic fragments that stop bleeding if vascular injury has occurred (see Chapter 22).

The cells and platelets carry out their roles with the assistance of three major plasma protein systems (the complement, clotting, and kinin systems) and immunoglobulins. The complement system not only activates and assists inflammatory and immune processes but also plays a major role in the direct destruction of cells (especially bacteria). The clotting system traps bacteria in injured tissues and interacts with platelets to prevent hemorrhage. The kinin system helps to control vascular permeability. Immunoglobulin is the fourth type of plasma protein that participates in inflammatory processes.

All of these cells and protein systems, along with the substances they produce, act at the site of tissue injury to kill microorganisms and remove the debris of "battle," including exudate and dead cells. This prepares the lesion for tissue regeneration or repair, the process known as resolution.

Like inappropriate immune processes, inappropriate or exaggerated inflammatory processes have deleterious effects on the host. Even appropriate inflammation can be painful and harm healthy tissues. Furthermore, because it is complex, nonspecific, and can be triggered and maintained by a great variety of stimuli, inflammation is often difficult to control with drugs. (See Chapter 8 for a discussion of exaggerated, deficient, or inappropriate immune and inflammatory processes.)

The function of acute inflammation and the stages by which it proceeds are not difficult to understand. The difficulty occurs when one asks, "How are the various stages initiated, regulated, and ended?" The biochemical mediators and cellular components of the acute inflammatory response form a complex system of interactions that frequently begins with degranulation of mast cells and ends with healing.

THE MAST CELL

The mast cell is probably the most important activator of the inflammatory response (Fig. 7-4). **Mast cells,** first described by Paul Ehrlich in 1877, are cellular bags of granules located in the loose connective tissues close to blood vessels (Ehrlich, 1877). **Basophils** are found in the blood and probably function in the same way as tissue mast cells. Mast cells activate the inflammatory response in two ways. The first is **degranulation,** by which they

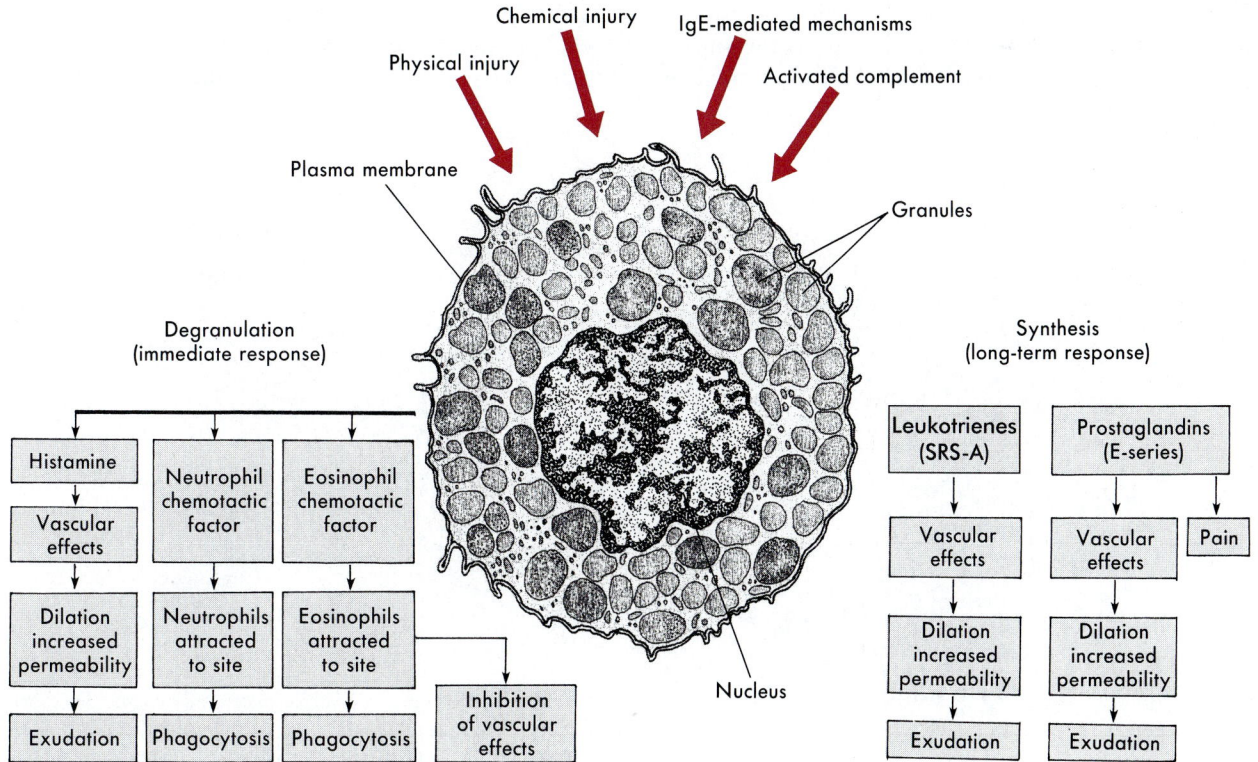

FIG. 7-4 **Effects of degranulation** *(left)* **and synthesis** *(right)* **by mast cells.** The electron micrograph of a tissue mast cell shows darkly stained granules in the cytoplasm (×9200).

release preformed granular contents into the extracellular matrix. The second is synthesis of certain mediators in response to a stimulus.

Degranulation of Vasoactive Amines and Chemotactic Factors

Mast cell degranulation is stimulated by (1) physical injury, such as heat, mechanical trauma, ultraviolet light, or x-rays; (2) chemical agents, such as toxins, snake and bee venoms, tissue proteases (enzymes), dextran, or a cationic protein released from neutrophils; or (3) immunologic means, such as the triggering of IgE-mediated hypersensitivity reactions (see Chapter 8), or direct processes, such as activation of complement components (see p. 240). Preformed biochemical mediators found in the granules, including histamine, neutrophil chemotactic factor, and eosinophil chemotactic factor of anaphylaxis, are released in seconds and exert their effects immediately. Serotonin, another potent mediator, is released by platelets.

Histamine and serotonin are both vasoactive amines. They cause temporary, rapid constriction of the smooth muscle of large vessel walls; dilation of the postcapillary venules, resulting in increased blood flow into the microcirculation; and increased vascular permeability resulting from retraction of endothelial cells lining the capillaries (see Fig. 7-3).

Two chemotactic factors, neutrophil chemotactic factor and eosinophil chemotactic factor of anaphylaxis (ECF-A), are also released during mast cell degranulation. A **chemotactic factor** is a biochemical substance that attracts a specific type of leukocyte to the site of inflammation. **Chemotaxis** is directional movement of cells along a chemical gradient formed by a chemotactic factor (Fig. 7-5). Neutrophil chemotactic factor attracts neutrophils to the site of inflammation. Neutrophils are the predominant leukocytes at work during early phases of acute inflammation.

Eosinophil chemotactic factor attracts eosinophils to the inflamed site. Eosinophils are leukocytes that have several functions in the inflammatory response. They are phagocytic and are the body's primary defense against some parasites. Their most important role, however, is to control the mediators of acute inflammation released from mast cells. As with most defense systems of the body, the acute inflammatory response is usually only needed in a circumscribed area and for a limited time. Therefore, control mechanisms are necessary to prevent biochemical mediators from evoking more inflammation than is needed. Eosinophils contain several enzymes that degrade the vasoactive amines, thereby controlling the vascular effects of inflammation. These enzymes include histaminase, which mediates the degradation of histamine, and arylsulfatase B, which mediates the degradation of leukotrienes.

Synthesis of Leukotrienes and Prostaglandins

Leukotrienes and prostaglandins are mediators synthesized by mast cells (see Fig. 7-4). **Leukotrienes (slow-reacting substances of anaphylaxis [SRS-A])** are acidic, sulfur-containing lipids that produce effects similar to those of histamine, namely, smooth muscle contraction, increased vascular permeability, and perhaps neutrophil and eosinophil chemotaxis. Leukotrienes appear to be important in the later stages of the inflammatory re-

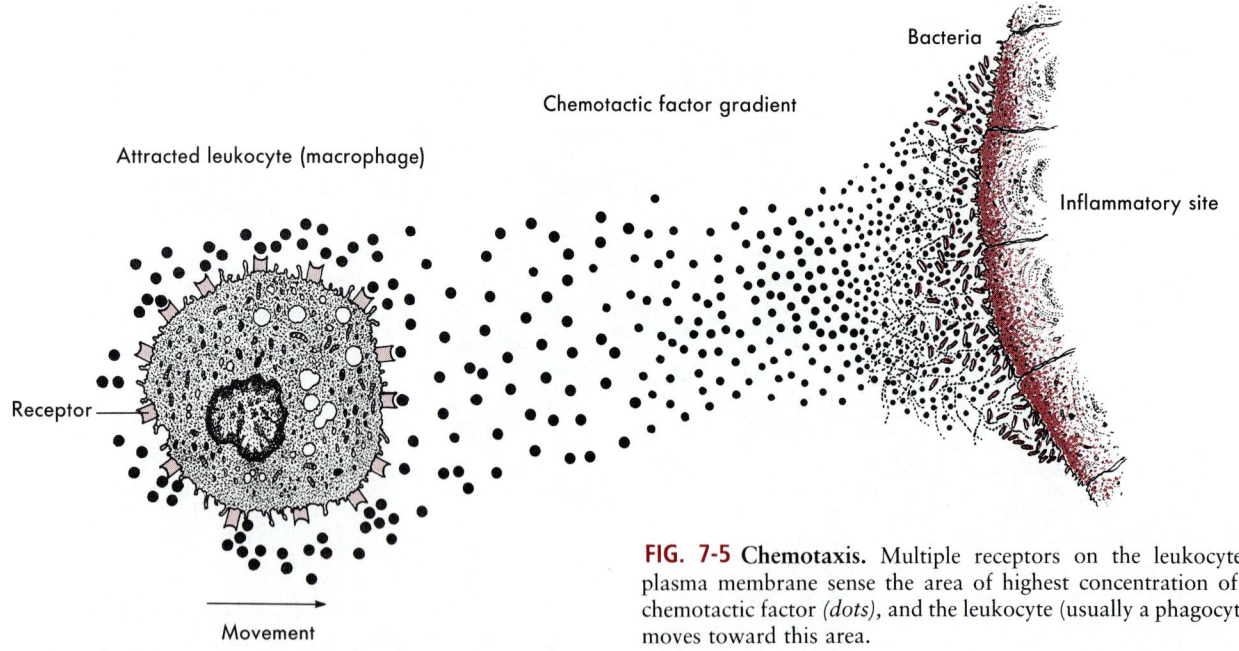

Chemotactic factor gradient

Bacteria

Inflammatory site

Attracted leukocyte (macrophage)

Receptor

Movement

FIG. 7-5 Chemotaxis. Multiple receptors on the leukocyte's plasma membrane sense the area of highest concentration of a chemotactic factor *(dots)*, and the leukocyte (usually a phagocyte) moves toward this area.

sponse, as they stimulate slower and more prolonged responses than do histamines. Leukotrienes are produced from a lipid, arachidonic acid, that is released from mast cell membranes by an intracellular phospholipase that acts on membrane phospholipids.

The mast cell also synthesizes **prostaglandins,** which, like leukotrienes, cause increased vascular permeability and neutrophil chemotaxis. Prostaglandins also induce pain. Prostaglandins are long-chain, unsaturated fatty acids produced from arachidonic acid by the action of the enzyme cyclooxygenase. They are classified into groups (E, A, F, and B) according to their structure. Prostaglandins E_1 and E_2 probably cause increased vascular permeability and smooth muscle contraction; they appear to act directly on postcapillary venules. They can also inhibit some aspects of inflammation by such actions as suppressing both the release of histamine from mast cells and the release of lysosomal enzymes (enzymes responsible for killing and digesting microorganisms) from neutrophils. Enhancement or suppression of

the inflammatory response may be related to concentrations of prostaglandins. Aspirin and some other nonsteroidal anti-inflammatory agents block the synthesis of prostaglandins of the E series and other arachidonic acid derivatives, thereby inhibiting inflammation.

PLASMA PROTEIN SYSTEMS

Inflammation is mediated by three key plasma protein systems: the complement system, the clotting system, and the kinin system. These systems have several characteristics in common. Each consists of a series of inactive enzymes, or **proenzymes.** When the first proenzyme in the series is converted to an active enzyme, it initiates a cascade in which the substrate of the activated enzyme is the next component of the system. Therefore, the entire cascade is activated upon activation of the first component. Activation usually involves the enzymatic cleavage of the inactive precursor (proenzyme) into two or

FIG. 7-6 Pathways of activation of the complement cascade. Complement components are cleaved into fragments, or subcomponents (denoted by *lowercase letters*), during activation. Many of the subcomponents are biochemical mediators of inflammation. The classic pathway is usually activated by antigen-antibody complexes through component C1, whereas the alternative pathway is activated by many agents, such as bacterial polysaccharides, through component C3. (*Bb* is the activated form of *factor B.*)

more components. The larger one is an active enzyme whose substrate is the next component in the system. The smaller component is usually a potent biochemical mediator of the inflammatory response. Most of these components are short-lived, since they are inactivated rapidly by other naturally occurring plasma proteins.

The Complement System

The complement system consists of at least 10 proteins and makes up 10% of the serum proteins in the circulation (Fig. 7-6). The complement system is perhaps the most important of the plasma protein systems of inflammation because, once activated, its components participate in virtually every inflammatory response. In addition, the last few proteins in the complement cascade are capable of killing microorganisms directly.

The complement system can be activated by antigen-antibody complexes, as well as by products released from invading bacteria and by components of the other plasma protein systems (Fig. 7-7). The complement system is a nonspecific mechanism of self-defense. Even when it is activated by a specific mechanism, namely antigen-antibody complexes (the immune system), it mediates inflammation, which is nonspecific. Thus proteins of the complement system (sometimes called complement components) are among the body's most potent defenders against bacterial infection.

The two routes by which the **complement cascade** is activated are shown in Fig. 7-6. The **classic pathway** is activated when an antigen-antibody complex containing IgG or IgM interacts with the first component of the complement cascade, C1. The **alternative pathway** can be activated by several biologic substances, chiefly bacterial and fungal cell wall polysaccharides (especially endotoxin on gram-negative bacteria). (Bacterial endotoxins are described in Chapter 2.)

FIG. 7-7 Immunologic mechanisms that activate the inflammatory response. Immunologic factors may affect inflammation through three mechanisms: (1) IgE can bind to the surface of a mast cell and, after binding antigen, induce the cell's degranulation; (2) antigen and antibody can form immune complexes that activate the complement cascade releasing small polypeptide fragments, primarily C5a, that have potent biologic activities resulting in mast cell degranulation and neutrophil chemotaxis; and (3) antigen may also react with T lymphocytes resulting in the production of lymphokines that may contribute to the development of either acute or chronic inflammation.

Activation of components Cl through C5 produces subunits that enhance inflammation by (1) opsonizing bacteria, (2) attracting leukocytes by chemotaxis, and (3) acting as **anaphylatoxins,** that is, inducing degranulation of mast cells. Components C6 through C9 form complexes capable of creating pores in bacterial cell walls. The pores disrupt the bacterium's rigid outer membrane, permitting the influx of water and ions. This causes the bacterium to burst or at least prevents its reproduction. (Cellular injury is discussed in Chapter 2.)

Classic Pathway

Activation of the classic pathway is preceded by formation of an **antigen-antibody complex (immune complex).** Because antigens tend to be multivalent (to have more than one antigenic determinant), multiple antibodies are bound in the complex. Complement activation occurs as a result of antibody Fc regions being held in close proximity. The Fc contains a site that binds Cl. The first component of the classic complement cascade, Cl, has six sites that can bind to the Fc region and is "fixed" to adjacent antibody molecules that are attached to the antigen. The complex formed by antigen-antibody-complement binding is shown in Fig. 7-8.

Activation of C1 results in the sequential enzymatic activation of all other components of the cascade. Although the cascade continues through the terminal components C6, C7, C8, and C9, whose activation results in the lysis of bacteria, the importance of the complement system resides in the activities of the small fragments, or subcomponents, generated during the activation of C4, C2, C3, and C5. C3b, a subcomponent that adheres to the surface of a target cell (e.g., bacterium) is an efficient opsonin. C4a, C2a, C3a, and C5a, which are soluble, low–molecular weight fragments, are potent activators of the acute inflammatory response. C2a affects smooth muscle, causing vasodilation and increased vascular permeability. C3a, C5a, and to a limited extent C4a are anaphylatoxins; that is, they induce the rapid degranulation of mast cells, with release of histamine (see Fig. 7-4).

The anaphylatoxins C3a and C5a, small polypeptides, are also chemotactic for neutrophils, although C5a is approximately 1000 times more anaphylatoxic and chemotactic than C3a. The dual functions, as a chemotaxic factor and an anaphylatoxin, are not needed simultaneously or to the same degree. Anaphylatoxic activity is necessary early in inflammation and close to the

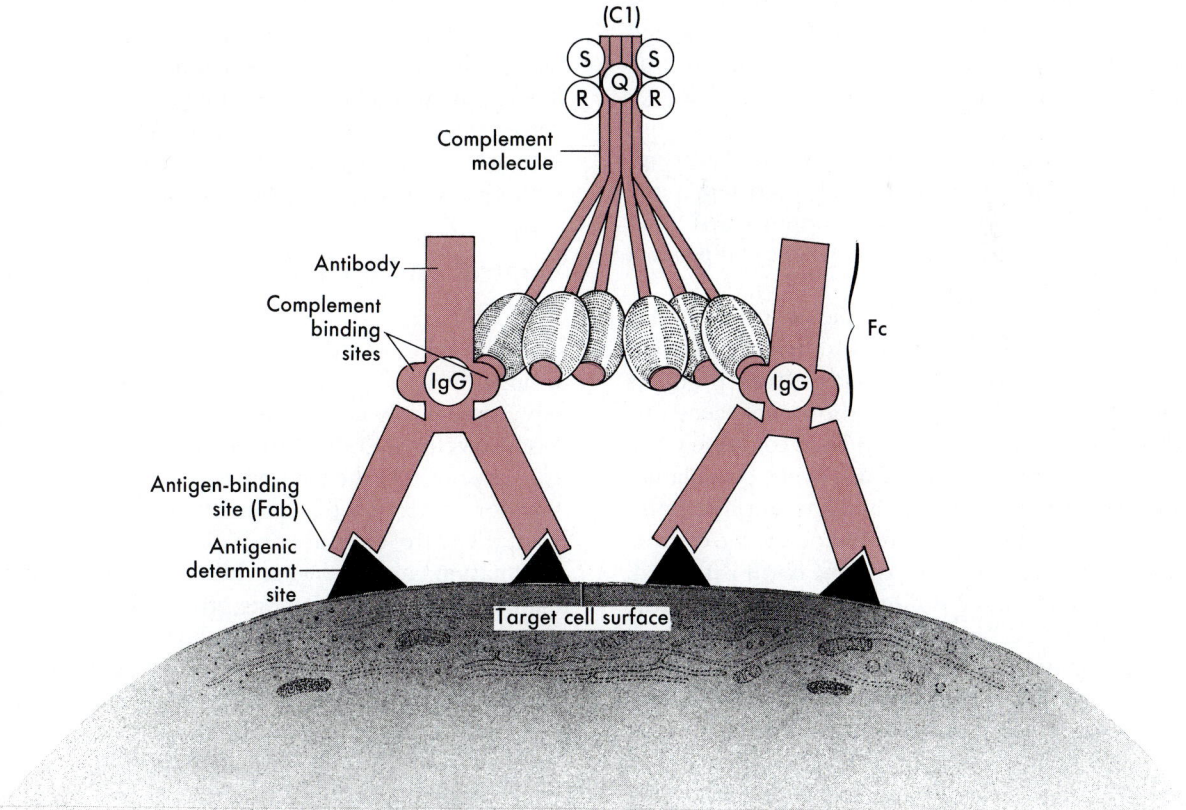

FIG. 7-8 Activation of the first component of complement (Cl). It takes two IgG molecules to activate one complement component. Activation of complement cannot occur unless (1) antigen-antibody binding has occurred, placing two Fc regions of the antibody molecule into close proximity, and (2) the complement component can span the gap between two adjacent Fc portions.

inflammatory site to induce local mast cell degranulation and increase the number of soluble mediators available to enhance vascular permeability. Degranulation of mast cells away from the site of injury would be contrary to the protective nature of the inflammatory response because the substances released would affect healthy neighboring tissues needlessly. Chemotactic activity, on the other hand, is required for a much longer period and distal to the inflammatory site to attract leukocytes from the circulation.

The anaphylatoxic activities of C3a and C5a are inactivated by a naturally occurring enzyme, plasma carboxy-peptidase B, which removes a terminal arginine, producing C3a des Arg and C5a des Arg. The removal of the arginine does not affect chemotactic activity.

Alternative Pathway

There are several non–antibody-mediated (alternate) avenues of entrance into the complement cascade. (Both pathways are shown in Fig. 7-6.) The components of the alternative pathway include those listed in Fig. 7-6.

Clotting System

The clotting (coagulation) system is a plasma protein system that forms a fibrinous exudate, or meshwork, at the inflamed site to trap exudates, microorganisms, and foreign bodies. This (1) prevents the spread of infection and inflammation to adjacent tissues, (2) keeps microorganisms and foreign bodies at the site of greatest phagocytic activity, and (3) forms a clot that stops bleeding and provides a framework for future repair and healing. The main substance in this fibrinous mesh is an insoluble protein called fibrin, which is the end product of the coagulation cascade.

Like the complement cascade, the coagulation cascade can be activated through two different pathways that converge at the point where each pathway produces the same substance (Fig. 7-9). In the complement cascade the classic and alternative pathways converge when each has activated C5 (see Fig. 7-6). In the coagulation cascade, the **extrinsic pathway** and the **intrinsic pathway** converge at factor X. From that point, the cascade proceeds on a common pathway until fibrin is formed. (The coagulation cascade is discussed further and illustrated in Chapter 22.)

The clotting system can be activated by many substances released during tissue destruction and infection, including collagen, proteases, kallikrein, plasmin, and bacterial endotoxins. In addition, activation of the clotting cascade produces subcomponents that enhance the inflammatory response. The two low–molecular weight fibrinopeptides released from fibrinogen during fibrin production (especially fibrinopeptide B) are chemotac-

tic for neutrophils and increase vascular permeability by enhancing the effects of bradykinin (formed from the kinin system).

Kinin System

The third plasma protein system with a role in inflammation is the kinin system. The primary kinin is **bradykinin**, which, at low doses, causes dilation of vessels, acts with prostaglandins to induce pain, causes extravascular smooth muscle contraction, increases vascular permeability, and may increase leukocyte chemotaxis. Bradykinin induces smooth muscle contraction more slowly than histamine and may be more important during the prolonged phase of inflammation. Bradykinin, along with prostaglandins of the E series, is probably responsible for endothelial cell retraction and increased vascular permeability in the later phases of inflammation (endothelial cell retraction is shown in Fig. 7-3).

The kinin system is activated by stimulation of the **plasma kinin cascade** (Fig. 7-10). The conversion of plasma prekallikrein to kallikrein is induced by a subunit, *prekallikrein activator,* that is generated during the activation of Hageman factor (factor XII) by the coagulation cascade. Kallikrein then converts kininogen to kinin, the primary kinin being bradykinin. Another source of kinin is the tissue kallikreins in saliva, sweat, tears, urine, and feces. These kallikreins convert serum kininogens to kallidin (lys-bradykinin), which may be converted to bradykinin by plasma aminopeptidase. Kinins are rapidly degraded and, therefore, controlled by kininases, which are enzymes present in plasma and tissues.

Control and Interaction of Plasma Protein Systems

The activation of the plasma protein systems involved in inflammation produces a large number of very potent, biologically active substances that protect the host from infection. Control of this process is essential for two reasons: (1) the inflammatory process is so important for protection that its activation must be guaranteed; therefore, there are multiple means of initiating inflammation; and (2) the activities of the biochemical mediators generated during this process are so potent and potentially detrimental to the host that their actions must be confined to injured or infected tissues; therefore, multiple mechanisms are available to inactivate or regulate the inflammatory mediators.

Control is apparent at many levels. Many components of inflammation are rapidly destroyed within seconds by enzymes from the plasma. Two components of the complement cascade, C3a and C5a, are inactivated by the plasma enzyme carboxypeptidase, and histamine

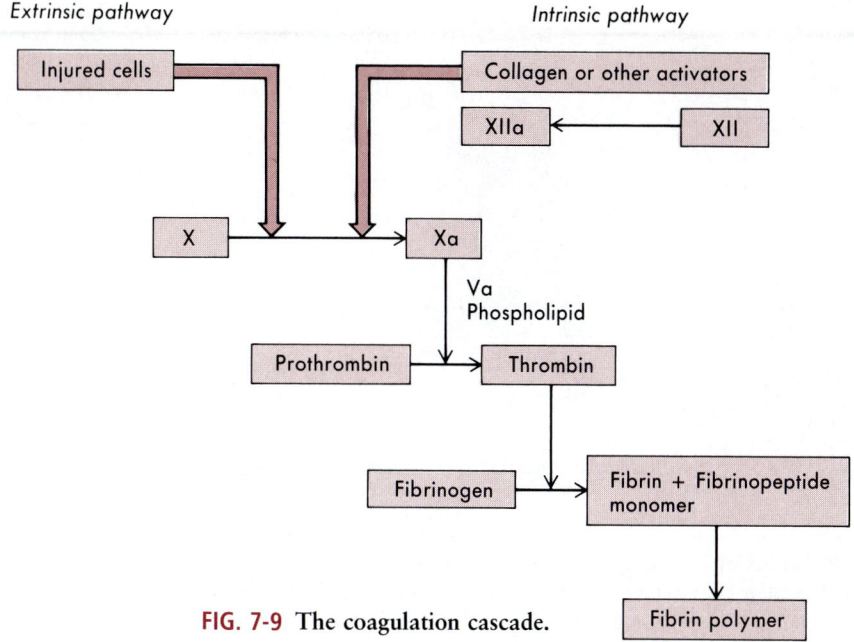

FIG. 7-9 The coagulation cascade.

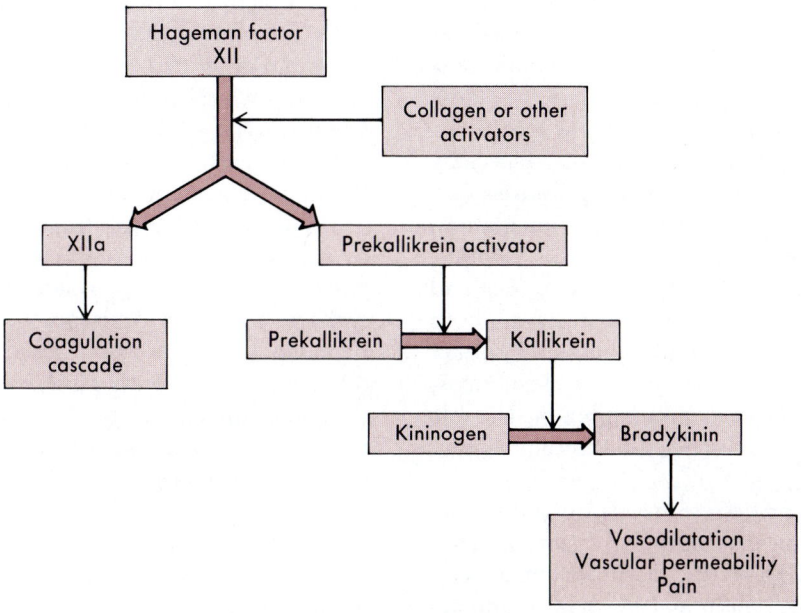

FIG. 7-10 The plasma kinin cascade.

FIG. 7-11 **Effects of histamine through H1 and H2 receptors.** Effects depend on (1) density and affinity of H1 and/or H2 receptors on the target cell and (2) the identity of the target cell. *GTP*, Guanosine triphosphate; *cGMP*, cyclic guanosine monophosphate; *ATP*, adenosine triphosphate; *cAMP*, cyclic adenosine monophosphate.

and leukotrienes are inactivated by the eosinophilic enzymes histaminase and arylsulfatase. Many other natural inhibitors are present, including antagonists for histamine, kinins, complement components, kallikrein, and plasmin.

Histamine activity is controlled, in part, by histamine receptors on the host's target cells. At least two types of receptors exist for histamine: H1 and H2 receptors (Fig. 7-11). The H1 receptor is responsible for promoting inflammation, whereas inflammation is generally inhibited through the H2 receptor by suppression of leukocyte function and mast cell degranulation. The H1 receptor is thought to be present on cells of smooth muscle, especially those of the bronchi, and to cause bronchial smooth muscle to contract (bronchoconstriction) when stimulated. The H2 receptor is especially abundant on parietal cells of the stomach mucosa and induces the secretion of gastric acids upon stimulation. The distribution of both types of receptors is variable, and frequently they are present on the same cells and may act in an antagonistic fashion. For instance, both receptors are present on neutrophils. Stimulation of H1 receptors results in the augmentation of chemotaxis, whereas H2 stimulation results in its inhibition. The role of H1 and H2 receptors is discussed further in Chapter 8 (allergic reactions).

Most of the control processes interact, so that the activation or control of one plasma system results in a similar effect on others (Fig. 7-12). Plasmin controls clot formation (by degrading fibrin and fibrinogen) and activates the complement cascade through C1, C3, and C5, as does thrombin. Plasmin also activates the plasma

kinin cascade by activating Hageman factor and producing prekallikrein activator. The activation of Hageman factor has four effects: (1) activation of the clotting cascade through factor XI; (2) activation of the fibrinolytic systems through conversion of plasminogen proactivator to plasminogen activator, resulting in the generation of plasmin; (3) activation of the kinin system by a Hageman factor fragment, prekallikrein activator; and (4) activation of C1 in the complement cascade. Plasmin itself exists as a proenzyme, plasminogen, which is activated by several factors, including plasminogen activator generated from the kallikrein system; thrombin generated from the clotting system; bacterial factors, such as streptokinase (produced by hemolytic streptococci); plasminogen activators produced by endothelial cells; and several cellular enzymes released during tissue destruction.

The interaction of control mechanisms is exemplified by the effects of C1 esterase inhibitor. Hereditary angioneurotic edema is an autosomal dominant disease characterized by a deficiency of C1 esterase inhibitor. In individuals with this disease, emotional stress and other stimuli frequently result in recurrent edema in the gastrointestinal tract, respiratory tract, and skin, with death occurring in some cases because of laryngeal swelling. The mechanism appears to be one of episodic, uncontrolled activation of plasmin, resulting in Hageman factor activation, bradykinin production, and C1 activation. C1 esterase inhibitor blocks several steps in the activation of all three cascades, including C1 esterase of the complement system, the effects of activated Hageman factor on the kinin system, and the effects of

FIG. 7-12 Interaction of the complement, clotting, kinin, and fibrinolytic (plasmin) systems. Bold arrows denote the activation of factors within a system. Thin arrows denote where a particular factor activates another system.

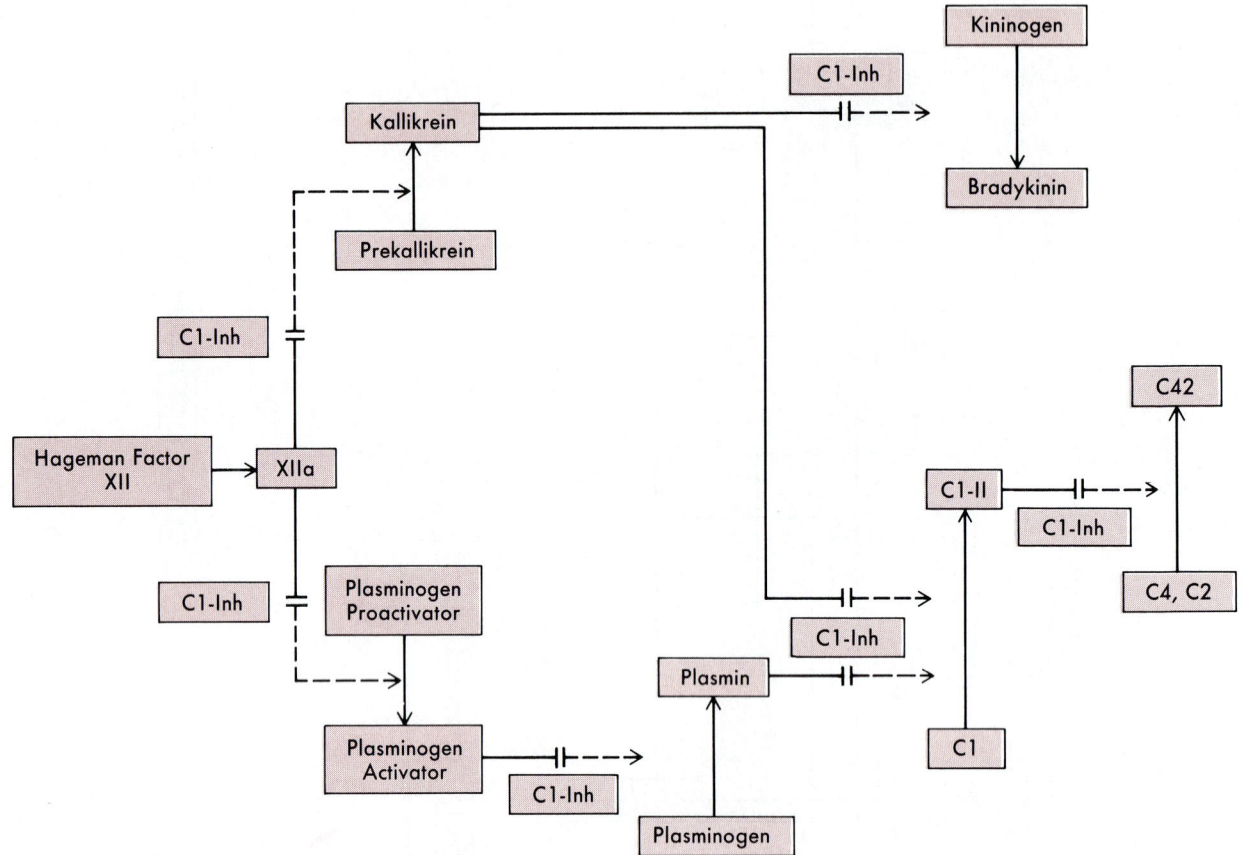

FIG. 7-13 Common control of the complement, clotting, and kinin systems by C1 esterase inhibitor (*C1-Inh*).

kallikrein and plasmin, as shown in Fig. 7-13. That activation of plasmin may be the most important single cause of hereditary angioneurotic edema is indicated by the fact that attacks are prevented by ε-aminocaproic acid, which prevents the conversion of plasminogen to plasmin.

CELLULAR COMPONENTS OF INFLAMMATION

The two main classes of leukocytes to carry out inflammatory processes are the granulocytes and the monocytes/macrophages. The granulocytes, so called because of the many enzyme-containing lysosomal granules in their cytoplasm, include the neutrophils, eosinophils, and basophils. Monocytes (the immature form in the blood) and macrophages (the mature cell in the tissues) have fewer and larger lysosomes in their cytoplasm than do granulocytes. All of these cells are phagocytes (capable of phagocytosis, the ingestion of unwanted matter), but the most important of the phagocytes are the neutrophils and macrophages. Lymphocytes also partic-

ipate in inflammation, primarily by producing soluble mediators (see the section on immunity).

The other cellular component important to inflammation is the platelet. Platelets are cytoplasmic fragments that circulate in the bloodstream until vascular injury occurs. After injury platelets (1) interact with components of the coagulation cascade to stop bleeding and (2) degranulate, releasing biochemical mediators, such as serotonin, which has vascular effects similar to those of histamine. Their activation is stimulated by many products of inflammation, including collagen, platelet-activating factor (PAF) released from mast cells, and antigen-antibody complexes. (Platelet function is described in detail in Chapter 22.)

Function of Phagocytes

The neutrophils and macrophages have essentially the same characteristics and functions. Each normally circulates in the bloodstream and is stimulated by inflammation to migrate through vessel walls near an inflammatory lesion. Once in the exudate, each is attracted to the lesion by specific chemotactic factors and kept there by the meshwork formed by fibrinous exudate. Once at the site, each type of cell phagocytoses (ingests) foreign or dead cells until its life span is over. The dead phagocyte then becomes part of the purulent exudate, or *pus*, which leaves the body through the lymphatic system or through the epithelium. Neutrophils and monocytes/ macrophages differ chiefly in (1) the speed with which they arrive at the site, the neutrophils arriving first; (2) the length of time they remain active, the macrophages being longer-lived; (3) the chemotactic factors capable of attracting them; (4) the enzymatic content of their lysosomes, or digestive vacuoles; and (5) their participation in the immune response, the macrophages being involved in antigen processing.

The phagocytes' role begins when the inflammatory response causes them to stick avidly to capillary and venule walls in a process called **margination,** or **pavementing** (Fig. 7-14). Margination is caused by increased stickiness of the phagocytes and increased adsorption by the endothelial cells lining the vessels as a result of the production of adhesion proteins on the surface of each

Basement membrane   Endothelial cell

Phagocytes in circulation

Intercellular junction

Margination (pavementing)

Diapedesis

Retracted intercellular junction

Exudation into inflamed tissue

FIG. 7-14 Diapedesis of a phagocyte. Phagocytes are capable of ameboid movement, which allows them to squeeze through intercellular junctions and migrate to inflammatory lesions.

cell. This is followed by **diapedesis,** or emigration through the retracting endothelial junctions and the basement membrane and out into the surrounding tissues (see Fig. 7-3).

Once they enter the inflammatory exudate, the phagocytes are attracted to the inflammatory site by chemotaxis. They respond to chemotactic factors because they can detect simultaneously, through chemoreceptors at multiple locations on their plasma membrane, where chemotactic factors are most highly concentrated (see Fig. 7-5). They then migrate in the direction of highest concentration. The primary chemotactic factors for neutrophils, eosinophils, and monocytes include many bacterial products, complement components C5a and C3a, kallikrein and plasminogen activator, fibrinopeptides, products of fibrin degradation, prostaglandins, the activated C567 complex from the complement system, the eosinophil and neutrophil chemotactic factors released from mast cells, and a monocyte chemotactic factor released from the neutrophil. Histamine, though not chemotactic itself, may facilitate chemotaxis. Some bacte-

rial toxins, such as streptococcal streptolysins, inhibit neutrophil chemotaxis.

Phagocytosis, the engulfment and destruction of microorganisms, dead cells, and foreign particles, begins when the phagocytic cell enters the inflammatory site. The process of phagocytosis involves four steps: (1) recognition of the target and its adherence to the phagocyte, (2) engulfment (ingestion, or endocytosis), (3) fusion with lysosomes within the phagocyte, and (4) destruction of the target by lysosomal enzymes (lysosomes are described in Chapter 1). Throughout the process both target and digestive enzymes are isolated within membrane-bounded vesicles. Isolation protects the phagocyte from the harmful effects of target microorganisms and its own enzymes. Phagocytosis of an opsonized bacterium is illustrated in Fig. 7-15.

Most phagocytes can trap and engulf bacteria that have not been "coated" with an opsonin, but the process is slow and inefficient. Opsonization, usually by antibody or complement component C3b, greatly enhances both recognition and binding (also called *adher-*

FIG. 7-15 Phases of phagocytosis. Opsonized microorganisms bind to the surface of a phagocyte *(1)* and are ingested *(2)* into a phagocytic vacuole, or phagosome *(3)*. Lysosomes fuse with the phagosome *(4)*, releasing their digestive enzymes into the vacuole. This results in the formation of a phagolysosome *(5)*, within which the microorganism is killed and digested.

ence). Opsonins function as "glue" between the phagocyte and the target cell because receptors on the phagocyte are specific for sites on the opsonin (Fc receptors for antibody, C3b receptors for C3b). This enables the phagocyte to bind opsonized bacteria very tightly to its surface. Although antibody forms a stronger attachment, C3b facilitates phagocytosis to a greater extent.

Engulfment is carried out by small pseudopods that extend from the plasma membrane and surround the adhered microorganism (Fig. 7-16), forming an intracellular phagocytic vacuole, or **phagosome.** The membrane that surrounds the phagosome consists of inverted plasma membrane. After the formation of the phagosome, lysosomes converge, fuse with the phagosome, and discharge their contents, creating a **phagolysosome.** Destruction of the bacterium takes place within the phagolysosome (see Fig. 7-15).

Phagocytosis is accompanied by a burst of metabolic activity in the phagocyte, resulting in the production of several oxygen-containing molecules that are reactive and highly damaging to cells. This is known as an oxygen-dependent killing mechanism. The principal oxygen-dependent mechanism of killing is hydrogen peroxide, especially in conjunction with the lysosomal enzyme myeloperoxidase and halide anions (I^-, Cl^-, and Br^-). Myeloperoxidase probably kills by iodination or the formation of toxic chloramines and aldehydes on the target cell's surface. The oxygen-independent mechanisms of killing are (1) acid pH (3.5 to 4.0) of the phagolysosome caused by lactic acid production; (2) the cationic proteins, which bind to and damage target cell membranes; (3) lysozyme and elastase, which attack mucopeptides in the target cell wall; and (4) lactoferrin, which inhibits bacterial growth by binding iron.

When the phagocyte dies at the inflammatory site, it lyses (breaks open) and its cytoplasmic contents, including the lysosomal enzymes, are released. Enzymes released from lysosomes can digest the connective tissue matrix, causing much of the tissue destruction associated with inflammation. α-1-Antitrypsin, a plasma protein produced by the liver, inhibits the destructive ef-

FIG. 7-16 Steps in phagocytosis. This scanning electron micrograph shows the progressive steps in phagocytosis. **A,** Red blood cells *(R)* attach to the surface of a macrophage *(M).* **B,** Part of macrophage *(M)* membrane starts to enclose the red cell *(R).* **C,** The red blood cells are almost totally engulfed by the macrophage. (From King, Fenoglio, & Lefkowitch, 1983.)

fects of many enzymes released by dead phagocytes. An inherited deficiency of α-1-antitrypsin often results in chronic lung damage and emphysema as a result of inflammation. (The pulmonary effects of α-1-antitrypsin deficiency are described in Chapter 30.)

Released lysosomal products contribute to other aspects of inflammation. These include increased vascular permeability, chemotaxis for monocytes, breakdown of connective tissues, and activation of the complement and kinin systems.

Polymorphonuclear Neutrophils

The **neutrophil**, or **polymorphonuclear neutrophil** (**PMN**), is the predominant phagocytic cell in the early inflammatory response, entering the inflammatory site within 6 to 12 hours after the initial injury. Neutrophils arrive first because they are attracted by the immediately generated chemotactic factors, such as complement subcomponents. Macrophages and lymphocytes, on the other hand, enter the site later, usually after 24 hours, and gradually replace the neutrophils.

Because the neutrophil is a mature cell incapable of division and is sensitive to the acidic environment of inflammatory lesions, it is short-lived in the inflammatory site. The primary roles of the neutrophil are removal of debris in sterile lesions, such as burns, and phagocytosis of bacteria in nonsterile lesions.

Monocytes and Macrophages

The **monocyte** is the largest normal blood cell (14 to 20 μm in diameter). Its single nucleus is usually indented or horseshoe-shaped. It is produced in the bone marrow, enters the circulation, and migrates to the inflammatory site, where it develops into a macrophage. The **macrophage** is generally larger (20 to 40 μm) and is a more active phagocyte than the monocyte (see Fig. 7-16). Monocytes also appear to be the precursors of macrophages that are fixed in tissues (tissue macrophages), including those of the mononuclear phagocytic system (formerly known as the reticuloendothelial system), including Kupffer cells of the liver and alveolar macrophages of the lungs. (Tissue macrophages are discussed in Chapter 6.)

Macrophage and lymphocyte infiltration is characteristic of chronic rather than acute inflammation. Macrophages may appear at the inflammatory site soon after the initial neutrophil infiltration (within 24 hours of injury) but usually arrive 3 to 7 days later. They migrate to the site slowly because (1) many of the chemotactic factors that attract them, such as macrophage chemotactic factor, are released by neutrophils and (2) monocytes, the immature macrophages, move somewhat sluggishly.

Macrophages are better suited than neutrophils to long-term defense against infectious agents because macrophages can survive and divide in the acidic inflam-

matory site, whereas neutrophils cannot. Macrophages can also fuse into larger cells capable of phagocytosing larger targets.

Macrophages have several roles in inflammation and immunity. They are responsive to the soluble products (lymphokines) secreted by T cells, participate in activating the immune response by processing antigen for presentation to lymphocytes (see Figs. 6-8, 6-14, and 6-16), and are a source of a soluble factor (colony-stimulating factor) that stimulates the growth and differentiation of granulocytes and monocytes in the bone marrow. Macrophages also secrete substances that promote regrowth of tissues during wound healing (see p. 262).

Several bacteria can survive and even thrive inside macrophages. Microorganisms such as *Mycobacterium tuberculosis*, *Mycobacterium leprae*, *Salmonella typhi*, *Brucella abortus*, and *Listeria monocytogenes* can remain dormant or multiply inside the phagolysosomes of macrophages. This occurrence is prevented or ameliorated with the help of the immune system, which is active by the time macrophages have infiltrated the inflammatory site (see Fig. 7-7). Macrophages are further activated, or "turned on," by lymphokines secreted by T cells. Lymphokines increase the killing capacity of the macrophage by increasing its phagocytic activity, size, plasma membrane area, glucose metabolism, and number of lysosomes (Fig. 7-17).

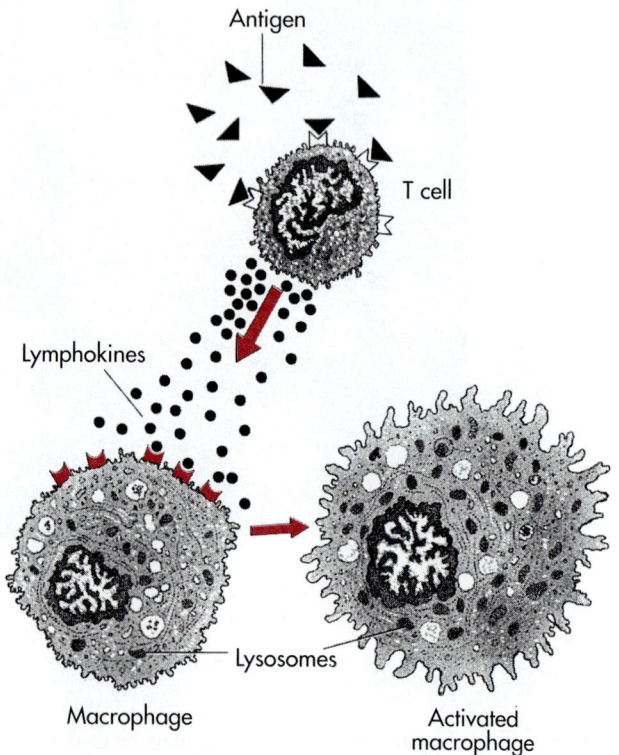

FIG. 7-17 Activation of a macrophage by a lymphokine (macrophage-activating factor, or MAF). Lymphokine is produced by T cells that have been stimulated by an antigen. The ruffled plasma membrane indicates macrophage activation.

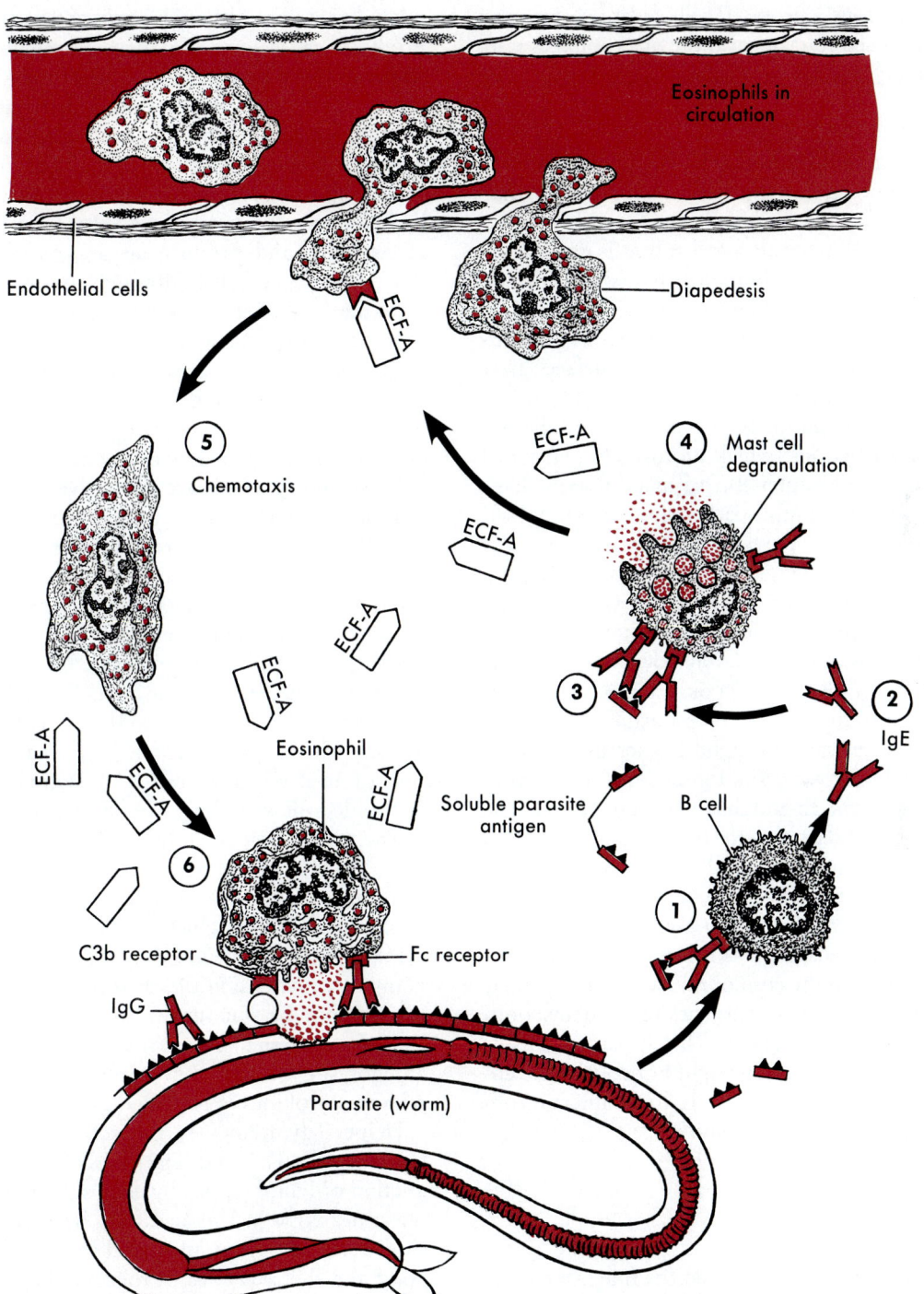

FIG. 7-18 IgE-mediated destruction of a parasite by an eosinophil. Soluble antigen from a parasite binds to an IgE-bearing B cell *(1)*, stimulating the B cell to produce IgE *(2)*, which binds to Fc receptors on a mast cell. Soluble antigen also binds to IgE on the mast cell *(3)*, causing the mast cell to degranulate *(4)*. ECF-A released from the mast cell granules attracts eosinophils out of the circulation and toward the site of inflammation *(5)*. IgG and complement component C3b are the opsonins that bind the eosinophil to the parasite. Once bound to the parasite, the eosinophil tries to ingest it and in the process releases its lysosomal enzymes onto the parasite, damaging its outer membrane *(6)*.

Failure of macrophages to turn on has been traced to defective T cell responses to certain microorganisms. For example, a form of leprosy called lepromatous leprosy is characterized by the survival of *M. leprae* that have been phagocytosed by macrophages. In individuals with lepromatous leprosy, T cells fail to secrete the lymphokines needed to transform the macrophages into cells more highly dedicated to killing.

Eosinophils

Eosinophils are granulocytes that have large numbers of lysosomes containing (1) biochemical mediators that control the vascular effects of serotonin and histamine (see p. 238) and (2) a caustic protein that is capable of dissolving the surface membranes of parasites. Eosinophils do not phagocytose parasites, many of which are multicellular organisms. Rather they bind to and degranulate onto the parasite, damaging its surface. This is preceded by the processes shown in Fig. 7-18.

IgE is the chief immunoglobulin involved in allergic hypersensitivity reactions, which are usually detrimental to the host (see Chapter 8). IgE may also mediate normal defenses against some pathogenic organisms (see Fig. 7-7). Multicellular parasites, particularly worms, elicit an IgE-mediated allergic response that benefits the host by destroying the parasite. As in allergic reaction, IgE mediates degranulation of mast cells in the presence of soluble antigens. Degranulation releases eosinophil chemotactic factor of anaphylaxis, ECF-A, which attracts eosinophils to the site of parasitic infestation. ECF-A also induces the eosinophil to increase the density of its membrane receptors for two opsonins, complement component C3b and the Fc portion of IgG. The increased density of receptors for these opsonins enables the eosinophil to bind very tightly to the parasite. The eosinophil is unable to phagocytose the large parasite. Instead of ingesting the organism and enclosing it in a phagolysosome, the eosinophil's lysosomal granules migrate to the surface of the eosinophil and discharge their contents, including highly caustic cationic proteins, onto the parasite's outer membrane. This causes extensive damage to the parasite, and the tight fit between the eosinophil and its target prevents lysosomal contents from damaging neighboring host tissues.

CELLULAR PRODUCTS

Some host cells produce soluble factors that contribute to nonspecific mechanisms of defense by affecting other, neighboring host cells. In general, these factors are referred to as cytokines, but have been subdivided into monokines (produced by macrophages) or lymphokines (produced by lymphocytes). (Cytokines are also discussed in Chapter 6.) This division has recently become very artificial because most cytokines are also produced by other cells, such as endothelial cells, fibroblasts, mast cells, and many others. The majority of cytokines that are relevant to immunology and inflammation are grouped into interleukins, interferons, and a few other related proteins. Although some of these factors may be produced in response to specific antigenic stimulation (especially the lymphokines), all of them act in a nonspecific manner to enhance the inflammatory response.

Many cells cooperate in producing an effective immune or inflammatory response. The interactions of those cells are governed by cytokines that are produced by cells, secreted from those cells, bind to appropriate target cells, and produce an appropriate response in those stimulated cells. Although most of the effects of cytokines are over short distances (e.g., between cells that are in contact), some effects are mediated over long distances within the body (e.g., the induction of fever by cytokines that are produced at an inflammatory site and act directly on the brain). The specific binding of cytokines to a particular cell is mediated through specific receptors, which are themselves under the regulation of cytokines. For instance, as discussed in Chapter 6, helper T cells (Th) are influenced by interleukin-1 (IL-1) produced by antigen-presenting cells. IL-1 acts in a paracrine manner and mediates neighboring Th cell function by binding to specific IL-1 receptors on the Th cell surface. The Th cell responds by production of another cytokine, interleukin-2 (IL-2). IL-2 will act in an autocrine manner, binding to IL-2 receptors on the same Th cell. The Th cell responds by increasing the production of IL-2 receptor and IL-2. (Paracrine, autocrine, and endocrine signalling are discussed in Chapter 1.)

The actions of cytokines are pleiotropic. This indicates that the same cytokine may have a large variety of different biological activities depending on the particular target cell to which it binds. In addition, the same cytokine may be produced by a large spectrum of cells, many of which are not part of the immune system. Cytokines may be synergistic (so that their combined activity exceeds the sum of their individual activities) or antagonistic (so that they inhibit each other). A list of relevant cytokines is provided in Table 7-1.

Helper T lymphocytes have recently been divided into two subsets (Th1 and Th2) based on differential production of lymphokines by each subset. Most of the pioneering work in this area has been performed using cloned Th cells from mice, and their significance in the body and the relevance of those findings to human Th cells has not yet been fully confirmed. Th1 cells more actively produce interferon (INFγ), tumor necrosis factor (TNFγ), and IL-2, whereas Th2 cells produce IL-4, IL-5, IL-6, IL-9, and IL-10. Both subsets produce IL-3 and granulocyte/macrophage–colony-stimulating factor (GM-CSF).

TABLE 7-1

List of Relevant Cytokines

Cytokine	Producers	Targets	Biologic activities
IL-1α, IL-1β (interleukin-1-alpha, interleukin-1-beta)	T, B, and NK cells, macrophages, endothelial cells, fibroblasts, and others	Th, B, and NK cells, endothelial cells, neutrophils, macrophages	↑ Th cell activation; ↑ IL-6, INF-β, and IL-8 production; ↑ B cell activation and proliferation; ↑ NK activity; chemotactic for neutrophil and macrophage; ↑ endothelial cell "stickiness" and procoagulant activity; ↑ activation and proliferation of fibroblasts, smooth muscle, keratinocytes, endothelial cells, osteoclasts, hepatocytes, and bone marrow cells; ↑ inflammation; fever
IL-2 (interleukin-2)	Th (Th1) cells, NK cells	Th, Tc, and NK cells	↑ Th, Tc, and B cell antigen-induced proliferation; activation of NK cells (resulting in lymphokine-activated killer cells; LAK); ↑ INF-γ and IL-4; ↓ TNF-β and IL-1
IL-3 (interleukin-3)	Th and NK cells, activated mast cell	Myeloid stem cells	↑ Proliferation and differentiation of Th and NK cells; ↑ mast cell growth and histamine secretion
IL-4 (interleukin-4)	Th (Th2) cells, mast cell	B and T cells, macrophage, mast cell, endothelial cell	↑ B cell proliferation and differentiation of antigen-activated cells (induces class switch to IgG4 and IgE, ↑ B cell surface IgM and ↓ differentiation to IgA-producing plasma cells); ↑ T cell proliferation, especially ↑ Tc activity; ↑ MHC classes I and II expression on macrophages; ↑ antigen presentation by macrophages; ↑ macrophage and neutrophil phagocytosis; ↓ endothelial cell stickiness for neutrophils, but ↑ endothelial cell stickiness for lymphocytes; ↑ mast cell growth; ↓ IL-1, IL-6, IL-8, IL-10, and TNF-α production
IL-5 (interleukin-5)	Th (Th2) cells	B cells, eosinophils, basophils	↑ B cell proliferation and differentiation (↑ class switch to IgA and IgM); ↑ IgE production (in cooperation with IL-4); ↑ eosinophil proliferation and differentiation; ↑ T cell production of IL-2 receptor; synergistic with IL-1 in Tc cell maturation
IL-6 (interleukin-6)	Th (Th2) and B cells, macrophages, fibroblasts, endothelial cells	B and T cells, myeloid stem cells	↑ Differentiation into plasma cells; ↑ T cell differentiation and proliferation; ↑ differentiation of granulocyte/monocyte stem cell; ↑ macrophage cytotoxic activity; ↑ inflammation; fever
IL-7 (interleukin-7)	Bone marrow stromal cells	Lymphoid stem cells, T cells	↑ Differentiation of lymphoid stem cells into B stem cell; ↑ IL-2 and IL-2 receptor production by T cells; ↑ proliferation of early T cells
IL-8 (interleukin-8)	Macrophage, endothelial cell, many others	PMN, T cells	↑ Chemotactic activity for neutrophils and T cells; ↑ neutrophil activation and adherence to endothelium

Data from Golub & Green, 1991; Kline, 1990; Kuby, 1992.   *Continued.*

TABLE 7-1

List of Relevant Cytokines—cont'd

Cytokine	Producers	Targets	Biologic activities
IL-9 (interleukin-9)	Th (Th2) cell	Th cells, mast cells	↑ T cell proliferation without antigen; ↑ mast cell proliferation
IL-10 (interleukin-10)	Th (Th2) and B cells	Th (Th1) and Tc cells, antigen presenting cells	↓ Cytokine production; ↑ Tc cell differentiation (in cooperation with IL-2)
TNF-α (tumor necrosis factor-alpha)	Macrophage and others	Tumors, endothelial cells	Cytotoxic to tumor cells, ↑ cytokine production by many types of cells; vascular shock; ↑ endothelial cell stickiness, procoagulant activity, and contraction; ↑ production of INF-β, IL-8, and IL-6
TNF-β (tumor necrosis factor-beta; lymphotoxin)	Th (Th1) and Tc cells	Tumors, macrophages, B cells	Cytotoxic to tumor cells, ↑ phagocytosis by macrophage and neutrophil; ↑ macrophage terminal differentiation; ↑ macrophage cytotoxicity; ↑ B cell proliferation
INF-γ (interferon-gamma; major component of MAF)	Th, Tc, and NK cells	Tc, Th, and NK cells, macrophages, tumors	↑ Class switch to IgG2a production; blocks class switch to IgE and IgG1; ↓ IL-4 induced class switch; ↓ tumor cell proliferation; ↑ class I and II antigen expression; ↑ Tc cell differentiation; ↓ IL-1; augments TNF action
INF-α (interferon-alpha)	T and B cells, macrophages	B, NK, and Tc cells, tumors	↓ Tumor growth; ↑ tumor antigen expression; ↓ B cell proliferation; ↑ NK, Tc, and macrophage activation; ↓ IL-8 production
INF-β (interferon-beta)	Fibroblasts	NK cells	Antiviral activity; ↑ NK cell activity; ↑ IL-6 production; ↓ IL-8 production
TGF-β (transforming growth factor-beta)	Platelets, macrophages, lymphocytes	Macrophages, B cells, fibroblasts	Chemotactic for macrophages, ↑ IL-1 production, ↑ class switch to IgA production, ↑ wound healing; inhibits activity of IL-2 and TNF; ↓ IL-4 production

Interleukins

The **interleukins (ILs)** are biochemical messengers sent from one leukocyte to another. The interleukins described in Chapter 6 are produced by macrophages or lymphocytes in response to stimulation by an antigen or by products of inflammation (Lachman & Maizel, 1983; Milanese, Richardson, & Reinherz, 1986). The function of this series of hormones is to enhance the response of lymphocytes and other cells to antigens and other foreign substances. Interleukins have effects on many other cells, frequently independent of antigen stimulation.

Interleukin-1 (IL-1) is produced mostly by phagocytes and antigen-presenting cells that have been stimulated by substances associated with tissue injury, including bacteria, endotoxins (bacterial pyrogens), interferon, antigen-antibody complexes, and antigen. IL-1 is a lymphocyte-activating factor that, among other functions, probably augments antibody production by enhancing the production of IL-2 by T helper cells (see Chapter 6). Macrophage-produced IL-1 promotes the growth and function of almost every cell on which it has been tested. It has several effects on neutrophils, including induction of neutrophilia (proliferation that increases the number of circulating neutrophils), chemotaxis, increased hexose-monophosphate shunt activity (i.e., cellular metabolism), and increased lysosomal enzyme activity.

Lymphokines

Lymphokines, which are produced by T cells in response to antigenic stimulation, are also biochemical mediators

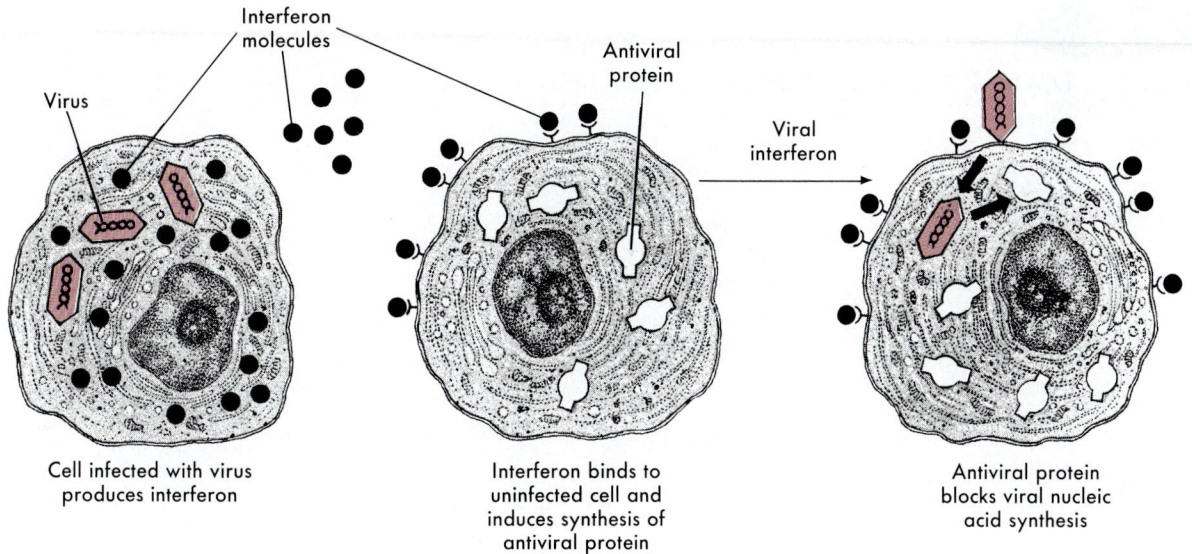

FIG. 7-19 The action of interferon.

that affect other cells of the immune and inflammatory responses (see Fig. 7-7). Although they are produced by cells of the immune system—a specific mechanism of self-defense—lymphokines have nonspecific effects. Many of the lymphokines have been identified as being members of the interleukin or interferon groups.

Different lymphokines have different effects. One lymphokine, called **migration-inhibitory factor (MIF),** is a glycoprotein that inhibits macrophage migration from the inflamed site. Another, **macrophage-activating factor (MAF),** increases the phagocytic activities of macrophages (see Fig. 7-17). MAF activity is most attributable to interferon-gamma (INFγ). At least three other lymphokines affect macrophages by causing chemotaxis, promoting maturation of monocytes into macrophages, enhancing macrophage migration along chemotactic gradients, and stimulating macrophages to aggregate or fuse into giant cells (see p. 257). Some lymphokines are chemotactic for the other phagocytes: neutrophils and eosinophils.

Other lymphokines affect lymphocytes, inducing them to produce more lymphokines, proliferate, or diminish their activities. Lymphokines called lymphotoxins are nonspecific killers of nonlymphocytes. Tumor necrosis factor-beta (TNF-β) is thought to be the primary constituent of lymphotoxin. A lymphokine called transfer factor is a ribonucleoprotein that, when extracted from leukocytes and inoculated into another individual, can transfer immunity from an immunocompetent donor to an immunoincompetent recipient and may be involved in the recruiting of other lymphocytes.

Interferon

One of the body's defenses against viral infection is the production of interferon. (Mechanisms of viral infection are described in Chapter 2.) Interferon does not kill viruses, but it can prevent them from infecting healthy cells. **Interferon** consists of small, low–molecular weight proteins produced and released by host cells that have been invaded by a virus. Once released, interferon molecules attach themselves to receptors on neighboring host cells. If a neighboring cell is uninfected, the interferon stimulates it to produce an antiviral protein (Fig. 7-19). Interferon has no effect on a cell that is already infected by the virus.

Slightly different kinds of interferon are produced by different types of cells. All types are host-specific but not virus-specific; therefore, human interferon is only effective in humans, but it is effective against almost all viruses.

SYSTEMIC MANIFESTATIONS OF ACUTE INFLAMMATION

The three primary systemic changes associated with the acute inflammatory response are fever, leukocytosis (a transient increase in circulating leukocytes), and increase in circulating plasma proteins. Fever appears to be induced by a mediator, endogenous pyrogen, which is identical to IL-1 and is released from neutrophils and macrophages. Endogenous pyrogen (a fever-causing chemical) acts directly on the hypothalamus, the portion of the brain that controls the body's thermostat. The release of endogenous pyrogen activity occurs after phagocytosis or after exposure of the cell to bacterial endotoxin or to antigen-antibody complexes. (Mechanisms of temperature regulation are discussed in Chapter 13.)

The generation of a febrile response can be beneficial

TABLE 7-2

Circulating Levels of Acute-Phase Reactants During Inflammation

Function	Increased	Decreased
Coagulation components	Fibrinogen Prothrombin Factor VIII Plasminogen	None
Protease inhibitors	α-1-Antitrypsin α-1-Antichymotrypsin	Inter-α-antitrypsin
Transport proteins	Haptoglobin Hemopexin Ceruloplasmin Ferritin	Transferrin
Complement components	C1s, C2, C3, C4, C5, C9, factor B, C1 inhibitor	Properdin
Miscellaneous proteins	α-1-Acid glycoprotein Fibronectin Serum amyloid A (SAA) C-reactive protein (CRP)	Albumin Prealbumin α-1-Lipoprotein β-Lipoprotein

to the defense of the host because the microorganisms that cause some conditions (e.g., syphilis, gonococcal urethritis) are very sensitive to small increases in body temperature. On the other hand, fever may have some harmful side effects, for it may enhance the host's susceptibility to the effects of endotoxins associated with gram-negative bacterial infections (bacterial toxins are described in Chapter 2).

During many infections numbers of circulating leukocytes, primarily neutrophils, increase. This increase is usually accompanied by a "left shift" in the ratio of immature to mature neutrophils, so that the more immature forms of neutrophils, such as band cells, metamyelocytes, and, occasionally, myelocytes, are present in greater than normal proportions. (See Chapter 22 for a discussion of the development and maturation of blood cells.) Leukocyte production increases because it is stimulated by several products of inflammation, including complement component C3a. Colony-stimulating factors produced by phagocytes also induce granulopoiesis (formation of granulocytes, namely, neutrophils, eosinophils, and basophils) in the bone marrow, primarily by the proliferation of committed precursors of granulocytes and monocytes (see Chapter 22).

Many plasma proteins, most of which are products of the liver, are increased during inflammation; these are referred to as **acute-phase reactants** (Table 7-2). Acute-phase reactants reach maximal circulating levels in 10 to 40 hours. Many are anti-inflammatory proteins whose rate of synthesis is increased in the liver (such as

inhibitors of proteases released during inflammation or proteins that are consumed during inflammation). Interleukin-1 may induce synthesis of acute-phase reactants directly by stimulating liver cells. Administration of IL-1 into animals leads to elevation of most acute-phase reactants, including fibrinogen, C-reactive protein, haptoglobin, α-1-antitrypsin, and ceruloplasmin.

A major systemic complication of infection is *septicemia*, or bacterial infection of the blood. (Septicemia is described briefly in Chapter 2. Its cardiovascular consequences, which include anaphylactic shock, are described in Chapter 27.)

Acute inflammation can be verified by hematologic tests, which are described in Chapter 22. An increase in blood levels of acute-phase reactants, primarily fibrinogen (see Table 7-2), is usually associated with an increased erythrocyte sedimentation rate. The alteration in plasma proteins probably leads to an enhanced erythrocyte rouleaux formation (stacking of erythrocytes, as in a stack of coins) and increased rates of sedimentation. Although a nonspecific reaction, increased erythrocyte sedimentation is considered a good indicator of an acute inflammatory response.

CHRONIC INFLAMMATION

Superficially, the difference between acute and chronic inflammation is purely one of duration, in that chronic inflammation lasts 2 weeks or longer, regardless of cause. There may also be characteristic histologic and mechanistic differences (Fig. 7-20). Chronic inflammation is sometimes preceded by an unsuccessful acute inflammatory response. For example, if bacterial contamination or foreign objects (e.g., dirt, wood splinter, glass) persist in a traumatic wound, an inflammatory response that is difficult to differentiate from the acute response will continue beyond 2 weeks. Suppuration, pus formation, and incomplete wound healing may characterize this type of chronic inflammation.

Chronic inflammation can also occur as a distinct process without much acute inflammation. Some microorganisms (e.g., mycobacteria) have cell walls with a very high lipid and wax content, making them relatively insensitive to degradation by phagocytes. The persistence of these bacteria continues to stimulate inflammation. Others, such as the microorganisms that cause tuberculosis, leprosy, syphilis, and brucellosis, can survive within the macrophage. In addition some microorganisms produce toxins that stimulate tissue-damaging reactions even after they are killed. Persistent inflammation can also be the result of prolonged irritation by chemicals, particulate matter, or physical irritants (e.g., inhaled dusts, wood splinters, or suture material).

Chronic inflammation is characterized by a dense infiltration of lymphocytes and macrophages. If macrophages are unable to protect the host from tissue damage, the body attempts to wall off and isolate the infected site, thus forming a **granuloma** (Fig. 7-21). Granulomas are formed if neutrophils and macrophages are unable to destroy microorganisms during the acute inflammatory response. Infections caused by some bacteria (listeriosis, brucellosis), fungi (histoplasmosis, coccidioidomycosis), parasites (leishmaniasis, schistosomiasis, toxoplasmosis), and perhaps large antigen-antibody complexes (rheumatoid arthritis) result in granuloma formation.

Granuloma formation begins when some of the macrophages differentiate into large **epithelioid cells:** cells that are incapable of phagocytosis but capable of taking up debris and other small particles. Other macrophages fuse into multinucleated **giant cells,** which are active phagocytes and can engulf particles too large to be engulfed by single macrophages. The granuloma itself is usually walled off (encapsulated) by fibrous deposits of collagen and may be hyalinized or calcified by deposits of calcium carbonate and calcium phosphate.

The classic granuloma associated with tuberculosis is

FIG. 7-20 The chronic inflammatory response. Inflammation usually becomes chronic because of the persistence of an infection, an antigen, or a foreign body in the wound. Chronic inflammation is characterized by the persistence of many of the processes of acute inflammation. In addition, large amounts of neutrophil degranulation and death, the activation of lymphocytes, and the concurrent activation of fibroblasts result in the release of mediators that induce the infiltration of more lymphocytes and monocytes/macrophages and the beginning of wound healing and tissue repair. The figure numbers refer to those in which more detailed information may be found on that portion of the response.

FIG. 7-21 Cross-section of a granuloma—granulomatous (de Quervain) thyroiditis. Outside the follicle (*lightly shaded*) are mononuclear inflammatory cells and fibrosis (×300). (From Kissane, 1990.)

characterized by a wall of epithelioid cells surrounding a center of dead and decaying tissue (caseous necrosis; see Chapter 2) and mycobacteria. Some of the epithelioid cells fuse into Langhans-type giant cells, with their nuclei distributed in a horseshoe pattern inside the plasma membrane (see Fig. 7-21). The epithelioid cells persist for 3 to 4 weeks, whereas the giant cells live only a few days.

The decay of cells within the granuloma results in the release of acids and the enzymatic contents of dead phagocytes' lysosomes. In this inhospitable environment the cellular debris is broken down into its basic constituents and a clear fluid (liquefaction necrosis; see Chapter 2) remains in the granuloma. Eventually this fluid diffuses out and leaves a hollow, thick-walled structure in the tissue that may remain for the life of the individual.

LOCAL MANIFESTATIONS OF INFLAMMATION

Because inflammation is a nonspecific defense mechanism, it generally proceeds in the same way, no matter what type of injury has occurred. All the local manifes-

tations of acute inflammation are caused by vascular changes and exudation. Swelling occurs as exudate accumulates. Swelling is usually accompanied by pain caused by pressure exerted by exudate accumulation and the presence of soluble biochemical mediators, such as prostaglandins and bradykinin. Heat and redness are the result of increased perfusion (increased blood flow through the area).

The function of vascular changes and exudation is to deliver leukocytes, plasma proteins, and their biochemical mediators to the site of injury. Exudate and its contents have three functions: (1) to dilute toxins produced by bacteria and toxic products released by dying cells, (2) to carry plasma proteins (including antibody) and leukocytes (both phagocytes and lymphocytes) to the site, and (3) to carry away bacterial toxins, dead cells, debris, and other products of inflammation. This third function occurs via channels through the epithelium (sinuses) or through lymphatic vessels. Drainage by lymphatic vessels facilitates the immune response because antigens in lymphatic fluid pass through the lymph nodes, where they stimulate B lymphocytes to become antibody-producing plasma cells or T lymphocytes to become effector T cells. (The lymphatic system is described in Chapter 26.)

Exudate varies in composition, depending on the stage of the inflammatory response and, to some extent, the injurious stimulus. In early or mild inflammation the exudate is watery, or a **serous exudate,** with very few plasma proteins or leukocytes, such as fluid in a blister. In more severe or advanced inflammation the exudate may be thick and clotted, or a **fibrinous exudate,** such as in the lungs of individuals with lobar pneumonia. If a large number of leukocytes accumulates, as in persistent bacterial infections, the exudate consists of pus and is called a **purulent (suppurative) exudate.** Purulent exudate is characteristic of walled-off lesions (**cysts** or **abscesses**). If bleeding occurs, the exudate is filled with erythrocytes and is described as a **hemorrhagic exudate.**

The local manifestations of inflammation can affect all vascularized tissues, but lesions vary, depending on the organ or tissue involved. The lesion resulting from widespread cellular death (necrosis), for example, differs in myocardial (heart muscle), brain, and hepatic (liver) tissue. Cellular death resulting from myocardial infarction (deprivation of oxygen caused by cessation of blood flow) causes a response that proceeds to replacement of the dead tissue with a fibrinous scar. The same injury to brain tissue is more likely to result in the formation of an abscess filled with necrotic tissue (types of necrosis are described in Chapter 2). Destruction of liver tissue stimulates the regrowth, or regeneration, of liver cells.

Because inflammation can occur only in vascularized and perfused tissues, perforative injuries, such as wounds or ulcers, and gangrene, in which an area of a limb or internal organ is killed by bacteria and lack of perfusion, result in inflammation at the *borders* of the lesion. (Gangrene is discussed in Chapter 2.)

Local manifestations of inflammation also accompany all types of nonlethal cellular and tissue injury, from fractures or strains of the musculoskeletal system to burn injuries (see Chapter 2). No matter what the cause or where the lesion, inflammation occurs without fail because without it, healing could not occur. Acute inflammation is so closely tied to healing that it is sometimes called the defense phase of healing.

RESOLUTION AND REPAIR

Destruction of tissue is followed by a period of healing that begins during acute inflammation and may not be complete for as long as 2 years. The most favorable outcome of healing is complete return to normal structure and function. This is possible if damage is minor, no complications occur, or destroyed tissues are capable of **regeneration** (mitotic proliferation of remaining cells; mitosis is described in Chapter 1). Restoration of original structure and physiologic function is called **resolution.**

If extensive damage is present (particularly in tissues incapable of regeneration), if infection results in abscess or granuloma formation, or if fibrin persists in the lesion, resolution is not possible and repair takes place instead. **Repair** is the replacement of destroyed tissue with scar tissue. Scar tissue is composed of **collagen.** It fills in the lesion and restores tensile strength but cannot carry out the physiologic functions of destroyed tissue.

Both regeneration and repair begin during inflammation with phagocytosis of particulate matter in the inflammatory exudate (fibrin from dissolved clots, microorganisms, erythrocytes, and dead tissue cells). This cleanup of the lesion, which also involves dissolution of fibrin clots (or scabs) by fibrinolytic enzymes, is called **débridement.** After débridement, exudate, toxic products, and particulate matter are drained away and vascular dilation and permeability are reversed, preparing the lesion for either regeneration or repair.

Repair, which ends in the formation of scar tissue, always involves processes that (1) fill in the wound, (2) cover or seal the wound, and (3) shrink the wound. These common denominators of wound healing vary in importance and duration among different types of wounds. A clean incision, such as a "paper cut" or a sutured surgical wound, heals primarily through the process of collagen synthesis. Because sealing of this type of wound has already been facilitated by minimal tissue loss and apposition (joining) of the wound edges,

very little sealing (epithelialization) and shrinkage (contraction) are required for healing. Wounds that heal under conditions of minimal tissue loss are said to heal by **primary intention** (Fig. 7-22).

Other wounds do not heal so neatly and easily. Healing of an open wound, such as a stage IV pressure sore (decubitus ulcer), requires a great deal more tissue replacement than healing of a surgical incision. With an open wound, epithelialization, scar formation, and contraction take longer, and healing occurs through **secondary intention** (Fig. 7-22). Healing by either primary or secondary intention may occur at different rates for different types of tissue and for different types of injury.

Resolution and repair occur in two overlapping phases. The first phase, called the **reconstructive phase,** begins 3 to 4 days after the initial injury and continues for up to 2 weeks. This phase is also known as the proliferative, fibroblastic, or connective tissue phase. During the reconstructive phase the lesion is characterized by fibroblast (connective tissue cell) proliferation, which is followed by collagen synthesis by the fibroblasts, epithelialization, and cellular differentiation.

The second phase, the **maturation phase,** begins several weeks post injury and is normally complete within 2 years. The maturation phase is also known as the differentiation, remodeling, or plateau phase. With maturation there is continuing differentiation of cells, contraction of the wound, scar formation, and remodeling of the scar.

Reconstructive Phase

Because surgical and perforative wounds exhibit all the phases of resolution and repair, they are useful models of both normal and abnormal (dysfunctional) healing. The wound is initially sealed off by a blood clot containing fibrin and trapped cells (erythrocytes and leukocytes). The cross-linked mesh of fibrin is created by activation of the coagulation cascade. The fibrin mesh traps platelets, which further seal damaged vessels by forming a platelet plug (see Chapter 22). Most surgical wounds are completely sealed with fibrin several hours after they have been closed. Sealing creates a barrier to bacterial invasion, although it does not always prevent it. The fibrin seal also helps to unite the wound edges. Fibrin provides a framework for the collagen molecules or regenerated tissue cells that will ultimately fill the wound.

For healing to proceed, the fibrin clot must be dissolved and replaced by normal tissue or scar tissue. Enzymatic digestion of the clot usually occurs after activation of the plasma fibrinolytic system (plasmin generation, see Chapter 22) or release of lysosomal enzymes from dead neutrophils. Macrophages invade the dissolving clot and clear away debris and dead cells by phagocytosis. Débridement by macrophages and remaining

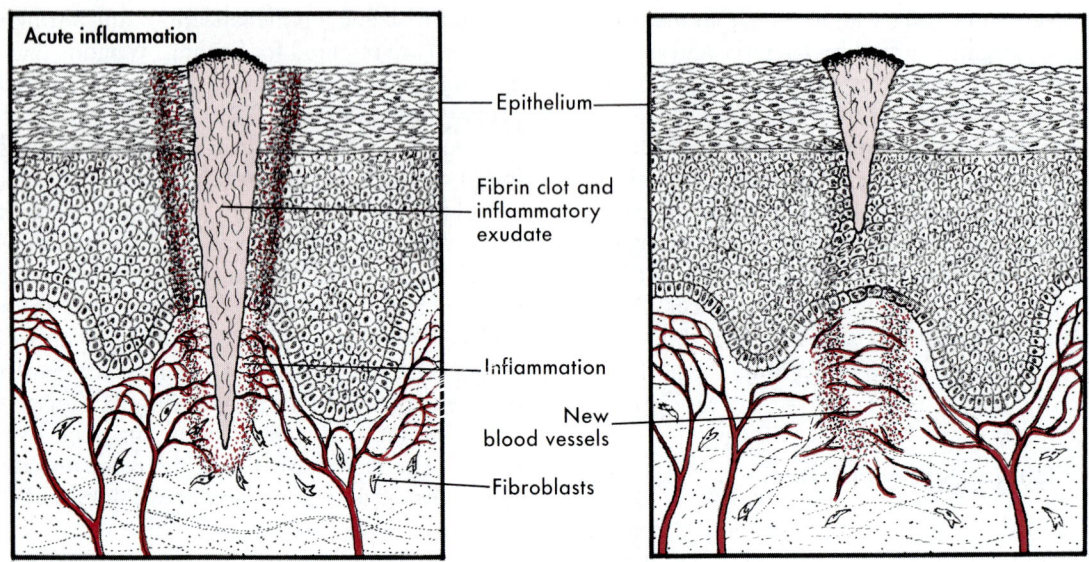

Present in inflammatory exudate:
Neutrophils
Macrophages
Bacteria and dead cells
Erythrocytes
Fibrin

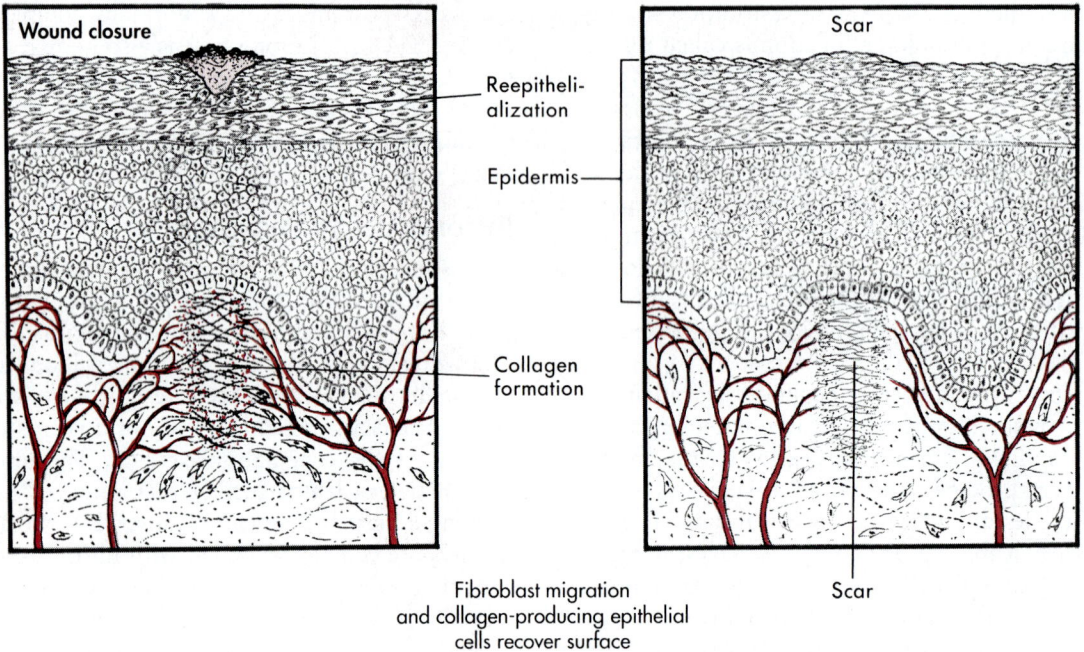

Fibroblast migration
and collagen-producing epithelial
cells recover surface

FIG. 7-22 Wound repair by primary or secondary intention.

neutrophils is followed by simple resolution with regeneration of destroyed cells or, if regeneration is not possible, by the process of repair that ends in scar formation (see Fig. 7-22).

Repair begins as tissue called **granulation tissue** grows inward from surrounding healthy connective tissue. Granulation tissue is filled with new capillaries that give

it a red, granular appearance and is surrounded by fibroblasts and macrophages. First, capillary buds sprout out of vascular endothelial cells around the wound and extend into the debrided areas. Loops form when the young capillaries join *(anastomose)*. The loops are more fragile and permeable than mature vessels, resulting in a leakage of erythrocytes and neutrophils. The erythro-

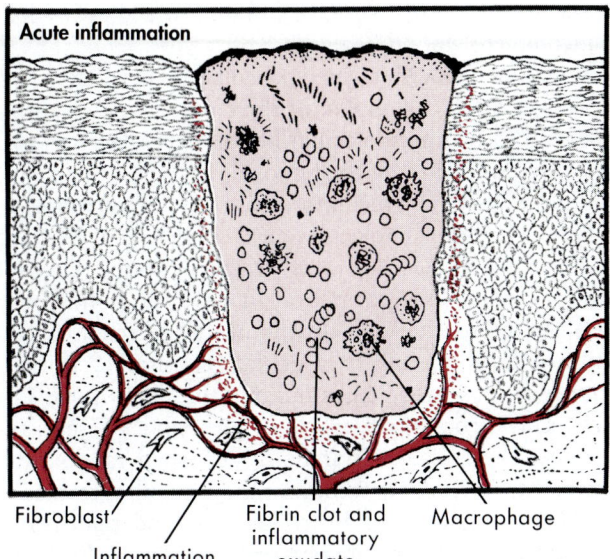

Fibroblast

Inflammation

Fibrin clot and inflammatory exudate

Macrophage

New blood vessels

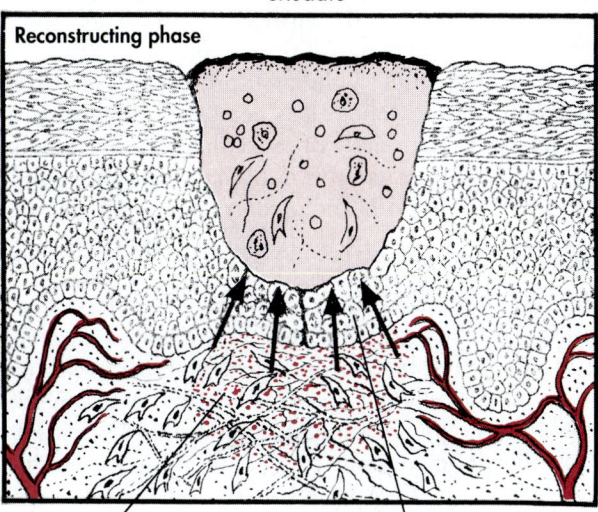

Granulation tissue   Epithelialization

Acute inflammation
  Present in inflammatory exudate: neutrophils, macrophages, bacteria, dead cells, and erythrocytes.
  Macrophages release (1) angiogenesis factor to attract epithelial cells and vascular endothelial cells (capillary and lymphatic buds) and (2) fibroblast-activating factor to attract fibroblasts.

Reconstructing phase
  Epithelialization includes formation of granulation tissue, inward migration of fibroblasts, and the beginning of collagen synthesis and secretion.
  Granulation tissue becomes scar tissue, contraction begins, and differentiation begins.

Maturation phase
  This phase includes completion of contraction, differentiation, and remodeling of scar tissue, and disappearance of capillaries from scar tissue.

Collagen fibers

Scar tissue

FIG. 7-22, cont'd Wound repair by primary or secondary intention.

cytes are phagocytosed by macrophages, and the neutrophils participate in further débridement of the inflammatory lesion. Many of the new capillaries differentiate into arterioles and venules as repair continues. New lymphatic vessels grow into the granulation tissue by a similar process.

The macrophage performs several functions in healing. Besides acting as the primary phagocyte of débridement, it secretes biochemical mediators that promote healing, namely (1) fibroblast-activating factor, which stimulates fibroblasts to enter the lesion and synthesize and secrete the collagen precursor, procollagen; (2) angiogenesis factor, which stimulates vascular endothelial cells to form capillary buds that grow into the lesion; and (3) an unidentified factor that stimulates epithelial cells to grow over and seal the wound's surface. Macrophages also secrete collagenase, which debrides injured collagen fibers in the wound.

As the clot or scab is being dissolved and granulation tissue is being formed, the healing wound must be protected. This is accomplished by **epithelialization**, the process by which epithelial cells grow into the wound from surrounding healthy tissue. Attracted by a factor secreted by macrophages, the epithelial cells migrate under the clot or scab, using proteolytic enzymes to sever the connection between the clot and the wound surface (see Fig. 7-22). Eventually the migrating epithelial cells contact similar cells from all sides of the wound, make contact, and seal the wound, after which migration and proliferation cease. The epithelial cells remain active, however, undergoing differentiation to give rise to the various epidermal layers (see Chapter 41). Epithelialization of a skin wound can be hastened if the wound is kept moist, preventing the fibrin clot from becoming a scab.

Fibroblasts are the most important cells during the reconstructive phase of wound healing because they synthesize and secrete collagen. Fibroblasts are stimulated by fibroblast-activating factor (from macrophages) to proliferate and enter the lesion. The collagen produced by fibroblasts is laid down in debrided areas about 6 days after fibroblasts have entered the lesion.

Collagen is the most abundant protein in the body and is the material of tissue repair. It is present in skin, bones, teeth, blood vessels, tendons, cartilage, and connective tissue. Collagen is produced in fibroblasts as a polypeptide of repeating sequences of the amino acids glycine, proline, hydroxyproline, lysine, and hydroxylysine. Proline and lysine are enzymatically hydroxylated after the polypeptide chain is synthesized, and their hydroxylation is absolutely necessary for collagen polymerization and function. Cofactors that are necessary for hydroxylation include iron, ascorbic acid (vitamin C), α-ketoglutarate (from the Krebs cycle), and mo-

lecular oxygen (O_2). Absence of these cofactors results in incomplete wound healing.

Immature collagen, termed **procollagen,** is secreted by the fibroblast as a complex of three polypeptide chains cross-linked by intermolecular bonds. Procollagen must be activated further by the removal of a small polypeptide sequence by a specific protease. As the scar tissue matures, collagen molecules are cross-linked by intramolecular bonds to form collagen fibrils. Cross-linking involves the formation of covalent bonds between lysine residues. At this point, the secreted collagen molecules are still of a gel-like consistency in the wound. With further cross-linking, the fibrils form fibers. This process occurs over a period of several months. The collagen is initially deposited randomly, but during remodeling of the scar tissue that has formed, the fibers are dissolved by collagenase and reformed. During this period the fibers reorient along the lines of mechanical stress and further cross-linking adds strength.

Wound **contraction** is the final process of the reconstructive phase of healing. It is necessary for closure of all wounds, but especially of those that heal by secondary intention. Contraction is noticeable 6 to 12 days after injury. In normal healing, contraction may amount to inward movement of the wound edge by approximately 0.5 mm per day.

The granulation tissue contains **myofibroblasts,** specialized cells that probably cause wound contraction. As the name implies, myofibroblasts have features of both smooth muscle cells and fibroblasts. Microscopically the myofibroblast appears similar to a fibroblast, but it differs in that its cytoplasm contains bundles of parallel fibers similar to those found in smooth muscle cells. These fibers exert a contractile force within the cell. Wound contraction occurs as structures extending from the plasma membrane of the myofibroblast establish connections with neighboring cells. Once connected, myofibroblasts can exert pull on neighboring cells and anchor themselves to the wound bed, promoting contraction.

Maturation Phase

Collagen deposition, tissue regeneration, and wound contraction all begin during the reconstructive phase. When this phase ends, about 2 weeks after injury, these processes are usually not complete. Therefore, they continue into the maturation phase, which can continue for years. During the maturation phase scar tissue is remodeled. Capillaries disappear, leaving an avascular scar. Within 2 to 3 weeks after maturation has begun, the scar tissue has gained about two thirds of its eventual maximum strength.

Epidermal wounds that heal by secondary intention

and unsutured internal lesions are seldom completely restored by healing. At best repaired tissue regains 80% of its original tensile strength. Only epithelial, hepatic (liver), and bone marrow cells are capable of the complete mitotic regeneration known as compensatory hyperplasia (hyperplasia is described in Chapter 2). In fibrous connective tissue, such as joints and ligaments, normal healing results in the replacement of the original tissue, but the new tissue does not have exactly the same structure as the original. Some damaged tissue heals without replacement. For instance, the damage resulting from myocardial infarction heals with a scar composed of fibrous tissue rather than replacing cardiac muscle. Although the composition of healed tissue may differ, the healing process of soft tissues is the same for all wounds.

Dysfunctional Wound Healing

Dysfunctional healing may occur during any phase of the wound-healing process and may involve insufficient repair, excessive repair, or infection. The etiologic cause of dysfunctional healing can be related to a predisposing disorder, such as diabetes mellitus, or to an acquired condition, such as hypoxemia (insufficient oxygen in arterial blood). Numerous drugs and nutrients can also affect wound healing. Wound repair delays healing by reactivating inflammatory processes.

Dysfunction During the Inflammatory Response

Healing may be prolonged if bleeding is not stopped during acute inflammation. Hemorrhage in a damaged area delays healing for several reasons. A clot increases the amount of space that granulation tissue has to fill and serves as a mechanical barrier to oxygen diffusion. The accumulation of excess blood cells resulting from hemorrhage prolongs the inflammatory process, since these cells must be cleared prior to repair. Accumulated blood, which is an excellent culture medium for bacteria, promotes infection and prolongs inflammation by increasing exudation and pus formation. In addition to slowing healing, sepsis can promote excessive scar formation or prevent healing completely.

Excessive amounts of fibrin are also detrimental to healing. The great amount of fibrin that is released in response to injury must eventually be reabsorbed so it will not organize into fibrous adhesions. Adhesions are seldom clinically significant unless they form in the pleural, pericardial, or abdominal cavities. Adhesions in these areas may bind organs together by fibrous bands, the shrinkage of which can distort or strangulate the affected organ.

Many factors may adversely affect the inflammatory process during wound healing. Hypovolemia-decreased blood volume inhibits inflammation. The physiologic response to hypovolemia is vessel constriction rather than the dilation required to deliver inflammatory cells to the site of injury. Anti-inflammatory steroids prevent macrophages from migrating to the site of injury and inhibit their release of collagenase and plasminogen activator (Alvarez et al., 1984). Anti-inflammatory steroids also inhibit fibroblast migration into the wound during the reconstructive phase of healing.

Optimal nutrition is important during all phases of healing because metabolic needs are increased. During inflammation the substances most essential for healing are glucose, oxygen, and protein. Because leukocytes need glucose to produce the adenosine triphosphate 5'(ATP) needed for chemotaxis, phagocytosis, and intercellular killing, the wounds of diabetics who receive insufficient insulin heal poorly, mainly because of infection. Diabetics are at risk for ischemic wounds because they are likely to have both small-vessel diseases that impair the microcirculation and altered (glycosylated) hemoglobin, which has an increased affinity for oxygen and thus does not readily release oxygen in tissues. (Hemoglobin's function as the oxygen-carrying component of blood is described in Chapter 22.) Oxygen delivery is also compromised by hypoxemic states. Ischemic tissue is susceptible to infection, which prolongs inflammation. Hypoproteinemia also prolongs inflammation because it impairs fibroblast proliferation.

Wound sepsis is treated in several ways. Most important is the removal or débridement of necrotic tissue and foreign bodies. Débridement is accomplished by surgery or use of absorbent dressings. Wound irrigation and antibiotic therapy also combat infection.

Dysfunction During the Reconstructive Phase
Impaired collagen synthesis

A number of factors may interfere with the production of collagen in healing tissues. Most of these factors are nutritional. Scurvy, for example, is a condition caused by lack of ascorbic acid. Ascorbic acid is one of the cofactors required for the hydroxylation of the amino acids proline and lysine. Without hydroxylation these amino acids cannot be incorporated into collagen monomers; therefore, procollagen is not secreted from the fibroblast. The results of scurvy are poorly formed connective tissue and greatly impaired healing.

Other nutrients play a cofactor role in enzyme systems required for collagen synthesis. These include iron, oxygen, α-ketoglutarate, manganese, copper, and calcium. Usually such minute amounts of these substances are required as cofactors that deficiencies are not clinically significant.

Protein is essential for collagen synthesis. Especially important is the amino acid methionine, which is converted to cystine. The role of cystine in collagen synthe-

FIG. 7-23 Keloid (scar) formation. Scar caused by excessive synthesis of collagen. Keloid from suture marks in a black individual. (From Habif, 1990.)

sis is twofold: (1) it functions as an important cofactor in enzyme systems required for collagen synthesis; and (2) it contains sulfur, which contributes to the formation of strong disulfide bonds in cross-linked collagen fibrils.

Collagen synthesis may be impaired during the processes of polymerization and cross-linking. After procollagen is secreted from the fibroblast, it must be activated by cleavage of its terminal peptides. Cleavage does not occur, for example, in individuals with Ehlers-Danlos syndrome (type VII). This disease prevents formation of normal connective tissue, causing the skin to be thin and fragile. All forms of Ehlers-Danlos syndrome are characterized by defects in collagen cross-linking. (The role of collagen in bone formation is described in Chapter 38.)

Dysfunctional collagen synthesis may also involve excessive production of collagen. This causes surface overhealing, which is manifested by a keloid or a hypertrophic scar (Fig. 7-23). Both keloid and hypertrophic scars are caused by an imbalance between collagen synthesis and collagen lysis in which synthesis is increased and lysis (degradation) is decreased. A **keloid** is a raised scar that extends beyond the original boundaries of the wound. It invades surrounding tissue and is likely to recur after surgical removal. A familial tendency to keloid formation has been observed, with a greater incidence in blacks than whites. A **hypertrophic scar** is raised but remains within the original boundaries of the wound. Hypertrophic scars tend to regress over time.

Impaired epithelialization

Epithelialization is suppressed by anti-inflammatory steroids, hypoxemia, ionizing radiation, and zinc deficiencies. Wound care technique may greatly influence epithelial cell migration.

External wounds that are draining or healing by secondary intention are often debrided and protected with dressings. The ideal dressing is one that absorbs some drainage without being incorporated into the clot or granulation tissue. Because epithelial cells must migrate across the wound during healing, dressings that debride healthy epithelial cells along with necrotic tissue prolong epithelialization.

Many solutions that have traditionally been used to clean or irrigate wounds are deleterious to the fragile new cells in the wound bed. Normal saline is the most innocuous solution that can be used to cleanse or irrigate a wound that is healing primarily by epithelialization. Solutions such as povidone-iodine and hydrogen peroxide are very desiccating (drying) and subsequently inhibit rather than promote epithelial cell migration.

Wound disruption

A potential complication of wounds that are sutured closed is **dehiscence,** in which the wound pulls apart at the suture line. The greatest incidence of dehiscence occurs 5 to 12 days after suturing. Paradoxically, this is the time when collagen synthesis is at its peak. Approximately 50% of the time dehiscence is associated with wound sepsis. It may also occur when sutures break because of excessive strain. Obesity increases the risk for dehiscence because adipose tissue is difficult to suture. Wound dehiscence is usually heralded by an increase in serous drainage from the wound. Additionally, the individual may report a feeling that "something gave way." Prompt surgical attention is required.

Impaired contraction

Wound contraction is necessary for healing. This process may become pathologic when there is excessive contraction resulting in a deformity or **contracture.**

Burns are especially susceptible to the development of contractures. Internal contracture may occur in cirrhosis of the liver. Scar tissue that becomes contracted constricts vascular flow, which may contribute to the development of portal hypertension and esophageal varices. Other types of internal contraction deformity include duodenal strictures caused by dysfunctional healing of an ulcer and esophageal strictures caused by lye burns.

Proper positioning and range-of-motion exercises and surgery are among the physical means used to overcome myofibroblast pull and prevent contractures. Biochemical means include control of myofibroblast contraction by the administration of smooth muscle inhibitors (e.g., colchicine) and attempts to inhibit collagen synthesis with drugs that prevent collagen cross-linking or collagenase activity. This treatment is based on the knowledge that collagen can "lock" contracted myofibroblasts into position. Clinical use of pharmacologic methods for control of wound contracture is still largely experimental.

AGING and Mechanisms of Self-Defense

Besides immature or depressed immune function, neonates frequently have transiently depressed inflammatory function. For example, neutrophils and perhaps monocytes may not be capable of chemotaxis. Insufficient response to chemotactic factors appears to be due to lack of fluidity in the phagocyte's plasma membrane, so that it cannot form pseudopods and migrate. Neonates are prone to infections associated with chemotactic defects, including cutaneous abscesses caused by staphylococci and cutaneous candidiasis. Furthermore, neutrophils in neonates stressed by in utero infection or respiratory insufficiency have diminished oxidative and bacterial responses. (Acquired phagocytic defects, which may be induced by a variety of infections, metabolic disorders, nutrition deficiencies, or drugs, are described in Chapter 8.)

Neonates are also partially deficient in complement, especially components of the alternative pathway. They tend to have a relative deficiency of factor B and to develop severe, overwhelming sepsis and meningitis when infected with bacteria against which there is no transferred maternal antibody.

The elderly population is at risk for impaired wound healing. There is no concrete evidence that impaired wound healing is a consequence of normal aging, however. Often impaired healing is associated with chronic illnesses, such as diabetes mellitus or cardiovascular disease. Additionally, many elderly persons require medications, such as anti-inflammatory steroids, that interfere with healing.

Because of impaired sensation or mobility and physiologic changes in the skin, the elderly are at increased risk for sustaining various wounds. With aging subcutaneous fat is lost, diminishing a layer of protection. Collagen fibers become thicker and less elastic, thus further contributing to loss of protection.

Diminished immune function may interfere with the elderly person's natural ability to ward off infection in a wound. The regenerative capability of the skin is maintained with aging, but the epidermis undergoes some atrophy that includes atrophy of underlying capillaries. The consequent decrease of perfusion makes the elderly more susceptible than others to the adverse effects of hypoxia (insufficient oxygen) in the wound bed.

SUMMARY REVIEW

The Acute Inflammatory Response

1 Inflammation is a rapid and nonspecific protective response to cellular injury from any cause. It can occur only in vascularized tissue.
2 The macroscopic hallmarks of inflammation are redness, swelling, heat, pain, and loss of function of the inflamed tissues.
3 The microscopic hallmark of inflammation is an accumulation of fluid and cells at the inflammatory site.

The Mast Cell

1 The most important activator of the inflammatory response is the mast cell, which initiates inflammation by releasing biochemical mediators (histamine, chemotactic factors) from preformed cytoplasmic granules and synthesizing other mediators (prostaglandins, leukotrienes) in response to a stimulus.
2 Histamine and serotonin are the major vasoactive amines of inflammation. Both cause constriction of vascular smooth muscles, dilation of capillaries, and retraction of endothelial cells lining the capillaries, which increases vascular permeability.

Plasma Protein Systems

1 Inflammation is mediated by three key plasma protein systems: the complement system, the clotting system, and the kinin system. The components of all three systems are a series of inactive proteins (proenzymes) that are activated in cascade fashion.
2 The complement system can be activated by antigen-antibody reactions (through the classic pathway) or by other products, especially bacterial polysaccharides (through the alternative pathway), resulting in the production of biologically active (anaphylatoxic or chemotactic) fragments and target cell lysis.
3 The clotting system stops bleeding, localizes microorganisms, and provides a meshwork for repair and healing.
4 Bradykinin is the most important kinin protein and causes vascular permeability, smooth muscle contraction, and pain.

Cellular Components of Inflammation

1 The cells involved in the inflammatory process include phagocytic leukocytes (neutrophils, macrophages, and eosinophils), platelets, and lymphocytes.
2 Phagocytic cells engulf and destroy microorganisms by enclosing them in phagocytic vacuoles (phagolysosomes), within which toxic products (especially metabolites of oxygen) and degradative lysosomal enzymes kill and digest the microorganisms.
3 Opsonins, such as antibody and complement component C3b, coat microorganisms and make them more susceptible to phagocytosis by binding them more tightly to the phagocyte.
4 The polymorphonuclear neutrophil (PMN), the predominant phagocytic cell in the early inflammatory response, exits the circulation by diapedesis through the retracted endothelial cell junctions and moves to the inflammatory site by chemotaxis.
5 The macrophage, the predominant phagocytic cell in the late inflammatory response, is highly phagocytic, responsive to lymphokines, and responsible for antigen processing and presentation to lymphocytes.
6 Eosinophils release products that control the inflammatory response and are induced by IgE-mediated mechanisms of hypersensitivity to kill parasitic organisms directly.

Cellular Products

1 The cells involved in immunity and inflammation stimulate other cells by secreting lymphokines, interferons, or interleukins.
2 Lymphokines are produced by T cells and have their most important effects on macrophages. These effects include chemotaxis, inhibition of migration once the macrophage has entered the inflammatory site, and activation of the macrophage, which makes it a more powerful phagocyte.

3 Interferons are produced by host cells that are already infected by viruses. Once released from infected cells, interferons can stimulate neighboring healthy cells to produce substances that prevent viral penetration.
4 Interleukins are produced by leukocytes that have been stimulated by an antigen. Interleukins stimulate other leukocytes to proliferate or otherwise increase their immune functions. The chief effect of interleukins is to accelerate the immune response.

Systemic Manifestations of Acute Inflammation

1 The systemic effects of inflammation are fever and increases in levels of circulating leukocytes and plasma proteins.

Chronic Inflammation

1 Chronic inflammation lasts 2 weeks or longer. It can occur as a distinct process without much acute inflammation.
2 Chronic inflammation is characterized by a dense infiltration of lymphocytes and macrophages. The body walls off and isolates the host from tissue damage, forming a granuloma.

Local Manifestations of Inflammation

1 Local manifestations of inflammation all involve the same hallmarks of inflammation, but types of exudate and necrosis vary with the injury and the tissue or organ affected.

Resolution and Repair

1 Inflammatory lesions proceed to resolution if little tissue has been lost or injured tissue is capable of regeneration. This is called healing by primary intention.
2 Inflammatory lesions that involve extensive damage or tissues incapable of regeneration heal by repair. This process is called healing by secondary intention.

Aging and Mechanisms of Self-Defense

1 Neonates frequently have transiently depressed inflammatory function. The eldery person is at risk for impaired wound healing.
2 Diminished immune function may interfere with the elderly person's natural ability to ward off infection in a wound.

KEY TERMS

Abscess, 258
Acute-phase reactant, 256
Alternative pathway, 240
Anaphylatoxin, 241
Antigen-antibody complex (immune complex), 241
Basophil, 237
Bradykinin, 242
Chemotactic factor, 238
Chemotaxis, 238
Classic pathway, 240
Collagen, 259
Complement cascade, 240
Contraction, 262
Contracture, 264
Cyst, 258
Débridement, 259
Degranulation, 237
Dehiscence, 264
Diapedesis, 248
Eosinophil, 252
Epithelialization, 262
Epithelioid cell, 257

Extrinsic pathway, 242
Exudate, 234
Fibrinous exudate, 258
Fibroblast, 262
Giant cell, 257
Granulation tissue, 260
Granuloma, 257
Hemorrhagic exudate, 258
Hypertrophic scar, 264
Interferon, 255
Interleukin (IL), 254
Intrinsic pathway, 242
Keloid, 264
Leukotriene (slow-reacting substance of anaphylaxis [SRS-A]), 238
Lymphokine, 254
Macrophage, 250
Macrophage-activating factor (MAF), 255
Margination (pavementing), 247
Mast cell, 237
Maturation phase, 259
Migration-inhibitory factor (MIF), 255

Monocyte, 250
Myofibroblast, 262
Neutrophil, 250
Phagocytosis, 248
Phagolysosome, 249
Phagosome, 249
Plasma kinin cascade, 242
Platelet, 237
Polymorphonuclear neutrophil (PMN), 250
Primary intention, 259
Procollagen, 262
Proenzyme, 239
Prostaglandin, 239
Purulent (suppurative) exudate, 258
Reconstructive phase, 259
Regeneration, 259
Repair, 259
Resolution, 259
Secondary intention, 259
Serous exudate, 258

REFERENCES

Alvarez, O. M., Levendorf, K. D., Smerbeck, R. V., Mertz, P. M., & Eaglstein, W. H. (1984). Effect of topically applied steroidal and nonsteroidal anti-inflammatory agents on skin repair and regeneration. *Federation Proceedings, 43,* 2793-2798.

Habif, T. P. (1990). *Clinical dermatology.* (2nd ed.). St. Louis: Mosby–Year Book.

King, D. W., Fenoglio, C. M., & Lefwitch, J. H. (1983). *General pathology: Principles and dynamics.* Philadelphia: Lea & Febiger.

Kissane, J. M. (1990). *Anderson's pathology* (9th ed.). St. Louis: Mosby–Year Book.

Lachman, L. B., & Maizel, A. L. (1983). The interleukins: Immunoregulatory molecules. *Clinical Immunology Newsletter, 4,* 113-115.

Milanese, C., Richardson, N. E., & Reinherz, E. L. (1986). Identification of a T helper cell-derived lymphokine that activates resting T lymphocytes. *Science, 231*(4742), 1118-1122.

Dinarello, C. A., & Mier, J. W. (1987). Current concepts: Lymphokines. *New England Journal of Medicine, 317,* 940-945.

Ehrlich, P. (1877). Dietbage zur Kenntnis der Anilinsfarb und Ihrer Verwendung nin ungen der Mikroskopichen technik. *Arch Mikr Anat, 13,* 263-277.

Gallin, J. I., & Goldstein, R. S. (1992). *Inflammation: Basic principles and clinical correlates* (2nd ed.). New York: Raven Press.

Golub, E. S., & Green, D. R. (1991). *Immunology: A synthesis* (2nd ed.). Sunderland, MA: Sinauer Associates.

Henson, P. M. (1985). Mechanisms of tissue injury produced by immunologic reactions. In J. A. Bellanti (Ed.), *Immunology III* (p. 251). Philadelphia: W.B. Saunders.

Kline, J. (1990). *Immunology.* New York: Blackwell Scientific.

Kuby, J. (1992). *Immunology.* New York: Freeman.

Malech, H. L., & Gallen, J. I. (1987). Current concepts—immunobiology: Neutrophils in human diseases. *New England Journal of Medicine, 317,* 687-693.

Serafin, W. E., & Austen, K. F. (1987). Current concepts: Mediators of immediate hypersensitivity reactions. *New England Journal of Medicine, 317,* 30-34.

SUGGESTED READINGS

Ballow, M., Levinson, A. I., & Insel, R. A. (Eds.). (1992). Symposium: Future directions of cytokine and immunoglobulin therapy. *Clinical Immunology and Immuno Pathology, 62,*. S1-S97.

Alterations in Immunity and Inflammation

Neal S. Rote

Chapter Outline

The immune system is a finely tuned network that protects the host against foreign antigens, particularly infectious agents. Sometimes this network breaks down, causing the immune system to react inappropriately. Inappropriate immune responses may be (1) exaggerated against environmental antigens (allergy), (2) misdirected against the host's own cells (autoimmunity), (3) directed against beneficial foreign tissues, such as transfusions or transplants (isoimmunity), or (4) insufficient for protection (immune deficiency). All of these can be serious or life-threatening. Exaggerated immune responses (allergy) are the most common and usually the least life-threatening.

HYPERSENSITIVITY: ALLERGY, AUTOIMMUNITY, AND ISOIMMUNITY

The first three types of inappropriate responses listed above can be collectively classified as **hypersensitivity.** Hypersensitivity is an altered immunologic reactivity to an antigen that results in a pathologic immune response after reexposure. Allergy, autoimmunity, and isoimmunity are differentiated by the source of the antigen against which the hypersensitivity response is directed (Table 8-1). The term **allergy** originally denoted both facets of the immune response: immunity, which is beneficial, and hypersensitivity, which is harmful. Allergy has come to mean the deleterious effects of hypersensitivity to environmental (exogenous) antigens, and immunity the protective responses to antigens expressed by disease-causing agents.

Autoimmunity is a disturbance in the immunologic tolerance of self-antigens. A great variety of clinical disorders are associated with autoimmunity and are referred to as **autoimmune diseases** (Table 8-2). Autoimmune diseases occur when the immune system reacts against self-antigens and destroys host tissues. Antibodies against self-antigens, termed **autoantibodies,** are also produced by healthy individuals, particularly the elderly. In fact, part of the aging process may, in part, represent a deterioration of tolerance to self-antigens. Healthy individuals of all ages may produce autoantibodies, without concurrent overt autoimmune disease, in response to tissue damage. Therefore, the presence of low quantities of autoantibodies does not necessarily indicate a disease state.

Isoimmune diseases occur when the immune system of one individual produces an immunologic reaction against tissues of another individual. **Isoimmunity** can be observed during immunologic reactions against transfusions, grafted tissue, or the fetus during pregnancy.

The pathogenesis of hypersensitivity, whether it consists of allergy, autoimmunity, or isoimmunity, is not completely understood. It is generally accepted that genetic, infectious, and possibly environmental factors contribute to hypersensitivity. Most diseases caused by hypersensitivity evolve because of the interactions of at least three variables: (1) an original insult, which alters **immunologic homeostasis** (a steady state of tolerance to self-antigens; more important in autoimmunity than in isoimmunity or allergy); (2) the individual's genetic makeup, which determines susceptibility to the effects of the insult; and (3) an immunologic process that amplifies the insult.

Mechanisms of Hypersensitivity

Diseases caused by hypersensitivity are also characterized by immune mechanisms that initiate inflammation and result in the destruction of healthy tissue (see Table 8-1). These mechanisms are apparent in most hypersensitivity reactions and have been divided into four distinct types: (1) type I (IgE-mediated allergic reactions), (2) type II (tissue-specific reactions), (3) type III (immune-complex–mediated reactions), and (4) type IV (cell-mediated reactions) (Gell, Coombs, & Lachman, 1975) (Table 8-3). This classification is artificial and seldom is a particular disease associated with a single

TABLE 8-1

Relative Incidences and Examples of Hypersensitivity Reactions*

Target antigen	Mechanism			
	Type I (IgE-mediated)	Type II (Tissue-specific)	Type III (Immune-complex)	Type IV (Cell-mediated)
Allergy Environmental antigens	++++ Hay fever	+ Hemolysis in drug allergies	+ Gluten (wheat) allergy	++ Poison ivy allergy
Autoimmunity Self-antigens	± May contribute to some type III reactions	++ Autoimmune thrombocytopenia	+++ Systemic lupus erythematosus	+ Hashimoto thyroiditis
Isoimmunity Other person's antigens	± May contribute to some type III reactions	++ Hemolytic disease of the newborn	+ Anaphylaxis to IgA in IV γ-globulin	++ Graft rejection

*The frequency of each reaction is indicated in a range from rare (±) to very common (++++). An example of each reaction is given.

TABLE 8-2

Disorders Associated with Autoimmunity

System disease	Organ or tissue	Probable self-antigen
Endocrine system		
Hyperthyroidism (Graves disease)	Thyroid gland	Receptors for thyroid-stimulating hormone on plasma membrane of thyroid cells
Autoimmune thyroiditis	Thyroid gland	Thyroglobulin; microsomes
Primary myxedema	Thyroid gland	Microsomes
Insulin-dependent diabetes	Pancreas	Islet cells, insulin, insulin receptors on pancreatic cells
Addison disease	Adrenal gland	Surface antigens on steroid-producing cells; microsomes of adrenal cortex
Premature gonadal failure	Ovary	Interstitial cells; corpus luteum
Male infertility	Testis	Surface antigens on spermatozoa
Orchitis	Testis	Germinal epithelium
Female infertility	Ovary	Zona pellucida
Idiopathic hypoparathyroidism	Parathyroid gland	Surface antigens on chief cells (epithelial cells of gland)
Partial pituitary deficiency	Pituitary gland	Prolactin-producing cells; growth–hormone–producing cells
Skin		
Pemphigus vulgaris	Skin	Intercellular substances in stratified squamous epithelium
Bullous pemphigoid	Skin	Basement membrane
Dermatitis herpetiformis	Skin	Basement membrane (IgA)
Vitiligo	Skin	Surface antigens on melanocytes (melanin-producing cells)
Neuromuscular tissue		
Polymyositis (dermatomyositis)	Muscle	Nuclear materials; myosin
Multiple sclerosis	Neural tissue	Unknown
Myasthenia gravis	Neuromuscular junction	Acetylcholine receptors; striations of skeletal and cardiac muscle
Polyneuritis	Nerve cell	Peripheral myelin
Rheumatic fever	Heart	Cardiac tissue (subsarcolemmal membrane); cross-reaction with group A streptococcal antigen
Cardiomyopathy	Heart	Cardiac muscle
Postvaccinal or postinfectious encephalitis	Central nervous system	Central nervous system myelin or basic protein
Gastrointestinal system		
Celiac disease (gluten-sensitive enteropathy)	Intestine	Gluten
Ulcerative colitis	Colon	Mucosal cells
Crohn disease	Ileum	Unknown
Pernicious anemia	Stomach	Surface antigens of parietal cells; intrinsic factor
Atrophic gastritis	Stomach	Parietal cells
Primary biliary cirrhosis	Liver	Mitochondria; cells of bile duct
Chronic active hepatitis	Liver	Surface antigens, nuclei, microsomes, mitochondria or hepatocytes; smooth muscle
Eye		
Sjögren syndrome	Lacrimal gland	Antigens of lacrimal gland, salivary gland, thyroid, and nuclei of cells; IgG
Uveitis	Uveal structures	Antigens of the iris, ciliary body, and choroid

TABLE 8-2

Disorders Associated with Autoimmunity—cont'd

System/disease	Organ or tissue	Probable self-antigen
Connective tissue		
Ankylosing spondylitis	Joints	Sarcoiliac and spinal apophyseal joint
Rheumatoid arthritis	Joints	IgG, collagen
Systemic lupus erythematosus	Multiple sites	Numerous antigens in nuclei, organelles, and extracellular matrix
Mixed connective tissue disease	Multiple sites	Ribonucleoprotein and numerous others
Polyarteritis nodosa (necrotizing vasculitis)	Arterioles (small arteries)	Unknown
Scleroderma (progressive systemic sclerosis)	Multiple organs	Nuclear antigens; IgG
Felty syndrome	Joints	IgG
Renal system		
Immune-complex glomerulonephritis	Kidney	Numerous immune complexes
Goodpasture disease	Kidney	Glomerular basement membrane
Hematologic system		
Idiopathic neutropenia	Neutrophil	Surface antigens on polymorphonuclear neutrophils
Idiopathic lymphopenia	Lymphocytes	Surface antigens on lymphocytes
Autoimmune hemolytic anemia	Erythrocytes	Surface antigens on erythrocytes
Autoimmune thrombocytopenic purpura	Platelets	Surface antigens on platelets
Respiratory system		
Goodpasture disease	Lung	Septal membrane of alveolus

TABLE 8-3

Immunologic Mechanisms of Tissue Destruction

Type	Name	Rate of development	Class of antibody involved	Principal effector cells involved	Complement participation	Examples of disorders
I	IgE-mediated reaction	Immediate	IgE	Mast cells	No	Seasonal allergic rhinitis
II	Tissue-specific reaction	Immediate	IgG IgM	Macrophages in tissues	Frequently	Autoimmune thrombocytopenic purpura, Graves disease, autoimmune hemolytic anemia
III	Immune-complex–mediated reaction	Immediate	IgG IgM	Neutrophils	Yes	Systemic lupus erythematosus
IV	Cell-mediated reaction	Delayed	None	Lymphocytes Macrophages	No	Contact sensitivity to poison ivy and metals

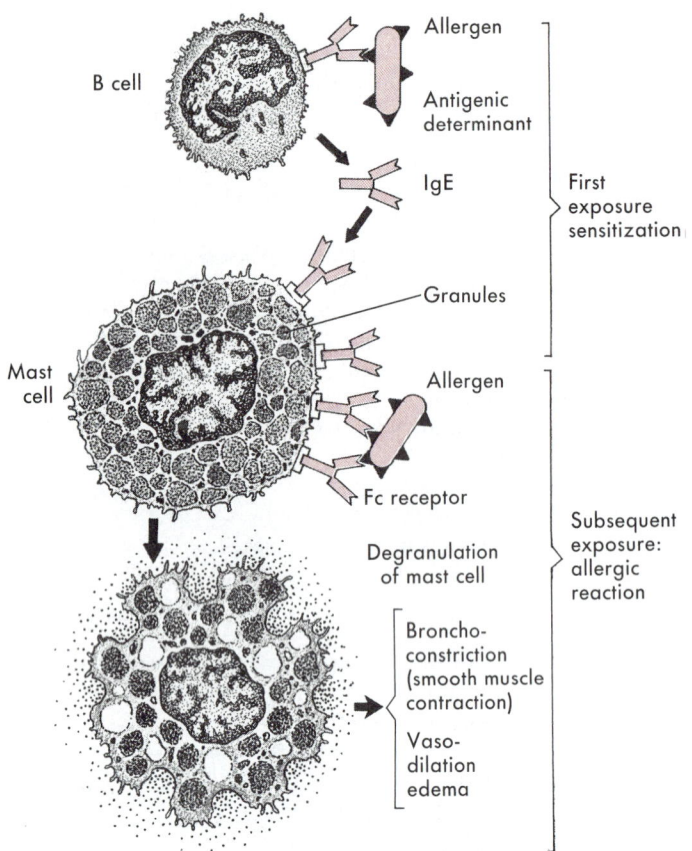

FIG. 8-1 Mechanism of type I IgE-mediated reactions. Initial sensitization to an allergen stimulates B cells to produce IgE. The IgE coats the surface of the mast cell by binding with IgE-specific Fc receptors on the mast cell's plasma membrane. Further exposure to the same allergen cross-links the surface-bound IgE and causes degranulation of the mast cell.

mechanism only. The four mechanisms are interrelated and, in most hypersensitivity reactions, several are at work simultaneously. Some of them are secondary to disease, whereas others are pathognomonic (diagnostic of) and the primary cause of tissue destruction.

Hypersensitivity reactions are immediate or delayed, depending on the time required to elicit the secondary immune response (i.e., for the reaction to appear after reexposure to the antigen). Reactions that occur within minutes are termed **immediate hypersensitivity reactions. Delayed hypersensitivity reactions** may take several hours to appear and are at maximum severity days after reexposure to the antigen.

The most rapid immediate hypersensitivity reaction is anaphylaxis. **Anaphylaxis** is a rapid and severe response that occurs within minutes of reexposure to the antigen and can be either systemic (generalized) or cutaneous (localized) (Portier & Richet, 1902). Symptoms of sys-

temic anaphylaxis include itching, erythema, vomiting, abdominal cramps, diarrhea, and breathing difficulties. In severe cases, laryngeal edema and vascular collapse may result in respiratory distress, decreased blood pressure, shock, and death. Cutaneous anaphylaxis causes the less severe symptoms of local inflammation.

IgE-Mediated Reactions

Type I reactions are characterized by the production of antigen-specific immunoglobulin E (IgE) after exposure to an antigen. Most common allergic reactions are mediated by IgE and therefore are type I reactions. In addition, most type I reactions are against environmental antigens and are, therefore, allergic. Antigens that cause allergic responses are called **allergens.** It is not known why some antigens are allergens and others are not, but most allergens appear to be proteins that enter the host from the environment.

Role of IgE

In some individuals, exposure to an allergen causes IgE production by selected B cells. Repeated exposure to relatively large doses of allergen usually is required to elicit enough IgE so that the person is "sensitized." IgE binds to Fc receptors on the plasma membranes of mast cells (Fig. 8-1). The Fc region of IgE and the subclass IgG4 have binding sites specific for receptors on the mast cell. Antibody that binds to mast cells is termed **cytotropic** (able to bind to cell surfaces). **Reagin,** or skin-sensitizing antibody, has been used interchangeably with the term *cytotropic antibody*. The Fc receptors on mast cells bind with IgE that has not previously interacted with antigen.

After the individual is sensitized, and with further exposure to the allergen, the allergen's antigenic determinants bind to two molecules of mast-cell–bound IgE, cross-linking two IgE-Fc receptor complexes and initiating degranulation of the mast cell and the release of a plethora of mast cell products (see Chapter 6). Sometimes the IgE-mediated allergic response is beneficial to the host, as is the case with IgE-mediated destruction of parasites. (This mechanism is described in Chapter 7 and illustrated in Fig. 7-18.)

Mechanisms of IgE-mediated hypersensitivity

The products of mast cell degranulation can modulate almost all aspects of an acute inflammatory response. (The effects of biochemical mediators released by mast cells are illustrated in Fig. 7-4.) The most potent mediator of IgE-mediated hypersensitivity is histamine, which has effects on key target cells. Acting through certain histamine receptors (H1 receptors) on target cells in the host tissue, histamine contracts bronchial smooth muscles causing bronchial constriction, increases vascular permeability causing edema, and causes vasodilation increasing blood flow into the affected area (see Fig. 7-11). The interaction of histamine with H2 receptors on target cells results in increased gastric secretion and a decrease of histamine released from mast cells and basophils. (Basophils are granulocytes in the blood that are thought to be similar to mast cells.) The action of histamine through H2 receptors suggests an important negative-feedback loop that stops degranulation. That is, the released histamine inhibits release of additional histamine by interacting with H2 receptors on the mast cells. Histamine also may affect control of the immune response through H2 receptors on most T suppressor cells. Another important activity of histamine is its function as a chemotactic factor for eosinophils. In conjunction with eosinophil chemotactic factor of anaphylaxis (ECF-A), the histamine enhances attraction of eosinophils into sites of allergic inflammatory reactions, and also deactivates and prevents them from migrating out of the inflammatory site. (The role of the eosinophil in inflammation is discussed in Chapter 7.)

Although some control of the allergic response is mediated through histamine receptors, the primary mechanism of control is the autonomic nervous system. The autonomic nervous system includes biochemical mediators (e.g., epinephrine and acetylcholine) that, like the mediators of the inflammatory response, have profound effects on the behavior of target cells in the host tissue. The nervous system mediators bind to appropriate receptors on both mast cells and the target cells of inflammation, thereby controlling (1) release of inflammatory mediators from mast cells and (2) the degree to which target cells respond to inflammatory mediators (see Chapters 1 and 12).

Clinical Manifestations

The clinical manifestations of type I reactions are mostly attributable to the biologic effects of histamine released during mast cell degranulation. The target tissues of the type I response contain large numbers of mast cells and are sensitive to the effects of histamine released from them. These tissues are found in the gastrointestinal tract, the skin, and the respiratory tract (Fig. 8-2 and Table 8-4).

Gastrointestinal allergy is primarily caused by allergens that enter through the mouth, usually foods. Hypersensitivity is frequently manifested by vomiting, diarrhea, or abdominal pain and may be severe enough to result in malabsorption or protein-losing enteropathy. Foods most frequently implicated in gastrointestinal allergies are milk, chocolate, citrus fruits, eggs, wheat, nuts, peanut butter, and fish. When food is the allergen, the active immunogen may be an unidentifiable product of food breakdown by digestive enzymes. Sometimes the allergen is a drug, additive, or preservative in the food. For example, cows treated for mastitis

with penicillin yield milk containing trace amounts of this antibiotic. Thus hypersensitivity apparently caused by milk proteins may instead be the result of an allergy to penicillin.

Urticaria, or **hives,** is a dermal (skin) manifestation of allergic reactions. The underlying mechanism is the localized release of histamines and increased vascular permeability, resulting in limited areas of edema. Urticaria is characterized by white fluid-filled blisters (wheals) surrounded by areas of erythema, or redness (flares). The wheal and flare reaction is usually accompanied by itching. Not all urticarial symptoms are caused by allergic (immunologic) reactions. Some, termed *nonimmunologic urticaria,* result from exposure to cold temperatures, emotional stress, drugs, systemic diseases, hyperthyroidism, or malignancies (e.g., lymphomas).

Effects of allergens on the mucosa of the eyes, nose, and respiratory tract include conjunctivitis (inflammation of the membranes lining the eyelids), rhinitis (inflammation of the mucous membranes of the nose), and asthma (constriction of the bronchi). Clinical manifestations are caused by vasodilation, hypersecretion of mucus, edema, and swelling of the respiratory mucosa. Because the mucous membranes lining the respiratory tract (accessory sinuses, nasopharynx, and upper and lower respiratory tract) are continuous, they are all adversely affected by the allergic reaction. The degree to which each is affected determines the clinical manifestations of the disease.

The central defect in allergic diseases of the lung, such as asthma, is obstruction of the lumen of the large and small airways (bronchi) of the lower respiratory tract by bronchospasm (constriction of smooth muscle in airway walls), edema, thick secretions, and hyperplasia of smooth muscle and mucus-secreting glands. This leads to ventilatory insufficiency, wheezing, and difficult or labored breathing. Asthma is acute, intermittent, and reversible. Extrinsic asthma is an allergic reaction caused by a known exogenous allergen, whereas intrinsic asthma has no known cause. (Asthma is described further in Chapter 30.)

Genetic predisposition

Certain individuals appear to be "prone" to allergies, or are **atopic.** Atopic individuals tend to produce higher concentrations of IgE and to have more Fc receptors on their mast cells. Subtle defects in T lymphocyte function (e.g., a deficiency in IgE-specific suppressor cells) may account for heightened IgE production. The airways and the skin of atopic individuals are also more responsive to a wide variety of both specific and nonspecific stimuli than the airways and skin of normal individuals. There appears to be a genetic basis for the state; some individuals are genetically predisposed to become sensi-

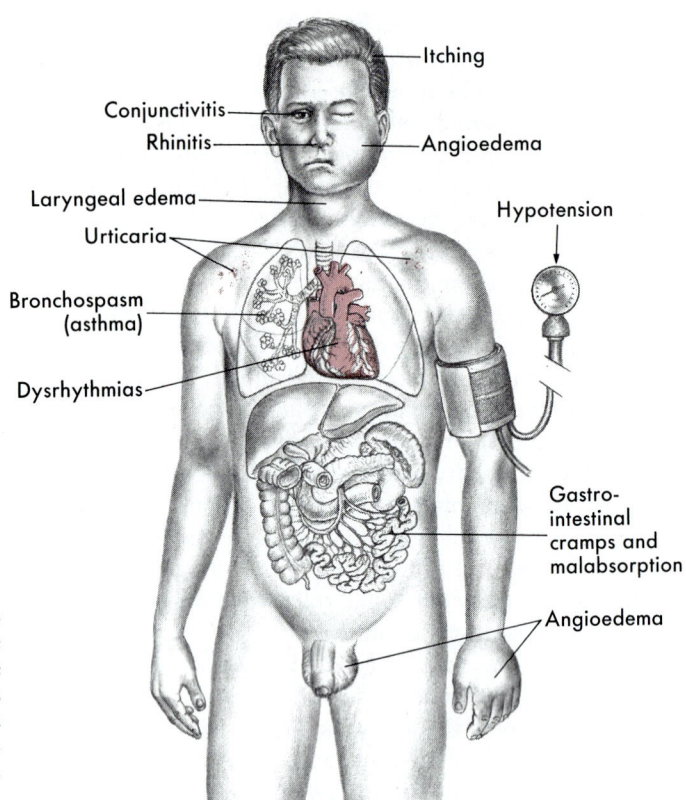

FIG. 8-2 Type I hypersensitivity reactions. Local manifestations of allergic reactions as a result of type I hypersensitivity include itching, angioedema (swelling caused by exudation), edema of the larynx, urticaria (hives), bronchospasm (constriction of airways in the lungs), hypotension (low blood pressure) and dysrhythmias (irregular heartbeat) because of anaphylactic shock, and gastrointestinal cramping caused by inflammation of the gastrointestinal mucosa.

TABLE 8-4

Causes of Clinical Manifestations of Allergy

Typical allergen	Mechanism of hypersensitivity	Clinical manifestation
Ingestants		
Foods	Type I	Gastrointestinal allergy
Drugs	Types I, II, III	Urticaria, immediate drug reaction, hemolytic anemia, serum sickness
Inhalants		
Pollens, dust, molds	Type I	Allergic rhinitis, bronchial asthma
Aspergillus fumigatus	Types I, III	Allergic bronchopulmonary aspergillosis
Thermophilic actinomycetes*	Types III, IV	Extrinsic allergic alveolitis
Injectants		
Drugs	Types I, II, III	Immediate drug reaction, hemolytic anemia, serum sickness
Bee venom	Type I	Anaphylaxis
Vaccines	Type III	Localized Arthus reaction
Serum	Types I, III	Anaphylaxis, serum sickness
Contactants		
Poison ivy, metals	Type IV	Contact dermatitis

Modified from Bellanti, J. A. (1985). *Immunology III*. Philadelphia: Saunders.
*An order of fungi that is stimulated by warmth to grow and proliferate.

tized against allergens. In families in which one parent has an allergy, allergies develop in about 40% of the offspring. If both parents have atopic disease, the incidence in offspring is approximately 80%. (Principles of genetic inheritance are discussed in Chapter 4.)

Tests of IgE-mediated hypersensitivity

Allergic reactions can be life-threatening; therefore, it is essential that severely allergic individuals be made aware of the specific allergen against which they are sensitized and instructed to avoid contact with that material. Several tests are available to determine the specific allergen. These tests include skin tests with allergens and laboratory tests for total IgE and allergen-specific IgE.

On injection of an allergen into (intradermal) or onto (epicutaneous or prick test) the skin of a sensitized individual, a local anaphylactic reaction occurs within a few minutes. It consists of a localized swelling and redness; a **wheal and flare reaction.** The diameter of the flare reaction is usually indicative of the individual's sensitivity to that allergen. In the most severely allergic individuals, even the extremely small amounts of allergen used for the skin test may evoke a systemic anaphylaxis.

There are a variety of laboratory tests for the detection of IgE antibodies. **Radioimmunosorbent (RIST) testing** measures circulating levels of total IgE, atopic individuals usually having elevated levels. **Radioallergosorbent (RAST) testing** has been used to measure circulating levels of specific IgE antibodies against many allergens and the amount of IgE has been found to correlate well with the degree of positive skin test and the severity of clinical symptoms.

Desensitization

Clinical desensitization to allergens can be achieved in some individuals. Minute quantities of the allergen to which the person is sensitive are injected in increasing doses over a prolonged period. This procedure may reduce the severity of the allergic reaction in the treated individual. Desensitization may work by inducing the production of large amounts of so-called blocking antibodies. A **blocking antibody** presumably competes in the tissues or in the circulation for binding with antigenic determinants on the allergen. Thus neutralized, the antigen is unable to bind with IgE on mast cells. In serum, blocking antibodies are predominantly IgG. The role of blocking antibodies has not been firmly established. Desensitization injections also may stimulate the generation of clones of suppressor T lymphocytes, which inhibit hypersensitivity by suppressing the production of IgE.

Tissue-Specific Reactions

Type II hypersensitivity reactions are generally characterized by the destruction of a target cell through the action of antibody against an antigen on the cell's plasma membrane. In addition to histocompatibility (HLA) antigens, most tissues have other antigens. These other antigens are generally called **tissue-specific antigens,** because they are only expressed on the plasma membranes of certain cells. Platelets, for example, have groups of self-antigens that are found on no other cells of the body. Because of limited distribution of tissue-specific antigens, type II diseases are limited to those tissues or organs that express the particular antigen. Environmental antigens (e.g., drugs or their metabolites) also may bind to the plasma membranes of cells (especially erythrocytes and platelets) and function as targets of type II reactions.

There are four mechanisms by which type II, or tissue-specific, hypersensitivity reactions can destroy or alter cells (Fig. 8-3). All of these mechanisms begin with antibody binding to tissue-specific antigens.

The first mechanism, complement-mediated lysis of cells, occurs by the same mechanism described and illustrated in Chapter 7 for foreign antigens (see Fig. 7-6). Antibody that is bound to the target cell "fixes" complement, initiating the complement cascade and ultimately dissolving (lysing) the plasma membrane of the cell. Circulating erythrocytes, for example, are destroyed by complement-mediated lysis in individuals with autoimmune hemolytic anemia (see Chapter 23) or isoimmune reactions to transfused blood cells from a donor (see p. 282).

A second mechanism of type II cell destruction is phagocytosis by macrophages of the mononuclear phagocyte system. The Fc receptors on the macrophage recognize and bind the antibody on the opsonized cell. Phagocytosis of the target cell follows. (Phagocytosis is illustrated in Fig. 7-15.) Antibodies against platelet-specific antigens or against red blood cell antigens of the Rh system will coat those cells at low density, resulting in their preferential removal by phagocytosis in the spleen, rather than by complement-mediated lysis.

Antibody-dependent cell-mediated cytotoxicity (ADCC) is the third mechanism of type II host cell destruction. This mechanism involves cell destruction by a subpopulation of cytotoxic cells, which are not antigen-specific. Antibody on the target cell is recognized by and bound to Fc receptors on the cytotoxic cells, which release toxic substances that destroy the cell.

The fourth mechanism does not destroy the target cell, but rather causes it to "malfunction." In this mechanism of type II injury, the damage is done by antibody binding alone. The antibody binds to the target cell, occupying and altering receptors that would bind with the various molecules (ligands) required for normal cellular function. For example, in hyperthyroidism (excessive thyroid activity) caused by Graves disease, autoantibody

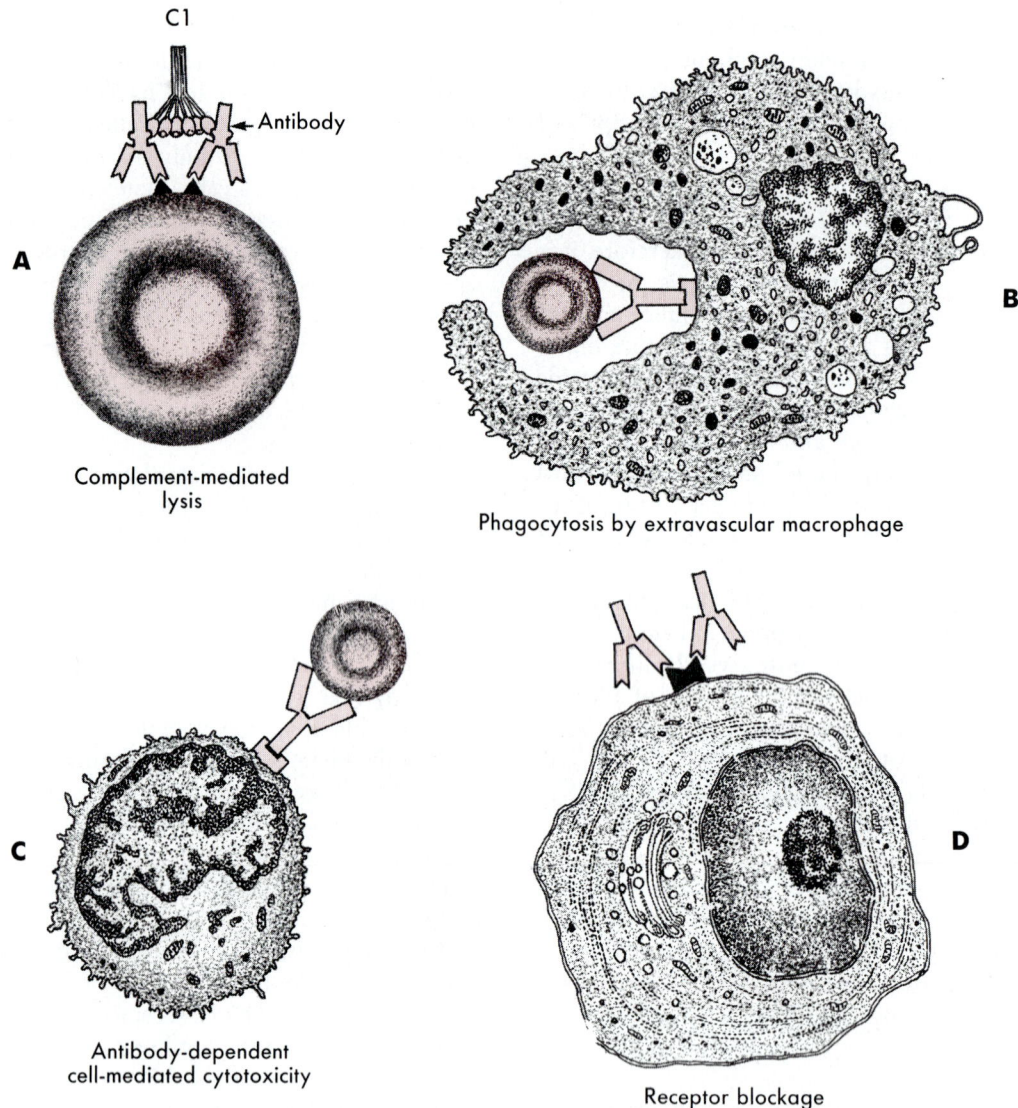

C1

Antibody

A

Complement-mediated
lysis

B

Phagocytosis by extravascular macrophage

C

Antibody-dependent
cell-mediated cytotoxicity

D

Receptor blockage

FIG. 8-3 **Mechanisms of type II, tissue-specific reactions.** Antigens on the target cell bind with antibody and are destroyed or prevented from functioning by, **A,** complement-mediated lysis; **B,** clearance by macrophages in tissues; **C,** antibody-dependent cell-mediated cytotoxicity (ADCC); or **D,** the modulation or blockage of receptors on the target cell.

activates receptors for thyroid-stimulating hormone (TSH) (a pituitary hormone that controls the production of the hormone thyroxine by the thyroid). The antibody-activated receptors stimulate the thyroid cells to continue producing thyroxine despite decreasing amounts of TSH (see Chapter 18).

Immune-Complex—Mediated Injury
Mechanisms

Most type III hypersensitivity diseases are caused by antigen-antibody (immune) complexes that are formed in the circulation and deposited later in vessel walls or extravascular tissues (Fig. 8-4). Type III, immune-complex—mediated reactions, therefore, are not organ

specific, and symptoms have very little to do with the antigenic target of the antibody (Rote, 1985). In some instances, immune-complex disease begins with the deposition of antigen in the tissues, and is followed by local interactions with antibody and complement. Regardless of whether immune complexes are formed in the circulation or in the tissues, their harmful effects are caused by complement activation, particularly the generation of complement fragments that are chemotactic for neutrophils. The neutrophils attempt to ingest the immune complexes, but are frequently unsuccessful because the complexes are bound to the tissues. During the neutrophil's attempts to phagocytose the immune complexes, large quantities of lysosomal enzymes are re-

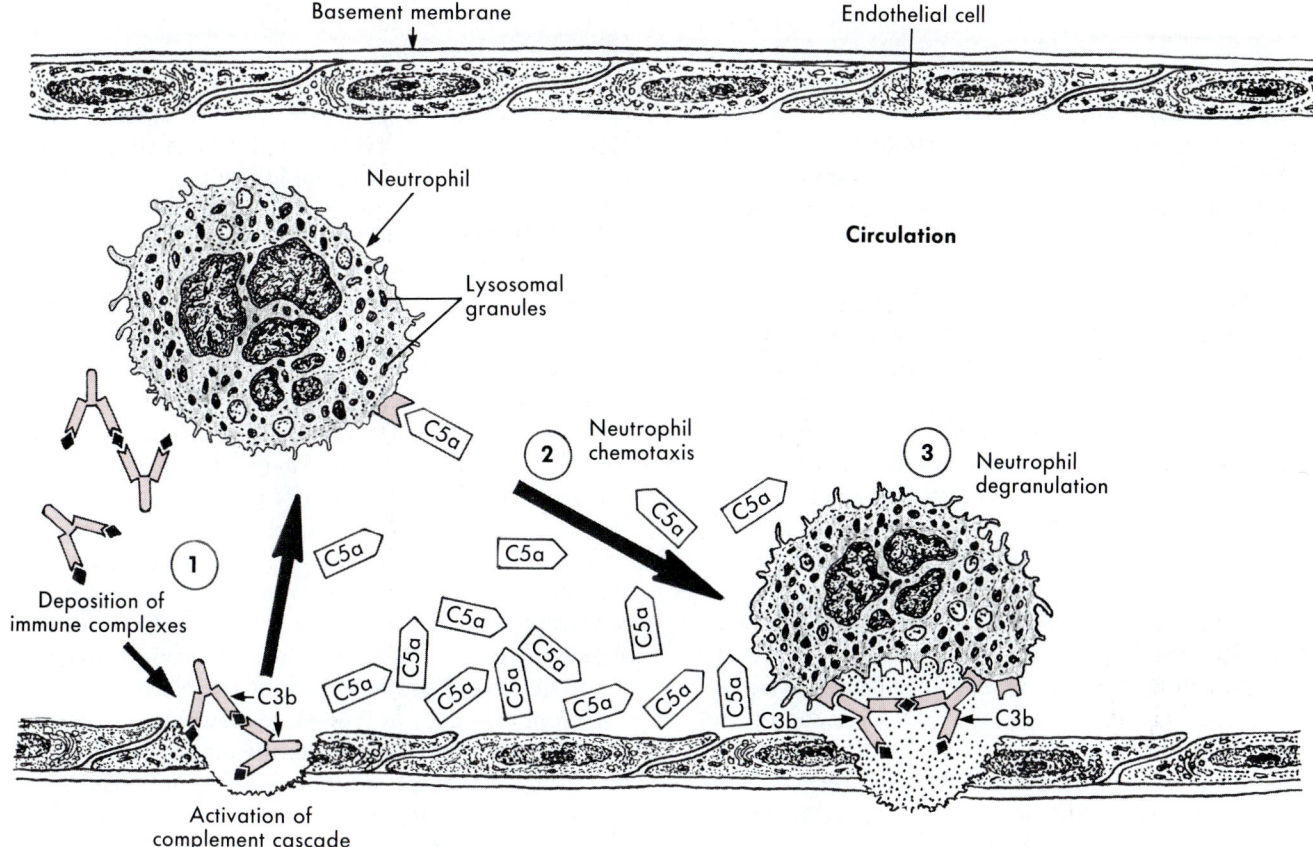

FIG. 8-4 Mechanism of type III, immune-complex—mediated reactions. Immune complexes are deposited in the vessels or other healthy tissue, where they activate the complement cascade and generate complement fragments including C5a (1). C5a is chemotactic for neutrophils and attracts many degradative enzymes that destroy healthy tissues (3).

leased into the inflammatory site instead of into phagolysosomes. The attraction of neutrophils and the subsequent release of lysosomal enzymes cause most of the resulting tissue damage.

The fate of circulating immune complexes depends on the ratio of antigen to antibody and other variables in the components of the immune complex. Other variables that influence immune-complex clearance are the inclusion of complement in the complex, the class or subclass of the antibody, and the nature and size of the antigen. Fairly large immune complexes are rapidly cleared from the circulation by the tissue macrophages of the mononuclear phagocyte system, whereas very small complexes are eventually filtered from blood through the kidneys, without any pathologic consequences. Intermediate-sized immune complexes (formed at a ratio of antigen to antibody that has a slight excess of antigen) are likely to be deposited in the tissues, where they have severe pathologic consequences, such as glomerulonephritis or degenerative joint disease (arthritis).

Immune-complex disease

The nature of the immune complexes may change and result in changes in severity of the symptoms. Variations in the ratio of antigen to antibody, the class and subclass of antibody, and the quantity and quality of circulating antigen cause the disease activity to be in constant flux.

Because some immune complexes activate complement very effectively and covalently bind some complement components, complement levels in the blood are also in flux. In many conditions in which immune complexes are formed, the individual's blood becomes **hypocomplementemic** (i.e., contains decreased amounts of complement activity). In conditions caused by the other three mechanisms of hypersensitivity (types I, II, and IV) complement levels are unaffected or some components of the complement cascade, such as C3, may even be increased. The interaction of complement with some immune complexes results in the dissolution of the complex and an alteration in its harmful effects.

Immune-complex formation is dynamic: immune

complexes formed early in a disease may be totally different from those formed later in the disease. At any one time, several types of immune complexes may be present simultaneously. With the tremendous potential heterogeneity of immune complexes, it is not surprising that these diseases are characterized by a variety of symptoms and periods of remission or exacerbation of symptoms.

Serum sickness. The systemic form of immune-complex–mediated disease is called **serum sickness** because it was initially described as being caused by the therapeutic administration of foreign serum, such as horse antitetanus toxin (Pirquet & Schick, 1905). Foreign serum is generally not administered to individuals today, although serum sickness reactions can be caused by the repeated intravenous administration of other antigens, such as drugs. Serum sickness is caused by the generalized deposition of immune complexes and inflammation. Typically affected are the blood vessels, joints, and kidneys. Other manifestations include fever, enlarged lymph nodes, rash, and pain at sites of inflammation. Laboratory findings may include decreased levels of circulating lymphocytes, granulocytes, and platelets.

A form of serum sickness is **Raynaud phenomenon,** an autoimmune condition caused by the temperature-dependent deposition of immune complexes in the peripheral circulation. (Immune complexes that precipitate at temperatures below normal body temperature are called cryoglobulins.) The symptoms of Raynaud phenomenon are localized pallor and numbness (usually in the fingers and toes), followed by cyanosis (a bluish tinge resulting from oxygen deprivation) and gangrene or by pain and redness. These signs and symptoms are caused by the temperature-dependent precipitation of immune complexes in the capillary beds of the peripheral circulation and the resulting inflammatory processes.

Arthus reaction. An **Arthus reaction** is an example of a localized immune-complex–mediated inflammatory response (Arthus & Breton, 1903). It is caused by repeated local exposure to exogenous antigen that reacts with preformed antibody in the walls of blood vessels. Symptoms of an Arthus reaction begin within an hour of exposure and peak 6 to 12 hours later. The lesions are characterized by a typical inflammatory reaction, with increased vascular permeability, an accumulation of neutrophils, edema, hemorrhage, clotting, and tissue damage.

Arthus reactions are observed after injection, ingestion, or inhalation of exogenous antigens. Skin reactions can follow subcutaneous or intradermal inoculation with drugs, fungal extracts, or antigens used in skin tests. Gastrointestinal reactions, such as gluten-sensitive enteropathy (celiac disease), follow ingestion of antigen, usually gluten from wheat products (see Chapter 36). Allergic alveolitis (farmer's lung; pigeon breeder's disease) is an Arthus-like acute hemorrhagic inflammation of the air sacs (alveoli) of the lung (see Chapter 30). Allergic alveolitis is caused by inhalation of fungal antigens, usually particles from moldy hay.

Cell-Mediated Tissue Destruction

Whereas hypersensitivity reactions I, II, and III are mediated by antibody, type IV (cell-mediated) reactions are mediated by specifically sensitized T lymphocytes and do not involve antibody (Fig. 8-5). Type IV mechanisms occur as one of two types involving either cytotoxic T lymphocytes (Tc cells) or lymphokine-producing T cells (Td cells). Cytotoxic T cells (Tc) can attack and destroy cellular targets directly. Td cells produce lymphokines, which affect various types of cells and can recruit and activate phagocytic cells, especially macrophages, at the inflammatory site. Tissue destruction is usually caused by direct killing by toxins from cytotoxic T cells or the release of soluble factors, such as lysosomal enzymes and toxic oxygen products from macrophages.

Clinical examples of type IV hypersensitivity include graft rejection, tumor rejection, the tuberculin reaction, and allergic reactions resulting from contact with such substances as poison ivy and metals. A type IV component also may be present in many autoimmune diseases such as rheumatoid arthritis, in which the self-antigen is apparently type II collagen (a protein present in joint tissues); autoimmune thyroiditis (Hashimoto disease), in which the self-antigen is a protein on thyroid cells; and insulin-dependent diabetes mellitus, in which the self-antigen is a protein on the beta cell of the pancreas (the cell that normally produces insulin).

A type IV hypersensitivity in the skin was first thoroughly described in 1891 and led to the development of a diagnostic skin test for tuberculosis (Koch, 1891). The reaction in the skin that follows intradermal injection of antigen into a suitably sensitized individual is called delayed hypersensitivity because of its slow onset—24 to 72 hours to reach maximal intensity. The reaction site is also infiltrated with T lymphocytes and macrophages. One of the characteristics of delayed hypersensitivity is that it can be transferred to an unreactive recipient by cells but not by antiserum. This demonstrates that type IV hypersensitivity is mediated by lymphocytes rather than by antibody.

Allergic type IV reactions are elicited by some environmental antigens that are too small to be immunogenic by themselves (haptens). (Immunogenicity is described in Chapter 6.) Antigens with a molecular weight of less than 1000 daltons are not usually immunogenic but become so after binding with a carrier protein in the host. In cases of allergic contact dermatitis, the carrier protein is in the skin of the host. The best-known

FIG. 8-5 **Mechanism of type IV, cell-mediated reactions.** Self-antigens from target cells stimulate T cells to produce cytotoxic T cells *(Tc)*, which have direct cytotoxic activity, and T cells involved in delayed hypersensitivity *(Td)*. Td cells produce lymphokines, some of which attract and activate macrophages. The macrophages and enzymes released by them are responsible for most of the tissue destruction.

Self-antigen

Tc

Lymphokines

Porphyrin

Lysosomal enzymes and toxic oxygen products

Activated macrophage

Catechol molecules

Skin protein

7-10 days

1-2 days

T cells → T memory cells

T memory cells → Many active cells

No dermatitis

Dermatitis

Catechols combined with skin proteins

Primary contact

Secondary contact

FIG. 8-6 **Development of allergic contact dermatitis, a delayed hypersensitivity reaction.** Shown here is the development of allergy to catechols from poison ivy. No dermatitis results from the primary contact because the antigens (catechols) are catabolized before any sensitized T cells are produced. Secondary contact, however, quickly activates a type IV, cell-mediated reaction that causes dermatitis.

FIG. 8-7 **Contact dermatitis.** Contact dermatitis caused by a delayed hypersensitivity reaction to shoes. (From Habif, 1990.)

example of allergic contact dermatitis is the delayed reaction caused by contact with poison ivy (Fig. 8-6). The antigen in this instance is a plant catechol, urushiol, that reacts with normal skin proteins and evokes a cell-mediated immune response. Skin reactions to industrial chemicals, cosmetics, detergents, clothing, food, metals, and topical medicines (such as penicillin) are elicited by the same mechanism.

Whether a skin reaction is caused by immediate or delayed hypersensitivity may be determined by the distribution of the lesions. The immediate reaction, termed **atopic dermatitis,** is manifested by widely distributed lesions, whereas **contact dermatitis** consists of lesions only at the site of contact (Fig. 8-7).

Targets of Hypersensitivity
Allergy

Allergens are environmental antigens that cause atypically exorbitant immunologic responses in genetically predisposed individuals. Typical allergens include pollens (e.g., ragweed, timothy), molds and fungi (e.g., *Penicillium notatum*), foods (e.g., milk, eggs, fish), animals (e.g., cat dander, dog dander), cigarette smoke, and components of house dust (e.g., fecal pellets of house mites). Frequently, the allergen is contained within a particle that is too large to be phagocytosed or is surrounded by a protective nonallergenic coat. The actual allergen is released after enzymatic breakdown (e.g., by lysozyme in secretions) of the larger particle. Most allergens are either haptens that have the capacity to react with proteins or small–molecular weight immunogenic proteins.

In certain situations an allergen complexes with components of host tissue. The **neoantigen,** or new antigenic determinant, is recognized as foreign and the tissue is destroyed. This occurs in allergic reactions to drugs (e.g., penicillin, sulfonamides), in which the drug binds to proteins on the plasma membranes of host cells. The drugs, which are usually haptens, become immunogenic

after binding to the host cell's proteins. The immune system attacks the neoantigen on the host cell's membrane and destroys the cell as well. In allergic reactions to penicillin, the immunogenic antigen is a metabolite of penicillin catabolism that binds to the plasma membranes of erythrocytes and induces an antibody response that destroys the cells, causing anemia.

The allergens that induce contact hypersensitivity, a type IV allergic reaction, are also haptens (e.g., metals such as nickel, acetylates and chemicals in rubber, resins in poison ivy and poison oak), which react with normal self-proteins in the skin. When presented in this fashion, these antigens induce a cell-mediated response.

Autoimmunity
Breakdown of tolerance

Self-antigens usually are tolerated by the host's own immune system. Immunologic tolerance, or immunologic homeostasis, develops in humans during the embryonic period, during which any autoreactive lymphocytes are either eliminated or suppressed. Autoimmunity is a breakdown of tolerance in which the body's immune system begins to recognize self-antigens as foreign. The mechanisms of breakdown are many and vary among autoimmune diseases, although in most such diseases the mechanism is unknown. Some of the mechanisms that have been implicated in the development of autoimmunity include (1) exposure within the body of a previously sequestered antigen, (2) the development of a neoantigen, (3) the complications of an infectious disease, (4) the emergence of a previously controlled or "forbidden" clone of lymphocytes with specificity for self-antigens, and (5) an alteration of suppressor T cell or anti-idiotypic antibody function. (Anti-idiotypic antibody is discussed in Chapter 6.)

Sequestered antigen. To be tolerated after birth, a self-antigen must be present in the fetus and exposed to the developing fetal immune system. Some self-antigens are not normally encountered in either fetal or adult life. Certain self-antigens, for example, in the cornea of the eye and in the testicles, are in areas of the body that are not drained by the lymphatics. Therefore, these self-antigens never encounter antigen-processing cells in the draining lymph nodes or other lymphoid organs. They are sequestered or hidden from the immune system in **immunologically privileged sites,** so named because foreign tissues can be transplanted into these sites without danger of immunologic rejection. Immunologically privileged sites are vascular, however, so that if an immunologic reaction should occur, antibodies and lymphocytes can enter the site and cause immunologic rejection of the tissue. In some situations, especially trauma, the structure of an immunologically privileged site is disturbed and the previously **sequestered antigens** are released from the damaged tissue and enter the lymphatics. The immune system recognizes these antigens as foreign, and a primary immune response occurs that can inflict extensive immunologic damage to the untraumatized site. An example of this occurrence is sympathetic uveitis, an ocular disease in which physical trauma to one eye results in immunologic injury to the other eye.

Neoantigen. In certain situations, a neoantigen that induces an allergic reaction may lead also to autoimmunity. Many neoantigens are haptens, which become immunogenic after binding to host proteins. The immune reaction against the neoantigen may lead to an immunologic reaction against the unaltered host protein. Many experimental autoimmune diseases (e.g., experimental autoimmune thyroiditis) can be initiated by this mechanism.

Infectious disease. Foreign antigens from infectious microorganisms can initiate autoimmune disease by (1) forming immune complexes that precipitate in host tissues, causing inflammatory disease; or (2) so closely resembling a particular self-antigen (cross-reacts with the self-antigen) that they stimulate production of antibodies that also recognize the self-antigen as foreign. Group A streptococci are capable of initiating both of these mechanisms, usually as sequelae to streptococcal pharyngitis.

The first mechanism, deposition of immune complexes, is the cause of poststreptococcal glomerulonephritis (inflammation of the kidney). Deposition elicits an inflammatory response that destroys tissues in the glomeruli of the kidney. (In Fig. 8-4 this mechanism is illustrated in a blood vessel.) The second mechanism, in which the foreign antigen mimics the molecular structure of a self-antigen, occurs in rheumatic fever. In rheumatic fever, streptococcal antigens so closely resemble self-antigens on the heart valve that antibodies produced to incapacitate the streptococci also damage cells of the heart valve.

Forbidden clone. One theory that explains tolerance is that maturing lymphocytes in the central lymphoid organs encounter self-antigen during embryogenesis and, as lymphocytes reactive against self-antigen develop, their clones are prevented, or "forbidden," from maturing. Autoimmunity may result from the survival of a **forbidden clone** and its proliferation later in life. No known autoimmune disease has been shown to be caused by this mechanism, but the pathogenesis of most autoimmune diseases has not yet been discovered. Most likely the only autoreactive clones that are deleted in the central lymphoid organs are those against self-HLA antigens.

Suppressor cell dysfunction. Despite the normal development of tolerance, sometimes clones of lymphocytes against self-antigens develop in healthy adults. One of the roles of suppressor T cells is to suppress the immune responses that these clones activate. Suppressor T cell dysfunction can, therefore, result in autoimmune disease. If a single antigen-specific population of suppressor cells is affected, a tissue-specific autoimmune disease results. A generalized autoimmune reaction occurs if many suppressor cell populations are dysfunctional. Systemic lupus erythematosus (SLE), which is characterized by the production of a large array of autoantibodies, may be caused by a general breakdown in the suppressor cell network.

Original insult

The cause of some immune diseases is quite apparent. For example, in drug-induced anemia or thrombocytopenia (decreased numbers of circulating platelets), there is ample evidence that immunologic destruction of erythrocytes or platelets follows the integration of a drug or its metabolite (product of catabolism) into the plasma membranes of the host cells. This causes the immune system to recognize the altered plasma membranes as new and foreign cellular antigens. B cells are stimulated to produce antibody against the drug-cell complex, and immune processes destroy the host cells. Viruses can induce autoimmune reactions by altering the plasma membranes of host cells. In rubella infections, for example, encephalitis can ensue when cells of the nervous system become infected and express virally derived antigens on their plasma membranes. Like the antigenic alterations caused by drug metabolism, virus-induced changes result in the destruction of infected cells by the host's immune system.

The causes of other immune diseases, such as rheumatoid arthritis and SLE, are less clear. Most autoimmune diseases are probably sequelae of preexisting infections that leave no traces to facilitate their identification.

Genetic factors

Genetic factors that contribute to autoimmunity are easier to identify than pathogenic agents. It is fairly well established that autoimmune diseases are familial. Affected family members may not all develop the same disease, but several members may have different disorders characterized by hypersensitivity.

The association of diseases with specific HLA antigens (see Chapter 6) has been recognized only recently and is a relatively nebulous phenomenon. The HLA types of susceptible and resistant individuals have been analyzed for almost every known disease and, almost universally, individuals with certain diseases are more likely than the general population to have a specific HLA allele or alleles. Some associations are strong; others are more tenuous. The reason why some HLA alleles are associated with inappropriate immune function is unclear, but it may directly involve the products of the HLA locus or the histocompatibility-complex—

linked immune response (Ir) genes. These genes may determine an individual's susceptibility to specific infectious agents or the capacity of that individual to mount an immune response against specific antigens. Therefore, an individual of a specific HLA type may have inappropriate or exaggerated immune responses against a microorganism, resulting in a hypersensitivity reaction.

Isoimmunity

Isoimmunity occurs when an individual's immune system reacts against antigens on the tissues of other members of the same species. There are two clinically relevant examples of this reactivity: (1) transient neonatal diseases (in which the maternal immune system becomes sensitized against antigens expressed by the fetus) and (2) transplant rejection and transfusion reactions (in which the immune system of a recipient of an organ transplant or blood transfusion reacts against antigens on the donor cells).

Because the fetus is a hybrid between the mother and father, it expresses paternal antigens that are not found in the mother. Occasionally, these fetal antigens cross the placenta and elicit an immune response in the mother. Maternal antibody may be transported into the fetal circulation to produce isoimmune disease in the fetus. The mother's immune system produces the antibody, but because her cells do not express the target antigen, she has no manifestations of the disease.

Isoimmune disease may be in conjunction with maternal autoimmune diseases. The mother may be producing an IgG autoantibody specific for maternal self-antigens that are found on fetal cells as well. Therefore, symptoms of the same autoimmune disease may affect both mother and child, even though the autoantibody is being produced only by the mother's immune system. This form of disease usually occurs only in association with type II (tissue-specific) reactions. It does not occur in association with IgE-mediated (type I) reactions, immune-complex–mediated (type III) reactions, or cell-mediated (type IV) reactions, because the immunologic products of these reactions do not readily cross the placenta and enter the fetal circulation in sufficient quantity.

At birth, the source of the antibody in the fetal circulation is removed. Although symptoms of the isoimmune disease may be manifested in utero or immediately after birth and may be fatal to the fetus or neonate, if symptoms are successfully treated at birth the disease will disappear as the maternal antibody is catabolized.

Examples of immunologic diseases in which the child can be affected include such antibody-mediated diseases as the following:

1. Graves disease, an autoimmune disease in which maternal antibody against the receptor for thyroid-stimulating hormone causes neonatal hyperthyroidism.

2. Myasthenia gravis, an autoimmune disease in which maternal antibody binds with receptors for neural transmitters on muscle cells, causing neonatal muscular weakness (see Chapter 15).
3. Immune thrombocytopenic purpura, in which maternal antiplatelet antibody destroys platelets in the neonate (see Chapter 25).
4. Isoimmune neutropenia, in which maternal antibody against neutrophils destroys neutrophils in the neonate.
5. Systemic lupus erythematosus (SLE), in which diverse maternal autoantibodies induce anomalies (e.g., congenital heart defects) in the fetus.
6. Rh and ABO isoimmunization (e.g., erythroblastosis fetalis) in which maternal antibody against erythrocyte antigens induces anemia in the child (see Chapter 25).

Autoimmune and Isoimmune Diseases

Autoimmunity and isoimmunity are exemplified by two disease states, SLE (an autoimmune disease) and transplant rejection (an isoimmune phenomenon). Most of the classic autoimmune diseases, including disorders of the endocrine system (autoimmune thyroiditis and Graves disease), hematologic system (the hemolytic and pernicious anemias), nervous system (myasthenia gravis), and connective tissue in joints (rheumatoid arthritis) are discussed in Unit II of this book.

Systemic Lupus Erythematosus

Systemic lupus erythematosus (SLE), which is a chronic, multisystem, inflammatory disease, is one of the most common, complex, and serious of the autoimmune disorders. Systemic lupus erythematosus is characterized by the production of a large variety of autoantibodies against nucleic acids, erythrocytes, coagulation proteins, phospholipids, lymphocytes, platelets, and many other self-components. The most characteristic autoantibodies produced in SLE are against nucleic acids: single-stranded DNA, double-stranded DNA, histones, ribonucleoproteins, and other nuclear materials.

Deposition of circulating immune complexes containing antibody against host DNA produces tissue damage in individuals with SLE. DNA and DNA-containing immune complexes have a high affinity for glomerular basement membranes and therefore may be selectively deposited in the glomerulus. (Kidney structures are described in Chapter 33.) The presence of DNA in the circulation increases from cellular damage in response to trauma, drugs, or infections; it is usually removed in the liver, but removal of circulating DNA is slowed in the presence of immune complexes, thereby increasing the potential for deposition in the kidney. (The liver's role in removing waste products from the blood is discussed in Chapter 35.) Deposition of immune complexes composed of DNA and antibody also causes inflammatory lesions in the renal tubular basement membranes, brain (choroid plexus), heart, spleen, lung, gastrointestinal tract, skin, and peritoneum.

Systemic lupus erythematosus, as with most autoimmune diseases, is seen more frequently in women, especially in the 20- to 40-year-old age group. Blacks are affected more frequently than whites. A genetic predisposition for the disease has been implicated on the basis of increased incidence in twins and the existence of autoimmune disease in the families of individuals with SLE.

A transient lupuslike syndrome that is indistinguishable both clinically and in the laboratory from spontaneously occurring SLE also can develop from the prolonged use of drugs. The drugs most often implicated are hydralazine (an antihypertensive agent) and procainamide (an antiarrhythmic drug). In genetically susceptible individuals, certain environmental agents, such as ultraviolet light, and several infectious agents may trigger lupuslike immune reactions.

Clinical manifestations of SLE include arthralgias or arthritis (90% of individuals), vasculitis and rash (70% to 80% of individuals), renal disease (40% to 50% of individuals), hematologic abnormalities (50% of individuals, with anemia being the most common complication), and cardiovascular diseases (30% to 50% of individuals). As with most autoimmune diseases, SLE is characterized by frequent remissions and exacerbations. Because the signs and symptoms affect almost every body system and tend to come and go, SLE is extremely difficult to diagnose. This has led to the development of a list of 11 clinical findings. The serial or simultaneous presence of at least four of them indicates that the individual has SLE. The 11 findings are as follows (Fritzler & Tan, 1985):

1. Facial rash confined to the cheeks (malar rash)
2. Discoid rash (raised patches, scaling)
3. Photosensitivity (skin rash in sunlight)
4. Oral or nasopharyngeal ulcers
5. Nonerosive arthritis of at least two peripheral joints
6. Serositis (pleurisy, pericarditis)
7. Renal disorder (proteinuria of 0.5 g/day or cellular casts)
8. Neurologic disorders (seizures or psychosis)
9. Hematologic disorders (hemolytic anemia, leukopenia, lymphopenia, or thrombocytopenia)
10. Immunologic disorders (positive SLE cell preparation, anti-nDNA, anti-Smith [Sm] antigen, or false-positive serologic test for syphilis)
11. Presence of anti-nuclear antibody (ANA)

Graft Rejection

Transplantation of organs is commonly complicated by an immune response against antigens—primarily HLA antigens—on the donated tissue. Most knowledge on the transplantation of organs, and the emphasis here, is from renal transplant studies. The primary mechanism of the rejection of transplanted organs is a type IV, cell-mediated reaction. Two randomly chosen individuals are almost certainly antigenically different to some degree. Organ transplants between them are rejected in approximately 2 weeks without the extensive use of immunosuppressive drugs.

Because HLA antigens are the principal targets of the rejection reaction, HLA matching of donor and recipient greatly enhances the probability of acceptance of the graft. Matching at each HLA locus is of differential importance; matching at the HLA-D/DR locus appears to be the most critical for graft acceptance and at HLA-A, B, and C of lesser importance. (These loci are discussed in Chapter 6.)

Transplant rejection is classified as hyperacute, acute, or chronic, depending on the amount of time that elapses between transplantation and rejection. Hyperacute rejection is immediate and rare. When the circulation is reestablished to the grafted area, the graft may immediately turn white (the so-called white graft) instead of a normal pink color. Hyperacute rejection usually occurs in recipients with preexisting antibody to antigens in the graft. As circulation to the graft is established, antibody binds to the grafted tissue and activates the inflammatory response, including the coagulation cascade, which results in stasis of blood flow into the tissue. (Coagulation is described in Chapters 7 and 22.) Biopsies of the graft frequently show deposits of antibody (IgG and IgM), complement, and neutrophils.

Acute rejection is a cell-mediated immune response that occurs approximately 2 weeks after the transplant. This type of rejection occurs when the recipient develops an immune response against unmatched HLA antigens after transplantation. Immunosuppressive drugs may delay or lessen the intensity of acute rejection. A biopsy of the rejected organ shows an infiltration of lymphocytes and macrophages characteristic of a type IV reaction.

Chronic rejection may occur after a period of months or years of normal function. It is characterized by slow, progressive organ failure. Chronic rejection may be caused by inflammatory damage to endothelial cells lining blood vessels as a result of a weak immunologic reaction against minor histocompatibility antigens on the grafted tissue.

DEFICIENCIES IN IMMUNITY AND INFLAMMATION

Disorders resulting from immune deficiency are the clinical sequelae (results) of impaired function of one or more components of the immune or inflammatory response, including B cells, T cells, phagocytic cells, and

TABLE 8-5

Congenital Defects of Phagocytosis and Complement Function

Type of defect	Characteristic	Clinical manifestation
Defects of phagocytosis		
Quantitative defects	Neutropenia (decreased granulocyte number)	General increase in bacterial infections
Chemotactic defects	Decreased neutrophil response to chemotactic factors	General increase in bacterial infections
Bacterial killing defects	Decreased bacterial killing because of insufficient H_2O_2 or lysosomal enzymes	Increased bacterial infections—especially with catalase+ organisms
Complement defects		
Defects in early classic pathway	Decreased activity of C1, C2, or C4	Mild bacterial infections; SLE-like syndrome
Defects in alternative pathway	Decreased activity of alternative pathway components—especially factor B	Increased infections with encapsulated bacteria
Defects in C3	Decreased production of C3b	Severe infections mostly with encapsulated bacteria
Defects in late pathway	Decreased activity of C5, C6, C7, or C8	Recurrent disseminated *Neisseria gonorrhoeae* or *N. meningitidis* infections

complement (Table 8-5 lists defects in phagocytic cells and complement). An **immune deficiency** is the failure of these mechanisms of self-defense to function at their normal capacity. **Congenital (primary) immune deficiency** is caused by a genetic anomaly, whereas **acquired (secondary) immune deficiency** is caused by another illness, such as cancer or viral infection, or by normal physiologic changes, such as aging. Acquired forms of immune deficiency are far more common than the congenital forms.

Whether congenital or acquired, the chief cause of immune deficiency is disruption of lymphocyte function. A stem cell defect may prevent normal lymphocyte development and cause total failure of the immune system, a central lymphoid organ dysfunction may prevent maturation of stem cells into B or T cells, or the final stages of B cell maturation may be disrupted, precluding the production of a specific class of immunoglobulin. Other defects may interfere with intercellular cooperation. For example, hyperactive suppressor T cells may prevent a normal immune response from taking place or helper T cells may be unable to mediate immune interactions. Sometimes enzymatic defects in lymphocytes cause a general accumulation of toxic metabolites. Alterations in the inflammatory response, particularly the chemotactic and phagocytic activities of neutrophils and macrophages, or the activity of complement, also can result in impaired host resistance.

The clinical hallmark of immune deficiency is a tendency to develop unusual or recurrent, severe infections. Preschool and school-aged children normally have 6 to 12 infections per year, and adults have 2 to 4 per year. Most of these are not severe and are limited to viral infections of the upper respiratory tract or recurrent streptococcal pharyngitis. Potential immune deficiencies are considered if the individual has had severe, documented bouts of pneumonia, otitis media, sinusitis, bronchitis, septicemia, or meningitis, or infections with microorganisms that are not normally pathogenic (e.g., *Pneumocystis carinii*). Deficiencies in T cell immune responses are suggested when recurrent infections are caused by certain viruses (e.g., varicella, vaccinia, herpes, cytomegalovirus), fungi and yeasts (e.g., *Candida, Histoplasma*), or certain atypical organisms (e.g., *P. carinii*). B cell deficiencies, however, are suggested if the individual has documented, recurrent infections with microorganisms that require opsonization (e.g., encapsulated bacteria) or viruses against which humoral immunity is normally effective (e.g., rubella).

Many immune deficiencies also are associated with other defects; some of these appear to be unrelated to the immune defect, yet may be life-threatening by themselves. Examples include eczema and thrombocytopenia (in Wiskott-Aldrich syndrome); cardiac anomalies, low levels of calcium in the blood, and structural anomalies of the face (in DiGeorge syndrome); and a severe lack of muscular coordination and dilation of the small blood vessels (in ataxia telangiectasia). The association of these other symptoms can sometimes clarify the pathophysiology of the disease. For instance, in DiGeorge syndrome the defects are the partial or complete absence of a thymus (resulting in depressed T cell immunity), partial or complete absence of the parathyroid gland (resulting in decreased blood calcium levels), and structural defects in the heart. Each of these anatomic structures originates from the same region in the embryo during the 12th week of gestation; therefore, the defect in DiGeorge syndrome can be traced to an abnormal development at a specific time and in a specific region during embryogenesis.

Routine care of individuals with immune deficiencies must be tempered with the knowledge that the immune system may be totally ineffective. It is unsafe to administer conventional immunizing agents or blood products to many of these individuals because of the risk that the immunizing agent will cause an uncontrolled infection. Uncontrolled infection is particularly a problem when attenuated vaccines that contain live, but weakened, microorganisms are used (e.g., vaccinia virus used for im-munization against smallpox). Although the virus is attenuated enough to be destroyed by a normal immune system, it can survive, multiply, and cause severe disease in an immune-deficient recipient. Furthermore, even simple procedures, such as penetrating the skin for routine blood tests, may lead to fatal septicemia (bacterial infection of the blood) in the immune-deficient person.

Individuals with immune deficiencies are also at risk for graft-versus-host (GVH) disease. This occurs if T cells in a graft (e.g., transfused blood) are mature and are therefore capable of the cell-mediated destruction of tissues in the graft recipient. If the recipient's immune system is normal, the grafted T cells are controlled and no tissue destruction occurs. If, however, the recipient's immune system is deficient, the grafted T cells remain unchecked and attack the recipient's tissues.

Congenital Immune Deficiencies

Congenital, or primary, immune deficiency occurs if lymphocyte development is arrested or disrupted in the fetus or embryo (Fig. 8-8). Defects that occur at different stages of stem cell, T cell, or B cell maturation cause different immune deficiency diseases. Some diseases are primarily caused by a defect in one or the other of the

FIG. 8-8. Lymphocyte development defects. Defects in lymphocyte development that may account for congenital immune deficiencies: *(1)* reticular dysgenesis, *(2)* severe combined immune deficiency (SCID), *(3)* DiGeorge syndrome, *(4)* Bruton agammaglobulinemia, *(5)* chronic mucocutaneous candidiasis, and *(6)* selective IgA deficiency.

cell lines, although both T and B cell lines may be deficient in some respect. Other congenital immune deficiency diseases affect stem cells of both cell lines, disrupting both cell-mediated and humoral immune processes. A defect in B cell development results in lower levels of circulating immunoglobulin. The condition in which immunoglobulins are present in insufficient amounts is termed **hypogammaglobulinemia**. The condition in which they are totally or nearly absent is termed **agammaglobulinemia**. (Normal lymphocyte development is discussed in Chapter 6.)

Although most congenital immune deficiency diseases are rare, much of our current understanding of the development of the immune system and the interactions of the cells in the immune response was developed by studying congenital immune deficiencies or, as they have been called, "experiments of nature." The immune systems of experimental animals have been studied in the laboratory by specifically altering or removing one component of the system and observing the effect of that manipulation on the remainder of the immune response. Studying congenital immune deficiencies allows us the opportunity to make similar observations in humans.

The role of bone marrow stem cells in the evolution of the immune system was elucidated by studying children with the most severe deficiencies, **severe combined immune deficiencies (SCID)**. The most severe form of SCID is **reticular dysgenesis** (failure of blood cells to develop), in which a common stem cell for all white blood cells is absent; therefore, T cells, B cells, and phagocytic cells never develop (Fig. 8-8). Most children with reticular dysgenesis die in utero or very soon after birth.

The common stem cell normally matures into more developed stem cells for individual populations of white blood cells. Most individuals with SCID are deficient only in a stem cell for lymphocyte development, and therefore have normal numbers of all other white cells and few, if any, detectable lymphocytes. T and B lymphocytes are few or totally absent in both the circulation and secondary lymphoid organs (spleen, lymph nodes). The thymus is usually hypoplastic (underdeveloped) because of the absence of T cells. Immunoglobulin levels, especially of IgM and IgA, are absent or greatly reduced, although IgG levels may be almost normal because of the presence of maternal antibodies.

Two forms of SCID are caused by autosomal recessive enzymatic defects that result in the accumulation of toxic metabolites to which rapidly dividing cells, like lymphocytes, are especially sensitive. Deficiencies in adenosine deaminase (**ADA deficiency**) or purine nucleoside phosphorylase (**PNP deficiency**) result in the accumulation of toxic purine metabolism.

Stem cells mature in the central or primary lymphoid organs (thymus and bursal equivalence tissue). The importance of these organs was determined by studying

children who failed to develop them during embryogenesis. These children presented with either a defective thymus (DiGeorge syndrome) or a defective bursal-equivalent tissue (Bruton agammaglobulinemia).

DiGeorge syndrome (congenital thymic aplasia or hypoplasia) is caused by the lack, or more commonly partial lack, of the thymus, resulting in lymphopenia with greatly decreased T cell numbers and function (DiGeorge, 1968) (see Fig. 8-8).

Bruton agammaglobulinemia is caused by blocked development of B cell precursors into mature B cells because of the lack of normal bursal-equivalent tissue (see Fig. 8-8). There are few or no circulating B cells, although T cell number and function are normal. At 6 months, the approximate normal serum concentrations of immunoglobulins are IgG, 400 mg/dl; IgM, 40 mg/dl; and IgA, 30 mg/dl. In 6-month-old children with Bruton agammaglobulinemia, serum IgG levels are well below 100 mg/dl, and IgM and IgA are almost absent.

Even if nearly adequate numbers of B and T cells are produced, their cooperation may be defective. The **bare lymphocyte syndrome** is an immune deficiency characterized by an inability of lymphocytes and macrophages to produce HLA class I or class II antigens. Several forms of this syndrome have been reported: type I, in which class I HLA antigen expression is deficient; type II, in which class II HLA antigen is not expressed; and type III, in which both class I and class II HLA antigen expression is defective. Without HLA antigen expression, antigen presentation and intercellular cooperation cannot effectively occur. Children with this deficiency develop serious, life-threatening infections and usually die before the age of 5.

Some immune deficiencies involve a defect that results in depressed development of a small portion of the immune system and, therefore, provide us with information about the function of that portion. For instance, an individual can be unable to produce a certain class of antibody. An example is **Wiskott-Aldrich syndrome** (an X-linked recessive disorder), in which IgM antibody production is greatly depressed and, therefore, antibody responses against antigens that elicit primarily an IgM response, such as polysaccharide antigens from bacterial cell walls (e.g., of *P. aeruginosa, S. pneumoniae, H. influenzae,* and other microorganisms with polysaccharide outer capsules), are deficient.

Another defect in which a particular class of antibody is affected is **selective IgA deficiency.** This is the most common type of immune deficiency, having an incidence of between 1 in 700 and 1 in 400 individuals. Individuals with selective IgA deficiency are able to produce other classes of immunoglobulins, but fail to produce IgA. This suggests a disruption of terminal processes of differentiation, so that immature B cells that are committed to IgA production fail to mature into IgA-producing plasma cells (see Fig. 8-8). Many individuals are asymptomatic, although others manifest a history of severe recurring sinus, lung, and gastrointestinal infections. Individuals with IgA deficiency frequently present with chronic intestinal candidiasis (infection with *C. albicans*). (The secretory, or mucosal, immune system is described in Chapter 6.)

Complications of IgA deficiency include severe atopic disease and autoimmune diseases; selective IgA deficiency is two or three times more common in atopic individuals than in others. As a result of studying these individuals, we can conclude that secretory IgA may normally prevent the uptake of allergens from the environment. Therefore, IgA deficiency may lead to increased allergen uptake and a more intense challenge to the immune system because of prolonged exposure to environmental antigens. One of the most severe complications of IgA deficiency is an anaphylactic reaction that can follow administration of IgA-containing blood products. Serious anaphylactic reactions can occur in individuals totally lacking IgA because the immune system recognizes donor IgA as a foreign antigen. Initial sensitization can occur in fetal life through exposure to maternal IgA or later through the ingestion of maternal IgA in breast milk or bovine IgA in cow's milk. Sensitization also can occur with initial administration of blood products containing IgA. The individual's primed immune system then acts against donor IgA on subsequent exposure.

Other immune deficiencies are characterized by a defect in the capacity to produce an immune response against a particular antigen. In **chronic mucocutaneous candidiasis,** the defect is the inability of T lymphocytes to respond against a specific infectious agent, *Candida albicans* (see Fig. 8-8). Individuals with chronic mucocutaneous candidiasis usually have mild to extremely severe recurrent *Candida* infections that involve the mucous membranes and skin. Systemic candidiasis is extremely rare, although infection of the mucosal lining of the esophagus may develop.

Acquired Deficiencies

Acquired, or secondary, immune and inflammatory deficiency develops after birth and is not related to genetic defects. The following physiologic or pathophysiologic conditions are known to be associated with acquired deficiencies:

Pregnancy

Infancy

Infections, such as rubella (congenital), cytomegalovirus (congenital), measles, leprosy, tuberculosis, coccidioidomycosis

Down syndrome

Malignancies, such as Hodgkin disease, acute or chronic leukemia, nonlymphoid malignancy, or myeloma

Stress caused by surgery or emotional trauma

Malnutrition caused by insufficient intake of protein, calories, iron, or zinc

Aging

Diabetes

Alcoholic cirrhosis

Sickle cell anemia

Immunosuppressive treatment with corticosteroids, cytotoxic drugs, or ionizing radiation

Anesthesia

Nutritional Deficiencies

Nutritional status can have a profound effect on immune function. Severe deficits in calorie or protein intake lead to deficiencies in T cell function and numbers. The humoral immune response is less affected by starvation, although complement activity, neutrophil chemotaxis, and bacterial killing within neutrophils are frequently depressed, resulting in infections with organisms that are normally disabled by opsonization and phagocytosis.

Deficient zinc intake can profoundly depress both T and B cell function. Zinc is required as a cofactor for at least 70 different enzymes, some of which are found in lymphocytes and are necessary for their function. Secondary zinc deficiencies may be associated with malabsorption syndrome (failure to absorb zinc), chronic renal disease (loss of zinc in the urine), chronic diarrhea (loss of zinc through the gut), or burns or severe psoriasis (loss of zinc through the skin). Other enzyme cofactors, such as vitamins (pyridoxine, pantothenic acid, folic acid, vitamin A, or vitamin E) also may result in severe depressions of both B and T cell function.

Iatrogenic Deficiencies

Iatrogenic disorders are caused by some form of medical treatment (e.g., iatrogenic neutropenia is usually caused by drugs). Some drugs (e.g., cancer chemotherapeutic agents) profoundly suppress blood cell formation in the bone marrow. Other drugs induce immunologic responses that destroy mature granulocytes. The list of drugs having this effect is ever increasing and includes analgesics, antithyroid medications, anticonvulsants, antihistamines, antimicrobial agents, and tranquilizers.

Many drugs also affect B and T cell function, especially against antigens that require the interaction of T helper and B cells for antibody production. These complications have been observed since the advent of potent immunosuppressive (e.g., corticosteroids) and chemotherapeutic drugs as treatment for individuals with transplants, cancer, or autoimmune diseases. Depression of B and T cell formation is manifested as a progressive increase in infections with opportunistic microorganisms (especially *P. carinii,* cytomegalovirus, *C. al-*

bicans, and other fungi), the extent and location of which are unusual.

The immunosuppressive effects of chemotherapeutic drugs are exacerbated by concurrent treatment with ionizing radiation (x-rays). Most cytotoxic drugs and x-rays destroy cells that are proliferating or are in susceptible stages in their cell cycles. Therefore, these therapies mainly suppress the primary immune response, which involves proliferation of clones of B and T cells.

Surgery and anesthesia also can suppress both T and B cell function. Transient, severe lymphopenia is a common postoperative condition that can last for up to 1 month. Surgery to remove the spleen (splenectomy) results in a depressed humoral response against encapsulated bacteria (especially *S. pneumoniae, H. influenzae, S. aureus,* the group A streptococci, and *N. meningitidis*), depressed serum IgM levels, and decreased levels of opsonins.

Deficiencies Caused by Trauma

Burn victims are susceptible to severe bacterial infections. Thermal burns appear to be associated with decreased neutrophil function (especially chemotaxis), decreased complement levels, decreased cell-mediated immunity, and decreased primary humoral responses, although secondary humoral responses are normal. The mechanism of this immunosuppression may be twofold. Sera from burned individuals contain nonspecific immunosuppressive factors (will suppress all immune responses, regardless of the antigen involved). In addition, burn victims also have increased suppressor cell function, which may increase antigen-specific suppression.

Deficiencies Caused by Stress

The relationship between emotional stress and depressed immune function recently has become an area of intense research interest. For many decades there were anecdotal reports of increased incidence of infection and malignancy associated with periods of both intense stress (e.g., the loss of a loved one, divorce) and relatively minor stress (e.g., final examination periods at colleges and universities). In addition, early studies showed that immune function, as demonstrated by delayed hypersensitivity skin test results, could be depressed through posthypnotic suggestion.

Only recently have the mechanisms of this interaction begun to be investigated. Many of the lymphoid organs are innervated and can be affected by nerve stimulation. In addition, lymphocytes have receptors for many hormones (i.e., sex hormones, neurotransmitters, and neuropeptides) and can respond to changing levels of these chemicals with increased or decreased function. (Further discussion of the effects of stress on susceptibility to disease can be found in Chapter 9.)

Acquired Immune Deficiency Syndrome (AIDS)

AIDS, or **acquired immune deficiency syndrome,** is currently the best-known example of an acquired dysfunction of the immune system. It represents one of the most frightening diseases to appear in modern times because of its extremely high mortality rate (more than 98% of individuals who develop the most severe form of the disease die within 5 years of diagnosis, and as of 1992, approximately 150,000 have died in the United States); the possibility of transmission by asymptomatic individuals who apparently incubate the disease over a period of years; the rapid increase in the number of clinical cases (more than 240,000 AIDS cases in the United States as of this writing and increasing logarithmically at almost 100% per year); and the relatively uncontrollable modes of transmission (which include transplacental or perinatal routes and blood products or semen transmitted through homosexual and heterosexual contact, intravenous drug abuse, or the medical use of blood or blood products). It is estimated that in 1991 alone, 55,000 AIDS patients died, the same number of men and women who died during the entire Vietnam war. In 1992, that number will probably increase to almost 70,000. In New York City, AIDS is the leading cause of death for men between the ages of 25 and 44 and for women between the ages of 25 and 34.

Acquired immune deficiency syndrome is a viral disease that probably arose in central Africa in the 1950s, but is now found throughout the world. As of 1992, almost every country or territory has reported cases of AIDS. The estimated number of AIDS cases, worldwide, exceeds 1 million in at least 180 countries. As of 1988, 73% of reported cases were in the Americas, 13% in Europe, 13% in Africa, and 1% in Asia ("Update: Acquired Immunodeficiency Syndrome [AIDS]," 1988). Since then, the number of reported cases in Africa and Asia has increased considerably, so that more than half of AIDS cases are in Africa and almost 10% in Asia. More than 80% of AIDS in women is found in Africa. The virus infects and depletes a portion of the immune system, making the individuals extremely susceptible to life-threatening infections and malignancies.

Epidemiology

In the United States the groups at highest risk for developing AIDS include homosexual and bisexual men. In 1989, approximately 74% of the reported cases were in men who reported a history of sexual activity with other men, and an additional 8% were homosexual or bisexual intravenous drug users. The remaining patients consisted of heterosexual abusers of injected drugs (19%), female sexual partners of people in AIDS risk groups (1%), and children born of mothers at risk (<1%). The incidence of AIDS was approximately 8%

in women (52% were intravenous drug abusers and 17% were sexual partners of intravenous drug abusers) and 2% in children under the age of 13 ("Quarterly Report," 1988). It is estimated that more than 50% of homosexual men in some urban areas, such as New York City, are infected (Piot et al., 1988). With increased education, however, the incidence among homosexual men may be stabilizing. In more recent reports, only 60% of new cases are found in homosexual or bisexual men ("Update: CD4+," 1992). In some metropolitan areas, the incidence rates among intravenous drug abusers are beginning to surpass those of the homosexual population.

Although the incidence of apparently heterosexual transmission of AIDS in the United States is currently rather low (approximately 7% of the total AIDS cases, but more than 25% of cases in women), this route is becoming increasingly more common. Since 1981, the percentage of AIDS patients in the United States who are women has risen from 3% to almost 12%. Women make up more than half of all new AIDS cases in high school and college students and in health care providers. It is currently the most prevalent route in Africa, where the male-to-female ratio is near 1:1 (Adler, 1987). It is estimated that almost 100% of prostitutes in Kenya are infected (Piot et al., 1988), that 10% of the entire population of Uganda is HIV infected, and that 25% of the women attending prenatal clinics in Zambia are infected. Heterosexual transmission of AIDS is also rapidly rising in Asia, especially Thailand and India. In Thailand, much of the tourist trade is centered around certified HIV-free "tea houses," where prostitutes reside; almost 80% of these women are, in fact, HIV infected. It is estimated by the World Health Organization that by the year 2000 approximately 90% of AIDS will occur by heterosexual transmission.

Recipients of blood products or of semen for artificial insemination also have developed AIDS, but AIDS tests for screening donors of these products have greatly reduced this risk. Approximately 3% of AIDS patients have been transfusion recipients or had received blood products for coagulation disorders. The incidence of HIV seropositivity in hemophiliacs is 70% in individuals with hemophilia A (factor VIII deficiency) and 35% in individuals with hemophilia B (factor IX deficiency), mostly because of pre-1985 exposure ("Human Immunodeficiency," 1987).

Almost 4000 cases of AIDS have been reported in children. Three quarters of pediatric AIDS cases are newborns who contract the virus from their mothers across the placenta or through the milk during breastfeeding. The remaining patients are hemophiliacs or transfusion recipients. Symptoms usually develop within 6 months, and the life expectancy is generally less than 3 years. Certain aspects of pediatric AIDS remain enigmatic. Although the fetus is in direct contact with human immunodeficiency virus (HIV)-infected maternal blood during the entire pregnancy and HIV can cross the placenta as early as the eighth week of gestation, the incidence of pediatric AIDS is relatively low. Most studies report incidences of infection of approximately 30%, or even less.

The disease appears to be especially prevalent in the black and Hispanic communities. As of January 1992, AIDS cases nationally were distributed 54% in non-Hispanic whites, 29% in blacks, and 17% in Hispanics ("Unexplained CD4+," 1992). Blacks and Hispanics accounted for more than 70% of cases in heterosexual men, 70% of cases in women, and 75% of cases in children in the United States. Most were associated with intravenous drug abuse or heterosexual transmission.

The first reported health care provider to become occupationally infected with HIV was an emergency room nurse who became infected in 1986. The route of infection was probably through cuts in her hand that were exposed to contaminated blood through a gauze pad she was holding on a patient's open wound. As of 1992, more than 40,000 health care workers are infected with HIV. At least 40 were infected while caring for patients. These were primarily health care workers who had been accidentally stuck with needles containing virus-contaminated blood or had broken areas of skin exposed to large quantities of contaminated blood. Nurses are, by far, the most commonly exposed health care workers. As of March 14, 1988, 2586 health care workers in the United States had been diagnosed as having AIDS, of which 95% fall into known risk groups; however, most of the remaining 5% are still under investigation. As of December 31, 1987, 901 health care workers had been exposed through sticks (needles or other sharp objects); of these, 870 were exposed to blood and the rest to other fluids and four were infected (all through blood), and 169 were exposed through mucous membrane, open wound, or nonintact skin and none were infected. More recent reports on health care workers who are infected without other risks, however, include 15 cases in which workers have seroconverted and 7 in which they have not. The seroconverted individuals include four nurses, one home health care provider, one phlebotomist, one technologist, one research laboratory worker, and seven not specified ("Update: Acquired Immunodeficiency Syndrome and Human Immunodeficiency," 1988). Because of the potential risk, all health care personnel should routinely follow the guidelines for Universal Precautions published for the Centers for Disease Control ("Update: Universal Precautions," 1988).

Cause

Acquired immune deficiency syndrome is caused by a virus, currently named human immunodeficiency virus or HIV, that has been isolated by researchers at the National Institutes of Health as the human T-lymphotropic virus type III or HTLV-III (Gallo et al., 1984) and the Pasteur Institute as the lymphadenopathy/AIDS virus or LAV (Barre-Sinoussi et al., 1983). At least one other AIDS virus (HIV-2) has been identified (Clavel et al., 1987).

HIV is a retrovirus carrying genetic information in RNA rather than DNA (Fig. 8-9). Retroviruses infect cells by binding to the surface of a target cell through a receptor and inserting their RNA into the target cell (Fig. 8-10). Through the use of a viral enzyme, reverse transcriptase, the viral RNA is converted to DNA and inserted into the infected cell's genetic material. If the cell is activated, viral proliferation may occur, resulting in the lysis and death of the infected cell. If, however, the cell remains relatively dormant, the viral genetic material is integrated into the infected cell's DNA, may remain latent for years, and is probably present for the life of the individual (Ho, Pomerantz, & Kaplan, 1987).

CD4 is an antigen on the surface of T-helper cells that acts as a receptor for the HIV. The virus primarily infects CD4-positive T-helper lymphocytes, but also may infect various other cells of the central nervous system that also express the CD4 antigen (Funke et al., 1987).

Once activated, the virus infects other CD4-positive cells and kills them, causing a marked decrease in CD4 cells.

A second virus, HIV-2, has recently been identified in West Africa. The first case of HIV-2 in the United States was diagnosed in December 1987 in a recent visitor from West Africa ("Update: Acquired Immunodeficiency Syndrome [AIDS]," 1988). HIV-2 is very similar to HIV-1 in route of infection and clinical diagnosis, although it may be less destructive to the immune system and more slowly growing than HIV-1.

Origins of the virus

Acquired immune deficiency syndrome may have been around for considerably longer than we first suspected. The first unequivocal case in the United States was identified from stored blood samples. The patient was a 15-year-old boy who died in 1969 of AIDS. Antibodies against HIV-1 also have been detected from stored serum samples collected on patients who died of undetermined illnesses in the early 1960s.

It has been proposed that the AIDS virus developed in Africa as a result of genetic mutation from a monkey or chimpanzee virus. The African green monkey does carry an AIDS virus (SIV-agm) that is very similar to HIV-2. Genetic analysis of homology shows that SIV-agm and HIV-2 share approximately 80% of their genetic material. The SIV-agm virus is only about 50% related to HIV-1, however.

FIG. 8-9 Close-up of human immunodeficiency virus (HIV). Human immunodeficiency virus released from infected CD4 cells (particles spherical in shape) spread over adjacent CD4 cells, infecting them in turn. The individual AIDS particles are very tiny; more than 200 million would fit on the period at the end of this sentence.

FIG. 8-10 **Infection and cellular outcomes of the HIV.** HIV infection begins *(1)* when a virion, or virus particle, *(2)* binds to the outside of a susceptible cell and fuses with it, *(3)* injecting the core proteins and two strands of viral RNA. Uncoating occurs, during which the core proteins are removed and the viral RNA is released into the infected cell's cytoplasm. *(4)* The double-stranded DNA (provirus) migrates to the nucleus, *(5)* uncoats itself, and *(6)* is integrated into the cell's own DNA. The provirus then can do a couple of things: *(7A)* remain latent or *(7B)* activate cellular mechanisms to copy its genes into RNA, some of which is translated into viral proteins or ribosomes. The proteins and additional RNA then are assembled into new virions that bud from the cell. The process can take place slowly, sparing the host cell *(7B)*, or so rapidly that the cell is lysed or ruptured *(7C)*.

Clinical Manifestations

At the time of diagnosis, the individual may manifest one of four different conditions: serologically negative, serologically positive but asymptomatic, early stages of HIV disease, or AIDS. The currently accepted Centers for Disease Control (CDC) definition of AIDS relies on both laboratory tests and clinical symptoms. The most common laboratory test is for antibodies against HIV. Without a positive test for antibodies (seropositive), however, individuals can be diagnosed as having AIDS if they have a lymphoma of the brain and are younger than 60 years of age or if they have lymphoid interstitial pneumonitis and are younger than 13 years of age. If they are seropositive, the diagnosis of AIDS is made in association with a variety of clinical symptoms. These include disseminated coccidioidomycosis or histoplasmosis, extrapulmonary tuberculosis, persistent isosporiasis, recurrent salmonella septicemia, recurrent bacterial infections, HIV encephalopathy, HIV wasting syndrome, lymphoma of the brain at any age, and non-Hodgkin lymphoma. Other clinical symptoms of AIDS include persistent lymphadenopathy, weight loss, recurrent fevers, neurologic abnormalities, recurrent pulmonary infiltrates, and the development of opportunistic infections (such as *Pneumocystis carinii* pneumonia) and other atypical malignancies (such as Kaposi sarcoma) (Fig. 8-11).

The major immunologic finding in AIDS is the striking decrease in the number of T-helper cells (CD4-positive cells). Suppressor cells, which have the CD8 antigen, are usually normal or slightly elevated in number. This results in a reversal of the normal helper-to-suppressor T cell ratio, which is about 1.9. Most individuals with AIDS have ratios much lower than 0.9 and frequently near 0. In contrast, B cell numbers are usually normal. More recently, the CDC has added decreased CD4 T cell numbers and a variety of other clinical complications, including cervical cancer, as indicators of AIDS. These additional criteria most certainly will increase the number of reportable AIDS cases dramatically.

HIV virus also infects the central nervous system, resulting in AIDS dementia complex in the late stages of the disease (Price et al., 1988). Dementia is present in most individuals because of atrophy of cells of the cerebrum and degeneration of the nerve endings. Symptoms include lack of motor coordination and behavioral changes, including psychosis in the most extreme cases.

An intermediate stage of development used to be identified as AIDS-related complex (ARC). This description, however, has recently been dropped from the definition of AIDS and is now referred to as the early stages of HIV disease. Individuals with early stage disease present with relatively mild symptoms that may resemble influenza, such as night sweats, swollen lymph glands, diarrhea, or fatigue. AIDS, however, is characterized by severe symptoms and an increase in infections and malignancies. This stage may last for as long as 10 years.

The presence of circulating antibody against the AIDS virus apparently indicates infection by the virus, although many of these individuals are asymptomatic. Antibody appears rather rapidly after infection through blood products, usually within 4 to 7 weeks. After sex-

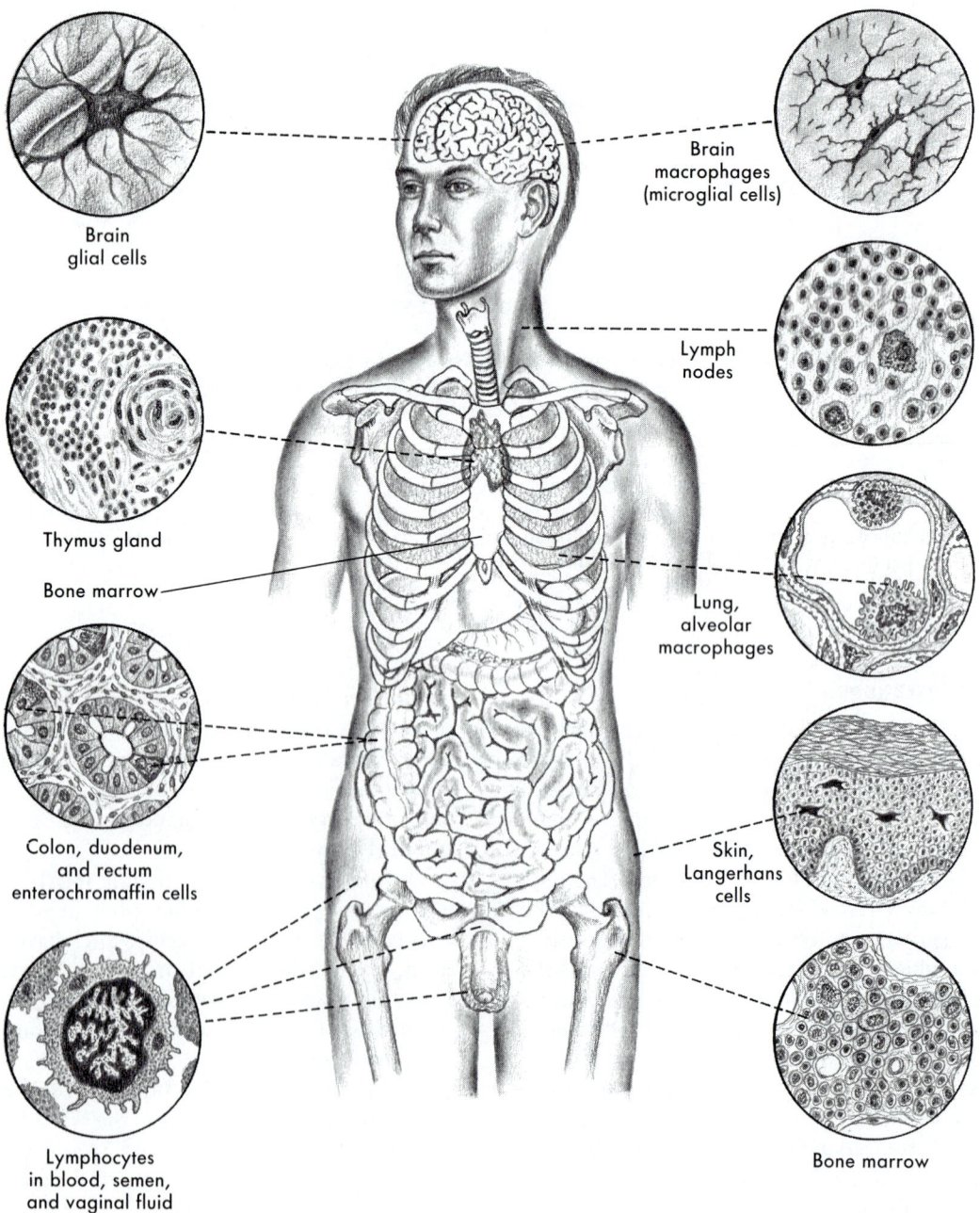

FIG. 8-11 **Distribution of tissues that can be infected by the HIV.** Infection is closely linked to the presence of CD4 receptors on host tissue, with the possible exceptions of glial cells in the brain and chromaffin cells in the colon, duodenum, and rectum. (Modified from Weber & Weiss, 1989.)

ual exposure, however, the individual can be infected yet seronegative for 6 to 14 months. In addition, in the late stages of the disease, some individuals become seronegative because of a deficient immune system.

Estimates are that for every diagnosed case of AIDS, approximately 100 others are HIV infected. It is also estimated that diagnosed cases of AIDS are underestimated by 10% to 15%. The incidence of antibody detected in asymptomatic individuals suggests that more than 2 million people in the United States are infected at the time of this writing, and this will double by the year 2000. Worldwide, approximately 40 million people will become HIV infected and from 10 to 13 million people will develop AIDS by 2000.

The period between infection and the appearance of antibody is referred to as the **window period**. Although the patient may not have antibody, he or she may have virus growing, be viremic, and be infectious to others within 2 weeks of being infected. The average time from infection to AIDS has been estimated at just under 10 years. Some estimates are that approximately 99% of

HIV-infected individuals eventually progress to AIDS.

A very recent development is the description of individuals who appear to have AIDS but are negative for any indication of HIV-1 or HIV-2 infection ("Update: CD4+," 1992). Thirty cases were reported that met all criteria for AIDS, including decreased numbers of CD4 T cells and AIDS-defining illnesses. Whether these individuals represent a new form of the disease is currently under investigation.

Treatment and Prevention

Both treatment of ongoing HIV infection and prevention of the initial infection have been very difficult to address. HIV has certain characteristics that frustrate attempts to develop effective treatments and vaccines.

There are two approaches to treatment for AIDS: restoration of immune function and prevention of viral replication. Restoration of immune function has been attempted with bone marrow transplants, transfusions of white blood cells from healthy donors, and the injection of soluble mediators (e.g., interleukin-2, interfer-

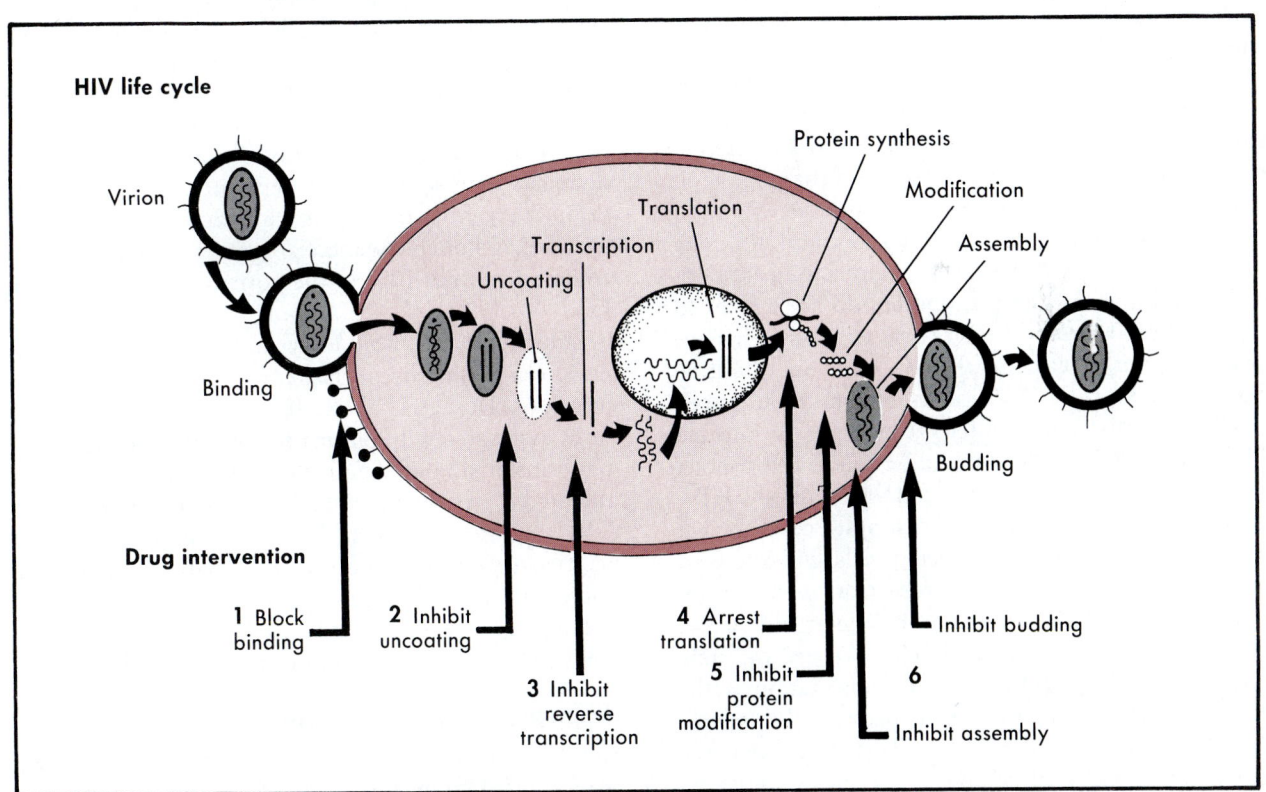

FIG. 8-12 HIV is subject to attack by drugs at several stages. Certain agents could block the binding of the HIV to CD4 receptors on the surface of helper T cells *(1)*. Other agents might keep viral RNA and reverse transcriptase from leaving their protein coat *(2)*. Drugs such as *AZT* and other *dideoxynucleosides* prevent the reverse transcription of viral RNA into viral DNA *(3)*. Later, *antisense oligonucleotides* could block the translation of mRNA into viral proteins *(4)*. Certain compounds could interfere with viral assembly by modifying such processes *(5)*, and finally, antiviral agents such as *interferon* could keep the virus from assembling itself and budding out of the cell *(6)*. (Modified from Yarchoan, Metsuya, & Broder, 1989.)

ons). Attempts at restoration have met with little or no success because the virus very quickly infects the donor cells.

Several antibiotics have been tried to prevent viral replication (Fig. 8-12). Some of these agents are designed to block reverse transcriptase activity, and some have been successful as antibiotics against other viruses or parasites (e.g., suramin against trypanosomiasis; ribavirin against cold and flu viruses; acyclovir against herpes simplex virus; and azidothymidine [AZT], which suppresses retrovirus-induced leukemia in mice). Although most of these agents are effective in preventing AIDS virus replication in vitro, their efficacy in individuals has not been generally good. One promising therapy has been AZT, and more recently its less toxic analog cyanothymidine (CNT), which has shown remarkable effects in extremely advanced AIDS cases with recurrent *P. carinii* infections.

Drug therapy for AIDS is difficult because, like most retroviruses, the AIDS virus incorporates into the genetic material of the host and may never be removed by antibiotic therapy. Therefore, drug administration may have to continue for the lifetime of the individual.

The development of an effective AIDS vaccine has been slowed by several major difficulties. *First,* the AIDS virus is genetically and antigenically variable, in a fashion similar to the influenza virus, so that a vaccine created against one variant may not provide protection against another variant. As many as 30 to 40 different genetic variants have been isolated from the same individual during the progression of the disease. Many of these may coexist in the individual. *Second,* although AIDS individuals have high levels of circulating antibodies against the virus, these antibodies do not appear to be protective. Therefore, even if an antibody response can be induced by vaccine, that response might not be effective. *Third,* the AIDS virus is transmitted from cell to cell and initially may enter the body in an infected cell. Microorganisms that spread by cell-to-cell contact are usually not susceptible to circulating antibody. HIV-infected cells also tend to fuse with other cells, so that infection can spread to uninfected cells without viral particles being produced. It is problematic whether antibodies against HIV prevent intercellular fusion between infected and uninfected cells. *Fourth,* the only good animal model for AIDS experimentation is the chimpanzee, which is a protected species and relatively unavailable for medical research. This means that the efficacy and toxicity of candidate vaccines cannot easily be evaluated.

Clinical Evaluation of Immunity

Individuals with immune deficiencies first go to the health provider with one common symptom, recurrent infections. To delineate the pathophysiology of a par-

ticular deficiency, certain observations and tests of the immune system are made. Significant information on the specific immune deficiency can be obtained by noting certain characteristics of the individual, including the presence of any associated anomalies, age, sex, and the types of infections (bacterial, viral, or fungal, and the specific organisms involved). Laboratory evaluation of immune deficiencies is presented in Table 8-6.

Replacement Therapies for Immune Deficiencies
Gamma Globulin Therapy

Individuals with B cell deficiencies that cause hypogammaglobulinemia or agammaglobulinemia usually can be treated successfully with administration of gamma globulin. Commercial gamma globulin preparations are usually administered intramuscularly once a month at dosages determined by body weight (0.2 to 0.6 ml/kg). Schedule and dosage are also determined according to titers of circulating immunoglobulins and the incidence of infections in the individual. In a 70-kg adult, a monthly dose can be as high as 42 ml, in which case it may be divided into smaller doses injected weekly at different sites to minimize discomfort. Complications of treatment include anaphylactic reactions caused by aggregated immunoglobulins in the preparations (aggregated immunoglobulins, although not immune complexes, can activate inflammation as immune complexes do) and inadvertent intravenous (IV) administration. Individuals with selective IgA deficiency occasionally develop allergic reactions to IgA in gamma globulin preparations, although commercial gamma globulins usually contain less than 10% of the normal levels of IgM and IgA.

Individuals who need larger amounts of IgM or IgA are given fresh frozen plasma in monthly intravenous infusions. Dosage is about 10 to 15 ml/kg. Complications associated with plasma therapy include the potential transmission of hepatitis or AIDS. The plasma is irradiated to destroy immunocompetent T cells and avoid GVH disease in individuals with accompanying T cell deficiencies. Administration of fresh frozen plasma is successful in individuals with Wiskott-Aldrich syndrome (IgM deficient), ataxia telangiectasia (IgA deficient), or complement component deficiencies.

Transplantation and Transfusion

In SCID caused by a lack of stem cells, bone marrow is transplanted from a HLA-matched donor. Other diseases involving depletion of the bone marrow (i.e., aplastic anemia, leukemia requiring eradication of tumor cells in the marrow) are also treated by bone marrow transplantation. At least 75% of bone marrow transplants between individuals who are matched for HLA-A, B, C, and DR, and whose lymphocytes are non-

TABLE 8-6

Laboratory Evaluation of Immune Deficiencies

Function tested	Laboratory test	Interpretation of test
Tests of humoral immune function		
Antibody production	Total immunoglobulin levels	Presence of antibody-producing B cells
	Levels of isohemagglutinins	Capacity to produce specific IgM antibodies
	Levels of antibodies against vaccines—especially diphtheria and tetanus toxoids	Capacity to produce specific IgG antibodies
B cell numbers	Numbers of lymphocytes with surface immunoglobulin	Presence of circulating B cells
Tests of cellular immune function		
Delayed hypersensitivity skin test	Skin test reaction against previously encountered antigens—especially *C. albicans* or tetanus toxoid	Presence of antigen-responsive T cells and cellular interactions (e.g., lymphokine activity and macrophage function)
T cell numbers	Numbers of T cells forming rosettes with sheep erythrocytes or expressing membrane CD3 or CD11 antigen	Presence of circulating T cells
T cell proliferation in vitro	Proliferative response to nonspecific mitogens (e.g., phytohemagglutinin)	Capacity of all T cells to divide in response to nonspecific stimulation (mitogens)
	Proliferative response to antigens (e.g., tetanus toxoid)	Capacity of antigen-reactive T cells to respond to antigen

stimulatory in one-way mixed lymphocyte reactions (matched at HLA-D), are accepted. Most rejections of HLA-matched transplants are because of recognition of minor histocompatibility antigens by individuals who have received multiple transfusions and are, as a result, sensitized against those antigens, which are not evaluated in tissue typing.

Graft-versus-host (GVH) disease may develop if the recipient's cells express histocompatibility antigens not found on the donor's cells. GVH disease occurs when immunocompetent T lymphocytes in the grafted material recognize foreign antigens in the recipient, initiating a type IV hypersensitivity reaction against the recipient's tissues. The main target tissues of the reaction are the skin, gastrointestinal mucosa, and the liver. Symptoms of a GVH reaction usually appear within 10 to 30 days after the transplant, develop as a skin rash, hepatomegaly, and diarrhea, and may lead to death of infections. GVH disease is not a problem when the recipient is immunocompetent, that is, has an immune system that can control the donor's lymphocytes.

Several attempts have been made to prevent GVH disease by removing mature immunocompetent T lymphocytes from grafts. One procedure is to infuse the graft with monoclonal antibody against plasma membrane antigens found only on mature T cells. Another is to use fetal tissue as the graft. For example, fetal liver, which contains stem cells but not immunocompetent lymphocytes, is sometimes grafted in place of bone marrow if an HLA-matched donor cannot be found. Usually, fetal liver transplants are only successful over the short term.

Reconstitution of thymic function is one therapy for deficiency diseases in which the individual lacks a thymus or thymic function (i.e., DiGeorge syndrome, ataxia telangiectasia, or chronic mucocutaneous candidiasis). The procedure is to transplant fetal thymus tissue, which lacks immunocompetent T cells, or thymic epithelial cells (the cells that produce the thymic hormones) from which mature T cells have been removed. In some individuals, transplantation increases the number of circulating mature T cells, but in most cases improvement is only temporary.

Enzymatic defects that cause SCID (e.g., adenosine deaminase deficiency) are sometimes treated successfully with transfusions of glycerol frozen-packed erythrocytes. The donor erythrocytes contain the needed enzyme and can, at least temporarily, provide sufficient enzyme for normal lymphocyte function.

The administration of soluble materials that affect lymphocyte function can restore T cell function, especially in individuals with Wiskott-Aldrich syndrome or chronic mucocutaneous candidiasis. Transfer factor, a low-molecular-weight nucleoprotein prepared from lymphocyte lysates, can confer specific reactivity against certain antigens and has been used successfully in some individuals. Thymosin, a thymic hormone, has also been used, although with limited success.

Gene Therapy

The first attempt at therapeutic replacement of defective genes has been made in a little girl with SCID caused by an ADA deficiency. The normal gene for ADA had been cloned and inserted into a retroviral vector. The gene for ADA had replaced some of retroviral genes, resulting in a virus that carried the normal human gene but did not cause disease. The virus was used to infect bone marrow stem cells from the child. The retrovirus inserted the normal ADA gene into the patient's genetic material. The genetically altered stem cells were infused into the child resulting in apparent reconstitution of her immune system.

SUMMARY REVIEW

Hypersensitivity: Allergy, Autoimmunity, and Isoimmunity

1 Hypersensitivity is an inappropriate immune response misdirected against the host's own tissues (autoimmunity); directed against beneficial foreign tissues, such as transfusions or transplants (isoimmunity); or exaggerated responses against environmental antigens (allergy).

2 Mechanisms of hypersensitivity are classified as type I (IgE-mediated) reactions, type II (tissue-specific) reactions, type III (immune-complex–mediated) reactions, and type IV (cell-mediated) reactions.

3 Hypersensitivity reactions can be immediate (developing within seconds or hours) or delayed (developing within hours or days).

4 Anaphylaxis, the most rapid immediate hypersensitivity reaction, is an explosive reaction that occurs within minutes of reexposure to the antigen and can lead to cardiovascular shock.

5 Allergens are antigens that cause allergic responses.

6 Type I (IgE-mediated) reactions are mediated through the binding of IgE to Fc receptors on mast cells and cross-linking of IgE by antigens that bind to the Fab portions of IgE. Cross-linking causes mast cell degranulation and the release of histamine and other inflammatory substances.

7 Type II (tissue-specific) reactions are caused by four possible mechanisms: complement-mediated lysis, opsonization and phagocytosis, antibody-dependent cell-mediated cytotoxicity, and modulation of cellular function.

8 Type III (immune-complex–mediated) reactions are caused by the formation of immune complexes that are deposited in target tissues, where they activate the complement cascade, generating chemotactic fragments that attract neutrophils into the inflammatory site.

9 Immune-complex disease can be a systemic reaction, such as serum sickness, or localized, such as the Arthus reaction.

10 Type IV (cell-mediated) reactions are caused by specifically sensitized T cells, which either kill target cells directly or release lymphokines that activate other cells, such as macrophages.

11 Allergies can be mediated by any of the four mechanisms of hypersensitivity.

12 Clinical manifestations of allergic reactions are usually confined to the areas of initial intake or contact with the allergen. Ingested allergens induce gastrointestinal symptoms, airborne allergens induce respiratory or skin manifestations, and contact allergens induce allergic responses at the site of contact.

13 Atopic individuals are genetically predisposed to the development of allergies.

14 Autoimmunity is a breakdown of immunologic homeostasis, the immune system's tolerance of self-antigens.

15 Autoimmune disease can be caused by the exposure of a previously sequestered antigen, the development of a neoantigen, the complications of infectious disease, the emergence of a forbidden clone of lymphocytes, or an alteration of suppressor T cell function.

16 Isoimmunity is the immune system's reaction against antigens on the tissues of other members of the same species.

17 Isoimmune disorders include transient neonatal disease, in which the maternal immune system becomes sensitized against antigens expressed by the fetus, and transplant rejection and transfusion reactions, in which the immune system of the recipient of an organ transplant or blood transfusion reacts against foreign antigens on the donor's cells.

Deficiencies in Immunity and Inflammation

1 Immune deficiency is the failure of mechanisms of self-defense to function in their normal capacity.

2 Immune deficiencies are either congenital (primary) or acquired (secondary). Congenital immune deficiencies are caused by genetic defects that disrupt lymphocyte development, whereas acquired immune deficiencies are secondary to disease or other physiologic alterations.

3 The clinical hallmark of immune deficiency is a propensity to unusual or recurrent severe infections. The type of infection usually reflects the immune system defect.

4 The most common infections in individuals with defects of cell-mediated immune response are fungal and viral, whereas infections in individuals with defects of the humoral immune response or complement function are primarily bacterial.

5 Severe combined immune deficiency (SCID) is a total lack of T cell function and a severe (either partial or total) lack of B cell function.

6 DiGeorge syndrome (congenital thymic aplasia or hypoplasia) is characterized by complete or partial lack of the thymus (resulting in depressed T cell immunity), the parathyroid glands (resulting in hypocalcemia), and cardiac anomalies.

7 Defects in B cell function are diverse, ranging from a complete lack of the human bursal equivalent, the lymphoid organs required for B cell maturation (as in Bruton agammaglobulinemia), to deficiencies in a single class of immunoglobulins (e.g., selective IgA deficiency).

8 Defects in phagocyte function, which include insufficient numbers of phagocytes or defects of chemotaxis, phagocytosis, or killing, can result in recurrent, life-threatening infections, such as septicemia and disseminated pyogenic lesions.

9 Acquired immune deficiencies are caused by superimposed conditions, such as malnutrition, medical therapies, physical or psychologic trauma, or infections.

10 AIDS is an acquired dysfunction of the immune system caused by a retrovirus (HIV) that infects and destroys T4-positive lymphocytes (helper T cells).

11 Immune deficiency syndromes are usually treated by replacement therapy. Deficient antibody production is treated by replacement of missing immunoglobulins with commercial gamma globulin preparations. Lymphocyte deficiencies are treated with the replacement of host lymphocytes with transplants of bone marrow, fetal liver, or fetal thymus from a donor.

KEY TERMS

Acquired (secondary) immune deficiency, 284
Acquired immune deficiency syndrome (AIDS), 288
ADA deficiency (adenosine deaminase deficiency), 286
Agammaglobulinemia, 286
Allergen, 272
Allergy, 269
Anaphylaxis, 272
Arthus reaction, 278
Atopic dermatitis, 280
Atopic individual, 273
Autoantibody, 269
Autoimmune disease, 269
Autoimmunity, 269
Bare lymphocyte syndrome, 286
Blocking antibody, 275
Bruton agammaglobulinemia, 286
Chronic mucocutaneous candidiasis, 287

Congenital (primary) immune deficiency, 284
Contact dermatitis, 280
Cytotropic, 272
Delayed hypersensitivity reaction, 272
DiGeorge syndrome, 286
Forbidden clone, 281
Hypersensitivity, 269
Hypocomplementemia, 277
Hypogammaglobulinemia, 286
Immediate hypersensitivity reaction, 272
Immune deficiency, 284
Immunologically privileged site, 280
Immunologic homeostasis (tolerance), 269
Isoimmune disease, 269
Isoimmunity, 269
Neoantigen, 280

PNP deficiency (purine nucleoside phosphorylase deficiency), 286
Radioallergosorbent (RAST) testing, 275
Radioimmunosorbent (RIST) testing, 275
Raynaud phenomenon, 278
Reagin, 272
Reticular dysgenesis, 286
Selective IgA deficiency, 286
Sequestered antigen, 280
Serum sickness, 278
Severe combined immune deficiency (SCID), 286
Systemic lupus erythematosus (SLE), 282
Tissue-specific antigen, 275
Urticaria (hives), 273
Wheal and flare reaction, 275
Window period, 293
Wiskott-Aldrich syndrome, 286

REFERENCES

Adler, M. W. (1987). ABC of AIDS: Development of the epidemic. *British Medical Journal, 294,* 1083-1085.

Arthus, M. & Breton, M. (1903). Lésions cutanées produites par les injections de sérum. *Comptes Rendus Societe de Biologie, 55,* 817-820.

Barre-Sinoussi, F., Chermann, J. C., Rey, F., Nugeyre, M. T., Chamaret, S., Gruest, J., Dauguet, C., Axler-Blin, C., Vezinet- Brun, F., Rouzioux, C., Qozenbaum, W., & Montagnier, L. (1983). Isolation of a T-lymphocyte retroviruses from a patient at risk for acquired immune deficiency syndrome (AIDS). *Science, 220,* 868-871.

CDC surveillance summaries: Report on selected racial/ethnic groups. (1988). *Morbidity and Mortality Weekly, 37,* 1-10.

Clavel, F., Mansinho, K., Chamaret, S., Guetard, D., Favier, V., Nina, J., Santos-Ferreira, M-O, Champalimaud, J-J., & Montagnier, L. (1987). Human immunodeficiency virus type 2 infection associated with AIDS in West Africa. *New England Journal of Medicine, 316,* 1180-1185.

DiGeorge, A. M. (1968). Congenital absence of the thymus and its immunologic consequences. In D. Bergsma & F. A. McKusick (Eds.), *Immunologic deficiency diseases in man.* Baltimore: National Foundation—March of Dimes Original Article Series: Williams & Wilkins.

Fritzler, M. J. & Tan, E. M. (1985). Antinuclear antibodies and the connective tissue diseases. In A. S. Cohen (Ed.), *Laboratory diagnostic procedures in the rheumatic diseases* (p. 213). Orlando, FL: Grune and Stratton, Inc.

Funke, I., Hahn, A., Reiber, E. P., Weiss, E., & Riethmüller, G. (1987). The cellular receptor (CD4) of the human immunodeficiency virus is expressed on neurons and glial cells in human brain. *Journal of Experimental Medicine, 165,* 1230-1235.

Gallo, R. C., Salahuddin, S. Z., Popovic, M., Shearer, G. S., Kaplan, M., Haynes, B. F., Kaplan, M., Palker, T. J., Redfield, R., Oleske, J., Safai, B., White, G., Foster, P. & Markham, P. D. (1984). Frequent detection and isolation of cytopathic retroviruses (HTLV-III) from patients with AIDS. *Science, 224,* 500-503.

Gell, P. G. H., Coombs, R. R. A., & Lachman, P. T. (1975). *Clinical aspects of immunology.* Oxford: Blackwell Scientific Publications.

Habif, T. P. (1985). *Clinical dermatology: A color guide to diagnosis and therapy.* St. Louis: Mosby—Year Book.

Ho, D. D., Pomerantz, R. J., & Kaplan, J. C. (1987). Pathogenesis of infection with human immunodeficiency virus. *New England Journal of Medicine, 317,* 278-286.

Human immunodeficiency virus infection in the United States: A review of current knowledge. (1987). *Morbidity and Mortality Weekly, 36,* 1-48.

Koch, R. (1891). Fortsetzung der mitteilungen über ein heilmittel gegen tuberkulose. *Deutsche Medizinische Wochenschrift, 9,* 101-102.

Piot, P., Plummer, F. A., Mhalu, F. S., Lamboray, J-L., Chin, J., & Mann, J. M. (1988). AIDS: An international perspective. *Science, 239,* 573-579.

Pirquet, C. & Schick, B. (1905). *Serum sickness.* Leipzig: Franz Denticke.

Portier, P. & Richet, C. (1902). De l'action anaphylactique de certains venins. *Comptes Rendus Societie de Biologie (Paris), 54,* 170-172.

Price, R. W., Brew, B., Sidtis, J., Rosenblum, M., Schenk, A. C., & Cleary, P. (1988). The brain in AIDS: Central nervous system HIV-1 infection and AIDS dementia complex. *Science, 239,* 586-592.

Quarterly report to the domestic policy council on the prevalence and rate of spread of HIV and AIDS in the United States. (1988). *Morbidity and Mortality Weekly, 37,* 223-227.

Rote, N. S. (1985). Immune complex disorders and vasculitis. In N. Gleicher (Ed.), *Principles of medical therapy in pregnancy.* New York: Plenum, pp. 981-989.

Unexplained CD4+ T-lymphocyte depletion in persons without evident HIV infection—United States. (1992). *Morbidity and Mortality Weekly, July 31, 41,* 541-545.

Update: Acquired immunodeficiency syndrome (AIDS)—Worldwide. (1988). *Morbidity and Mortality Weekly, 37,* 286-295.

Update: Acquired immunodeficiency syndrome and human immunodeficiency virus infection among health-care workers. (1988). *Morbidity and Mortality Weekly, 37,* 229-239.

Update: CD4+ T-lymphocytopenia in persons without evident HIV infection—United States. (1992) *Morbidity and Mortality Weekly, August 7, 41,* 578-579.

Update: Universal precautions for prevention of transmission of human immunodeficiency virus, hepatitis B virus, and other bloodborne pathogens in health-care settings. (1988). *Morbidity and Mortality Weekly, 37,* 377-388.

Weber, J. N., & Weiss, R. A. (1989). HIV infection: The cellular picture. In *The science of AIDS: readings from Scientific American.* New York: W. H. Freeman.

Yarchoan, R., Mitsuya, H., & Broder, S. (1989). AIDS therapies. In *The science of AIDS: readings from Scientific American.* New York: W. H. Freeman.

SUGGESTED READINGS

Bruton, O. C. (1952). Agammaglobulinemia. *Pediatrics, 9,* 722-728.

Church, J. A. & Schlegel, R. J. (1985). Immune deficiency disorders. In J. A. Bellanti (Ed.), *Immunology III.* Philadelphia: W.B. Saunders, p. 493.

Frank, M. M. (1987). Current concepts: Complement in the pathophysiology of human disease. *New England Journal of Medicine, 316,* 1525-1530.

Schlegel, R. J., Bernier, G. M., Bellanti, J. A., Maybee, D. A., Osborne, G. B., Stewart, J. L., Peralman, D. S., Ouelette, J., & Biehusen, F. C. (1970). Severe candidiasis associated with thymic dysplasia, IgA deficiency, and plasma antilymphocyte effects. *Pediatrics, 45,* 926.

Stine, G. J. (1993). *Acquired immune deficiency syndrome.* Englewood Cliffs, NJ: Prentice-Hall.

CHAPTER 9

Stress and Disease

Kathryn L. McCance

Jane Shelby

T he notion that prolonged emotional or psychologic stress can contribute to or even cause the
development of physical illness has a long history.
For example, Galen (200 AD) stated that "melan-
cholic" women developed breast cancer more often
than did "sanguine" women (Bieliauskas, 1982).

It is often reported that the use of the term stress
in a biologic sense began with Hans Selye in 1946.
In 1914, however, Walter B. Cannon used the term
in both a physiologic and a psychologic sense in a paper reporting his psychoendocrine studies (Cannon,
Bringer, & Fritz, 1914). In his report, Cannon used
such phrases as "great emotional stress" and "times
of stress" (Cannon, et al., 1914). In 1935, Cannon
published another paper, called "Stresses and Strains
of Homeostasis." In it he applied the engineering
concept of stress and strain in a physiologic context

(Cannon, 1935). Cannon also thought that stress involved psychologic factors; he stated in his paper that
physical as well as emotional stimuli can cause stress.
The popularization of the term, however, began with
Hans Selye's work.

The concept that stress may influence immunity
and resistance to disease has been the subject of several investigations since the middle of the century.
Studies reporting psychosocial factors relating to infectious diseases appeared in the literature in the
1950s. Rene Dubos (1965) emphasized that a multitude of factors cause disease, including prior exposure to a microorganism and development of immunity, nutritional status of the individual, presence of
other disease, and many genetic factors.

Meyer and Haggarty (1962) reported that during
the course of 1 year, the significant factor that deter-

299

mined whether an individual acquired a respiratory tract infection was acute or chronic family stress. Jacobs and colleagues reported that psychologic stimuli characterized by failure, unresolved role crisis, and social isolation in students were frequently associated with respiratory infections (Jacobs, Spilken, & Norman, 1969; Jacobs, Spilken, Norman, & Andersson, 1970). Overall, studies in the 1970s found that life changes or emotions resulting from life changes occurring for a prolonged time were associated with decreases in one or more immune functions. The past decade for the first time in history has demonstrated the interactions among social, psychologic, and biologic factors in the causes and courses of many diseases. Molecular biologists, immunologists, neurologists, clinicians, and behavioral scientists have begun to explore the role of the neglected half of the mind-body (dualistic) model—the mind. What is emerging is a more holistic and complex model involving biochemical relationships of the central and autonomic nervous systems, the endocrine system, and the immune system. Discoveries of these links have, in fact, created the new field of psychoneuroimmunology.

CONCEPTS OF STRESS

The term *stress* has been used persistently and widely in specialties such as biology, health sciences, and social sciences, despite numerous disagreements over its definition. Nevertheless, acceptance in recent years is that stress is more usefully defined as a *transactional or interactional concept* (Ostell, 1991). Transactionally, stress is viewed as the state of affairs arising when a person relates to (i.e., interacts or transacts with) situations in certain ways. People are not disturbed by situations *per se*, but by the ways they appraise and react to situations (Ostell, 1991). Important to this definition is that stress is a condition in which a demand *exceeds* a person's coping abilities. Various stress reactions include disturbances of cognition, emotion, and behavior that can adversely affect a person's well-being.

General Adaptation Syndrome

Selye (1946) originally sought to discover a new sex hormone when he discovered the biologic syndrome of stress. In his attempts to discover the new hormone, Selye injected crude ovarian extracts into rats. Repeatedly, he found that the following triad of structural changes occurred: (1) enlargement of the cortex of the adrenal gland, (2) atrophy of the thymus gland and other lymphoid structures, and (3) development of bleeding ulcers of the stomach and duodenal lining. Selye soon discovered that this triad of manifestations was not specific for his ovarian extracts, but also occurred after he

exposed the rats to other noxious stimuli, such as cold, surgical injury, and restraint. He called these stimuli **stressors.** Selye concluded that this triad or syndrome of manifestations represented a nonspecific response to noxious stimuli. Because many diverse agents caused the same syndrome, Selye suggested that it be called the **general adaptation syndrome** (GAS). In 1959, Selye wrote:

Specific homeostatic mechanisms for the maintenance of body temperature, blood sugar, etc., have been under study since Claude Bernard. The principal contribution of stress research was precisely to show that if we abstract from three specific reactions, there remains a common residual response that is nonspecific in regard to its cause and can be elicited with such diverse agents as cold, heat, x-rays, adrenalin, insulin, tubercle bacilli, or muscular exercise. This is so despite the coexistence of highly specific adaptive reactions to any one of these agents.

Selye later defined three successive stages in development of the GAS: (1) the **alarm stage,** in which the central nervous system is aroused and the body's defenses are mobilized (e.g., "flight or fight"); (2) the **stage of resistance or adaptation,** during which mobilization contributes to "flight or fight"; and (3) the **stage of exhaustion,** in which continuous stress causes the progressive breakdown of compensatory mechanisms (acquired adaptations) and homeostasis. The stage of exhaustion, Selye believed, marked the onset of certain diseases he called **diseases of adaptation.**

The nonspecific physiologic response identified by Selye consists of interaction among the sympathetic branch of the autonomic nervous system (see Chapter 12) and two glands, the pituitary gland and the adrenal gland (see Chapter 17). The alarm phase of the GAS begins when a stressor triggers the actions of the pituitary gland and the sympathetic nervous system (Fig. 9-1). The resistance or adaptation phase begins with the actions of the adrenal hormones cortisol, norepinephrine, and epinephrine. Exhaustion occurs if stress continues and adaptation is not successful. The ultimate signs of exhaustion are impairment of the immune response, heart failure, and kidney failure, leading to death.

After further experimentation, Selye defined **physiologic stress** as a chemical or physical disturbance in the cells or tissue fluid produced by a change, either in the external environment or within the body itself, that requires a response (i.e., begins the GAS) to counteract the disturbance. On the basis of this definition, Selye identified three components of physiologic stress: (1) the exogenous or endogenous stressor initiating the disturbance, (2) the chemical or physical disturbance produced by the stressor, and (3) the body's counteracting (adaptational) response to the disturbance (Selye, 1946).

Psychologic Mediators and Specificity

Although Selye's identification of the GAS is regarded as tremendously important and the cornerstone of stress research, the idea that stress is a purely physiologic response is oversimplified. In the mid-1950s, studies showed that activation of the adrenal cortex occurred in humans in response to psychologic stressors (Hill et al., 1956); in monkeys with conditional emotional responses (Mason & Brady, 1956); and in humans subjected to a stressful interview technique (Hetzel, Schottsteadt, Grace, & Wolff, 1955). In the early 1960s, researchers found that plasma cortisol levels in groups of subjects increased while they watched war movies and decreased while they viewed Walt Disney nature films (Handlon et al., 1962; Wadeson, Mason, Hamburg, & Handlon, 1963). Later, Mason (1971) demonstrated in a series of experiments that occurrence of the GAS depended on psychologic factors surrounding the stressors. Mason demonstrated that several factors, including degrees of discomfort, unpleasantness, or suddenness of the stress, could account for the presence or absence of the physiologic stress response.

Another challenge to Selye's concept of the GAS focused on his idea that stressors cause a general or nonspecific response (Bieliauskas, 1982). The triad of adrenal cortical enlargement, thymus and lymphoid shrinkage, and gastrointestinal ulceration may not be as nonspecific as Selye believed it to be (Mason, 1975).

Research done in the past 25 years has shown the remarkable sensitivity of the pituitary gland and adrenal cortex to emotional, psychologic, and social influences. Thus it is difficult to know when it is the way an individual thinks and feels about a physical stressor or the stressor itself that produces the neuroendocrine responses. In experiments in which psychologic reactions were minimized, physical stressors did not appear to stimulate the pituitary or adrenal cortex in a nonspecific fashion. For example, fasting monkeys who were given nonnutritive placebo food to minimize the discomfort of an empty gastrointestinal tract did not secrete adrenal cortical hormones (Mason, 1972). In another experiment, in which precautions were taken to avoid discomfort, exposure of human subjects to heat actually suppressed adrenal cortical hormone levels (Mason, 1974).

Many physiologists resist Selye's concept of nonspecificity because it appears to be incompatible with the principles of physiologic homeostasis (Cannon, 1963; Mason, 1975). W. B. Cannon defined **homeostasis** as the sum of the processes by which the body maintains itself at a relatively constant composition (Cannon, 1935). Adaptive bodily responses are selective and are organized to counteract the specific bodily changes that elicit them. It is difficult, then, to explain how any nonspecific physiologic or biochemical response could help

the body adapt, for example, to both cold and heat (Mason, 1975). Physiologically, the body adapts to cold by conserving heat (peripheral vasoconstriction) and producing more heat (shivering), and to heat by losing heat (peripheral vasodilation and sweating) and decreasing heat production. To support Selye's concept of nonspecificity, hard evidence is needed that increased adrenal cortical or medullary activity can promote adaptations to both cold and heat. In fact, no single hormone responds to all stressful stimuli in the absolutely nonspecific fashion implied in Selye's definition of the GAS.

Homeostasis as a Dynamic Steady State

Another source of confusion in the literature about stress is the concept of homeostasis. Selye used Cannon's definition of homeostasis (the sum of the processes by which the body maintains itself at a relatively constant composition) and expanded it to mean also that the body's need determines body responses and that adaptive responses are necessary to maintain body stability. Both Cannon's definition and Selye's extrapolation were oversimplified. Research with a variety of radioisotopes has since demonstrated that homeostasis does not mean "constant composition." Much more accurate is the concept of homeostasis as a **dynamic steady state.** For example, the fat or protein content of the body may not vary much from day to day, but the substances that make up the fat and protein—fatty acids and amino acids—can vary widely (Dickman, 1988). The enzymes in a healthy person are constantly synthesizing fat and proteins and also constantly breaking them down. The process of synthesis and breakdown of all bodily substances is known as **turnover.** Homeostasis, then, is more accurately defined as a dynamic steady state representing the net effect of all the turnover reactions.

Stressors cause a series of reactions that alter the dynamic steady state. This alteration may be either short-term or long-term. For example, the normal concentration of glucose in the blood is 80 ± 10 mg/100 ml. The concentration of glucose increases with acute stress, such as a burn injury, and then slowly returns to normal. If blood glucose remains high in the absence of a known stressor, it is diagnosed as a sign of disease, probably diabetes mellitus. Prolonged, unrelenting stress can cause a chronic elevation of glucose levels that leads to diabetes mellitus.

THE STRESS RESPONSE

Psychoneuroimmunologic Regulation

Psychoneuroimmunology is the study of the interaction of consciousness (psycho), brain and central nervous system (neuro), and the body's defense against external

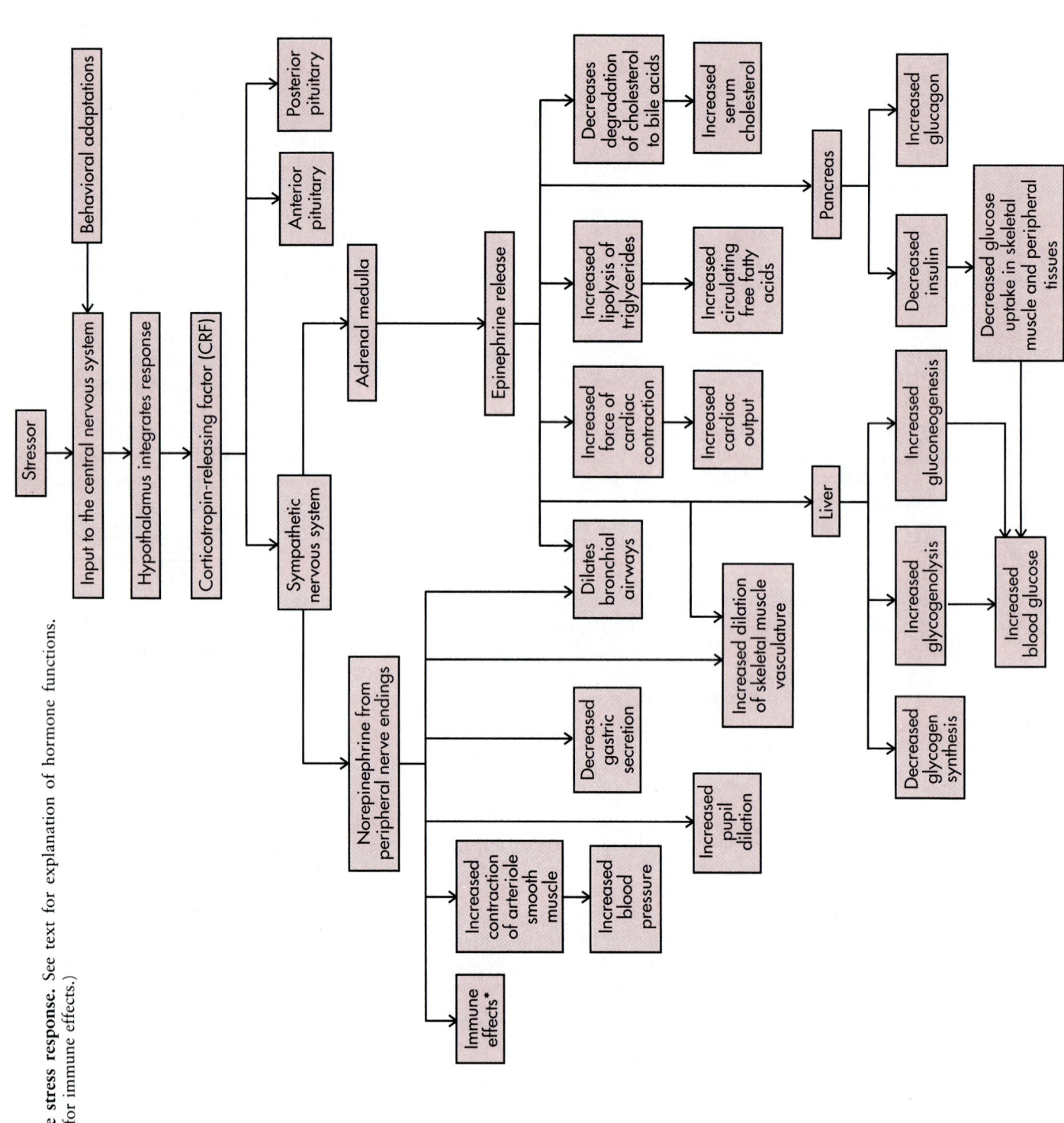

FIG. 9-1 The stress response. See text for explanation of hormone functions. (*See p. 308 for immune effects.)

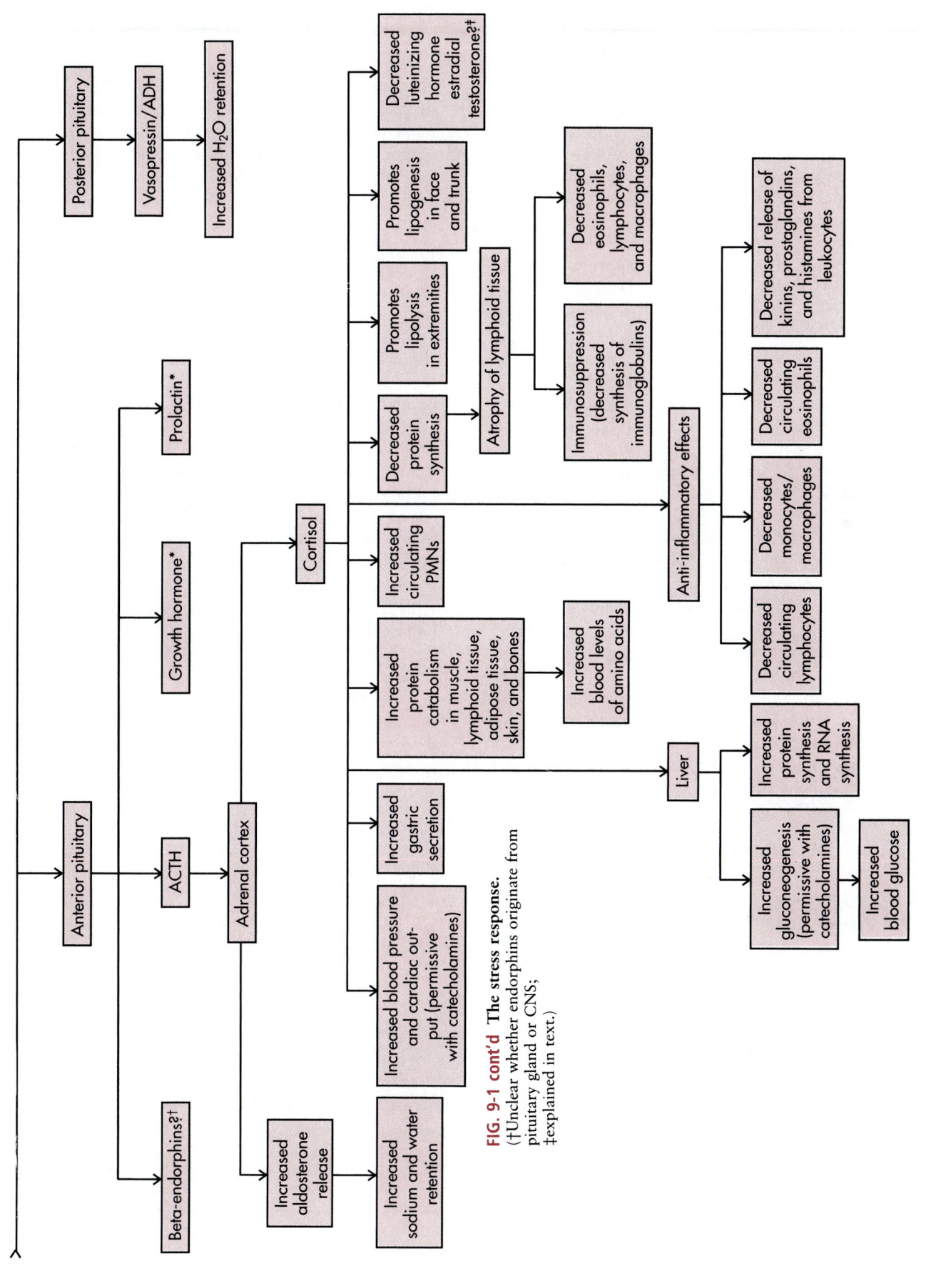

FIG. 9-1 cont'd The stress response.
(†Unclear whether endorphins originate from pituitary gland or CNS; ‡explained in text.)

infection and abnormal cell division (immunology) (Pelletier & Herzing, 1988). Psychoneuroimmunology assumes that all disease is multifactorial—the result of interrelationships—among psychosocial, emotional, genetic, neurologic, endocrine, and immune systems and behavioral factors. Evidence from the last decade suggests that the immune system is integrated with other physiologic processes and is sensitive to changes in central nervous system and endocrine functioning, such as those that accompany psychologic states (Houldin, Lev, Prystowsky, Redei, & Lowery, 1991). Stressors, such as infection, noise, decreased oxygen supply, pain, malnutrition, heat, cold, trauma, prolonged exertion, responses to life events, including anxiety, depression, anger, fear, excitement, and radiation, obesity, old age, drugs, disease, surgery, and medical treatment can elicit the stress response.

The **stress response** is initiated by the nervous and endocrine systems, specifically corticotropin-releasing factor (CRF) from the hypothalamus, the locus ceruleus-norepinephrine/autonomic (sympathetic) nervous system (LC-NE), the pituitary gland, and the adrenal gland (see Fig. 9-1) (Chrousos & Gold, 1992). The activation of these systems redirects adaptive energy to the central nervous system and stressed body sites. The LC-NE system is located in the brainstem and stimulates the release of norepinephrine throughout the brain, promoting arousal, increased vigilance, increased anxiety, and other protective emotional responses. Reproduction, growth, and thyroid hormone are suppressed during stress and may conserve energy during stress. The adrenocortical hormones and the sympathetic nervous system have been postulated as mediators of enhancement or suppression of immune functioning (Ader & Cohen, 1975; Houldin et al., 1991; Vollhardt, 1991).

Neuroendocrine Regulation

The sympathetic nervous system is aroused during the stress response and causes the medulla of the adrenal gland to release catecholamines (epinephrine, norepinephrine, and dopamine) into the bloodstream. The adrenal medulla is actually an extension of the sympathetic nervous system because preganglionic fibers from the splanchnic nerve terminate in the medulla, where they innervate the chromaffin cells that produce the catecholamine hormones. Simultaneously, hypothalamic corticotropin-releasing factor stimulates the pituitary gland to release a variety of hormones, including antidiuretic hormone, from the posterior pituitary gland, and prolactin, growth hormone, and adrenocorticotropin hormone (ACTH) from the anterior pituitary gland. ACTH stimulates the cortex of the adrenal gland to release cortisol. (Relationships between the neuroendocrine and immune systems are discussed on p. 308.)

Catecholamines

Epinephrine released from the adrenal medulla goes to the liver and skeletal muscle, but is then rapidly metabolized. Very little adrenal norepinephrine reaches distal tissue; thus, the effects caused by norepinephrine during the stress response are primarily from the sympathetic nervous system (Dimsdale & Zeigler, 1981; Herd, 1991). Catecholamines cannot cross the blood-brain barrier; hence, they are synthesized locally in the brain (Granner, 1988). Catecholamines circulate in plasma in a loose association with albumin (Granner, 1988).

The catecholamines act by stimulating two major classes of receptors: α-adrenergic receptors and β-adrenergic receptors. These two classes are divided further into two subclasses: (1) α_1 and α_2 and (2) β_1 and β_2. Table 9-1 summarizes the actions of the two

---

TABLE 9-1

Summary of the Physiologic Actions of the Alpha and Beta Receptors

Receptor	Physiologic actions
Alpha$_1$	Increased glycogenolysis; smooth muscle contraction (blood vessels, genitourinary tract)
Alpha$_2$	Smooth muscle relaxation (gastrointestinal tract); smooth muscle contraction (some vascular beds); inhibition of lipolysis, renin release, platelet aggregation, and insulin secretion
Beta$_1$	Stimulation of lipolysis; myocardial contraction (increased rate, increased force of contraction)
Beta$_2$	Increased hepatic gluconeogenesis; increased hepatic glycogenolysis; increased muscle glycogenolysis; increased release of insulin, glucagon, and renin; smooth muscle relaxation (bronchi, blood vessels, genitourinary tract, gastrointestinal tract)

From Granner, 1988.

subclasses of adrenergic receptors. (A thorough discussion of receptors can be found in Chapters 1, 17, and 26.) Epinephrine binds to and activates both α and β receptors. Norepinephrine at physiologic concentrations primarily binds to α receptors (Granner, 1988).

The circulating catecholamines have essentially the same effects as direct sympathetic stimulation. (Sympathetic function is described in Chapter 12.) Norepinephrine regulates blood pressure because it is the primary constrictor of smooth muscle in all blood vessels. During stress, norepinephrine raises blood pressure by constricting peripheral vessels. It also inhibits gastrointestinal activity and dilates the pupil of the eye (see Fig. 9-1).

Epinephrine causes some of the same effects as norepinephrine, yet it has greater influence on cardiac action and is the principal catecholamine involved in metabolic regulation. Epinephrine enhances myocardial contractility (inotropic effect), increases the heart rate (chronotropic effect), and increases venous return to the heart, all of which increase cardiac output and blood pressure. Epinephrine dilates blood vessels of skeletal muscle. Metabolically, epinephrine causes transient hyperglycemia (high blood sugar) by activating enzymes whose actions promote glucose formation (gluconeogenesis and glycogenolysis in the liver) while inhibiting glucose breakdown. Epinephrine decreases glucose uptake in the muscle and other organs and decreases insulin release from the pancreas. The decrease in insulin release prevents glucose from being taken up by peripheral tissue and thus preserves it for the central nervous system. Epinephrine also mobilizes free fatty acids and cholesterol by stimulating lipolysis, freeing triglycerides and fatty acids from fat stores, and inhibiting the degradation of circulating cholesterol to bile acids. The metabolic actions of epinephrine aid the metabolic actions of cortisol, which are similar. Table 9-2 summarizes other well-known effects of adrenal catecholamines. All of these effects prepare the body to take physical action: to "fight or flee." Stressors commonly associated with catecholamine release by the adrenal medulla include exercise, thermal changes, and acute emotional states.

Cortisol

The adrenal cortex is activated during stress by adrenal corticotropin hormone (see Fig. 9-1). Activation increases adrenal cortical secretion of glucocorticoid (steroid) hormones, primarily cortisol. (Cortisol is also known as hydrocortisone.) Cortisol circulates in the plasma, both protein bound and free. The main plasma-binding protein is called **transcortin** or **corticosteroid-binding globulin**. The unbound, or free, fraction is approximately 8% of the total plasma cortisol and is the most biologically active fraction of cortisol (Granner,

TABLE 9-2

Physiologic Effects of the Catecholamines*

Organ	Process or result
Brain	Increased blood flow Increased glucose metabolism
Cardiovascular system	Increased rate and force of contraction Peripheral vasoconstriction
Pulmonary system	Increased oxygen supply Bronchodilation Increased ventilation
Muscle	Increased glycogenolysis Increased contraction Increased dilation of skeletal muscle vasculature
Liver	Increased glucose production Increased gluconeogenesis Increased glycogenolysis Decreased glycogen synthesis
Adipose tissue	Increased lipolysis Increased fatty acids and glycerol
Skin	Decreased blood flow
Skeleton	Decreased glucose uptake and utilization (decreases insulin release)
Gastrointestinal and genitourinary tracts	Decreased protein synthesis
Lymphoid tissue	Increased protein breakdown (lymphoid tissue shrinks)

From Granner, 1988.
*Some of these responses require glucocorticoids (e.g., cortisol) for maximal activity (see text for explanation).

1988). Cortisol mobilizes substances needed for cellular metabolism. One of the primary effects of cortisol is the stimulation of gluconeogenesis, or the formation of glycogen from noncarbohydrate sources, such as amino or free fatty acids in the liver. In addition, cortisol enhances the elevation of blood glucose promoted by other hormones, such as epinephrine, glucagon, and somatotropic growth hormone. This action by cortisol is said to be **permissive** for the actions of other hormones. Cortisol also inhibits the uptake and oxidation of glucose by many body cells. The overall action of cortisol on carbohydrate metabolism results in an elevation of blood glucose.

Cortisol also affects protein metabolism. It has an anabolic effect, or increases the rate of synthesis, of proteins and RNA in liver, and catabolic effects in muscle, lymphoid tissue, adipose tissue, skin, and bone (Granner, 1988). The overall breakdown effect of proteins results in a negative nitrogen balance and an increase in circulating amino acids. There is some evidence that cortisol depresses transport of amino acids into muscle cells, while enhancing their uptake into the liver, where they are converted to glucose. Cortisol also can promote lipolysis in some areas of the body (the extremities) and lipogenesis in others (the face and trunk). The lipid effects of tissue are specific because not all areas show increased fat deposition or lipolysis (Granner, 1988).

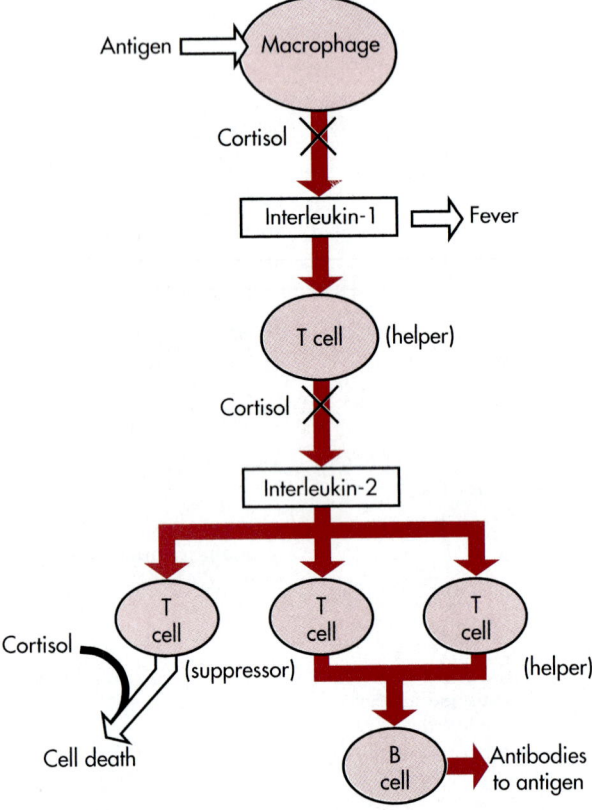

FIG. 9-2 Cortisol effects on cell-mediated immunity. Cortisol inhibits antigen-stimulated production of the peptide interleukin-1 macrophages, decreasing the initial recruitment of T lymphocytes. Cortisol also inhibits production of interleukin-2, reducing secondary proliferation of helper and suppressor T lymphocytes. Depending in part on the ratio of these two cell populations, production of antibody to the original antigen may be either facilitated or retarded. In some species, large doses of cortisol are also lymphocytotoxic, causing cell death. (Modified from Berne, R. M., & Levy, M. N. [Eds.]. [1988]. *Physiology* [2nd ed.]. St. Louis: Mosby–Year Book.)

Cortisol acts as an immunosuppressant by suppressing protein synthesis, including synthesis of immunoglobulin. Cortisol also reduces peripheral blood populations of eosinophils, lymphocytes, and macrophages (Fauci, 1975; Granner, 1988; Stein, 1985). Large doses of cortisol are known to promote atrophy of lymphoid tissue in the thymus, spleen, and lymph nodes (Granner, 1988). This action of cortisol could account for the lymphoid atrophy observed by Selye.

Cortisol directly influences immune responses to antibodies (Berne & Levy, 1990). The mechanisms of inhibition of the immune response are multifactorial (Fig. 9-2). When an antigen intrudes into the body, it is picked up by a macrophage. The macrophage presents the antigen to thymus-derived lymphocytes (T cells) and simultaneously produces and releases interleukin-1 (IL-1), a protein lymphokine that activates a subset of T cells with helper function. Likewise, T-helper cells secrete interleukin-2 (IL-2), a protein that stimulates the proliferation of still more T cells. These T cells can either activate or suppress bursa-derived lymphocytes (B cells). These B cells then produce antibodies directed against the original invading antigen. Cortisol inhibits the production of both IL-1 and macrophages and IL-2 by helper T cells, thus decreasing T cell responses, as well as the generation of fever. The diminished helper T cells cause a decrease in B-cells and antibody production (see Chapter 6). Once antibodies are present, neither their degradation nor their specific reaction with antigen molecules is affected by cortisol (Berne & Levy, 1990).

The ability of cortisol and other glucocorticoids to suppress the inflammatory response is well documented and provides the basis for the major therapeutic use of these steroids. Cortisol decreases the number of circulating lymphocytes, monocytes/macrophages, and eosinophils because these cells are shifted from the vascular compartment to other sites, including the bone marrow, lymphoid tissue, and spleen (Granner, 1988). Cortisol enhances the release of polymorphonuclear leukocytes from bone marrow, thus increasing their number in blood, although their effectiveness decreases. Glucocorticoids inhibit the accumulation of leukocytes at the site of inflammation and inhibit the release of substances involved in the inflammatory response (e.g., kinins, plasminogen-activating factor, prostaglandins, and histamine) from the leukocytes (Granner, 1988). Cortisol inhibits fibroblast proliferation and function at the site of an inflammatory response. This inhibition accounts for the poor wound healing, increased susceptibility to infection, and decreased inflammatory response that are often seen in individuals with chronic glucocorticoid excess. Glucocorticoids are necessary for the maintenance of normal blood pressure and cardiac output. This is another example of how cortisol maximizes the action of the catecholamines (the "permissive effect").

In the gastrointestinal tract, cortisol promotes gastric secretion. This is opposite to the effect of norepinephrine, which reduces gastric secretion. Excessive cortisol may stimulate gastric secretion enough to cause ulceration of the gastric mucosa. This could account for the gastrointestinal ulceration observed by Selye.

Cortisol exerts inhibiting effects by suppressing levels of release of luteinizing hormone, estradiol, and possibly testosterone (Chrousos & Gold, 1992). The inhibitory effects also render target tissues of sex steroids resistant to these hormones, resulting in hypogonadism.

It is not entirely clear why cortisol secretion during stress is beneficial. It has been suggested that gluconeogenesis promoted by cortisol ensures an adequate source of glucose (energy) for body tissues, and nerve cells in particular. The pooling of amino acids from catabolized proteins may ensure amino acid availability for protein synthesis in certain cells. The redistribution of protein to sites where replacement is critical, such as muscle or cells of damaged tissue, would be beneficial. Short-term, cortisol-induced alterations in immune cell distribution (e.g., traffic) patterns may be adaptive, with a decrease in peripheral blood cell numbers as effector cells locate to sites of injury or inflammation. In addition, decrease of immune cell activity by cortisol may be beneficial in some situations because it prevents immune-mediated tissue damage by prolonged cell exposure to high levels of certain cytokines. Whether cortisol-induced effects are adaptive or destructive may depend on the intensity, type, and duration of the stressor, and the subsequent concentration and length of cortisol exposure that target cells of the individual experience. The biologic effects of cortisol are summarized in Table 9-3.

TABLE 9-3

Physiologic Effects of Cortisol

Functions affected	Physiologic effects
Carbohydrate and lipid metabolism	Diminishes peripheral uptake and utilization of glucose; promotes gluconeogenesis in liver cells; enhances the gluconeogenic response to other hormones; promotes lipolysis in adipose tissue
Protein metabolism	Increases protein synthesis in the liver and depresses protein synthesis (including immunoglobulin synthesis) in muscle, lymphoid tissue, adipose tissue, skin, and bone; increases plasma level of amino acids; stimulates deamination in the liver
Inflammatory effects	Decreases circulating eosinophils, lymphocytes, and monocytes; increases release of polymorphonuclear leukocytes from the bone marrow; decreases accumulation of leukocytes at the site of inflammation; delays healing; permissive for vasoconstrictive action of norepinephrine
Lipid metabolism	Lipolysis in the extremities and lipogenesis in the face and trunk
Immune reserve	Decreases the tissue mass of all lymphoid tissues (e.g., decreases protein synthesis); promotes rapid decrease in circulating lymphocytes, eosinophils, basophils, and macrophages; inhibits the production of interleukin-1 and interleukin-2; consequently, also blocks cell-mediated immunity and the generation of fever
Digestive function	Promotes gastric secretion
Urinary function	Enhances urinary excretion
Connective tissue function	Decreases proliferation of fibroblasts in connective tissue (thus delaying healing)
Muscle function	Maintains normal contractility and maximal work output for skeletal and cardiac muscle
Bone function	Decreases bone formation
Vascular system and myocardial function	Maintains normal blood pressure; permits increased responsiveness of arterioles to the constrictive action of adrenergic stimulation; optimizes myocardial performance
Central nervous system function	Somehow modulates perceptual and emotional functioning, essential for normal arousal and initiation of daytime activity

Other Hormones
Endorphins

β-Endorphins (endogenous opiates) are released into the blood as part of the response to stressful stimuli (Guillemin et al., 1977). The secretion of ACTH and β-endorphin is stimulated by corticotropin-releasing factor; it is unclear if β-endorphins come from the pituitary gland or the central nervous system. Evidence is accumulating that β-endorphins can regulate ACTH secretion and, with ACTH, inhibit hypothalamic CRF secretion, a possible down-regulation pathway of the stress response (Calogero, Gallucci, Gold, & Chrousos, 1988).

Increased β-endorphin levels are associated with a parallel increase in pain threshold, i.e., stress-induced analgesia (Cohen, Pickar, Dubois, & Bunney, 1982; JungKunz, Engel, King, & Kuss, 1983). In a number of conditions or activities in which there is increased endogenous opiate activity, subjects not only experience insensitivity to pain but also report increased feelings of excitement, positive well-being, or euphoria (Rose, 1985). For example, vigorous running increases β-endorphin levels (Colt, Wardlaw, & Franz, 1981). Endorphins may play a role in the excitement and exhilaration produced by dancing, contact sports, and combat. There is little direct evidence, however, documenting the endorphin system in most of these activities.

Growth hormone

Somatotropin. Growth hormone is released from the anterior pituitary gland and affects protein, lipid, and carbohydrate metabolism. Growth hormone levels increase in the blood after a variety of stressful stimuli, such as cardiac catheterization, electroshock therapy, gastroscopy, surgery, fever, and physical exercise (Berne & Levy, 1990; Schalach, 1967). Psychologic stimuli associated with increased levels of growth hormone include examinations, viewing of violent or sexually arousing films, anticipation of exhausting exercise, and certain psychologic performance tests. In most circumstances, the increase in growth hormone occurs only with a parallel rise in cortisol secretion. Prolonged activation of the stress response (chronic stress) leads to suppression of growth hormone and other growth factor effects on target tissues (Burguera, Muruais, Penalva, Dieguez, & Casaneuva, 1990).

Prolactin

Prolactin is released from the anterior pituitary gland and is necessary for lactation and breast development (Shiu & Friesen, 1980). Prolactin levels in plasma increase from a variety of stressful stimuli, including such procedures as gastroscopy, proctoscopy, pelvic examination, and during surgery (Noel, Suh, Stone, & Frantz,

1972). Prolactin also rises during parachute jumping, during motion sickness, and after examinations (Rose, 1985). Unlike growth hormone, prolactin levels show little change after exercise. Like growth hormone, however, prolactin appears to require more intense stimuli than those leading to increases in catecholamine or cortisol levels. Prolactin levels also increase in the plasma after a variety of sexual stimuli, for example, stimulation of the nipple or areola in women.

Testosterone

Testosterone, a hormone secreted by Leydig cells, regulates male secondary sex characteristics and libido. Testosterone levels decrease after stressful stimuli. The decrease in testosterone occurs after such stimuli as ether or anesthesia, surgery, marathon running, and mountain climbing (Matsumoto, Takeyasu, Mizutani, Hamanaka, & Uozumi, 1970). The mechanism causing decreased levels of testosterone is thought to be exerted by cortisol.

Psychologic stimuli also lead to a decrease in testosterone levels. Men engaged in rigorous combat training and those engaged in the first several weeks of Officer Candidate School experience significant drops in testosterone levels (Aakvaag et al., 1978; Kreuz, Rose, & Jennings, 1972). Individuals with acute illness, such as respiratory failure, burns, and congestive heart failure, show a marked reduction in plasma testosterone (Rose, 1985).

Role of the Immune System

Many immune-related conditions and diseases are associated with stress. The specific stress-induced mechanisms causing these illnesses are not clearly defined. Recent research is focused on the regulatory interactions between the immune system and the nervous and endocrine systems, which may represent mechanistic pathways for stress-associated immune-mediated diseases, including infection, some forms of cancer, allergy, and autoimmunity (Greer & Brady, 1988) (Table 9-4).

Evidence thus far suggests that the immune, nervous, and endocrine systems "communicate" through pathways involving hormones, neurotransmitters, neuropeptides, and immune cell products. Various components of immune system responses are potentially affected by all of the known neuroendocrine-produced factors involved in the stress reaction. Conversely, immune-cell–derived cytokines and other products have effects on neurocrine and endocrine cells (Aoki, Ohno, & Imamura, 1990; Khansari, Murgo, & Faith, 1990; Rabin, Cohen, Ganguli, Lysle, & Cunnick, 1989). Several pathways appear to regulate communication between these systems with both direct and indirect patterned effects (Fig. 9-3).

Direct influence of the stress response on immune system functioning may occur through hypothalamic and pituitary peptides, and by products of the sympathetic branch of the autonomic nervous system. These factors include corticotropin-releasing factor (CRF), ACTH, endorphins, substance P, epinephrine, norepinephrine, dopamine, serotonin, histamine, growth hormone (GH), vasoactive intestinal polypeptide (VIP), β-endorphin, methionine-enkephalin, leucine-enkephalin, and somatostatin (Dunn, 1989; Jankovic, 1989; Rabin et al., 1989). Evidence has accumulated that suggests that CRF may be a primary mediator of many stress-induced alterations in immune functions, in part because of its role as an initiator of biologic responses within the brain in response to stress, which result in activation of the hypothalamic-pituitary-adrenal (HPA) axis and autonomic nervous system (ANS). Direct suppressive effects of CRF, however, have been reported also on two immune cell types processing CRF receptors, the monocyte-macrophage and CD4 (T-helper) lymphocyte (Jain et al., 1991). Release of endogenous opiates occurs during stress, and these peptides have been shown to have concentration-dependent, enhancing, and suppressive effects on various immune cells (Dunn, 1989). Immune cells have been shown to have surface β-adrenergic and serotoninergic receptors, as well as receptors for ACTH, CRF, endorphins, GH, and steroids (Boranic et al., 1990; Borboni et al., 1989; De Souza, Webster, Grigoriadis, & Tracey, 1989; Weigent, Carr, & Blalock, 1989).

Products of the sympathetic branch of the ANS also influence immune cell behavior. It has been known for some time that there is direct innervation of the thymus, spleen, lymph nodes, and bone marrow (Rabin et al., 1989). Histochemical studies have verified the presence of cholinergic, adrenergic, and peptinergic nerve terminals in the lymphoid organs and tissues. There is evidence for interaction of norepinephrine released from nerve endings with lymphocytes and macrophages in the spleen, implicating the presence of a route of communication between the ANS and immune system through direct delivery of chemical mediators that alter immune cell behavior in a paracrine (cell-to-adjacent-cell) fashion in the microenvironment of the lymphoid organ.

The pineal gland has a role in regulation of immune response and mediates the apparent effects of circadian rhythm on immunity. Blockage of production of melatonin (by continuous light or by pharmacologic means) results in suppression of immune response, while administration of melatonin reverses these effects (Maestroni & Conti, 1991). This pathway of immunomodulation may be operative in immune changes observed in sleep disturbance and in other settings where the circadian rhythm is dysregulated.

Indirect effects of the central nervous system (CNS) on immune function involve the HPA axis. This is the

TABLE 9-4

Examples of Stress-Related Diseases and Conditions

Target organ or system	Disease or condition
Cardiovascular system	Coronary artery disease Hypertension Stroke Disturbances of heart rhythm
Muscles	Tension headaches Muscle contraction backache
Connective tissues	Rheumatoid arthritis (autoimmune disease) Related inflammatory diseases of connective tissue
Pulmonary system	Asthma (hypersensitivity reaction) Hay fever (hypersensitivity reaction)
Immune system	Immunosuppression or deficiency Autoimmune diseases
Gastrointestinal system	Ulcer Irritable bowel syndrome Diarrhea Nausea and vomiting Ulcerative colitis
Genitourinary system	Diuresis Impotence Frigidity
Skin	Eczema Neurodermatitis Acne
Endocrine system	Diabetes mellitus Amenorrhea
Central nervous system	Fatigue and lethargy Type A behavior Overeating Depression Insomnia

most extensively studied pathway, with original interest stemming from early studies showing profound effects of prolonged severe stress on immunologic structures (Ader, Felten, & Cohen, 1990). It was noted that the adrenal gland enlarged with simultaneous involution of the thymus and lymph nodes. Increased levels of circulating glucocorticoids (GCS) are thought to be an important mechanism, both in the stress-related alterations

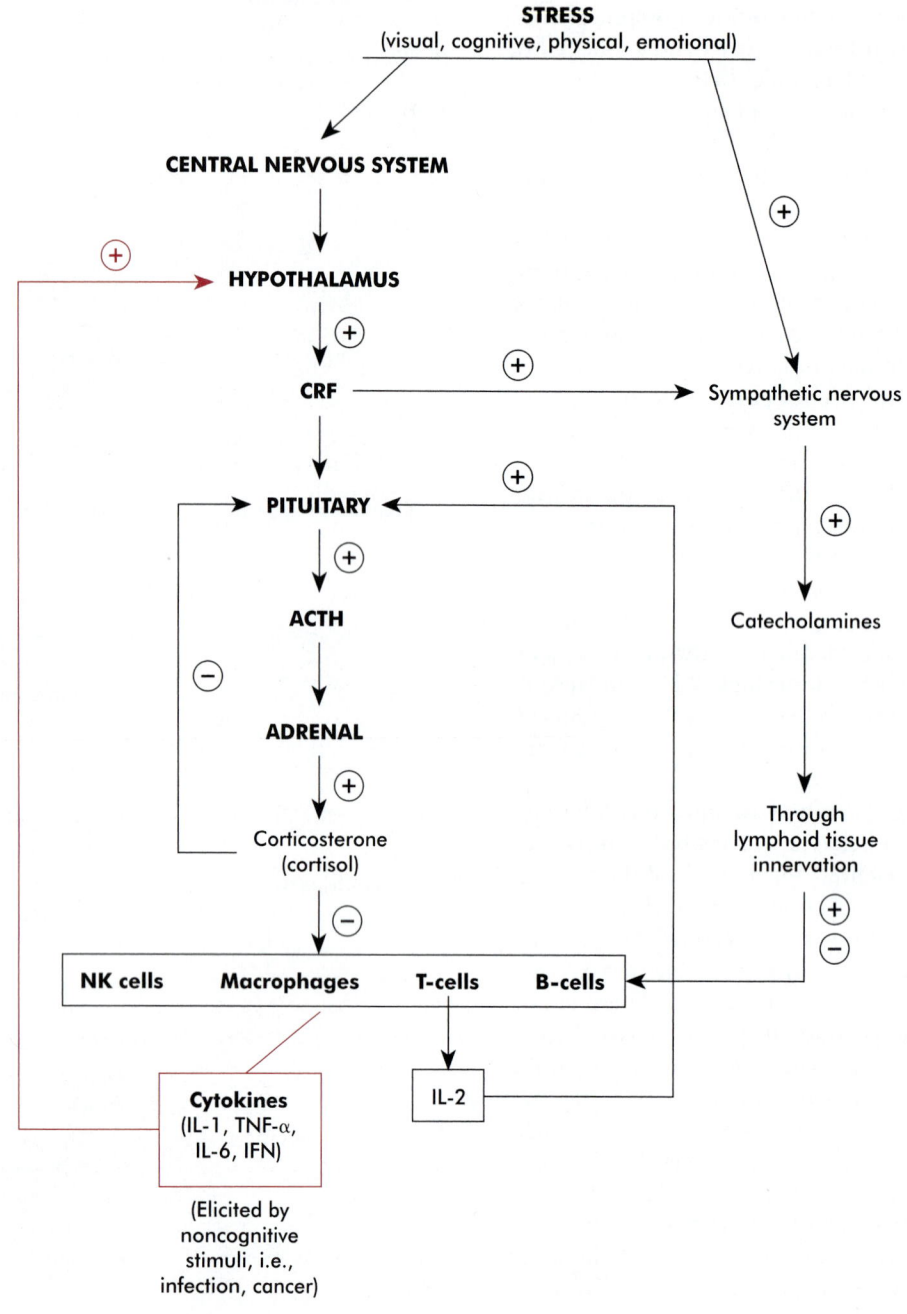

FIG. 9-3 Nervous system/endocrine system/immune system interactions.

in immune structures and in suppression of immune response (Ader et al., 1990). The increase in GCS level is attributable to signaling by pituitary ACTH production. Enhanced production of ACTH by the pituitary is a result of increased hypothalamic CRF. The production of CRF is initiated by a number of stress factors, including high levels of IL-1. Production of IL-1 by activated macrophages and monocytes is inhibited by GCS, suggesting a feedback loop with IL-1, CRF, ACTH, and GCS secretion (Su, London, & Jaffe, 1988; Sundar, Cierpial, Kilts, Ritchie, & Weiss, 1990).

The observation that IL-1 can elicit changes in the nervous and endocrine systems by stimulating CRF production in the hypothalamus is a part of a growing body of evidence demonstrating immune-induced regulation of the CNS. The release of immune inflammatory mediators IL-6, tumor necrosis factor β (TNF-β), and interferon is triggered by bacterial or viral infections, cancer, and tissue injury that, in turn, initiate a stress response through the HPA pathway as described previously. Enhanced systemic production of these cytokines also induces other CNS and behavior changes seen frequently during the acute phase of an infectious episode, acting either directly in a distant systemic "endocrine" fashion or through the mediation of neuropeptides (Aoki et al., 1990; Busbridge & Grossman, 1991; Hori et al., 1991; Navarra et al., 1991). These effects include pyrogenesis (fever), induction of slow wave sleep, and anorexia. These are adaptive responses to infection and possibly cancer, hyperthermia resulting in an inhospitable environment for many microorganisms and tumor cells (by slowing bacterial and tumor growth, and viral replication). Slow wave sleep is associated with enhanced release of GH, which is beneficial for tissue repair and enhances antibody production by B cells (Hall & O'Grady, 1989). There is some animal evidence that anorexia is beneficial in the early phase of infection because of the reduction in the availability of nutrients essential for the growth of the microorganisms (Hori et al., 1991).

Lymphocytes also are known to produce ACTH and endorphins in small amounts, which probably influence immune response in an autocrine (same cell stimulation) or paracrine (cell to cell) manner in the local microenvironment of an ongoing immune response (Weingent, Carr, & Blalock, 1990). There is also new evidence that the T cell growth factor, IL-2, can upregulate pituitary ACTH. It appears that the cytokines mentioned above, produced in response to infectious challenge and acting in a distant systemic fashion, have the greatest influence on neuroendocrine function, with evidence for direct and indirect cytokine effects on nervous and adrenal cell functions. These effects on neuroendocrine function by immune cells indicate an adaptive role for the immune system as a "signal" organ to alert other systems of inner threatening stimuli (i.e., infection, tissue damage, tumor cells) that may upset the dynamic steady state.

The stress-induced alterations in the equilibrium of various neuropeptides and hormones have a significant effect on the immune response. Whether this impact on immune function is suppressive or potentiating depends on the type of immunomodulating factor that is secreted, with some factors known to have enhancing or suppressing activities, or both, depending on the concentration and length of exposure, the target cell, and the specific immune function studies (Aoki et al., 1990). The immunomodulatory activity of neuropeptides and neuroendocrine hormones may involve the direct control of biochemical events affecting cell proliferation, differentiation, and function. These factors also may indirectly control immune cell behavior by affecting the production or activity of cytokines (Khansari et al., 1990).

In summary, there is a significant body of evidence that now supports a linkage between the nervous, endocrine, and immune systems. The bidirectional communication between these systems involves common usage of signal molecules and their receptors that, in turn, regulates the behavior of cells in each system. Thus, the most recent findings are that (1) there are direct effects of CNS and ANS neuropeptides on immune cells; (2) neuro-induced endocrine products influence immune cell and neuro-cell function; and (3) immune cell products (cytokines) affect nervous and endocrine cell function through both direct and indirect pathways.

STRESS, COPING, AND ILLNESS

Extreme physiologic stressors, such as severe burn injury, represent a predictable stimulus for the stress responses described previously. A less severe and defined event or situation, however, can be a stressor for one person and not for another. The studies already described have demonstrated that many stressors, such as fasting or temperature changes, do not necessarily cause a physiologic stress response if psychologic factors are minimized. It has become apparent that stress itself is not an independent entity but a system of interdependent processes that are moderated by the nature, intensity, and duration of the stressor and the perception, appraisal, and coping efficacy of the affected individual, all of which in turn mediate the psychologic and physiologic response to stress.

In the past two decades, many investigators have reported that psychosocial distress may be predictive of psychologic and physical health outcomes. **Psychologic distress** has been defined as a general state of unpleasant arousal after life events with the subsequent responses to these events in the distressed individual manifest as physiologic, emotional, cognitive, and behavior changes (Thoits, 1983). Numerous studies have shown that periods of depression and emotional upheaval many times are associated with adverse life events and place the affected individual at risk for immunologic deficits and, subsequently, increase the risk of ill health (Baker, 1987). Adverse life events resulting in depression and emotional upheaval have been associated with transient immune deficiency. Psychosocial variables studied have included bereavement, academic pressures (including examinations), and life events (positive and negative changes) (Baker, 1987). Adverse life events that have been shown to have the most negative effect on immunity have been characterized as uncontrollable, undesirable, and overtaxing the individual's ability to cope (Irwin, Daniels, Smith, Bloom, & Weiner, 1988; Kiecolt-Glaser, Glaser, Strain et al., 1986; Laudenslager, Ryan, Drugan, Hyson, & Maier, 1984; Perez & Ferrant, 1988; Workman & La Via, 1987a, 1987b).

The clinical significance of studies linking distress with transient immune dysfunction is not clear. Recent studies, however, have strengthened the association of stress with potential for illness in humans. One study examined medical students who were immunized with hepatitis B vaccine on the third day of a stressful examination period, and the time to seroconversion and level of antibody titer to the vaccine were measured later. The students with the most rapid seroconversion and the highest titers also reported being less stressed and had a good social support system (which may reduce stress) (Glaser et al., 1992). These results suggest that stress does modulate immune response in humans and may potentiate the risk for disease. Even more convincing is a study in which the psychologic stress status was determined in healthy individuals after experimentally controlled exposure to respiratory virus by nasal inoculation. Individuals reporting more stress had an increased incidence of clinical cold and respiratory symptoms compared with subjects reporting less stress (Cohen, Tyrrell, & Smith, 1991).

Stressful life events and mood also have been reported to be possibly important factors preceding onset or exacerbation of symptoms in AIDS infection, diabetes, and multiple sclerosis (Solomon, Kemeny, & Temoshok, 1991; Warren, Greenhill, & Warren, 1982). In addition, the interaction with health care providers in a clinical setting, the diagnosis of a major illness, and various medical procedures (blood draws, injections, examinations, surgical procedures, etc.) may represent a significant negative life event to many individuals (Fig. 9-4). These additional stresses may affect the course of illness in these individuals, possibly interfering with the efficacy of the medical intervention. The identification and reduction of stress in the clinical setting, therefore,

are an important area of concern and have particular applicability to clinicians, in both prevention and illness management.

One factor proposed to have a beneficial influence during stressful experiences is the use of adaptive coping strategies, especially those that are problem-focused and those that encourage seeking social support (Folkman & Lazarus, 1988a; Lazarus & Folkman, 1987; Vitaliano, Katon et al., 1987; Vitaliano, Maiuro, Russo, & Becker, 1987). Coping is defined as the process of managing stressful demands and challenges that are appraised as taxing or exceeding the resources of the person (Folkman & Lazarus, 1988b). The extent to which an individual responds to distress, using effective positive coping strategies, determines the degree of successful moderation of the stress challenge. Conversely, ineffective negative coping attempts may exacerbate the effects of distress on health, thus augmenting the potential for illness (Folkman & Lazarus, 1988b). An individual experiencing distress may draw on internal, as well as external, resources to meet the demands. Mediating factors that may influence stress susceptibility or resilience include age, social economic status, gender, social support status, personality, self-esteem, genetics, life events, past experiences, and current health status. Although an individual may not be able to avoid stressors and cannot change many of these factors, there is evidence for effective intervention resulting in greater stress resilience and improved psychologic and physiologic outcomes. In a study of nursing home residents, randomly assigned to control or social support intervention groups, improved psychologic measures and immune function (natural killer cell activity) was observed in the experimental group at 6 weeks (Kiecolt-Glaser, Glaser, Williger et al., 1985). In another study, women with recurrent metastatic breast cancer were given routine follow-up or routine care and weekly support group sessions (extended treatment) to explore their concerns. Survival in the extended treatment group was an average of 19 months longer than in the routine care group, suggesting a mediating influence of additional support for these women (Spiegel, Bloom, Kraemer, & Gottheil, 1989).

The importance of social support for seriously ill individuals has focused attention on the health and well-being of family members who function as caregivers. Significant stress manifested as depression, anxiety, and fatigue has been noted in family caregivers of those with cancer, Alzheimer disease, and burn trauma. These studies demonstrated significant suppression of various measures of immune function with improved function being associated with better perceived social support (Baron, Cutrona, Hicklin, Russell, & Lubaroff, 1990; Kiecolt-Glaser, Glaser, Dyer et al., 1987; Shelby, Sullivan, Groussman, Gray, & Saffle, 1992).

Potential interventions for prevention or management of stress-related psychologic or physical problems include both short- and long-term coping strategies. Stress management consists of educational components specific to the individual's problems and relaxation techniques, which may include meditation, imagery, and biofeedback. These approaches may be used on an individual or support group basis. Incorporation of these approaches into clinical training facilitates the use of stress-reducing methodology in the clinical arena. There is a need for future research to focus on efficacy of such approaches with various populations.

A POTENTIAL EFFECTS IN HEALTHY INDIVIDUALS

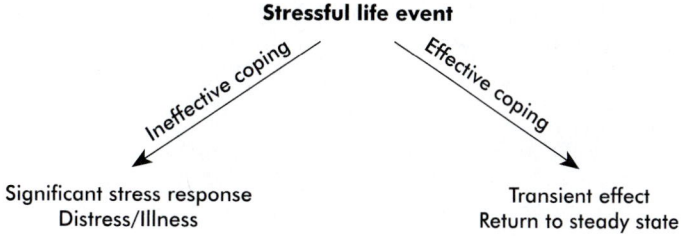

B POTENTIAL EFFECTS IN SYMPTOMATIC INDIVIDUALS

FIG. 9-4 Health outcome determination in stressful life situations is moderated by numerous factors. Whether a life-challenged individual experiences distress or illness depends on the subject's appraisal of the event and the coping strategies used during the stressful period. Models **A** and **B** reflect possible outcomes in stressed healthy and symptomatic individuals. Model **C** illustrates the dynamic clinical setting in which the diagnosis of a serious illness and subsequent medical interventions may be perceived as stressful challenges and have potentially detrimental influences on physical outcome.

C POTENTIAL EFFECTS DURING MEDICAL INTERVENTION

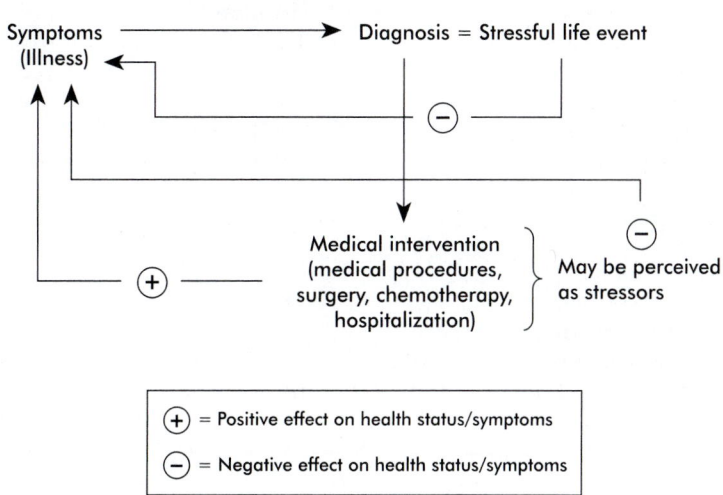

SUMMARY REVIEW

Concepts of Stress

1 Stress has recently been defined as the state of affairs arising when a person relates to (i.e., interacts or transacts with) situations in a certain way. Important is how they "appraise" and "react" to situations.

2 Hans Selye identified three structural changes in rats subjected repeatedly to noxious stimuli (stressors): enlargement of the cortex of the adrenal gland, atrophy of the thymus gland and other lymphoid tissues, and gastrointestinal ulceration.

3 Selye believed that the three changes were caused by nonspecific physiologic response to any long-term stressor. He called this response the general adaptation syndrome (GAS).

4 The GAS occurs in three stages: the alarm stage, the stage of resistance or adaptation, and the stage of exhaustion. Diseases of adaptation develop if the stage of resistance or adaptation does not restore homeostasis.

5 Selye identified three components of physiologic stress: the stressor, the physiologic or chemical disturbance produced by the stressor, and the body's adaptational response to the stressor.

6 Other investigators have shown that the physiologic stress response also occurs in response to psychologic or emotional stress.

7 There is disagreement on the nonspecific nature of the stress response because different processes occur in response to specific stimuli, such as exposure to cold or heat.

8 W. B. Cannon defined homeostasis as the sum of the processes by which the body maintains itself at a relatively constant composition. This definition has since been modified. Homeostasis is now considered to mean the sum of the processes by which the body maintains itself in a dynamic steady state.

9 The function of the physiologic stress response is to maintain the body's dynamic steady state.

The Stress Response

1 The stress response involves the nervous system (sympathetic branch of the autonomic nervous system), the endocrine system (pituitary and adrenal glands), and the immune system.

2 The stress response is initiated when a stressor is present in the body or perceived by the mind.

3 The neuroendocrine response to stress consists of sympathetic stimulation of the adrenal medulla to secrete catecholamines (norepinephrine and epinephrine) and stressor-induced stimulation of the pituitary to secrete ACTH, which, in turn, stimulates the adrenal cortex to secrete steroid hormones, particularly cortisol.

4 In general, the catecholamines prepare the body to act, and cortisol mobilizes energy (glucose) and other substances needed to fuel the action.

5 Epinephrine exerts its chief effects on the cardiovascular system. Epinephrine increases cardiac output and increases blood flow to the heart, brain, and skeletal muscles by dilating vessels that supply these organs. It also dilates the airways, thereby increasing delivery of oxygen to the bloodstream.

6 Norepinephrine's chief effects complement those of epinephrine. Norepinephrine constricts blood vessels of the viscera and skin; this has the effect of shifting blood flow to the vessels dilated by epinephrine. Norepinephrine also increases mental alertness.

7 Cortisol's chief effects involve metabolic processes. By inhibiting the use of metabolic substances while promoting their formation, cortisol mobilizes glucose, amino acids, lipids, and fatty acids, and delivers them to the bloodstream. Cortisol also suppresses immune and inflammatory function.

8 The nervous, endocrine, and immune systems communicate through the common use of signal molecules and their receptors, which in turn regulate the behavior of cells in each system during stress challenge.

9 There are direct and indirect pathways of influence between the nervous, endocrine, and immune systems. Neuropeptides have direct effects on immune cells, as well as indirect influences through neuro-mediated endocrine modulation of immune function. Endocrine products (cortisol) also influence neuro-cell behavior. Immune cell products affect both nervous and endocrine cell function, reflecting an adaptive role for the immune system as a "signal" organ to alert other systems of threatening stimuli.

10 Other hormones are affected by the stress response and include increased circulating levels of β-endorphins, growth hormone, prolactin, and antidiuretic hormone. Testosterone decreases during the stress response.

Stress, Coping, and Illness

1 Stress is a system of interdependent processes that are moderated by the nature, intensity, and duration of the stressor, and coping efficacy of the affected individual, all of which, in turn, mediate the psychologic and physiologic response to stress.

2 Many studies have linked psychologic distress with altered immune function, and there is now evidence that strengthens the association of stress with potential for illness in humans.

KEY TERMS

REFERENCES

Aakvaag, A., Bentdal, O., Quigstad, K., Walstad, P., Rohnningen, H., & Fonnum, F. (1978). Testosterone and testosterone-binding globulin (TeBG) in young men during prolonged stress. *International Journal of Andrology, 1,* 22-31.

Ader, R., & Cohen, N. (1975). Behaviorally conditioned immunosuppression. *Psychosomatic Medicine, 37,* 333-340.

Ader, R., Felten, D., & Cohen, N. (1990). Interactions between the brain and the immune system. *Annual Review of Pharmacology and Toxicology, 30,* 561-602.

Aoki, N., Ohno, Y., & Imamura, M. (1990). Physiological interactions between the immune and endocrine systems: Are cytokines hormones? *Medical Science Research, 18,* 195-201.

Baker, G. H. B. (1987). Invited review: Psychological factors and immunity. *Journal of Psychosomatic Research, 31,* 1-10.

Baron, R. S., Cutrona, C. E., Hicklin, D., Russell, D. W., & Lubaroff, D. M. (1990). Social support and immune function among spouses of cancer patients. *Journal of Personality and Social Psychology, 59,* 344-352.

Berne, R. M., & Levy, M. N. (Eds.). (1990). *Principles of physiology.* St. Louis: Mosby–Year Book.

Bieliauskas, L. A. (1982). *Stress and its relationship to health and illness.* Boulder, CO: Westview Press.

Boranic, M., Pericic, D., Blazi, M. P., Manev, H., Svenko, V., Gabrilovac, J., Radacic, M., Pivac, N., & Miljenovic, G. (1990). Immune response of stressed rats treated with drugs affecting serotoninergic and adrenergic transmission. *Biomedicine and Pharmacotherapy, 44,* 381-387.

Borboni, P., Di Cola, G., Sesti, G., Marini, M. A., Del Porto, P., Saveria, M., Montani, G., Lauro, R., & De Pirro, R. (1989). β-endorphin receptors on cultured and freshly isolated lymphocytes from normal subjects. *Biochemical and Biophysical Research Communications, 163*(1), 642-648.

Burguera, B., Muruais, C., Penalva, A., Dieguez, C., & Casanueva, F. (1990). Dual and selective actions of glucocorticoid upon basal and stimulated growth hormone release in man. *Neuroendocrinology, 51,* 51-58.

Busbridge, N. J., & Grossman, A. B. (1991). Stress and the single cytokine: Interleukin modulation of the pituitary-adrenal axis. *Molecular and Cellular Endocrinology, 82,* C209-C214.

Calogero, A., Gallucci, W. T., Gold, P. W., & Chrousos, G. P. (1988). Multiple regulatory feedback loops in hypothalamic corticotropin-releasing hormone secretion. *Journal of Clinical Investigation, 82,* 767-774.

Cannon, W. B., Bringer, C. A. L., & Fritz, R. (1914). Experimental hyperthyroidism. *American Journal of Physiology, 36,* 363.

Cannon, W. B. (1935). Stresses and strains of homeostasis. *American Journal of Medical Science, 189,* 1-14.

Cannon, W. B. (1963). *The wisdom of the body.* New York: W. W. Norton & Co.

Chrousos, G. P., & Gold, P. S. (1992). The concepts of stress and stress system disorders: Overview of physical and behavioral homeostasis. *Journal of the American Medical Association, 267*(9), 1244-1252.

Cohen, M. R., Pickar, D., Dubois, M., & Bunney, W. E., Jr. (1982). Stress-induced plasma beta-endorphin immunoreactivity may predict post-operative morphine usage. *Psychiatry Research, 6,* 7-12.

Cohen, S., Tyrrell, D. A., & Smith, A. D. (1991). Biological stress in humans and susceptibility to the common cold. *New England Journal of Medicine, 325,* 606-612.

Colt, E. W. D., Wardlaw, S. L., & Franz, A. G. (1981). The effect of running on plasma β-endorphin. *Life Science, 28,* 1637-1640.

De Souza, E. B., Webster, E. L., Grigoriadis, D. E., & Tracey, D. E. (1989). Corticotropin-releasing factor (CRF) and interleukin-1 (IL-1) receptors in the brain-pituitary-immune axis. *Psychopharmacology Bulletin, 25*(3), 299-305.

Dickman, S. R. (1988). *Pathways to wellness.* Champaign, IL: Life Enhancement Publishers.

Dimsdale, J. E., & Ziegler, M. H. (1991). What do plasma and urinary measures of catecholamines tell us about human response to stressors? *Circulation, 83*(Supp. II), 36-42.

Dubos, R. (1965). *Man adapting.* New Haven, CT: Yale University Press.

Dunn, A. J. (1989). Psychoneuroimmunology for the psychoneuroendocrinologist: A review of animal studies of nervous system-immune system interactions. *Psychoneuroendocrinology, 14,* 251-274.

Fauci, A. S. (1975). Corticosteroids and circulating lymphocytes. *Transplant Proceedings, 7,* 37-48.

Folkman, S., & Lazarus, R. S. (1988a). *Manual for the ways of coping questionnaire.* Palo Alto, CA: Consulting Psychologists Press.

Folkman, S., & Lazarus, R. S. (1988b). The relationship between coping and emotion: Implications for theory and research. *Social Sciences Medicine, 26,* 309-317.

Glaser, R., Kiecolt-Glaser, J. K., Bonneau, R. H., Malarkey, W., Kennedy, S., & Hughes, J. (1992). Stress induced modulation of the immune response to recombinant hepatitis B vaccine. *Psychosomatic Medicine, 54,* 22-29.

Granner, D. K. (1988). Hormones of the adrenal medulla. In R. K. Murray et al. (Eds.), *Harper's biochemistry* (21st ed.). New York: Lange Medical Books.

Greer, S., & Brady, M. (1988). Natural killer cells: One possible link between cancer and the mind. *Stress Medicine, 4,* 105-111.

Guillemin, R., Vargo, T., Rosier, J., Minick, S., Ling, N., Rivier, C., Valle, W., & Bloom, F. (1977). Beta-endorphin and adrenocorticotropin are secreted concomitantly by the pituitary gland. *Science, 197,* 1367-1369.

Hall, N. R. S., & O'Grady, M. P. (1989). Regulation of pituitary peptides by the immune system. *BioEssays, 11*(5), 141-144.

Handlon, J. H., Wadeson, R. W., Fishman, J. R., Sachar, E. J., Hamburg, D. A., & Mason, J. W. (1962). Psychological factors in 17-hydroxycorticosteroid concentration. *Psychosomatic Medicine, 24,* 535-542.

Herd, J. A. (1991). Cardiovascular response to stress. *Physiological Reviews, 71*(1), 305-330.

Hetzel, B. S., Schottstaedt, W. W., Grace, W. J., & Wolff, H. G. (1955). Changes in urinary 17-hydroxycorticosteroid excretion during stressful life situations in man. *Journal of Clinical Endocrinology, 15,* 1057-1068.

Hill, S. R., Goetz, F. C., Fox, H. M., Murawski, B. J., Krakauer, L. J., Reifenstein, R. W., Gray, S. J., Reddy, W. J., Hedberg, S. E., St. Marc, J. R., & Thorn, G. W. (1956). Studies on adrenocortical and psychological responses to stress in man. *Archives of Internal Medicine, 97,* 269-298.

Hori, T., Nakashima, T., Take, S., Kaizuka, Y., Mori, T., & Katafuchi, T. (1991). Immune cytokines and regulation of body temperature, food intake, and cellular immunity. *Brain Research Bulletin, 27,* 309-313.

Houldin, A. D., Lev, E., Prystowsky, M. B., Redei, E., & Lowery, B. J. (1991). Psychoneuroimmunology: A review of literature. *Holistic Nursing Practice, 5*(4), 10-21.

Irwin, M., Daniels, M., Smith, T., Bloom, E., & Weiner, H. (1988). Impaired natural killer activity during bereavement. *Brain, Behavior, and Immunity, 1,* 98-104.

Jacobs, M. A., Spilken, A., & Norman, M. M. (1969). Relationship of life change, maladaptive aggression, and upper respiratory infection in male college students. *Psychomatic Medicine, 33,* 33-42.

Jacobs, M. A., Spilken, A., Norman, M. M., & Andersson, L. S. (1970). Life stress and respiratory illness, *Psychosomatic Medicine, 32,* 233-242.

Jain, R., Zwickler, D., Hollander, C. S., Brand, H., Saperstein, A., Hutchinson, B., Brown, C., & Audhya, T. (1991). Corticotropin-releasing factor modulating the immune response to stress in the rat. *Endocrinology, 128,* 1329-1336.

Jankovic, B. D. (1989). Neuroimmunomodulation: Facts and dilemmas. *Immunology Letters, 21,* 101-118.

JungKunz, G., Engel, R. R., King, U. G., & Kuss, H. J. (1983). Endogenous opiates increase pain tolerance after stress in humans. *Psychiatry Research, 8,* 13-18.

Khansari, D. N., Murgo, A. J., & Faith, R. E. (1990). Effects of stress on the immune system. *Immunology Today, 11*(5), 170-175.

Kiecolt-Glaser, J., Glaser, R., Dyer, C., Shuttleworth, E. C., Ogrocki, P., & Speicher, C. E. (1987). Chronic stress and immune function in family caregivers of Alzheimers disease victims. *Psychosomatic Medicine, 45*(5), 523-535.

Kiecolt-Glaser, J., Glaser, R., Strain, E. C., Stout, J. C., Tarr, K. L., Holliday, J. E., & Speicher, C. E. (1986). Modulation of cellular immunity in medical students. *Journal of Behavioral Medicine, 9,* 5-21.

Kiecolt-Glaser, J., Glaser, R., Williger, D., Stout, J., Messick, G., Sheppard, S., Ricker, D., Romisher, S. C., Briner, W., & Bonnell, G., Donnerberg, R. (1985). Psychosocial enhancement of immunocompetence in a geriatric population. *Health Psychology, 4,* 25-41.

Kreuz, L. E., Rose, R. M., & Jennings, J. R. (1972). Suppression of plasma testosterone levels and psychological stress: A longitudinal study of young men in officer candidate school. *Archives of General Psychiatry, 26,* 479-482.

Laudenslager, M. L., Ryan, S. M., Drugan, R. C., Hyson, R. L., & Maier, S. R. (1984). Coping and immunosuppression: Inescapable but not escapable shock suppresses lymphocyte proliferation. *Science, 221,* 568-570.

Lazarus, R. S., & Folkman, S. (1987). Coping and adaptation. In W. D. Gentry (Ed.), *The handbook of behavioral medicine.* New York: Guilford.

Maestroni, G. J. M., & Conti, A. (1991). Anti-stress role of the immuno-opioid network: Evidence for a physiological mechanism involving T cell-derived, immunoreactive β-endorphin and metenkephalin binding to thymic opioid receptors. *International Journal of Neuroscience, 61,* 289-298.

Mason, J. W. (1971). A reevaluation of the concept of nonspecificity in stress theory. *Journal of Psychiatric Research, 8,* 323-333.

Mason, J. W. (1972). Organization of psychoendocrine mechanisms: A review and reconsideration of research. In N. S. Greenfield & R. A. Steinbach (Eds.), *Handbook of psychophysiology.* New York: Holt, Rinehart, & Winston, pp. 3-91.

Mason, J. W. (1974). Specificity in the organization of neuroendocrine response profiles. In P. Seeman & G. Brown (Eds.), *Frontiers in neurology and neuroscience research.* Toronto, Canada: University of Toronto.

Mason, J. W. (1975, March). A historical view of the stress field. *Journal of Human Stress, 1*(1), 6-12.

Mason, J. W., & Brady, J. V. (1956). Plasma 17-hydroxycorticosteroid changes related to reserpine effects on emotional behaviors. *Science, 124,* 983-984.

Matsumoto, K., Takeyasu, K., Mizutani, S., Hamanaka, Y., & Uozumi, T. (1970). Plasma testosterone levels following surgical stress in male patients. *Acta Endocrinology, 65,* 11-17.

Meyer, R. J. & Haggerty, R. J. (1962). Streptococcal infections in families: Factors altering individual susceptibility. *Journal of Pediatrics, 29,* 539-549.

Navarra, P., Tsagarakis, S., Faria, M. S., Rees, L. H., Besser, G. M., & Grossman, A. B. (1991). Interleukins-1 and -6 stimulate the release of corticotropin-releasing hormone-41 from rat hypothalamus *in vitro* via the eicosanoid cyclooxygenase pathway. *Endocrinology, 128*(1), 37-44.

Noel, G. L., Suh, H. K., Stone, J. G., & Frantz, A. G. (1972). Human prolactin and growth hormone release during surgery and other conditions of stress. *Journal of Clinical Endocrinology and Metabolism, 35,* 840-851.

Ostell, A. (1991). Coping, problem-solving, and stress: A framework for intervention strategies. *British Journal of Medical Psychology, 64,* 11-24.

Pelletier, K. R., & Herzing, D. L. (1988). Psychoneuroimmunology: Review. *Advances, 5*(1), 27-56.

Perez, M., & Farrant, J. (1988). Immune reaction and mental disorders. *Psychological Medicine, 18,* 11-13.

Rabin, B. S., Cohen, S., Ganguli, R., Lysle, D. T., & Cunnick, J. E. (1989). Bidirectional interaction between the central nervous system and the immune system. *Clinical Reviews in Immunology, 9*(4), 279-312.

Rose, R. M. (1985). Psychoendocrinology. In J. D. Wilson & D. W. Foster (Eds.), *Williams textbook of endocrinology* (7th ed.). Philadelphia: Saunders.

Schalach, D. S. (1967). The influence of physical stress and exercise on growth hormone and insulin secretion in man. *Journal of Laboratory and Clinical Medicine, 69,* 256-269.

Selye, H. (1946). The general adaptation syndrome and the diseases of adaptation. *Journal of Clinical Endocrinology, 6,* 117-230.

Shelby, J., Sullivan, J., Groussman, M., Gray, R., & Saffle, J. (1992). Severe burn injury: Effects on psychologic and immunologic function in noninjured close relatives. *Journal of Burn Care & Rehabilitation, 13*(1), 58-63.

Shiu, R. P. C., & Friesen, H. G. (1980). Mechanisms of action of prolactin in the control of mammary gland function. *Annual Review of Physiology, 42,* 83-96.

Solomon, G. F., Kemeny, M. E., & Temoshok, L. (1991). Psychoneuroimmunologic aspects of human immunodeficiency virus infection. In R. Alder, D. L. Felten, & N. Cohen (Eds.), *Psychoneuroimmunology* (2nd ed.). New York: Academic Press.

Spiegel, D., Bloom, J., Kraemer, H. C., & Gottheil, H. (1989). Effect of psychosocial treatment on survivors of patients with metastatic breast cancer. *Lancet, II,* 888-891.

Stein, N. (1985). Bereavement, depression, stress, and immunity. In R. Guillemin & M. Cohen (Eds.), *Neural modulation of immunity.* New York: Raven Press, pp. 29-44.

Su, T. P., London, E. D., & Jaffe, J. H. (1988). Steroid binding at ς receptors suggests a link between endocrine, nervous, and immune systems. *Science, 240,* 219-221.

Sundar, S. K., Cierpial, M. A., Kilts, C., Ritchie, J. C., & Weiss, J. M. (1990). Brain IL−1−induced immunosuppression occurs through activation of both pituitary-adrenal axis and sympathetic nervous system by corticotropin-releasing factor. *The Journal of Neuroscience, 10,* 3701-3706.

Thoits, P. A. (1983). Dimensions of life events that influence psychological distress: An evaluation and synthesis of the literature. In H. B. Kaplan (Ed.), *Psychosocial stress: Trends in theory and research*. Orlando, FL: Academic Press.

Vitaliano, P. P., Katon, W., Russo, J., Maiuro, R. D., Anderson, K., & Jones, M. (1987). Coping as an index of illness behavior in panic disorder. *Journal of Nervous and Mental Disease, 175*, 78-84.

Vitaliano, P. P., Maiuro, R. D., Russo, J., & Becker, J. (1987). Raw versus relative scores in the assessment of coping strategies. *Journal of Behavioral Medicine, 10*, 1-19.

Vollhardt, L. T. (1991). Psychoneuroimmunology: A literature review. *American Journal of Orthopsychiatric, 61*(1), 35-47.

Wadeson, R. W., Mason, J. W., Hamburg, D. A., & Handlon, J. H. (1963). Plasma and urinary 17-OHCS responses to motion pictures. *Archives of General Psychiatry, 9*, 146-156.

Warren, S., Greenhill, S., Warren, K. G. (1982). Emotional stress and the development of multiple sclerosis: Case-control evidence of a relationship. *Journal of Chronic Disease, 35*, 821-831.

Weigent D. A., Carr, D. J., & Blalock, J. E. (1990). Bidirectional communication between the neuroendocrine and immune systems: Common hormones and hormone receptors. *New York Academy of Science, 579*, 17-27.

Workman, E. A., & La Via, M. F. (1987a). T-lymphocyte polyclonal proliferation: Effects of stress and stress response style. *Psychological Reports, 60*, 1121-1122.

Workman, E. A., & La Via, M. F. (1987b). T-lymphocyte polyclonal proliferation: Effects of stress and stress response style on medical students taking national board examinations. *Clinical Immunology & Immunopathology, 43*(3), 308-313.

SUGGESTED READINGS

Kaplan, H. B. (1991). Social psychology of the immune system: A conceptual framework and review of the literature. *Social Science and Medicine, 33*(8), 909-923.

Selye, H. (1959). Perspectives in stress research. *Perspectives in Biology and Medicine, 2*(4), 403-416.

UNIT IV

Cellular Proliferation
Cancer

CANCER occurs in most if not all multicellular animals—mammals, fish, reptiles, and amphibians. Evidence from fossil records even shows bone cancer in dinosaurs, and sarcomas have been observed in bones from Egyptian mummies (Moodie, 1923). Hippocrates (460-375 BC) is given credit for the term "carcinoma," the Greek word for crab, possibly because of the invasive and spreading nature of the disease.

Theories about the dissemination of cancer began with a proposal by Galen (AD 131-203) that all tumors were disseminated by concentrations of black bile in areas of invasion.

Later, Marcello Morgagni (1682-1771) examined cancer tissue with a crude microscope and saw no black bile, but did see large amounts of blood and lymph. This observation led to the "lymph theory": that a drop of cancer lymph caused cancer when it moved to nearby nodes (Rusch, 1983). Not until the 19th century did Johannes Peta Muller, Karl Rokitansky, and Rudolf Virchow (1821-1902) demonstrate with improved microscopes a cancer cell's emergence from other nonlymphatic cells (Ewing, 1940). With this new cellular knowledge of cancer came several competing hypotheses:

A breast cancer cell illustrating protruding pseudopodia.
(Courtesy National Library of Medicine.)

- Excretion from cancer cells produced cancer in normal cells.
- Cells with abnormal membranes permitted uncontrolled epithelial growth.
- Retained embryo cells in the adult were responsible for later malignancy.
- Bacteria and parasites caused cancer.

With the discovery that cancer also develops in animals, transplantation experiments began, and cancer cells were implanted from one animal to another. Because of this significant procedure, investigators learned to induce tumor growth from biologic and chemical stimulation. The testing of chemicals as cancer-producing agents (carcinogens) started long after the dramatically astute observation made by Sir Percival Pott in 1775 (Pott, 1981). He proposed that scrotal cancer in young chimney sweeps may be caused by "the lodgment of soot in the rugae (folds) of the scrotum" (Pott, 1981). This was the first observation that linked an environmental agent, coal tar, to cancer growth. Not until 1918, however, did the first experiments using chemical derivatives, the polycyclic hydrocarbons, specifically benzo[*a*]pyrene found in coal tar, demonstrate skin cancer in rats. The first report that an infectious agent could cause cancer was made by Vilhelm Ellerman and Oluf Bang, two investigators from Denmark. In 1908 they reported on the transmission of a blood disease in domestic fowl that resembled human leukemia. Their experiments led to the observation that the cancer was caused by a virus. In 1911 Peyton Rous established a viral cause for another type of cancer in domestic fowl—sarcoma. The importance of his discovery was recognized 55 years later when he was awarded the Nobel Prize. Since these early studies, a number of cancer-causing viruses (oncogenic viruses) have been identified.

The harmful effects of radiation became known soon after Wilhelm Konrad Roentgen discovered the x-ray in 1896. Roentgen himself developed skin cancer. X-ray calibration procedures were unknown at this time, and proper radiation dosage was determined by taking repeated pictures of the operator's hand. Soon after, the first cancer of the hand was reported from these excessive doses. The most dramatic observations linking radiation and cancer occurred from the increase in bone cancers in radium watch dial painters and leukemias in people exposed to the Hiroshima atomic bomb. Currently, researchers are studying the effects of low-dose ionizing radiation and its potential carcinogenic effects.

Environmental hazards, such as solar radiation, also are known to cause cancer. Epidemiologic studies show a direct link between exposure to solar ultraviolet radiation and risk for developing basal and squamous cell skin cancers. These types of skin cancers are the most predominant form of human cancer, affecting one in three people in the United States. Furthermore, childhood sunburns are a risk factor for melanoma. Current awareness about depletion of atmospheric ozone levels, resulting in increased ultraviolet radiation energy at the Earth's surface, has raised concern about a potential future increase in skin cancer incidence. The use of sunscreen lotions and avoiding overexposure to solar ultraviolet radi-ation is advocated as one way to reduce the risk of skin cancer.

In 1932 Lacassagne reported that estrogen injections caused mammary cancer in mice. This stimulated research into the relationship between hormones and cancer.

Current research in cancer reflects its unique importance in cell biology. It is now known that to understand cancer and to devise ways to treat it, greater understanding is needed of both the inner workings of cells and their social interaction in the tissues of the body. Thus, basic cancer research has been the source of many advances in cellular biology. Byproducts of cancer research have provided important technical advances for studying cell biology. Examples include molecular biologic tools such as reverse transcriptase discovered in normal RNA tumor viruses and myeloma cell lines derived from cancerous B lymphocytes, which are used to make monoclonal antibodies (Alberts et al., 1989). Contributions directed toward improvements in cancer treatment, such as immunotherapy, have benefitted scientists in a large number of disciplines other than that of cancer alone.

CHAPTER 10

Tumor Biology

Kathryn L. McCance
Lee K. Roberts

Chapter Outline

Perhaps no other disease causes more concern, fear, and disability than cancer. The human responses to cancer are vast and profound, progressing from shock and disbelief to uncertainty and dread of recurrence, to hope and coping or possible cure. Cancer is, in reality, a variety of disorders with differing pathophysiology. Mechanisms of cancer development vary according to the site of the disease and the precipitating cause.

CANCER: A DISEASE OF GROWTH, DIVISION, AND CELL DIFFERENTIATION

Cells of multicellular organisms are specialized members of a society—*cellular society*. The goal of this cellular society is survival of the entire organism and not just the individual cell. Therefore, some cells must refrain from dividing even when the nutrients are plentiful (Alberts et al., 1989). Cell division proliferation and differentiation are strictly regulated under normal conditions. In this way, organ and tissue mass does not change because a balance is maintained between cell birth rate and cell death rate. When a need arises in an organ or tissue for new cells, however, as in the repair of damage, previously nondividing cells (e.g., resting cells) are rapidly triggered to reenter the division cycle (see Cell Cycle, p. 32). Resting cells must be "turned on" for division and proliferation and "turned off" after proliferation has been completed. The cellular control mechanisms that regulate cell birth and cell death are referred to as "social controls" and require "social control genes." Abnormal cells that disobey the social control mechanisms of normal cell division, proliferation, and differentiation proliferate to form tumors in the body. Virtually every cell in the body, if mutated, has the potential to form tumors.

Social Control Genes and Cellular Division

Cell division depends on complex social controls. Proliferation of different cell types is regulated by different combinations of protein growth factors (see Chapter 1). A cell that undergoes a mutation or set of mutations presumably disrupts the social control genes that give rise to growth-factor–regulated cell division. In other words, the protein growth factors of these genes "turn on" and "turn off" normal cell division and proliferation. Cancer is caused by the malfunction or mutation of these genes that regulate division and proliferation (Yarbro, 1992). The identification and characteristics of

many of these *genes* have been one of the great triumphs of molecular biology in the past decade (Alberts et al., 1989).

There are two mutational routes resulting in uncontrolled cell proliferation that is characteristic of cancer: (1) stimulation of a gene causing *hyperactivity* and (2) inhibition of a gene causing *inactivity*. The stimulation route has a dominant effect, because only one of the cell's two gene copies has mutated. The resulting hyperactivity, that is, overexpression of a growth-related gene product, causes tumor formation. In this case, the altered gene is called an **oncogene** (from the Greek *onkos*, a mass or tumor). Conversely, the unaltered normal allele of that gene in a healthy cell is called a **proto-oncogene** (see p. 337). In the inhibitory route, the mutation has a recessive effect. In this instance, both copies of the cell's particular differentiation gene are inactivated or deleted to free the cell of controlled growth inhibition. The lost gene is called a **tumor suppressor gene** (see p. 339).

In addition to ordinary mutation, there is another type of genetic change that can lead to cancer—that caused by **tumor viruses**. Several types of tumors are caused by viruses. The viruses shed from these tumors can infect normal cells and, as a result of the insertion of the RNA or DNA carried by the virus, transform them into tumor cells (see p. 335).

Cell Differentiation

Cancer cells are defined by two heritable properties, autonomy and anaplasia. **Autonomy** refers to the cancer cell's independence from normal cellular controls. **Anaplasia** is the loss of differentiation, the process of developing specialized functions, and organization, meaning literally "without form." In general, the cancer cell has lost its ability to function normally and to control its growth and division. In normal growth and development, cells become irreversibly more specialized or "committed" to a particular line of development, or pathway of differentiation. Thus *differentiation* is the process of acquiring specific new characteristics resulting in observable changes in cellular function.

Transformation is the process by which a normal cell becomes a cancer cell. It was previously thought that all cancer cells merged from fully differentiated, normal cells that had "dedifferentiated" because of transformation. It was thought also that cells regressed in the direction of their embryonic forms when "hit" by a carcinogen (Kupchella, 1990). Later, it was believed that cancer cells all came from the small number of undifferentiated cells already present in normal tissue.

Today, evidence shows that genes (proto-oncogenes) previously turned off during differentiation can be mutated or reactivated by carcinogenic agents. It is also possible experimentally to cause the cells at one level of

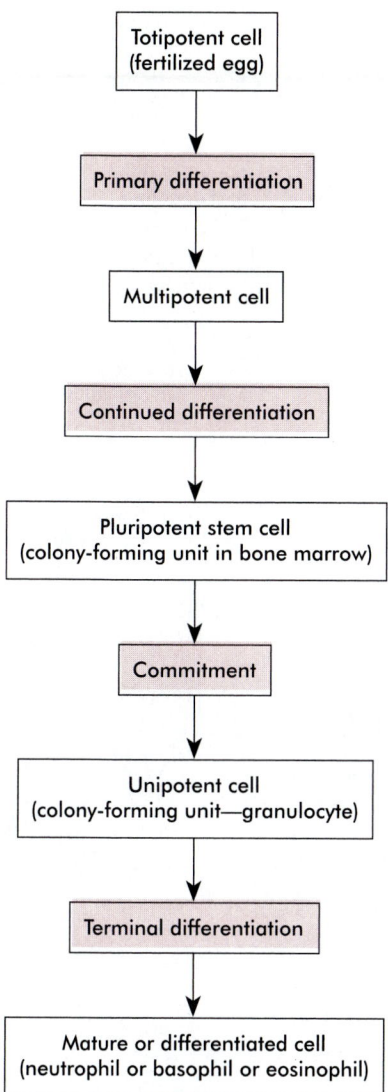

FIG. 10-1 Example of differentiation. Differentiation occurs several times in the lifetime of a granulocyte with each step further limiting the cell's potential. Eventually, the cell *terminally* differentiates and can no longer divide, and the mature cell dies. (Modified from Galucci, 1991.)

differentiation to become transformed into less well-differentiated cells by exposing them to carcinogenic agents (Kupchella, 1990).

As cells mature, they differentiate to perform the specific functions of the tissue they constitute. In the adult, *undifferentiated cells* (not totally committed to a specific function) are known as pluripotent cells, precursor cells, or *stem cells* (Galucci, 1991). In comparison, cells within a developing embryo display the least amount of differentiation. Cancer cells become more like embryonic cells and are less differentiated (thus, the observation that cancerous tissue resembles embryonic tissue). As a cell becomes more differentiated, it loses its ability to replicate. In some tissues, like the epidermis of the skin, the cell is destined to die (Fig. 10-1).

Cancer is considered a disorder of growth and differentiation because neoplasms resemble undifferentiated tissue. The less the tumor resembles normal tissue, the more undifferentiated or anaplastic the tumor is said to be. Tumor **grading**, which grades differentiation, is thus a gauge of the tumor's degree of malignancy (Table 10-1). As the malignant cells grow and divide, they often lose their mature characteristics and no longer resemble their tissue of origin.

Cancerous growth often depends on derangements of cell differentiation. Differentiation depends on the functioning of the stem cell. Cell populations are renewed by simple duplication by means of **stem cells** (Fig. 10-2, *A*). The defining properties of a stem cell are these: (1) it is not at the end of the pathway of differentiation; that is, it is not, itself, terminally differentiated; (2) it can divide without limit; and (3) when it divides, each daughter cell has a choice—it can remain a stem cell or it can become irreversibly committed to terminal differentiation (Fig. 10-2, *B*). Normally, each stem cell division generates one daughter stem cell and one cell (although it may be pluripotent, giving rise to several types of blood cells) that is committed to terminal differenti-

TABLE 10-1

Tumor Grading: Degrees of Differentiation

Grade	Tumor characteristics
Grade I: well differentiated	Tumor closely resembles tissue of origin and thus retains some specialized functions
Grade II: moderately differentiated	Tumor has less resemblance to tissue of origin; more variation in size and shape of tumor cells; increased mitoses
Grade III: poorly to very poorly differentiated	Tumor does not closely resemble tissue of origin; much variation in size and shape of tumor cells; greatly increased mitoses
Grade IV: very poorly differentiated	Tumor has no resemblance to tissue of origin; great variation in size and shape of tumor cells

Modified from Moosa, Robson, & Schimpff, 1986.

FIG. 10-2 **Differentiation of a stem cell. A,** When a stem cell divides, each daughter cell has a choice: it can either remain a stem cell or go on to become terminally differentiated. **B,** This pattern of cell renewal and proliferation of stem cells in the epithelium forms the lining of the small intestine. (Modified from Alberts et al., 1989.)

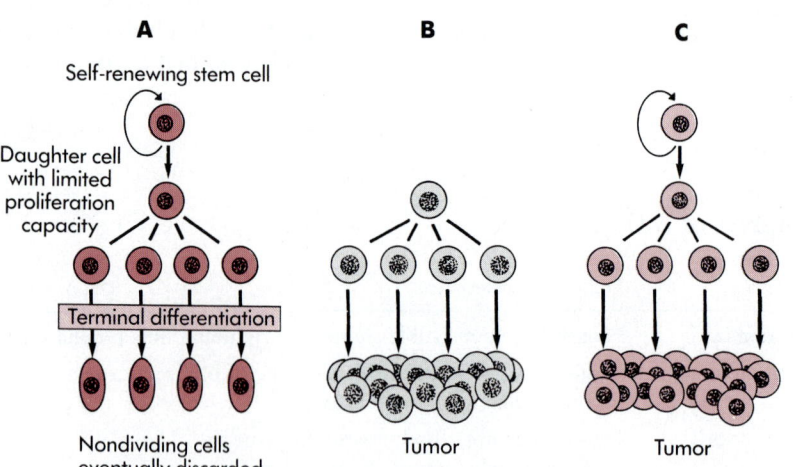

FIG. 10-3 **Differentiated cells and two types of derangements. A,** The normal stem cell pathway for producing new differentiated cells. **B,** Stem cell fails to produce one non–stem-cell daughter in each division and thus proliferates to form a tumor. **C,** Daughter cells fail to differentiate normally and thus proliferate to form a tumor. (Modified from Alberts et al., 1989.)

ation and a cessation of cell division. If the stem cell divides more rapidly, terminally differentiated cells are produced more rapidly. As already mentioned, regulation of stem cell proliferation with cell growth and terminal differentiation is required to maintain the balance of new cell production and cell destruction within a tissue. To produce a steadily growing tumor, however, a transformed stem cell must cause an imbalance in cell production and cell destruction. An excessive cell division rate for the stem cells will not by itself have this effect (Alberts et al., 1989). Two derangements in differentiation, however, could presumably cause an imbalance leading to tumor development (Fig. 10-3). First, more than 50% of the daughter cells must remain as stem cells, or second, the process of differentiation must be deranged so that the daughter cells committed to this route retain an ability to carry on indefinitely and avoid being discarded at the end of the production line (Alberts et al., 1989).

Tumor Classification and Nomenclature

Tumors are classified on the basis of cell type, tissue of origin, whether benign or malignant, degree of differentiation (well, moderately, or poorly), anatomic site, and function. Tumors are named according to the tissues from which they arise, generally with the suffix "oma." Cancers include those of epithelial tissue (**carcinomas**), connective tissue (**sarcomas**), lymphatic tissue (**lymphomas**), glial cells of the central nervous system (**gliomas**), and blood-forming organs, primarily the bone marrow (**leukemias**). The leukemias usually involve an abnormal growth or proliferation of blood-forming cells that infiltrate and replace normal bone marrow and lymphatic tissue. Table 10-2 presents the nomenclature and classification of tumors.

Carcinoma in situ refers to preinvasive epithelial tumors of glandular or squamous cell origin. These tumors have not broken through basement membranes of the squamous cells. Carcinoma in situ occurs in the cervix, skin, oral cavity, esophagus, and bronchus. In glandular epithelium, in situ lesions occur in the stomach, endometrium, and large bowel. These lesions may erroneously be confused with benign tumors, but both the squamous and glandular cell types show disorganization and atypical changes of epithelium. The time that such lesions remain in situ before becoming invasive is unknown. Some carcinomas of the cervix are known to be preinvasive lesions in situ for several years before they progress to invasive carcinoma or metastatic tumors (see Fig. 10-10, C).

TABLE 10-2

Nomenclature and Classification of Benign and Malignant Tumors

Tissue of origin	Benign tumor	Malignant tumor
Epithelial tissue	Papilloma	Carcinoma
Glandular epithelial	Adenoma	Adenocarcinoma
Epidermoid or squamous epithelial	Squamous papilloma	Squamous epithelium carcinoma
Basal layer of epidermis		Basal cell carcinoma
Hair sheath	Pilomatrixoma	
Melanocytes of basal layer	Nevi (mole)	Malignant melanoma
Epithelium of respiratory tract	Papilloma	Bronchogenic carcinoma
Renal tubular epithelium	Adenoma	Renal cell carcinoma or renal adenocarcinoma
Connective tissue or mesenchyme		
Fibrous tissue	Fibroma	Fibrosarcoma
Adipose tissue	Lipoma	Liposarcoma
Cartilage	Chondroma	Chondrosarcoma
Bone	Osteoma	Osteosarcoma
Blood vessels	Hemangioma	Hemangiosarcoma
Muscle		
Smooth	Leiomyoma	Leiomyosarcoma
Skeletal	Rhabdomyoma	Rhabdomyosarcoma

From Rubin, Bakemeier, & Krackov, 1984.

Continued.

TABLE 10-2

Nomenclature and Classification of Benign and Malignant Tumors—cont'd

Tissue of origin	Benign tumor	Malignant tumor
Hematopoietic tissue		
Leukocytes		Leukemias
Granular leukocytes and precursors		Granulocytic leukemia
		Myelocytic leukemias
		Myelogenous leukemias
Plasma cells		Multiple myeloma
Lymphoid		
Nongranular leukocytes and prelympho-cytes		Lymphomas
Proliferating lymphocytes and monocytes		Lymphocytic leukemia
Proliferating immature precursor mono-cytes		Lymphoblastic leukemia
Solid tumors of lymph tissue (thymus, spleen, lymph nodes)		Lymphoma or lymphosarcoma
Nerve tissue		
Nerve cell	Neuroma	
Glial tissue		Glioma or neuroglioma
Nerve sheaths	Neurilemoma	Neurilemic sarcoma
Meninges	Meningioma	Meningeal sarcoma
Neuroectoderm	Neurocytoma	Neuroblastoma
Retina		Retinoblastoma
Adrenal medulla mixed tissue	Pheochromocytoma	Pheochromocytoma
Breast	Fibroadenoma	Cystosarcoma phyllodes
Embryonic kidney		Nephroblastoma (Wilms tumor)
Uterus		Mixed mesodermal, leiomyosarcoma
Others difficult to classify		
Melanoblasts	Pigmented nevus	Melanoma
Placenta	Hydatidiform mole	Choriocarcinoma
Ovary	Granulosa-theca cell tumors	Carcinoma
	Brenner tumor	
	Arrhenoblastoma	
	Gynandroblastoma	
	Hilar cell tumor	
	Sex cord mesenchyme	
Testis	Interstitial cell tumor	Seminoma
		Carcinoma
		Choriocarcinoma
Thymus	Thymoma	Yolk sac

CHARACTERISTICS OF CANCER CELLS

Cancer cells differ according to the cell type from which they derive. To apply any definition to *all* cancer cells, however, would be presumptuous. Some tumors retain useful functions and closely mimic normal tissue, whereas others are so disorganized that the tissue of origin is unidentifiable.

The following cellular characteristics are standard features of cancerous tissue:

Local increase in cell number

Loss of normal arrangement of cells

Variation of cell shape and size

Increase in nuclear size and density of staining (reflects an increase in total DNA)

Increase in mitotic activity

Abnormal mitoses and chromosomes

Two types of disorganization are generally involved. The first is the chaotic nuclear changes and cytoplasmic changes, and second is the disordered relationship of the component cells to each other. Nuclear and cytoplasmic changes are characteristic of cells undergoing transformation. Cancer cells are disordered cells with pronounced cellular proliferation and great variation in size and shape. They divide in an uncoordinated fashion, invading and destroying neighboring tissue, a process termed **progression.** Cancer tumor progression is an increase of abnormal biologic properties and not necessarily a progression in tumor size. The biologic worsening is related to the tumor's malignant capabilities or its lack of differentiation.

A cancer is, therefore, a delinquent cell mass. Disorganized cellular relationships are caused by differences between the cell-surface properties of normal and cancerous cells (Fig. 10-4).

Cell-Surface Changes and Their Functional Importance
Glycolipids and Glycoproteins

In cancer cells, cell-surface glycoproteins and glycolipids are lost or modified. Overall, the protein content of the transformed cell is low, and the glycolipid content of transformed cell membrane is reduced. Terminal sugar residues are often missing. Changes in one type of glycolipid, the *glycosphingolipids,* are related to a number of important features of the transformed cell. The composition and metabolism of certain glycosphingolipids have been shown to change when normal cells

Lost or altered glycoproteins

Lost or altered glycolipids

Changed surface ions or surface charges

Altered component mobility

Altered surface enzymes

New antigens

Altered cytoskeleton control

Lost antigens

Altered cytoskeleton control

Altered transport or permeability

Impaired intercellular communication and density inhibition of growth

Nuclear modification

Secretion or shedding

Increased lectin agglutination

Altered phagocytosis or endocytosis

Virus integration

Changes in adhesion and contact inhibition of movement

FIG. 10-4 Cell surface changes reported in cancer cells.

are transformed. Glycosphingolipids, by interacting with receptor proteins, may decrease cell responsiveness to growth factors. Decreases or changes in glycosphingolipids may increase the cell's responsiveness to growth factors and promote cellular proliferation (Kupchella, 1990). The experimental addition of certain glycosphingolipids to proliferating cells has been shown to inhibit them (HaKomori, 1986; Kojima & HaKomori, 1991). In addition, glycosphingolipids are known to serve as surface markers involved in cell-to-cell recognition (HaKomori, 1986).

The effect of glycoprotein and glycolipid changes may be to alter receptor density or configuration of the cell surface, resulting in decreased communication or signalling between cells. Glycoprotein and glycolipid changes also may enhance the immune defense against cancer, because altered glycoproteins and glycolipids (as antigens) enable the cancer cells to be recognized by the immune system (Kupchella, 1990).

Altered Membrane Transport or Permeability

Substances are transported at generally higher rates across the membranes of transformed cells (Douglas & Shaw, 1990). Noteworthy are glucose, other sugars, and certain amino acids. A glucose transporter protein is thought to be responsible for increased transport of glucose (Burnbaum, Haspel, & Rosen, 1987). Because cancer cells exhibit a greater metabolic demand for certain substrates, it seems consistent that they would have enhanced transport. Increased transport of sugars and amino acids is, however, probably not an initial change responsible for the malignant state; it is more likely that whatever triggers malignant transformation also increases transport (Kupchella, 1990).

Among the most important cell surface changes is the *loss* of large glycoproteins, at first called large external transformation-sensitive protein, or LETS. It is now called **fibronectin**. Fibronectin is a large-molecular-weight glycoprotein found in the blood and on normal cell surfaces. Fibronectin is an anchoring molecule. Together with various proteoglycans (a family of protein-carbohydrate complexes), collagen, and elastin, fibronectin holds cells in place in tissue (Kupchella, 1990). It is thought to hold receptor molecules in particular arrangements. Fibronectin also contributes to the internal organization of the cell (e.g., cytoskeleton), apparently by interacting with actin filaments and proteins that span the cell membrane. This interaction may contribute to the overall shape of the cell.

Cancer cells may make a defective type of fibronectin or they may break down fibronectin as they make it (Kupchella, 1990). Functionally, the low levels of fibronectin in cancer cells are thought to cause changes in cellular organization, cell-to-cell adhesion, cellular migration, and cytoskeletal structure.

Protease

Plasma fibronectin levels rise in the blood of individuals with cancer. In the laboratory, fibronectin is shed into the medium in which transformed cells are growing (Kupchella, 1990). The sloughing of fibronectin could be caused by an increase in enzymes secreted by cancer cells that break up proteins or protease.

Cancer cells secrete "plasminogen-activating factor," which activates the inactive protease, plasminogen, into the active form, plasmin. In turn, protease secretion or activation may be necessary first to change the expression or phenotype of the malignant cell.

Altered Anchoring Junctions and Gap Junctions

Anchoring junctions connect the cytoskeleton of a cell to its neighbor cell or to the extracellular matrix (a loose meshwork of large, extracellular organic molecules that bind cells together) (Fig. 10-5 and see Fig. 1-26). Anchoring junctions are abundant in cardiac muscle, skin epithelium, and the neck of the uterus—tissues that are subjected to severe mechanical stress. Anchoring junctions are classified as two structurally and functionally different types: (1) *adherens junctions* and (2) *desmosomes* and *hemidesmosomes* (see Fig. 1-26). They join the cytoskeleton filaments through intracellular attachment proteins and transmembrane glycoproteins. Normal cells presumably do not divide and proliferate unless they are anchored (see Fig. 10-5).

Cancer cells exhibit **anchorage-independence**. Transformed cells have abnormal or decreased cell-cell and cell–extracellular-matrix attachments. Without anchorage, the transformed cell is allowed to **metastasize**, or grow in new environments. Unlike normal cells, tumor cells continue to divide when they are missing the necessary requirement for anchorage. Anchorage tends to inhibit, rather than to promote, the proliferation of transformed cells (Alberts et al., 1989). Cell division in normal cells is thought to occur when three things happen: (1) the cell is anchored to the extracellular matrix through anchoring junctions that enable the required cytoskeleton proteins to become organized inside the cell; (2) activation of this organized assembly occurs, typically by one or more growth factors, causing the release of an intracellular signal for cell division; and (3) as a necessary part of the process of releasing the signal, the cell-matrix attachments become partially disassembled (Alberts et al., 1989). Theoretically, in cancer cells, step 1 (anchorage to the extracellular matrix) is not required to generate the signal to proliferate. A theoretical model comparing anchorage and anchorage-independence and proliferation of cells is presented in Fig. 10-6. It is not known why tumor cells fail to make firm attachments to the extracellular matrix.

Gap junctions are actually narrow gaps or channels between adjacent cells, allowing inorganic ions and small water-soluble molecules to pass directly from the cytoplasm of one cell to the cytoplasm of the other (see Fig. 1-26). Gap junctions are important in regulating metabolic communication and cooperation among cells. Therefore, it is considered that altered gap-junctional intercellular communication (GJIC) may play an essential role in cancer development (Trosko, Chang, & Madhuker, 1990). Evidence for this includes (1) inhibition of GJIC by tumor-causing agents or by activated oncogenes; (2) selective lack of GJIC between transforming and neighboring normal cells; and (3) decrease of GJIC within tumor or transformed cells (Krutovskikh, Oyamada, & Yamasaki, 1991). Investigators have found that many tumor promoters, such as chemicals or growth factors, disrupt or block gap junction function (Albright et al., 1991; Konishi, Donovan, & Waro, 1990; Krutovskikh et al., 1991; Miki et al., 1990). Furthermore, tumor metastasis has been related to changes in intercellular communication—the more metastatic a tumor becomes, the greater the loss or decrease in intercellular communication (Hamada, Takeichi, & Kobayshi, 1988).

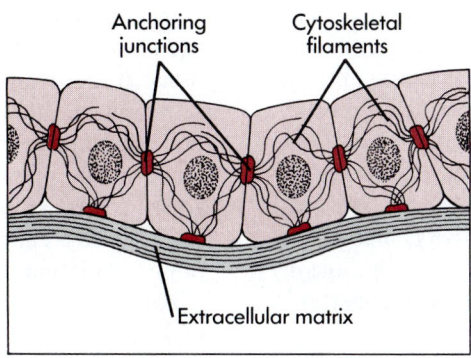

FIG. 10-5 Anchoring junctions. Schematized drawing of anchoring junctions joining cytoskeletal filaments from cell to cell or from cell to extracellular matrix. (Modified from Alberts et al., 1989.)

FIG. 10-6 Comparison of normal cell division and proliferation and that of a cancer cell. A hypothetical drawing comparing the normal process of cell division and proliferation (e.g., anchorage, activation of the cell through growth factors to release an intracellular signal for cell division) with that of a cancer cell. **A,** When an anchored cell (normal cell) is stimulated by growth factors, the signaling molecules are "turned on," signaling the cell to divide and weakening the extracellular adhesion so the cell can proliferate. **B,** Normal cells in suspension fail to divide in response to growth factors because very few of the intracellular signaling molecules are bound to the transmembrane protein, allowing them to be turned on. **C,** Cancer cells have reduced adherence and can divide even in suspension because somehow the signaling molecules can turn on the transmembrane proteins. (Modified from Alberts et al., 1989.)

Tumor Cell Markers

Tumor cell markers are substances produced by cancer cells that are found on tumor plasma membranes or in the blood, spinal fluid, or urine (Table 10-3). Tumor cell markers (also called biologic markers) have been associated with cancer for many decades (McIntire, 1985). They include hormones, enzymes, genes, antigens, and antibodies (Lovejoy, Thomas, Halliburton, & Mimvaugh, 1987). Tumor cell markers, which vary with the degree of tumor progression, are produced by the cancer cell's genetic material when it is activated during carcinogenesis.

Tumor cell markers can be used in three ways: (1) to screen and identify individuals at high risk for cancer; (2) to help diagnose the specific type of tumor in individuals with clinical manifestations relating to cancer; and (3) to follow the clinical course of cancer. Ideally, a tumor marker must demonstrate specificity, sensitivity, proportionality, predictability, and feasibility (Lovejoy et al., 1987). To demonstrate specificity, marker levels must increase or decrease in the presence of only one type of cancer. To demonstrate sensitivity, marker levels must increase or decrease before tumors are clinically palpable or detectable by current diagnostic methods. Proportionality is demonstrated if changes in marker levels are proportional to (or reflect) tumor growth or regression and stage of disease. Predictability requires that marker levels predict treatment response, metastatic disease, recurrent disease, and survival time. Feasibility depends on how well marker levels can be measured by a simple, cost-effective, commercially available, biochemical test that yields a high degree of specificity and sensitivity. Because tumor markers rarely meet all of these criteria, there are no ideal tumor markers. Therefore, tumor markers are known as "borderline" markers.

A significant problem in diagnosis of cancer from tumor marker assays is that many nonmalignant diseases are associated with tumor markers. The presence of a tumor marker may increase the suggestion of cancer, but is not used alone as a diagnostic test. The need for the identification of ideal tumor markers remains a high priority because improvement in cancer therapy will depend on earlier detection and tumor identification.

Hormones

Some tumors inappropriately produce hormones, such as adrenocorticotropic hormone (ACTH), insulin, human chorionic gonadotropin (hCG), parathyroid hormones, and erythropoietin. The phrase "ectopic hormone production" is used to describe the production of hormones by tumors of nonendocrine origin. Detection of certain tumors occurs through abnormally high serum levels of hormones and substrates produced in response to the hormone. Human chorionic gonado-

tropin, for example, is one of the best clinical detectors or tumor markers. Ectopic ACTH production by certain types of tumors causes the increased adrenal secretion of cortisol.

Enzymes

Cancer causes two types of enzymatic abnormalities: (1) the expression of an immature or fetal form of an enzyme and (2) the ectopic production of enzymes. Of current clinical interest are isoenzymes (variable forms of an enzyme). A partial listing of cancer-related isoenzymes is presented in Table 10-3.

Extensive research on enzymes and isoenzymes in cancer has clearly shown that cancers do not produce new or unique enzymes. The enzymes or isoenzymes found are normally produced by the noncancerous tissue from which the cancer arises (Moosa, Robson, & Schimpff, 1986). The tumor may cause the production of enzymes in different or abnormal proportions, however, decreases and increases in enzymes within a given cell type are associated with cancer (Weber, 1977). These enzyme changes occur mainly within the tumor itself and, unfortunately, are expressed in the circulation only when the tumor is very large or widespread metastases have occurred (Moosa et al., 1986).

Genes

Technologic advances have enabled researchers to search for tumor markers inside the cell, including chromosomes and oncogenes. The Philadelphia chromosome (Ph[1]) was the first chromosome marker identified. Because the Ph[1] is present in 95% of individuals with chronic myelocytic leukemia, it is used to establish the diagnosis of the disease (Lovejoy et al., 1987).

Oncogene probes and other technologies have enabled researchers to identify more than 20 oncogenes, including the phosphokinases (c-*src*, -*fps*, -*yes*, -*ros*), DNA-binding proteins (c-*myc*, -*myb*, -*fos*), and cellular growth factors (e.g., c-*sis*). The search for additional oncogenes is continuing.

Antigens

Cancer cells express "nonself" antigens. Some of these are antigens of tumor-inducing viruses. Others are simply *neo*antigens associated with the cell's transformed state. Although the evidence for the existence of unique tumor-*specific* antigens capable of causing tumor rejection in human tumors is weak, human tumors do exhibit tumor-*associated* neoantigens. Many of these antigens normally appear only during embryonic development. In tumors, such antigens are apparently expressed as a result of the reactivation of genes turned off at the end of fetal development. (See p. 353 for a complete discussion of tumor antigens.)

TABLE 10-3

Tumor Cell Markers

Marker	Tumor
Cytology	Aspirates, exudates, urine, brushings
Antigens	
Carcinoembryonic antigen	Many solid tumors
α-Fetoprotein	Liver, ovary, testis
Tumor-specific cell-mediated reactions	
Cytotoxicity tests	Many solid tumors
Delayed hypersensitivity reaction to tumor extracts	Many solid tumors
Ectopic hormones	
Human chorionic gonadotropin	Many tumors
Parathormone	Kidney, lung
Adrenocorticotropic hormone	Lung
Antidiuretic hormone	Lung
Melanin-stimulating hormone	Lung
Thyroid-stimulating hormone	Placenta (choriocarcinoma)
Insulin	Lung
Isoenzymes	
Acid phosphatase	Carcinoma of the prostate; breast cancer
Placental alkaline phosphatase	Choriocarcinoma; carcinomas of ovary, pancreas, colon, breast, uterus, bronchus; testicular cancers; reticulum cell sarcoma; Hodgkin disease; multiple myeloma
Nonplacental alkaline phosphatase	Osteogenic sarcoma; parathyroid carcinoma; cancers metastatic to bone from prostate, breast, multiple myeloma, infiltrative cancers of the liver, leukemia, reticulum cell sarcoma
Galactosyl transferase	Carcinomas of lung, breast, esophagus, stomach, pancreas, colon, gallbladder; chronic lymphocytic leukemia
Aminopeptidases	Carcinomas of pancreas, liver, stomach lining; carcinoma metastatic to liver
Gamma glutamyl transpeptidase	Carcinomas metastatic to liver
Ribonuclease	Carcinoma of pancreas
Sialyltransferase	Carcinomas of breast, colon, lung, prostate; leiomyosarcoma; leukemia; lymphoma; melanoma
Elevated normal substances	
Immunoglobulins	Multiple myeloma
Insulin	Islet cell tumors
Serotonin	Carcinoid tumors
Parathormone	Parathyroid tumors
Prolactin	Pituitary tumors
Gastrin	Islet cell tumors
Human chorionic gonadotropin	Choriocarcinoma
Calcium	Medullary carcinoma (thyroid), parathyroid tumors

Modified from King, Fenoglio, & Lefkowitch, 1983; Moosa, Robson, & Schimpff, 1986.

Antibodies

The development of monoclonal antibody (MAb) technology has made antibodies one of the most interesting and potentially rewarding categories of tumor markers. Monoclonal antibody technology produces hybrid cells that are able to secrete an antibody to a specific tumor antigen. (See the clinical commentary on p. 380 for a complete discussion of MAb technology.)

Intercellular Changes in Cancer Cells
Cytoskeleton

Internal structures that provide the "bones and muscles" of the cell constitute the *cytoskeleton*. The cytoskeleton maintains the cell's shape and internal organization, permits the movement of substances within the cell, and permits movement of external projections (cilia or microvilli) from the plasma membrane. The internal skeleton is composed of a network of protein filaments, two of the most important of which are microtubules and actin filaments (microfilaments) (see Fig. 1-7). Microfilaments and microtubules are not well organized in cancer cells or in normal cells during division.

In normal cells, bundles of actin filaments bind to the plasma membrane in a way that allows the filaments to pull on the extracellular matrix—at sites called *focal contacts* or adhesion plaques—or to another cell (Alberts et al., 1989). Stable arrangements of actin filaments give rise to persistent structures. In cancer cells, focal contacts are disrupted. Diminished adhesion to extracellular surfaces causes the cell to "round up," just as a normal cell does during mitosis.

Microtubules are important not only in controlling cell shape, but also in cell locomotion and cellular division. While the cell is not in the process of division, only a few microtubules are assembled. During cellular division (mitosis) or defense (phagocytosis), rapid assembly and disassembly of microtubules are induced within cells. Microtubules involved in cellular division are arranged in centrioles. Antimitotic drugs, such as vinblastine and vincristine, disrupt microtubular function preferentially, killing many rapidly dividing cells. The specific role that microtubules play in cancer cell mobility remains a controversial topic.

Cytoplasmic Organelles and Altered Metabolism

Investigators have written much about the cytoplasmic and metabolic differences between cancer cells and normal cells. Still unclear is which changes are a result of transformation and which initiate transformation.

The mitochondrial changes and the metabolism of glucose were among the first cellular systems to be investigated, beginning with Otto Warburg's writings in the 1920s and 1930s. Warburg suggested that neoplasms may originate from normal cells because of a defect in their respiratory pathways for which they compensate by increased use of lactic acid or anaerobic glycolysis. He found that cancer cells engage in anaerobic glycolysis and rapid use of glucose even in the presence of oxygen. Although it does seem to be generally true that cancer cells burn up sugar faster than their supposed normal counterparts, the "Warburg theory" has little agreement today (Kupchella, 1990). Increased glycolysis is most likely a *secondary* result of increased rates of cellular division and, presumably, *any* rapidly growing tissues require more glucose. Also, many normal tissues have been found to have glycolytic rates greater than those of tumors, and many kinds of neoplasms have since been found to have normal glycolytic rates (Kupchella, 1990).

Other metabolic observations have been reported, including changes in enzymatic patterns and relationships between enzyme patterns and growth rates in cancer cells and normal cells (Douglas & Shaw, 1990; Weber, 1977). Currently, however, there is no evidence of any *unique* metabolic change that accounts for the difference between normal cells and cancer cells. (Metabolic changes are also discussed further on p. 327.)

Density-Dependent Inhibition of Growth

In the laboratory, when two or more normal cells grown in monolayer (single-layer) culture come in contact with each other, they tend to stop dividing (proliferating) and form a single layer or sheet of cells called a confluent monolayer. The cells do not pile up on one another. This phenomenon is known as **density-dependent inhibition of growth.** Cancer cells, however, usually continue to grow and pile up on top of one another after they have formed a confluent monolayer (Fig. 10-7).

Such phenomena were originally described in terms of "contact inhibition of cell division"; this is now thought to be misleading. This lack of density-dependent inhibition of growth may be the result of two independent properties, mobility and the amount of growth factors in the medium (Alberts et al., 1989; Pitot, 1986; Watson, Hopkins, Roberts, Steitz, & Weiner, 1987). Thus, it is not just the coming in contact with each other that prevents cell proliferation. Confusing is the old term "contact inhibition of cell division," now replaced by density-dependent inhibition of growth, and "contact inhibition of movement." Contact inhibition of movement is an important feature of wound healing in animals. Sheets of epithelial cells at the margin of a wound move rapidly out over the wounded area and cease movement when the cells contact each other across the gap created by the wound (Alberts et al., 1989).

Transformed cells are more mobile and do not adhere to other cells as well as do normal cells (Galucci, 1991). This property is related to changes in the plasma membrane of the transformed cells, as well as to alteration

Contact-inhibited monolayer of normal cells

Multilayer of uninhibited cancer cells

Growth   Culture
medium   dish

FIG. 10-7 **Cancer cell uninhibited growth.** Cancer cells, unlike most normal cells, usually continue to grow and pile up on top of one another after they have formed a confluent monolayer. (Modified from Alberts et al., 1989.)

in the cytoskeleton. Normal cells form tight junctions and other areas of close contact with cells of their own type; transformed cells do not.

Growth Requirements: Inducers of Differentiation

Cell division in multicellular hosts depends on complex social controls, and the proliferation of different cell types is governed by different combinations of protein growth factors (see Chapter 1). These growth factors act at very low concentrations. Most serve as local chemical mediators—initiators and inhibitors—to help regulate cell population densities. Perhaps such factors are balanced in normal cells and unbalanced in cancer cells (Marx, 1986, 1988). Maybe some cancer cells are unable to respond to growth-suppressor factors; perhaps others are chronically stimulated.

Positive and negative regulatory factors that work only in certain types of cells have not been identified (Maniatis, Goodbrown, & Fischer, 1987). Transforming growth factor-β (TGF-β) inhibits the growth of most cells but stimulates the differentiation of fibroblasts (Kupchella, 1990). Inhibition occurs because the growth factor "turns off" genes. Investigators found that TGF-β is linked to the turning off of the *myc* gene in fibroblasts (Marx, 1988). Other agents known to inhibit growth include interferons and tumor necrosis factor. (Cytokines are discussed in Chapter 6.) The *myc* gene is an oncogene whose product is thought to regulate nuclear changes required for cell proliferation. When *myc* is ac-

tivated, cells become committed to proliferate indefinitely. Examples of growth factors and their physiologic actions are presented in Table 1-4 in Chapter 1.

Sachs (1987) and others have isolated and characterized both growth inducers and differentiation inducers and have found that:

1. Growth inducers and differentiation inducers are *different* proteins. Differentiation inducers inhibit growth, and growth inducers cannot cause stem cell progeny to mature.
2. Different growth inducers stimulate cells at different stages of differentiation to produce different inducers of differentiation at different times.

Thus the result is variable numbers of different *types* of differentiated cells derived from the same stem cell type. Because terminally differentiated cells usually no longer divide, differentiation must ultimately neutralize growth inducers (Kupchella, 1990). Investigators suggest that whereas normal cells depend on other cells for growth inducer, either cancer cells need little or no growth inducers, or they make their own (Sachs, 1987).

Autocrine Stimulation Hypothesis

The process by which transformed cells become independent of growth factors, because they produce their own, was conceptualized as *autocrine secretion*. Malignant and transformed cells have surface receptors for growth factors, as well as the ability to release growth factors. This discovery led to the hypothesis of **autostimulation,** or the **autocrine stimulatory hypothesis,** of cancer. Several mechanisms are proposed by which transformed and malignant cells become *autonomous* with respect to growth factors. Mechanisms of autonomy include (1) manufacture by transformed cells of their own growth factors; (2) reduction in the amount of growth factor necessary for division; (3) defects of the growth factor receptor on the plasma membrane; and (4) alteration of the receptor signal pathway for second messengers (Kahn & Graf, 1986). See Chapter 1 for a discussion of how growth factor binding to membrane receptors initiates a cascade of metabolic events leading to cell division.

All this evidence suggests that the normal processes of cell division and cell differentiation are driven and guided by growth factors, and that the cancer cell produces its own. Growth factors are the product of a highly organized sequence of gene activation and gene suppression. Unraveling the complex genetic sequences involved may lead to enormous breakthroughs in cancer therapy. For example, Kupchella (1990) suggests how exciting it would be to find differentiation inducers that could cause cancer cells to differentiate and stop dividing. Chemotherapeutic agents with some maturation effects on cancer cells include cytosine arabinoside (ARA C) (low doses), 6-thioguanine (low doses), hexamethylene bisacetamine (HMBA), and various hematopoietic growth factors.

Transformed cells, then, commonly have a complex syndrome of abnormalities. These abnormalities and their functional significance are summarized in Tables 10-4 and 10-5.

Changes in the Nucleus and Cell Protein

The nuclei of malignant cells are often *pleomorphic*, that is, enlarged and variably shaped. Clumping of chromatin is sometimes noted along the periphery of the nucleus. Alterations of the nuclear membrane can include projections, pockets, blebbing, and a diminished number of nuclear pores, which are associated with DNA replication sites. The rate of mitosis is frequently increased in cancerous tissues. Changes in chromosomes include breaks, deletions, ring forms, and abnormal chromosome karyotypes. For example, frequent changes are reported in chromosomes 1 and 17 in a number of hematologic cancers. A change in chromosome 22 (the Philadelphia chromosome), whereby the long arm is translocated to chromosome 9, is well known in chronic myelocytic leukemia (see Chapter 24).

Other genetic changes are phenotypic; that is, they are "translated and transcribed" into protein. Transfer RNA, for example, may have too few or too many methyl groups (CH_3) attached. Proteins that regulate genes and enzymes involved in nucleic acid synthesis may exhibit phenotypic changes. All of these phenotypic changes are potentially expressions of the malignant state. Although their actual significance is unknown, pathologists rely on phenotypic changes, along with functional and growth-requirement changes, to identify the transformed state and diagnose cancer. The evidence is strong that phenotypic and other changes result from a *change*—a defect in the genetic information of the cell.

TABLE 10-4

Comparison of Normal and Tumor Cells: Cellular Changes Commonly Observed

Growth characteristics	Normal cells	Tumor cells
Density-dependent inhibition of growth	Present	Absent
Growth factor requirements	High	Low
Anchorage dependence	Present	Absent
Proliferative life span	Finite	Indefinite
Adhesiveness	High	Low
Morphology	Flat	Rounded; various shapes; abnormal change
Fibronectin	Present	Reduced
Plasminogen activator	Present	Increased

TABLE 10-5

Functional Significance of Cellular Changes in Tumor Cells

Change	Functional significance
Decreased adhesion Disorganized actin filaments (cytoskeleton) Reduced fibronectin Increased production of plasminogen activator	Decreased cell-to-cell adherence, therefore, maintenance of a rounded morphology; increased plasminogen activation, therefore, increased extracellular proteolysis
Indefinite proliferative life span Lowered requirement for growth factors Less anchorage dependence Density-dependent inhibition of growth	Abnormalities of growth and mitotic division; increased potential for invasion and metastasis

THE GENETICS OF CANCER

Is cancer genetic? Does our genetic inheritance *determine* our susceptibility to certain cancers? The answer is yes and no! The genetics of cancer is complex. In attempts to understand it, researchers study inheritance patterns from one generation to the next (family studies), chromosomes, mutations, and the effects of lifestyle and environmental agents.

Gene-Environment Interaction

The causes of "common" cancers include environmental factors (see also Chapter 5). Reportedly, environmental agents cause cancer by increasing the frequency of mutations in somatic cells (White, 1993). Most carcinogens are **mutagens**, that is, chemicals that increase the frequency of mutations (see Chapter 4).

Two lines of evidence support the idea that exposure to environmental agents can increase an individual's risk of cancer. The first is based on the identification of environmental agents that have carcinogenic properties (White, 1993). Evidence from both epidemiologic and laboratory studies, for example, shows that cigarette smoke causes lung cancer. Environmental agents, such as chemical carcinogens, x-rays, and ultraviolet radiation, can cause certain types of cancer.

The second line of evidence is based on comparisons of populations of different lifestyles. Breast cancer, for example, is prevalent among northern Europeans and Americans but relatively rare among women in developing countries. The difficulty lies in determining whether these differences between populations are attributable to lifestyle factors or to genetics or both. The influence of environmental agents was demonstrated in studies of Japanese who emigrated to Hawaii and the United States mainland. Researchers studied the changes in incidence of colon and stomach cancer after emigration. In Japan, colon cancer is a rare form of cancer. Among the first Japanese emigrants (first generation) in Hawaii, colon cancer incidence rose severalfold, but not as high as overall incidence on the U.S. mainland. Among second-generation Japanese on the U.S. mainland, colon cancer rates rose to the U.S. average. Conversely, stomach cancer is common in Japan but relatively rare in the United States. Japanese on the U.S. mainland have the same low incidence of stomach cancer as the U.S. average. Although these observations implicate environment and lifestyle in the cause of colon and stomach cancer, they do not rule out genetic factors. The difference in incidence rates could be the result of predisposing genes. One could argue that these genes are less penetrating for colon cancer in Japan because of environmental differences (White, 1993).

Inherited Cancer Genes

Most human cancers appear to arise spontaneously. That is, they develop without any known prior exposure to a carcinogenic agent. To explain how these neoplasms arise, it was proposed that cancer is caused by genetic factors. It is now known that certain forms of cancer oncogenes (cancer-causing genes) can be introduced into the individual or inherited within some families. Examples of inherited human cancers include retinoblastoma, a childhood cancer of the eye; Wilms tumor, a childhood cancer of the kidney; neurofibromatosis, fibrosarcomas of nerves; and familial polyposis coli, adenomas of the colon. A specific oncogene has been isolated for each of these cancers. Colon and breast cancers show strong familial associations, suggesting that genetic factors are involved in their causation. Characterization of oncogenes and other genetic risk factors helps identify individuals who are prone to developing cancer. Early cancer detection and therapy result in better prognoses for at-risk individuals.

Oncogenic Viruses

Viruses were first isolated from certain types of tumors in the early 1900s. These viruses caused cancers when transferred into normal healthy animals. A number of **oncogenic viruses** (cancer-causing viruses) have been isolated, including several that cause human cancers. These oncogenic viruses are true pathogenic agents because they cause a specific type of malignant or benign tumor in susceptible individuals. From a genetic standpoint, these viruses represent an exogenous source of oncogenes. Cells infected by these viruses are transformed when the viral oncogene is activated.

Classification of oncogenic viruses

Oncogenic viruses are divided into two major groups, according to the nucleic acid content (DNA or RNA) of the viral particle (Table 10-6). The three main types of oncogenic DNA viruses are papovaviruses, adenoviruses, and herpesviruses. DNA viruses penetrate host cells by the action of their coat proteins. Inside the cell the viral DNA is uncoated and enters the cell's nucleus, where it is inserted (integrated) into the host's DNA. The integrated viral DNA then is transcribed into two "waves" to produce early and late mRNAs (messenger RNAs are described in Chapter 4). Early mRNAs encode for viral proteins that are involved in the replication of the viral DNA. Late mRNAs are transcribed after viral DNA replication and encode for the viral structural proteins. (Viral replication is discussed in Chapter 1 and RNA transcription is discussed in Chapter 4.)

Oncogenic DNA viruses cause tumors in a variety of tissues of different animals. Hepatitis B virus, Epstein-

TABLE 10-6

Classification and Examples of Oncogenic Viruses

Viral class	Virus	Species of isolation
Oncogenic DNA viruses		
Papovaviruses	Papilloma	Rabbit, human, others
	Polyoma	Mouse
	SV 40	Monkey
Adenoviruses[*]	Adenovirus 12	Human
Herpes viruses	Epstein-Barr	Human
	Frog herpesvirus	Frog
	Marek disease	Chicken
Oncogenic RNA viruses[†]		
Acute-acting type	Rous sarcoma	Chicken
	Maloney sarcoma	Mouse
	Harvey/Kirsten sarcoma	Rat
Subacute type	Avian leukosis	Chicken
	Mouse mammary tumor	Mouse
	Bovine leukemia	Cow
	Human T leukemia/lymphoma virus	Human

Modified from Ruddon, 1981.
*There are 31 types of adenovirus that have been isolated from man; three of these (types 12, 18, and 31) are highly oncogenic when inoculated into newborn rodents.
†The oncogenic RNA viruses are divided into two classes; the acute-acting types transform cells in vitro, induce rapid disease in vivo, and carry oncogenes in their genome; the subacute types do not cause cell transformation in vitro, have long latency periods for disease induction in vivo, do not possess oncogenes, and appear to be horizontally transmitted.

Barr virus, and human papilloma virus (HPV) are associated with about 15% of all human cancers worldwide (Hausen, 1991). Cancer of the cervix and hepatocellular carcinoma account for about 80% of virus-linked cancer. Hepatitis B virus infection is considered a high-risk factor for hepatocellular carcinoma. In immune-suppressed individuals, Epstein-Barr virus is the causative agent of Burkitt lymphoma, nasopharyngeal cancer, and B-lymphoma. Sixty different substrains of HPV have been isolated from benign and malignant human tumors. Certain strains of HPV cause warts, benign tumors of the skin, anus, and genitalia. Other strains of HPV cause anogenital carcinoma, oral carcinoma, laryngeal carcinoma, nasal and paranasal carcinomas, as well as conjunctival carcinoma. Except in individuals with the rare disease epidermodysplasia verruciformis, evidence is lacking that HPVs play a role in the induction of either squamous cell carcinoma or melanoma of the skin (Quan & Moy, 1991).

Two other types of DNA viruses have been implicated as causing cancers. These are human immunodeficiency virus (HIV) and the herpes simplex viruses (HSV). Human immunodeficiency virus is the causative agent of acquired immune deficiency syndrome (AIDS), a disease associated with a high incidence of B cell lymphoma and Kaposi sarcoma, a rare form of blood vessel cancer in the skin. Herpes simplex viruses are associated with anogenital and oral cancers. It appears, however, that neither HIV nor HSV is directly involved in the development of human cancers (Hausen, 1991).

Oncogenic RNA viruses are termed **retroviruses** because they contain a certain unique enzyme, **reverse transcriptase.** This enzyme is required for successful infection by the virus. Before viral replication can occur in the host cell, the viral genome (all the genetic information of the virus) must be transcribed from viral RNA to viral DNA by the reverse transcriptase enzyme (Fig. 10-8). Once the viral genome has been transcribed to viral DNA, it can be integrated into the host's DNA, where it is transcribed and replicated by the host's genetic machinery. Human T-cell leukemia-lymphoma virus (HTLV) is an oncogenic retrovirus. It is critical for development and progression of adult T cell leukemia-lymphoma (ATLL). HTLV is transmitted both vertically, that is, inherited by children from infected parents, and horizontally, by breastfeeding, sexual intercourse, blood transfusions, and exposure to infected needles.

Infection by an oncogenic virus is not enough to cause cancer. For example, in some industrialized regions,

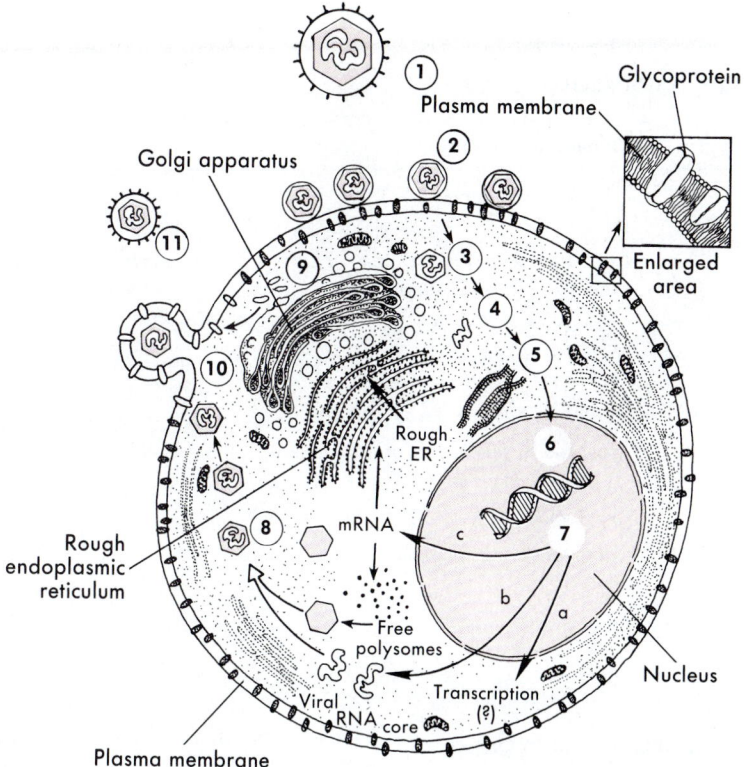

1 Oncogenic retrovirus

2 Absorption—virus binds to cell surface

3 Penetration—virus enters cytoplasm

4 Eclipse—viral RNA freed from core

5 Reverse transcriptase—viral RNA to viral DNA

6 Viral DNA incorporated into host DNA

7 Transcription of host DNA—virus replication
  a. Transcribed v-onc causes transformation
  b. Viral mRNA released to cytoplasm: core protein translated on free polysomes and coat proteins processed on rough endoplasmic reticulum and Golgi apparatus

8 Maturation—core and capsid are assembled in cytoplasm

9 Coat proteins are inserted into plasma membrane

10 Release—virus cores bind to coat proteins and "bud" from cell surface

11 Infectious virus particles

FIG. 10-8 Stages of oncogenic RNA viral infection.

Epstein-Barr virus can infect 90% of the adolescent and young adult population. Yet only a small percentage of these individuals develop cancer. Long latency periods, often lasting decades, the low number of infected individuals that eventually develop cancer, monoclonality of the tumors, and in some cases exposure to other carcinogenic or promoting agents before the appearance of cancer suggest that additional modifications are required to cause a virally infected cell to develop a malignant phenotype.

Oncogenes

In addition to the genes required by the virus to maintain its integrity as an infectious agent (i.e., virus core proteins, envelope glycoproteins, or reverse tran-

scriptase), the oncogenic virus also possesses specific oncogenes, termed **v-onc** (identifying them as viral oncogenes). In 1976, Stehelin showed that cellular oncogenes (termed **c-onc**) in normal, nontransformed chicken cells and v-onc of the avian sarcoma virus had virtually identical nucleic acid sequences. It is now known that cellular oncogenes, c-onc, are incorporated into the genomes of a variety of different organisms, including humans. Because normal, nontransformed cells carry c-onc, a number of conclusions have been drawn concerning the origin and function of these genes.

First, the existence of these c-onc throughout evolution in a variety of unrelated animal species suggests they play an important role in the normal function of the cell. The term *proto-oncogene* sometimes is used to

TABLE 10-7

Oncogenes and Tumor Suppressor Genes

Biochemical function	Identifying acronym*
Growth factors	int-2, hst-1, hst-2, bcl-1
Growth factor receptors	
GTP-binding proteins	ros, met, kit, sea, ret, eph, eck, neu, erb B-2, erb B-3, erb A
Cytoplasmic serine kinase	mos, raf-1, raf-2, pim-1, cdc
Plasma membrane tyrosine kinase	src, yes-1, yes-2, lck, fgr, hck, fyn, lyn, abl, fps
PKC-substrate	c-src
Tyrosine kinase modifier	crk
Cytoplasmic signal transducers	R-ras, H-ras, K-ras, N-ras, rho-1, rho-2, rho-3, ral-1, ral-2, ral-3, ral-4, rap/rev-1
Nuclear regulators	fos, fos B, fru-1, jun, jun B, c-myc, L-myc, N-myc, myb, ets-1, ets-2, rel, ski, sno-N, erg, evi-1
Suppressor genes	rb-1, p53, WT-1, NF-1, APC-1, DCC
Unknown	dbl, put-1, gli, flt, mel

*Abbreviated name of the proto-oncogene or suppressor gene.

refer collectively to the various c-onc. The term proto-oncogene also indicates that c-onc and v-onc genes were likely derived from a common prototype gene. It has been determined that proto-oncogenes encode for growth factors, growth-factor receptors, signal transducers, nuclear proteins, and tumor-suppressor proteins (Table 10-7). This suggests that the proto-oncogenes both are normal genetic components of the cell and encode for viral products or activities required for cell growth and differentiation. It is believed that many of the viral oncogenes thus originated from normal cellular DNA sequences.

Second, it is known that some viruses, especially the retroviruses, can incorporate infected host cell genes into their viral genome during their replication process. This would explain how oncogenic viruses obtained their proto-oncogenes. Although this suggests the origin of v-onc, it does not explain how these viruses transform cells into cancers.

A tremendous amount of research has been directed toward understanding the mechanism or mechanisms by which oncogenic viruses are able to cause cell transformation. This has led to the development of the "oncogene hypothesis." This hypothesis states that virtually all cells possess oncogenes. Because these c-onc are similar to the v-onc carried by oncogenic viruses, their activation during viral infections leads to transformation of the cell. These transformations can result in neoplastic cells that are able to form benign or malignant tumors. It is unknown, however, how oncogenes are activated in normal cells or their role in maintaining the transformed cell phenotype.

Mechanisms of viral carcinogenesis

Because oncogenic viruses act as intracellular parasites, a number of mechanisms for viral carcinogenesis are proposed. Several of these mechanisms are discussed here. It should be appreciated, however, that cancer is a complex disease process that can involve a multitude of factors. As with other diseases, the pathogenic agents may have either (1) a direct effect, in which the tumor cells are or were at some stage infected with the oncogenic virus; or (2) an indirect effect, in which the neoplastic cells were not altered by the virus but were stimulated to grow because of the viral infection.

Direct mechanisms. During the infection process, the virus may cause mutations in surviving cells that could lead to neoplastic changes. This process may not cause cellular transformation, although viral genes may persist within the noninfected tumor cells. Interestingly, viral genes appear to be incorporated into the host genome in a random manner, suggesting that the viral genes do not cause transformation directly.

It appears that most oncogenic viruses cause transformation by a mechanism termed **insertional mutagenesis.** In this process, the viral genes are incorporated into the host's genome at specific sites. Insertion of the v-onc within the host genome can lead to activation of the v-onc or c-onc genes that are associated with cell transformation. These inserted genes become an inherited trait of all the cancer cells derived from the original transformed cell.

Indirect mechanisms. Because viral infections lead to tissue damage, there is a burst of cell proliferations in the damaged tissue after the infection subsides that is associated with the normal repair and healing processes. Actively dividing cells are known to be at higher risk of mutation than resting cells. As a result, these cells would be more susceptible to both spontaneous mutagenesis and transformation by a physical or chemical carcinogen. Alternatively, during some viral infections, the host's immune system can become compromised. This reduced immunologic protection can allow neoplastic cells to emerge that would normally be rejected by the host. The role of the immune system in cancer is discussed in more detail on p. 353. In conclusion, viral infections may affect carcinogenesis by increasing the individual's risk for neoplasia induced by other means.

Tumor Suppressor Genes

By definition, oncogenes encode for proteins that cause cancer. Because most of the oncogene-derived proteins are cell growth and differentiation factors, it is thought that their unregulated overexpression plays a role in cell transformation. Thus an imbalance in positive growth signals received by the cell causes it to assume the transformed phenotype. Proliferation of normal cells may be regulated by growth-promoting oncogenes counterbalanced by growth-constraining tumor suppressor genes (Weinberg, 1991).

Early evidence of tumor suppressor genes came from cell hybridization experiments. When tumor cells were fused with normal cells, the resulting hybrids were not tumorigenic. Loss of the normal cells' chromosomes from these hybrids caused reversion to tumorigenic cells. This suggested that normal cells possess growth-regulating genes. These growth-regulating tumor suppressor genes could prevent the cancer potential of transformed cells.

Tumor suppressor genes encode for proteins that act as negative transducers of growth factor stimulation. The negative growth signals produced by tumor suppressor gene proteins block specific phases of the cell cycle, induce end-stage differentiation, and stimulate cell senescence or death. Carcinogenesis involves *inactivation* of tumor suppressor genes and activation of oncogenes. Examples of suppressor genes include the following: deleted in colon cancer (DCC) gene, neurofibromatosis (NF-1) gene, retinoblastoma (rb) gene, p53 gene, and Wilms tumor (WT-1) gene.

Several of these tumor suppressor genes are involved in inherited human cancers, for example, rb in retinoblastoma, NF-1 in neurofibromatosis, and WT-1 in Wilms tumor. These inherited genes are mutant forms of normal cell growth–regulating genes because of the mutation they encode for defective regulatory proteins that allow for cell transformation to occur. Thus, individuals inheriting these genes are prone to cancer development because of a loss in normal cell growth and differentiation controls. This concept was validated in a recent study. Donehower and colleagues (1992) developed a strain of mice that had defective p53 tumor suppressor genes. Animals that were homozygous for the defective p53 gene grew normally; however, they developed a variety of *spontaneous* tumors. These results point out the important role that normal tumor suppressor genes play in preventing neoplasia.

Genetic or Epigenetic Changes

The initial problem in understanding tumor development is to discover whether the inheritable aberration is attributable to a genetic change—an alteration in the cell's DNA sequence—or to an **epigenetic change**—a change in the pattern of gene expression without a change in the DNA sequence. The stability of the differentiated state is dependent on cell memory or heritable epigenetic change. One rare type of tumor, teratocarcinoma—an embryonic tumor containing many varieties of differentiated tissue (e.g., skin, bone, epithelium)—favors an epigenetic origin. Many investigators, however, think that most cancers are initiated by genetic change, yet epigenetic change may be important in the future development of the disease. The argument is that most of the agents known to cause cancer cause genetic change or agents that cause genetic change cause cancer. This relationship between carcinogenesis and **mutagenesis** is known for three classes of agents: chemical carcinogens (changes in the nucleotide sequence), ionizing radiation such as x-rays (typically cause chromosome breaks and translocations), and viruses (which insert foreign DNA into the cell). The role of these agents in cancer is discussed later in this chapter.

CARCINOGENESIS

Understanding of the process of tumor development, **carcinogenesis**, is very limited. Within the past couple of decades, several theories have greatly influenced our viewing of the carcinogenic process (see box below). These theories or proposed mechanisms of carcinogen-

---

THEORIES OR CONCEPTUAL MODELS OF CARCINOGENESIS

Initiation-promotion-progression model
   Oncogene and tumor-suppressor gene model
   Cancer as a disease of differentiation (blocked or partially unblocked ontogeny)
   Cancer as a stem cell disease
   Cancer as a disease of intercellular communication

esis, derived from experimental studies in animals, epidemiologic studies of human populations, and laboratory biochemical and molecular studies, have suggested that the formation of a cancerous tumor is not a "one-hit" event. Instead, *all* of the evidence supports, overwhelmingly, that there is an evolution of phenotypic and, hence, presumably genotoxic (DNA toxic) changes from the normal cell to the invasive, metastasizing cell.

The multistep process of cancer seems to involve the loss of the ability for the cell to terminally differentiate (see p. 323), to control growth, to travel to distal tissues, and to invade and colonize these tissues. The tumor, once formed, appears to be derived from a single "outlaw" stem cell.

Monoclonal Origin

Where evidence is available, it usually confirms that the cancer has a monoclonal origin. For example, the leukemic white blood cells of individuals with chronic myelogenous leukemia are distinguished from the normal cells by a specific chromosomal abnormality (Philadelphia chromosome) (see p. 882). It is doubtful that the genetic mistake responsible for this abnormality would have occurred in several cells at once in the same individual. It is more likely that all the leukemic cells are descendants of the same mutant cell. Other evidence of cancer having a monoclonal origin is from studies of X chromosome inactivation (see Chapter 4). The inactivation of one X chromosome in each cell occurs early in embryonic development and is observable in many interphase cells. Once the X chromosome is inactivated in a cell, all of the descendants of that cell have the same chromosome inactivated. Consequently, X chromosome inactivation can be used as a heritable marker to trace the lineage of cells in the body. In most tumors that have been studied, both benign and malignant, all the tumor cells have been found to have the same X chromosome inactivated. This strongly suggests that the tumor cells originated from a single aberrant cell (Alberts et al., 1989).

Many Cell Accidents Are Required to Cause Cancer

Many lines of evidence indicate that tumor development requires several *independent* rare accidents to occur together in one cell. The evidence involves the relationship of tumor development to age. If a single mutation were responsible, the chance of developing cancer in any given year would be independent of age. For most types of cancer, however, the change increases at a rapid rate with age (Fig. 10-9). Approximations of somewhere between three and seven independent random events are typically required to alter a normal cell into a cancer cell; the smaller numbers apply to leukemias, the larger to carcinomas (Alberts et al., 1989).

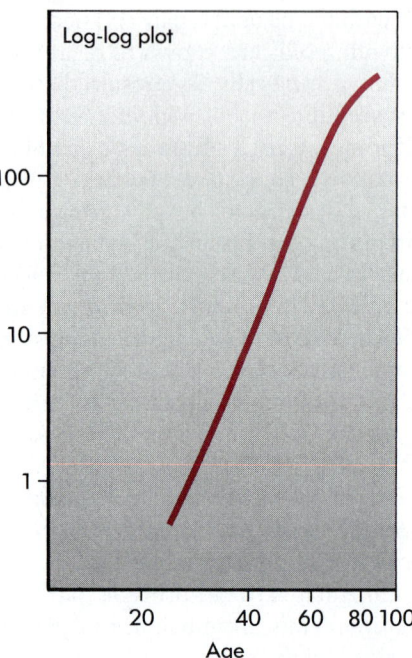

FIG. 10-9 Incidence of cancer rises steeply as a function of age. A cell must accumulate the abnormal effects of several independent accidents before it will give rise to a tumor. (Modified from Alberts et al., 1989.)

Cancers Develop in Slow Stages

Tumor development almost always involves a long delay between the initial causal event and the onset of the disease; for example, the incidence of lung cancer rises steeply after 10 or 20 years of heavy smoking. During this latent period, the cancer cells undergo multiple and successive changes. It appears for most cancers as though cells of the initial mutant clone undergo further mutation that enables them to divide more rapidly before they **terminally differentiate**, that is, come to the end of a pathway of specialization (see Fig. 10-2, *A*). Because of the rapid division and, therefore, proliferation of cells, the cancer cells begin to outnumber the normal cells as well as those with the primary mutation.

Cancers of the uterine cavity provide a clear example of the early steps in the development of a tumor. These cancers originate from the multilayered cervical epithelium, which is similar to the epidermis of the skin. Normally, proliferation occurs only in the basal layer, and the differentiating cells travel outward from their site of origin. It seems logical that among these basal cells is at least one cell whose line of descendants will not die out in one lifetime—an **immortal stem cell**. Cells moving out toward the surface differentiate into flattened, keratin-rich, nondividing cells as they go and, finally, are sloughed off from the surface (Fig. 10-10, *A*). Examination of Pap specimens from different women

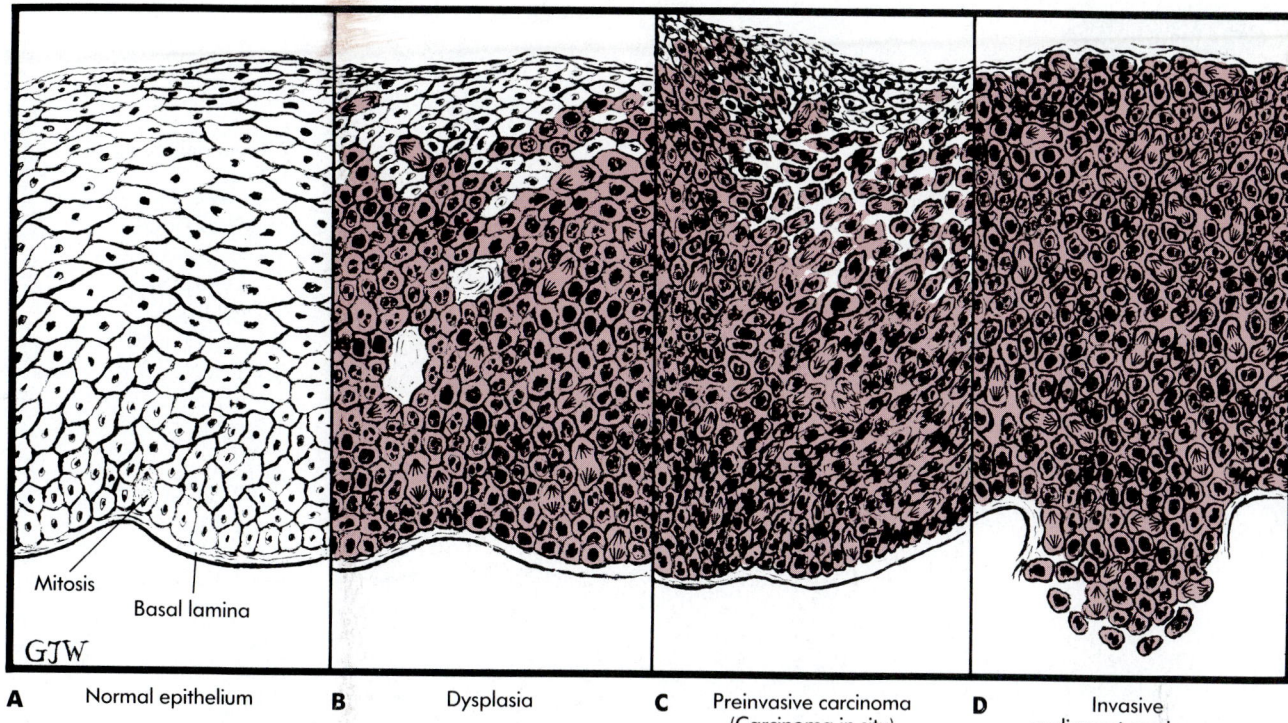

A   Normal epithelium   B   Dysplasia   C   Preinvasive carcinoma   D   Invasive
(Carcinoma in situ)   malignant carcinoma

FIG. 10-10 **Stages of progression.** Stages of progression of development of cancer of the epithelium of the uterine cervix. **A,** Normal. **B,** In dysplasia, the most superficial cells still show signs of differentiation, but this is incomplete, and proliferating cells are seen far above the basal layer. **C,** In carcinoma in situ, the cells in all the layers are proliferating and apparently undifferentiated. **D,** Malignancy begins when the cells cross the basal lamina and begin to invade the underlying connective tissue. Several years may elapse from the first signs of dysplasia to the onset of full-blown malignant cancer. (Modified from Alberts et al., 1989.)

shows patches of *dysplasia*, where dividing cells are no longer confined to the basal layer and there is disorder in the process of differentiation (Fig. 10-10, *B*). These cells, obtained by a "Pap smear," can be viewed under the microscope. If these cells are allowed to progress over a period of years, they give rise to *carcinoma in situ* (Fig. 10-10, *C*). In carcinoma in situ, the cells in all the layers are proliferating and apparently undifferentiated. Yet, the abnormal cells are still confined to the epithelial side of the basal lamina and are highly variable in size and karyotype. Without treatment, the carcinoma in situ cells may still remain harmless or over a period of several years give rise to a malignant clinical carcinoma whose cells cross the basal lamina (see p. 368) and begin to invade the underlying connective tissue (Fig. 10-10, *D*).

Oncogenes and Tumor Suppressor Genes

It is now known that proto-oncogenes represent an array of cell growth and differentiation regulatory genes. Oncogenes are generally considered to encode for factors that stimulate cell growth. In contrast, tumor suppressor genes encode for proteins that counteract cell growth signals. (Oncogenes and tumor suppressor genes

were introduced earlier on p. 322.) Mutations or gene activation of growth-promoting oncogenes and inactivation of tumor suppressor genes can lead to transformation. Because of the complexity of transformation processes, it is not surprising that cancers express multiple oncogenes and tumor suppressor genes. Oncogenes involved in human breast carcinoma include growth factors (*int*-2, *hst*, and *bcl*-1), growth factor-receptors (*erb*-2, *erb* A, and *erb* B-3), signal transducers (*ras*), nuclear regulators (*myc*, *myb*, and *fos*), and suppressors (rb and p53) (Leslie & Howard, 1992). Furthermore, it has been shown in experimental animals that synergy between specific oncogenes is required for tumor induction (Alberts & Cory, 1991). Collectively, these observations suggest that as transformed cells grow and metastasize, different growth and regulatory pathways are activated, as represented by oncogenes and tumor suppressor genes.

In addition to the complex interaction between oncogenes and suppressor genes, other genetic abnormalities occur in many cancers. These abnormalities include deletions, translocations, and inversions of genes, as well as terminal deletions, monosomy, and trisomy of specific chromosomes. Because these chromosome ab-

TABLE 10-8

Genetic Abnormalities Associated with Certain Cancers

Abnormality	Cancer type	Chromosomes/genes affected
Translocations*	Renal carcinoma	t(3;8)(p21;q24)
	Breast carcinoma	t(1)(q21-23)
	Ovarian carcinoma	t(6;14)(q21;q24)
	Melanoma	t(1)(q11-q12)
		t(1;6)(q11-12;q15-21)
		t(1;19)(q12;p13)
		t(6)(p11-q11)
		t(7)(q11)
Deletions†	Renal carcinoma	3p13-21
	Breast carcinoma	17q21(BTSG)
		1p11-13
		3p11-13(?)
		3q11-13(?)
		17p(p53)
		18q(DCC)
		11p(?)
		13q(?)
	Retinoblastoma	13q14(rb)
	Wilms tumor	11p13(PRAD-1)
	Bladder carcinoma	1q21-23
		Monosomy 9
	Colorectal carcinoma	17p(p53)
		18q(DCC)
	Adenomatous polyposis coli	6q21(APC)
Rearrangements‡		
(A)	Burkitt lymphoma	t(8;14)(q24;q32) *myc*
(B)	T-ALL	t(8;14)(q24;q11) *myc*
(C)	B-CLL	t(8;12)(q24;q22) BTG-1 deregulates *myc*
(D)	CML	t(9;22)(q34;q11) BCR-*abl*
(E)	Some lymphomas	11q13 *bcl*-1
Amplifications§	Breast carcinoma	17q21 c-*erb* B-2
		8q24 c-*myc*
		11q13 *int*-2/*hst*-1/*bcl*-1
	Esophageal carcinoma	17q21 c-*erb* B-2
		11q13 *hst*-1/*int*-2
	Acute leukemia	6q22-23p75-*myb*
	Small cell lung carcinoma	8q24 c-*myc*/N-*myc*

Modified from Solomon, 1991.

*Translocation of the affected chromosome is written as, for example, renal carcinoma—a translocation (t) of chromosome 3, band p21, and chromosome 8, band q24.

†Deletion is listed as, for example, renal carcinoma—a deletion affecting bands p13-21 of chromosome 3. Suggested suppressor gene(s) affected by the deletion are shown in parentheses. PRAD-1 is a suppressor gene associated with parathyroid adenomas. BTSG refers to the Breast Tumor Susceptibility Gene. Deletions where a suppressor gene is suspected, but not yet identified, are designated as (?).

‡Examples of rearrangements are (A) oncogene juxtaposed to immunoglobulin genes; (B) oncogene juxtaposed to T-cell receptor genes, (C) oncogene juxtaposed to some "other" genes, (D) fusion oncoproteins, and (E) site rearrangement of the *bcl*-1 oncogene. T-ALL, T-cell acute lymphocytic leukemia; B-CLL, B-cell chronic lymphocytic leukemia; CML, chronic myelogenous leukemia.

§Amplification refers to a condition in which more than one copy of the gene is present in the tumor cells. The affected chromosome and oncogenes are listed.

normalities are consistent for certain types of cancer, it is believed they are involved in the carcinogenesis process (Solomon, Borrow, & Goddard, 1991). Multiple genetic alterations have been well characterized in colorectal carcinoma (Hamilton, 1992), including expression of dominant-acting oncogenes (*ras, myc, src*), inactivation or deletion of suppressor genes (DCC, p53, APC), and deletions from chromosomes 1 and 22. A list of a few of the chromosome abnormalities associated with certain cancers is presented in Table 10-8. This provides further evidence for the role of genetic factors in carcinogenesis.

Stem Cell or Blocked Differentiation

The concept of cancer as a stem cell disease or a disease of differentiation was derived from several observations: (1) the ability of both the stem cell and the cancer cell to proliferate extensively; (2) cancer cells and stem cells both appear to self-renew or self-generate (see Fig. 10-2); (3) both types of cells act similarly with radiation therapy; and (4) terminal differentiation can be experimentally (in vitro) induced for both types of cells with natural differentiation factors.

Differentiation depends on the natural functioning of the stem cell progeny (see Fig. 10-2, *B*). A transformed stem cell causes an imbalance in the rates of cell production and cell destruction in a normal tissue. Two proposed derangements in differentiation, previously discussed, could possibly cause this imbalance and tumor development (see Fig. 10-3). Cancer as a disease of abnormal differentiation is discussed on p. 322.

Intercellular Communication

All cells that are part of a multicellular organism are able to "talk to" or influence each other by processes of cellular communication (see Chapter 1, p. 19). Normal tissue growth and differentiation depend on cellular feedback mechanisms that take place through intercellular communication.

In multicellular organisms, the delicate integration of the three major types of communication is required: *intercellular, intracellular,* and *extracellular* (Fig. 10-11). Extracellular communication involves signals from different molecules or ligands, such as neurotransmitters, chemicals, and hormones. These signals are received by specific cell receptors or directly taken into the cell through coated pits and carrier proteins. Intracellular communication occurs with the activation of second messengers inside the cell membrane, including cyclic-adenosine monophosphate (c-AMP), IP³-diocylglyceride (IP³-DG), phosphokinase C, Ca^{++} flux, and pH changes. Intercellular communication involves ions and other small molecules that directly communicate with neighboring cells through gap junctions (see Chapter 1 and Figs. 1-28 and 10-11). These three types of cell com-

munication are closely related and are capable of controlling cellular function.

Investigators propose that gap junction intercellular communication (GJIC) is either blocked or down-regulated in transforming cancer cells and, therefore, communication between the transformed cells and normal surrounding cells is lost (Hasler, Bennick, & Trosko, 1991; Trosko & Chang, 1989). This concept has been incorporated into other theories on carcinogenesis, including the initiation-promotion-progression theory (discussed in detail on p. 345), oncogene theory, and the stem cell theory. In fact, it is postulated that intercellular communication is the integrating factor to place the initiation-promotion-progression theory together with the idea that cancer is a disease of altered growth control and differentiation, involving oncogenes.

Investigators have reported that gap junctions can be down-regulated or blocked by many tumor promoters, such as chemicals or growth hormones. Phorbol esters are known to promote tumors in certain tissues (Miki et al., 1990). For example, 12-0-tetradecanoylphorbol-13-acetate (TPA) affects intercellular communication (Miki et al., 1990). These investigators demonstrated that TPA decreases communication between transformed and nontransformed cells. Interestingly, communication among transformed cells was less affected by TPA.

FIG. 10-11 Cellular communication. Proposed link between extracellular and intracellular communication. Schema shows the proposed link between extracellular communication and intercellular communication through various intracellular signaling mechanisms (e.g., transmembrane). It provides a holistic view (mind/body connection) of how the neuroendocrine immune system and other coordinations could occur. Although not shown here, activation or altered expression of various oncogenes and tumor suppressor genes could contribute to the regulation of gap junction function. (Modified from Trosko et al., 1990.)

FIG. 10-12 Multistage theory. Tumor development according to the multistage theory: initiation, promotion, progression.

Oncogenes produce abnormal proteins that can take the place of normal hormones, chemicals, or receptors (Trosko et al., 1990). These oncogene proteins are capable of blocking normal up- and down-regulation of intercellular communication and gap junction function and, therefore, stimulate tumor cell growth (Trosko et al., 1990). Investigators have studied oncogenes and chemical promoters and compared them in their ability to block intercellular communication. They found that both the oncogenes and the chemical promoters had "selective" communication between transformed cells but lacked communication with nontransformed cells. The investigators proposed that this "selective communication" allowed the transformed cells to maintain autonomous growth.

Much further research is needed on the relationship between intercellular communication and carcinogenesis. Many studies show that intercellular communica-

---

FIG. 10-13 Initiation and promotion. Procedure demonstrating initiation and promotion of tumors.

tion between transformed cells and normal cells is decreased or blocked and that transformed cells communicate with each other. The exact mechanisms are still unclear, however, and are being investigated.

Initiation-Promotion-Progression Theory of Carcinogenesis

In 1941 Rous and Kidd hypothesized a two-stage mechanism for the development of cancer. These were an initiation stage (transformation) induced by a mutagen followed by a promotion stage mediated by another agent (Rous & Kidd, 1941) (Fig. 10-12). In the late 1940s, Berenblum and Shubik devised a series of experiments that demonstrated the two-stage mechanism for skin cancer (Fig. 10-13). The initiating agent was methylcholanthrene and the promoting agent was croton oil. Neither agent alone would cause carcinogenesis (i.e., the cancer-causing process required both agents). When two such agents are required to initiate and promote carcinogenesis, they are called **cocarcinogens.**

Initiation or DNA damage (mutation) is the development stage of the cancer precursor cell after exposure to the carcinogen. Initiation is an irreversible step. The initiated cell may not be considered cancerous, however, until a promoting agent acts on that cell to produce an altered, autonomous phenotype. **Promotion** appears to involve cell proliferation and tumor development, thus accelerating the process by which the initiated cells become cancerous. Initiation and promotion mechanisms have not been experimentally shown for all cancers, but the process is most useful when applied to chemical agents, such as benzo[a]pyrene found in coal tar or cigarette smoke. Other carcinogens are part of the physical environment (e.g., ionizing and nonionizing radiation) or are biologic agents (e.g., viruses or hormones).

Initiators cause alterations in the DNA. The DNA changes can include one or more complete interruptions of the DNA chain, errors in DNA repair, or an elimination of a base pair (pyrimidine or purine) or sugar. (Normal DNA replication is discussed in Chapter 4.) Promoters may affect cell proliferation by altering cell-

to-cell communication or by the production of oxygen radicals (Ames, Magaw, & Gold, 1987; Trosko, Chang, & Mudhuker, 1990). Promoters include hormones, drugs, chemicals, plant products, and other environmental factors. These factors induce initiated cells to divide within a tissue. Several agents induce cell division, but only promoters induce tumor development. It is suggested that promoting agents may interfere with the process of differentiation, usually after division has occurred. In the early stages of epidermal carcinogenesis, the biologic effects of promotion are reversible and are modulated by diet, hormones, and related factors. Table 10-9 compares initiation and promotion substances.

Boutwell (1964) suggested that progression of a tumor may be a late phase of promotion. The biologic difference between promotion and progression is unknown, but progression is thought to depend on structural changes in the chromosome and, contrarily, promotion may not cause chromosome abnormalities.

Environmental Risk Factors

Because the exact biochemical cause of cancer is unknown, the traditional emphasis (as part of the initiation-promotion theory) is on those factors with suggested pathogenic mechanisms that increase the incidence of different cancerous tumors. (Methods of risk factor analysis are discussed in Chapter 5.)

Table 10-10 summarizes the estimated new cases and deaths, by gender, for specified sites. Although population trends in incidence rates of cancer are the focus of epidemiologists, laboratory scientists use experimental approaches to determine the effect and nature of environmental factors as initiators or promoters of carcinogenesis. To identify an agent as being an initiator, laboratory scientists must demonstrate that altered DNA changes occur in response to variable doses of that agent, a difficult task at best. Thus the relationship between lifestyle and carcinogenesis of a given human population can be explored and evaluated from two divergent but equally important approaches: epidemiologic and experimental. Each approach has strengths

---

TABLE 10-9

Initiation and Promotion Substances

Initiators	Promoters
Single exposure to alter cell	Contact after initiator and requires prolonged exposure
Irreversible process	Reversible during early stage
Metabolically converted to reactants that bind covalently to DNA	Neither metabolic conversion nor covalent binding necessary
High doses carcinogenic	Only weakly carcinogenic without prior treatment of initiator

Modified from Weinstein, 1976; King, Fenoglio, & Lefkowitch, 1983.

TABLE 10-10

Estimated New Cancer Cases and Deaths by Sex for Specified Sites, 1993

Types of cancer	Estimated new cases			Estimated deaths		
	Total	Female	Male	Total	Female	Male
Oral	29,800	9,500	20,300	7,700	2,725	4,975
Esophagus	11,300	3,200	8,100	10,200	2,600	7,600
Stomach	24,000	9,200	14,800	13,600	5,400	8,200
Pancreas	27,700	14,200	13,500	25,000	13,000	12,000
Colon (large intestine)	109,000	56,000	53,000	50,000	25,000	25,000
Rectum	43,000	19,000	24,000	7,000	3,200	3,000
Lung	170,000	70,000	100,000	149,000	56,000	93,000
Bone	2,000	900	1,100	1,050	450	600
Skin (melanoma)	32,000	15,000	17,000	6,800	2,600	4,200
Breast	183,000*	182,000*	1,000*	46,300	46,000	300
Cervix	13,500*	13,500*	—	4,400	4,400	—
Corpus, endometrium	31,000	31,000	—	5,700	5,700	—
Ovary	22,000	22,000	—	13,300	13,300	—
Prostate	165,000	—	165,000	35,000	—	35,000
Testis	6,600	—	6,600	350	—	350
Bladder	52,300	13,300	39,000	9,900	3,400	6,500
Brain and central nervous system	17,500	7,900	9,600	12,100	5,500	6,600
Thyroid	12,700	9,300	3,400	1,050	600	450
Leukemias	29,300	12,600	16,700	18,600	8,500	10,100
Hodgkin disease	7,900	3,400	4,500	1,500	600	900
TOTAL	1,170,000	570,000	600,000	526,000	249,000	277,000

From American Cancer Society, 1993.
*Invasive only.

and weaknesses, and each requires cautionary interpretations. These two perspectives, however, do indicate some agreement about particular agents or conditions that either cause cancer or are associated with an increase in cancer incidence rates.

Personal behaviors

Tobacco use. Both epidemiologic and experimental data support the conclusion that cigarette smoke is carcinogenic and remains the most important cause of cancer (Henderson, Ross, & Pike, 1991). Between 1920 and 1955, cigarette consumption in the United States increased fourfold for all persons 14 years of age or older. From 1976 to 1985, men smokers (20 years and older) decreased from 42% of the population to 32%, and women smokers decreased from 32% to 28%; however, the number of cigarettes smoked by young women, particularly teenagers, has increased (American Cancer Society [ACS], 1992). In both sexes, the average smoker

appears to be smoking more heavily (ACS, 1992). At the same time, respiratory cancer death rates in middle-aged women, which started to increase in the 1960s, are now increasing at an alarming rate.

By late middle age, cancer of the lung is more than 10 times greater in cigarette smokers than in lifelong nonsmokers. Accumulating evidence suggests that cigarette smoking increases the incidence of cancer of the bladder, pancreas, and to a lesser extent, of the kidney, larynx, oral cavity, and esophagus (Doll & Peto, 1981; Henderson et al., 1991). These correlations are not surprising, considering the chemical composition of cigarette smoke. These chemicals possess mutagenic capabilities, are absorbed from the lungs into the blood, through their distribution by the circulation gain access to distant organs, and are present in increased concentration in the urine of smokers.

The harmful effects of cigarette smoke are worse than smoke from pipes or cigars (Henderson et al., 1991).

This difference may be attributable to the increased alkalinity of pipe and cigar smoke, which may decrease nicotine absorption rates in the blood. Alkaline smoke is also more irritating than cigarette smoke and is therefore less readily inhaled into the lungs. The greatest risk among the numerous causes of cancer of the lung thus appears to be related to the inhalation of tobacco smoke (Henderson et al., 1991). Low-tar cigarettes do not reduce the risk of lung cancer (ACS, 1992).

There are hazards for nonsmokers who breathe the smoke of others' cigarettes (passive smoking). Passive smoking is associated with a modestly increased risk of lung cancers and possibly other cancers (Henderson et al., 1991).

There has been a recent resurgence in the use of forms of smokeless tobacco—plug, leaf, and snuff. "Dipping snuff," in which a coarse, moist powder is placed between the cheek and gum, and nicotine and other carcinogens are directly absorbed through the oral tissue, has caused the greatest concern. Oral cancer occurs more frequently among snuff dippers compared with nontobacco users (Henderson et al., 1991).

Diet. Perhaps no other area of cancer investigation has proven more difficult than identifying the carcinogenic nature of dietary practices. Reliable information is increasing, particularly about the cancer-causing effects of substances occurring naturally in food or produced during the processes of food storage, cooking, and digestion.

Diet seems also to function over time to place an individual at risk for cancer. In women, who have a much higher incidence of hormone-dependent cancer than men, diet has been suggested as the main single determinant in the cause of these cancers (Adlercreutz, 1990; Doll & Peto, 1981; Henderson et al., 1991). Studies have found a consistent relationship between increasing weight in women and the risk of cancer, although this has not been the case for men. Obesity is a consistent risk factor for endometrial cancer, possibly because "overnutrition" causes the excessive exposure to estrogen. After menopause, the only natural estrogens produced are those from adipose tissue, so that more adipose tissue causes more estrogen exposure. High consumption of dietary fat also has been linked to endometrial, breast, prostatic, ovarian, and rectal cancer (Adlercreutz, 1990; Carroll, 1991; Henderson et al., 1991; Kelsey & Gammon, 1991). Experiments on animals have indicated that polyunsaturated vegetable oils promote cancer more effectively than does saturated fat, whereas total dietary fat correlates more significantly with cancer incidence and mortality in the epidemiologic data (Carroll, 1991).

Much controversy concerns the need to limit the amount of preservatives added to foods. Food preservation is needed because food is grown in one part of the world and eaten in another, sometimes months or even years later. Advocates argue that preservatives allow people more dietary freedom and actually may encourage "better" diets. Consumers may ingest chemicals unknowingly, unnecessarily, and without judicious knowledge for making responsible choices, however. Most noteworthy among the preservatives and artificial additives under study are saccharin and nitrites.

Facts concerning saccharin are the following:
- Saccharin has been shown to cause bladder cancer in rats, more clearly in males than females, after very large quantities have been consumed.
- Cancer has not occurred in other organs or in other animals under the same conditions.
- The mechanism of action is unclear and obscure.
- Thus far, studies with humans have failed to show a relationship between cancer and saccharin intake.

Nitrites are used as preservatives in fish and meat and may concentrate in the soil and water of some regions. The reaction of nitrites to other nitro compounds causes cancer of the glandular stomach in animals. Potentially harmful nitrite reactions can occur when foods are cooked. For example, nitrite-cured bacon, when cooked, yields nitrous acid that then reacts with amines (derivative of ammonia present in many foods) in the meat to form dimethylnitrosamine (DMN). This reaction is favored at an acidic pH and therefore occurs when nitrites and secondary amines are ingested and encounter the acidic gastric juice. Dietary salts also seem to enhance this reaction. By decreasing the formation of carcinogenic nitrosamines, vitamins C and E (in lettuce and salad greens) exert a protective effect when ingested at the same time as salt and nitrites (Henderson et al., 1991). The inhabitants of countries with high rates of gastric cancer (e.g., China) ingest large quantities of salted fish and similarly preserved foods.

Three primary mechanisms whereby dietary factors may affect cancer production are suggested (Doll & Peto, 1981). These are (1) direct-acting carcinogens or their precursors, (2) indirect-acting carcinogens (those that affect the formation of body carcinogens), and (3) dietary factors that affect transport, activation, and deactivation of carcinogens.

Direct-acting carcinogens include dietary substances in natural foodstuffs, carcinogens produced by cooking, and carcinogens produced by microorganisms in stored foods. The thorough search for naturally occurring carcinogenic food substances is incomplete, especially for humans. Compounds such as hydrazines found in some mushrooms, aflatoxin produced by some food-related fungi, and other substances are known to cause cancer in experimental animals. Aflatoxin is also likely to be carcinogenic for humans because human liver cells contain the enzymes needed to activate the agent metabolically. High intake of aflatoxin by people in the tropics is associated with a high rate of liver cancer, at least among those chronically affected with the hepatitis B virus (Ames et al., 1987). Aflatoxin is found in contaminated peanuts and other staple carbohydrate foods stored in hot and humid climates. This association raises the possibility that other toxins in food may be carcinogenic.

Some carcinogens may be produced by cooking (Spingarn et al., 1980). Benzo[*a*]pyrene and other polycyclic hydrocarbons are produced when meat or fish is excessively smoked or broiled or when fat is used repeatedly to fry food. Food must be nearly charred or cooked at very high temperatures, however, to produce these potentially harmful substances.

Indirect-acting carcinogens provide necessary compounds for the formation of carcinogens in the body (e.g., the production of *N*-nitrosamine compounds). Animal studies have shown these compounds to be powerful carcinogenic agents; their carcinogenic effects in humans have not been verified, although they have been suggested. Nitrosable compounds can occur naturally in many foods such as fish and meat; they may be ingested as pesticide residues or drugs; and they may be formed in the colon from amino acids.

Certain ingested fats might contribute to the production of carcinogens in the body by increasing the amount of bile acids and cholesterol metabolites in the feces. These metabolites, which include deoxycholic and lithocholic acids, are found in greater quantities in populations that ingest a typical Western fatty diet and in whom colorectal cancer is common.

The most significant dietary factor affecting transport is fiber. Much work has been done to characterize the various components of dietary fiber. (Fiber refers to the remnants of the cell wall not hydrolyzed by human digestive enzymes.) Considerable data support the finding that a diet low in fiber is associated with an increased risk of cancer of the colon (Henderson et al., 1991). High fiber intake is associated with low levels of sex hormones in plasma (e.g., sex hormone–binding globulin, free estradiol, free testosterone), causing a reduction in the bioavailability of the hormones that, possibly, would reduce the risk of hormone-dependent cancers. It has been suggested recently that because fat intake is related to decreased excretion of biologically active sex hormones and fiber is also related to their levels in plasma, a ratio of fat:total fiber may be a better index of risk than either alone (Adlercreutz, 1990).

For many carcinogens, certain intermediate steps must happen before they can cause cellular damage. Some carcinogens must be oxidized, yielding metabolically activated intermediates. These activated metabolites are generated from the mechanisms of oxidation and peroxidation and include the short-lived intermediates, the oxidative free radicals (free radical OH^- and the superoxide radical O_2) (see Chapter 2). In animals, polyunsaturated fatty acids are readily oxidized to yield free radicals and peroxidates that are toxic to cells and

related to tumor development (Odeleye, Watson, Eskelson, & Mufti, 1990). Omega-3 fatty acids (e.g., fatty fish), a class of polyunsaturated fats, however, decrease the number and size of tumors and increase the time elapsed before appearance of tumors (Simopoulos, 1991). The destruction of toxic peroxides or radicals depends on selenium-containing enzymes. Levels of selenium have been found to be lower in individuals with cancer than individuals without cancer (Shamberger, Tytko, & Willis, 1976). High-selenium areas in the United States (Western plains regions) have the lowest colon cancer rates (Blott & Fraumeni, 1982).

Alcohol. Incidence rates for cancer of the mouth, pharynx, larynx, esophagus, and liver are higher in individuals who ingest large quantities of both alcohol and smoke (ACS, 1992; Henderson et al., 1991). (These cancers are discussed further in Chapter 36.) Wine, beer, and "hard liquor" seem to produce an equivalent effect on cancer risk (Henderson et al., 1991). Alcohol interacts with smoke, increasing the risk of malignant tumors, possibly by acting as a solvent for the carcinogenic smoke products. Alcohol consumption has been consistently linked to breast cancer and colorectal cancer (Henderson et al., 1991; Kelsey & Gammon, 1991; Rohan & McMichael, 1988; Willett et al., 1987; Young, 1989). The mechanisms for increasing the incidence of breast cancer caused by alcohol are unknown; however, suggestions include the liver's inability to rid the body of carcinogens, impairment of the immune system, or interference with cell-membrane permeability in breast tissue. Alcohol stimulates rectal cell proliferation in the rat, providing a possible mechanism for the observed association with large bowel cancer (Henderson et al., 1991). (Breast cancer is discussed further in Chapter 20.) The relationship between cancer risk and alcohol consumption is difficult to determine because of problems in accurately measuring the amount of alcohol ingested and in defining other behavioral habits, such as smoking, that further complicate or confound the clinical picture.

Sexual and reproductive behavior. The risk of developing cervical cancer is related to the age of first sexual intercourse and to the number of sexual partners (ACS, 1992). Women who have had one sexual partner are also at risk if that partner has had previous multiple partners. The possible mechanism may be a virus transmitted between partners. A number of viruses have been implicated, including herpes simplex virus type 2 (HSV-2) and human papillomavirus (HPV) (Brinton, 1984; Hausen, 1991). Cancer of the cervix is one of the most prevalent virus-linked cancers (Hausen, 1991).

HSV-2 has not been shown to be a causative agent, but antibodies to the virus increase with the severity of cervical dysplasia, and invasive carcinoma is associated with higher antibody titers. Studies have failed to provide evidence of HSVs in human cancers (Hausen, 1991).

HSV types 6 and 11 have been identified as the viruses present in condyloma acuminatum (genital warts), thought to be a precursor of squamous cell carcinoma of the genital tract (Hausen, 1991; Ostrow et al., 1986). The risk factors associated with the disorder include sexually active young women, multiple sexual partners, and a sexual partner with multiple partners. The most common cause of abnormal Papanicolaou smears is the HPV virus, followed by cervical dysplasia (Micha, 1984). Multiple other types of HPV are associated with cancers of the cervix, vulva, penis, and anus (Hausen, 1991).

The incidence of invasive cervical cancer is two and one-half times greater in black women than white women in the United States (ACS, 1992). Cervical malignancy is also found more often in women from lower socioeconomic groups (Devesa & Diamond, 1980). Cancers of the breast, ovary, and cervix account for 13% of all cancers and 29% of all female cancer deaths in the United States. (These cancers are discussed further in Chapter 20.)

Pregnancy and childbearing seem to be protective factors against cancers of the endometrium, ovary, and breast. Other factors related to a decreased risk of breast cancer are discussed in Chapter 20.

Air pollution

A person inhales about 20,000 L of air in 1 day; thus, even modest contamination of the atmosphere can result in inhalation of appreciable doses of pollutants (Ames et al., 1987). Concerns have recently focused on industrial emissions including arsenicals, benzene, chloroform, vinyl chloride, and acrylonitrile (Renard, Goydan, & Stolki, 1992). Proximity of residence to certain industries is a recognized cancer risk factor. It is difficult, however, to determine cancer risk from outdoor pollution because investigators must accurately control for smoking and radon. One team of investigators estimate that one must breathe Los Angeles smog for 1 year to inhale the same amount of burnt material that a two-pack-per-day smoker inhales in 1 day (Ames, 1983). Other studies that controlled or stratified for smoking demonstrate associations between excess lung cancer rates and heavy metal and aromatic hydrocarbon emissions in polluted air (Epstein & Swartz, 1981).

Indoor pollution is generally considered worse than outdoor pollution, partly because of cigarette smoke (Ames et al., 1987). Another significant indoor air pollutant may be radon gas. Radon is a natural radioactive gas that is present in soil, trapped in houses, and gives rise to radioactive decay products that are known to be carcinogenic to humans (Jenks, 1992). Estimated cases of lung cancer attributed to radon pollution in houses is 10% (Ames et al., 1987). The most hazardous houses can be identified and modified to prevent radon contamination. Radon increases the risk of lung cancer in smoking and nonsmoking underground miners (Vahakangas et al., 1992).

Occupation

One way of providing useful information (amid an avalanche of information) about occupational practices and exposures to subsequent cancer risk is to identify

TABLE 10-11

Occupational Exposures Related to Cancer

Cancer site and causal agent	Related occupation
Lung	
Bischloro-methylether	Ion exchange resin producers
Chromium	Ore and pigment manufacturers
Mustard gas	Poison gas producers
Lung, pleura	
Asbestos	Miners, insulation installers, shipyard workers
Lung and skin	
Arsenic	Smelter and pesticide workers
Lung and nasal	
Nickel	Nickel refiners
Lung and skin	
Polycyclic hydrocarbons	Workers using mineral oil and tar
Skin	
UV light	Outdoor workers, fishermen
Liver	
Vinyl chloride	Vinyl chloride workers
Alcohol	Brewery workers
Bladder	
Aromatic amines	Dye and rubber workers
Leukemia	
Benzene	Workers using glue and varnish
Nasal	
Isopropyl alcohol	Isopropyl alcohol manufacturers
Wood dusts	Furniture makers
Multiple sites	
Ionizing radiation	Radium dial painters, uranium miners

Modified from American Cancer Society, 1993.

cancers associated with occupational hazards. Table 10-11 identifies occupational hazards causally associated with cancers in humans.

A substantial percentage of cancers of the upper respiratory passages, lung, bladder, and peritoneum are attributed to occupational factors. One notable occupational factor is asbestos, which may cause as much as 5% of all lung cancers (Demers, 1991; Doll & Peto, 1981). Carcinoma of the bladder has been linked with the manufacture of dyes, rubber, paint, and aromatic amines, especially β-naphthylamine and benzidine. Benzol inhalation is linked to leukemia in shoemakers and in workers in the rubber cement, explosives, and dyeing industries.

Ultraviolet radiation

Ultraviolet (UV) sunlight or solar radiation *causes* basal cell carcinoma and squamous cell carcinoma, two common skin cancers found in white individuals. Basal cell carcinoma is commonly located on the head and neck. Individuals with these tumors generally have light complexions, light eyes, and fair hair, and they live in areas of high sunlight exposure. In general, these cancers arise on areas of the body that receive the greatest sun exposure, although they are not necessarily always restricted to these cancer sites. Squamous cell carcinoma is found more commonly in men who work outdoors. These tumors are distributed over the head, neck, and exposed areas of the upper extremities (see Chapter 41).

The incidence of melanoma, a malignant pigmented mole, *correlates* with the amount of exposure to UV light. Although the nonmelanoma skin cancers are related to cumulative exposure to UV radiation, melanoma is related to heavy, blistering overdoses at a young age (Henderson et al., 1991; Scotto, Fears, & Gori, 1976). The relatively recent worldwide increase in melanoma among white-skinned people is largely attributed to changes in clothing that promote greater exposure. The body areas receiving greater sun exposure vary between the sexes because of clothing differences. Malignant melanomas occur on the upper back and the dorsum of the hands of both sexes and the legs of females. There has been an alarming increase in the incidence of melanoma over the past four decades. Recently it has been suggested that by the year 2020 this trend will reverse and melanoma incidence will steadily decrease (Scotto, Pitcher, & Lee, 1991). It also has been suggested that changing habits of sun exposure along with the use of sunscreen lotions is responsible for this predicted decrease in melanoma incidence.

Xeroderma pigmentosum is a rare autosomal disease characterized by pigmentation abnormalities and malignancies. Persons with this disease demonstrate excessive skin damage caused by sun exposure at very young ages. People with xeroderma pigmentosum lack enzymes that repair sun-damaged DNA.

Ionizing radiation

Much knowledge of the effects of radiation and human cancer has stemmed from observations of the Hiroshima and Nagasaki atomic bomb exposures. These unfortunate exposures caused acute leukemias in adults and children and increased frequencies of thyroid and breast carcinomas. Lung, stomach, colon, esophageal, and urinary tract cancers and multiple myeloma have lately been added to the list. At Nagasaki and Hiroshima, leukemia incidence in individuals 15 years or younger reached its peak 6 to 7 years after the explosions and has steadily declined since 1952. Middle-aged people, 45 years and older at the time of exposure, had a latent period of 20 years before developing acute leukemia. Children conceived after the exposure of their parents to the atomic bombs have surprisingly suffered no increase in any cancer thus far. Human exposure to ionizing radiation includes emissions from x-rays, radioisotopes, and other radioactive sources.

Carcinogenesis. An important effect of ionizing radiation is thought to be inhibition of cell division. Cells of lymphoid tissue, bone marrow, and intestinal epithelium are normally short-lived, rapidly dividing cells. Symptoms and causes of death from exposure to large doses of whole-body radiation are related to the inability of these cells to divide. For example, the suppression of stem cell (primitive precursor cell) division in the bone marrow can cause the disappearance of granulocytes and cause the remaining stem cells, if there are any, to repopulate the tissues. Depending on how many cells are lost, repopulation may require days, weeks, or more, which may be too late to reverse the effects.

At low doses of radiation, a small percentage of the dividing cells may be damaged, and in some tissues this may lead to no detectable change in function. Smaller doses, however, can alter the developing fetus (del Regato, Spjut, & Cox, 1985). Organ development occurs early and extremely rapidly during pregnancy; exposure of the fetus to radiation can greatly alter cellular integrity and normal development. These effects depend on the number of stem cells available and the stage of fetal development.

Carcinogenesis can occur from mutation or cell transformation caused by radiation (see Chapter 2). Radiation can cause dominant and recessive mutations in the DNA and chromosome aberrations. To produce a carcinogenic effect, these DNA alterations must survive in cells capable of cell division. Radiation can directly damage macromolecules or carbohydrates, proteins, lipids, and nucleic acids. Indirectly, radiation interacts with substances (generally water) within the cell, producing reactive-free radicals that then interact and damage DNA.

Carcinogenesis also can be the result of gene-environment interactions. Host factors can influence the carcinogenic effects of radiation. For example, although

CLINICAL COMMENTARY   SOURCES OF RADIATION

Medical and dental procedures in which radiation is used for treatment and diagnosis account for the largest source of *deliberately* generated radiation in North America. It is estimated that more than 300,000 x-ray units (excluding portable units) are used by medical personnel for diagnosis and therapy. Of the total average annual dose of ionizing radiation, half is attributable to medical use.

The units of radiation dose and exposure include roentgen, rad, gray, and rem. Roentgen (R) is a measure of exposure that defines the intensity of a radiation beam or field. Exposure of 1 g of soft tissue or water to 1 R of x-ray results in a dose of around 1 rad, or 100 ergs of energy absorbed per gram of tissue. A millirad corresponds to absorption of 0.1 erg/g. The rem (rad-equivalent-mammal) is a unit accounting for differences in the relative biologic effectiveness of different types of ionizing radiation (1 rem = 1 rad times a correction factor to equalize biologic effects).

Large particle radiations (alpha rays and accelerated protons) are described as high-linear-energy-transfer (LET) radiations, whereas x-rays and gamma rays (electromagnetic radiations) are low-LET radiations. The biologic effects (e.g., a chromosome break) depend on the LET. More cellular damage occurs with high-LET than with low-LET radiation. Of major concern to the general public, however, is the effect of low-LET radiation to which individuals are repeatedly exposed by common x-ray procedures. The specific carcinogenic effects that are produced by low-LET radiation are unclear.

The major overall source of radiation exposure to humans is from natural sources in the environment. These sources come from extraterrestrial or cosmic radiation and terrestrial radiation from radionuclides in the earth. Cosmic radiation (whole-body) exposure, originating from the sun and stars, produces its effects because of the energetic particles that strike the earth. The atmosphere serves as a shield against cosmic radiation: the thinner the shield, the greater the dose-equivalent (DE) rate. Therefore, the cosmic radiation DE rate increases with altitude. The earth's magnetic field also modulates the exposure of cosmic rays. The average DE rate per person in North America is 28 mrem per year. Travel in airplanes slightly increases cosmic ray exposure.

Terrestrial radiation exposure varies with the concentration of radionuclides in the soil. People living in areas where foods are grown in soil with extensive deposits of uranium, thorium, or phosphates containing uranium will receive higher radiation doses. Foods grown in areas with high radioactivity also have increased concentrations of incorporated radionuclides.

The deposition of naturally occurring radionuclides in the human body results from inhalation and ingestion of these substances in air, food, and water. Lung cancer in miners has recently been linked to the inhalation of radon gas in the air of mines. Luminescent instrument dial painters who ingest paint that contains radium and mesothorium (by licking the paint brush to prepare the dials) have an increased incidence of osteogenic sarcomas. Radionuclides that are soluble salts, like radium and strontium, tend to invade bone, whereas potassium or iodine penetrate soft-tissue organs like the thyroid, and can cause cancer. Accidental injection is another mechanism for radionuclides or isotope exposure in an industrial setting.

Carcinogenic effects are associated with the half-lives of different nuclides. Longer half-lives are associated with longer exposure to radiation and therefore cause greater cellular damage.

---

cells can repair some lesions in DNA, some genetic abnormalities alter the repair mechanism, making the individual sensitive to ionizing radiation. Disturbances in the DNA repair mechanism affect the risk of radiation-induced genetic effects and the risk of cancer.

Many other biologic variables affect responses to radiation, including the part and percentage of the body exposed, the individual's age or developmental stage at time of exposure, hormonal balance (e.g., sex hormones regulate cellular growth), genetic integrity, drugs, and other disease processes. Certain drugs can inhibit the immune response by affecting the surveillance role of the lymphoid cells. In the presence of infections, viral nucleoproteins may be introduced into the DNA, rendering the cell susceptible to transformation. Ionizing radiation can cause leukemias and many solid tumors (e.g., thyroid, breast, and salivary gland) (Henderson et al., 1991). Compelling data exist that diagnostic x-rays to the trunk are related to risk of chronic myelogenous leukemia and that the risk increases with increasing x-ray dose to active bone marrow (Henderson et al., 1991). Solid tumors seldom appear before 10 years after radiation exposure and continue to appear for 30 years or more after exposure. Leukemia is an exception, appearing within a few years after radiation exposure.

Hormones

The relationship between hormones and human cancer has been extensively studied. Interest began in 1919 when Laek reported that the removal of the ovaries in female mice prevented the development of breast cancer. About one third of new cancer cases in 1990 were associated with hormones. Four notable types of human cancer—carcinoma of the breast, endometrium, ovary, and prostate—occur in target or hormone-responsive tissues. (These cancers are also discussed in Chapter 20.)

Much of the current research on hormones and cancer is centered on the direct actions of the sex steroids (estrogens, testosterone, and progesterone). Prolactin, a major pituitary hormone, has a direct role in rat mammary cancer growth but is not believed to be of primary importance in human breast cancer.

Oral contraceptives

Many epidemiologic studies have found that oral contraceptive use does not affect the risk of breast cancer in most women regardless of dose, brand, or type of estrogen or progestin (Kelsey & Gammon, 1991; Prentice & Thomas, 1987). Some studies, however, have identified subgroups of oral contraceptive users who have an increased risk of breast cancer. Such subgroups include women with many years of oral contraceptive use before the age of 25 or before the first full-term pregnancy; women who use oral contraceptives at age 45 or older; women with a history of biopsy-confirmed benign breast disorders; nulliparous, premenopausal women with an early menarche; women with only one child; and women with a family history of breast cancer (Kelsey & Gammon, 1991).

Ovarian cancer seems to develop from the epithelial cells on the surface of the ovary. The main stimulus for division of these cells is ovulation. After each ovulation, epithelial cells replicate to cover the exposed surface of the ovary. Those factors that *prevent* ovulation help protect against the development of ovarian cancer. Complete and incomplete pregnancies and oral contraceptive use all reduce the risk of ovarian cancer (Henderson et al., 1991). In women who have used oral contraceptives for 5 years, endometrial cancer risk is reduced about 55%, relative to that of nonusers (Henderson et al., 1991).

Male sex hormones, testosterone and its derivative 5-dihydrotestosterone (DHT), stimulate the growth of target tissues, such as the prostate. Men who take exogenous androgens, however, do not seem to have a higher risk of prostate cancer, whereas women who take estrogens without progestogens after menopause seem to have a higher risk for development of endometrial cancer.

The difficulty in understanding the carcinogenic nature of hormones has been the separation of the hormones as modulators of target tissue growth and function from their potential causative carcinogenic effects. More simply, do hormones cause cancer, or do they promote only tumor growth, or do they do both? Most of the evidence thus far supports their role as promoters of carcinogenesis in target tissues rather than as primary carcinogens. The sex steroids produce their actions by way of the receptor mechanism (see Chapters 1 and 19), sensitizing the cell to the carcinogenic insult, promoting the carcinogenic process, and modifying the growth of the established tumor. Hormones thus appear as promoters rather than primary carcinogens.

Estrogens

Estrogen replacement therapy has been prescribed for women to relieve perimenopausal symptoms (e.g., hot flashes) and to prevent osteoporosis. Chronic use of estrogens by these women has been linked to endometrial cancer (ACS, 1992; Henderson et al., 1991). Long-term use of postmenopausal estrogen replacement therapy is associated with a small increase (10%) in breast cancer risk. In only one study, so far, a significantly larger increase in breast cancer was found among women who used a progestogen along with estrogen than among women who used estrogen alone (Henderson et al., 1991). Breast cells proliferate in response to estrogens; the simultaneous intake of progesterone appears to further increase the *rate* of such cell division (Henderson et al., 1991).

The synthetic estrogen diethylstilbestrol (DES) has also been linked to cancer. Daughters of women treated with DES to avert habitual abortion have demonstrated a higher than expected percentage of clear cell adenocarcinomas of the vagina (Herbst, Ultelder, & Poskanzer, 1971; Kelsey & Gammon, 1991). Diethylstilbestrol has a low affinity for binding to its transporter protein, plasma steroid-binding globulin, which may in turn result in high free levels of circulating DES that cross the placenta to the fetus. The use of DES during pregnancy is associated with an increased risk for breast cancer (Kelsey & Gammon, 1991).

Progestogens and androgens

Endometrial cells divide in response to estrogen; however, the simultaneous presence of progestogens can decrease or even eliminate such mitotic activity (Henderson et al., 1991). Estrogen stimulation "unopposed" by progestogen increases endometrial cancer risk. The best evidence that increased levels of estrogen and progestogens, in combination (i.e., hormone replacement therapy), increase breast cancer risk is that early menarche and late menopause with associated increased hormone levels are such significant risk factors for this disease. Breast cancer risk is reduced 10% to 20% each year menarche is delayed. In addition, for any given age at menarche, rapid establishment of regular menstrual cycles with the associated increased hormone levels further increases risk (Henderson et al., 1991). Women who stop menstruating before age 45 have one-half the risk of breast cancer of women who continue to menstruate to age 55 or beyond (Henderson et al., 1991). Breast cancer is related to cumulative exposure to estrogens, an effect increased by progesterone.

IMMUNOBIOLOGY OF CANCER
Tumor Immune Surveillance Theory

One conclusion that can be drawn from the viral theory of carcinogenesis is that the induction of altered or abnormal cell products is not necessarily required for the development of cancer cells. It is conceivable that the only difference between normal and transformed cells is the amount, rather than the type, of cellular components (e.g., enzymes, cell surface receptors, plasma membrane-bound proteins) that each possesses. In this regard, the overall structural composition of the plasma membranes of normal and transformed cells may be quite similar, if not identical. Thus, any differences between normal and cancer cells may be both subtle and possibly imperceptible by the organism.

The immune system of higher organisms, such as humans, has evolved to recognize antigens that are considered to be "foreign," or "nonself," structures (see Chapter 6). Therefore, if the immune system is capable of recognizing and rejecting tumors, cancer cells must express "nonself" antigens. The **tumor immune surveillance theory** is based on this assumption.

For some time, investigators have been intrigued with the idea that the body could defend itself against the development of cancer. In 1908, Paul Ehrlich, the renowned biologist, proposed that the transformation process was a common event and, that as a result, cancer cells were constantly arising in normal animals. He went on to propose that most cancer cells express "foreign" antigens that make them susceptible to rejection by their host's immune system.

Since that time, a number of studies have supported Ehrlich's general concept. Based on this work, Sir Macfarlin Burnet formally proposed the tumor immune surveillance theory in 1970. In short, Burnet proposed that cell-mediated cytotoxicity (i.e., tumor cell killing by immunologic cells such as lymphocytes) evolved as an immunologic need to act as a primary surveillant for the emergence of cancer cells. Certain experimental and clinical observations support Burnet's theory. These include the identification of tumor antigens, increased risk of certain types of cancers in immune-suppressed individuals, identification of tumor-reactive antibodies in the serum of some individuals with cancer, and demonstration of tumor-specific T cell–mediated cellular immunity (mechanisms of cellular immunity are described in Chapter 6).

Tumor Antigens

Human cancer cells express numerous "foreign" molecules on their surface that can be recognized by the immune system as **tumor-specific antigens** (TSAs). Several types of molecules have been identified as TSAs. By the strictest definition, TSAs are expressed by tumor cells but not by normal cells. In reality, many of the TSAs expressed by human cancer cells are also expressed by normal cells. This is consistent with the preceding description of cancer. Because cancer is a disease of unregulated cell growth and differentiation, the differences between the molecules expressed on the surfaces of normal and cancer cells are subtle. Thus, the recognition of a molecule as a TSA results from a complex interaction between the tumor and its host's immune system.

In the early 1950s, Main and Prehn conducted a series of tumor transplantation experiments in mice. These experiments were the first to show that chemically induced mouse skin tumors express transplantation antigens that can immunize their host against the tumor. Furthermore, these antigens were truly TSAs, because they were not expressed by normal skin cells. It is now known that TSAs are expressed by most experimentally induced mouse tumors. These mouse tumor transplantation antigens are generally divided into two main groups: (1) tumor-specific transplantation antigens (TSTAs), which are unique for each tumor, and (2) cross-reactive tumor-associated transplantation antigens (TATAs), which are shared by a number of different tumors (Fig. 10-14). The TSTAs are generally the most immunogenic (i.e., they cause the strongest immune response) of the tumor antigens expressed by experimentally induced tumors.

Because transplantation studies cannot be performed with human tumors, there is much less known about their ability to elicit a tumor rejection response. Most of our knowledge of human TSAs has come from the study of tumor-reactive antibodies that are obtained from individuals' sera or experimental generation of monoclonal antibodies. Serologically defined human TSAs include viral antigens, oncofetal antigens, oncogene products, and "mutant" proteins and carbohydrates.

Viral antigens

The **viral antigens** are products expressed by virally transformed cells. Viral antigens are common to all tumors induced by the same virus.

Research suggests that Burkitt lymphoma and nasopharyngeal carcinoma are caused by Epstein-Barr virus (EBV) and produce EBV antigens. Individuals with Burkitt lymphoma have higher antibody titers to EBV antigens than do unaffected individuals of the same age, sex, and geographic location, evidence that these tumors express viral antigens. Antibody titers against EBV in individuals with nasopharyngeal carcinoma correlate with the stage of their disease. This suggests that viral antigens are continually expressed by the tumor cells. (Lymphomas are further discussed in Chapter 24.)

FIG. 10-14 Two general classes of tumor-specific antigens (TSAs).

Tumor 1

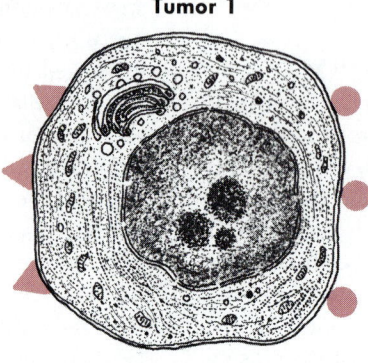

TSTA

Tumor specific transplantation antigens

1 Unique to individual tumors

2 Highly immunogenic

3 Function as rejection antigens after single immunization

4 Recognized by antibody and Tc-cells

5 Biochemical nature unknown

Common TATA

Tumor associated transplantation antigens

1 Shared by different tumors

2 Weakly immunogenic

3 Require multiple immunizations to function as rejection antigen

4 Recognized by antibody and Tc-cells

5 Viral gene products or onco-fetal/differentiation antigens

Tumor 2

Tumor 3

Other human cancers that appear to be caused by viruses include T-cell leukemias associated with human T-cell leukemia virus (HTLV) and cervical carcinomas associated with human papillomaviruses (HPV) (Hellstrom & Hellstrom, 1989). It is not known, however, whether these cancers express TSA of viral origin.

Oncofetal antigens

The **oncofetal antigens** represent molecules that are expressed by cells during certain stages of embryonic development but are absent or expressed at very low concentrations by normal adult cells. The two best characterized antigens in this group are alpha-fetoprotein and carcinoembryonic antigen.

The **α-fetoprotein (α-FP)** is a serum alpha-globulin that is secreted by embryonic liver cells. It is similar in size and structure to serum albumin (Wahren & Harmenbert, 1991). During the first trimester, α-FP constitutes about 90% of the total serum globulins in the blood of human embryos. These levels quickly decline after birth. Individuals with hepatic, pancreatic, and embryonal carcinomas (malignant tumors of epithelial cells) have high levels of α-FP in their serum. Although α-FP appears to be associated specifically with these types of tumors, increased α-FP levels in the blood of individuals with nonneoplastic diseases, such as acute viral hepatitis, also have been observed. It is now known that initial high levels of serum α-FP at the time of liver cancer diagnosis are correlated with a poor prognosis (Wahren & Harmenbert, 1991).

The **carcinoembryonic antigen (CEA)** is a glycoprotein that is part of the family of immunoglobulin-related proteins (Wahren & Harmenbert, 1991). This glycoprotein is a calcium-independent intercellular adhesion molecule. Carcinoembryonic antigen is associated with the mucous coating of the cells of the fetal gut, pancreas, and liver through the sixth month of gestation. Antibody titers to CEA have been found in the serum of individuals with various types of cancer. For example, 70% of colon, 90% of pancreas, and 35% of breast cancer patients have detectable CEA antibody titers, compared with normal individuals (about 5% of the normal human population have CEA-reactive antibody titers). As with α-FP, however, serologic titers to CEA have been found in a large percentage of specific groups of normal people (e.g., pregnant women and heavy cigarette smokers) and in individuals with noncancerous diseases. Because α-FP and CEA antigens are found in a large number of normal individuals, their use as sole diagnostic markers for cancer screening is not always reliable.

Other oncofetal-like antigens include pregnancy-specific β-1 glycoprotein (SP1), human chorionic gonadotropin (hCG), placental lactogen, and haptoglobin-related protein (Hrp) (Merino, Monteagudo, & Neumann, 1991). These antigens are expressed by women during pregnancy. They are also expressed by breast cancers.

Malignancies of hematopoietic tissues express a unique form of oncofetal or differentiation antigens (Vaickus, Ball, & Foon, 1991). Mature hematopoietic cells arise from a common stem cell population and differentiate through a number of well-defined, lineage-specific stages. For example, the stage of differentiation of T and B lymphocytes can be defined by the cell surface antigens they express. Virtually all cancerous lymphocytes retain and express the antigens from that stage of development in which they were transformed. Pathologists can determine the type and prognosis of the cancer by evaluating the patterns of antigens expressed by these cancers.

One of the best-recognized TSAs expressed by hematopoietic cancers is the common acute lymphoblastic leukemia-associated antigen, referred to as CALLA. It has been shown that CALLA is the lymphocyte differentiation antigen CD10. CD10 is expressed by normal bone marrow progenitor cells, bone marrow macrophages and megakaryocytes, germinal center B cells, and mature neutrophils. It also can be detected on a variety of nonhematopoietic cells such as mammary epithelium, fibroblasts, and solid tumors. CD10 expression is a valuable marker of non-B, non-T acute lymphoblastic leukemia (ALL). It has been found that individuals with CD10$^+$ ALL have a better prognosis than those with B cell, T cell, or CD10$^-$ non-B, non-T ALL.

Oncogene-related antigens

Numerous oncogene-encoded antigens are associated with individual tumors. This suggests that complex activation of certain oncogenes is required for transformation of normal cells (Leslie & Howard, 1992). A number of oncogene-encoded antigens are expressed by lung cancers (Gazdar, 1992). These include *ras*, *myc*, and *neu*. The oncogene-encoded proteins are associated with cellular growth and differentiation. The antigen *myc* is a nuclear phosphoprotein that binds DNA and regulates transcription. The *neu* protein is similar to epidermal growth factor receptor. Antibodies to the *neu* protein can affect cell proliferation in tumor cells that express this antigen.

A number of mutations are recognized to be associated with certain types of cancers (Urban & Schreiber, 1992). These mutations are summarized in Table 10-8. For example, 90% of chronic myelogenous leukemias have a translocation of the BCR gene (gene for guanosine triphosphate–activating protein) from chromosome 22 to the 5' end of the ABL proto-oncogene on chromosome 9.

Alternatively, proteins encoded by tumor-suppressor genes can be identified as TSA. For example, retinoblastoma (rb) gene, p53 gene, Wilms tumor gene, and deleted colon cancer (DCC) gene products are expressed as tumor antigens (Gazdar, 1992). The rb and p53 are nuclear phosphoproteins that can bind several viral oncogene-encoded proteins. Interestingly, both rb and p53 are expressed by lung carcinomas. The deleted colon cancer gene product is a TSA expressed by most colorectal cancers. Another interesting TSA that is a cell growth–regulatory protein is the MDR1 gene product. Multidrug resistance (MDR1) increased the excretion of cancer drugs. Neoplasms that express MDR1 are usually more resistant to drugs used for cancer chemotherapy than tumor cells that do not express MDR1.

Carbohydrate tumor antigens

The tumor-associated carbohydrate antigens arise from alterations in normal glycosylation of proteins or lipids (Hakomori, 1991). To some degree, carbohydrate TSAs are oncofetal antigens because many of these antigens are transiently expressed in normal tissues during development and re-expressed by neoplasia (Souhami, 1992). These antigens result from blocked synthesis of particular carbohydrate chains; increased synthesis of carbohydrate structures that are absent in normal cells; and changes in membrane organization, lipid composition, or associations between glycosphingolipids (GSL) and membranous proteins. Examples of these types of antigens include the lacto-series of Lewis blood group antigens expressed on GSL and glycoproteins; the core carbohydrate o-linked mucins expressed on glycoproteins; and precursor GSL molecules, such as GM3, GM2, and

9-o-acetyl-GD3 that are expressed by melanoma and other neuroectodermal cancers. Lewis blood group antigens Le[a] and Le[b] have been detected on gastrointestinal cancers regardless of the Le blood group type of the individual. Le[x] and G1 have been found on colorectal and lung cancers.

The expression of the blood group A antigen on lung cancers is associated with a worse prognosis. Most of these antigens are cellular adhesion molecules. These molecules help cells bind with target structures on other cells. Expression of these antigens is, thus, a prerequisite for metastatic cells to bind vascular endothelium and initiate tissue invasion. Carbohydrate antigen expression has been shown, in most cases, to correlate with tumor invasiveness and decreased patient survival.

Protein tumor antigens

Mouse tumor transplantation experiments conducted in the 1950s suggested that TSAs were new proteins that could only be synthesized and expressed by transformed cells. It is now known that these types of TSA are abnormally expressed proteins with normal function. These TSAs function in proliferation, in enzymatic processes, as receptors, and as cellular structures. These antigens can be located in the nucleus, cytoplasm, plasma membrane, or extracellular compartment. There are numerous examples of these types of TSA.

The major histocompatibility class II antigen, HLA-DR, is not usually expressed by normal epithelial cells. (HLA is discussed in Chapter 6.) However, HLA-DR is expressed, to varying degrees, by melanomas, gastric carcinomas, larynx carcinomas, lung carcinomas, colorectal carcinomas, and breast carcinomas (Ruiz-Cabello, Klein, & Garrido, 1991). Except for melanoma, HLA-DR expression is usually observed on tumors with a more favorable prognosis. This may be attributable to the role of class II antigens for stimulating helper T-lymphocyte responses (see Chapter 6).

Some protein and glycoprotein TSAs are expressed by tumors and found in the serum of individuals with cancer. The function of these proteins is unknown. Examples include TAG-72, which is expressed by breast, colon, ovary, pancreas, stomach, endometrium, and non–small cell lung carcinomas (Guadagni, Roselli, Schlom, & Greiner, 1991), and TA-4, an antigen expressed by squamous cell (skin) carcinomas (Campbell & DéAmbrosis, 1990). As mentioned previously, in combination with CEA, TAG-72 expression has diagnostic value for identifying adenocarcinoma. In contrast, TA-4 is elevated in the serum of individuals with squamous cell carcinoma, skin disorders (e.g., psoriasis and atopic dermatitis), and kidney failure. In this regard, TA-4 is of little diagnostic value.

There are several examples of protein TSA that are enzymes. Prostate-specific antigen (PSA) is expressed by prostate tumors (Cooper, 1991). Increased PSA serum levels are observed in individuals with increased tumor burdens. There is a strong correlation between PSA serum levels and tumor recurrence in individuals undergoing cancer therapy. CO17-1A is a nonsecreted glycoprotein expressed by colorectal carcinomas. It is a cell membrane calcium transporter that is similar in structure to epidermal growth factor and thymosin receptors (Wahren & Harmenbert, 1991). Monoclonal antibodies against CO17-1A have tumoricidal properties. These antibodies have been used in immunotherapeutic trials. Metastatic melanomas express a glycoprotein that is melanotransferrin (Naftzger & Houghton, 1991).

Recently, a new group of TSA proteins has been identified. These are the stress-induced or heat shock proteins (hsp) (Srivastana & Maki, 1991). A majority of the nonviral TSAs expressed by human cancers are related to hsp (Srivastana & Maki, 1991). These proteins can bind steroid receptors, immunoglobulin heavy chains, actin, oncogene proteins, and fatty acids.

The concepts about TSA have changed during the last century; that is, the idea that neoantigens are synthesized and expressed by transformed cells is probably incorrect. Based on our current understanding of carcinogenesis and knowledge of the biochemical nature of tumor antigens, clearly "TSA," per se, may not exist. Rather, it is more likely that tumor immune surveillance mechanisms respond to tumor-specific epitopes (e.g., antigenic determinants) associated with common cellular molecules. In this regard, a variety of modifications in normal molecular expression and association can account for the emergence of tumor-specific epitopes.

Immunologic Defense Against Tumors

When a tumor expresses cell surface TSA, the immune system of an immunologically competent host can reject the tumor. A number of clinical observations strongly support the concept of immunologic involvement in the tumor surveillance process. In the 1700s, it was noted that individuals with draining, abscessed tumors lived longer than those whose tumors did not appear to be inflamed. Berg, in 1959, reported that women with breast cancer tumors that were infiltrated with lymphocytes had a better prognosis than women whose tumors were free of lymphocytes. For certain types of neoplasia there is an increased risk (2% to 20% increase over the normal population) of developing cancer in individuals who are immunologically suppressed. Such individuals (Table 10-12) include (1) children with immunodeficiency diseases, (2) organ transplant recipients whose immune systems are suppressed with drugs (like cyclosporin A to block graft rejection), (3) individuals with cancer for whom cancer therapy results in the suppression of immune responsiveness (many of the current radiation and chemotherapies that are used to treat various forms of cancer depress the immune system, and these individuals have a high risk of developing secondary tumors), and (4) individuals with AIDS. These various clinical observations provide strong support for immune surveillance mechanisms and their role in the development of certain types of cancer.

Immune mechanisms for defense against cancer

As with other antigens, TSAs can elicit both protective and suppressive immune responses. Certain immune responses are more beneficial than others for protecting the individual against cancer. The various types of known cancer defense mechanisms are summarized in Fig. 10-15.

The main involvement of B lymphocytes in a host's defense against cancer is through the production of TSA-reactive antibodies. Many individuals develop antibodies to various TSAs on their tumors. Although antibodies are the basis for identifying and defining tumor antigens expressed by various human cancers, they do not play a major role in protecting the individual against tumor emergence and growth. When effective, antibodies can prevent cancer growth by one of two means. Cytotoxic antibodies can activate complement killing of tumor cells. Alternatively, noncytotoxic antibodies can kill tumors by a mechanism called antibody-dependent cell-mediated cytotoxicity (ADCC) (see Chapter 6).

Antibody-dependent cell-mediated cytotoxicity is a mechanism whereby lymphoid cells capable of killing tumor cells gain the ability to recognize TSA by binding antibodies to their cell surfaces. The TSA-specific antibodies are bound by the cells' Fc receptors (see Chapter 6). The ADCC cells use surface-bound antibody as antigen-specific receptors to bind tumor cells. Once bound to the tumor, ADCC cells deliver a tumor-killing signal (the lytic event). Monocytes, neutrophils, B cells, and certain null cells, called killer cells or K cells, possess ADCC function. Macrophages with ADCC activity are called "armed macrophages."

Unlike "armed macrophages," nonspecific tumor cell killing can be mediated by "activated macrophages." Macrophages can be activated in several ways to lyse tumor cells. One way is by injection of bacterial adjuvants, such as the bacterium *Corynebacterium parvum* and bacille Calmette-Guérin (BCG). Adjuvants have been used in immunotherapy (see Chapter 8). Immune T lymphocytes can release macrophage-activating factors that stimulate macrophages to kill tumor cells. Once activated, macrophages kill tumor cells in a localized, antigen-specific fashion.

Natural killer (NK) and K cells may be the first line of defense against cancer cells. Natural killer cells are present in normal, cancer-free individuals. In mice, a transient increase in NK cell activity occurs after TSA and adjuvant stimulation. Mouse strains with high lev-

TABLE 10-12

Correlation Between Immunodeficiency and Cancer Risk

Types of cancer	Increased risk over normal population
Lymphomas	14 times greater
Leukemias	6 times greater
Carcinomas	
Skin (low-sun geographic areas)	4-7 times greater
(high-sun geographic areas)	21 times greater
Uterine cervix	13 times greater
Stomach	11 times greater
Urinary bladder	2 times greater

Modified from Penn, 1981.

NOTE: There is an increased risk for developing specific types of cancer in individuals with various immunodeficiencies versus that of the normal population. The values presented are generalized to include the various immunodeficient conditions. There is no increased risk in immunodeficient individuals for specific cancers not listed.

els of NK cell activity appear to be more resistant to the growth of certain transplantable tumors. Similarly, many individuals with cancer have low levels of NK cell activity. This suggests that NK cells are involved in human tumor immune surveillance.

Cytotoxic T lymphocytes (CTLs) are the most effective mediators of tumor rejection. They are TSA specific and differentiated from resting T cells after antigen presentation by macrophages and activation by helper T lymphocytes. Once activated, CTLs can recognize and kill tumor cells that express the appropriate TSA. Activated CTLs cause tumor rejection by secreting lymphokines (soluble lymphocyte products) that directly lyse tumor cells, inhibit the growth of transformed cells, or stimulate noncommitted cells to join in an antitumor response. These **tumor-infiltrating lymphocytes (TILs)** have been used as a form of cancer immunotherapy. By isolating TILs, expanding them in tissue culture containing the appropriate interleukins, and injecting them back into the individual, oncologists have been successful in treating cancers such as melanoma.

Immune surveillance escape mechanisms

Although the immune system can reject tumors, individuals with normal immunologic function develop cancers. The host-tumor relationship during tumor emergence and progression is, thus, a complex process. Changes in host immunologic potential (i.e., range of antigenic responses) and characteristics of growing can-

1 Humoral immunity

Cytotoxic
antibodies
bind to TAA

Bound antibody fixes complement (C¹) to tumor
cell surface—cell dies

2 (ADCC) or armed macrophages

Fc

Fc

Lytic event

1, Monocytes, neutrophils, B cells, null cells, and macrophages bind to
tumor-bound antibody through Fc receptors. **2,** Bound ADCC cell
delivers the lytic event.

3 Activated macrophages

BCG   BCG   BCG

BCG

Lytic event

1, BCG injection activates and calls macrophages to the tumor site.
2, Activated macrophages deliver the lytic event.

4 Natural killer cells

Lytic event

NK cells bind to tumor cells and
deliver the lytic event.

5 Cytotoxic T lymphocytes

Lytic event

Th

APC

Tc

1, TAA stimulate the immune response: interactions among antigen plus
antigen-presenting cells plus T helper cells and T cytotoxic cell.
2, Tc cell binds to TAA (specifically) and delivers the lytic event.

FIG. 10-15 Tumor immune surveillance mechanisms.

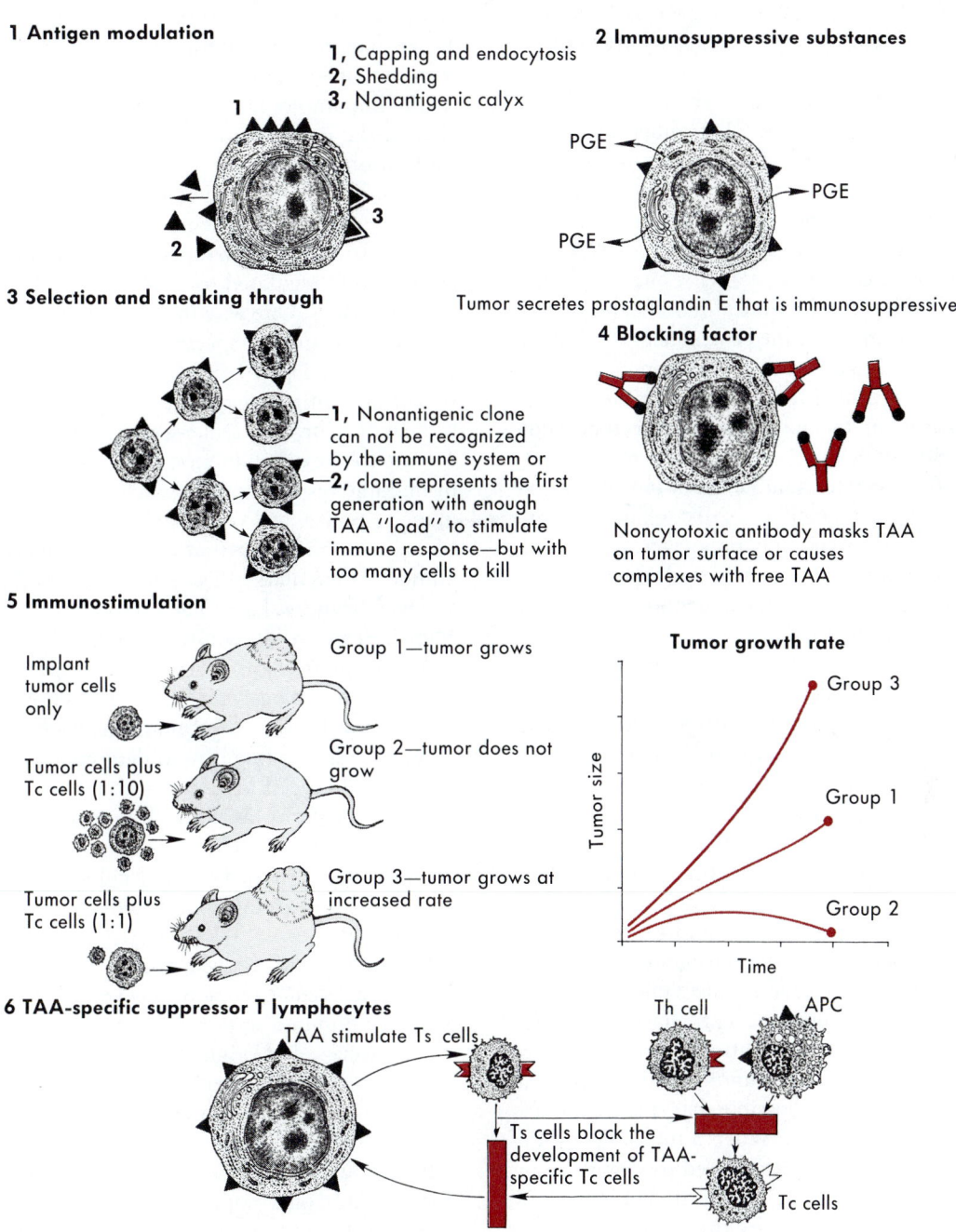

1 Antigen modulation

1, Capping and endocytosis
2, Shedding
3, Nonantigenic calyx

2 Immunosuppressive substances

PGE
PGE
PGE

Tumor secretes prostaglandin E that is immunosuppressive

3 Selection and sneaking through

1, Nonantigenic clone can not be recognized by the immune system or
2, clone represents the first generation with enough TAA "load" to stimulate immune response—but with too many cells to kill

4 Blocking factor

Noncytotoxic antibody masks TAA on tumor surface or causes complexes with free TAA

5 Immunostimulation

Implant tumor cells only

Group 1—tumor grows

Tumor cells plus Tc cells (1:10)

Group 2—tumor does not grow

Tumor cells plus Tc cells (1:1)

Group 3—tumor grows at increased rate

Tumor growth rate

Group 3
Group 1
Group 2

Tumor size

Time

6 TAA-specific suppressor T lymphocytes

TAA stimulate Ts cells

Th cell   APC

Ts cells block the development of TAA-specific Tc cells

Tc cells

FIG. 10-16 Potential immune surveillance escape mechanisms.

cer cells (e.g., TSA expression, growth rate, and metabolism) constantly occur. By taking advantage of these changes, many cancers can bypass the host's immune surveillance potential. Ways that tumors escape immunologic rejection include (1) antigenic modulation, (2) secretion of immunosuppressive substances, (3) escape and sneaking through, (4) blocking factor, (5) immunostimulation, and (6) TSA-reactive suppressor T lymphocytes (Ts cells). These escape mechanisms are summarized in Fig. 10-16.

Cancer cells can regulate their expression of cell surface molecules, including TSA. A number of agents, such as cyclic-AMP (cAMP), interferons, interleukins, growth factors, tumor promoters, and retinoic acid, can cause modulation of tumor antigens, such as CEA, TAG-72, and HLA-DR (Guadagni et al., 1991; McKeever, Davenport, & Shakui, 1991). Cancer cells also can mask their TSA by biochemical modifications. Human glioma cells (tumors of the central nervous system) can mask surface antigens with a hyaluronic acid–rich glycosaminoglycan coat. Modulated and masked TSAs are not recognized by the antibodies or cells that mediate effective antitumor immune responses.

Some tumors secrete soluble **immunosuppressive substances** like prostaglandins. Prostaglandin E increases cellular cAMP levels in lymphocytes. As a result, lymphocyte proliferation is blocked and clonal expansion of TSA-reactive T lymphocytes cannot occur. This weakens the overall immune response to the tumor.

Tumors arise from a single transformed cell. During progression, cancer cells are actively dividing to increase the tumor mass and changes to the original transformed cell phenotype occur. When a tumor reaches a detectable size, the cells within it are a heterogenous mixture of subclones. Such a process can facilitate **escape** from host defense mechanisms. This is especially true under conditions in which daughter cells lose or modify their TSA.

Experiments show that some tumors are rejected when a large number of cells are transplanted into a syngeneic host. When fewer cells of the same tumor are transplanted, however, tumors eventually grow in the syngeneic recipients. This observation led to the theory of **sneaking through.** Because tumors originate from a single transformed cell, it is possible that small amounts of TSA are not immunogenic. When a tumor reaches a size where enough antigen is expressed to stimulate an immune response, it is too large, with too many rapidly growing cells, to be eliminated by the immune system.

Blocking factor, or **blocking antibodies,** can be found in the sera of tumor-bearing animals and in some individuals with cancer. Blocking antibodies bind TSA but do not activate complement or function in ADCC responses. Blocking antibodies inhibit tumor rejection by (1) masking TSA, (2) forming antigen-antibody complexes that cannot be processed by antigen-presenting cells, and (3) inhibiting CTL interaction with the tumor.

Prehn (1971) has shown that a "little" **immunologic stimulation** enhances tumor cell growth. When mouse tumor cells were mixed with an optimal number of CTLs and transplanted to syngeneic hosts, the tumors were rejected. In contrast, when tumor cells were mixed with suboptimal numbers of CTL, the tumors grew faster than implants of tumor cells alone. Similar results were obtained when TSA-reactive antibodies were used as the immunologic stimulator. Prehn's studies suggest that in the early phases of an immune response, CTL infiltration into the tumor mass stimulates cancer cell growth. Tumor-infiltrating macrophages appear to have the same growth-enhancing effect.

The various effector functions of the immune system are carefully regulated to avoid potential destruction of normal tissues. One way that the immune system is controlled is by antigen-specific **suppressor T lymphocytes** (Ts cells) (see Fig. 10-16). These Ts cells can be elicited by various antigens expressed by progressively growing tumors (Naor & Duke-Cohan, 1986). Suppressor T-lymphocyte cells function by (1) blocking other types of immune responses, (2) switching off an ongoing immune response, or (3) modifying the magnitude or type of immune response that is elicited. Increases in the number of circulating Ts cells in the blood of individuals with cancer have been reported (Frentz, Bang, Munch-Petersen, & Wantzin, 1988).

Active suppression is an effective way for tumors to escape immunologic rejection. Induction of immune suppression by growing tumors may be caused by the immune system's inability to determine whether an actively dividing cell is detrimental (as with transformed cells) or beneficial (as with actively dividing bone marrow cells) to the host. This is a very complex problem because most cell surface molecules (antigens) present on tumor cells are also expressed by their normal cell counterparts.

In addition to antigen-specific Ts cells, **activated macrophages** can exert suppressive activity. Suppression of tumor immune response by macrophages is nonspecific, however, and results in a general depression of the immune system. The mechanism of suppression by macrophages is unknown but appears to be mediated by cytokines.

In conclusion, it appears that tumor growth or rejection depends on complex interactions between cancer cells and the immune system of their host. A range of immunologic protective mechanisms have been identified that cause tumor lysis. Transformation processes, however, can select for cancer cells that escape the host's tumor surveillance system. Furthermore, many carcinogenic agents can cause immune suppression, making individuals more susceptible to the growth of neoplasia.

Cancer: A Disease of Growth, Division, and Cell Differentiation

1 Abnormal cells that disobey the social control mechanisms of normal cell division proliferate to form tumors in the body.

2 Cell division is regulated by different combinations of protein growth factors presumably made by several "social control genes."

3 Two mutational routes result in uncontrolled cell proliferation: (1) stimulation of a gene causing *hyperactivity* and (2) *inhibition* of a gene causing inactivity. Hyperactivity is the result of a mutation causing overexpression of a growth gene. The gene is called an oncogene. Initiation or inactivation of the cell's particular differentiation gene frees the cell of controlled growth. The inactivated or deleted gene is called a tumor-suppressor gene.

4 Another type of genetic change can lead to cancer—those caused by tumor viruses.

5 Cancer cells are characterized by anaplasia, or loss of differentiation, and autonomy, or independence from normal cellular controls.

6 In the adult, undifferentiated cells (not totally committed to a specific function) are known as pluripotent cells, precursor cells, or stem cells. Cancer cells become more like embryonic cells and are less differentiated. Cancerous growth depends on derangements of cell differentiation.

Characteristics of Cancer Cells

1 The degree of disorganization varies among tumors, but disordered nuclear and structural components of cells are common.

2 Decreased communication or signalling between cells is the result of alterations in the surface. Because glycolipid and glycoprotein content is reduced, cellular communication is thought to be reduced.

3 Loss of fibronectin contributes to the overall loss in shape, cell-to-cell adhesion, and cellular migration.

4 Cancer cells exhibit anchorage independence with decreased cell-cell and cell–extracellular-matrix attachments. Without anchorage, cancerous cells are allowed to metastasize.

5 Tumor metastasis has been related to changes in intercellular communication. Gap junctions are important in regulating communication and are thought to be disrupted or blocked in cancer cells.

6 Tumor cell markers are substances, such as hormones, enzymes, genes, antigens, and antibodies, that denote specific tumors.

7 Several intercellular changes occur in cancer cells, including alterations in the cytoskeleton, density-dependent inhibition of growth, growth requirements, and changes in the nucleus and cell protein.

The Genetics of Cancer

1 In rare families, cancer is inherited in an autosomal dominant fashion. The mechanism by which environmental agents cause cancer is reportedly through increasing the frequency of mutation in somatic cells. Most human cancers, however, appear to arise without any known prior exposure to a carcinogenic agent.

2 Cancer-causing genes, oncogenes, can be introduced into an individual (e.g., by oncogenic viruses) or inherited within some families.

3 The three main types of oncogenic DNA viruses are papovaviruses, adenoviruses, and herpesviruses. An example of an oncogenic RNA virus is human T-cell leukemia-lymphoma virus.

4 Oncogenic viruses possess specific oncogenes called v-onc.

5 It is now known that cellular oncogenes, c-onc, are incorporated into the genomes of a variety of different organisms, including humans.

6 The term *proto-oncogene* is used to refer collectively to the various c-onc. The term proto-oncogene indicates that c-onc and v-onc genes were probably derived from a common prototype gene.

7 Proto-oncogenes encode for growth factors, growth factor receptors, signal transducers, nuclear proteins, and tumor-suppressor proteins.

8 Viruses may cause mutations in surviving (e.g., infected) cells that could lead to neoplastic changes. Most oncogenic viruses cause transformation by a mechanism called insertional mutagenesis. Here the viral genes are incorporated into the host's genome at specific sites. The inserted genes are associated with cell transformation.

9 During some viral infections, the host's immune system can become compromised, allowing neoplastic cells to emerge that would otherwise be rejected.

10 Tumor-suppressor genes encode for proteins that act as inhibitors of growth factor stimulation. Tumor-suppressor gene proteins block specific phases of the cell cycle, induce end-stage (e.g., terminal) differentiation, and stimulate cell senescence or death. Carcinogenesis involves inactivation of tumor-suppressor genes and activation of oncogenes.

11 Certain tumors are known to be caused by epigenetic changes—or change in the pattern of gene expression without a change in the DNA sequence.

Carcinogenesis

1 Carcinogenesis is the process of tumor development.

2 Most evidence confirms that cancer has a monoclonal origin.

3 Because of the complexity of transformation processes, it is not surprising that cancers express multiple oncogenes and tumor-suppressor genes.

4 Researchers propose that gap junction intercellular communication is either blocked or down-regulated in transforming cancer cells and, therefore, communication between the transformed cancer cells and normal surrounding cells is lost.

5 One theory of carcinogenesis suggests that cancer development is a two-stage process: (1) an initiation stage that causes irreversible changes in DNA after exposure to a carcinogen and (2) a promotion stage in which the initiated cells become cancerous.

6 Initiators and promoters include hormones, drugs, environmental agents, and a variety of personal behaviors. Because the precise biochemical cause of cancer is unknown, these are actually risk factors associated with increased incidence of cancer.

7 Personal behaviors associated with increased cancer risk include smoking and chewing smokeless tobacco, as well as sexual and reproductive behavior.

8 Smoking is associated with cancers of the lung, bladder, larynx, oral cavity, esophagus, and kidney; lung cancer is related to inhalation of tobacco smoke, which contains known carcinogenic compounds.

9 Oral cancer is associated with "dipping snuff."

10 Dietary factors can act as cancer-promoting or cancer-inhibiting agents.

11 Vitamin A is known to block tumor production in animals and cancerous transformation in tissue cultures.

12 Obesity is associated with endometrial cancer, and high-fat diets are associated with endometrial, breast, and colon cancer.

13 Artificial additives and preservatives in food may include some compounds that are carcinogenic; particularly controversial is the use of nitrites, which react to form direct- or indirect-acting carcinogens when food is cooked.

14 Three primary mechanisms by which dietary factors affect cancer production are direct-acting carcinogens or their precursors; indirect-acting carcinogens; and dietary factors that affect transport, activation, and deactivation of carcinogens.

15 Direct-acting carcinogens may occur in natural foodstuffs, may be produced by cooking, and may be produced by microorganisms in stored foods.

16 Indirect-acting carcinogens provide compounds that act to form carcinogens in the body. Compounds currently being studied include nitrites, fats, and cholesterol.

17 Dietary factors that affect transport, activation, or deactivation of carcinogens include dietary fiber, which probably promotes rapid passage of food through the digestive tract, and selenium, which appears to destroy cytotoxic radicals when reacting at low levels.

18 Age at first sexual intercourse and number of sexual partners are related to development of cervical cancer.

19 Human papillomavirus appears to be the causal agent of warts and cervical cancer.

20 Pregnancy and childbearing seem to be protective factors against cancer of the endometrium, ovary, and breast; other reproductive factors related to decreased risk for breast cancer include late onset of menstruation and early menopause.

21 Air pollution is a concern for causing cancer because of inhalation of emissions including arsenicals, benzene, chloroform, vinyl chloride, and acrylonitrite. Indoor pollution is considered worse than outdoor pollution because of cigarette smoke and possibly radon gas.

22 Cancers of the upper respiratory tract, lung, bladder, and peritoneum are often attributed to occupational exposures, including asbestos, fossil fuels, dyes, rubber, and paint.

23 Ultraviolet sunlight causes basal cell and squamous cell carcinomas, is associated with malignant melanoma, and is also implicated in increasing the severity of xeroderma pigmentosum.

24 Ultraviolet light damages DNA, inhibits cell division, and can lead to cell death. Damaged DNA can cause cancer by misrepairing itself and creating mutagenic cells that are susceptible to tumor development.

25 Exposure to ionizing radiation is caused by emissions from x-rays, radioisotopes, and other radioactive sources, some of which are industry- or occupation-related exposures.

26 Ionizing radiation inhibits cell division, especially in lymphoid tissue, bone marrow, and intestinal epithelium, which contain normally short-lived, rapidly dividing cells.

27 Carcinogenesis can occur from radiation-induced mutations or cell transformations; mutations may be dominant or recessive and also may cause chromosome aberrations.

28 Genetic factors can alter the repair mechanisms for DNA, so that an individual is particularly sensitive to the carcinogenic effects of ionizing radiation.

29 Biologic variables that affect responses to radiation include the part and percentage of the body exposed, the individual's age or stage of development at the time of exposure, genetic integrity, drugs, and other disease processes.

30 Radiation exposure in the neonate, infant, or child also can cause growth retardation; the younger the child, the more vulnerable the child is to the effects of radiation.

31 For cancers that occur in hormone-responsive target tissues, hormones probably act as promoters of carcinogenesis rather than as primary carcinogens.

Immunobiology of Cancer

1 Cancer cells express tumor-associated antigens, which are not found on normal, nontransformed cells.

2 Tumor-specific antigens (TSAs) may be caused by synthesis of new molecules, by unmasking of potential tumor-associated antigen, by loss of plasma membrane components, by biochemical modification, or by release of intracellular components.

3 Tumor-specific antigens are generally classified as tumor-specific transplantation antigens (TSTAs) or cross-reactive, tumor-associated transplantation antigens (TATAs).

4 Tumor-specific transplantation antigens are apparently more immunogenic than TATAs and therefore produce a stronger immune response.

5 Tumor antigens include viral antigens, oncofetal antigens (alpha-fetoprotein and carcinoembryonic antigen), oncogene-related antigens, carbohydrate, and protein tumor antigens.

6 When a developing tumor expresses TSA, an immunologically competent host can recognize these antigens and produce a range of immune responses to reject the tumor.

7 In spite of the immune system's ability to reject cancer cells, some cancer cells are apparently capable of bypassing the host's immune surveillance and by "escaping" can cause cancer.

8 Proposed "immune surveillance escape mechanisms" include antigenic modulation, secretion of immunosuppressive substances, escape and sneaking through, selective stimulation of suppressor cells, production of blocking antibodies, and immunostimulation.

KEY TERMS

α-Fetoprotein (α-FP), 354
Activated macrophage, 360
Anaplasia, 322
Anchorage-independence, 328
Anchoring junction, 328
Autocrine stimulatory hypothesis, 333
Autonomy, 322
Autostimulation, 333
Blocking antibody, 360
Blocking factor, 360
Carcinoembryonic antigen (CEA), 355
Carcinogenesis, 339
Carcinoma, 325
Carcinoma in situ, 325
Cocarcinogen, 345
c-onc, 337
Density-dependent inhibition of growth, 332

Epigenetic change, 339
Escape, 360
Fibronectin, 328
Gap junction, 328
Glioma, 325
Grading, 323
Immortal stem cell, 340
Immunologic stimulation, 360
Immunosuppressive substance, 360
Initiation, 345
Insertional mutagenesis, 338
Leukemia, 325
Lymphoma, 325
Metastasize, 328
Mutagen, 335
Mutagenesis, 339
Oncofetal antigen, 354
Oncogene, 322
Oncogenic virus, 335
Progression, 327

Promotion, 345
Proto-oncogene, 322
Retrovirus, 336
Reverse transcriptase, 336
Sarcoma, 325
Sneaking through, 360
Stem cell, 323
Suppressor T lymphocyte, 360
Terminally differentiate, 340
Transformation, 322
Tumor cell marker, 328
Tumor immune surveillance theory, 353
Tumor-infiltrating lymphocyte (TIL), 357
Tumor-specific antigen (TSA), 353
Tumor suppressor gene, 322
Tumor virus, 322
Viral antigen, 353
v-onc, 337

REFERENCES

Adlercreutz, H. (1990). Western diet and Western diseases: Some hormonal and biochemical mechanisms and associations. *Scandinavian Journal of Clinical Laboratory Investigation, 50*(Suppl. 201), 3-23.

Alberts, B., Bray, D., Lewis, J., Raff, M., Roberts, K., & Watson, J. D. (1989). *Molecular biology of the cell* (2nd ed.). New York: Garland Press.

Alberts, J. M., & Cory, S. (1991). Transgenic models of tumor development. *Science, 254,* 1161-1167.

Albright, C. D., Grimley, P. M., Jones, R. T., Fontana, J. A., Keenan, K. P., & Resau, J. H. (1991). Cell-to-cell communication: A differential response to TGF-B in normal and transformed human bronchial epithelial cells. *Carcinogenesis, 12*(11), 1993-1999.

American Cancer Society (ACS). (1992). *Cancer facts & figures 1992.* New York: American Cancer Society.

American Cancer Society (ACS). (1993). *Cancer facts & figures 1993.* New York: American Cancer Society.

Ames, B. N. (1983). Dietary carcinogens and anticarcinogens. *Science, 221,* 1256.

Ames, B. N., Magaw, R., & Gold, L. S. (1987). Ranking possible carcinogenic hazards. *Science, 236,* 271-280.

Berenblum, I., & Shubik, P. (1947). A new quantitative approach to the study of the stages of chemical carcinogenesis in the mouse's skin. *British Journal of Cancer, 1,* 383-391.

Blott, W. J., & Fraumeni, J. F., Jr. (1982). Geographic epidemiology of cancer in the United States. In D. Schottenfield & J. F. Fraumeni, Jr. (Eds.), *Cancer epidemiology and prevention* (pp. 179-193). Philadelphia: Saunders.

Boutwell, R. K. (1964). Some biological aspects of skin carcinogenesis. *Progress in Experimental Tumor Research, 4,* 207-250.

Brinton, L. A. (1984). Etiologic factors for invasive and noninvasive cervical abnormalities. In E. B. Gold (Ed.), *The changing risk of disease in women: An epidemiologic approach.* Lexington, Mass: The Collamore Press.

Burnbaum, M. J., Haspel, H. C., & Rosen, O. M. (1987). Transformation of rat fibroblasts by FSV rapidly increases glucose transporter gene transcription. *Science, 235,* 1495-1497.

Campbell, B., & DéAmbrosis. (1990). Squamous cell carcinoma antigen in patients with cutaneous disorders. *Journal of the American Academy of Dermatology, 22,* 639-642.

Carroll, K. K. (1991). Dietary fats and cancer. *American Journal of Clinical Nutrition, 53*(4), 10654-10675.

Cooper, E. H. (1991). Tumor markers in prostatic cancer. *Scandinavian Journal of Clinical Laboratory Investigation, 206,* 42-51.

del Regato, J. A., Spjut, H. J., & Cox, J. D. (1985). *Ackerman and del Regato's cancer: Diagnosis, treatment, and prognosis* (6th ed.). St. Louis: Mosby–Year Book.

Demers, R. (1991). Overview of radon, lead, and asbestos exposure. *American Family Physician, 44*(5 Suppl.), 51S-52S, 55S-61S.

Devesa, S. S., & Diamond, E. L. (1980). Association of breast cancer and cervical cancer incidences with income and education among whites and blacks. *National Cancer Institute, 65,* 515-528.

Doll, R., & Peto, R. (1981). *The causes of cancer.* New York: Oxford University Press.

Donehower, L. A., Harvey, M., Slagle, B. L., McArthur, M. J., Montgomery, C. A., Jr., Butel, J. S., & Bradley, A. (1992). Mice deficient for p53 are developmentally normal but susceptible to spontaneous tumors. *Nature, 356,* 215-221.

Douglas, R. G., & Shaw, J. H. F. (1990). Metabolic effects of cancer. *British Journal of Surgery, 77,* 246-254.

Epstein, S. S., & Swartz, J. B. (1981). Fallacies of lifestyle cancer theories. *Nature, 289,* 127.

Ewing, J. (1940). *Neoplastic disease.* Philadelphia: Saunders.

Frentz, G., Bang, F. D. C., Munch-Petersen, B., & Wantzin, G. L. (1988). Increased number of circulating suppressor T-lymphocytes in sun-induced multiple skin cancer. *Cancer, 61,* 294-297.

Galucci, B. B. (1991). Cancer biology: Molecular and cellular aspects. In S. B. Baird, R. McCorkle, & M. Grant (Eds.), *Cancer nursing: A comprehensive textbook.* Philadelphia: Saunders.

Gazdar, A. F. (1992). Molecular markers for the diagnosis and prognosis of lung cancer. *Cancer, 69,* 1592-1599.

Guadagni, F., Roselli, M., Schlom, J., & Greiner, J. W. (1991). Regulation of human tumor antigen expression by biological response modifiers (BMRs). *Annual Ist Super Sanita, 27,* 71-78.

Hakomori, S. (1986). Glycosphingolipids. *Scientific American, 254,* 44-53.

Hakomori, S. (1991). Possible functions of tumor-associated carbohydrate antigens. *Current Opinions in Immunology, 3,* 646-653.

Hamada, J., Takeichi, N., & Kobayshi, H. (1988). Metastatic capacity and intercellular communication between normal cells and metastatic cell clones derived from a rat mammary carcinoma. *Cancer Research, 48*(18), 5129-5132.

Hamilton, S. R. (1992). Molecular genetic alterations as potential prognostic indicators in colorectal carcinoma. *Cancer, 69,* 1589-1591.

Hasler, C. M., Bennick, M. R., & Trosko, J. E. (1991). Inhibition of gap junction–mediated intercellular communication by alpha-linolenate. *Journal of Physiology, 261*(1pt1), 161-168.

Hausen, H. Z. (1991). Viruses in human cancers. *Science, 254,* 1167-1173.

Hellstrom, K. E., & Hellstrom, I. (1989). Oncogene associated tumor antigens as targets for immunotherapy. *Federation of the American Society of Experimental Biology Journal, 3,* 1715-1722.

Henderson, B. E., Ross, R. K., & Pike, M. C. (1991). Toward the primary prevention of cancer. *Cancer Science, 254,* 1131-1137.

Herbst, A. L., Ulteder, H., & Poskanzer, D. C. (1971). Adenocarcinomas of the vagina: Association of maternal stilbestrol therapy with tumor appearance in young females. *New England Journal of Medicine, 284,* 878-881.

Jenks, S. (1992). Researchers open a molecular window on radon damage in lung cancer. *Journal of the National Cancer Institute, 84*(7), 473-474.

Jorde, L. B., Carey, J. B., & White, R. L. (1995). *Medical genetics.* St. Louis: Mosby–Year Book (in press).

Kahn, P., & Graf, T. (Eds.). (1986). Malignant transformation as a multistep process. In *Oncogenes and growth control* (pp. 292-293). New York: Springer-Verlag.

Kelsey, J., & Gammon, M. D. (1991). The epidemiology of breast cancer. *CA—A Cancer Journal for Clinicians, 41*(3), 146-165.

Kojima, N., & HaKomori, S. (1991). Cell adhesion, spreading, and motility of GM3-expressing cells based on glycolipid-glycolipid interaction. *Journal of Biological Chemistry, 226*(26), 17552-17558.

Konishi, N., Donovan, P. J., & Waro, J. M. (1990). Differential effects of renal carcinogenesis tumor promoter on growth promotion and inhibition of gap junctional communication. *Carcinogenesis, 11*(6), 903-908.

Krutovskikh, V. A., Oyamada, M., & Yamasaki, H. (1991). Sequential changes of gap-junctional intercellulars during multistage rat liver carcinogenesis: Direct measure of communication in vivo. *Carcinogenesis 12*(9), 1701-1706.

Kupchella, C. E. (1990). Cellular biology of cancer. In S. L. Groenwald et al. (Eds.), *Cancer nursing: Principles and practice* (2nd ed.). Boston: Jones & Bartlett.

Lacassagne, A. (1932). Appartition de cancers de la mamelle dez la souvis male soumis a des injections de folliculine. *Comptes Rendus Academie des Sciences, 195,* 630-632.

Leslie, K. O., & Howard, P. (1992). Oncogenes and antioncogenes in human breast carcinoma. *Pathology Annual, 27* (Pt. 1), 321-342.

Lovejoy, N. C., Thomas, M. L., Halliburton, P., & Mimvaugh, L. (1987). Tumor markers: Relevance to clinical practice. *Oncology Nursing Forum, 14*(5), 75-82.

Maniatis, T., Goodbrown, S., & Fischer, J. A. (1987). Regulation of inducible and tissue-specific gene expression. *Science, 236,* 1244.

Marx, J. L. (1986). The yin and yang of cell growth. *Science, 232,* 1093-1096.

Marx, J. L. (1988). Cell growth control takes balance. *Science, 239,* 975-976.

McCance, K. L., & Huether, S. E. (1990). *Pathophysiology: The basis for disease in adults and children.* St. Louis: Mosby–Year Book.

McIntire, K. R. (1985). Tumor markers. In V. T. DeVita, S. Hellman, & S. A. Rosenberg (Eds.), *Cancer: Principles and practice of oncology* (vol. 1, 2nd ed.). Philadelphia: Lippincott.

McKeever, P. E., Davenport, R. D., & Shakui, P. (1991). Patterns of antigenic expression of human glioma cells. *Critical Review of Neurobiology, 6,* 119-147.

Merino, M. J., Monteagudo, C., & Neumann, R. D. (1991). Monoclonal antibodies for radioimmunoscintigraphy of breast cancer. *Nuclear Medicine and Biology, 18,* 437-443.

Micha, J. P. (1984). Genital warts: Treatable warning of cancer. *The Female Patient, 9,* 31-34.

Miki, H., Yamadori, I., Ursula, I. H., Kenney, S., Riggs, C. W., & Rice. J. W. (1990). Effect of TPA on intercellular communication in various clones of mouse epidermal cells. *Cancer Research, 50,* 1323-1329.

Moodie, R. L. (1923). *Paleopathology.* Urbana: University of Illinois Press.

Moosa, A. R., Robson, M. C., & Schimpff, S. C. (Eds.). (1986). *Comprehensive textbook of oncology.* Baltimore: Williams & Wilkins.

Naftzger, C., & Houghton, A. N. (1991). Tumor immunology. *Current Opinions in Oncology, 3*(1), 93-99.

Naor, D., & Duke-Cohan, J. S. (1986). Suppressor cells and malignancy. I. Suppressor macrophages and suppressor T-cells in experimental animals. In P. K. Ray (Ed.), *Advances in immunity and cancer therapy* (pp. 1-130). New York: Springer-Verlag.

Odeleye, O. E., Watson, R. R., Eskelson, C. D., & Mufti, S. I. (1990). Dietary polyunsaturated fatty acid promoter peroxidation and its role in the promotion of cancer. *Advances in Experimental Medical Biology, 283,* 789-791.

Ostrow, R. S., Zachow, K. R., Niimura, M., Okagaki, T., Muller, S., Bender, M., & Faras, A. J. (1986). Detection of papilloma virus DNA in human semen. *Science, 231,* 731-733.

Penn, I. (1981). Depressed immunity and the development of cancer. *Clinical and Experimental Immunology, 46,* 459-474.

Pitot, H. C. (1986). *Fundamentals of oncology* (3rd ed., p. 532). New York: Dekker.

Pott, P. (Reprinted, 1981). Chirugical observations relative to the cataract, polyps of the nose, the cancer of the scrotum, the different kinds of rupture and the mortification of the toes and feet [London, 1775]. In R. Doll & R. Peto (Eds.), *Causes of cancer.* New York: Oxford University Press.

Prehn, R. T. (1971). Perspectives on oncogenesis: Does immunity stimulate or inhibit neoplasia? *Journal of the Reticuloendothelial Society, 10,* 1.

Prentice, R. L., & Thomas, D. B. (1987). On the epidemiology of oral contraceptives and disease. *Advances in Cancer Research, 49,* 285-401.

Quan, M. B., & Moy, R. L. (1991). The role of human papillomavirus in carcinoma. *Journal of the American Academy of Dermatology, 25,* 698-702.

Renard, E. P., Goydan, R., & Stolki, T. (1992). Permeation of multifunctional acrylates through selected protective glove materials. *American Indiana Hygiene Association Journal, 53*(2), 117-123.

Rohan, T. E., & McMichael, A. J. (1988). Alcohol consumption and risk of breast cancer. *International Journal of Cancer, 41,* 695-699.

Rous, P., & Kidd, J. G. (1941). Conditional neoplasms and subthreshold neoplastic states. *Journal of Experimental Medicine, 73,* 365.

Rubin, P., Bakemeier, R. F., & Krackov, S. K. (Eds.). (1984). *Clinical oncology for medical students and physicians: A multidisciplinary approach* (6th ed.). New York: American Cancer Society.

Ruddon, R. (1981). *Cancer biology.* New York: Oxford University Press.

Ruiz-Cabello, F., Klein, E., & Garrido, F. (1991). MHC antigens on human tumors. *Immunology Letters, 29,* 181-190.

Rusch, H. P. (1983). History of research on cancer causation. In S. B. Kahn, R. R. Love, C. Sherman, & R. Chakravarty (Eds.), *Concepts in cancer medicine.* New York: Grune & Stratton.

Sachs, L. (1987). The molecular control of blood cell development. *Science, 238,* 1374-1379.

Scotto, J., Fears, T. R., & Gori, G. B. (1976). *Measurements of ultraviolet radiation in the United States and comparisons with skin cancer data* (DHEW Publication No. NIH 76-1029, pp. 3.1-3.10). Washington, DC: U.S. Government Printing Office.

Scotto, J., Pitcher, H., & Lee, J. A. H. (1991). Indications of future decreasing trends in skin-melanoma mortality among whites in the United States. *International Journal of Cancer, 49,* 390-407.

Shamberger, R. J., Tytko, S. A., & Willis, C. E. (1976). Antioxidants and cancer VI: Selenium and age adjusted human cancer mortality. *Archives of Environmental Health, 31,* 231-235.

Simopoulos, A. P. (1991). Omega-3 fatty acids in health and disease and in growth and development. *American Journal of Clinical Nutrition, 54*(3), 438-463.

Solomon, E., Borrow, J., & Goddard, A. D. (1991). Chromosome aberrations and cancer. *Science, 254,* 1153-1160.

Souhami, R. L. (1992). The antigens of lung cancer. *Thorax, 47,* 153-156.

Spingarn, N. E., Slocum, L. A., & Weisburger, J. H. (1980). Formation of mutagens in cooked foods II: foods with high starch content. *Cancer Letters, 9,* 7-12.

Srivastava, P. K., & Maki, R. G. (1991). Stress-induced proteins in immune response to cancer. *Current Topics in Microbiology and Immunology, 167,* 109-123.

Trosko, J. E., & Chang, C. C. (1989). Stem cell theory of carcinogenesis. *Toxicology Letters, 4*(2-3), 283-295.

Trosko, J. E., Chang, C. C., & Madhuker, B. V. (1990). Symposium: Cell communication in normal and uncontrolled growth. Modulation of intercellular communication during radiation and chemical carcinogens. *Radiation Research, 123,* 241-251.

Urban, J. L., & Schreiber, H. (1992). Tumor antigens. *Annual Review of Immunology, 10,* 617-644.

Vahakangas, K. H., Samet, J. M., Metcalf, R. A., Welsh, J. A., Bennett, W. P., Lane, D. P., & Harris, C. C. (1992). Mutations of p53 and ras genes in radon-associated lung cancer from uranium miners. *Lancet, 339* (8793), 576-580.

Vaickus, L., Ball, E. D., & Foon, K. A. (1991). Immune markers in hematologic malignancies. *Critical Review of Oncology and Hematology, 11,* 267-297.

Wahren, B., & Harmenbert, U. (1991). Tumour markers in gastrointestinal cancer. *Scandinavian Journal of Clinical Laboratory Investigation, 206* [Suppl.], 21-27.

Watson, J. D., Hopkins, N. H., Roberts, J. W., Steitz, J. A., & Weiner, A. M. (1987). *Molecular biology of the gene: Vol. II, Specialized aspects* (4th ed., pp. 747-1163). Menlo Park, CA: Benjamin/Cummings.

Weber, G. (1977). Enzymology of cancer cells I. *New England Journal of Medicine, 296,* 486-492.

Weinberg, R. A. (1991). Tumor suppressor genes. *Science, 254,* 1138-1146.

White, R. L. (1995). Cancer genetics. In L. B. Jorde, J. B. Carey, & R. L. White, *Medical Genetics.* St. Louis: Mosby (in press).

Willett, W. C., Stampfer, M. J., Colditz, G. A., Rosner, B. A., Hennekens, C. H., & Speizer, F. E. (1987). Fat and the risk of breast cancer. *New England Journal of Medicine, 316*(1), 22-28. St. Louis: Mosby (in press).

Yarbro, J. W. (1992). Oncogenes and tumor suppressor genes. *Seminars in Oncology Nursing 8*(1), 30-39.

Young, T. B. (1989). A case-control study of breast cancer and alcohol consumption habits. *Cancer, 64,* 552-558.

SUGGESTED READINGS

American Association of Dermatologists (AAD). (1991). Guidelines for care of squamous cell carcinoma. *AAD Bulletin, 9,* 6-9.

Colcher, D., Milenic, D. E., Ferroni, P., Roselli, M., & Schlom, J. (1991). In vivo and in vitro clinical applications of monoclonal antibodies against TAG-72. *Nuclear Medicine and Biology, 18,* 395-401.

Epstein, S. S., & Swartz, J. B. (1988). Technical comments: Carcinogenic risk estimates. *Science, 240,* 1043-1045.

Williams, G. M. (1987). DNA reactive and epigenetic carcinogens. In J. C. Barrett (Ed.), *Mechanisms of environmental carcinogenesis* (vol. 1, p. 113). Boca Raton, FL: CRC Press.

Tumor Metastasis in Adults and Cancer in Children

Kathryn L. McCance

Lee K. Roberts

Kathleen Hardin Mooney

Chapter Outline

The major cause of illness and death as a result of most human malignant diseases is metastasis. Approximately 40% to 50% of malignant tumors are cured by current therapies (Liotta, 1991). However, most individuals who have malignant tumors suffer from multiple metastases, too small to be detected, at the time the primary tumor is treated. Consequently, an important goal is to develop new therapies or analytic approaches that can be used for accurate prediction of the metastatic potential of a tumor. The hope is that such therapies will be derived from cell-molecular research into the mechanism of invasion and metastases. Basic research in this important field has lagged behind attention to cancer prob-

lems such as carcinogenesis and cancer genetics. Because of the complexities of the metastatic process, investigators only recently have attempted to study the biochemical mechanisms of cancer invasion (Liotta, 1991).

HISTORICAL THEORIES OF CANCER INVASION

Critical to understanding current research approaches to invasion and metastasis is knowing, historically, where we have been. Table 11-1 reviews the evolution of research on cancer invasion and metastasis.

TUMOR SPREAD

Tumor spread throughout the body can take several forms: (1) direct invasion of contiguous organs or local spread, (2) metastasis to distant organs by lymphatics and veins, and (3) metastases by implantation (del Regato, Spjut, & Cox, 1985). Spreading of a tumor depends on its rate of growth, its degree of differentiation, the anatomic presence or absence of barriers, and other unknown biologic factors.

Local Spread

Invasion, or local spread, is a prerequisite for metastasis and the first step in the metastatic process. In its earliest stages, local invasion may occur as a function of direct tumor extension (Hubbard & Liotta, 1991). Eventually, however, cells or clumps of cells become detached from the primary tumor and invade the surrounding interstitial spaces. Possible mechanisms thought to be important in local invasion include (1) cellular multiplication, (2) mechanical pressure, (3) release of lytic enzymes, (4) decreased cell-to-cell adhesion (making cancer cells "slippery"), and (5) increased motility of individual tumor cells (Fidler, Gersten, & Hart, 1978; Franks & Teich, 1986; Hubbard & Liotta, 1991; Liotta, 1991).

TABLE 11-1

Historical Development of the Cellular Theory of Cancer Invasion and Metastasis

Time frame	Theory proposal
Hippocrates (460-370 B.C.)	First theory on cancer invasion; cancer was a disease of black bile leakage into tissue; black bile diffusion theory (imbalance)
Galen (A.D.131-203)	Rejected the notion of an imbalance of black bile; proposed black bile concentrated in areas of invasion (humoral theory)
Paracelsus (1493-1541)	Revised humoral theory that cancer invasion was caused by diffusion of mineral salts
Morgagni (1682-1771)	Performed numerous deposits and described cancer deposits in the liver
Müller (1828)	Established cellular origin of cancer
Recamier (1829)	First to propose that invasion and metastasis were the result of translocation of cells; first to use the term *metastasis*—Recamier was not properly acknowledged for this finding
Virchow (1821-1902)	Was convinced of the cellular nature of tumors but retained the humoral diffusion theory
Thiersch (1822-1895)	Refuted the humoral concept, demonstrated that invasion was a process starting from the primary tumor; reported that cancer cells reached the lymph nodes by cellular embolism (cellular-embolic theory); by the end of the 19th century, the cellular theory had become firmly established
Paget (late 1800s)	First to speculate about the factors that promote cellular "seeding" or tumor cells (seed versus soil theory)
Tyzzer (early 1900s)	First scientist to develop an experimental model of metastasis
1900s-1970s	Tumor invasion and metastasis thought to be the result of passive growth pressure and low tumor cell cohesiveness
1960s-1970s	Active mechanisms of tumor growth were investigated (e.g., what mechanisms facilitated the movement of tumor cells through host barriers); possible mechanisms included tumor cell mobility, lytic enzymes, and secretions of other factors
1980s-present	Continuation of mechanisms of tumor growth with a recent emphasis on the *biochemical mechanisms*

Cellular Multiplication

The aforementioned mechanisms are not mutually exclusive, and it is likely that in a given tumor any combination of the five may be involved. Invasion depends on the rate of cellular multiplication, which is a function of the cell generation time (through the cell cycle), the number of cells that are dividing (growth fraction), and the cell loss from the tumor. Cells from malignant lesions thus can divide rapidly, but the tumor may not grow because a number of cells are rapidly dying. (The cell cycle is discussed in Chapters 1 and 10.)

Mechanical Invasion

Invasion, in relation to mechanical pressure, is analogous to the way in which plants force their roots through the soil (i.e., by building up pressure that forces sheets, fingerlike projections, along the lines of least mechanical resistance). Pressure from the growing mass blocks local blood vessels, leading to local tissue death and a reduction in mechanical resistance that further aids the spread.

Lytic Enzymes

Areas of normal host tissue adjacent to areas of tumor invasion show considerable amounts of lytic damage. Because many animal and human tumors have higher levels of hydrolases (e.g., proteases and collagenases, plasminogen activators, and lysosomal enzymes) than do corresponding normal tissue, the concept that malignant tumors produce and secrete lytic enzymes that destroy normal tissue has become firmly established. Tumor cells can either release collagenase (e.g., digest collagen) or secrete collagenolytic substances in latent forms that are converted to activate collagenase by lysosomal proteases such as plasmin (Hubbard & Liotta, 1991). Collagens are the major structural elements of the extracellular matrices where invasion begins (see p. 370). Tumor-derived collagenases that break down interstitial collagen types I, II, and III have been identified by several investigators (Liotta, 1991). However, type IV collagen, the structural element of the vascular basement membrane, is resistant to interstitial collagens. A type IV–specific collagenase that is increased in the cells of many highly metastatic tumors has been identified (Garbisa et al., 1987). Expression of this collagenase can be induced experimentally by interaction with the *ras*[H] oncogene (see Chapter 10). These data provide additional support for the hypothesis that metastatic phenotypes can be induced by the action of certain oncogenes.

A number of other proteases that are attached to or released from the cell surface appear to increase tumor invasion through proteolysis, including heparinases and serine proteases such as plasminogen activator. Plasminogen activator is increased in tumor cells (Hubbard & Liotta, 1991). Plasminogen activator converts the serum proenzyme plasminogen into the protease plasmin, which can degrade a variety of proteins. It is believed that plasminogen activator plays an important role in the degradation of the extracellular matrix during tumor cell invasion. Protease inhibitors can be produced by the host or by the tumor cells themselves (Liotta, 1991).

Decreased Cell Adhesion

Cancer cells do not adhere to one another as well as normal cells. The "slippery" trait has partially been related to fibronectin. Fibronectin can regulate cell attachment, spreading, phagocytosis, and various effects on cell structure. It also stimulates cell movement. Cancer cells may make a defective type of fibronectin or they may break down fibronectin as they make it (Kupchella, 1990). Low levels or loss of this anchoring molecule, fibronectin, may help cancer cells "slip" between normal cells in the process of invasion.

Increased Motility

Cell movement is key for tumor cells to invade and traverse necessary stages in the invasion process. Such stages include the detachment and subsequent infiltration of cells from the primary tumor into adjacent tissue, as well as the migration of cells through the vascular wall into the circulation (intravasation) and out of the vascular wall (extravasation) into a secondary site (Fig. 11-1). Data suggest that tumor cells actually may move under their own power by means of chemotactic factors referred to as *autocrine motility factors*. Investigators have identified motility factors from melanoma (a type of skin cancer) cells (Liotta et al., 1986). Thus the **autocrine motility factor hypothesis** specifies that the tumor cell secretes a factor that binds to a specific receptor on the cell surface and stimulates motility. In this way the tumor cell acquires independent and continuous stimulation of its motile behavior, which is necessary for invasion (Liotta, 1991).

The Three-Step Theory of Invasion

A three-step theory has been proposed to describe the sequence of biochemical events during tumor cell invasion of the extracellular matrix (Fig. 11-2). The three steps include tumor cell attachment to the matrix, degradation or dissolution of the matrix, and locomotion into the matrix. The first step, attachment, is mediated by specific attachment factors such as laminin, a complex glycoprotein that is a major constituent of all basement membranes. Membrane vesicles on the cell surface of tumor cells are rich in laminin receptors that enable their attachment to basement membrane (Liotta, 1991). Laminin forms a bridge between the cell-surface **laminin receptor** and type IV collagen (see Fig. 11-2). Once

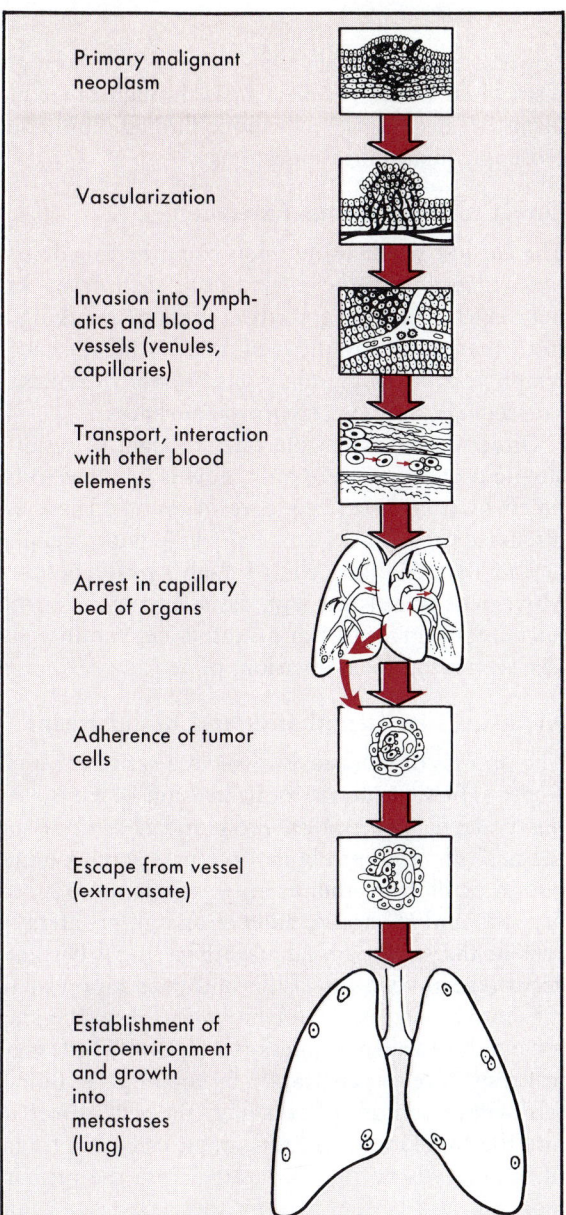

Primary malignant
neoplasm

Vascularization

Invasion into lymph-
atics and blood
vessels (venules,
capillaries)

Transport, interaction
with other blood
elements

Arrest in capillary
bed of organs

Adherence of tumor
cells

Escape from vessel
(extravasate)

Establishment of
microenvironment
and growth
into
metastases
(lung)

FIG. 11-1 Pathogenesis of metastasis. Initial neoplastic transformation of susceptible cells gives rise to a small population of tumor cells. Vascularization of this initial neoplastic lesion allows further proliferation of tumor cells and enlargement of the primary tumor. Malignant cells within the primary tumor next begin to invade the surrounding host tissue(s). Entry of invading tumor cells into lymphatics or blood vessels serves to transport them to distant sites in the body, where they lodge and become arrested in the capillary beds of various organs. For illustrative purposes, this figure shows arrest of malignant cells in the lung capillary bed. The arrested cells then exit from capillaries into the surrounding lung parenchyma where, subject to provision of a suitable environment, they proliferate to form metastases. (From Poste & Fidler, 1980.)

1. Attachment   2. Dissolution   3. Locomotion

Tumor cell

Basement
membrane

Laminin
receptor   Laminin   Type IV   Type IV
collagen   collagenase

FIG. 11-2 The three-step hypothesis of tumor invasion: attachment, dissolution, and locomotion. Step 1 is tumor cell attachment to the extracellular matrix. Surface receptors on the tumor cell (laminin receptors) bind to parts of the basement membrane (laminin) in the extracellular matrix. Step 2 is degradation of the matrix by tumor cell proteases (collagenase IV). The anchored tumor cell either secretes proteolytic enzymes or causes the host cell to secrete the proteolytic enzymes that degrade the matrix in a region very close to the tumor cell surface. Step 3 is the migration (locomotion) of the tumor cell through the degraded basement membrane. During this phase, pseudopodia (fingerlike projections) of the tumor cell cross the basement membrane, enabling the cell to extravasate from the blood vessel into the interstitial tissue. (Modified from Hubbard & Liotta, 1991.)

FIG. 11-3 **Pseudopodia.** Photograph of electron microscopy of a breast cancer cell with fingerlike projections called *pseudopodia*. (Source: National Library of Medicine.)

anchored, the tumor cell in the second step either secretes proteolytic enzymes or induces host cells to produce them, and degradation of the matrix, or step two, begins. Such enzymes may degrade both the attachment proteins and the structural collagenous proteins of the matrix. **Type IV collagenase,** a powerful proteolytic enzyme, may outnumber the natural protease inhibitors present in the matrix. The third step is tumor cell locomotion into the degraded region of the matrix. Fingerlike projections called *pseudopodia*, which extend from the tumor cell (Fig. 11-3), facilitate movement by attaching to blood vessel walls that traverse the basement membrane. The tumor cells then extravasate from the vasculature into the interstitial stroma. Theoretically, invasion occurs by cyclic repetition of these steps. The direction of locomotion may be influenced by chemotactic factors (see autocrine motility factors, p. 368).

Patterns of Spread: Metastasis

Metastasis, the spread of cancer cells from a primary site of origin to a distant site, is the life-threatening characteristic of malignancy. Local invasion is a condition of metastases. Methods exist for successfully eradicating **primary tumors** (original sites of tumor origin); yet the real challenge for reducing cancer mortality is controlling metastasis because removal of the primary tumor does not affect the proliferating growth at other sites. Often the primary tumor is not even diagnosed before secondary spread occurs. Three basic mechanisms of metastasis exist: direct or continuous extension, lymphatic spread, and bloodstream dissemination. These mechanisms, however, are not mutually exclusive. Tumor cell spread or dissemination through one mecha-

nism often facilitates metastasis through other mechanisms because tumor cells move through numerous microscopic anatomic connections.

Direct or Continuous Extension

The earliest result of invasion could be called *continuous extension* (Kupchella, 1990). Cancerous tumors may extend into several areas without breaking away from the parent tumor, including (1) tissue spaces, (2) lymph vessels, (3) blood vessels, (4) body cavities (serosal seeding), and (5) cerebrospinal spaces.

Direct tumor extension, once thought to result from simple growth pressure only, now is believed to be initiated by a complex sequence of events. These events, discussed earlier, are initiated by loss of intracellular adhesion that enables cells to "slip" past one another. Movement of cells through tissue barriers is further influenced by proteases and (autocrine) motility factors (see section on local invasion, p. 367).

Metastasis by Lymphatics and Bloodstream

The process of metastasis involves a series of sequential steps: (1) extension or local invasion of the surrounding tissue; (2) penetration into blood vessels or lymphatics, or both, and into body cavities; (3) release into the lymph or blood circulation; (4) transport to a secondary site; and (5) arrest, adherence, and proliferation of cells at the secondary site (see Fig. 11-1). Distant cancer spread involves invasion and penetration of tumor cells into blood vessels or lymphatics, or both. Lymphatics and thin-walled venules offer relatively little mechanical resistance to penetration by tumor cells. Blood vessels within tumors offer malignant cells direct access into the circulation. Clusters, single cells, and fragments of tumor cells become separated from the primary tumor site and disseminate by these routes. Clumps of cells have a better chance of successful metastasis than do single cells. Those that arise close to a serous surface can invade through that surface, implant, and become distant metastases. These effusions, also known as *seeding*, occur in the pleural space surrounding the lung and in the peritoneal space surrounding the abdominal cavity.

The most common route for distant metastases is through the lymphatics. Tumors generally lack a well-formed lymphatic network (Hubbard & Liotta, 1991). Lymphatic channels occur at the periphery of the tumor and not within the tumor mass. Tumor cells entering the lymphatic vessels are carried to regional lymph nodes. For many types of cancer, the first evidence of distant spread is a mass in the regional lymph node. An enlarged axillary lymph node, for example, may signal breast cancer; an enlarged inguinal node may indicate a malignant melanoma; an enlarged mesenteric node may be caused by cancer of the gastrointestinal tract.

Initially, regional lymph nodes may exert a barrier effect, preventing the further spread of tumor cells into the lymphatic system. Host defenses, such as macrophages and natural killer cells, play an important role in the elimination of circulating tumor cells (Hubbard & Liotta, 1991). Several events can occur in a cancer cell that becomes lodged in lymph nodes, including (1) death as a result of local inflammatory reaction, (2) death because of an incompatible local environment, (3) growth into a discernable lump, (4) sustained dormancy for unknown reasons, or (5) detachment from the nodes and entrance into the efferent lymphatics.

Penetrance of small lymphatic vessels causes the release of tumor cell emboli into these lymphatic vessels and is responsible for lymphatic metastasis. Shedding of emboli is influenced by changes in vessel pressure, by turbulent alterations in lymphatic flow, and by movements or manipulation of the tumor during diagnostic tests or surgery. Tumor cells eventually move into the regional or systemic venous drainage because of numerous venolymphatic communications.

Hematogenous spread is a complex process that requires tumor cells to penetrate and detach from blood vessels and spread to distant organs. Yet it is known that vascularized tumors shed malignant cells constantly as they grow, often releasing millions of cells without producing metastases (Fidler et al., 1978; Liotta, Kleinerman, & Saidel, 1974). To establish metastasis, tumor cells must "escape" host defenses, survive mechanical trauma in the bloodstream, and lodge in the vascular bed of the target organ (Hubbard & Liotta, 1991). About 80% of the tumor cells circulate as single cells and attach directly to the endothelial surface or to pre-existing regions of exposed subendothelial basement membrane (Liotta, 1991). Emboli or tumor cells that contain leukocytes, fibrin, or platelets can cause direct embolization in the precapillary venules by mechanical action. The formation of a fibrin-platelet complex is thought to protect tumor cells within the emboli from host defenses and to assist successful attachment to the vascular epithelium (Hubbard & Liotta, 1991). Once arrested in a blood vessel, tumor cells can actively invade the vascular wall and interstitial stroma and invade the parenchyma of the target organ. Growth in the target organ parenchyma requires the development of a vascular network (angiogenesis) and continued escape of host defenses.

Angiogenesis and Angiogenesis Factors

Growth of cancerous colonies probably depends on an adequate blood supply. Investigators have demonstrated that tumor implants cannot grow more than a few millimeters in diameter without developing new blood vessels to "feed" them, a process called **angiogenesis** (Folkman, Merler, Abernathy, & Williams, 1971). It has been suggested that development of blood vessels is the result of diffusible substances, *tumor-angiogenesis factor* (TAF), secreted by the tumor (see Fig. 11-1). Two different angiogenesis factors have been identified, a heparin-binding endothelial mitogen (an endothelial cell growth factor) and angiogenin (Fett et al., 1985; Shing et al., 1984). Researchers believe that angiogenin and the heparin-binding proteins may be members of a family of factors that induce and regulate the growth of new blood vessels. The development of a new capillary network involves many steps and is similar to the blood coagulation cascade in that one event triggers the next through the action of specific mediators.

The rate of spread, as well as the growth of the tumor, is correlated with tumor vascularity in clinical situations. For example, small-cell carcinoma of the lung arises in highly vascularized capillary beds and spreads easily and widely to other vascular organs such as the brain.

Growth of Metastases and Metastatic Potential

As noted earlier, the ability of a metastasis to grow and develop requires the development of a vascular network, evasion of host defenses, and a compatible environment ("the soil"). The metastatic potential of many common carcinomas is related to the size of the primary tumor. Although the reasons are unclear, it is likely that more aggressive tumor cells evolve into larger tumors (Hubbard & Liotta, 1991). Larger tumors also may overwhelm host defense mechanisms, thus favoring a survival of disseminated malignant cells. Breast cancer, colorectal carcinoma, transitional carcinoma of the bladder, carcinoma of the stomach, and squamous carcinoma of the lung all show a relationship between size and probability of metastases (Sugarbaker, 1981).

Distribution and Frequent Sites of Distant Metastases

Distant metastasis in many types of cancer appears to be the first capillary bed encountered by the circulating cells (Schirrmacher, 1985; Sugarbaker, 1981). Table 11-2 summarizes frequent sites of distant metastases in some types of cancer. Patterns of metastasis for certain other tumors, however, are not related to patterns of blood flow and the location of capillary beds (Dudjak, 1992; Goldfarb & Brunson, 1989). Ocular melanoma, for example, frequently metastasizes to the liver, and clear cell kidney carcinomas often spread to bone and the thyroid. Several mechanisms have been proposed to explain preferential growth in specific organs, collectively called *organ tropism*. These mechanisms include local growth factors or hormones present in the target organ, preferential adherence to the surface of certain target organs, and the presence of chemotactic factors that diffuse from the target organ and cause circulating

TABLE 11-2

Frequent Sites of Distant Metastasis in Some Types of Cancer

Primary tumor	Major anatomic pathways	Frequent site of distant metastasis
Lung	Pulmonary vein, left ventricle	Multiple organs, including brain
Colorectal	Mesenteric lymphatics, portal venous system	Liver
	Inferior vena cava, right ventricle, pulmonary artery	Lungs
Testicular	Lymphatics to the periaortic area to the subclavian veins to the right ventricle	Lungs, liver
Prostate	Batson plexus of paravertebral veins; ilium, lumbar spine	Bones, lung, liver, endocrine glands, central nervous system
Breast	Batson plexus of paravertebral veins, lymph nodes, superior vena cava	Bony skeleton, lungs
Head and neck	Direct extension, Batson plexus	Lymphatics, liver, bone
Ovarian	Direct extension	Peritoneal surfaces, diaphragm
	Omentum and mesenteric veins	Omentum, liver
Sarcoma (extremity)	Inferior vena cava, right ventricle, pulmonary artery	Lungs

tumor cells to extravasate from the vessel and aggregate in the target organ (Hubbard & Liotta, 1991). Evidence exists that organ tropism is determined genetically and that tumor cells contain organ-specific receptors that can discriminate between various vascular beds and preferentially "locate" to certain organs (Hubbard & Liotta, 1991).

CLINICAL MANIFESTATIONS OF CANCER

Pain

Usually little or no pain is associated with the early stages of malignant disease, but pain occurs in 60% to 80% of those who are terminally ill with cancer. Pain is strongly influenced by fear, anxiety, sleep loss, fatigue, and overall physical deterioration. Pain is known to occur through an interaction among psychogenic, cultural, and physiologic components. (The neurophysiology of pain is discussed in Chapter 13.)

General mechanisms that cause pain associated with cancer include pressure, obstruction, invasion of a sensitive structure, stretching of visceral surfaces, tissue destruction, and inflammation. Although the pain may be directly related to the malignancy, it can result from other problems such as infection. A common cause of pain is bone metastasis, but the pain may be referred away from the involved bone and might, for example, manifest as back pain. Bone pain can be caused by peri-

osteal irritation, medullary pressure, and pathologic fractures.

Abdominal pain often is caused by severe stretching from the tumor invasion of the hollow viscus. Tumors that obstruct and distend the bowel cause pain. Small-bowel obstructions in persons with known malignant disease are commonly the result of recurrent cancer, surgical adhesions, or new primary tumors. Surgery often is needed to obtain symptomatic relief. Enlargement of the liver from hepatic malignancies stretches the liver, resulting in a dull pain or a feeling of fullness over the right upper quadrant of the abdomen.

Tumor compression of nerve endings against a firm surface creates pain. Brain tumors have very little space to grow without compressing blood vessels and nerve endings between the tumor and the cranial vault. Tissue destruction from infection and necrosis can cause pain. A frequent site of infection is the oral area, in which a common cause of pain is ulcerative lesions of the mouth and esophagus.

Cachexia

The syndrome of **cachexia** includes anorexia, early satiety (filling), weight loss, anemia, asthenia (marked weakness), taste alterations, and altered protein, lipid, and carbohydrate metabolism (Fig. 11-4). Cachexia is the most severe form of malnutrition associated with cancer and results in wasting, emaciation, and decreased quality of life. Anorexia, or loss of appetite, frequently can be attributed to pain, depression, chemotherapy, or

FIG. 11-4 **Cachexia.** Sunken appearance of the eyes, cheeks, and temporal areas; sharp nose; dry rough skin. (From Seidel, Ball, Dains, & Benedict, 1987.)

radiotherapy. Alterations in taste also can account for the anorexia of cancer. Reductions in sensitivities to sweet, sour, and salty tastes make moderately seasoned foods seem bland. Persons with cancer, especially involving the liver, commonly have an aversion to red meat. Other aversions include coffee and chocolate. The process that produces such aversions is unknown, although several mechanisms have been suggested, including the following:

1. Poor use of glucose, resulting in an elevation of blood sugar that may depress appetite
2. A decreased supply of insulin, resulting in and causing an elevation of blood sugar, which may depress appetite
3. Increased mobilization of proteins and elevated amino acid level in the blood, which stimulates the satiety center and results in reduced appetite
4. Stimulation of visceral receptors from decreased peristalsis caused by surgery and other treatments, which stimulates the satiety center
5. A reduction in the emotional pleasures of eating or alterations in smell or taste of food, which can depress appetite

Anorexia leads to a protein-energy malnutrition (PEM), which has been classified according to three types: (1) similar to kwashiorkor, (2) marasmus, and (3) a combination of the two. Kwashiorkor is a form of malnutrition that evolves from a protein-deficient diet, in which calories are gained primarily from carbohydrates. Because the onset usually is rapid, anthropometric measurements tend to be normal, but serum proteins (transferrin, albumin) are decreased. This protein serum decrease (hypoalbuminemia) causes the serum colloid osmotic pressure to decrease, so that fluid escapes to the interstitium and causes edema. Marasmus is a form of

malnutrition resulting from a decreased intake of calories and proteins. It is characterized by decreased anthropometric measurements caused by a prolonged and gradual wasting of muscle mass and normal serum albumin. A combination of kwashiorkor and marasmus results in hypoalbuminemia, edema, diminished immunologic competence (which depends on normal protein stores), and an overall physical deterioration. (Malnutrition is discussed in detail in Chapter 36.)

Progressive weight loss in the person with cancer occurs despite normal or increased food intake. Starvation usually decreases the basal metabolic rate (BMR), but metabolic rates in persons with cancer are high. The relationship between increased BMR and weight loss resulting in a breakdown of protein and nitrogen loss or negative nitrogen balance is unclear. This increase may be a result of accelerated metabolic activity of the tumor itself. Malignant cells replicate more rapidly than normal cells and require more food for their growth, but at the expense of the normal tissue. The normal tissue, over time, is sacrificed, and waste begins to occur. Alterations in protein, lipid, and carbohydrate metabolism undoubtedly play a role.

Carbohydrate metabolism is altered, causing a syndrome that resembles diabetes mellitus. Hyperinsulinemia is present, and many individuals show insulin resistance, hyperglycemia, and an abnormal glucose tolerance test result. These disturbances cause an increased gluconeogenesis, which produces glucose from amino acids. In starvation, protein usually is spared to protect vital structures, but in cancer, protein and fatty acids are used for meeting energy needs. Fatty acids are released from the breakdown of adipose tissue.

An unusual and frustrating component of cancer care is the person's early satiety, or a sense of filling. The individual initially may feel hungry but experiences fullness after a few mouthfuls of food. Researchers have investigated tumor metabolites that could be responsible for the cachectic state. Several factors have been identified, including serotonin, bombazine, and lipolytic factors; however, they have been measured only in a small number of cancers (Langstein & Norton, 1991). What seems to be more important in inducing cancer cachexia is a group of cytokines (e.g., tissue hormones) produced by the body in response to the presence of cancer. One of the most significant cytokines is the activated macrophage-produced tumor necrosis factor (TNF), also called *cachectin* because of its role in the cachexia syndrome. Natural induction of TNF is protective; that is, it plays an important role in the defense against viral, bacterial, and parasitic infections; in autoimmune responses; and in the selective destruction of malignant cells (Fiers, 1991). Its overproduction, however, may be detrimental to the host. Cerami (1992) has studied for many years the severe wasting that often accompanies chronic parasitic, bacterial, or viral infection found in persons with cancer. Thus many cell types may become highly susceptible to the cytotoxic effect of TNF (Fiers, 1991). Currently TNF is being investigated as an inducer of septic shock (see Chapter 27). Other implicated cytokines include interleukin-1, interleukin-6, and interferon-γ. (Cytokines are discussed in detail in Chapter 7.)

Anemia

Anemia is a common disorder associated with malignancy. Most persons with cancer usually have a mild anemia, although 20% may have hemoglobin concentrations below 9 g/dl (normal value = 15 g/dl). Several mechanisms cause anemia in persons with cancer; these include chronic bleeding resulting in iron deficiency, severe malnutrition, medical therapies, or malignancy in blood-forming organs. Chronic bleeding and iron deficiency can accompany colorectal or genitourinary malignancy. Iron also is malabsorbed in persons with gastric, pancreatic, or upper intestinal cancer. In addition, anorexia can cause iron deficiency, although folate deficiency is more common with anorexia.

Generally, anemia is not a common consequence of chemotherapy, but normochromic (normal hemoglobin concentration) and normocytic (average red cell size) anemias can occur after prolonged administration of alkylating agents or nitrosoureas, both classes of chemotherapeutic agents. Megaloblastic (large red cell) anemias may develop after treatment with methotrexate, which causes abnormal folate metabolism.

Malignancy of the blood-forming organs is associated with a number of hemolytic anemias. An autoimmune hemolytic anemia occasionally develops in persons with chronic lymphocytic leukemia. (Anemia associated with leukemia is discussed in Chapter 23.)

The anemia in persons with cancer is not characterized by low levels of erythropoietin, a hormone (cytokine) produced in the peritubular interstitial cells of the kidney and a small amount in the liver and bone marrow macrophages (Lange, Bragger, Rosenthal, Kanz, & Lindemann, 1991). Erythropoietin acts on specific erythroid progenitor cells in the bone marrow to stimulate the release of immature red blood cells (e.g., reticulocytes). Erythropoietin, however, has been effective in correcting the anemia in several persons with cancer who participated in a study (Lange et al., 1991); fewer red blood cell transfusions were required in most of the subjects. In addition, anemias that occurred after chemotherapy or radiotherapy also were treated successfully by erythropoietin.

Leukopenia and Thrombocytopenia

Direct tumor invasion to the bone marrow causes both leukopenia (a decreased leukocyte count) and thrombo-

cytopenia (a decreased number of platelets). Chemotherapeutic drugs are toxic to the bone marrow, often causing both granulocytopenia and thrombocytopenia. Leukopenia is usually the result of chemotherapy, but radiotherapy of areas of the bone marrow also causes leukopenia. Thrombocytopenia, reduction in number of platelets, is a major cause of hemorrhage in persons with cancer. It usually results from chemotherapy or bone marrow involvement by the malignancy. Thrombocytopenia is an accompanying disorder of disseminated intravascular coagulation, which occurs in persons with acute promyelocytic leukemia (see Chapter 23) and prostate cancer (see Chapter 20).

Infection

Infection is the most significant cause of complications and death in persons with malignant disease. A reduction in the absolute granulocyte or lymphocyte count increases the risk of infection development, and persons with cancer are highly susceptible to infection because of reductions in immunologic functions, debility with advanced disease, and immunosuppression from radiotherapy and chemotherapy. (Factors that predispose persons to infection are summarized in Table 11-3.) Surgery also can lower resistance to infection because removal of large quantities of tissue, together with hemorrhage, dead spaces, and poor tissue perfusion, creates favorable sites for infection. The incidence of hospital-related (nosocomial) infections is increased because of indwelling medical devices, quality of wound care, and the introduction of microorganisms from visitors and other patients.

Leukopenia from bone marrow radiation dramatically increases the risk of infection. Mucous membranes and other rapidly dividing cells in the radiation field are prone to irritation and ulceration. Radiation also can lead to fistula formation or abnormal passages between tissue cavities. Fistula formations can result from radiation of the cervix, bladder, and intestinal tract. Surgery often is required to repair the fistula and eliminate continuous infectious cross-contaminations.

CANCER TREATMENT

Cancer is treated with chemotherapy, radiotherapy, surgery, immunotherapy, and combinations of these modalities (Table 11-4).

Chemotherapy

Several classes of chemotherapeutic agents are used concurrently to treat different types of cancer tumors (Table 11-5). The mechanism by which each drug acts to eradicate tumor cells depends largely on its effect on the cell cycle (described in Chapter 1). Malignant tumors

TABLE 11-3

Factors Predisposing Cancer Patients to Infection

Factor	Basis
Age	Many common malignancies occur mostly in older age.
	Immunologic functions decline with age.
	General debility reduces immunocompetence.
	Immobility predisposes to infection.
	Far-advanced cancer often results in immobility and general debility that worsens with age.
	Elderly persons are predisposed to nutritional inadequacies.
	Malnutrition impairs immunocompetence.
Tumor	Nutritional derangements can be caused.
	Sites and circumstances favorable to growth of microorganisms (obstruction, serous or blood effusion, ulceration) can be created.
	Far-advanced disease predisposes patients to debility and immobility.
	Humoral or cellular immune defects may be caused.
	Metastasis to bone marrow may cause leukopenia or other defects in immunity.
Leukemias	Inadequate granulocyte production (impaired phagocytosis) results.
	Thrombocytopenia (bleeding, breaks in skin integrity) can occur.
	Late effect: Chronic lung disease from *Pneumocystis carinii* pneumonia can develop during therapy.
Lymphomas and other reticuloen- dothelial malig- nancies	Humoral and cellular immune defects (anergy, altered immunoglobin production) result.
	Late effect: Splenectomy in children can cause increased susceptibility to infection.
Treatment: surgery	Invasive procedure interrupts first lines of defense.
	Radical nature of surgery (removal of large blocks of tissue in lengthy procedures) causes hemorrhage, decreased tissue perfusion, creation of dead spaces, devitalization of tissues.
	Procedure may be "dirty" surgery (bowel, infected or contaminated areas).
	Surgery patients are often older and at poor risk.
	Long preoperative hospitalization often precedes surgery.
	Patients may have had previous adrenocorticosteroid therapy.
	Patients may have infections at sites remote from operative area.
	Nutritional derangements (especially important in head and neck surgery) may result.
	Lymph node dissection may predispose patient to local infection and impair containment to area.
	Gynecologic surgery may result in fistulas.
	Lung surgery may cause bronchopleural fistulas.
	Debility and immobility may be caused.

From Donovan & Girton, 1984.

TABLE 11-4

Examples of Treatment of Site-Specific Cancers

Usual treatment	Site
Surgery	Colon
	Breast
	Ovary
	Lung
	Thyroid
	Skin
	Uterus
Chemotherapy	Lymphoma
	Leukemia
	Choriocarcinoma
	Ovary
	Breast
Radiation	Breast (all have been combined with surgery)
	Uterus or cervix
	Lymphomas
	Lung
	Combined with surgery in many sites
Hormones	Breast
	Prostate
	Endometrium

Modified from King, Fenoglio, & Lefkowitch, 1983; Baird et al., 1991.

TABLE 11-5

Classes of Chemotherapeutic Drugs

Class	Drug
Antimetabolites	Methotrexate
	Cytosine arabinoside
	Aminopterin
	Bromouridyldeoxyriboside (BUDR)
	Fluorouridyldeoxyriboside (FUDR)
	Hydroxyurea
	Thymidine
Alkylating agents	Nitrogen mustard
	Cyclophosphamide
	Chlorambucil
	Mechlorethamine
	Melphalan
	Busulfan
Antibiotics	Daunorubicin
	Doxorubicin (Adriamycin)
	Actinomycin D
	Bleomycin
	Mitomycin C
Hormones	Estrogens
	Androgens
	Steroids
	Tamoxifen
Mitotic inhibitors	Vincristine
	Vinblastine
	Etoposide
	Teniposide
Nitrosoureas	Lomustine
	Semustine
	Streptozocin

TABLE 11-6

Mechanisms of Action of Common Chemotherapeutic Drugs

Drug	Mechanism
Actinomycin D	Prevents transcription; inhibits tRNA, mRNA synthesis
	Inhibits protein synthesis
Bleomycin	Breaks and fragments single strands of DNA
	Damages nonproliferating as well as proliferating cells
Cytosine arabinoside	Decreases production of DNA replicating units
	Inhibits transcription
	Prematurely terminates nucleic acid chains
Doxorubicin	Binds to DNA
	Uncoils DNA helix
	Inhibits DNA-directed RNA polymerase
Mitomycin	Produces cross-linking of DNA strands

have three cellular compartments: (1) cells undergoing mitosis and cytokinesis, (2) cells capable of entering the cell cycle in the G_1 phase (see Fig. 1-23), and (3) cells that do not divide and have irreversibly left the cell cycle (dying malignant cells, differentiated malignant cells, nonmalignant support cells). Cells in compartment 3 will die a natural death without chemotherapy. The specific aim of chemotherapy, therefore, is to kill cells from compartments 1 and 2—cells that are dividing and cells that are in interphase. Table 11-6 summarizes the mechanisms of action of certain common chemotherapeutic drugs.

To be curative, chemotherapy must eradicate enough tumor cells so that the body's own defenses can eradicate the remaining cells. Smaller tumors have a faster growth rate and generally are more sensitive to chemotherapy. Few cells in a large tumor are dividing and, as a result, these are largely insensitive to chemotherapy.

Radiation

Ionizing radiation is a common approach to the treatment of malignant disease. The goals are (1) to eradicate cancer without producing excessive toxicity during treatment and (2) to avoid damage to normal structures. The application of radiation therefore requires precision and skillful application.

Ionizing radiation leads to damage of important macromolecules, especially DNA. Damage resulting from radiation is divided into three categories: (1) lethal damage, in which the cell is killed by radiation; (2) potentially lethal damage, in which the cell is so severely affected by radiation that modifications in its environment will cause it to die; and (3) sublethal damage, in which the cell is damaged but subsequently can repair itself. Cellular compartments with rapidly renewing cells are, in general, more radiosensitive. (Cellular effects of ionizing radiation are discussed in Chapter 2.)

Surgery

Surgical therapy is used when the tumor has not yet spread beyond the limits of surgical excision. Surgeons are generally in agreement that if there is any chance of regional lymph node involvement and there is no evidence of distant disease, the lymph nodes also should be removed. In some circumstances the removal of adjacent tissues has increased survival and enhanced cure. However, in more than half the cases, surgery may reveal evidence of micrometastatic disease or solid tumors.

Curative resections are performed if distant metastasis is not evident. The goals of palliative surgery (alleviation without cure) are (1) prevention of symptoms that would have occurred if the individual were not treated and (2) relief of symptoms that are present. Surgery also is indicated for benign tumors that could

progress into malignant tumors. Premalignant and in situ tumors of epithelial tissues, such as skin, mouth, and cervix, therefore are removed.

Immunotherapy

Chemotherapy and radiation treatments are the most common methods for managing cancer. Although effective treatments for certain types of cancer, these therapies have drawbacks. In general, both therapies act by eliminating mitotically or metabolically active cells. Within a tumor mass, however, a significant portion of cells is in a part of the cell cycle that is not affected by either metabolic inhibitors or mitotic poisons. In addition, these therapies have numerous side effects because they affect normal cell populations that, like transformed cells, have high rates of cell division. Cells of the gut epithelium, hair follicles, bone marrow, and gonads are affected by radiation and chemotherapy.

Because cancer is a dynamic disease in which the transformed cells in a tumor mass can adapt to changes in their environment, a single form of cancer therapy that is effective against all types of cancer may not be possible. More specific methods, however, eventually may eliminate transformed cells without damaging normal tissues.

In this regard, immunotherapy (immunologic treatment) holds great promise. (The immune system is discussed in detail in Chapter 6.) First, the immune system has specificity for antigen recognition and is highly regulated; thus antitumor immune rejection responses (described in Chapter 10) can selectively eliminate cancer cells while sparing normal tissues. Second, immune memory cells are long-lived and capable of providing extended protection against the emergence of recurrent primary tumor cells and foci of metastatic cancer cells. Third, numerous immunologic mechanisms are able to cause rejection of various types of cancer. Although tumor-immune surveillance provides protection against cancer, certain evasive mechanisms allow tumor cells to escape immune rejection. (Tumor-immune surveillance is described in Chapter 10.) Therefore current research efforts for establishing effective anticancer immunotherapies focus on characterizing the immunogenic properties of various tumor-specific antigens and developing methods to selectively enhance tumor rejection immune responses.

Immunotherapies for the treatment of cancer generally are referred to as **biologic response modifiers (BRMs)** (Talmadge, 1992). BRMs are defined as mammalian gene products, agents, and clinical protocols that affect biologic responses in host-tumor interactions. Three mechanisms describe the activities of BRMs: (1) a direct cytotoxic effect on cancer cells; (2) the initiation or augmentation of the host's tumor-immune rejection response; and (3) the modification of cancer cell

TABLE 11-7

Classification of Biologic Response Modifiers

Major classification	Specific examples
Immunomodulating agents	Alkyl lysophospholipids BCG Bestatin *C. parvum* Endotoxin Levamisole Muramyldipeptide Picibanil (OK432) Tuftsin
Interferons and interferon inducers	Interferons (alpha, beta, and gamma) Poly IC-LC *Brucella abortus* Viruses
Thymosins	Thymosin alpha-1 Other thymosin factors Thymosin factor V
Antigens	Tumor-associated antigens Hapten-modified tumor antigens Vaccines
Effector cells	Macrophages Natural killer cells Cytotoxic T cells LAK cells
Lymphokines and cytokines	Colony-stimulating factors (CSF) Lymphotoxin Interleukins (IL-1, IL-2, IL-3, etc.)
Monoclonal antibodies	Cytotoxic antibodies Immunotoxins Phototoxins

Modified from Oldham & Smalley, 1985.

susceptibility to the lytic or tumor-static effects of the immune system. The major classifications of BRMs are presented in Table 11-7. The basis of action and clinical applications of specific BRMs, selected from among the major classifications, are briefly discussed in the remainder of this section.

Immunomodulating Agents

Nonspecific stimulation of the immune system by an adjuvant (a substance that enhances the immune response) has been attempted in individuals with a variety of different cancers (Fig. 11-5). This therapy consists of the administration of an adjuvant (a bacterium), such as *Corynebacterium parvum* or bacille Calmette-Guérin (BCG), an attenuated strain of *Mycobacterium bovis*.

Bacterial cell wall extracts, live BCG, or nonviable *C. parvum* is injected at the tumor site. Retardation of tumor growth results through the activation of macrophages, augmentation of natural killer cells, or by some degree of antigenic cross-reactivity between the organism (BCG) and the antigen produced by certain human cancers, such as melanomas.

Some success has been observed in the treatment of genitourinary and lung cancer, usually through combined adjuvant treatments and chemotherapies. The most effective use of this type of immunotherapy, however, has been in the treatment of skin cancers.

Interferons

The interferons are a family of cell-derived proteins that have antiviral and immune modulating activities. The most successful clinical trials have come from the use of α-interferon. α-Interferon is a 20 to 25 kd molecular-weight glycoprotein made by activated leukocytes. In addition to its antiviral activity, α-interferon inhibits tumor growth, enhances natural killer cell activity, and increases cancer cell expression of tumor antigens, thus making them more immunogenic (i.e., eliciting stronger tumor-immune rejection responses). Used either alone or in combination with other treatment modalities, α-interferon has been effective in the treatment of hairy-cell leukemia, Kaposi sarcoma (a common cancer of persons with AIDS), and renal cell carcinoma. Similarly, α-interferon is effective for treating ovarian carcinoma when used after surgical removal of the tumor mass (Colombo et al., 1992). The use of interferons in cancer therapy is greatly enhanced by the ability to produce these biologic agents by recombinant gene-cloning techniques.

Antigens

Some success in treating skin tumors has been obtained by the application of contact sensitizing agents (materials that cause a hypersensitivity response in the skin), such as dinitrochlorobenzene (DNCB) (Fig. 11-6). With this approach the individual is first sensitized to DNCB through topical application to normal skin, and the tumor is subsequently painted with DNCB.

Tumor regression is thought to occur by inducing a contact hypersensitivity response to the DNCB at the tumor site. (Hypersensitivity reactions are discussed in Chapter 8.) Tumor cells probably are killed because DNCB has become associated with their cell surface and functions as an antigen. This type of therapy, however, is restricted to superficial tumors of the skin.

Research efforts are under way to identify tumor-specific antigens (the various types of antigens are described in Chapter 10) that could be used to develop anticancer vaccines. Ideally, common tumor-antigens expressed by a wide range of cancers could be devel-

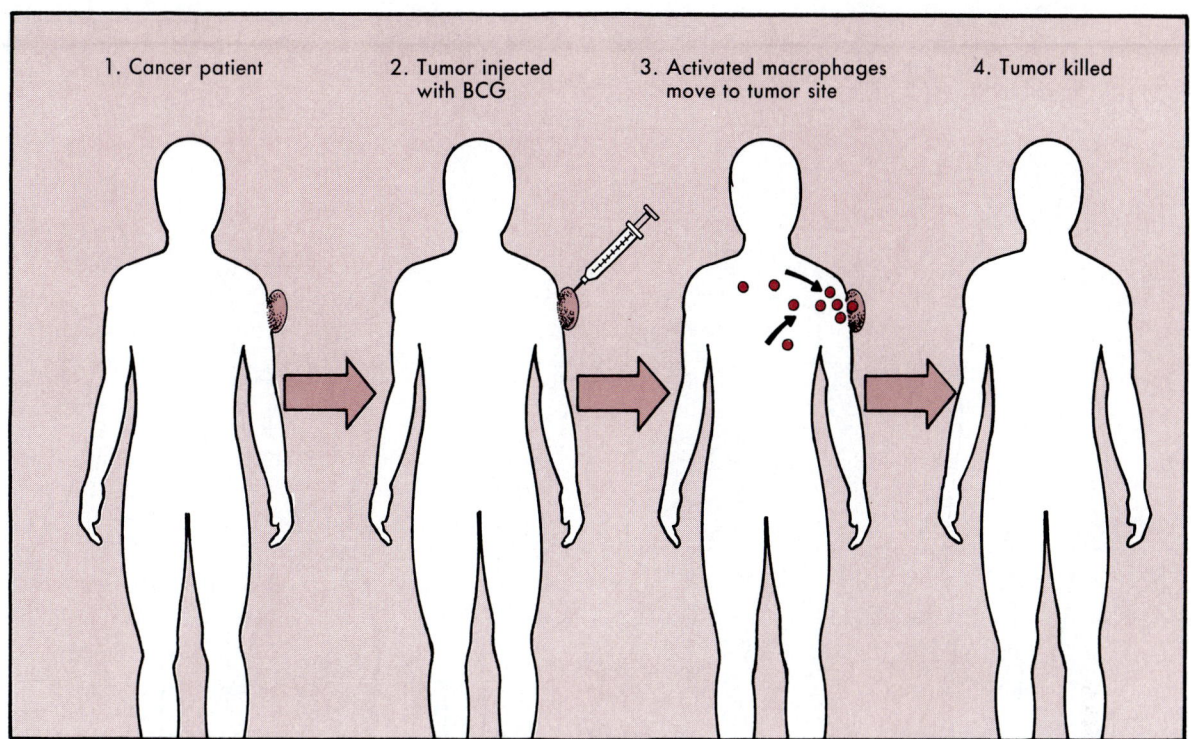

FIG. 11-5 Immunostimulation in cancer therapy.

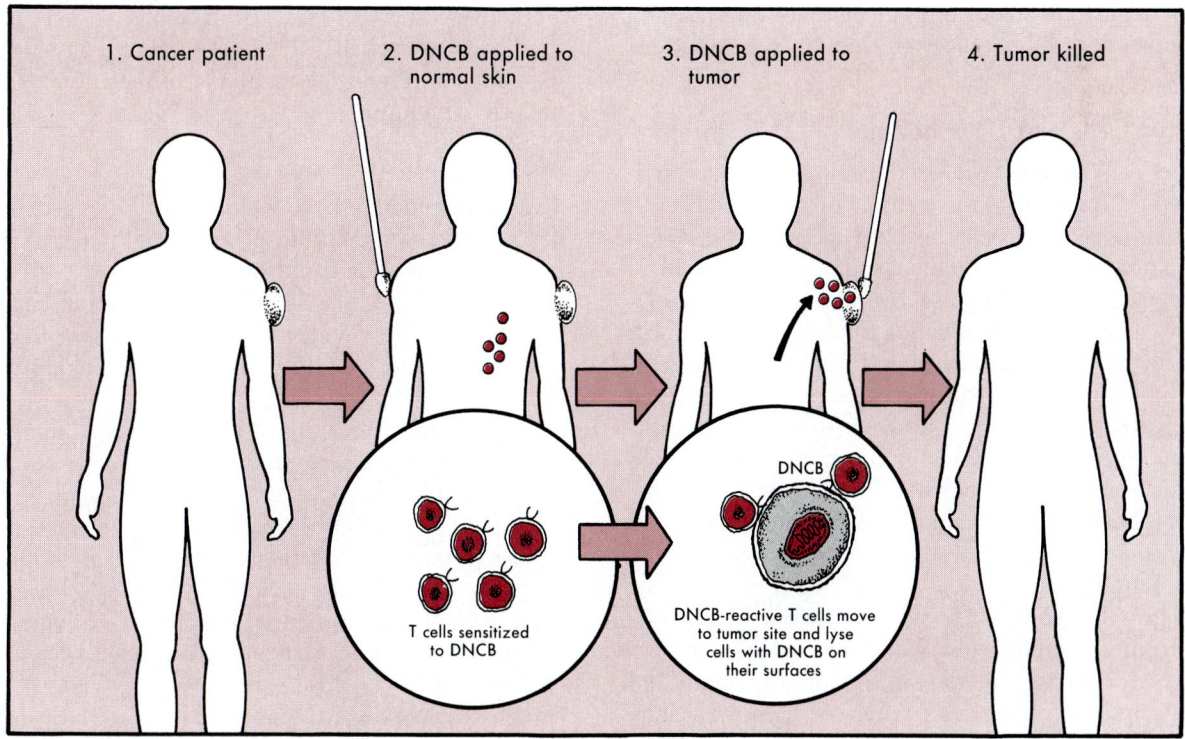

FIG. 11-6 Cancer therapy through antigen modification with dinitrochlorobenzene (DNCB).

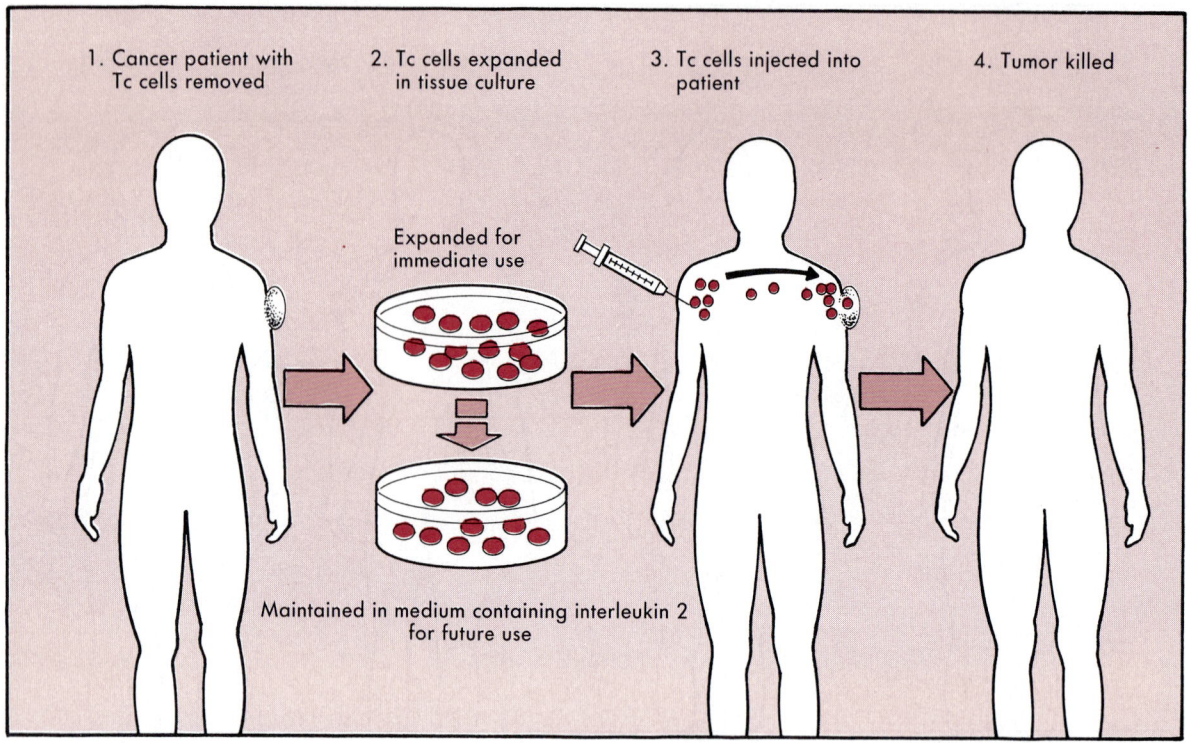

1. Cancer patient with Tc cells removed

2. Tc cells expanded in tissue culture

Expanded for immediate use

Maintained in medium containing interleukin 2 for future use

3. Tc cells injected into patient

4. Tumor killed

FIG. 11-7 Development of cytotoxic T cell (Tc cell) lines for cancer immunotherapy.

oped as vaccines. These vaccines could be used either as immunotherapies to augment the host's immune response against the tumor or as preventive immunization techniques to inhibit cancer emergence in populations at risk.

Effector Cells and Lymphokines

Theoretically an effective form of cellular immunotherapy would result from the transfer or augmentation of cytotoxic T cells (Tc cells) that are specific for the antigens expressed by the individual's tumor cells (Fig. 11-7) (Appelbaum, 1992). Because this represents such an attractive form of immunotherapy for cancer, a treatment protocol has been established and is undergoing extensive clinical trials. It is known as lymphokine-activated killer (LAK) cell therapy. The idea is to establish tumor-specific cytotoxic cell lines in tissue culture that can mediate tumor rejection when injected back into the cancer patient. The procedure takes advantage of the ability to expand LAK cells in vitro by growing them in tissue culture medium that contains interleukin-2, the T-cell growth factor. LAK cells are phenotypically distinct from T lymphocytes. When injected into the patient, LAK cells are able to infiltrate into the tumor and mediate lysis of cancer cells. LAK cell therapy usually is combined with interleukin-2 treatment, which is believed both to maintain LAK cell activity and to enhance

other antitumor immune rejection mechanisms. Some success has been obtained by interleukin-2 treatment alone (Melioli et al., 1992) or in combination with chemotherapy (Mitchell, 1992). LAK cell therapy has been used successfully in the treatment of melanoma and renal cell carcinoma.

Monoclonal Antibodies

The development of monoclonal antibody technology has provided a method to generate highly specific antibody reagents that could not be obtained with traditional antisera. (Monoclonal antibodies are discussed in Chapter 6.) These reagents have a promising future in both the diagnosis and the treatment of human cancer (Fig. 11-8).

In the past, clinicians have relied on a number of methods to diagnose human cancers. For example, in the case of most skin cancers, the diagnosis can be made by visual examination of the lesion. In contrast, the diagnosis of various soft tissue cancers, such as lung tumors, may require the identification of certain clinical signs (e.g., obstruction, bleeding, pain). Cytologic methods (e.g., Pap smear) or histologic analysis of cells also can be used to diagnose various types of cancer. These diagnoses generally are confirmed by tissue biopsies and pathologic evaluations. The major problems associated with these diagnostic methods are that some tests can

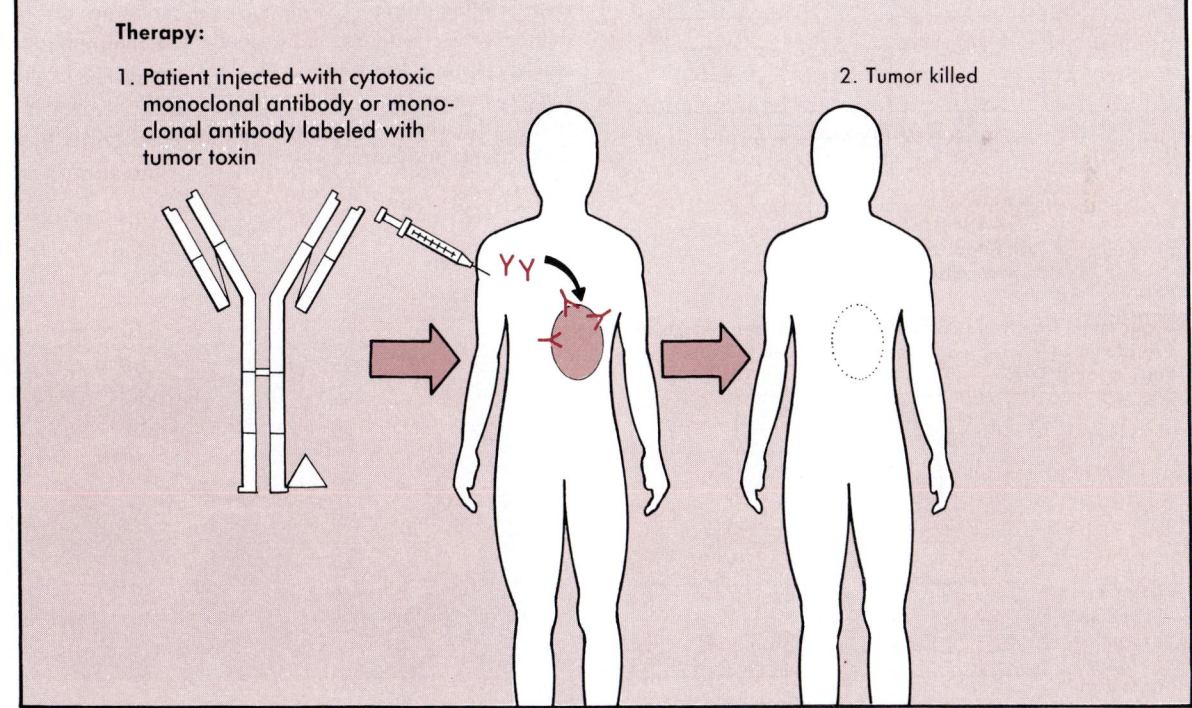

FIG. 11-8 **Monoclonal antibodies.** **A,** Tumor immunodiagnosis and, **B,** cancer immunotherapy with monoclonal antibodies. *TAA,* Tumor-associated antigen.

In 1975 Kohler and Milstein described their method for fusing mouse myeloma cells (transformed antibody-producing cells) with normal antibody-secreting cells from the spleens of immunized mice. The resulting hybridoma cells (fused or "hybridized" cancer cells) possessed characteristics of both the myeloma cells and the B lymphocytes used for fusion. These hybridoma cells were both immortal (characteristic of the myeloma cells) and capable of secreting antigen-specific antibody (characteristic of the normal B lymphocyte). Because these hybridoma cells can be cloned (generate a cell line from a single cell) and maintained in tissue culture indefinitely, investigators are able to select individual hybridoma cell lines that produce large amounts of highly specific monoclonal antibody (a single species of antibody protein). Since the development of this technology, the use and potential application of monoclonal antibodies have reached virtually every field of applied science. As a result, Kohler and Milstein received the Nobel Prize in 1984 for their contributions.

The basic monoclonal antibody technology is quite simple. First, animals are immunized with the antigen to which a monoclonal antibody is desired. Second, spleen cells (B lymphocytes) from the immunized animal are fused with hypoxanthine, aminopterin, and thymidine (HAT)–sensitive myeloma cells and grown in tissue culture medium that contains HAT. This strategy is based on the following criteria: normal B lymphocytes cannot survive in long-term tissue culture; myeloma cells, selected because they lack the necessary enzyme required for the nucleotide salvage pathway, are killed when cultured in HAT-containing medium because purine synthesis is blocked; and only hybrid cells (immortalized by the myeloma cells and capable of nucleotide reutilization) grow in HAT medium. Third, supernatants from the wells of tissue culture plates that contain hybridoma cells are screened for antigen-specific antibody activity. Fourth, hybridomas secreting the appropriate antibody are cloned (to generate a homogenous cell line), and large amounts of monoclonal antibody are produced in expanded tissue culture or ascites fluids (i.e., hybridoma cells grown as an ascites tumor in mice). Finally, purified monoclonal antibodies can be obtained for experimental or clinical use. Monoclonal antibodies have the following advantages over conventional antiserum: (1) a single antibody species of known antigen specificity is generated rather than a mixture of different antibody molecules; (2) monoclonal antibodies have a single, constant binding affinity; (3) monoclonal antibodies can be diluted to a constant titer because the actual antibody concentration is known; and (4) the antibody can be purified to homogeneity. The application of monoclonal antibodies for cancer diagnosis and therapy has a potentially significant future.

Technique for developing monoclonal antibodies. *Inset,* Hybridoma that is dividing. (From Raven, 1992.)

give false results or may detect only tumor masses that have become too large to be removed surgically, that have invaded and destroyed surrounding tissues and organs, or that have metastasized to secondary sites.

The reason for the development and use of monoclonal antibodies as diagnostic reagents for detecting cancer is that their high specificity for antigen could reduce the number of false results. Coupled with the appropriate laboratory or clinical assay system, monoclonal antibodies may provide methods for earlier detection of neoplastic disease. For example, highly purified monoclonal antibodies could be used to detect circulating tumor antigens in the individual's serum and thus provide a method for periodic screening of persons at high risk for the development of a specific type of cancer. Monoclonal antibodies, when bound to a radionuclide (radioactive material), also could be used for radiologic imaging (a diagnostic process for detecting radioactive deposits in tissues). Such techniques could help in diagnosing both primary tumors and metastases in persons suspected of having disease.

Another goal is to develop monoclonal antibodies specific for tumor antigens that would mediate tumor rejection without affecting normal tissues. In recent studies, monoclonal antibodies against specific antigens expressed by gastric carcinoma and ricin have been highly effective in causing regression of human tumors grown in experimental mice (Pimm, Robins, & Baldwin, 1992). The ability to couple cytotoxic substances or cell poisons, such as the alpha chain of ricin (immunotoxins) and porphyrins (phototoxins), to monoclonal antibodies could greatly enhance the efficacy of these reagents as immunotherapy for cancer. The major problems currently faced in the attempt to use monoclonal antibodies in cancer therapy are (1) developing functional reagents with the appropriate antigen specificities, (2) overcoming clinical complications that are associated with injecting large amounts of foreign antibodies (currently, most monoclonal antibodies can be made only in rodents), and (3) controlling immunoregulatory mechanisms that would eliminate their efficacy. Certainly the potential use of monoclonal antibodies, as well as other forms of immunotherapy, has generated new interest in immune surveillance mechanisms as possible methods for development of immunotherapies for cancer treatment.

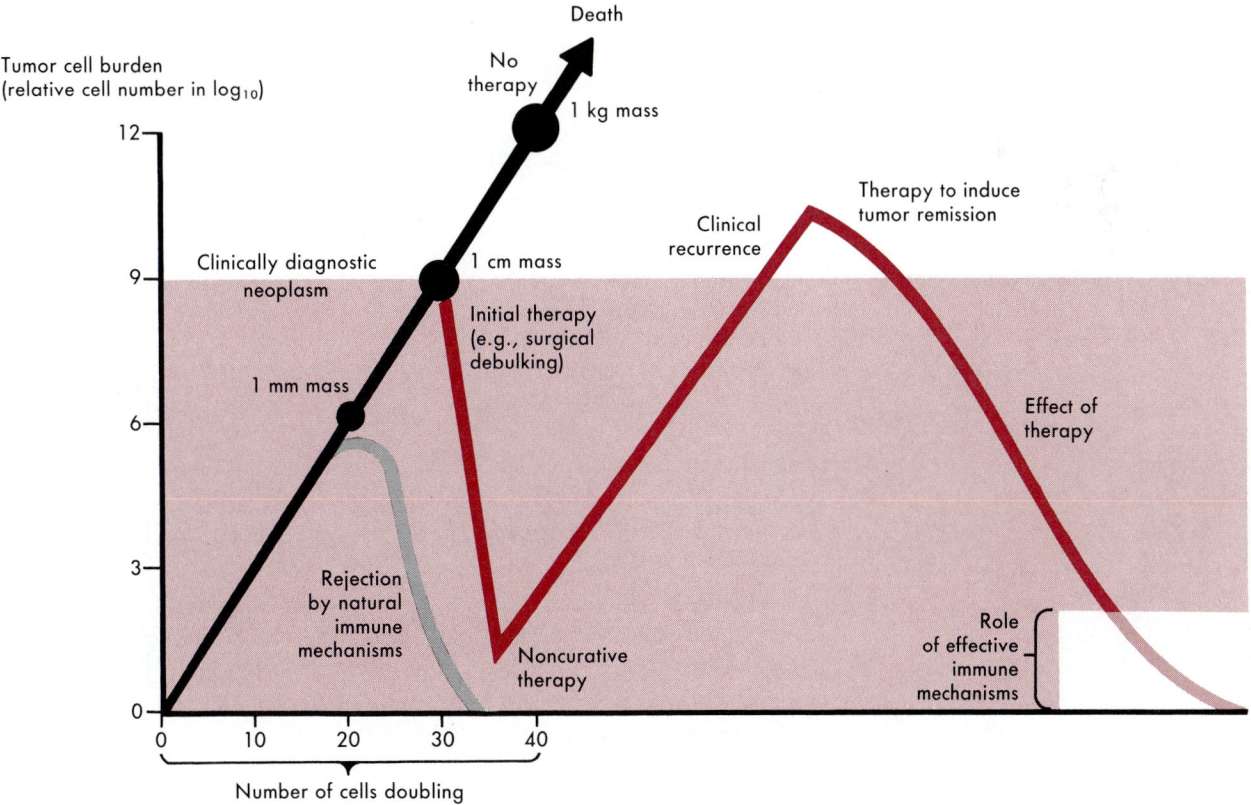

FIG. 11-9   **Relationship between tumor cell burden and phases of cancer treatment.** (Modified from Bakemeier, 1978.)

Applications and Clinical Complications of Immunotherapies

Immunotherapy represents the so-called fourth modality of cancer treatment. Although some immunotherapy protocols are designed to be used as a single method of cancer treatment, it should be appreciated that, like other types of cancer treatment (i.e., surgery, radiation therapy, and chemotherapy), the efficacy of immunotherapy may be increased when used as part of a combined treatment modality. The typical effects of cancer treatment on the growth of a tumor are summarized in Fig. 11-9. Typically, a solid tumor is not clinically detectable until it has reached a size of 1 cm, approximately 30 doublings of a transformed cell. Surgery often is used as a method to remove or debulk (partially reduce) the tumor mass. Other forms of therapy (i.e., radiation, chemical, or immunologic) would be used to prevent clinical recurrence of the tumor mass or growth of metastatic tumor foci. This type of combined modality approach can lead to a successful cancer cure.

As with other forms of cancer treatment, numerous side effects are associated with various immunotherapies. In general, during the administration of the immunotherapy (regardless of type) the patients usually manifest flulike symptoms (i.e., fever, chills, nausea, vomiting, and headache). Urticaria and skin rashes often occur during the treatment. Associated with the LAK cell therapy is a condition referred to as *vascular-leak syndrome*. This condition appears to result from the effect of interleukin-2 that causes increased vascular permeability. Thus, in addition to the symptoms listed, severe edema and cardiovascular hypotension occur. Although immunotherapies produce some adverse side effects and require extensive administration and clinical management, their potential benefit in cancer treatment demands their continued use and further development.

TABLE 11-8

Comparison of Usual Childhood and Adult Cancers

Factor	Childhood cancers	Adult cancers
Incidence	Rare, <1% of all cancers	Common, >99% of all cancers
Sites	Involves tissue (e.g., mononuclear phagocyte system, CNS, muscle, bone)	Involves organs (e.g., lung, breast, colon, prostate)
Histology	Most common type—nonepithelial: sarcomas, embryonal, leukemia, lymphoma	Most common type—epithelial: carcinomas
Latency (from initiation to diagnosis)	Relatively short period	Long period; can be well over 20 years
Influence of environmental factors in causation	Some environmental factors known, few life-style factors; overall not strong influence shown; more likely an interaction of genetic alterations and environmental factors, called ecogenetics	Strong relationship to environmental exposures and life-style factors
Prevention	Minimal strategies known to date	80% estimated to be preventable
Early detection	Generally accidental; small percentage known to be genetically at high risk can be monitored more closely	Possible with adherence to early detection and screening recommendation
State at diagnosis	80% have metastasized	Local or regional
Response to treatment	Very responsive to chemotherapy; tolerate higher doses	Less responsive to chemotherapy
Treatment side effects	Less difficulty with acute toxicity but more significant long-term consequences	More difficulty with acute toxicity but less long-term consequences
Prognosis	>60% cure	<60% cure

Modified from Fernbach & Vietti, 1991.

CANCER IN CHILDREN

Cancer in children is rare, but, because so many diseases of childhood have been successfully conquered, cancer is the second leading cause of death in children who have survived their first year (Bleyer, 1990). (Trauma remains the leading killer of children and adolescents.) The unique feature of childhood cancer is the short latency time, a sharp contrast to adult tumors, which usually involve a long latent period. Table 11-8 summarizes the differences between childhood and adult cancers.

Incidence and Types of Childhood Cancers

Both incidence rates and types of cancer that develop vary between children and adults (Table 11-9). For example, approximately 7800 children up to the age of 15 years and 3500 adolescents and young adults between the ages of 15 to 19 years were diagnosed with cancer in 1992, whereas approximately 1,100,000 adults were diagnosed with cancer during the same year (American Cancer Society [ACS], 1992). The incidence of cancer in children between birth and the age of 15 years is estimated to be 14 cases per 100,000 per year and increases to 20 cases per 100,000 per year for adolescents between 15 and 19 years of age. This translates to the development of cancer in 1 in every 475 children before the age of 15 years and 1 in every 333 children by the age of 19 years (Bleyer, 1990).

Most childhood cancers originate from the mesodermal germ layer that gives rise to connective tissue, bone, cartilage, muscle, blood, blood vessels, gonads, kidney, and the lymphatic system. Thus the more common childhood cancers are leukemias, sarcomas, and embryonic tumors. Embryonic tumors originate during intrauterine life. These tumors contain abnormal cells that appear to be immature embryonic tissue unable to mature or differentiate into fully developed functional cells. Embryonic tumors are diagnosed early in life (usually by 5 years of age) and therefore are very rare in adults. Embryonic tumors often are named with the term *blast*, which refers to the immature nature of the cells.

Sarcomas and lymphoreticular cancers seen in childhood also occur in adults, but most adult cancers involve epithelial tissue (and are therefore carcinomas). Carcinomas almost never occur in children because these cancers most commonly result from environmental carcinogens and require a long period from exposure to the appearance of the carcinoma. However, epithelial tumors begin to increase between the ages of 15 to 19 years and become the most frequent cancer tissue type after adolescence (Miller & Myers, 1983).

By far the most common malignancy in children is leukemia, which accounts for more than one third of childhood cancers. The second most common group of cancers is tumors of the nervous system, primarily brain tumors. All other pediatric malignancies occur much less frequently. Neuroblastoma and Wilms tumor are both embryonic tumors. Neuroblastoma is a tumor of the sympathetic nervous system. Wilms tumor is a malignancy of the kidney (named after Max Wilms, who identified the tumor); the histologic name is *nephroblastoma*. Rhabdomyosarcoma is a soft tissue sarcoma of striated muscle. Two major bone tumors also occur in children. These are osteosarcoma and Ewing sarcoma (named after James Ewing, who identified this tumor type).

Childhood cancers most often are diagnosed during peak times of physical growth and maturation. In general, they are extremely fast-growing cancers, with 80% having distant spread (metastases) at diagnosis. Many childhood cancers have a peak incidence before the child is 5 years of age. Among these are the leukemias and the embryonic tumors: neuroblastomas, Wilms tumor, and retinoblastoma. Central nervous system tumors are more common from ages 5 to 10 years, and bone tumors, soft tissue sarcomas, and lymphomas are more likely to occur from 10 to 15 years of age.

Cancer is 10% to 25% more common in white than in black children. This is due primarily to the lower incidence of acute lymphocytic leukemia, lymphomas, and Ewing sarcoma in black children (ACS, 1992; Miller, 1989). Some geographic differences also are found. These include increases in Burkitt lymphoma in Nige-

TABLE 11-9

Childhood Cancers by Age

Site	Percentage of each tumor in three age groups		
	0-5 years	5-10 years	10-15 years
Leukemia	39.6*	35.7	22.1
Lymphoma	3.7	13.3	16.4*
Central nervous system	15.0	27.1*	18.9
Neuroblastoma	13.0*	2.2	0.5
Soft tissue sarcoma	3.7	3.5	6.0*
Wilms tumor	9.2*	6.1	2.0
Bone tumor	0.6	5.0	10.5*
Retinoblastoma	6.4*	1.3	0.0
Other	8.6	5.9	23.7
TOTAL	100.0	100.0	100.0

*Peak incidence for tumor.

ria, intestinal lymphomas in Israel, Hodgkin disease in Colombia, and retinoblastoma in India (Miller, 1989). In the United States, childhood cancer also is slightly more common in boys than in girls. The male to female ratio for childhood cancers is 1.2:1.0, respectively (Young, Reis, & Silverberg, 1986).

Etiology

As in adult cancer, the causes of cancer in childhood are largely unknown. Some environmental and host factors are known to predispose a child to cancer, but causal factors have not been established for most childhood cancers. A number of host factors, many of which are genetic risk factors or congenital conditions, have been implicated in the development of childhood cancer (Table 11-10). The cause of childhood cancer most likely is attributed to the complex interaction of both genetic and environmental factors, now an important area of study called *ecogenetics*.

Most childhood cancers, however, do not lend themselves to early cancer warning signs. Certainly the American Cancer Society's seven warning signs of cancer do not apply because they describe adult, environmentally caused carcinomas. Although host factors are important in identifying populations of children at risk for cancer, most children who are diagnosed with cancer do not demonstrate any predisposing environmental or host factors.

Genetic Factors

Genetic factors may involve chromosome aberrations or single-gene defects. These chromosome abnormalities

TABLE 11-10

Host Factors Associated with Childhood Cancer

Syndrome	Associated risk factors
Chromosome alterations	
Down syndrome	Acute leukemia
13q syndrome	Retinoblastoma
Chromosome instability	
Ataxia-telangiectasia	Lymphoma
Bloom syndrome	Acute leukemia
Fanconi anemia	Nonlymphocytic leukemia
Hereditary syndromes	
Beckwith-Wiedemann syndrome	Wilms tumor, sarcoma, brain tumors
Neurofibromatosis	Brain tumors, sarcomas, neuroblastoma, Wilms tumor, nonlymphocytic leukemia
Tuberous sclerosis	Brain tumors
Immune deficiency disorders	
Congenital:	
Agammaglobulinemia	Lymphoma, leukemia, brain tumors
IgA deficiency	Lymphomas, leukemia, brain tumors
Wiskott-Aldrich syndrome	Leukemia, lymphoma
Acquired:	
Aplastic anemia	Leukemia
Organ transplantation	Leukemia, lymphoma
Congenital malformation syndromes	
Aniridia, hemihypertrophy, hamartoma, genitourinary anomalies	Wilms tumor
Cryptorchidism	Testicular tumor
Gonadal dysgenesis	Gonadoblastoma
Family susceptibility	
Twin or sibling with leukemia	Leukemia

include aneuploidy, deletions, translocations, and fragility. Some congenital malformations herald the onset of pediatric malignancies. For example, certain syndromes involve easily diagnosed abnormalities, and the children can then be carefully followed and screened for tumor development. One of the more recognized syndromes is the association of trisomy 21 (Down syndrome) with an increased susceptibility to acute leukemia. For children with Down syndrome, the risk of developing leukemia is 10 to 18 times greater during the first 10 years of life than the risk in healthy children (Miller, 1970). After a child reaches 10 years of age, the evidence shows no increase in susceptibility.

Wilms tumor is particularly recognized for its association with a number of malformations, including genitourinary anomalies—for example, horseshoe kidney, cryptorchidism (undescended testicles), and collecting system malformation; aniridia (congenital absence of the iris of the eye); and hemihypertrophy (muscular overgrowth of one half of the body or face). Approximately 15% of children diagnosed with Wilms tumor demonstrate one of these congenital abnormalities. Retinoblastoma, a malignant embryonic tumor of the eye, occurs as an inherited defect or as an acquired mutation (see p. 616).

More than 150 single-gene defects have been associated with the subsequent development of both childhood and adult cancers (Mulvihill, 1975). For instance, two autosomal recessive diseases involving increased chromosome fragility, Fanconi anemia and Bloom syndrome, are risk factors that evidently predispose the child to acute nonlymphocytic leukemia.

The relative ineffectiveness of the immune surveillance system during intrauterine life may explain the occurrence of embryonic tumors (the immune surveillance system is discussed in Chapter 10). Because this period requires rapid proliferation and differentiation of cells in the developing fetus, cell mutation theoretically could result in embryonic tumors.

Children with immunodeficiencies experience a striking 100-fold increased risk of subsequent cancer over healthy children (Lenarsky, 1983). These conditions may be either congenital, generally involving X-linked recessive inheritance, or acquired, generally caused by therapeutic immunosuppression after organ transplantation or treatment for aplastic anemia (see Table 10-12).

Although not determined to be genetically transmitted, a few malignancies seem to demonstrate a familial tendency, suggested by the clustering of specific cancers in a particular family. A child who has a sibling with leukemia has a risk for the development of leukemia that is four times greater than for children with normal siblings (Robinson, Mertens, & Neglia, 1991). A strong association for subsequent leukemia also is apparent in children with monozygous twins who have leukemia. The degree of risk appears to be age-related. If the twin with leukemia was diagnosed at younger than 1 year of age, the probability is nearly 100%; if diagnosed between the ages of 1 and 4 years, the risk drops to 15%; after 4 years of age the risk is equal to that of other siblings.

Environmental Factors

Although many adult cancers are associated with environmental agents, few childhood tumors share a strong association. Because of the lengthy latency period required between exposure and development of cancer, early exposure to carcinogens does not result in a tumor until the child is an adult.

Prenatal exposure

Prenatal exposure to some drugs and to ionizing radiation has been linked to subsequent cancers. Perhaps the most well-known such drug is diethylstilbestrol (DES), a drug taken to avert early abortion. In 1971, DES was identified as a transplacental chemical carcinogen. Adenocarcinoma of the vagina has developed in a small percentage of the daughters of mothers who had taken DES while pregnant. Most of these cancers appeared when the daughters were between 14 and 23 years of age. Other potential transplacental carcinogens have been identified but await further study before any conclusion can be drawn (Robinson, Mertens, & Neglia, 1991).

A recent area of intense study has been the role of parental occupational exposures and subsequent childhood cancers in children. The exposure could lead to genetic changes of the egg or sperm or to transplacental transfer of the carcinogen. Several associations have been consistently found in more than one study, including parental occupations with hydrocarbon exposure, petroleum and chemical exposure, and paint exposure. Further study is needed because this is a difficult area to study and conflicting results are common (Savitz & Chen, 1990).

Intrauterine radiation by obstetric x-ray exposure may increase risk of all childhood cancers. A British study reported a 1.4- to 1.5-fold increase in cancers in children who had experienced x-rays in utero (Bithell & Stewart, 1975). Studies of children who were in utero when their mothers were exposed to atomic fallout, however, showed no increase in childhood cancers (Jablon & Kato, 1970).

Childhood exposure

Childhood exposures to drugs, ionizing radiation, and viruses have been implicated as risk factors that increase susceptibility to specific cancers. In addition to those drug and environmental agents that are known to cause cancer in adults and therefore also are risks for exposure during childhood, a few drugs may particularly increase cancer risk during childhood. These drugs include (1) anabolic androgenic steroids, which are used in the treatment of aplastic anemia or used illegally by teenage athletes for body development and have been associated with subsequent hepatocellular carcinoma, (2) cytotoxic agents used in the treatment of pediatric cancers, which may predispose the child to leukemia in later years, and (3) immunosuppressive agents, particularly those used for transplant surgeries, which have been shown to increase the risk of lymphoma.

Current areas of study focus on the role of childhood environmental exposures to radon gas in the home and electromagnetic fields from residential power lines and the operation of small household appliances. Thus far, results suggest there may be an association, but further study is needed to determine the significance of any associations (Ahlbom, 1988; Henshaw, Eatough, & Richardson, 1990; London et al., 1991).

Although viruses have been implicated in childhood cancers, research has not yet proved a strong association. Viruses have been shown to affect cancer development in some animal models, but causal evidence is only suggestive in humans. (The viral theory of carcinogenesis is discussed in Chapter 10.) In children, the strongest carcinogenic relationship has been shown between the Epstein-Barr virus (EBV) and Burkitt lymphoma. Most African children with Burkitt lymphoma have high titers of antibodies against EBV. Up to 50% of American children with Burkitt lymphoma, however, do not have elevated EBV titers (Hirschaut, Cohen, & Stevens, 1974). Therefore, although EBV can induce lymphocyte transformation in laboratory studies, evidence has not yet shown whether the relationship is causal. Investigators are examining the role of viruses in the development of neuroblastomas, Wilms tumor, and osteosarcoma.

Prognosis

Today, childhood cancer should not be considered an inevitably fatal illness. Significant progress has been made in the last 10 years so that more than 60% of children diagnosed with cancer can now be expected to survive. Overall, children have a more favorable prognosis than do adults (American Cancer Society, 1992). Children appear to be both more responsive to available treatments and better able to tolerate the immediate side effects of therapies.

Because of the progress made in successful treatment of childhood cancers, health care providers are now grappling with a system to determine length of treatment needed and the point at which cure has been achieved. In adults a general rule-of-thumb is a 5-year survival rate, although a number of cancers (e.g., breast cancer) can recur well after the 5-year time frame. For children a unique method has been suggested to determine when a cure has been achieved (Fernbach & Vietti, 1991). Because a pediatric cancer could not have been present any longer than the age of the child at diagnosis, plus 9 months of intrauterine life, it could be assumed that, if the cancer were to recur, it would grow to its size at the initial diagnosis in the same amount of time. This time period is called the **period of risk**. This theory does not take into account alterations in the growth curves of tumors caused by the effect of treatment, but other cancer specialists have found the period of risk to be clinically accurate. A 2-year disease free period after cancer treatment is completed also has been compared with the period of risk and found to be of equal value for predicting cure (Platt & Linden, 1964). This 2-year disease-free period is useful for older children diagnosed with cancer because a much shorter period of time is required to determine cure than with the period of risk.

Because childhood cancer should be viewed as a chronic disease instead of a fatal illness, the focus of treatment is on the quality of life. Even those cancers that cannot be cured generally can be treated, resulting in a significant period of quality time. With increasing survival periods, the long-term effects of treatment are under careful investigation. More effective yet less toxic chemotherapy and radiation treatments must be found. Cured children still face residual and late effects of treatment. These late effects are more significant in children than in adults because childhood treatment occurs in a physically immature, growing individual. Potential effects that need further attention include physical impairments, reproductive dysfunction, soft tissue and bone atrophy, learning disabilities, secondary cancers, and psychologic sequelae. More must be learned about the genetic factors associated with childhood malignancies and about the genetic consequences of treatment. Genetic counseling is appropriate for children cured of cancers known to be transmitted genetically (e.g., retinoblastoma).

Historical Theories of Cancer Invasion

1 Historical analysis of theories of cancer invasion and metastasis began with Hippocrates' black bile diffusion theory and later included such theories as the cellular-embolic theory and the seed versus soil theory. Today the emphasis is on the biochemical mechanisms of metastasis.

Tumor Spread

1 Tumor spread takes several forms: (1) direct invasion, (2) metastasis to distant organs by lymphatics and veins, and (3) metastasis by implantation.

2 Invasion is the first step in the metastatic process. Mechanisms of local invasion include (1) cellular multiplication, (2) mechanical pressure, (3) release of lytic enzymes, (4) decreased adhesion (slipperiness), and (5) increased motility.

3 The three-step theory of invasion includes (1) tumor cell attachment to the matrix, (2) degradation or dissolution of the matrix, and (3) tumor cell locomotion.

4 Metastasis is the life-threatening charateristic of malignancy. The three mechanisms of metastasis include (1) direct or continuous extension, (2) lymphatic spread, and (3) bloodsteam dissemination. These mechanisms are not mutually exclusive.

5 Tumor growth is supported by the development of new blood vessels, a process called *angiogenesis*. Two angiogenic factors thought to be secreted by the tumor include a heparin-binding endothelial mitogen (a cell-growth factor) and angiogenin.

Clinical Manifestations of Cancer

1 Clinical manifestations of cancer include pain, cachexia, anemia, leukopenia, thrombocytopenia, and infection.

2 Pain generally is associated with the late stages of cancer. It can be caused by pressure, obstruction, invasion of a structure sensitive to pain, stretching, tissue destruction, and inflammation.

3 Cachexia (loss of appetite, weakness, inability to maintain weight, taste alterations, and altered metabolism) leads to protein-calorie malnutrition and progressive wasting.

4 Anemia associated with cancer usually occurs because of malnutrition, chronic bleeding and resultant iron deficiency, chemotherapy, and malignancies in the blood-forming organs.

5 Leukopenia is usually a result of chemotherapy, which is toxic to bone marrow, or radiation, which kills circulating leukocytes.

6 Thrombocytopenia is usually the result of chemotherapy or malignancy in the bone marrow.

7 Infection may be caused by leukopenia, immunosuppression, or debility associated with advanced disease.

Cancer Treatment

1 Cancer is treated with surgery, radiation therapy, chemotherapy, immunotherapy, and combinations of these modalities.

2 The theoretic basis of chemotherapy is the vulnerability of tumor cells in various stages of the cell cycle. The goal of chemotherapy is to eradicate enough tumor cells so that the body's natural defenses can eradicate remaining cells.

3 Ionizing radiation causes cell damage, so that the goal of radiation therapy is to damage the tumor without causing excessive toxicity or damage to undiseased structures.

4 Surgical therapy is used for nonmetastatic disease, for which cure is possible by removing the tumor, and as a palliative measure to alleviate symptoms.

5 Immunotherapy is appropriate for cancers that cannot be effectively managed by chemotherapy or radiation, usually because enough tumor cells are inactive and invulnerable to these modalities.

6 Forms of immunotherapy known as *biologic response modifiers* include immunomodulating agents, interferons, antigens, effector cells, lymphokines, and monoclonal antibodies.

7 The use of effector cells and lymphokines provides a form of cellular immunotherapy that involves the transfer of cytotoxic T cells (Tc cells) that are specific for tumor cell antigens.

8 The use of immunomodulating agents provides the nonspecific stimulation of the immune system by means of an adjuvant; it is most effective in treating skin cancers.

9 The use of antigens causes regression in skin tumors by producing a hypersensitivity response that affects the antigenic properties of the cell surface.

10 Monoclonal antibodies ultimately may be used both as diagnostic reagents for detecting cancer and as a form of cancer therapy in which antibodies specific for tumor antigens would mediate tumor rejection.

Cancer in Children

1 Although childhood cancer is rare, it is still the second leading cause of death in children.

2 The unique feature of childhood cancers is the short period of latency, which contrasts sharply with the long latency period common in adults.

3 Common childhood cancers include leukemias, sarcomas, and embryonic tumors that contain immature fetal tissue that has not differentiated into fully developed cells.

4 Embryonic tumors almost always are diagnosed early and are very rare in adults.

5 Because most carcinomas are caused by environmental exposure, these cancers are extremely rare in children, who have not lived long enough to be affected.

6 Host factors are especially important in identifying a child at risk for cancer because environmental risk factors have had less effect on the child's short lifetime.

7 Genetic factors that place a child at risk for cancer include some congenital malformations that are chromosome aberrations or single-gene defects.

8 A familial tendency is evident for a few childhood cancers, including leukemia.

9 Environmental risk factors associated with childhood cancer include prenatal exposure to some drugs and ionizing radiation and postnatal exposure to certain drugs (particularly anabolic steroids and some cytotoxic and immunosuppressive agents), to radiation, and possibly to certain viruses.

10 Improved survival for children with cancer has led to investigations for less toxic treatments that minimize residual effects and for more research into the genetic factors associated with cancer in childhood.

KEY TERMS

Angiogenesis, 371
Autocrine motility factor hypothesis, 368
Biologic response modifier (BRM), 377
Cachexia, 372
Invasion, 367
Laminin receptor, 368
Metastasis, 370
Primary tumor, 370
Type IV collagenase, 370

REFERENCES

Ahlbom, A. (1988). A review of the epidemiological litrature on magnetic fields and cancer. *Scandinavian Journal on Work and Environmental Health, 14,* 337-343.

American Cancer Society (ACS). (1992). *Cancer facts & figures 1992.* New York: American Cancer Society.

Appelbaum, J. W. (1992). The role of the immune system in the pathogenesis of cancer. *Seminars in Oncological Nursing, 8,* 51-62.

Bakemeier, R. F. (1978). Principles of medical oncology and cancer chemotherapy. In P. Rubin (Ed.), *Clinical oncology for medical students and physicians: A multidisciplinary approach* (p. 43). New York: American Cancer Society.

Bithell, J., & Stewart, A. (1975). Prenatal irradiation and childhood malignancy: A review of British data from the Oxford survey. *British Journal of Cancer, 31,* 271-287.

Bleyer, W. A. (1990). The impact of childhood cancer on the United States and the world. *CA: A Cancer Journal for Clinicians, 40*(6), 355-367.

Cerami, A. (1992). Inflammatory cytokines. *Clinical Immunology and Immunopathology, 62*(1 Pt 2), S3-S10.

Colombo, N., Peccatori, F., Paganin, C., Bini, S., Brandely, M., Mangioni, C., Mantovani, A., & Allavena, P. (1992). Antitumor and immunomodulatory activity of intraperitoneal IFN-gamma in ovarian carcinoma patients with minimal residual tumor after chemotherapy. *International Journal of Cancer, 51,* 42-46.

del Regato, J. A., Spjut, H. J., & Cox, J. D. (1985). *Ackerman and del Regato's cancer: Diagnosis, treatment, and prognosis* (2nd ed.). St. Louis: Mosby–Year Book.

Donovan, M. I., & Girton, S. F. (1984). *Cancer care nursing* (2nd ed.). New York: Appleton-Century-Crofts.

Dudjak, L. A. (1992). Cancer metastasis. *Seminars in Oncology Nursing, 8*(1), 40-50.

Fernbach, D. J., & Vietti, T. (1991). General aspects of childhood cancer. In D. J. Fernbach & T. Vietti (Eds.), *Clinical pediatric oncology* (4th ed., p. 2). St. Louis: Mosby–Year Book.

Fett, J. W., Strydom, D. J., Lobb, R. R., Alderman, E. M., Bethune, J. L., Riordan, J. F., & Vallee, B. L. (1985). Isolation and characterization of angiogenin, an angiogenic protein from carcinoma cells. *Biochemistry, 24*(20), 5480-5486.

Fidler, I. J., Gersten, D. M., & Hart, I. R. (1978). The biology of cancer invasion and metastasis. *Advances in Cancer Research, 28,* 149-160.

Fiers, W. (1991). Review: Tumor necrosis factor: Characterization of the molecular, cellular, and in vivo level. *FEBS Letters, 285*(2), 199-212.

Folkman, J., Merler, E., Abernathy, C., & Williams, G. (1971). Isolating a tumor factor responsible for angiogenesis. *Journal of Experimental Medicine, 133,* 275.

Franks, L. M., & Teich, N. (1986). *Introduction to the cellular and molecular biology of cancer.* New York: Oxford University Press.

Garbisa, S., Pozzatti, R., Muschel, R. J., Saffiotti, U., Ballin, M., Goldfarb, R. H., Khoury, G., & Liotta, L. A. (1987). Secretion of type IV collagenolytic protease and metastatic phenotype: Induction by transfection with c-Ha-ras but not c-Ha-ras plus AD2-E1A. *Cancer Research, 47,* 1523-1528.

Goldfarb, R. H., & Brunson, K. W. (1989). Overview of current understanding of tumor spread. In R. H. Goldfarb (Ed.), *Fundamental aspects of cancer.* Dordrecht, Netherlands: K. Power Academic.

Henshaw, D. L., Eatough, J. P., & Richardson, R. B. (1990). Radon as a causative factor in induction of myeloid leukaemia and other cancers. *Lancet, 335,* 1008-1012.

Hirschaut, Y., Cohen, N. M., & Stevens, D. A. (1974). Letter: Epstein-Barr virus and Burkitt's lymphoma. *Lancet, 1,* 742.

Hubbard, S. M., & Liotta, L. A. (1991). The biology of metastases. In S. B. Baird, R. McCorkle, & M. Grant (Eds.), *Cancer nursing: A comprehensive textbook.* Philadelphia: W. B. Saunders.

Jablon, S., & Kato, H. (1970). Childhood cancer in relation to prenatal exposure to atomic bomb radiation. *Lancet, 2,* 1000-1003.

King, D. W., Fenoglio, C. M., & Lefkowitch, J. H. (1983). *General pathophysiology: Principles and dynamics.* Philadelphia: Lea & Febiger.

Kupchella, C. E. (1990). Cellular biology of cancer. In S. L. Groenwald, M. H. Frogge, & M. Goodman (Eds.), *Cancer nursing: Principles and practice* (2nd ed.). Boston: Jones & Bartlett.

Lange, W., Bragger, W., Rosenthal, F. M., Kranz, L., & Lindemann, A. (1991). The role of cytokines in oncology. *International Journal of Cell Cloning, 9,* 252-273.

Langstein, J., & Norton, J. (1991). Mechanisms of cancer cachexia. *Hematology/Oncology Clinics of North America, 5*(1), 103-123.

Lenarsky, C. (1983). Etiology of childhood malignancy. In P. Lanzkowsky (Ed.), *Pediatric oncology.* New York: McGraw-Hill.

Liotta, L. A. (1991). Overview of the biology of cancer invasion and metastasis. In S. A. Rosenberg (Ed.), *Surgical treatment of metastatic cancer.* Philadelphia: J. B. Lippincott.

Liotta, L. A., Kleinerman, J., & Saidel, G. M. (1974). Quantitative relationships of intravascular tumor cells, tumor vessels, and pulmonary metastases following tumor implantation. *Cancer Research, 34,* 997.

Liotta, L. A., Mandler, R., Murano, G., Katz, D. A., Gordon, R. K., Chiang, P. K., & Schiffmann, E. (1986). Tumor cell autocrine motility factor. *Proceedings of the National Academy of Sciences of the United States of America, 83*(10), 3302-3306.

London, S. J., Thomas, D. C., Bowman, J. D., Sobel, E., Cheng, T., & Peters, J. M. (1991). Exposure to residential electric and magnetic fields with risk of childhood leukemia. *American Journal of Epidemiology, 134*(9), 923-937.

Melioli, G., Margarino, G., Scala, M., Mereu, P., Bertoglio, S., Schenone, G., Barbaresi, M., Machi, A. M., Santi, L., Badellino, F., et al. (1992). Perilymphatic injections of recombinant interleukin-2 (rIL-2) partially correct the immunologic defects in patients with advanced head and neck squamous cell carcinoma. *Laryngoscope, 102*(5), 572-578.

Miller, R. W. (1989). Frequency and environmental epidemiology of childhood cancer. In P. A. Pizzo & D. G. Poplack (Eds.), *Principles and practices of pediatric oncology.* Philadelphia: J. B. Lippincott.

Miller, R. W., & Myers, M. H. (1983). Age distribution of epithelial cancers. *Lancet, 2,* 1250.

Mitchell, M. S. (1992). Chemotherapy in combination with biomodulation: A 5-year experience with cyclophosphamide and interleukin-2. *Seminars in Oncology, 19,* 80-87.

Mulvihill, J. (1975). Congenital and genetic diseases. In J. Fraumeni, Jr. (Ed.), *Persons at high risk of cancer: An approach to cancer etiology and control.* New York: Academic Press.

Oldham, R., & Smalley, R. (1985). Biologicals and biological response modifiers. In V. DeVita, S. Hellman, & S. Rosenberg (Eds.), *Cancer principles and practices of oncology.* Philadelphia: J. B. Lippincott.

Pimm, M. V., Robins, R. A., & Baldwin, R. W. (1992). Capture of recombinant recin A chain by a bispecific anti-RTA:anti-CEA monoclonal antibody pretargeted to a human gastric carcinoma xenograft in nude mice. *Journal of Cancer Research and Clinical Oncology, 118,* 367-370.

Platt, B., & Linden, G. (1964). Wilms' tumor—A comparison of 2 criteria for survival. *Cancer, 17,* 1573-1578.

Poste, G., & Fidler, I. J. (1980). The pathogenesis of cancer metastasis. *Nature, 20,* 139-145.

Robinson, L., Mertens, A., & Neglia, J. (1991). Epidemiology and etiology of childhood cancer. In D. J. Fernbach & T. Vietti (Eds.), *Clinical pediatric oncology* (4th ed.). St. Louis: Mosby–Year Book.

Savitz, D. A., & Chen, J. H. (1990). Parental occupation and childhood cancer: Review of epidemiologic studies. *Environmental Health Perspectives, 88,* 325-337.

Schirrmacher, V. (1985). Cancer metastasis: Experimental approaches, theoretical concepts, and impacts for treatment strategies. *Advanced Cancer Research, 43,* 1-71.

Seidel, H. M., Ball, J. W., Dains, J. E., & Benedict, G. W. (1991). *Mosby's guide to physical examination* (2nd ed.). St. Louis: Mosby–Year Book.

Shing, Y., Folkman, J., Sullivan, R., Butterfield, C., Murray J., & Klagsbrun, M. (1984). Heparin affinity: Purification of a tumor-derived capillary endothelial cell growth factor. *Science, 223*(4642), 1296-1299.

Sugarbaker, E. V. (1981). Patterns of metastasis in human malignancies. *Cancer Biology, (2),* 235-245.

Talmadge, J. E. (1992). Development of immunotherapeutic strategies for the treatment of malignant neoplasms. *Biotherapy, 4,* 215-236.

Young, J., Jr., Reis, L. G., & Silverberg, E. (1986). Cancer incidence, survival, and mortality for children younger than age 15 years. *Cancer, 8,* 598-602.

SUGGESTED READINGS

Foley G., Fochtman, D., & Mooney, K. (1993). *Nursing care of the child with cancer* (2nd ed.). Philadelphia: W.B. Saunders.

Groenwald, S.L., & Kupchella, C.E. (Eds). (1992). Biology of cancer. *Seminars in Oncology Nursing* 8(1), 1-70.

PART TWO

Pathophysiologic Alterations
Organs and Systems

UNIT V

The Neurologic System

TREATMENT OF NEUROLOGIC DISEASE dates back to the time before written history. Trephination, the process of cutting away a piece of the skull, was performed as long ago as the Neolithic Age (about 7000 to 3000 BC), although no written record exists to provide a rationale for the procedure. Evidence of such procedures has been found in France, Peru, and other widespread geographic areas. The earliest written record of the study and treatment of neurologic disease, known as the Edwin Smith papyrus, consists of 48 hypothetical cases of neurologic disease and dysfunction with prognosis and management; it dates back to 1600 BC and represents a copy of an older work.

Although the Greeks believed the heart was the source of human thought and feelings and that animal spirit was made in the ventricles and resided there to be distributed by hollow nerve fibers to the body, Hippocrates (born 460 BC) was fairly accurate in his written descriptions of facial paralysis, sciatica, and the complex of headache, visual disturbance, and vomiting. He accurately described signs associated with disorders of the brain, such as aphasia, unconsciousness, pupillary inequality, ophthalmoplegia, and respiratory and cardiovascular irregularities. This Greek physician was aware that injury to one side of the head could be followed by convulsions or paralysis of the contralateral extremities, that

NERVE ENDINGS

Wood engraving.
(Courtesy National Library of Medicine.)

compression of the spinal cord had functional effects, and that dural lacerations had a poor prognosis. His writings contain the first recorded description of trephination and vertebral dislocation reduction.

Galen, a noted Greek physician of the second century AD, having studied brain structure through animal dissection and brain function and injury while he served as physician to gladiators in Rome, tried, with limited success, to refute the belief that the heart (and not the brain) was the center of human thought. Little progress was made for centuries. What would become the fields of neuroanatomy, neurophysiology, and neuropathology began to advance slightly in the fourteenth century when Italian medical schools were permitted to authorize the dissection of human cadavers. Laws gradually became so liberalized that nonphysicians, such as Leonardo DaVinci could conduct dissections. Although DaVinci's neurophysiology was wanting (he declared that the first ventricle mediated imagination and common sense, the second ventricle mediated reasoning, and the third mediated memory), his

drawings and the drawings of others in Europe and Britain during the 1600s and 1700s were amazingly accurate and detailed. Willis, in 1664, was the man who finally retired the belief that the ventricles were more important than the brain, itself a pivotal point in the emergence of modern neuroscience. The door was opened for study of the localization of function within the nervous system, although this emergence had to wait two centuries while the search for localization of the soul in the brain was pursued and the theory of phenomenology overshadowed attempts to study the relation- ship between neuroanatomy and neural function.

Broca, a general surgeon, initiated work in the area of localization with his basic discovery of the motor speech area named after him in 1861. Neurologists and neurosurgeons, such as Wernicke, Foerster, and Penfield, along with other neuroscientists and histologists, advanced the science of neurophysiology.

Neuropathology had its true birth in the latter part of the 1800s and the early 1900s. Charcot is viewed as one of the principal founders of the field. Using simple staining techniques, Charcot established the histologic basis of a number of nervous system diseases. Charcot and his pupils—Marie, Dejerine, and Babinski—established the anatomic and clinical classification of neurologic processes. Cajal, a Spaniard, provided early knowledge of synapses and supported von Waldeyer's neuron theory, and German neuroscientists—Nissl, Alzheimer, Spiermeyer, and Weigert—established the basic neurohistopathology of nervous system disorders. The study of the neuropathology of specific diseases and the origin and pathogenesis of specific features, such as ischemia, inflammation, and edema, were clearly launched. Technologic advances in this century, including the electron microscope, histochemistry, computed tomography (CT) scanning, positron emission tomography (PET), magnetic resonance imaging (MRI), and magnetic resonance angiography (MRA), are facilitating rapid progress in the field.

CHAPTER 12

Structure and Function of the Nervous System

Peter M. Sunderland

Chapter Outline

The human nervous system is a remarkable structure responsible for the body's ability to interact with the environment and for the regulation of activities involving internal organs. The nervous system literally drives the other systems of the body. It is a network composed of complex structures that transmit signals—both electrically and chemically—between the body's many organs and tissues and the brain.

OVERVIEW AND ORGANIZATION OF THE NERVOUS SYSTEM

Although the nervous system functions as a unified whole, structures and functions have been divided to facilitate understanding. Structurally the nervous system is divided into the central nervous system and the peripheral nervous system. The **central nervous system (CNS)** consists of the brain and spinal cord, enclosed within the rigid cranial vault and the bony spine. The **peripheral nervous system (PNS)** is composed of the **cranial nerves,** which communicate with the brain through foramina (openings) in the skull, and the **spinal nerves,** which communicate with the spinal cord through intervertebral foramina in the bony spine. Peripheral nerve pathways are differentiated into **afferent pathways (ascending pathways),** which carry sensory impulses toward the CNS, and **efferent pathways (descending pathways),** which innervate skeletal muscle or effector organs by transmitting motor impulses away from the CNS.

Functionally, the PNS can be divided into the somatic nervous system and the autonomic nervous system. The **somatic nervous system** consists of pathways that regulate voluntary motor control (e.g., skeletal muscle). The **autonomic nervous system (ANS)** is involved with regulation of the body's internal environment (viscera) through involuntary control of organ systems. The ANS is further divided into sympathetic and parasympathetic divisions. Organs innervated by specific components of the nervous system are called **effector organs.**

CELLS OF THE NERVOUS SYSTEM

Two basic types of cells comprise nervous tissue, neurons and supporting cells. The **neuron** is the primary cell of the nervous system. Working alone or as units, neurons detect environmental changes and initiate body responses to maintain a dynamic steady state. The sup-

porting cells, such as the **neuroglial cells** of the CNS and the **Schwann cells** of the PNS, provide structural support and nutrition for the neurons.

The Neuron

Neuronal structure varies markedly, so that each neuron is adapted to perform specialized functions. Neurons share many of the same metabolic activities and constituents as other types of cells. The fuel source for the neuron is predominantly glucose; insulin, however, is not required for cellular glucose uptake in the CNS. Neurons also have unique cellular constituents, that is, microtubules, neurofibrils, microfilaments, and Nissl substances. **Microtubules, microfilaments,** and **neurofibrils** are believed to be involved in transport of cellular products. **Nissl substances** are involved in protein synthesis. Because of the lack of centrosomes, an entire neuron does not have the ability to regenerate. Cell division stops at the time of birth, and further replication ceases.

A neuron (Fig. 12-1) has three components: a cell body (soma) and the thin processes of the cell, the dendrites, and the axons. Most cell bodies are located within the CNS. Cell bodies in the PNS usually are found in groups called **ganglia.** The **dendrites** are extensions that carry nerve impulses toward the cell body. The **dendritic zone** is the receptive portion of a neuron that receives a stimulus and continues further conduction. **Axons** are long, conductive projections from the cell body that carry nerve impulses away from the cell body. The **axon hillock** is the cone-shaped process where the axon leaves the cell body. The initial segment of the axon hillock has the lowest threshold for stimulation, and as a result, action potentials begin here. A typical neuron has only one axon. The axon may be covered with a segmented layer of lipid material called **myelin,** which acts as an insulating substance. This entire membrane is referred to as the **myelin sheath,** and the thin membrane between the myelin sheath and the **endoneurium** is the **neurilemma (Schwann sheath).** The neurilemma and the myelin sheath are interrupted at regular intervals by the **nodes of Ranvier.** Axons are capable of extensive branching, which occurs at the nodes of Ranvier. The principle of divergence refers to the ability of these branches to influence many different neurons. *Convergence* is the term applied to branches of various numbers of neurons "converging" on and influencing a single neuron. Exchange of nutrients is not possible through the myelin sheath, although nutrient exchange can occur at the nodes of Ranvier. The presence of myelin is associated with an increase in the velocity of nerve impulses. Myelin acts as an insulator that allows ions to flow between segments rather than along the entire length of the membrane, resulting in this increased velocity. This mechanism is referred to as **salta-**

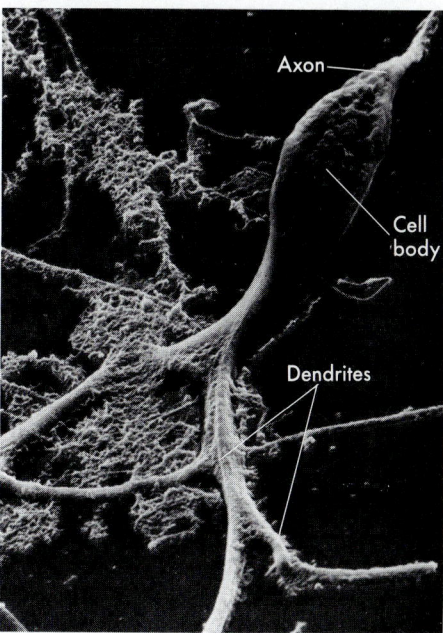

FIG. 12-1 Neuron with composite parts. **A,** Diagram. **B,** Scanning electron micrograph. (**A,** from Rudy, 1984; **B,** from Thibodeau & Patton, 1993.)

tory conduction. Disorders of the myelin sheath (demyelinating diseases), such as multiple sclerosis and Guillain-Barré syndrome, demonstrate the important role myelin plays in nerve function (see Chapter 14). Conduction velocities depend not only on the myelin coating but also on the diameter of the axon. Larger axons transmit impulses at a faster rate.

Neurons are structurally classified on the basis of the number of processes (projections) extending from the cell body. There are three basic types of cell configuration: (1) unipolar, (2) bipolar, and (3) multipolar. **Unipolar neurons** have one process that branches shortly after leaving the cell body. One process extends away from the CNS whereas the other projects into the CNS. The configuration is typical of sensory neurons in both cranial and spinal nerves. **Bipolar neurons** have two distinct processes arising from the cell body. This type of neuron connects the rod and cone cells of the optic system, as well as the auditory and vestibulocochlear systems to the CNS. **Multipolar neurons** are the most common and have multiple processes capable of extensive branching. A motor neuron is typically multipolar (Fig. 12-2).

Functionally there are three types of neurons (with their direction of transmission and typical configuration noted in parentheses): (1) sensory (afferent, mostly unipolar), (2) associational (interneurons, multipolar), and (3) motor (efferent, multipolar). **Sensory neurons** carry impulses from peripheral sensory receptors to the CNS (see the box above). **Associational neurons (interneurons)** transmit impulses from neuron to neuron, that is, sensory to motor neurons. They are located solely within the CNS. **Motor neurons** transmit impulses away

---

MAJOR TYPES OF SENSORY RECEPTORS

1. Nociceptors (pain)
2. Mechanoreceptors (touch, pressure, and mechanical deformation)
3. Photochemical (light on the retina)
4. Chemoreceptors (flavors, odors, oxygen levels, osmolarity of body fluids, and carbon dioxide levels in the blood)
5. Thermoreceptors (heat and cold)

---

from the CNS to an effector (i.e., skeletal muscle or organ). In skeletal muscle the end processes form a **neuromuscular (myoneural) junction.**

Neuroglia and Schwann Cells

Neuroglia ("nerve glue") are cells that support the neurons of the CNS. They comprise approximately half of the total brain and spinal cord volume and are five to ten times more numerous than neurons. Different types of neuroglia serve different functions. **Astrocytes,** for example, form points of contact between the nervous and circulatory systems; **oligodendroglia** function to deposit myelin within the CNS. Schwann cells are the PNS counterpart of oligodendroglia. Ependymal cells line the cerebrospinal fluid–filled cavities (ventricles). Microglia function to remove debris (phagocytosis) in the CNS. (Characteristics of neuroglia and Schwann cells are summarized in Fig. 12-3 and Table 12-1.)

FIG. 12-2 **Neuronal transmission and synaptic cleft.** Electrical impulse travels along axon of first neuron to synapse. Chemical transmitter is secreted into synaptic space to depolarize membrane (dendrite or cell body) of next neuron in pathway. *Cell A* represents unipolar cell; *cell B* represents multipolar cell. (From Thompson et al., 1993.)

Ependymal cell   Astrocyte

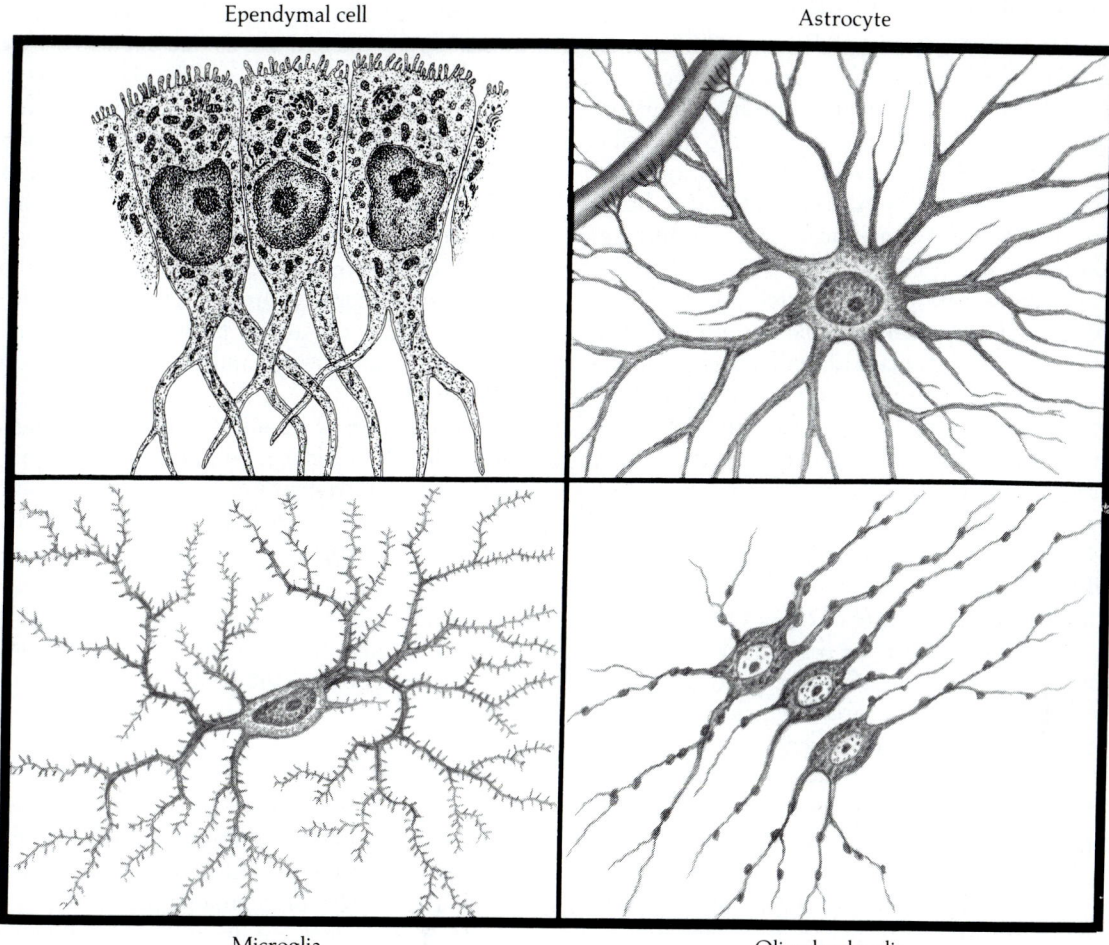

Microglia   Oligodendroglia

FIG. 12-3 Types of neuroglia cells. (From Thompson et al., 1993.)

TABLE 12-1

Support Cells of the Nervous System

Cell type	Primary functions
Astrocytes	Form specialized contacts between neuronal surfaces and blood vessels
	Provide for rapid transport for nutrients and metabolites
	Believed to form an essential component of the blood-brain barrier
	Appear to be the scar-forming cells of the CNS, which may be the foci for seizures
	May play a role in segregating postsynaptic receptor surfaces from other regions
Oligodendroglia	Deposition of myelin within the CNS
Schwann's cells (neurolemmocytes)	Formation of the myelin sheath and neurilemma in the PNS
Microglia	Responsible for clearing cellular debris (phagocytic properties)
Ependymal cells	Serve as a lining for the ventricles and choroid plexuses involved in the production of cerebro-spinal fluid

Nerve Injury and Regeneration

When an axon is severed, a typical sequence of events, known as *Wallerian degeneration*, occurs in the distal axon: (1) a characteristic swelling appears within the portion of the axon distal to the cut, (2) the neurofilaments hypertrophy, (3) the myelin sheath shrinks and disintegrates, and (4) the axon degenerates and disappears. The neurilemma (Schwann sheath) usually remains intact.

At the proximal end of the injured axon similar changes occur, but only a short segment is affected. The cell body responds to trauma with an increase in metabolic activity, protein synthesis, and mitochondrial activity. Approximately 7 to 14 days after the injury, new neurofibrils project from the proximal segment and may enter the remaining neurilemma. This process, however, is limited to myelinated fibers and generally occurs only in the PNS. The regeneration of axonal constituents in the CNS is limited by an increased incidence of scar formation and the different nature of myelin formation by the oligodendrocyte (see Fig. 12-4 for a more detailed representation of these events). Surgical repair of injured peripheral nerves must be performed quickly to prevent degenerative processes from occurring.

Nerve regeneration depends on many factors, such as location of the injury, type of injury, the inflammatory responses, and the process of scarring. The closer to the cell body the nerve is injured, the greater the chances that the nerve cell will die and not regenerate. A crushing type of injury affects recovery more significantly than does a cut that severs the nerve. A crushed nerve may fully recover, whereas a severed or even partially cut nerve quickly forms a connective tissue scar, blocking the regenerating axonal branches.

THE NERVE IMPULSE

The neuron's basic role is the generation and conduction of electrical and chemical impulses. This is accomplished by selectively changing the electrical potential of its plasma membrane and influencing other nearby neurons by the release of chemicals (neurotransmitters). A neuron in its unexcited state maintains a resting membrane potential (see Chapter 1). When the membrane potential is raised, an action potential is generated and the nerve impulse then flows to all parts of the neuron. The action potential of a neuron is not a graded response. The stimulus either is strong enough to induce an action potential or is too weak and the membrane remains in its unexcited state. This property is sometimes termed the *all or none response*.

Synapses

Neurons are not physically continuous with one another. The region between elements of adjacent neurons is called a **synapse** (see Fig. 12-2). Transmission of impulses across the synapse is accomplished by chemical and electrical conduction (see Fig. 12-2); however, only chemical conduction is discussed here. The neurons that participate in conduction of a nerve impulse are named according to whether they relay impulses toward the synapse (**presynaptic neurons**) or away from the synapse (**postsynaptic neurons**). Four basic types of connections occur in regions of contact between the presynaptic and postsynaptic neurons. These are between axons (axoaxonic), axon to cell body (axosomatic), axon to dendrite (axodendritic), and dendrite to dendrite (dendodendritic).

Transmission of impulses across the synapse is accomplished by chemical conduction. When an impulse originates in a presynaptic neuron, the impulse reaches the vesicles, where chemicals (**neurotransmitters**) are stored in the terminal end of the axon (called the **synaptic terminal**). Once released from the vesicles, the neurotransmitters diffuse across the **synaptic cleft** (the space between the neurons) and bind to receptor sites on the plasma membrane of the postsynaptic neuron (see Fig. 12-2).

Neurotransmitters

More than 30 substances are thought to be neurotransmitters. Most noted are norepinephrine, acetylcholine, dopamine, histamine, and serotonin. Many of these transmitters have more than one function. For example, norepinephrine in the brain probably is involved in the regulation of mood, in dreaming sleep, and in the maintenance of arousal. Several amino acids are thought to be neurotransmitters, including γ-aminobutyric acid (GABA), glutamic acid, and aspartic acid. Small chains of amino acids also are known to be neurotransmitters, such as enkephalins and endorphins. These neuropeptides are involved in the perception and integration of pain as well as in emotional experiences. Noback, Strominger, and Demarest (1991) define a neurotransmitter as a chemical that "must be synthesized in the neuron, become localized in the presynaptic terminal, be released into the synaptic cleft, bind to a receptor site (binding site) on the postsynaptic membrane of another neuron or effector where it affects ion channels and, lastly, be removed by a specific mechanism from its site of action." Neurotransmitter and/or neuromodulator substances are listed in Table 12-2.

Because the neurotransmitter is stored on one side of the synaptic cleft and the receptor sites are on the other side, chemical synapses operate in only one direction. Action potentials therefore are transmitted along a multineuronal pathway in only one direction. The binding of the neurotransmitter at the receptor site changes the permeability of the postsynaptic neuron and consequently its membrane potential. Two possible scenarios can then follow: (1) the postsynaptic neuron may be ex-

TABLE 12-2

Substances That Are Neurotransmitters and/or Neuromodulators

Substance	Location	Effect	Clinical example
Acetylcholine	Many nuclei scattered throughout the brain and spinal cord. Nerve tracts from the nuclei extend to many areas of the brain and spinal cord. Also found in the neuromuscular junction of skeletal muscle and many ANS synapses.	Excitatory or inhibitory	Alzheimer disease (a type of senile dementia) is associated with a decrease in acetylcholine-secreting neurons. Myasthenia gravis (weakness of skeletal muscles) results from a reduction in acetylcholine receptors.
Monoamines			
Norepinephrine	A small number of small-sized nuclei in the brainstem. Nerve tracts extend from the nuclei to many areas of the brain and spinal cord. Also in some ANS synapses.	Excitatory or inhibitory	Cocaine and amphetamines,* resulting in overstimulation of postsynaptic neurons.
Serotonin	A small number of small-sized nuclei in the brainstem. Nerve tracts extend from the nuclei to many areas of the brain and spinal cord.	Generally inhibitory	Involved with mood, anxiety, and sleep induction. Levels of serotonin are elevated in schizophrenia (delusions, hallucinations, and withdrawal).
Dopamine	Confined to a small number of nuclei and nerve tracts. Distribution is more restricted than that of norepinephrine or serotonin. Also found in some ANS synapses.	Generally excitatory	Parkinson disease (depression of voluntary motor control) results from destruction of dopamine-secreting neurons. Drugs used to increase dopamine production induce vomiting and schizophrenia.
Histamine	Hypothalamus, with nerve tracts to many parts of the brain and spinal cord.	Generally inhibitory	No clear indication of histamine-associated pathologies. Histamine apparently is involved with arousal, pituitary hormone secretion, control of cerebral circulation, and thermoregulation.
Amino acids			
Gamma-aminobutyric acid (GABA)	GABA-secreting neurons mostly control activities in their own area and are not usually involved with transmission from one part of the CNS to another. Most neurons of the CNS have GABA receptors.	Majority of postsynaptic inhibition in the brain; some presynaptic inhibition in the spinal cord	Drugs that increase GABA function have been used to treat epilepsy (excessive discharge of neurons).
Glycine	Spinal cord and brain. Like GABA, glycine predominantly produces local effects.	Most postsynaptic inhibition in the spinal cord	Glycine receptors are inhibited by strychnine.

From Seeley, Stephens, & Tate, 1992.   *Continued.*
*Increase the release and block the re-uptake of norepinephrine.

TABLE 12-2

Substances That Are Neurotransmitters and/or Neuromodulators—cont'd

Substance	Location	Effect	Clinical example
Amino acids—cont'd			
Glutamate and aspartate	Widespread in the brain and spinal cord, especially in nerve tracts that ascend or descend the spinal cord or in tracts that project from one part of the brain to another.	Excitatory	Drugs that block glutamate or aspartate are under development. These drugs might prevent seizures and neural degeneration from overexcitation.
Neuropeptides			
Endorphins and enkephalins	Widely distributed in the CNS and PNS.	Generally inhibitory	The opiates morphine and heroin bind to endorphin and enkephalin receptors on presynaptic neurons and reduce pain by blocking the release of neurotransmitter.
Substance P	Spinal cord, brain, and sensory neurons associated with pain.	Generally excitatory	Substance P is a neurotransmitter in pain transmission pathways. Blocking the release of substance P by morphine reduces pain.

From Seeley, Stephens, & Tate, 1992.

cited (depolarized) or (2) the postsynaptic neuron's plasma membrane may be inhibited (hyperpolarized). These effects on the plasma membrane of the postsynaptic neuron are referred to as **excitatory postsynaptic potentials (EPSPs)** and **inhibitory postsynaptic potentials (IPSPs).** (Chapter 1 contains a review of electrical impulses and membrane potentials.)

A single EPSP is not generally capable of inducing a neuron's action potential and the propagation of the nerve impulse. Whether this occurs depends on the number and frequency of potentials the postsynaptic neuron receives. This concept is referred to as **summation. Temporal summation** (time relationship) refers to the effects of successive impulses received at the same synapse. **Spatial summation** (spacing effect) is the combined effects of impulses a single neuron transmits to different synapses at the same time. **Facilitation** is a term that refers to the effect of EPSP on the plasma membrane potential. The plasma membrane is said to be facilitated when summation has brought the membrane closer to the threshold potential and the stimulus required to induce an action potential is then less. The effect that a chemical neurotransmitter has on the plasma membrane potential depends on the balance of these effects. The mechanisms of convergence, divergence, summation, and facilitation allow for the integrative processes of the nervous system.

THE CENTRAL NERVOUS SYSTEM
The Brain

The human brain is credited with a multitude of tasks that make reason, intellectual function, personality, mood, and interaction with the environment possible. The brain is a pinkish gray organ that weighs approximately 3 pounds. It receives approximately 15% to 20% of the total cardiac output. On the basis of embryologic origin, the three major divisions of the brain are (1) the forebrain, which includes the two cerebral hemispheres; (2) the midbrain, including the corpora quadrigemina, tegmentum, and cerebral peduncles; and (3) the hindbrain, which forms the cerebellum, pons, and medulla (Table 12-3). The midbrain, together with the medulla and pons, comprises the **brainstem,** which connects the hemispheres of the brain, cerebellum, and spinal cord. A collection of nerve cell bodies (nuclei) within the brainstem also comprises the **reticular formation** (Fig. 12-5). The reticular formation is a large network of connected tissue and contains portions of vital reflexes, such as those controlling cardiovascular function and respiration. The reticular formation is essential for maintaining wakefulness and therefore is referred to as the **reticular activating system** (Fig. 12-5). Some nuclei within the reticular formation have been shown to cause specific motor movements.

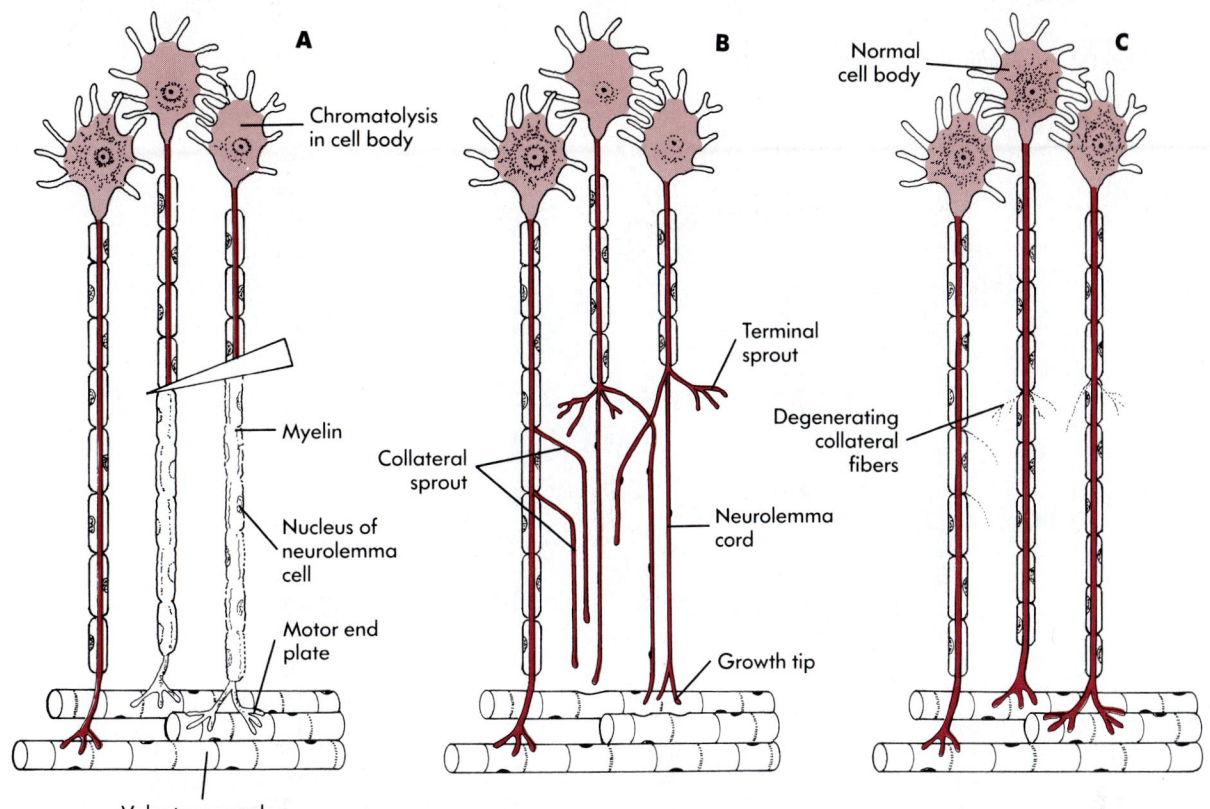

FIG. 12-4 **Degeneration and regeneration of peripheral somatic motor nerve fibers. A,** Several days after transection (at the wedge). Note the chromatolysis and eccentric nuclei, increase in number of neurolemma cells, and fragmentation of myelin sheaths. **B,** Several weeks later, the neurilemma cord receives regenerating axis cylinders from the transected fibers and collateral branches from the adjacent normal fiber. **C,** Several months later, collateral branches of axis cylinders that failed to innervate motor endplates degenerate. The regenerated portions of the fibers contain more internodes than before; hence they conduct nerve impulses more slowly.

TABLE 12-3

Division of the Central Nervous System

Primary vesicles	Secondary vesicles	Associated structures
Forebrain (prosencephalon)	Telencephalon	Cerebral hemispheres
		Cerebral cortex
		Rhinencephalon
		Basal ganglia
	Diencephalon	Epithalamus
		Thalamus
		Hypothalamus
		Subthalamus
Midbrain (mesencephalon)	Mesencephalon	Corpora quadrigemina
		Tegmentum
		Cerebral peduncles
Hindbrain (rhombencephalon)	Metencephalon	Cerebellum
		Pons
	Myelencephalon	Medulla oblongata
Spinal cord	Spinal cord	Spinal cord

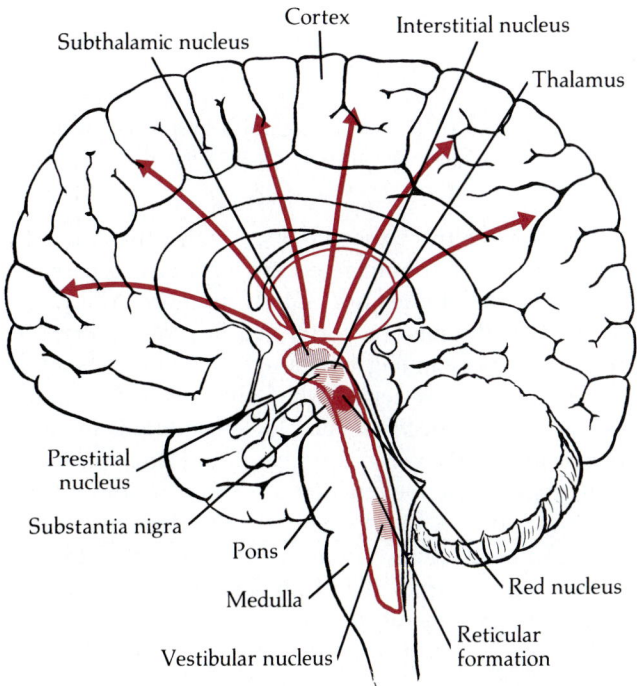

FIG. 12-5 **The reticular activating system.** (From Rudy, 1984.)

FIG. 12-6 **The cerebral hemispheres. A,** Principal functional subdivisions of cerebral hemisphere. **B,** Functional areas of specific cortical areas. (From Rudy, 1984.)

Divisions of the brain are associated with different functions, but attributing specific functions to definite regions of the brain is not entirely accurate. Many activities actually may be performed in several different regions. Understanding functional destinations is very useful, however, especially when one tries to determine or localize the effects of pathologic conditions in various regions of the nervous system. Many attempts have been made to ascribe function to various regions of the cerebral cortex. A neuropsychiatrist (Brodmann) is credited with postulating various activities to many regions of the cerebral cortex. (Fig. 12-6 illustrates these regions and describes some of the areas.)

Forebrain
Telencephalon

The **telencephalon** consists of the **cerebrum** (the largest portion of the brain), the limbic system, and **basal ganglia** composed of several "nuclei." The surface of the cerebrum (cerebral cortex) is characterized by many convolutions called *gyri* (Fig. 12-7). This irregular structural arrangement increases the surface area in which the nerve cell bodies can lie and thereby maximizes their function. Grooves between adjacent gyri are termed **sulci.** Deeper grooves are referred to as **fissures.** The cerebral cortex contains the cell bodies of neurons, a substance termed **gray matter. White matter** lies beneath the

FIG. 12-7 Lateral view of cerebral hemisphere (showing lobes and principal fissures, cerebellum, pons, and medulla oblongata). (From Rudy, 1984.)

cerebral cortex and is composed of myelinated nerve fibers.

The two cerebral hemispheres are separated by the longitudinal fissure. The surface of each hemisphere is divided into lobes that take their names from the region of the skull under which each of them lies. The **frontal lobe** has its posterior margin on the **fissure of Rolando (central fissure)**, and it borders inferiorly on the **sylvian fissure (lateral fissure)** (Fig. 12-7). The **prefrontal area** is responsible for goal-oriented behavior (e.g., ability to concentrate), short-term or recall memory, and the elaboration of thought. It also exerts an inhibitory influence over the limbic and vegetative areas of the cerebrum. The **premotor area** contains motor programs for fine repetitive motor movements. This area contains the cell bodies that form part of the **extrapyramidal system** (efferent pathways outside the pyramidal pathway that connect the cerebral cortex with spinal nerve pathways). The term *pyramidal* originates from a pyramid-shaped structure in the medulla, where these pathways converge. The pyramids are also the location where motor pathways cross over. Cerebral impulses control function in the opposite side of the body, a phenomenon called **contralateral control** (see Fig. 12-9).

The **primary motor area** is located along the **precentral gyrus** and forms the **primary voluntary motor pathway.** The axons traveling from the cell bodies in this region are projection fibers that form the **pyramidal system** that descends into the spinal cord. At the inferior edge of the precentral gyrus (usually in the left hemisphere) is **Broca's speech area.** It is responsible for

the motor aspects of speech. Damage to this area, commonly as a result of a cerebrovascular accident (stroke), results in speech difficulty or even inability to form words (expressive aphasia or dysphasia) (see Chapter 14).

The **parietal lobe** lies between the borders of the central, parietooccipital, and lateral fissures. This lobe contains the major area for somatic sensory input, primarily located along the **postcentral gyrus,** which is adjacent to the primary motor area. Communication between the motor and sensory areas (and among other regions in the cortex) is provided by **association fibers.** The remainder of this region is involved in sensory association (storage, analysis, and interpretation of sensory stimuli). (Fig. 12-6, *A,* shows the distribution of function associated with both the primary motor area and the primary sensory area of the cerebral cortex.)

The **occipital lobe** lies behind the parietooccipital sulci and above the cerebellum. The primary visual cortex (visual receptive area) is located in this region. The remainder of this lobe is involved primarily in visual association. The **temporal lobe** lies below the lateral fissure. Primary auditory and secondary associational areas account for the primary functional aspects of this region. **Wernicke's area** lies in the superoposterior portion of this region and extends up into the parietal lobe. This area is responsible for reception and interpretation of speech, and dysfunction may result in receptive aphasia or dysphasia. The temporal lobe also is involved as a major area for long-term memory, as well as secondary functions such as balance, taste, and smell.

Another lobe, the **insula,** lies hidden from view in the lateral fissure (see Fig. 12-7). The deepest groove in the cerebrum, the longitudinal fissure, divides the cerebrum into two hemispheres. Lying directly beneath the longitudinal fissure is a mass of white matter pathways called the **corpus callosum (transverse or commissural fibers).** The corpus callosum connects the two cerebral hemispheres and is essential in the coordination of activities between hemispheres, especially specific tasks that may be present in only one hemisphere (see Fig. 12-15).

The large interior of the cerebrum consists mainly of white matter made of numerous tracts. Some gray matter, however, lies deep inside the white matter. Collectively these areas of gray matter are called **basal ganglia.** Since gray matter within the CNS is normally called *nuclei* instead of ganglia, this group of nuclei should be called **cerebral nuclei.** The cerebral nuclei include the **caudatus nucleus** and the **lentiform nucleus.** A structure associated with the cerebral nuclei is the **internal capsule.** It is located between the caudatus and lentiform nuclei. Collectively the caudatus nucleus, internal capsule, and lentiform nucleus constitute the **corpus striatum.** The corpus striatum appears striped because of the connections between its gray matter and the white matter of the internal capsule.

The cerebral nuclei are part of the extrapyramidal system. They contain multiple connections to various regions of the CNS and are believed to exert a fine-tuning effect on motor movements. Parkinson disease and Huntington disease (chorea) are conditions associated with defects of the cerebral nuclei, or basal ganglia. They are characterized by various involuntary or exaggerated motor movements (see Chapters 14 and 15).

The **limbic system** (emotional brain) primarily is composed of a group of structures surrounding the corpus callosum, as well as parts of the diencephalon. It has primary connections with other parts of the brain, notably the thalamus, fornix, septal nucleus, **amygdaloid nucleus** (the tip of the caudatus nucleus, one of the cerebral nuclei), and the hypothalmus. The limbic system's principal effects are believed to be involved with primitive behavioral responses, visceral reaction to emotion, feeding behaviors, biologic rhythms, and the sense of smell. Expression of affect (emotional and behavioral states) is mediated by extensive connections with the limbic system and prefrontal cortex.

Diencephalon

The **diencephalon,** surrounded by the cerebrum, is made up of four divisions: **epithalamus, thalamus, hypothalamus,** and **subthalamus** (see Table 12-3 and Fig. 12-8). The epithalamus forms the roof of the third ventricle (a brain cavity) and composes the most superior portion of the diencephalon. It has connections and functions closely associated with those of the limbic system. For example, the hormones of the pineal body have been shown to influence reproductive ability, and the secretion of melatonin is associated with circadian rhythms (see Chapter 17).

The largest component of the diencephalon is the thalamus. It borders and surrounds the third ventricle, and it is a major integrating center for afferent impulses to the cerebral cortex. The perception of various sensations occurs at this level but requires cortical processing for interpretation. The thalamus also serves as a relay center for information from the basal ganglia and cerebellum that is sent to the appropriate portion of the motor area.

The hypothalamus forms the base of the diencephalon. Hypothalamic function falls into two major areas: (1) maintenance of a constant internal environment and (2) behavioral patterns. Integrative centers control ANS function, regulation of body temperature, endocrine function, and regulation of emotional expression. (Temperature regulation is discussed in Chapter 13.) The hypothalamus exerts its influence through the endocrine system as well as neural pathways (see box below for a more detailed description). (For endocrine functions of the hypothalamus and pituitary, see Chapter 17.)

The subthalamus flanks the hypothalamus laterally. It serves as an important extrapyramidal center for motor activities.

Midbrain

The midbrain (**mesencephalon**) is composed of three structures: the **corpora quadrigemina,** also known as the **tectum,** (composed of the superior and inferior colliculi); the **tegmentum** (containing the red nucleus and substantia nigra); and the cerebral peduncles.

The **superior colliculi** are involved with voluntary and involuntary visual motor movements (e.g., the ability of the eyes to *track* moving objects in the visual field). The **inferior colliculi** accomplish similar motor activities but involve movements that affect the auditory system (such as positioning of the head to improve hearing). The **red**

FUNCTIONS OF THE HYPOTHALAMUS

Visceral and somatic responses
Affectual responses
Hormone synthesis
Autonomic nervous system activity
Temperature regulation
Feeding responses
Physical expression of emotions
Sexual behavior
Pleasure-punishment centers
Level of arousal or wakefulness

FIG. 12-8 The diencephalon (thalamus and hypothalamus) and cranial nerves. (From Rudy, 1984.)

nucleus and **substantia nigra** are extensions of the extrapyramidal system. The substantia nigra synthesizes **dopamine**, a neurotransmitter and precursor of norepinephrine. Its dysfunction also is associated with Parkinson disease (see Chapter 15). The **cerebral peduncles** consist of efferent fibers of the corticospinal tract.

Other notable structures of this region are the nuclei of the third and fourth cranial nerves. The **cerebral aqueduct** (aqueduct of Sylvius), which carries cerebrospinal fluid, also traverses this structure.

Hindbrain
Metencephalon

The major structures of the **metencephalon** are the cerebellum and the pons. The **cerebellum** (see Figs. 12-7 and 12-8) is composed of gray and white matter and its cortical surface is convoluted like the surface of the cerebrum. It also is divided by a central fissure into two lobes that are connected by a midline structure called the **vermis.**

The cerebellum is responsible for reflexive, involuntary fine-tuning of motor control and for maintaining balance and posture. This is accomplished by means of extensive neural connections with the medulla through the inferior cerebellar peduncle and with the midbrain

through the superior cerebellar peduncle. The two hemispheres are connected to the pons by the middle cerebellar peduncle. These connections allow extensive sampling of visual, vestibular, and proprioceptive data from other regions of the CNS and periphery. Damage to the cerebellum is characterized by a loss of equilibrium, balance, and motor coordination.

The **pons** (bridge) is easily recognized by its bulging appearance. It lies below the midbrain and above the medulla. Its primary function is the transmission of information from the cerebellum to the brainstem and between the two cerebellar hemispheres. The pons is an important center for the control of respiration (i.e., rate and relationship of inspiration to expiration). The nuclei of the fifth through eighth cranial nerves are located in this structure.

Myelencephalon

The **myelencephalon** usually is called the **medulla oblongata** and forms the lowest portion of the brainstem. Reflex activities, such as heart rate, respiration, blood pressure, coughing, sneezing, swallowing, and vomiting, are controlled in this area. The nuclei of cranial nerves IX through XII (see p. 422 for discussion) also are located in this region.

The medulla is the point at which a major portion of the descending motor pathways (i.e., corticospinal tracts) cross to the other side, or decussate (Fig. 12-9). These pathways, together with other areas of decussation in the CNS, are the basis for the phenomenon of contralateral control. Sleep-wake rhythms also are processed by neural influences from lower brain centers and are associated with a complex group of diffuse structures and functions (see Chapter 13). Among these structures is the reticular activating system, a system of cells that receives collateral signals from the afferent sensory pathways and projects the signals to the higher brain centers, thus controlling CNS activity.

The Spinal Cord

The **spinal cord** is the portion of the CNS that lies within the vertebral canal and is surrounded and protected by the **vertebral column.** The spinal cord essentially functions as a large nerve cable that connects the brain and body. It extends from the medulla and ends at the level of the first or second lumbar vertebra in adults (Fig. 12-10). The end of the spinal cord is cone-shaped and is termed the **conus medullaris.** Spinal nerves continue from the end of the spinal cord and form a nerve bundle called the **cauda equina.**

A cross section of the spinal cord (Fig. 12-11) is characterized by a butterfly-shaped inner core of gray matter (containing nerve cell bodies). In the center of this region lies the **central canal,** which extends through the spinal cord from its origin in the fourth ventricle. The gray matter of the spinal cord is divided into three regions and displays specific functional characteristics. These regions include the **dorsal horn (posterior horn),** which primarily is composed of interneurons and axons from sensory neurons whose cell bodies lie in the **dorsal root ganglion.** At the tip of the dorsal horn is the **substantia gelatinosa,** a structure involved in transmission of pain (see Chapter 13). The **lateral horn** contains cell bodies involved with the ANS, as well as interneurons to connect the dorsal horn cells to the ventral horn. The **ventral horn (anterior horn)** contains the nerve cell bodies for efferent pathways leaving the spinal cord by way of spinal nerves.

Surrounding the gray matter is white matter that forms ascending and descending pathways called **spinal tracts.** Spinal tracts are named to denote their beginning and ending points. For example, the **spinothalamic tract** carries nerve impulses from the spinal cord to the thalamus in the diencephalon. Numerous spinal tracts are grouped into columns according to their location within the white matter. These consist of the **ventral column, lateral column,** and **dorsal column.** (Fig. 12-12 identifies the location and principal activities of the major spinal tracts.)

Neural circuits in the spinal cord, when activated, dis-

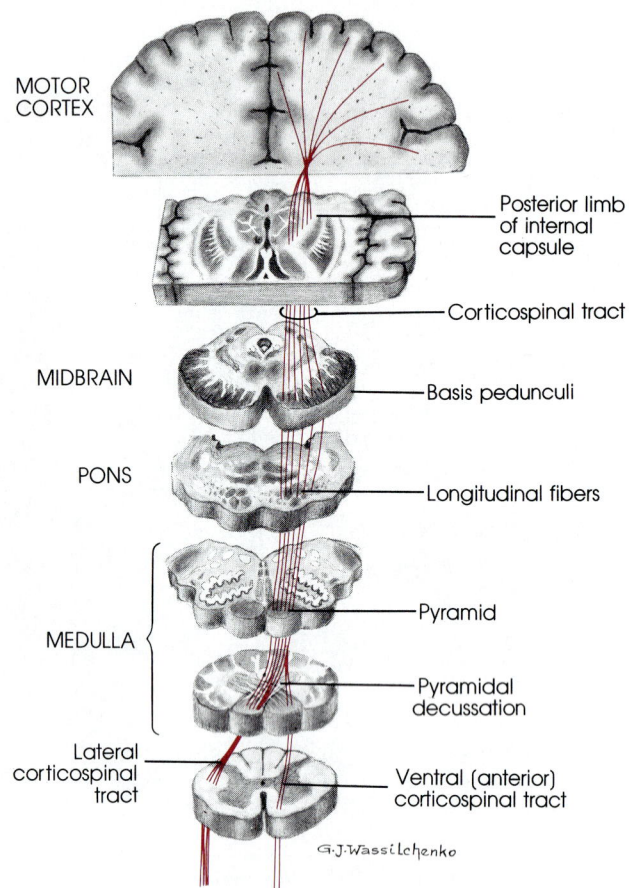

FIG. 12-9 Schematic drawing of decussation of pyramids at level of medulla. (From Rudy, 1984.)

play specific sets of motor responses. **Reflex arcs** form basic units that respond to stimuli and provide protective circuitry for motor output. Structures mandatory for a reflex arc are a receptor, an **afferent (sensory) neuron,** an **efferent (motor) neuron,** and an effector muscle or gland. A simple reflex arc may contain only two neurons. (Fig. 12-13 illustrates a simple reflex arc.)

Much of the regulation of the internal environment is mediated by reflex activity involving the ANS. The motor effects of reflex arcs generally occur before perception of the event in the higher centers of the brain.

Afferent pathways transmit information from peripheral receptors and eventually terminate in the cerebral or cerebellar cortex or both. Efferent pathways primarily relay information from the cerebrum to the brainstem or spinal cord. **Upper motor neurons** are the classification of motor pathways that are completely contained within the CNS. Their primary role is influencing and modifying spinal reflex arcs and circuits. Generally, upper motor neurons form synapses with interneurons, which then form synapses with lower motor neurons before projecting into the periphery. **Lower**

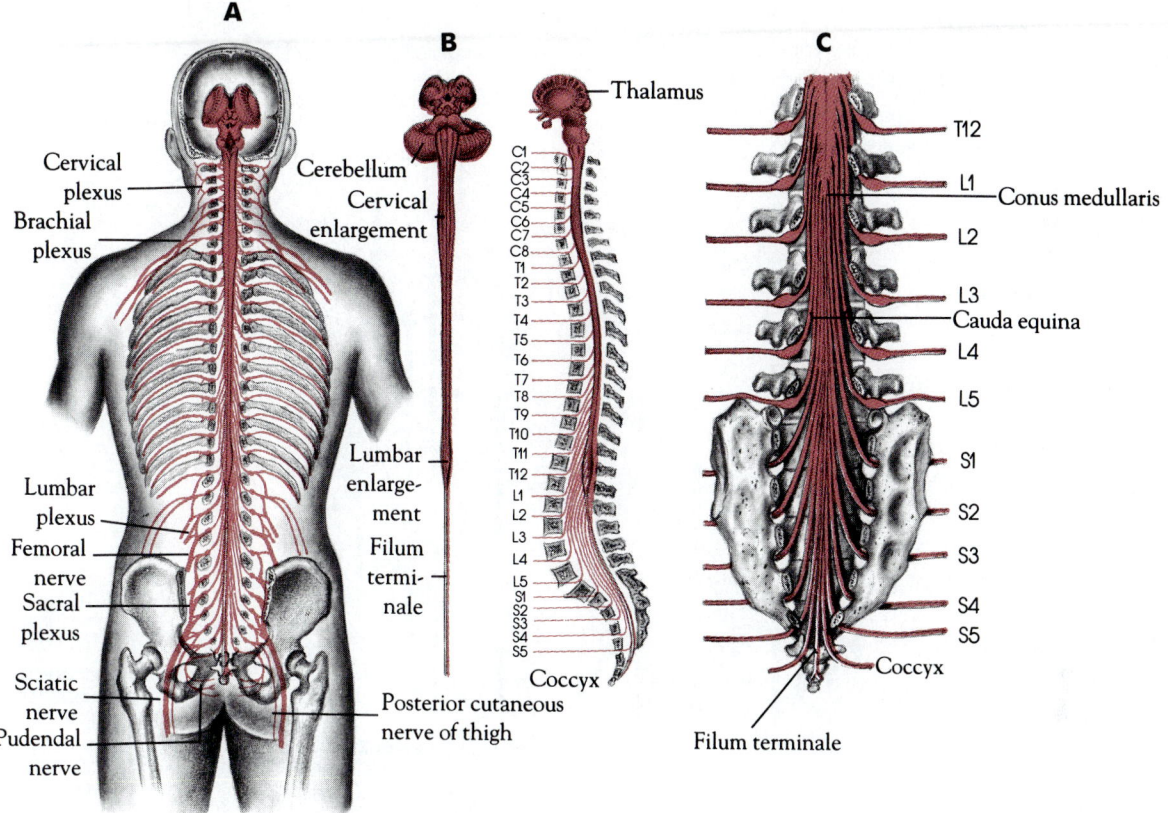

FIG. 12-10 **Spinal cord within vertebral canal and exiting spinal nerves. A,** Posterior view of brainstem and spinal cord in situ with spinal nerves and plexus. **B,** Anterior view of brainstem and spinal cord. **C,** Enlargement of caudal area showing termination of spinal cord (conus medullaris) and group of nerve fibers constituting the cauda equina. (From Rudy, 1984.)

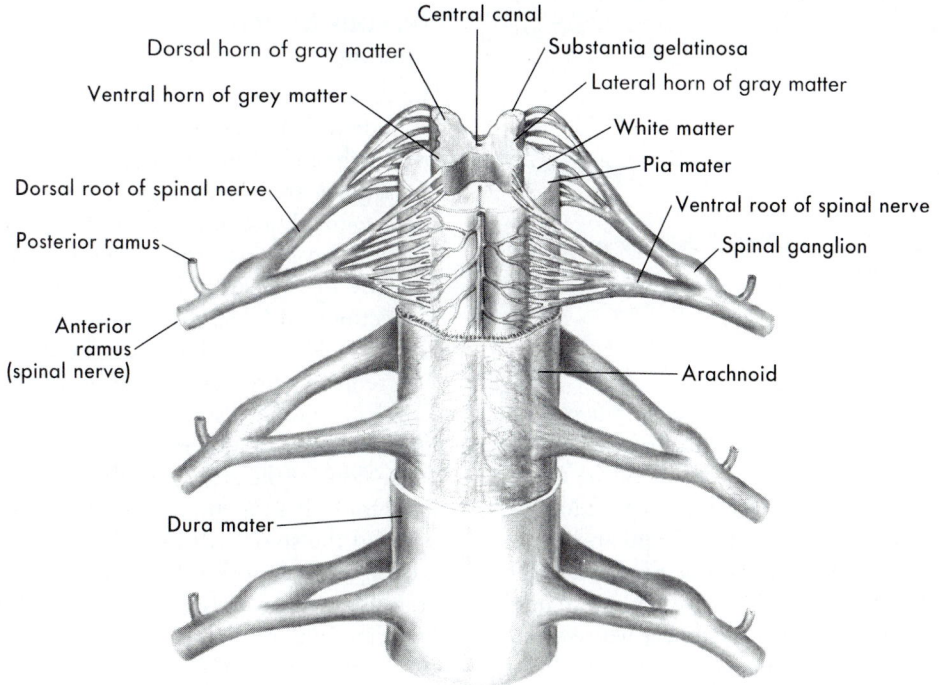

FIG. 12-11 Cross section of spinal cord showing attachments of spinal nerves.

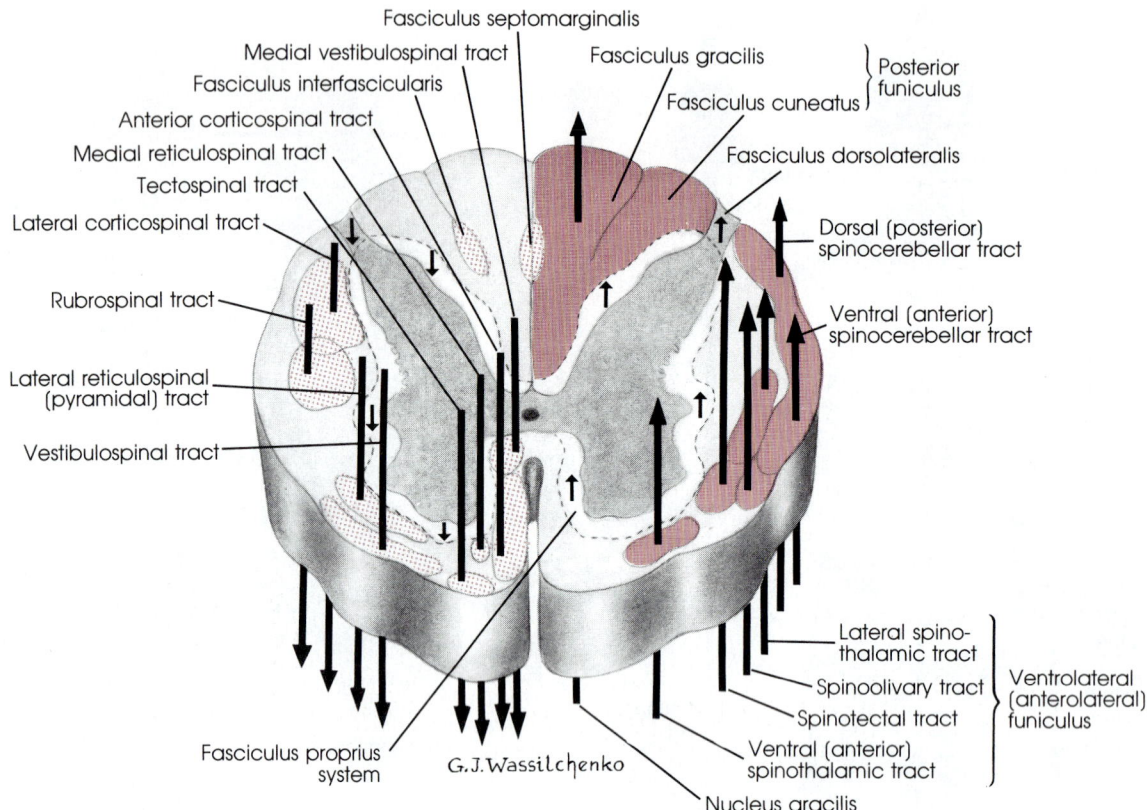

FIG. 12-12 Spinal cord tracts. Cross section of upper thoracic cord. Tracts and their placement at various levels of the cord. (From Rudy, 1984.)

FIG. 12-13 Cross section of spinal cord showing simple reflex arc. (From Rudy, 1984.)

motor neurons are responsible for direct influence to muscles. Their cell bodies lie in the gray matter of the spinal cord, but their processes extend out of the CNS.

Muscle activity (i.e., stimulation and contraction) is regulated by nerve impulses. Motor neurons innervate one or more muscle cells, forming **motor units** that consist of a neuron and the skeletal muscles it stimulates. The junction between the axon of the motor neuron and the plasma membrane of the muscle cell is called the **neuromuscular (myoneural) junction** (Fig. 12-14). (Injury to motor neurons is discussed in Chapter 14.)

Protective Structures of the Central Nervous System
Cranium

The cranium is composed of eight bones that fuse early in childhood. The cranial vault functions to enclose and protect the brain and its associated structures.

The **galea aponeurotica,** which is a thick fibrous band of tissue overlying the cranium between the frontal and occipital muscle, affords added protection to the bony structure of the skull. The subgaleal space has venous connections with the dural sinuses and, with increased intracranial pressure, blood can be shunted to the space, thus reducing pressure in the intracranial cavity. The subgaleal space is also a common site for wound drains after intracranial surgery.

The floor of the cranial vault is irregular and contains many foramina (openings) for cranial nerves, blood vessels, and the spinal cord to exit. The cranial floor is divided into three fossae (depressions). The frontal lobes lie in the **anterior fossa,** the temporal lobes and base of the diencephalon lie in the **middle fossa** (temporal fossa), and the cerebellum lies in the **posterior fossa.** These terms are commonly used anatomic landmarks to describe the location of intracranial lesions.

FIG. 12-14 **Neuromuscular junction. A,** Diagram of neuromuscular junction. **B,** Neuron axons typically branch as they connect with skeletal muscle as shown here. Each connection at a neuromuscular junction ends in a motor end-plate. (**A** from Thompson et al., 1993; **B** from Raven & Johnson, 1991.)

Meninges

Surrounding the brain and spinal cord are three protective membranes: the dura mater, the arachnoid membrane, and the pia mater. Collectively they are called the **meninges** (Fig. 12-15). The **dura mater** (meaning literally "hard mother") is composed of two layers, with the venous sinuses formed between them. The outermost layer forms the **periosteum (endosteal layer)** of the skull. The **inner dura (meningeal layer)** is responsible for the formation of rigid plates that serve to support and separate various brain structures.

One of these membranous plates, the **falx cerebri,** dips between the two cerebral hemispheres along the longitudinal fissure. The falx cerebri is anchored anteriorly to the base of the brain at the crista galli of the ethmoid bone. The **tentorium cerebelli** is a membrane that surrounds the brainstem and separates the cerebellum below from the cerebral structures above. The tentorium is also a common landmark used to describe intracranial lesions. For example, supratentorial means above the tentorium and infratentorial means below the tentorium. The tentorium may become involved during periods of increased intracranial pressure caused by an injury to the brain. An injury within the cranial cavity tends to shift intracranial contents, and as structures shift, they tend to be compressed against these rigid membranes, resulting in damage or destruction. A common example is tentorial herniation.

Below the dura mater lies the **arachnoid membrane,** characterized by its spongy weblike structure. It loosely follows the contours of the cerebral structures.

The space between the dura and arachnoid membrane is the **subdural space.** Many small bridging veins that have little support traverse the subdural space. Their disruption results in a subdural hematoma (see Chapter 15). The **subarachnoid space** lies between the arachnoid membrane and the pia mater and contains cerebrospinal fluid (see Fig. 12-15). Disruption of intracranial vessels can lead to a condition called subarachnoid hemor-

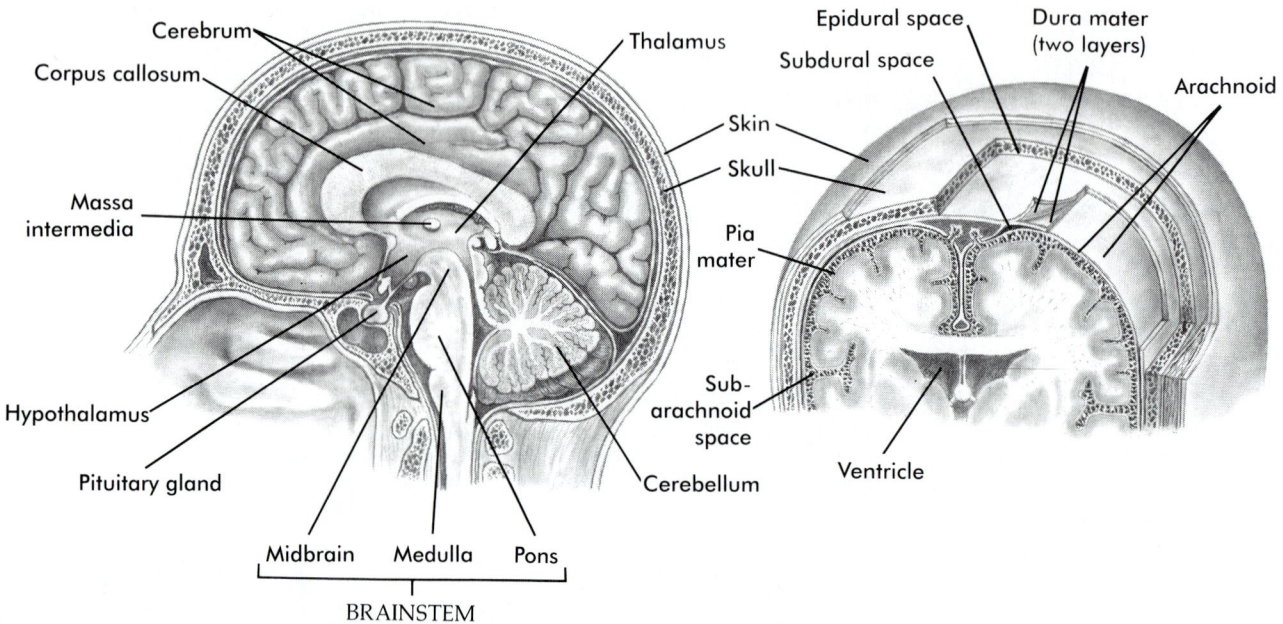

FIG. 12-15 Meninges of brain. (From Thompson et al., 1993.)

rhage. This occult location of blood frequently results in signs of meningeal irritation.

Unlike the dura mater and arachnoid membrane, the delicate pia mater follows the contours of the brain and spinal cord very closely. It provides support for blood vessels serving brain tissue. The **choroid plexuses,** structures that produce cerebrospinal fluid, arise from the pial membrane (see Fig. 12-15). The spinal cord is anchored to the vertebrae by extension of the meninges. The meninges continue beyond the end of the spinal cord to the lower portion of the sacrum. Cerebrospinal fluid, contained within the subarachnoid space, also circulates down to about the second sacral vertebra.

The meninges form potential and real spaces important to understanding functional and pathologic mechanisms. For example, between the dura mater and skull lies a potential space termed the **epidural space** (see Fig. 12-15). The arterial supply to the meninges consists of blood vessels that lie within grooves in the skull. As a result of trauma, the skull can be fractured and the blood vessels disrupted. The ruptured vessels can lead to an accumulation of blood within the epidural space, called an *epidural hematoma* (see Chapter 15). An inflammation of the meninges (meningitis) also can have serious implications because of the relative proximity to the brain. (Disorders of the CNS are discussed in Chapter 15.)

Cerebrospinal Fluid and the Ventricular System

Cerebrospinal fluid (CSF) is a clear, colorless fluid similar to that of blood plasma and interstitial fluid. It cushions the CNS by protecting soft tissue from jolts and blows. The intracranial and spinal cord structures float in CSF. The buoyant properties of the CSF protect the delicate structures of the brain and prevent the brain from tugging on meninges, nerve roots, and blood vessels. (Constituents of CSF are listed in Table 12-4.) Between 125 and 150 ml of CSF is circulating within the **ventricles** (small cavities) and subarachnoid space at any given time. Approximately 600 ml of CSF is produced daily.

The choroid plexuses in the lateral, third, and fourth ventricles produce the major portion of CSF. (Ventricles are illustrated in Fig. 12-15.) These plexuses are characterized by a rich network of blood vessels, supplied by the pia mater, that lie in close contact with the ependymal cells of the ventricles.

The CSF exerts pressure within the brain and spinal cord. With a person in a recumbent position, CSF pressure is approximately 120 to 180 mm of water pressure, or approximately 9 to 14 mm Hg pressure. CSF flow is a result of a pressure gradient between the arterial system and the CSF-filled cavities. Beginning in the lateral ventricles, the CSF flows through the **interventricular foramen (foramen of Monro)** into the third ventricle. From the third ventricle it passes through the cerebral aqueduct (aqueduct of Sylvius) into the fourth ventricle. From the fourth ventricle the CSF may pass through either the paired **foramen of Luschka** or **foramen of Magendie** before communicating with the subarachnoid spaces of the brain and spinal cord. The CSF does not, however, accumulate. Instead, it is reabsorbed into the venous circulation through the arachnoid villi. The **arachnoid villi** are structures that protrude from the

TABLE 12-4

Composition of Cerebrospinal Fluid

Constituent	Normal value
Na^+	148 mM
K^+	2.9 mM
Cl^-	125 mM
HCO_3^-	22.9 mM
Glucose (fasting)	50-75 mg/dl (60% of serum glucose)
pH	7.3
Protein	15-45 mg/dl
Albumin	80%
Gamma globulin	6%-10%
Cells	
White (lymphocytes)	0-6/mm^3
Red	0/mm^3

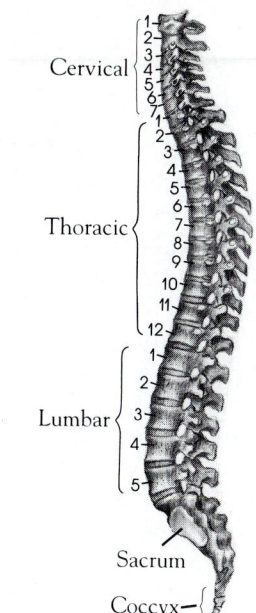

FIG. 12-16 **Vertebral column.** (From Rudy, 1984.)

FIG. 12-17 **Vertebra and intervertebral disk.** (From Rudy, 1984.)

G.J.Wassilchenko

arachnoid space, through the dura mater, and lie within the blood flow of the venous sinuses. CSF is reabsorbed by means of a pressure gradient between the arachnoid villi and the cerebral venous sinuses. The villi function as one-way valves directing CSF outflow into the blood but preventing blood flow into the subarachnoid space. Thus CSF is formed from the blood, and after circulating throughout the CNS, it returns to the blood.

Samples of CSF are withdrawn for diagnostic purposes by inserting a needle between the third and fourth lumbar vertebrae into the subarachnoid space—a procedure called **lumbar puncture**—or from an intraventricular catheter. Spinal anesthesias (blocks) are administered in a similar manner.

Vertebral Column

The vertebral column (Fig. 12-16) is composed of 33 vertebrae: 7 cervical, 12 thoracic, 5 lumbar, 5 fused sacral, and 4 fused coccygeal. Between each interspace (except the fused sacral and coccygeal vertebrae) is an **intervertebral disk** (Fig. 12-17). At the center of the intervertebral disk is the **nucleus pulposus**, a pulpy mass of elastic fibers. The intervertebral disk functions to absorb shocks, preventing damage to the vertebrae. The intervertebral disk is also a common source of back problems. If too much stress is applied to the vertebral column, the disk contents may rupture and protrude into the spinal canal, causing compression of the spinal cord or nerve roots.

Blood Supply of the Central Nervous System

Blood Supply to the Brain

The brain receives approximately 20% of the cardiac output, or 800 to 1000 ml of blood flow per minute. Carbon dioxide serves as a primary regulator for blood flow within the CNS. Carbon dioxide is a potent vasodilator in the CNS, and its effects ensure an adequate blood supply.

The brain derives its arterial supply from two systems: the **internal carotid arteries** and the **vertebral arteries** (Fig. 12-18). The internal carotid arteries supply a proportionately greater amount of blood flow. They take their origin from the common carotid arteries, enter the cranium through the base of the skull, and pass through the **cavernous sinus.** After giving off some small branches, they divide into the anterior and middle cerebral arteries. The vertebral arteries originate at the subclavian arteries and pass through the transverse foramina of the cervical vertebrae, and enter the cranium

through the framen magnum. They join at the junction of the pons and medulla to form the **basilar artery.** The basilar artery divides at the level of the midbrain to form paired posterior cerebral arteries. The large arteries on the surface of the brain and their branches are called **superficial arteries (conducting arteries).** The small branches that project into the brain are termed **projecting arteries (nutrient arteries).**

The **circle of Willis** (Fig. 12-19) is a structure credited with the ability to compensate for reduced blood flow from any one of the major contributors (collateral blood flow). The circle of Willis is formed by the posterior cerebral arteries, posterior communicating arteries, internal carotid arteries, anterior cerebral arteries, and anterior communicating artery. The anterior cerebral, middle cerebral, and posterior cerebral arteries leave the circle of Willis and extend to various brain structures. (Table 12-5 and Fig. 12-20 illustrate structures served, functional relationships, and pathologic considerations related to occlusion of cerebral arteries.)

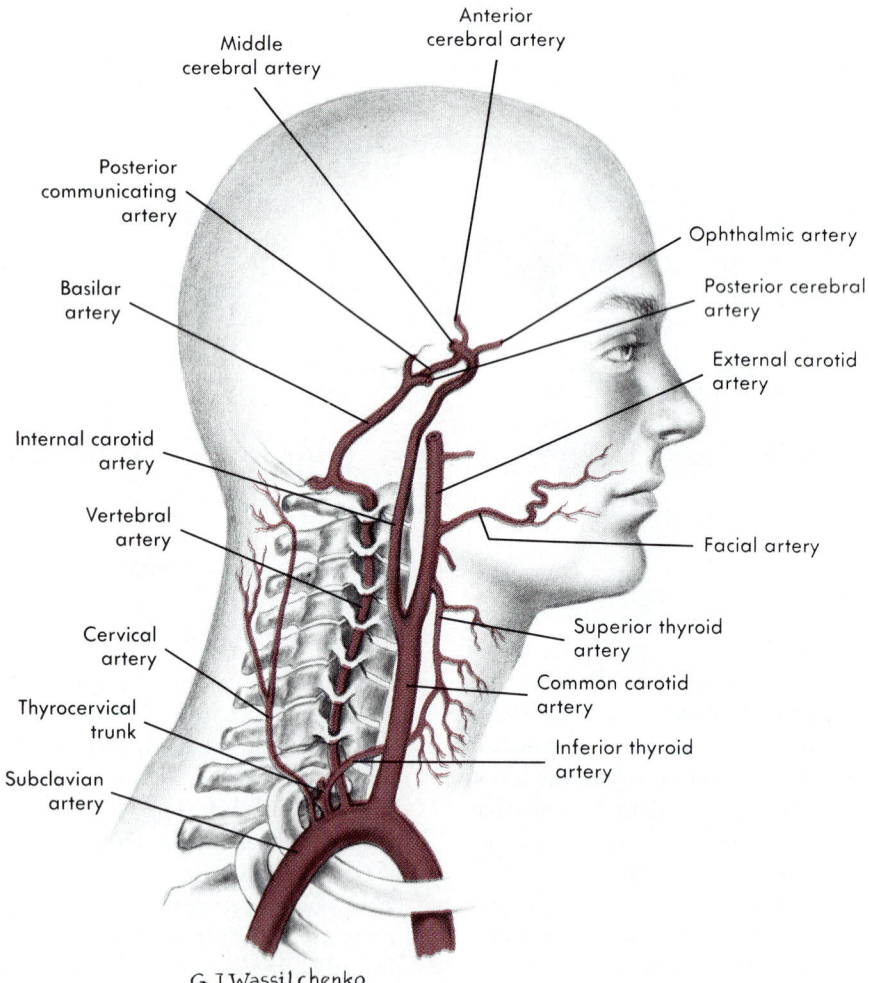

G.J.Wassilchenko

FIG. 12-18 Anatomic diagram of circle of Willis. (Chipps, Clanin, & Campbell, 1992.)

FIG. 12-19 Blood supply of the brain. (From Rudy, 1984.)

The venous drainage of the cerebrum is not parallel (side by side) to the arterial supply, whereas the venous drainage of the brainstem and cerebellum is parallel to the arterial supply. The cerebral veins are classified as superficial veins and deep cerebral veins. The veins drain into venous plexuses and dural sinuses (formed between the dural layers) and eventually drain into the internal jugular veins at the base of the skull (Fig. 12-21). Adequacy of venous outflow can have a significant effect on intracranial pressure. For example, in individuals with head injury, turning or letting the head fall to the side partially occludes venous return and can increase intracranial pressure because of decreased flow through the jugular veins.

Blood Supply to the Spinal Cord

The spinal cord derives its blood supply from branches off the vertebral arteries and from branches from various regions of the aorta (Fig. 12-22). The **anterior spinal arteries** and the paired **posterior spinal arteries** branch off the vertebral artery at the base of the cranium and descend alongside the spinal cord. Arterial branches from vessels exterior to the spinal cord follow the spinal nerve through the intervertebral foramina, pass through the dura, and divide into the anterior and posterior radicular arteries.

> ### CLINICAL COMMENTARY
> ### BLOOD-BRAIN BARRIER
>
> The *blood-brain barrier* is a term used to describe cellular structures that selectively inhibit certain substances in the blood from entering the interstitial spaces of the brain or CSF. This term emphasizes the impermeability of the nervous system to large and potentially harmful molecules. It is thought that the supporting cells (neuroglia), particularly the astrocytes, and tight junctions between endothelial cells of brain capillaries (see Chapter 1) are involved in the formation of the blood-brain barrier. The exact nature of this mechanism is controversial, but it appears that certain metabolites, electrolytes, and chemicals have differing abilities to cross into the brain. This has substantial implications for drug therapy because certain types of antibiotics and chemotherapeutic drugs show a greater propensity than others for crossing the barrier.

Arterial Systems Supplying the Brain

Arterial origin	Structures served	Conditions caused by occlusion
Anterior cerebral artery	Basal ganglia; corpus callosum; medial surface of cerebral hemispheres; superior surface of frontal and parietal lobes	Hemiplegia on the contralateral side of the body, greater in the lower than in the upper extremities
Middle cerebral artery	Frontal lobe; parietal lobe; temporal lobe (primarily the cortical surfaces)	Aphasia in dominant hemisphere and contralateral hemiplegia (see Chapter 14)
Posterior cerebral artery	Part of the diencephalon and temporal lobe; occipital lobe	Contralateral hemiplegia greater in the face and upper extremities than in the lower extremities; sensory loss; visual loss

FIG. 12-20 Areas of the brain effected by occlusion of the anterior, middle, and posterior cerebral artery branches. **A,** Cross section. **B,** Lateral view. (From Rudy, 1984.)

FIG. 12-21 **Large veins of the head. Deep veins and dural sinuses are projected on the skull.** Note connections (emissary veins) between the superficial and deep veins. (From Rudy, 1984.)

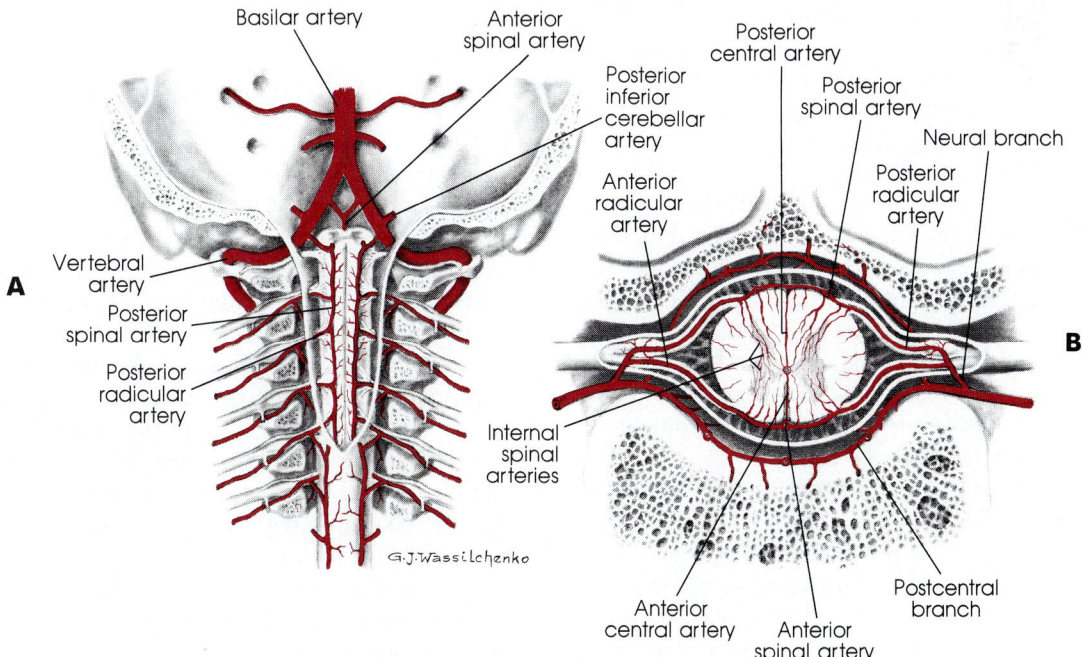

FIG. 12-22 **Arteries of the spinal cord. A,** Arteries of cervical cord exposed from the rear. **B,** Arteries of spinal cord diagrammatically shown in horizontal section. (From Rudy, 1984.)

The radicular arteries eventually reconnect to the spinal arteries. Branches from the radicular and spinal arteries form plexuses whose branches penetrate the spinal cord, supplying the deeper tissues. Venous drainage parallels the arterial supply closely and drains into venous sinuses located between the dura and periosteum of the vertebrae.

THE PERIPHERAL NERVOUS SYSTEM

The cranial and spinal nerves, including their branches and ganglia, constitute the PNS. A peripheral nerve (cranial or spinal) is composed of individual axons wrapped in a myelin sheath. These individual fibers are arranged in bundles called **fascicles** (Fig. 12-23). The coverings supply structural support, a blood supply, and interstitial compartments necessary for the supply of essential electrolytes to support nerve impulse conduction.

The 31 pairs of spinal nerves derive their names from the vertebral level from which they exit. There are eight cervical spinal nerves. The first cervical nerve exits above the first cervical vertebra and the rest of the spinal nerves exit below their corresponding vertebrae. From the thoracic region (and interiorly) nerves correspond to the vertebral level above their exit.

Spinal nerves contain both sensory and motor neurons and are called **mixed nerves** that arise as rootlets from the ventral and dorsal horn cells of the spinal cord. These two spinal nerve roots converge in the region of the intervertebral foramen to form the spinal nerve trunk. Shortly after converging, the spinal nerve divides into anterior and posterior rami (branches). The anterior rami (except the thoracic) initially form **plexuses** (networks of nerve fibers), which then branch into the peripheral nerves. Instead of forming plexuses, the thoracic nerves pass through the intercostal spaces and innervate regions of the thorax.

The main spinal nerve plexuses innervate the skin and the underlying muscles of the limbs. The **brachial plexus,** for example, is formed by the last four cervical nerves (C_5 to C_8) and the first thoracic nerve (T_1). The brachial plexus extends downward and laterally to innervate the nerves of the arm, wrist, and hand. The **lumbar plexus** (L_2 to L_4) and **sacral plexus** (L_5 to S_5) contain nerves that innervate the anterior and posterior portions of the lower body, respectively.

The posterior rami of each spinal nerve, with their many processes, are distributed to a specific area in the body. Sensory signals thus arise from specific sites associated with a specific spinal cord segment. Specific areas of cutaneous innervation at these spinal cord segments are called **dermatomes.** The dermatomes of various spinal nerves are distributed in a fairly regular pattern, although adjacent regions between dermatomes can be innervated by more than one spinal nerve.

Like spinal nerves, cranial nerves are categorized as peripheral nerves. Most of these are mixed nerves (like the spinal nerves), although some are purely sensory or purely motor. Cranial nerves arise from nuclei in the brain and brainstem. (Fig. 12-8 illustrates their structure, and Table 12-6 describes structural and functional characteristics.)

THE AUTONOMIC NERVOUS SYSTEM

Components of the autonomic nervous system (ANS) are located in both the PNS and CNS; however, the ANS is considered part of the efferent division of the PNS. Many neurons of the ANS travel in the spinal nerves and certain cranial nerves. The widespread activity of this system indicates that its components are distributed all over the body. The peripheral autonomic nerves are mainly efferent fibers, but not purely motor or secretory. The motor component of the ANS is a two-neuron system consisting of **preganglionic** and **postganglionic neurons.** This arrangement contrasts with the somatic nervous system, in which a single motor neuron travels from the CNS to the structure innervated.

The ANS coordinates and maintains a steady state among visceral (internal) organs, such as regulation of cardiac muscle and the glands of the body. This system is mostly an involuntary system, whereby one *generally* cannot "will" these functions to happen. The ANS is separated both structurally and functionally into two divisions: (1) the **sympathetic nervous system** (Fig. 12-24) and (2) the **parasympathetic nervous system** (Fig. 12-25).

Anatomy of the Sympathetic Nervous System

The sympathetic nervous system functions to mobilize energy stores in times of need (e.g., in the "fight or flight response") (see Fig. 9-1; see also Chapter 9). The sympathetic division receives its innervation from cell bodies located from the first thoracic (T1) through the second lumbar (L2) regions of the spinal cord and therefore is called the **thoracolumbar division.** The preganglionic axons of the sympathetic division form synapses shortly after leaving the cord in the **sympathetic (paravertebral) ganglia.** At this point the impulse may travel several ways: (1) directly across the same ganglion level and form a synapse with the cell bodies of the postganglionic neuron, (2) up or down the sympathetic chain before forming synapses with a higher or lower postganglionic neuron, or (3) passage through the chain ganglion without synapsing (see Fig. 12-24). Some of the preganglionic axons form pathways called **splanchnic nerves,** which lead to **collateral ganglia** located on the front of the aorta. The collateral ganglia are named ac-

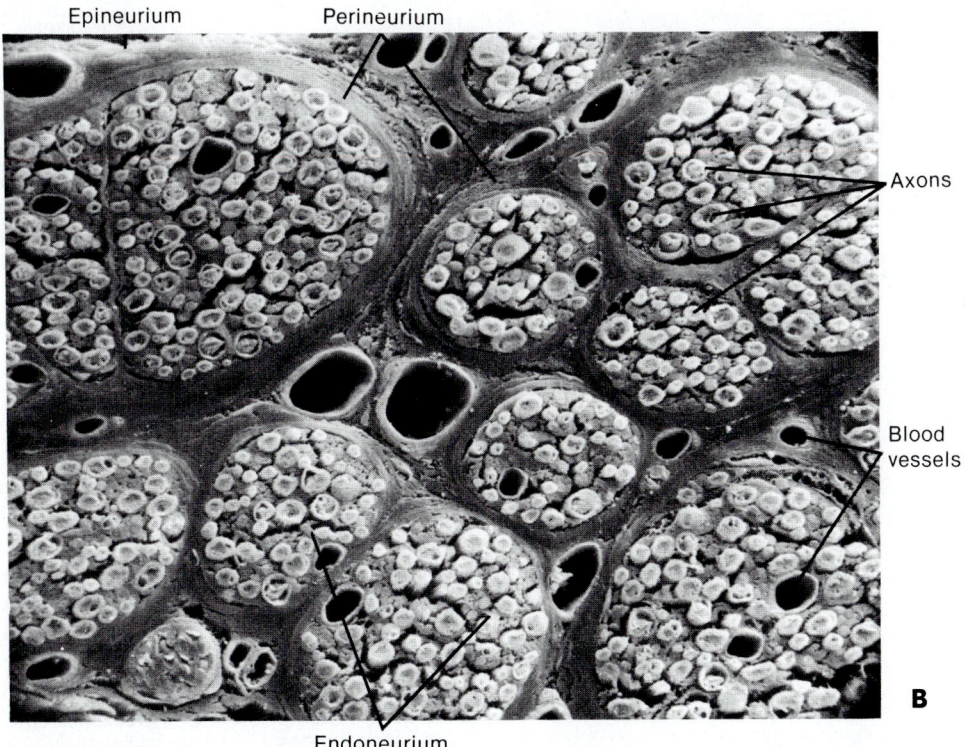

FIG. 12-23 **Peripheral nerve. A,** Peripheral nerve trunk and coverings. **B,** Scanning electron micrograph of a freeze-fractured preparation of peripheral nerve. (**A** from Thompson et al., 1993; **B** from Nolte, 1991.)

TABLE 12-6

The Cranial Nerves

Number and name	Origin and course	Function	How tested
I. Olfactory	Fibers arise from the nasal olfactory epithelium and form synapses with the olfactory bulbs, which transmit impulses to the temporal lobe of the cerebral cortex	Purely sensory; carries impulses for sense of smell	Person is asked to sniff aromatic substances, such as oil of cloves and vanilla, and to identify them
II. Optic	Fibers arise from the retina of the eye to form the optic nerve, which passes through the sphenoid bone; the two optic nerves then form the optic chiasma (with partial crossover of fibers) and continue on to the occipital cortex as the optic tracts	Purely sensory; carries impulses for vision	Vision and visual field are tested with an eye chart and by testing the point at which the person first sees an object (finger) moving into the visual field; the inside of the eye is viewed with ophthalmoscope to observe blood vessels of the eye interior
III. Oculomotor	Fibers emerge from midbrain and exit from skull to run to eye	Contains motor fibers to the superior, inferior, and medial rectus muscles that direct the eyeball to the muscles of the eyelid, and to the iris and smooth muscle controlling lens shape; contains proprioceptor fibers from the external eye muscles to the brain	Pupils are examined for size and shape, and equality; pupillary reflex is tested with a pen light (pupils should constrict when illuminated); ability to follow moving objects
IV. Trochlear	Fibers emerge from the midbrain and exit from skull to run to eye	Proprioceptor and motor fibers for superior oblique muscle of the eye (external eye muscle)	Tested in common with cranial nerve III relative to the ability to follow moving objects
V. Trigeminal	Fibers emerge from pons and form three divisions that exit from skull and run to face	Both motor and sensory for face; conducts sensory impulses from mouth, nose, and surface of eyes; also contains motor fibers that stimulate chewing muscles	Sensations of pain, touch, and temperature are tested with safety pin and hot and cold objects; corneal reflex tested with a wisp of cotton; motor branch tested by asking the subject to clench teeth, open mouth against resistance, and move jaw from side to side
VI. Abducens	Fibers leave inferior pons and exit from skull to run to eye	Contains motor fibers to lateral rectus muscle and proprioceptor fibers from same muscle to brain	Tested in common with cranial nerve III relative to the ability to move each eye laterally

TABLE 12-6

The Cranial Nerves—cont'd

Number and name	Origin and course	Function	How tested
VII. Facial	Fibers leave pons and travel through temporal bone to reach face	Mixed: (a) Supplies motor fibers to muscles of facial expression and to lacrimal and salivary glands and (b) carries sensory fibers from taste buds of anterior part of tongue	Anterior two thirds of tongue is tested for ability to taste sweet (sugar), salty, sour (vinegar), and bitter (quinine) substances; symmetry of face is checked; subject is asked to close eyes, smile, whistle, and so on; tearing is tested with ammonia fumes
VIII. Vestibulocochlear (acoustic)	Fibers run from inner ear (hearing and equilibrium receptors in temporal bone) to enter brainstem just below pons	Purely sensory; vestibular branch transmits impulses for sense of equilibrium; cochlear branch transmits impulses for sense of hearing	Hearing is checked by air and bone conduction by use of a tuning fork
IX. Glossopharyngeal	Fibers emerge from midbrain and leave skull to run to throat	Mixed: (a) Motor fibers serve pharynx (throat) and salivary glands and (b) sensory fibers carry impulses from pharynx, posterior tongue (taste buds), and pressure receptors of the carotid artery	Gag and swallowing reflexes are checked; subject is asked to speak and cough; posterior one third of tongue may be tested for taste
X. Vagus	Fibers emerge from medulla, pass through skull, and descend through neck region into thorax and abdominal region	Fibers carry sensory and motor impulses for pharynx; a large part of this nerve is parasympathetic motor fibers, which supply the smooth muscles of abdominal organs; transmits sensory impulses from the viscera	Same as for cranial nerve IX (IX and X are tested in common because they both serve muscles of the throat)
XI. Spinal accessory	Fibers arise from medulla and superior spinal cord and travel to the muscles of neck and back	Provides sensory and motor fibers for sternocleidomastoid and trapezius muscles and muscles of soft palate, pharynx, and larynx	Sternocleidomastoid and trapezius muscles are checked for strength by asking subject to rotate head and shrug shoulders against resistance
XII. Hypoglossal	Fibers arise from medulla and exit from skull to travel to tongue	Carries motor fibers to muscles of tongue and sensory impulses from tongue to brain	Subject is asked to stick out tongue, and any position abnormalities are noted

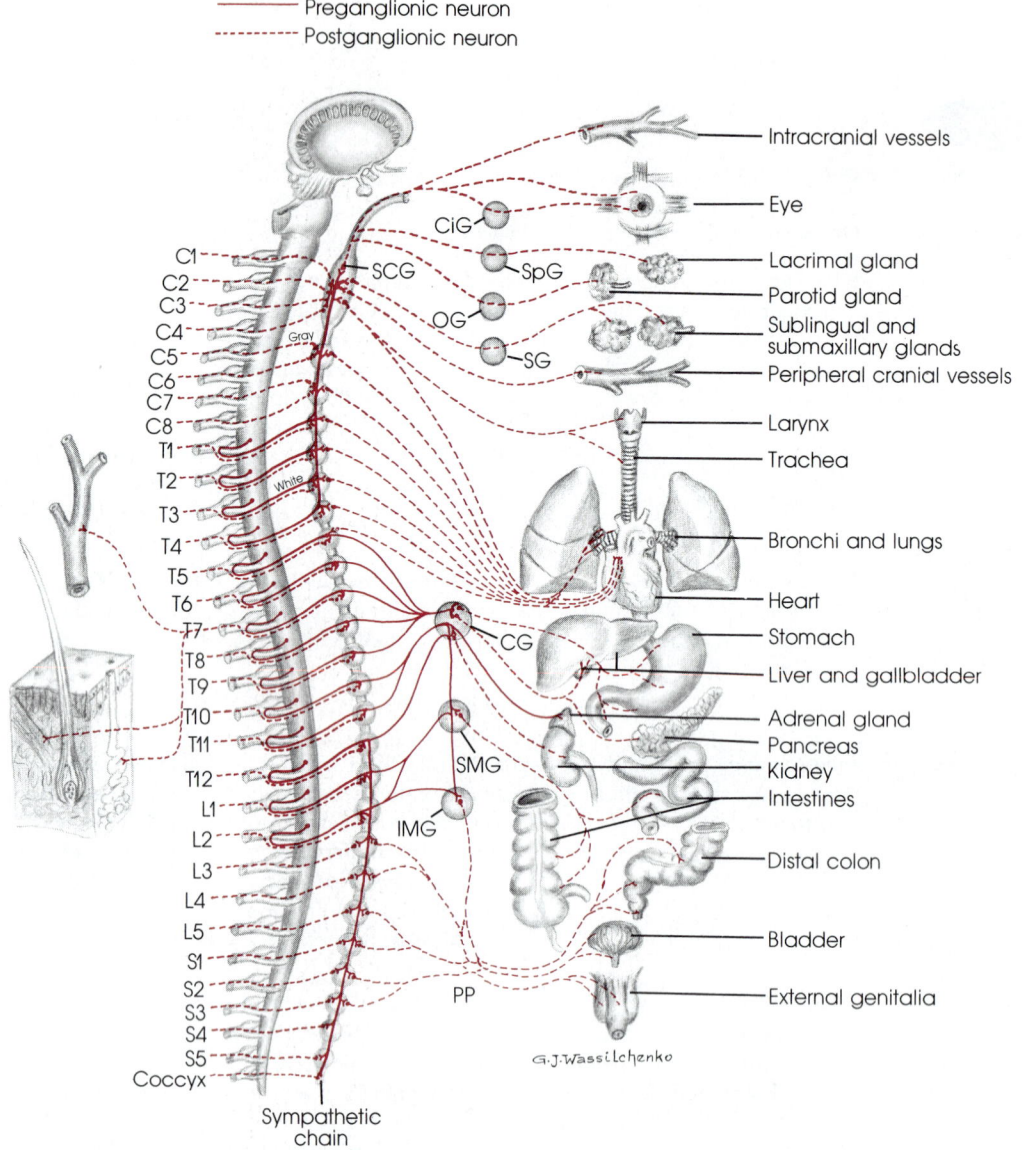

Preganglionic neuron
Postganglionic neuron

C1
C2
C3
C4
C5
C6
C7
C8
T1
T2
T3
T4
T5
T6
T7
T8
T9
T10
T11
T12
L1
L2
L3
L4
L5
S1
S2
S3
S4
S5
Coccyx

Gray
White

SCG
CiG
SpG
OG
SG
CG
SMG
IMG
PP

Sympathetic
chain

Intracranial vessels
Eye
Lacrimal gland
Parotid gland
Sublingual and
submaxillary glands
Peripheral cranial vessels
Larynx
Trachea
Bronchi and lungs
Heart
Stomach
Liver and gallbladder
Adrenal gland
Pancreas
Kidney
Intestines
Distal colon
Bladder
External genitalia

G.J.Wassilchenko

FIG. 12-24 **Sympathetic division of the autonomic nervous system.** *CiG,* Ciliary ganglion; *SpG,* sphenopalatine ganglion; *SCG,* superior cervical ganglion; *OG,* otic ganglion; *SG,* submandibular ganglion; *CG,* celiac ganglion; *SMG,* superior mesenteric ganglion; *IMG,* inferior mesenteric ganglion; *PP,* pelvic plexus. (From Rudy, 1984.)

cording to the branches of the aorta nearest them, the **celiac, superior mesenteric,** and **inferior mesenteric.** The preganglionic neurons synapse with postganglionic neurons within the collateral ganglia. These postganglionic neurons leave the collateral ganglia and innervate the viscera below the diaphragm.

Preganglionic sympathetic neurons that innervate the adrenal medulla also travel in the splanchnic nerves and *do not* synapse before reaching the gland. There is no postganglionic sympathetic component to the adrenal medulla; thus it is the only exception to the usual two-neuron chain in the autonomic afferent pathway. Because preganglionic sympathetic fibers are all myeli-

nated, travel to the adrenal medulla is quick, and innervation causes the rapid release of epinephrine and norepinephrine. Epinephrine and norepinephrine are mediators of the "fight or flight response" (see Chapter 9).

Anatomy of the Parasympathetic Nervous System

The parasympathetic nervous system (PNS) functions to conserve and restore energy. The nerve cell bodies of this division are located in the cranial nerve nuclei and in the sacral region of the spinal cord and therefore con-

FIG. 12-25 **Parasympathetic division of the autonomic nervous system.** *CiG*, Ciliary ganglion; *SpG*, sphenopalatine ganglion; *OG*, otic ganglion; *SG*, submandibular ganglion; *VN*, vagus nerve; *CG*, celiac ganglion; *SMG*, superior mesenteric ganglion; *PP*, pelvic plexus; *PN*, pelvic nerve. Fibers of the parasympathetic system pass through the CG and SMG, but these ganglia are not part of the parasympathetic system. (From Rudy, 1984.)

stitute the **craniosacral division.** Unlike the sympathetic branch, the preganglionic fibers in the parasympathetic division travel close to the organs they innervate before forming synapses with the relatively short postganglionic neurons (see Fig. 12-25). Parasympathetic nerves arising from nuclei in the brainstem travel to the viscera of the head, thorax, and abdomen within cranial nerves—including the oculomotor (III), facial (VII), glossopharyngeal (IX), and vagus (X) nerves.

Preganglionic parasympathetic nerves that originate from the sacral region of the spinal cord run either separately or together with some spinal nerves. The preganglionic axons join together to form the **pelvic nerve,** which innervates the viscera of the pelvic cavity. These preganglionic axons synapse with postganglionic neu-

rons in terminal ganglia located close to the organs they innervate.

Neurotransmitters and Neuroreceptors

Sympathetic preganglionic fibers and parasympathetic preganglionic and postganglionic fibers release **acetylcholine**—the same neurotransmitter released by somatic efferent neurons (Fig. 12-26). These fibers are characterized by **cholinergic transmission.** Most postganglionic sympathetic fibers release **norepinephrine** (adrenaline) and thus are considered to function by **adrenergic transmission.** A few postganglionic sympathetic fibers release acetylcholine, such as those that innervate the sweat glands.

The action of catecholamines varies with the type of

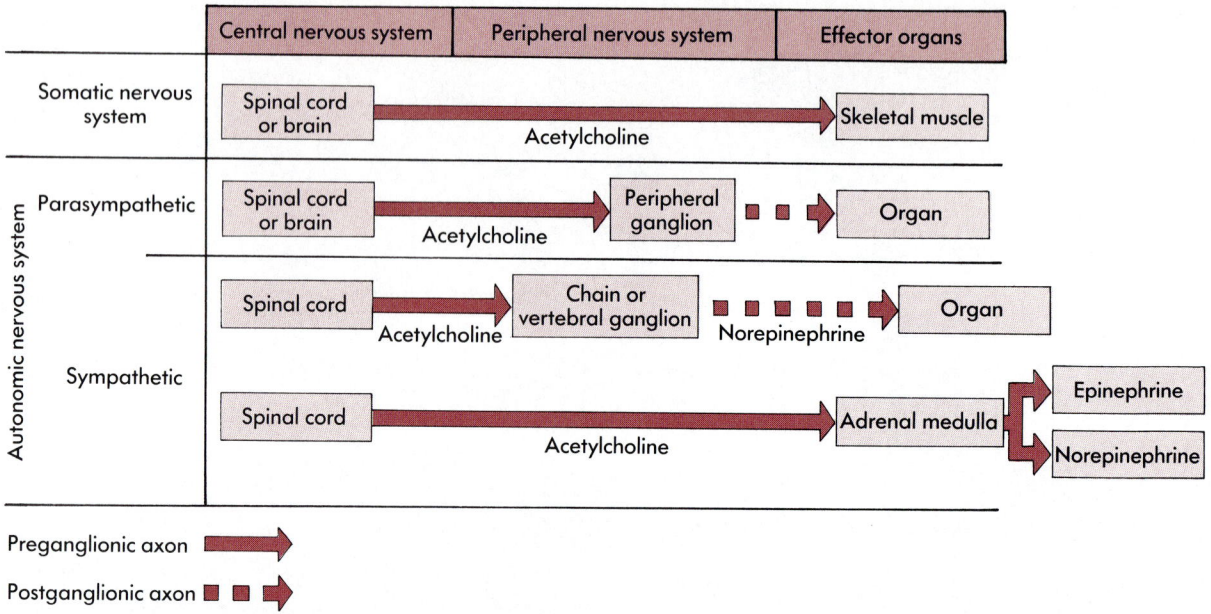

FIG. 12-26 The autonomic nervous system and the type of neurotransmitters secreted by preganglionic and postganglionic fibers. A somatic nerve is used for comparison.

TABLE 12-7

Actions of the Autonomic Nervous System of Neuroreceptors

Effector organ or tissue	Receptor	Adrenergic effect	Cholinergic effect
Eye, iris			
Radial muscle	α_1	Contraction (mydriasis)	—
Sphincter muscle	—	—	Contraction (miosis)
Eye, ciliary muscle	β	Relaxation for far vision	Contraction for near vision
Lacrimal glands	—	—	Secretion
Nasopharyngeal glands	—	—	Secretion
Salivary glands	α_1	Secretion of K and water	Secretion of K and water
	β	Secretion of amylase	—
Heart			
SA node	β_1	Increase heart rate	Decrease heart rate; vagus arrest
Atria	β_1	Increase contractility and conduction velocity	Decrease contractility; shortened action-potential duration
AV junction	β_1	Increase automaticity and propagation velocity	Decrease automaticity and propagation velocity
Purkinje system	β_1	Increase automaticity and propagation velocity	—
Ventricles	β_1	Increase contractility	—
Arterioles			
Coronary	α, β_2	Constriction, dilatation	Dilatation
Skin	α_2	Constriction, dilatation	Dilatation
Mucosa	α	Constriction	Dilatation
Skeletal muscle	α, β_2	Constriction, dilatation	Dilatation
Cerebral	α	Constriction (slight)	—
Pulmonary	α, β_2	Constriction, dilatation	—
Mesenteric	α	Constriction	—
Renal	$\alpha_1, \beta_1, \beta_2, d_1, D^*$	Constriction, dilatation	—
Salivary glands	α	Constriction	Dilatation

Modified from Vick, 1984.
D, Dopaminergic.

Continued.

neuroreceptor stimulated. Remember, catecholamines also are released by the adrenal medulla gland that physiologically and biochemically resembles the sympathetic nervous system. Two types of adrenergic receptors exist, α and β. Cells of the effector organs may have only one or both types of adrenergic receptors. The **α-adrenergic receptors** have been further subdivided according to the action produced. α_1-Adrenergic activity is associated mostly with excitation or stimulation; α_2-adrenergic activity is associated with relaxation or inhibition. Most of the α-adrenergic receptors on effector organs belong to the α_1 class. The **β-adrenergic receptors** are classified as β_1-adrenergic receptors (which fa-

cilitate increased heart rate and contractility and cause the release of renin from the kidney) and β_2-adrenergic receptors (which facilitate all of the remaining effects attributed to β receptors) (Berne & Levy, 1993). Norepinephrine stimulates all α_1 and β_1 receptors and only certain β_2 receptors. The primary response from norepinephrine, however, is stimulation of the α_1-adrenergic receptors that cause vasoconstriction. Epinephrine strongly stimulates all four types of receptors and induces general vasodilation because of the predominance of β receptors in muscle vasculatures. (Table 12-7 summarizes the effects of neuroreceptors on their effector organs.)

TABLE 12-7

Actions of the Autonomic Nervous System of Neuroreceptors—cont'd

Effector organ or tissue	Receptor	Adrenergic effect	Cholinergic effect
Veins, systemic	α_1,β_2	Constriction, dilatation	—
Lung			
Bronchial muscle	β_2	Relaxation	Contraction
Bronchial glands	α_1,β_2	Decreased secretion; increased secretion	Stimulation
Stomach			
Motility	α_1,β_2	Decrease (usually)	Increase
Sphincters	α	Contraction (usually)	Relaxation (usually)
Secretion	—	Inhibition (?)	Stimulation
Liver			
	α,β_2	Glycogenolysis and gluconeogenesis	Glycogen synthesis
Gallbladder and ducts	—	Relaxation	Contraction
Pancreas			
Acini	α	Decreased secretion	Secretion
Islet cells	α_2,β_2	Decreased secretion, increased secretion	—
Intestine			
Motility and tone	α_1,β_1,β_2	Decrease	Increase
Sphincters	α	Contraction (usually)	Relaxation (usually)
Secretion	—	Inhibition (?)	Stimulation
Adrenal medulla	—	—	Secretion of epinephrine and norepinephrine (nicotinic effect)
Kidney	β_1	Secretion of renin	—
Ureter			
Motility and tone	α	Increased	Increased
Urinary bladder			
Detrusor	β	Relaxation (usually)	Contraction
Trigone and sphincter	α	Contraction	Relaxation
Sex organs, male	α	Ejaculation	Erection
Skin			
Pilomotor muscles	α	Contraction	—
Sweat glands	α	Localized secretion	Generalized secretion
Fat cells	α,β_1	Lipolysis	—
Pineal gland	β	Melatonin synthesis	—

Functions of the Autonomic Nervous System

Many body organs are innervated by both the sympathetic and parasympathetic nervous systems. The two divisions frequently cause opposite responses; for example, sympathetic stimulation of the stomach causes decreased peristalsis, whereas parasympathetic stimulation of the intestine increases peristalsis. In general, sympathetic stimulation promotes responses that are concerned with the protection of the individual. For example, sympathetic activity increases blood sugar levels, temperature, and raises the blood pressure. In emergency situations, a generalized and widespread discharge of the sympathetic system occurs. This process is accomplished by an increase in the firing frequency of sympathetic fibers and by activation of sympathetic fibers normally silent and at rest (fibers to the sweat glands, pilomotor muscles, and the adrenal medulla, as well as vasodilator fibers to muscle). Regulation of vasomotor tone is considered the single most important function of the sympathetic nervous system. (Fig. 12-27 illustrates some of the most important functions of the sympathetic nervous system; also see Fig. 9-1.)

Increased parasympathetic activity promotes rest and tranquility and is characterized by reduced heart rate and enhanced visceral functions concerned with digestion. Stimulation of the vagus nerve in the gastrointestinal tract increases peristalsis and secretion, as well as relaxation of sphincters. Activation of parasympathetic fibers in the head, provided by cranial nerves III, VII, and IX, causes constriction of the pupil, tear secretion, and increased salivary secretion. Stimulation of the sacral division of the parasympathetic system contracts the urinary bladder and facilitates the process of genital erection.

The parasympathetic system lacks the generalized and widespread response of the sympathetic system. Specific parasympathetic fibers are activated for the regulation of particular functions. Although the actions of the parasympathetic and sympathetic systems usually are antagonistic, there are exceptions. Peripheral vascular resistance, for example, is increased dramatically by sympathetic activation but is not appreciably altered by activity of the parasympathetic system. Most of the blood vessels involved in the control of blood pressure are innervated by sympathetic nerves. To decrease blood pressure, therefore, it is more important to block or paralyze the continuous (tonic) discharge of the sympathetic system than to promote parasympathetic activity.

❑ AGING and the Nervous System

The CNS mechanisms involved in the aging process are extremely complex, and many questions concerning the neurologic effects of aging have yet to be answered.

Some of the identified mechanisms associated with aging are pathologically induced, but the distinction between these mechanisms and those that are a part of the normal aging process remains somewhat cloudy.

Structural Changes with Aging

The CNS demonstrates many structural changes during the aging process. The primary mechanism responsible for most of these structural changes is a decrease in the number of neurons. Predominant external features of the aging brain include decreased brain weight and size (primarily the frontal hemispheres), increased adherence of the dura mater to the skull, fibrosis and thickening of the meninges, narrowed gyri, and widened sulci with a corresponding increase in the size of the subarachnoid space. The basal ganglia and ventricular system are internal structures that commonly reveal changes with aging. The basal ganglia reveal aberrations in vascular structures, and the ventricles (primarily the lateral and third ventricles) are enlarged.

Cellular Changes with Aging

Practically every cell type within the CNS reflects specific responses to aging. Characteristic of aging is a decrease in the number of neurons. Although neuronal cell loss is a general feature of aging, these losses are not consistently related to deteriorating mental function or age of the individual (Scheibel & Scheibel, 1975). Controversy regarding the effects of neuronal cell loss still exists.

Principal cellular changes associated with aging include dendrite structure, lipofuscin deposition, and the presence of neurofibrillary tangles, senile plaques, and Lewy bodies. Hirano and Llena (1983) described a decreased number of dendritic processes and their multiple synaptic connections. Lipofuscin, a yellow-brown fatty pigment, is found to be deposited intracellularly in increased amounts with age. Controversy still exists concerning whether increasing intracellular quantities of lipofuscin might be associated with disruption of cytoplasmic function, that is, protein synthesis (Sellcoe, 1992).

Senile plaques (areas of nerve degeneration) are found in the interstitial spaces of the cerebral cortex associated with tissue degeneration. **Neurofibrillary tangles** involve degenerative changes in neural protein fibers. These entities also are common in Alzheimer disease and some other forms of dementia. At present, however, little definitive evidence directly links quantitative presence of the cellular changes and nervous system function in aging individuals.

Closely paralleling cell function is a selective alteration in neurotransmitter function. One potentially fruitful area of research is correlating the effects of ace-

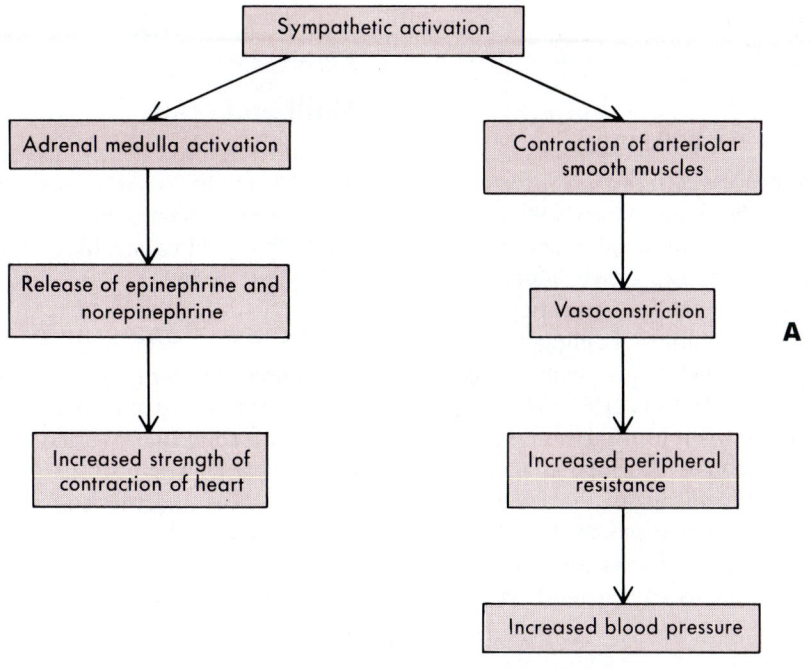

FIG. 12-27 Some important functions of the sympathetic nervous system. **A,** Regulation of vasomotor tone. **B,** Regulation of strenuous muscular exercise ("fight or flight response"). (See also Chapter 9 and Fig. 9-1 for more detail of the stress response.)

tylcholine (i.e., cholinergic transmission) and defects of memory and cognitive function associated with aging (Sellcoe, 1992).

Functional Changes with Aging

Because of integrative processes in the CNS, the consequences of aging have widespread implications for critical steady state, psychologic, and social function. Many theories have been proposed to explain the observations of progressive slowing of neurologic responses seen in aging persons (Table 12-8). Studies of changes in brain electrical activity have been helpful in determining alterations in neural function. Timiras (1972, p. 516) described the relationship between transmission of neural signals and slowing of responses observed in aging persons: "It is evident that the efficacy of the signals may be disturbed not only by irregularities in the action of cells carrying the signals but also by the amount of random background activity." This background activity is termed *neural noise.*

TESTS OF NERVOUS SYSTEM FUNCTION

Skull and Spine Roentgenograms

Roentgenograms (x-ray films) of the skull or spine, from multiple angles (views), are used primarily to localize bony defects, bone density, erosion, or calcified structures. X-ray films are likely the most commonly used radiologic studies.

Computer Tomography

Computer tomography (CT) creates two-dimensional reconstructions from multiple radiologic images by means of computer-assisted analysis. It is capable of demonstrating fine distinctions in densities of a variety of tissues. CT imaging is a safe and noninvasive procedure used in evaluating cranial and spinal structures. A variety of contrast mediums also are commonly used in conjunction with this procedure to aid in enhanced delineation of selected structures.

TABLE 12-8

Common Neurologic Signs in Aging

Neurologic sign	Examples	Change in response
Reflexes	Ankle reflex	Usually the first tendon reflex to be lost in elderly persons
	Superficial reflex	Decreased or absent responsiveness
Primitive reflexes (reflexes seen normally in infancy but that subside with maturity)	Suck and grasp	Reappearance with aging
Sensation	Taste and smell	Progressive deficit
	Pain	Increased pain threshold, although subjective complaints increase
	Vibratory sense	Decreased
	Vision	Decreased visual color sense in a significant percentage of the aged; pupils commonly smaller; slowing of pupillary relaxation and accommodation
Motor function	Physiologic tremor	Exaggeration of normally unnoticeable resting tremor that is present at all ages
	Neuromuscular control	Decreased, resulting in postural effects
	Posture	Stance commonly shows increased flexion of hips and knees; swaying motion while standing in one position more common
	Gait	Shuffling or shortened stride; loss of arm movement with walking
	Muscular atrophy	Age-associated loss of muscle fibers

Magnetic Resonance Imaging

A new development in diagnostic medicine is magnetic resonance imaging (MRI). Instead of radiation, it uses a static magnetic field to orient physiologic atomic particles. Disruption of this orientation by excitation of the particles through serial radio-frequency pulsations provides the image data. The specific tissue reaction is computer analyzed to give an image of exquisite detail, similar to that provided by CT. The MRI also provides reconstruction of images in three views at right angles (i.e., axial, sagittal, and coronal) (Fig. 12-28). The MRI is reported to have no adverse effects, particularly the associated side effects of radiation examinations.

Magnetic Resonance Angiography

A newer addition to MRI is magnetic resonance angiography (MRA). Special imaging techniques allow the visualization of blood vessels in great detail. MRA undoubtedly will be indispensable alone or in conjunction with traditional percutaneous angiography in detecting and localizing pathologic lesions of the circulatory system of the brain.

Positron Emission Tomography Scan

The positron emission tomography (PET) scan uses CT imaging to detect the emission of positive electrons from radioactive substances. These substances are injected into the bloodstream or administered as inhaled gases. As they are distributed in tissues, they display characteristic patterns that indicate physiologic and metabolic processes, for example, glucose and oxygen uptake, cerebral blood flow, neural and neurotransmitter function, and the effects of drugs.

Brain Scan

The brain scan images radionuclide substances (technetium [Tc 99m]) that have been introduced into the bloodstream. For example, visualization of tissue uptake of the radioactive agent provides an indication of blood-brain barrier integrity (increased uptake of the agent indicates disruption). This scanning technique also can identify abnormalities in blood flow dynamics and cellular metabolic function. The brain scan is particularly helpful in detecting abnormal vascularity resulting from the presence of neoplasms, abscesses, and vascular lesions.

Isotope cisternography is another radionuclide imaging technique that uses brain scan imaging to detect CSF flow, CSF resorption, and integrity of CSF pathways. The radionuclide agent in this case is injected directly into the subarachnoid space. Under normal conditions the agent passes over the cortical surface and is resorbed through the arachnoid villi. Demonstration of the agent in the ventricular system after a specific period of time indicates CSF obstruction.

FIG. 12-28 Midsagittal MRI image. Demonstrates the extraordinary anatomic detail possible with this technique. (From Nolte, 1993.)

TABLE 12-9

Cerebrospinal Fluid Analysis

Parameters	Normal	Abnormal	Possible cause
Pressure (initial readings)	120-180 mm H_2O (9-14 mm Hg)	<60 mm	Faulty needle placement Dehydration Spinal block along subarachnoid space Block of foramen magnum
		>200 mm	Muscle tension Abdominal compression Brain tumor Subdural hematoma Brain abscess Brain cyst Cerebral edema (any cause) Hydrocephalus
Color	Clear, colorless	Cloudy	Increased cell count Increased microorganisms
		Yellow	Xanthochromic (due to RBC pigments) High protein content
		Smoky	Presence of RBCs
Red blood cells	None	Blood-tinged	Traumatic tap
		Grossly bloody	Traumatic tap Subarachnoid hemorrhage

White blood cells	0-6 mm³	>10 mm³
		(Cell counts range from below 100 to many thousands depending on causative factor; all are abnormal findings.)
			Occurs in many conditions:
			  Bacterial infections of meninges
			  Viral infections of meninges
			  Neurosyphilis
			  Tuberculous meningitis
			  Metastatic neoplastic lesions
			  Parasitic infections
			  Acute demyelinating diseases
			  Following introduction of air or blood into subarachnoid space

Protein*	15-45 mg/100 ml (1% of serum protein)	<10 mg/100 ml	Little clinical significance

		>60 mg/100 ml	Occurs in many conditions:
			  Complete spinal block
			  Guillain-Barré syndrome
			  Carcinomatosis of meninges
			  Tumors close to pial or ependymal surfaces, or in cerebellopontine angle
			  Acute and chronic meningitis
			  Meningeal hemorrhage
			  Demyelinating disorders
			  Degenerative diseases

Modified from Rudy, 1984.
*NOTE: If CSF contains blood this will raise the protein level.

TABLE 12-9

Cerebrospinal Fluid Analysis—cont'd

Parameters	Normal	Abnormal	Possible cause
Glucose	50-75 mg/100 ml (approximately 60% of blood glucose level)	<40 mg/100 ml	Acute bacterial meningitis Tuberculous meningitis Meningeal carcinomatosis
		>100 mg/100 ml	Diabetes
Chloride	700-750 mg/100 ml; 125 mM	<625 mg/100 ml	Hypochloremia Tuberculous meningitis
		>800 mg/100 ml	Not of neurologic significance; correlate with blood levels of chloride

Cerebral Angiography

Angiography is a radiologic technique that demonstrates cerebrovascular blood flow. This technique is commonly performed by the introduction of a small catheter into the femoral artery. The catheter is then passed to the level of the cerebral circulation and a contrast dye is injected. Serial x-ray films are then taken. These films demonstrate flow of the dye through the cerebral vasculature and provide information on patency, location, and size of the vessels. Another technique used in cerebral angiography is the retrograde (reverse flow) injection of the dye through catheterization of a brachial, axillary, subclavian, or femoral vein.

Myelography

A myelogram demonstrates intraspinal anatomy by the introduction of a radiographic dye into the lumbar subarachnoid space or the cisterna magna. The dye is allowed to flow in a cephalic direction, as in the case of a lumbar injection, or caudally in a cisterna magna puncture. X-ray films are then obtained. The distribution of the dye delineates spinal cord and nerve root structure and integrity.

Echoencephalography (Ultrasound)

Echoencephalography, or ultrasound, is a safe, noninvasive procedure using sound waves that are deflected at differing rates, depending on the density of the tissue. Information is processed and displayed on an oscilloscope screen. The procedure is useful primarily in the detection of structural characteristics of intracranial space-occupying mass lesions and the determination of ventricular dimensions, especially in newborns.

Electroencephalography

The electroencephalograph (EEG) is a recording of electrical impulses, arising from the cortical surface of the brain, that is detected by scalp electrodes. The recording of brain-wave patterns is analyzed for alterations or localization of specific electrical activity, or both. This test is especially useful in detecting and localizing foci that initiate seizure activity.

Evoked Potentials

Evoked potentials (EPs) provides a method of detecting electrical brain activity that results from a stimulus—primarily auditory, visual, or peripheral sensory. Electrical activity is computer-formatted to display changes in trends. The primary uses of EPs include perioperative detection of sensory pathway integrity and disease- or drug-related sensory dysfunction.

Cerebrospinal Fluid Analysis

Cerebrospinal fluid (CSF) generally is obtained from the lumbar or cisternal subarachnoid space by means of a hollow needle that allows passive flow. The lumbar puncture is performed most often at the L3-4 interspace (below the level of the spinal cord at L1-2). Cisternal puncture is performed by the insertion of a needle into the cisterna magna, with an approach from the back of the neck in the region of the foramen magnum. CSF pressure also is commonly measured during these procedures. In addition, the CSF can be analyzed for gross characteristics and constituents (color, blood cells, electrolytes, and protein). The cerebrospinal fluid also may be cultured for microorganisms (Table 12-9).

SUMMARY REVIEW

Overview and Organization of the Nervous System

1 The divisions of the nervous system have been categorized as either structural (central nervous system [CNS] and peripheral nervous system [PNS]) or functional (somatic nervous system and autonomic nervous system [ANS]).

2 The CNS is contained within the brain and spinal cord.

3 The PNS is composed of cranial and spinal nerves, which carry impulses toward the CNS (afferent) and away from the CNS (efferent) to target organs or skeletal muscle.

Cells of the Nervous System

1 The neuron and neuroglial cells comprise nervous tissue. The neuron is specialized to transmit and receive electrical and chemical impulses, whereas the neuroglial cell provides supportive functions. The neuron is further divided into unipolar, bipolar, and multipolar categories, according to its structure and particular mechanics of impulse transmission.

2 The neuron is composed of a cell body, dendrite(s), and an axon. A myelin sheath around selected axons forms an insulation that allows quicker nerve impulse conduction.

The Nerve Impulse

1 The region between the neurons is the synapse and the region between the neuron and muscle is the myoneural junction. Neurotransmitters are responsible for chemical conduction across the synapse, and myoneural junction nerve impulse is regulated predominantly by a balance of inhibitory postsynaptic potentials (IPSP) and excitatory postsynaptic potentials (EPSP), temporal and spatial summation, and convergence and divergence.

The Central Nervous System

1 The brain is contained within the cranial vault and is divided into three distinct regions: (1) forebrain, (2) hindbrain, and (3) midbrain.

2 The forebrain comprises the two cerebral hemispheres and allows conscious perception of internal and external stimuli, thought and memory processes, and voluntary control of skeletal muscles. The deep portion of the forebrain is termed the *diencephalon* and processes incoming sensory data. The center for voluntary control of skeletal muscle movements is located along the precentral gyrus in the frontal lobe, whereas the center for perception is along the postcentral gyrus in the parietal lobe. Broca's area (inferior edge of the postcentral gyrus) and Wernicke's area (superoposterior temporal lobe) are major speech centers.

3 The hindbrain allows sampling and comparison of sensory data, which are received from the periphery and motor impulses of the cerebral hemispheres, for the purpose of coordination and refinement of skeletal muscle movement.

4 The midbrain is primarily a relay center for motor and sensory tracts, as well as a center for auditory and visual reflexes.

5 The spinal cord contains most of the nerve fibers that connect the brain with the periphery. Reflex arcs are completed in the spinal cord and influenced by the higher centers in the brain.

6 The CNS is protected by the scalp, bony cranium, meninges, vertebral column, and the cerebrospinal fluid (CSF). CSF is formed from blood components in the choroid plexuses of the ventricles and is reabsorbed in the arachnoid villi (located in the dural venous sinuses) after circulating through the brain and spinal cord.

7 The paired carotid and vertebral arteries supply blood to the brain and connect to form the circle of Willis. The major branches projecting from the circle of Willis are the anterior, middle, and posterior cerebral arteries. Drainage of blood from the brain is accomplished through the venous sinuses and jugular veins.

8 Blood supply to the spinal cord originates from the vertebral arteries and branches arising from the aorta.

The Peripheral Nervous System

1 The PNS functions to relay information from the CNS to muscle and effector organs through cranial and spinal nerve tracts arranged in fascicles (multiple fascicles bound together form the peripheral nerve).

The Autonomic Nervous System

1 The ANS is responsible for the maintenance of a steady state in the internal environment. Two opposing systems comprise the ANS: (1) the sympathetic nervous system responds to stress by mobilizing energy stores and prepares the body to defend itself and (2) the parasympathetic nervous system conserves energy and the body's resources.

Aging and the Nervous System

1 Major structural changes with aging include a decrease in number of neurons and a decrease in brain weight and size.

2 Deposition of lipofuscin and the presence of senile plaques, multiple neurofibrillary tangles, and Lewy bodies are common cellular changes with aging.

3 A progressive slowing of neurologic function occurs with advancing age.

Tests of Nervous System Function

1 Tests of nervous system function include x-ray films, computer tomography, magnetic resonance imaging and angiography, positron emission tomography, brain scan, cerebral angiography, myelography, echoencephalography, electroencephalography, evoked potentials, and analysis of the cerebrospinal fluid.

KEY TERMS

Acetylcholine, 425
α-Adrenergic receptor, 427
β-Adrenergic receptor, 427
Adrenergic transmission, 425
Afferent (sensory) neuron, 410
Afferent pathway (ascending pathway), 398
Amygdaloid nucleus, 408
Anterior fossa, 412
Anterior spinal artery, 417
Arachnoid membrane, 413
Arachnoid villi, 414
Association fiber, 407
Associational neuron (interneuron), 399
Astrocyte, 399
Autonomic nervous system (ANS), 398
Axon, 398
Axon hillock, 398
Basal ganglia, 406, 408
Basilar artery, 416
Bipolar neuron, 399
Brachial plexus, 420
Brainstem, 404
Broca's speech area, 407
Cauda equina, 410
Caudatus nucleus, 408
Cavernous sinus, 416
Celiac, 424
Central canal, 410
Central nervous system (CNS), 398
Cerebellum, 409
Cerebral aqueduct (aqueduct of Sylvius), 409
Cerebral cortex, 406
Cerebral nuclei, 408
Cerebral peduncle, 409
Cerebrospinal fluid (CSF), 414
Cerebrum, 406
Cholinergic transmission, 425
Choroid plexus, 414
Circle of Willis, 416
Collateral ganglia, 420
Contralateral control, 407
Conus medullaris, 410
Corpora quadrigemina (tectum), 408
Corpus callosum (transverse fibers or commissural fibers), 408
Corpus striatum, 408
Cranial nerves, 398
Craniosacral division, 425
Dendrite, 398
Dendritic zone, 398
Dermatome, 420
Diencephalon, 408

Dopamine, 409
Dorsal column, 410
Dorsal horn (posterior horn), 410
Dorsal root ganglion, 410
Dura mater, 413
Effector organ, 398
Efferent (motor) neuron, 410
Efferent pathway (descending pathway), 398
Endoneurium, 398
Epidural space, 414
Epithalamus, 408
Excitatory postsynaptic potential (EPSP), 404
Extrapyramidal system, 407
Facilitation, 404
Falx cerebri, 413
Fascicle, 420
Fissure, 406
Fissure of Rolando (central fissure), 407
Foramen of Luschka, 414
Foramen of Magendie, 414
Frontal lobe, 407
Galea aponeurotica, 412
Ganglia, 398
Gray matter, 406
Hypothalamus, 408
Inferior colliculi, 408
Inferior mesenteric, 424
Inhibitory postsynaptic potential (IPSP), 404
Inner dura (meningeal layer), 413
Insula, 408
Internal capsule, 408
Internal carotid artery, 416
Interventricular foramen (foramen of Monro), 414
Intervertebral disk, 415
Lateral column, 410
Lateral horn, 410
Lentiform nucleus, 408
Limbic system, 408
Lower motor neuron, 410
Lumbar plexus, 420
Lumbar puncture, 415
Meninges, 413
Mesencephalon (midbrain), 408
Metencephalon, 409
Microfilament, 398
Microtubule, 398
Middle fossa (temporal fossa), 412
Motor neuron, 399
Motor unit, 412
Multipolar neuron, 399

Myelencephalon (medulla oblongata), 409
Myelin, 398
Myelin sheath, 398
Neurilemma, 398
Neurofibril, 398
Neurofibrillary tangle, 428
Neuroglia, 399
Neuroglial cell, 398
Neuromuscular (myoneural) junction, 399, 412
Neuron, 398
Neurotransmitter, 402
Nissl substance, 398
Node of Ranvier, 398
Norepinephrine, 425
Nucleus pulposus, 415
Occipital lobe, 407
Oligodendrocyte (pl. = oligodendroglia), 399
Parasympathetic nervous system, 420
Parietal lobe, 407
Pelvic nerve, 425
Periosteum (endosteal layer), 413
Peripheral nervous system (PNS), 398
Plexus, 420
Pons, 409
Postcentral gyrus, 407
Posterior fossa, 412
Posterior spinal artery, 417
Postganglionic neuron, 420
Postsynaptic neuron, 402
Precentral gyrus, 407
Prefrontal area, 407
Preganglionic neuron, 420
Premotor area, 407
Presynaptic neuron, 402
Primary motor area, 407
Primary voluntary motor pathway, 407
Projecting artery (nutrient artery), 416
Pyramidal system, 407
Red nucleus, 408
Reflex arc, 410
Reticular activating system, 404
Reticular formation, 404
Sacral plexus, 420
Saltatory conduction, 398
Schwann cell, 398
Schwann sheath, 398
Senile plaque, 428
Sensory neuron, 399
Somatic nervous system, 398
Spatial summation, 404

REFERENCES

Berne, R. M., & Levy, M. N. (1993). *Physiology* (3rd ed.). St. Louis: Mosby–Year Book.

Chipps, E., Clanin, N., & Campbell, V. (1992). *Neurologic disorders*. St. Louis: Mosby–Year Book.

Hirano, A., & Llena, J. F. (1983). Degenerative diseases of the central nervous system. In R. N. Rosenburg (Ed.), *The clinical neurosciences: Neuropathology* (Vols. 1 and 2, pp. 285-324). New York: Churchill Livingstone.

Noback, C. R., Strominger, N. L., & Demarest, R. J. (Eds.). (1991). *The human nervous system: Introduction and review* (4th ed.). Malvern, PA: Lea & Febiger.

Nolte, J. (1993). *The human brain: An introduction to its functional anatomy* (3rd ed.). St. Louis: Mosby–Year Book.

Raven, P. H., & Johnson, G. B. (1991). *Biology* (3rd ed.). St. Louis: Mosby–Year Book.

Rudy, E. B. (Ed.). (1984). *Advanced neurological and neurosurgical nursing*. St. Louis: Mosby–Year Book.

Scheibel, E. S., & Scheibel, B. S. (1975). Structural changes in the aging brain. In H. Brody, D. Harman, & J. M. Ordy (Eds.), *Clinical, morphological, and neurochemical aspects of the aging nervous system* (pp. 11-37). New York: Raven Press.

Seeley, R., Stevens, T. D., & Tate, P. (1992). *Anatomy and physiology* (2nd ed.). St. Louis: Mosby–Year Book.

Sellcoe, D. J. (1992). Aging brain, aging mind. *Scientific American, 267*(3), 134-143.

Thompson, J. M., McFarland, G. K., Hirsch, J. E., & Tucker, S. M. (1993). *Mosby's clinical nursing* (3rd ed.). St. Louis: Mosby–Year Book.

Timiras, P. S. (Ed.). (1972). *Development physiology and aging*. New York: Macmillan.

SUGGESTED READINGS

Dayan, A. D., & Lewis, P. D. (1985). The central nervous system—Neuropathology of aging. In J. C. Brocklehurst (Ed.), *Textbook of geriatric medicine and gerontology* (3rd ed.). New York: Churchill Livingston.

Gilman, S., & Winans, S. (Eds.). (1987). *Manter and Gatz's essentials of clinical neuroanatomy and neurophysiology* (7th ed.). Philadelphia: Davis.

Hickey, J. V. (1986). *The clinical practice of neurological and neurosurgical nursing* (2nd ed.). Philadelphia: Lippincott.

Larson, E. (1980). The epidemiology of brain tumors. *Journal of Neurosurgical Nursing, 12*(3), 121-127.

Noback, C. R., & Demarst, R. J. (1986). *The human nervous system. Basic principles of neurobiology*. New York: McGraw-Hill.

Pathy, M. S. (1985). The central nervous system—Clinical presentations and management of neurological disorders in old age. In J. C. Brocklehurst (Ed.), *Textbook of geriatric medicine and gerontology* (pp. 391-426). New York: Churchill Livingstone.

Piel, J. (Ed.). (1992). Mind and brain: Special Issue. *Scientific American, 267*(3).

Restak, R. M. (1984). *The brain*. New York: Bantam.

Rossor, M. N. (1985). The central nervous system—Neurochemistry of the aging brain and dementia. In J. C. Brocklehurst (Ed.), *Textbook of geriatric medicine and gerontology* (pp. 294-308). New York: Churchill Livingstone.

Snyder, S. H. (1985, October). The molecular basis of communication between cells. *Scientific American, 253*, 4.

Timiras, P. S., & Vernadakis, A. (1972). Structural, biochemical, and functional aging of the nervous system. In P. S. Timiras (Ed.), *Developmental physiology and aging* (pp. 502-526). New York: Macmillan.

Vick, R. L. (1984). *Contemporary medical physiology*. Menlo Park, CA: Addison-Wesley.

Willis, W. D., & Grosman, R. G. (1981). *Medical neurobiology: Neuroanatomical and neurophysiological practices basic to clinical neuroscience* (3rd ed.). St. Louis: Mosby–Year Book.

CHAPTER 13

Pain, Temperature Regulation, Sleep, and Sensory Function

Patti Ludwig-Beymer

Sue E. Huether

Mary Schoessler*

Chapter Outline

*Contributing author to the first edition.

A lterations in sensory function may involve dysfunctions of the general or the special senses. Dysfunctions of the general senses include chronic pain, abnormal temperature regulation, tactile dysfunction, and proprioceptive dysfunction. Dysfunctions of the special senses include visual, auditory, vestibular, olfactory, and gustatory (taste) dysfunction.

The special senses of vision, hearing, touch, smell, and taste are the means by which individuals perceive stimuli that are essential in interacting with the environment. Special sensory receptors are connected to specific areas of the cerebral cortex through the afferent pathways of the central nervous system (CNS). Each of the special senses thus involves a connected system of organs and tissues that receives stimuli and portions of the CNS, where sensory stimuli are processed.

All definitions of pain suggest that it is a complex phenomenon composed of sensory experiences that include time, space, intensity, emotion, cognition, and motivation. Pain is an unpleasant phenomenon that is uniquely experienced by each individual; it cannot be adequately defined, identified, or measured by an observer. McCaffery (1980) defines pain as "whatever the experiencing person says it is, existing whenever he says it does."

Unlike pain, which is a subjective experience without a precise form of measurement, temperature regulation is measured by clearly defined normal limits. Like pain, however, variations in temperature can signal disease. Fever is a common manifestation of dysfunction and is often the first symptom observed in an infectious or inflammatory condition. If the body's temperature regulatory mechanism is out of balance, the result may be death.

Sleep is a normal cyclical process that restores the body's energy and maintains normal functioning. Sleep is so essential to both physiologic and psychologic function that sleep deprivation causes a wide range of clinical manifestations. Prolonged deprivation or disruption of sleep ultimately leads to serious dysfunction.

PAIN

The Experience of Pain

Three systems interact to produce pain. They are (1) the sensory/discriminative system, (2) the motivational/affective system, and (3) the cognitive/evaluative system

(Sanders, 1979). The **sensory/discriminative system** processes information about the strength, intensity, and temporal and spatial aspects of pain. These sensations are mediated through afferent nerve fibers, the spinal cord, the brainstem, and the higher brain centers, and result in prompt withdrawal from the painful stimulus. The **motivational/affective system** determines the individual's conditioned or learned approach/avoidance behaviors. These behaviors are mediated through the interaction of the reticular formation, limbic system, and brainstem.

The **cognitive/evaluative system** overlies the individual's learned behavior concerning the experience of pain. The individual's interpretation of appropriate pain behavior is learned in several ways, among them cultural preferences, male and female roles, and past experience. The influence of the cognitive/evaluative system may block, modulate, or enhance the perception of pain.

Somatogenic Versus Psychogenic Pain

Attempts to categorize pain have suggested two common classes: (1) somatogenic and (2) psychogenic. **Somatogenic pain,** such as the pain of a crushed finger or a heart attack, is pain with a cause. In contrast, **psychogenic pain** is pain for which there is no known physical cause. Psychogenic pain, however, is *not* imaginary pain. It may be just as intense as somatogenic pain and just as distressing. The labels somatogenic and psychogenic provide some basis for describing pain, but pain is only *primarily* somatogenic or psychogenic; it is rarely, if ever, purely one type or the other (McCaffery, 1980).

Acute Versus Chronic Pain

The pain experience may be functionally divided into acute and chronic types. **Acute pain** is a protective mechanism that alerts the individual to a condition or experience that is immediately harmful to the body. The onset of acute pain is usually sudden, and the pain is relieved after the chemical mediators that stimulate the nociceptors are removed. Acute anxiety is always associated with acute pain. Anxiety is a response to the threat inherent in the painful experience, including issues surrounding the cause of pain, its treatment, and prognosis. Hope of recovery is also associated with acute pain. Acute pain mobilizes the individual to take prompt action to relieve it (Melzack & Wall, 1983).

Chronic pain is persistent, usually defined as lasting at least 6 months. The cause of chronic pain is often unknown, and if the cause is known, the pain does not respond to usual therapy. The onset may be sudden, but chronic pain often develops insidiously so that the individual generally experiences more suffering over time. Individual behavior is adaptive and directed toward modifying the pain. Chronic pain is very often associated with a sense of hopelessness and helplessness as the cure becomes more elusive and the timeframe protracted. The pain is perceived as meaningless. Depression often results. (Table 13-1 compares the characteristics of chronic and acute pain.)

Pain Threshold and Pain Tolerance

The **pain threshold** is the point at which a stimulus is perceived as pain. The threshold does not vary significantly among people or in the same person over time. Intense pain at one location, however, may cause an increase in the threshold in another location. For example, a person with severe pain in one knee is less likely to experience chronic back pain that is less intense. This phenomenon is called **perceptual dominance.** Because of perceptual dominance, an individual with many painful sites may report only the most painful one. Then, when the dominant pain is diminished, the individual identifies other painful areas (Berlin, Boodell, & Wolff, 1958).

Pain tolerance is the duration of time or the intensity of pain that an individual will endure before initiating overt pain responses. It is the amount of pain the person will tolerate before outwardly responding to it. Pain tolerance is influenced by the person's cultural prescriptions, expectations, role behaviors, and physical and mental health. Pain tolerance is generally decreased with repeated exposure to pain. Tolerance is decreased also by fatigue, anger, boredom, apprehension, and sleep deprivation. Tolerance may be increased by alcohol consumption, medication, hypnosis, warmth, distracting activities, and strong beliefs or faith (McCaffery, 1980).

Pain tolerance varies greatly among people and in the same person over time, because of the body's ability to respond differently to noxious stimuli. No direct relationship exists between the intensity of painful stimuli and an individual's perception of pain or response to pain.

❏ AGING and the Perception of Pain

Children and the elderly may experience or express pain differently than adults. Children and infants have anatomic and functional ability to perceive pain. Pain pathways and cortical and subcortical centers for pain perception, as well as neurochemicals associated with pain transmission and modulation, are functional in the preterm and newborn (Anand, 1990).

Change in facial expression, crying, and body movements are the most consistent expression of pain in infants. The painful facial expression includes lowered brows drawn together; presence of a vertical bulge and furrows in the forehead between the brows; broadened nasal root; tightly closed, scourged eye fissures; and an-

---

TABLE 13-1

Comparison of Acute and Chronic Pain

Characteristic	Acute pain	Chronic pain
Experience	An event	A situation, state of existence
Source	External agent or internal disease	Unknown; if known, treatment is prolonged or ineffective
Onset	Usually sudden	May be sudden or develop insidiously
Duration	Transient (up to 6 months)	Prolonged (months to years)
Pain identification	Painful and nonpainful areas generally well identified	Painful and nonpainful areas less easily differentiated; change in sensations becomes more difficult to evaluate
Clinical signs	Typical response pattern with more visible signs	Response patterns vary; fewer overt signs (adaptation)
Significance	Significant (informs person something is wrong)	Person looks for significance
Pattern	Self-limiting or readily corrected	Continuous or intermittent; intensity may vary or remain constant
Course	Suffering usually decreases over time	Suffering usually increases over time
Actions	Leads to actions to relieve pain	Leads to actions to modify pain experience
Prognosis	Likelihood of eventual complete relief	Complete relief usually not possible

Modified from Black, R.G. (1975). The chronic pain syndrome. *Surgical Clinics of North America*, 999-1011.

Vertical bulge and
furrows in the
forehead

Lowered brows
drawn together

Tightly closed
scourged eye
fissures

Broadened
and bulging nasal root

Angular, squarish
mouth

FIG. 13-1 Painful facial expression of infants.

gular, squarish mouth and chin quiver (Fig. 13-1) (Beyer & Wells, 1989). Physiologic responses include an increase in heart rate, blood pressure, and respiratory rate. There may be flushing or pallor, sweating, and decreased oxygen saturation. Toddlers also express pain with crying, facial expression, and body language (body tenses, guarding, and hands holding body [Davis, 1990]). Older children, between the ages of 5 and 18 years, tend to have a lower pain threshold than do adults (Haslam, 1969). Children, like adults, have very individual responses to pain.

Studies on pain perception in the elderly have yielded conflicting evidence. Some studies show an increase in the pain threshold with aging (Sherman & Mitchell, 1974); others show no change (Birren, Shapiro, & Miller, 1950; Harkins & Warner, 1977). The varied results are probably a function of independent variation in the sensory/discriminative, motivational/affective, and cognitive/evaluative components of the pain experience. In general, studies confirm that an increase in the pain threshold occurs in some elderly people. This change is probably caused by peripheral neuropathies and changes in the thickness of the skin (Kenshalo & Hall, 1974). (Neuropathies are discussed in Chapter 15.) A decrease in pain tolerance is also evident in the elderly, and women appear to be more sensitive to pain than men (Woodrow, Friedman, & Siegelaub, 1972).

Neuroanatomy of Pain

The portions of the nervous system responsible for the sensation and perception of pain may be divided into three areas: (1) the afferent pathways, (2) the central nervous system, and (3) the efferent pathways. The afferent portion of the system is composed of **nociceptors** (pain receptors) in the tissues. (As Chapter 12 describes, afferent nerves carry signals to the spinal cord, and the spinal cord network that transmits the signal to the brain.) Afferent pathways terminate in the dorsal horn of the spinal cord, which contains the substantia gelatinosa at the tip of the horn and layers of ganglia called laminae. Some laminae have only nociceptor-specific function. Both incoming and descending stimuli modulate pain patterns in the dorsal horn cells. The portions of the CNS involved in the interpretation of the pain signals are the limbic system, reticular formation, thalamus, hypothalamus, medulla, and cortex. The ventroposterior and medial thalamic nuclei facilitate discrimination and localization of pain. The limbic and reticular tracts are probably involved in alerting, arousal, and motivational behaviors related to pain. The medulla and hypothalamus activate coping responses, such as "fight-or-flight," the release of corticosteroids, and cardiovascular responses. The various regions of the brain that modulate spinal pain transmission are complex and integrated. The efferent pathways, composed of the fibers connecting the reticular formation, midbrain, and substantia gelatinosa, are responsible for modulating pain sensation.

The Role of the Afferent and Efferent Pathways

The nociceptors are at the ends of the small unmyelinated and lightly myelinated afferent neurons. The ends of these neurons respond to chemical, mechanical, and thermal stimuli (Table 13-2). Mild stimulation, such as gentle touch or warmth, may produce a positive, pleasurable sensation. Deep pressure or extreme heat generally produces pain. The differences in the interpretation of these stimuli are a result of the frequency and amplitude of the afferent signal. In addition to distal stimulation, nociceptors may be activated more proximally as they pass through areas of entrapment in the spinal column. Heat injury and inflammation associated with rheumatic disease appear initially to lower the threshold and increase the intensity of response to additional painful stimuli. Repeated noxious stimulation

TABLE 13-2

Stimuli That Activate Nociceptors (Pain Receptors)

Location of receptor	Provoking stimuli
Skin	Pricking, cutting, crushing, burning, freezing
Gastrointestinal tract	Engorged or inflamed mucosa, distention or spasm of smooth muscle, traction on mesenteric attachment
Skeletal muscle	Ischemia, injuries of the connective tissue sheaths, necrosis, hemorrhage, prolonged contraction, injection of irritating solutions
Joints	Synovial membrane inflammation
Arteries	Piercing, inflamed
Headache	Traction and displacement of arteries and meningeal structures, arterial pulsation

FIG. 13-2 Nociceptors and spinal segment. A, Nociceptive and other afferent and efferent pathways in a spinal nerve at the dorsal horn. **B,** Small A-delta and C fibers from synapses primarily with cells in lamina V but also with cells in laminae IV and VI.

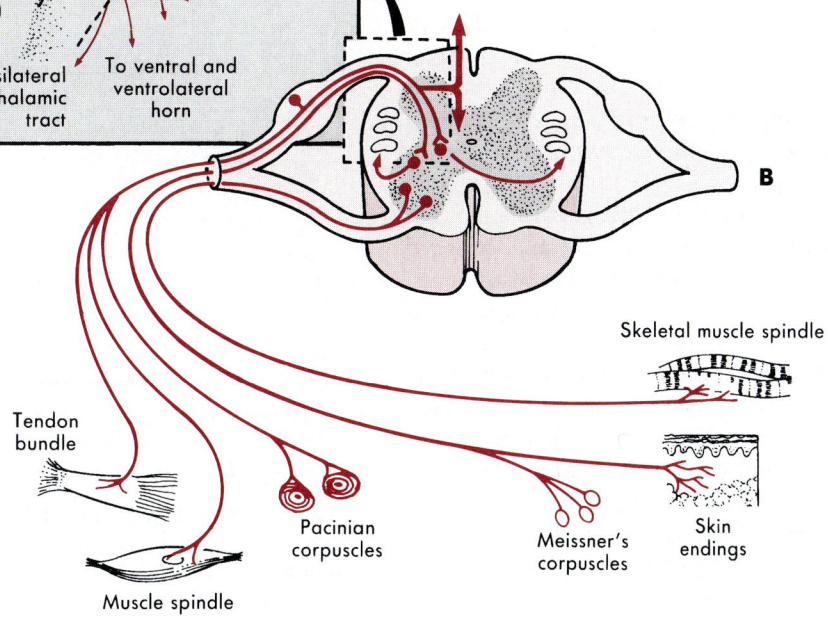

to inflamed joints results in an eventual decrease in sensitivity, however (Smukler, 1985). In some instances, physiologic states, such as increased skeletal muscle tone, enhance excitability of nociceptors (Brena, 1985).

Nociceptors may be found in the muscles, tendons, subcutaneous tissue (as nerve endings termed **pacinian corpuscles**), and epidermis (as **Meissner's corpuscles**). They also appear as bare endings in the skin. They are not evenly distributed in the body. For example, the skin has many more nociceptors than the internal structures, and the eye has many more than the arm. This maldistribution of nociceptors affects the relative sensitivity to pain of different areas of the body.

As Fig. 13-2 illustrates, stimulation of nociceptors produces impulses that are transmitted through small A-delta fibers and C fibers to the spinal cord, where they form synapses with neurons in the dorsal horn. From the dorsal horn, the nociceptive impulses are transmitted to various parts of the spinal cord and to the rest of the central nervous system.

The small unmyelinated C neurons are responsible for the transmission of diffuse burning or aching sensations. Because of the size of the fiber and the lack of a myelin sheath, transmission through C fibers is relatively slow. Transmission through the slightly larger, myelinated A fibers occurs much more quickly. A fibers carry well-localized, sharp pain sensations. The reflex arc to and from the spinal cord is much faster than the transmission of the pain stimulus. Therefore, the retraction of the injured body part occurs before the individual perceives the pain.

Most afferent pain fibers terminate in the dorsal horn of the spinal segment that they enter. Some, however, extend toward the head or the foot for several segments before terminating. The A fibers terminate in the substantia gelatinosa; some large A-delta fibers and small C fibers terminate in the laminae. The laminae then transmit specific information. For example, lamina I neurons specifically transmit information about burned or crushed skin, and lamina IV neurons transmit information about gentle pressure.

Secondary neurons transmit the impulse from the substantia gelatinosa and laminae to the ventral and lateral horn, crossing, in the same or adjacent spinal segments, to the other side of the cord. From there the impulse is carried through the spinothalamic tracts to the brain (Fig. 13-3). The two divisions of the spinothalamic tract that carry pain information to the brain are (1) the neospinothalamic tract (acute pain) and (2) the paleospinothalamic tract (dull and burning pain). The neospinothalamic tract carries information to the midbrain, postcentral gyrus (where pain is perceived), and cortex. The paleospinothalamic tract carries information to the reticular formation, pons, limbic system, and midbrain.

The efferent pathway is responsible for modulation or inhibition of afferent pain signals. Afferent stimulation of the **periaqueductal gray (PAG)** (gray matter surrounding the cerebral aqueduct) in the midbrain stimulates the efferent pathway. Efferent neurons located in the PAG form synapses with structures in the medulla that inhibit pain through a noradrenergic system (Yaksh, 1985). From there the impulse is transmitted through the spinal cord to the dorsal horn. The dorsolateral funiculus (a cordlike structure lying between the dorsal root ganglion and ventral root ganglion) contains efferent inhibitory fibers that make contact with cells in laminae I, II, and V to impair or block transmission of nociceptive impulses.

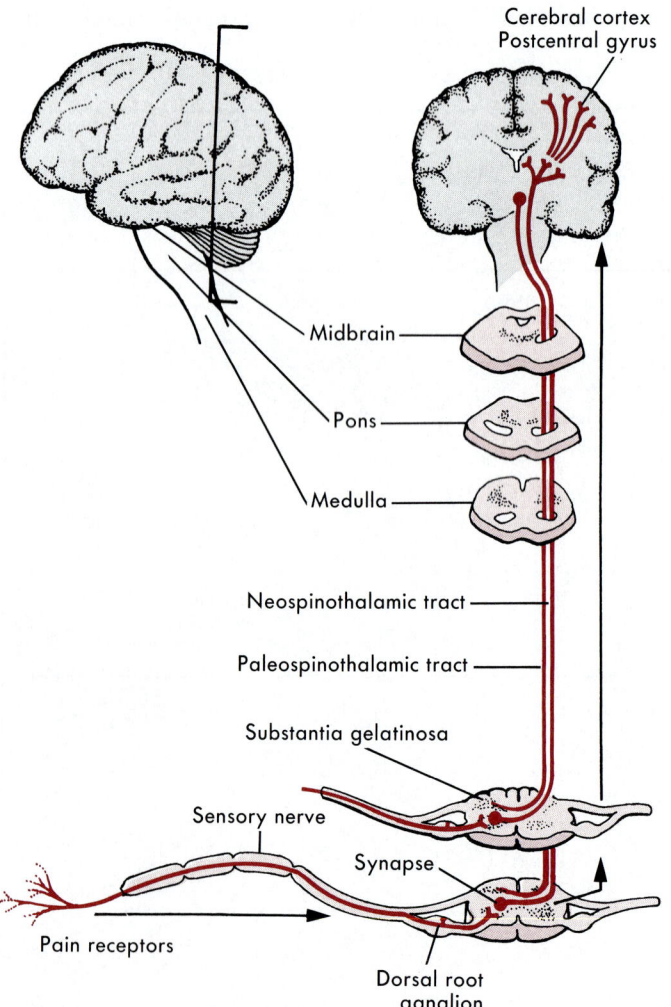

FIG. 13-3 Spinal cord and CNS pathway. Stimuli are transmitted from pain receptors through sensory nerves into the dorsal root ganglia. The impulse enters the spinal cord, forms a synapse, crosses the cord, and rises to the spinothalamic tract.

Neurophysiology of Pain
Theories of Pain

Several theories have been proposed to describe the mechanisms of pain, including the specificity theory, the intensity theory, the pattern theory, and the gate control theory. The **specificity theory** proposes four major categories of cutaneous sensation: (1) touch, (2) warmth, (3) cold, and (4) pain. Each cutaneous sensation is the result of stimulation of specific receptor sites on the skin. Stimulation of the nerve endings of the pain receptors precipitates transmission of the painful stimuli (through A-δ and C fibers) to the spinal cord. The pain neurons form synapses in the substantia gelatinosa and cross to the opposite side of the spinal cord, ascending to the brain through the spinothalamic tract. The perception of pain then occurs in special areas of the thalamus and cerebral cortex.

According to the specificity theory, there is a direct relationship between the stimulus and the perception of pain. Although this theory postulates the existence of specific skin receptors for pain and explains why actual tissue damage causes pain, it fails to account for adaptation to pain and effects of psychosocial factors on pain perception (Melzack & Wall, 1965).

The **intensity theory** proposes that pain results from excessive stimulation of sensory receptors. Pain occurs if the stimulus is applied with enough intensity. Excessive stimulation of receptors or pathology that promotes summation of impulses produced by non-noxious stimuli can cause pain (Bonica, 1990). The theory does not account for intense stimulation of some sites that produce no pain.

The **pattern theory** suggests that the perception of pain is the result of stimulus intensity (a function of the length of time and the amount of tissue involved) and the summation of the impulses. According to the pattern theory, nonspecific receptors transmit patterns of nerve impulses from the skin to the spinal cord. Certain patterns of impulses then are perceived as pain. Theorists disagree about where the summation occurs. According to some, summation occurs in the spinal cord; according to others, it occurs in the brain. Although the pattern theories do not account for adaptation to pain, they do allow for the many factors that contribute to pain perception (Melzack & Wall, 1965).

Melzack and Wall proposed the **gate control theory** in 1965 (Fig. 13-4). According to this theory, nociceptive impulses are transmitted from specialized skin receptors to the spinal cord through large A and small C fibers (see Fig. 13-4). These fibers terminate in the substantia gelatinosa, in the dorsal horn of the spinal cord. Cells in the substantia gelatinosa function as a gate, regulating transmission of impulses to the central nervous system. Stimulation of larger fibers causes the cells in the substantia gelatinosa to "close the gate." A closed gate decreases stimulation of trigger cells, decreases transmission impulses, and diminishes pain perception. Persistent stimulation of the large fibers, however, allows adaptation. When adaptation to impulses from large fibers occurs, the result is a relative increase in small neuron activity. Adaptation to larger fibers thus may "open the gate." Scratching and vibration prevent large neuron adaptation and keep the gate closed over prolonged periods.

Small fiber input inhibits cells in the substantia gelatinosa and opens the gate. An open gate increases the stimulation of trigger cells, increases transmission of impulses, and enhances pain perception. In addition to

FIG. 13-4 Schematic diagram of the gate control theory of pain mechanism.

gate control through large- and small-fiber stimulation, the central nervous system, through efferent pathways, may close, partially close, or open the gate.

Cognitive functioning thus may modulate pain perception. Interaction of the cognitive/evaluative, motivational/affective, and sensory/discriminative systems determines the individual's pain response (Melzack, 1975; Melzack & Casey, 1968; Melzack & Wall, 1965, 1970).

Neuromodulation

Neuromodulators of pain are found in the pathways that mediate information about painful stimuli, including the periphery; ascending and descending spinal tracts; the cortex; and the gastrointestinal tract (Aimone, 1992). Tissue injury results in the release of prostaglandins (PGE_2 and PGI_2), bradykinins, and histamine, which depolarize adjacent nociceptors causing pain. Lymphokines released from lymphocytes in chronic inflammatory lesions may contribute to some types of chronic pain. Substance P, neurokinin A, and calcitonin-gene–related peptide are released from peripheral pain receptors and promote the spread of pain locally. Norepinephrine and 5-hydroxytryptamine contribute to pain modulation (inhibition) in the medulla and pons. Substance P and other neurotransmitters contribute to the modulation of pain in both the afferent and efferent fibers of the spinal cord.

Endorphins (endogenous morphines) are a family of neuropeptides that inhibit transmission of pain impulses in the spinal cord and brain (Go & Yaksh, 1989). The three classifications of endorphins are: (1) β-lipotrophin, (2) enkephalin, and (3) dynorphin. **β-Lipotrophin** (β-, γ-, and α-endorphin) is a potent endorphin located in the hypothalamus and the pituitary gland. These endorphins may be responsible for general sensations of well-being. **Enkephalin,** found in the neurons of the brain and spinal cord, is a weaker analgesic than other endorphins but is more potent and longer lasting than morphine. **Dynorphin** (a powerful endorphin) is 50 times more potent than β-endorphin. Dynorphin reportedly originates in the neural lobe of the pituitary (Henry, 1986).

All endorphins act by attaching to **opiate receptors** on the plasma membrane of the afferent neuron (Fig. 13-5). The combination of the opiate receptor and endorphin inhibits the release of excitatory neurotransmitters, i.e., substance P, thus blocking the transmission of the painful stimulus. In much the same way, exogenous opiates relieve pain by attaching to the opiate receptors and augmenting the natural endorphin response (West, 1981). The enkephalin-endorphin receptors also have been identified as specific cellular attachment sites for morphine and other exogenous narcotic molecules.

Stress, excessive physical exertion, acupuncture, intercourse, and other factors increase the levels of circulating endorphins, serotonin, norepinephrine, and other neurotransmitters, raising the pain threshold (Henry, 1986). Although still controversial, there is some evidence to suggest that high levels of circulating endorphins may play a role in so-called painless myocardial ischemia and infarction (Sheps et al., 1987; Van Rijn & Rabkin, 1981).

Clinical Manifestations of Pain
Acute Pain

Three types of acute pain are (1) somatic, (2) visceral, and (3) referred. **Somatic pain** is superficial (coming from the skin or close to the surface of the body) and is either sharp and well localized or dull, aching, poorly localized, and accompanied by nausea and vomiting. **Visceral pain** refers to pain in internal organs, the abdomen, or skeleton. It is poorly localized because of the lesser number of mechanoreceptors in the visceral structures. It is associated with nausea and vomiting, hypotension, restlessness, and, in some cases, shock. Visceral pain often radiates (spreads away from the actual site of the pain) or is referred. **Referred pain** is pain that is present in an area removed or distant from its point of origin. The area of referred pain is supplied by the same spinal segment as the actual site of pain. Impulses from many cutaneous and visceral neurons converge on the same ascending neuron and the brain cannot distinguish between the two. Because there are more receptors in the skin, the painful sensation is experienced there (Seeley, Stephens, & Tate, 1992). (Common areas of referred pain and their associated sites of origin appear in Fig. 13-6.)

Physiologic response

Acute pain is a warning of actual or impending tissue injury. Physiologic responses therefore include increased heart rate, increased respiratory rate, elevated blood pressure, pallor or flushing, dilated pupils, and diaphoresis. Blood sugar is elevated; gastric acid secretion and motility are decreased; and blood flow to the viscera and skin is decreased. Nausea occasionally occurs.

Psychologic and behavioral response

Individuals often psychologically respond to acute pain with fear (e.g., fear of diagnosis, fear of continued pain), anxiety, and a general sense of unpleasantness or unease. The stress of fear may in turn contribute to the physiologic signs of pain. Individuals do not always discuss their pain. One study, for example, showed that 70% of hospitalized persons with acute pain did not like to discuss it with others, either because of negative social connotations or because they believed their pain to be insignificant when measured against others' problems. More than two thirds of these individuals would

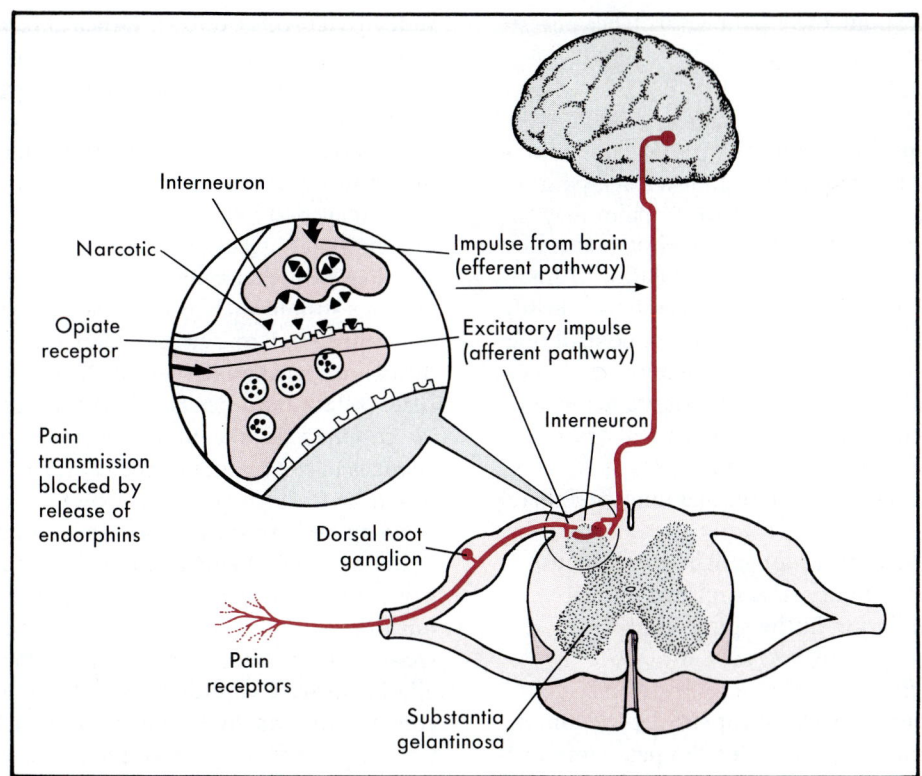

FIG. 13-5 **Descending pathway and endorphin response.** The biologic receptors of the enkephalins and endorphins are located close to known pain receptors in the periphery, ascending, and descending pain pathways.

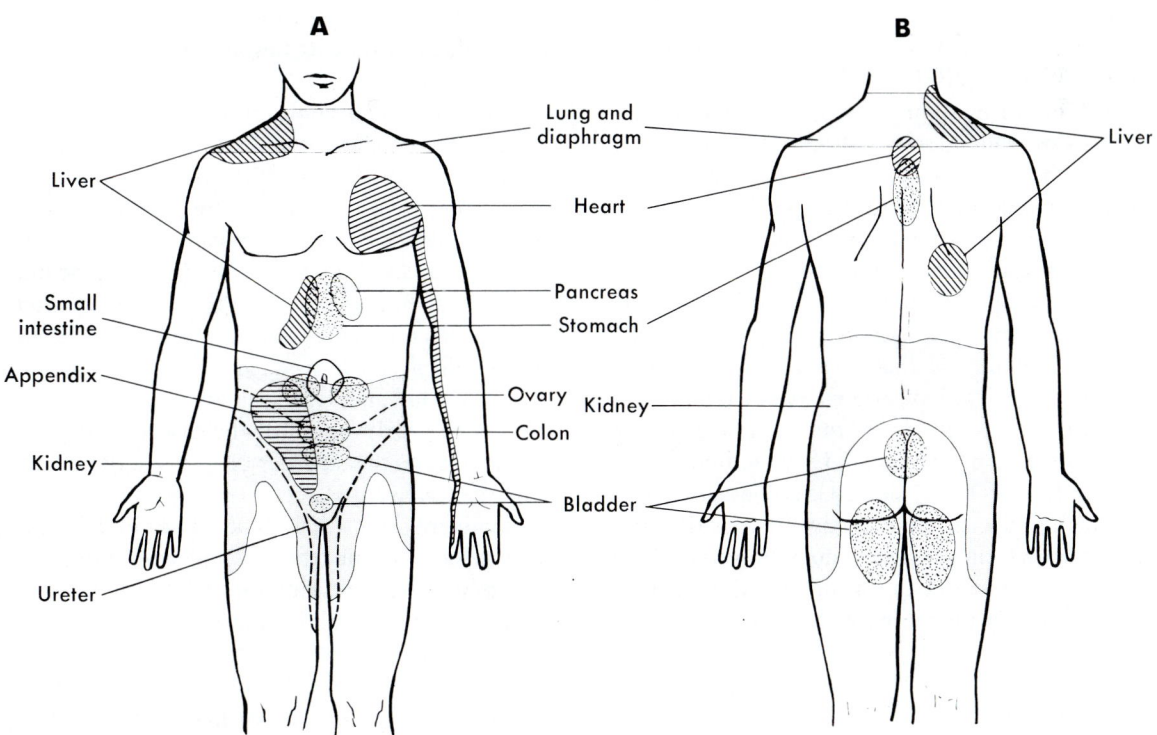

FIG. 13-6 **Sites of referred pain. A,** Front. **B,** Back. (From Phipps, Long, & Woods, 1987.)

not communicate about their pain until it became severe (Jacox, 1979).

Chronic Pain

Chronic pain is prolonged pain (lasts longer than 6 months) that may be persistent (e.g., low back pain) or intermittent (e.g., migraines). Chronic pain may be caused or aggravated by a decreased level of endorphins or a predominance of a C neuron stimulation (Almay, Johansson, Knorring, Sedvall, & Terenius, 1980). Chronic pain is more difficult to manage or control than acute pain (see Table 13-1). Changes in nerve terminals, afferent fibers, and the CNS may contribute to chronicity of pain (Whitehead & Kuhn, 1990):

Changes in sensitivity of neurons

Spontaneous impulses from regenerating peripheral nerves

Alterations in the dorsal root ganglion in response to peripheral nerve injury in neurotransmitters

Loss of pain inhibition in the spinal cord

Physiologic response

Physiologic responses to chronic pain depend on the persistent or intermittent nature of the pain. Intermittent pain produces a physiologic response similar to that of acute pain, whereas persistent pain allows for physiologic adaptation. Adaptation produces normal heart and respiratory rates and normal blood pressure. Other physiologic responses to acute pain also become normal, but even though the physiologic responses are normal, the pain is not relieved.

Psychologic and behavioral response

Chronic pain produces significant behavioral and psychologic changes. Individuals with chronic pain often are depressed, have difficulty sleeping and eating, and may become preoccupied with the pain (Sternbach, 1974). Living with chronic pain requires constant attention to the earliest signs of pain so that the pain-provoking stimuli can be identified and avoided. Persons with chronic pain generally attempt to keep pain-related behavior to a minimum so that they appear as normal as possible. They need to have someone understand that the pain and the need to hide it are usually conflicting drives for those with chronic pain. They tend not to report pain for fear of being labeled complainers. They often deny pain and sometimes engage in activities that provoke pain so that they can keep up with others. Even in learning to pace themselves through the day's activities, they may aggravate the pain (Strauss & Glasser, 1975).

Chronic pain conditions

The most common chronic pain condition is persistent low back pain. This, like many other conditions, is a result of poor muscle tone, inactivity, muscle strain, or sudden vigorous exercise. Other chronic conditions include neuralgias, hyperesthesias, myofascial pain syndrome, and hemiageusias. Chronic pain is associated with cancer in some instances.

Neuralgias are painful conditions that result from an infection or disease that damages a peripheral nerve. Causalgias and reflex sympathetic dystrophies are types of neuralgias. **Causalgia** is a condition causing severe burning pain that may be triggered by normally non-noxious stimuli such as light touch, sound, or cold. The pain appears 1 to 2 weeks after injury to the brachial plexus, the median nerves, or the sciatic nerves. The severe, diffuse, and persistent pain occurs in the extremity supplied by the injured nerve. Discoloration and changes in the texture of the skin may appear in the affected area. Excessive nail growth may be noted, and swelling and stiffness of proximate joints may occur.

Reflex sympathetic dystrophies occur after peripheral nerve injury and are characterized by continuous severe, burning pain. The pain often is associated with vasospasm and vasomotor changes. Vasomotor changes usually begin with vasodilation and are followed by vasoconstriction and cool cyanotic and edematous extremities. As muscle wasting occurs, amputation of the involved extremity may be required.

Hyperesthesias are chronic pain conditions characterized by increased sensitivity and decreased pain threshold to tactile and painful stimuli. Stimuli that usually do not produce pain thus become painful. The pain is usually diffuse, modified by fatigue and emotion, and mixed with other sensations. The hyperesthesia may be the result of chronic irritation of the thalamus and other central areas.

Myofascial pain syndromes are the second most common cause of chronic pain. These conditions include myositis, fibrositis, myofibrositis, myalgia, and muscle strain; they involve injury to the muscle and fascia. The pain is a result of muscle spasm, tenderness, and stiffness. These conditions lead to muscle guarding, a behavior that limits muscle motion. In turn, limited motion causes muscle weakness, stiffness, tenderness, and spasm, all of which produce more pain. The pain is described as dull and aching and may be mild to disabling. During the early stages of the disorder, the pain is localized, but as the disorder progresses, the pain becomes more generalized.

Hemiagnosia is a loss of ability to identify the source of pain on one side (the affected side) of the body. Application of painful stimuli to the affected side thus produces discomfort, anxiety, moaning, agitation, and distress but no attempt to withdraw from or push aside the offending stimulus because of an inability to locate the site through normal sensory pathways. Hemiagnosia is associated with stroke that produces paralysis and a hypersensitivity to pain in the affected side.

Phantom limb pain is pain that an individual feels in

an amputated limb after the stump has completely healed. It is more likely to appear in individuals who experienced pain in the limb before amputation. If the neuronal pathway from the amputated limb is stimulated at any point along the pathway, action potentials are propagated toward the cortex. Central nervous system integration results in the perception of pain from the receptors in the amputated limb even though it is no longer there. The pain suppression effect of other sensations, such as touch, pressure, and proprioception, from the amputated limb may be a factor in the intensity of phantom limb pain.

Phantom limb pain may be influenced by emotions and sympathetic stimulation and may be associated also with trigger points. **Trigger points** are small hypersensitive regions in the muscle or connective tissue. They may be close to or removed from the area of pain, but stimulation of the trigger point produces pain in a specific area.

Cancer often is associated with chronic pain. Studies done at Memorial Sloan-Kettering Cancer Center indicate three major categories of pain syndromes that result in chronic pain in the individual with cancer (Foley, 1984). The categories are (1) pain attributed to the advance of the disease, (2) pain associated with treatment of the disease, and (3) pain attributed to coexisting entities (e.g., osteoarthritis) that are unrelated to the disease.

By far the most common cause of chronic pain in the individual with cancer is that attributed to the advance of the disease (Foley, 1984). Pain can be caused by infection and inflammation, increasing pressure of a growing tumor on nerve endings, stretching of visceral surfaces, or obstruction of ducts and intestine. This pain may be acute, intermittent, or continuous. Therapeutic approaches are partially effective in controlling the pain. Pain from tumor infiltration of nerve tissue; trauma or chemical injury to the nerve; damage from radiation, chemotherapy, or surgical sectioning of the nerve produces another form of chronic pain referred to as deafferentation pain. (Deafferentation refers to a loss of sensory input from a portion of the body.) Deafferentation pain is described as a constant dull ache, "viselike," with paroxysms of burning or electrical-shock–like sensations. It may lead to hyperactivity of neurons in the spinal cord and thalamus. Deafferentation pain is poorly controlled by peripheral and epidural analgesia (Foley, 1985; Payne, 1987).

Some individuals experience chronic pain after treatment (see Chapter 10). Chronic postoperative pain occurs in a small percentage of individuals after the following:

1. Thoracotomy, with pain often caused by tumor recurrence or invasion of the chest wall
2. Radical mastectomy, with pain resulting from interruption of the intercostobrachial nerve (which

branches from the brachial plexus to the thoracic region)
3. Radical neck dissection, with pain attributable to surgical injury or interruption of the cranial nerves
4. Surgical amputation, which may be followed by phantom limb pain

Chemotherapy, especially treatment with vinca alkaloids, may be associated with a variety of neuropathies producing painful dysesthesias (needles and pins sensations) in the feet and hands. Radiation therapy may result in connective tissue fibrosis and secondary nerve injury that produces pain (Foley, 1984).

TEMPERATURE REGULATION

In all homeothermic animals, temperature regulation is achieved through precise balancing of heat production, heat conservation, and heat loss. In humans, body temperature is maintained in a range around 37° C (98.6° F). The normal range is considered to be 36.2° to 37.7° C (96.2° to 99.4° F), but all parts of the body do not have the same temperature. The extremities, for example, are generally cooler than the trunk. The temperature at the core of the body (as measured by rectal temperature) is generally 0.05° C higher than at the surface (as measured by oral temperature). The internal temperature varies normally in response to activity, environmental temperature, and daily fluctuation of **circadian rhythm** (the pattern of each 24-hour day). Oral temperatures generally fluctuate within 0.02° to 0.05° C over a 24-hour period. Women tend to have wider fluctuations that follow the menstrual cycle, with a sharp rise in temperature just before ovulation. In both sexes the daily fluctuating temperature peaks around 6:00 in the evening and is at its lowest during sleep (Dinarello & Wolff, 1978). Maintenance of body temperature within the normal range is necessary for life.

Hypothalamic Control of Temperature

Temperature regulation is mediated hormonally by the hypothalamus. Peripheral thermoreceptors in the skin and central thermoreceptors in the hypothalamus, spinal cord, abdominal organs, and other central locations provide the hypothalamus with information about skin and core temperatures. If these temperatures are low, the hypothalamus responds by triggering heat production and heat conservation mechanisms.

Increased heat production is initiated by a series of hormonal mechanisms involving the hypothalamus and its connections with the endocrine system (see Chapter 17). The heat-producing mechanism begins with a hypothalamic hormone, thyrotropin-stimulating hormone-releasing hormone (TSH-RH). In turn, TSH-RH stimulates the anterior pituitary to release thyroid-stimulating hormone (TSH), which acts on the thyroid gland, stimulating release of thyroxine (T_4), one of the thyroid hormones. This hormone then acts on the adrenal medulla, causing the release of epinephrine (a catecholamine and vasopressive hormone) into the bloodstream (see Chapter 17). Epinephrine causes vasoconstriction, stimulates glycolysis, and increases metabolic rates, thus increasing heat production.

The hypothalamus also triggers heat conservation. The mechanisms of heat conservation involve stimulating the sympathetic nervous system, which is responsible for stimulating the adrenal cortex, increasing skeletal muscle tone, initiating the shivering response, and producing vasoconstriction. The hypothalamus also functions in raising body temperatures by relaying information to the cerebral cortex. Awareness of cold provokes voluntary responses such as increased body movement.

The hypothalamus responds to warmer core and peripheral temperatures by reversing the same mechanisms. The TSH-RH pathway is shut down. The sympathetic pathway is prompted to produce vasodilation, decreased muscle tone, and increased sweat production. Hypothalamic stimulation of the cerebral cortex provokes voluntary measures to reduce heat production and promote heat loss.

Mechanisms of Heat Production

Body heat is produced by the chemical reactions of metabolism, skeletal muscle tone and contraction, and chemical thermogenesis.

Chemical reactions of metabolism

The chemical reactions that occur during the ingestion and metabolism of food and those required to maintain the body at rest (basal metabolism) require energy and give off heat. These processes occur in the body core (liver) and are in part responsible for the maintenance of core temperature.

Skeletal muscle contraction

Skeletal muscles produce heat through two mechanisms: (1) gradual increase in muscle tone and (2) rapid muscle oscillations (shivering). Both increasing muscle tone and shivering are controlled by the hypothalamus and occur in response to cold. As peripheral temperature drops, muscle tone increases, and shivering begins. Shivering is a fairly effective method for increasing heat production, because no work is performed and all the energy produced is retained as heat.

Chemical thermogenesis

Chemical thermogenesis, also called nonshivering thermogenesis, results from the release of epinephrine. Epinephrine produces a rapid, transient increase in heat production by raising the body's basal metabolic rate.

Chemical thermogenesis seems to be different from hormone-triggered increases in the basal metabolic rate. Chemical thermogenesis—through epinephrine—produces a quick, brief rise in basal metabolic rate, whereas the hormone thyroxine triggers a slow, prolonged rise (Himms-Hagen, 1980). Chemical thermogenesis occurs in brown adipose tissue present mainly in small newborn mammals that have high surface-to-volume ratios. Like other small newborn mammals, human infants lose more heat through **conduction** and **convection** than they are capable of generating through normal metabolic mechanisms. Brown adipose tissue, therefore, plays an important role in maintaining body temperature in the newborn. As with most mammals reared in a temperature-controlled environment, humans gradually lose the capacity for chemical thermogenesis as brown adipose cells dedifferentiate. This can occur as early as 4 weeks after birth (Benito, 1985). Because of the decrease in brown adipose tissue in the adult, the role of this mechanism of heat production in adults is unknown (Heaton, 1972).

Mechanisms of Heat Loss

Heat loss is achieved through several mechanisms: (1) radiation, (2) conduction, (3) convection, (4) vasodilation, (5) decreased muscle tone, (6) evaporation, (7) increased respiration, (8) voluntary measures, and (9) adaption to warmer climates.

Radiation

Radiation refers to heat loss through electromagnetic waves. These waves emanate from surfaces with temperatures higher than the surrounding air. Thus if the temperature of the skin is higher than that of the air, the skin and therefore the body lose heat to the air.

Conduction

Conduction refers to heat loss by direct molecule-to-molecule transfer from one surface to another. Through conduction the warmer surface loses heat to the cooler surface. Thus the skin loses heat through direct contact with cooler air, water, or another surface. In the same manner the core of the body loses heat to the cooler body surface.

Convection

Convection is the transfer of heat through currents of gases or liquids. It greatly aids heat loss through conduction by exchanging warmer air at the surface of the body with cooler air in the surrounding space. Convection occurs passively as warmer air at the surface of the body rises away from the body and is replaced by cooler air, but the process may be aided by fans or wind. (The combined effect of conduction and convection by wind is conventionally measured as the "wind-chill factor.")

Vasodilation

Peripheral vasodilation increases heat loss by diverting core-warmed blood to the surface of the body. As the core-warmed blood passes through the periphery, heat is transferred by conduction to the skin surface and from the skin to the surrounding environment. Because heat loss through conduction depends on the temperature of the surrounding medium, heat loss through conduction is minimal to nonexistent if the surrounding air is warmer than the body surface.

Vasodilation occurs in response to autonomic stimulation under the control of the hypothalamus. It is useful in instances of moderate temperature elevation. As core temperature increases, vasodilation increases until maximal dilation is achieved. At that point the body must use additional heat loss mechanisms.

Decreased muscle tone

To decrease heat production, muscle tone may be moderately reduced and voluntary muscle activity curtailed. These mechanisms explain in part the "washed-out" feeling associated with high temperatures and warm weather. Both decreased muscle tone and reduced activity have a limited effect on decreasing heat production, however, because muscle tone and heat production cannot be reduced below basal body requirements.

Evaporation

Evaporation of body water from the surface of the skin and the linings of the mucous membranes is a major source of heat reduction. Insensible water loss (in the absence of perceptible sweating) accounts for a loss of about 600 ml water per day. Heat is lost as surface fluid is converted to gas, so that heat loss by evaporation is increased if more fluids are available at the body surface. To speed this process, fluids are actively secreted through the sweat glands. Up to 4 L fluid per hour may be lost by sweating. Electrolytes are lost with the water. Therefore, loss of large volumes through sweating may result in decreased plasma volume, decreased blood pressure, weakness, and fainting. (Alterations in fluid balance are discussed in Chapter 3.)

Like other heat reduction mechanisms, stimulation of sweating occurs in response to sympathetic neural activity and depends on a favorable temperature difference between the body and the environment. In addition, heat loss through evaporation is affected by the relative humidity of the air. If the humidity of the air is low, sweat evaporates quickly, but if the humidity is high, sweat does not evaporate and instead remains on the skin or drips off.

Increased respiration

Exchanging air with the environment through the normal respiratory process provides some heat loss, although it is minimal. As air is inhaled, the air draws heat from the upper respiratory tract. The air is further warmed in the alveoli by blood in the microcirculation. This warmed air then is exhaled into the environment. This normal process occurs faster at higher body temperatures through an increase in respiratory rates. Thus hyperventilation is associated with hyperthermia. (Normal pulmonary function is discussed in Chapter 29.)

Voluntary mechanisms

In response to high body temperatures, people typically "stretch out," thereby increasing the body surface area available for heat loss. They also "slow down" or "take it easy," thereby decreasing skeletal muscle work, and they "dress for warm weather." The most efficient dress for warm weather is a light-colored, loose-fitting garment, because light colors reflect heat from the body and loose-fitting garments allow free air movement for convection, conduction, and evaporation to occur.

Adaptation to warmer climates

When individuals move from cooler to much warmer climates, their bodies undergo a period of adjustment, a process that takes several days to weeks. At first the individual experiences feelings of lassitude, weakness, and faintness with even moderate activity. Body temperatures rise with any work. Within several days, however, the individual experiences an earlier onset of sweating; the volume of sweat is increased; and the sodium content is lowered. Heart rate is decreased and stroke volume increased so that cardiac output remains unchanged. Extracellular fluid volume increases, as does plasma volume. These physiologic adaptations result in improved warm weather functioning and decreased symptoms of heat intolerance. People's work output, endurance, and coordination increase, while their subjective feelings of discomfort decrease (Yousef, 1987).

Mechanisms of Heat Conservation

The body conserves heat and protects core temperature through two important mechanisms: (1) involuntary vasoconstriction and (2) voluntary mechanisms. To preserve core temperature, the skin and periphery are used as an insulating cover (Yousef, 1987).

Vasoconstriction

By constricting peripheral blood vessels, centrally warmed blood is shunted away from the periphery (where radiation, conduction, and convection would allow heat loss) to the core of the body, where heat can be retained. This mechanism takes advantage of the insulating layers of the skin and subcutaneous fat to protect core temperature.

Voluntary mechanisms

In response to lower body temperatures, individuals typically "bundle up," "keep moving," or "curl up in a ball." Bundling up involves dressing with several layers of clothes that allow air to be trapped between the skin and the clothing, thus providing an additional layer of insulation. Keeping moving, stamping feet, clapping hands, jogging, and other types of physical activity increase skeletal muscle activity and thus promote heat production. Curling up in a ball decreases the amount of skin surface available for heat loss through radiation, convection, and conduction.

AGING and Changes in Temperature Regulation

Infants and the elderly require special attention to maintenance of body temperature. Infants produce sufficient body heat but are unable to conserve heat produced. The poor heat conservation is caused by the infant's small body size and greater ratio of body surface to body weight, which give the infant more surface area for heat loss. Infants also have a very thin layer of subcutaneous fat and thus are not as well insulated as adults (Hammarlund, Stromberg, & Sedin, 1986). The elderly have poor responses to environmental temperature extremes as a result of slowed blood circulation, structural and functional changes in the skin, and overall decrease in heat-producing activities. Other factors affecting thermal regulation in the elderly include decrease in shivering response (delayed onset and decreased effectiveness), slowed metabolic rate, sedentary lifestyle, decreased vasoconstrictor response, diminished or absent sweating, desynchronization of circadian rhythm, undernutrition, and decreased perception of heat and cold (Collins & Exton-Smith, 1983; Fellows, MacDonald, & Bennett, 1985).

Both infants and elderly people have difficulty regulating body heat through physiologic mechanisms of heat production and conservation. Health care providers need to be aware of these particular developmental differences, because infants cannot adjust to the environment to compensate for heat loss, and the elderly, because of decreased peripheral sensation, may not be alerted to the need to do so.

Pathogenesis of Fever

Fever is not the result of a failure of the normal thermoregulatory mechanism but is thought to be a "resetting of the hypothalamic thermostat" to a higher level. The thermoregulatory mechanisms adjust heat production, conservation, and loss to maintain body core temperature at a normal level. During fever this level is raised so that the thermoregulatory center now adjusts heat production, conservation, and loss to maintain the core temperature at the new, higher temperature, which

functions as a new "set point" (Boulant, 1991).

The pathophysiology of fever begins with the introduction of **exogenous pyrogens,** or endotoxins (Fig. 13-7). The most frequently encountered exogenous pyrogens are the lipopolysaccharide complex in the cell wall of gram-positive bacteria and viruses (Cooper & Veale, 1987). The production and release of interleukin-1 (IL-1) occur as exogenous bacteria are destroyed and absorbed by phagocytic cells within the host. Tumor necrosis factor (TNF) and IL-1 act on the brain to cause fever. The action of IL-1 appears to be due in part to release of the prostaglandin E series. Interleukin-6, interferons, and other mechanisms are known to be involved in fever. As the set point is raised, the hypothalamus signals an increase in heat production and conservation to raise body temperature to the new level. Peripheral vasoconstriction occurs; epinephrine release increases metabolic rate; and muscle tone increases. Shivering also may occur. The individual feels colder, dresses more warmly, decreases body surface area by curling up, and may go to bed in an effort to get warm. Body temperature is maintained at the new level until the fever "breaks."

During fever, arginine vasopressin (AVP), alpha-melanocyte–stimulating hormone, and corticotropin-releasing factor are released and can act as **endogenous antipyretics** to help diminish the febrile response. This antipyretic effect constitutes a negative feedback loop (see Fig. 13-7) (Clark, 1991). The antipyretic effect may help to explain fluctuations in the febrile response.

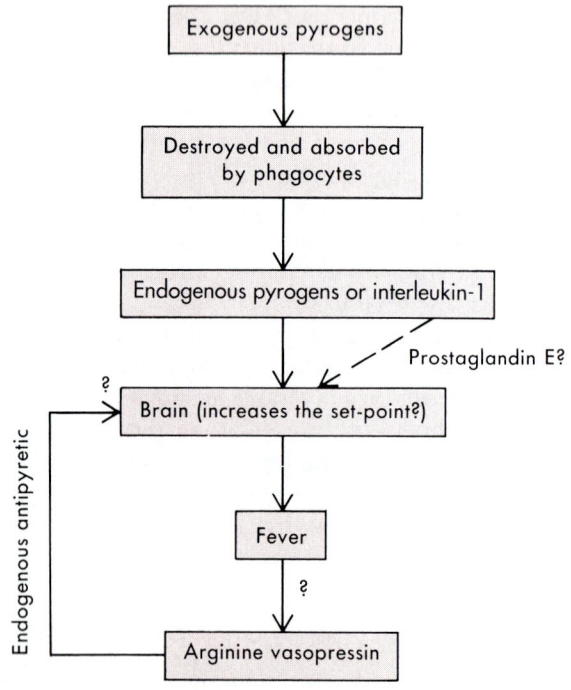

FIG. 13-7 **Pathophysiology of fever.** (See text for explanation.)

When the fever breaks, the set point is returned to normal. The hypothalamus responds by signaling a decrease in heat production and an increase in heat reduction mechanisms. The result is decreased muscle tone, peripheral vasodilation, flushing of the skin, and sweating. The individual feels very warm, replaces warm clothing with cooler clothes, throws off the covers, and stretches out. Once the body has returned to a normal temperature, the individual feels more comfortable, and the hypothalamus adjusts thermoregulatory mechanisms to maintain the new temperature.

Benefits of Fever

Fever production aids responses to infectious processes through several mechanisms (Roberts, 1991). Simple raising of body temperature kills many microorganisms and has adverse effects on the growth and replication of others. Higher body temperatures decrease serum levels of iron, zinc, and copper, all of which are needed for bacterial replication. Increased temperature also causes lysosomal breakdown and autodestruction of cells, thus preventing viral replication in infected cells. Heat increases lymphocytic transformation and motility of polymorphonuclear neutrophils, thus facilitating the immune response. Phagocytosis is enhanced, and production of antiviral interferon may be augmented (Dinarello & Wolff, 1982).

Because fever is a beneficial response to infection, suppression of fever by treatment with antipyrogenic medications should be carefully reviewed (Bruce & Grove, 1992). Such treatment should be employed only if the fever produces or is high enough to produce serious side effects such as nerve damage or convulsion (Cunha, Digamon-Beltran, & Gobbo, 1984; Gurevich, 1985).

Infection and fever responses in the elderly and in children may vary from those in the normal adult. The elderly may have decreased or no fever response to infection. The absence of fever responses to infection and, therefore, the beneficial aspects of fever production may explain the increase in morbidity and mortality seen in the very elderly (Jones, 1991; Norman, Grahn, & Hoshikawa, 1985). In contrast to the very elderly, children develop higher temperatures than adults for relatively minor infections. Febrile seizures may occur with temperatures above 39° C (102.2° F), although most children do not develop febrile seizures until temperatures are much higher. Febrile seizures are more predominant in male children before the age of 5. Febrile seizures are generally brief and self-limiting, lasting less than 5 minutes in 40% of children and less than 20 minutes in 75% of children. Authorities differ over the significance of febrile seizures. Although in most instances there appears to be no long-term effect on the child, a very few children (1% to 2%) may develop epilepsy (Fruthaler, 1985; Wright, 1987).

Disorders of Temperature Regulation
Hyperthermia

Hyperthermia (marked warming of core temperature) can produce nerve damage, coagulation of cell proteins, and death. At 41° C (106° F) nerve damage produces convulsions in the adult. At 43° C (109° F), death results. Hyperthermia is not mediated by pyrogens and there is no resetting of the hypothalamic set point. Hyperthermia may be accidental or therapeutic. Therapeutic hyperthermia is a form of local or general body-induced hyperthermia. Its purpose is to destroy pathologic microorganisms or tumor cells by facilitating the host's natural immune process through fever production. As a form of treatment, it is generally controversial. The four forms of accidental hyperthermia are (1) heat cramps, (2) heat exhaustion, (3) heatstroke, and (4) malignant hyperthermia.

Heat cramps

Heat cramps are severe, spasmodic cramps in the abdomen and extremities that follow prolonged sweating and associated sodium loss. Heat cramps usually appear in individuals who are not accustomed to heat or in those who are performing strenuous work in very warm climates. Fever, rapid pulse, and increased blood pressure often accompany the cramps. Treatment involves administration of dilute salt solutions through oral or parenteral routes.

Heat exhaustion

Heat exhaustion, or collapse, is a result of prolonged high core or environmental temperatures. These high temperatures cause the appropriate hypothalamic response of profound vasodilation and profuse sweating. Over a prolonged period, the hypothalamic responses produce dehydration, decreased plasma volumes, hypotension, decreased cardiac output, and tachycardia. The individual feels weak, dizzy, nauseated, and faint. The symptoms of heat exhaustion cause the individual to stop work, lie down, and rest. Ceasing activity decreases muscle work, causing decreased heat production. Lying down redistributes vascular volume. The individual should be encouraged to drink warm fluids to replace fluid lost through sweating.

Heatstroke

Heatstroke is a potentially lethal result of a breakdown in control of an overstressed thermoregulatory center. The brain cannot tolerate temperatures over 40.5° C (105° F). When core temperature reaches or exceeds 40.5° C (105° F), the brain may be preferentially cooled by maximal blood flow through the veins of the head and face, specifically the forehead. Sweat production on the face is maintained even during dehydration. Evaporation of the sweat cools the blood in the veins of the face and forehead; the blood then is returned to the endocranial venous network and sinus cavernosus, cooling the blood in the cerebral arterial vessels that lie in close proximity. Fanning the face enhances this mechanism. In this way the brain can be temporarily maintained at 40° C (105° F), even when core temperatures are higher (Cabanac & Brinnell, 1987; Yousef, 1987). In instances of very high core temperatures (40° to 43° C [104° to 109.4° F]), the regulatory center may cease to function appropriately. Sweating ceases, and the skin becomes dry and flushed. The individual may be irritable, confused, stuporous, or comatose. Visual disturbances may occur.

As heat loss through the evaporation of sweat ceases, core temperatures increase rapidly. High core temperatures and vascular collapse produce cerebral edema, degeneration of the central nervous system, swollen dendrites, and renal tubular necrosis. Death results unless immediate, effective treatment is initiated (Clowes & O'Donnell, 1974).

Treatment includes removing the person from the warm environment, if possible, and using a cooling blanket or cool water bath. Care must be taken to prevent too rapid cooling of the surface, which causes peripheral vasoconstriction and prevents core cooling. Individuals who recover from heat stroke may have permanent damage to the thermoregulatory center and thus may have difficulty tolerating environmental temperature changes.

Children are more susceptible to heat stroke than adults because (1) they produce more metabolic heat when exercising, (2) they have a greater surface area to mass ratio, and (3) their sweating capacity is less than that of adults (Committee on Sports Medicine, 1982).

Malignant hyperthermia

Malignant hyperthermia is a potentially lethal complication of an inherited muscle disorder. The condition is precipitated by the administration of volatile anesthetics and neuromuscular blocking agents. About 1 in 200 individuals may be at risk for the muscle disorder. Malignant hyperthermia is caused by either increased calcium release or decreased calcium uptake with muscle contraction. This allows intracellular calcium levels to rise, producing sustained, uncoordinated muscle contractions, which in turn increase muscle work, oxygen consumption, and lactic acid production. As a result of these contractions, acidosis develops and temperature rises (body temperature may rise 1° C [1.8° F] every 5 minutes); approximately 20% of those who develop malignant hyperthermia do not survive. Malignant hyperthermia occurs most often in children and young adults immediately after the induction of anesthesia.

Sympathetic responses and acidosis produce tachycardia and cardiac arrhythmias, followed by hypotension, decreased cardiac output, and, eventually, cardiac arrest. Increasing temperature, acidosis, hyperkalemia, and hypoxia produce comalike symptoms in the central nervous system (including unconsciousness, absent reflexes, fixed pupils, apnea, and, sometimes, a flat electroencephalogram [EEG]). Oliguria and anuria are common, probably resulting from shock, ischemia, and low cardiac output (Rogers & Sturgeon, 1985).

Treatment includes withdrawal of the provoking agents and administration of dantrolene sodium (a skeletal relaxant that inhibits calcium release during muscle contraction). Procainamide (Pronestyl) is used to treat cardiac arrhythmias. Sodium bicarbonate also may be used. Body temperature can be decreased through use of ice bags, cooling blanket, and iced saline lavage (Rogers & Sturgeon, 1985).

Hypothermia

Hypothermia (marked cooling of core temperature) produces vasoconstriction, alterations in microcirculation, coagulation, and ischemic tissue damage. In a controlled situation, such as a surgical procedure, most tissues can tolerate temperatures as low as 7° C. In severe hypothermia, ice crystals forming on the inside of the cell cause cells to rupture and die. Tissue hypothermia slows the rate of chemical reactions (tissue metabolism), increases the viscosity of the blood, slows blood flow through the microcirculation, facilitates blood coagulation, and stimulates profound vasoconstriction. Hypothermia may be accidental or therapeutic.

Accidental hypothermia

Accidental hypothermia (i.e., temperature below 35° C [95° F]) is generally the result of sudden immersion in cold water or prolonged exposure to cold environments. At particular risk for accidental hypothermia are the young and the elderly, because thermoregulatory mechanisms are altered in these two groups (Reuler, 1978). Also at risk are individuals with conditions that diminish the ability to generate heat. Such conditions include hypothyroidism, hypopituitarism, malnutrition, Parkinson disease, and rheumatoid arthritis. Other risk factors include chronic increased vasodilation and decreased thermoregulatory control caused by cerebral injuries, ketoacidosis, uremia, and drug overdoses (DeLapp, 1983).

In acute hypothermia, peripheral vasoconstriction shunts blood away from the cooler skin to the core in an effort to decrease heat loss. This peripheral vasoconstriction produces peripheral tissue ischemia. Intermittent reperfusion of the extremities (the Lewis phenomenon) helps preserve peripheral oxygenation. Intermittent peripheral perfusion continues until core temperatures drop dramatically.

The hypothalamic center stimulates shivering in an effort to increase heat production. Severe shivering occurs at core temperatures of 35° C (95° F) and continues until core temperature drops to about 30° to 32° C (86° to 89.6° F). Thinking becomes sluggish and coordination is decreased at 34° C (93.2° F). As hypothermia deepens, paradoxical undressing may occur as hypothalamic control of vasoconstriction is lost and vasodilation occurs with loss of core heat to the periphery. The hypothermic individual, therefore, feels suddenly warm and begins to remove clothing (DeLapp, 1983).

At 30° C (86° F), the individual becomes stuporous; heart rate and respiratory rates decline; and cardiac output is diminished. Cerebral blood flow is decreased. Metabolic rate declines, further decreasing core temperature. Sinus node depression occurs with slowing of conduction through the atrioventricular node. In severe hypothermia (core temperature of 26° to 28° C [78.8° to 82.4° F]), pulse and respirations may be undetectable. Acidosis is moderate to severe. Ventricular fibrillation and asystole are common (Cabanac & Brinnel, 1987).

If hypothermia is mild, passive rewarming may be sufficient. Passive rewarming includes provision of warm, dry clothes and warm drinks and performance of isometric exercises to increase heat production and minimize heat loss. Core temperature should be checked as soon as possible.

If core temperature is above 30° C (86° F), active rewarming also may be required. Active rewarming employs warm water baths, warm blankets, heating pads, and warm oral fluids when the individual is fully alert. Active core rewarming is performed when core temperatures have dropped below 30° C (86° F) or when severe cardiovascular abnormalities appear. Core rewarming may be accomplished through administration of warm intravenous solutions, warm gastric lavage, warm peritoneal lavage, inhalation of warmed gases,

and, in extreme cases, exchange transfusions, warming blood in a pump oxygenator circuit, and mediastinal lavage (Dean, 1987).

Rewarming generally should proceed at no faster than a few degrees per hour. (Short-term complications of rewarming are listed in Table 13-3.) Long-term complications include congestive heart failure, hepatic and renal failure, abnormal erythropoiesis, myocardial infarction, pancreatitis, and neurologic dysfunctions.

Therapeutic hypothermia

Therapeutic hypothermia is used to slow metabolism and thus preserve ischemic tissue during surgery or limb reimplantation. The actual mechanism of tissue preservation has been recently debated (Osterman et al., 1984). It was originally believed that the slowed metabolism in hypothermic tissues preserved adenosine triphosphate (ATP), but recent evidence suggests that ATP is not preserved in hypothermia. Regardless of the mechanism, however, it is clear that hypothermic ischemic cells remain viable long after normothermic ischemic cells have died. Survival from accidental hypothermia has been reported in individuals with core temperatures at 16° C (60.8° F) and from therapeutic hypothermia with temperatures at 9° C (48.2° F) (Cabanac & Brinnel, 1987).

The temperature changes of hypothermia place a great deal of stress on the heart. Moderate to severe hypothermia may lead to ventricular fibrillation and cardiac arrest. (This may be the desired outcome in open heart surgery when the heart must be stopped during portions of the surgical procedure) (Shaver, Camarata, Taleisnik, & Gazzaniga, 1984.) Prolonged hypothermia may precipitate exhaustion of liver glycogen stores by prolonged shivering. Surface cooling may cause burns, frostbite, and fat necrosis.

TABLE 13-3

Accidental Hypothermia: Complications of Rewarming

Complication	Mechanism
Acidosis	Rewarming stimulates peripheral vasodileution; peripheral blood, returning to the core from the ischemic peripheral tissues, causes a reduction in the pH of core blood
Rewarming shock	As rewarming and vasodilation progress, the body is unable to maintain blood pressure because of reduced fluid volume (from "cold diuresis"), catecholamine depletion (prolonged shivering), and myocardial injury
Deep-ended hypothermia	As colder surface blood is returned to the core, core temperatures may drop; this is also referred to as "after fall" or "after drop"
Dysrhythmia	Rewarming places an additional stress on an already severely stressed myocardium

Trauma

Major body trauma has varying effects on temperature regulation, depending on the body systems involved. Five types of traumatic injury that usually affect temperature regulation are (1) central nervous system trauma (discussed in Chapter 15), (2) accidental injury, (3) hemorrhagic shock, (4) major surgery, and (5) thermal burns.

Central nervous system trauma

Central nervous system trauma that causes CNS damage, inflammation, increased intracranial pressures, or intracranial bleeding typically produces a fever of greater than 39° C (102° F). This temperature, often referred to as a "central fever," appears with or without relative bradycardia. The temperature is sustained, does not induce sweating, and is very resistant to antipyretic therapy (Cunha et al., 1984).

Accidental injuries

Mild accidental injuries may produce a slight elevation in core temperature. Moderate to severe injuries result in peripheral vasoconstriction with decreased surface and core temperatures. Core temperature seems inversely related to the severity of the injury and may be a result of decreased oxygen transport to the tissues. In severe injuries, shivering is absent and some alteration in thermoregulation is evident (Little & Stoner, 1981).

Hemorrhagic shock

Loss of blood volume in hemorrhage triggers peripheral vasoconstriction and a slight increase in core temperature. Subsequent decreases in core temperature have been demonstrated in individuals with hemorrhagic shock treated with unwarmed volume-expanding solutions and surgical repair. Volume expansion with warmed solutions is recommended to prevent the deleterious effects of hypothermia on cardiac output, cardiac rhythm, and the immune system (Shaver et al., 1984).

Major surgery

Because many victims of trauma undergo major surgical repair, the effect of the surgical procedure on temperature regulation needs to be considered by health care providers. Major surgery often induces significant hypothermia through exposure of body cavities to the relatively cool operating room environment. Other mechanisms that contribute to intraoperative hypothermia include irrigation of body cavities with room temperature solutions, infusion of room temperature intravenous solutions, use of drugs that impair thermoregulatory mechanisms, and inhalation of unwarmed anesthetic agents (Shaver et al., 1984). Use of warmed irrigating and intravenous solutions may reduce intraoperative hypothermia.

Thermal burns

Large burn injuries produce significant hypothermia because of the loss of the skin barrier to fluid evaporation and the loss of control of the microcirculation in the skin. Severe burns also compromise the normal insulation of the skin and subcutaneous tissues. (Burns are discussed in Chapter 40.)

SLEEP

Sleep is an active multiphase process. Although brain activity during sleep varies from wakeful states, an equal amount of energy is consumed during both states (Schauf, Moffett, & Moffett, 1990). Normal sleep has two phases that can be documented by EEG: REM (rapid eye movement) sleep and non-REM, or slow wave, sleep. Non-REM sleep is divided into four stages based on changes in the EEG pattern (Fig. 13-8).

Stage 1—Light sleep, alpha waves are interspersed with low-frequency theta waves; slow eye movements

Stage 2—Further slowing of the EEG with the presence of sleep spindles and slow eye movements

Stage 3—Low-frequency delta waves with occasional sleep spindles; no slow eye movements

Stage 4—Delta waves

Non-REM Sleep

Non-REM (slow wave) sleep is initiated by the withdrawal of neurotransmitters from the reticular formation and by the inhibition of arousal mechanisms in the

FIG. 13-8 EEG stages of wakefulness and sleep. *Awake,* low-voltage fast activity; *stage 1,* falling asleep; *stage 2,* light sleep with sleep spindles; *stage 3,* moderately deep sleep; *stage 4,* deep sleep with slow delta waves. REM sleep looks similar to awake and stage 1.

cerebral cortex. During non-REM sleep, respiration is controlled by metabolic processes (Phillipson, 1978). The basal metabolic rate is decreased by 10% to 15%. Temperature is decreased 0.5° to 1° C (1° F). Heart rate decreases by 10 to 30 beats per minute. Respiration, blood pressure, and muscle tone all decrease. Knee jerk reflexes are absent. Pupils are constricted. During stages I and II, cerebral blood flow to the brainstem and cerebellum is decreased. During stages III and IV, cerebral blood flow to the cortex is decreased (Sakai, Meyer, Karacan, Derman, & Yamamoto, 1980). Growth hormone is released during stage IV, and levels of corticosteroids and catecholamines are depressed.

REM Sleep

REM (rapid eye-movement) sleep is characterized by desynchronized, low-voltage fast activity that occurs about every 90 minutes beginning after 1 or 2 hours of non-REM sleep. This sleep is also known as "paradoxical sleep" because the EEG pattern is similar to the normal awake pattern. Alternating periods of REM and non-REM sleep occur throughout the night, with lengthening intervals of REM sleep and fewer intervals of deeper stages of non-REM sleep toward morning. REM sleep is characterized by bursts of conjugate rapid eye movement; atonia of antigravity muscles; loss of temperature regulation; alteration in heart rate, blood pressure, and respiration; penile erection in men and clitoral engorgement in women; and a high rate of memorable dreams. Steroids are released in short bursts. During REM sleep, respiratory control appears largely independent of metabolic requirements and oxygen variation. Loss of normal voluntary muscle control in the tongue and upper pharynx may produce some respiratory obstruction. Cerebral blood flow to both hemispheres is increased. About 20% to 25% of sleep time is represented by REM sleep in the adult. REM sleep is controlled by the pontine reticular formation.

Many neurotransmitters are associated with excitatory and inhibitory sleep mechanisms, including catecholamines, acetylcholine, serotonin, histamine, L-tryptophan, and adenosine. Their mechanism of action is complex and not clearly understood. The reticular formation is primarily responsible for generating REM sleep, and projections from the reticular formation and other areas of the mesencephalon and brainstem produce non-REM sleep (Siegel, 1990).

While asleep, an individual progresses through REM and non-REM sleep in a predictable cycle. Each cycle lasts approximately 90 to 100 minutes, with the individual's passing through four to five cycles per night. The first cycle of the night begins with stage I. The individual then progresses through stages II, III, IV, III, II, and REM sleep. A new cycle, beginning with stage II, follows each REM sleep. With each successive cycle, the amount of time spent in stage IV sleep decreases,

and the amount of time spent in REM increases (Fig. 13-9). The individual who is awakened begins the next cycle with stage I. Forced awakenings in the middle of the night may result in increased difficulty returning to sleep or may alter the normal progression of sleep, or both (Campbell, 1987; Kedas, Lux, & Amodeo, 1989). The purpose of sleep is unknown, although restorative processes have been proposed because growth hormone peaks are associated with slow wave sleep. It is an important enough need that we spend about one third of our lives sleeping.

❑ AGING and Sleep Patterns
Sleep Patterns in Children

The sleep patterns of the newborn and young child vary from those of the adult in total sleep time, cycle length, and percentage of time spent in each sleep cycle. Newborns sleep about 16 to 17 hours per day. About 53% of that time is spent in active sleep (REM sleep), 23% in quiet sleep (non-REM sleep), and the remainder in

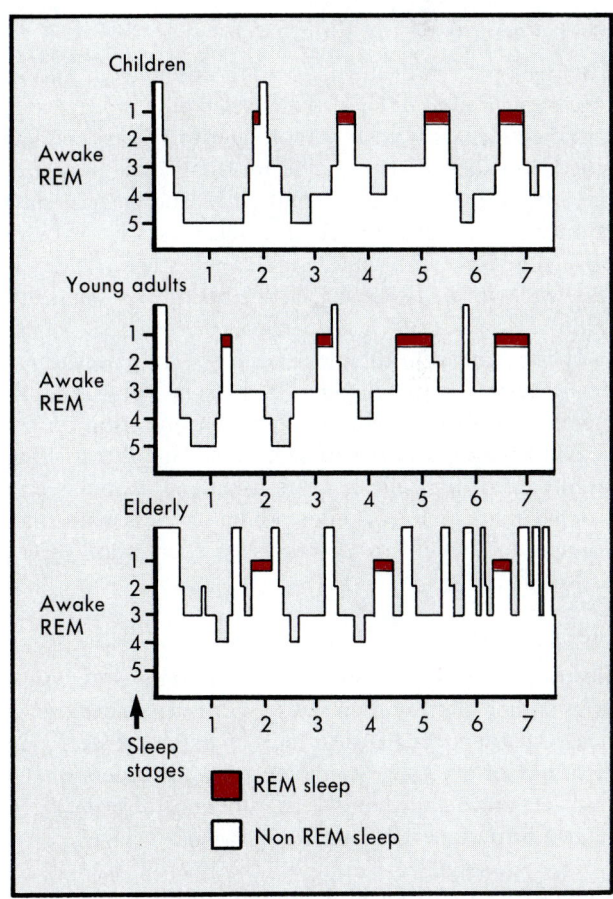

FIG. 13-9 Normal sleep cycles. REM sleep occurs cyclically throughout the night at intervals of approximately 9 minutes in all age groups. REM sleep shows little variation in the different age groups, whereas stage IV sleep decreases with age. In addition, the elderly awaken frequently and show a marked increase in total time awake.

an indeterminate phase. The infant sleep cycle is approximately 50 to 60 minutes in length, with 20 minutes of non-REM sleep and 10 to 45 minutes of REM sleep, in contrast to the adult sleep cycle. Newborns enter REM sleep immediately on falling asleep (Anders & Keener, 1985; Keefe, 1987). At about 1 year of age the infant spends approximately 45% of total sleep time in quiet sleep and 41% in REM sleep. Total sleep time decreases slightly from birth to 1 year. In the American culture, where infants are bottle fed and do not share sleeping space with the mother, infants increase maximum sleep time from 4 to 5 hours to 8 to 10 hours by 4 months of age. They begin to "sleep through the night." In other cultures, where infants are breast fed for up to 2 years and share sleeping space with the mother, they continue to sleep in short bouts and waken frequently to nurse (Elias, Nicholson, Bora, & Johnston, 1986).

In the young child, the sleep cycle length is 45 to 60 minutes, in contrast to 90 to 100 minutes in the adult. The child assumes the adult sleep pattern at some point during the first 2 to 5 years of life (Kales & Kales, 1970).

Sleep Patterns of the Elderly

The sleep pattern of the older adult differs from that of the younger adult or child. Total sleep time is decreased, and the older individual takes longer to fall asleep. The elderly awaken earlier in the morning and more frequently during the night. Total REM and stage II time is unchanged, but stage IV sleep decreases by 15% to 30%. On EEG, the spindle indicating stage II sleep is less well formed (Guazzelli, Feinberg, & Aminoff, 1986).

These changes in the older adult's sleep pattern may be associated with changes in lifestyle, physical ailments, lack of daily routine, desynchronization of circadian rhythm, and use of sedatives. The alteration in sleep pattern typically appears about 10 years later in women than in men. Older adults are less able than younger individuals to tolerate sleep deprivation (Kales & Kales, 1970).

Sleep Disorders

Sleep disorders are classified by their signs and symptoms rather than by their cause. Four classifications of sleep disorders are (1) disorders of initiating sleep, (2) disorders of excessive somnolence, (3) disorders of the sleep-wake schedule, and (4) dysfunctions of sleep, sleep stages, or partial arousals.

Disorders of Initiating Sleep: Insomnia

Insomnia is defined as the inability to fall or stay asleep. Insomnia may be transient, lasting a few days, and related to travel across time zones or caused by acute stress. Long-term insomnia is associated with drug or alcohol abuse, chronic pain disorders, or chronic depression. Drugs known to produce insomnia include amphetamines, steroids, central adrenergic blockers, bronchodilating agents, and caffeine.

Disorders of Excessive Somnolence

Two disorders of excessive somnolence, or excessive daytime sleepiness, are **pickwickian syndrome** and **hypersomnia sleep apnea (HSA) syndrome.** Substantially more men than women are affected by these syndromes. One hypothesis is that the female hormone progesterone (a respiratory stimulant) may protect premenopausal women from sleep-disordered breathing (Block, 1980). Both pickwickian syndrome and HSA syndrome are associated with periodic breathing and episodes of apnea appearing in stages I, II, and REM sleep. The periodic breathing is associated with decreased arterial oxygen saturation, which eventually produces arousal. Each arousal causes an interruption in the sleep cycle, reducing total sleep time and producing sleep and REM deprivation (Long, 1982).

Sleep apnea (lack of breathing during sleep) is absence of air flow through the nose or mouth for at least 10 seconds during sleep. It may result from one of three mechanisms: (1) central apnea, which is apparently the result of altered chemosensitivity and cerebral respiratory control; (2) obstructive apnea, which is caused by partial or complete obstruction of the upper airway during sleep; and (3) mixed apnea, which results from both central and obstructive causes (Guilleminault, Tilkian, & Dement, 1976). In pickwickian syndrome, sleep is frequently interrupted by apneic periods lasting 10 seconds or longer. The apneic periods are generally a result of obesity, decreased chemosensitivity to carbon dioxide and oxygen tensions, or upper airway obstruction occurring during sleep. The apnea that results is a combination of CNS dysfunction (decreased O_2 and CO_2 sensitivity) and upper airway obstruction. The sleep apnea produces low oxygen saturation and eventually produces polycythemia, pulmonary hypertension, right-sided congestive heart failure, liver congestion, cyanosis, and peripheral edema. Cardiac arrhythmias during sleep are common.

Because the apnea is due in part to an alteration of CNS control of respiration, daytime hypercapnia also occurs. Individuals exhibit excessive daytime sleepiness, often falling asleep when driving a car, working, or even in the middle of a conversation. Treatment includes weight loss, controlled oxygen therapy, administration of a respiratory stimulant, and treatment of congestive heart failure. When medical treatment fails, surgical approaches are considered, including uvulopalatopharyngeoplasty or tracheostomy (Kales, Vela-Bueno, & Kales, 1987).

Hypersomnia sleep apnea syndrome is primarily a result of upper airway obstruction occurring during sleep. Persons with HSA syndrome may experience hundreds of apneic episodes each night; these are followed by excessive daytime sleepiness. Their spouses often observe excessive snoring or snorting and thrashing about during sleep. Some individuals may sleepwalk or experience **enuresis.** Profound personality changes, depression, and impotence can occur. Physiologic changes include polycythemia and right-sided heart failure. Daytime respirations, PO_2, and PCO_2 are normal. Treatment involves relief of the upper airway obstruction during sleep, including continuous positive airway pressure (CPAP) or surgery (Block, 1980).

Disorders of the Sleep-Wake Schedule

Common disorders of the sleep-wake schedule include rapid time-zone change (or "jet-lag syndrome"), changing sleep schedule with an advance or a delay of 3 hours or more in sleep time, or a change in total sleep time from day to day. These changes in the timing of established sleep schedules have been shown to desynchronize circadian rhythm. Degree of vigilance, performance of psychomotor tasks, and subjective reports of levels of arousal are markedly depressed after alterations in the sleep-wake schedule. Individuals may experience short sleep episodes called microsleeps without being aware of decreased vigilance (Monk, 1989).

It is well established that industrial shift workers exhibit a decrease in accuracy and increased accident proneness (Taub & Berger, 1976). For similar reasons persons suffering from jet lag require several days to adapt to the new time zone. Travel across time zones requires 2 days to adjust the sleep-wake schedule, 5 days to adjust the body temperature cycle, and 8 days to adjust cortisol secretion. Transmeridian travel requires up to 10 days to adjust the body clock when traveling from east to west. Czeisler's experiments with timed bright-light stimulation have had some success in retiming or resetting the body clock after time zone shifts (Long, 1982).

Dysfunctions of Sleep, Sleep Stages, or Partial Arousals

Three dysfunctions of sleep are common in children. They are **somnambulism** (sleepwalking), **night terrors** (dream anxiety attacks), and **enuresis** (bedwetting).

Somnambulism

Somnambulism is primarily a disorder of childhood and appears to resolve itself within several years of the onset of the sleepwalking episodes. Sleepwalking occurs in stages III and IV and is therefore not associated with dreaming. During the sleepwalking episode, the child functions at a very low level of arousal and has no memory of the event on awakening.

The greatest concern is for the safety of the child, because some children leave home or in some way injure themselves during sleepwalking episodes. If the child does not "outgrow" the disorder or grave safety risks arise, drugs to suppress stage IV sleep are sometimes administered.

Night terrors

Night terrors are characterized by "sudden apparent arousals in which the child expresses intense fear or emotion" (Kales & Kales, 1970). The child, however, is not awake and is very difficult to arouse. Once awakened, the child has no memory of the night terror event. Night terrors occur during stage IV sleep and are not associated with the dreams of REM sleep. Although night terrors occur most often in children, adults may experience them as well. Unlike children, however, adults often display corresponding daytime anxiety (Long, 1982).

Enuresis

Enuresis is possibly the most disturbing of the childhood sleep dysfunctions, because of the stress society places on nighttime continence and the misconception that children are bedwetting to act out against parents. Bedwetting incidents also are associated incorrectly with dreaming. Laboratory studies of sleep have demonstrated that very few incidents of bedwetting occur when the child is dreaming and that by far most incidents occur during non-REM sleep and during the first one third of the night when the child is most difficult to arouse (Kales & Kales, 1970). If the bed is not changed, however, the child may incorporate the feeling of wetness with the next REM dream cycle and therefore may incorrectly associate the enuresis with the dream. Children do eventually "outgrow" the enuretic episodes.

Relation Between Sleep and Disease

Sleep and disease are interrelated. Some diseases produce alterations in the quantity and quality of sleep or affect sleep stages. These are referred to as **secondary sleep disorders.** In some instances sleep stages produce alterations in certain disease states. These are referred to as **sleep-provoked disorders.** Other entities, such as sudden infant death syndrome (SIDS) and sudden unexplained nocturnal death syndrome (SUNDS), produce unexplained death almost exclusively during sleep (Long, 1982).

Secondary Sleep Disorders

The most common causes of secondary sleep disorders are depression, alterations in thyroid hormone secretion (hypothyroidism or hyperthyroidism), pain, and sleep apnea syndromes. Depressed persons have difficulty falling asleep and exhibit less slow-wave sleep, less time spent in REM sleep, early awakening, and less total sleep time. In addition, depressed individuals move through the sleep stages more quickly than do individuals who are not depressed. Sleep deprivation paradoxically relieves depression (Long, 1982).

Changes in thyroid hormone secretion produce changes in stage III and IV sleep. An increase in thyroid secretion produces an increase in stage III and IV activity, whereas a decrease in thyroid hormone produces a decrease in both stage III and IV sleep.

Chronic pain is a cause of insomnia. Chronic pain inhibits sleep, increases arousals during sleep, and causes prolonged awake intervals during the night. Individuals with chronic pain report not only a decrease in the quantity of sleep but also a decrease in its quality.

Sleep-Provoked Disorders

Some diseases are provoked by certain aspects of sleep. Signs and symptoms of the disease appear during, or are enhanced by, sleep. Diseases that are affected by sleep include coronary artery disease, bronchial asthma, chronic obstructive pulmonary disease (COPD), diabetes, and duodenal ulcers.

Coronary artery disease is most affected during REM sleep. During REM, dreams may provoke nocturnal angina, increased heart rate, and electrocardiogram (ECG) changes. In adults, attacks of bronchial asthma may occur at any time during the night. The attacks cause the individual to spend more of the sleep period awake and thus cause a decrease in stage IV sleep. In children, bronchial asthma attacks are uncommon during the first one third of the night, when stage IV sleep predominates, and occur more frequently during the final two thirds of the night. Stage IV sleep is decreased overall in the child with bronchial asthma. In addition to these changes asthmatics may experience bronchial spasm during REM sleep (Kales & Kales, 1970).

Persons with COPD experience significantly lowered oxygen tension and increases in carbon dioxide retention during sleep (Calverly, Brezinova, Douglas, Catterall, & Flenley, 1982). The lowered oxygen tension is most significant in the tonic phase of REM sleep when voluntary neuromuscular control, including intercostal muscle function, is depressed. Pulmonary spasm and transient pulmonary hypertension result. These changes are particularly evident in the so-called blue bloater individual and may contribute to early pulmonary hypertension and cor pulmonale in these persons (Block, 1981).

Because blood glucose levels vary during sleep, individuals with uncontrolled diabetes may need careful attention to blood sugar levels during sleep. Studies show that people with duodenal ulcers secrete 3 to 20 times more gastric acid during REM sleep than people without duodenal ulcers. This increased gastric acid secretion often produces nocturnal epigastric pain (Kales & Kales, 1970).

Sudden infant death syndrome (SIDS) affects children primarily in the first 2 years of life and may be related to central sleep apnea episodes. (For further discussion of SIDS, see Chapter 31.) Sudden unexplained nocturnal death syndrome (SUNDS) occurs in previously healthy Asian men in the second, third, or fourth decade of life. Postmortem studies have demonstrated abnormalities of the cardiac conduction system and, frequently, left ventricular hypertrophy or cardiomyopathy. The relationship between the SUNDS event and sleep is unclear but may involve cardiac arrhythmias occurring during REM sleep (Kirschner, Eckner, & Baron, 1986; Melles, 1987).

THE SPECIAL SENSES

Vision

The eyes are complex sense organs responsible for vision. Within a protective casing, each eye has receptors, a lens system for focusing light on the receptors, and a system of nerves for conducting impulses from the receptors to the brain (Ganong, 1991). Visual dysfunction may be caused by abnormal ocular movements or alterations in visual acuity, refraction, color vision, or accommodation. Visual dysfunction also may be the secondary effect of another neurologic disorder.

The External Eye Structures

The external structures protecting the eye include the eyelids (palpebrae), conjunctiva, and lacrimal apparatus (Fig. 13-10). Infection and inflammatory responses are the most common conditions affecting the supporting structures of the eyes. **Blepharitis** is an inflammation of the eyelids caused by staphylococcus or seborrheic dermatitis. Redness, edema, and itching are common symptoms. A **hordeolum** (stye) is an infection of the sebaceous glands of the eyelids, and a **chalazion** is an infection of the meibomian (oil-secreting) gland. These conditions are treated symptomatically (Moses & Hart, 1987).

Conjunctivitis

Conjunctivitis is an inflammation of the conjunctiva (mucous membrane covering the front part of the eyeball). Conjunctivitis may be caused by bacteria, viruses, allergies, or chemical irritations. The inflammatory response produces redness, edema, pain, and lacrimation. Treatment is related to cause.

Acute bacterial conjunctivitis (pinkeye) is highly contagious and is often caused by gram-positive organisms (*Staphylococcus, Haemophilus, Proteus*) although other bacteria may be involved. The onset is acute, characterized by mucopurulent drainage from one or both eyes. Preventing spread of the organism with meticulous hand washing and use of separate towels is important. The

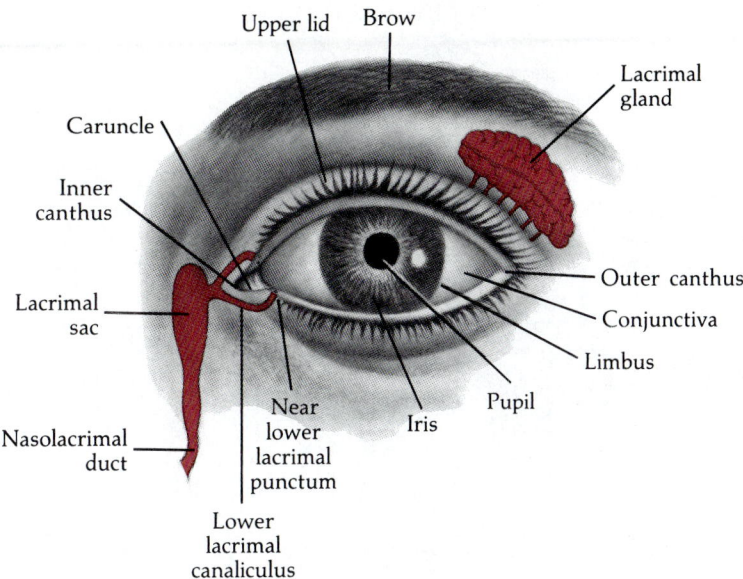

FIG. 13-10 **External eye structures.** (From Thompson et al., 1993.)

disease is frequently self-limiting and resolves spontaneously in 10 to 14 days. Antibiotic eyedrops are usually effective.

Viral conjunctivitis is caused by an adenovirus. Symptoms vary from mild to severe. Some strains of virus cause conjunctivitis and pharyngitis (pharyngoconjunctival fever), and others cause keratoconjunctivitis. Both diseases are contagious, with watering, redness, and photophobia. Treatment is symptomatic.

Allergic conjunctivitis is associated with a variety of antigens, including pollens. There is ocular itching associated with photophobia, burning, and gritty sensations in the eye. Treatment is symptomatic and may include antihistamines, steroids, and vasoconstrictors.

Chronic conjunctivitis is the result of any persistent conjunctivitis. The cause requires identification for effective treatment.

Trachoma (chlamydial conjunctivitis) is caused by *Chlamydia trachomatis.* It is often associated with poor hygiene and is the leading cause of preventable blindness in the world. The severity of the disease varies but can involve inflammation and vascularization of the cornea with scarring of the conjunctiva and eyelids, leading to blindness. Chlamydial organisms are sensitive to local or systemic antibiotics.

Keratitis

Keratitis is an infection of the cornea that can be caused by bacteria or viruses. Bacterial infections often cause corneal ulceration and require intensive antibiotic treatment. Type I herpes simplex virus can involve both the cornea and conjunctiva. Common symptoms include photophobia, pain, and lacrimation. Severe ulcerations with residual scarring require corneal transplantation.

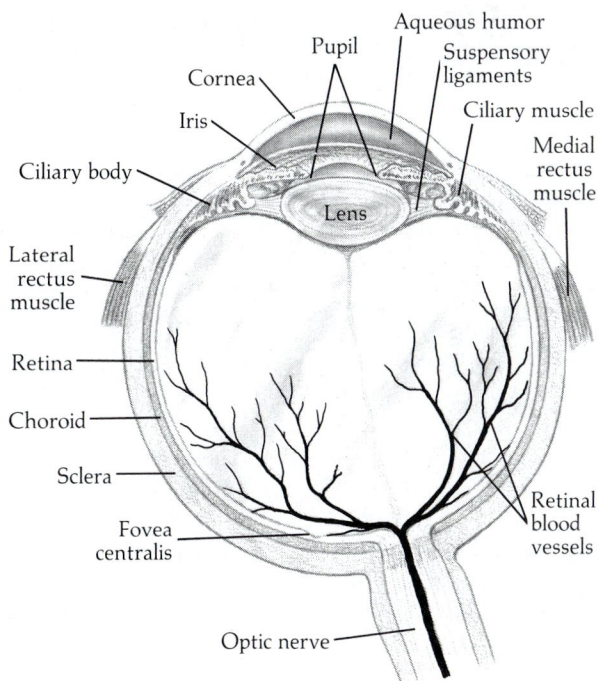

FIG. 13-11 **Internal anatomy of the eye.** (From Thompson et al., 1993.)

The Eye

The wall of the eye is formed of three layers: (1) sclera, (2) choroid, and (3) retina (Fig. 13-11). The **sclera** is the thick, white, outermost layer. It becomes transparent at the **cornea,** the portion of the sclera in the central anterior region that allows light to enter the eye. The **choroid** is the deeply pigmented middle layer that prevents

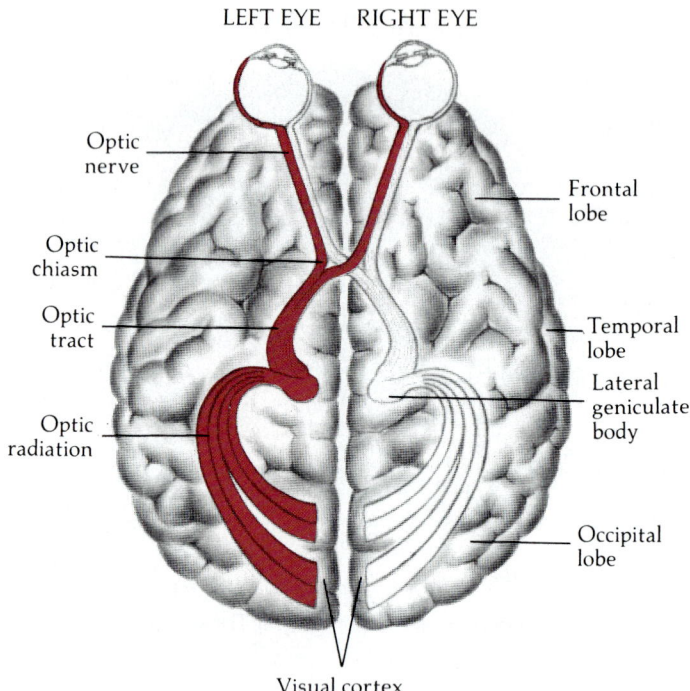

LEFT EYE RIGHT EYE

Optic nerve

Optic chiasm

Optic tract

Optic radiation

Frontal lobe

Temporal lobe

Lateral geniculate body

Occipital lobe

Visual cortex

FIG. 13-12 **Visual pathway.** (From Thompson et al., 1993).

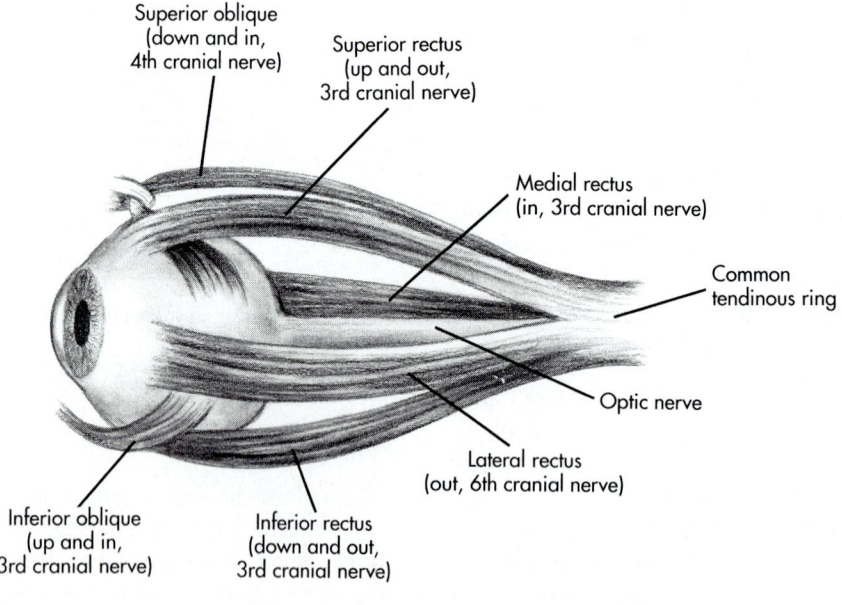

Superior oblique
(down and in,
4th cranial nerve)

Superior rectus
(up and out,
3rd cranial nerve)

Medial rectus
(in, 3rd cranial nerve)

Common
tendinous ring

Optic nerve

Lateral rectus
(out, 6th cranial nerve)

Inferior oblique
(up and in,
3rd cranial nerve)

Inferior rectus
(down and out,
3rd cranial nerve)

FIG. 13-13 **Extraocular muscles.** (From Rudy, 1984.)

light from scattering inside the eye. The **iris,** part of the choroid, has a round opening, the **pupil,** through which light passes. Smooth muscle fibers control the size of the pupil so that in close vision and bright light the pupil constricts and in distant vision and dim light the pupil dilates.

The innermost layer of the eye, the **retina,** contains millions of rods and cones, special photoreceptors that convert light energy into nerve impulses. In the retina **rods** mediate peripheral and dim light vision and are densest at the periphery. **Cones,** densest in the center of the retina, are color and detail receptors. The photoreceptive rods and cones are distributed over the entire retina, except where the optic nerve leaves the eyeball. Lack of rods and cones in this area results in the **optic disc,** or blind spot. Lateral to each optic disc is the **fovea centralis,** a tiny area that contains only cones and provides the greatest visual acuity (Fig. 13-11).

As shown in Fig. 13-12, nerve impulses pass through the optic nerves after leaving the retinas. At the optic chiasm, the fibers from the inner (nasal) halves of the retinas cross to the opposite side, where they join fibers from the outer (temporal) halves of the retinas to form the optic tracts. The fibers of the optic tracts synapse in the dorsal lateral geniculate nucleus, and from there the geniculocalcarine fibers pass by way of the optic radiation (or geniculocalcarine tract) to the primary visual cortex in the occipital lobe of the brain (Guyton, 1992).

Light entering the eye is focused on the retina by the **lens:** a flexible, biconvex, crystal-like structure. In youth the lens is transparent and has the consistency of hardened jelly. With age the lens becomes increasingly hard and opaque. The lens divides the anterior chamber into (1) the aqueous chamber and (2) the vitreous chamber. **Aqueous humor,** which fills the aqueous chamber, helps to maintain the pressure inside the eye and provides nutrients to the lens and cornea. Aqueous humor is free-flowing fluid, secreted by the ciliary processes, and reabsorbed into the canal of Schlemm. If drainage is blocked, pressure within the eye increases (as it does with glaucoma). The vitreous chamber is filled with a gel-like substance called **vitreous humor.** Vitreous humor helps to prevent the eyeball from collapsing inward.

The central retinal artery provides blood to the inner retinal surface. Nutrients are supplied to the outer surface of the retina by the choroid. Six extrinsic eye muscles, attached to the outer surface of each eye, allow gross eye movements and permit eyes to follow a moving object (Fig. 13-13).

❑ AGING and Vision

Changes in the structural components of the eye caused by aging begin at an early age, particularly in the lens of the eye. Changes caused by aging are summarized in Table 13-4. The combined structural changes result in a decline in visual acuity (Pathy, 1991).

TABLE 13-4

Changes in the Eye Caused by Aging

Structure	Change	Consequence
Cornea	Thicker and less curved	Increase in astigmatism
	Formation of a gray ring at the edge of the cornea (arcus senilis)	Not detrimental to vision
Anterior chamber	Decrease in size and volume caused by thickening of lens	Occasionally exerts pressure on Schlemm canal and may lead to increased intraocular pressure and glaucoma
Lens	Increase in opacity	Decrease in refraction with increased light scattering and decreased color vision (green and blue); can lead to cataracts
	Increased firmness and loss of elasticity	Decrease in accommodation for near vision; presbyopia develops by age 50-55 years
Ciliary muscles	Reduction in pupil diameter, atrophy of radial dilation muscles	Persistent constriction (senile miosis); decrease in critical flicker frequency*
Retina	Reduction in number of rods at periphery, loss of rods and associated nerve cells	Increase in the minimum amount of light necessary to see an object

*The rate at which consecutive visual stimuli can be presented and still be perceived as separate.

Visual Dysfunction
Alterations in ocular movements

Abnormal ocular movements occur as a result of oculomotor, trochlear, or abducens cranial nerve dysfunction (see Table 12-6). The three types of eye movement disorders are (1) strabismus, (2) nystagmus, and (3) paralysis of individual extraocular muscles.

Strabismus is the deviation of one eye from the other when the person is looking at an object caused by weak or hypertonic muscle in one of the eyes. The deviation may be upward, downward, inward, or outward. Strabismus in children requires early intervention to prevent the development of **amblyopia** (reduced vision in the affected eye often caused by cerebral blockage of the visual stimuli). The primary symptom of strabismus is **diplopia** (double vision). Strabismus may be caused by a neuromuscular disorder of the eye muscle, diseases involving the cerebral hemispheres, or thyroid disease.

Nystagmus is an involuntary unilateral or bilateral rhythmic movement of the eyes. It may be present at rest, or it may occur with eye movement. The two major forms of nystagmus are pendular nystagmus and jerk nystagmus. **Pendular nystagmus** is characterized by a regular to-and-fro movement of the eyes in which both phases of the movement are equal in length. In **jerk nystagmus,** one phase of the eye movement is faster than the other. Nystagmus may be caused by an imbalance in the normally coordinated reflex activity of the inner ear, **vestibular** nuclei (connecting the vestibular nerve with vestibulospinal tracts), cerebellum, medial longitudinal fascicle (connecting the mesencephalon with the upper portion of the spinal cord), or nuclei of the oculomotor, trochlear, and abducens cranial nerves (see Table 12-5). Drugs, retinal disease, and diseases involving the cervical cord also may produce nystagmus.

Paralysis of specific extraocular muscles may cause a variety of abnormalities, including limited abduction, abnormal closure of the eyelid, ptosis (drooping of the eyelid), and diplopia. The abnormalities occur as a result of unopposed muscle activity. Trauma or pressure in the area of the cranial nerves may cause paralysis of specific extraocular muscles. Diseases such as diabetes mellitus and myasthenia gravis also may affect specific extraocular muscles.

Alterations in visual acuity

Visual acuity is the ability to see objects in sharp detail. With advancing age, the lens of the eye becomes less flexible and less adjustable. In addition, the sclera changes shape, causing light to fall on the macula (an opaque portion of the cornea). Thus, visual acuity declines with age. In addition, visual acuity may change or diminish for many other reasons. Specific causes of visual acuity changes are (1) amblyopia, (2) scotoma, (3) cataracts, (4) papilledema, (5) **dark adaptation**, and (6) glaucoma.

Amblyopia is a reduction or dimness of vision for unknown reasons. It does not result from a change in refraction (i.e., deviation of light rays) or from any visible changes in the eye. Amblyopia is associated with such diseases as diabetes mellitus, renal failure, and malaria and with toxic substances such as alcohol and tobacco.

A **scotoma** is a circumscribed defect of the central field of vision. It is most often a sequel to **retrobulbar neuritis,** an inflammatory lesion of the optic nerve frequently associated with multiple sclerosis (see Chapter 15). Less common causes include the compression of one optic nerve by a retroorbital tumor, neuromyelitis optica (inflammation of the optic nerve), pernicious anemia, and toxic/metabolic causes such as methyl alcohol poisoning and use of tobacco. The precise mechanisms for these conditions causing a scotoma are uncertain, but the result is always a serious impairment in visual acuity.

A **cataract** is a cloudy or opaque area in the ocular lens. The incidence of cataracts increases with age as the lens enlarges. Cataracts develop because of alterations of metabolism and transport of nutrients within the lens. Although the most common form of cataract is degenerative, cataracts also may occur congenitally as a result of infection, radiation, trauma, drugs, or diabetes mellitus. Cataracts cause decreased visual acuity, blurred vision, glare, and decreased color perception. Cataracts are treated by removal of the entire lens and replacement with an artificial lens.

Papilledema is edema and inflammation of the optic nerve at its point of entrance into the eyeball. Generally, papilledema is caused by some obstruction to the venous return from the retina. An early symptom is distention of the retinal vein. Obliteration of the physiologic cup (a bright area normally located in the center of the optic disc) follows. Later the optic disc becomes raised above the level of the surrounding retina, and the margins become blurred and indistinct. With severe swelling, hemorrhage and patches of white exudate develop around the disc margins. The three principal causes of papilledema are (1) increased intracranial pressure, (2) retrobulbar neuritis, and (3) changes in the retinal blood vessels. Retinal blood vessel changes are especially prevalent in individuals with diabetes mellitus or hypertension. Such changes account for a large percentage of individuals newly affected with blindness each year. Typically the blood vessels narrow, and hemorrhages and white exudate appear. Ultimately papilledema occurs.

Dark adaptation also affects visual acuity. Low illumination causes impaired visual acuity, particularly in the elderly. The average 80-year-old needs more than twice as much light as 20-year-olds to see equally well. Changes in the quantity and quality of rhodopsin, a substance found in the rods and responsible for low-light vision, are thought to be responsible for reduced dark adaptation in older adults. Vitamin A deficiencies can cause the same phenomenon in individuals of any age.

Glaucoma is characterized by intraocular pressures above the normal pressures of 12 to 20 mm Hg maintained by the aqueous fluid. The mechanisms of intraocular fluid accumulation are summarized in Fig. 13-14. Chronic increased intraocular pressure first causes loss of peripheral vision, which is followed by central vision impairment and blindness. Extremely high pressures can cause blindness within days or hours (Guyton, 1992). Loss of visual acuity results from pressure on the optic nerve, which is believed to block the flow of cytoplasm from neuronal bodies in the retina to peripheral optic nerve fibers entering the brain. Lack of nutrients leads to death of the involved neurons. Acute pain may result (Yanofsky, 1988). The types of glaucoma are summarized in Table 13-5. Glaucoma is often treated with eye drops to reduce secretion or increase absorption of aqueous humor. Surgery may be needed to open the spaces of the trabeculae (Moses & Hart, 1987).

Alterations in accommodation

Accommodation is the process whereby the thickness of the lens changes. Accommodation is needed for clear vision and is mediated through the oculomotor nerve. Pressure, inflammation, and disease of the oculomotor nerve may alter accommodation. Symptoms include diplopia, blurred vision, and headache. Accommodation is also affected by the decreased flexibility of the lens that occurs with aging. By the age of 60, the lens has become so inelastic that accommodation is not possible.

Loss of accommodation in the elderly is termed **presbyopia**, a condition in which the ocular lens becomes larger, firmer, and less elastic. The major symptom is reduced near vision, causing the holding of reading material at arm's length. Correction is accomplished through reading glasses or bifocal lenses.

Alterations in refraction

Alterations in refraction are the most common visual problem. Errors in refraction are due to irregularities of the corneal curvature, the focusing power of the lens, and the length of the eye. The major symptoms of refraction alterations are blurred vision and headache. Three types of refraction alterations are (1) myopia, (2) hyperopia, and (3) astigmatism (Fig. 13-15).

In **myopia** (nearsightedness), light rays are focused in front of the retina when the person is looking at a distant object. A concave lens is needed for correction. Myopia requires frequent changes of eyeglasses while the eyeball is lengthening in childhood.

In **hyperopia** (farsightedness), light rays are focused behind the retina when the person is looking at a near object. Hyperopia is corrected with a convex lens. **Astigmatism** is caused by an unequal curvature of the cornea. In astigmatism, light rays are bent unevenly and do not come to a single focus on the retina. Astigmatism may coexist with myopia, hyperopia, or presbyopia. Correction is accomplished with a cylinder lens.

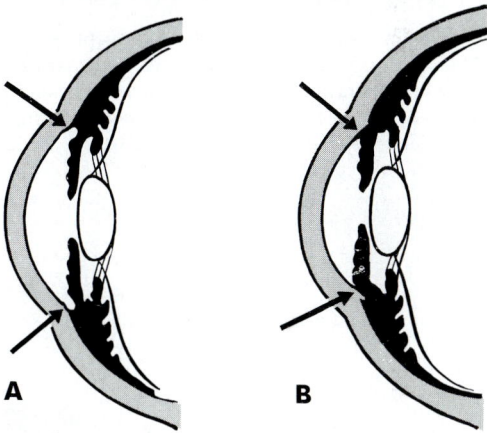

FIG. 13-14 Glaucoma. **A**, Open-angle glaucoma. The obstruction to aqueous flow lies in the trabecular meshwork. **B**, Closed-angle glaucoma. The trabecular meshwork is covered by the root of the iris. (From Stein, Slatt, & Stein, 1988.)

TABLE 13-5

Types of Glaucoma

Type	Mechanism of increased pressure
Open-angle glaucoma	Obstruction to the outflow of aqueous humor at the trabecular meshwork or Schlemm canal
Narrow-angle glaucoma (angle closure)	Forward displacement of the iris toward the cornea with narrowing of the iridocorneal angle and obstruction to the outflow of aqueous humor from the anterior chamber
Acute angle closure glaucoma	Acute closure of the iridocorneal angle with a sudden rise in intraocular pressure, producing nerve pain and visual disturbances

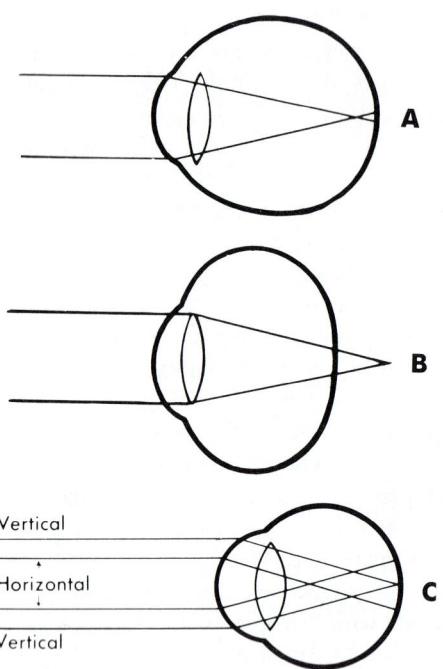

FIG. 13-15 Alterations in refraction. A, Myopic eye. Parallel rays of light are brought to a focus in front of the retina. **B,** Hyperopic eye. Parallel rays of light come to a focus behind the retina in the unaccommodative eye. **C,** Simple myopic astigmatism. The vertical bundle of rays is focused on the retina; the horizontal rays are focused in front of the retina. (From Stein et al., 1988.)

Alterations in color vision

Normal sensitivity to color diminishes with age because of the progressive yellowing of the lens that occurs with aging. All colors become less intense, although color discrimination for blue and green is most greatly affected. Color vision deteriorates more rapidly for individuals with diabetes mellitus than for the general population. The deterioration is thought to be an accelerated version of senile color vision deterioration.

Abnormal color vision also may be caused by **color blindness,** an inherited trait. Color blindness is generally an X-linked, recessive characteristic affecting 8% of the male population and 0.5% of the female population. Although many forms of color blindness exist, most commonly the affected individual cannot distinguish red from green.

Neurologic disorders causing visual dysfunction

Various neurologic disorders may cause visual dysfunction. Vision may be disrupted at many points along the visual pathway, causing a variety of defects in fields of vision. Visual changes do not always cause defects or blindness in the entire visual field; **hemianopia** is the term that describes defective vision in half a visual field. (Fig. 13-16 illustrates the many areas along the visual pathway that may be damaged and the associated visual changes.)

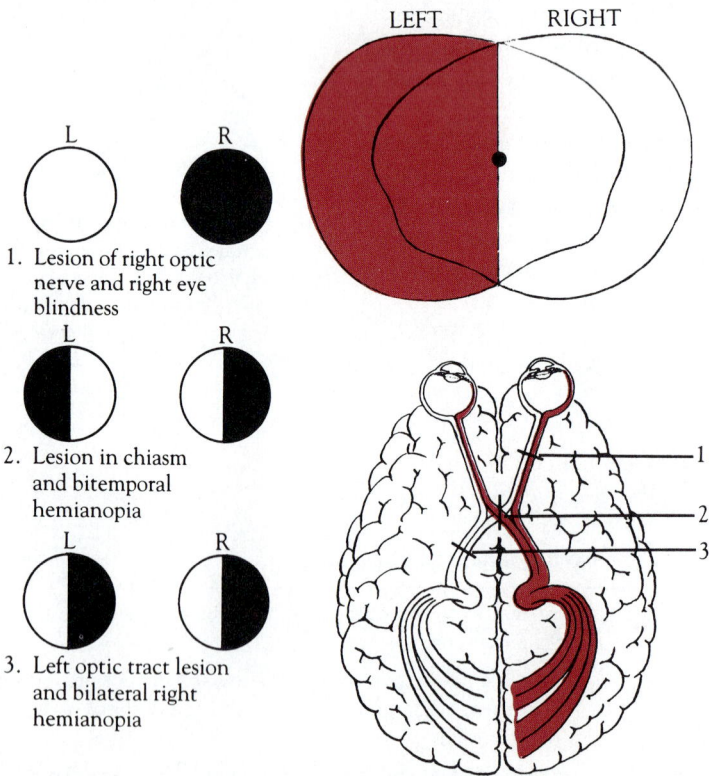

FIG. 13-16 Visual pathway defects. (From Thompson et al., 1993.)

Because of the anatomy of the optic nerves, injury to the optic nerve causes ipsilateral (same side) blindness, but a normal contralateral (opposite side) visual field. Injury to the **optic chiasm** (the X-shaped crossing of the optic nerves), often caused by atherosclerotic ischemia or external compression from trauma or aneurysm, can cause a variety of defects, depending on the location of injury. These defects vary because at the optic chiasm, nerve fibers from the medial half of each retina separate from the lateral half and enter the opposite optic tract.

Because of the normal structure of the visual pathways, destruction of one optic tract causes **homonymous hemianopsia** (complete loss of vision in the inner half of one eye and the outer half of the other). Thus, if an injury to the left optic tract occurs, the individual is blind in the right eye's medial (inner) field and the left eye's lateral (outer) field. If the compression of the optic tract is asymmetric, an incongruous (or uneven) homonymous defect results. Injury to one optic radiation (an ocular pathway in the internal capsule, temporal lobe, or occipital lobe) also causes a homonymous (same field) defect. A major injury in the optic radiation causes homonymous hemianopsia. A lesser injury may cause an upper quadrant homonymous defect. Generally the defects are the same size in both eyes. When the homonymous hemianopsia is caused by an occipital lobe lesion, the area of hemianopsia is split. Although visual acuity may remain unimpaired, reading is difficult because of the inability to group words.

Hearing

The external auditory canal is surrounded by the bones of the cranium. Its opening (meatus) is just above the **mastoid process,** which contains air-filled sinuses called **mastoid air cells.** These promote conductivity between the external and the middle ear.

The Normal Ear

The ear is divided into three areas: (1) the external ear, involved only with hearing; (2) the middle ear, involved only with hearing; and (3) the inner ear, involved with both hearing and equilibrium.

The external ear is composed of the **pinna** (auricle), which is the visible portion of the ear, and the **external auditory canal,** a tube that leads to the middle ear (Fig. 13-17). Sound waves entering the external auditory canal hit the **tympanic membrane** (eardrum) and cause it to vibrate. The tympanic membrane separates the external ear from the middle ear.

The middle ear is composed of the **tympanic cavity,** a small chamber in the temporal bone. Three ossicles (small bones) transmit the vibration of the tympanic membrane to the inner ear. The three ossicles are termed the **malleus** (hammer), **incus** (anvil), and **stapes** (stirrup).

When the tympanic membrane moves, the malleus moves with it and transfers the vibration to the incus, which passes it on to the stapes. The stapes presses against the **oval window,** a small membrane of the inner ear. The movement of the oval window sets the fluids of the inner ear in motion (Fig. 13-18).

The **eustachian (pharyngeotympanic) tube** connects the middle ear with the thorax. Normally flat and closed, the eustachian tube opens briefly when a person swallows or yawns, and it equalizes the pressure in the

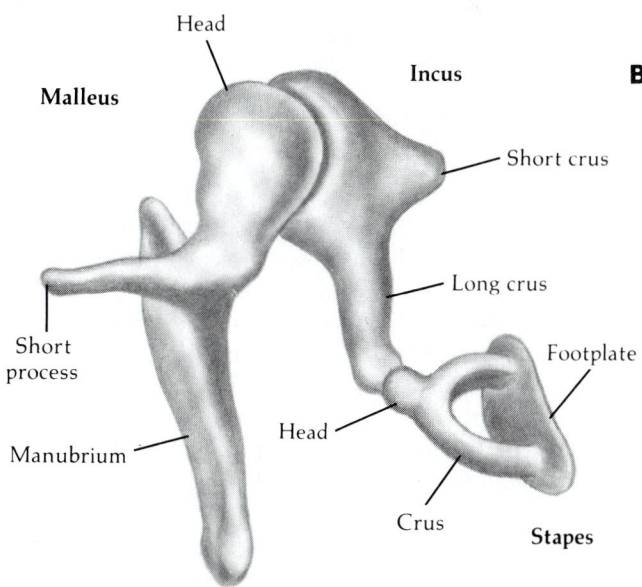

FIG. 13-17 Ear structures. A, Relationship of external, middle, and inner ear. **B,** Ossicles of right middle ear. (From Thompson et al., 1993.)

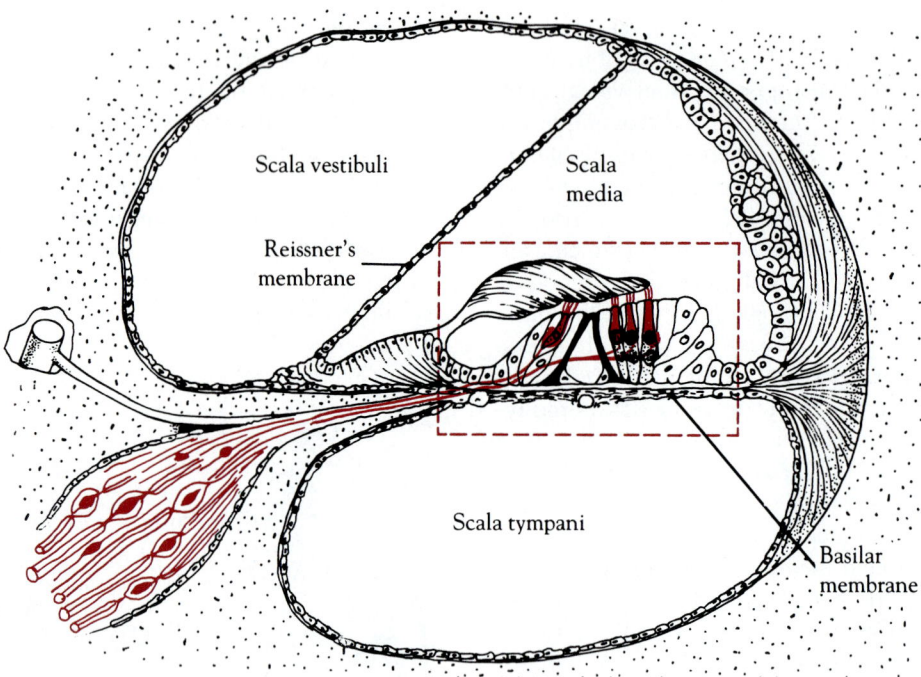

FIG. 13-18 Scalae of the cochlea, separated by Reissner's membrane and basilar membrane. (From Thompson et al., 1993.)

middle ear with atmospheric pressure. Equalized pressure permits the tympanic membrane to vibrate freely. Through the eustachian tube the mucosa of the middle ear is continuous with the mucosal lining of the throat.

The inner ear is a system of osseous labyrinths (bony, mazelike chambers) filled with a fluid called **perilymph.** The bony labyrinth is divided into the **cochlea,** the **vestibule,** and the **semicircular canals** (see Fig. 13-17). Suspended in the perilymph is a membranous labyrinth that basically follows the shape of the bony labyrinth. The membranous labyrinth is filled with a thicker fluid called **endolymph.**

Within the cochlea is the **organ of Corti,** which contains **hair cells** (hearing receptors). Sound waves that reach the cochlea through vibrations of the tympanic membrane, ossicles, and oval window set the cochlear fluids into motion. Receptor cells on the basilar membrane are stimulated when their hairs are bent or pulled by the movement. Once stimulated, hair cells transmit impulses along the cochlear nerve (a division of the vestibulocochlear nerve) to the auditory cortex of the temporal lobe in the brain (see Fig. 13-18). There interpretation of the sound occurs.

The semicircular canals and vestibule of the inner ear contain **equilibrium receptors.** In the semicircular canals the dynamic equilibrium receptors respond to changes in direction of movement. Within each semicircular canal is the **crista ampullaris,** a receptor region composed of a tuft of hair cells covered by a gelatinous cupula. When the head is rotated, the endolymph in the canal lags behind and moves in the direction opposite to the head's movement. The hair cells are stimulated, and impulses are transmitted through the vestibular nerve (a division of the vestibulocochlear nerve) to the cerebellum.

The vestibule in the inner ear contains **maculae,** receptors essential to the body's sense of static equilibrium. As the head moves, **otoliths** (small pieces of calcium salts) move in a gel-like material in response to changes in the pull of gravity. The otoliths pull on the gel, which in turn pulls on the hair cells in the maculae. Nerve impulses in the hair cells are triggered and transmitted to the brain (see Fig. 13-18). Thus the ear not only permits the hearing of a large range of sounds but also assists with maintaining balance through the sensitive equilibrium receptors.

❑ AGING and Hearing

Auditory changes caused by aging are common and incremental. Changes in hearing with aging are summarized in Table 13-6. Approximately one third of people older than age 65 have hearing loss (Timiras, 1988). Changes may occur in both the structural and functional components of the peripheral or central auditory system. Loss of hearing for sounds in the high-frequency range (**presbycusis**) is most common and interferes with

TABLE 13-6

Changes in Hearing Caused by Aging

Change in structure	Change in function
Cochlear hair cell degeneration	Inability to hear high-frequency sounds (sensory/neural loss)
Loss of auditory neurons in spiral ganglia of organ of Corti	Inability to hear high-frequency sounds (sensory/neural loss)
Degeneration of basilar (cochlear) conductive membrane of cochlea	Inability to hear at all frequencies but more pronounced at higher frequencies (cochlear conductive loss)
Decreased vascularity of cochlea	Equal loss of hearing at all frequencies (strial loss)
Loss of cortical auditory neurons	Diminished hearing and speech comprehension

understanding speech, particularly high-frequency consonant sounds (e.g., *s*, *sh*, and *f*). Hearing may be lost in both ears but not at the same time. Elderly individuals from rural areas have less hearing loss than those in noisy cities. The ability to discriminate localization of sound varies with high and low frequencies and diminishes with age. In the low-frequency range, sound localization is a function of the timing of sound arrival between the two ears; localization of high-frequency sounds is a function of sound intensity. Because the elderly tend to lose high-frequency hearing first, they may have difficulty localizing high-frequency sounds.

Auditory Dysfunction

Between 5% and 10% of the general population have a hearing impairment. The major categories of auditory dysfunction are conductive hearing loss, sensorineural hearing loss, mixed hearing loss, and functional hearing loss.

Conductive hearing loss

A **conductive hearing loss** occurs when a change in the outer or middle ear impairs the sound from being conducted from the outer to the inner ear. Conductive hearing loss occurs when there is interference in air conduction. Conditions that commonly cause a conductive hearing loss include impacted cerumen, foreign bodies lodged in the ear canal, benign tumors of the middle ear, carcinoma of the external auditory canal or middle ear, eustachian tube dysfunction, otitis media, acute viral otitis media, chronic suppurative otitis media, cholesteatoma, and otosclerosis.

Symptoms of conductive hearing loss include diminished hearing and soft speaking voice. The voice is soft because often the individual hears his or her voice, conducted by bone, as loud. In addition, although the cause is unknown, the individual often hears better in a noisy environment than in a quiet one (a condition called par-

acusia willisiana). Treatment of the underlying cause generally eliminates the hearing loss (Glasscock & Shambaugh, 1990). A hearing aid is used if the hearing loss is greater than 40 to 50 decibels.

Sensorineural hearing loss

A **sensorineural hearing loss** is caused by impairment of the organ of Corti or its central connections. The hearing loss may be gradual or sudden. Conditions that commonly cause sensorineural hearing loss include congenital and hereditary factors, noise exposure, aging, **Ménière disease**, ototoxicity, and systemic disease (syphilis, Paget disease, collagen diseases, diabetes mellitus). Congenital and neonatal sensorineural hearing loss may be caused by maternal rubella, ototoxic drugs, prematurity, traumatic delivery, erythroblastosis fetalis, and congenital hereditary malfunction. Diagnosis is often made when delayed speech development is noted.

Presbycusis is the most common form of sensorineural hearing loss and is especially common in the elderly. Presbycusis may occur because of atrophy of the basal end of the organ of Corti, a loss in the number of auditory receptors, vascular changes, or stiffening of the basilar membranes. Because of the slow progression of hearing loss, onset of symptoms is gradual. In addition, drug ototoxicities (drugs that cause destruction of auditory function) have been observed after exposure to a variety of chemicals. Antibiotics such as streptomycin, neomycin, gentamicin, and vancomycin; diuretics such as ethacrynic acid and furosemide; and chemicals such as salicylate, quinine, carbon monoxide, nitrogen mustard, arsenic, mercury, gold, tobacco, and alcohol are considered ototoxic. Because of increased concentrations of antibiotics in the endolymph, these drugs generally cause damage to the cells of the cristae and maculae (located in the inner ear) or the cells of the organ of Corti. The increased concentration of drugs in the endolymph is preferentially toxic to the cells.

Diuretics affect hearing primarily by altering the sodium-potassium balance, causing extracellular fluid accumulation and changes in the microstructure of secretory cells. Quinine, mercury, and lead affect the neural pathways of hearing, including the spinal ganglia, the eighth cranial nerve, and the cochlear nucleus. The site of action for the other chemicals, including alcohol and tobacco, has not yet been determined. In most instances the drugs and chemicals listed previously initially cause **tinnitus** (ringing in the ear), followed by a progressive high-tone sensorineural hearing loss. Care is aimed at prevention of further hearing loss because the loss is usually permanent.

Mixed hearing loss

A **mixed hearing loss** is caused by a combination of conductive and sensorineural losses.

Functional hearing loss

A **functional hearing loss** occurs for no organic reason. The individual does not respond to voice and appears not to hear. Functional hearing loss is thought to be caused by emotional or psychologic factors. It occurs only rarely.

Olfaction and Taste

Olfaction (smell) and taste (gustation) dysfunctions may occur separately or jointly. The strong relationship between smell and taste creates the sensation of flavor. If either sensation is impaired, the perception of flavor is altered. (Olfactory structures are illustrated in Fig. 13-19.)

Olfactory cells, located in the olfactory epithelium, are the receptor cells for smell. Several different theories attempt to explain the function of the receptor cells (Elain, 1991). Seven different primary classes of olfactory stimulants have been identified: (1) camphoraceous, (2) musky, (3) floral, (4) peppermint, (5) ethereal, (6) pungent, and (7) putrid. The primary sensations of taste are (1) sour, (2) salty, (3) sweet, and (4) bitter. Taste buds sensitive to one of the primary sensations are located in specific areas of the tongue (Bartoshuk, 1989).

☐ AGING and Olfaction and Taste

Olfaction

Sensitivity to odors declines steadily with aging (Stevens & Cain, 1986). A recent study of odor identification indicates an increasing ability from childhood to adolescence and then a decline after age 60 years. The most significant impairments develop after 80 years (Doty, 1989). Women generally have better olfactory abilities than men, but the patterns of decline are similar (Cain & Stevens, 1989).

The sense of smell begins to degenerate with loss of

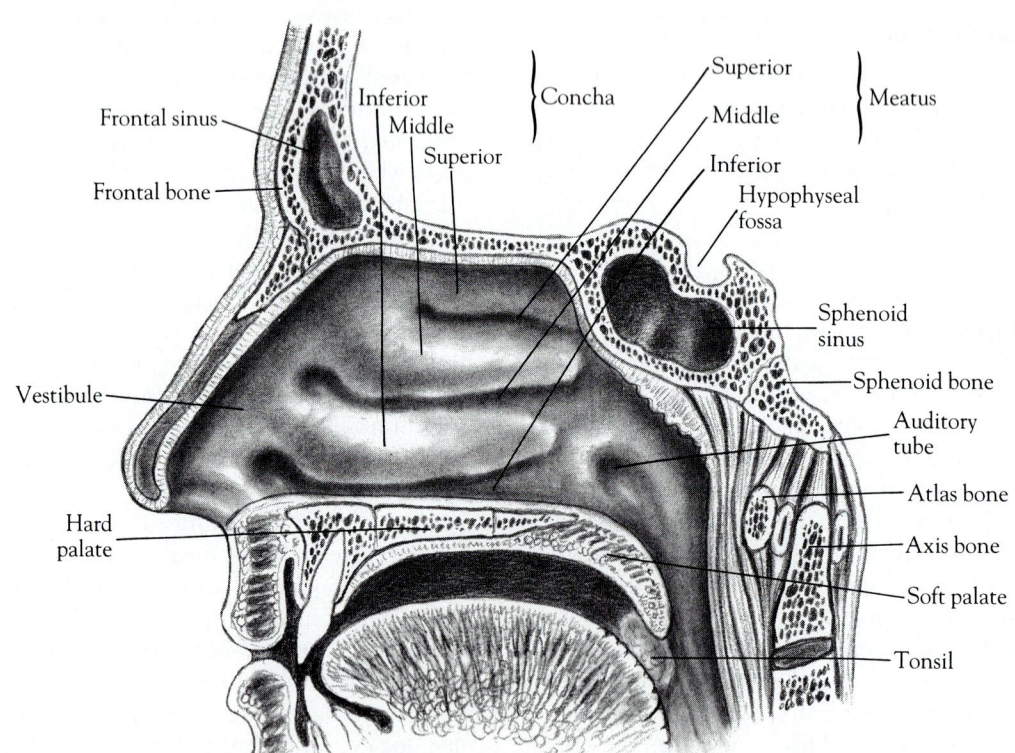

FIG. 13-19 **Lateral wall of nose.** (From Thompson et al., 1993.)

olfactory sensory neurons and loss of cells from the olfactory bulbs (Bhatnagar, Kennedy, Baron, & Greenberg, 1987). Loss of olfactory sensitivity and odor identification may diminish appetite and food selection and thus may lead to malnutrition. Safety also may be compromised with an inability to smell toxic or hazardous gases.

Taste

The decline in taste sensation is more gradual than that of smell. Higher concentrations of flavors are required, and the elderly have difficulty differentiating combinations of flavors (Cain, Reid, & Stevens, 1990). The best-known changes with aging are the decline in the number of fungiform papillae on the tongue, which decrease by 50% by about 50 years of age (Pathy, 1991). Taste also may be affected by decreased salivary gland secretion. Amylase, contained in saliva, facilitates perception of sweet sensations and is also reduced with aging.

Olfactory Dysfunction

Olfactory dysfunctions include hyposmia, anosmia, hallucinations, and parosmia. **Hyposmia** is the impaired sense of smell, whereas **anosmia** is the complete loss of smell. When hyposmia or anosmia occurs bilaterally, it is usually the result of rhinitis (inflammation of the nasal mucosa), severe coryza (head cold), or excessive smoking. Unilateral hyposmia or anosmia may indicate compression of one olfactory bulb (a bulblike portion of the olfactory nerves) or nerve tract (olfactory nerve pathway), possibly by tumor. **Olfactory hallucinations** arise from hyperactivity in cortical neurons and involve the smelling of odors that are not really present. They are associated with temporal lobe seizures and rarely with schizophrenia. **Parosmia,** an abnormal or perverted sense of smell, may occur with severe depression (Scott, 1989).

Taste Dysfunction

The sense of taste can be impaired by injury or by aging. An alteration in taste also may be attributable to impairment of smell associated with injury near the hippocampus.

Hypogeusia is the decrease in taste sensation, whereas **ageusia** is the absence of taste. Ageusia affecting the entire tongue may follow head injury. Damage to the glossopharyngeal nerve (cranial nerve IX, which innervates the posterior one third of the tongue) causes the loss of the ability to detect bitterness. This loss occurs because the receptors for bitter are located on the base of the tongue. Damage to the facial nerve (cranial nerve VII, which innervates the anterior two thirds of the tongue) causes loss of the ability to detect sour, sweet, and salt tastes. Only bitter tastes can be detected. These losses occur because sour, sweet, and salt receptors are located

on the anterior portion of the tongue. **Parageusia** is a perversion of taste in which substances possess an unpleasant flavor. Parageusia occasionally develops for no apparent reason in the elderly and also is common in individuals receiving chemotherapy for cancer. In both cases, parageusia often leads to anorexia.

SOMATOSENSORY FUNCTION

Touch

Touch is not a uniform sensory experience. The sensation of touch involves the fusion of several qualities, including modality, intensity, location, and duration of the sensory stimulus. Receptors sensitive to touch are present in the skin. Meissner's and pacinian corpuscles are rapidly adapting receptors, whereas Merkel's disks and Ruffini's endings are slowly adapting touch receptors. Touch receptors are most numerous in the skin of the fingers and lips, and are more scarce in the skin of the trunk. Research suggests that four afferent fiber types mediate tactile sensation (Bolanowski, Gescheider, Verrillo, & Checkosky, 1988). Specific sensory input is carried to the higher levels of the central nervous system by the dorsal column of the spinal cord and the anterior spinothalamic tract.

Much of the development of the cutaneous senses takes place before birth, but structural growth of the cutaneous senses continues into early adulthood at a reduced rate. Then a gradual decline occurs. Studies have documented loss in tactile sensitivity with advancing age (Balin & Klingman, 1989; Stevens, 1992). This occurs simultaneously with an increase in the size of pacinian corpuscles and a decrease in the number of corpuscles.

Abnormal tactile perception may be caused by alterations at any level of the nervous system, from the receptor to the cerebral cortex. Any factor that interrupts or impairs reception, transmission, perception, or interpretation of touch also alters tactile sensation. Trauma, tumor, infection, metabolic changes, vascular changes, and degenerative diseases thus may cause tactile dysfunction, which may involve heightened or diminished tactile perceptions.

In addition, most tactile sensations evoke affective responses that determine whether the sensation is unpleasant, pleasant, or neutral. Cerebral and hypothalamic centers influence this response. Sedative drugs and prefrontal injury, which interrupt connections between the prefrontal cortex and subcortical centers, diminish the interpretation of the sensations.

Proprioception

The perception and awareness of the position of the body and its parts depend on impulses from the inner ear and from receptors in joints and ligaments. The role of muscle, tendon, and cutaneous receptors is indefinite. Sensory data are transmitted to higher centers, primarily through the dorsal columns and the spinocerebellar tracts, with some data passing through the medial lemnisci and thalamic radiations to the cortex. Some evidence suggests that proprioceptive information passes to consciousness in the anterolateral columns of the spinal cord (Ganong, 1991). These stimuli are necessary for the coordination of movements, the grading of muscular contraction, and the maintenance of equilibrium.

A progressive loss of proprioception has been reported in the elderly (Pathy, 1991). Proprioceptive dysfunction may be caused by alterations at any level of the nervous system. As with tactile dysfunction, any factor that interrupts or impairs the reception, transmission, perception, or interpretation of proprioceptive stimuli also alters proprioception. Two frequent causes of proprioceptive dysfunction are vestibular dysfunction and neuropathy.

Specific vestibular dysfunctions are vestibular nystagmus and vertigo. **Vestibular nystagmus** is the constant, involuntary movement of the eyeball caused by ear disturbances. This condition occurs when the semicircular canal system is overstimulated. **Vertigo** is the sensation of spinning that occurs with inflammation of the semicircular canals in the ear. The individual may feel either that he or she is moving in space or that the world is revolving. Vertigo often causes loss of balance. Vertigo and nystagmus may occur in a variety of conditions, including labyrinthitis, vestibular neuritis, acute toxic labyrinthitis, and Ménière disease.

Ménière disease is a vestibular disorder that can cause proprioceptive dysfunction. The pathologic basis of Ménière disease is still unclear. The individual with Ménière disease may experience loss of proprioception during an acute attack, so that standing or walking is impossible.

Peripheral neuropathies also can cause proprioceptive dysfunctions. Neuropathies may be caused by a variety of conditions and are commonly associated with renal disease and diabetes mellitus. Although the exact sequence of events is unknown, neuropathies are thought to be caused by a metabolic disturbance of the neuron itself. The result is a diminished or absent sense of body position or position of body parts. Gait changes often occur. (Neuropathies are further discussed in Chapter 15.)

SUMMARY REVIEW

Pain

1 Pain is a complex phenomenon composed of sensory experiences (time, space, intensity) and emotion, cognition, and motivation.

2 Categories of pain include somatogenic pain (with a known physiologic cause), psychogenic pain (without a physiologic cause), acute pain (signal to the person of a harmful stimulus), and chronic pain (persistence of pain of unknown cause or unusual response to therapy).

3 Pain threshold is the point at which pain is perceived. Pain threshold does not vary significantly among people or within the same person over time.

4 Pain tolerance is the duration of time or the intensity of pain that an individual will endure before initiating overt pain response. Tolerance varies widely among individuals and in the same individual over time.

5 Newborns and young children have anatomic and functional ability to perceive pain. Older individuals tend to have a slightly higher pain threshold, probably because of changes in the thickness of the skin and peripheral neuropathies. In all age groups, women appear to be more sensitive to pain than men.

6 The portions of the nervous system responsible for the sensation and perception of pain may be divided into three areas: (1) the afferent fibers, (2) the central nervous system, and (3) the afferent pathways.

7 The afferent system is composed of nociceptors, A and C fibers, the dorsal horn of the spinal column, and afferent neurons in the spinothalamic tract.

8 Efferent pathways from the periaqueductal gray are responsible for modulation or inhibition of afferent pain signals.

9 The thalamus, cortex, and postcentral gyrus perceive, describe, and localize pain. The reticular formation and limbic system control the emotional and affective response to pain.

10 The specificity theory of pain proposes that pain is caused by stimulation of nerve endings in the skin, transmission of the painful stimuli through A and C fibers to the spinal cord, and ascent of impulses to the brain, causing a direct relationship between the stimulus and the perception of pain.

11 Endorphins inhibit transmission of the pain impulse. They are present in varying concentration in the neurons in the brain, spinal cord, and gastrointestinal tract.

12 According to the gate control theory, there are specialized cells within the substantia gelatinosa that act as a gate, opening and closing the afferent pathways to transmission of painful stimuli.

13 The intensity theory proposes that pain results from excessive stimulation of sensory receptors with summation of impulses.

14 According to the pattern theory of pain, pain perception is the result of stimulus intensity and summation of the impulses.

15 Acute pain may be (a) somatic (superficial), (b) visceral (internal), or (c) referred (present in an area distant from its origin). The area of referred pain is supplied by the same spinal segment as the actual site of pain.

16 Physiologic responses to acute pain include increased heart rate, respiratory rate, and blood pressure; pallor or flushing; dilated pupils; and diaphoresis. Blood sugar is elevated; gastric secretion and motility are decreased; and blood flow to the viscera and skin is decreased.

17 Psychologic, behavioral, and physiologic responses to chronic pain include depression, difficulty in sleeping, preoccupation with pain, lifestyle changes, and physiologic adaptation.

18 Chronic pain may be a result of decreased levels of endorphins, predominance of C neuron stimulation, or leukokinin.

19 Chronic pain conditions include lower back pain, neuralgias, reflex sympathetic dystrophies, hyperesthesias, myofascial pain syndrome, pain hemiagnosia, phantom limb pain, and chronic pain associated with cancer.

Temperature Regulation

1 Temperature regulation is achieved through precise balancing of heat production, heat conservation, and heat loss. Body temperature is maintained in a range around 37° C (98.6° F).

2 Temperature regulation is mediated by the hypothalamus. Peripheral thermoreceptors in the skin and central thermoreceptors in the hypothalamus, spinal cord, and abdominal organs provide the hypothalamus with information about skin and core temperatures.

3 Heat is produced through chemical reactions of metabolism, skeletal muscle contraction, and chemical thermogenesis.

4 Heat is lost through radiation, conduction, convection, vasodilation, decreased muscle tone, evaporation of sweat, increased respiration, and voluntary mechanisms.

5 Heat conservation is accomplished through vasoconstriction and voluntary mechanisms.

6 Infants and the elderly require special attention to maintenance of body temperature. Because of their greater body-surface-to-mass ratio and decreased subcutaneous fat, infants do not conserve heat well. The elderly have poor responses to environmental temperature extremes as a result of slowed blood circulation, structural and functional changes in skin, and overall decrease in heat-producing activities.

7 Fever is triggered by the release of pyrogens from leukocytes, bacteria, and other cells involved in the immune response. Fever is both a symptom of a disease and a normal immunologic mechanism.

8 Fever involves the "resetting of the hypothalamic thermostat" to a higher level. When the fever breaks, the "set point" is returned to normal.

9 Fever production aids responses to infectious processes. Higher temperatures kill many microorganisms and decrease serum levels of iron, zinc, and copper that are needed for bacterial replication.

10 Hyperthermia (marked warming of core temperature) can produce nerve damage, coagulation of cell proteins, and death. Forms of accidental hyperthermia include heat cramps, heat exhaustion, heatstroke, and malignant hyperthermia. Heatstroke and malignant hyperthermia are potentially lethal developments.

11 Hypothermia (marked cooling of core temperature) slows the rate of chemical reaction (tissue metabolism), increases the viscosity of the blood, slows blood flow through the microcirculation, facilitates blood coagulation, and stimulates profound vasoconstriction. Hypothermia may be accidental or therapeutic.

Sleep

1 Sleep may be divided into REM and non-REM stages, each of which has its own series of stages. While asleep, an individual progresses through REM and non-REM (slow wave) sleep in a predictable cycle.

2 Sleep is initiated by the withdrawal of neurotransmitters from the afferent formation and by the inhibition of arousal mechanisms in the cerebral cortex. Rapid-eye-movement sleep is controlled by mechanisms in the pontine reticular formation.

3 The sleep patterns of the newborn and young child vary from those of the adult in total sleep time, cycle length, and percentage of time spent in each sleep cycle. The elderly experience a total decrease in sleep time.

4 During sleep the body is actively engaged in restoring and repairing itself. Sleep deprivation can cause profound changes in personality and functioning.

5 The restorative, reparative, and growth processes occur during slow wave sleep.

6 Sleep disorders include (a) disorders of initiating sleep (insomnia), (b) disorders of excessive somnolence (pickwickian syndrome and hypersomnia sleep apnea syndrome), (c) disorders of the sleep-wake

schedule (jet lag, shift work), and (d) dysfunctions of sleep, sleep stages, or partial arousals (somnambulism, night terrors, or enuresis).

7 Ingestion of alcohol and some medications can alter or suppress sleep stages, producing sleep disorders.

8 Sleep and disease are interrelated. Some diseases may produce alterations in the quantity and quality of sleep or affect sleep stages. These are referred to as secondary sleep disorders. In some instances sleep stages produce alterations in certain disease states. These are referred to as sleep-provoked disorders.

The Special Senses

1 The eyelids, conjunctiva, and lacrimal apparatus protect the eye. Infections are the most common disorders; they include blepharitis, conjunctivitis, chalazion, and hordeolum.

2 Conjunctivitis can be acute or chronic, bacterial, viral, or allergic. Redness, edema, pain, and lacrimation are common symptoms. Chlamydial conjunctivitis is the leading cause of blindness in the world and is associated with poor sanitary conditions.

3 Keratitis is a bacterial or viral infection of the cornea that can lead to corneal ulceration. Photophobia, pain, and tearing are common symptoms.

4 The wall of the eye has three layers: sclera, choroid, and retina. The retina contains millions of baroreceptors known as rods and cones that receive light through the lens and then convey signals to the optic nerve and subsequently to the visual cortex of the brain.

5 The eye is filled with vitreous and aqueous humor that prevents it from collapsing.

6 Structural eye changes caused by aging result in decreased visual acuity.

7 The major alterations in ocular movement include strabismus, nystagmus, and paralysis of the extraocular muscles.

8 Alterations in visual acuity can be caused by amblyopia, scotoma, cataracts, papilledema, macular degeneration, and glaucoma.

9 Alterations in accommodation develop with increased intraocular pressure, inflammation, and disease of the oculomotor nerve. Presbyopia is loss of accommodation caused by loss of elasticity of the lens with aging.

10 Alterations in refraction, including myopia, hyperopia, and astigmatism, are the most common visual disorders.

11 Trauma or disease of the optic nerve pathways, or optic radiations, can cause blindness in the visual fields. Homonymous hemianopsia is caused by damage of one optic tract.

12 The ear is composed of external, middle, and inner structures. The external structures are the pinna, auditory canal, and tympanic membrane. The tympanic cavity (containing three bones: the malleus, the incus, and the stapes), oval window, eustachian tube, and fluid compose the middle ear and transmit sound vibrations to the inner ear.

13 The inner ear includes the bony and membranous labyrinths that transmit sound waves through the cochlea to the division of the eighth cranial nerve. The semicircular canals and vestibule help maintain balance through the equilibrium receptors.

14 Approximately one third of all people older than age 65 have hearing loss.

15 Hearing loss can be classified as conductive, sensorineural, mixed, and functional.

16 Conductive hearing loss occurs when sound waves cannot be conducted through the middle ear.

17 Sensorineural hearing loss develops with impairment of the organ of Corti or its central connections.

18 A combination of conductive and sensorineural loss is a mixed hearing loss.

19 Loss of hearing with no known organic cause is a functional hearing loss.

20 The perception of flavor is altered if olfaction or taste dysfunctions occur. Sensitivity to odor and taste decreases with aging.

21 Hyposmia is a decrease in the sense of smell, and anosmia is the complete loss of smell. Inflammation of the nasal mucosa and trauma or tumors of the olfactory nerve lead to diminished sense of smell.

22 Hypogeusia is a decrease in taste sensation, and ageusia is the absence of taste. Loss of taste buds or trauma to the facial or glossopharyngeal nerves decreases taste sensation.

Somatosensory Function

1 Tactile sensation is a function of receptors present in the skin (pacinian corpuscles), and the sensory response is conducted to the brain through the dorsal column and anterior spinothalamic tract.

2 Alterations in touch can result from disruption of skin receptors, sensory transmission, or central nervous system perception.

3 Proprioception is the position and location of the body and its parts. Proprioceptors are located in the inner ear, joints, and ligaments. Proprioceptive stimuli are necessary for balance, coordinated movement, and grading of muscular contraction.

4 Disorders of proprioception can occur at any level of the nervous system with impaired balance and lack of coordinated movement.

KEY TERMS

Acute bacterial conjunctivitis (pink-eye), 458
Acute pain, 438
Ageusia, 469
Allergic conjunctivitis, 459
Amblyopia, 462
Anosmia, 469
Aqueous humor, 461
Astigmatism, 463
Blepharitis, 458
Cataract, 462
Causalgia, 446
Chalazion, 458
Choroid, 459
Chronic conjunctivitis, 459
Chronic pain, 438
Circadian rhythm, 447
Cochlea, 466
Cognitive/evaluative system, 438
Color blindness, 464
Conduction, 448
Conductive hearing loss, 467
Cone, 461
Convection, 448
Cornea, 459
Crista ampullaris, 466
Dark adaptation, 462
Diplopia, 462
Dynorphin, 444
Endogenous antipyretic, 450
Endolymph, 466
Enkephalin, 444
Enuresis, 457
Equilibrium receptor, 466
Eustachian (pharyngeotympanic) tube, 465
Exogenous pyrogen, 450
External auditory canal, 465
Fovea centralis, 461
Functional hearing loss, 468
Gate control theory, 443
Glaucoma, 463
Hair cell, 466
Heat cramp, 451
Heat exhaustion, 451
Heatstroke, 451
Hemiagnosia (to pain), 446
Hemianopia, 464
Homonymous hemianopsia, 465
Hordeolum (stye), 458
Hyperesthesia, 446
Hyperopia, 463
Hypersomnia sleep apnea (HSA) syndrome, 456
Hyperthermia, 451

Hypogeusia, 469
Hyposmia, 469
Hypothermia, 452
Incus (anvil), 465
Insomnia, 456
Intensity theory, 443
Iris, 461
Jerk nystagmus, 462
Lens, 461
β-Lipotrophin, 444
Macula, 466
Malignant hyperthermia, 452
Malleus (hammer), 465
Mastoid air cell, 465
Mastoid process, 465
Meissner's corpuscle, 442
Ménière disease, 467, 470
Mixed hearing loss, 468
Motivational/affective system, 438
Myofascial pain syndrome, 446
Myopia, 463
Neuralgia, 446
Night terrors, 457
Nociceptor, 440
Non-REM (slow wave) sleep, 454
Nystagmus, 462
Olfactory hallucination, 469
Opiate receptor, 444
Optic chiasm, 465
Optic disc, 461
Organ of Corti, 466
Otolith, 466
Oval window, 465
Pacinian corpuscle, 442
Pain threshold, 439
Pain tolerance, 439
Papilledema, 462
Parageusia, 469
Parosmia, 469
Pattern theory, 443
Pendular nystagmus, 462
Perceptual dominance, 439
Periaqueductal gray (PAG), 442
Perilymph, 466
Phantom limb pain, 446
Pickwickian syndrome, 456
Pinna, 465
Presbycusis, 466, 467
Presbyopia, 463
Psychogenic pain, 438
Pupil, 461
Radiation, 448
Referred pain, 444
Reflex sympathetic dystrophy, 446

REM (rapid eye movement) sleep, 455
Retina, 461
Retrobulbar neuritis, 462
Rod, 461
Sclera, 459
Scotoma, 462
Secondary sleep disorder, 457
Semicircular canal, 466
Sensorineural hearing loss, 467
Sensory/discriminative system, 438
Sleep-provoked disorder, 457
Somatic pain, 444
Somatogenic pain, 438
Somnambulism, 457
Specificity theory, 443
Stapes (stirrup), 465
Strabismus, 462
Tinnitus, 468
Trachoma, 459
Trigger point, 447
Tympanic cavity, 465
Tympanic membrane, 465
Vertigo, 470
Vestibular nuclei, 462
Vestibular nystagmus, 470
Vestibule, 466
Viral conjunctivitis, 459
Visceral pain, 444
Vitreous humor, 461

REFERENCES

Aimone, L. D. (1992). Neurochemistry and modulation of pain. In R. S. Sinatra, A. H. Hord, B. Ginsberg, & L. M. Preble (Eds.), *Acute pain: Mechanisms and management*. St. Louis: Mosby–Year Book.

Almay, G. L., Johansson, F., Knorring, L., Sedvall, G., & Terenius, L. (1980). Relationships between CSF levels of endorphins and monoamine metabolites in chronic pain patients. *Psychopharmacology, 67*, 139-142.

Anand, K. J. S. (1990). The biology of pain perception in newborn infants. In D. C. Tyler & E. J. Krane (Eds.), *Advances in pain research and therapy* (Vol. 15). New York: Raven Press.

Anders, T. F., & Keener, M. (1985). Developmental course of nighttime sleep-wake patterns in full-term and premature infants during the first year of life. *Sleep, 8*(3), 173-192.

Balin, A. K., & Klingman, A. M. (Eds.). (1989). *Aging and the skin*. New York: Raven Press.

Bartoshuk, L. M. (1989). The functions of taste and olfaction. *Annals of the New York Academy of Science, 575*, 353-361.

Benito, M. (1985). Contribution of brown fat to the neonatal thermogenesis. *Biology of the Neonate, 48*(4), 245-249.

Berlin, L., Boodell, H., & Wolff, H. G. (1958). Relation of pain perception and central inhibitory effects of noxious stimulation to phenomenon of excitation of pain. *Archives of Neurology, 80*, 533-543.

Beyer, J. E., & Wells, N. (1989). The assessment of pain in children. *Pediatric Clinics of North America, 36*(4), 837-854.

Bhatnagar, K. P., Kennedy, R. C., Baron, G., & Greenberg, R. A. (1987). Number of mitral cells and the bulb volume in the aging human olfactory bulb: A quantitative morphological study. *Anatomical Record, 218*, 73-87.

Birren, J. E., Shapiro, H. B., & Miller, J. H. (1950). The effect of salicylate upon pain sensitivity. *Journal of Pharmacological Experimental Therapy, 100*, 67-71.

Block, A. J. (1980, November-December). Respiratory disorders during sleep. Part I. *Heart and Lung*, 1011-1024.

Block, A. J. (1981, January-February). Respiratory disorders during sleep. Part II. *Heart and Lung*, 90-96.

Bolanowski, S. J., Gescheider, G. A., Verrillo, R. T., & Checkosky, C. M. (1988). Four channels mediate the mechanical aspects of touch. *Journal of Acoustical Society of America, 85*(5), 1680-1694.

Bonica, J. J. (1990). *The management of pain* (vol 1, 2nd ed.). Philadelphia: Lea & Febiger.

Boulant, J. (1991). Thermoregulation. In P. Mackowiak (Ed.), *Fever: Basic mechanisms and management*. New York: Raven Press.

Brena, S. F. (1985). Nerve blocks and chronic pain states—an update. *Post Graduate Medicine, 78*(4), 77-86.

Bruce, J. L., & Grove, S. K. (1992). Fever: Pathology and treatment. *Critical Care Nurse, 12*(1), 40-49.

Cabanac, M., & Brinnel, H. (1987). The pathology of human temperature regulation: Thermiatrics. *Experimentia, 43*(1), 19-27.

Cain, W. S., Reid, F., & Stevens, J. C. (1990). Missing ingredients: Aging and the discrimination of flavor. *Journal of Nutrition for the Elderly, 9*(3), 3-15.

Cain, W. S., & Stevens, J. C. (1989). Uniformity of olfactory loss in aging. *Annals of the New York Academy of Sciences, 561*, 29-38.

Calverly, P. M., Brezinova, V., Douglas, N. J., Catterall, J. R., & Flenley, D. C. (1982). The effect of oxygenation on sleep quality in chronic bronchitis and emphysema. *American Review of Respiratory Disease, 126*, 206-210.

Campbell, S. S. (1987). Evolution of sleep structure following brief intervals of wakefulness. *Electroencephalography and Clinical Neurophysiology, 66*(2), 175-184.

Clark, W. G. (1991). Antipyretics. In P. Mackowaik (Ed.), *Fever: Basic mechanisms and management*. New York: Raven Press.

Clowes, G. H., & O'Donnell, T. F. (1974). Heat stroke. *New England Journal of Medicine, 291*, 564-567.

Collins, K. J., & Exton-Smith, A. N. (1983). Thermal homeostasis in old age. *Journal of the American Geriatrics Society, 31*(9), 519-524.

Committee on Sports Medicine. (1982). Climatic heat stress and the exercising child. *Pediatrics, 69*, 808-809.

Cooper, K. E., & Veale, W. L. (1987). Effects of endotoxins on heat tolerance and exercise performance. In J. R. S. Hales & D. A. B. Richards (Eds.), *Heat stress: Physical exertion and environment*. New York: Elsevier Science Publications.

Cunha, B. A., Digamon-Beltran, M., & Gobbo, P. N. (1984). Implications of fever in the critical care setting. *Heart and Lung, 13*, 460-465.

Davis, L. K. (1990). Postoperative pain in toddlers: Nurses' assessment and intervention. In D. C. Tyler & E. J. Krane (Eds.), *Advances in pain research and therapy* (vol. 15, pp. 53-61). New York: Raven Press.

Dean, N. C. (1987). Hypothermia. *Post Graduate Medicine, 82*(8), 48-58.

DeLapp, T. D. (1983, January). Accidental hypothermia. *American Journal of Nursing*, 63-67.

Dinarello, C. A., & Wolff, S. M. (1978, March). Pathogenesis of fever in man. *New England Journal of Medicine*, 607-612.

Dinarello, C. A., & Wolff, S. M. (1982). Molecular basis of fever in humans. *The American Journal of Medicine, 72*, 799-810.

Doty, R. L. (1989). Influence of age and age-related diseases on olfactory function. *Annals of the New York Academy of Science, 565*, 76-86.

Elain, M. (1991). Olfactory impairment in motor neuron disease: A pilot study. *Journal of Neurology, Neurosurgery, and Psychiatry, 54*(10), 927-928.

Elias, M. F., Nicholson, N. A., Bora, C., & Johnston, J. (1986). Sleep/wake patterns of breast-fed infants in the first 2 years of life. *Pediatrics, 77*(3), 322-329.

Fellows, I. W., MacDonald, I. A., & Bennett, T. (1985). The effect of undernutrition on thermoregulation in the elderly. *Clinical Science, 69*(5), 525-532.

Foley, K. M. (1984, Summer). A review of pain syndromes in patients with cancer. *Symposium on the Management of Cancer Pain*, 7-16.

Foley, K. M. (1985). The treatment of cancer pain. *The New England Journal of Medicine, 313*, 84-95.

Fruthaler, G. J. (1985). Fever in children: Phobia vs. facts. *Hospital Practice, 20*(11A), 49-53.

Ganong, W. F. (1991). *Review of medical physiology* (15th ed.). Norwalk, CT: Appleton & Lange.

Glasscock, M. E., & Shambaugh, G. E. (1990). *Surgery of the ear* (4th ed.). Philadelphia: Saunders.

Go, V. L. L. U., & Yaksh, T. L. (1987). Release of substance P from the cat spinal cord. *Journal of Physiology, 391*, 141-167.

Guazzelli, M., Feinberg, I., & Aminoff, M. (1986). Sleep spindles in the normal elderly: Comparison with young adult patterns and relation to nocturnal awakening, cognitive function, and brain atrophy. *Electroencephalography and Clinical Neurophysiology, 63*(6), 526-539.

Guilleminault, C., Tilkian, A., & Dement, W. C. (1976). The sleep apnea syndromes. *Annual Review of Medicine*, 465-484.

Gurevich, I. (1985). Fever: When to worry about it. *RN, 48*, 14-19.

Guyton, A. C. (1992). *Human physiology and mechanisms of disease* (5th ed.). Philadelphia: Saunders.

Hammarlund, K., Stromberg, B., & Sedin, G. (1986). Heat loss from the skin of preterm and full-term newborn infants during the first weeks after birth. *Biology of the Neonate, 50*(1), 1-10.

Harkins, S. W., & Warner, M. H. (1977). Age and pain. *Behavioral and Social Sciences*, 121-129.

Haslam, D. R. (1969). Age and the perception of pain. *Psychonomic Science, 15*, 86.

Heaton, J. M. (1972). The distribution of brown adipose tissue in the human. *Journal of Anatomy, 112*, 35-39.

Henry, J. L. (1986). Role of circulating opioids in the modulation of pain. *Annals of the New York Academy of Sciences, 467*, 169-181.

Himms-Hagen, J. (1980). Current status of nonshivering thermogenesis. In Ross Laboratories, *Assessment of energy metabolism in health and disease: A report of the first Ross conference in medical research*. Columbus, OH: Ross Laboratories.

Jacox, A. K. (1979, May). Assessing pain. *American Journal of Nursing, 895-900.*

Jones, S. R. (1991). Fever in the elderly. In P. Mackowiak (Ed.), *Fever: Basic mechanisms and management.* New York: Raven Press.

Kales, A., & Kales, J. D. (1970, September). Evaluation, diagnosis, and treatment of clinical conditions related to sleep. *Journal of the American Medical Association, 2229-2235.*

Kales, A., Verla-Bueno, A., & Kales, J. D. (1987). Sleep disorders, sleep apnea, and narcolepsy. *Annals of Internal Medicine, 106, 434.*

Kedas, A., Lux, W., & Amodeo, S. (1989). A critical review of aging and sleep research. *Western Journal of Nursing Research, 11(2), 196-206.*

Keefe, M. R. (1987). Comparison of neonatal nighttime sleep-wake patterns in nursing versus rooming-in environments. *Nursing Research, 36(3), 140-144.*

Kenshalo, D. R., & Hall, E. C. (1974). Thermal thresholds of the rhesus monkey. *Journal of Comparative Physiology and Psychology, 86, 902-910.*

Kirschner, R. N., Eckner, F. A., & Baron, R. C. (1986). The cardiac pathology of sudden unexplained nocturnal death in southeast Asian refugees. *Journal of the American Medical Association, 256(19), 2700-2705.*

Little, R. A., & Stoner, H. B. (1981). Body temperature after accidental injury. *British Journal of Surgery, 68, 221.*

Long, M. E. (1982). Sleep. *National Geographic, 172(6), 786-821.*

McCaffery, M. (1980, September). Understanding your patient's pain. *Nursing 80, 26-31.*

Melles, R. B. (1987). Sudden, unexplained nocturnal death syndrome and night terrors. *Journal of the American Medical Association, 257(21), 2918-2919.*

Melzack, R. (1975). The McGill pain questionnaire: Major properties and scoring methods. *Pain, 1, 277-299.*

Melzack, R., & Casey, K. L. (1968). Sensory, motivational, and central control determinants of pain: A new conceptual model. In D. Kenshalto (Ed.), *The skin senses.* Springfield, Ill.: Charles C Thomas.

Melzack, R., & Wall, P. (1965). Pain mechanisms: A new theory. *Science, 150, 971-979.*

Melzack, R., & Wall, P. (1970). Psychophysiology of pain. *International Anesthesiology Clinics, 8, 3-33.*

Melzack, R., & Wall, P. (1983). *The challenge of pain.* New York: Basic Books.

Monk, T. H. (1989). Shift work. In M. H. Kryger, T. Roth, & W. C. Dement (Eds.), *Principles and practice of sleep medicine.* Philadelphia: Saunders.

Moses, R. A., & Hart, W. M. (Eds.). (1987). *Adler's physiology of the eye. Clinical applications* (8th ed.). St. Louis: Mosby–Year Book.

Norman, D. C., Grahn, D., & Hoshikawa, T. T. (1985). Fever and aging. *Journal of the American Geriatrics Society, 33, 859-863.*

Osterman, A. L., Heppenstall, R. B., Sapega, A. A., Katz, M., Chance, B., & Sokolow, D. (1984). Muscle ischemia and hypothermia: A bioenergetic study using phosphorus nuclear magnetic resonance spectroscopy. *The Journal of Trauma, 24(9), 811-817.*

Pathy, M. S. J. (Ed.). (1991). *Principles and practices of geriatric medicine.* (2nd ed.). New York: John Wiley & Sons.

Payne, R. (1987). Anatomy, physiology, and neuropharmacology of cancer pain. *Medical Clinics of North America, 71(2), 153-167.*

Phillipson, E. A. (1978). State-of-the-art control of breathing during sleep. *American Review of Respiratory Disease, 118, 909-939.*

Phipps, W. J., Long, B. C., & Woods, W. F. (1987). *Medical surgical nursing: Concepts and clinical practice* (p. 306). St. Louis: Mosby–Year Book.

Reuler, R. (1978). Hypothermia: Pathophysiology, clinical settings, and management. *Annals of Internal Medicine, 89, 519-527.*

Roberts, N. J. (1991). The immunological consequences of fever. In P. Mackowiak (Ed.), *Fever: Basic mechanisms and management.* New York: Raven Press.

Rogers, A. L., & Sturgeon, C. L. (1985). Malignant hyperthermia. *AORN Journal, 41, 369-374.*

Rudy, E. B. (1984). *Advanced neurological and neurosurgical nursing.* St. Louis: Mosby–Year Book.

Sakai, F., Meyer, J. S., Karacan, I., Derman, S., & Yamamoto, M. (1980, May). Normal human sleep: Regional cerebral hemodynamics. *Annals of Neurology, 7(5), 471-478.*

Sanders, S. H. (1979). Behavioral assessment and treatment of clinical pain: Appraisal of current status. *Progress in Behavior Modification, 8, 249-285.*

Schauf, C., Moffet, D., & Moffett, S. (1990). *Human physiology.* St. Louis: Mosby–Year Book.

Scott, A. E. (1989). Clinical characteristics of taste and smell disorders. *Ear, Nose & Throat Journal, 68(4), 297-298, 301.*

Seeley, R. R., Stephens, T. D., & Tate, P. (1992). *Anatomy and physiology* (2nd ed.). St. Louis: Mosby–Year Book.

Shaver, J., Camarata, G., Taleisnik, A., & Gazzaniga, A. B. (1984). Changes in epicardial and core temperatures during resuscitation of hemorrhagic shock. *The Journal of Trauma, 24(11), 957-963.*

Sheps, D. S., Adams, K. F., Hinderliter, A., Price, C., Bissette, J., Orlanda, G., Margolis, B., & Koch, G. (1987). Endorphins are related to pain perception in coronary artery disease. *The American Journal of Cardiology, 59, 523-527.*

Sherman, A. D., & Mitchell, C. L. (1974). Effect of morphine on regional levels of gamma hydroxybutyrate in mouse brain. *Neuropharmacology, 13, 239-243.*

Siegel, J. M. (1990). Mechanisms of sleep control. *Journal of Clinical Neurophysiology, 7, 49.*

Smukler, N. M. (1985). Pain perception. *Bulletin of the Rheumatic Diseases, 35(1), 1-8.*

Stein, H. A., Slatt, B. J., & Stein, R. M. (1988). *The ophthalmic assistant: Fundamentals in clinical practice.* St. Louis: Mosby–Year Book.

Sternbach, R. A. (1974). *Pain patients: Traits and treatment.* New York: Academic Press.

Stevens, J. C. (1992). Age and spatial acuity of touch. *Journal of Gerontology, 47(1), 35-40.*

Stevens, J. C., & Cain, W. S. (1986). Aging impairs the ability to perceive gas odor. *Chemical Senses and Nutrition, 11, 679.*

Strauss, A. L., & Glasser, B. G. (1975). *Chronic illness and the quality of life.* St. Louis: Mosby–Year Book.

Taub, J. M., & Berger, R. J. (1976). The effects of changing the phase and duration of sleep. *Journal of Experimental Psychology: Human Perception and Performance, 2(1), 30-41.*

Thompson, J. M., McFarland, G. K., Hirsch, J. E., & Tucker, S. M. (1993). *Mosby's clinical nursing* (3rd ed.). St. Louis: Mosby–Year Book.

Timiras, P. S. (1988). *Physiological basis of geriatrics.* New York: Macmillan, p. 163.

Van Rijn, T., & Rabkin, S. W. (1981). Effect of naloxone, a specific opioid antagonist on exercise-induced angina pectoris. *Circulation, 64 (IV), 149.*

West, A. B. (1981, February). Understanding endorphins: Our natural pain relief system. *Nursing 81, 50-53.*

Whitehead, III, W., & Kuhn, W. F. (1990). Chronic pain: An overview. In T. W. Miller (Ed.), *Chronic pain* (vol. 1, pp. 5-48). Madison, WI: International Universities Press.

Woodrow, K. M., Friedman, G. D., & Siegelaub, A. B. (1972). Pain tolerance: Differences according to age, sex, and race. *Psychosomatic Medicine, 34, 548-556.*

Wright, S. W. (1987). The child with febrile seizures. *American Family Physician, 36(5), 163-167.*

Yaksh, T. L. (1985). Pharmacology of spinal adrenergic systems which modulate spinal nociceptive processing. *Pharmacology, Biochemistry, and Behavior, 22, 845-858.*

Yanofsky, N. M. (1988). The acute painful eye. *Emergency Medicine Clinics of North America, 6(1), 21-42.*

Yousef, M. K. (1987). Effects of climactic stresses on thermoregulatory processes in man. *Experientia, 43(1), 14-19.*

SUGGESTED READINGS

Adams, R., & Victor, M. (1993). *Principles of neurology* (5th ed.). San Francisco: McGraw-Hill.

Bernheim, H. A., Blosck, L. H., & Atkins, E. (1979). Fever: Pathogenesis, pathophysiology, and purpose. *Annals of Internal Medicine, 91*, 261-270.

Bliwise, D. (1993). Sleep in normal aging and dementia. *Sleep, 16*(1), 40-81.

Cailliet, R. (1993). *Pain: Mechanisms and management.* Philadelphia, PA: Davis.

Dowling, J. E. (1992). *Neurons and networks: An introduction to neuroscience.* Cambridge: Belknap Press of Harvard University.

Ferrell, B. A. (1991). Pain management in elderly people. *Journal of the American Geriatric Society, 39*, 64-73.

Johnson, C. C., Stevens, B., Craig, K. D., & Grunau, R. V. (1993). Developmental changes in pain expression in premature, full-term, two- and four-month old infants. *Pain, 52*(2), 201-208.

Kluger, M. J. (1992). Fever revisited. *Pediatrics, 90*(6), 846-850.

LaRocca, H. (1992). A taxonomy of chronic pain syndromes. *Spine, 17*(10 Suppl.), S344-355.

McCaffery, M. (1989). *Pain: Clinical manual for nursing practice.* St. Louis: Mosby–Year Book.

Schechter, N. L., Berde, C. B., & Yaster, M. (1993). *Pain in infants, children and adolescents.* Baltimore: Williams & Wilkins.

Shapiro, C. M., & Flanigan, M. J. (1993). ABC of sleep disorders: Function of sleep. *British Medical Journal, 306*(6874), 383-385.

Warfield, C. A. (1993). *Principles and practice of pain management.* New York: McGraw-Hill.

Weinberg, A. D. (1993). Hypothermia. *Annals of Emergency Medicine, 22,*370-377.

Zeltzer, L. K., Barr, R. G., McGrath, P. A., & Schechter, N. L. (1992). Pediatric pain: Interacting behavioral and physical factors. *Pediatrics, 90*(5 Pt. 2), 816-821.

CHAPTER 14

Concepts of Neurologic Dysfunction

Barbara J. Boss

Chapter Outline

A person achieves functional adequacy (competence) through complex integrated processes. Three major neural systems account for this functional adequacy: cognitive systems, sensory systems, and motor systems. Alterations in any or all of these affect functional adequacy. Alterations in cognitive and motor systems are discussed in this chapter.

The neural systems basic (core) to the cognitive sphere are attentional systems that provide arousal and maintenance of attention over time, memory and language systems by which information is communicated, and affective or emotive systems that mediate feeling tone. These core systems are fundamental to the processes of abstract thinking and reasoning. The products of abstraction and reasoning are organized and made operational through the executive system. The normal functioning of the aforementioned systems manifests through the motor system in a behavioral array viewed by others as appropriate to human activity and successful living.

477

ALTERATIONS IN COGNITIVE SYSTEMS

Full consciousness in its broadest sense is both a state of awareness of oneself and the environment and a set of responses to that environment. Full consciousness implies that the individual responds to external stimuli with a wide array of responses. Any decrease in this state of awareness and varied responses is, thus, a decrease in consciousness.

Consciousness often is viewed as having two distinct components, arousal and content of thought. Arousal, an attentional system, is the state of awakeness that an individual exhibits. Level of arousal is mediated by the reticular activating system that extends from midpons to the diencephalon. The reticular activating system provides arousal to the cerebral hemispheres (see Fig. 12-5). When cerebral function is lost, the reticular activating system and brainstem can maintain a crude waking state known as a **vegetative state**. Cognitive cerebral functions, however, cannot occur without a functioning reticular activating system. **Content of thought** encompasses all cognitive functions that embody awareness of self, environment, and affective states (i.e., moods). Content of thought is mediated by attentional systems, memory systems, language systems, concept and reasoning systems, and the executive system.

Alterations in Arousal (Coma)

Possible causes of an altered level of arousal with acute onset may be separated into three major groups: **structural, metabolic,** and **psychogenic.** Structural causes are divided according to original location of the pathologic condition: supratentorial (above the tentorium cerebelli), infratentorial (subtentorial, below the tentorium cerebelli), subdural (below the dura mater), extracerebral (outside the brain tissue), and intracerebral (within the brain tissue).

Causes of altered level of arousal also are grouped according to a pathologic process: infectious, vascular, neoplastic, traumatic, congenital (developmental), degenerative, polygenic, and metabolic. Metabolic causes may be further divided into hypoxia, electrolyte disturbances, hypoglycemia, drugs, and toxins (both endogenous and exogenous). All the systemic diseases that eventually produce nervous system dysfunction are part of this metabolic category.

Pathophysiology

Supratentorial processes produce a decreased level of arousal by one of three mechanisms: (1) diffuse bilateral cortical dysfunction, (2) bilateral subcortical dysfunction, or (3) localized hemispheric dysfunction. Disease processes may produce diffuse bilateral cortical dysfunction (e.g., encephalitis) and actually may occur in either the cerebral cortex or the underlying subcortical white matter. Bilateral subcortical dysfunction involves destructive disease that compromises the reticular activating system (e.g., brainstem trauma or cerebral vascular accident) and probably surrounding structures. Localized hemispheric dysfunction generally is caused by masses that directly impinge on deep diencephalic structures or that secondarily compress these structures in the process of herniation. Such localized destructive processes directly impair function of the thalamic or hypothalamic activating systems.

Extracerebral disorders also can produce diffuse bilateral cortical dysfunction. Extracerebral disorders include neoplasms, closed-head trauma with subsequent bleeding, and subdural empyema (accumulation of pus). Intracerebral disorders (those within the brain substance) primarily function as masses. These disorders include bleeding, infarcts and emboli, and tumors.

Infratentorial processes produce a reduction in arousal in one of two ways: (1) there may be direct destruction of the reticular activating system and its pathways or (2) the brainstem may be destroyed either by direct invasion or by indirect impairment of its blood supply. The most common cause of direct destruction is cerebrovascular disease, but demyelinating diseases, neoplasms, granulomas, abscesses, and head injury also may cause brainstem destruction. In addition, decreased level of consciousness may result from compression of the reticular activating system by a disease process. This compression may occur because of (1) direct pressure on the pons and midbrain, producing ischemia and edema of the neurons of the reticular activating system, (2) upward herniation of the cerebellum through the tentorial notch, thus compressing the upper midbrain and diencephalon, and (3) downward herniation of the cerebellum through the foramen magnum, compressing and displacing the medulla oblongata. Specific causes of compression of the brainstem include hematomas, hemorrhage, and aneurysm; cerebellar hemorrhage, infarcts, abscesses, and neoplasms; and demyelinating disorders.

A wide spectrum of diseases may produce a metabolically induced alteration in arousal. In encephalopathic conditions, widespread direct or indirect interference with neuronal metabolism occurs throughout much of the brain (see Chapter 15). Psychogenic unresponsiveness, although uncommon, may signal general psychiatric disorders. Despite apparent unconsciousness, the person actually is physiologically awake.

Clinical Manifestations and Evaluation

Evaluating an altered level of arousal requires distinguishing between organic and functional causes. A further distinction between metabolic and structural causes then is made (Table 14-1). If the cause is structural, the pathologic condition must be localized.

Patterns of clinical manifestations and their evolution

TABLE 14-1

Clinical Manifestations of Metabolic and Structural Causes of Comas

Manifestation	Metabolically induced coma	Structurally induced coma
Blink to threat (cranial nerves II, VII)	Equal	Asymmetric
Disks (cranial nerve II)	Flat, good pulsation	Papilledema
Extraocular movement (cranial nerves III, IV, VI)	Roving eye movements; normal doll's eyes and calorics	Gaze paresis, nerve III palsy, MLF syndrome (internuclear ophthalmoplegia)
Pupils (cranial nerves II, III)	Equal and reactive, may be large (i.e., atropine), pinpoint (i.e., opiates), or midposition and fixed (i.e., glutethimide [Doriden])	Asymmetric and/or nonreactive; may be midposition (midbrain injury), pinpoint (pons injury), large (tectal injury)
Corneal reflex (cranial nerve V, VII)	Symmetric response	Asymmetric response
Grimace to pain (cranial nerve VII)	Symmetric response	Asymmetric response
Motor function movement	Symmetric	Asymmetric
Tone	Symmetric	Paratonic, spastic, flaccid, especially if asymmetric
Posture	Symmetric	Decorticate, especially if symmetric; decerebrate, especially if asymmetric
Deep tendon reflexes	Symmetric	Asymmetric
Babinski's sign	Absent or symmetric response	Present
Sensation	Symmetric	Asymmetric

Modified from Heilman, Watson, and Greer, 1977.
MLF, Medial longitudinal fasciculus.

TABLE 14-2

Differential Characteristics of States Causing Coma

Mechanism	Manifestations
Supratentorial mass lesions compressing or displacing the diencephalon or brainstem	Initiating signs usually of focal cerebral dysfunction Signs of dysfunction progress rostral to caudal Neurologic signs at any given time point to one anatomic area (e.g., diencephalon, mesencephalon, medulla) Motor signs often asymmetric
Infratentorial mass of destruction causing coma	History of preceding brainstem dysfunction or sudden onset of coma Localizing brainstem signs precede or accompany onset of coma and always include oculovestibular abnormality Cranial nerve palsies usually manifest "bizarre" respiratory patterns that appear at onset
Metabolic coma	Confusion and stupor commonly precede motor signs Motor signs usually are symmetric Pupillary reactions usually are preserved Asterixis, myoclonus, tremor, and seizures are common Acid-base imbalance with hyperventilation or hypoventilation is frequent
Psychiatric unresponsiveness	Lids close actively Pupils reactive or dilated (cycloplegics) Oculocephalic reflexes are unpredictable; oculovestibular reflexes are physiologic (nystagmus is present) Motor tone is inconsistent or normal Eupnea or hyperventilation is usual No pathologic reflexes are present Electroencephalogram (EEG) is normal

Modified from Plum & Posner, 1980.

have been identified. The patterns of clinical manifestation are important because they help in determining the extent of brain dysfunction, and they serve as indexes for identifying increasing or decreasing central nervous system function. The specific clusters of manifestations of abnormal function and their evolution suggest whether the cause of the altered arousal state is supratentorial, infratentorial, metabolic, or psychogenic (Table 14-2). Five categories of neurologic function are critical to the evaluation process: (1) level of consciousness, (2) pattern of breathing, (3) size and reactivity of pupils, (4) eye position and reflexive responses, and (5) skeletal muscle motor responses.

Level of consciousness

Level of consciousness is the most critical clinical index of nervous system function or dysfunction. An alteration in consciousness indicates either improvement or deterioration of the individual's condition. A person who is alert and oriented to self, others, place, and time is considered to be functioning at the highest level of consciousness, which implies full use of all the person's cognitive capacities.

Because many different terms are used to indicate level of consciousness, definition becomes necessary. The term *unconscious*, for example, has no specific clinical definition and signifies different things to different people. From the normal alert state, levels of consciousness diminish in stages, each of which is clinically defined (Table 14-3).

Pattern of breathing

Several characteristic respiratory patterns are helpful in evaluating level of brain dysfunction and level of coma.

Among these characteristics are rate, rhythm, and pattern of breathing. The breathing patterns can be categorized as hemispheric or brainstem breathing patterns (Table 14-4).

With normal breathing, a neural center believed to be located in the forebrain (cerebrum) produces a rhythmic breathing pattern despite lowered arterial carbon dioxide pressure ($Paco_2$). When neural control at this center is lost as consciousness decreases, the lower brainstem centers regulate the breathing pattern by responding only to changes in $Paco_2$ levels. The result is the irregular breathing associated with posthyperventilation apnea (PHVA).

The pathophysiology of Cheyne-Stokes respirations (CSR) involves an increased ventilatory response to carbon dioxide stimulation, causing hypercapnia and a diminished ventilatory stimulus. The neural center that causes PHVA thus is related to the CSR, as changes in $Paco_2$ produce irregular breathing that contributes to overbreathing when stimulated by carbon dioxide. As a result, the $Paco_2$ level decreases to below normal, and because of the cerebral brain dysfunction, breathing stops until the carbon dioxide reaccumulates to bring the $Paco_2$ level to normal. In cases of opiate or sedative drug overdose, the respiratory center is depressed and the rate of breathing gradually decreases until respiratory failure occurs.

Certain motor activities related to breathing signify the level of brain dysfunction. Yawning, vomiting, and hiccups are complex reflexlike motor responses that are integrated by neural mechanisms in the lower brainstem. These responses may be produced by compression or diseases that involve tissues in the medulla oblongata. Such disorders include infection, neoplasm, or infarct.

TABLE 14-3

Levels of Coma

State	Definition
Confusion	Loss of ability to think rapidly and clearly; impaired judgment and decision making
Disorientation	Beginning loss of consciousness; disorientation to time followed by disorientation to place and impaired memory; lost last is recognition of self
Lethargy	Limited spontaneous movement or speech; easy arousal with normal speech or touch; may or may not be oriented to time, place, or person
Obtundation	Mild to moderate reduction in arousal (awakeness) with limited response to the environment; falls asleep unless stimulated verbally or tactilely; questions answered with minimum response
Stupor	A condition of deep sleep or unresponsiveness from which the person may be aroused or caused to make a motor or verbal response only by vigorous and repeated stimulation; response is often withdrawal or grabbing at stimulus
Coma	No motor or verbal response to the external environment or to any stimuli, even noxious stimuli such as deep pain or suctioning; no arousal to any stimulus

TABLE 14-4

Patterns of Breathing

Breathing pattern	Description	Location of injury
Hemispheric breathing patterns		
Normal	After a period of hyperventilation that lowers the arterial carbon dioxide pressure ($Paco_2$), the individual continues to breathe regularly but with a reduced depth.	Response of the nervous system to an external stressor—not associated with injury to the CNS
Posthyperventilation apnea (PHVA)	Respirations stop after hyperventilation has lowered the Pco_2 level below normal. Rhythmic breathing returns when the Pco_2 level returns to normal.	Associated with diffuse bilateral metabolic or structural disease of the cerebrum
Cheyne-Stokes respirations (CSR)	The breathing pattern has a smooth increase (crescendo) in the rate and depth of breathing (hyperpnea), which peaks and is followed by a gradual smooth decrease (decrescendo) in the rate and depth of breathing to the point of apnea when the cycle repeats itself. The hyperpneic phase lasts longer than the apneic phase.	Bilateral dysfunction of the deep cerebral and/or diencephalic structures, seen with supratentorial injury and metabolically induced coma states
Brainstem breathing patterns		
Central neurogenic hyperventilation (CNH)	A sustained deep rapid, but regular pattern (hyperpnea) occurs, with a decreased $Paco_2$ and a corresponding increase in pH and increased Po_2.	May result from CNS damage or disease that involves the midbrain and upper pons; seen after increased intracranial pressure and blunt head trauma
Apneusis	A prolonged inspiratory cramp (a pause at full inspiration) occurs. A common variant of this is a brief end-inspiratory pause of 2 or 3 seconds often alternating with an end-expiratory pause.	Indicates damage to the respiratory control mechanism located at the pontine level; most commonly associated with pontine infarction but documented with hypoglycemia, anoxia, and meningitis
Cluster breathing	A cluster of breaths has a disordered sequence with irregular pauses between breaths.	Dysfunction in the lower pontine and high medullary areas
Ataxic breathing	Completely irregular breathing occurs, with random shallow and deep breaths and irregular pauses. Often the rate is slow.	Originates from a primary dysfunction of the medullary neurons controlling breathing
Gasping breathing pattern	A pattern of deep "all-or-none" breaths is accompanied by a slow respiratory rate.	Indicative of a failing medullary respiratory center

Similar responses are produced by dysfunction in the lower brainstem through direct stimulation.

Most central nervous system (CNS) disorders produce both nausea and vomiting. Vomiting with no associated nausea indicates direct involvement of the central neural mechanism. Vomiting is particularly associated with CNS injuries that (1) involve the vestibular nuclei (located in the lower pons and medulla oblongata) or its immediate projections, particularly when double vision (diplopia) also is present, (2) impinge directly on the floor of the fourth ventricle, or (3) produce brainstem compression secondary to increased intracranial pressure.

Pupillary changes

Anatomically, brainstem areas that control arousal are adjacent to areas that control pupils. Pupillary changes thus are a valuable guide to evaluating the presence and level of brainstem dysfunction (Fig. 14-1).

Certain drugs that affect pupils must be considered in the evaluation of pupillary response in comatose states. Atropine and scopolamine in large concentrations fully dilate and fix pupils. Glutethimide (Doriden) in amounts sufficient to produce a coma causes the pupils to become midposition or moderately dilated (4 to 8 mm in diameter), unequal, and frequently fixed to light. Opiates (heroin and morphine) cause pinpoint pupils. Severe barbiturate intoxication may produced fixed pupils.

Severe ischemia and hypoxia produce bilaterally wide and fixed pupils in most instances. Occasionally the pupils remain small or midposition even in the presence of profound hypoxia. Hypothermia also may cause fixed pupils.

Oculomotor responses

Resting, spontaneous, and reflexive eye movements (oculocephalic [doll's head, doll's eyes] and oculovestibular [caloric] reflexes) undergo change at various levels of brain dysfunction (Table 14-5). Persons with metabolically induced coma, except in cases of barbiturate-hypnotic and phenytoin (Dilantin) poisoning, generally do retain ocular reflexes, however, even when other signs of brainstem damage, such as central neurogenic hyperventilation, are present.

The presence of brisk oculocephalic reflexes and roving eye movements, as well as the failure to elicit nystagmus with instillation of cold or warm water into the

Metabolic imbalance

Small reactive, regular

Diencephalic dysfunction
Small and reactive

Dysfunction of tectum (roof)
of the midbrain
Large "fixed" hippus

Dysfunction of third cranial nerve
Sluggish, dilated, and fixed

Pontine dysfunction
Pinpoint

Midbrain dysfunction
Midposition and fixed

FIG. 14-1 Pupils at different levels of consciousness.

external ear canal, indicates a decrease in consciousness (loss of cortical influence) but an intact brainstem (Figs. 14-2 and 14-3).

Destructive or compressive injury to the brainstem causes specific abnormalities of the oculocephalic and oculovestibular reflexes. For example, a skewed devia-

tion, in which one eye diverges downward and the other looks upward, indicates brainstem dysfunction. Destructive or compressive disease processes that involve an oculomotor nucleus or nerve cause the involved eye to deviate outward, producing a resting dysconjugate lateral position of the eyes. Unilateral abducens paraly-

---

TABLE 14-5

Changes in Oculomotor Responses

State	Resting and spontaneous eye movements	Reflexive eye movements
Full consciousness	Eyes at rest, still (cortical gaze centers inhibit spontaneous roving eye movements)	Eyes move as the head turns Oculocephalic responses not elicited or inconsistently elicited (frontal gaze centers inhibit brainstem reflexes that fix gaze straight ahead) Oculovestibular (caloric) stimulation produces nystagmus
Cortical dysfunction or disruption of efferent pathways	Roving eye movements may well be present (cortical gaze centers no longer inhibit these brainstem-generated roving eye movements)	Gaze fixed straight ahead regardless of head position—positive doll's eyes reaction (normal oculocephalic reflexes are no longer inhibited by frontal gaze centers) Nystagmus is no longer induced by caloric stimulation (normally a cold water stimulus produces deviation of the eyes opposite the irrigated ear; a warm water stimulus deviates the eyes to the same [ipsilateral] side) With an injury that depresses cortical gaze center function, the eyes (and often the entire head) will deviate, or appear to look toward the side of the injured hemisphere With an injury that irritates (stimulates) the neurons of the cortical gaze center, the eyes (and often the entire head) will deviate away from the injured hemisphere (all fibers from the frontal gaze centers decussate and therefore control the function of the contralateral pontine gaze center, which moves the eyes in the ipsilateral direction)
Mesencephalon dysfunction	Roving eye movements cease, and the eyes become immobile and directed ahead (roving eye movements require an intact brainstem)	Oculovestibular reflexes become inconsistent and abnormal Loss of Bell's phenomenon (upward deviation of eyes on stimulation) (required intact eye movement pathways from the mesencephalon to pons)
Pontine dysfunction	Loss of spontaneous blinking (requires an intact pons)	

G. J. Wassilchenko

FIG. 14-2 Test for oculocephalic reflex response (doll's eyes phenomenon). **A,** Normal response—eyes turn together to side opposite from turn of head. **B,** Abnormal response—eyes do not turn in conjugate manner. **C,** Absent response—eyes do not turn as head position changes. (From Rudy, 1984.)

FIG. 14-3 **Test for oculovestibular reflex (caloric ice water test). A,** Normal response—conjugate eye movements. **B,** Abnormal response—dysconjugate or asymmetric eye movements. **C,** Absent response—no eye movements. (From Rudy, 1984.)

FIG. 14-4 **Pathologic reflexes. A,** Grasp reflex. **B,** Snout reflex. **C,** Palmomental reflex. **D,** Suck reflex.

sis (paralysis of cranial nerve VI) results in an upward deviation of the ipsilateral eye. With bilateral abducens paralysis, the eyes come together (converge).

Motor responses

Motor responses contribute both to evaluating the level of brain dysfunction and to determining the side of the brain that is maximally damaged. The pattern of response is described to be (1) purposeful, a defensive or withdrawal movement to noxious stimuli, (2) inappropriate (i.e., not purposeful), generalized motor movement, grimacing, or groaning, and (3) not present (i.e., no motor response).

Motor signs indicating loss of cortical inhibition that are commonly associated with decreased consciousness include contralateral or bilateral (depending on whether the process is localized or diffuse) reflex grasping, reflex sucking, snout reflex, palmomental reflex, and rigidity (paratonia) (Fig. 14-4). Abnormal flexor and extensor responses in the upper and lower extremities are defined in Table 14-6 and illustrated in Fig. 14-5.

Outcomes

Two forms of neurologic death, cerebral death and brain death, result from severe pathologic conditions and are associated with coma. **Cerebral death** (irreversible coma) is death of the cerebral hemispheres exclusive of the brainstem and cerebellum. Brain damage is permanent and sufficiently severe that the individual is unable forever to respond behaviorally in any significant way to the environment. The brain, however, may continue to maintain internal homeostasis (normal respiratory and cardiovascular functions, normal temperature control, and normal gastrointestinal function).

Brain death occurs when irreversible brain damage is so extensive that the brain has no potential for recovery and no longer can maintain the body's internal homeostasis. Destruction of the neuronal contents of the intracranial cavity includes the brainstem and cerebellum. On postmortem the brain is autolyzing (self-digesting) or already autolyzed.

General agreement holds that brain death has occurred in the absence of discernible evidence of cerebral hemisphere function or function of the brainstem's vital centers for an extended period. In addition, the abnormality of brain function must result from structural or known metabolic disease and *not* be caused by a depressant drug, alcohol poisoning, or hypothermia. An isoelectric, or flat, electroencephalogram (EEG) (electrocerebral silence) for a period of 6 to 12 hours in a person who is not hypothermic and has not ingested depressant drugs indicates that no mental recovery is possible and usually means that the brain is already dead.

The following clinical criteria determine brain death (Plum & Posner, 1980; Walker, 1985):

1. Completion of all appropriate and therapeutic procedures
2. Unresponsive coma (absence of motor and reflex movements)
3. No spontaneous respiration (apnea)—a Pa_{CO_2} that rises above 60 mm Hg without breathing efforts, providing evidence of a nonfunctioning respiratory center
4. Absent cephalic reflexes (no ocular responses to head turning or caloric stimulation) with dilated, fixed pupils
5. Isoelectric (flat) EEG (electrocerebral silence)
6. Persistence of the aforementioned signs for 30 minutes to 1 hour and for 6 hours after onset of coma and apnea
7. Confirming test indicating absence of cerebral circulation (optional)

FIG. 14-5 Decorticate and decerebrate responses. A, Decorticate response. Flexion of arms, wrists, and fingers with adduction in upper extremities. Extension, internal rotation, and plantar flexion in lower extremities. **B,** Decerebrate response. All four extremities in rigid extension, with hyperpronation of forearms and plantar extension of feet. **C,** Decorticate response on right side of body and decerebrate response on left side of body. (From Rudy, 1984.)

Vegetative states. Cerebral function is lost in the vegetative state, but sleep-wake cycles are present. The person's eyes open spontaneously in response to external stimuli such as voice or touch. The individual maintains blood pressure and breathing without support, and brainstem reflexes (pupillary, oculocephalic, chewing, swallowing) are intact. No discrete localizing motor responses are present, and the individual does not speak any comprehensible words or follow commands.

A vegetative state is distinctly different from **locked-in syndrome.** With locked-in syndrome, both the content of thought and level of arousal are intact but the efferent pathways are disrupted. Thus the individual cannot communicate either through speech or through body movement but is fully conscious, with intact cognitive function. The upper cranial nerves (I through IV) often are preserved, however, so that the person possesses vertical eye movement and blinking as a means of communication.

Seizures

A **seizure** is a sudden, explosive, disorderly discharge of cerebral neurons and is characterized by a sudden, transient alteration in brain function, usually involving motor, sensory, autonomic, or psychic clinical manifestations and an alteration in level of arousal. Seizure disorders, the second most common neurologic disorder,

represent a syndrome, however, and not a specific disease entity. The alteration in level of arousal is temporary.

The term *convulsion,* sometimes applied to seizures, refers to the clonic-tonic (jerky, contract-relax) movement associated with some seizures. The term *epilepsy,* meaning "to be seized by a force from without," generally is applied to conditions in which no underlying correctable cause for the seizures is found so that the seizure activity recurs without treatment. **Epilepsy** therefore is a general term for the primary condition that causes seizures.

Conditions associated with seizure disorders

Any disorder that alters the neuronal environment may cause seizure activity, so that theoretically anyone may experience a seizure. Some persons, however, have a genetic predisposition toward seizure activity; their "seizure threshold" in neuronal tissues apparently is lower.

A seizure disorder can be produced by a variety of pathologic processes, including medical diseases, that can extend to involve the nervous system. The onset of a seizure disorder also may indicate the presence of an ongoing primary neurologic disease. Persons with organic brain injury have greater tendencies toward seizure activity than do persons with normal CNS function. Etiologic factors in seizures generally include (1)

TABLE 14-6

Abnormal Motor Responses with Decreased Responsiveness

Motor response	Description of motor responses	Location of injury*
Abnormal motor responses, upper extremity flexion with or without extensor responses in the leg (decorticate rigidity)	Slowly developing flexion of the arm, wrist, and fingers with adduction in the upper extremity and extension, internal rotation, and plantar flexion of the lower extremity	Suggest mostly cortical damage and less severe hemispheric dysfunction
Extensor responses in the upper and lower extremities (decerebrate posturing, decerebrate rigidity)	Opisthotonus (hyperextension of the vertebral column) with clenching of the teeth; extension, adduction, and hyperpronation of the arms; and extension of the lower extremities In acute brain injury, shivering and hyperpnea may accompany unelicited recurrent decerebrate spasms	Associated with severe hemispheric damage
Extensor responses in the upper extremities accompanied by flexion in the lower extremities		Indicates pontine level dysfunction
Flaccid state with little or no motor response to stimuli		Damage to lower pons and upper myelencephalon

*A less fully developed response has the same localizing significance but reflects a smaller, less-damaging injury.

cerebral lesions, (2) biochemical disorders, (3) cerebral trauma, and (4) epilepsy, which can result from the following conditions:

Metabolic defects
Congenital malformation
Genetic predisposition
Perinatal injury
Postnatal trauma
Motor syndromes
Infection
Brain tumor
Vascular disease

Causes of recurrent seizures also are age-related (Table 14-7).

In persons with seizure disorders, seizure activity may be precipitated by hypoglycemia, fatigue or lack of sleep, emotional or physical stress, febrile illness, large amounts of water ingestion, constipation, use of stimulant drugs, withdrawal from depressant drugs (including alcohol), hyperventilation (respiratory alkalosis), and some environmental stimuli such as blinking lights, a poorly adjusted television screen, loud noises, certain music, certain odors, or merely being startled. Women may have increased seizure activity immediately before or during menses.

Types of seizure disorders

Seizures are classified in different ways—by clinical manifestations, site of origin, EEG correlates, or response to therapy. A simplified version of the interna-

tional classification of epileptic seizures is presented in Table 14-8. **Generalized seizures** involve neurons bilaterally, often do not have a local (focal) onset, and usually originate from a subcortical or deeper brain focus. With a generalized seizure, consciousness always is impaired or lost. **Partial seizures (focal seizures)** involve neurons only unilaterally, often have a local (focal) onset, and usually originate from cortical brain tissue, thereby having a superficial focus. Consciousness usually is maintained as long as the seizure activity is limited to one hemisphere, but partial seizures may become generalized to involve neurons of the other hemisphere and the deeper brain nuclei. This process is called **secondary generalization**. Consciousness is lost at the point of generalization.

Status epilepticus is the experience of a second, a third, and often subsequent seizures before the person has fully regained consciousness from the preceding seizure. The person is still in a **postictal state** (state that follows a seizure) when the next seizure begins. Status epilepticus most frequently results from abrupt discontinuation of antiseizure medications but also may occur in untreated or inadequately treated persons with seizure disorders. The situation is a medical emergency because of the resulting cerebral hypoxia. Mental retardation, dementia, and other brain damage, and even death, are serious threats. Aspiration also is a great risk. (Terminology associated with seizure activity is defined in Table 14-9.)

Pathophysiology. An **epileptogenic focus** appears to

TABLE 14-7

Causes of Recurrent Seizures in Different Age-Groups

Age of onset	Probable cause
Neonatal	Congenital maldevelopment, birth injury, metabolic disorders (hypocalcemia, hypoglycemia), vitamin B deficiency, phenylketonuria
Infancy (1-6 months)	As above Infantile spasms
Early childhood (6 months-3 yr)	Infantile spasms, febrile convulsions, birth injury and anoxia, infections, trauma
Childhood, 3-10 yr	Perinatal anoxia, injury at birth or later, infections, thrombosis of cerebral arteries or veins, indeterminant cause ("idiopathic" epilepsy)
Adolescence, 10-18 yr	Idiopathic epilepsy, including genetically transmitted types, trauma
Early adulthood, 18-35 yr	Trauma, neoplasm, idiopathic epilepsy, withdrawal from alcohol or other sedative-hypnotic drugs
Middle age, 35-60 yr	Neoplasm, trauma, vascular disease, alcohol or other drug withdrawal
Late life, over 60 yr	Vascular disease, tumor, degenerative disease, trauma

From Adams, 1985.

TABLE 14-8

International Classification of Epileptic Seizures

Traditional terminology	New nomenclature
	I. Partial seizures (seizures beginning locally)

Focal motor; jacksonian seizures (occasionally become secondarily generalized)	A. Simple (without impairment of consciousness)
	   1. With motor symptoms
	   2. With special sensory or somatosensory symptoms
	   3. With autonomic symptoms
	   4. With psychic symptoms

Temporal lobe or psychomotor seizures	B. Complex (with impairment of consciousness)
	   1. Simple partial onset followed by impaired consciousness—with or without automatisms
	   2. Impaired consciousness at onset—with or without automatisms
	C. Secondarily generalized (partial onset evolving to generalized tonic-clonic seizures)

	II. Generalized seizures (bilaterally symmetric and without local onset)
Petit mal	A. Absences
Minor motor	B. Myoclonic seizures
Limited grand mal	C. Clonic seizure
	D. Tonic seizure
Grand mal	E. Tonic-clonic seizure
Drop attacks	F. Atonic seizure
	G. Infantile spasms
	III. Unclassified seizures (because of incomplete data)
	IV. Status epilepticus (prolonged partial or generalized recovery between attacks)

TABLE 14-9

Terminology Applied to a Seizure Disorder

Term	Definition
Aura	A peculiar sensation immediately preceding the onset of a seizure that may take the form of gustatory, visual, or auditory experience or a feeling of dizziness, numbness, or just "a funny feeling"
Prodroma	Early clinical manifestations, such as malaise, headache, or a sense of depression, that may occur hours to a few days before the onset of a seizure
Tonic phase	A state of muscle contraction in which there is excessive muscle tone
Clonic phase	A state of alternating contraction and relaxation of muscles
Postictal state	The time period immediately following the cessation of seizure activity

be a group of neurons that have lost their afferent stimulation. The plasma membranes of neuronal cells seem more permeable, making them more easily activated by hyperthermia, hypoxia, hypoglycemia, hyponatremia, repeated sensory stimulation, and certain sleep phases. These neurons are hypersensitive and may even remain in a chronic partially depolarized state.

The firing of involved epileptogenic neurons becomes increasingly greater in frequency and amplitude. When the intensity of the neuronal discharge reaches a threshold point, the discharge spreads to adjacent normal neurons through corticocortical synapses. If uninhibited at this point, the cortical excitation spreads through interhemispheric tracts to the contralateral cortex and through projection pathways to the subcortical areas of the basal ganglia, thalamus, and brainstem. The excitation spread to the subcortical, thalamic, and brainstem areas corresponds to the **tonic phase** (phase of muscle contraction with increased muscle tone) and is associated with loss of consciousness. Autonomic clinical manifestations also may emerge at this point, and apnea may be present for a few seconds. The excitation is further projected downward to the spinal cord neurons through the corticospinal and reticulospinal pathways.

The **clonic phase** (phase of alternating contraction and relaxation of muscles) begins as inhibitory neurons in the cortex, anterior thalamus, and basal ganglia begin to inhibit the cortical excitation. This inhibition causes an interruption in the seizure discharge, producing an intermittent contract-relax pattern of muscle contractions. The intermittent clonic bursts gradually become more and more infrequent until they finally cease. At this point the epileptogenic neurons are exhausted and the neuronal membranes also may be hyperpolarized.

The maintenance of seizure activity demands a 250% increase in adenosine triphosphate (ATP). Cerebral oxygen consumption is increased by 60%. Although cerebral blood flow also increases approximately 250% during seizure activity, available glucose and oxygen are readily depleted. With a severe seizure, the brain tissue may require more ATP than can be produced by the tissues from the available oxygen and glucose. A deficiency of ATP, phosphocreatine, and glucose then occurs, and lactate accumulates in the brain tissues. Severe seizures thus may produce secondary hypoxia, acidosis, and lactate accumulation, all of which are imbalances that may result in progressive brain tissue injury and destruction. Cellular exhaustion and destruction are consequences of these events.

If a seizure focus is active for a prolonged period, a secondary focus, called a **mirror focus,** may develop in normal tissue. This process apparently is caused by the interhemispheric communication, inasmuch as the mirror focus is located in the contralateral cortical area.

Clinical Manifestations

The clinical manifestations associated with seizure depend on the type of seizure (see Table 14-13). Two types of symptoms often signal an impending seizure. These are an **aura,** a peculiar sensation that immediately precedes the onset of a seizure, and a **prodroma,** an early manifestation that may occur hours to days before a seizure (Table 14-10). Both manifestations may become familiar to the person experiencing recurrent seizures and so may help in preventing injuries during the seizure.

Evaluation and Treatment

The health history is the most critical aspect in diagnosing a seizure disorder and establishing the cause. The health history is supplemented by the physical examination and laboratory tests of blood and urine (blood glucose, serum calcium, blood urea nitrogen, urine sodium, and creatinine clearance) to identify any systemic diseases known to have seizures as a clinical manifestation. Skull x-ray films, computed tomography (CT) scan, and cerebrospinal fluid examination are useful to identify any neurologic diseases associated with seizures. The electroencephalogram is useful in assessing the type of seizure and may help to determine its focus.

Treatment for a seizure disorder is first to correct or control its cause, if possible. If this is not possible, the major means of management is the judicious administration of antiseizure medications. The therapeutic goal is complete suppression of seizure activity without intolerable side effects of the drug. Other medical therapies may include prescription of a ketogenic diet, biofeedback, and surgery. In severe cases, psychologic, social, educational, and vocational counseling is often appropriate for the individual and family.

Alterations in Content of Thought (Cognition)

Selective attention, a second attentional system, refers to the ability to select from available, competing environmental and internal stimuli specific information to be consciously processed. Certain brainstem structures have been demonstrated to contribute to selective attention. Thus any of the etiologic factors previously discussed under coma have the potential to alter selective attention, but clinical recognition of the alteration is difficult because the decreased level of arousal masks the clinical signs and symptoms. Selective attention also has been demonstrated to be mediated in part by the parietal lobes, especially the right parietal lobe. An isolated (pure) **selective attention deficit,** which manifests as a neglect syndrome, rarely, if ever, occurs clinically because typically other parietal lobe deficits also are present, including concept formation deficits and higher cortical sensory deficits. A neglect syndrome may appear

TABLE 14-10

Clinical Manifestations Related to Seizure Types

Type	Clinical manifestations	Site
I. Partial seizures		
A. Simple		
1. With motor symptoms:		
a. Without jacksonian march (focal motor seizure—the motor movements do not extend into adjacent areas)	Motor activity is usually clonic. Motor movement elicited by the seizure activity depends on the anatomic-physiologic portion of the irritated cortex, but motor seizures most often begin in the face and hands. Focal seizures begin with slow, repetitive jerking of the body part, which increases in strength and rate over a period of 5 to 15 seconds. The seizure can cease spontaneously, with a gradual decrease in clonic movement.	Primary motor area
b. With jacksonian march (jacksonian seizure—the seizure activity spreads in an orderly fashion of adjacent areas)	Seizure activity spreads to adjacent areas after the initial clonic movement increases; motor movements, for example, would begin in the fingers of one side and spread to the hand, wrist, forearm, arm, face, and finally the lower extremity on the same side of the body. After spreading, the jerking movements in all areas would spontaneously stop.	Primary motor area
c. Adversive seizure	Turning movement of hand and eyes to the side opposite the irritative focus occurs. Often it is associated with contractions of the trunk and extremities. It may remain local or develop into a generalized seizure.	Frontal lobe anterior to the primary motor area
2. With special sensory or somatosensory symptoms (focal sensory seizure); less common than focal motor seizures; any age may be affected	Sensory experience is subjective and confined to the primary sensory modalities (somesthetic, visual, auditory-vestibular, or olfactory). If sensory seizure begins on the hand area of the sensory cortex, the patient experiences numbness, tingling, or "pins and needles" phenomena. Other sensory experiences include burning, a crawling sensation, or a feeling of movement of the body part. Most frequent areas affected include lips, fingers, and toes. May remain local or develop into a generalized seizure.	Sensory cortex Postcentral gyrus (parietal lobe) with involvement of the primary sensory area

Modified from Hickey, 1992.

Continued.

TABLE 14-10

Clinical Manifestations Related to Seizure Types—cont'd

Type	Clinical manifestations	Site
I. Partial seizures—cont'd		
B. *Complex (temporary lobe or psychomotor seizure)*		
1. Simple partial onset followed by impairment of consciousness—with or without automatisms; common seizures found in both children and adults but in most persons occur before the age of 20	The person is able to interact with the environment with purposeful, although inappropriate, movements; although the body muscles stiffen, the person does not fall and may even continue the complex activity in which he/she was involved, such as driving; the person may appear "wide eyed." A wide variety of sensory experiences precede the automatism and include illusions, hallucinations, and primitive visceral, olfactory, and gustatory sensations. Most characteristic event of a temporal lobe seizure is the automatism; common examples of automatism are lipsmacking, chewing, facial grimacing, swallowing movements, and patting, picking, or rubbing oneself or one's clothing. Temporal lobe seizures generally last from 1 to 4 minutes and are followed by several minutes of postictal confusion.	Temporal lobe and its connections
2. Impaired consciousness at onset—with or without automatisms	See above	
C. *Secondarily generalized*	Unconsciousness appears. General symptoms are produced.	
II. Generalized seizures		
A. *Absences (petit mal seizure), always occur in children after the age of 4 years and before puberty*	Characterized by an abrupt cessation of activity with a momentary arrest of consciousness lasting about 5 to 10 seconds, whereas a few last 30 seconds; the eyes become vacant and roll or the child may stare straight ahead; the lips may droop or twitch. The child is responsive if spoken to during the seizure. The child resumes previous activity after a seizure.	Multifocal
B. *Myoclonic*	Characterized by sudden, uncontrollable jerking movements of one or more extremities or the entire body. Seizures usually occur in the morning. Usually momentary loss of consciousness is followed by postictal confusion.	Multifocal

TABLE 14-10

Clinical Manifestations Related to Seizure Types—cont'd

Type	Clinical manifestations	Site
	Person often is flung violently to the ground so that injury is a real possibility. Myoclonic seizures can occur in clusters. If the frequency and amplitude of the seizures are severe, mental retardation can result.	
C. Clonic	Characterized by repetitive clonic jerks of constant amplitude and diminishing frequency.	
D. Tonic (affects infants and children)	Loss of postural tone without evidence of clonicity, with flexion of the upper limbs and extension of the lower limbs. Child assumes an abnormal posture for seconds or minutes without losing consciousness.	
E. Tonic-clonic (grand mal seizure) (affects both children and adults)	A prodromal period of irritability and tension may precede a tonic-clonic seizure by several hours or days; however, in most persons, seizures begin without warning. Characteristically tonic-clonic seizures begin with a sudden loss of consciousness and generalized tonic muscle contractions; the person falls to the ground and the body stiffens in an opisthotonus position with legs and, usually, arms extended; the jaw snaps shut; a shrill cry may be heard as a result of forceful exhalation of air through the closed vocal cords as the thoracic muscles initially contract; the bladder and, less often, the bowel may evacuate; during the tonic phase, the person is apneic with subsequent cyanosis; pupils are dilated and unresponsive to light. The tonic phase lasts less than 1 minute (average 15 seconds). The clonic phase is characterized by violent, rhythmic, muscular contractions accompanied by strenuous hyperventilation; the face is contorted; the eyes roll, and there is excessive salivation with frothing from the mouth; profuse sweating and a rapid pulse are evident. The clonic jerking subsides in frequency and amplitude over a period of about 30 seconds.	Multifocal

Continued.

TABLE 14-10

Clinical Manifestations Related to Seizure Types—cont'd

Type	Clinical manifestations	Site
II. Generalized seizures—cont'd		
E. *Tonic-clonic (grand mal seizure)(affects both children and adults)—cont'd*	The tonic-clonic seizure lasts from 2 to 5 minutes. After the clonic phase, the person is in a stupor or coma for about 5 minutes; the extremities are limp; breathing is quiet; and the pupils begin to respond to light. When the person awakens, he/she may be confused and disoriented and complains of headache, muscle aching, and fatigue. There is no recollection of the attack. Tonic-clonic seizures may occur at any time of the day or night, whether the person is awake or asleep. The frequency of recurrence may vary from hours, weeks, months, or years.	
F. *Atonic (drop attack, akinetic seizure)*	Characterized by sudden loss of postural muscle tone.	Multifocal
G. *Infantile spasms (affects 3-month to 2-year age-group)*	Characterized by flexor spasms of the extremities and the head (have been described as jackknife seizures). Seizure lasts a few seconds and often appears in clusters with several clusters occurring daily. Infantile spasms associated with metabolic, degenerative, or structural illness in 50% of cases; in other 50% no correlation is noted. Most victims are mentally retarded.	

temporary as a result of seizure activity or a postictal state. Temporary or permanent deficits may occur with parietal lobe contusions or subdural hematomas, encephalitis, and ischemic parietal lobe stroke. Progressive neglect deficits may be found with parietal lobe gliomas or metastatic tumor and in Alzheimer and Pick diseases.

Dysmnesia is a disorder of the **recent memory system** defined as the loss of past memories (retrograde amnesia) coupled with an inability to form new memories (anterograde amnesia) despite intact attentional systems. Isolated (pure) dysmnesia is caused by only a limited number of conditions, such as transient global dysmnesia (episodic global dysmnesia), amnesic stroke, and Korsakoff psychosis (amnestic or dysmnestic syndrome), as well as after temporal lobectomy. Many disorders may temporarily or permanently produce dys-

mnesia that accompanies other deficits of the cognitive systems. A temporary dysmnesia is found during complex partial seizures that persist for a time in the postictal state, in postconcussive states, and in mild posttraumatic brain injury states. A permanent dysmnesia may be seen after subarachnoid hemorrhage or moderate or severe posttraumatic brain injury states, in carbon dioxide poisoning and other hypoxic/anoxic states, in Wernicke encephalopathy, viral encephalitis, and granulomatous meningitides, in tumors, and in Alzheimer and Pick diseases.

Remote memory, in which permanent memories are stored, is located in the association areas of the temporal, occipital, and parietal lobes. A pure auditory or visual remote memory deficit manifests as an isolated agnosia (see p. 498 for etiologic factors). An isolated (pure) **remote memory deficit** of tactile sensations rarely occurs clinically because selected attention and concept formation would likely be affected as well. A temporary auditory, visual, or tactile remote memory deficit may appear as a result of seizure activity or a postictal state. A temporary or permanent deficit can occur with temporal, occipital, or parietal lobe contusion; subdural hematoma or ischemic stroke; and in encephalitis. A progressive remote memory deficit may occur in temporal, occipital, or parietal gliomas or metastatic tumors, and in Alzheimer and Pick diseases.

Concept formation is the capacity to analyze the relationships between objects and their properties to reach a generalization. Concept formation is fundamental to the ability to abstract. Concept formation and abstraction generally are believed to be mediated predominantly by the parietal lobes. Etiologic factors in **concept and abstract formation deficit** are similar to those discussed previously under selective attention deficits caused by parietal lobe dysfunction.

The prefrontal areas mediate several cognitive functions, including vigilance, reasoning, and executive functions. The vigilance system provides the person with an ability to concentrate over time or to maintain sustained attention, that is, to be attentive. Reasoning is the ability to understand relationships, identify essential parts, synthesize the parts, and arrive at a common theme. Reasoning skill is the ability to organize or categorize concepts. Executive functions, or overseer functions, comprise a system of programming, verification, and correction. Specific executive functions include anticipation (motivation), goal selection or formulation, planning, initiating (programming), self-monitoring, and self-correction.

Isolated (pure) vigilance, reasoning, and executive system deficits have been discussed only rarely in the literature, and their occurrence is uncommon because these deficits invariably are present simultaneously. **Vigilance, reasoning,** and **executive system deficits,** accompanied by other deficits of the cognitive systems, are much more common. Whether the deficits are temporary or permanent depends on the cause and severity of injury. Deficits caused by CNS depressant drugs and seizure activity, and it is hoped, by neurosurgical procedures involving retraction of the frontal lobes are temporary. Deficits in postconcussive and mild traumatic brain injury states may prove to be temporary and resolve over time. Permanent deficits are more likely to be found with frontal lobe contusions, moderate or severe posttraumatic brain injury states, ischemic frontal lobe stroke, and neurosurgery that requires frontal lobe resection. Progressive deficits in vigilance, reasoning, and executive system functions are caused by frontal lobe gliomas, frontal lobe infarcts associated with hypertensive vascular disease, and Alzheimer and Pick diseases.

Pathophysiology

Disorders of selective attention, at least as they relate to visual orienting behavior, are produced by disease that involves portions of the midbrain. Persons with a disease affecting the superior colliculi have a disturbance in the "move" operation of selective attention, which manifests as a slowness in orienting attention. Persons with parietal lobe disease may experience selective attention deficits related to disengagement from a stimulus. Persons with parietal lobe dysfunction, especially the right parietal lobe, also may experience a unilateral neglect syndrome, the prototype of a selective attention disorder. Perhaps some of the other agnosias could be classified as selective attention deficits.

A disorder in vigilance (concentration over time) may be produced by disease in the prefrontal areas. A pathologic condition in the prefrontal areas also may produce impaired problem-solving and executive system deficits. Impaired concept formation and abstraction may result from a pathologic process in the cortical association areas of the parietal, temporal, and occipital lobes.

The exact pathophysiology of the various disorders of cognitive systems is not fully known. Researchers currently are studying the defects in the elementary operations (components) of each cognitive system. Pathophysiology related to the memory systems has been the most studied. Dysmnesia/amnesia, which originates from pathologic conditions in the hippocampus and related temporal lobe structures, is the result of a failure to transfer information from working (short-term) to long-term memory, as well as a failure to consolidate or retrieve long-term memory stores.

As a very general statement, the primary pathophysiologic mechanisms that operate in cognitive systems disorders are (1) direct destruction because of direct ischemia and hypoxia or indirect destruction as a result of compression and (2) the effects of toxins and chemicals. Disinhibition resulting in overactivity, such as seen in some drug withdrawal states, is a pathologic mechanism that can produce vigilance deficits. The pathophysiologic processes are very generally presented in Fig. 14-6.

Clinical Manifestations

Clinical manifestations of attention deficits, memory deficits, impaired concept formation, impaired reasoning, and executive function deficits are presented in Table 14-11.

Evaluation and Treatment

Immediate medical management is directed at diagnosing the cause and treating reversible factors. Rehabilitative measures for cognitive system deficits generally are either compensatory in nature or restorative in nature and have of late been greatly facilitated by com-

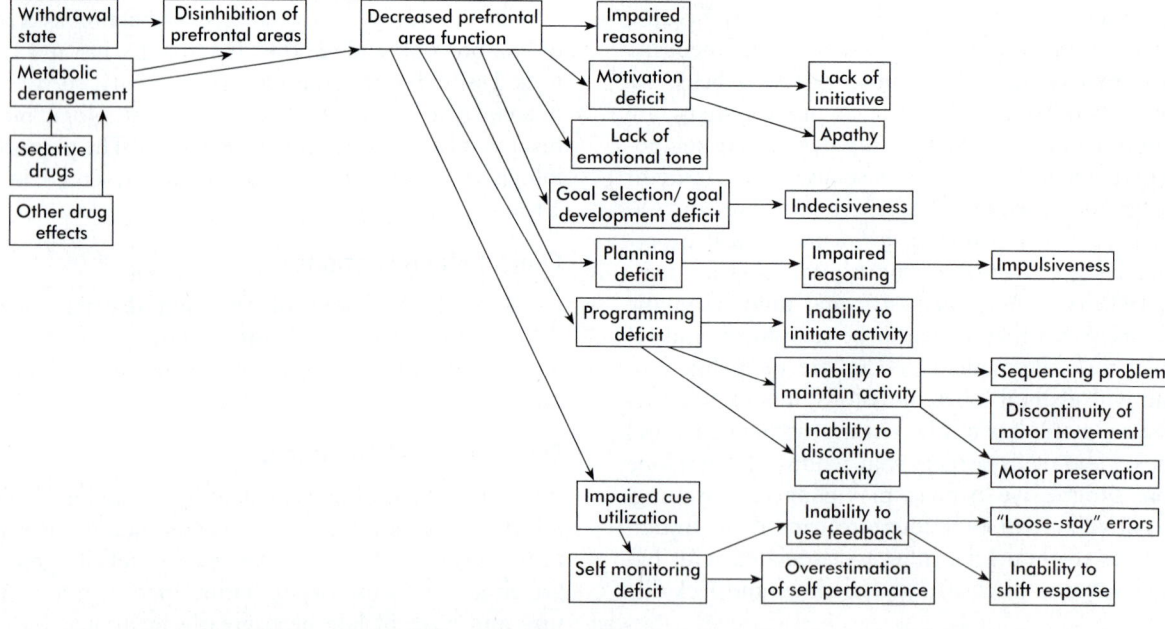

FIG. 14-6 **Cognitive system deficits.** General pathophysiologic mechanisms underlying cognitive system deficits.

TABLE 14-11

Clinical Manifestations of Cognitive System Deficits

Deficit	Clinical signs	Symptoms
Attention		
Selective attention	Inability to focus attention; decreased eye, head, and body movements associated with focusing on the stimuli; decreased search and scanning; faulty orientation to stimuli causing safety problems; inability to screen out distractions; distractibility	Person reports distractibility, inability to focus attention, inability to screen out distraction, failure to perceive objects and other stimuli (history of injuries, falls, and safety problems)
Vigilance	Distractibility/inattentiveness; inability to concentrate; impulsiveness	Person reports distractibility; inability to concentrate; poor memory/forgetfulness; reports by others of inattentiveness or impulsiveness (associated with apathy, laziness, and lack of motivation)
Memory		
Recent (anterograde memory)	*Left hemisphere:* disorientation to time, situation, place, name, person (verbal identification); impaired language memory (e.g., names of objects); impaired semantic memory *Right hemisphere:* disorientation to self, person (visual), place (visual); impaired episodic memory (personal history); impaired emotional memory. *Either or both hemispheres:* confusion; behavioral change	Person reports disorientation, confusion, "not listening," "not remembering"; reports by others of person being disoriented, not able to remember, not able to learn new information
Remote	*Left hemisphere:* inability to retrieve personal history, past medical history; unaware of recent current events *Right hemisphere:* inability to recognize persons, places, objects, music, etc., from past	Person reports remote memory problems; others report that person cannot recall formerly known information
Concept formation	Inability to categorize (identify similarities and differences), sort; inability to form concepts; inability to analyze relationships; misinterpretation; inability to interpret proverbs	Reports by others of frequent misinterpretation of data, failure to conceptualize or generalize information
Reasoning	Inability to perform deductive reasoning (convergent reasoning); inability to perform inductive reasoning (divergent reasoning); inability to abstract; concrete reasoning demonstrated; delusions	Reports by others of predominantly concrete thinking; lack of understanding of everyday situations, health care regimens, and such; delusional thinking
Executive functions		
Motivation	Lack of initiative (anergy); lack of ambition; lack of motivation; flat affect; no awareness of feelings; appears depressed, apathetic, and emotionless; fails to appreciate deficit; disinterested in appearance; lacks concern about childish or crude behavior	Reports by others of laziness or apathy, flat affect or lack of emotional expression, failing to exhibit or be aware of feelings
Mild	Responds to immediate environment but no new ideas; grooming and social graces are lacking	Reports by others of lack of ambition, motivation, or initiative, failure to carry out adult tasks, lack of social graces and new ideas
Severe	Motionless, lack of responding to even internal cues, does not respond to physical needs, does not interact with surroundings	Reports by others of failure to groom or toilet self, unawareness of surroundings and own physical needs

Continued.

TABLE 14-11

Clinical Manifestations of Cognitive System Deficits—cont'd

Deficit	Clinical signs	Symptoms
Executive functions—cont'd		
Goal formation	Slow to orient; inability to set goals or form goals; indecisiveness	Reports by others of failure to set goals, indecisiveness
Planning	Failure to make plans; inability to produce a complete line of reasoning; inability to make up a story; appears impulsive	Reports by others of failure to plan, impulsiveness, "does not think things through"
Programming	Failure to initiate behavior; failure to maintain behavior; failure to discontinue behavior; slowness to alternate response for the next step; motor perseveration	Reports by others of not knowing where to begin, inability to carry out sequential acts (maintain a behavior), inability to cease a behavior
Self-monitoring	Inability to use feedback regarding behavior; failure to recognize omissions and errors in self-care, speech, writing, and arithmetic; impaired cue utilization; overestimation of performance	Reports by others of not changing behavior when requested; unawareness of limitations; does not recognize and correct errors in dressing, grooming, toileting, eating, and such; fails to recognize speech and arithmetic errors; careless speech
Incorporation of feedback	Failure to shift response set; failure to change behavior when conditions change; cue utilization may be impaired	Reports by others of failure to use feedback; inability to incorporate feedback (does not correct when feedback is given)

puter technology and other electronic-assisted devices. Approaches based on behavioral techniques tend to be compensatory, whereas process-oriented approaches, it is hoped, are restorative.

Attention deficit masquerades as other cognitive deficits. Differential diagnosis of other cognitive deficits is blocked, and learning potential is largely obscured by the presence of an attention deficit. Therefore the diagnosis and treatment of attention deficits are fundamental.

Specific Cognitive Disorders
Agnosia

Agnosia is a defect of recognition, a failure to recognize the form and nature of objects. The disorder involves the loss of recognition through one sense, although the object or person may still be recognized by other senses. Agnosia can be tactile, visual, or auditory. For example, an individual may be unable to identify a safety pin by touching it with a hand but is able to name it when looking at it. Agnosia may be as minimal as a finger agnosia (failure to identify by name the fingers of one's hand) or as devastating as complete denial of hemiplegia.

Agnosia is produced by dysfunction in the primary sensory area or in the interpretive areas of the cerebral cortex (see Fig. 12-5). (The types of agnosia and the associated area that is most commonly involved with each are presented in Table 14-12.) Although agnosia most commonly is associated with cerebrovascular accidents,

agnosia may arise from any pathologic process that injures these specific areas of the brain.

Sensory inattentiveness is a mild form of agnosia and may be visual, auditory, or tactile. The person with sensory inattentiveness is able to recognize individual sensory input from the dysfunctional side when called on to do so but ignores (i.e., neglects, extinguishes) the sensory input from the dysfunctional side when stimulated from both sides. This phenomenon is called **extinction.** The entire complex of denial of dysfunction, loss of recognition of one's own body parts, and extinction sometimes is referred to as the **neglect syndrome.**

Dysphasia

Dysphasia is impairment of comprehension or production of language. With dysphasia, comprehension or use of symbols, in either written or verbal language, is disturbed or lost. **Aphasia** is *loss* of the comprehension or production of language.

Dysphasias usually are associated with cerebrovascular accident involving the middle cerebral artery or one of its many branches. The language disorders, however, may arise from a variety of injuries and diseases—vascular, neoplastic, traumatic, degenerative, metabolic, or infectious. Dysphasia results from dysfunction in the left cerebral hemisphere, most commonly in the frontotemporal region, particularly around the insulae (Fig. 14-7; see also Fig. 12-5). Most language disorders are due to acute processes that either resolve or cause a chronic residual deficit. Some language disorders are due to de-

TABLE 14-12

Types of Agnosia

Type of agnosia	Definition	Location of injury
Tactile agnosia (astereognosis)	Inability to recognize objects by touch	Parietal lobe
Spatial agnosia	Incapacity to find one's way around familiar places	Parietal lobe
Body image agnosias		
Anosognosia	Ignorance or denial of the existence of the disease	Right parietal lobe
Autotopagnosia	Loss of ability to identify the body, in whole or in part, or to recognize relationships among various parts	Right parietal lobe
Prosopagnosia	Inability to recognize human faces	Temporooccipital region
Visual agnosia	Inability to recognize objects, pictures, and human faces	Temporoparietooccipital area
Word blindness (alexia)	Inability to recognize written symbols	Left parietotemporal region
Color agnosia	Inability to understand colors as qualities of objects, faulty color concepts, and inability to evoke color images in the absence of color blindness	Occipital lobe; posterior corpus callosum
Auditory agnosia (pure word deafness)	Inability to recognize speech sounds	Superior temporal area
Amusia (music deafness)	Loss of capacity to recognize tones and melodies	Right superior temporal area
Gertsmann syndrome		Left angular gyrus
Finger agnosia	Inability to identify the names of one's fingers	
Right-left confusion	Inability to distinguish right from left	
Agraphia	Inability to write	
Acalculia	Inability to perform mathematic calculations	

FIG. 14-7 Development of dysphasia. Portion of the left cerebral hemisphere considered most important in the development of dysphasia. (From Thompson et al., 1993.)

TABLE 14-13

Major Types of Dysphasia

Type	Expression	Verbal comprehension	Repetition
Expressive (Broca dysphasia, motor)	Nonfluent; impairment of ability to find words, difficulty in writing	Relatively intact	Impaired
Receptive			
Wernicke dysphasia, sensory	Fluent: able to produce verbal language but language is meaningless; words are often inappropriate; words with similar sounds or words with similar meaning are substituted for the correct words; words that are not part of the language may be present; these neologisms may be so extensive as to make the speech entirely incomprehensible; because the person has no means to monitor the language for correctness, errors are not recognized; intonation, accent, cadence, rhythm, and articulation are normal	Impaired (disturbance in understanding all language)	Impaired
Word deafness or auditory verbal agnosia, sensory	Fluent; self-initiated speech is normal	Impaired; hears noise rather than language; language has no meaning and is perceived as foreign	Impaired, unable to repeat what is said
Global (sensory—motor, receptive—expressive)	Nonfluent; produces little speech; at best speaks a few words or phrases	Impaired or completely lost; person understands only the simplest things said	Impaired; not able to repeat
Conduction	Fluent but with paraphrasia in self-initiated speech and writing or reading aloud	Relatively intact	Impaired; not able to repeat
Normal (anomia)	Fluent but impaired ability to name objects, persons, qualities, or characteristics; knows what he or she wants to say but cannot find words; may even use desired word in another context but still cannot isolate word when needed	Relatively intact; able to recognize word when it is given	Intact
Transcortical motor	Nonfluent	Relatively intact	Intact
Transcortical sensory	Fluent	Impaired	Intact

Modified from Mancall, 1981.

Name	Reading comprehension	Writing	Location of lesion	Cause of lesion
Impaired	Variable	Impaired	Posteroinferior frontal lobe (Broca's area)	
Impaired	Impaired	Impaired	Posterosuperior temporal lobe (Wernicke's area)	Occlusion of inferior division of left middle cerebral artery
Impaired	Intact; able to read	Intact; able to write	Pathways connecting the primary auditory cortex and the auditory association areas in the middle third of the left superior temporal gyrus	Small, superficial injury typically associated with occlusion of a branch of the middle cerebral artery
Impaired	Impaired or completely lost	Impaired: produces little written language	Frontotemporal lobe; anterior and posterior speech areas extensively impaired	Occlusion of the left middle cerebral artery of left internal carotid artery; tumors, other mass lesions, and hemorrhage may cause
Impaired	Variable	Impaired	Arcuate fasciculus, supramarginal gyrus, disruption of the large bundle of fibers that arise from the temporal lobe and pass posteriorly around the sylvian fissure and then project anteriorly to the premotor area	Typical cause is embolic occlusion of the ascending parietal or posterior temporal branch of the middle cerebral artery
Impaired	Variable	Variable	Angular gyrus— posterosuperior temporal lobe	
Impaired	Variable	Impaired	Anterior presylvian fissure	
Impaired	Impaired	Impaired	Posterior presylvian fissure	

TABLE 14-14

Examples of Language Disturbances

Disorder		Example
Verbal paraphrasia	Question:	What did the car do?
	Patient:	The car would spit sweetly down the road. (The car sped swiftly down the road.)
Literal paraphrasia	Request:	Say "persistence is essential to success."
	Patient:	Mesastence is instans to success.
Neologism	Question:	What do you call this? (Pointing to a plant.)
	Patient:	It's a logper.
Circumlocution	Question:	What do you call this? (Pointing to a plant.)
	Patient:	Something that grows.
Anomia	Question:	What do you call this? (Pointing to a plant.)
	Patient:	It's . . .
		or
	Question:	What did you do this morning?
	Patient:	Reading.
	Question:	Were you reading a book or a newspaper?
	Patient:	One of those.
Telegraphic style	Question:	Where is your daughter?
	Patient:	New Orleans . . . home . . . Monday.

From Boss, 1984.

generative disorders that make the dysfunction progressive.

Dysphasias have been classified both anatomically and functionally. Other classifications are linguistic and describe fluency, volume, or quantity of speech. Pure forms of any language dysfunction, however, are rare. **Expressive dysphasias** are characterized primarily by expressive deficits, but a verbal comprehension (auditory-receptive element) deficit may be present. Receptive dysphasias may have expressive deficits. (Table 14-13 compares types of dysphasias; Table 14-14 illustrates some of the language disturbances.)

Dysphasias referred to as **transcortical dysphasias, (transcortical sensory dysphasia, mixed transcortical dysphasia, isolated speech center)** involve the ability to repeat (called **echolalia**) and to recite. Speech is fluent but with striking paraphrases. The individual is unable to read and write, and comprehension is impaired.

Transcortical dysphasias are caused by hypoxia from prolonged hypotension, carbon monoxide poisoning, or other mechanisms that destroy the border zone (watershed area) between the anterior, middle, and posterior cerebral arteries (see Fig. 12-18). Blood supply is marginal in this region. Hypoxia in this area occasionally may isolate the posterior speech areas or all the speech areas from the remainder of the cortex, although both areas remain intact. The sensory and motor speech areas, therefore, are functional, but connections with other sensory or motor areas are impaired. Information from the remaining areas of the cortex cannot be transmitted to Wernicke's area to be transformed into language.

Acute Confusional States

Acute confusional states result from cerebral dysfunction secondary to such causes as drug intoxication or nervous system disease. A common cause of an acute confusional state is withdrawal from alcohol, barbiturate, or other sedative drug ingestion. Acute confusional states of toxic origin may have either sudden or gradual onset, depending on the amount of exposure to the toxin. These states often occur with febrile illnesses, with systemic diseases such as heart failure, or after head injury or anesthesia.

Pathophysiology

Three pathophysiologic mechanisms probably underlie the development of acute confusional states associated with delirium. These are (1) injury to nervous tissue, (2) action of exogenous chemicals on neuronal cells, and (3) overactivity of a previously depressed brain center. Destructive injuries directly affect the nervous tissues and disturb the function of the neurons. In states of intoxication, the direct action of toxins or chemicals on neuronal cells produces dysfunction of the involved cells. In states of withdrawal, the lower brain centers are over-

TABLE 14-15

Differences Between Organic and Functional Confusion

Factor	Organic confusion	Functional confusion
Memory impairment	Recent, more impaired than remote	No consistent difference between recent and remote
Disorientation		
Time	Within own lifetime or reasonably near future	May not be related to patient's lifetime
Place	Familiar place or one where patient might easily be	Bizarre or unfamiliar places
Person	Sense of identity usually preserved	Sense of identity diminished
	Misidentification of others as familiar	Misidentification of others based on delusion system
Hallucinations	Visual, vivid	Auditory more frequent
	Animals and insects common	Bizarre and symbolic
Illusions	Common	Not prominent
Delusions	Concerns everyday occurrences and people	Bizarre and symbolic
Confused	Spotty confusion	More consistent
	Clear intervals mixed with confused episodes	No tendency to become worse at night
	Worse at night	

From Morris & Rhodes, 1972.

active after the depressant action of the drug wears off, and this overactivity accounts for the development of the acute confusional state.

Clinical Manifestations

The predominant features of an acute confusional state are impaired or lost vigilance. Because of dysfunction of the prefrontal cortex (see Fig. 12-6), the ability to sustain attentional focus is seriously impaired or completely lost. The person is highly distractible and unable to concentrate on incoming sensory information or on any one particular mental or motor task.

The onset of an acute confusional state usually is abrupt rather than insidious. Memory impairments, distractibility and disorientation, misperception and misinterpretation of sensory stimuli (illusion), and frank delusions are all manifestations of acute confusional states. Intellectual functioning also is inadequate, and judgment is impaired. Anxiety and restlessness appear, and obsessions, compulsive behavior, and rituals may be evident.

In acute confusional states with associated underactivity, the individual exhibits decreases in mental function. Alertness is decreased, as are attention span, accurate perception, and interpretation of the environment. Forgetfulness is prominent. Reactions to the environment are slowed and indecisive. The individual dozes frequently.

Delirium, an acute confusional state associated with overactivity, typically develops over a period of 2 to 3 days. Early clinical manifestations include difficulty in concentrating, restlessness, irritability, insomnia, tremulousness, and poor appetite. Some persons experience seizures. Unpleasant, even terrifying, dreams may occur.

In a fully developed delirium state, the individual is completely inattentive, and perceptions are grossly altered. Misperception and misinterpretation are predominant. Hallucinations may be present. The person appears distressed and often very perplexed. Conversation is incoherent. Frank tremor is evident, and a great deal of restless movement is common. Violent behavior may be present. The individual cannot sleep, is flushed, and has dilated pupils, a rapid pulse (tachycardia), temperature elevation, and perfuse sweating (diaphoresis). Delirium typically abates suddenly or gradually in 2 to 3 days, although occasional delirium states persist for several weeks.

Evaluation and Treatment

The initial goal is to establish that the individual is confused, and the cause must be distinguished as organic or functional (Table 14-15). Next, the goal is to determine whether the confusion is delirium, an acute confusional state with associated underactivity, or an underlying dementia. The precise cause of an acute confusional state is established through the complete history and physical examination. Laboratory tests include an electrocardiogram and blood, urine, cerebrospinal fluid, and radiologic studies.

Once the cause is established, treatment is directed at controlling the primary disorder. In an acute confusional state, all drugs that may be contributing to or causing the condition are discontinued unless the problem is due to drug withdrawal. Supportive measures are designed to enhance coping skills and to minimize the individual's need for drug-altered cortical functions. Supportive management also involves maintaining the person's intact cortical functions by promoting use of these functions.

Dementing Processes

The dementias are characterized by reduction in cognitive functions (intellectual function). Mental abilities are impaired in the dementing process. The result may be a decrease in orientation, general knowledge and information, vigilance, recent memory, remote memory, concept formation, abstraction, reasoning, executive functions, judgment, insight, and interpretation. Because of declining intellectual ability, the individual exhibits alterations in behavior.

Dementias can be classified according to etiologic factors (e.g., trauma, tumors, vascular disorders, infections) and according to associated clinical and laboratory signs. Most recently, dementing processes have been grouped according to types of memory disorders, **attentional dementia** (loss of arousal), **amnestic dementia** (loss of recent memory), **cognitive dementia** (loss of remote memory), and **intentional dementia** (loss of vigilance and executive functions). The culmination of a progressive dementing process is nerve cell degeneration and brain atrophy.

Pathophysiology

Mechanisms in dementing processes include tissue destruction, compression, inflammation, and biochemical imbalances. For example, persons with Alzheimer disease have a lack of acetylcholine, a neurotransmitter, the first biochemical abnormality that has been demonstrated consistently (Danison, 1986; Sims et al., 1983). Acetylcholine is needed for recent memory at the biochemical level. As the level of acetylcholine is reduced, the individual is able to store less and less information until all recent memory is lost. The cause for the failure of the enzyme system that produces acetylcholine is not known, but a defect in amyloid metabolism is highly suspected. Slow-growing viruses are probably associated with some unexplained dementias, such as Jakob-Creutzfeldt disease.

A genetic predisposition probably is a contributing factor to the dementing process. In some instances, a familial history of dementia increases by four times the likelihood that dementia will develop. Environmental influences also may play a role in the pathogenesis of dementia. The exact nature of the influence of environmental factors, such as aluminum, is not clearly understood as yet.

Clinical Manifestations

A summary of the clinical manifestations of the dementias is presented in Table 14-16.

Evaluation and Treatment

Establishing the cause for a dementing process may be complicated, but all persons evidencing the clinical manifestations of dementia should be evaluated with laboratory and neuropsychologic testing to identify underlying conditions that may be treatable.

If a specific treatable cause is identified, the appropriate treatment is initiated. For example, an infectious process requires the appropriate antibiotic, and a potentially resectable mass may require neurosurgery. Nutritional deficiencies are corrected. If the cause is metabolic, the imbalance is corrected or the metabolic disorder is treated, or both.

Unfortunately, no specific treatment or cure exists for most progressive dementias. In such instances, therapy is directed at maintaining and maximizing use of the remaining capacities, restoring functions if possible, and accommodating to lost abilities. Assisting the family to understand the dementing process and to learn ways to assist the demented individual is an essential component of supportive management.

Alzheimer Disease

Alzheimer disease (**senile disease complex**) is a commonly occurring neurologic disorder. Formerly believed to occur mostly in persons younger than 65 years of age, Alzheimer disease has now been demonstrated to be one of the most common causes of severe cognitive dysfunction in older persons. Its more prevalent forms are late-onset familial Alzheimer dementia (FAD) and nonhereditary, or sporadic, late-onset AD (70% of cases).

Pathophysiology

The exact cause of Alzheimer disease is unknown. Several possible theories are under investigation, including loss of neurotransmitter stimulation by choline acetyltransferase, mutation for encoding amyloid precursor protein, and alteration in apolipoprotein E, which binds beta amyloid (Golde, Estus, Younkin, Selkoe, & Younkin, 1992; Hardy & Higgins, 1992). Early-onset FAD includes at least three gene defects on chromosomes 14, 19, and possibly 21 or another gene not yet mapped. Late-onset FAD is linked to a defect on chromosome 19 (Strittmatter et al., 1992; VanBroeckhoven et al., 1992). Each of these mechanisms may be linked

TABLE 14-16

Clinical manifestations of dementia

Type	Location	Manifestation
Amnestic dementia	Temporal lobe	Difficulty with naming
		Decreased language comprehension
		Loss of recent memory
		Development of a vegetative state
Intentional dementia	Frontal lobe	Distraction
		Failure to achieve specific goals (executive functions)
		Can follow simple commands but not able to carry out sequential intellectual functions (executive functions)
		Loss of attention span (vigilance)
		Inability to make decisions or judgments (reasoning)
		Accident prone
		Personality changes and inappropriate affect
		Loss of motor function: wide shuffling gait with small steps, muscle rigidity, flexion posturing, tendency to fall, abnormal reflexes, bowel and bladder incontinence, immobility
Cognitive dementia	Cerebral cortex	Loss of remote memory
		Decreased language comprehension
		Decreased mathematic skill
		Altered visuospatial relationships

to aggregation and precipitation of insoluble amyloid (senile plaques) in brain tissue and blood vessels. Alzheimer disease also has been linked to a lysosomal pathway in the breakdown of amyloid precursor protein to yield beta amyloid, a neurotoxic substance. A reduction in protein kinase C (PKC) and the scavenging of phospholipid from the cell membrane are being studied as the cause for the lysosomal pathway taking precedence (Hooper, 1992). A link between the pathology of Alzheimer disease and aluminum has not been established (Chipps, Clanin, & Campbell, 1992). Researchers have not yet been able to isolate a virus that causes the disease (Mozar, Bal, & Howard, 1987), but submicroscopic proteinaceous infectious particles ("prions") have been isolated. These prions already have been linked to at least one other form of degenerative brain disease. Antibrain antibodies may account for Alzheimer disease, and an autoimmune cause also is being investigated. In addition, aging and injury also may result in changes that contribute to the development of this disease. Such changes could include decreased oxygen and glucose transport, loss of the blood-brain barrier, and mitochondrial defects that alter cell metabolism and processing of proteins, including amyloid. Familial risk appears to be greatest in families affected by the classic early onset of Alzheimer disease (Kolata, 1981). The risk for a sibling older than 70 years of age does not differ from that of the general population.

Microscopically the protein in the neurons becomes distorted and twisted, forming a tangle called a **neurofibrillary tangle** (Fig. 14-8). An accumulation of these bundles of paired helical abnormal protein fibers (filaments) occurs within the neurons. Groups of nerve cells, especially terminal axons, degenerate and coalesce around an amyloid core. Microscopic examination of these areas of degeneration reveals plaquelike material known as **senile plaques.** These plaques disrupt nerve-impulse transmission. Senile plaques and neurofibrillary tangles are more concentrated in the cerebral cortex and hippocampus. The greater the number of senile plaques and neurofibrillary tangles, the more dysfunction is present (Coyle, Price, & Delong, 1983; Kolata, 1983).

Clinical Manifestations

Initial clinical manifestations are insidious and often attributed to forgetfulness, emotional upset, or other illness. The individual becomes progressively more forgetful over time, particularly in relation to recent events. Memory loss increases as the disorder advances and the person become disoriented and confused. The ability to concentrate declines. Abstraction, problem solving, and judgment gradually deteriorate. A failure in mathematic calculation ability, language, and visuospatial orientation occurs. Dyspraxia may appear. The mental status changes induce behavioral changes including irritability, agitation, and restlessness. Mood changes also result

FIG. 14-8 Pathologic changes in Alzheimer disease. **A,** Neuritic (senile) plaques and neurofibrillary tangles in Alzheimer disease. (Hortega silver carbonate stain; ×135.) **B,** Neurofibrillary change in cell of locus ceruleus in individual with parkinsonism. (Hematoxylin-eosin stain; ×600.) (**A,** From Kissane, 1993; **B,** from Kissane, J. M. [1985]. *Anderson's pathology* [8th ed.]. St. Louis: Mosby–Year Book.)

from the deterioration in cognition. The person may become anxious, depressed, hostile, emotionally labile, and prone to mood swings. Motor changes may occur if the posterior frontal lobes are involved. The individual exhibits rigidity (paratonia, gegenhalten), with flexion posturing, propulsion, and retropulsion. Great variability in age of onset, intensity and sequence of symptoms, and location and extent of brain abnormalities occurs among individuals with the disease.

Evaluation and Treatment

The diagnosis of Alzheimer disease is made by ruling out other causes of a dementing process. The history, including the mental status examination and the course of the illness, is used for diagnosis. The course of the disorder is highly variable, usually developing over 5 years or more.

The treatment of Alzheimer disease is directed at decreasing the need for the impaired cognitive function by a compensation technique, such as memory aids, maintaining those cognitive functions that are not impaired, and maintaining or improving the general state of hygiene, nutrition, and health. Environmental manage-

ment, counseling, education, pharmacotherapy, and health promotion measures provide the foundation on which a comprehensive treatment program is built.

ALTERATIONS IN CEREBRAL HOMEOSTASIS

Increased Intracranial Pressure

Intracranial pressure normally is 5 to 15 mm Hg, or 60 to 180 cm H_2O. **Increased intracranial pressure** may result from an increase in intracranial content (as occurs with tumor growth), edema, excess cerebrospinal fluid, or hemorrhage. A rise in intracranial pressure necessitates an equal reduction in volume of the other contents. The most readily displaced content of the cranial vault is cerebrospinal fluid (CSF). If intracranial pressure remains high after CSF displacement out of the cranial vault, cerebral blood volume is altered, which causes *stage 1* of intracranial hypertension. Vasoconstriction and external compression of the venous system occur in an attempt to further decrease the intracranial pressure. Thus, during the first stage of intracranial hypertension, intracranial pressure may not change because of the effective compensatory mechanisms. Cerebrospinal fluid is reduced through increased reabsorption. Blood volume is reduced by compression of intracranial veins. Small increases in volume, however, cause an increase in pressure and the pressure may take longer to return to baseline. Clinical manifestations at this stage usually are subtle and often transient and include episodes of confusion, drowsiness, and slight pupillary and breathing changes.

If intracranial pressure is still high, a state of intracranial hypertension occurs. With continued expansion of the intracranial content, the resulting increase in intracranial pressure may exceed the brain's compensatory capacity to adjust to the increasing pressure. In this state, the pressure begins to compromise neuronal oxygenation, and systemic arterial vasoconstriction occurs in an attempt to elevate the systemic blood pressure sufficiently to overcome the increased intracranial pressure. This stage is called *stage 2* of intracranial hypertension.

As intracranial pressure begins to approach arterial pressure, the brain tissues begin to experience hypoxia and hypercapnia, and the individual's condition rapidly deteriorates. Clinical manifestations include decreasing levels of arousal, Cheyne-Stokes respirations and/or central neurogenic hyperventilation, pupils that become sluggish and dilated, widened pulse pressure, and bradycardia.

Dramatic sustained rises in intracranial pressure are not seen until all the compensatory mechanisms have been exhausted. Once decompensation begins, dramatic rises in intracranial pressure occur over a very short period of time. **Autoregulation**, the compensatory alteration in the diameter of the intracranial blood vessels designed to maintain a constant blood flow during changes in cerebral perfusion pressure, is lost with progressively increased intracranial pressure. Accumulating carbon dioxide may still cause vasodilation at the local tissue level, but now without autoregulation this vasodilation causes the hydrostatic (blood) pressure in the vessels to drop and blood volume to increase. The brain volume is thus further enhanced and intracranial pressure continues to rise. This is called *stage 3* of intracranial hypertension. Small increases in volume cause dramatic increases in intracranial pressure, and the pressure takes much longer to return to baseline. As the intracranial pressure begins to approach systemic blood pressure, cerebral perfusion pressure falls and cerebral perfusion slows dramatically. The brain tissues experience severe hypoxia and acidosis.

Increased intracranial pressure in one compartment of the cranial vault is not evenly distributed throughout the other vault compartments. In the last stage of intracranial hypertension, called *stage 4* of intracranial hypertension, brain tissue shifts (herniates) from the compartment of greater pressure to a compartment of lesser pressure (Fig. 14-9). With this shift in brain tissue, the herniating brain tissue's blood supply is compromised, causing further ischemia and hypoxia in the herniating tissues. The herniated brain tissues increase the volume of content within the lower pressure compartment, exerting pressure on the brain tissue that normally occupies that compartment, thus impairing that tissue's blood supply. Small hemorrhages frequently develop in the involved brain tissue. Obstructive hydrocephalus may develop. The herniation process markedly and rapidly increases intracranial pressure. Mean systolic arterial pressure soon equals intracranial pressure, and cerebral blood flow ceases at this point.

Herniation Syndromes
Supratentorial Herniation

The three types of supratentorial herniation syndromes are (1) uncal (temporal lobe, lateral transtentorial) herniation, (2) central (transtentorial) herniation, and (3) cingulate gyrus herniation. **Uncal herniation** occurs when the uncus or hippocampal gyrus, or both, shifts from the middle fossa through the tentorial notch into the posterior fossa, compressing the ipsilateral third cranial nerve, then the contralateral third cranial nerve, and finally the mesencephalon. Uncal herniation generally is caused by an expanding mass in the lateral region of the middle fossa. The classic manifestations of uncal herniation are a decreasing level of consciousness, pupils that become sluggish before fixing and dilating (first the ipsilateral, then the contralateral pupil), Cheyne-Stokes respirations (which later shift to central neurogenic hyperventilation), and the appearance of decorticate, then later decerebrate, posturing.

Central herniation is the straight downward shift of the diencephalon through the tentorial notch. Causes of central herniation are injuries or masses located around the outer perimeter of the frontal, parietal, or occipital lobes, extracerebral injuries around the central apex (top) of the cranium, bilaterally positioned injuries or masses, and unilateral cingulate gyrus herniation. The individual experiencing transtentorial herniation rapidly passes from a conscious to an unconscious state; from Cheyne-Stokes respirations to apnea; from small, reactive pupils to dilated and fixed pupils; and from decortication to decerebration.

Cingulate gyrus herniation occurs when the cingulate gyrus shifts under the falx cerebri. Little is known about the clinical manifestations of this type of herniation.

Infratentorial Herniation

Two types of infratentorial herniation syndromes may occur. In the most common infratentorial herniation syndrome, a cerebellar tonsil shift through the foramen magnum because of increased pressure within the pos-

FIG. 14-9 Herniation. A, Normal relationship of intracranial structures. **B,** Shift of intracranial structures. **C,** Downward herniation of the cerebellar tonsils into the foramen magnum.

FIG. 14-10 Brain edema. Intercellular lakes of high protein content fluid. (Hematoxylin-eosin stain; ×90.) (From Kissane, 1993.)

terior fossa. The clinical manifestations of this downward infratentorial herniation are an arched stiff neck, paresthesias in the shoulder area, decreased consciousness, respiratory abnormalities, and pulse rate variations. Occasionally the pressure force is such that an upward transtentorial herniation of a cerebellar tonsil or the lower brainstem results. No specific set of clinical manifestations is associated with this infratentorial herniation syndrome.

Cerebral Edema

Cerebral edema is an increase in the fluid content of brain tissue (Fig. 14-10). Cerebral edema causes an increase in extracellular or intracellular tissue volume after brain insult from trauma, infection, hemorrhage, tumor, ischemia, infarct, or hypoxia. The harmful effects of cerebral edema are caused by the distortion of blood vessels, the displacement of brain tissues, and the eventual herniation of brain tissue from one brain compartment to another.

Four types of cerebral edema are (1) vasogenic edema, (2) cytotoxic (metabolic) edema, (3) ischemic edema, and (4) interstitial edema. **Vasogenic edema** is clinically the most important type. It is caused by the increased permeability of the capillary endothelium of the brain after injury to the vascular structure. The result is a disruption in the blood-brain barrier. Plasma proteins leak into the extracellular spaces, drawing water to them, and the water content of the brain parenchyma increases. Vasogenic edema starts in the area of injury and spreads with preferential accumulation in the white matter of the ipsilateral side because the parallel myelinated fibers separate more easily. Edema then promotes more edema because of ischemia from increasing pressure.

Clinical manifestations of vasogenic edema include focal neurologic deficits, disturbances of consciousness, and a severe increase in intracranial pressure. Vasogenic edema resolves by slow diffusion.

In **cytotoxic (metabolic) edema**, toxic factors directly affect the cellular elements of the brain parenchyma (neuronal, glial, and endothelial cells), causing failure of the active transport systems. The cells lose their potassium and gain larger amounts of sodium. Water follows by osmosis into the cell, so that the cells swell. Cytotoxic edema principally occurs in the gray matter and may increase vasogenic edema.

Ischemic edema follows cerebral infarction. The ischemia has components of both vasogenic and cytotoxic edema. Soon after the onset of ischemia, the initial edema is confined to the intracellular compartment. During the following hours and then over several days, brain cells begin to undergo necrosis and die, releasing lysosomes. In this autodigestive process, the blood-brain barrier's permeability is increased.

Interstitial edema is seen most often with noncommunicating hydrocephalus (see Chapter 15). The edema is caused by transependymal movement of cerebrospinal fluid from the ventricles into the extracellular spaces of the brain tissues. The brain fluid volume thus is increased predominantly around the ventricles. The hydrostatic pressure within the white matter increases, and the size of the white matter is reduced because of the rapid disappearance of myelin lipids.

ALTERATIONS IN EMOTIONS AND EMOTIONAL CONTROL

Emotions such as anger, hostility, envy, fear, and love all guide behavior and are largely mediated by the limbic system. Alterations in emotions or emotional control arise from dysfunction in the limbic system, in the hypothalamus, which choreographs the behaviors that accompany emotional states, or in the cerebral cortex, especially the neural tracts of the frontal lobes that project to the limbic system to exert inhibiting and modulating effects. Changes in the physical, chemical, or electrical status of the frontal lobes, limbic system, or hypothalamus may be associated with significant changes in emotions and behavior. Changes in emotions and behavior can result from abscesses, tumors, hemorrhages, metabolic disorders, and intoxication states.

Pathophysiology

Damage to the frontal lobes and frontolimbic tracts that project inhibitory influences to the limbic system frees the limbic system and leaves it unchecked to generate an array of emotions. Behavior then becomes erratic and unpredictable. Pathologic processes within the limbic system itself may produce a deficiency in emotional response, either a lack of arousability (as in the depressive disorder) or excessive arousability, as in certain psychomotor seizures or acute anxiety states.

Hypothalamic dysfunction may excessively arouse the limbic system by supplying too much epinephrine, the fear-producing hormone and neurotransmitter, to the limbic system, resulting in an acute anxiety state or producing associated behaviors without inducing the feelings. For example, tumors that involve the tracts projecting from the hypothalamus are associated with raging behaviors, but the feeling of anger or rage is not present.

Clinical Manifestations

Common among all types of frontal lobe damage is a change in the experience and expression of emotion. The clinical manifestations associated with frontal lobe dysfunction range from excessive, seemingly purposeless activity to spontaneity. Irritability, impulsiveness, mood swings, mood shifts, inability to tolerate frustration, and loss of control occur frequently. Clinical manifestations can include depression, mania, hyperactivity, acute anxiety, acute confusional states, and dementia.

Evaluation and Treatment

Evaluation of alterations in emotion include several strategies: physical and psychologic examinations, CT scans, magnetic resonance imaging (MRI), EEG, and obtaining appropriate blood chemistries. Treatment is directed at preventing injury, including suicide, medically or surgically treating the underlying cause, instituting appropriate drug therapy and psychotherapy, and providing support and guidance to the family. Drugs used to achieve symptomatic control alter the levels of neurotransmitters within the brain tissues. For example, diazepam (Valium) and other drugs compete for the receptors ordinarily occupied by epinephrine so that level of arousal is decreased.

ALTERATIONS IN MOTOR FUNCTION

Movements are complex patterns of activity controlled by the CNS. Movements are influenced by the cerebral cortex, the pyramidal system, the extrapyramidal sys-

TABLE 14-17

Alterations in Muscle Tone

Alterations	Characteristics	Cause
Hypotonia	Passive movement of a muscle mass with little or no resistance	Thought to be caused by decreased muscle spindle activity as a result of decreased excitability of neurons
Flaccidity	Muscles may be rapidly moved without resistance Associated with limp, atrophied muscles and paralysis	Occurs typically when nerve impulses necessary for muscle tone are lost
Hypertonia	Increased muscle resistance to passive movement May be associated with paralysis May be accompanied by muscle hypertrophy	Results when the lower motor unit reflex arc continues to function but is not mediated or regulated by higher centers
Spasticity	A gradual increase in tone causing increased resistance until tone suddenly is reduced, which results in clasp-knife phenomenon	Exact mechanism unclear; appears to arise from an increased excitability of the alpha motor neurons to any input because of absence of the descending inhibition of the pyramidal systems
Gegenhalten (paratonia)	Resistance to passive movement, which varies in direct proportion to force applied	Exact mechanism unclear: associated with frontal lobe injury
Dystonia	Sustained involuntary twisting movement	Produced by slow muscular contraction
Rigidity	Muscle resistance to passive movement of a rigid limb that is uniform in both flexion and extension throughout the motion	Occurs as a result of constant, involuntary contraction of muscle
Plastic, or lead-pipe	Increased muscular tone relatively independent of degree of force used in passive movement; does not vary throughout the passive movement	Associated with basal ganglion damage
Cogwheel	The uniform resistance may be interrupted by a series of brief jerks resulting in movements much like a rachet, "cogwheel" phenomenon	Associated with basal ganglion damage
Gamma	Characterized by extensor posturing (decerebrate rigidity)	Loss of excitation of extensor inhibitory areas by the cerebral cortex decreasing the inhibition of alpha and gamma motor neurons
Alpha		Loss of cerebellum input to lateral vestibular nuclei

tem, and the motor units. Dysfunction in any of these areas can cause motor dysfunction. General motor dysfunctions may produce changes in muscle tone, movement, and complex motor performance.

Alterations in Muscle Tone

Normal muscle tone involves a slight resistance to passive movement. The resistance is smooth, constant, and even throughout the range of motion. The abnormalities of muscle tone are presented in Table 14-17.

Hypotonia

In **hypotonia** (decreased muscle tone) passive movement of a muscle occurs with little or no resistance. Hypotonia is thought to be due to decreased muscle spindle activity secondary to decreased excitability of neurons. Hypotonia is caused by pure pyramidal tract damage (a rare occurrence) and cerebellar damage. A pure pyramidal tract injury produces hypotonia and weakness. The hypotonia contributes to the ataxia and intention tremor in cerebellar damage and manifests with minimal weakness, with normal or slightly exaggerated reflexes. Hypotonia, often described as flaccidity (a state in which the muscle may be rapidly moved without resistance), occurs when nerve impulses necessary for muscle tone are lost, such as in spinal cord injury or cerebrovascular accident.

Individuals with hypotonia report that they tire easily (asthenia) or are weak, signs that can be observed during their activity attempts. They may have difficulty rising from a sitting position, sitting down without using arm support, and walking up and down stairs, as well as an inability to stand on their toes. Because of their weakness, accident proneness during locomotion and self-care activities is commonplace. Inasmuch as the joints become hyperflexible in hypotonic states, persons with hypotonia may be able to assume positions that require extreme joint mobility. The joints may appear loose, and the knee jerks are pendulous.

The muscle mass atrophies because of decreased input entering the motor unit. Muscle cells gradually are replaced by connective tissue and fat. The muscles are flabby on palpation and are flat in appearance. Fasciculations may be present in some cases.

Hypertonia

In **hypertonia** (increased muscle tone) passive movement of a muscle occurs with resistance. Four types of hypertonia are described: spasticity, gegenhalten (paratonia), dystonia, and rigidity.

Spasticity results from hyperexcitability of the stretch reflexes (overactivation of the alpha motor neurons) and is associated with damage to the motor, premotor, and supplementary motor areas, as well as lateral corticospinal tract damage. Spasticity is accompanied by increased deep tendon reflexes (hyperflexia) and the spread of reflexes (**clonus**).

Gegenhalten (**paratonia**) manifests as resistance to passive movement that varies in direct proportion with the force applied and is associated with frontal lobe injury. **Dystonia** manifests as sustained, involuntary twisting movements caused by slow muscle contraction and may be due to a failure in appropriate reciprocal inhibition of the muscles. Injury to the putamen or its outflow tracts also is associated with hemidystonia.

Rigidity produced by tonic reflex activity mediated by gamma motor neurons may be continuous or intermittent in nature. The involved muscles are firm and tense; the increase in muscle movement is even and uniform throughout the range of passive movement. Four types of rigidity are described: plastic or lead-pipe rigidity, cogwheel rigidity, gamma rigidity, and alpha rigidity (see Table 14-17).

Individuals with hypertonia may report that they tire easily (asthenia) or are weak. Passive and active movement is equally affected, except in paratonia, in which

more active than passive movement is possible. As a result of hypertonia and weakness, accident proneness during locomotion and self-care activities is commonplace.

The muscles may atrophy because of decreased use of the muscles. However, hypertrophy occasionally may occur in some diseases. Hypertrophy results from overstimulation of muscle fibers. Overstimulation occurs when the motor unit reflex arc remains intact and functioning but is not inhibited by higher centers. The loss of inhibition and the constant state of excitation cause continual muscle contraction, resulting in enlargement of the muscle mass. The muscles are firm on palpation.

Alterations in Movement

Movement requires a change in the contractile state of muscles. Abnormal movements may occur when a variety of CNS dysfunctions alter muscular innervation. Movement disorders are not well understood. Current knowledge has come predominantly from the areas of neuropharmacology and experimental therapeutics. The neurotransmitter dopamine has an apparent role in motor function. Some movement disorders (such as the akinesias) result from too little dopaminergic activity, whereas others (such as chorea, ballism, and tardive dyskinesia) result from too much dopaminergic activity. Still others are not primarily related to dopamine function. Movement disorders are not necessarily associated with mass, strength, or tone but are neurologic dysfunctions with either a decreased amount of movement or an excess of movement.

Muscle strength is quantitatively evaluated on a scale of 0 to 4+, in which 4+ is normal and 0 indicates an inability to move against gravity. Degrees of abnormal muscle strength range from **paresis** (weakness) to **paralysis** (inability of a muscle group to overcome gravity). Sites of paresis and paralysis are named in different ways. **Hemiparesis** refers to weakness on one side of the body; **hemiplegia** indicates paralysis on one side of the body. These conditions result from dysfunction, such as a tumor or cerebral vascular accident, in the brain or brainstem.

Paraplegia refers to paralysis of the lower extremities, whereas **quadriplegia** refers to paralysis of all four extremities. Both paraplegia and quadriplegia may be caused by dysfunction of the spinal cord. Upper cord damage results in quadriplegia, and lower cord damage preserves upper extremity function and causes paraplegia (spinal cord injury is discussed in Chapter 15).

Hyperkinesia

Hyperkinesia (excessive movements) represents the second broad category of abnormal movements. Within this category are a number of specific dysfunctions (Table 14-18). Also included under the general category of

TABLE 14-18

Types of Hyperkinesia

Type	Characteristics	Causes
Chorea*	Nonrepetitive muscular contractions, usually of the extremities of face; random pattern of irregular, involuntary rapid contractions of groups of muscles; disappears with sleep, decreases with resting; increases with emotional stress and attempted voluntary movement	Associated with excess concentration of or a supersensitivity to dopamine within basal ganglia
Athetosis*	Disorder of distal-muscle postural fixation; slow, sinuous, irregular movements most obvious in the distal extremities, more rhythmic than choreiform movements and always much slower; movements accompany characteristic hand posture; slowly fluctuating grimaces	Occurs most commonly as a result of injury to the putamen of the basal ganglion; exact pathophysiologic mechanism is not known
Ballism	Disorder of proximal-muscle postural fixation with wild flinging movement of the limbs; movement is severe and stereotyped, usually lateral; does not lessen with sleep; ballism is most common on one side of the body, a condition termed *hemiballism*	Results from injury to subthalamus nucleus (one of the nuclei that comprise the basal ganglia); thought to be due to reduced inhibitory influence in the nucleus, a release phenomenon; hemiballism results from injury to the contralateral subthalamic nucleus
Hyperactivity	State of prolonged, generalized, increased activity that is largely involuntary but may be subject to some voluntary control; not highly stereotyped but rather manifests as continuous changes in total body posture or in excessive performance of some simple activity, such as pacing under inappropriate circumstances	May be due to frontal and reticular activating system injury
Wandering	Tendency to wander without regard for environment	"Release" phenomenon; associated with bilateral injury to globus pallidus or putamen
Akathisia	Special type of hyperactivity; mild compulsion to move (usually more localized to legs); severe frenzied motion possible; movements are partly voluntary and may be transiently suppressed; carrying out the movement brings a sense of relief; a frequent complication of antipsychotic drugs	Dopaminergic transmission may be involved
Tremor at rest	Rhythmic, oscillating movement affecting one or more body parts	Caused by regular contraction of opposing groups of muscles
Parkinsonian tremor	Regular, rhythmic, slow flexion-extension contraction; involves principally the metacarpophalangeal and wrist joints; alternating movements between thumb and index figure described as "pill rolling"; disappears during voluntary movement	Loss of inhibitory influence of dopamine in the basal ganglia, causing instability of basal ganglial feedback circuit within the cerebral cortex

*Choreoathetosis involves both chorea and athetosis; precise pathophysiology unknown.

TABLE 14-18

Types of Hyperkinesia—cont'd

Type	Characteristics	Causes
Postural tremor		
Asterixis (tremor of hepatic encephalopathy)	Irregular flapping movement of the hands accentuated by outstretching arms	Exact mechanisms responsible unknown; thought to be related to accumulation of products normally detoxified by the liver
Metabolic	Rapid, rhythmic tremor affecting fingers, lips, and tongue; accentuated by extending the body part	Occurs in conditions associated with disturbed metabolism or toxicity, as in thyrotoxicosis (hyperthyroidism), alcoholism, and chronic use of barbiturates; exact mechanism responsible unknown
Essential (familial)	Tremor of fingers, hands, and feet; absent at rest, but accentuated by extension of body part, prolonged muscular activity, and stress	Not associated with any other neurologic abnormalities; cause unknown
Intentional tremor		
Cerebellar	Tremor initiated by movement, maximal toward end of movement	Occurs in disease of the dentate nucleus (one of the deep cerebellar nuclei responsible for efferent output) and the superior cerebellar peduncle (a stalklike structure connected to the pons); caused by errors in feedback from the periphery and errors in preprogramming goal-directed movement
Rubral	Rhythmic tremor of limbs that originates proximally by movement	Results from lesions involving the dentatorubrothalamic tract (a spinothalamic tract connecting the red nucleus in the reticular formation and the dentate nucleus in the cerebellum)
Myoclonus	Series of shocklike contractions that cause throwing movements of a limb; usually appear at random but frequently triggered by sudden startle; do not disappear during sleep	Associated with an irritable nervous system and spontaneous discharge of neurons; structures associated with myoclonus include the cerebral cortex, cerebellum, reticular formation, and spinal cord

hyperkinesias are dyskinesias, that is, abnormal involuntary movements.

Paroxysmal dyskinesias are abnormal, involuntary movements that occur as spasms. The type of dyskinesia varies depending on the specific disorder.

Tardive dyskinesia is the involuntary movement of the face, trunk, and extremities. Although the condition occurs occasionally in individuals with Parkinson disease, it usually occurs as a side effect of prolonged phenothiazine drug therapy. The antipsychotic drugs bind to the dopamine receptor, somehow altering the receptor so that it mimics the effect of too much dopamine. The most common symptom of tardive dyskinesia is rapid, repetitive, stereotypic movements. Most characteristic is continual chewing with intermittent protrusions of the tongue. Stereotypic movements are believed to be a form of excessive dopaminergic activity.

Other movement disorders under this category are (1) complex repetitive movements, including automatism, stereotype, complex tics, compulsions, perseverations, and mannerisms; (2) positivism (excessive reactions to certain stimuli); and (3) paroxysmal excessive activity, including cataplexy and excessive startle reaction.

Hypokinesia

Hypokinesia (decreased movement) is loss of voluntary movement despite preserved consciousness and normal peripheral nerve and muscle function. Types of hypokinesia include paresis/paralysis, akinesia, bradykinesia, and loss of associated movement.

Paresis/Paralysis

Paresis (weakness) is impairment of motor function, that is, partial paralysis with incomplete loss of muscle power. **Paralysis** is loss of motor function, that is, inability of a muscle group to overcome gravity. Two subtypes of paresis/paralysis are described: upper motor neuron paresis/paralysis and lower motor neuron paresis/paralysis (Table 14-19).

TABLE 14-19

Upper and Lower Motor Neuron Syndromes

Factor	Upper motor neuron syndromes*	Lower motor neuron syndromes†
Distribution of affected muscles	Muscle groups are affected; when movement is possible, the proper relationship among agonists, antagonists, synergists, and fixators is preserved	Individual muscles may be affected
	Synkinesias (residual movements) are present; attempts to move paralyzed part causes a variety of associated movements; movements of normal limb may cause imitative or mirror movements in the paralyzed limb	Individual muscles may be affected
Muscle tone	Hypertonia, specifically spasticity	Hypotonia, flaccidity
Tendon reflexes	Hyperreflexia with extensor plantar reflex present	Hyporeflexia, no abnormal reflexes present
Atrophy	Slight, caused by disuse	Pronounced atrophy
Fasciculations	Absent	May be present

*Pyramidal motor syndromes.
†All are motor unit syndromes.

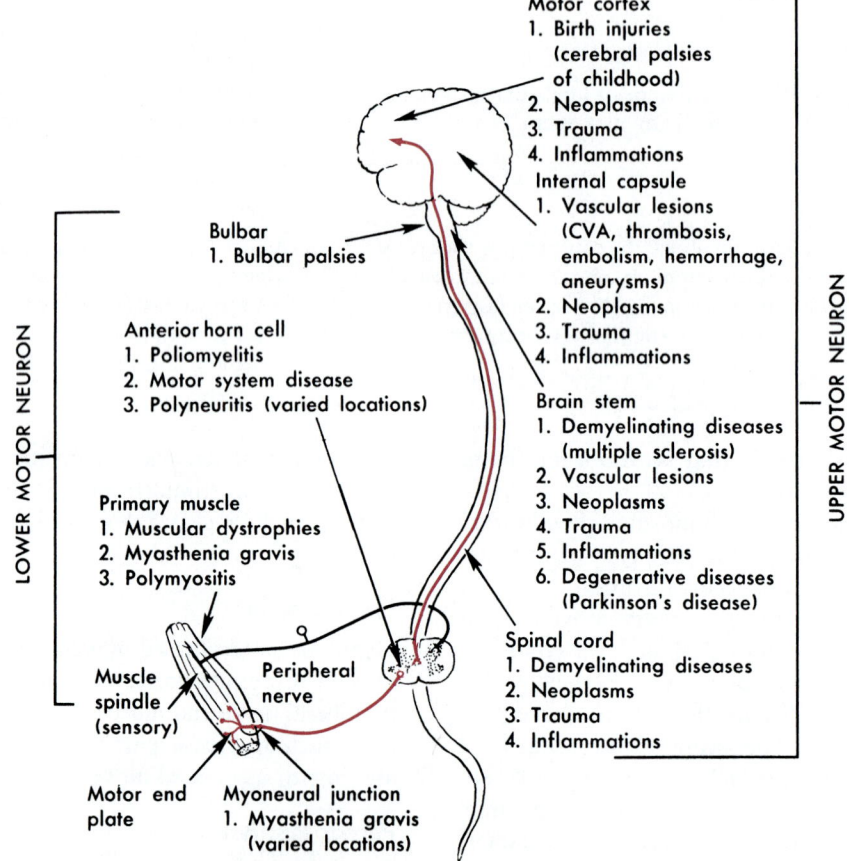

FIG. 14-11 Disturbances in motor function. Disturbances in motor function are classified pathologically along upper and lower motor neuron structures. It should be noted that the same pathologic condition occurs at more than one site in upper motor neuron, *above right.* A few pathologic conditions involve both upper and lower motor neuron structures, as in amyotrophic lateral sclerosis, for example. Other lesion sites include myoneural junction and primary muscle, making it possible to classify conditions as neuromuscular and muscular, respectively. (Modified from Chusid, 1985.)

Upper motor neuron syndromes. Upper motor neuron paresis/paralysis is known also as spastic paresis/paralysis, and many different terms are used to describe a specific paresis/paralysis. **Hemiparesis/hemiplegia** is paresis/paralysis of the upper and lower extremities on one side. **Diplegia** is the paralysis of both upper or lower extremities as a result of cerebral hemisphere injuries. **Paraparesis/paraplegia** refers to weakness/paralysis of the lower extremities. **Quadriparesis/quadriplegia** refers to paresis/paralysis of all four extremities. Both paraparesis/paraplegia and quadriparesis/quadriplegia may

be caused by dysfunction of the spinal cord. Upper cord damage results in quadriparesis/quadriplegia, and lower cord damage preserves upper extremity function and causes paraparesis/paraplegia (spinal cord injury is discussed in Chapter 15).

Upper motor neuron paresis/paralysis is associated with a pyramidal motor syndrome. The **pyramidal motor syndrome** is a series of motor dysfunctions that result from interruption of the pyramidal system (Figs. 14-11 and 14-12). The injury may be in the cerebral cortex, the subcortical white matter, the internal capsule,

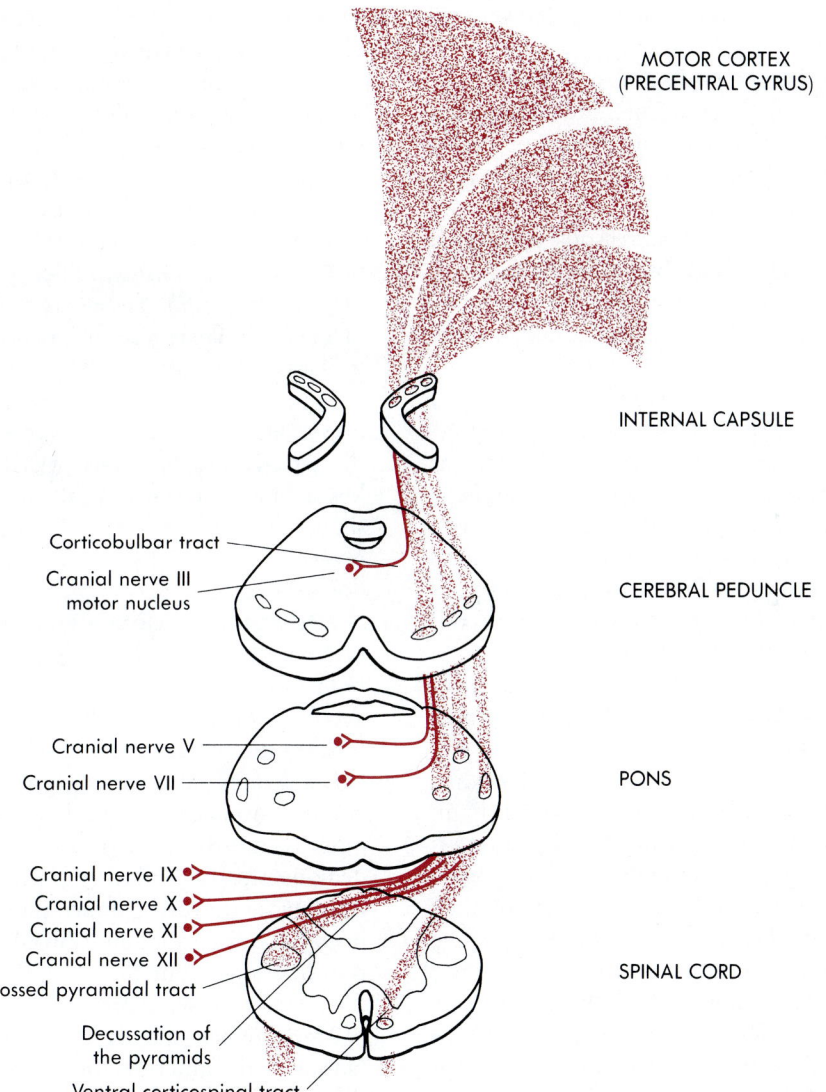

FIG. 14-12 Structures making up upper motor neuron, or pyramidal system. Pyramidal system fibers are shown to originate primarily in cells in precentral gyrus of motor cortex; to converge at internal capsule; to descend to form central third of cerebral peduncle; to descend further through pons, where small fibers are given off to cranial nerve motor nuclei along the way; to form pyramids at medulla, where most of the fibers decussate; and then to continue to descend in lateral column of white matter of spinal cord. A few fibers descend without crossing at medulla level. (Modified from original painting by Frank H. Netter, M.D.; from Ciba Collection of Medical Illustrations. Copyright by Ciba Pharmaceutical Co., Division of Ciba-Geigy Corp. All rights reserved.)

the brainstem, or the spinal cord. The clinical manifestations of a pure pyramidal injury without other damage are not known, but bilateral interruption of the pyramidal system in monkeys causes hypotonic paralysis, although much control of movement eventually returns. In human beings, however, injury generally involves more than merely the interruption of the pyramidal system, so that an upper motor neuron paralysis occurs, which indicates involvement of several motor pathways.

The distribution of clinical manifestations varies, depending on the location of the lesion, although certain features are constant. Excessive movements such as clonus and spasms occur regularly, and much variation exists depending on the suddenness of onset and the age of the individual.

When the pyramidal system is destroyed below the level of the pons, spinal shock occurs. **Spinal shock** is the complete cessation of spinal cord functions below the lesion. It is characterized by complete flaccid paralysis, absence of reflexes, and marked disturbances of bowel and bladder function. The reasons for spinal shock are not fully understood, but a major factor is the sudden destruction of the efferent pathways. If destruction occurs more slowly, spinal shock may not develop (see Chapter 15).

If the pyramidal system is interrupted above the level of the pons, the hand and arm muscles are greatly affected. Paralysis rarely involves all the muscles on one side of the body, however, even when the hemiplegia results from complete damage to the internal capsule. Bilateral movements, such as those of the eye, jaw, and larynx, are affected only slightly if at all. The limbs are predominantly affected. Because of their bilateral control, trunk muscles are much less influenced.

Paralysis associated with a pyramidal motor syndrome rarely remains flaccid for a prolonged length of time. After a few days or weeks, a gradual return of spinal reflexes marks the end of spinal shock. Reflexes then become hyperactive, and muscle tone is significantly increased, particularly in antigravity muscles. Spasticity is common, although rigidity occasionally occurs. Most often, passive range-of-motion causes the "clasp-knife" phenomenon, probably because of the activation of the two varieties of stretch receptors: (1) the muscle spindles and (2) the Golgi tendon organ. (Muscle function is discussed in Chapter 38.) With pyramidal motor syndrome, the flexors of the arms and extensors of the legs are predominantly affected.

Lower motor neuron syndromes. Lower (primary, alpha) motor neurons are the large motor neurons in the anterior (or ventral) horn of the spinal cord, the motor nuclei of the brainstem, and the axons that originate from these nerve cell bodies (to course in the anterior spinal roots and the spine or in the cranial nerves to reach skeletal muscles) (Fig. 14-13). Dysfunction in this motor system impairs movement, both voluntary and involuntary. The degree of paralysis or paresis is proportional to the number of lower motor neurons affected. If only a portion of the motor units that supply a muscle are affected, only partial paralysis (or paresis) results. If all the motor units are affected, a complete paralysis results. Other clinical manifestations also are proportional to the degree of dysfunction, but the precise manifestations depend on the location of the dysfunction in the motor unit and in the CNS.

Small motor (gamma) neurons, which function to maintain muscle tone and protect the muscle from injury, also are necessary for normal motor movement. These neurons depend on input from the muscle spindle (arriving through an afferent limb rising to the cord). Dysfunction in this motor system impairs tone and reduces the tendon reflexes, causing hyporeflexia. The muscle is lax and soft, with a decrease in normal tone, or hypotonia, which impairs voluntary and involuntary motor movements. The muscles become susceptible to damage from hyperextensibility because the normal protective mechanisms, which prevent muscle fiber injury, are impaired. The degree of tone loss and the loss of tendon reflexes are proportional to the dysfunction in these reflex motor units.

Generally, in a pathologic process the large and small motor neuron systems are equally affected. Therefore the paresis and paralysis caused by a disorder of the lower motor neurons is called a **flaccid paresis/paralysis** because the muscle has reduced or absent tone and is accompanied by hyporeflexia or **areflexia** (loss of tendon reflexes).

A few **gamma neuropathies** (small motor neuron disorders) affect only the gamma motor system. A manifestation of these disorders is a marked reduction in the deep tendon reflexes, which are strikingly out of proportion to the degree of muscle weakness present.

Denervated muscles (i.e., muscles that have lost their nervous system input) undergo atrophy over weeks to months, mostly from disuse. Denervated muscles also demonstrate fasciculations, which are seen as muscle rippling or quivering under the skin. Occasionally, denervated muscles cramp. **Fibrillation** (isolated contraction of a single muscle fiber) also may occur, although this manifestation is not visible clinically.

Amyotrophies. Lower motor neuron syndromes originating in the anterior horn cells or the motor nuclei of the cranial nerves are called **amyotrophies.** Paralytic poliomyelitis is the prototype of these disorders. It involves a severe inflammatory reaction in motor neurons, some of which do not survive, leaving a permanent lower motor neuron syndrome.

Several pathologic processes may give rise to an amyotrophy. A virally induced or postinfectious/postvaccination inflammatory process may injure or destroy an

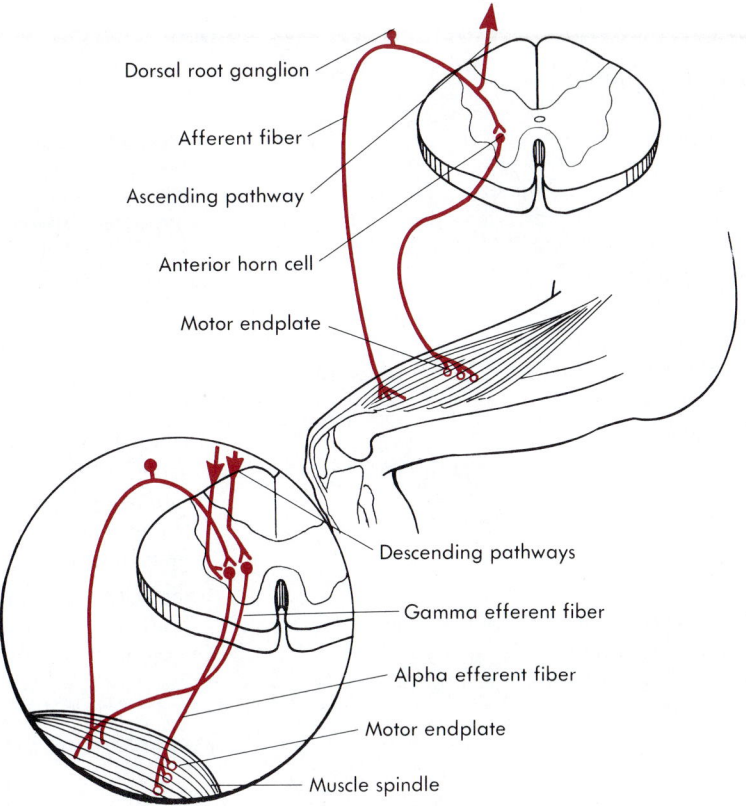

Dorsal root ganglion
Afferent fiber
Ascending pathway
Anterior horn cell
Motor endplate

Descending pathways
Gamma efferent fiber
Alpha efferent fiber
Motor endplate
Muscle spindle

FIG. 14-13 **Structures making up lower motor neuron, including motor (efferent) and sensory (afferent) elements.** *Top,* *Anterior horn cell* (in anterior gray column of spinal cord and its axon), terminating in motor end plate as it innervates extrafusal muscle fibers in quadriceps muscle. *Detailed enlargement,* Sensory and motor elements of γ-loop system. γ-Efferent fiber is shown innervating polar, or end, region of muscle spindle (sensory receptor of skeletal muscle). Contraction of muscle spindle fibers stretches central portion of spindle and causes afferent spindle fiber to transmit impulse centrally to cord. Muscle spindle afferent fibers in turn synapse on anterior horn cell and are transmitted by way of γ-efferent fibers to skeletal (extrafusal) muscle, causing it to contract. Muscle spindle discharge is interrupted by active contraction of extrafusal muscle fibers. (Modified from Truex & Carpenter. [1969]. *Human neuroanatomy* [6th ed.]. Baltimore: Williams & Wilkins.)

terior horn cells or cranial nerve cell bodies. Most of these inflammatory processes are mild and are followed by rapid cellular recovery.

In the amyotrophies, muscle strength, muscle tone, and muscle bulk are affected in the muscles innervated by the involved motor neurons. The paresis and paralysis associated with anterior horn cell injury are segmental, but because each muscle is supplied by two or more roots, the segmental character of the weakness may be difficult to recognize. When cranial nerve motor nuclei are affected (these lack nerve roots and have only small rootlets near the point of exit from the brainstem), the distribution of the motor weakness follows that of the peripheral nerve. The weakness may involve distal muscles, proximal muscles, and the muscles of midline structures. Hypotonia and hyporeflexia/areflexia are present.

The atrophy associated with amyotrophy is segmental when the anterior horn cells of the spinal cord are involved and follows the distribution of the peripheral

nerve when the motor nuclei of the cranial nerves are affected. The atrophy may be in distal, proximal, or midline muscles. Fasciculations are particularly associated with primary motor neuron injury, and muscle cramps are common. Mild fatigue is a frequent complaint. If the pathologic process is limited to the primary motor neuron, no sensory changes are evident.

Because degenerative disorders cause loss of nerve cells in the anterior horn or motor nuclei, the surviving cells are small, shrunken, and filled with lipofuscin. Lost neurons are replaced by astrocytes. The roots or rootlets are thin and the muscles show denervation and atrophy.

Several brainstem syndromes involve damage to one or more of the cranial nerve nuclei. These are called **nuclear palsies** (Table 14-20) and may be caused by vascular occlusion, tumor, aneurysm, tuberculosis, or hemorrhage.

The anterior horn cells and the motor nuclei of the

TABLE 14-20

Examples of Nuclear Palsy Syndromes

Type of nuclear palsy	Causes	Associated clinical manifestations
Ocular	Upper brainstem tumor Cerebrovascular disease in the vertebrobasilar system Aneurysm Intramedullary bleeding	Other cranial nerve signs Contralateral spastic hemiparesis/hemiplegia Contralateral hyperreflexia Contralateral extensor plantar reflex
Facial	Pontine tumor Cerebrovascular disease in the vertebrobasilar system	Paresis/paralysis of both the upper and lower facial muscles for both voluntary movement and emotionally induced movement
Vagal	Intramedullary tumor Cerebrovascular disease in the vertebrobasilar system	Ipsilateral loss of pain and temperature sensations of the face Contralateral spastic arm and leg paresis/hemiplegia Ipsilateral cerebellar signs
Hypoglossal	Intramedullary tumor Cerebrovascular disease in the vertebrobasilar system	Contralateral loss of position sense and vibration in the arm and leg Contralateral spastic hemiparesis/hemiplegia

cranial nerves may be secondarily affected in many severe pathologic processes that primarily involve the peripheral nerves. The condition may extend proximally to affect the nerve roots or rootlets and the motor neurons themselves, a process commonly seen, for example, in Guillain-Barré syndrome. If sufficient numbers of motor neurons are destroyed, permanent loss of motor function results because regeneration of the damaged axons requires a living neuronal cell body.

A group of degenerative disorders principally cause progressive motor cell atrophy. One of these is **progressive spinal muscular atrophy** in which the anterior horn cells of the spinal cord are the affected motor neurons. This disorder occurs in adults and closely resembles the familial progressive muscular atrophies that occur in infants and children and are considered inherited metabolic disorders (see Chapter 40). If the motor nuclei of the cranial nerves are affected instead of the anterior horn cells, the disorder is labeled **progressive bulbar palsy,** so named because the myelencephalon originally was called the bulb and a degenerative process causes a progressively more serious condition. When any lower motor neuron syndrome involves the cranial nerves that arise from the bulb (i.e., cranial nerves IX, X, and XII), the dysfunction is called a **bulbar palsy.**

The clinical manifestations of bulbar palsy include paresis or paralysis of the jaw, face, pharynx, and tongue musculature. Articulation is affected, especially articulation of the lingual (r, n, l), labial (b, m, p, f), dental

(d, t), and palatal (k, g) consonants. Modulation is impaired, making the voice rasping or nasal. Pharyngeal reflexes are diminished or lost. Palate and vocal cord movement during phonation is impaired, and chewing and swallowing are affected. The facial muscles are weak, and the face appears to droop. The jaw jerk is decreased. Atrophy eventually becomes apparent, as do fasciculations. All these manifestations become progressively worse, leading to aspiration, malnutrition, possible dehydration, and an inability to communicate verbally.

Akinesia

Akinesia is a decrease in associated and voluntary movements. There is a disturbance in the time it takes to perform a movement. Akinesia is related to dysfunction of the extrapyramidal system, as in parkinsonism. Pathogenesis is related to either a deficiency of dopamine or a defect of the postsynaptic dopamine receptors, which occurs in parkinsonism (see Chapter 15).

Bradykinesia

Bradykinesia is slowness of voluntary movements. There is a disturbance in the time it takes to perform a movement. In bradykinesia, all voluntary movements become slow, labored, and deliberate. Bradykinesia consists of (1) difficulty in initiating movements, (2) difficulty in continuing movements smoothly, and (3) difficulty in performing synchronous (at the same time) and consecutive tasks. Difficulty in initiating movements ranges from slight hesitancy to severe **freezing** (transient, helpless immobility). Each intended movement requires effort. Difficulty in continuing motions smoothly causes jerky, irregular, rapid movements, which then decrease in rate and amplitude until they stop. The individual is scarcely aware of the cessation. Difficulty in performing synchronous and consecutive tasks means that each motor act is performed separately. The individual is unable to integrate two acts or to change from one motor pattern to the next with a single smooth motion.

Loss of associated neuron syndromes

In hypokinesia the normal, habitually associated movements that provide skill, grace, and balance to voluntary movements are lost. Decreased associated movements accompanying emotional expression cause an expressionless face, a statuelike posture, absence of speech inflection, and absence of spontaneous gestures. Decreased associated movements accompanying locomotion cause reduction in arm and shoulder movements, in hip swinging, and in rotary motion of the cervical spine.

Alterations in Complex Motor Performance

The alterations in complex motor performance include disorders of posture (stance), disorders of gait, and disorders of expression.

Disorders of Posture (Stance)

An inequality of tone in muscle groups because of a loss of normal postural reflexes results in a posturing of limbs. Many reflex systems govern tone and posture, but the most important factor in posture control is the stretch reflex, in which stretching of extensor (antigravity) muscles causes increased extensor tone and inhibited flexor tone. Four types of disorders of postures are described: (1) dystonic posture, (2) decerebrate posture, (3) basal ganglion posture, and (4) senile posture. Equilibrium and balance are disrupted when postural disorders are present.

Dystonia is the maintenance of an abnormal posture through muscular contractions. When muscular contractions are sustained for several seconds, they are called **dystonic movements,** such as in choreoathetoid movements associated with high levels of L-dopa; when contractions last for longer periods, they are called **dystonic postures,** such as in torticollis. Dystonic postures may last for weeks, causing permanent fixed contractures. Dystonia has been associated with basal ganglia abnormality, but the exact pathophysiologic mechanisms are unknown. One particularly relevant dystonic posture already discussed in this chapter is decorticate (striatal posture or upper motor neuron dysfunction

posture), which may be unilateral or bilateral in occurrence. **Decorticate posture** (also referred to as **antigravity posture** or **hemiplegic posture**) is characterized by upper extremities flexed at the elbows and held close to the body and by lower extremities that are externally rotated and extended. Decorticate posture is believed to occur when the brainstem, which facilitates the antigravity position, is not inhibited by the motor function of the cerebral cortex. Upper motor neuron posture is more commonly described as the arm flexed at the elbow with a wrist drop, the leg inadequately bent at the knee, with the hip excessively circumabducted, and the presence of a foot drop.

Decerebrate posture refers to increased tone in extensor muscles and trunk muscles, with active tonic neck reflexes. When the head is in a neutral position, all four limbs are rigidly extended. The decerebrate posture is caused by severe injury to the brain and brainstem, resulting in overstimulation of the postural righting and vestibular reflexes.

Basal ganglion posture refers to a stooped, hyperflexed posture with a narrow-based, short-stepped gait. This posture abnormality results from the loss of normal postural reflexes and not from defects in proprioceptive, labyrinthine, or visual function. Dysfunctional equilibrium results from the loss of postural stability, and thus the individual is unable to make the appropriate postural adjustment to tilting or loss of balance and falls instead. Dysfunctional righting is the inability to right oneself when changing from a lying or crouching to a standing position or when rolling from the supine to the lateral or prone position. Dysfunctional postural fixation is the involuntary flexion of the head and neck, causing the person difficulty in maintaining an upright trunk position while standing or walking. Basal ganglion dysfunction accounts for this posture.

Senile posture is characterized by an increasingly flexed posture similar to that caused by basal ganglion dysfunction. The posture is associated with frontal lobe dysfunction, but the primary pathophysiology is not well described.

Disorders of Gait

Four predominant types of gait are: (1) upper motor neuron dysfunction gait, (2) cerebellar (ataxic) gait, (3) basal ganglion gait, and (4) senile gait (pseudoparkinsonian gait). As with posture, equilibrium and balance are affected with gait disturbances.

Several upper motor neuron gaits exist. In the presence of mild upper motor neuron dysfunction, a foot drop may appear only with fatigue. The individual may complain of hip and leg pain. A **spastic gait,** which is associated with unilateral injury, manifests by a shuffling gait with the leg extended and held stiff, causing a scraping over the floor surface. There is an impaired leg swing around the body rather than an appropriate lifting and placing of the leg. The foot may drag on the ground, and the person tends to fall to the affected side. A **scissors gait** is associated with bilateral injury and spasticity. The legs are abducted, causing them to touch each other. As the person walks, the legs are still swung around the body but then cross in front of each other because of adduction. Injury to the pyramidal system accounts for these gaits.

A **cerebellar gait** manifests as a wide-based gait with the feet apart and often turned outward or inward for greater stability. The pelvis is held stiff, and the trunk seems to be independent of the trunk. The individual staggers when walking. Cerebellar dysfunction accounts for this particular gait.

A **basal ganglion gait** and a **senile gait** are both broad-based gaits. The person walks with small steps and a decreased arm swing. The head and body are flexed and the arms semiflexed and abducted while the legs are flexed and rigid in more advanced states. Basal ganglion and frontal lobe dysfunction, respectively, account for these two gaits.

Disorders of Expression

Disorders of expression involve the motor aspects of communication and include (1) hypermimesis, (2) hypomimesis, and (3) dyspraxias/apraxias. Hypermimesis is a disinhibition phenomenon that most commonly manifests as pathologic laughter or crying. Pathologic laughter is associated with right hemisphere injury, and pathologic crying is associated with left hemisphere injury. The exact pathophysiology is not known. Hypomimesis manifests as aprosody, the loss of emotional language. Receptive aprosody involves an inability to understand emotion in speech and facial expression, whereas expressive aprosody involves the inability to express emotion in speech and facial expression. Aprosody is associated with right hemisphere damage.

Dyspraxia/apraxia is the inability to perform purposeful or skilled motor acts in the absence of paralysis, sensory loss, abnormal posture and tone, abnormal involuntary movement, incoordination, or inattentiveness. Dyspraxia/apraxia is associated with vascular disorders, trauma, tumor, degenerative disorders, infections, and metabolic disorders. Because the performance of any activity is composed of three parts—(1) the development of the idea, (2) the formulation of the plan of execution, and (3) the motor performance of the activity—three types of dyspraxia have been described (Table 14-21).

True dyspraxias occur when the connecting pathways between the left and right cortical areas are interrupted (Fig. 14-14). Dyspraxias may result from any pathologic process that disrupts the cortical areas necessary for the conceptualization and execution of a complex motor act or the communication pathways within the left hemisphere or between the hemispheres.

FIG. 14-14 Pathways disrupted in dyspraxias. Formulation of the idea of the motor act is believed to originate in the region of the supramarginal gyrus in the inferior left parietal lobe. This area is connected via associational pathways to the left premotor cortex. The left premotor cortex is connected through the corpus callosum to the right premotor and motor areas. An injury that interrupts the pathways between the left supramarginal gyrus and the premotor region produces a dyspraxia that involves the entire body. An injury that disrupts the callosal pathways produces a dyspraxia of the left side of the body only.

TABLE 14-21

The Dyspraxias

Types	Description	Location
Dyspraxias describing the components of a motor act		
Ideational	Impairment in ability to comprehend, grasp an idea, or retain the idea of the described act	Diffuse cortical injury
Ideomotor	Impairment in ability to perform a given motor act correctly (but habitual motor acts may be performed spontaneously or repetitiously)	Associated with left hemisphere dysfunction in the posterosuperior area of temporal lobe and in the inferior areas of parietal and frontal lobes
Motor (limb kinetic)	Impairment in use of kinesthetic memory patterns (engrams) necessary to perform a motor act; automatic tone and position changes necessary for action do not occur	Associated with premotor area dysfunction
Dyspraxias related to specific types of motor activity		
Constructional	Impairment in ability to draw or use shapes and designs accurately	May occur with visual association area dysfunction and with posterior parietal lobe injury; more severe when right posterior hemisphere is involved rather than left hemisphere because right parietooccipital area controls visuospatial orientation
Dressing	Impairment in ability to clothe oneself correctly; agnosia and neglect syndrome contribute to dressing dyspraxia and may be entirely responsible for its occurrence	Associated with right parietal injury
Speech	An articulation disorder resulting from impairment of capacity to program positioning of speech musculature and sequencing of muscle movements for volitional production of speech sounds (phonemes); a motor dyspraxia	Associated with dysfunction in Broca's area in left hemisphere
	When involvement is more extensive than just the muscles used in speech articulation, the dysfunction is called *facial dyspraxia*	Associated with dysfunction in Broca's area and premotor areas controlling the facial muscles
Gait (frontal lobe ataxia, frontal lobe gait)	Impairment in ability to use extremities effectively and in coordinated manner during ambulation, producing a low, shuffling gait with small, hesitant steps	Associated with loss of integration between cortex and basal ganglion related to stance and locomotion; not a true dyspraxia because dysfunction is not purely cortical
Callosal	An ideomotor dyspraxia in which right arm and leg use is normal but with impairment in ability to perform the same movements with left arm and leg	Associated with anterior corpus callosum injury

Extrapyramidal Motor Syndromes

Because the extrapyramidal system encompasses all the motor pathways except the pyramidal system, two types of motor dysfunction make up the **extrapyramidal motor syndromes**: (1) the basal ganglia motor syndromes and (2) the cerebellar motor syndromes. Unlike pyramidal motor syndromes, both extrapyramidal motor syndromes result in movement or posture disturbance without significant paralysis, along with other distinctive symptoms (Table 14-22).

Basal Ganglia Motor Syndromes

Basal ganglia motor syndromes are movement disorders that involve either a paucity or an excess of movements. Stress and nervous tension typically worsen the symp-

toms, whereas relaxation improves motor performance. Akinesia may occur despite normal strength. Involuntary movements, such as tremor, chorea, ballism, athetosis, and dystonia, also may occur and probably are caused by the loss of the normal modulating effects of the corpus striatum and other parts of the basal ganglia.

Basal ganglia motor syndromes also are characterized by alterations in muscle tone and posture. Rigidity, together with the cogwheel phenomenon, is present in all muscle groups but is most prominent in those that maintain flexed position. Postural abnormalities result from the loss of normal postural reflexes. Dysfunctional equilibrium results from the loss of postural stability.

The symptoms of basal ganglia motor syndromes are

TABLE 14-22

Pyramidal Versus Extrapyramidal Motor Syndrome

Manifestations	Pyramidal motor syndrome	Extrapyramidal motor syndrome
Unilateral movement	Paralysis of voluntary movement	Little or no paralysis of voluntary movement
Tendon reflexes	Increased tendon reflexes	Normal or slightly increased tendon reflexes
Involuntary movements	Absence of involuntary movements	Presence of tremor, chorea, athetosis, or dystonia
Muscle tone	General spasticity in muscles (e.g., clasp phenomenon) Hypertonia present in flexors of arms and extensors of legs	May have rigidity or intermittent rigidity (cogwheel rigidity)

TABLE 14-23

Cerebellar Motor Syndromes

Syndrome	Location of dysfunction	Characteristics
Lateral	Intermediate and lateral corticonuclear zone of anterior and posterior lobes	Muscles of the extremities on the side of the injury become hypotonic with decreased resistance to passive movement Reflexes hypoactive Ataxia (uncoordination) of extremities is prevalent during voluntary movement, causing some degree of gait disturbance Dysmetria (extremity overshooting its target) occurs Intentional and postural tremors present
Medial	Medical corticonuclear zone and flocculonodular lobe	Disequilibrium of head and trunk during static posture and locomotion Posture and gait are normal Oculomotor disturbances are common Muscle tone is normal Extremities are not ataxic in voluntary movement

explained as an imbalance of dopaminergic and cholinergic activity in the corpus striatum. A relative excess of cholinergic activity produces akinesia and hypertonia. A relative excess of dopaminergic activity produces hyperkinesia and hypotonia. The precise mechanisms by which imbalances of these striatal neurotransmitters cause specific symptoms are unknown.

Cerebellar Motor Syndromes

Cerebellar motor syndromes involve the cerebellum and may result in (1) loss of muscle tone, (2) difficulty with coordination of voluntary movements, (3) minor degrees of muscle weakness, tendency toward fatigue, and impairment of associated movements, and (4) disorders of equilibrium and gait. Cerebellar effects are chiefly ipsilateral (primarily affecting the same side of the body), so that damage to the right cerebellum generally causes symptoms on the right side of the body. Predominant symptoms depend on the area of damage within the cerebellum. The two cerebellar syndromes are the lateral syndrome and the medial syndrome (Table 14-23).

Diagnosis of a cerebellar motor syndrome is based on the symptoms, but these may vary because of the individual's attempts at compensation. Furthermore, the nervous system often can operate well despite destruction of parts of the cerebellum, although the mechanisms responsible for this retained function are not fully understood.

SUMMARY REVIEW

Alterations in Cognitive Systems

1 Full consciousness is an awareness of oneself and the environment with an ability to respond to external stimuli with a wide variety of responses.

2 Consciousness has two components, arousal and content of thought.

3 Decreased level of arousal occurs by diffuse bilateral cortical dysfunction, bilateral subcortical (reticular formation, brainstem) dysfunction, and localized hemispheric dysfunction.

4 An alteration in breathing pattern and level of coma reflects the level of brain dysfunction.

5 Pupillary changes reflect changes in level of brainstem function, drug action, and response to hypoxia and ischemia.

6 Abnormal eye movements, including nystagmus and divergent gaze, reflect alterations in brainstem function.

7 Level of brain function manifests by changes in generalized motor responses or no responses.

8 Loss of cortical inhibition associated with decreased consciousness includes abnormal flexor and extensor movements.

9 Cerebral death or irreversible coma represents permanent brain damage, with an ability to maintain cardiac, respiratory, and other vital functions.

10 Brain death results from irreversible brain damage, with an inability to maintain internal homeostasis.

11 Arousal returns in vegetative states, but content of thought is absent.

12 Seizures represent a sudden, chaotic discharge of cerebral neurons, with transient alterations in brain function. Seizures may be generalized or focal and can result from cerebral lesions, biochemical disorders, trauma, or epilepsy.

13 With a deficit in selective attention, mediated by brainstem and parietal lobe structures, the individual cannot focus on selective stimuli and thus neglects those stimuli.

14 In dysmnesia and amnesia, some past memories are lost and new memories cannot be stored.

15 Concept formation, predominantly mediated by the parietal lobe, is fundamental to abstraction.

16 Prefrontal areas mediate vigilance, reasoning, and executive system functions.

17 With a vigilance deficit, the person cannot concentrate and is distractible.

18 With reasoning deficits, the person cannot analyze sufficiently to problem solve.

19 With executive system deficits, the person is unmotivated, unable to set goals, plan, initiate and carry out a plan, or self-evaluate and use the feedback.

20 Some specific disorders of content of thought (cognition) are agnosias, dysphasias, acute confusional states, and dementias, including Alzheimer disease.

21 Agnosias are a defect of recognition and may be tactile, visual, or auditory. They are due to dysfunction in the primary sensory area or the interpretive areas of the cerebral cortex.

22 Dysphasia is an impairment of comprehension or production of language. Dysphasia may be expressive or sensory.

23 Aphasia is loss of language comprehension or production.

24 Wernicke dysphasia is a disturbance in understanding all language, both verbal and reading comprehension.

25 Conductive dysphasias result from disruption of temporal lobe fibers, with a failure to repeat words but an ability to initiate speech, writing, and reading aloud.

26 Anomic dysphasia is an inability to name objects, persons, or qualities.

27 Transcortical dysphasias involve an inability to repeat and recite.

28 Broca aphasia is an expressive dysphasia of speech and writing but with retention of comprehension.

29 Global aphasia involves both anterior and posterior speech areas, with both expressive and receptive aphasia.

30 Acute confusional states are characterized chiefly by a loss of the vigilance system and, in the case of delirium, an intense autonomic nervous system hyperactivity.

31 Alzheimer disease is a chronic irreversible dementia that can be related to beta amyloid metabolism.

Alterations in Cerebral Homeostasis

1 Increased intracranial pressure may result from edema, excess cerebrospinal fluid, hemorrhage, or tumor growth. When intracranial pressure approaches arterial pressure, hypoxia and hypercapnia produce brain damage.

2 Cerebral edema is an increase in the fluid content of the brain resulting from infection, hemorrhage, tumor, ischemia, infarct, or hypoxia.

3 The shifting or herniation of brain tissue from one compartment to another disrupts the blood flow of both compartments and damages brain tissue.

4 Supratentorial herniation involves temporal lobe and hippocampal gyrus shifting from the middle fossa to posterior fossa; transtentorial herniation with a downward shift of the diencephalon through the tentorial notch; and shifting of the cingulate gyrus herniation under the falx.

5 The most common infratentorial herniation is a shift of the cerebellar tonsils through the foramen magnum.

Alterations in Emotions and Emotional Control

1 Disorders of the frontal lobes, limbic system, or hypothalamus may be associated with a broad range of changes in emotion and behavior.

Alterations in Motor Function

1 Motor dysfunction may be characterized as alterations of motor tone, movement, and complex motor performance.

2 Hypotonia and hypertonia are the main categories of altered tone.

3 Four types of hypertonia exist: spasticity, gegenhalten, dystonia, and rigidity.

4 Hyperkinesia and hypokinesia are the main categories of altered movement.

5 Included in the category of hyperkinesia are chorea, athetosis, ballism, akathisia, tremor, and myoclonus.

6 Types of hypokinesia include paresis/paralysis, akinesia, bradykinesia, and loss of associated movements.

7 Two subtypes of paresis/paralysis are described: upper motor neuron paresis/paralysis and lower motor neuron paresis/paralysis.

8 An upper motor neuron syndrome is characterized by paresis/paralysis, hypertonia, and hyperreflexia.

9 Interruption of the pyramidal tract below the pons results in spinal shock.

10 Lower motor neuron syndromes manifest by impaired voluntary and involuntary movements.

11 Partial paralysis occurs with only partial loss of alpha motor neurons, and total paralysis is complete loss of alpha motor neurons. Loss of gamma motor neurons impairs muscle tone and decreases tendon reflexes.

12 Amyotrophy (e.g., poliomyelitis) is a lower motor neuron syndrome involving the anterior horn cells, with loss of muscle tone and strength resulting in segmental paresis and hyporeflexia.

13 Nuclear palsies involve damage to the cranial nerve nuclei.

14 Bulbar palsies involve cranial nerves IX, X, and XII.

15 Alterations in complex motor performance include disorders of posture (stance), disorders of gait, and disorders of expression.

16 Disorders of posture include dystonic posture, decerebrate posture, basal ganglion posture, and senile posture.

17 Disorders of gait include upper motor neuron gaits, cerebellar gait, basal ganglion gait, and senile gait.

18 Disorders of expression include hypermimesis, hypomimesis, and dyspraxia/apraxia.

19 Dyspraxia is an impairment of the conceptualization or execution of a complex motor act.

20 Extrapyramidal motor syndromes include basal ganglia and cerebellar motor syndromes.

21 Basal ganglia disorders manifest by alterations in muscle tone and posture, including rigidity, involuntary movements, and loss of postural reflexes.

22 Cerebellar motor syndromes result in loss of muscle tone, difficulty with coordination, and disorders of equilibrium and gait.

KEY TERMS

Abstract formation deficit, 495
Acute confusional state, 502
Agnosia, 498
Akinesia, 518
Alzheimer disease (senile disease complex), 504
Amnestic dementia, 504
Amyotrophy, 516
Aphasia, 498
Apraxia, 520
Areflexia, 516
Attentional dementia, 504
Aura, 490
Autoregulation, 507
Basal ganglia motor syndrome, 522
Basal ganglion gait, 520
Basal ganglion posture, 519
Brain death, 486
Bulbar palsy, 518
Central herniation, 507
Cerebellar gait, 520
Cerebellar motor syndrome, 523
Cerebral death, 486
Cerebral edema, 508
Cingulate gyrus herniation, 507
Clonic phase, 490
Clonus, 511
Cognitive dementia, 504
Concept formation deficit, 495
Content of thought, 478
Cytotoxic (metabolic) edema, 509
Decerebrate posture, 519
Decorticate posture (antigravity posture, hemiplegic posture), 519
Diplegia, 515
Dysmnesia, 494
Dysphasia, 498
Dyspraxia, 520
Dystonia, 511, 519
Dystonic movement, 519
Dystonic posture, 519
Echolalia, 502
Epilepsy, 487
Epileptogenic focus, 488
Executive system deficit, 494
Expressive dysphasia, 502
Extinction, 498
Extrapyramidal motor syndrome, 522
Fibrillation, 516
Flaccid paresis/paralysis, 516

Freezing, 519
Gamma neuropathy, 516
Gegenhalten (paratonia), 511
Generalized seizure, 488
Hemiparesis, 511, 515
Hemiplegia, 511, 515
Hyperkinesia, 511
Hypertonia, 511
Hypotonia, 510
Increased intracranial pressure, 506
Intentional dementia, 504
Interstitial edema, 509
Intracranial pressure, 506
Ischemic edema, 509
Isolated speech center, 502
Locked-in syndrome, 487
Metabolic arousal alteration, 478
Mirror focus, 490
Mixed transcortical dysphasia, 502
Neglect syndrome, 498
Neurofibrillary tangle, 505
Nuclear palsy, 517
Paralysis, 511, 513
Paraparesis, 515
Paraplegia, 511, 515
Paresis, 511, 513
Paroxysmal dyskinesia, 513
Partial seizure (focal seizure), 488
Postictal state, 488
Prodroma, 490
Progressive bulbar palsy, 518
Progressive spinal muscular atrophy, 518
Psychogenic arousal alteration, 478
Pyramidal motor syndrome (upper motor neuron syndrome), 515
Quadriparesis, 515
Quadriplegia, 511, 515
Reasoning deficit, 495
Recent memory system, 494
Remote memory deficit, 494
Rigidity, 511
Scissors gait, 520
Secondary generalization, 488
Seizure, 487
Selective attention deficit, 490
Senile gait, 520
Senile plaque, 505
Senile posture, 519
Sensory inattentiveness, 498
Spastic gait, 519

Spasticity, 511
Spinal shock, 516
Status epilepticus, 488
Structural arousal alteration, 478
Tardive dyskinesia, 513
Tonic phase, 490
Transcortical dysphasia, 502
Transcortical sensory dysphasia, 502
Uncal herniation, 507
Vasogenic edema, 508
Vegetative state, 478
Vigilance deficit, 495

REFERENCES

Adams, R. D. (1985). The convulsive state and idiopathic epilepsy. In G. W. Thorn et al. (Eds.), *Harrison's principles of internal medicine,* New York: McGraw-Hill.

Boss, B. J. (1984). Dysphasia, dyspraxia, and dysarthria: Distinguishing features (Part I). *Journal of Neurosurgical Nursing, 16*(3), 151-160.

Chipps, E., Clanin, N., & Campbell, V. (1992). *Neurologic disorders.* St. Louis: Mosby–Year Book.

Chusid, J. G. (1970). *Correlative neuroanatomy and functional neurology* (15th ed.) (p. 793). Los Altos, CA: Lange Medical Publications.

Coyle, J. T., Price, D. L., & DeLong, M. R. (1983). Alzheimer disease: A disorder of cortical cholinergic innervation. *Science, 217,* 1184-1189.

Danison, A. N. (1986). New concepts in relation to the pathophysiology of Alzheimer disease. In M. Briley, A. Kato, & M. Weber (Eds.), *New concepts in Alzheimer disease.* London: Macmillan Press, Ltd.

Golde, T. E., Estus, S., Younkin, L. H., Selkoe, D. J., & Younkin, S. G. (1992). Processing of amyloid protein precursor to potentially amyloidogenic derivatives. *Science, 255,* 728.

Hardy, J. A., & Higgins, G. A. (1992). Alzheimers disease: The amyloid cascade hypothesis. *Science, 256,* 184.

Heilman, D. M., Watson, R. T., & Greer, M. (1977). *Handbook for differential diagnosis of neurologic signs and symptoms.* New York: Appleton-Century-Crofts.

Hickey, J. V. (1992). *The clinical practice of neurological and neurosurgical nursing.* Philadelphia: J. B. Lippincott.

Hooper, C. (1992). Researchers say Alzheimer protein is ubiquitous. *Journal of NIH Research, 4*(10), 29-30.

Kissane, J. M. (Ed.). (1993). *Anderson's pathology* (9th ed.). St. Louis: Mosby–Year Book.

Kolata, G. B. (1981, March). Clues to the causes of senile dementia. *Science, 211,* 1032-1033.

Kolata, G. B. (1983). Clues to Alzheimer disease emerge. *Science, 219,* 941-942.

Mancall, E. L. (1981). *Alper's and Mancall's essentials of the neurologic examination.* Philadelphia: F. A. Davis.

Morris, M., & Rhodes, M. (1972). Guidelines for the care of confused patients. *American Journal of Nursing, 72*(9), 1632.

Mozar, H. N., Bal, D. G., & Howard, J. T. (1987). Perspectives on the etiology of Alzheimer disease. *Journal of the American Medical Association, 257,* 1503-1507.

Plum, F., & Posner, J. B. (1980). *The diagnosis of stupor and coma.* Philadelphia: F. A. Davis.

Rudy, E. B. (1984). *Advanced neurological and neurosurgical nursing.* St. Louis: Mosby–Year Book.

Sims, N. R., Bowen, D. M., Allen, S. J., Smith, C. C. T., Neary, D., Thomas, D. J., & Daniston, A. N. (1983). Presynaptic cholinergic dysfunction in patients with dementia. *Journal of Neurochemistry, 40,* 503-509.

Strittmatter, W. J., Saunders, A. M., Schmeckel, D., Pericak-Vance, M., Enghild, J., Salvensen, G. S., & Roses, A. D. (1993). Apolipoprotein E: High affinity binding to β-amyloid and increased frequency of type 4 allele in familial Alzheimer's. *Proceedings of the National Academy of Science, 90* (5), 1977-1981.

Thompson, J. M., McFarland, G. K., Hirsch, J. E., & Tucker, S. M. (1993). *Mosby's clinical nursing* (3rd ed.). St. Louis: Mosby–Year Book.

VanBroeckhoven, C., Backhoven, H., Cruts, M., DeWinter, G., Bruyland, M., Cras, P., & Martin, J. J. (1992). Mapping of a gene predisposing to early-onset Alzheimer's disease to chromosome 14q24.3. *Nature Genetics, 2.*

Walker, A. E. (1985). *Cerebral death* (3rd ed.). Baltimore: Urban & Schwarzenberg.

SUGGESTED READINGS

Adams, R. D., & Victor, M. (1989). *Principles of neurology.* New York: McGraw-Hill.

Andrus, C. (1991). Intracranial pressure: Dynamics and nursing management. *Journal of Neuroscience Nursing, 23*(2), 85-92.

Barlow, H. B., & Mollon, J. D. (Eds.). (1982). *The senses.* Cambridge: Cambridge University Press.

Barnes, D. M. (1987). Defect in Alzheimer is on chromosome 21. *Science, 235,* 846-847.

Boss, B. J. (1982). Acute mood and behavior disturbances of neurological origin: Acute confusional states. *Journal of Neurosurgical Nursing, 14*(2), 61-68.

Boss, B. J. (1983). The dementias. *Journal of Neurosurgical Nursing, 15*(2), 87-97.

Boss, B. J. (1989). *Head injury, part III: Motor status.* Skokie, IL: Rehabilitation Nurses' Foundation.

Boss, B. M. (1991). Attention and memory systems: Nursing assessment. *Axon, 12*(4), 89-94.

Boss, B. M. (1991). Cognitive systems: Nursing assessment and management in the critical care environment. *AACN Clinical Issues in Critical Care Nursing, 2*(4), 685-698.

Brown, M. M., & Hachjinski, V. C. (1991). Acute confusional states, amnesia, and dementia. In J. D. Wilson, E. Braunwald, K. J. Isselbacher, R. G. Petersdorf, J. B. Martin, A. S. Fauci, & R. K. Root (Eds.), *Harrison's principles of internal medicine* (pp. 183-193). New York: McGraw-Hill.

Drachman, D.B. (Ed.). (1991). Myasthenia gravis. In J. D. Wilson, E. Braunwald, K. J. Isselbacher, R. G. Petersdorf, J. B. Martin, A. S. Fauci, & R. K. Root (Eds.), *Harrison's principles of internal medicine* (pp. 2118-2121). New York: McGraw-Hill.

Ezzell, C. (1992, March 7). Alzheimer alchemy. *Science News, 141*(10), 152-153.

Gilman, S. (1991). Ataxia and disorders of balance and gait. In J. D. Wilson, E. Braunwald, K. J. Isselbacher, R. G. Petersdorf, J. B. Martin, A. S. Fauci, & R. K. Root (Eds.), *Harrison's principles of internal medicine* (pp. 169-173). New York: McGraw-Hill.

Griggs, R. G., Bradley, W. G., & Shahani, B. (1991). Approach to the patient with neuromuscular disease. In J. D. Wilson, E. Braunwald, K. J. Isselbacher, R. G. Petersdorf, J. B. Martin, A. S. Fauci, & R. K. Root (Eds.), *Harrison's principles of internal medicine* (pp. 2088-2096). New York: McGraw-Hill.

Growdon, J. H., & Fink, J. S. (1991). Paralysis and movement disorders. In J. D. Wilson, E. Braunwald, K. J. Isselbacher, R. G. Petersdorf, J. B. Martin, A. S. Fauci, & R. K. Root (Eds.), *Harrison's principles of internal medicine* (pp. 157-169). New York: McGraw-Hill.

Michael, J. E. (1992). Vagal nerve stimulation in the treatment of intractable partial seizures: Nursing implications. *Journal of Neuroscience Nursing, 24*(1), 19-25.

Ropper, A. H., & Martin, J. B. (1991). Coma and other disorders of consciousness. In J. D. Wilson, E. Braunwald, K. J. Isselbacher, R. G. Petersdorf, J. B. Martin, A. S. Fauci, & R. K. Root (Eds.), *Harrison's principles of internal medicine* (pp. 193-200). New York: McGraw-Hill.

Rusy, K. L. (1991). Temporal lobectomy: A promising alternative. *Journal of Neuroscience Nursing, 23*(5), 320-324.

Sohlberg, M. M., & Mateer, C. A. (1989). *Introduction to cognitive rehabilitation: Theory and practice.* New York: Guilford Press.

Wassenberg, C. (1981). Common visual disorders in children. *Nursing Clinics of North America, 16*(3), 479-485.

Wilson, B. A. (1987). *Rehabilitation of memory.* New York: Guilford Press.

Wilson, B. A., & Moffat, N. (1984). *Clinical management of memory.* London: Croom Helm.

CHAPTER 15

Alterations of Neurologic Function

Barbara J. Boss
Peter M. Sunderland*
Joleen Heath*

Chapter Outline

*Contributing authors to first edition.

Alterations in central nervous system function are caused by traumatic injury, vascular disorders, tumor growth, infectious and inflammatory processes, metabolic derangements (including those arising from nutritional deficiencies and drugs/chemicals), and degenerative processes. Alterations in peripheral nervous system function involve the nerve roots (radiculopathies), a nerve plexus, or the nerves themselves (neuropathies). Disorders of the neuromuscular junction also occur.

CENTRAL NERVOUS SYSTEM (CNS) DISORDERS

Trauma
Head Trauma

Head injury is defined by the National Head Injury Foundation as a traumatic insult to the brain capable of producing physical, intellectual, emotional, social, and vocational changes. Persons at highest risk for traumatic brain injury (TBI) are young persons 15 to 24 years of age, infants 6 months to 2 years, young school-aged children, and the elderly. The male-to-female ratio for such injury is 2:1. Traumatic brain injury is highest among blacks and in the lower socioeconomic groups. Persons living in high-crime areas are at greater risk.

Traumatic brain injuries are broadly categorized into **blunt (closed) trauma** and **open (penetrating) trauma.** Blunt trauma, the more common, involves the head striking a hard surface or a rapidly moving object striking the head. The dura remains intact and brain tissues are not exposed to the environment. Blunt trauma may result in both focal brain injuries and diffuse axonal injuries (Table 15-1). When a break in (penetration of) the dura results in exposure of the cranial contents to the environment, open trauma has occurred, which results in focal brain injuries.

The most common types of traumatic brain injury are mild concussion and classical cerebral concussion (see p. 534). Seventy-five percent to 90% of head injuries are less than severe head injuries (Table 15-1). Focal brain injury and diffuse axonal injury (DAI) each account for one half of all injuries. Focal brain injury accounts for more than two thirds of head injury deaths; DAI, for fewer than one third. However, DAI accounts for the greatest number of severely disabled survivors, including persons who persist in an unresponsive state (Table 15-2).

In recent years, the surviving traumatic head injury population has changed, mostly because of focus on reducing severity of injury (e.g., passive seat restraints and air bags), reduced transport time, and improved on-the-scene medical management. Improved management of secondary and tertiary injury is also influencing the situation; acute care health professionals are beginning to

---

TABLE 15-1

Severity of Trauma Related to Trauma Injury, Onset of Clinical Manifestations, and Persistence of Clinical Manifestations

Severity of trauma	Trauma state induced		Onset of clinical manifestations	Persistence of DAI clinical manifestations
	Focal injury	DAI		
Mild blunt trauma		Mild concussion	Immediate	Hours to days
Moderate blunt trauma		Classic cerebral concussion	Immediate	Up to 6 months or longer
	Paraplegia (associated with injury to top of head)		Immediate	
	Blindness (associated with occipital injury)		Immediate	
	Delayed development of unresponsiveness (vaso-motor or vasovagal syncopal episode)		Delayed	
Severe blunt trauma		Mild DAI	Immediate	Permanent
		Moderate DAI	Immediate	Residual
		Severe DAI	Immediate	
	Acute epidural hemorrhage		Immediate to delayed (2 to 3 hours)	
	Acute contusional swelling		Delayed onset (few hours after injury)	
	Acute subdural hematoma		Delayed onset (few hours to 1 week after injury)	
	*Subacute subdural hematoma		Delayed onset (1 to few weeks)	
	Subdural hygroma		Delayed onset	
	*Traumatic cerebral hemorrhage		Delayed onset (as late as a week after injury)	

*May be seen after moderate head injury, especially in the elderly.

focus more on morbidity than mortality. As a result, persons with more severe traumatic brain injuries are being admitted to rehabilitation programs.

Cause

Most traumatic brain injuries are caused by transportation-related events and falls. Sports-related events and crime also account for a portion of traumatic brain injuries.

Related to focal brain injuries, objects (e.g., baseball bat or weapon) striking the front of the head usually produce only coup injuries (contusions and fractures) because the inner skull in the occipital area is smooth. Objects striking the back of the head usually result in both **coup** (directly below the point of impact) and **contrecoup** (on the pole opposite the site of impact) injuries because of the irregularity of the inner surface of the frontal bones (Fig. 15-1). Objects striking the side

of the head may produce coup or contrecoup injuries. The same is true for the head striking an immovable object with little velocity (e.g., a short fall).

Extradural hematomas are caused most commonly by vehicular accidents, and occasionally by minor falls and sporting accidents. A temporal fracture is the cause of 90% of temporal lobe extradural hematomas. Direct frontal lobe trauma is associated with frontal extradural hematomas. Posterior extradural hematomas are associated with a fracture across the transverse sinus from an occipital blow.

Vehicular accidents are the most common cause of subdural hematomas; 50% of subdural hematomas are associated with skull fractures. Falls, especially in the elderly or in persons with chronic alcohol abuse, are associated with chronic subdural hematomas.

Intracerebral hemorrhage is associated with the presence of contusions. This hemorrhage is caused by force-

---

TABLE 15-2		
Prognosis Related to DAI		
	1 Month	**3 Months**
Mild DAI		78% good recovery or moderate disability
		3% severe disability
		15% die, usually of secondary infection complications or associated extracranial injuries
		4% unaccounted for
Moderate DAI	26% good or moderate disability	38% good recovery
		20% moderate disability
	50% severe disability	18% severe disability
	24% succumb to complications	
Severe DAI		15% good recovery
		27% moderate to severe disability

FIG. 15-1 Coup and contrecoup head injury following blunt trauma. *1,* Coup injury: impact against object; *a,* site of impact and direct trauma to brain; *b,* shearing of subdural veins; *c,* trauma to base of brain; *2,* contrecoup injury: impact within skull; *a,* site of impact from brain hitting opposite side of skull; and *b,* shearing forces through brain. These injuries occur in one continuous motion—the head strikes the wall (coup), then rebounds (contrecoup). (From Rudy, 1984.)

G.J. Wassilchenko

ful impact, usually associated with vehicular accidents and falls from some distance.

Compound fractures are caused by objects striking the head with great force or by the head striking an object forcefully. The comments regarding contusion hold true for compound fractures. Temporal blows, related to basilar skull fractures, may produce a fracture involving the middle fossa. An occipital blow may result in a basilar fracture down the occipital bone and across the petrous pyramid. The cervical vertebrae upwardly impacting the base of the skull can produce a posterior fossa **basilar skull fracture.**

Causes of penetrating injuries are missiles (most commonly bullets fired from rifles and handguns) and sharp projectiles (such as knives, ice picks, axes, and screwdrivers). Most through-and-through injuries are from high-velocity bullets.

Related to diffuse axonal injury, mild concussion and classic cerebral concussion are particularly associated with a moving head striking a hard, unyielding object. A concussion may result from a moving object striking a stationary head, however. Moderate DAI is usually sustained by vehicular occupants and pedestrians. Sagittal or horizontal (torsional) head motion produces mild or moderate DAI. Severe DAI occurs only in coronal (lateral) head motion and is caused by vehicular injuries.

Pathophysiology

Damage originates from three mechanisms: primary, secondary, and tertiary injury. Primary injury is caused by the impact and involves neural injury, primary glial injury, and vascular response.

In primary glial injury, oligodendroglia are affected by axon injury and by direct mechanical disruption caused by debris and leakage. The vascular response is immediate at the time of injury and involves increased capillary endothelial permeability to solutes.

Secondary injury includes cerebral edema, brain swelling, hemorrhage, infection, and increased cranial pressure. Significant to secondary injury is tissue hypoxia arising from cerebral ischemia (inadequate perfusion and tissue hypoxia). Consequences of ischemia are that (1) ischemic neurons release substances that produce glial permeability to sodium (cytotoxic edema); (2) with energy failure, influxes of calcium through incompetent channels produce electrophysiologic consequences and activation of phospholipases to release free fatty acids with reoxygenation, prostaglandins, and free radicals; and (3) lactic acidosis occurs. Secondary injury occurs from compromise of circulation or brain shift.

Tertiary injury is caused by apnea, hypotension, change in pulmonary resistance, and change in electrocardiogram (ECG; specifically ST and T wave changes).

Primary injury. Insight into the nature of the injury and its potential effects can be obtained from information about the causal agent and from the nature, extent, and site of damage. Knowledge of the cellular biology of head injury has progressed dramatically over the past 15 years. Previously, no explanation existed for why persons with similar CT scans had different clinical pictures or for the electrophysiologic changes in concussion, and outcome was totally unexplained and unpredictable. Technological advances set the stage for research to uncover different, more satisfactory explanations.

Grennarelli and his associates (1982) led the way and reconceptualized traumatic brain injury. Their research and that of others have led to the position that two types of injury may occur—focal and diffuse brain injury.

Focal brain injury. Focal brain injury is specific, grossly observable brain lesions—cortical contusions, epidural hemorrhage, subdural hematoma, and intracerebral hematoma. The force of impact (translational acceleration) typically produces **contusions** from direct contact (as well as injury to the vault, vessels, and supporting structures) that, in turn, produces epidural hemorrhage, and subdural and intracerebral hematomas. The mechanisms of injury are depicted in Fig. 15-1. Damage results from compression of the skull at the point of impact and rebound effect. Contusion and bleeding occur because of small tears in blood vessels resulting from these forces. The severity of contusion is associated with the amount of energy transmitted by the skull to underlying brain tissue. In addition, the smaller the area of impact, the greater the severity of injury because the force is concentrated into a smaller area. The focal injury may be coup or contrecoup. Brain edema forms around and in damaged neural tissues, contributing to the increasing intracranial pressure. Within the contused areas are infarction and necrosis, multiple hemorrhages, and edema. The tissue has a pulpy quality. The maximum effects of injury related to contusion, bleeding, and edema peak from 18 to 36 hours after severe head injury.

Contusions (Fig. 15-2) are most commonly found in the frontal lobes, particularly at the poles and along the inferior orbital surfaces; in the temporal lobes, especially in the anterior poles and along the inferior surface; and at the frontotemporal junction. They result in changes in attention, memory, executive function (motivation; goal selection or formation; planning; maintenance and termination of motor acts; self-motivating; and use of feedback), affect, emotion, and behavior. Less commonly, contusions occur in the parietal lobes and the occipital lobes. Focal cerebral contusions are superficial, involving just the gyri. Hemorrhagic contusions may coalesce into a large confluent intracranial hematoma.

FIG. 15-3 Acute epidural hematoma. Skull fracture with tear of middle meningeal artery and vein. (From Kissane, 1993.)

FIG. 15-2 Recent contusions of frontal and temporal lobes. There is displacement of cingulate gyrus and lateral ventricles. Secondary hemorrhages have occurred in lower midbrain and upper pons. (From Kissane, 1993.)

Extradural hematomas (epidural hematomas or epidural hemorrhages) represent 1% to 2% of major head injuries and occur in all age-groups, but most commonly in 20- to 40-year-olds. An artery is the source of bleeding in 85% of extradural hematomas (Fig. 15-3); 15% result from injury to the meningeal vein or dural sinus. The temporal fossa is the most common site of extradural hematoma caused by injury to the middle meningeal artery or vein. The resulting shift of the temporal lobe medially precipitates uncal and hippocampal gyrus herniation through the tentorial notch. Extradural hemorrhages are found occasionally in the subfrontal area, especially in the young and elderly, caused by injury to the anterior meningeal artery or a venous sinus, and in the occipital-suboccipital area, which results in herniation of the posterior fossa contents through the foramen magnum.

Subdural hematomas arise in 10% to 20% of persons with traumatic brain injury. Acute subdural hematomas rapidly develop, usually within hours, and are usually located at the top of the skull (the cerebral convexities). Bilateral hematomas occur in 15% to 20% of persons. Subacute subdural hematomas develop more slowly, often over 1 or more weeks. Chronic subdural hematomas, commonly found in the elderly and alcohol abusers having some degree of brain atrophy with a subsequent increase in the extradural space, develop over weeks to months. Tearing of the bridging veins is the major cause of rapidly developing and subacutely developing subdural hematomas, although torn cortical veins or venous sinuses and contused tissue may be the source. These subdural hematomas act as expanding masses, giving rise to increased intracranial pressure that eventually compresses the bleeding vessels (Figs. 15-4 and 15-5). The displacement of brain tissue can result in a herniation syndrome.

The pathogenesis of a chronic subdural hematoma is different. The existing subdural space gradually fills with blood. A vascular membrane forms around the hematoma in approximately 2 weeks. Further enlargement takes place in some persons, but the mechanism of this enlargement is unclear.

Intracerebral hematomas occur in 2% to 3% of persons with head injuries, may be single or multiple, and are associated with contusions. Although most commonly located in the frontal and temporal lobes, intracerebral hematomas may occur in the hemispheric deep white matter. Small blood vessels are traumatized by shearing forces. The intracerebral hematoma then acts as an expanding mass, resulting in increased intracranial pressure and compression of brain tissues with resultant edema (Fig. 15-6). The pathogenesis is unclear for delayed intracerebral hematomas that may appear 1 week or more after the head injury.

Open trauma produces discrete (focal) injuries and includes compound fractures and missile injuries. A compound fracture opens a communication between the cranial contents and the environment and should be investigated whenever there are lacerations of the scalp, tympanic membrane, a sinus, eye, or mucous membranes. Such fractures may involve the cranial vault or the base of the skull (basilar skull fracture). The injury incurred from bone fragments is mainly a tangential injury (injury caused by direct contact), and occasionally, a penetrating injury. Bone fragments may lacerate or contuse brain tissues or blood vessels. In addition, cranial nerves may be damaged with a basilar skull fracture.

Missiles include bullets, rocks, shell fragments, knives, and blunt instruments. The injury incurred from a missile is a tangential injury to the coverings and the

FIG. 15-4 **Subdural hematoma.** Dura has been reflected downward, exposing neomembrane and hematoma in situ, and normal underlying pia-arachnoid and brain are exposed in upper part of field. (Courtesy Dr. H. G. Schwartz, St. Louis, MO. From Rosai, 1989.)

FIG. 15-5 **Chronic subdural hematoma.** Compression of underlying brain and lateral ventricle. Note bone formation in falx and uncal herniation on side of hematoma. (From Kissane, 1993.)

FIG. 15-6 **Hematomas.** Recent hematomas, resulting from trauma, in frontal lobes. (From Kissane, J. M.: *Anderson's pathology,* (8th ed.). St. Louis, 1985, Mosby–Year Book.)

brain (scalp lacerations), skull fractures, laceration of the meninges, and cerebral lacerations. Projectiles and debris from scalp and skull injury, when driven into the brain substance, produce a penetrating brain injury. Occasionally, projectiles are so forceful that they exit the cranial vault in addition to entering it, producing a through-and-through injury. Primary damage is localized along the path of the penetrating object and direct tissue disruption along the projectile tract results. A high-velocity bullet produces contusions at the site of entry caused by bone striking the brain tissue on impact. Bone fragments are driven inward. Air compressed in front of the bullet exerts an explosive effect on entry, producing extreme distant tissue damage and an immediate increase in intracranial pressure; a cavity many times greater than the bullet is produced because the brain tissue is propelled away from the track. The cavity and pressure produce contrecoup injuries. The intracranial volume is directly increased by the projectile and the debris. The temporary cavity collapses back onto itself, leaving a smaller, permanent cavity. Intracranial bleeding occurs into the permanent cavity and may cause the cavity to expand. Edema in and around the injured brain tissue rapidly develops; edema and bleeding contribute markedly to intracranial pressure. Because of acute ischemic damage to the tract, necrosis of tissue begins. Within hours after bullet-induced injury, tissue within 1 cm adjacent to the tract disintegrates. Demyelination of white matter affected by hemorrhage and edema occurs by the second day.

Diffuse brain injury. **Diffuse brain injury** (diffuse axonal injury, DAI) results from a shaking effect (inertial effects of mechanical input to head associated with high levels of acceleration and deceleration, effects of head motion). Rotational acceleration (twisting movement) is the primary mechanism of injury producing strains and distortions within the brain (see Fig. 15-1). The brain tissues experience shearing stresses that are set up by the rotational forces that operate when a freely moving head is struck because of the skull's motion from its attachment to the neck. Shearing, tearing, or stretching of

nerve fibers with subsequent axonal damage results. Forces applied axially as a result of centrifugal acceleration of the head establish a gradient of injury severity from the hemispheres to the brainstem (Simon & Sayre, 1987). The most severe axonal injuries are located more peripheral to the brainstem, thus accounting for the tremendous cognitive and affective impairments seen in survivors of traumatic brain injury from vehicular accidents. The frontal and temporal axonal tracts are particularly vulnerable. Damage reduces the speed of informational processing and responding, as well as disrupts attention.

The common pathologic substrate in diffuse brain injury is axonal damage (disruption). Pathophysiologically, at the time of injury, the damage can be seen only with an electron microscope and involves either numerous axons alone or axonal injury in conjunction with actual tissue tears. Areas where axons and small blood vessels are torn appear as small hemorrhages, particularly located in the corpus callosum and dorsolateral quadrant of the rostral brainstem at the superior cerebellar peduncle.

Progressively increasing numbers of damaged axons are visible 12 hours to several days after the injury. Chromatolysis of the neurons involving eccentric relocation of the nucleus, swelling of the axon hillock, and redistribution of the rough endoplasmic reticulum in the cell body is evident. During this time the torn axons, which resemble dilated sausage links, also regress into round balls called retraction balls. These retraction balls are visible with light microscopy.

The number of retraction balls increases during the first week or two but begins to diminish in 2 to 3 weeks. Clusters of microglia appear in their place. Lastly, astrocytosis (gliosis, equivalent to scarring) occurs at the sites of axonal damage. Demyelination is particularly seen in the long axon tracts of the upper brainstem.

Severity of the diffuse injury correlates with the direction and velocity of rotation, that is, how much shearing force was applied to the brainstem. Figure 15-7 illustrates the spectrum of the diffuse injury as the mag-

As magnitude increases, progress from:

FIG. 15-7 Spectrum of diffuse brain injury.

nitude increases. Diffuse axonal injury is not associated with intracranial hypertension soon after injury, but acute brain swelling (increased intravascular blood within the brain, vasodilation, and increased cerebral blood volume) frequently is seen.

Several categories of diffuse brain injury exist: mild concussion, classic concussion, mild DAI, moderate DAI, and severe DAI. An organic component is present within each category, in contrast to the previous conceptualization that concussion had no structural injury component.

Mild concussion involves temporary axonal disturbances. Cerebral cortical dysfunction related to attentional and memory systems results, but consciousness is not lost. Three forms have been described:

Grade I Confusion and disorientation accompanied by amnesia (momentary)

Grade II Momentary confusion and retrograde amnesia that develops after 5 to 10 minutes (memory loss involves only events occurring several minutes before injury)

Grade III Confusion and retrograde amnesia present from impact (also anterograde amnesia) (persists for several minutes)

Classic cerebral concussion (*Grade IV*) involves diffuse cerebral disconnection from the brainstem reticular activating system and is a phenomenon of physiologic neurologic dysfunction without substantial anatomic disruption. Evidence of this disconnection is the immediate loss of consciousness, which lasts less than 6 hours. Retrograde and anterograde (posttraumatic) amnesia is present. This type of diffuse injury frequently is associated with focal pathology, especially cerebral contusions that yield focal signs, not loss of consciousness. Two forms of classic cerebral contusion exist: uncomplicated classic cerebral concussion (without focal injury) and complicated classic cerebral concussion (accompanied by focal injury).

Diffuse axonal injury (DAI) produces prolonged traumatic coma lasting more than 6 hours because of axonal disruption. Three forms of DAI exist: mild, moderate, and severe. In **mild DAI,** posttraumatic coma lasts 6 to 24 hours. Death is uncommon, but residual cognitive, psychologic, and sensorimotor deficits may persist. Mild DAI is a relatively uncommon lesion, occurring in 8% of all severe head injuries and 19% of all cases of DAI.

In **moderate DAI,** widespread physiologic impairment exists throughout the cerebral cortex and diencephalon. Actual tearing of some axons in both hemispheres occurs. Basal skull fracture, a focal injury, is commonly associated with moderate DAI. Prolonged coma lasting more than 24 hours is present but prominent brainstem signs do not exist with moderate DAI. Recovery is often incomplete in those individuals who survive. Mod-

---

TERMS DESCRIBING PROLONGED TRAUMATIC COMA (DAI)

More commonly used terms

Brainstem contusion
Cerebral concussion (grade V, prolonged, severe)
Closed head injury
Diffuse degeneration of white matter
Diffuse injury
Edema
Shearing injury

Less commonly used terms

Central cerebral trauma
Contusion cerebri
Diffuse brain damage of immediate impact type
Diffuse neuronal injury
Diffuse white matter shearing injury
Inner cerebral trauma
Strich injury
Unspecified head injury

---

erate DAI is the most common type of DAI and is found in 20% of severe head injuries and 45% of all cases of DAI.

Severe DAI, formerly called primary brainstem injury or brainstem contusion, involves severe mechanical disruption of many axons in both cerebral hemispheres and those extending to the diencephalon and brainstem. Additional synonyms for severe DAI are listed in the box above. Severe DAI represents 16% of all severe head injuries and 36% of all cases of DAI.

Clinical Manifestations, Evaluation, and Treatment

Focal brain injury. The clinical manifestations of a contusion may include immediate loss of consciousness (generally accepted to last no longer than 5 minutes), loss of reflexes with which the individual falls to the ground, transient cessation of respiration, brief period of bradycardia, and decrease in blood pressure (lasting 30 seconds to a few minutes). A momentary increase in cerebrospinal fluid pressure and ECG and electroencephalographic (EEG) changes have been demonstrated to occur on impact. Vital signs may stabilize to normal values in a few seconds. Reflexes return next, and the person begins to regain consciousness. Returning to being fully awake and alert takes variable periods, from minutes to days. Regaining a full level of consciousness may be extremely slow, and residual deficits may persist. In some persons, full level of consciousness never really returns. Evaluation should include a complete history and physical examination. Skull and spinal x-ray films are frequently taken, and a computed tomography

(CT) scan or magnetic resonance imaging (MRI) may be done. Large contusions and lacerations with hemorrhage may be surgically excised. Otherwise treatment is directed at controlling intracranial pressure and managing symptoms.

Individuals with classic temporal extradural hematomas (i.e., over the temporal lobe) have a period of loss of consciousness at the time of injury followed by a lucid period that lasts from a few hours to a few days (if a vein is bleeding). As the hematoma accumulates, a headache of increasing severity, vomiting, drowsiness, confusion, seizure, and hemiparesis may develop. Level of consciousness may be rapidly lost as the temporal lobe herniation begins. Clinical manifestations of temporal lobe herniation also include ipsilateral pupillary dilatation and contralateral hemiparesis.

The diagnosis of an extradural hematoma is usually made with a CT scan or MRI. In some instances diagnosis is made by history and clinical findings, because time for a CT scan or MRI is not available. The prognosis is usually good if intervention is initiated before bilateral dilatation of the pupils.

Surgical therapy is evacuation of the hematoma through burr holes, which is followed by ligation of the bleeding vessel or vessels. Extradural hematomas are almost always medical emergencies.

In acute, rapidly developing subdural hematomas, the expanding clots directly compress the brain, giving rise to the clinical manifestations. As the intracranial pressure rises, the bleeding veins are compressed, and thus bleeding is self-limiting, although cerebral compression and displacement of brain tissue can cause temporal lobe herniation.

An acute subdural hematoma classically begins with headache, drowsiness, restlessness or agitation, slowed cognition, and confusion. These symptoms worsen over time and progress to loss of consciousness, respiratory pattern changes, and pupillary dilatation (i.e., the symptoms of temporal lobe herniation). These manifestations are more pronounced than focal manifestations such as dysphasia, dyspraxia, or hemiparesis. Other clinical manifestations may include homonymous hemianopia (defective vision in either the right or the left field), dysconjugate gaze, and gaze palsies.

Presenting manifestations of chronic subdural hematomas are varied. Of persons affected, 80% have chronic headaches and tenderness over the hematoma on percussion. Most persons appear to have a progressive dementia accompanied by generalized rigidity (paratonia).

Whereas most acute and subacute subdural hematomas are treated with clot evacuation through a burr hole, chronic subdural hematomas (and some that are subacute) require a craniotomy to evacuate the gelatinous blood. The membrane around a chronic subdural hematoma is then dissected away from the dura mater and arachnoid membranes. A technique for percutaneous drainage for chronic subdural hematomas has recently proved successful.

A decreasing level of consciousness is associated with an intracerebral hematoma. Coma or a confusional state from other injuries, however, can make the cause of this increasing unresponsiveness difficult to detect. Contralateral hemiplegia also may occur. As the intracranial pressure rises, clinical manifestations of temporal lobe herniation may appear. In delayed intracerebral hematoma, the presentation is similar to that of a hypertensive brain hemorrhage: sudden, rapidly progressive decreased level of consciousness with pupillary dilatation, breathing pattern changes, hemiplegia, and bilateral positive Babinski reflexes.

History and physical examination help to establish the diagnosis. CT scan, MRI, and cerebral angiography confirm the diagnosis. Evacuation of a singular intracerebral hematoma has only occasionally been helpful, mostly for subcortical white matter hematomas. Otherwise treatment is directed at reducing the intracranial pressure and allowing the hematoma to reabsorb slowly.

With open-head injury, most persons lose consciousness. The depth of the coma and the length of the unresponsive state are related to the location of injury, extent of damage, and amount of bleeding.

Open-head injury often requires surgery to debride the traumatized tissues to prevent infection and to remove blood clots to help reduce the intracranial pressure. Intracranial pressure is also managed with steroids, dehydrating agents, osmotic diuretics, or a combination of these drugs. Broad-spectrum antibiotics are administered.

The diagnosis of a compound fracture is made through physical examination, skull x-ray films, or both. The diagnosis of a basilar skull fracture is made on the basis of clinical findings. Skull x-rays often do not demonstrate the fracture, although intracranial air or air in the sinuses on x-ray film, CT scan, or MRI is indirect evidence of a basilar skull fracture.

A compound linear fracture is debrided nonsurgically in cooperative adults and surgically in children and uncooperative adults. Cranioplasty with insertion of bone or an artificial graft may be necessary. Antibiotics are administered after surgery.

Bed rest and close observation for meningitis and other complications are prescribed for a basilar skull fracture. Use of prophylactic antibiotics is controversial because studies have failed to demonstrate that they reduce the rate of infection.

Diffuse brain injury. Diffuse axonal injury is associated with physical, cognitive, psychologic/behavioral, and social consequences. Spastic paralysis, peripheral nerve injury, swallowing disorders, dysarthria, visual and hearing impairments, and taste and smell deficits are some of the physical consequences. Common cognitive deficits include disorientation and confusion, short attention span, memory deficits, learning difficulties, dysphasia, poor judgment, and perceptual deficits. Behavioral disorders that emerge include agitation, impulsiveness, blunted affect, social withdrawal, and depression.

Mild concussion is characterized by an immediate onset of clinical manifestations at time of injury and the transitory nature of clinical manifestations. A momentary rise in CSF pressure and ECG and EEG changes have been demonstrated to occur on impact in the laboratory. No loss of consciousness is experienced. The initial confusional state exists for a moment to several minutes. Amnesia for events preceding the trauma (retrograde amnesia) may be experienced. Anterograde amnesia may exist transiently. Persons may experience head pain and complain of nervousness and "not being oneself" for a short time up to a few days.

In classic cerebral concussion, loss of consciousness is up to 6 hours and there is a loss of reflexes, causing falls. Reflexes are regained as responsiveness returns. Transient cessation of respiration, brief periods of bradycardia, and a decrease in blood pressure lasting 30 seconds or less occur. Vital signs stabilize within a few seconds to within normal limits. Retrograde and anterograde amnesia exists. A confusional state persists for hours to days. There is head pain and complaint of nausea and fatigue. Attentional and memory system impairments may persist for weeks to months and may include inability to concentrate and forgetfulness. Mood and affect changes may persist for weeks to months and may include nervousness, anxiety reactions, depression, irritability, fatigability, and insomnia.

Some of the effects of a concussion may persist for weeks or months, depending on the severity of the injury. A **postconcussive syndrome** that includes headache, nervousness or anxiety, irritability, insomnia, depression, inability to concentrate, forgetfulness, and fatigability may develop.

Treatment entails reassurance and symptomatic relief. A period of 24 hours of close observation by a reliable individual is indicated, so that immediate intervention can be obtained if delayed effects become severe.

In mild DAI, 30% of persons display decerebrate or decorticate posturing; they may experience prolonged periods of stupor or restlessness (see Fig. 14-5).

In moderate DAI, the Glasgow Coma Score (GCS) is 4 to 8 initially, 6 to 8 by 24 hours. Thirty-five percent of victims have transitory decerebration or decortication. The person often remains unconscious for days or weeks and on awakening is confused. He or she experiences a long period of posttraumatic anterograde and retrograde amnesia, and often has permanent deficits in memory, attention, abstraction, reasoning, problem-solving, executive functions, visual or perceptual deficits, language deficits, and mood and affect changes ranging from mild to severe.

Severe DAI is associated with brainstem signs that disappear in a few weeks. The person experiences immediate autonomic dysfunction that disappears in a few weeks. Increased intracranial pressure appears 4 to 6 days after injury. Pulmonary complications occur frequently, with profound sensorimotor and cognitive system deficits. Severely compromised coordinated movements and verbal and written communication, inability to learn and reason, and inability to modulate behavior are also found.

Diagnosis of focal and diffuse injury is determined by high-resolution CT scan and MRI. Medical management must include management of endocrine and metabolic derangement. Early and late seizures must be prevented and controlled.

Spinal Cord Trauma

Each year 15,000 to 20,000 persons suffer serious spinal cord injury. Most are men between the ages of 16 and 30 years who sustain their injuries from car and motorcycle accidents (48%), sports activities (14%), and penetrating injuries (gunshot or stab wounds) (15%). The elderly, because of preexisting degenerative vertebral disorders, are particularly at risk for minor trauma resulting in serious spinal cord injury; 21% of injuries are attributable to falls.

Pathophysiology

Spinal cord injuries most commonly occur because of vertebral injuries, which are the result of acceleration, deceleration, or deformation forces most frequently applied at a distance. These forces injure the vertebral or neural tissues by compressing the tissues, pulling or exerting a traction (tension) on the tissues, or shearing tissues so that they slide into one another. These forces may be exerted on the vertebral and neural tissues by hyperextension, hyperflexion, vertical compression, or rotation of the spine (Figs. 15-8 to 15-11). The bones, ligaments, and joints of the vertebral column may be damaged. The vertebral column may incur fracture and often compression of one or more elements, dislocation of its elements, or both fracture and dislocation. Vertebral injuries can be classified as (1) simple fracture, a single break usually affecting transverse or spinous processes; (2) compressed (wedged) vertebral fracture, vertebral body compressed anteriorly; (3) comminuted (burst) fracture, vertebral body shattered into several fragments; and (4) dislocation.

The vertebrae fracture readily with both direct and indirect trauma. When the supporting ligaments are

FIG. 15-8 **Hyperextension injuries of the spine.** (From Rudy, 1984.)

FIG. 15-9 **Flexion injury of the spine.** (From Rudy, 1984.)

G. J. Wassilchenko

FIG. 15-10 Compression injuries of the spine. (From Rudy, 1984.)

FIG. 15-11 Flexion-rotation injuries of the spine. (From Rudy, 1984.)

torn, the vertebrae move out of alignment and dislocations occur. A horizontal force moves the vertebrae straight forward; if the individual is in a flexed position at the time of injury, the vertebrae are then in an angulated position. Flexion and extension injuries may result in dislocations. (The bone, ligament, and joint injuries are presented in Table 15-3.)

Vertebral injuries occur mostly at vertebrae C1 to C2 (cervical), C4 to C7, and T12 (thoracic) to L2 (lumbar) (see Fig. 12-10). These are the most mobile portions of the vertebral column. The cord occupies most of the vertebral canal in the cervical and lumbar regions. The size makes the cord in these areas more easily injured. (Injuries to the cord are summarized in Table 15-4.)

Within a few minutes after injury, microscopic hemorrhages appear in the central gray matter and pia-arachnoid that increase in size until the entire gray matter is hemorrhagic and necrotic. Edema progresses into the white matter, impairing the microcirculation of the cord. Localized hemorrhaging and edema therefore are followed by reduced vascular perfusion and development of ischemic areas. Oxygen tension in the tissue at the injury site is decreased. The microscopic hemorrhages and edema are maximal at the level of injury and for two cord segments above and below it.

Cellular and subcellular alterations and tissue necrosis occur. Chemical and metabolic changes in spinal cord tissues include increased tissue lactate and increased norepinephrine concentration. The elevated norepinephrine levels may produce further ischemia,

TABLE 15-3

Mechanisms of Vertebral Injury

Mechanisms of injury	Vertebral injury	Forces of injury	Location of injury
Hyperextension	Fracture and dislocation of posterior elements such as spinous processes, transverse processes, laminae, pedicles, or posterior ligaments	Results from forces of acceleration-deceleration and the sudden reduction in the anteroposterior diameter of the spinal cord	Cervical area
Hyperflexion	Fracture or dislocation of the vertebral bodies, disks, or ligaments	Results from sudden and excessive force that propels the neck forward or causes an exaggerated lateral movement of the neck to one side	Cervical area
Vertical compression	Shattering fractures	Results from a force applied along an axis from the top of the cranium through the vertebral bodies	T12 to L2
Rotational forces	Rupture support ligaments in addition to producing fractures	Adds shearing force to acceleration—acceleration forces	Cervical area

TABLE 15-4

Spinal Cord Injuries

Injury	Description
Cord concussion	Results in a temporary disruption of cord-mediated functions
Cord contusion	Bruising of the neural tissue causing swelling and temporary loss of cord-mediated functions
Cord compression	Pressure on the cord causing ischemia to tissues; must be relieved (decompressed) to prevent permanent damage to the spinal cord
Laceration	Tearing of the neural tissues of the spinal cord; may be reversible if only slight damage sustained by the neural tissues; may result in permanent loss of cord-mediated functions if spinal tracts are disrupted
Transection	Severing of the spinal cord, causing permanent loss of function
Complete	All tracts in the spinal cord completely disrupted; all cord-mediated functions below the transection are completely and permanently lost
Incomplete	Some tracts in the spinal cord remain intact, together with functions mediated by these tracts; has the potential for recovery although function is temporarily lost
Hemorrhage	Bleeding into the neural tissue due to blood vessel damage; usually no major loss of function
Damage or obstruction of spinal blood supply	Causes local ischemia

vascular damage, and necrosis of tissues. Cord swelling increases the individual's degree of dysfunction, so that distinguishing the functions to be permanently lost from those that are just temporarily impaired becomes difficult. In the cervical region, cord swelling may be life-threatening because of the possibility of resulting impairment of the diaphragm function (phrenic nerves exit C3 to C5) and vegetative functions mediated by the medulla oblongata.

Circulation in the white matter tracts of the spinal cord returns to normal in about 24 hours, but gray matter circulation remains altered. Phagocytes appear in 36 to 48 hours after injury. There is proliferation of microglia and changes in astrocytes. Red cells then begin to disintegrate and resorption of hemorrhages begins. Degenerating axons are engulfed by macrophages in the first 10 days after injury. The traumatized cord is replaced by acellular collagenous tissue, usually in 3 to 4 weeks. Meninges thicken as part of the scarring process.

Clinical Manifestations

Normal activity of the spinal cord cells at and below the level of injury ceases because of loss of the continuous tonic discharge from the brain or brainstem and inhibition of suprasegmental impulses immediately after cord injury, thus causing spinal shock. *Spinal shock* (neurogenic shock) is characterized by a complete loss of reflex function in all segments below the level of the lesion. This condition involves all skeletal muscles, bladder, bowel, sexual function, and autonomic control. Severe impairment below the level of the lesion is obvious; it includes paralysis and flaccidity in muscles, absence of sensation, loss of bladder and rectal control, transient drop in blood pressure, and poor venous circulation. The condition also results in disturbed thermal control because the sympathetic nervous system is damaged. This damage causes faulty control of sweating and radiation through capillary dilatation. The hypothalamus cannot regulate body heat through vasoconstriction and increased metabolism; therefore, the individual assumes the temperature of the air.

Spinal shock may last for 7 to 20 days after onset; it may persist for as short a time as a few days or as long as 3 months. Indications that spinal shock is terminating include the reappearance of reflex activity, hyperreflexia, spasticity, and reflex emptying of the bladder.

Loss of motor and sensory function depends on the level of injury. All motor, sensory, reflex, and autonomic functions cease below any transected area and also may cease below concussive, contused, compressed, or ischemic areas (Table 15-5). Paralysis of the lower half of the body with both legs involved is termed paraplegia. Paralysis involving all four extremities is termed quadriplegia (tetraplegia). In complete quadriplegia, the level of injury is above C6, and all upper extremity func-

tion is lost. In incomplete quadriplegia, function at or above C6 is preserved, leaving the shoulder, upper arm, and some forearm muscle control intact. With acceleration injuries, the greatest stress point is C4-C5. With a deceleration force, the greatest stress point is at C5-C6.

Return of spinal neuron excitability occurs slowly. Either motor, sensory, reflex, and autonomic functions return to normal, or autonomic neural activity in the isolated segment develops, depending on the degree of damage. The sequence of hyperactivity phases, which vary in length, may include (1) minimal reflex activity, (2) flexor spasms, (3) alternation between flexor and extensor spasms, and (4) predominant extensor spasms.

The initial clinical manifestations associated with acute spinal cord injury are rapid loss of (1) voluntary movement in body parts below the level of injury, (2) sensations in the lower extremities and possibly lower trunk (depending on the level of injury), and (3) spinal and autonomic reflexes below the level of injury. The duration of this areflexic state is highly variable. In most persons, reflex activity returns in 1 to 2 weeks.

Gradually reflexes return and become increasingly easier to elicit. A pattern of flexion reflexes emerges, first involving the toes and later the feet and legs. Reflex voiding and bowel elimination appear. Flexor spasms accompanied by profuse sweating, piloerection, and automatic bladder emptying (together called a **mass reflex**) may develop. The ability to sweat when overheated may be disrupted, and extensor spasms may develop, usually after full development of flexor spasms. Sometimes after several months episodes of autonomic hyperreflexia are elicited.

Autonomic hyperreflexia (dysreflexia) is a syndrome that may occur at any time after spinal shock resolves. The syndrome is associated with a massive, uncompensated cardiovascular response to stimulation of the sympathetic nervous system (Fig. 15-12). The condition is life-threatening and requires immediate treatment. Individuals most likely to be affected have lesions at the T6 level or above. Autonomic hyperreflexia is characterized by paroxysmal hypertension (up to 300 mm Hg, systolic), a pounding headache, blurred vision, sweating above the level of the lesion with flushing of the skin, nasal congestion, nausea, piloerection caused by pilomotor spasm, and bradycardia (30 to 40 beats per minute). The symptoms may develop singly or in combination (syndrome) and are often associated with a distended bladder or rectum.

Pathophysiology of hyperreflexia involves the stimulation of sensory receptors below the level of the cord lesion. The intact autonomic nervous system reflexively responds with an arteriolar spasm that increases blood pressure. Baroreceptors in the cerebral vessels, the carotid sinus, and the aorta sense the hypertension and stimulate the parasympathetic system. The heart rate de-

TABLE 15-5

Clinical Manifestations of Spinal Cord Injury

Stage	Manifestations
Spinal shock stage	

Complete transection	Loss of motor function
	  a. Quadriplegia with injuries of the cervical spinal cord
	  b. Paraplegia with injuries of the thoracic spinal cord
	Muscle flaccidity
	Loss of all reflexes below the level of injury
	Loss of pain, temperature, touch, pressure, and proprioception below the level of injury
	Pain at the site of injury caused by a zone of hyperesthesia above the injury
	Atonic bladder and bowel
	Paralytic ileus with distention
	Loss of vasomotor tone in the lower body parts, low and unstable blood pressure
	Loss of perspiration below the level of injury
	Loss or extreme depression of genital reflexes such as penile erection and bulbocavernous reflex
	Dry and pale skin, possible ulceration over bony prominences
	Respiratory impairment

Partial spinal cord transection	Asymmetric flaccid motor paralysis below the level of injury
	Asymmetric reflex loss
	Preservation of some sensation below the level of injury
	Vasomotor instability less severe than with complete cord transection
	Bowel and bladder impairment less severe than that seen with complete cord transection
	Preservation of ability to perspire in some portions of the body below the level of injury
	Brown-Séquard syndrome (associated with penetrating injuries, arises from a relative hemisection of the cord)
	  a. Ipsilateral paralysis or paresis below the level of injury
	  b. Ipsilateral loss of touch, pressure, vibration, and position sense below the level of injury
	  c. Contralateral loss of pain and temperature sensations below the level of injury
	Central cord syndrome (associated with hyperextension or interruption of blood supply)
	  a. Motor deficit in the upper extremities denser than in the lower extremities
	  b. Varying degrees of bladder dysfunction
	Anterior cord syndrome (compromise of the anterior spinal artery by occlusion or the pressure effect of bone fragments or disk)
	  a. Loss of motor function below the level of injury
	  b. Loss of pain and temperature sensations below the level of injury
	  c. Touch, pressure, position, and vibration senses intact
	Horner syndrome (injury to preganglionic sympathetic trunk or postganglionic sympathetic neurons of the superior cervical ganglion)
	  a. Ipsilateral pupil smaller than contralateral pupil
	  b. Sunken ipsilateral eyeball
	  c. Ptosis of the affected eyeball
	  d. Lack of perspiration on the ipsilateral side of the face

Heightened reflex activity stage	Emergence of Babinski reflexes, possibly progressing to a triple reflex; possible development of still later flexor spasms Reappearance of ankle and knee reflexes, which become hyperactive Contraction of reflex detrusor muscle leading to urinary incontinence Appearance of reflex defecation Mass reflex with flexion spasms, profuse sweating, piloerection, and bladder and occasional bowel emptying may be evoked by an autonomic stimulation of skin or from a full bladder Episodes of hypertension Defective heat-induced sweating Eventual development of extensor reflexes, first in muscles of hip and thigh, later in leg Possible paresthesias below the level of transection: dull, burning pain in the lower back, abdomen, buttocks, and perineum

Modified from Boss, 1984.

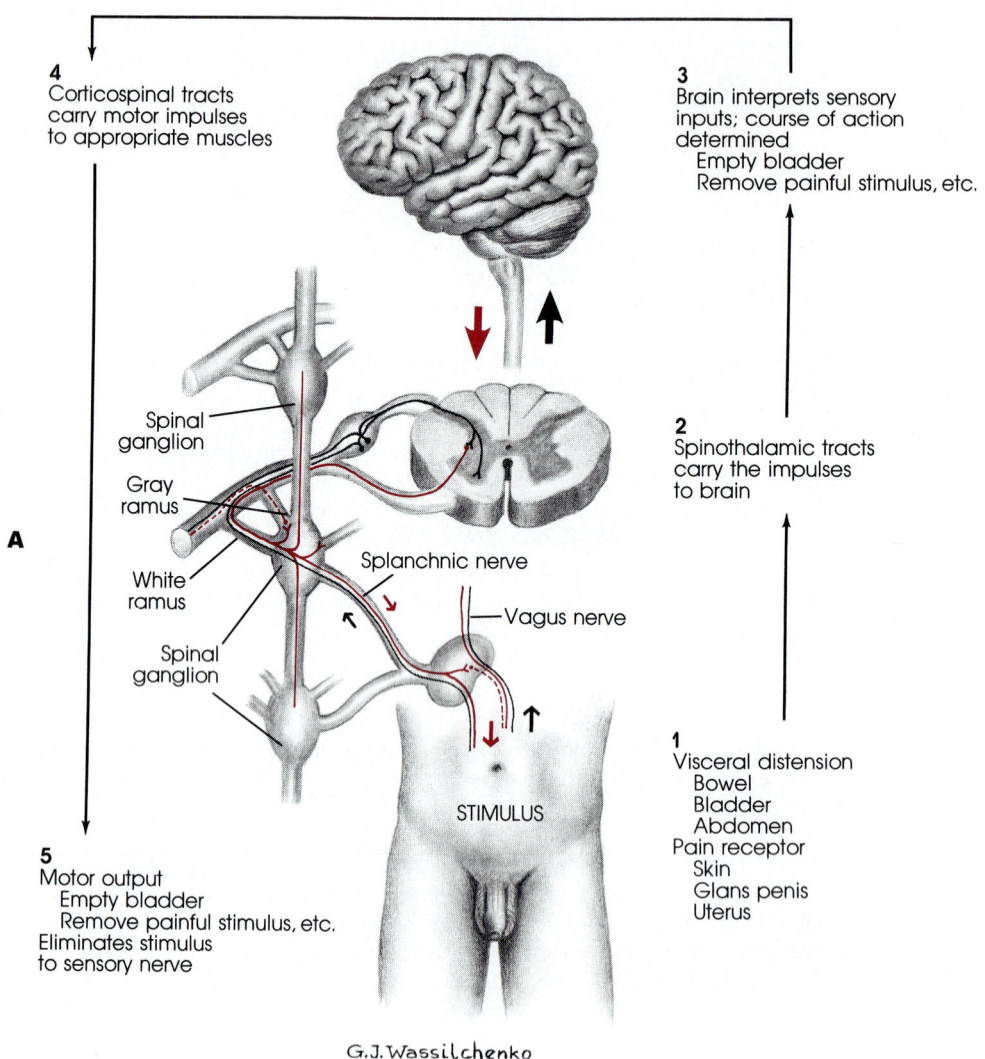

4
Corticospinal tracts
carry motor impulses
to appropriate muscles

3
Brain interprets sensory
inputs; course of action
determined
  Empty bladder
  Remove painful stimulus, etc.

Spinal
ganglion

Gray
ramus

White
ramus

Spinal
ganglion

A

Splanchnic nerve

Vagus nerve

2
Spinothalamic tracts
carry the impulses
to brain

STIMULUS

5
Motor output
  Empty bladder
  Remove painful stimulus, etc.
Eliminates stimulus
to sensory nerve

1
Visceral distension
  Bowel
  Bladder
  Abdomen
Pain receptor
  Skin
  Glans penis
  Uterus

G.J.Wassilchenko

FIG. 15-12 **Autonomic hyperreflexia. A,** Normal response pathway. (From Rudy, 1984.)

creases, but the visceral and peripheral vessels do not dilate because efferent impulses cannot pass through the cord.

The most common precipitating cause is a distended bladder or rectum, but any sensory stimulation can elicit autonomic hyperreflexia. Stimulation of the skin or stimulation of the pain receptors may cause autonomic hyperreflexia. Emptying of the bladder or bowel usually relieves the syndrome, and this may be facilitated by drugs, such as phenoxybenzamine.

Evaluation and Treatment

Diagnosis of spinal cord injury is made on the basis of physical examination, radiologic examination, CT scan, MRI, and myelography. For a suspected or confirmed vertebral fracture or dislocation, regardless of the presence or absence of spinal cord injury, the immediate intervention is immobilization of the spine to prevent further injury. Decompression and surgical fixation may be necessary. Large single doses of corticosteroids are given at the time of injury to decrease secondary cord injury. Nutrition, lung function, skin integrity, and bladder and bowel management must be addressed. Plans for rehabilitation need early consideration.

In cases of autonomic hyperreflexia, intervention must be prompt because cerebrovascular accident is possible. The head of the bed should be elevated, and the stimulus should be found and removed. Medications may be used if these measures do not effectively reduce blood pressure.

5
Ninth cranial nerve stimulated by carotid; receptors send message to vasomotor center of medulla, vagus nerve stimulated; impulse sent to S-A node; results in bradycardia

Carotid sinuses

Glossopharyngeal nerve (IX)

4
Increased blood pressure stimulates carotid sinus receptors

Medulla

Carotid sinus nerve

Vagus nerve (X)

S-A node

6
Autonomic response to hypertension down to level of cord lesion.
    Arterial dilation
    Flushed skin
    Headache
    Sweating

B

Lesion

3
Reflex stimulus to major sympathetic outflow resulting in:
→ Vasospasm
→ Hypertension
→ Pallor of skin
→ Pilomotor spasms

2
Spinothalamic tracts carry sensory impulses to level of lesion (T6 and above)

1
Visceral distention
    Bowel
    Bladder
    Abdomen
Pain receptors
    Skin
    Glans penis
    Uterus

STIMULUS

FIG. 15-12 —cont'd Autonomic hyperreflexia. B, Autonomic dysreflexia pathway.

Low Back Pain

Low back pain affects the area between the lower rib cage and gluteal muscles and often radiates into the thighs. About 1% of individuals with acute low back pain have sciatica, pain in the distribution of a lumbar nerve root (Frymoyer, 1988). Sciatica is often accompanied by neurosensory and motor deficits, such as weakness.

The incidence of, or percentage of population affected with, low back pain at some point in their lives is 60% to 90%, and the annual incidence is 5% (Frymoyer, 1988). Men and women are equally affected; however, women report low back symptoms more often after the age of 60.

Pathogenesis

Most cases of low back pain are idiopathic, and clinicians are unable to provide a precise diagnosis for most individuals suffering from this disorder. The local processes involved in low back pain range from tension caused by tumors or disk prolapse, bursitis, synovitis, rising venous and tissue pressure (found in degenerative joint disease), abnormal bone pressures, problems with spinal mobility, inflammation caused by infection (as in osteomyelitis), bony fractures, or ligamentous sprains to pain referred from viscera or the posterior peritoneum. General processes resulting in low back pain include bone diseases such as osteoporosis or osteomalacia and hyperparathyroidism.

Several risk factors have been identified in the pathogenesis of low back pain. They include involvement caused by occupations that require repetitious lifting in the forward bent-and-twisted position, exposure to vibrations caused by vehicles or industrial machinery, and cigarette smoking (Frymoyer, 1988). Osteoporosis increases the risk of spinal compression fractures and may be the reason why elderly women report more symptoms than men. Genetic predispositions for low back pain include isthmic spondylolisthesis (vertebra slides forward or slips in relation to a vertebra below), spinal osteochondrosis, and spinal stenosis associated with achondroplasia. Variations in posture, such as lordosis and scoliosis of less than 60 degrees, do not appear to increase the risk of low back pain or sciatica (Pope, Bevins, Wilder, & Frymoyer, 1985; Weinstein, 1986). Differences in weight, height, and leg length are controversial (Pope et al., 1985).

Anatomically, low back pain must come from innervated structures, but deep pain is widely referred and varies from person to person. The nucleus pulposus has no intrinsic innervation; however, when extruded or herniated through a diskal prolapse, it irritates the dural membranes and is responsible for pain referred to the segmental area (Fig. 15-13). The interspinous bursae can be a source of low back pain between L3, L4, L5, and S1, but also may affect L1, L2, and L3 spinous processes, depending on the closeness of the adjacent pair of spines. The anterior and posterior longitudinal ligaments of the spine and the interspinous and supraspinous ligaments are abundantly supplied with pain receptors, as is the ligamentum flavum. All of these ligaments are vulnerable to traumatic tears (sprains) and fracture. The role of muscle injury in the production of low back pain remains uncertain, even though sprains and strains are the most common diagnoses (Frymoyer, 1988). The muscle spasms that are often produced during sieges of low back pain are thought to be produced by as yet unknown sensory or motor-reflex pathways (Frymoyer, 1988). The most commonly encountered causes of low back pain include lumbar disk herniation, degenerative disk disease, spondylolysis, spondylolisthesis, and spinal stenosis. (For a discussion of disk herniation and rupture, see p. 545.)

Degenerative disk disease. **Degenerative disk disease** is a common finding in individuals 50 years of age and older; however, only a small percentage of people with degenerative disk disease have any functional incapacity because of pain (Spengler, 1982). The cause of degenerative disk disease includes biochemical and biomechanical alterations of the tissue of intervertebral disk. Fibrocartilage replaces the gelatinous mucoid material of the nucleus pulposus as the disk changes with aging, and the narrowing disk results in variable segmental instability. The process seems to stabilize when segmental fibrosis results, and often the incidence of back pain decreases (Spengler, 1982).

Spondylolysis. **Spondylolysis** is a structural defect of the spine involving the lamina or neural arch of the vertebra. The most common site affected is the lumbar spine. This defect occurs in the portion of the lamina between the superior and inferior articular facets called the pars interarticularis. Mechanical pressure may cause a forward displacement of the deficient vertebra, called spondylolisthesis.

Heredity plays a significant role, and spondylolysis is associated with an increased incidence of other congenital spinal defects. As a result of torsional and rotational "stress," "microfractures" occur at the affected site and eventually cause dissolution of the pars interarticularis.

Spondylolisthesis. **Spondylolisthesis** is caused when a vertebra slides forward in relation to the vertebra below, commonly occurring at L5-S1. Spondylolisthesis is graded from 1 to 4 on the basis of the percentage of slip that has occurred. Individuals with grade 3 or 4 are

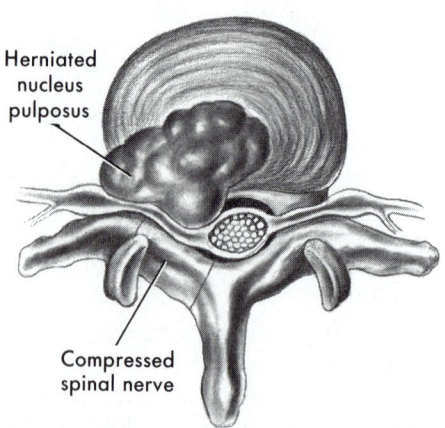

FIG. 15-13 Herniated nucleus pulposus. (From Thompson et al., 1993.)

Herniated nucleus pulposus

Compressed spinal nerve

considered for operative decompression or stabilization, or both. Grades 1 and 2 are usually managed symptomatically and by nonsurgical methods.

Spinal stenosis. Spinal stenosis may represent several conditions ranging from entrapment of a single nerve root in the lateral recess to diffuse central stenosis involving many roots. It is classified as acquired (more common) or developmental (such as occurs in achondroplastic dwarfs). Surgical decompression is recommended for those with chronic symptoms and those who remain unresponsive to medical management.

Evaluation and Treatment

Diagnosis of low back injury is made on the basis of physical examination, electromyelography, CT with or without myelography, MRI, nerve conduction studies, discogram, and epidurography. Most individuals with acute low back pain benefit from a nonspecific short-term treatment regimen including bed rest, analgesic medications, exercises, physical therapy, and education. Surgical treatments may be indicated if individuals do not respond to medical management. Surgical treatments include diskectomy and spinal fusions. Individuals with chronic low back pain can be treated with antiinflammatory and muscle relaxant medications and exercise programs. Aerobic exercises are a popular treatment and seem to be more effective than traction or low back exercises (Frymoyer, 1988). Spinal surgery has a limited role in curing chronic low back pain.

Herniated Intervertebral Disk

Herniation of an intervertebral disk is a protrusion of part of the nucleus pulposus (like stepping on an ice cream sandwich) through a tear in the posterior rim of the annulus fibrosus (the fibrous capsule enclosing the gelatinous center of the disk) (see Fig. 15-13). Rupture of an intervertebral disk is usually caused by trauma, degenerative disk disease, or both. Lifting with the trunk flexed and sudden straining when the back is in an unstable position are the most common causes. Men are more affected than women, with the highest incidence in the 30- to 50-year age group. Most commonly affected are the lumbosacral disks, that is, L5-S1 and L4-L5. Disk herniation occasionally occurs in the cervical area, usually at C5-C6 and C6-C7. Herniations at the thoracic level are extremely rare. The injury may have an immediate onset or an onset within a few hours, or the manifestations of injury may take months to years to develop.

Pathophysiology

In a herniated disk, the ligament and posterior capsule of the disk are usually torn, allowing the gelatinous material (the nucleus pulposus) to extrude. This extrusion compresses the nerve root. Occasionally the injury tears the entire disk loose, and it protrudes onto the nerve root or compresses the spinal cord. One or more nerve roots may be compressed. This multiple nerve root compression is especially found at the L5-S1 level, where the cauda equina may be compressed. Large amounts of extruded nucleus pulposus or complete disk herniation (that is, of both the capsule and the nucleus pulposus) may compress the spinal cord.

Clinical Manifestations

The location and size of the herniation into the spinal canal, together with the amount of space that exists inside the spinal canal, determine the clinical manifestations associated with the injury (Fig. 15-14). A herniated disk in the lumbosacral area is associated with pain that radiates along the sciatic nerve course over the buttock and into the calf or ankle. The pain occurs with straining, including coughing and sneezing, and usually on straight leg raising. Other clinical manifestations include limited range of motion of the lumbar spine; tenderness on palpation in the sciatic notch and along the sciatic nerve; impaired pain, temperature, and touch sensation in the L5-S1 or L4-L5 dermatomes of the leg and foot; decreased or absent ankle jerk; and mild weakness of the foot.

With the herniation of a lower cervical disk, paresthesias and pain are present in the upper arm, forearm, and hand in the affected nerve root distribution. Neck and nerve root pain may be increased by neck motion and straining, including coughing and sneezing. Neck range of motion is diminished. Slight weakness and atrophy of biceps or triceps may occur; the biceps or triceps reflex may decrease. Occasionally signs of corticospinal and sensory tract impairments appear. These include motor weakness of the lower extremities, sensory disturbances in the lower extremities, and presence of a Babinski reflex.

Evaluation and Treatment

Diagnosis of a herniated intervertebral disk is made through the history and physical examination, spinal x-ray films, electromyelography, CT scan, MRI, myelography, discography, and nerve conduction studies. Multiple avenues of therapy are available. The conservative approach comprises traction, bed rest, heat and ice to the affected areas, and an effective analgesic regimen. The surgical approach is indicated if there is evidence of severe compression (weakness, decreased deep tendon reflexes and bladder/bowel reflexes) or if the conservative approach is unsuccessful. The newest therapy is injection of the enzyme chymopapain into the disk to dissolve it. Chymopapain injections, however, have numerous side effects and are rarely used now.

FIG. 15-14 Clinical features of a herniated lumbar nucleus pulposus.

Cerebrovascular Disorders

Cerebrovascular disease is the most frequently occurring neurologic disorder. More than 50% of the persons admitted to general hospitals with neurologic problems have cerebrovascular disease. Any abnormality of the brain caused by a pathologic process in the blood vessels is referred to as a cerebrovascular disease. Included in this category are lesions of the vessel wall, occlusion of the vessel lumen by thrombus or embolus, rupture of the vessel, and alteration in vessel permeability such as increased blood viscosity.

The brain abnormalities induced by cerebrovascular disease are of two types: (1) ischemia with or without infarction (death of brain tissues) and (2) hemorrhage. The common clinical manifestation of cerebrovascular disease is a **cerebrovascular accident** (CVA, stroke): a sudden, nonconvulsive focal neurologic deficit.

Cerebrovascular Accidents

Cerebrovascular accidents (CVAs) are the third leading cause of death in the United States. The highest incidence of stroke is among those older than 65 years of age. Strokes, however, do occur in a 3 to 10 ratio in individuals younger than age 65. Stroke tends to run in families and is more frequent in women. The incidence is greater in blacks than whites, presumably because of the greater incidence of hypertension in blacks. In its mildest form, a CVA is so minimal as to be almost unnoticed. In its most severe state, hemiplegia, coma, and death result.

Cerebrovascular accidents are classified according to pathophysiology and thus are thrombotic, embolic, or hemorrhagic.

Thrombotic stroke

Thrombotic strokes arise from arterial occlusions caused by thrombi formed in the arteries supplying the brain or in the intracranial vessels. The risk factors for cerebrovascular occlusive disease are the following:

Arteriosclerosis, which includes the following risk factors: hypertension, cigarette smoking, elevated blood cholesterol or triglyceride levels, lipoprotein ratio, diabetes mellitus, sedentary lifestyle
Hypothyroidism
Use of oral contraceptives
Sickle cell disease
Coagulation disorders
Polycythemia vera
Arteritis
Subclavian steal syndrome
Chronic hypoxia
Dehydration, especially when combined with any of the preceding conditions

The development of a cerebral thrombosis is most frequently attributed to atherosclerosis and inflammatory disease processes (arteritis) that damage arterial walls. Increased coagulation can lead to thrombus formation. Conditions causing inadequate cerebral perfusion (such as dehydration, hypotension, and prolonged vasoconstriction from malignant hypertension) increase the risk of thrombosis. Over 20 to 30 years, atheromatous plaques tend to form at branchings and curves in the cerebral circulation. Degeneration or bleeding into the vessel wall may cause endothelial damage. Platelets and fibrin adhere to the damaged wall and delicate clots form. Small thrombi collect over time, with gradual occlusion of the artery. Once the artery is occluded, the thrombus may enlarge both distally and proximally in the vessel.

Thrombotic strokes may be further subdivided on the basis of clinical manifestations into transient ischemic attacks, strokes-in-evolution, and completed strokes. **Transient ischemic attacks** (TIAs) probably represent thrombotic particles causing an intermittent blockage of circulation or spasm. In a true TIA all the neurologic deficits must be completely clear within 24 hours, leaving no residual dysfunction. Approximately 35% of completed thrombotic strokes are preceded by TIAs.

The symptoms of thrombotic strokes occasionally have an abrupt onset but tend to be slowly progressive, evolving in a step-by-step fashion over minutes to hours. The typical development of thrombotic stroke causes the clinical syndrome known as a **stroke-in-evolution** (progressive stroke). An intermittent progression of a neurologic deficit over hours to days is characteristic of thrombotic stroke or slow hemorrhage. The **completed stroke** is a cerebrovascular accident that has reached its maximum destructiveness in producing neurologic deficits, although cerebral edema may not have reached its maximum.

Embolic stroke

An **embolic stroke** involves fragments that break from a thrombus formed outside the brain, in the heart, aorta, common carotid, or thorax. Emboli infrequently arise from the ascending aorta or common carotid artery. The embolus usually involves small vessels and obstructs at a bifurcation or other point of narrowing, thus causing ischemia. An embolus may plug the lumen entirely and remain in place or break into fragments and move up the vessel. Conditions associated with the onset of an embolic stroke include atrial fibrillation, myocardial infarction, endocarditis, rheumatic heart disease, valvular prostheses, atrial-septal defects and disorders of the aorta, carotids, or vertebral-basilar circulation. Less common contributors to embolic stroke are air, fat, and tumors. Fat emboli sometimes develop with fractures of long bones. Air emboli also can develop after certain types of surgery. In persons who experience an embolic stroke, usually a second stroke follows at some point because the source of emboli continues to exist. Embolization is usually in the distribution of the middle cerebral artery.

Hemorrhagic stroke

Hemorrhagic stroke (intracranial hemorrhage) is the third most frequent cause of cerebrovascular accident. The most common causes of hemorrhagic stroke are hypertension, ruptured aneurysms or arteriovenous malformation, and hemorrhage associated with bleeding disorders.

A hypertensive hemorrhage is associated with a significant increase in systolic-diastolic pressure over several years and usually occurs within the brain tissue. A mass of blood is formed, and its volume increases. Adjacent brain tissue is displaced and compressed. Rupture or seepage into the ventricular system occurs in many of the cases. Hemorrhages are described as massive, small, slit, or petechial. Massive hemorrhages are several centimeters in diameter; small hemorrhages are 1 to 2 cm in diameter; a slit hemorrhage lies in the subcortical area, whereas petechial hemorrhage is the size of a pinhead bleed. The most common sites for hypertensive hemorrhages are in the putamen of the basal ganglia (a portion of the lentiform nucleus) (55%), the thalamus (10%), cortex and subcortex (15%), the pons (10%), and cerebellar hemispheres (10%).

Lacunar stroke

Lacunar strokes (lacunar infarcts) are infarcts smaller than 1 cc in size and involve the small perforating arteries predominantly in the basal ganglia, internal capsules, and brainstem. Lacunar infarcts are associated with hypertension. Because of the subcortical location and small area of infarction, these strokes may have pure motor and sensory deficits.

Pathophysiology

Cerebral infarction. Cerebral infarction results when an area of the brain loses blood supply because of vascular occlusion. Proposed pathogenesis may include (1) abrupt vascular occlusion (e.g., embolus), (2) gradual vessel occlusion (e.g., atheroma), and (3) vessels that are stenosed but not completely occluded. Cerebral thrombi and cerebral emboli are the most common causes of occlusion, but atherosclerosis and hypotension are the dominant underlying processes.

Cerebral infarctions are ischemic or hemorrhagic. In ischemic infarcts, the affected area becomes slightly discolored and softens in about 6 to 12 hours after the occlusion. Necrosis, swelling around the insult, and mushy disintegration have appeared by 48 to 72 hours after infarction. At a microscopic level, neuronal cell bodies change, myelin sheaths and axis cylinders are interrupted and disintegrate, and there is loss of oligodendrites and astrocytes.

In hemorrhagic infarcts, bleeding occurs into the infarcted area as a result of restoration of blood flow. Reperfusion occurs when the embolus fragments, or lysis or compressive forces lessen, allowing blood flow to be reestablished into the infarcted area. Most hemorrhagic infarcts are located in the cerebral cortex.

Cerebral hemorrhage. The primary cause of cerebral hemorrhage is hypertension. Aneurysms and arteriovenous malformations are discussed on p. 550.

The pathogenesis of hypertensive cerebral hemorrhage is not fully understood. Hypertension primarily involves smaller arteries and arterioles, resulting in thickening of the vessel walls, and increased cellularity of the vessels and hyalinization. Necrosis is sometimes present. Many experts believe that microaneurysms in these smaller vessels or arteriolar necrosis precipitate the bleeding.

A mass of blood is formed as bleeding continues into the brain tissue. Adjacent brain tissue is displaced and compressed, producing ischemia and subsequent vasogenic edema. Increased intracranial pressure results. Rupture or seepage of blood into the ventricular system occurs in many cases.

The cerebral hemorrhage resolves through reabsorption. Macrophages and astrocytes appear to clear away the blood. A cavity forms surrounded by a dense gliosis after removal of the blood.

Clinical Manifestations

Because neurons surrounding the ischemic or infarcted areas undergo changes that disrupt plasma membranes, cellular edema results, causing further compression of capillaries. Cerebral edema reaches its maximum in about 72 hours and takes about 2 weeks to subside. Most persons survive an initial hemispheric ischemic stroke unless massive cerebral edema develops. Massive brainstem infarcts, caused by basilar thrombosis or embolism, are almost always fatal, however.

Clinical manifestations of thrombotic stroke vary, depending on the artery obstructed. Different sites of obstruction create different occlusion syndromes (see box on p. 549).

With hemorrhagic stroke, clinical manifestations vary, depending on the location and size of the bleed. Once a deep unresponsive state occurs, the person rarely survives. The immediate prognosis is grave. If, however, the person survives, recovery of function is frequently possible.

Individuals experiencing intracranial hemorrhage from a ruptured or leaking aneurysm have one of three sets of symptoms: (1) onset of an excruciating generalized headache with an almost-immediate lapse into an unresponsive state, (2) headache but with consciousness maintained, and (3) sudden lapse into unconsciousness. If the hemorrhage is confined to the subarachnoid space, there may be no local signs. If bleeding spreads into the

CLINICAL MANIFESTATIONS ASSOCIATED WITH CEREBROVASCULAR OCCLUSIVE SYNDROMES

I. CVA involving the anterior cerebral artery

Mental status impairments
- Confusion
- Amnesia
- Perseveration
- Personality changes: flat affect, apathy
- Cognitive changes: short attention span, slowness
- Deterioration of intellectual function

Urinary incontinence (long duration)

Contralateral hemiparesis or hemiplegia; sensory impairments; foot and leg deficits greater than arm deficits

Footdrop

Apraxia on affected side

Expressive aphasia (for left hemisphere involvement)

Deviation of eyes and head toward affected side

Abulia (inability to make decisions or perform voluntary acts)

Gait dysfunction

II. CVA involving the middle cerebral artery

Dysphasia (left hemisphere involvement), dyslexia, dysgraphia

Contralateral hemiparesis or hemiplegia

Contralateral hemisensory disturbances

Rapid deterioration in consciousness from confusion to coma

Vomiting

Homonymous hemianopia

Denial or lack of recognition of a paralyzed extremity

Inability to turn eyes toward affected side

III. CVA involving the posterior cerebral artery

Peripheral signs
- Visual disturbances
  Homonymous hemianopia
  Cortical blindness
  Lack of depth perception
  Failure to see objects not centered in the field of vision
  Visual hallucinations
- Memory deficits
- Perseveration
- Dyslexia

Central Signs
- Thalamic or subthalamic nuclei involvement: diffuse sensory loss, mild hemiparesis, intentional tremor
- Cerebral peduncle involvement: contralateral hemiplegia, oculomotor nerve deficits
- Brainstem involvement: pupillary dysfunction, nystagmus, loss of conjugate gaze (Hickey, 1981)

IV. CVA involving the internal carotid artery

Contralateral hemiparesis with facial asymmetry

Contralateral sensory deficits, especially paresthesia

Hemianopia

Ipsilateral episodes of visual blurring or amaurosis fugax (temporary blindness)

Dysphasia (left hemisphere involvement)

Carotid bifurcation bruit

Mild Horner syndrome

V. CVA involving the vertebral-basilar system

Dysarthria, dysphagia

Vertigo, nausea, and syncope

Memory loss, disorientation

Ataxic gait

Dysmetria

Visual symptoms: double vision, homonymous hemianopia

Tinnitus, hearing loss

Ocular signs: nystagmus, conjugate gaze paralysis, ophthalmoplegia

Akinetic mutism (locked-in syndrome when basilar artery occlusion occurs)

Numbness of tongue

Facial weakness, alternating motor paresis

Drop attacks

VI. CVA involving the anterior inferior cerebellar artery (inferior lateral pontine syndrome)

Contralateral signs
- Horizontal nystagmus
- Sensory impairments, mainly of trunk and limbs

Ipsilateral signs
- Horner syndrome
- Tinnitus and deafness
- Ataxia and nystagmus
- Facial paralysis and loss of tactile sensation

VII. CVA involving the posterior inferior cerebellar artery

Dysarthria, dysphagia, dysphonia

Vertigo, nystagmus, unsteady gait

Ipsilateral Horner syndrome

Sensory changes—ipsilateral face and contralateral body

Hiccoughs, vomiting

Paralysis of larynx and soft palate

Wallenberg syndrome: sudden onset of:
- Vertigo, horizontal nystagmus, ataxia
- Nausea and vomiting
- Dysphagia
- Horner syndrome (ipsilateral)
- Pain and temperature loss on trunk and limbs (contralateral)
- Balance loss on affected side
- Pain and temperature loss on face (ipsilateral)

From Kneisl & Ames, 1986.

brain tissue, hemiparesis/paralysis, dysphasia, or homonymous hemianopia may be present. Warning signs of an impending aneurysm rupture may include headache, transient unilateral weakness, transient numbness and tingling, and transient speech disturbance. Warning signs, however, are often not present.

Evaluation and Treatment

In thrombotic strokes, treatment is directed at supportive management to control cerebral edema and increased intracranial pressure. Ancrod (Arvin), a drug, is being tested experimentally to achieve defibrinogenation to increase local cerebral blood flow in the ischemic areas. Later surgical intervention to restore blood supply may be indicated. Arresting the disease process by control of risk factors is critical. In embolic strokes, treatment is directed at preventing further embolization by instituting anticoagulation therapy and correcting the primary problem. Rehabilitation is indicated in both thrombotic and embolic stroke. Treatment of an intracranial bleed, regardless of cause, is focused on stopping or reducing the bleeding, controlling the increased intracranial pressure, preventing a rebleed, and preventing vasospasm. Occasionally an attempt is made to evacuate or aspirate the blood.

Intracranial aneurysm

Intracranial aneurysms may result from arteriosclerosis, congenital abnormality, trauma, inflammation, or infection. Cocaine has recently been linked to aneurysm formation (Willis & Harbit, 1990). The size may vary from 2 mm to 2 or 3 cm. Most aneurysms are located at bifurcations in or near the circle of Willis or in the vertebrobasilar arteries, or within the carotid system (see Fig. 12-19). Aneurysms may be single, but in 20% to 25% of the cases, more than one aneurysm is present. In these instances, the aneurysms may be unilateral or bilateral. Peak incidence is 35 to 60 years of age. Women have a slightly greater incidence.

Pathophysiology

No single pathologic mechanism exists. Aneurysms may be classified on the basis of shape and form. **Saccular aneurysms** (berry aneurysms) occur frequently (in approximately 2% of the population) and are probably the result of congenital abnormalities in the media of the arterial wall. The sac gradually grows over time. A saccular aneurysm may be (1) round with a narrow stalk connecting it to the parent artery, (2) broad-based without a stalk, or (3) cylindrical (Fig. 15-15). Saccular aneurysms are rare in childhood; their highest incidence of rupturing or bleeding is among persons 35 to 65 years of age (Fig. 15-16).

Fusiform aneurysms (giant aneurysms) occur as a result of diffuse arteriosclerotic changes and are found most commonly in the basilar arteries or terminal portions of the internal carotid arteries (see Fig. 15-15, *B*). They act as space-occupying lesions. **Mycotic aneurysms** result from arteritis due to bacterial emboli; these aneurysms are uncommon. **Traumatic aneurysms** are caused by a weakening of the arterial wall by a fracture line, a penetrating missile, or after neurosurgical procedures.

Aneurysms rupture because their walls are thin, causing hemorrhage into the subarachnoid space with rapid spread, producing localized changes in the cerebral cortex and focal irritation of nerves and arteries (see Laplace's law, p. 965). Bleeding ceases with the formation of a fibrin-platelet plug at the point of rupture and because of compression. Blood undergoes reabsorption through arachnoid villi within 3 weeks.

Clinical Manifestations

Aneurysms are frequently asymptomatic. Of all persons undergoing routine autopsy, 2% are found to have one or more intracranial aneurysms. Clinical manifestations may arise from cranial nerve compression, but the signs vary, depending on the location and size of the aneurysm. Most often, cranial nerves III, IV, V, and VI are affected (see Table 12-6). Unfortunately the most common first indication of the presence of an aneurysm is an acute subarachnoid hemorrhage, intracerebral hemorrhage, or combined subarachnoid-intracerebral hemorrhage (see p. 552).

Evaluation and Treatment

Diagnosis before a bleeding episode is made through arteriography. After a subarachnoid or intracerebral hemorrhage, a tentative diagnosis of an aneurysm is based on clinical manifestations, history, CT scan, and MRI. The treatment of choice for an aneurysm is surgical management. The location and size of the aneurysm and the person's clinical status determine whether invasive therapy is feasible.

Arteriovenous Malformation

An **arteriovenous malformation** (AVM) is a tangled mass of dilated blood vessels creating abnormal channels between the arterial and venous systems (arteriovenous fistula). Arteriovenous malformations may occur in any part of the brain. Their size is highly variable, from those of a few millimeters to large malformations that extend from the cortex to the ventricle, and they are usually cone-shaped. The large AVMs also may involve the dura mater, including the falx cerebri and the tentorium cerebelli. Arteriovenous malformations occur as frequently in males as in females, and they occasionally occur in families. Although usually present at birth, AVMs exhibit a delayed age of onset, and symptoms most commonly occur between the ages of 10 and 20.

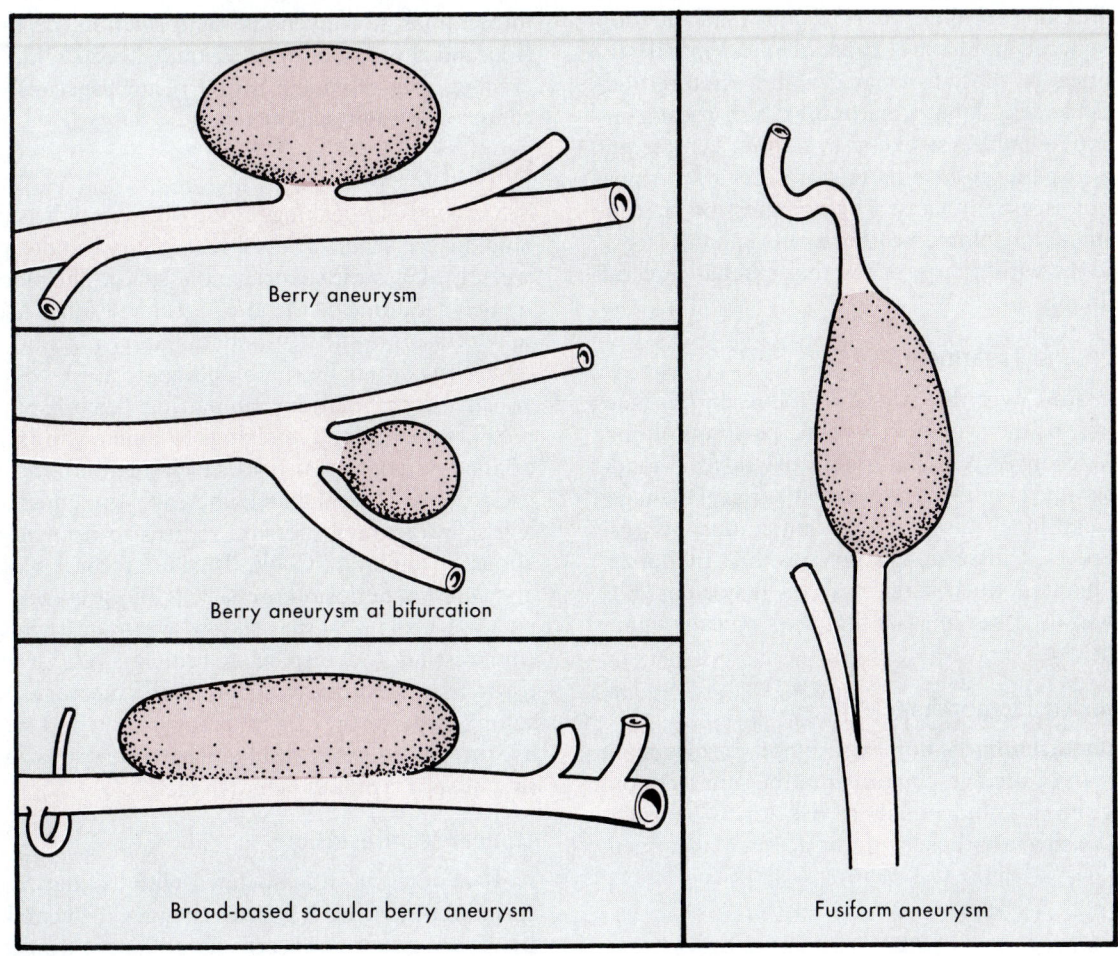

FIG. 15-15 Types of aneurysms.

Pathophysiology

Arteriovenous malformations, developmental abnormalities that represent persistence of embryonic patterns of blood vessels, do not have a normal blood vessel structure and are abnormally thin. The involved vessels are thought by some to enlarge over time. The arteriovenous malformation may be fed by one or several arteries. These feeder vessels become tortuous over time and often dilated. With moderate to large AVMs, sufficient blood is shunted into the malformation to deprive surrounding tissue of adequate blood perfusion.

Clinical Manifestations

Clinical manifestations vary. Twenty percent of persons with an AVM have a characteristic chronic nondescript headache, although some experience migraine. Thirty percent of persons experience seizure disorders caused by compression. Initially, the seizures tend to be focal or Jacksonian; generalization often occurs over time. (Seizures are discussed in Chapter 14.) The other 50% suffer an intracerebral, subarachnoid, or subdural hem-

FIG. 15-16 **Ruptured berry aneurysms.** Larger aneurysm is at terminal portion of basilar artery. Smaller aneurysm is in bifurcation angle of middle cerebral artery on right. (From Kissane, 1993.)

orrhage. Bleeding from an arteriovenous malformation into the subarachnoid space causes clinical manifestations identical to those associated with a ruptured aneurysm. If bleeding is into the brain tissue, focal signs that develop resemble a stroke-in-evolution. Ten percent of persons experience hemiparesis or other focal signs. Hemiparesis is usually caused by compression or rupture. At times, noncommunicating hydrocephalus (see p. 576) develops with a large AVM that extends into the ventricle lining.

Evaluation and Treatment

A systolic bruit over the carotid in the neck, the mastoid process, or the eyeball in a young person is almost diagnostic of an AVM. Confirming diagnosis is made by arteriogram. Treatment of choice is surgical management through block dissection or obliteration by ligation of feeders if dissection is not possible. Embolization may be used when surgical access is not possible. Radiation is also used in cases that are surgically unapproachable.

Subarachnoid Hemorrhage

With a **subarachnoid hemorrhage**, blood escapes from a defective or injured vasculature into the subarachnoid space (Fig. 15-17). Individuals at risk for a subarachnoid hemorrhage are those with intracranial aneurysm,

FIG. 15-17 Recent diffuse subarachnoid hemorrhage. Subarachnoid hemorrhage in individual with massive intracerebral hemorrhage. (From Kissane, 1993.)

intracranial arteriovenous malformation, or hypertension and those who have sustained head injuries. Subarachnoid hemorrhages often recur, especially from a ruptured intracranial aneurysm.

Pathophysiology

When a vessel is leaking, blood oozes into the subarachnoid space. When a vessel tears, blood under pressure is pumped into the subarachnoid space. The blood is extremely irritating to the meningeal and other neural tissues and so produces an inflammatory reaction in these tissues. Additionally the blood coats nerve roots, clogs arachnoid granulations (impairing cerebrospinal fluid [CSF] reabsorption), and clogs foramina within the ventricular system (impairing CSF circulation). Intracranial pressure (ICP) immediately increases to almost diastolic levels. Intracranial pressure returns to near baseline in about 10 minutes (Cook, 1991). Cerebral blood flow and cerebral perfusion pressure (CPP) decrease. The expanding hematoma acts like a space-occupying lesion, compressing and displacing brain tissue. Granulation tissue is formed and scarring of the meninges with resulting impairment of CSF reabsorption and secondary hydrocephalus often results. There is a 50% mortality rate in subarachnoid hemorrhage.

Clinical Manifestations

Early manifestations associated with leaking vessels are episodic headache, transient changes in mental status, transitory visual or speech disturbances, transient motor weakness, and transitory numbness and tingling. A ruptured vessel is often accompanied by a sudden throbbing, "explosive" headache. The headache is associated with nausea and vomiting, visual disturbances, motor deficits, and loss of consciousness. These signs all can be related to a dramatic rise in ICP. Meningeal irritation and inflammation often occur, causing neck stiffness (nuchal rigidity), photophobia, blurred vision, irritability, restlessness, and low-grade fever. A positive **Kernig sign** (in which straightening the knee with the hip and knee in a flexed position produces pain in the back and neck regions) and **Brudzinski sign** (in which passive flexion of the neck produces neck pain and increased rigidity) may appear. No localizing signs are present if the bleed is confined completely to the subarachnoid space.

The Hunt and Hess subarachnoid hemorrhage (SAH) grading system is based on description of the clinical manifestations (Table 15-6). Rebleeding is a significant risk with a high mortality rate (up to 70%). The period of greatest risk is the first 3 weeks, with the peak incidence of rebleed during the first 24 hours after the initial bleed. Rebleeding is manifested by a sudden increase in blood pressure and ICP, along with a deteriorating neurologic status.

TABLE 15-6

Subarachnoid Hemorrhage Classification Scale

Category	Description
Grade I	Neurologic status intact; mild headache, slight nuchal rigidity
Grade II	Neurologic deficit evidenced by cranial nerve involvement; moderate to severe headache with more pronounced meningeal signs (e.g., photophobia, nuchal rigidity)
Grade III	Drowsiness and confusion with or without focal neurologic deficits; pronounced meningeal signs
Grade IV	Stuporous with pronounced neurologic deficits (e.g., hemiparesis, dysphasia); nuchal rigidity
Grade V	Deep coma state with decerebrate posturing and other brainstem functioning

From Cook, 1991.

Delayed cerebral ischemia, a syndrome of progressive neurologic deterioration, is associated with cerebral artery vasospasm. Forty percent to 60% of persons with a subarachnoid hemorrhage experience vasospasms in adjacent and sometimes in nonadjacent vessels. The pathophysiology of vasospasm is unclear. Vasospasm is thought to occur because of the effects of vasoactive substances, such as calcium, prostaglandins, serotonin, and catecholamines, on the arteries of the subarachnoid space. Edema, medial necrosis, and proliferation of the intima have been found. Vasospasm causes decreased cerebral blood flow, ischemia, and may produce infarct. The peak time of occurrence is 4 to 12 days after the initial bleed, but vasospasm may persist for several weeks.

Seizures occur in 25% of persons with an SAH. The incidence of hydrocephalus after a bleed is 20%. Hypothalamic dysfunction, manifested by salt wasting, hyponatremia, and ECG changes, is common.

Evaluation and Treatment

The diagnosis of a subarachnoid hemorrhage is based on the clinical presentation, a CT scan, MRI, and a lumbar puncture. Arteriography is the definitive diagnostic measure for identifying an aneurysm or arteriovenous malformation. Treatment is directed at control of intracranial pressure, prevention of ischemia and hypoxia of neural tissues, and prevention of rebleeding episodes. Calcium channel blockers, such as nifedipine, are used to prevent or reverse vasospasm. Hemodilutional hyper-

perfusion through continuous or bolus administration of hetastarch and plasma protein factors to maintain a hematocrit of 33% is used to expand blood volume and augment cerebral perfusion (Cook, 1991). Cerebral angioplasty is being tested for vasospasm. The primary problem must be diagnosed and corrected as well.

Tumors of the Central Nervous System

No proven causative agents have been established. Carcinogenesis is discussed in Chapter 10.

Cranial Tumors

Tumors within the cranium can be either primary or metastatic. Primary tumors are classified as primary intracerebral tumors or primary extracerebral tumors. Primary intracerebral tumors originate from brain substance, neuroglia, neurons, cells of the blood vessels, and connective tissue. Primary extracerebral tumors originate outside the substance of the brain and include meningiomas, acoustic nerve tumors, and tumors of the pituitary and pineal glands. Metastatic tumors, or secondary tumors, can be found inside or outside the brain substance. Sites of intracranial tumors are illustrated in Fig. 15-18.

Central nervous system tumors include both brain and spinal cord tumors. The incidence of CNS tumors seems to increase up to age 70, then decreases. These tumors represent the second most common group of tumors in children (Fischer, Linggood, & Recht, 1986). Approximately 70% of all intracranial tumors in children are located infratentorially, and in adults 70% are located supratentorially (Chipps, Clanin, & Campbell, 1992). Peripheral nerve tumors are rare in children and common in adults.

Cranial tumors cause local and generalized clinical manifestations. The local effects are caused by the destructive action of the tumor itself on a particular site in the brain and compression causing decreased cerebral blood flow. The effects are varied and include seizures, visual disturbances, unstable gait, and cranial nerve dysfunction.

The generalized effects result from increased ICP (Fig. 15-19). Increased ICP may occur because of obstruction of the ventricular system, hemorrhages occurring in and around the tumor, or cerebral edema caused by tumors.

Intracranial brain tumors do not metastasize as readily as tumors in other organs because there are no lymphatic channels within the brain substance. If metastasis does occur, it is usually through seeding of cerebral blood, or cerebrospinal fluid, or during cranial surgery, or through artificial shunts (Willis, 1992).

Primary intracerebral tumors

Primary intracerebral tumors, also called **gliomas**, comprise both encapsulated and nonencapsulated or inva-

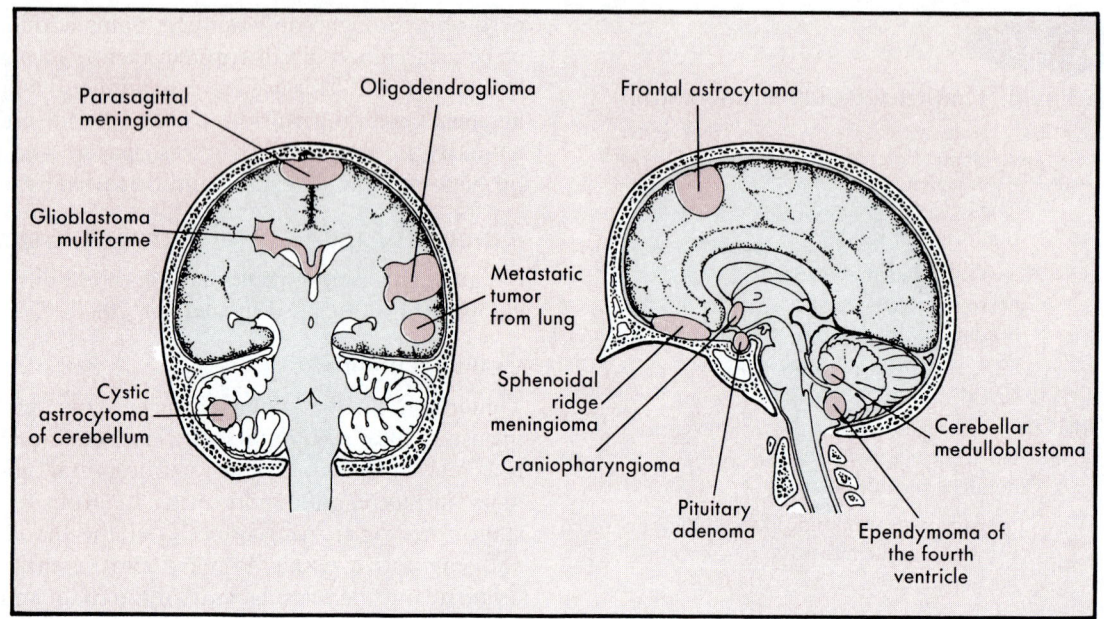

FIG. 15-18 Common sites of intracranial tumors.

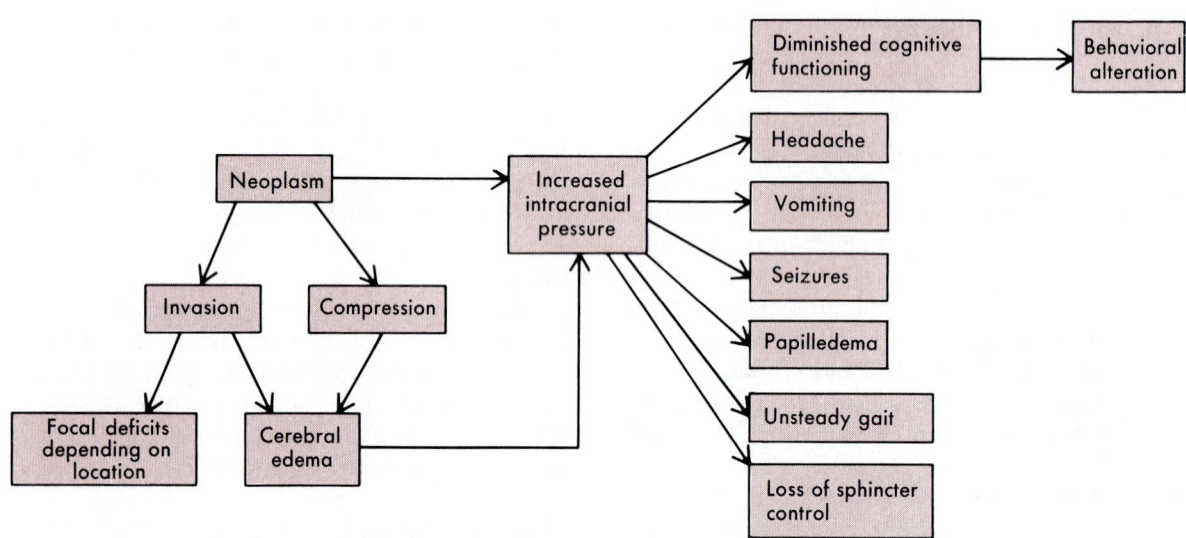

FIG. 15-19 Origin of clinical manifestations associated with an intracranial neoplasm.

sive tumors (Table 15-7). Typically the invasive tumors invade and destroy adjacent normal CNS tissue, whereas more distal neural and vascular tissues are displaced and compressed, causing ischemia, edema, and increased intracranial pressure. Encapsulated tumors generally do not invade adjacent tissues but displace and compress adjacent and distal CNS tissues and vascula-

ture. As with invasive tumors, encapsulated tumors produce ischemia, edema, and increased pressure. Normal function of the neurons is ultimately impaired by the invasion or compression.

The principal treatment for cerebral tumors is surgical or radiosurgical excision or surgical decompression if total excision is not possible. Chemotherapy and ra-

TABLE 15-7

Brain and Spinal Cord Tumors

Neoplasm	Location	Characteristics	Cell of origin
Gliomas			
Astrocytoma	Anywhere in brain or spinal cord	Slow-growing, invasive	Astrocytes
Glioblastoma multiforme	Predominantly in cerebral hemispheres	Highly invasive and malignant	Thought to arise from mature astrocytes
Oligodendrocytoma	Most commonly in frontal lobes deep in white matter; may arise in brainstem, cerebellum, and spinal cord	Relatively avascular, tends to be encapsulated; more malignant form called an oligodendroblastoma	Oligodendrites
Ependymoma	Intramedullary: wall of the ventricles, may arise in caudal tail of the spinal cord	More common in children, variable growth rates; more malignant, invasive form is called ependymoblastoma; may extend into the ventricle or invade brain tissue	Ependymal cells
Neuronal cell			
Medulloblastoma	Posterior cerebellar vermis, roof of fourth ventricle	Well-demarcated, rapid-growing, fills fourth ventricle	Embryonic cells
Mesodermal tissue			
Meningioma	Intradural, extramedullary: sylvian fissure region, superior parasagittal surface of frontal and parietal lobes, olfactory groove, wing of sphenoid bone, superior surface of cerebellum, cerebellopontine angle, spinal cord	Slow-growing, circumscribed, encapsulated, sharply demarcated from normal tissues, compressive in nature	Arachnoid cells, may be from fibroblast
Choroid plexus			
Papillomas	Choroid plexus of the ventricular system, lateral ventricle in children, fourth ventricle in adults	Usually benign, slow expansion inducing hemorrhage and hydrocephalus; malignant tumor is rare	Epithelial cells
Cranial nerves and spinal nerve roots			
Neurilemmoma	Cranial nerves (most commonly vestibular division of cranial nerve VIII)	Slow-growing	Schwann cells
Neurofibroma	Extramedullary—spinal cord	Slow-growing	Neurilemma, Schwann cells

Continued.

TABLE 15-7

Brain and Spinal Cord Tumors—cont'd

Neoplasm	Location	Characteristics	Cell of origin
Pituitary tumors	Pituitary gland; may extend to or invade floor of the third ventricle	Age-linked, several types, slow-growing, macro- and microadenomas	Pituitary cells, pituitary chromophobes, basophils, eosinophils
Pineal region	Pineal region; pineal parenchyma	Several types (germinoma, pineocytoma, teratoma)	Several types with different cell origins
Blood vessel tumors			
Angioma	Predominantly in posterior cerebral hemispheres	Slow-growing	Arising from congenitally malformed arteriovenous connections
Hemangioblastomas	Predominantly in cerebellum	Slow-growing	Embryonic vascular tissue

TABLE 15-8

Classification Systems for Astrocytomas

	Kernohan et al. system	Rigertz system
Astrocytoma		Well-differentiated astrocytoma
Grade I	Well-differentiated astrocytoma	
Grade II	More cellular and anaplastic astrocytoma	
Glioblastoma		Malignant anaplastic astrocytoma
Grade III	Poorly differentiated astrocytoma	
Grade IV	Poorly differentiated astrocytoma (glioblastoma multiforme)	Glioblastoma multiforme

diotherapy also may be used. Supportive treatment is directed at reducing edema. (Cancer treatment is discussed in Chapter 10.)

Astrocytoma. Astrocytomas are the most common primary CNS tumors (30% of all gliomas) and are graded by one of two predominant classification systems (Table 15-8). Developed from astrocytes, astrocytomas grow by expansion and infiltration into the normal surrounding brain tissues. These tumor cells are believed to have lost normal growth restraint and, thus, proliferate uncontrollably.

One third of astrocytomas are classified at diagnosis as grade I or grade II astrocytoma. These slow-growing but infiltrative gliomas tend to form cavities (pseudocysts); however, some are firm, noncavitating, avascular, gray-white masses that are difficult to distinguish from normal white matter of the brain. Although these tumors may occur anywhere in the brain or spinal cord, they most commonly are located in the cerebellum, temporal lobes, frontal lobes, and parietal lobes (Fig. 15-20). Low-grade astrocytomas in adults tend to have a lateral or supratentorial location, and they tend to be midline or near midline in position in children.

Headache may be an early symptom. Approximately half of persons with low-grade astrocytomas experience a focal or generalized seizure. Onset of a focal seizure disorder between the second and sixth decade of life is suggestive of an astrocytoma. Other general or focal neurologic manifestations develop gradually. Increased intracranial pressure is usually a late clinical manifestation.

FIG. 15-20 Astrocytoma. **A,** External appearance of astrocytoma of pons, illustrating symmetric enlargement of structure often seen in this tumor. **B,** Cross section of astrocytoma of pons, showing hemorrhagic tumor of ill-defined margins partially obliterating fourth ventricle. (Courtesy Dr. J. E. Olivera-Rabiela, Mexico City, Mexico. From Rosai, 1989.)

Conventional surgery or radiosurgery is the treatment of choice, often followed by radiotherapy. Survival time from diagnosis is often 6 to 10 years. Grade I and II astrocytomas commonly undergo anaplasia at some point, progressing to a higher-grade tumor. (Anaplasia is discussed in Chapter 10.)

Grade III and IV astrocytomas are found predominantly in the temporal and frontal lobes, as well as in the basal ganglia. These tumors also may be located in the brainstem, cerebellum, and spinal cord. They are found twice as frequently in men as in women and the 45- to 55-year age group has the highest incidence. Grade III and IV astrocytomas are often large and well circumscribed with a variegated pattern. The peripheral rim is pinkish-gray and solid with a soft yellow necrotic center and points of hemorrhage. Microscopically, there is increased cellularity, vascular proliferation, cellular pleomorphism, and necrosis. Necrosis is the principal histologic difference between an anaplastic grade III tumor and a grade IV glioblastoma multiforme.

Grade IV astrocytomas, glioblastoma multiforme, are highly vascular and extensively infiltrative. They may become large enough to extend from the meningeal surface through the ventricular wall. Fifty percent of glioblastomas are bilateral or at least occupy more than one lobe at the time of death.

The typical clinical presentation for a glioblastoma multiforme is that of diffuse, nonspecific clinical manifestations, such as headache, irritability, and "personality changes" that progress to more clear-cut manifestations of increased intracranial pressure, such as head-ache on position change, papilledema, or vomiting. Of persons affected, 30% to 40% experience seizure activity. Symptoms may progress to definite focal signs, such as hemiparesis, dysphasia, dyspraxia, cranial nerve palsies, and visual field deficits in addition to the generalized signs from increased intracranial pressure.

Diagnosis of high-grade astrocytomas most commonly takes 3 to 6 months from onset of the first clinical manifestations because the person does not recognize the need to consult a health care provider. The treatment of choice is conventional surgical or radiosurgical resection, which is commonly followed by radiotherapy and then chemotherapy. Immunotherapy using ImuVert and interstitial hyperthermia are currently under investigation as adjunctive therapies. Fewer than one fifth of persons survive 12 to 18 months beyond the onset of clinical manifestations with a grade IV tumor; fewer than 10% live beyond 2 years. Adding radiotherapy to the conventional surgical regimen has extended mean survival time after surgery from 14 to 36 weeks in grade IV tumors. Adding chemotherapy has increased this mean survival time to more than 1 year.

Oligodendroglioma. A far less commonly occurring glioma is the **oligodendroglioma**, comprising perhaps 5% to 7% of all intracranial gliomas. A typically slow-growing tumor, most oligodendrogliomas are macroscopically indistinguishable from other gliomas (Fig. 15-21). Of oligodendrogliomas, 40% to 70% develop in the frontal lobes, often in the deep white matter. They may also be found in other parts of the cerebrum, third ventricle, brainstem, cerebellum, and spinal cord. A high

FIG. 15-21 Oligodendroglioma with operative hemorrhage. There is ventricular displacement and cingulate gyrus herniation. (From Kissane, J. M.: *Anderson's pathology,* ed 8, St. Louis, 1985, Mosby–Year Book.)

FIG. 15-22 Large septal ependymoma. With secondary hydrocephalus. (Courtesy Dr. J. E. Olivera-Rabiela, Mexico City, Mexico. From Rosai, 1989.)

FIG. 15-23 Parasagittal meningioma, fibrous type. There are small, remote anemic infarcts in internal capsules and left putamen. (From Kissane, 1993.)

incidence of this tumor is found in young adults with a history of temporal lobe epilepsy. Approximately one half of these tumors generally classified as oligodendrogliomas are actually a mixed type of oligodendroglioma and astrocytoma. Malignant degeneration occurs in approximately one third of persons with oligodendrogliomas, and the tumors are then referred to as **oligodendroblastomas.** The tumor rarely becomes a glioblastoma. If there is extension to the pia mater or ependymal wall (see Fig. 12-14), oligodendrogliomas may metastasize to distant CNS sites through the ventriculoarachnoid spaces.

More than 50% of individuals experience a focal or generalized seizure as the first clinical manifestation. Only approximately one half of persons with an oligodendroglioma have experienced increased intracranial pressure at the time of diagnosis and surgery, and only one third develop any focal manifestations. The time from first clinical manifestation to surgical intervention often ranges from 2 to 6 years. Mean survival time after operation is approximately 5 years, and recurrences are common after surgery.

Ependymoma. Ependymomas are gliomas that arise from ependymal cells that form the walls of the ventricles and grow either into the ventricle or into adjacent brain tissue; they are not encapsulated (see Fig. 15-22 and Table 15-8). They comprise about 5% of all intracranial gliomas in adults and 20% in children and adolescents. Of ependymomas, 70% occur in the fourth ventricle. Other common sites for ependymomas are the third ventricle, lateral ventricles, and caudal portion of the spinal cord. Approximately 40% of the infratentorial ependymomas occur in children younger than 10 years of age. Occurrence of cerebral (supratentorial) ependymomas is distributed among all ages.

Ependymomas in the cerebrum resemble other gliomas in their clinical presentation. In approximately one third of persons, seizures occur. In fourth ventricle ependymomas, two thirds of persons have increased intracranial pressure. Other clinical manifestations may include vomiting, vertigo, difficulty swallowing, head tilt, and paresthesias of the extremities.

Clinical manifestations and progression of dysfunction associated with ependymomas may follow a short or long course. The interval between first manifestations and surgery may be as short as 4 weeks with some ependymoblastomas to as long as 7 to 8 years with others.

Surgery is the treatment of choice. Ependymomas are not very radiosensitive. Some persons benefit from a shunting procedure when the ependymoma has caused a noncommunicating hydrocephalus (see p. 576).

Primary extracerebral tumors

Meningioma. Meningioma constitutes 15% of all intracranial tumors. They are considered benign because they are encapsulated and usually do not invade the surrounding brain (Fig. 15-23). These tumors originate from the dura mater or arachnoid membranes. Rarely do meningiomas arise from arachnoid cells of the choroid plexus of the ventricles. Meningiomas most commonly are located in the olfactory grooves, on the wings of the sphenoid bone (at the base of the skull), in the tuberculum sellae (a structure next to the sella turcica), on the superior surface of the cerebellum, and in the cerebellopontine angle and spinal cord.

Small meningiomas (less than 2.0 cm in diameter) are often found on postmortem examination in middle-aged and elderly individuals who had experienced no clinical manifestations and died of totally unrelated causes. The cause of meningiomas is unknown.

A meningioma is a sharply circumscribed mass that derives its shape from the space it occupies. A meningioma may extend to the dural surface and erode the cranial bones or produce an osteoblastic reaction. A few meningiomas exhibit malignant, invasive qualities.

Only when meningiomas reach a certain size, at which time they begin to indent the brain parenchyma, do they begin to produce clinical manifestations. Focal seizures are frequently the first manifestation. Other clinical manifestations depend on the tumor's location. Because of the extremely slow-growing nature of most meningiomas, increased intracranial pressure is less common than with gliomas.

Surgical excision results in a cure if all the tumor and its meningeal stem are accessible. If only partial resection is possible, the tumor recurs.

Neurilemmoma. Neurilemmoma (neuromas, schwannomas) arise from the sheath of Schwann cells sur-

FIG. 15-24 External appearance of neurilemmoma of cerebellopontine angle. Tapered end of acoustic nerve on one side and compression of pons and medulla on other are well appreciated. (Courtesy Dr. J. E. Olivera-Rabiela, Mexico City, Mexico. From Rosai, 1989.)

rounding the axons of the cranial nerves. The tumors most commonly affect persons older than 50 years of age, and both sexes are affected equally. The vestibular division of cranial nerve VIII is most commonly affected, although neurilemmomas of the acoustic division of cranial nerve VIII, cranial nerve V, and cranial nerve IX are found (Fig. 15-24).

The tumor most commonly originates just distal to the junction between the nerve root and the brainstem. As the tumor grows, it extends into the posterior fossa to occupy the cerebropontine angle and compress adjacent nerves. Eventually the brainstem is displaced, and the CSF flow is obstructed.

Initial clinical manifestations may include headache, tinnitus, hearing loss, impaired balance, unsteady gait, facial pain, and loss of facial sensations. Later, vertigo with nausea and vomiting, a sense of pressure in the ear, and moderate to severe unsteadiness with rapid position changes may appear.

CT scan or MRI can establish the diagnosis. Posterior fossa dye studies may be required. Treatment is by surgical excision of the neurilemmoma.

Pituitary tumors are discussed in Chapter 18 and cerebral tumors in children are discussed in Chapter 16.

Metastatic carcinoma. An estimated 25% of persons with cancer develop metastasis to the brain. One third of metastatic brain tumors arise from the lung, approximately one sixth from the breast, and a lesser number from the gastrointestinal tract and kidney. Melanoma and carcinoma of the gallbladder, liver, thyroid, testes, uterus, ovary, and pancreas also may metastasize to the brain. Other tumors, besides carcinomas, that metastasize only occasionally are rhabdomyosarcomas, Ewing tumors, chorioepithelioma, lymphoma, and carcinoma.

Carcinomas are disseminated to the brain from the circulation. In more than three fourths of persons, the metastases are multiple and found in both the cerebrum and cerebellum in a scattered distribution. The metastatic tumors are often located in the meninges and near the brain surface in the gray matter and subcortical white matter. These tumors produce little glial cell reaction in the brain tissue but do cause vasogenic edema in the surrounding brain tissue.

The clinical manifestation of a metastatic brain tumor usually resembles that of a glioblastoma, although several unusual syndromes do exist. Carcinomatous encephalopathy causes headache, nervousness, depressed mood, trembling, confusion, and forgetfulness. In carcinomatosis of the cerebellum, headache, dizziness, and ataxia are found. Carcinomatosis of the craniospinal meninges (carcinomatous meningitis) manifests with headache, confusion, and manifestations of cranial or spinal nerve root dysfunction.

Metastatic brain tumors carry a poor prognosis. If a solitary tumor is found, surgery or radiation therapy is used, but if multiple tumors exist, symptomatic relief only is pursued.

Spinal Cord Tumors

Spinal cord tumors are named to reflect their cell type, growth rate, and structure of origin. Spinal cord tumors are classified as **intramedullary tumors** (originating within the neural tissues) or **extramedullary tumors** (originating from tissues outside the spinal cord). Extramedullary tumors arise from the meninges or roots (forming **intradural tumors**) or from epidural tissue or vertebral structure (forming **extradural tumors**). About 5% of spinal cord tumors seen in general hospital settings are intramedullary; 40% are intradural-extramedullary; and 55% are extradural.

Metastatic spinal cord tumors are usually carcinomas, lymphomas, or myelomas. Their location is often extradural. Of extradural tumors 50% are metastatic and have spread to the spine through direct extension from tumors of the vertebral structures or from extraspinal sources extending through the interventricular foramen or through the bloodstream.

The most common primary extramedullary spinal cord tumors are neurofibromas and meningiomas. These tumors are intradural more often than extradural. Neurofibromas are found most commonly in the thoracic region. Meningiomas are more evenly distributed through the spine. Other extramedullary tumors in order of frequency of occurrence are sarcomas, vascular tumors, chordomas, and epidermoid and similar tumors. Of intradural-extramedullary tumors, 70% are meningiomas, neurofibromas, or sarcomas.

Intramedullary tumors have the same cellular origins as brain tumors. Ependymomas account for 40% of intramedullary spinal cord tumors. Astrocytomas, glioblastomas, oligodendrogliomas, ganglioneuromas, medulloblastomas, hemangiomas, and hemangioblastomas are more or less equally distributed in frequency of occurrence.

Pathophysiology

Extramedullary spinal cord tumors produce dysfunction by compression of adjacent tissue, not by direct invasion. The spinal cord is compressed by the tumor from without, and destruction of the white matter tracts occurs. The spinal canal around the cord becomes filled by tumor.

Intramedullary spinal cord tumors produce dysfunction by both invasion and compression. The cord enlarges from the tumor that is enlarging inside the cord. Additionally, distortion of adjacent white matter tracts occurs. Metastases from spinal cord tumors occur from seeding through the cerebrospinal fluid; medulloblastomas and ependymomas establish distant implants in this manner.

Clinical Manifestations

The acute onset of clinical manifestations suggests a vascular insult caused by thrombosis of vessels supplying the spinal cord. Clinical manifestations that are gradual and progressive suggest compression. The clinical manifestations associated with spinal cord tumors fall into three major categories: (1) a compressive syndrome (sensorimotor syndrome), (2) an irritative syndrome (radicular syndrome), and (3) rarely, a syringomyelic syndrome.

The **compressive syndrome** is associated with compression and is less frequently caused by invasion and destruction of the spinal cord tracts. Symptoms are usually gradual and progressive, and initial manifestations may be asymmetric. With tumors located in the cervical area, the motor dysfunction usually has the following pattern: ipsilateral arm involvement, followed by ipsilateral and contralateral leg involvement, and finally involvement of the opposite arm. With thoracic tumors, the pattern of motor involvement is paresis and spasticity of one leg, followed by involvement of the opposite leg. The sensory clinical manifestations of tingling paresthesias have a similar pattern to that of the motor signs. Pain and temperature dysfunctions are more commonly found than touch, vibration, and proprioceptive changes, although posterior column signs are also frequently found. Pain is less well localized than with an irritative syndrome caused by root involvement. Initially the pain and temperature changes are contralateral to the motor deficit (Brown-Séquard syndrome). Bladder and bowel deficits usually appear when paresis develops in the legs.

The **irritative syndrome** combines the clinical manifestations of a cord compression with radicular pain, which is pain in the sensory root distribution and indicates root irritation. The segmental manifestations associated with root irritation include segmental sensory changes that include paresthesias and impaired pain and touch perception; motor disturbances, including cramps, atrophy, fasciculations, and decreased or absent deep tendon reflexes; and ache in the spine. Tenderness of the spinous processes over the tumor is present in about one half of persons with extramedullary tumors. The segmental changes may appear months and sometimes years before the clinical manifestations of compression in benign tumors. The compressive clinical manifestations include an asymmetric spastic paresis of the lower extremities with tumors in the thoracic or lumbar region, paresis of the arms and legs with tumors in the cervical area, decreased or absent pain and temperature perception below the tumor site, posterior column signs, and spastic bladder.

Because they involve the central gray matter of the cord, intramedullary spinal cord tumors, notably ependymomas, may produce **syringomyelic syndrome**, or inflammation of the spinal cord. Inflammation results in the development of tubular (syrinx) cavities in the spinal cord. Occasionally an extramedullary tumor may produce the same effect, although the mechanisms are unknown.

Evaluation and Treatment

The diagnosis of a spinal cord tumor is made through spinal roentgenograms, cerebrospinal fluid studies, CT scan, MRI, myelogram (EMG), and spinal angiography. Involvement of specific cord segments is established. Any metastases are also identified.

Treatment varies, depending on the nature of the tumor and the person's clinical status. Intradural-extramedullary tumors are surgically removed or decompressed through laminectomy. Laminectomy with decompression and excision is used for gliomas and is followed by radiotherapy. Extradural metastatic tumors are often managed by radiation therapy, chemotherapy, hormonal therapy, or pain management protocols.

Infection and Inflammation of the Central Nervous System

The CNS may be affected directly by bacteria, viruses, fungi, protozoans, and rickettsiae. The resulting infection is pyogenic, or pus producing. Bacterial toxins also may affect the CNS. The meninges, neural tissues, and vasculature also may be involved in the inflammatory process.

Meningitis

Meningitis (infection of the meninges) may be caused by bacteria, viruses, fungi, parasites, or other toxins. The infections are classified as acute, subacute, or chronic processes, and the pathophysiology, clinical manifestations, and treatment are different for each type of organism.

Bacterial meningitis is primarily an infection of the pia mater and arachnoid, the subarachnoid space, the ventricular system, and the CSF. A systemic or bloodstream infection or a direct extension from an infected area is the access route to the subarachnoid space. Meningococcus (*Neisseria meningitidis*), pneumococcus (*Streptococcus pneumoniae*), and *Haemophilus influenzae* are the common causes of bacterial meningitis.

Meningococcus has been identified worldwide. Meningococcal meningitis occurs predominantly in men and boys and in the fall, winter, and spring of the year. Epidemics of meningococcal meningitis occur in approximately 10-year cycles. Children and adolescents are affected predominantly. With pneumococcal meningitis, the young and those older than 40 years of age are mostly affected. *Haemophilus influenzae* occurs almost exclusively in children 2 months to 7 years of age.

Less frequent causes are staphylococcus, streptococcus, gonococcus, and gram-negative bacteria.

Aseptic meningitis (viral meningitis, nonpurulent meningitis) is an inflammation believed to be limited to the meninges. Aseptic meningitis produces a variety of symptoms and is caused by a variety of infectious agents, most of which are viruses. Enteroviral viruses (echovirus, Coxsackievirus, and nonparalytic poliomyelitis), mumps, herpes simplex (type I), adenoviruses, and California virus are the most common causes of aseptic meningitis. Bacterial infections not adequately treated are another cause of aseptic meningitis.

Fungal meningitis is a chronic, much less common condition than bacterial or viral meningitis. The most common fungal infections of the nervous system are cryptococcosis, coccidioidomycosis, mucormycosis, candidiasis, and aspergillosis. Fungal meningitis most frequently occurs in persons with impaired immune responses or alterations in normal body flora. Fungal meningitis develops insidiously, usually over days or weeks.

Pathophysiology

The bacteria that commonly cause bacterial meningitis are common inhabitants of the nasopharynx, but a predisposing factor such as a prior upper respiratory infection must be present before the bacteria become blood borne. The method of CNS entry is still unclear. The bacteria or their toxins do, however, function as irritants and induce an inflammatory reaction by the meninges (pia and arachnoid), the CSF, and the ventricles. The meningeal vessels undergo change, becoming hyperemic and increasingly permeable. Blood cells (neutrophils) migrate into the subarachnoid space, producing an exudate that thickens the CSF and interferes with normal CSF flow around the brain and spinal cord. The exudate has the potential to obstruct arachnoid villi and produce hydrocephalus. This purulent exudate increases rapidly, causing further inflammation. The exudate increases, especially around the base of the brain, and extends into the sheaths of the cranial and spinal nerves, and into the perivascular spaces of the cortex. Meningeal cells become edematous. The exudate and edematous cells increase intracranial pressure. The small and medium-sized subarachnoid arteries, veins, and choroid plexuses undergo inflammatory changes and become engorged, disrupting blood flow and potentially producing thrombosis. Secondary infection of the brain may occur. The cortical neurons also show some changes, including an increase in the number of microglia and astrocytes.

Fungi in the nervous system usually produce a granulomatous reaction with formations of granulomas or gelatinous masses. These usually develop in the meninges at the base of the brain. Fungi also may extend along the perivascular sites in the subarachnoid space and into the brain tissue, producing arteritis with thrombosis, infarction, and communicating hydrocephalus. Meningeal fibrosis develops later in the inflammatory process. Cranial nerve dysfunction, caused by compression, often results from the granulomas and fibrosis.

Clinical Manifestations

The clinical manifestations of a bacterial meningitis that arise from the meningeal inflammation are a generalized throbbing headache that becomes very severe, forceful flexion of the neck onto the chest, causing Brudzinski sign (flexion of the legs and thighs), and Kernig sign (inability to extend the leg with the hip flexed at a right angle). The irritation and damage to the cranial nerve produced by the inflamed sheaths are manifested in photophobia, which becomes extreme; diplopia; and tinnitus. Neck stiffness, pain with nuchal rigidity, and possibly head retraction reflect the irritability of the spinal accessory and cervical spinal nerves. Often the vomiting center is irritated, causing projectile vomiting. Confusion and decreasing responsiveness are evidence of the cortical involvement. Fever is usually present. With meningococcal meningitis, there is a petechial or purpuric rash involving the skin and mucous membranes. As intracranial pressure increases, papilledema may develop and delirium may progress so that the individual reaches an unconscious state.

The clinical manifestations of aseptic meningitis are mild compared with those associated with bacterial meningitis. Mild generalized throbbing headache, mild photophobia, mild neck pain, stiffness, fever, and malaise are all manifestations of aseptic meningitis.

Fungal meningitis develops slowly and insidiously. The first manifestations are often those of dementia (see Chapter 14) or communicating hydrocephalus (see p. 576). The individual is characteristically afebrile.

Evaluation and Treatment

Diagnosis of bacterial meningitis is based on physical examination and cultures of blood and CSF. Bacterial meningitis and fungal meningitis are treated with appropriate antibiotic therapy and other supportive measures. Aseptic meningitis is sometimes managed pharmacologically with antibiotics, antiviral drugs, and steroids.

Abscess

Abscesses are localized collections of pus within the parenchyma of the brain and spinal cord. The incidence of abscesses is about 1 per 100,000 hospital admissions. Men experience abscesses more frequently than women, with a 2:1 ratio. The median age for abscess formation is 30 to 40 years of age. Abscesses occur (1) after open trauma and during neurosurgery; (2) in association with a contiguous focus of infection, such as the middle ear, mastoid cells, nasal cavity, and nasal sinuses; (3) through metastatic or hematogenous spread from distant foci, such as the heart, lungs, pelvic organs, skin, tonsils, abscessed teeth, osteomyelitis in other than cranial bones, and dirty needles (especially in compromised hosts); and (4) cryptogenically, arising without other associative areas of infections. Streptococci, staphylococci, and *Bacteroides*, often in combination with anaerobes, are the most common bacteria that cause abscesses; however, yeast and fungi have also been found in CNS abscess. *Toxoplasma gondii* is producing an ever-increasing number of CNS abscesses in persons with acquired immune deficiency syndrome (AIDS). Eighty percent of abscesses are located in the cerebrum, and 20% are cerebellar. The frontal and temporal lobes are the most common sites. The abscesses are in more than one site in 5% to 20% of cases. Immunosuppressed persons are particularly at risk for abscesses.

Brain abscesses are classified as extradural or intracerebral. **Extradural brain abscesses** are associated with osteomyelitis in a cranial bone. Unlike **intracerebral brain abscesses,** they rarely arise from a vascular source. **Spinal cord abscesses** are classified as epidural or intramedullary. Individuals with diabetes mellitus show an increased incidence of **spinal epidural abscesses** (which form in the epidural space), whereas debilitated individuals with sepsis more frequently develop **intramedullary spinal cord abscesses** (those within the spinal cord). Epidural spinal abscesses usually originate as osteomyelitis in a vertebra; the infection then spreads into the epidural space. (Osteomyelitis is discussed in Chapter 39.)

Pathophysiology

Organisms gain entrance to the CNS from adjacent sites by direct extension from osteomyelitis or spread along the wall of a vein. Infective emboli carry the organisms from distant sites. Initially, a localized inflammatory process (focal cerebritis) develops, leading to edema, hyperemia, softening, and petechial hemorrhage. There is exudate formation, septic thrombosis of vessels, and aggregates of degenerating leukocytes. The surrounding tissues are edematous (Fig. 15-25). The veins are filled with fibrin and polymorphonuclear leukocytes (white blood cells [WBCs]). After a few days the intense reaction abates, and fibroblasts from capillaries adjacent to the focal cerebritis deposit collagen fibers to contain and encapsulate the purulent focus. The infection becomes delimited with a center of pus and a wall of granular tissue. Encapsulation takes about 2 to 3 weeks. A free (nonencapsulated) abscess is associated with a higher mortality rate. A mature abscess has three layers: (1) a center of polymorphonuclear leukocytes, (2) a collagenous capsule, and (3) peripheral gliosis. Existing abscesses also tend to spread and form daughter abscesses.

FIG. 15-25 Chronic brain abscesses in temporal lobe and insula. Surrounding brain shows swelling and edema. There are compression and displacement of lateral and third ventricles. Cingulate gyrus and uncal herniations are also present. (From Kissane, 1993.)

Abscesses arising from the ear are frequently located in the middle or inferior temporal lobe or in the anterolateral cerebellar hemispheres. Abscesses originating from the oral and nasal area most commonly are located in the frontal and temporal lobes. Abscesses from distant foci often occur in multiple numbers in the distal portion of the middle cerebral arteries. In extradural abscesses, pus and granulation tissue accumulate in the extradural space.

Clinical Manifestations

Clinical manifestations of brain abscesses are associated with (1) intracranial infection, such as fever and increased sedimentation rate; or (2) an expanding intracranial mass, such as headache, nausea, vomiting, decreasing cognitive abilities, paresis, and seizures. Early clinical manifestations of brain abscesses are low-grade fever, headache, neck pain and stiffness with mild nuchal rigidity, confusion, drowsiness, sensory deficits, and communication deficits. Headache is the most frequent early symptom. Later clinical manifestations may include inattentiveness (distractibility), memory deficits, decreased visual acuity and narrowed visual fields, papilledema, ocular palsy, ataxia, and dementia. Symptoms depend on the location of the abscess. The development of symptoms may be very insidious, often making an abscess difficult to diagnose.

Extradural brain abscesses are associated with localized pain, purulent drainage from the nasal passages or auditory canal, fever, localized tenderness, and neck stiffness. Occasionally the individual experiences a focal seizure.

Clinical manifestations of spinal cord abscesses have four stages: (1) spinal aching; (2) root pain, which is usually severe, accompanied by spasms of the back muscles and limited vertebral movement because of pain and spasm; (3) weakness caused by progressive cord compression; and (4) paralysis.

Evaluation and Treatment

The diagnosis is suggested on the basis of clinical features and confirmed by CT scan. Magnetic resonance imaging is helpful when the CT scan does not show a strongly suggested abscess. Aspiration through a burr hole or excision through craniotomy accompanied by

FIG. 15-26 Chronic necrotizing encephalitis caused by herpes simplex. There is necrosis of temporal lobes, insula, and cingulate gyri. (From Kissane, J. M. (1985). *Anderson's pathology,* (8th ed.). St. Louis: Mosby–Year Book.)

antibiotic therapy is the recommended but somewhat controversial treatment for brain abscesses. In addition, intracranial pressure may have to be managed.

Because decompression is necessary, spinal cord abscesses are treated with surgical excision or aspiration. Antibiotic and support therapy is also instituted.

Encephalitis

Encephalitis is an acute febrile illness, usually of viral origin, with nervous system involvement. The most common encephalitides are caused by arthropod-borne (mosquito-borne) viruses and herpes simplex, almost exclusively herpes simplex type I (Fig. 15-26). Referred to as infectious viral encephalitides, encephalitis also may occur as a complication of systemic viral diseases such as poliomyelitis, rabies, or mononucleosis, or it may arise after recovery from some viral infection such as rubella or rubeola. Encephalitis also may follow vaccination with a live attenuated virus vaccine, if the vaccine has an encephalitis component. Such vaccines include measles, mumps, and rubella. Typhus, trichinosis, malaria, and schistosomiasis also are associated with encephalitis. Toxoplasmosis may acutely reactivate in immunosuppressed persons when the once dormant parasite in cyst form disseminates in brain tissues (see p. 567).

With the exception of the California viral encephalitis, which is endemic, the arthropod-borne encephalitides occur in epidemics, varying in geographic and seasonal incidence (Table 15-9). Eastern equine encephalitis is the most serious but least common of the encephalitides.

TABLE 15-9

Viral Encephalitis

Type	Geographic incidence	Seasonal incidence
Arthropod-borne:		
Eastern equine encephalitis	Eastern United States	Autumn
Western equine encephalitis	Uniform distribution, throughout the United States	Summer and early fall
St. Louis encephalitis	Widespread distribution; in the far west occurs in rural areas, elsewhere in urban areas	Late summer
Venezuelan equine encephalitis	Southwestern United States	Year round
California virus encephalitis	Midwestern states	Early fall
Herpes simplex encephalitis	No particular geographic distribution	No seasonal incidence
Poliovirus poliomyelitis	Sporadic distribution where nonimmunized persons cluster	Summer and early fall
Rabies	Sporadic distribution throughout the United States	Bites more common in late spring and throughout the early fall

From Boss, 1984.

Pathophysiology

Evidence of meningeal involvement appears in all encephalitides. The arthropod-borne viral encephalitides cause widespread nerve cell degeneration. Edema and areas of necrosis with or without hemorrhage develop. Increased intracranial pressure develops and may progress to herniation. Large degenerative injuries are found in Eastern equine encephalitis, whereas the other arthropod-borne viral encephalitides have microscopic areas of injury and degeneration.

Infectious encephalitis may result from a postinfectious autoimmune response to the virus or from direct invasion of the CNS by the virus. Herpes simplex type I has a tendency to infect the inferomedial surfaces of the temporal and frontal lobes and causes hemorrhagic necrosis.

Clinical Manifestations

Encephalitis may be a mild infectious disease to a severe disorder that is life-threatening. The dramatic clinical manifestations of encephalitis are fever, delirium, or confusion progressing to unconsciousness, seizure activity, cranial nerve palsies, paresis and paralysis, involuntary movement, and abnormal reflexes. Signs of marked intracranial pressure may be present.

Evaluation and Treatment

Diagnosis is made by history and clinical presentation aided by CSF examination and culture, serology, WBC count, CT, or MRI. Until very recently no definitive treatment was available for the viral encephalitides, but herpes encephalitis is now being treated with antiviral agents such as acyclovir. Supportive therapy is initiated, and measures to control intracranial pressure are paramount.

Neurologic Complications of AIDS

Approximately 40% to 60% of all persons with AIDS have neurologic complications of AIDS. On postmortem examination, 75% of AIDS victims have nervous system pathology. The CNS pathologies found in persons with AIDS result from (1) the primary human immunodeficiency virus (HIV) infection, (2) opportunistic infections, (3) neoplasms, and (4) systemic illness. Cerebrovascular complications and complications from the therapeutic drugs used to treat AIDS also may involve the CNS.

A variety of CNS complications of AIDS exist (Table 15-10). Multiple CNS pathologies may be experienced by one person. The most common neurologic disorder is HIV encephalopathy. Other common neurologic disorders are peripheral neuropathies, vacuolar (spongy softening) myelopathy, opportunistic infections of the CNS, and neoplasms.

Although HIV has been isolated in the CSF and brain/spinal cord tissues, the mechanism by which HIV infects the CNS is not known. The virus can be isolated in the CSF at approximately the time of seroconversion.

Pathologically, there may be (1) diffuse CNS involvement that produces a variety of clinical manifestations, (2) focal lesions that act as space-occupying lesions, and (3) obstructive hydrocephalus.

HIV encephalopathy

HIV encephalopathy (subacute encephalitis, AIDS encephalopathy, AIDS dementia complex, or AIDS-related dementia) may affect both adults and children and is characterized by progressive cognitive dysfunction in conjunction with motor and behavioral alterations. The syndrome typically develops later in the disease but may be an early or singular manifestation in some persons.

The viral route of entry into the CNS is unclear but it is believed that HIV encephalopathy is the result of direct brain tissue infection by the virus. Human immunodeficiency virus is found mostly in white matter subcortical areas, but there is some viral replication in some of the glial cells and, occasionally, within neurons. Multiple small nodules containing inflammatory cells are found scattered throughout the white matter and in subcortical gray matter, such as the basal ganglia and thalami. Multinucleated giant cells are present, as is perivascular inflammation. There are focal and diffuse demyelination of white matter and spongy changes of the spinal cord. Factors other than direct cell damage also may be involved, such as toxins, lymphokines, or other substances.

HIV encephalopathy is insidious in onset and unpredictable in its course. Most persons experience a steady progression of signs over several months to more than one year, although some individuals experience an abrupt onset or an accelerated course.

Early clinical manifestations of HIV encephalopathy may be vague. Impaired concentration and memory deficits commonly occur. Apathy and lack of motivation may appear. Later difficulties with language and visual construction appear. Some persons manifest an organic psychosis with agitation, inappropriate behavior, and hallucinosis.

There are generalized cognitive system deficits later in the course of HIV encephalopathy, often accompanied by psychomotor slowing and decreased speech spontaneity and fluency. Ataxia, spastic paraparesis or paralysis, and generalized hyperreflexia are common motor signs. Tremor, myoclonus, and seizure are less commonly seen.

Diagnosis is difficult, especially in early stages. History with physical examination findings and supporting CSF and CT and MRI data helps establish the diagno-

TABLE 15-10

Neurologic Manifestations of HIV Infection (Ordered by Prevalence)

Neurologic disorder	Prevalence	Clinical features	Treatment
HIV encephalopathy	60%-70%	Memory/concentration impairment, apathy, depressive symptoms, psychomotor slowing, incontinence	Symptomatic ?AZT
Toxoplasmosis	up to 30%	Focal neurologic deficits, fever, altered mental status, seizures	Pyrimethamine and sulfadiazine
Painful sensory neuropathy	30%	Painful dysesthesias, numbness, paresthesias	Amitriptyline
Myelopathy	20%	Gait ataxia, spastic paraparesis, incontinence	None
Cryptococcal meningitis	10%	Headache, meningismus, altered mental status	Amphotericin B and flucytosine
Acute aseptic meningitis	5%-10%	Fever, headache, meningismus, cranial nerve palsies	Symptomatic
Herpes simplex/zoster encephalitis	5%	Fever, focal neurologic deficits, seizures	Acyclovir
CMV retinitis	5%	Blurred vision, hemorrhage on ophthalmoscopy	DHPG
Herpes zoster radiculitis	3%	Pain, paresthesias over trunk, face, or limb, weakness	Amitriptyline or carbamazepine
Progressive multifocal leukoencephalopathy	2%	Focal neurologic deficits, altered mental status, headache, weakness, gait abnormalities	None
Chronic inflammatory demyelinating polyneuropathy	1%-2%	Progressive weakness, areflexia	Plasmapheresis, steroid therapy
Myositis	Rare	Myalgias, proximal weakness	?Immunosuppressive therapy
Neurosyphilis	Rare	Headache, meningeal signs, fever, nausea, and vomiting	IV penicillin
Lymphoma	Rare <2%	Change in mentation, apathetic, abulic, psychomotor slowing	Radiation with supplemental chemotherapy

From McArthur, J. H., Palenicek, J. G., & Bowersox, L. L. (1988). Human immunodeficiency virus and the nervous system. *Nursing Clinics of North America, 23*(4), 824-825.

sis. Antiviral agents have not been demonstrated to be effective but may be used. Otherwise, treatment is supportive.

Vacuolar myelopathy

Myelopathy involving diffuse degeneration of the spinal cord may occur in persons with AIDS. The most common myelopathy is a **vacuolar myelopathy** that affects the lateral and posterior columns of the spinal cord and is associated with HIV encephalopathy in 60% of individuals. The exact timing of the development of the myelopathy is unknown.

Researchers believe that the pathology is a direct consequence of HIV. Other agents also may be involved in the pathogenesis. Vacuolation in the lumbar cord develops.

A progressive spastic paraparesis with ataxia is the predominant clinical manifestation. Leg weakness, upper motor neuron signs, incontinence, and posterior column sensory loss may be present.

Diagnosis is made on the basis of history, physical findings, and supporting data from diagnostic procedures. Treatment is supportive in nature.

Peripheral neuropathy

The peripheral nervous system may sustain injury in AIDS, manifesting as a peripheral neuropathy. The most common neuropathy is a sensory neuropathy that most commonly occurs later in the disease and is unresponsive to treatment.

Human immunodeficiency virus has been isolated from peripheral nerves, so it is believed that the virus may directly infect nerves. Persons experience painful dysesthesias and paresthesias, typically in the extremities. Weakness and decreased or absent distal reflexes may be present.

Diagnosis is established through history, physical findings, and laboratory data.

Aseptic viral meningitis

Some persons develop an acute aseptic meningitis at approximately the time of seroconversion. This may well represent the initial infection of the nervous system by the HIV. Symptoms include headache, fever, and meningismus. Cranial nerve involvement, especially V and VII, may appear, but the disease is self-limiting and requires only symptomatic treatment.

Opportunistic viral and nonviral infections

Opportunistic viral infections may produce nervous system disease. Cytomegalovirus encephalitis is increasing among persons with AIDS. Persons with cytomegalovirus encephalitis may experience altered cognitive functions, tremor, focal neurologic deficits, and sensory deficits. Herpes encephalitis and herpes varicella zoster radiculitis may develop. Papovavirus (especially JC virus) in the immunocompromised person with AIDS may produce a demyelinating disorder called progressive multifocal leukoencephalopathy (PML). This virus is found in 90% of healthy persons, but is dormant. The virus reactivates to cause PML in the person with AIDS.

Opportunistic nonviral infections also may cause nervous system disease. **Toxoplasmosis** is the most common CNS disorder associated with AIDS and accounts for almost 50% of CNS disease in some studies. Central nervous system toxoplasmosis typically manifests as a focal encephalitis.

Toxoplasma gondii, a protozoan, is thought to reactivate from latent lesions to produce a well-demarcated necrotizing process. Inflammatory infiltrates, thrombotic lesions, and fibrinoid vascular walls are present at the necrotic edge. Marked edema is present adjacent to necrotic areas. Lesions may be multiple and exist throughout the cerebral hemispheres.

Clinical manifestations of CNS toxoplasmosis are highly variable and include clumsiness to hemiplegia, aphasia, seizures, ataxia, cognitive changes, and constitutional symptoms. Toxoplasmosis is difficult to diagnose but is effectively treated with pyrimethamine and sulfadiazine. Allergic response to sulfadiazine is a problem and other drugs can be substituted. Persons with AIDS may develop meningitis, encephalitis, or brain abscesses of fungal, mycobacterial, and bacterial origin.

CNS neoplasms

CNS neoplasms associated with AIDS include CNS lymphoma, systemic non-Hodgkin lymphoma, and metastatic Kaposi sarcoma. The precise mechanism of tumor development is not known. Primary CNS lymphoma is a large cell lymphoma that presents as rapidly developing and expanding multicentric intracranial mass lesions. There is invasion of the meninges and, possibly, the cranial nerves and spinal cord in systemic non-Hodgkin lymphoma. Metastasis to the CNS of a Kaposi sarcoma is uncommon.

Other CNS complications

Persons with AIDS may develop multifocal ischemic infarctions, hemorrhagic infarctions, hemorrhage into tumors, subdural hematomas, and epidural hemorrhage. The precise mechanism of these cardiovascular complications is not yet known. Reported neurologic symptoms produced by AIDS therapeutics include extrapyramidal movements, myoclonus, dysphasia, delirium, and acute myelopathy.

Degenerative Diseases
Parkinson Disease

Parkinson disease is a commonly occurring degenerative disorder of the basal ganglia (corpus striatum) involving the dopaminergic (dopamine-secreting) nigrostriatal pathway. Nigrostriatal disorders produce a syndrome of abnormal movement called **parkinsonism** (**Parkinson syndrome, parkinsonian syndrome**) (Fig. 15-27).

Etiologic classification of parkinsonism includes primary Parkinson disease and secondary parkinsonism. Secondary parkinsonism is parkinsonism caused by disorders other than Parkinson disease (i.e., trauma, infection, neoplasm, atherosclerosis, toxins, and drug intoxication). Drug-induced parkinsonism, particularly that caused by phenothiazines, is the most common cause of the secondary form and is usually reversible. Illegal "designer drugs" containing the chemical MPTP have recently produced a parkinsonian syndrome in users.

The onset of Parkinson disease is after the age of 40, with peak age of onset in the early 60s (Duvoisin, 1984). Men and women appear to be equally affected (Duvoisin, 1984). Parkinson disease is one of the most prevalent of the primary CNS disorders and a leading cause of neurologic disability in individuals older than age 60 (Chipps et al., 1992). The prevalence rate is 130 per 100,000 persons (Chipps et al., 1992). An estimated half-million persons in the United States are affected.

Pathophysiology

The pathogenesis of Parkinson disease is unknown. The disease does not show a hereditary pattern or familial tendency. Epidemiologic data suggest vascular, viral, and metabolic factors as possible causes. One hypothe-

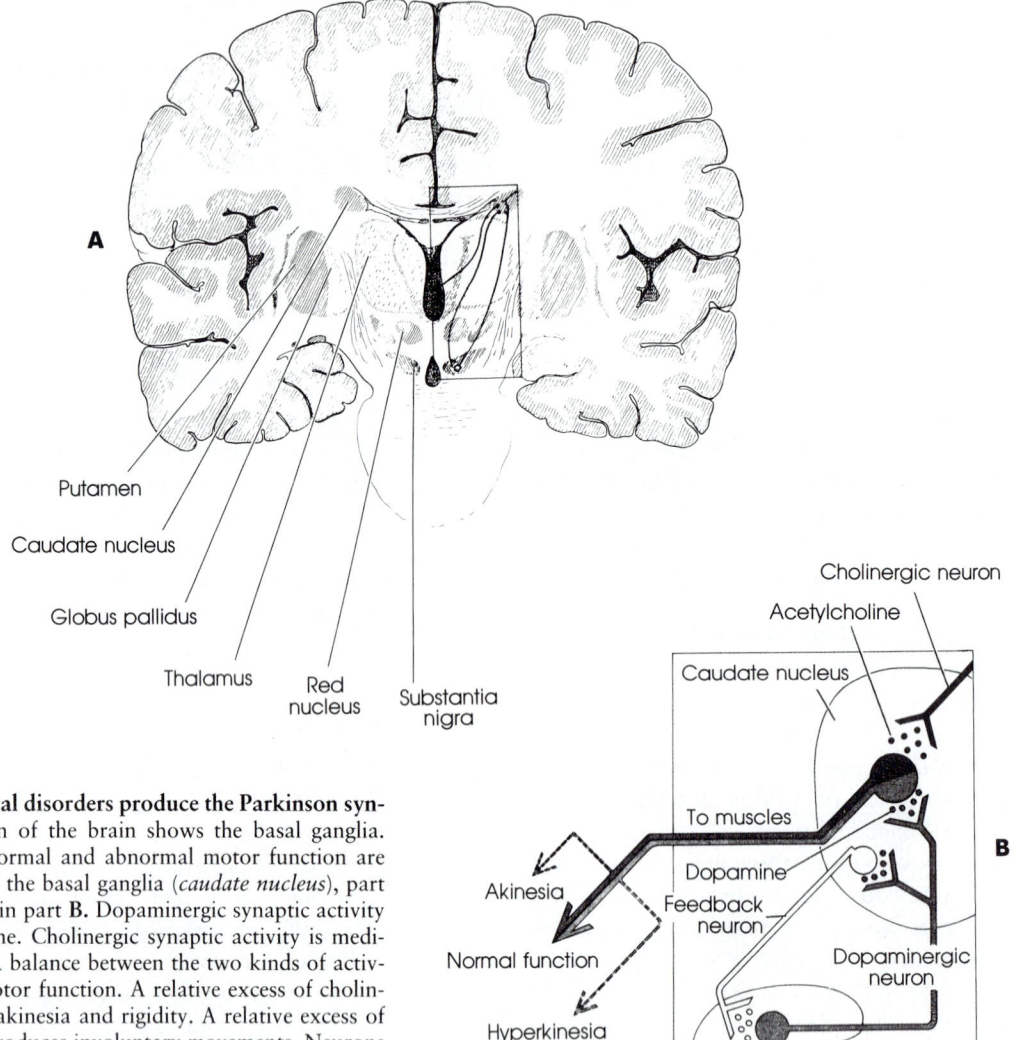

Putamen

Caudate nucleus

Globus pallidus

Thalamus Red Substantia
nucleus nigra

Cholinergic neuron

Acetylcholine

Caudate nucleus

To muscles

Akinesia

Dopamine

Feedback
neuron

Normal function

Dopaminergic
neuron

Hyperkinesia

Substantia nigra

GABA

B

FIG. 15-27 Nigrostriatal disorders produce the Parkinson syndrome. Coronal section of the brain shows the basal ganglia. Pathways controlling normal and abnormal motor function are depicted in a portion of the basal ganglia (*caudate nucleus*), part **A**, and shown enlarged in part **B**. Dopaminergic synaptic activity is mediated by dopamine. Cholinergic synaptic activity is mediated by acetylcholine. A balance between the two kinds of activity produces normal motor function. A relative excess of cholinergic activity produces akinesia and rigidity. A relative excess of dopaminergic activity produces involuntary movements. Neurons in the caudate nucleus contain gamma-aminobutyric acid (GABA) and possibly control dopaminergic neurons in the substantia nigra through a feedback pathway. (From Cutler, 1983.)

sis is that age predisposes the nigrostriatal pathway to damage by viruses or toxins. Isolation of the neurotoxic chemical MPTP, demonstration of its ability to produce an irreversible parkinsonian syndrome, and selective destruction of substantia nigra cells have produced a research focus on toxins as an causative agent.

Atrophy and neuronal loss are found in the cerebral cortex in more than one half of individuals with Parkinson disease (Duvoisin, 1984). The principal pathologic feature of Parkinson disease is degeneration of the dopaminergic nigrostriatal pathway, which is composed of neurons of the substantia nigra ("black substance"), with fibers synapsing in the caudate and putamen basal ganglia (Fig. 15-27, *A*). Signs of inflammation or infection are absent. The severity of Parkinson disease seems to correlate with the degree of neuronal loss in the substantia nigra. Another pathologic feature is significant

reduction in certain dopamine receptors (D_1 receptors) in the basal ganglia.

Nigral and basal ganglial depletion of dopamine, an inhibitory neurotransmitter, is the principal biochemical alteration in Parkinson disease (Fig. 15-27, *B*). Symptom development in basal ganglial disorders is explained as an imbalance of dopaminergic (inhibitory) and cholinergic (excitatory) activity in the caudate and putamen of the basal ganglia. Dopaminergic-cholinergic balance produces normal motor function. In Parkinson disease, degeneration of the dopaminergic nigrostriatal pathway causes dopamine depletion in the basal ganglia and relative excess of cholinergic activity in the feedback circuit involving the cerebral cortex, basal ganglia, and thalamus. A relative excess of cholinergic activity in this circuit, as in Parkinson disease, is manifested by hypertonia (tremor and rigidity) and akinesia.

FIG. 15-28 Production of the tremor in Parkinson disease. Feedback cycles of motor outflow. (Redrawn from Riley & Massey, 1980; from Rudy, 1984.)

Clinical Manifestations

The classic manifestations of Parkinson disease are tremor at rest (resting tremor), rigidity (muscle stiffness), and akinesia (poverty of movement). They may develop alone or in combination, but as the disease progresses, all three are usually present to at least some degree. There is no true paralysis. The symptoms are always bilateral but usually develop asymmetrically. Because of the insidious onset, the beginning of symptoms is difficult to document. In early stages of the disease, reflex, sensory, and mental status is usually normal. Postural abnormalities, autonomic-neuroendocrine symptoms, and, in some cases, dementia are also part of the syndrome.

Parkinsonian tremor, rigidity, and akinesia. Parkinsonian tremor is usually the first symptom to appear. It is an asymmetric, regular, rhythmic, low-amplitude tremor, with slowly alternating flexion-extension contraction (4 to 8 cycles per second). Later the tremor becomes symmetric at 7 to 12 cycles per second. It is a tremor at rest, disappearing briefly during the course of a voluntary movement and reappearing when the limb is held in a stationary position. Intensity and amplitude of the tremor vary.

Parkinsonian tremor appears to result from instability of feedback from the basal ganglia to the cerebral cortex caused by loss of the inhibitory influence of dopamine in the basal ganglia. Oscillation in the normal feedback cycles of the motor outflow feedback circuit when the muscles are at rest produces the tremor (Fig. 15-28). When the individual performs voluntary movements, the tremor becomes temporarily blocked, presumably because other motor control signals arriving in

the thalamus override the abnormal basal ganglial signals. As the disorder worsens, tremor may lessen as rigidity supervenes.

Rigidity, a state of involuntary contraction of all skeletal muscles, impedes active and passive movement. The first symptoms of rigidity may be painful muscle cramps in the toes or hands. More commonly the limb feels stiff, heavy, tired, or aching. Rigidity is felt by the examiner as lead-pipe resistance during passive movement that may be interrupted by brief jerks palpable as a cogwheel sensation. The mechanism underlying rigidity is increased resting muscle activity.

Akinesia is poverty of associated and voluntary movements. It is the most prevalent and crippling symptom and is often overlooked in the early stages. All striated muscles—extremity, trunk, ocular, facial—are eventually affected, including muscles of mastication (chewing), deglutition (swallowing), and articulation. Extreme underactivity in the individual with Parkinson disease makes the person appear stiff, even when resistance to passive movement cannot be felt. Akinesia is a separate phenomenon from rigidity and may be severe even in the presence of rigidity. Individuals state that they feel "wooden" as though moving "against resistance" and complain of rapid, severe fatigue. Akinesia is attributed to failure of the mechanism programming movement patterns manifested as a defect in the voluntary production of smooth motions at different speeds.

Akinetic symptoms are hypokinesia and bradykinesia. Hypokinesia, decreased frequency or absence of associated movements, is one of the earliest akinetic symptoms. Individuals with Parkinson disease sit and lie motionless for long periods without the little shifts a normal person makes to prevent discomfort and stiffness. Bradykinesia, slowness of voluntary movements, is characterized by difficulty initiating, continuing, or synchronizing movements. Both associated and voluntary movements are interspersed by freezing. Freezing may be precipitated by (1) increasing the effort to move, (2) turning, and (3) initiating certain types of tactile and visual contact.

Postural abnormalities. Postural abnormalities are caused by a loss of normal postural reflexes. Three types of postural abnormalities occur in individuals with Parkinson disease: (1) disorders of postural fixation, (2) disorders of equilibrium, and (3) disorders of righting.

The disorder of postural fixation associated with Parkinson disease is involuntary flexion of the head and neck. The individual is unable to maintain an upright position of the trunk while standing or walking. The stooped (flexed, forward leaning) posture is characteristic (Fig. 15-29). Postural abnormalities of the hands and feet also occur.

Disorders of equilibrium result from loss of postural stability. The person with Parkinson disease is unable to make the appropriate postural adjustment to tilting or falling and falls like a post when starting to tilt. The festinating gait (short, accelerating steps) of the individual with Parkinson disease is an attempt to maintain an upright position while walking (Fig. 15-29). Individu-

FIG. 15-29 Characteristic shuffling gait of individual with Parkinson disease. (From Rudy, 1984.)

als are also unable to right themselves when changing from a reclining or crouching position to a standing position and when rolling over from a supine to a lateral or prone position.

Autonomic and neuroendocrine symptoms. Autonomic and neuroendocrine dysfunctions in Parkinson disease produce symptoms that are distressing but not incapacitating. The basal ganglia influence hypothalamic function (autonomic and neuroendocrine) through pathways connecting the hypothalamus with the basal ganglia and cerebral cortex. Common autonomic symptoms in Parkinson disease include inappropriate diaphoresis, orthostatic hypotension, gastric retention, constipation, and urinary retention. A symptom attributed to neuroendocrine dysfunction is seborrhea. Hypothalamic hypersecretion of hormone-releasing factors acting on the anterior pituitary causes hypersecretion of androgenotropic hormones. The androgen excess produces sebum hypersecretion by sebaceous glands. The resulting seborrhea is characterized by oily skin with seborrheic dermatitis along the hairline and in chin-nasal creases.

Late symptoms. Progressive dementia may be associated with the advanced stages of the disease and is manifested on the EEG as diffuse slowing and disorganization. The person's mental status may be further compromised by the side effects of the medication taken to control symptoms.

The combination of all the parkinsonian symptoms gives the individual a characteristic appearance: a wide-eyed, unblinking, staring expression with the facial muscles smoothed out and almost immobile. Saliva frequently drools from the corners of the slightly open mouth. The skin of the face is frequently greasy. The gait is pathognomic: the individual walks with slow, short, shuffling steps; the arms are flexed, abducted, and held stiffly at the side; and the trunk is bent slightly forward. The person may break into a run spontaneously or when pushed forward or backward. Because of the disorder of postural fixation, the tendency is to fall to the side.

Evaluation and Treatment

The diagnosis of Parkinson disease is based on the history and physical examination. Causes of secondary parkinsonism are first excluded. No specific diagnostic tests are available. Treatment of Parkinson disease is symptomatic. Drug therapy includes administration of dopaminergic drugs, such as levodopa (L-dopa), a precursor of dopamine (dopamine does not cross the blood-brain barrier), and dopamine agonists. These drugs are used to decrease akinesia. Because of troublesome side effects, however, drug therapy is not started until the symptoms become incapacitating. So far, adrenal medullary transplantation has not proven effective. Dysphagia and general immobility are special problems of the person with Parkinson disease, requiring preventive, symptomatic, supportive, and rehabilitative management.

Parkinson disease takes a slowly progressive course for 15 to 20 years before producing total invalidism (Duvoisin, 1984). The course shows much variation among individuals. The prognosis is better since the advent of levodopa, but the disorder still shortens life substantially. Pneumonia is the leading cause of death.

Huntington Disease

Huntington disease (HD), also known as chorea, is a relatively rare, hereditary-degenerative disorder diffusely involving the basal ganglia and cerebral cortex. The onset of Huntington disease is usually between 40 and 50 years of age when the trait may already have been passed to the victim's children. The disorder has a prevalence rate of approximately 5 per 100,000 persons and occurs in all races (Kandel & Schwartz, 1985).

Pathophysiology

Huntington disease is inherited as an autosomal dominant trait with high penetrance. (Mechanisms of genetic inheritance are discussed in Chapter 4.) The principal pathologic feature of Huntington disease is severe degeneration of the basal ganglia, particularly the caudate and putamen nuclei, and the frontal cerebral cortex (Fig. 15-30). The basal ganglia normally contain a preponderance of GABA-nergic (γ-aminobutyric-acid–secreting) neurons, including the pathway between the basal ganglia and substantia nigra (pallidonigral pathway). Basal ganglia and nigral depletion of GABA, an inhibitory neurotransmitter, is the principal biochemical alteration in Huntington disease. Degeneration of the GABA-nergic pallidonigral pathway causes GABA depletion in the substantia nigra with decreased inhibitory GABA activity on dopaminergic neurons in the substantia nigra and relative excess of dopaminergic activity in the basal ganglial feedback circuit with the cerebral cortex. A relative excess of dopaminergic activity in this circuit, as in Huntington disease, is manifested by hypotonia and hyperkinesia (involuntary, fragmentary movements such as chorea).

Clinical Manifestations

The classic manifestations of Huntington disease are abnormal movement and progressive dysfunction of intellectual processes (dementia) and thought processes. Any one of these features may mark the onset of the disease. Chorea is the most common type of abnormal movement affecting individuals with Huntington disease. Choreiform movements begin in the face and arms, eventually affecting the entire body. Consistent signs of intellectual dysfunction are impaired memory and judg-

ment. Individuals with Huntington disease are prone to a wide variety of thought disturbances, including delusions and depressive disorders.

Evaluation and Treatment

The diagnosis of Huntington disease is based on family history and clinical presentation of the disorder. No known treatment is effective in halting the degeneration or progression of symptoms. The discovery in 1983 of the Huntington disease marker, called G8, on chromosome 4 paves the way for presymptomatic diagnosis of the disorder and isolation of the Huntington disease gene. Recombinant genetic techniques may someday prevent or control the disorder.

Multiple Sclerosis

Multiple sclerosis (MS) is a relatively common dysimmune disorder diffusely involving CNS myelin. The peripheral nervous system is not involved. Multiple sclerosis is one of many CNS demyelinating disorders. They are acquired conditions and are characterized by degeneration of previously normal myelin with relative preservation of axons. Central nervous system demyelinating disorders are subclassified as primary and secondary. Multiple sclerosis and its variants are primary demyelinating disorders. In secondary disorders, CNS demyelination is caused by disorders other than multiple sclerosis.

The onset of multiple sclerosis is usually between 20 and 40 years of age (Adams & Victor, 1989). Male-to-female ratio is about 1 to 2 (Adams & Victor, 1989). Multiple sclerosis is the most prevalent CNS demyelin-

FIG. 15-30 Huntington disease. Atrophy of caudate nuclei and putamina is diagnostic. Cortical atrophy is moderate. There is compensatory internal and external hydrocephalus. (From Kissane, 1993.)

ating disorder and a leading cause of neurologic disability in early adulthood. The disease is most prevalent in areas far from the equator. In the United States and Canada, the prevalence rate ranges from 30 to 80 per 100,000 persons (Adams & Victor, 1989). Multiple sclerosis occurs in all races, but it is chiefly a disorder of caucasians. Although the disorder does not exhibit a defined inheritance pattern, it is 5 to 15 times more likely to occur in first-degree relatives of affected persons than in the population at large (Adams & Victor, 1989).

Pathophysiology

The pathogenesis of multiple sclerosis is unknown. (A theoretic pathogenic model is shown in Fig. 15-31.) Although controversial, most theories suggest an immunogenetic-viral cause for multiple sclerosis. The disease is associated with a possible genetic predisposition and interaction with environmental risk factors (see Chapter 5). Possible genetically determined susceptibility is suggested by a pattern (haplotype) of histocompatibility antigens (HLA-DR2, DR3, B_7, A_3) found more frequently in persons with multiple sclerosis than in normal individuals (Adams & Victor, 1989). (Histocompatibility antigen is discussed in Chapter 6.) According to theory, this haplotype is a marker for a multiple sclerosis susceptibility gene that alters the body's immune response to viral infection (Adams & Victor, 1989). The central component of the pathogenic model is the demyelinating process. Pathologic features of this process are (1) interaction between the systemic immune system and the CNS and (2) demyelinating lesions (plaques and diffuse lesions) (Fig. 15-32). (The systemic immune system is discussed in Chapter 6.)

The interaction between the systemic immune system and the CNS is a complex and incompletely understood process. An immune response, possibly to chronic viral infection, causes initial and recurring mild inflammatory reactions in the form of a venular vasculitis. The vasculitis causes focal, limited intermittent breakdown of the blood-brain barrier. Some B-lymphocyte clones that migrate into the CNS during the inflammatory episodes of onset and exacerbation are trapped there when the inflammation subsides. In response to constant antigenic stimulation, these B-lymphocyte clones colonize the CNS. Within the brain and spinal cord they form plasma cells that secrete immunoglobulin G (IgG) against unknown viruses. IgG synthesis against these antigens persists throughout the disease and is increased during exacerbations. CNS-produced IgG causes an oligoclonal electrophoretic pattern in which several IgG bands in the CSF are not seen in the serum, indicating immunologic activity in the brain. Systemic-produced IgG causes a polyclonal electrophoretic pattern in which IgG bands in the CSF correspond with those in the se-

rum, indicating a systemic immune response to the antigens. Neither elevated CSF IgG nor oligoclonal IgG bands, however, are specific for multiple sclerosis. These findings are also seen in other conditions, such as neurosyphilis. T-suppressor cell function is altered but the precise role of these cells is yet to be established.

The demyelinating lesions (plaques and diffuse lesions) are the second pathologic feature of the demyelinating process. Virus(es) or other antigens may directly attack the myelin or provoke a hypersensitivity reaction, destroying myelin or the oligodendrogliocytes.

Plaques characteristically involve the CNS white matter, but occasionally they may extend into the adjacent gray matter. They often coalesce into much larger plaques. In established disease the multifocal, multistaged feature of plaques gives rise to the aphorism that the lesions are "scattered in space and time." Symptoms therefore are multiple and variable. Whether plaques are multiple from the onset of the disease is not known. In many individuals the initial symptoms suggest a single lesion.

The acute (early) stage of plaque formation is characterized by the process of perivenular demyelination. Most of the neurologic deficits in the acute stage are attributed to inflammatory edema in and around the plaque and to partial demyelination. Symptoms usually remit, partially or completely, weeks after the onset of an early episode (Adams & Victor, 1989).

The chronic stage of demyelination and plaque formation is characterized by the process of **gliosis** (glial scarring with late degeneration of axons). Progressive loss of function leads to permanent disability, usually over 20 years or more (Adams & Victor, 1989).

Although plaques are considered diagnostic of multiple sclerosis, diffuse lesions are common pathologic findings in actively progressive cases. Diffuse lesions are small, widespread areas of perivenular demyelination that do not progress through gliosis. These lesions are sometimes accompanied by edema of surrounding normal brain tissue. The relationship of plaques to diffuse lesions is unknown.

Clinical Manifestations

A variety of events occurring immediately before the onset or exacerbation of symptoms are regarded as precipitating factors related to MS. Infection, physical injury, pregnancy, emotional stress, and fatigue are the most important. Most of the pregnancy-related exacerbations occur 3 months postpartum, suggesting a relation to the stresses of labor and the increased fatigue during the postpartum period rather than to the pregnancy itself (Adams & Victor, 1989).

The major manifestations of MS are initial syndromes followed by remissions and established syndromes with no remissions. Usually persons with early multiple scle-

FIG. 15-31 An etiopathogenic model for MS. The initiating or trigger event in MS is presumed to be invasion by a virus with a prolonged incubation period, causing an altered immune response. The resulting chronic viral infection or other environmental insult becomes active in early adulthood, provoking the demyelinating process.

FIG. 15-32 Multiple sclerosis. Multiple sclerosis of chronic relapsing type with numerous plaques. Plaques occur in all characteristic areas. (From Kissane, 1993.)

rosis predominantly have one of the initial syndromes—spinal, brainstem, cerebellar, or cerebral—that occur in the order of frequency indicated. The initial syndrome depends on the portion of the CNS that is most involved (see box at right). After about 15 years, almost all individuals appear to have established syndromes of mixed involvement (Scheinberg, 1983).

Corticospinal syndrome. The corticospinal syndrome is most common, chiefly involving the corticospinal tracts and dorsal column. Subjective corticospinal (upper motor neuron) symptoms—stiffness, slowness, weakness—are a component of fatigability. Corticospinal signs are usually symmetric, with lower limbs more often and more severely affected than upper limbs; spastic paraparesis is probably the most common single neurologic finding in multiple sclerosis.

Bladder and bowel symptoms occur with major spinal cord involvement. Urgency and hesitancy generally precede incontinence. Bladder dysfunction most often involves a small, spastic bladder, although occasionally a large, flaccid bladder may result. Neurogenic impotence is often present when sphincter symptoms are present. Bowel incontinence is rare, but constipation is common with severe disease. Subjective dorsal column symptoms are symmetric paresthesias (tingling and numbness) in an unpredictable pattern, but with a predilection for lower extremities over upper extremities. Dorsal column signs are vibration, position, and two-point discrimination deficits. Sensory complaints are often not substantiated by objective findings.

Brainstem syndrome. The brainstem syndrome reflects lesions of cranial nerves III through XII at the root, nuclear, or corticobulbar (upper motor neuron) level. Intranuclear ophthalmoplegia, nystagmus, and dysarthria are the most common brainstem symptoms, followed by vertigo, tinnitus, facial weakness, and facial sensory deficit. Intranuclear ophthalmoplegia is lateral gaze paralysis caused by involvement of the medial longitudinal fasciculus, the brainstem pathway that coordinates eye movement. Diplopia and eyeball pain are the common complaints. Bilateral intranuclear ophthalmoplegia in a young adult is virtually diagnostic of MS.

Cerebellar syndrome. Cerebellar syndrome deficits are usually symmetric, with all four limbs involved. With combined corticospinal and cerebellar involvement, the individual has a spastic ataxic gait and ataxia of the arms. Pure cerebellar symptoms are those of motor ataxia, hypotonia, and asthenia (weakness). Manifestations of motor ataxia are decomposition of movement, inability to perform rapid alternating movements (dysdiadochokinesis), dysmetria, and Charcot triad (a combination of dysarthria, intention tremor, and nystagmus). Hypotonia is manifested by decreased resistance to passive movement, hypoactive deep tendon reflexes, and pendular knee jerk.

INITIAL SYNDROMES OF MULTIPLE SCLEROSIS

Cerebral syndrome
Optic neuritis (ON)
Intellectual-emotional changes
Seizures
Hemiparesis, hemisensory loss, dysphasia

Cerebellar syndrome
Motor ataxia
Hypotonia
Asthenia

Brainstem syndrome
Intranuclear ophthalmoplegia (INO)
Nystagmus
Dysarthria

Spinal syndrome
Spastic paresis
Bowel and bladder dysfunction
Paresthesias

Cerebral syndrome. The cerebral syndrome is characterized by optic neuritis, the manifestation of optic nerve demyelination. Although not as common as other symptoms, it is highly suggestive of MS. Involvement may be unilateral or bilateral. Subjective symptoms are impaired central vision (blurring, fogginess, haziness) and impaired color perception. Signs are decreased central visual acuity; central or paracentral scotoma (area of diminished vision); acquired color vision deficit, especially to red and green; and defective pupillary reaction to light. In the acute phase, these symptoms may reflect optic papillitis (inflammation and swelling of the optic disc) or retrobulbar neuritis with a normal disc. Later pallor of the temporal half of the disc occurs from demyelination of a portion of the optic nerve. (Normal visual function is discussed in Chapter 13.)

Intellectual and emotional changes also occur. Depression is more common than euphoria, although euphoria is sometimes associated with dementia. Other less common symptoms of cerebral involvement include seizures, hemiparesis, hemisensory loss, and dysphasia.

Within the overall course of multiple sclerosis, short-lived and paroxysmal attacks may occur. Symptoms of the attack tend to subside as the inciting event is removed.

Short-lived attacks are the temporary appearance or worsening of symptoms. The mechanism of these attacks is complete, reversible conduction block in partially demyelinated axons. Conditions that cause short-lived attacks include (1) minor increases in body temperature or serum Ca^{++} concentration and (2) functional demands exceeding conduction capacity. An increase in body temperature or serum Ca^{++} level increases current leakage through demyelinated neurons. Persons with multiple sclerosis may become dramatically worse when body temperature is raised. Hypercalcemia induced by decreased serum pH may aggravate symptoms of multiple sclerosis. Physical and emotional stress imposes functional demands that may exceed conduction capacity of affected neurons.

Paroxysmal attacks are sensory or motor symptoms of abrupt onset and short duration (few seconds or minutes). These symptoms include paresthesias, dysarthria and ataxia, and tonic head turning. The mechanism of paroxysmal attacks is nonsynaptic transmission in which nerve impulses are directly transmitted between adjacent demyelinated axons. These impulses arise focally and spuriously in the cervical portion of the spinal cord or in the brainstem. A common paroxysmal symptom, called Lhermitte sign, is the momentary paresthesia (shocklike or tingling sensation) that shoots down the trunk or limbs during active or passive flexion of the neck. Bending the neck evokes nonsynaptic impulses in demyelinated axons of the dorsal column in the spinal cord. A person with multiple sclerosis may have many paroxysmal attacks each day. Inciting events include sensory stimulation, voluntary movement, hyperventilation, and emotional stress. Paroxysmal attacks tend to persist for weeks or months and may be followed by progressive symptoms of multiple sclerosis.

Evaluation and Treatment

The diagnosis of multiple sclerosis (definite, probable, or possible) is based on the history and physical examination supported by findings from CSF examination, evoked response (ER) studies, CT scans of the head, and MRI. Persistently elevated CSF IgG is found in about two thirds of individuals with multiple sclerosis (Adams & Victor, 1989), and oligoclonal IgG bands on electrophoresis are found in more than 90% (Poser, 1985). Evoked response studies aid diagnosis by detecting decreased conduction velocity in visual, auditory, and somatosensory pathways. In the study reported by Kirshner, Tsai, Runge, and Price (1985), positive MRI scans in 27 individuals with "definite" multiple sclerosis suggest that MRI is the most sensitive available method of detecting the disease as compared with oligoclonal banding, ER studies, or CT scanning (Kirshner et al., 1985). Magnetic resonance imaging, which is not subject to bone artifacts, shows brainstem lesions not detected by CT. Optic nerve and spinal cord lesions, however, are not detected by current MRI techniques. When MRI is normal, ER studies are useful in confirming suggested multiple sclerosis.

No treatment is available to alter the overall course of MS. Adrenocorticotropic hormone and prednisone are used to shorten the duration of acute exacerbations. Special problems requiring preventive and symptomatic management are weakness; spasticity; bladder, bowel, and sexual dysfunction; pain; tremor and ataxia; depression; and heat intolerance. Supportive and rehabilitative management is directed toward preventing the complications of immobility, especially pressure sores and infections of the pulmonary and genitourinary systems. Estimates suggest that current therapies and management will permit a normal life span for approximately 85% of individuals (Slater & Yearwood, 1980).

Amyotrophic Lateral Sclerosis

Amyotrophic lateral sclerosis (ALS, sporadic motor neuron disease, or sporadic motor system disease) is a relatively rare degenerative disorder diffusely involving lower and upper motor neurons. The term *amyotrophic* (without muscle nutrition or progressive muscle wasting) refers to the predominant lower motor neuron component of the syndrome. Lateral sclerosis, scarring of the corticospinal tract in the lateral column of the spinal cord, refers to the upper motor neuron component of the syndrome. Amyotrophic lateral sclerosis differs from other motor neuron disorders in that both upper and lower motor neurons are involved.

Classic ALS (Lou Gehrig disease) may begin at any time from the fourth decade of life; its peak occurrence rate is in the early 50s (Chipps et al., 1992). Male-to-female ratio is 2 or 3 to 1 (Chipps et al., 1992). The disorder has a prevalence rate of approximately 1 per 100,000 persons (Chipps et al., 1992). Variants of ALS include primary lateral sclerosis, progressive bulbar palsy, and progressive muscular atrophy.

Pathophysiology

The pathogenesis of ALS is unknown. Current data suggest viral-immune factors as a possible cause. A genetic or external agent is thought to be the agent in Guam. Metabolic, nutritional, and systemic stimuli, such as infection or trauma, have been investigated as causative agents. Serum immune complexes are elevated in ALS, but the nature of the complexes is unknown.

The principal pathologic feature of ALS is lower and upper motor neuron degeneration, although without inflammation. There is a reduction in the number of large motor neurons in the spinal cord, brainstem, and cerebral cortex (premotor and motor areas), with ongoing degeneration in the remaining motor neurons. The nuclei of cranial nerves III, IV, and VI are not involved. Death of the motor neuron results in axonal degeneration and secondary demyelination with glial proliferation and sclerosis (scarring).

Lower motor neuron degeneration denervates motor

units. Adjacent, still-viable lower motor neurons attempt to compensate by a process of distal intramuscular sprouting, reinnervation, and enlargement of motor units. The initial symptoms of the disease may be related to lower and upper motor neuron dysfunction or to both.

Clinical Manifestations

Weakness may begin in any or all muscles of the body. Muscle weakness in ALS exhibits the following characteristics:

1. Paresis usually begins in a single muscle group.
2. Corresponding muscle groups are asymmetrically affected in a mottled distribution.
3. Gradual involvement occurs in all striated muscles except extraocular muscles and heart and progresses to paralysis with no remissions.
4. Flaccid and spastic paresis may coexist in a single muscle group; flaccid paresis may mask spasticity, which is usually mild.
5. Urethral and anal sphincter weakness is uncommon.
6. No associated mental, sensory, or autonomic symptoms are present. Normal intellectual and sensory functions are sustained until death.

The lower motor neuron syndrome of flaccid paresis consists of weakness of individual muscles, progressing to paralysis, associated with hypotonia and primary muscle atrophy (i.e., atrophy caused by denervation). Hypotonic is manifested by (1) decreased resistance to passive movement, (2) hypoactive or absent deep tendon reflexes, (3) absent abdominal and cremasteric reflexes, and (4) absent Babinski sign. Primary atrophy is manifested by (1) severe, irreversible muscular wasting; (2) fasciculations; (3) metabolically related changes in the skin and appendages; and (4) specific electromyelographic findings. Fasciculations, along with fibrillations, are prominent features of ALS. Metabolic changes include (1) thinning of the skin, (2) thickening of the nails, (3) loss of body hair, and (4) decreased perspiration.

The upper motor neuron syndrome of spastic paresis consists of weakness of movement patterns, progressing to paralysis, associated with spasticity and, in some cases, atrophy secondary to disuse. Spasticity is manifested by (1) clasp-knife phenomenon, evident with passive movement; (2) hyperactive deep tendon reflexes and clonus with severe spasticity; (3) absent abdominal and cremasteric reflexes; and (4) presence of Babinski sign.

Evaluation and Treatment

The diagnosis of the syndrome is based predominantly on the history and physical examination. Electromyography and muscle biopsy verify lower motor neuron degeneration and denervation. Muscle biopsy usually is not needed to confirm the diagnosis. No treatment is available to alter the overall course of the ALS syndrome. Special problems requiring preventive and symptomatic management are communication difficulty caused by dysphonia and dysarthria; dehydration and weight loss resulting from dysmasesis and dysphagia; and dyspnea caused by diaphragmatic and intercostal weakness. Supportive and rehabilitative management is directed toward preventing complications of immobility. Psychologic support of the affected individual and the family is extremely important in this disorder.

The average duration of life is approximately 2 to 3 years from the appearance of symptoms, but the course of the disease may run from a few months to 15 years. Twenty percent of persons survive 5 to 20 years (Chipps et al., 1992).

Hydrocephalus

The term **hydrocephalus** refers to a variety of conditions characterized by an excess of fluid within the cranial vault, subarachnoid space, or both. Hydrocephalus occurs because of interference with cerebrospinal fluid flow caused by increased fluid production, obstruction within the ventricular system, or defective reabsorption of the fluid. A papilloma (i.e., epithelial tumor) may, in rare instances, cause overproduction of cerebrospinal fluid.

Types of Hydrocephalus

Obstruction within the ventricular system, called **noncommunicating hydrocephalus** or internal (intraventricular) hydrocephalus, may result from congenital abnormalities in the ventricular system or mass lesions such as a tumor that compresses one of the structures of the ventricular system (see Pediatrics, Chapter 16, for additional discussion). Impaired absorption of cerebrospinal fluid from the subarachnoid space occurs when an obstructive process disrupts the flow of cerebrospinal fluid through the subarachnoid space. The fluid is prevented from reaching the convex portion of the cerebrum, where the arachnoid granulations are located.

Hydrocephalus from impaired absorption may be caused by adhesions from inflammation, as with a meningitis or subarachnoid hemorrhage; compression of the subarachnoid space by a mass, such as a tumor; congenital abnormalities of the subarachnoid space; or high venous pressure within the sagittal sinus. This type of hydrocephalus is termed **communicating (extraventricular) hydrocephalus**. The most common causes of communicating hydrocephalus are subarachnoid hemorrhage, developmental malformation, head injury, and neoplasm.

One form of communicating hydrocephalus is **hydrocephalus ex vacuo**, which arises from cerebral atrophy. Cerebrospinal fluid fills the unoccupied space. The amount of cerebrospinal fluid is increased, but the fluid is not under pressure. Another form of communicating hydrocephalus is **normal-pressure hydrocephalus** (low-pressure, adult, or occult hydrocephalus), which occurs mostly in late middle age. The cause is thought to be arachnoid adhesions that obstruct the subarachnoid space. This form of hydrocephalus is most frequently seen as a complication of head injury and subarachnoid hemorrhage.

Course of the Disease

Hydrocephalus may develop from infancy through adulthood. Congenital hydrocephalus (i.e., ventricular enlargement before birth) is rare. Noncommunicating hydrocephalus is more commonly seen in children. The more frequent type of hydrocephalus in adults is the "communicating" type. (Hydrocephalus in children is discussed in Chapter 16.)

Most hydrocephalus develops gradually and insidiously over time. **Acute hydrocephalus**, however, may develop in a couple of hours in persons who have sustained head injuries. Acute hydrocephalus contributes significantly to increased intracranial pressure.

Pathogenesis

The obstruction of cerebrospinal fluid flow associated with hydrocephalus produces dilation of the ventricles proximal to the obstruction. Obstructed cerebrospinal fluid is under pressure, causing atrophy of the cerebral cortex and degeneration of the white matter tracts. There is selective preservation of gray matter. When excess cerebrospinal fluid fills a defect caused by atrophy, a degenerative disorder, or a surgical excision, this fluid is not under pressure; therefore, atrophy and degenerative changes are not induced.

Clinical Manifestations

The presentation of acute hydrocephalus is one of rapidly developing increased intracranial pressure. The person deteriorates rapidly into a deep coma if not promptly treated. Normal-pressure hydrocephalus has a chronic presentation and develops slowly over time. The individual or family complains of declining memory and cognitive function. An unsteady, broad-based gait with a history of falling is common. Additional clinical manifestations are apathy, inattentiveness, and indifference to self, family, and the environment. Urinary incontinence is present.

Evaluation and Treatment

The diagnosis is made on the basis of physical examination, CT scan, and MRI. A radioisotopic cisternogram may be performed to diagnose normal-pressure hydrocephalus. Hydrocephalus can be treated by surgery to resect cysts, neoplasms, or hematomas, or by ventricular bypass into the normal intracranial channel or into an extracranial compartment using a shunt. Excision or coagulation of the choroid plexus is occasionally needed when a papilloma is present. In normal-pressure hydrocephalus, reduction in cerebrospinal fluid through a diuresis regimen is often used.

PERIPHERAL NERVOUS SYSTEM AND NEUROMUSCULAR JUNCTION DISORDERS

Peripheral Nervous System Disorders

The axons traveling to and from the brainstem and spinal cord neuronal cell bodies may be injured by a multitude of disease processes. Distinct anatomic areas of the axon may be injured, or the spinal nerves may be affected at the spinal roots, at the plexus before peripheral nerve formation, or at the peripheral nerves themselves. The cranial nerves do not have roots or plexuses so are only affected within the nerves themselves. Autonomic nerve fibers may be injured as they travel within certain cranial nerves or emerge through the ventral root and plexuses to travel in the peripheral nerves of the body.

Radiculopathies

As the spinal roots emerge from or enter into the vertebral canal, they may be injured or damaged by compression, inflammation, or direct trauma whereby the roots are stretched or torn. **Radiculopathies** are disorders of roots of spinal nerves. **Radiculitis** (radiculoneuritis) refers to an inflammatory disorder of the spinal nerve roots. One or more roots may be affected.

Pathophysiology

Many different pathologic conditions may cause compression, inflammation, or tearing of nerve roots. Roots may be traumatized by a forceful tearing of a nerve, termed *avulsion*, often associated with injuries to the head and shoulders. An acute intervertebral disk prolapse (herniated disk) or a benign tumor may compress nerve roots. Metastatic tumors of the lung, breast, and gastrointestinal tract may produce a carcinomatous meningitis, causing compression and inflammatory changes in nerve roots. Other causes of inflammatory changes in nerve roots are chronic meningitis, neurosyphilis, sarcoidosis, and **inflammatory arachnoiditis** produced by myelography and lumbar punctures.

Clinical Manifestations

The strength, tone, and bulk of the muscles innervated by the involved roots are affected. The pattern and distribution of weakness and atrophy are similar to those of the amyotrophies. Tone and deep-tendon reflexes are decreased but rarely absent because the involved muscles usually are innervated by two or more spinal roots. Fasciculations are often present, and mild fatigue may be experienced. Because pathologic processes usually affect both the ventral and dorsal roots, sensory alterations are common.

Diseases that involve spinal roots typically produce local pain; pain on local percussion; pain and paresthesias in the sensory root distribution (called **radicular pain** and **radicular paresthesia**); increased pain with movement, stretching of the root, and maneuvers that transiently increase cerebrospinal fluid pressure; sensory loss in a radicular pattern; and spasms of the muscles surrounding the vertebral column (i.e., paravertebral muscle spasms).

Evaluation and Treatment

Diagnostic measures may include spinal films, electromyography, lumbar puncture with cerebrospinal fluid examination, myelography, and biopsy of tumor masses. Treatment is directed at the cause of the injury and may take the form of surgery, antibiotics, removal of the injurious agent, steroids, and radiation therapy and chemotherapy. Supportive management may include control of the discomfort, protection from further injury, prevention of complications, and rehabilitation where appropriate.

Plexus Injuries

Plexus injuries involve the nerve plexus distal to the spinal roots but proximal to the formation of the peripheral nerves. Such injuries may be caused by trauma, compression, or infiltration, or they may be iatrogenic, caused by positioning during surgery or by an intramuscular injection. Clinical manifestations include motor weakness, muscle atrophy, and sensory loss in affected areas. Paralysis can occur with complete plexus lesions.

The diagnosis is made on the basis of history and clinical manifestations. Therapeutic treatment is directed at removal of the cause, repair and approximation of nervous tissue, prevention of further injury, control of discomfort, prevention of complications, and rehabilitation where appropriate.

Neuropathies

Where the peripheral nerves themselves are affected, whether cranial nerves, nerves arising from spinal roots and plexuses, or autonomic nervous system fibers, the resulting syndrome is a neuropathy or **neuritis** when an inflammatory process is involved. Most neuropathies are classified as **sensorimotor neuropathies** because motor, sensory, and reflex changes are generally present, although some neuropathies are predominantly motor or sensory. **Sensory neuropathies** are predominantly caused by leprosy, some industrial solvents, chloramphenicol, and hereditary mechanisms. **Motor neuropathies** are predominantly caused by Guillain-Barré syndrome, infectious mononucleosis, viral hepatitis, acute porphyria, lead, mercury, and triorthocresylphosphates

(TCP). Autonomic fibers may be involved in either a motor or a sensorimotor neuropathy.

Pathophysiology

Although distinct pathophysiologic processes are recognized in a neuropathy, these are not disease specific and may exist simultaneously in any one neuropathy. Wallerian degeneration, in which the axon and myelin distal to the site of axonal interruption degenerate, may be present (see Chapter 12). This type of degeneration is characteristic of a traumatic nerve injury in which the nerve is severed. In some neuropathies the axon may be spared and only the myelin degenerates. Such polyneuropathies are called **segmental demyelinating neuropathies**. This type of degeneration is especially seen in the early phases of many neuropathies. In **axonal degeneration** distal degeneration of the axon occurs first and is followed by degeneration of the myelin and the axis cylinder. Many pathologic processes may give rise to neuropathy and one or more nerves may be involved.

Clinical Manifestations

When the axons are affected, muscle strength, muscle tone, and muscle bulk are also affected. Whole muscles or groups of muscles are paretic or paralyzed, and the muscles of the feet and legs are often affected first and more severely. These long, large axons are thought to (1) be more vulnerable to injury because of their size and length, (2) have more Schwann cells available to be injured, and (3) exhibit a "dying back" phenomenon caused by difficulty of the nerve cell body in maintaining the terminal portion of the axon. If unchecked, the pathologic process tends to involve the hands and arms because these are the next longest and largest axons.

Tone and the deep tendon reflexes in the affected muscles are generally decreased in a neuropathy. Atrophy is distributed according to the peripheral nerves involved. The degree and distribution of the atrophy probably depend on the extent of the injury. Fasciculation may be present, especially with associated ventral root or motor neuron changes, or both as in Guillain-Barré syndrome, diabetic neuropathy, and porphyric neuropathy. Mild fatigue may be experienced. A few disorders, notably Guillain-Barré syndrome, produce a pattern of paresis and paralysis that involves all limbs, the trunk, and the neck. Peripheral bifacial and other cranial nerve palsies may be seen with a variety of disorders. Tenderness of the nerve trunks and associated sensory alterations help to distinguish neuropathy from amyotrophy. These include paresthesias and dysesthesias as well as decreased or absent primary sensations, such as temperature, touch, light pain, position sense, or vibratory sense. Ataxia of gait or limb may arise from the loss of position and vibratory sensations (i.e., proprioceptive sensory loss) and may be enhanced by motor weakness.

Reflexes may be altered. Reflex-mediated autonomic nervous system functions, such as sweating and pupillary size, may be affected. Neuropathies associated with autonomic disturbances include diabetes mellitus, alcoholism and related nutritional neuropathies, amyloidosis, porphyria, Guillain-Barré syndrome, Riley-Day syndrome, and familial sensory neuropathy. In many chronic polyneuropathies, the feet, hands, and spine become deformed. Metabolic changes may arise secondary to nerve dysfunction.

Evaluation and Treatment

The diagnostic workup to determine the cause of a neuropathy is often extensive. Early diagnosis and treatment before irreversible neuronal cell damage ensues are of paramount importance. Although axonal regrowth and recovery of function may take months, many neuropathies can be reversed. The therapeutic management is directed first and foremost at elimination of the cause, if possible. At least the primary disorder, such as diabetes mellitus, should be controlled. Further damage to the axon must be prevented by avoiding trauma from too-early demand for reuse of the nerve and accidents that cause tissue damage, and by avoiding hypoxia and ischemia or other deprivation of essential substrates.

Guillain-Barré Syndrome

Guillain-Barré syndrome (idiopathic polyneuritis, acute inflammatory demyelinating polyradiculopathy, postinfectious polyneuritis) is characterized by the acute onset of a motor paralysis usually of an ascending nature. This neurologic disorder, first described by Landry in 1859, occurs throughout the world, affects children and adults of both sexes and all age groups equally, and occurs in all seasons of the year. Precipitating, or at least preceding, events include a mild respiratory or gastrointestinal viral infection 1 to 4 weeks before onset of neurologic manifestations, surgical procedures, viral immunizations, and lymphomatous disease.

Pathophysiology

The neurologic dysfunctions in Guillain-Barré syndrome are caused by a cell-mediated immunologic reaction directed at the peripheral nerves. Lymphocytes migrate into the areas adjacent to the nerve and attack the myelin sheath surrounding the nerve fibers, causing demyelination of nerve segments. As the process continues, the axons themselves are interrupted. The muscle innervated by the damaged peripheral nerves undergoes denervation and atrophy. If the cell body survives, regeneration of the peripheral nerve takes place, and recovery of motor function is likely. If the cell body dies from intense ventral root involvement in the inflammatory-degenerative process, then no regeneration is possible. Collateral reinnervation from surviving axons and re-

generating axons may take place. In this case motor recovery is less complete, and residual deficits persist.

Clinical Manifestations

Clinical manifestations may vary from paresis of the legs to complete quadriplegia, respiratory insufficiency, and autonomic nervous system instability. The individual may have a symmetric weakness or paralysis involving the legs, the trunk, and possibly the neck and face. Hypotonia of the involved muscles is present, and the deep tendon reflexes are absent. The person may complain of paresthesias that began in the legs and ascended upward. Position and vibratory sensations may be decreased. Autonomic nervous system dysfunction may be manifested as sinus tachycardia, hypertension, hypotension, or loss of sweating. Ventilatory capacity is often decreased, and the individual may complain of shortness of breath. Persons may experience a respiratory arrest or cardiovascular collapse.

Evaluation and Treatment

The individual's clinical history helps to diagnose the disorder. The significant signs include paresthesias, paralysis, and CSF findings. The major diagnostic tests are the examination of the CSF and nerve conduction tests. The CSF findings include an unusually high protein level (600 mg/ml) without cellular abnormality. Ventilatory support and management of the autonomic nervous system dysfunction are two dominant aspects of the therapeutic management. During the acute phase, steroid therapy may be initiated. Data support the use of plasmapheresis within the first 2 weeks of onset of clinical manifestations (McKhann & Griffin, 1987). After the disorder begins to remit, aggressive rehabilitation should be instituted.

Neuromuscular Junction Disorders

Transmission of the nerve impulse at the neuromuscular junction requires the release of adequate amounts of neurotransmitter from the presynaptic terminals of the axon and effective binding of the released transmitter to the receptors on the membranes of muscle cells (see Fig. 12-14). Nutritional deficits, certain drugs (e.g., reserpine or Aldomet), and certain disorders that interfere with the synthesis or packaging of the neurotransmitter or its release into the synaptic cleft may result in weakness. Likewise, any pathologic process or drug that interferes with the binding of the neurotransmitter to the receptor may cause weakness.

Marked weakness results from interference with neuromuscular transmission. The distribution of affected muscles is mainly in the bulbar, respiratory, and proximal muscle groups. Botulism toxin has a predilection for the cranial nerves. Eaton-Lambert syndrome affects limb musculature, whereas myasthenia gravis predominantly involves ocular, bulbar, and proximal upper extremity muscles. There is marked fatigability. Muscle tone may be slightly reduced, as may deep tendon reflexes, but the muscle cells are not denervated. Atrophy, if present, is only mild, probably because the small motor system is intact so that tone is maintained to a large degree. Fasciculations or sensory alterations are not present.

The weakness associated with presynaptic dysfunction, as in botulism or Eaton-Lambert syndrome, and that associated with postsynaptic dysfunction, as in myasthenia gravis, are difficult to distinguish clinically, although theoretically some difference should be evident.

Myasthenia Gravis

Myasthenia gravis is a disorder of voluntary (striated) muscles characterized by muscle weakness and fatigability. In 15% of persons with myasthenia gravis, thymic tumors are found. Of persons with myasthenia gravis, 70% to 80% have pathologic changes in the thymus (Adams & Victor, 1989). Such tumors are more common in males than in females. Myasthenia gravis is an autoimmune disease associated with an increased incidence of other autoimmune diseases, including systemic lupus erythematosus, rheumatoid arthritis, polymyositis, and thyrotoxicosis. (Autoimmune mechanisms are discussed in Chapter 8.) Transitory signs of myasthenia gravis are present in 10% to 15% of infants born to mothers with myasthenia gravis.

The three types of myasthenia gravis are ocular, generalized, and bulbar myasthenia. **Ocular myasthenia,** which is more common in males, involves muscle weakness that is confined to the eye muscles. **Generalized myasthenia** involves the proximal musculature throughout the body and has several courses: (1) a course with periodic remissions, (2) a slowly progressive course, (3) a rapidly progressive course, or (4) a fulminating course. **Bulbar myasthenia** involves the muscles innervated by cranial nerves IX, X, XI, and XII, and tends to be rapidly progressive or fulminating.

Pathophysiology

Myasthenia gravis results from a defect in nerve impulse transmission at the neuromuscular junction. The postsynaptic acetylcholine receptors on the muscle cell's plasma membrane for an unknown reason are no longer recognized as "self" and therefore elicit an antigenic effect. IgG antibody is secreted against the acetylcholine receptors. These antibodies fix onto the receptor sites and block the binding of acetylcholine. Eventually the antibody action causes the destruction of receptor sites and the number of receptors on the plasma membrane is reduced. The destruction of receptor sites causes diminished transmission of the nerve impulse across the neuromuscular junction. Muscle depolarization is not achieved.

The cause of this autosensitization is not known. Evidence supports the autoimmune theory. Clinical and laboratory data show the following:

1. Receptor-binding antibodies are present in 85% to 90% of persons with myasthenia gravis.
2. Passive transfer of myasthenia gravis to animals is possible by injecting serum and IgG from humans with myasthenia gravis.
3. Myasthenia gravis is frequently associated with other autoimmune disorders, such as rheumatoid arthritis and systemic lupus erythematosus.
4. Transitory neonatal myasthenia gravis occurs.
5. A strong association between myasthenia gravis and thymus gland hyperplasia exists.
6. Steroid therapy, antimetabolite drugs, plasma exchange, and thoracic duct drainage all improve the clinical status of the person who has myasthenia gravis.

Clinical Manifestations

Myasthenia gravis typically has an insidious onset. Clinical manifestations may first appear during pregnancy, during the postpartum period, or in conjunction with the administration of certain anesthetic agents. The person often complains of fatigue after exercise and has a recent history of recurring upper respiratory tract infections. The muscles of the eyes, face, mouth, throat, and neck are usually affected first. The extraocular (eye) muscles and the levator muscles are most affected. Manifestations include diplopia, ptosis, and ocular palsies.

The muscles of facial expression, mastication, swallowing, and speech are the next most involved. The results are facial droop and an expressionless face; difficulty chewing and swallowing associated with dietary changes and weight loss; drooling, episodes of choking and aspiration; and a nasal, low-volume but high-pitched monotonous speech pattern.

The muscles of the neck, shoulder girdle, and hip flexors are less frequently affected. When these muscles do become involved, however, the person experiences fatigue requiring periods of rest, weakness of the arms and legs that improves with rest, and difficulty in maintaining head position. The respiratory muscles of the diaphragm and chest wall become weak and ventilation is impaired. Impairment in deep breathing and coughing predispose the individual to atelectasis and congestion. In the advanced stage of the disease all the muscles are weak.

Myasthenic crisis occurs when severe muscle weakness causes extreme quadriparesis or quadriplegia, respiratory insufficiency with shortness of breath and a markedly decreased tidal volume and vital capacity, and extreme difficulty in swallowing. The individual in myasthenic crisis is in danger of respiratory arrest.

Cholinergic crisis may arise from anticholinesterase drug toxicity. The clinical picture is like that of myasthenic crisis, but other symptoms are also present. Intestinal motility increases and is associated with episodes of diarrhea and complaints of cramping; fasciculation, bradycardia, pupillary constriction, increased salivation, and increased sweating are present. These clinical manifestations are caused by the smooth muscle hyperactivity secondary to excessive accumulation of acetylcholine at the neuromuscular junctions and excessive parasympathetic-like activity. As in myasthenic crisis, the individual is in danger of respiratory arrest.

Evaluation and Treatment

The diagnosis of myasthenia gravis is made on the basis of a response to edrophonium chloride (Tensilon), electromyography (EMG), and serum anti-AChR (acetylcholine receptor) antibody titer. With the intravenous administration of the drug immediate demonstrable improvement in muscle strength usually persists for several minutes. On EMG, the amplitude of the action potentials of stimulated muscles rapidly declines. Mediastinal tomography is used to determine whether a thymoma is present. The progression of myasthenia gravis is highly variable. In some individuals it is mild and spontaneously remits. There is usually a series of relapses with symptom-free intervals ranging from weeks to months. Over time the disease can progress, leading to death.

Ocular myasthenia has a very good prognosis.

Anticholinesterase drugs, steroids, and immunosuppressant drugs are used to treat myasthenia gravis and myasthenic crisis. Plasmapheresis may be lifesaving during myasthenic crisis, before and after thymectomy, and at the start of immunosuppressant therapy. For individuals with cholinergic crisis, treatment is to withhold anticholinergic drugs until blood levels fall out of the toxic range, while providing ventilatory support and preventing respiratory complications. Thymectomy is the treatment of choice in individuals with a thymoma.

Myopathies

Myopathy is the term applied to a primary muscle disorder. Many pathologic processes affect muscles and cause loss of functional muscle cells. Within myopathies, muscle strength, tone, and bulk are affected.

Primary muscle disease is invariably associated with weakness, usually marked weakness. The distribution of the weakness in myopathy is usually symmetric and proximal, although occasionally the weakness is predominantly distal, such as in myotonic dystrophy. The weakness is associated with mild fatigue. Tone is decreased as are the tendon reflexes. Atrophy may be present. Some myopathies are associated with muscle hypertrophy as in cretinism and the familial progressive muscular dystrophies of childhood, in which hypertrophied muscles are rubbery and weak. Fasciculations are not present with myopathy because no denervation is present. No sensory changes are found. (Specific myopathies are discussed in Chapter 14.)

SUMMARY REVIEW

Central Nervous System (CNS) Disorders

1 Motor accidents are the major cause of traumatic CNS injury. Traumatic injuries are classified as closed-head trauma (blunt) or open-head trauma (penetrating). Closed-head trauma is the more frequent type of trauma.

2 Different types of focal brain injury include contusion (bruising of the brain), laceration (tearing of brain tissue), extradural hematoma (accumulation of blood above the dura mater), subdural hematoma (blood between the dura mater and arachnoid membrane), intracerebral hematoma (bleeding into the brain), and open-head trauma.

3 Open-head trauma involves a skull fracture with exposure of the cranial vault to the environment. The types of open-head trauma (compound fracture, per-forated fracture) are linear, comminuted, compound, and basilar skull fracture (in the cranial vault or at the base of the skull).

4 Diffuse brain injury (DAI) results from the effects of head rotation. The brain experiences shearing stresses resulting in axonal damage manifested as concussion to a severe DAI state.

5 Spinal cord injuries occur most frequently in men between 16 and 30 years of age who sustain different kinds of injuries (recreational or travel-related) and the elderly because of preexisting degenerative vertebral disorders.

6 Spinal cord injury involves damage to vertebral or neural tissues by compressing tissue, pulling or exerting tension on tissue, or shearing tissues so that they slide into one another.

7 Spinal cord injury often causes spinal shock with cessation of all motor, sensory, reflex, and autonomic functions below any transected area. Loss of motor and sensory function depends on the level of injury.

8 Paralysis of the lower half of the body with both legs involved is called paraplegia. Paralysis involving all four extremities is called quadriplegia.

9 Return of spinal neuron excitability occurs slowly. Reflex activity can return in 1 to 2 weeks in most persons with acute spinal cord injury. A pattern of flexion reflexes emerges, involving first the toes, then the feet and the legs. Eventually reflex voiding and bowel elimination appear, and mass reflex (flexor spasms accompanied by profuse sweating, piloerection, and automatic bladder emptying) may develop.

10 Immobilization of the spine is the immediate intervention for a suggested or confirmed vertebral fracture.

11 Low back pain is pain between the lower rib cage and gluteal muscles and often radiates into the thigh.

12 Low back pain has a high prevalence, affecting 60% to 90% of the population at some point in their lifetime. Sciatica affects about 1% of those with low back pain.

13 Most causes of low back pain are unknown; however, some secondary causes are disk prolapse, tumors, bursitis, synovitis, degenerative joint disease, osteoporosis, fracture, inflammation, and sprain.

14 The role of muscle injury in low back pain remains uncertain; however, muscle spasms often accompany low back pain.

15 Diagnosis of injury to the lower back is made on the basis of physical examination, electromyography, myelography, computerized tomography, and magnetic resonance imaging.

16 Treatment for low back pain includes bed rest, use of analgesics and anti-inflammatory agents, exercise, physical therapy, education, and surgery.

17 Herniation of an intervertebral disk is a protrusion of part of the nucleus pulposus. Herniation most commonly affects the lumbosacral disks (L5-S1 and L4-5). The extruded pulposus compresses the nerve root, causing pain that radiates along the sciatic nerve course.

18 The conservative approach to treatment of an intervertebral rupture is traction and bed rest. Surgery is indicated if there is evidence of severe compression (weakness, chronic pain, decreased deep tendon reflexes, and bladder/bowel reflexes).

19 Cerebrovascular disease is the most frequently occurring neurologic disorder. Any abnormality of the blood vessels of the brain is referred to as a cerebrovascular disease.

20 Cerebrovascular disease is associated with two types of brain abnormalities: (a) ischemia with or without infarction and (b) hemorrhage.

21 The most common clinical manifestation of cerebrovascular disease is a cerebrovascular accident (CVA, stroke).

22 Cerebrovascular accidents are classified according to pathophysiology and include thrombotic (arterial occlusions caused by thrombi), embolic (fragments that break from a thrombus outside the brain), hemorrhagic (intracranial hemorrhage), and lacunar strokes.

23 Treatment for an ischemic CVA includes anticoagulant therapy and supportive management for cerebral edema and increased intracranial pressure. Surgical intervention may be needed to restore blood supply.

24 Intracranial aneurysms result from defects in the vascular wall and are classified on the basis of form and shape. They are frequently asymptomatic, but the signs vary, depending on the location and size of the aneurysm.

25 In cerebral aneurysms, surgical intervention is the treatment of choice before rupture.

26 An arteriovenous malformation (AVM) is a tangled mass of dilated blood vessels. Although sometimes present at birth, AVM exhibits a delayed age of onset.

27 Clinical manifestations of AVM range from headache and dementia to seizures and intracerebral or subarachnoid hemorrhage.

28 A subarachnoid hemorrhage occurs when blood escapes from defective or injured vasculature into the subarachnoid space. When a vessel tears, blood under pressure is pumped into the subarachnoid space. The blood produces an inflammatory reaction in these tissues.

29 Clinical manifestations of a subarachnoid hemorrhage include headache, changes in mental status, transient motor weakness, and numbness and tingling. Vasospasm is a serious complication and may cause ischemia and infarct. Treatment of vasospasm includes use of calcium channel blockers to prevent or reverse vasospasm and augmenting cerebral perfusion by hemodilutional hyperperfusion.

30 Two main types of tumors occur within the cranium: primary and metastatic. Primary tumors are classified as intracerebral tumors or extracerebral tumors. Metastatic tumors can be found inside or outside the brain substance.

31 CNS tumors cause local and generalized manifestations. The effects are varied and local manifestations include seizures, visual disturbances, loss of equilibrium, and cranial nerve dysfunction.

32 The principal treatment for brain tumors is surgical or radiosurgical excision or decompression if total excision is not possible. Chemotherapy and radiation therapy also are used.

33 Spinal cord tumors are classified as intramedullary tumors (within the neural tissues) or extramedullary

tumors (outside the spinal cord). Metastatic spinal cord tumors are usually carcinomas, lymphomas, or myelomas.

34 Extramedullary spinal cord tumors produce dysfunction by compression of adjacent tissue, not by direct invasion. Intramedullary spinal cord tumors produce dysfunction by both invasion and compression.

35 The onset of clinical manifestations of spinal cord tumors is gradual and progressive, suggesting compression. Specific manifestations depend on the location of the tumor; for example, there may be paresis and spasticity of one leg with thoracic tumors, followed by involvement of the opposite leg.

36 Spinal cord tumors are treated by surgery, radiation therapy, chemotherapy, and hormonal therapy.

37 Infection and inflammation of the CNS can occur by bacteria, viruses, fungi, protozoans, and rickettsiae. The resulting infection of bacterial infections is pus-producing, or pyogenic.

38 Meningitis (infection of the meninges) is classified as bacterial, aseptic (nonpurulent), or fungal. Bacterial meningitis is primarily an infection of the pia mater and arachnoid, and of the fluid of the subarachnoid space. Aseptic meningitis is believed to be limited to the meninges. Fungal meningitis is a chronic, less common type of meningitis.

39 The meningeal vessels become hyperemic and neutrophils migrate into the subarachnoid space with bacterial meningitis. An inflammatory reaction occurs and exudate is formed and increases rapidly.

40 The variety of clinical manifestations depends on the type of meningitis and ranges from throbbing headache to neck stiffness and rigidity and decreasing responsiveness. Specific cranial nerve dysfunction is a common occurrence.

41 Bacterial meningitis and fungal meningitis are treated with appropriate antibiotic therapy; aseptic meningitis is treated with antibiotics, antiviral drugs, and steroids.

42 Brain abscesses often originate from infections outside the CNS. Organisms gain access to the CNS from adjacent sites or spread along the wall of a vein. A localized inflammatory process develops with exudate formation, thrombosis of vessels, and degenerating leukocytes. After a few days the infection becomes delimited with a center of pus and wall of granular tissue.

43 Clinical manifestations of brain abscesses include headache, nuchal rigidity, confusion, drowsiness, and sensory and communication deficits. Treatment includes antibiotic therapy and surgical excision or aspiration.

44 Encephalitis is an acute, febrile illness of viral origin with nervous system involvement. The most common encephalitides are caused by arthropod-borne viruses and herpes simplex. Meningeal involvement appears in all encephalitides.

45 Clinical manifestations of encephalitis include fever, delirium, confusion, seizures, abnormal and involuntary movement, and increased intracranial pressure.

46 Herpes encephalitis is treated with antiviral agents. No definitive treatment exists for the other encephalitides.

47 The common neurologic complications of AIDS are HIV encephalopathy, peripheral neuropathies, vacuolar myelopathy, opportunistic infections of the CNS, and neoplasms. Pathologically, there may be diffuse CNS involvement, focal pathology, and obstructive hydrocephalus.

48 Parkinson disease is a commonly occurring degenerative disorder of the basal ganglia (corpus striatum) involving degeneration of the dopamine-secreting nigrostriatal pathway. The pathogenesis of Parkinson disease is unknown, but researchers suggest vascular, viral, and metabolic factors as possible causes.

49 Degeneration of the dopaminergic nigrostriatal pathway causes dopamine depletion in the basal ganglia and excess of cholinergic activity in the cortex, basal ganglia, and thalamus. Tremor and rigidity are caused by the excess cholinergic activity. Progressive dementia may be associated with an advanced stage of the disease.

50 Treatment of Parkinson disease is symptomatic, involving levodopa (L-dopa), a precursor of dopamine. The disease takes a slowly progressive course for 15 to 20 years before producing complete invalidism.

51 Huntington disease (chorea) is a rare hereditary disease involving the basal ganglia and cerebral cortex. It is inherited as an autosomal dominant trait and commonly manifests between 40 and 50 years of age.

52 The major pathologic feature of Huntington disease is severe degeneration of the basal ganglia and the frontal cerebral cortex. The basal ganglia and the substantia nigra exhibit a depletion of γ-aminobutyric acid (an inhibitory neurotransmitter) secreting neurons. This depletion leads to an excess of dopaminergic activity that causes involuntary, fragmentary movements.

53 No known treatment is effective in halting the degenerative process in Huntington disease.

54 Multiple sclerosis (MS) is a relatively common degenerative disorder involving CNS myelin. Although the pathogenesis is unknown, the demyelination is thought to result from an immunogenetic-viral cause. Viruses or other antigens may directly attack the myelin or provoke a hypersensitivity reaction.

55 The clinical manifestations of MS involve different syndromes: corticospinal (corticospinal tract and dorsal column), brainstem (cranial nerves), cerebellar (corticospinal tract or cerebellum), and cerebral (optic neuritis). Persons with early MS usually have one of the initial syndromes; over time individuals eventually have mixed involvement.

56 No treatment is available to alter the course of MS. Steroid therapy is used to shorten the duration of acute exacerbations.

57 Amyotrophic lateral sclerosis (ALS) is a rare degenerative disorder diffusely involving lower and upper motor neurons. The pathogenesis of ALS is unknown; however, there is lower and upper motor neuron degeneration.

58 Clinical manifestations of ALS may include weakness in all muscles. Flaccid paresis progressing to paralysis is characteristic of the lower motor neuron syndrome. No treatment is currently available to alter the overall course of the ALS syndrome.

59 Hydrocephalus comprises a variety of disorders characterized by an excess of fluid within the cranial vault, subarachnoid space, or both. Hydrocephalus occurs because of interference with cerebrospinal fluid flow caused by increased fluid production or obstruction within the ventricular system or by defective reabsorption of the fluid.

60 Hydrocephalus can be treated by reducing CSF in the ventricles through the use of shunts and diuretic therapy if resection of the cause is not possible.

Peripheral Nervous System and Neuromuscular Joint Disorders

1 Radiculopathies are disorders of the roots of spinal cord nerves. The roots may be compressed, inflamed, or torn. Clinical manifestations include local pain or paresthesias in the sensory root distribution. Treatment may involve surgery, antibiotics, steroids, radiation therapy, and chemotherapy.

2 Plexus injuries involve the plexus distal to the spinal roots. Paralysis can occur with complete plexus involvement.

3 Neuropathies are the resulting syndrome when the peripheral nerves are affected. Axon and myelin degeneration may be present. Neuropathies are classified as sensorimotor, sensory, or motor. The neuropathies are characterized by varying degrees of paresis and paralysis, and secondary atrophy may be present.

4 Therapy for the neuropathies is directed at the primary cause, such as diabetes mellitus. Axonal regrowth and recovery of function may take months but many neuropathies can be reversed.

5 Guillain-Barré syndrome is a demyelinating disorder caused by a cell-mediated immunologic reaction directed at the peripheral nerves. The clinical manifestations may vary from paresis of the legs to complete quadriplegia, respiratory insufficiency, and autonomic nervous system instability. Steroid therapy and plasmapheresis may be used during the acute phase and followed by aggressive rehabilitation.

6 Myasthenia gravis is a disorder of voluntary muscles characterized by muscle weakness and fatigability. It is considered an autoimmune disease and is associated with an increased incidence of other autoimmune diseases.

7 Myasthenia gravis results from a defect in nerve impulse transmission at the neuromuscular junction. IgG antibody is secreted against the "self" acetylcholine receptors and blocks the binding of acetylcholine. The antibody action destroys the receptor sites, causing decreased transmission of the nerve impulse across the neuromuscular junction.

8 Clinical manifestations of myasthenia gravis include weakness of the muscles of the face and throat and may involve muscles of the diaphragm and chest wall.

9 Treatment of myasthenia gravis involves symptom relief. The progression of the disease is highly variable; in some individuals it is mild and spontaneously remits.

10 Primary disorders with weakness and atrophy are known as myopathies.

KEY TERMS

Acute hydrocephalus, 577

Amyotrophic lateral sclerosis (ALS, sporadic motor system disease, sporadic motor neuron disease), 575

Arteriovenous malformation (AVM), 550

Aseptic meningitis (viral meningitis, nonpurulent meningitis), 562

Autonomic hyperreflexia (autonomic dysreflexia), 540

Axonal degeneration, 578

Bacterial meningitis, 561

Basilar skull fracture, 530

Blunt trauma (closed-head trauma), 528

Brain abscess, 563

Brudzinski sign, 552

Bulbar myasthenia, 580

Cerebrovascular accident (CVA, stroke), 547

Cholinergic crisis, 581

Classic cerebral concussion, 534

Classic ALS (Lou Gehrig disease), 575

Communicating hydrocephalus (extraventricular hydrocephalus), 576

Completed stroke, 547

Compound fracture, 530

Compressive syndrome (sensorimotor syndrome), 561

Contrecoup injury, 529

Contusion, 530

Coup injury, 529

Degenerative disk disease, 544

Embolic stroke, 547

Encephalitis, 564

Ependymoma, 559

Extradural brain abscess, 563

Extradural hematoma, 531

Extradural tumor, 560

REFERENCES

Adams, R. D., & Victor, M. (1989). *Principles of neurology*. New York: McGraw-Hill.

Chipps, E., Clanin, N., & Campbell, V. (1992). *Neurologic disorders*. St. Louis: Mosby–Year Book.

Cook, H. A. (1991). Aneurysmal subarachnoid hemorrhage: Neuroscience frontiers and nursing challenges. In C. Winkelman (Ed.), *AACN clinical issues in critical care nursing* (pp. 665-674). Philadelphia: Lippincott.

Cutler, W. P. (1983). *Degenerative and hereditary diseases* (7th ed.). Washington, DC: Scientific American Medicine.

Duvoisin, R. C. (1984). *Parkinson's disease, a guide for patient and family* (2nd ed.). New York: Raven Press.

Fischer, E. G., Linggood, R. M., & Recht, L. D. (1986). Cancers of the central nervous system. In *Cancer manual*. Boston, Mass.: American Cancer Society.

Frymoyer, J. W. (1988, February). Back pain and sciatica. *New England Journal of Medicine, 318*(5), 291-300.

Grennarelli, T. A., Spielman, G. M., Langfitt, T. W., Gildenberg, P. L., Harrington, T., Jane, J. A., Marshall, L. E., Miller, J. D., & Pitts, L. H. (1982). Influence of the type of intracranial lesion on outcome from severe head injury. *Journal of Neurosurgery, 56*(1), 26.

Kandel, E. R., & Schwartz, J. H. (1985). *Principles of neural science*. New York: Elsevier Science Publishing.

Kirshner, H. S., Tsai, S. I., Runge, V. M., & Price, A. C. (1985). Magnetic resonance imaging and other techniques in the diagnosis of multiple sclerosis. *Archives of Neurology, 42*, 859.

Kissane, J. M. (ed.). (1985). *Anderson's pathology* (8th ed.). St. Louis: Mosby–Year Book.

Kissane, J. M. (ed.). (1989). *Anderson's pathology* (9th ed.). St. Louis: Mosby–Year Book.

Kneisl, C. R., & Ames, S. A. (1986). *Adult health nursing: A biopsychosocial approach*. Reading, MA: Addison-Wesley.

McArthur, J. H., Palenicek, J. G., & Bowersox, L. L. (1988). Human immunodeficiency virus and the nervous system. *Nursing Clinics of North America, 23*(4), 823.

McKahn, G. M., & Griffin, J. W. (1987). Plasmapheresis and the Guillain-Barré syndrome. *Annals of Neurology, 22*(60), 762.

Pope, M. H., Bevins, T., Wilder, D. G., & Frymoyer, J. W. (1985). The relationship between anthropometric, postural, muscular, and mobility characteristics of males ages 18-55. *Spine, 10*, 644-648.

Poser, C. M. (1985). MRI and CT scan in multiple sclerosis [Letter]. *Journal of the American Medical Association, 253*(22), 3250.

Rosai, J. (1989). *Ackerman's surgical pathology* (7th ed.). St. Louis: Mosby–Year Book.

Rudy, E. B. (1984). *Advanced neurological and neurosurgical nursing*. St. Louis: Mosby–Year Book.

Scheinberg, L. C. (Ed.). (1983). *Multiple sclerosis, a guide for patients and their families*. New York: Raven Press.

Simon, R. H., & Sayre, J. T. (1987). *Strategy in head injury management*. Norwalk, CT: Appleton & Lange.

Slater, R. J., & Yearwood, A. C. (1980). MS: Facts, faith, and hope. *American Journal of Nursing, 80*, 276.

Spengler, D. M. (1982). *Low back pain, assessment, and management*. New York: Grune & Stratton.

Thompson, J. M., McFarland, G. K., Hirsch, J. E., & Tucker, S. M. (1993). *Mosby's clinical nursing* (3rd ed.). St. Louis: Mosby–Year Book.

Weinstein, S. L. (1986). Idiopathic scoliosis: Natural history. *Spine, 11*, 780-783.

Willis, D. (1992). Intracranial astrocytoma: Pathology, diagnosis, and clinical presentation. *Journal of Neuroscience Nursing, 23*(1), 171.

Willis, D., & Harbit, M. D. (1990). Transcatheter arterial embolization of cerebral arteriovenous malformation. *Journal of Neuroscience Nursing, 22*(5), 280.

SUGGESTED READINGS

Adams, B. A., Clancey, J. K., & Eddy, M. (1991). Malignant glioma: Current treatment perspectives. *Journal of Neuroscience Nursing, 23*(1), 15.

Aita, J. F. (1982). Why patients with Parkinson's disease fall. *Journal of the American Medical Association, 247*(4), 515.

Ashbury, A. K. (1991). Diseases of the peripheral nervous system. In J. D. Wilson, E. Braunwald, K. J. Isselbacher, R. G. Petersdorf, J. B. Martin, A. S. Fauci, & R. K. Root (Eds.), *Harrison's principles of internal medicine* (pp. 2096-2108). New York: McGraw-Hill.

Bell, J. (1989). Understanding and managing myasthenia gravis. *Focus on Critical Care Nursing, 16*(1), 57.

Bradbury, K., & Bauer, M. (1990). Brain graft surgery: A new treatment for Parkinson's disease. *Critical Care Nursing, 10*(8), 15.

Bronstein, K. S., Popovich, J. M., & Stewart-Amidei, C. (1991). *Promoting stroke recovery: A research-based approach for nurses.* St. Louis: Mosby–Year Book.

Chipps, E. (1991). Myasthenia gravis: The patient in crisis. *Critical Care Nursing, 11*(1), 18.

Flaskerud, J. (1987). AIDS: Neuropsychiatric complications. *Journal of Psychosocial Nursing, 25*(12), 17.

Gee, G., & Moran, T. (1988). *AIDS: Concepts in nursing practice.* Baltimore: Williams & Wilkins.

Grabbe, L. L., & Frown, L. B. (1989). Identifying neurologic complications of AIDS. *Nursing, 15*(5), 66.

Marshall, S. B., Marshall, L., Vos, H., & Chestnut, R. (1990). *Neuroscience critical care: Pathophysiology and patient management.* Philadelphia: Saunders.

Morgante, L., Madonna, M., & Pokoluk, R. (1989). Research and treatment in multiple sclerosis: Implications for nursing practice. *Journal of Neuroscience Nursing, 21*(5), 285.

Raney, D. J. (1991). Malignant spinal cord tumors: A review and case presentation. *Journal of Neuroscience Nursing, 23*(10), 44.

Shatkin, J., Bolt, B., & Norton, D. (1987). Teaching program for patients with low back pain. *Journal of Neuroscience Nursing, 19*, (5), 240.

Twomey, C. R. (1992). Brain abscess: An update. *Journal of Neuroscience Nursing, 24*(1), 34.

CHAPTER 16

Alterations of Neurologic Function in Children

Judith A. Farley
Kathleen Hardin Mooney
Margaret M. Andrews*

Chapter Outline

C*entral nervous system (CNS) malformations are responsible for 75% of fetal deaths and 40% of deaths during the first year of life. During the perinatal period, CNS malformations account for one third of all apparent congenital malformations, and 90% of CNS malformations are defects of neural tube closure. Although embryology is a highly complex and often difficult science, the process of embryonic development explains many of the malformations that occur in children.*

Environmental influences also play a significant role in nervous system development. Nutrition, hormones, oxygen levels, and external stimulation all affect normal growth. The proper proportions of essential nutrients are necessary for proliferation of the nervous system tissue. Maternal lifestyle, nutrition, and state of health also have a crucial impact on nervous system development at certain critical periods of maturation.

STRUCTURE AND FUNCTION OF THE NERVOUS SYSTEM IN CHILDREN

The central nervous system develops from a dorsal thickening of the ectoderm known as the **neural plate.** This plate appears around the middle of the third gestational week and unfolds to form a **neural groove** and **neural folds.** During the fourth gestational week, the neural groove deepens; its folds develop laterally; and it closes dorsally to form the **neural tube,** epithelial tissue that ultimately becomes the CNS. The neural tube closes first in the cervical region and then "zippers" in two directions, cranially and caudally (Fig. 16-1).

In the developmental process, some neuroectodermal cells separate from the neural tube but remain between the tube and the surface ectoderm, creating what is called the **neural crest.** This cellular band develops into the cranial and spinal ganglia, more commonly referred to as the peripheral nervous system. Other structures associated with the nervous system arise from mesoderm (**somite**) and include blood vessels, microglial cells, dura and arachnoid layers of the meninges, the capsule of some peripheral sensory nerve endings, and peripheral nerve coverings.

The cranial end of the neural tube forms the brain, and the remainder develops into the spinal cord. The lumen of the neural tube becomes the ventricles of the brain and the central canal of the spinal cord (Fig. 16-2). On either side of the neural tube's inner surface is a longitudinal groove (**sulcus limitans**). Anterior to this region (**basal plate**) the gray matter differentiates into the nuclei of the lower motor neurons. The region posterior to the sulcus (**alar plate**) differentiates into the sensory nuclei of the spinal cord.

Embryonic development of the nervous system occurs in six stages: (1) dorsal (posterior) induction, (2) ventral (anterior) induction, (3) proliferation, (4) migration, (5) organization, and (6) myelination. (Fig. 16-3 summarizes the embryonic development of the nervous system and identifies disorders associated with interference in any of these stages.) Many different events happen simultaneously, and critical periods must pass uninterrupted if the vulnerable fetus is to develop normally.

In the newborn the bones of the skull are separated, but definite **sutures** (bands of connective tissue) form shortly thereafter. The edges are several millimeters wide to allow for normal growth. At the junctions of the sutures are wider spaces of unossified membranous tissue called **fontanelles.** Sutures and fontanelles close as the skull and brain grow and develop.

On average the posterior fontanelle closes within the first 3 months of life. By 6 months of age, a fibrous union of suture lines occurs, and serrated edges interlock. By approximately 20 to 24 months, the anterior fontanelle is closed (Fig. 16-4). At approximately 8 years of age, ossification of the cranial bones is complete and the sutures usually are completely fused and cannot be separated by 12 years of age, even in the presence of increased intracranial pressure.

Myelin Sheath

Axons are wrapped in concentric layers of myelin, a lipid-protein sheath (see Chapter 12). Specialized connective tissue cells, which in the peripheral nervous system are called **Schwann's cells,** form membranes that wrap around the axon during embryonic development, laying down the lipoprotein lamellae of the myelin sheath. These axons are myelinated, whereas the axons that lack a sheath are thinner, unmyelinated fibers and conduct nerve impulses more slowly. During the first year of life, the presence or absence of various reflexes is indicative of the myelination that has occurred with growth of the infant.

Normal Growth and Development

Human neurologic functioning is primarily at a subcortical level at birth (impulses are handled by the brainstem and spinal cord). Many reflex patterns mediated by brainstem and spinal cord mechanisms are present at birth and disappear at predictable times during infancy. Table 16-1 summarizes the age at which reflexes appear and disappear.

Absence of expected reflex responses at the appropriate age indicates general depression of central or peripheral motor functions. Asymmetric responses may indicate lesions in the motor cortex or may occur with fractures of bones after traumatic delivery or postnatal injury. As the infant matures, the neonatal reflexes disappear in a predictable order as voluntary motor functions supersede them. Abnormal persistence of these reflexes is seen in infants with developmental delays or with central motor lesions.

Several differences between adults and children help one to understand the pathophysiology of the nervous system in children. First, the head of a normal infant accounts for approximately one fourth of the total height, whereas an adult's head is one eighth of the total body height. Second, the bones of the infant's skull are separated at the suture lines, thus forming two fontanelles or "soft spots," one diamond-shaped anterior fontanelle and one triangular-shaped posterior fontanelle. The posterior fontanelle may be open until 2 to 3 months of age, whereas the anterior fontanelle normally closes by 18 months. Although the adult's cranium is a closed cavity with sutures firmly holding the cranial bones together, the infant's cranium has room for expansion through the fontanelles. An adult's head size will not expand, regardless of intracranial events such as trauma or increased production of cerebrospinal fluid. The infant's head circumference, on the other

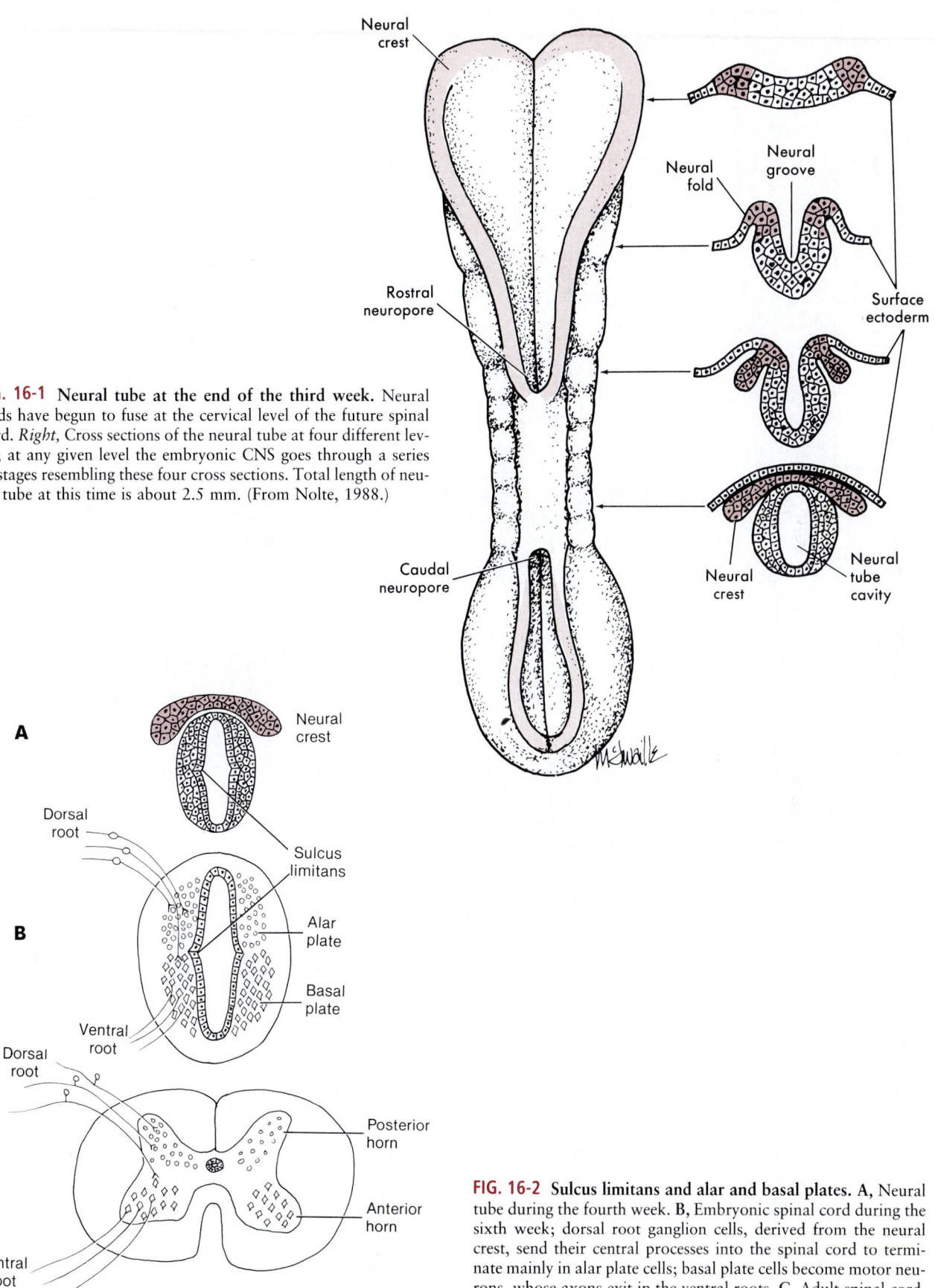

FIG. 16-1 **Neural tube at the end of the third week.** Neural folds have begun to fuse at the cervical level of the future spinal cord. *Right,* Cross sections of the neural tube at four different levels; at any given level the embryonic CNS goes through a series of stages resembling these four cross sections. Total length of neural tube at this time is about 2.5 mm. (From Nolte, 1988.)

FIG. 16-2 **Sulcus limitans and alar and basal plates. A,** Neural tube during the fourth week. **B,** Embryonic spinal cord during the sixth week; dorsal root ganglion cells, derived from the neural crest, send their central processes into the spinal cord to terminate mainly in alar plate cells; basal plate cells become motor neurons, whose axons exit in the ventral roots. **C,** Adult spinal cord. (From Nolte, 1988.)

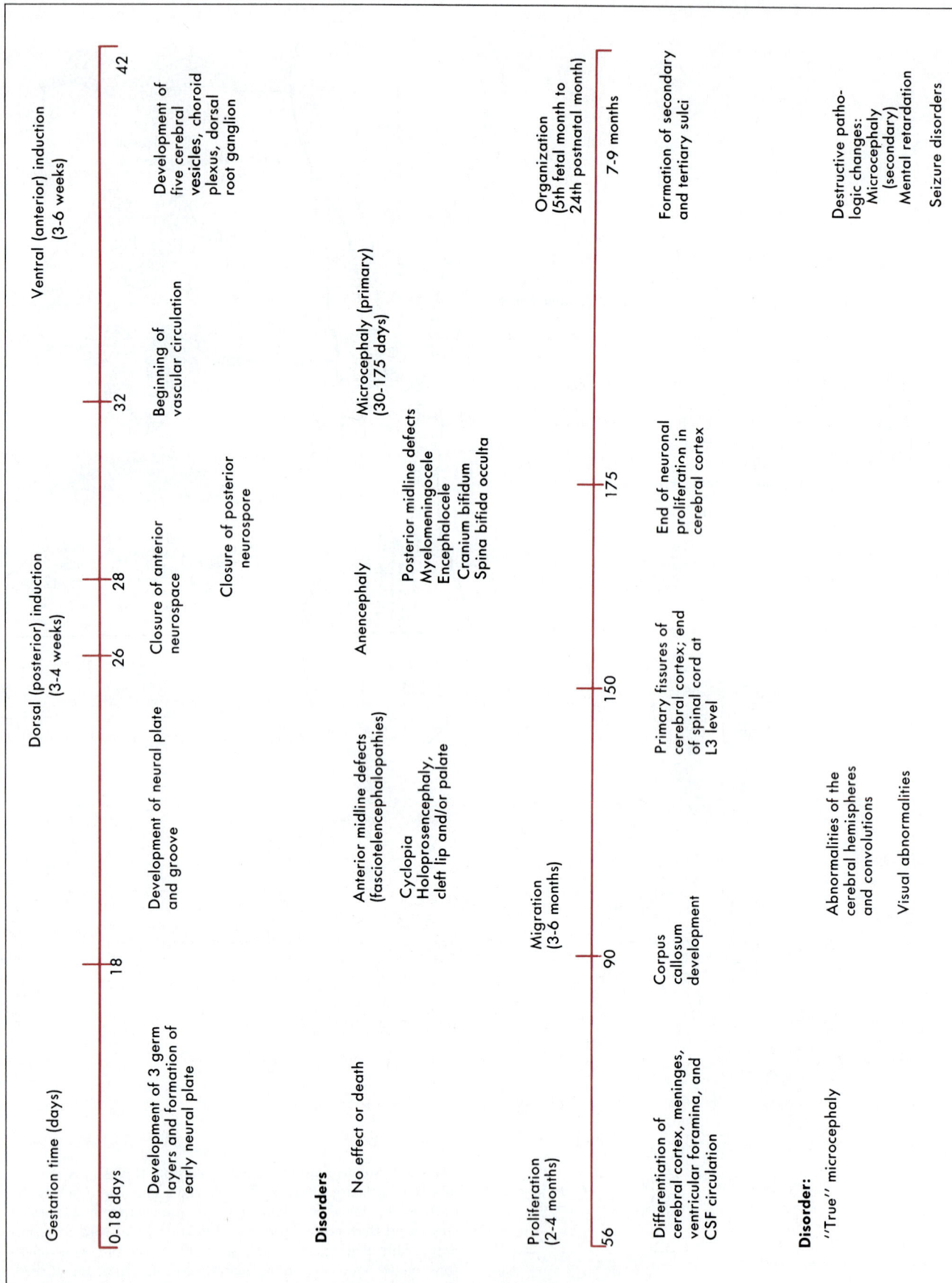

FIG. 16-3 Disorders associated with specific stages of embryonic development.

6 months
Development of myelin wrapping

Myelination
(6 months gestation to adulthood)

Adulthood

Disorder:
Schilder disease
Childhood multiple sclerosis
Leukodystrophies

FIG. 16-4 **Cranial sutures and fontanelles in infancy.** Fibrous union of suture lines and interlocking of serrated edges (occurs by 6 months; solid union requires approximately 12 years). (From Whaley & Wong, 1991.)

Frontal suture
Anterior fontanel
Frontal bone
Coronal suture
Sagittal suture
Parietal bone
Posterior fontanel
Occipital bone
Lambdoidal suture

TABLE 16-1

Reflexes of Infancy

Reflex	Age at appearance of reflex	Age at which reflex should no longer be obtainable
Moro	Birth	3 months
Stepping	Birth	6 weeks
Sucking	Birth	4 months awake 7 months asleep
Rooting	Birth	4 months awake 7 months asleep
Palmar grasp	Birth	6 months
Plantar grasp	Birth	10 months
Tonic neck	2 months	5 months
Neck righting	4-6 months	24 months
Landau	3 months	24 months
Parachute reaction	9 months	Persists for life

hand, increases in size as a result of normal growth up to age 5 years. The head is the fastest growing body part during infancy. Abnormal intracranial conditions, such as those characterized by increased intracranial pressure, also may result in an increased head circumference in excess of that expected with normal growth. Health care providers carefully monitor head growth during the first 5 years of life by measuring head circumference and comparing the results with a standardized growth chart.

STRUCTURAL MALFORMATIONS
Defects of Neural Tube Closure

Neural tube defects, which are caused by an arrest of the normal developmental process, have an incidence rate of approximately 0.7 to 1.0 for every 1000 live births in the United States each year (Hobbins, 1991; Wallander, Feldman, & Varni, 1989). There is a strong association of fetal death with neural tube defects, reducing the actual prevalence of neural defects at birth (Lemire, 1986). Defects of neural tube closure are divided into two categories: (1) posterior defects and (2) anterior midline defects.

Posterior defects are more common. These include **anencephaly** (an = without; enkephalos = brain) and a group of disorders collectively referred to as the **myelodysplasias** (dys = bad; plassein = to form). Although myelodysplasia is defined as a defective formation of the spinal cord, the term is used to refer to anomalies of both the vertebral column and the spine.

Anterior midline defects are less common because the inductive processes occur in a relatively short period, 2 to 3 days. These developmental defects may cause brain and skull abnormalities. The most extreme form is **cyclopia,** in which the child has a single midline orbit and eye with a protruding noselike appendage above the orbit.

Anencephaly

Anencephaly is an anomaly in which the soft, bony component of the skull and part of the brain are missing. This is a relatively common disorder, with an incidence rate of approximately 0.36 per 1000 total live births in the United States each year (Wiswell, Tuttle, Northam, & Simonds, 1990). When development is arrested early in anterior closure of the neural tube, the cerebral hemispheres, diencephalon, mesencephalon, cerebellum, brainstem, or spinal cord may be affected. At birth the infant's head, viewed face-on, has a froglike appearance. These infants are stillborn or die within a few days after birth.

Encephalocele

Encephalocele refers to a herniation or protrusion of brain and meninges through a defect in the skull, result-

ing in a saclike structure. The incidence rate is approximately 0.14 per 1000 live births in the United States each year (Wiswell et al., 1990). When the defect contains only meninges, it is referred to as a **cranial meningocele.** Most encephaloceles occur in the occipital area, with the remainder found in the frontal, parietal, or nasopharyngeal regions.

Clinical Manifestations

Encephalocele usually is seen at birth as a midline skull defect through which a large mass protrudes (Fig. 16-5). If the defect is located in the nasopharynx, no external anomaly is visible, but the child may experience nasal airway obstruction. On examination with a nasal speculum, a smooth, round mass will be visible in the nasal passages. A frontal encephalocele may extend into the orbit of the eye and produce proptosis on the affected side.

Evaluation and Treatment

Diagnosis is based on clinical manifestations and examination of the meningeal sac. With cranial meningocele, surgical repair of the cranial defect affords a good prognosis for most affected infants whose intellectual and motor functioning is normal. An occipital encephalocele may be associated with other findings, such as blindness and cognitive impairment. The size, location, and involvement of the encephalocele help determine the child's development and intellectual outcome.

Meningocele

Meningocele, which is a saclike cyst of meninges filled with spinal fluid, occurs when the neural tube fails to close completely (Fig. 16-6). This cystic dilation of me-

FIG. 16-5 Newborn with frontal, nasal, interocular encephalocele. (Courtesy Dr. Charles Linder, Medical College of Georgia.)

ninges protrudes through the vertebral defect and around the malformed tube. This defect does not involve the spinal cord. Meningoceles occur with equal frequency in the cervical, thoracic, and lumbar spine areas.

Clinical Manifestations

At birth the infant has a protruding sac on the back at the level of the defect. The sac may be covered by a thin layer of muscle and skin and usually appears as raw, fluid-filled tissue. Abnormal neurologic function sometimes is present. Talipes equinovarus (clubfoot), gait disturbance, bladder dysfunction, and upper extremity weakness also have been associated with meningocele. Hydrocephalus commonly is associated with this diagnosis.

Evaluation and Treatment

The diagnosis is made on the basis of clinical manifestations and examination of the meningeal sac. In an effort to preserve neuronal function and minimize potential damage that may occur from infection and manipulation of the fragile sac, surgical closure is optimal during the first 72 hours of life. Functional implications depend on the level and severity of the defect (Table 16-2).

FIG. 16-6 Normal spine, meningocele, and myelomeningocele. Diagram showing section through normal spine (**A**), meningocele (**B**), and myelomeningocele (**C**). (Modified from Farley & Dunleavy, 1991.)

TABLE 16-2

Functional Alterations in Myelodysplasia Related to Level of Lesion

Level of lesion	Functional implications
Thoracic	Flaccid paralysis of lower extremities; variable weakness in abdominal trunk musculature; high thoracic level may mean respiratory compromise; absence of bowel and bladder control
High lumbar	Voluntary hip flexion and adduction; flaccid paralysis of knees, ankles, and feet; may walk with extensive braces and crutches; absence of bowel and bladder control
Midlumbar	Strong hip flexion and adduction; fair knee extension; flaccid paralysis of ankles and feet; absence of bowel and bladder control
Low lumbar	Strong hip flexion, extension, and adduction and knee extension; weak ankle and toe mobility; may have limited bowel and bladder function
Sacral	Normal function of lower extremities; normal bowel and bladder function

Modified from Farley & Dunleavy, 1991.

Myelomeningocele

Myelomeningocele (meningomyelocele; spina bifida cystica) is a hernial protrusion of a saclike cyst (containing meninges, spinal fluid, and a portion of the spinal cord with its nerves) through a defect in the posterior arch of a vertebra. Eighty percent of myelomeningoceles are located in the lumbar and lumbosacral regions, the last regions of the neural tube to close. Being one of the most common developmental anomalies of the nervous system, myelomeningocele has an incidence rate ranging from 0.2 to 0.4 per 1000 live births (Behrman & Vaughan, 1983).

Clinical Manifestations

A myelomeningocele is the failure of the neural tube to close, resulting in a cystic dilation of meninges and protuberance of the spinal cord through the vertebral defect. A myelomeningocele is evident at birth as a pronounced skin defect on the infant's back (see Fig. 16-6). The bony prominences of the unfused neural arches can be palpated at the lateral border of the defect. The defect usually is covered by a transparent membrane that may have neural tissue attached to its inner surface. This membrane may be intact at birth or may leak cerebrospinal fluid, thereby increasing the risks of infection and neuronal damage. Until it is surgically closed, cerebrospinal fluid may accumulate, resulting in further dilation and enlargement of the sac that may risk further damage to neuronal function.

The actual involvement of the spinal cord has greater implications for the overall function of the infant throughout childhood (see Table 16-2). An absence of neurologic function may occur in some infants with myelomeningocele. Function may be attained if underlying fluid or pus accumulation is prevented from stretching and applying pressure to the neural tissue or if the biochemical alterations do not cause neural tissue to die. Residual neural tissue also may be temporarily or permanently lost at birth because of trauma to the tissue during delivery.

One serious, potentially life-threatening problem associated with myelodysplasia is the **Arnold-Chiari II malformation**. This deformity involves the downward displacement of the cerebellum, cerebral tonsils, brainstem, and fourth ventricle (Fig. 16-7). Arnold-Chiari II malformation compresses and essentially stretches the posterior region of the cerebellum and brainstem downward through the foramen magnum and into the cervical space. The brainstem houses the 12 cranial nerves. Pressure on this region may result in altered function of these nerves or actual palsies. Dysfunction of the lower cranial nerves is common, and the displacement of this area of the brain results in the compression and elongation of nerves and tissue that, in turn, restrict neuronal performance in varying degrees (Lemire, 1986).

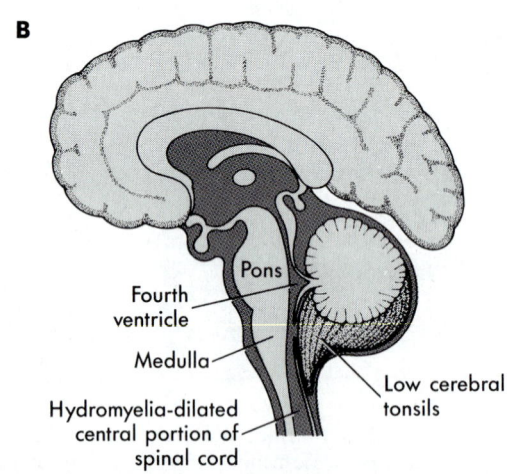

FIG. 16-7 Normal brain and Chiari malformation. Diagram showing normal brain (**A**), and brain with Arnold-Chiari malformation (**B**). (Modified from Farley & Dunleavy, 1991, p. 376.)

Hydrocephalus occurs in 95% of these infants. Seizures also occur in 15% of those with myelodysplasia. Visual and perceptual problems, including ocular palsies, astigmatism, and visuoperceptual deficits, occur in approximately 80% (Lemir, 1986; McLaughlin & Shurtleff, 1979). Motor and sensory functions below the level of the lesions are altered. This dysfunction may include degrees of weakness, paralysis, spasticity, and bowel and bladder dysfunction. Often these problems worsen as the child grows and the cord ascends within the vertebral canal, pulling primary scar tissue and tethering the cord (Venes & McGuire, 1986).

Several musculoskeletal deformities are related to this diagnosis, including clubfoot, dislocation of hip or hips, and poor spinal alignment. Spinal deformities, such as scoliosis and kyphosis, occur in approximately 90% of affected children (Park, Cail, Maggio, & Mitchell, 1985).

Tethering of the spinal cord may develop in children with myelodysplasia. The cord becomes caught or tethered from scar tissue as it transcends the vertebral canal with growth. Symptoms related to this problem can include scoliosis, altered gait pattern, changes in muscle strength at or below the lesion, disturbance in urinary and bowel patterns, and back pain.

Evaluation and Treatment

Diagnosis is based on clinical manifestations and examination of the meningeal sac. However, because the pathophysiology of myelodysplasia is determined early in gestation, prenatal diagnosis is possible through ultrasonography. In addition, the presence of a neural tube defect may result in an elevated amniotic fluid alpha-fetoprotein (AFP) level and subsequent maternal serum AFP levels. Antenatal diagnosis offers the parents the option to terminate the pregnancy. If they choose to continue with the pregnancy, prenatal diagnosis provides the family and the health care team the opportunity to prepare both physically and emotionally for the birth of the child. Delivery by cesarean section may be recommended to minimize trauma to the open myelomeningocele (Luthy et al., 1991).

Treatment for the infant with myelomeningocele is early surgical closure of the defect. Because myelodysplasia affects several other body systems, such as the renal, the gastrointestinal, and the musculoskeletal systems, these infants require a lifetime of comprehensive multidisciplinary approach to treatment. The prognosis depends on the extent of the involvement at birth and the success of prophylactic and acute treatment for potential and actual complications that affect the many body systems.

Malformations of the Axial Skeleton
Spina Bifida Occulta

When defects of neural tube closure occur, such as meningocele and myelomeningocele, an accompanying vertebral defect allows the protrusion of the neural tube contents. Such a defect is called **spina bifida.** It also is possible for a defect to occur without any visible exposure of meninges or neural tissue. Because the defect is not apparent to the naked eye (i.e., it is "occult" or hidden), the term **spina bifida occulta** is used. In spina bifida occulta, the posterior vertebral laminae have failed to fuse. Extremely common, the defect occurs to some degree in 10% to 25% of infants. Approximately 80% of these vertebral defects are located in the lumbosacral regions, most commonly in the fifth lumbar vertebra and the first sacral vertebra, and may be detected prenatally with ultrasonic scanning and AFP testing. About

3% of normal adults have spina bifida occulta of the atlas (cervical vertebra 1).

Certain cutaneous or subcutaneous abnormalities suggest underlying spina bifida, including the following:

1. Abnormal growth of hair along the spine, which often is either very coarse or very silky
2. A midline dimple with or without a sinus tract
3. A cutaneous angioma, usually of the "port wine" variety
4. A subcutaneous mass, usually representing a lipoma or dermoid cyst

Spina bifida occulta usually causes no serious neurologic dysfunctions. The spinal cord and spinal nerves generally are anatomically and functionally normal. When dysfunctions occur, the common lumbosacral defects cause gait abnormalities, positional deformities of the feet as a result of muscle weakness, or sphincter disturbances of the bladder and bowel. These dysfunctions become evident during periods of rapid growth.

Cranial Deformities

Skull malformations range from minor, insignificant defects to major defects that are incompatible with life.

Acrania

In **acrania** the cranial vault is almost completely absent, and an extensive defect of the vertebral column often is present. Acrania associated with anencephaly (absence of brain and spinal column) occurs in approximately 1 per 1000 live births and is incompatible with life. The malformation results from a failure of the cranial end of the neural tube to close during the fourth gestational week. Subsequently, the cranial vault fails to form.

Craniosynostosis

Craniosynostosis (craniostenosis) is the premature closure of one or more of the cranial sutures during the first 18 to 20 months of the infant's life. The incidence of craniosynostosis is 5 per 10,000 live births. Males are affected twice as often as females. Craniosynostosis prevents normal skull expansion and causes asymmetric skull growth. Premature closure of a suture causes failure of the growth of the bone located at a right angle to the involved suture. Compensatory growth occurs in regions where the sutures are patent, and this causes the various cosmetic deformities. In the absence of adequate sutures, cerebral growth may exceed the space present. Brain growth may be restricted, and compression may cause neurologic dysfunction from brain damage after age 6 months (Fig. 16-8).

Pathophysiology

The exact causes of craniosynostosis are unknown, but the condition represents more than a single disorder of embryonic development. One possible explanation is a

Sagittal suture   Coronal suture

NORMAL SKULL

MICROCEPHALY AND CRANIOSTENOSIS

SCAPHOCEPHALY OR DOLICHOCEPHALY

BRACHYCEPHALY

OXYCEPHALY OR ACROCEPHALY

PLAGIOCEPHALY

FIG. 16-8 Craniosynostosis. Abnormal head configuration resulting from premature closing of cranial sutures. *Normal skull,* Bones separated by membranous seams until sutures gradually close. *Microcephaly and craniostenosis,* Microcephaly is head circumference more than 2 standard deviations below the mean for age, sex, race, and gestation and reflecting a small brain; craniosynostosis is premature closure of sutures. *Scaphocephaly or dolichocephaly* (frequency 56%), Premature closure of sagittal suture resulting in restricted lateral growth. *Brachycephaly,* Premature closure of coronal suture resulting in excessive lateral growth. *Oxycephaly or acrocephaly* (frequency 5.8%/12%), Premature closure of all coronal and sagittal sutures, resulting in accelerated upward growth and small head circumference. *Plagiocephaly* (frequency 13%), Unilateral premature closure of coronal suture resulting in asymmetric growth. (From Whaley & Wong, 1991.)

germ layer disturbance involving the mesenchyma (embryonic connective tissue that gives rise to the connective tissues, blood vessels, and lymphatics). This mesenchymal defect may be due to a deficiency in enzyme inhibition of ossification. A number of metabolic disorders are accompanied by premature or delayed ossification of cranial bones, suggesting a metabolic mechanism. A genetic defect of hormonal or mineral metabolism may create ossification centers at abnormal sites. Mechanical factors also appear to play a role in craniosynostosis because secondary premature fusion of sutures occurs in microcephaly and after shunting in hydrocephalus.

Clinical Manifestations

Craniosynostosis is classified according to head contour or suture involvement. Final skull contour is determined by the sutures that close, the duration and order of closure, and the ability of other sutures to compensate by expansion. (The frequency and types of craniosynostosis are depicted in Figs. 16-8 and 16-9.)

Premature closure of the sagittal suture, the most common form of craniosynostosis, causes elongation of the skull in the anteroposterior direction. Other anomalies are seen in 25% of these children. When the coronal suture fuses prematurely, the brain expands in a lateral direction. This type of craniosynostosis is associated with a 33% to 66% incidence of associated anomalies. Approximately half of these children are mentally retarded.

Evaluation and Treatment

Diagnosis is made on the basis of physical examination, head circumference measurements, and radiologic examination. Surgical treatment is indicated when closure of multiple sutures causes chronic increased intracranial pressure. Surgery then limits the extent of brain damage. In children with craniosynostosis of one suture, surgery often is performed for cosmetic purposes to limit the appearance of deformity.

FIG. 16-9 Dolichoscaphocephaly in 14-year-old boy. One of the less threatening of the craniosynostoses. (From Siedel, Ball, Dains, & Benedict, 1991.)

Microcephaly

Microcephaly is a defect in brain growth as a whole (see Fig. 16-8). The word *microcephaly* is derived from the Greek *(mikrow* = small; *kephale* = head). Cranial size is significantly below average for the infant's age, sex, race, and gestation. The small size of the skull reflects a small brain, except in infants with premature closure of the sutures. The condition is not treatable.

True (primary) microcephaly can be caused by an autosomal recessive disorder, by a chromosomal abnormality, or by toxin exposure during the period of induction and major cell migration (Table 16-3). Radiation, maternal infection, or chemical exposure may be the initiating factor. Secondary microcephaly is associated with a variety of causes. Infection, trauma, meta-bolic disorders, and anorexia experienced during the third trimester of pregnancy, the perinatal period, or early infancy may be responsible.

Brain weight may be as low as 25% of normal in the microcephalic brain. Both the number and the size of the cortical gyri may be diminished. Growth of the frontal lobes is severely stunted, and the cerebellum often is disproportionately large. In microcephaly caused by perinatal or postnatal disorders, neuronal loss and gliosis may be present in the cerebral cortex. The neurologic manifestations of microcephaly range from decerebrate posture, complete unresponsiveness, and autistic behavior to mild motor impairment, **mental retardation,** and hyperkinesis.

Congenital hydrocephalus

Congenital hydrocephalus is characterized by an increased volume of cerebrospinal fluid (CSF). This increase in volume may be caused by a blockage within the ventricular system in which the CSF flows, an imbalance in production of the CSF, or a reduced reabsorption of the CSF that tesults in ventricular enlargement and increased intracranial pressure. The pressure within the ventricular system pushes and compresses the brain tissue against the skull cavity. When hydrocephalus develops before fusion of the cranial sutures, the skull has the capacity to increase its effort to accommodate this additional space-occupying volume and to preserve neuronal function. The overall incidence of hydrocephalus is approximately 2 per 1000 live births. The incidence of hydrocephalus, excluding the hydrocephalus associated with myelomeningocele, is approximately 0.5 to 1 per 1000 live births, with aqueductal stenosis as the cause for approximately one third of these cases (Jackson, 1992; Wiswell et al., 1990). (Types of hydrocephalus are discussed in Chapter 14.)

TABLE 16-3

Causes of Microencephaly

Defects in brain development	Intrauterine infections	Perinatal and postnatal disorders
Hereditary (recessive) microcephaly	Congenital rubella	Intrauterine or neonatal anoxia
Down syndrome and other trisomy syndromes	Cytomegalovirus infection	Severe malnutriton in early infancy
Fetal ionizing radiation exposure	Congenital toxoplasmosis	Neonatal herpesvirus infection
Maternal phenylketonuria	Congenital syphilis	
Seckel syndrome		
Cornelia de Lange syndrome		
Rubinstein-Taybi syndrome		
Smith-Lemli-Opitz syndrome		
Fetal alcohol syndrome		

Adapted from Behrman & Vaughan, 1983.

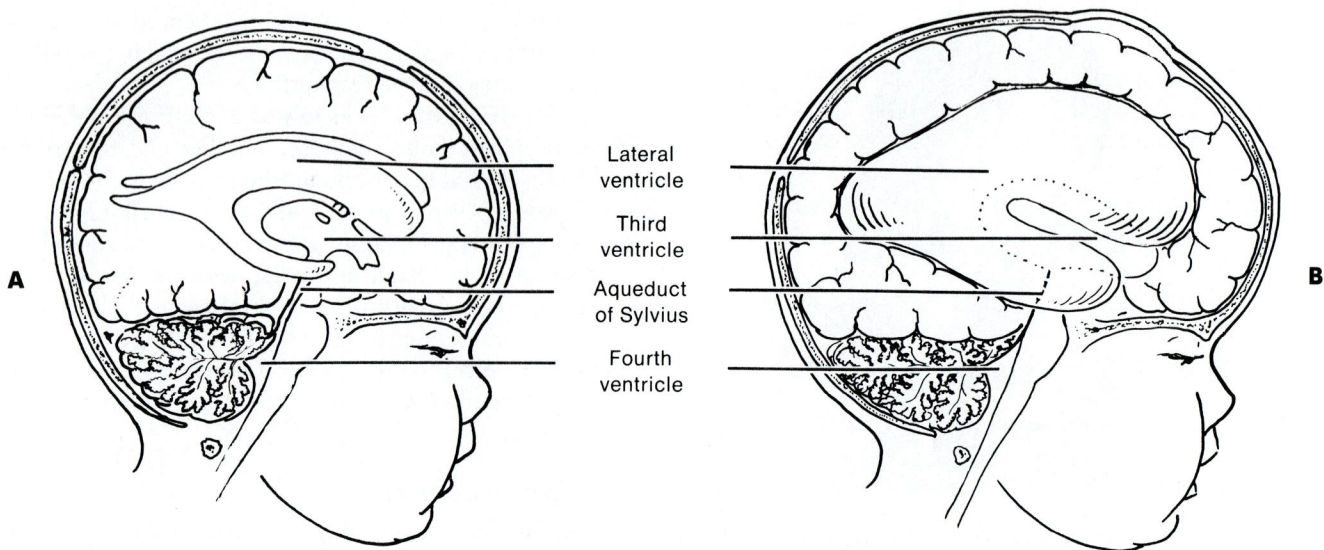

FIG. 16-10 **Hydrocephalus.** A block in flow of cerebrospinal fluid. **A,** Patent cerebrospinal fluid circulation. **B,** Enlarged lateral and third ventricles caused by obstruction of circulation—stenosis of aqueduct of Sylvius. (From Whaley & Wong, 1991.)

FIG. 16-11 **Child with enlarged head caused by hydrocephalus.** (From Whaley & Wong, 1991.)

Pathophysiology

Obstructive hydrocephalus is caused most commonly by congenital aqueduct stenosis. The cerebral aqueduct is narrowed or replaced by multiple channels, or "forks," that end blindly. In a small number of children, the stenosis is transmitted as an X-linked recessive trait. The **Dandy-Walker deformity** is a congenital defect of midline cerebellar structures in which hydrocephalus is caused by atresia of the foramina of Luschka or Magendie, leading the ventricular flow of CNS into a "blind pouch." Other causes of obstructions within the ventricular system that can result in hydrocephalus include brain tumors, cysts, trauma, arteriovenous malformations, blood clots, and infections.

CSF travels throughout the ventricular system, surrounds the brain, and is reabsorbed into the venous system by the arachnoid villi. Blockage of the arachnoid villi may occur in conditions such as bacterial or viral meningitis, intraventricular hemorrhage, and subarachnoid hemorrhage or may result from congenital malformations within this area. In this instance CSF flows or communicates effectively but is unable to be reabsorbed, resulting in hydrocephalus.

Clinical Manifestations

Congenital hydrocephalus may cause fetal death in utero, or the increased head circumference may require delivery of the infant by cesarean section. Symptoms of this condition depend directly on the cause and rate of hydrocephalus development. Infants may have no symptoms at birth. During the early weeks of life, the head begins to grow at an abnormal rate. Significant dilation of the ventricles may occur before an abnormal increase in head growth develops. The fontanelles enlarge and become full and bulging (Figs. 16-10 and 16-11). The separation of the cranial sutures leads to a resonant note when the skull is tapped, a manifestation termed **Macewen sign** or **"cracked-pot" sign.** The eyes may assume a staring expression, with sclera visible above the cornea, called "sunsetting."

The infant may have difficulty holding the head upright. The scalp skin is thin and shiny, and scalp veins may become prominent. The large cranial vault and the face are disproportionate, and frontal bossing may be present. The infant's cry becomes high-pitched as intracranial pressure rises; irritability, lethargy, vomiting, and other signs of increased intracranial pressure may develop. Dramatic head growth and enlargement, compression of the optic nerves, and optic chiasm occur in chronic, untreated hydrocephalus. Fortunately, these signs of hydrocephalus rarely are seen because of early surgical intervention. When hydrocephalus develops late in childhood, the head may not have the capacity to enlarge and evidence of increased intracranial pressure is present (see Chapter 14).

The relationship between hydrocephalus and mental retardation has been heavily debated. Correlation between the degree of hydrocephalus and impaired cognitive function often is a result of additional complications, such as severe congenital malformations, acute or chronic infections, or progressive brain tumors. Approximately two thirds of children with uncomplicated congenital hydrocephalus treated successfully with shunting may have normal to borderline intelligence (Amacher & Wellington, 1984; McCollough & Balzar-Martin, 1982).

Evaluation and Treatment

The definitive diagnostic tool for hydrocephalus is computed tomography (CT), and magnetic resonance imagery (MRI) may add information about the specific cause of the hydrocephalus. In infancy, head circumference measurements also are obtained and monitored. The treatment is surgical placement of a shunt to divert the excess CSF from the ventricular cavity to other areas of the body. Several types of shunts are available. The main objective of any shunt system is to decrease intracranial pressure and preserve neuronal function. With neurosurgical intervention and follow-up, the 5-year survival usually is greater than 80%. Most deaths that occur

within this category result from severe congenital malformations and/or progressive disorders such as brain tumors. Children with hydrocephalus are dependent on the internal shunt system to maintain safe intracranial pressures and therefore are forever at risk for sudden failure of this system, which leads to acute increased intracranial pressure and death.

ENCEPHALOPATHIES

Encephalopathy, a disorder involving the brain, is a general category that includes a number of syndromes and diseases (see Chapter 14). Encephalopathies in children are associated with a great variety of known and suspected causes. These disorders may be acute or chronic and static or progressive.

Static Encephalopathies

Brain injury may occur during gestation or birth or at any time during childhood growth and development, causing a static, nonprogressive disorder. The clinical manifestations depend on the site and extent of the injury, as well as the age of the child and stage of development at the time of injury. Varying degrees of impairment may result from diffuse or localized injury to the cortex. For example, cerebral palsy results when the motor areas of the brain are injured. Injury to the occipital lobe of the cerebral cortex early in gestation can interfere with normal cerebral maturation and result in future blindness. Cognitive impairment may follow diffuse cerebral injury. Seizures also may develop from cortical injury, particularly if scar tissue remains.

Prenatal factors that affect the developing nervous system may be endogenous or exogenous. The fetus may be affected by impaired embryo implantation, chromosomal abnormalities, infection, trauma, radiation, and toxic substances. Maternal toxemia, diabetes mellitus, and maternal nutritional deficiencies can produce neurologic damage in the fetus. The developing nervous system is most susceptible to injury occurring during the first trimester of pregnancy. Anoxia, trauma, and infections are the most common factors that cause injury to the nervous system in the perinatal period. Infections, metabolic disturbances (acute or a result of inborn errors), trauma, toxins, and vascular disease may injure the nervous system in the postnatal period.

Cerebral Palsy

Cerebral palsy is the *term* given to a diverse group of nonprogressive syndromes that affect the brain and cause motor dysfunction beginning in early infancy. Cerebral palsy can be classified on the basis of neurologic signs and symptoms. The major types are spasticity, ataxia, dyskinesia, and a mix of one or more of the three. Although cerebral palsy is, by definition, nonpro-

TABLE 16-4

Cerebal Palsy: Predisposing Factors and Known Causes

Risk factors	Associated causes
Prenatal	
Maternal	Metabolic diseases
	Nutritional deficiencies (e.g., anemia)
	Twin or multiple births
	Bleeding
	Toxemia
	Blood imcompatibilities
	Exposure to radiation
	Infection (e.g., rubella, toxoplasmosis, cytomegalic inclusion disease)
	Premature labor
Prematurity	Asphyxia leading to cerebral hemorrhage
Genetic factors	Absence of corpus callosum, aqueductal stenosis, cerebellar hypoplasia
Congenital anomalies of the brain	Unknown causes not evident on clinical examination
Perinatal	Anesthesia or analgesia during labor and delivery
	Mechanical trauma during delivery
	Immaturity at birth
	Metabolic disorders (hyperbilirubinemia, hypoglycemia, amino acid disorders, hyperosmolality)
	Electrolyte disturbances (e.g., hypernatremia, hypoglycemia)
Postnatal	Head trauma
	Infections (e.g., meningitis, encephalitis)
	Cerebrovascular accidents
	Toxicosis
	Environmental toxins (lead ingestion, methylmercury ingestion from contaminated fish)

gressive, its clinical manifestations change with growth and maturation of the child.

Cerebral palsy is one of the most common crippling disorders of childhood, affecting nearly 400,000 children in the United States alone. Although the exact incidence is unknown, studies suggest that the incidence is 1.5 to 5 cases of cerebral palsy per 1000 live births (Paneth, 1986). Causes of cerebral palsy are numerous, and both genetic and environmental factors may be responsible. These factors can occur during the prenatal, perinatal, or postnatal periods (Table 16-4).

Pathophysiology

Several factors, alone or in combination, can produce brain damage that leads to cerebral palsy. Prenatal cerebral hypoxia can be responsible for systemic degeneration of immature areas of the brain and can interfere with cell maturation. The severity of the damage depends on the gestational age at the time of the injury and the degree of injury sustained.

Low birth weight and birth asphyxia are commonly identified risk factors for cerebral palsy (Hensleigh,

Fainstat, & Spencer, 1986). Hypoxia and asphyxia are known to cause edema in the brain. Lack of oxygen and the incorporation of amino acids during protein synthesis lead to acidosis. Carbon dioxide and lactic acid accumulate with acidosis, causing osmotic pressure changes. This condition contributes to generalized cerebral swelling and CNS damage.

Vascular abnormalities, arterial or venous stasis, and thrombosis can occur as a result of tissue hypoxia or as an unrelated structural alteration. These anomalies may result in direct brain trauma that leads to infarction, intraventricular hemorrhage, and subarachnoid hemorrhage. Intraventricular hemorrhage is a common cause of death in newborn infants. Such injuries contribute to CNS damage.

Physical trauma to the central or peripheral nervous system can occur during the birthing process. Linear and depressed fractures are seen in newborn infants when head molding is extreme, with resultant hemorrhages and tears of the tentorium or falx cerebri. Tearing of the superficial cerebral veins is a relatively common occurrence and causes a thin layer of blood over the cerebral convexity. This blood may irritate the brain and result in CNS dysfunction. The infant's position during delivery may cause stretching and damage to nerves. Breech deliveries can cause traumatic injury to the brainstem or spinal cord, resulting in a more localized area of impairment. Malformations of the CNS play an important role in brain injury from perinatal trauma, and they predispose the infant to greater probability of sustained injury to the CNS. Both faulty maturation of the nervous system and a greater vulnerability to perinatal trauma and hypoxia are responsible for a high incidence of neurologic dysfunction in the preterm infant. Genetic, teratogenic, and early pregnancy influences on the development of cerebral palsy are not yet fully understood.

Clinical Manifestations

The syndromes associated with cerebral palsy are classified according to the predominant clinical manifestations. **Spastic cerebral palsy** is associated with increased muscle tone, prolonged primitive reflexes, exaggerated deep tendon reflexes, clonus, rigidity of the extremities, scoliosis, and contractures. This results from motor neuron involvement and injury to the cerebral cortex in either one or both hemispheres and accounts for approximately 65% to 75% of cerebral palsy cases.

Dyskinetic cerebral palsy is associated with extreme difficulty in fine motor coordination and purposeful movements. Movements are jerky, uncontrolled, and abrupt, resulting from injury to the basal ganglia or extrapyramidal tracts. This form of cerebral palsy accounts for approximately 20% to 25% of cases. **Ataxic cerebral palsy** manifests with gait disturbances and instability. The infant with this form of cerebral palsy may have hypotonia at birth, but stiffness of the trunk muscles develops by late infancy. This lack of flexibility exaggerates the infant's inability to balance body position without support. Persistence of this increased tone in truncal muscles affects the child's gait and ability to maintain equilibrium. This form of cerebral palsy accounts for approximately 5% of cases. A child may have symptoms of each of these cerebral palsy types, which leads to a mixed variety and disorder and accounts for approximately 13% of cases.

Children with cerebral palsy often have associated neurologic disorders, such as seizures (35% to 50%), intellectual impairment ranging from mild to severe (50% to 75%), and visual impairment (50%). Because standardized intelligence tests do not allow for the physical handicaps of cerebral palsy, the incidence of associated cognitive impairment is uncertain. Other associated complications include but are not limited to hearing impairment, communication disorders, respiratory problems, bowel and bladder problems, and orthopedic disabilities (Steele, 1992).

Evaluation and Treatment

Diagnosis of cerebral palsy is made on the basis of neurologic examination and history. The management of children with cerebral palsy varies with age, type and severity of involvement, and associated disorders. Thus the scope of care required by the child and family includes social and educational intervention and a multidisciplinary team approach.

Although the brain injury is static, the clinical picture of cerebral palsy may change with growth and development. Therefore a fundamental component to an effective treatment regimen includes ongoing assessment, evaluation, and revision of the child's overall management plan.

Inherited Metabolic Disorders of the CNS

A large number of inherited metabolic disorders have been identified. Because these disorders are inherited, their manifestations usually occur in infancy and childhood. Typically these metabolic disorders damage the entire CNS so extensively that these children do not survive to adulthood. The clinical syndromes of the inherited metabolic disorders depend on the nature of the biochemical defect and the stage of nervous system maturation. (Table 16-5 lists some of these inherited metabolic disorders.) Defects in amino acid and lipid metabolism are more common than rarely occurring defects in carbohydrate metabolism.

Defects in amino acid metabolism

Biochemical defects in amino acid metabolism may be classified as (1) those in which the transport of amino acid is impaired, (2) those involving an enzyme or cofactor deficiency, and (3) those grouped around certain chemical components such as sulfur-containing amino acids (Farmer, 1983). Most of the disorders in the literature described to date suggest that the absence of enzymatic activity most often is caused by the genetically determined absence of the enzyme protein.

Diseases caused by an enzymatic deficiency are associated with increased blood concentrations of the amino acid whose degradation pathway is impaired and with the presence of the amino acid in the urine. Because the normal pathway is blocked, small amounts of certain metabolites are found in the blood. Thus in certain diseases, an increase of compromised amino acids and unusual metabolites may appear in blood and urine concentrates (Swaiman, 1989).

Phenylketonuria. Phenylketonuria (PKU) is an inborn error of metabolism characterized by the inability of the body to convert the essential amino acid phenylalanine to tyrosine (Fig. 16-12). PKU is caused by phenylalanine hydroxylase deficiency and has an incidence of 1:10,000 worldwide (Schmidt, Kaufman, & Woo, 1989). Because of its genetic component and distribution, this statistical inci-

TABLE 16-5

Inherited Metabolic Disorders of the Central Nervous System

Age of onset	Disorder
Neonatal period	Pyridoxine dependency, galactosemia, maple syrup urine disease and its variant, phenylketonuria (PKU)
Early infancy	Tay-Sachs disease and its variants, infantile Gaucher disease, infantile Niemann-Pick disease, Krabbe disease (leukodystrophy), Farber lipogranulomatosis, Pelizaeus-Merzbacher disease and other sudanophilic leukodystrophies, spongy degeneration, Alexander disease, Alpers disease, Leigh disease (subacute necrotizing encephalomyelopathy), congenital lactic acidosis, Zellweger encephalopathy, Lowe disease (oculocerebrorenal disease)
Late infancy and early childhood	Disorders of amino acid metabolism, metachromatic leukodystrophy, late infantile GM1 gangliosidosis, late infantile Gaucher and Niemann-Pick diseases, neuroaxonal dystrophy, mucopolysaccharidosis, mucolipidosis, fucosidosis, mannosidosis, aspartylglycosaminuria, amaurotic idiocy (Jansky-Bielschowsky disease, Batten disease, Vogt-Spielmeyer disease, neuronal ceroid lipofuscinosis), Cockayne syndrome
Later childhood and adolescence	Progressive cerebellar ataxias of childhood and adolescence, hepatolenticular degeneration (Wilson disease), Hallervorden-Spatz disease, Lesch-Nyhan syndrome and other uremic states, familial calcification of vessels in basal ganglia and cerebellum, familial polymyoclonus, chronic familial leukodystrophy, homocystinuria, Fabry disease

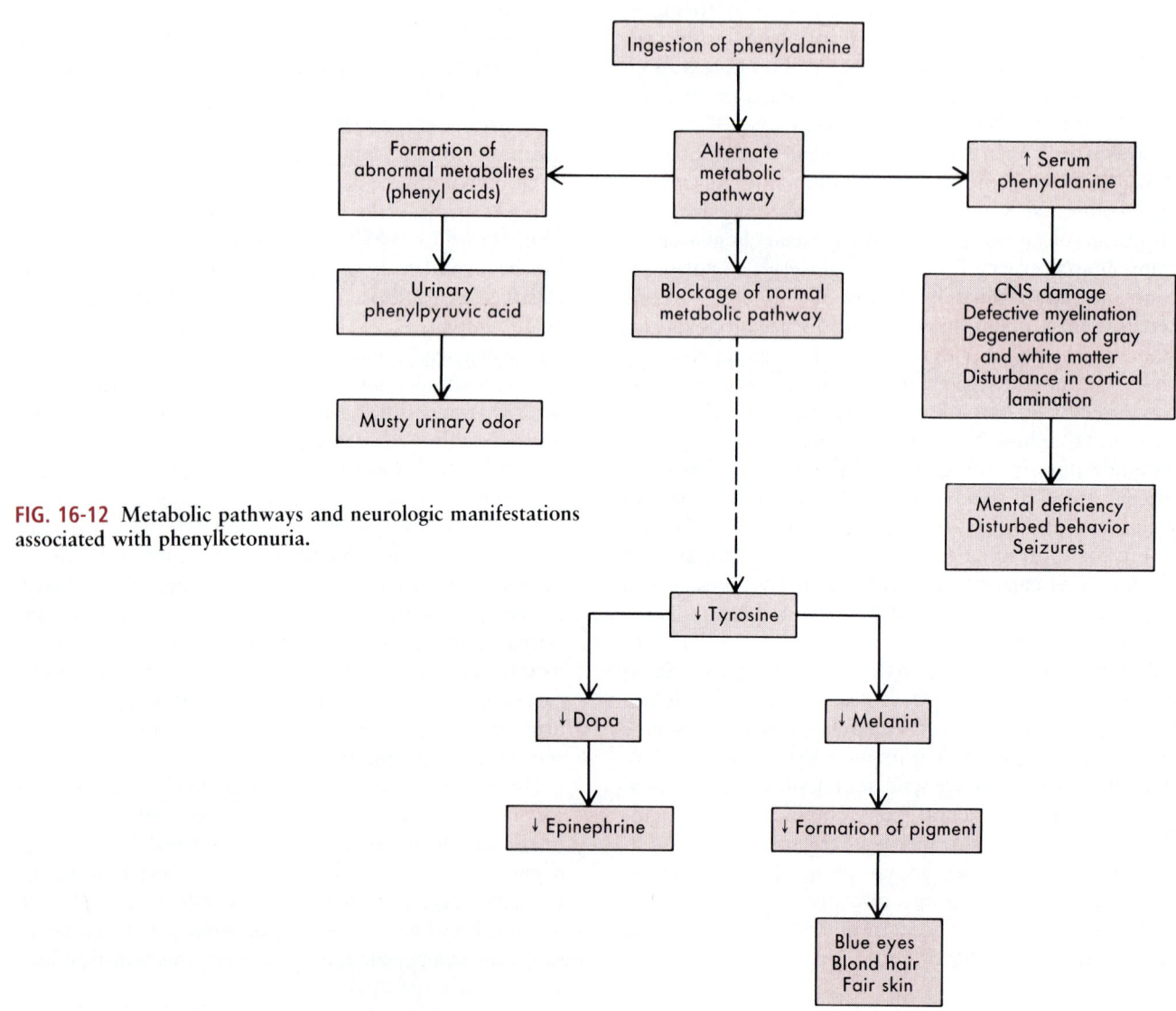

FIG. 16-12 Metabolic pathways and neurologic manifestations associated with phenylketonuria.

dence varies widely on the basis of geographic and ethnic differences (Schmidt, 1992). Most natural food proteins contain about 15% phenylalanine, an essential amino acid. Phenylalanine hydroxylase controls the conversion of this essential amino acid to tyrosine in the liver. The body uses tyrosine in the biosynthesis of protein, melanin, thyroxine, and the catecholamines in the brain and adrenal medulla. Phenylalanine hydroxylase deficiency causes an accumulation of phenylalanine in the serum and, subsequently, in the urinary excretion of abnormal metabolites called *phenyl acid*. One of these phenyl acids, phenylpyruvic acid, gives the urine a characteristic musty odor and is responsible for the name given to the disorder. Such high blood levels of phenylalanine prevent sufficient neutral amino acid entry into the brain, which contributes to the neuropathologic process of PKU (Kaufman, 1989). Abnormalities occur, such as anomalous development of the CNS, defective myelination, cystic degeneration of the gray and white matter, and disturbances in cortical layers. Unfortunately, brain damage occurs before the metabolites can be detected in the urine, and damage continues as long as phenylalanine levels remain high. Clinical manifestations related to CNS damage range from mild to severe behavioral disturbances, self-abusive tendencies, and seizures. Because of the lack of tyrosine and its relationship to the biosynthesis of melanin, children with PKU have a characteristic phenotype that includes blond hair, blue eyes, and fair skin. Children with genetically darker complexions may be red-haired or brunette. Less severe variants of this disorder are caused by defects in the phenylalanine hydroxylase *system* rather than the phenylalanine hydroxylase itself. This related disorder, known as **hyperphenylalaninemia (HPA)**, occurs when plasma phenylalanine levels rise above normal but do not elevate as high as in PKU (Schmidt et al., 1989). Most children develop normally on a regular diet. Nonselective newborn screening is used to detect PKU and HPA in the United States and in more than 30 countries. Such programs are the greatest source of referrals and allow for accurate interpretation and follow-up of test results, including appropriate genetic and nutrition counseling (Schmidt, 1992). Treatment for PKU involves restriction of phenylalanine in the diet to maintain a nontoxic level. The diet must be supplemented with adequate sources of energy, protein, and nutrients to allow for optimum growth and brain development. Supplementation of tyrosine also may be required if plasma levels are low. The child benefits from ideal management that begins at birth and continues throughout the life span, especially before conception and throughout the mother's pregnancy (Schmidt, 1992).

Defects in lipid metabolism

Disorders of lipid metabolism are termed **lysosomal storage diseases** because each disorder in this group can be traced to a missing lysosomal enzyme. (Lysosomes,

the vesicles within the cell whose primary function is to degrade the breakdown products of cellular metabolism, are discussed in Chapter 1.) An estimated 25 to 30 enzymes within the lysosomes participate in the breakdown of lipids, carbohydrates, proteins, and proteolipids (see Chapter 2). A missing or defective enzyme causes an excessive accumulation of a particular cell function. The enzyme defect may occur in the brain, liver, spleen, bone, and lung, thus involving several organ systems. Therapy has been unsuccessful to date.

Tay-Sachs disease. Perhaps the best known of the lysosomal storage disorders is **Tay-Sachs disease,** an autosomal recessive disorder. Approximately 80% of individuals diagnosed are of Jewish ancestry, although sporadic cases appear in the non-Jewish population (Swaiman, 1989).

In Tay-Sachs disease, the pathologic changes predominate in the CNS, but neurons throughout the body contain characteristic changes in the cytoplasm. With time, neurons become distorted and balloon, and microglial cells, which also are swollen and filled with large granules, proliferate. Cystic degeneration of the cerebral white matter and atrophy of the cerebellar hemispheres often occur. The number of neurons is diminished. Changes in the spinal cord, particularly in the motor cells of the anterior horn of the cord, also are characteristic. Involvement of this region of the spinal cord results in hypotonia, hyporeflexia, and overall weakness.

Onset of this disease usually occurs when the infant is 3 to 6 months old. A loss of milestones is associated with an excessive startle response. Seizures, muscular rigidity, and blindness become prominent after the first year of life, and head size may increase. Death usually occurs by 2 to 5 years of age. No beneficial therapy has been developed. Genetic counseling programs are available, and some states require screening techniques for couples and those at risk who may be carriers. One in 25 Ashkenazi Jews are carriers of this recessive gene.

Seizure Disorders in Children
Epilepsy

Seizures are the abnormal discharge of electrical activity within the brain. When a sufficient number of neurons become overexcited, they discharge abnormally, which sometimes results in clinical manifestations. If clinical manifestations do occur, the specific physical activity that occurs may depend on the origin of the electrical activity and its extent within the brain. Repeated recurrence of seizure activity is known as **epilepsy.** Seizures may result from an underlying disorder of the CNS or a disorder that directly or indirectly affects normal CNS function. Certain types of seizures may have a genetic component or familial predisposition, or they can result from maternal diseases or congenital structural anomalies of the CNS. During the newborn period, asphyxia, intracranial hemorrhage, CNS infections, injury, electrolyte imbalances, and inborn errors of metabolism may cause seizures. Etiologic factors of seizures in older infants and children generally are the same as during the first month of life. Often the cause of seizures is unknown.

Seizures and seizure patterns may change as a child grows and develops. The differences between the immature and mature nervous systems may help to explain the changing patterns of clinical seizures with age. The immature nervous system has a reduced capacity for sustaining well-organized seizures. Intracortical connections are poorly developed, and the sending of impulses throughout the cortex is limited. At the cellular level, neurons are less capable of firing in repetitive high-frequency bursts. The excitatory output of a seizure focus is further diminished because the affected neurons do not act synchronously. In addition, changing neurotransmitters, immaturity of cells, and ongoing postnatal factors affect seizure expression in children.

The incidence of epilepsy varies greatly with age. The incidence is greatest in the population of infants younger than 1 year of age, averaging roughly 1 per 1000 in the United States. Infants are particularly susceptible during the first 12 months of life. The incidence decreases with age; 75% to 80% of epilepsy cases initially occur before 20 years of age, with 30% of the cases initially occurring within the first 4 years of life. Approximately 50 per 500,000 persons in the United States are newly affected each year (Holmes, 1986; Penry, 1986).

Clinical Manifestations

The clinical manifestations at the time of diagnosis vary depending on the primary cause and the extent and involvement of abnormal electrical discharges within the neuronal tissue. Because of the diversities and complexities that seizure activity invariably displays, an international classification system was adopted. This classification system groups seizures with similar clinical manifestations. Its general purpose is to assist the clinician with the assessment of the clinical course, the identification of the most appropriate treatment, and the evaluation of the individual's response to treatment (see Table 14-13).

The international classification system of epilepsy contains three major groupings: (1) partial seizures, (2) generalized seizures, and (3) unclassified epileptic seizures. Each major grouping is then divided into subsets on the basis of clinical manifestations and electroencephalograph (EEG) findings.

Partial seizures are characterized by seizure activity that begins in and usually is limited to one part of either the left or right hemisphere. A *simple partial seizure* refers to seizure activity that occurs without loss of consciousness. A *complex partial seizure* refers to a seizure activity that occurs with impairment of consciousness. The clinical activity displayed by the individual is contingent on the particular part of the cortex from which the seizure is generated. For example, partial seizures may result in abnormal motor activity, such as twitching or loss of tone, or sensory changes, such as tingling or numbness (Holmes, 1986; Penry, 1986).

Simple partial seizures generally are confined to one hemisphere, whereas a complex partial seizure involves both cerebral hemispheres. A simple or complex partial seizure may evolve into a generalized tonic-clonic, tonic, or clonic convulsion. Partial seizures are less common in children than in adults, accounting for approximately 45% of all childhood seizure disorders.

Generalized seizures are those in which the first clinical manifestations indicate that the seizure activity starts in or involves both cerebral hemispheres. Consciousness may be impaired in this grouping of seizures. The clinical manifestations may include convulsive activity (tonic-tonic, tonic, or clonic activity) or nonconvulsive activity (absence seizures). Because both hemispheres are involved, the clinical manifestations almost always are bilateral. Generalized seizures occur with greater frequency in children than in adults, representing about 55% of all seizures in childhood.

Not all seizure disorders fit neatly into a classified grouping. These seizures are referred to as **unclassified epileptic seizures** and characteristically have a wide variety of abnormal clinical activity. Examples of this activity include rhythmic eye movements, chewing, and swimming movements. These activities are commonly seen in the neonatal seizures (Holmes, 1986; Penry, 1986).

In addition to the seizures classified by the international system, there are several types of epileptic syndromes. These are seizure disorders that display a group of signs and symptoms that occur collectively and that characterize or indicate a particular condition. Several syndromes associated with epilepsy occur in infants and children. The three syndromes that occur most often are infantile spasms, Lennox-Gastaut syndrome, and juvenile myoclonic epilepsy.

Infantile spasms are a form of epilepsy characterized by a variety of clinical manifestations. The infant may have episodes of sudden flexion or extension movements involving the neck, trunk, and extremities. Clinical manifestations of the resulting spasms may range from subtle head nods to violent body contractions, commonly referred to as "jackknife seizures." Onset of infantile spasms usually is between 3 and 12 months of age and may be idiopathic or may occur in response to a CNS insult. An EEG will display the classic hypoarrhythmic pattern of epileptic spike and wave discharges on a slow disorganized background (Lombroso, 1983). Infantile spasm manifests a typical clinical course. The "spasms" usually happen in clusters and occur 5 to 150 times a day. They usually are worse when the infant is waking up or falling asleep. Once begun, the seizure activity increases in intensity and severity over time. Invariably a loss of developmental milestones is associated with this syndrome.

Lennox-Gastaut syndrome is an epileptic syndrome characterized by an onset of seizures early in childhood, usually around 1 to 5 years of age. This syndrome includes a variety of generalized seizures—predominantly tonic-clonic, atonic (drop attacks), akinetic, absence, and myoclonic activity. Mental retardation and delayed psychomotor development often are associated with this syndrome (Holmes, 1986).

Juvenile myoclonic epilepsy is a primary generalized epilepsy that usually affects adolescents and young adults. This is a relatively benign form of epilepsy involving myoclonic jerks of the neck, shoulders, and arms. The seizures may occur singularly or repetitively. This form of epilepsy commonly is associated with a normal neurologic examination, normal intelligence, and a positive family history of seizures (Dreifuss, 1989).

Evaluation and Treatment

Diagnosis of epilepsy and seizure classification are based on history, clinical presentation, physical and developmental examination, and record of milestone achievement. Evaluation and testing include an EEG to isolate the focus or origin and involvement of seizure activity, CT scan, and/or MRI of the brain to investigate the presence of a lesion or abnormal tissue. A complete metabolic workup must be reviewed to explore the possibility of deficiency or malabsorption.

Specific treatment for epilepsy is directed at the particular clinical manifestations or syndrome of seizure activity and its underlying causes. Treatment usually begins with the use of anticonvulsant medications. Often the epileptic pattern and clinical course require the use of more than one drug to control the abnormal discharges.

Surgery provides treatment for some forms of epilepsy. As with medical interventions, surgical therapy focuses on the particular clinical manifestations of seizure activity. Surgical interventions include resection of brain tissue, that is, partial or complete severing of the corpus callosum. Some seizures are managed through a ketogenic diet.

Prognosis for epilepsy depends greatly on the type and severity of the disorder, the age of onset, coexisting factors, and the type and success of medical, surgical, and nutritional therapy. Several studies have estimated that approximately 40% to 50% of children diagnosed with epilepsy will be seizure free.

Benign febrile seizures

Benign febrile seizures occur in 3% to 4% of children younger than 5 years of age. These seizures usually are brief and self-limited and occur most frequently between the ages of 6 months and 3 years.

Clinical Manifestations

Characteristic features distinguish benign febrile seizures from seizures precipitated by fever: (1) benign febrile seizures are rare before 6 months or after 5 years of age; (2) the convulsion occurs with a rise in temperature greater than 38° C; (3) an acute respiratory or ear infection usually is present, with no evidence of CNS infection or inflammation; (4) most seizures occur during the first 24 hours of the illness; (5) the convulsion is short (15 minutes or less), generalized, and predominantly tonic; (6) interictal EEG is normal; (7) the seizure usually does not recur during the same infection; and (8) no acute systemic metabolic disorder is present.

Complex febrile seizures have similar characteristic features except that (1) they have a longer duration than do benign febrile seizures, usually longer than 15 minutes; (2) they have focal characteristics; and (3) they usually occur more than once in a 24-hour period. Complex features of febrile seizures are considered a risk factor for the development of epilepsy.

The pathogenesis of benign febrile seizures is unknown. A familial incidence of benign febrile seizures indicates a genetic predisposition to the problem. Factors that contribute to susceptibility include age, degree and rate of temperature elevation, and nature of particular fever-inducing illness. Any disorder producing a high fever may provoke benign febrile seizures in susceptible children.

Evaluation and Treatment

Reduction of elevated body temperature usually controls benign febrile seizures without anticonvulsant medication. In selected individuals, phenobarbital is the most effective medication for preventing recurrence of benign febrile seizures.

Status epilepticus

Status epilepticus is defined as the state of continuing or recurring seizure activity in which the recovery from seizure activity is incomplete. Seizure activity is unrelenting and usually lasts for 30 minutes or more. Any one of the seizure activities discussed can evolve into status epilepticus. Status epilepticus should be considered a medical emergency and requires immediate intervention.

Acute Encephalopathies
Reye Syndrome

Reye syndrome is characterized by encephalopathy and fatty changes in a variety of organs, especially the liver.

The incidence of Reye syndrome has declined sharply over the past 20 years, coinciding with increased public awareness of the association between ingestion of aspirin during illness and subsequent development of Reye syndrome. Twenty-five cases of Reye syndrome were reported to the National Reye Syndrome Surveillance System of the Centers for Disease Control (CDC). Results from 1990 and preliminary results from 1991 surveillance indicate a continuing decline.

Although Reye syndrome is becoming increasingly rare in the population, a brief overview of it is important for the following reasons: (1) it may be considered a prototype for acute hepatic encephalopathies, (2) the potential for recurrence is a factor, (3) the use of acetaminophen over aspirin should be considered important and discussed with the parents when obtaining a history, (4) it stresses the importance of teaching parents to use acetaminophen instead of aspirin.

Pathophysiology

Reye syndrome usually is associated with influenza B or varicella virus infections, although a wide variety of associated viral infections have been reported. A rather distinct clinical syndrome is apparent. The profound hypoglycemia, hyperammonemia, and an increase in short-chain fatty acids in the serum after liver involvement are responsible for the cerebral manifestations. The liver shows diffuse deposits of lipids and absence of any inflammatory reaction or necrosis. Fatty degeneration of the kidneys leads to azotemia (excess urea in the blood). The brain is extremely edematous.

The cause of Reye syndrome and its pathogenesis remain unclear. The development of Reye syndrome has been linked to the administration of salicylates (aspirin). The American Association of Pediatrics has recommended not administering aspirin to children who have varicella or flulike symptoms. Clearly, a direct relationship exists between this recommendation and the overall decrease in incidence of Reye syndrome.

Clinical Manifestations

Typically, Reye syndrome develops in a previously healthy child who is recovering from varicella, influenza B, upper respiratory infection, or gastroenteritis. The manifestations of the various clinical states are:

Stage I Vomiting, lethargy, drowsiness
Stage II Disorientation, delirium, aggressiveness and combativeness, central neurologic hyperventilation, shallow breathing, hyperactive reflexes, and stupor
Stage III Obtundation, coma, hyperventilation, and decorticate rigidity
Stage IV Deepening coma, decerebrate rigidity, loss of ocular reflexes, large fixed pupils, and divergent eye movements
Stage V Seizures, loss of deep tendon reflexes, flaccidity, and respiratory arrest

Evaluation and Treatment

According to the CDC, the following conditions must be present for consideration of a Reye syndrome diagnosis:

1. Acute, noninflammatory encephalopathy documented by (a) alteration in level of consciousness and, if available, (b) a record of CSF containing leukocytes ($8/mm^3$) and (c) a histologic specimen demonstrating cerebral edema without perivascular or meningeal irritation

2. Hepatomegaly documented either by a liver biopsy or by autopsy

3. No more reasonable explanation for cerebral and hepatic abnormalities

The severity of the condition is inversely related to the age of the child at the onset of the illness. The management of children with Reye syndrome ranges from simple monitoring to extremely complex neurointensive care. Treatment and outcome vary depending on the stage of involvement and the individual child's symptoms.

Intoxications of the CNS

Drug-induced encephalopathies always must be considered a possibility in the child with unexplained neurologic changes. Such encephalopathies may result from accidental ingestion, therapeutic overdosage, intentional overdose, or ingestion of environmental toxins (the most commonly ingested poisons are listed in Table 16-6). About 2 million childhood poisonings that require medical attention occur each year. Approximately 1000 children die each year of poisonings.

High blood levels of lead occur in lead poisoning. If untreated, lead encephalopathy will result and is responsible for serious and irreversible neurologic damage (Fig. 16-13). Those at great risk are 2- to 3-year-olds and

TABLE 16-6

Commonly Ingested Poisons

Pharmacologic agents	Heavy metals		Miscellaneous agents
Acetaminophen	Lead		Botulism
Amphetamines		Acute	Carbon monoxide
Anticonvulsants		Chronic	Ethyl alcohol
Antidepressants	Mercury		Organophosphates
Antihistamines	Thallium		Petroleum distillates
Atropine			
Barbiturates			**Venoms**
Methadone			
Phencyclidine			Snakebite
Salicylates			Tick paralysis
Tranquilizers			

From Swaiman & Wright, 1989.

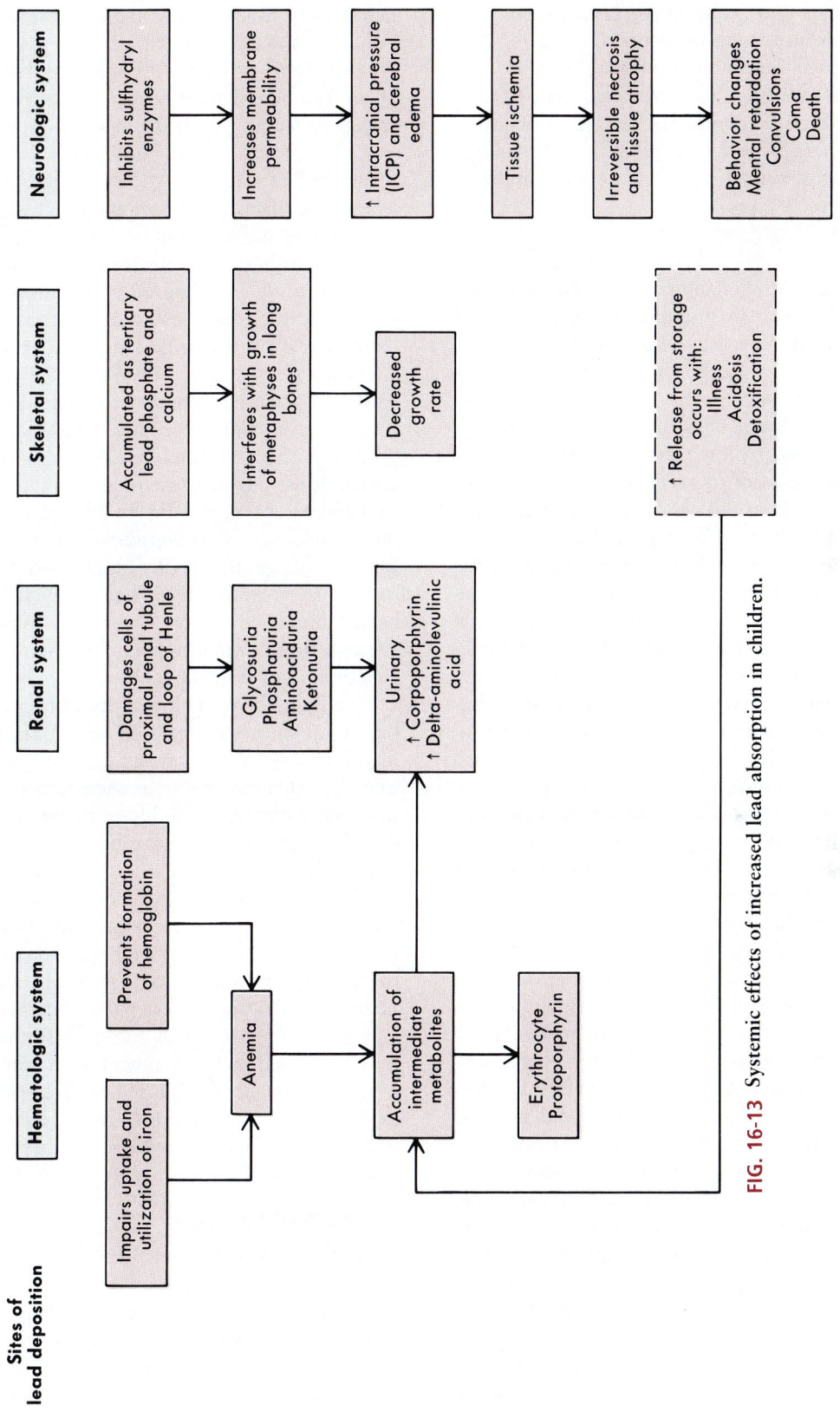

FIG. 16-13 Systemic effects of increased lead absorption in children.

children prone to picas. **Pica** is the habitual, purposeful, and compulsive ingestion of nonfood substances such as clay, dirt, and paint chips. Lead intoxication also may occur from chronic exposure to smelters, sniffing of gasoline, and ingestion of airborne lead.

An estimated 225,000 children in the United States and 4% of children 6 months to 5 years of age have excessive amounts of lead in their blood. Black children have a 6 times greater incidence of symptoms than white children.

Meningitis

Meningitis refers to the inflammation of the meningeal coverings of the brain. The origin of such inflammation and acute encephalopathy can be bacterial or viral.

Bacterial meningitis

Bacterial meningitis is one of the most serious infections to which infants and children are susceptible. Nearly 70% of all reported cases of bacterial meningitis occur in children younger than 5 years of age. Three microorganisms account for most of the reported cases of bacterial meningitis in the United States: *Haemophilus influenzae, Neisseria meningitidis,* and *Streptococcus pneumoniae.* Despite the availability of antibiotics capable of killing each of these microorganisms, the general incidence of bacterial meningitis remains unchanged.

In general, bacterial meningitis affects males more frequently than females and is most prevalent during infancy (Klein, Feigin, & McCracken, 1986). Conditions associated with increased incidence of respiratory infection heighten the occurrence of bacterial meningitis.

Haemophilus influenzae type B is the most common pathogen of bacterial meningitis in children younger than 5 years of age. Otitis media or sinusitis may be a precursor because the infections almost always are associated with a bacterium in the blood.

The second most common organism is *Neisseria meningitidis* (meningococcus). Approximately 2% to 5% of healthy children are carriers of *N. meningitidis.* The risk of meningitis in day-care center contacts of children with meningococcal disease is 1 per 1000. During epidemics among military personnel, nasal and oral secretions from as many as 90% reveal *N. meningitidis,* suggesting a high rate of infectious transmission.

The third organism is *Streptococcus pneumoniae,* which is likely to be found in children older than 4 years of age. Staphylococcal or streptococcal meningitis can occur in children of any age but shows a predilection for children who have had neurosurgery, skull fracture, or a complication of systemic bacterial infection. Infections that originate in the middle ear, sinuses, or mastoid cells also may lead to *S. pneumoniae* in children. In addition, this microorganism tends to occur in children with sickle cell disease or splenectomy. One in every 24 children with sickle cell disease develops pneumococcal meningitis by the age of 4 years. This incidence is 36 times greater than that found in the black population without sickle cell disease and 314 times greater than in white children. *Escherichia coli* and group B β-hemolytic streptococci are the most common causes of meningitis in the newborn period.

Pathogenesis

The cause of bacterial meningitis is related to the age of the child and to a number of factors that predispose the child to bacterial infection or that alter the child's response to an invading microorganism. Any microorganism may be pathogenic under the appropriate circumstances in a given individual.

During the first 2 months of life, the causative organisms are those that reflect the maternal flora or the environment in which the infant has been placed (e.g., gram-negative intestinal bacilli and group B streptococci). Most bacterial meningitis in children 2 months to 12 years of age is due to *H. influenzae* type B, *S. pneumoniae,* or *N. meningitidis.* In children older than 12 years of age, meningitis usually is due to *S. pneumoniae* or *N. meningitidis.* When the child's response has been compromised or when anatomic defects are present, other organisms may be responsible, including *Pseudomonas,* staphylococci, salmonellae, and *Serratia.*

Meningitis may follow bacterial infections of the paranasal sinuses or mastoid cells. Bacterial meningitis in children with otitis media generally follows bacteremia. Direct invasion of the meninges is rare. Infection may spread through the blood to the meninges in children with infective endocarditis, pneumonia, or thrombophlebitis.

Direct invasion of the CNS occurs with fracture of the paranasal sinus, dermoid sinus tracts, or myelomeningoceles if direct communication occurs between the skin and meninges. Meningitis also may occur after neurosurgical procedures, particularly those involving CSF diversion such as shunting. Infection of the CNS may be caused by environmental contamination or manipulation. Meningitis caused by *Staphylococcus aureus* or *Pseudomonas aeruginosa* may develop in the child with cystic fibrosis or with severe burns. (For further discussion, see Chapter 15.)

Clinical Manifestations

Acute bacterial meningitis often is preceded by an upper respiratory or gastrointestinal infection. Fever, headache, vomiting, irritability, photophobia, and nuchal and spinal rigidity develop and can progress rapidly to a decreased level of consciousness and seizures. Irritation of the meninges and spinal roots causes pain and resistance to neck flexion (nuchal rigidity), a positive Kernig sign (resistance to knee extension in the supine position with the hips and knees flexed against the body), and a positive Brudzinski sign (flexion of the knees and hips when the neck is flexed forward rapidly). With severe meningeal irritation, the child may demonstrate opisthotonic posturing (rigid arching of the back with the head extended). Meningococcal meningitis can produce a characteristic petechial rash. Increased intracranial pressure is caused by cerebral edema and may be increased further by obstruction to the CSF circulation. Thickened meninges and fibrous exudate in the subarachnoid space at the base of the brain obstruct the CSF, resulting in communicating hydrocephalus.

Evaluation and Treatment

A definitive diagnosis is made *only* by examination of CSF obtained from a lumbar puncture. The principles of treatment are similar to those followed for adults (see Chapter 14) and are based on the culture results in which the causative organism is identified. The vaccines against *H. influenzae*, however, do not affect antibody production in children younger than 2 years of age.

The factors that influence outcomes are the age of the child (mortality is highest in infants younger than 1 year old), the infective organism (the lowest mortality is in meningococcal meningitis and the highest in meningitis caused by gram-negative enteric organisms), and the duration and extent of inflammation before treatment. Approximately 8% of children with *H. influenzae* meningitis die; 35% of the survivors have serious and permanent sensory or motor dysfunction caused by pressure on the peripheral nerves during the early phases of the illness. Approximately 5% of the children who survive meningitis have hearing deficits; 10% to 15% have cerebral damage, hydrocephalus, motor deficits, or sensory impairments.

Viral meningitis

The hallmark of viral meningitis, or aseptic meningitis, is a mononuclear response in the CSF and the presence of normal sugar as well. In some cases the findings with aseptic meningitis are consistent with bacterial meningitis.

Clinical Manifestations

The clinical manifestations are similar to those in bacterial meningitis, although usually milder.

Evaluation and Treatment

Isolation of the virus is difficult and often impossible. Treatment usually begins with aggressive administration of antibiotics (potential bacterial meningitis) until the diagnosis is confirmed. Treatment may include use of antiviral agents.

HUMAN IMMUNODEFICIENCY VIRUS AND CNS INVOLVEMENT

The human immunodeficiency virus (HIV) subjects the body to multiple, repeated infections. The end stage of this infectious process is called *acquired immunodeficiency syndrome (AIDS)*. Through a process of replication, HIV perpetuates and integrates itself into the genetic materials of the organism it infects. The primary pathologic condition of HIV causes specific immunodeficiency that destroys the host's ability to withstand infection. The HIV directly invades most major organ systems, including the CNS (Demmler & Taber, 1990; Fahrner, 1992). (HIV and AIDS are discussed in Chapter 8.)

Infants and children have become infected with HIV through a variety of sources. Transmission may occur perinatally through the placenta, by exposure to infected maternal blood and vaginal secretions, and by postpartum ingestion of breast milk. This method of transmission accounts for approximately 84% of pediatric AIDS cases in the United States. Infection also can occur from contaminated blood products, although new safeguards with blood products have lessened this risk considerably over the past few years. The incidence of infection before these changes has been reported to be as high as 95% for children receiving contaminated blood products (AIDS, 1991).

The actual incidence of pediatric HIV is not known because no national statistics have been compiled. The CDC estimates that 10,000 to 20,000 infants and children in this country currently have HIV. This incidence continues on a rapid increase.

Clinical Manifestations

The clinical diagnosis of HIV in children very often is a difficult task. The CDC developed a classification for HIV infection in children younger than 13 years (see box, p. 610). The HIV infection may be identified by viral culture of blood or tissue, and the diagnosis is confirmed by the presence of specific antibodies to the virus. However, the presence of passive maternal antibody limits the use of HIV antibody testing in infants in the high-risk category up to 15 months of age. Therefore, two definitions of infection in children are necessary: one for prenatally exposed infants up to 15 months of age and one for older children (Fahrner, 1991).

HIV affects all body systems. Therefore the clinical manifestations vary greatly from child to child. The initial signs and symptoms may be nonspecific and subtle, and they may progress slowly or rapidly to an acute, life-threatening condition.

The largest site for HIV infection in children and infants is the CNS (Epstein et al., 1987). Many children

CDC CLASSIFICATION FOR HIV INFECTION IN CHILDREN LESS THAN 13 YEARS OLD

Class P-0 indeterminate infection

Perinatal exposure up to 15 months of age that cannot be classified definitively, due to presence of maternal antibody

Class P-1 asymptomatic infection
Subclass A: normal immune function

Without abnormalities in quantitative immunoglobulins, complete blood cell count with differential, T-lymphocyte subsets

Subclass B: abnormal immune function

One or more common abnormalities, including hypergammaglobulinemia, decreased T4/T8 ratio, decreased T4 count, and absolute lymphopenia

Subclass C: immune function not tested

Class P-2 symptomatic infection
Subclass A: nonspecific findings

Two or more of the following persisting for more than 2 months: fever, failure to thrive, or weight loss greater than 10%, hepatosplenomegaly, lymphadenopathy, parotitis, or diarrhea

Subclass B: progressive neurologic disease

Loss of milestones or intellectual ability, impaired brain growth, or progressive motor deficits

Subclass C: lymphoid interstitial pneumonitis
Subclass D: secondary infectious diseases

Category D-1
Specified secondary infectious diseases listed in the CDC surveillance definition for AIDS
Category D-2
Recurrent serious bacterial infections: sepsis, meningitis, pneumonia, abscess, or bone or joint infections
Category D-3
Other specified secondary infectious diseases: oral *Candida* persisting 2 months or more, two or more episodes of herpes stomatitis, or disseminated herpes zoster virus (HZV)

Subclass E: secondary cancers

Category E-1
Specified secondary cancers listed in the CDC surveillance definition for AIDS
Category E-2
Other malignancies possibly associated with HIV

Subclass F: other diseases

Conditions possibly caused by HIV such as hepatitis, cardiopathy, nephropathy, hematologic disorders, and dermatologic diseases

From Centers for Disease Control, 1987.

---

function well or with minimal delay despite this consideration. Classic signs and symptoms of a progressive encephalopathy may occur throughout the course of illness with a worsening in severity at the end stage of the disease. These include but are not limited to deterioration of fine and gross motor skills, intellectual impairment, language delay and impairment, cognitive and developmental delay, behavioral manifestations (such as irritability, lethargy, confusion), and onset of seizures. The onset of progressive encephalopathy may be a prognostic indicator of a poor outcome (Epstein, Sharer, & Goudsmit, 1988). Infants exposed to the virus during the perinatal period may have acquired microcephaly. Confirmation of diagnosis, obtained by CT scanning and MRI, includes the presence of diffuse cerebral atrophy.

It may be difficult to completely differentiate the impact of HIV infection on the CNS from the impact of prenatal and perinatal exposure. In addition, other insults probably accompany HIV in a young child and af-

fect growth and development, such as drug exposure, prematurity, chronic illness, and a chaotic social atmosphere (Fahrner, 1991).

Evaluation and Treatment

A definite diagnosis of HIV is made by history, viral culture, and clinical manifestations, and a growing number of investigational protocols are available for treatment of children with HIV. In general, treatment is focused on the preservation and maintenance of the immune system, aggressive response to opportunistic infections, and support and relief of symptomatic occurrences (HIV treatment is discussed in Chapter 8).

Acquired immunodeficiency syndrome (AIDS) is one of the 10 leading causes of death in children today and most likely will be rated among the top five causes of death in children within the next few years (Pizzo, 1990). Outcomes may depend on the child's age at diagnosis and subsequent onset of symptoms and complications of AIDS.

CEREBROVASCULAR DISEASE IN CHILDREN

Cerebrovascular disease in children differs from that in adults in three ways: (1) an absence of predisposing factors, such as high blood pressure and arteriosclerosis, (2) significant differences in the clinical response related to the developing nervous system and thus a greater capacity for the pediatric brain to recover from vascular insult, and (3) the anatomic site of the pathologic condition. Cerebrovascular disease can be divided into two categories: occlusive and hemorrhagic.

Occlusive Cerebrovascular Disease

Occlusive disease may result from embolism, thrombosis, or congenital or iatrogenic narrowing of vessels, which leads to a decreased flow of blood and oxygen to areas of the brain. Cardiac anomalies are the most common disorders that lead to complications of cerebral occlusion. Examples include cyanotic and congenital heart disease.

Moyamoya disease is a chronic progressive vascular disease that results in the progressive stenosis of arterial flow to the brain. The Japanese term means "puff of smoke," which describes its appearance on CT examination. The vascularity may be a congenital anomaly or can develop as a result of cranial radiation. Treatment is surgical bypass of the occluded region. Regardless of the cause, failure of blood flow to the brain results in an ischemic stroke. Strokes are relatively rare in the pediatric population, with an incidence of approximately 0.63 per 100,000 annually in the United States.

Hemorrhagic Cerebrovascular Disease

Hemorrhagic disease may result from vascular anomalies that lead to rupture, such as aneurysm, or from congenital arteriovenous malformation. The rupture and symptomatic development of a cerebral aneurysm are rare in children younger than 19 years of age. Treatment is surgical repair of the weakened vessel and does not differ from that for the adult population (see Chapter 15).

Congenital arteriovenous malformations are the most common cause of intracranial bleeding and hemorrhagic stroke in children. Malformations vary in size, location, and symptoms, and these factors determine treatment. Options include surgery, radiation, and occlusion of the malformation (see Chapter 15).

Clinical Manifestations

The extent of the pathologic condition usually is less extensive in children than in adults. Symptoms may include degrees of hemiplegia (flaccid, spastic), weakness, seizures, high fever, nuchal rigidity, hemianopia, sensory changes, facial palsy, and temporary aphasia.

Evaluation and Treatment

Diagnosis of cerebrovascular disease is made through a series of tests, including CT, MRI, MRI angiogram (MRA), angiogram, and echocardiogram. History of evolving symptoms and past medical history are of vital importance in accurate diagnosis. Causative factors in the change in vascular flow often are not determined. Treatment varies on the basis of diagnosis.

Excellent collateral circulation in the child's brain allows for more rapid recovery of motor function. The developing brain, however, may suffer more global, long-term effects, leading to mental retardation, behavior disorders, and seizures.

CHILDHOOD TUMORS

Brain Tumors

Brain tumors are the most common solid tumor and the second most common primary neoplasm in children, second only to leukemia. Overall, brain tumors account for nearly 20% of all childhood cancers, with an annual incidence of 2.4 per 100,000 in the United States; approximately 1300 cases are diagnosed in each year. Brain tumors remain the leading cause of death from disease in children ages 1 to 15 years (Bleyer, 1990; Robinson, Mertens, & Neglia, 1991).

The cause of brain tumors is largely unknown, although genetic, environmental, and immune factors have been implicated in some tumor development. Other considerations and factors that have been investigated in the cause of brain tumors include familial tendencies, radiation, oncologic viruses, and chemical carcinogens. An important area of study has been the relationship of parental occupation to subsequent brain tumors in offspring. Associations have been found with tumors and parental employment, for example, parental exposure to hydrocarbons and employment in the aircraft and paper/pulp industries. Alterations in embryologic development also may play a part in the development of childhood brain tumors. This theory suggests that tumors arise from cells that are "misplaced" during embryonic development, never maturing but later proliferating in this immature form. None of these factors, however, has proved significant.

Most childhood brain tumors arise from glial tissue, the supportive tissue of the brain. Tumors also may originate in other tissue such as nerve cells, cranial nerves, the pineal and pituitary glands, blood vessels, or neuroepithelium. Brain tumors are classified by the tissue and location from which they arise. Because a uniform pathologic nomenclature has yet to be established, inconsistencies occur when statistical data are compared.

Two thirds of all pediatric brain tumors are found in

TABLE 16-7

Treatment Strategies for Childhood Brain Tumors

Tumor type	Treatment and prognosis
Cerebellar astrocytoma	Surgery; possibly curative Radiation and chemotherapy not proved successful but may delay recurrence Survival rate of more than 5 years in 50%-75%; if tumor recurs, it does so very slowly
Medulloblastoma	Surgery, primarily as a partial resection to relieve increased intracranial pressure and "debulk" the tumor Radiation as the primary treatment; may include spinal radiation Chemotherapy showing some promise 35% 5-year survival rate
Brainstem glioma	Surgery, resection occasionally possible Radiation, primarily palliative treatment Chemotherapy not yet proved beneficial, but new protocols being studied 20% to 40% 5-year survival rate
Ependymoma	Tumor possibly indolent for many years Surgery rarely curative; risk of resecting an infratentorial tumor too great Radiation for palliation (current controversy whether local or craniospinal radiation is best) Chemotherapy used for recurrent disease but with disappointing results
Craniopharyngioma	Surgery possibly successful when a complete resection is performed (partial resection usually requires further treatment) Radiation after partial surgical resection Chemotherapy not commonly used 75% to 85% 5-year survival rate
Optic nerve glioma	Initial treatment controversial Surgery used for diagnosis or relief of hydrocephalus Radiation useful, particularly if the tumor not treated by surgery
Cerebral astrocytoma	Surgery used if resection is possible Radiation useful for all grades of astrocytoma Chemotherapy beneficial in higher grade tumors, but further study required

the posterior fossa region of the brain. This area also may be referred to as *infratentorial* because it is located below the tentorium. The tentorium is the layer of dura that separates the cerebellum from the cortex or cerebrum. Thus the area above the tentorium is referred to as the *supratentorial region.* Approximately one third of childhood brain tumors are located in the supratentorial space. On the other hand, in the adult population two thirds of brain tumors are located in the supratentorial region and only one third in the infratentorial region. The types and characteristics of childhood brain tumors are summarized in Table 16-7.

Brain tumors, by virtue of their location, have unique characteristics that distinguish them from tumors found elsewhere in the body. A number of brain tumors in children may be considered histologically benign yet clinically malignant and life-threatening because of their location. For example, a tumor located in the brainstem region may appear benign under the microscope but the clinical presentation threatens and all too often overrides the vital functions of the brainstem.

Types of Brain Tumors

Medulloblastoma, ependymoma, astrocytoma, brainstem glioma, craniopharyngioma, and optic nerve glioma make up approximately 75% to 80% of all pediatric brain tumors. The location of brain tumors in children is illustrated in Fig. 16-14; specific characteristics, treatment strategies, and prognosis are listed in Tables 16-7 and 16-8.

Clinical Manifestations

The actual location of the brain tumor dictates the presenting signs and symptoms (discussed in greater detail with each particular brain tumor type). In addition to tumor location and cell type, the rate of growth of the tumor also determines the presenting signs and symptoms. The ability of the brain and intracranial cavity to compensate for tumor growth is directly related to the rate of its growth. This compensatory mechanism allows the components of the intracranial space (blood, brain, and cerebrospinal fluid) to adapt temporarily to slow changes in intracranial pressure. Therefore slow-

TABLE 16-8

Brain Tumors in Children

Type	Characteristics
Astrocytoma	Arises from astrocytes, often in the cerebellum or lateral hemisphere Slow growing, solid or cystic Often very large before diagnosed Varies in degree of malignancy
Optic nerve glioma	Arises from optic chiasm or optic nerve Slow-growing, low-grade astrocytoma
Medulloblastoma (infil- trating glioma)	Often located in cerebellum, extending into fourth ventricle and spinal fluid pathway Rapidly growing malignant tumor Can extend outside of CNS
Brainstem glioma	Arises from pons or myeloencephalon Numerous cell types Compresses cranial nerves V through X
Ependymoma	Arises from ependymal cells lining ventricles Circumscribed, solid, nodular tumors
Craniopharyngioma	Arises near pituitary gland, optic chiasm, and hypothalamus Cystic and solid tumors that affect vision, pituitary, and hypothalamic functions

FIG. 16-14 Location of brain tumors in children.

growing tumors can grow to enormous size before signs and symptoms are apparent. Conversely, fast-growing tumors allow little time for compensation of the space-occupying lesion, and clinical symptoms occur.

Signs and symptoms of brain tumors in children vary from generalized and vague to those that are localized and related specifically to the anatomic area. If the tumor is located in the posterior fossa region, the fourth ventricle may become blocked, which leads to hydrocephalus and signs of increased intracranial pressure (IICP). IICP also may occur because of the additional mass volume within the fixed container of the skull vault. The symptoms of IICP include headache, vomiting, lethargy, and irritability. If a young child complains of a headache, a thorough investigation should take place because headache is an uncommon complaint in young children. Headache caused by IICP usually is worse in the morning and gradually improves during the day when the child is upright and venous drainage is enhanced. Frequency of headache and other symptoms worsens as the tumor grows. A headache related to IICP generally occurs because of expansion of the lateral ventricle and cerebral hemisphere, which causes a stretching of the pain-sensitive dura mater. Irritability or possible apathy and increased somnolence also may result from IICP. Like headache, vomiting occurs more commonly in the morning. It is frequently not preceded by nausea and may become projectile, differing from a gastrointestinal disturbance in that the child may be ready to eat immediately after vomiting. Other signs and symptoms that can accompany IICP include increased head circumference with bulging fontanelle in the child younger than 2 years of age, cranial nerve palsies, and papilledema.

Localized findings relate to the degree of disturbance in physiologic functioning in the area where the tumor is located (see Table 14-6). Infratentorial tumors exhibit localized signs of impaired coordination and balance, including ataxia, gait difficulties, truncal ataxia, and loss of balance. The **medulloblastoma** occurs as an invasive malignant tumor that develops in the vermis of the cerebellum and may extend into the fourth ventricle. The **ependymoma** develops in the fourth ventricle and arises from the ependymal cells that line the ventricular system. The histology of the ependymoma varies, which makes the treatment course and prognosis difficult to establish. Because both tumors are located in the posterior fossa region along the midline, presenting signs and symptoms are similar. In addition to those already described, they may obstruct the fourth ventricle, resulting in hydrocephalus and generalized IICP, headache, nausea and vomiting, and nystagmus (involuntary eye movement).

In contrast, **cerebellar astrocytomas** are located on the surface of the right or left cerebellar hemisphere and cause unilateral symptoms (occurring on the same side of the tumor), such as head tilt, limb ataxia, and nystagmus when the eyes are turned toward the tumor.

Brainstem gliomas often cause a combination of cranial nerve involvement, cerebellar signs of ataxia, and corticospinal tract dysfunction. A common clinical pattern includes unilateral paralysis of cranial nerves with contralateral paralysis of the arm and leg, hyperreflexia, and extensor plantar responses. ICP generally does not occur.

The area of the sella turcica, the structure containing the pituitary gland, is the site of several childhood brain tumors; most common of this group is the **craniopharyngioma**. These tumors may originate from the pituitary gland or the hypothalamus. Usually slow-growing tumors, they may be quite large by the time of diagnosis. Symptoms include headache, seizures, diabetes insipidus, early onset of puberty, and growth delay. Other tumors located in this region of the brain include **optic gliomas**. Tumors that involve the optic tract may cause complete unilateral blindness and hemianopia of the other eye. Optic atrophy is another common finding.

Supratentorial tumors of the cerebral hemispheres in children are not very common. Tumors located in the cortex may cause focal cerebral dysfunction, weakness, hemiparesis, seizures, and visual changes. Involvement of particular lobes may result in more specific localized symptoms. For example, a tumor located in the frontal lobe may cause changes in affect and behavior, and a tumor in the occipital lobe may cause cortical blindness or blindness in one half of the visual field.

Evaluation and Treatment

A child with signs and symptoms of a brain tumor requires a complete workup, including a neurologic, developmental, and ophthalmic examination. CT with contrast enhancement allows direct visualization of the tumor mass. MRI now provides advanced dramatic examination of the brain and neoplasms. Small, low-grade tumors not seen on CT may be detected by MRI. Although less commonly used, MRA is most helpful in assessing vascularity of the tumor and its relationship to major blood vessels (Black, 1991). Myelographic examination may be used to evaluate tumor dissemination along the spinal column. Lumbar puncture to examine cerebrospinal fluid for tumor cells also is an option. Tumors more likely to spread throughout the neuroaxis include medulloblastomas and ependymomas.

The most useful treatment for brain tumors is surgical resection. Surgery to establish the diagnosis by biopsy or to excise the tumor is part of the initial treatment for most brain tumors. Some brain tumors may be cured with complete resection alone, such as low-grade cerebellar astrocytomas. Contraindications to such interventions are tumors in which surgical resection and biopsy carry a high risk of mortality or serious morbidity (brainstem gliomas). In these instances diagnosis is made on radiologic evidence and clinical manifestations.

Most brain tumors require additional radiation and chemotherapy. Although these treatments are essential for potential eradication of the brain tumor, radiation to the child's brain is associated with significant morbidity, including both acute and long-term sequelae. Enormous amounts of research, persistence, and investigations are directed at uncovering the secrets to successful treatment of this disease. Prognosis varies according to the type and location of the brain tumor. Historically, survival rates have been low; however, advances have been made with the combination of surgery, radiation, and chemotherapy. Now, nearly 50% of children with brain tumors are surviving (Bleyer, 1990). Comprehensive care and management of these children and their families are vital. Multidisciplinary teams composed of neurosurgeons, neurologists, neuropathologists, radiation therapists, oncologists, nurses, social workers, physical therapists, and other providers are absolutely necessary to provide the continuity and consistency needed to care for these children.

Embryonal Tumors
Neuroblastoma

Neuroblastoma is an embryonal tumor that originates in neural crest cells that normally give rise to the sympathetic ganglia and the adrenal medulla. The primitive neural crest cells (also called *sympathogonia*) are pluripotential (i.e., they give rise to several cell types). They mature into ganglion cells, pheochromocytes (which are found in the sympathetic nervous system), or neurofibrous tissue. Thus tumors that develop from neural crest cells reflect the varying degrees of differentiation of the cells. **Ganglioneuroblastomas** are tumors of intermediate level of cellular differentiation. The most differentiated tumor is a **ganglioneuroma,** which is considered benign and does not metastasize.

Because neuroblastoma involves a defect of embryonal tissue, it most commonly is diagnosed in young children and infants. Most tumors are diagnosed during the first 2 years of life, and 75% are found before the child is 5 years old. Occasionally, these tumors have been diagnosed at birth with metastasis apparent in the placenta. Slightly more than 500 cases are diagnosed each year in the United States (Bleyer, 1990). It is seen more commonly in white children (9.6 per million) than in black children (7 per million). Although it accounts for 6% to 8% of pediatric malignancies, neuroblastoma causes 15% of cancer deaths in children.

Pathogenesis

Neuroblastoma is the most primitive, or immature, form of the sympathetic nervous system tumors. Areas of necrosis and calcification often are present in the tumor.

Neuroblastoma, more than any other cancer, has been associated with spontaneous remission, commonly in infants who have liver, bone marrow, or skin involvement in addition to the primary site. Remission has been estimated to occur in approximately 7% of cases, but it may occur much more frequently. Neuroblastoma in situ (i.e., noninvasive tumor) has been found during autopsies of infants who died of other causes.

The cause of neuroblastoma is elusive. The tumor has been associated with a number of conditions, including neurofibromatosis and Hirschsprung disease, but most children with neuroblastoma have neither of these conditions. Although familial tendency has been noted in individual cases, a nonfamilial or sporadic pattern occurs in most children with neuroblastoma. Familial cases of neuroblastoma are considered to have an autosomal dominant pattern of inheritance (mechanisms of inheritance are discussed in Chapter 4).

Intense genetic study of neuroblastoma cells has led to some interesting findings. Often these cells show a deletion of the short arm of chromosome 1, which is believed to represent the loss of a tumor-response gene. In addition, an oncogene, the n-*myc* oncogene, is present and amplified in neuroblastoma. There is an association between the number of n-*myc* copies present in the neuroblastoma cells and the child's prognosis. The greater the number of copies of the n-*myc* oncogene, the more rapidly progressive and lethal the disease is (Brodeur, 1990). Further, a gene, the human multidrug-resistant gene (MDR1), has been identified and is associated with chemotherapy failure. The MDR1 gene has been found to be amplified in some neuroblastoma cells after initial treatment with chemotherapy, and the increased presence of MDR1 is associated with chemotherapy resistance (Goldstein et al., 1990).

Clinical Manifestations

The clinical manifestations of neuroblastoma depend on the location of the tumor. Because neuroblastoma originates where there are elements of sympathetic nervous tissue, the tumor can arise in the sympathetic chain (column of sympathetic ganglia that parallels the spinal column), ganglia of effector organs, peripheral ganglia, adrenal medulla, bladder, and inner genitalia. The most common location is in the retroperitoneal region (65% of cases) and most frequently the adrenal medulla. The tumor is evident as an abdominal mass and may cause anorexia, bowel and bladder alteration, and sometimes spinal cord compression.

The second most common location of neuroblastoma is the mediastinum (area separating the lungs) (15% of cases). There the tumor may cause dyspnea or infection related to airway obstruction. If it is large, compression of the trachea, bronchi, lymphatic vessels, and mediastinal veins often results. Neck and facial edema may then be caused by superior vena cava syndrome. Less commonly, neuroblastoma may arise from the cervical sympathetic ganglion (3% to 4% of cases). Cervical neuroblastoma often causes Horner syndrome, which consists of miosis (pupil contraction), ptosis (drooping eyelid), enophthalmos (backward displacement of the eyeball), and anhidrosis (sweat deficiency).

The initial signs and symptoms of neuroblastoma often are related to metastatic disease. Two thirds of children have metastatic disease at the time of diagnosis. Common sites of metastasis include the skin, with characteristic blue or purple nodules; the liver, causing enlargement; bone, causing pain and pathologic fracture; and bone marrow infiltration, occurring in more than 50% of children. A unique but uncommon site of metastasis is the orbit of the eye, causing an ecchymotic discoloration of the upper and lower eyelids and a "raccoon" eye appearance.

A number of systemic signs and symptoms are characteristic of neuroblastoma, including weight loss, irritability, fatigue, and fever. Intractable diarrhea occurs in 7% to 9% of children and is due to tumor secretion of a hormone called *vasoactive intestinal polypeptide (VIP)*.

More than 90% of children with neuroblastoma have increased amounts of catecholamines and associated metabolites in their urine. High levels of urinary catecholamines and serum ferritin are associated with a poorer prognosis.

Evaluation and Treatment

Initial diagnostic studies are dictated by the location of the site of the primary tumor. Diagnosis begins with a complete physical and neurologic examination. Radiologic examination, including intravenous pyelogram, CT scan, and MRI of the primary site, provides further information. Investigation of metastatic disease includes skeletal survey, bone scan, liver scan, and bone marrow aspiration and examination. Newer nuclear medicine imaging studies for neuroblastoma, such as ^{131}I-metaiodobenzylguanadine (^{131}I-MIBG) and tumor-specific monoclonal antibody scan, may be helpful. Urinary catecholamine levels are measured by two metabolites, vanillylmandelic acid (VMA) and homovanillic acid (HVA). Measurement of these levels requires a 24-hour urine collection. Other laboratory analysis is likely to include ferritin; serum neuron-specific enolase (NSE), an enzyme produced by neuronal tissues; and gangliosides, lipid molecules that may be shed from the surface of tumor cells.

The diagnosis of neuroblastoma is confirmed by surgical biopsy. Occasionally the biopsy may be avoided if bone marrow aspiration shows tumor infiltration and significant elevation of urinary catecholamines. For many years, there was no agreement on a staging system for neuroblastoma. Finally in 1986, an international group proposed a single staging system that was adopted in 1987 (Brodeur et al., 1988). A special stage (IV-S) is designated for infants who otherwise would be classified as having early-stage disease but who also have metastatic disease involving the liver, skin, or bone.

Treatment is based on the extent of the disease and prognostic markers, such as age, n-*myc* copy numbers, and high serum ferritin or NSE levels. Early-stage disease is treated by primary excision of the tumor. Because neuroblastoma is a radiosensitive tumor, postoperative radiation may be given for residual disease. The success of radiation in early-stage disease, however, is controversial. Chemotherapy has not proved beneficial.

More extensive disease is treated by surgical debulking of as much tumor as possible. Radiation is directed at residual disease at the primary site. Systemic chemotherapy is used to control remaining disease, and many drugs have been tried over the past 20 years. Other more recent experimental approaches to treatment include bone marrow transplantation or monoclonal antibodies paired with internal radiation or used as targeted immunotherapy.

Stage IV-S disease requires very little treatment, primarily because of the high rate of spontaneous regression. Low-dose radiation treatment or single-course chemotherapy may be used to reduce large tumors.

Retinoblastoma

Retinoblastoma is a rare congenital eye tumor of young children that originates in the retina of one or both eyes (Fig. 16-15). It has been highly studied and is of much interest to geneticists. Retinoblastoma demonstrates both an inherited and acquired form. Retinoblastoma rarely is diagnosed after the child is 5 years of age. The inherited form of the disease generally is diagnosed during the first year of life and often involves multiple tumors and sometimes both eyes. The acquired disease most commonly is diagnosed in children 2 to 3 years of age and involves unilateral disease. Although retinoblastoma is the most common pediatric intraocular tumor, only 200 children are diagnosed each year in the United States.

FIG. 16-15 Retinoblastoma. Prominent white reflex (caused by retinoblastoma) in dilated pupil of left eye. (From Kissane, 1990.)

Pathogenesis

Approximately 40% of retinoblastomas are inherited, and the remaining 60% are acquired. In the early 1970s, Knudson (1971) proposed the "2-hit" hypothesis to explain the occurrence of both hereditary and acquired forms of the disease. This hypothesis predicts that two separate transforming events or "hits" must occur in a normal retinoblast cell to cause the cancer. Further it proposes that in the inherited form the first "hit" or mutation occurs in the germ cell (inherited from either parent) and the mutation is contained in every cell of the child's body. Only a second, random mutation in a retinoblast cell is necessary to transform that cell into cancer. Multiple tumors are observed in the inherited form because these second mutations are likely to oc-

cur in several of the approximately 1 to 2 million retinoblast cells. In contrast, the acquired form of retinoblastoma requires two independent "hits" or mutations to occur in the same somatic cell (after the egg is fertilized) for transformation to cancer. This is much less likely to happen. Fig. 16-16 illustrates the two-mutation model for these two patterns of mutation.

The gene location in which the initial retinoblastoma mutation occurs is on the long arm of chromosome 13, band q14. The gene responsible for retinoblastoma, a tumor-suppressor gene, is called the *Rb gene*. The first "hit" inactivates one allele of the Rb gene, and the second "hit" inactivates the other allele of the gene. Without the normal functioning of the Rb gene, production of protein growth regulators that control retinal cell

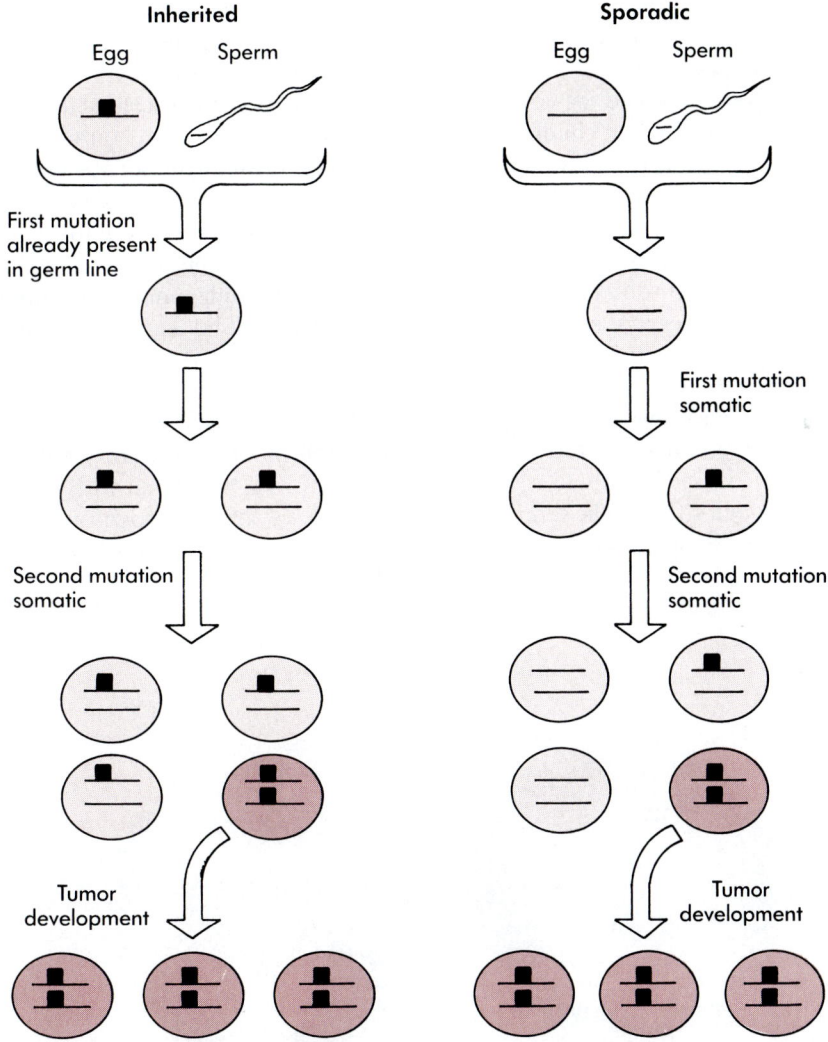

FIG. 16-16 The two-mutation model of retinoblastoma development. In inherited retinoblastoma, the first mutation is transmitted through the germ line of an affected parent. The second mutation occurs somatically in a retinal cell, leading to development of the tumor. In sporadic retinoblastoma, development of a tumor requires two somatic mutations.

growth is lacking. Because the gene is inactivated, lack of cell growth control results in unregulated proliferation and tumor development.

The Rb gene also has been implicated in other cancers, and survivors of hereditary retinoblastoma may be at increased risk for second cancers, particularly osteosarcoma but also cancer of the lung, breast, prostate, and bladder. Although retinoblastoma occurs in the very young child, second tumors can develop when survivors are in their 20s and 30s; such tumors are generally resistant to therapy.

Clinical Manifestations

Retinoblastoma grows as one or more tumors in the retina and extends into the vitreous humor. Free-floating, small tumors in the vitreous humor may attach to the surface of the retina in multiple areas and proliferate (Fig. 16-17). The tumor also can invade the optic nerve by infiltrating through the cribriform plate of the ethmoid bone (see Fig. 12-17) or can spread through the sheath around the nerve. In either case the tumor can gain access to the subarachnoid space and the CNS. The tumor spreads into the choroid in 25% of children with retinoblastoma. Because the choroid is highly vascular, metastasis by means of hematogenous spread is possible. When hematogenous spread occurs, metastatic sites include the bone marrow, long bones, lymph nodes, and liver. Should the tumor invade the orbit, lymphatic spread is possible. Spontaneous regression occurs, although infrequently, and may be due to the tumor outgrowing its blood supply.

The primary sign of retinoblastoma is leukokoria, a white pupillary reflex also called *cat's eye reflex*, that is due to the mass behind the lens (see Fig. 16-15). At this point the tumor is large enough that a light shone into the eye is reflected back by the tumor, making the pupil appear white. Other signs and symptoms include strabismus, a red, painful eye, and limited vision. Any of these signs and symptoms in a child younger than 4 years of age warrants careful ophthalmic examination of both eyes. Similarly, any newborn child with a known genetic risk for retinoblastoma should have routine ophthalmologic examinations.

Evaluation and Treatment

Diagnostic evaluation for retinoblastoma includes documentation of family history, complete ophthalmic examination, and metastatic studies that include bone marrow aspiration, lumbar puncture for spinal fluid examination, bone scan, and additional radiologic and CT studies of the orbit and brain. Because of the potential hereditary risk to a child's siblings, all siblings younger than 4 years of age also should receive ophthalmologic evaluations.

Because retinoblastoma is a treatable tumor, dual priorities are saving the child's life and restoring useful vision. Radiation therapy is the primary treatment for small tumors. Photocoagulation therapy that destroys the blood vessels to the tumor may be used after radiation therapy if the tumor has failed to completely regress or recurs. Cryotherapy that destroys the tumor by causing intracellular ice crystal formation and disrupting microcirculation may be used as an alternate approach. Large or multiple tumors, indicating more advanced disease, may require enucleation (removal) of the eye. Every attempt is made to preserve vision in at least one eye without jeopardizing the child's survival.

The prognosis for most children with retinoblastoma is excellent and has a greater than 90% long-term survival, although children with metastatic disease at diagnosis have a poor prognosis. Approximately 75% of children have useful vision in the treated eye.

FIG. 16-17 Bilateral retinoblastoma. Presence of white mass consisting of detached retina and neoplastic tissue immediately behind lens in each eye. (From Kissane, 1985.)

Structure and Function of the Nervous System in Children

1 The central nervous system develops from the neural tube, which is ectodermal in origin. The cranial end of the tube forms the brain, and the spinal cord is formed from the remainder of the tube.
2 The cranial and spinal ganglia form the neural crest.
3 There are six stages to the development of the nervous system, and disruption of any of the stages can lead to malfunction of the nervous system.
4 The bones of the skull are joined by sutures, and the wide membranous junctions of the sutures are known as *fontanelles* that close by 20 months of age.
5 Myelin is a sheath that develops around axons to facilitate speed of nerve impulse conduction. Progressive development of reflexes corresponds to normal maturation of nerve tissue.

Structural Malformations

1 Defects of neural tube closure include anencephaly, encephalocele, meningocele, and myelomeningocele.
2 Failure of the vertebra to close with protrusion of neural tube contents is known as *spina bifida occulta*.
3 Acrania is nearly complete absence of the cranial vault.
4 Premature closure of the cranial sutures causes craniosynostosis and prevents normal skull expansion and compression of growing brain tissue.
5 Microcephaly is lack of brain growth and retarded mental and motor development.
6 Congenital hydrocephalus results from an imbalance between the production and reabsorption of cerebrospinal fluid.

Encephalopathies

1 Static encephalopathies are nonprogressive disorders of the brain that can occur during gestation, birth, or childhood and can be caused by endogenous or exogenous factors.
2 Cerebral palsy can be caused by prenatal cerebral hypoxia or perinatal trauma with symptoms of mental retardation, seizure disorders, or developmental disabilities.
3 Inherited metabolic disorders that damage the nervous system include defects in amino acid metabolism (phenylketonuria) and lipid metabolism (Tay-Sachs disease) and result in abnormal behavior, seizures, and deficient psychomotor development.
4 Seizure disorders are associated with numerous nervous system disorders and more often are a generalized rather than a partial type of seizure.

5 Generalized forms of seizures include tonic-clonic, myoclonic, atonic, akinetic, and infantile spasms.
6 Partial seizures suggest more localized brain dysfunction.
7 Febrile seizures usually are limited to the ages of 6 months to 3 years with a pattern of one seizure per febrile illness.
8 Reye syndrome is associated with influenza B and varicella viruses and symptoms of hypoglycemia, hyperammonemia, and increased serum short-chain fatty acids. Progressive manifestations include lethargy, stupor, rigidity, seizures, and respiratory arrest.
9 Accidental poisonings from a variety of toxins can cause serious neurologic damage.
10 Bacterial meningitis is commonly caused by *Haemophilus influenzae*, *Neisseria meningitidis*, or *Streptococcus pneumoniae* and may result from respiratory or gastrointestinal infections, with symptoms of fever, headaches, photophobia, seizures, rigidity, and stupor.

Human Immunodeficiency Virus and CNS Involvement

1 HIV may be transmitted to infants and children through the placenta, by exposure to infected blood or vaginal secretions, or by ingestion of infected breast milk.
2 The incidence of HIV among children is increasing. The classic symptoms are related to progressive encephalopathy.
3 AIDS is one of the 10 leading causes of death among children.

Cerebrovascular Disease in Children

1 Cyanotic and congenital heart disease can be complicated by cerebrovascular occlusion that causes cerebral infarction and brain damage.

Childhood Tumors

1 Brain tumors are the most common tumors of the nervous system and the second most common type of childhood cancer.
2 Tumors in children most frequently are located below the tentorial membrane.
3 Fast-growing tumors produce symptoms early in the disease, whereas slow-growing tumors may become very large before symptoms appear.
4 Symptoms of brain tumors may be generalized or localized. The most common general symptom is increased intracranial pressure (headache, irritability, vomiting, somnolence, and bulging of fontanelles).

5 Localized signs of infratentorial tumors in the cerebellum include impaired coordination and balance. Cranial nerve signs occur with tumors near the brainstem.

6 Supratentorial tumors may be located near the cortex or deep in the brain. Symptoms depend on the specific location of the tumor.

7 Neuroblastoma is an embryonal tumor of the sympathetic nervous system and can be located anywhere there is sympathetic nervous tissue. Symptoms are related to tumor location and size of metastasis.

8 Retinoblastoma is a congenital eye tumor that has both a hereditary and a nonhereditary form.

KEY TERMS

Acquired immunodeficiency syndrome (AIDS), 610
Acrania, 595
Alar plate, 588
Anencephaly, 592
Arnold-Chiari II malformation, 594
Ataxic cerebral palsy, 601
Basal plate, 588
Benign febrile seizure, 605
Brainstem glioma, 614
Cerebellar astrocytoma, 614
Cerebral palsy, 599
Cranial meningocele, 592
Craniopharyngioma, 614
Craniosynostosis, 595
Cyclopia, 592
Dandy-Walker deformity, 598
Dyskinetic cerebral palsy, 601
Encephalocele, 592
Encephalopathy, 599
Ependymoma, 614

Epilepsy, 603
Fontanelle, 588
Ganglioneuroblastoma, 615
Ganglioneuroma, 615
Generalized seizure, 604
Hyperphenylalaninemia (HPA), 603
Infantile spasm, 604
Juvenile myoclonic epilepsy, 605
Lennox-Gastaut syndrome, 605
Lysosomal storage disease, 603
Macewen sign (cracked-pot sign), 599
Medulloblastoma, 614
Meningocele, 592
Mental retardation, 597
Microcephaly, 597
Moyamoya disease, 611
Myelodysplasia, 592
*Neisseria meningitidi*s, 608

Neural crest, 588
Neural fold, 588
Neural groove, 588
Neural plate, 588
Neural tube, 588
Neuroblastoma, 615
Optic glioma, 614
Partial seizure, 604
Phenylketonuria (PKU), 601
Pica, 608
Retinoblastoma, 616
Reye syndrome, 605
Schwann cell, 588
Somite, 588
Spastic cerebral palsy, 601
Spina bifida, 595
Spina bifida occulta, 595
Streptococcus pneumoniae, 608
Sulcus limitans, 588
Suture, 588
Tay-Sachs disease, 603
Unclassified epileptic seizure, 604

REFERENCES

AIDS. (1991). *Statistics from the Centers of Disease Control, 5,* 1279-1281.

Amacher, A. L., & Wellington, J. (1984). Infantile hydrocephalus: Long-term results of surgical therapy. *Child Brain, 11,* 217-229.

Bare, M. A. (1989). Hemispherectomy for seizures. *Journal of Neuroscience Nursing, 21,* 18-23.

Behrman, R. E., & Vaughan, V. C. (1983). *Nelson textbook of pediatrics* (12th ed.). Philadelphia: Saunders.

Black, P. McL. (1991). Brain tumors. *New England Journal of Medicine, 324*(22), 1555-1564.

Bleyer, W. A. (1990). The impact of childhood cancer in the United States and the world. *CA: A Cancer Journal for Clinicians, 40*(6), 355-367.

Brewer, K., & Sperling, M. R. (1988). Neurosurgical treatment of intractable epilepsy. *Journal of Neuroscience Nursing, 20,* 366-372.

Brodeur, G. M. (1990). Molecular biology and genetics of human neuroblastoma. In C. Pochedly (Ed.), *Neuroblastoma: Tumor biology and therapy* (pp. 31-50). Boca Raton, FL: CRC Press.

Brodeur, G. M., Seeger, R. C., Barrett, A., Berthold, G., Castleberry, R. P., D'Angio, G., DeBernardi, B., Evans, A. E., Favrot, M., Freeman, A. I., et al. (1988). International criteria for diagnosis, staging, and response to treatment in patients with neuroblastoma. *Journal of Clinical Oncology, 6*(12), 1874-1881.

Centers for Disease Control (CDC). (1987). *Morbidity and Mortality Weekly Report, 36,* 225-236.

Demmler, G. J., & Taber, L. H. (1990). Virology of HIV-1. *Seminars in Pediatric Infectious Diseases, 1,* 17-20.

Dreifuss, F. E. (1989). Juvenile myoclonic epilepsy: Characteristics of a primary generalized epilepsy. *Epilepsia, 30,* S1-S7.

Edwards, M. S., & Derechin M. (Eds.). (1986). *About hydrocephalus: A book for parents* (p. 21). San Francisco: University of California.

Epstein, L. G., Goudsmit, J., Paul, D. A., Morrison, S. H., Connor, E. M., Oleske, J. M., & Holland, B. (1987). Expression of human immunodeficiency virus in cerebrospinal fluid of children with progressive encephalopathy. *Annals of Neurology, 21,* 397-401.

Epstein, L. G., Sharer, L. R., & Goudsmit, J. (1988). Neurological and neuropathological features of human immunodeficiency virus infection in children. *Annals of Neurology Journal, 23*(Suppl.), S19-S23.

Evans, A., D'Angio, G., & Randolph, J. (1971). A proposed staging for children with neuroblastoma. *Cancer, 27,* 374-378.

Fahrner, R. (1992). Pediatric HIV Infections and AIDS. In P. L. Jackson & J. A. Vessey (Eds.), *Primary care of the child with a chronic condition* (pp. 408-425). St. Louis: Mosby–Year Book.

Farley, J. A., & Dunleavy, M. J. (1992). Myelodysplasia. In P. L. Jackson & J. A. Vessey (Eds.), *Primary care of the child with a chronic condition* (pp. 373-374, 376). St. Louis: Mosby–Year Book.

Farmer, T. H. (Ed.). (1983). *Pediatric neurology* (3rd ed.). Hagerstown, Md: Harper & Row.

Goldstein, L. J., Fojo, A. T., Ueda, K., Crist, W., Green, A., Brodeur, G., Pastan I., & Gottesman, M. M. (1990). Expression of the multidrug resistance, MDR1, gene in neuroblastomas. *Journal of Clinical Oncology, 8*(1), 128-136.

Hensleigh, P. A., Fainstat, T., & Spencer, R. (1986). Perinatal events and cerebral palsy. *American Journal of Obstetrics and Gynecology, 154,* 978-981.

Hobbins, J. C. (1991). Diagnosis and management of neural tube defects today. *New England Journal of Medicine, 324*(10), 690-691.

Holmes, G. L. (1986). *Diagnosis and management of seizures in children.* Philadelphia: Saunders.

Jackson, P. L. (1992). Hydrocephalus. In P. L. Jackson & J. A. Vessey (Eds.), *Primary care of the child with a chronic condition* (pp. 303-317). St. Louis: Mosby–Year Book.

Kaufman, S. (1989). An evaluation of the possible neurotoxicity of metabolites of phenylalanine. *Journal of Pediatrics, 114,* 895-900.

Kissane, J. M. (Ed.). (1985). *Anderson's pathology* (8th ed.). St. Louis: Mosby–Year Book.

Klein, J. O., Feigin, R. D., & McCracken, G. H. (1986). Report of the task force on treatment and management of meningitis. *Pediatrics (Suppl.), 78*(5), 959-982.

Knudson, A. G. (1971). Mutation and cancer: A statistical study of retinoblastoma. *Proceedings of the National Academy of Sciences of the United States of America, 68,* 620-623.

Lee, W. H., Bookstein, R., Hong, F., Young, L. J., Stew, J. Y., & Lee, E. Y. (1987). Human retinoblastoma susceptible gene: Cloning, identification, and sequela. *Science, 235,* 1394-1399.

Lemire, R. J. (1986). Causes of neural tube defects. In R. L. McLaurin (Ed.), *Spina bifida: A multidisciplinary approach* (pp. 2-7). New York: Praeger.

Lombroso, C. T. (1983). A prospective study of infantile spasms: Clinical and therapeutic correlations. *Epilepsia, 24,* 135.

Luthy, D. A., Wardinsky, T., Shurtleff, D. B., Hellenbach, K. A., Hickok, D. E., Nyberg, D. A., & Benedetti, T. J. (1991). Cesarean section before the onset of labor and subsequent motor function in infants with myelomingocele diagnosed internally. *New England Journal of Medicine, 324*(10), 662-666.

McCollough, D., & Balzar-Martin, L. A. (1982). Current prognosis in overt neonatal hydrocephalus. *Journal of Neurosurgery, 57,* 378-383.

McLaughlin, J. F., & Shurtleff, D. B. (1979). Management of the newborn with myelodysplasia. *Clinical Pediatrics, 8,* 463-480.

Nolte, J. (1988). *The brain: An introduction to its functional anatomy* (2nd ed.). St. Louis: Mosby–Year Book.

Paneth, N. (1986). Etiologic factors in cerebral palsy. *Pediatric Annals, 15*(3), 191-201.

Park, T. S., Cail, W. S., Maggio, W. M., & Mitchell, D. C. (1985). Progressive spasticity and scoliosis in children with myelomeningocele. *Journal of Neurosurgery, 62,* 367-375.

Penry, J. K. (1986). *Epilepsy: Diagnosis, management, quality of life* (2nd ed.). New York: Raven Press.

Pizzo, P. A. (1990). Pediatric AIDS: Problems within problems. *Journal of Infectious Diseases, 161,* 316-325.

Reye syndrome surveillance—United States, 1989. (1989). *Journal of the American Medical Association, 265*(8), 960.

Robinson, L. L., Mertens, A., & Neglia, J. P. (1991). Epidemiology and etiology of childhood cancer. In D. J. Fernbach & T. T. Vietti (Eds.), *Clinical pediatric oncology* (4th ed.). St. Louis: Mosby–Year Book.

Schmidt, K. (1991). Phenylketonuria. In P. L. Jackson & J. A. Vessey (Eds.), *Primary care of the child with a chronic condition* (pp. 426-445). St. Louis: Mosby–Year Book.

Schmidt, K., Kaufman, S., & Woo, S. L. C. (1989). The hyperphenylalaninemias. In C. R. Scriver, A. Beaudet, D. W. Sly, & D. Valle (Eds.), *The metabolic basis of inherited disease* (Vol. 1, 6th ed.). New York: McGraw-Hill.

Seidel, H. M., Ball, J. W., Dains, J. E., & Benedict, G. W. (1987). *Mosby's guide to physical examination.* St. Louis: Mosby–Year Book.

Spencer, D. D., & Spencer, S. S. (1989). Corpus callosotomy in the treatment of medically intractable secondarily generalized seizures of children. *Cleveland Clinic Journal of Medicine 56,* 69-78.

Steele, S. (1991). Cerebral palsy. In P. L. Jackson & J. A. Vessey (Eds.), *Primary care of the child with a chronic condition* (pp. 148-168). St. Louis: Mosby–Year Book.

Swaiman, K. F., & Wright, F. S. (1982). *The practices of pediatric neurology: Principles and practice.* St. Louis: Mosby–Year Book.

Venes, J. L., & McGuire, L. (1986). Progressive urological dysfunction in the child with repaired meningocele: A reversible sequela of cord tethering. In R. L. McLaurin (Ed.), *Spinal bifida: A multidisciplinary approach* (pp. 62-69). New York: Praeger.

Wallander, J. L., Feldmen, W. S., & Varni, J. W. (1989). Physical status and psychosocial adjustment in children with spina bifida. *Journal of Pediatric Psychology, 14,* 89-102.

Whaley, L. F., & Wong, D. L. (1987). Nursing care in childhood cancer: Retinoblastoma. *Journal of Nursing, 82,* 425-431.

Wiswell, T. E., Tuttle, D. J., Northam, R. S., & Simonds, G. R. (1990). Major congenital neurologic malformations. *American Journal of Diseases in Children, 144,* 61-67.

SUGGESTED READINGS

Annest, J. L., et al. (1982). Blood lead levels for persons 6 months-74 years of age: U.S. 1976-80. Vital and health statistics, National Center for Health Statistics. *Advance Data, 79,* 1-24.

Barabas, G., & Taft, L.T. (1986). Early signs and differential diagnosis of cerebral palsy. *Pediatric Annals, 15*(3), 203-214.

Baron, M. C. (1991). Advances in the care of children with brain tumors. *Journal of Neuroscience Nursing, 23*(1), 39-43.

Beckwith, J., & Perrin, E. (1963). In situ neuroblastoma: A contribution to the natural history of neural crest tumors. *American Journal of Pathology, 43,* 1089-1104.

Bigner, S. H., Mark, J., Burger, P. C., Mahaley, S., Bullard, D. E., Mahlbaier, L. H., & Bigner, D. D. (1988). Specific chromosomal abnormalities in malignant human gliomas. *Cancer Research, 88,* 405-411.

Bigner, S. H., Wong, A. J., Mark, J., Muhlbaier, L. H., Kinzler, K. W., Vogelstein, R., & Bigner, D. D. (1987). Relationship between gene amplification and chromosomal deviations in malignant human gliomas. *Cancer Genetics and Cytogenetics, 29,* 165-170.

Bonner, K., & Siegal, K. R. (1988). Pathology, treatment and management of posterior fossa brain tumors in childhood. *Journal of Neuroscience Nursing, 20*(2), 84-93.

Bruce, J. L., & Grove, S. K. (1992). Fever: Pathology and treatment. *Critical Care Nurse, 12*(1), 40-49.

Brumback, L. (1992). *Hydrocephalus: Current clinical concepts.* St. Louis: Mosby–Year Book.

Childhood Brain Tumor Consortium. (1988). A study of childhood brain tumors based on surgical biopsies from ten North American institutions: Sample description. *Journal of Neurooncology, 6,* 9-23.

Committee on Infectious Diseases. (1982). Aspirin and Reye syndrome. *Pediatrics, 62,* 810-812.

Crist, W. M., & Kun, L. E. (1991). Common solid tumors of childhood. *New England Journal of Medicine, 324*(7), 461-471.

Diamond, M. (1986). Rehabilitation strategies for the child with cerebral palsy. *Pediatric Annals, 15*(3), 230-236.

Dobbing, J. (Ed.). (1983). *Prevention of spina bifida and other neural tube defects.* New York: Academic Press.

Edwards, M. S. B., Hudgins, R. J., Wilson, C. B., Levin, V. A., & Wara, W. M. (1988). Pineal region tumors in children. *Journal of Neurosurgery, 68,* 689-697.

Hauser, W. A. (1992). Seizure disorders: The changes with age. *Epilepsia, 33*(4), 56-514.

Healy, M., & Aslam, M. (1982, March). Lead poisoning: Something in the air. *Nursing Mirror, 31,* 42-44.

Holtzhauer, R. J., Campbell, R. J., Hall, L. J., & Halpin, T. J. (1986). Reye's syndrome: An epidemiologic analysis of mild disease. *American Journal of Diseases of Children, 140*(12), 1231-1236.

Horowitz, J. M. (1993). Regulation of transcription by the retinoblastoma protein. *Genes Chromosomes & Cancer 6*(2), 124-131.

Kondziolka, D., Humphreys, R. P., Hoffman, H. J., Hendrick, E. B., & Drake, J. M. (1992). Arteriovenous malformations of the brain in children: A forty year experience. *Canadian Journal of Neurological Sciences, 19,* 40-45.

Lopez-Ibor, B., & Schwartz, A. (1985). Neuroblastoma. *Pediatric Clinics of North America, 32,* 755-778.

Malik, G. M., Sadasivan, B., Knighton, R. S., & Ausman, J. (1991). The management of arteriovenous malformations in children. *Child's Nervous System, 7,* 43-47.

Pizzo. P. A. & Poplack, D. G. (Eds.). (1993). *Principles and practice of pediatric oncology* (2nd ed.) Philadelphia: J. B. Lippincott.

Reye, R. D., Morgan, G., & Baral, J. (1963, October 12). Encephalopathy and fatty degeneration of the viscera: A disease entity in childhood. *Lancet, 2,* 749-752.

Schmidt, K. (1989). Primer to the inborn errors of metabolism for perinatal and neonatal nurses. *Journal of Perinatal and Neonatal Nursing, 2,* 60-71.

Sell, S. H. W. (1984). Long-term sequelae of bacterial meningitis in children. *Pediatric Infectious Diseases, 2,* 90-93.

Shiminski-Maher, T. (1990). Brain tumors in childhood: Implications for nursing practice. *Journal of Pediatric Health Care, 4*(3), 122-130.

Silver, L. (1986). Controversial approaches to treating learning disabilities and attention deficit disorders. *American Journal of Diseases of Children, 140*(10), 1045-1052.

So, E. L. (1993). Update on epilepsy. *Medical Clinics of North America (77)*1:203-204.

Spanos, A., Harrell, F. E., & Durack, D. T. (1989). Differential diagnosis of acute meningitis. *Journal of the American Medical Association, 262*(19), 2700-2707.

Tapley, N., Strong, L., & Sutow, W. (1991). Retinoblastoma. In W. Sutow, D. Fernbach, & T. Vietti (Eds.), *Clinical pediatric oncology* (4th ed.). St. Louis: Mosby–Year Book.

Volpe, J. J. (1987). *Neurology of the newborn.* Philadelphia: Saunders.

Voute, P. (1991). Neuroblastoma. In D. J. Fernbach & T. T. Vietti (Eds.), *Clinical pediatric oncology* (4th ed., pp. 559-587). St. Louis: Mosby–Year Book.

Waskerwitz, M., & Ruccione, K. (1985). An overview of cancer in children in the 1980s. *Nursing Clinics of North America, 20,* 5-29.

Whaley, L. F., & Wong, D. L. (1991). *Nursing care of infants and children* (4th ed.). St. Louis: Mosby–Year Book.

Wong, D., & Dornan, L. (1982). Nursing care in childhood cancer: Retinoblastoma. *American Journal of Nursing, 82,* 425-431.

Young, J. L., Ries, L. G., Silverberg, E., Horn, J. W., & Miller, R. W. (1986). Cancer incidence, survival, and mortality for children younger than age 15 years. *Cancer, 58*(2), 598-602.

UNIT VI

The Endocrine System

ENDOCRINE DYSFUNCTION is indicated by numerous examples. Goiters were described as early as the time of the Roman Empire, and it appears that people in early times recognized the anatomic and physiologic effects of castration in males, although the mechanisms for the effects were not understood. An Egyptian papyrus, dated 1500 BC, described a person producing excessive amounts of sweet urine. Despite these descriptions the surviving written records do not reflect an understanding of the endocrine system as such until the 1700s.

In 1766, A. V. Haller identified the thymus, thyroid, spleen, and ductless glands that pour special substances into the veins and thus into the general secretion. The term *internal secretions* as a descriptor for the special substances was introduced in 1855 by Claude Bernard. The term *hormone* was first used in 1905 by two British physiologists, W. M. Bayliss and E. H. Starling. The word *hormone* is derived from a Greek word meaning "I arouse to activity."

THE ENDOCRINE SYSTEM

A woman with exophthalmic goiter.
(From Curshmann, 1984; courtesy National Library of Medicine.)

One of the first endocrine deficiencies to be treated successfully was a case of hypothyroidism in 1891. G. R. Murray administered extract from the thyroid gland of a freshly killed sheep to his patient, and the symptoms of hypothyroidism subsequently improved. Hyperthyroidism was the first condition described as a result of the overproduction of an endocrine secretion. Surgical removal of the thyroid gland was performed in the mid-1800s and resulted in improvement of symptoms. The procedure was neither a common nor a successful treatment until after the development of surgical anesthesia and the implementation of surgical asepsis.

By the late 1890s and early 1900s, several endocrine glands and their functions had been identified. The substances secreted by the endocrine glands were not identified until much later. The parathyroid glands were discovered in 1855 and their function was determined in 1896, but parathyroid hormone was not isolated until 1925. The endocrine functions of the pancreas were identified in 1889, and in 1928 insulin was developed in a pure enough form for use in human beings; 25 years were to pass before Sanger established its amino acid sequence. The subspecialty of endocrinology was established in the 1930s, with H. D. Rolleston's definition of endocrinology as the clinical and biochemical study of all aspects of the ductless glands. In the 1940s through the 1970s a number of technologic advances contributed to dramatic strides in knowledge about the endocrine system; the development of paper and column chromatography, completely automated amino acid analyzers, and solid phase peptide synthesis are some examples. Recent advances include the development of assays to determine hormonal levels, including radioimmunoassay and enzyme-linked immunosorbent assays, and genetic engineering techniques to manufacture human insulin. These techniques have contributed to further discoveries in the area of endocrinology. The intricate relationships among the endocrine, immunologic, and nervous systems are just beginning to be explored, offering the possibilities for the emergence of many new ideas about endocrine homeodynamics.

CHAPTER 17

Mechanisms of Hormonal Regulation

Sue E. Huether
D. Patricia Gray*

Chapter Outline

The endocrine system is composed of various glands located throughout the body (Fig. 17-1). These glands are capable of synthesizing and releasing special chemical messengers called **hormones.** The endocrine system has five general functions: (1) differentiation of the reproductive and central nervous systems in the developing fetus, (2) stimulation of sequential growth and development during childhood and adolescence, (3) coordination of the male and female reproductive systems, which makes sexual reproduction possible, (4) maintenance of an optimal internal environment throughout the lifespan, and (5) initiation of corrective and adaptive responses when emergency demands occur. Hormones convey specific regulatory information among cells and organs.

MECHANISMS OF HORMONAL REGULATION

The endocrine glands respond to specific signals by synthesizing and releasing hormones into the circulation. Although a wide variety of hormones function within the body, they share certain general characteristics:

1. Hormones have specific rates and patterns of secretion. Three basic secretion patterns are (a) diurnal patterns, (b) pulsatile and cyclic patterns, and (c) patterns that depend on levels of circulating substrates (e.g., calcium, sodium, potassium, or the hormones themselves). Diurnal, pulsatile, and cyclic patterns of hormone release involve consistent patterns of secretion.
2. Hormones operate within feedback systems, either positive or negative, to maintain an optimal internal environment.
3. Hormones affect only cells with appropriate receptors and then act on these cells to initiate specific cell functions or activities.
4. Hormones are constantly excreted by the kidneys or deactivated by the liver or by other cellular mechanisms.

Hormones may be classified according to structure, gland of origin, effects, or chemical composition. (Table 17-1 categorizes known hormones by structural category.) The secretion and mechanisms of action of hormones represent an extremely complex system of integrated responses. Although much has been learned about these complex systems, many of the specific mechanisms of action are not yet understood. The endocrine and nervous systems work together to regulate responses to the internal and external environment. Both secrete regulatory substances into the bloodstream, and both can generate electrical potentials (Berne & Levy, 1993).

Regulation of Hormone Release

The release of hormones occurs either in response to an alteration in the cellular environment or in the process of maintaining a regulated level of certain hormones or certain substances. The common processes that regulate endocrine gland secretion include negative feedback, endocrine regulation (a hormone from one endocrine gland controlling another endocrine gland), and neural control of endocrine glands.

Hormone secretion may be regulated by one or several regulatory mechanisms. For example, insulin is secreted in response to increased glucose levels (a chemical stimulus); to direct stimulation of the insulin-secreting cells of the pancreas by the autonomic nervous system (a neural stimulus); and to the secretion of cortisol by the adrenal medulla, a form of endocrine regulation.

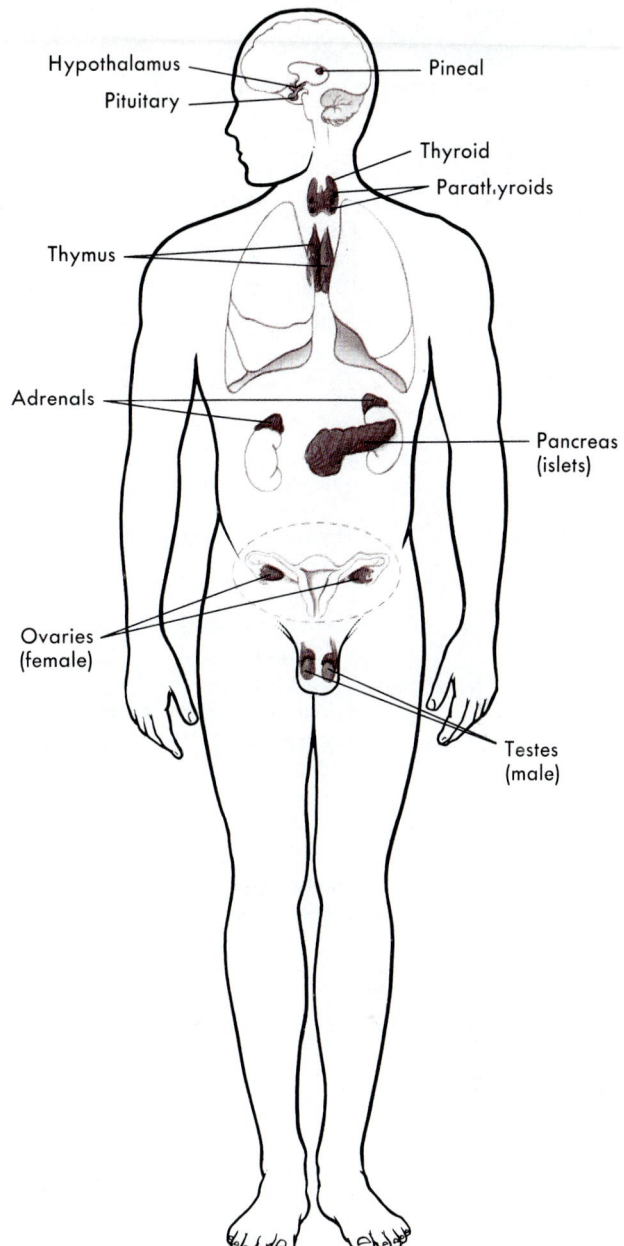

FIG. 17-1 The endocrine system. (From Thibodeau & Patton, 1993.)

Regulation of hormone secretion is achieved by a variety of feedback systems that provide precise monitoring and control of the cellular environment. **Negative feedback** is the most common feedback system. The feedback is negative because the rising hormone level negates the initiating change that triggered the release of the hormone. For example, if serum calcium levels fall (the initiating change), parathyroid hormone (PTH) secretion is increased. PTH causes an increase in serum calcium. The increase in calcium then serves to decrease PTH secretion, or to "turn off" the system. In this man-

TABLE 17-1

Structural Categories of Hormones

Structural category	Examples	Structural category	Examples
Proteins	Growth hormone Prolactin Insulin Parathyroid hormone	Amino acid derivatives	Epinephrine Norepinephrine Thyroxine (both T_4 and T_3) Melatonin

Glycoproteins	Follicle-stimulating hormone
	Luteinizing hormone
	Thyroid-stimulating hormone
		Lipids
		  Steroids (cholesterol is a
		    precursor for all steroids)
			Estrogens
			Progestins (progesterone)
			Testosterone
			Mineralocorticoids (aldosterone)
			Glucocorticoids (cortisol)

Polypeptides	Thyrotropin-releasing hormone Oxytocin Antidiuretic hormone Calcitonin Glucagon Adrenocorticotropic hormone Endorphins Thymosin Melanocyte-stimulating hormone Hypothalamic hormones Lipotropins Somatostatin	Fatty acids	Prostaglandins Thromboxanes Prostacyclins Leukotrienes

From Seeley, Stephens, & Tate, 1992.

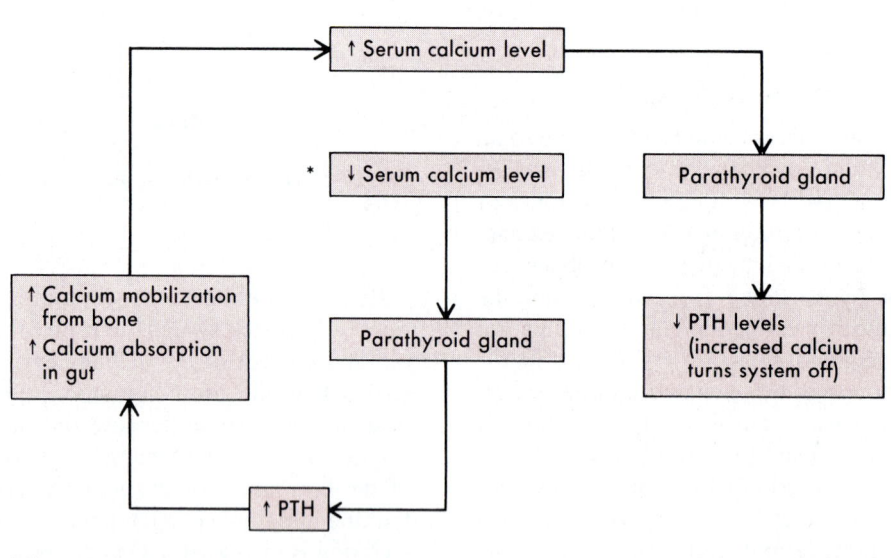

FIG. 17-2 Negative feedback for calcium regulation.

ner, serum calcium levels are maintained (Fig. 17-2). **Positive feedback,** which occurs when hormone secretion continues to trigger additional hormone secretion, rarely is seen in the endocrine system.

Feedback also is described in terms of ultra-short, short, and long feedback loops. The feedback loops are used to describe regulation of hormone secretion by hormones themselves (endocrine regulation). (These regulatory systems are diagrammed in Fig. 17-3.)

An example of neural regulation is the release of epinephrine from the adrenal medulla as a result of activation of the sympathetic division of the autonomic nervous system in response to stress. When the stress is removed, the nervous stimulation decreases and less epinephrine is released.

Hormone Transport

Once hormones are released into the circulatory system by the endocrine glands, they are distributed throughout the body. The protein hormones (insulin, pituitary, hypothalamic, and PTH) are water soluble and generally circulate in free (unbound) forms. This process immediately exposes these water-soluble hormones to circulating enzymes, giving them an expected half-life of seconds to minutes. Because of their composition, lipid-soluble hormones are transported primarily by carrier or binding proteins. The amount of bound hormone generally is determined by the amount of circulating binding protein. Water-soluble hormones pass through pores in the walls of capillaries, and lipid-soluble hormones diffuse through the walls of capillaries. Because

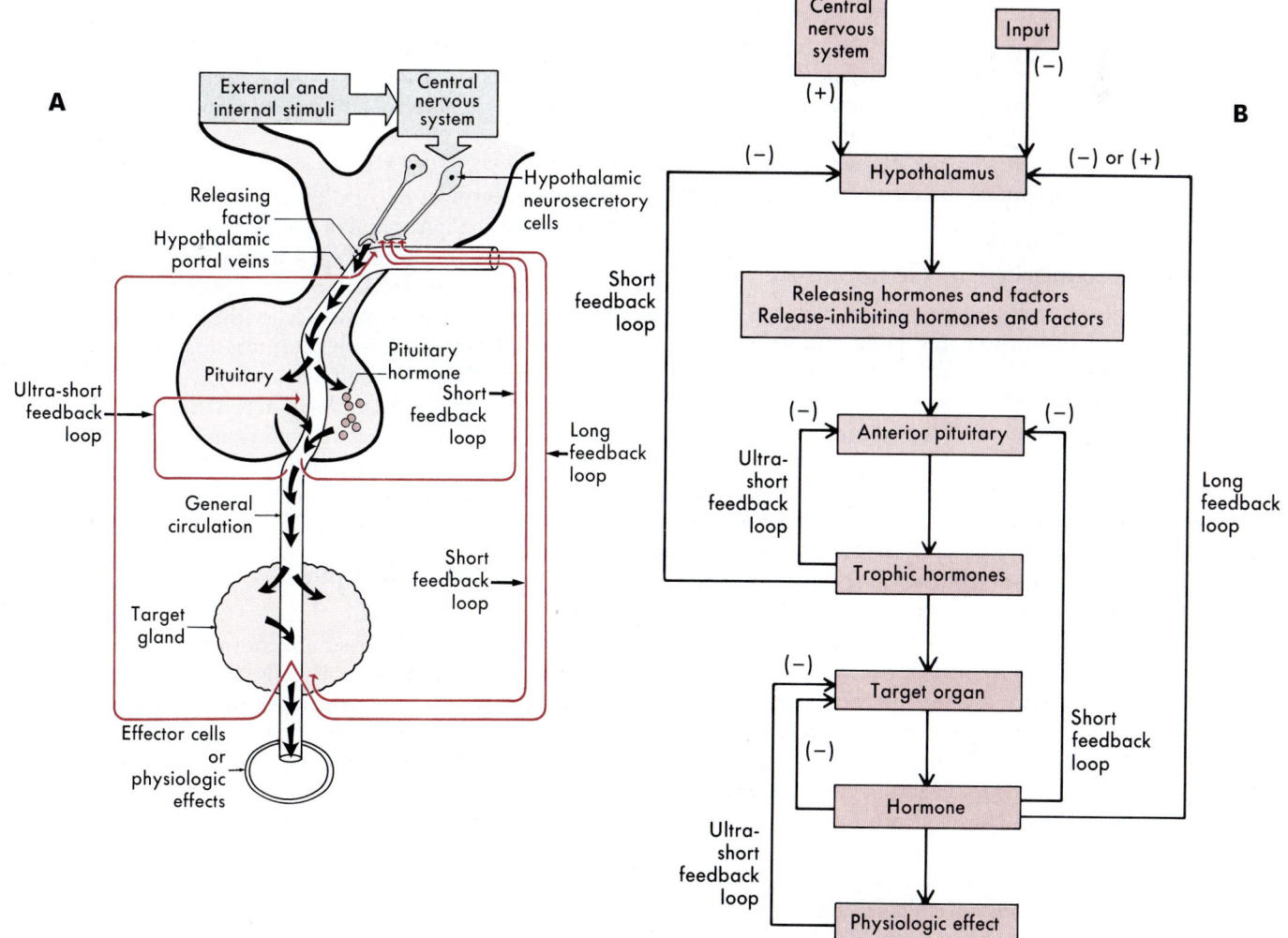

FIG. 17-3 Feedback loops. A, Endocrine feedback loops involving the hypothalamus—pituitary gland and end organs (endocrine regulation). **B,** General model for control and feedback to hypothalamic-pituitary target organ systems.

TABLE 17-2

Binding Proteins, Their Hormones, and Variables That Affect Their Circulating Levels

Binding protein	Hormone	Factors that increase binding protein	Factors that decrease binding protein
Corticosteroid-binding globulin	Cortisol Progesterone	Estrogen	Liver disease
Sex hormone–binding globulin	Dihydrotestosterone Testosterone Estradiol	—	Androgens Hypothyroidism Liver disease
Thyroid-binding globulin	T_4 T_3	Estrogen Hyperthyroidism	Testosterone Glucocorticoids Liver disease
Albumin	All lipid-soluble hormones	Estrogen	Liver disease Malnutrition Renal disease

T_4, Thyroxine; T_3, triiodothyronine.

an equilibrium exists between free hormones and hormones bound to plasma proteins, a large change in the concentration of binding proteins can affect the concentration of free hormones in the plasma (Table 17-2). (Mechanisms of hormone binding are discussed in Chapter 1.)

Cellular Mechanisms of Hormone Action

When a hormone is released into the circulatory system, it is distributed throughout the body, but only those cells with appropriate receptors for that hormone are affected. The **target cell** *hormone receptors* have two main functions: (1) to recognize and bind with high affinity to their particular hormones and (2) to initiate a signal to appropriate intracellular effectors.

Hormones have two general types of effects on target cells: direct and permissive. **Direct effects** are the obvious changes in cell function that specifically result from stimulation by a particular hormone. **Permissive effects** are less obvious hormone-induced changes that facilitate the maximal response or functioning of a cell. For example, insulin has a direct effect on skeletal muscle cells with insulin receptors, causing increased glucose transport into these cells. Insulin also has a permissive effect on mammary cells, facilitating the response of these cells to the direct effects of prolactin.

If hormones are excreted at supraphysiologic levels or are administered exogenously in high doses, a pharmacologic effect occurs. **Pharmacologic effects** are those cell responses seen only at extremely high hormone levels and may not reflect the actions of the hormone at usual or physiologic levels. For example, usual levels of antidiuretic hormone (ADH) affect the renal tubules, in-

creasing water absorption. At supraphysiologic, or pharmacologic, levels ADH acts as a vasoconstrictor.

Hormone Receptors

Hormone receptors may be located on the plasma membrane or in the intracellular compartment of the target cell. Water-soluble hormones, which include the protein hormones and the catecholamines, have a high molecular weight and cannot pass across the cell membrane. They interact or bind with receptors located in or on the cell membrane. Fat-soluble steroid, vitamin D, and thyroid hormones diffuse freely across the plasma and nuclear membranes and bind with primarily nuclear receptors (Fig. 17-4). (Types of hormones, their corresponding receptors, and the mechanisms by which they affect the cell are summarized in Table 17-3.)

Plasma Membrane Receptors
First messenger

Receptors for most water-soluble hormones are located in the plasma membranes of cells. The hormones are called **first messengers.** The receptors on the plasma membranes are continuously synthesized and degraded, so that changes in receptor concentration may occur within hours. In addition, the receptor's affinity for the hormone may vary. Both receptor affinity and receptor concentration are regulated by intracellular and extracellular mechanisms, which include the following:

Physicochemical environment
   pH
   Temperature
   Calcium concentration
   Sodium concentration

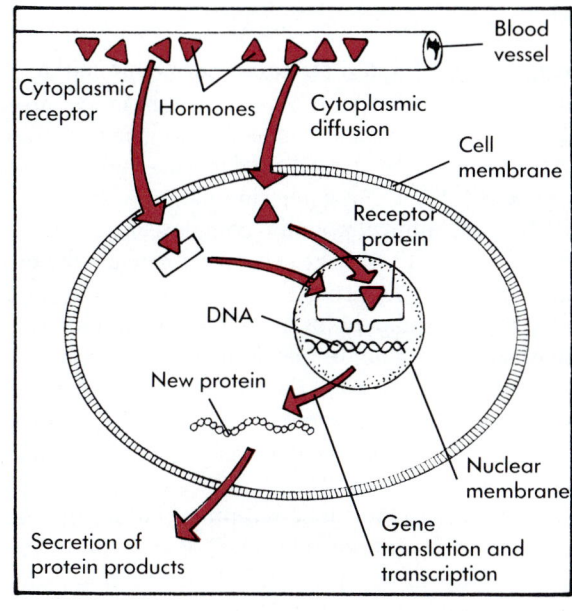

FIG. 17-4 Hormone receptors. **A,** Calcium as a second messenger. **B,** cAMP as second messenger. **C,** Receptors for lipid-soluble hormones are located in the nucleus. See text for more detailed explanation.

Urea concentration
   Levels of cyclic AMP (a "second messenger")
Lipid matrix of the plasma membrane
   Cholesterol content
   Saturation of fatty acid side chains
   Polar groups or phospholipids
   Alterations of the plasma membrane
Circulating levels of hormones
Stage of growth and development
Diet
Exercise
Drugs

The receptors for the water-soluble hormones serve first to recognize the hormone on the plasma membrane and then bind with the hormone. The receptor may span the membrane or weave in and out of it, drawing interaction with more than one signal-generating mechanism. Once recognition and binding have occurred, the hormone-receptor complex initiates the transmission of an intracellular signal by way of a "second messenger."

Second messenger

The signals initiated by hormone-receptor binding are transmitted into the cell by the action of a **second mes-**

TABLE 17-3

Types of Hormones, Their Receptors, and Their Mechanisms of Action

Hormone	Type of receptor	Mechanism of action
Water-soluble hormones		
Glycoproteins, amines, small peptides and proteins (except insulin)	Plasma membrane receptors	Second messenger, cAMP, cGMP, Ca^{++}, others
Insulin	Plasma membrane receptors	Second messenger other than cAMP, cGMP, or Ca^{++}
Lipid-soluble hormones		
Steroid hormones	Nuclear receptors	Nuclear translocation and altered genome transcription
Thyroid hormones (iodothyronines)	Nuclear receptors Cytosolic receptors	Altered genome transcription

From Lefkowitz, 1982.
cAMP, Cyclic adenosine monophosphate; *cGMP*, cyclic guanosine monophosphate.

TABLE 17-4

Second Messengers Identified for Specific Hormones

Second messenger	Associated hormones
Cyclic AMP	Adrenocorticotropic hormone (ACTH)
	Luteinizing hormone (LH)
	Human chorionic gonadotropin (HCG)
	Follicle-stimulating hormone (FSH)
	Thyroid-stimulating hormone (TSH)
	Antidiuretic hormone (ADH)
	Thyrotropin-releasing hormone (TRH)
	Parathyroid hormone (PTH)
	Glucagon
Cyclic GMP	Atrial natriuretic peptide
Calcium-calmodulin	Angiotensin II
	Gonadotropin-releasing hormone (GnRH)
Unidentified	Insulin
	Growth hormone
	Prolactin

senger (see Chapter 1). Some hormones initiate reactions by coupling with plasma membrane G proteins. They stimulate effector molecules to generate a second messenger, such as cyclic adenosine monophosphate (cyclic AMP), cyclic guanosine monophosphate (cyclic GMP), calcium-calmodulin complex, and prostaglandins (see Fig. 17-4). The second messengers for insulin, growth hormone, prolactin, and others have yet to be identified. Insulin binds to a tyrosine-kinase receptor that regulates glucose metabolism by phosphorylation or dephosphorylation. Evidence suggests that second messengers for these hormones do exist. (The hormones and their associated second messengers are listed in Table 17-4.)

Cyclic AMP. Hormone-receptor binding initiates an increase in the intracellular level of the second messenger. For this to occur a series of interactions within the plasma membrane must take place. For cells having cyclic AMP as a second messenger, the purpose of these interactions is to activate the intracellular cyclic nucleotides, adenylate or guanylate cyclase. Adenylate cyclase is an enzyme that converts adenosine triphosphate (ATP) to cyclic AMP, whereas **guanylate cyclase** enzymatically converts guanosine triphosphate (GTP) to cyclic GMP.

An example of the function of cyclic AMP as a second messenger can be seen with the action of the hormone epinephrine. Epinephrine stimulates breakdown of glycogen to glucose in the liver. Once activated by the epinephrine-receptor complex, adenylate cyclase catalyzes the synthesis of cyclic AMP. Cyclic AMP, in turn, activates the enzyme protein kinase, which then catalyzes the phosphorylation (addition of a phosphate group) to yet another enzyme, phosphorylase kinase. Activated phosphorylase kinase phosphorylates (and thus activates) another enzyme that catalyzes the breakdown of glycogen to glucose. Thus an elaborate cascade emerges in which inactive enzymes are converted in sequence to active enzymes, leading to glycogen breakdown.

Calcium. Like cAMP, calcium ions within the cell function as a second messenger for certain hormones, such as angiotensin II and gonadotropin-releasing hormone. Hormone-receptor binding through a G protein results in an influx of calcium ions into the cytoplasm, either from the extracellular fluid or from internal cellular stores (see Fig. 17-4). With the rise in intracellular calcium, calcium ions bind with an intracellular regulatory protein, calmodulin. The calcium-calmodulin complex mediates the effects of calcium on intracellular activities. These effects are similar to the actions of the cyclic nucleotides on intracellular protein kinases. The calmodulin-dependent protein kinases are involved in control of intracellular contractile components, alteration of plasma membrane permeability, and regulation of intracellular enzyme activity. Calcium-calmodulin and the cyclic nucleotides appear to interact in regulating the cell's metabolic and physiologic response to hormonal stimulation. These second messengers may act synergistically with each other or as antagonists to each other in achieving their effects.

Steroid Hormones (Lipid Soluble)

The lipid-soluble hormones are classified as steroid hormones (including androgens, estrogens, progestins, glucocorticoids, and mineralocorticoids) and thyroid hormones. Because steroid hormones are relatively small hydrophobic molecules (synthesized from cholesterol), they can cross the plasma membrane by simple diffusion (see Chapter 1). Some hormones bind to receptor molecules in the cytoplasm and then diffuse into the nucleus. Hormones without cytoplasmic receptors diffuse directly into the nucleus and bind with an acceptor molecule. Once activated by hormones, the receptor is thought to bind to specific sites on the chromatin of the target cell, causing RNA transcription and increased synthesis of specific proteins (discussed in Chapter 4).

STRUCTURE AND FUNCTION OF THE ENDOCRINE GLANDS

Hypothalamic-Pituitary System

The hormones of the pituitary gland regulate several other endocrine glands and affect a number of diverse bodily functions. Part of the pituitary gland is directly connected to the brain, and the pituitary gland also is closely related to the nervous system. Some of the hormones secreted by the pituitary gland act directly on organs of the reproductive system (see Unit VII). Other hormones act in conjunction with the thyroid and adrenal glands and with the endocrine pancreas.

The hypothalamic-pituitary unit forms the structural and functional basis for central integration of the neurologic and endocrine systems (Figs. 17-5 and 17-6). The hypothalamus, containing special neurosecretory cells and located at the base of the brain, is connected to the pituitary gland by a stalklike structure, the **infundibular stem.** The special cells of the hypothalamus are like other neurons in that they have similar electrical properties, organelles, membranes, and synapses. Neurosecretory cells, however, are able to synthesize and to secrete the hypothalamic-releasing hormones and to synthesize the hormones of the posterior portion of the pituitary gland.

The **pituitary gland** is located in the sella turcica (a saddle-shaped depression on the superior surface of the body). The pituitary gland weighs approximately 0.5 g, except during pregnancy when its weight approaches 1 g. It is composed of two distinctly different lobes: (1) the posterior pituitary, or neurohypophysis, and (2) the anterior pituitary, or adenohypophysis. These two lobes differ in their embryonic origins, cell types, and functional relationship to the hypothalamus.

The embryonic posterior pituitary (neurohypophysis) is derived from the hypothalamus and comprises three parts: (1) the median eminence located at the base of the hypothalamus, (2) the infundibular stem, and (3) the infundibular process, also known as the pars nervosa or neural lobe. The **median eminence** is composed largely of the nerve endings of axons that arise primarily in the ventral hypothalamus. The median eminence often is designated as part of the posterior pituitary but contains at least 10 biologically active hypothalamic-releasing hormones, as well as the neurotransmitters dopamine, norepinephrine, serotonin, acetylcholine, and histamine. The median eminence therefore might be more appropriately considered part of the hypothalamus. The infundibular stem contains the axons of neurons that originate in the supraoptic and paraventricular nuclei of the hypothalamus. The infundibular stem thus connects the pituitary gland to the brain. Axons originating in the hypothalamus terminate in the **infundibular process,** which secretes the hormones of the posterior pituitary.

The anterior pituitary (adenohypophysis) accounts for 75% of the total weight of the pituitary gland. It is composed of three regions: (1) the pars distalis, (2) the pars tuberalis, and (3) the pars intermedia. The **pars distalis** is the major component of the anterior pituitary and the source of the anterior pituitary hormones. The **pars tuberalis** is a thin layer of cells on the anterior and lateral portions of the infundibular stem. The **pars in-**

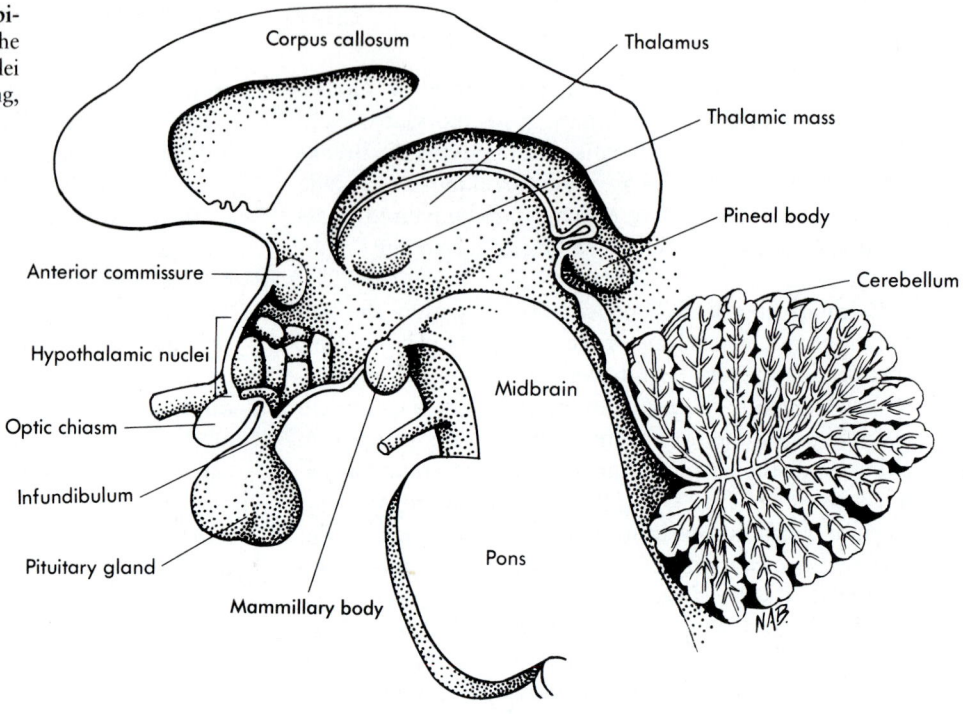

FIG. 17-5 **Hypothalamic nuclei and pituitary gland.** Sagittal section through the brain showing the hypothalamic nuclei and pituitary gland. (From Phipps, Long, Woods, & Cassmeyer, 1991.)

Corpus callosum

Thalamus

Thalamic mass

Pineal body

Cerebellum

Anterior commissure

Hypothalamic nuclei

Optic chiasm

Infundibulum

Pituitary gland

Mammillary body

Midbrain

Pons

FIG. 17-6 **Anterior pituitary hormones and their target hormones:** adrenocorticotropic hormone *(ACTH)*; thyroid-stimulating hormone *(TSH)*; follicle-stimulating hormone *(FSH)*; luteinizing hormone *(LH)*; male analogue of LH *(interstitial cell–stimulating hormone [ICSH])*; melanocyte-stimulating hormone *(MSH)*. (From Thibodeau & Patton, 1993.)

Anterior pituitary gland (adenohypophysis)

MSH (stimulates pigmentation)

Skin

ACTH

GH (STH) (stimulates protein anabolism, growth)

Prolactin

Gonadotropins (FSH, LH, ICSH)

Adrenal cortex

Breast

Bone

Muscle

TSH

Testis

Ovary

Thyroid

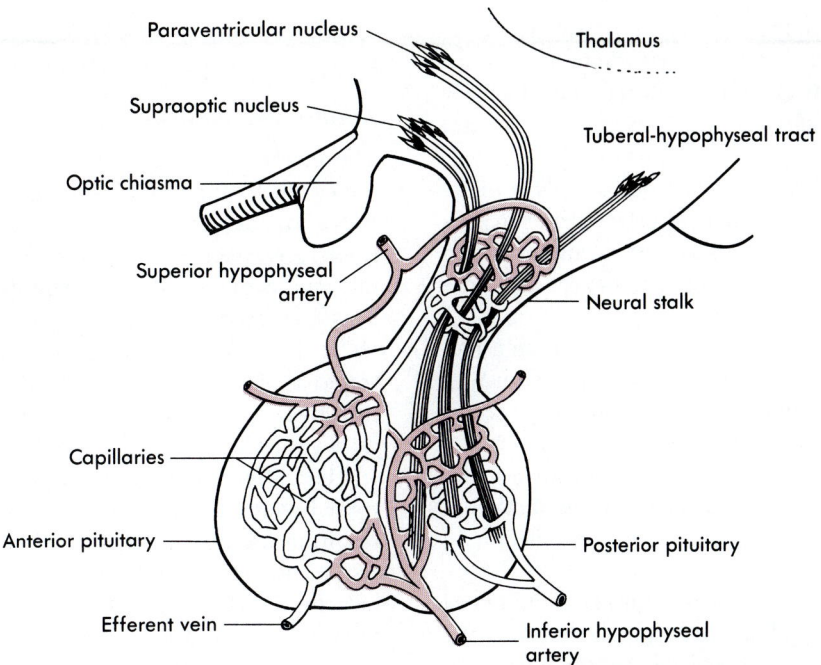

FIG. 17-7 **Blood supply to the anterior pituitary and posterior pituitary.** (From Phipps, Long, Woods, & Cassmeyer, 1991.)

TABLE 17-5

Hypothalamic Hormones

Hormone	Target tissue	Action
Thyrotropin-releasing hormone (TRH)	Anterior pituitary	Stimulates release of thyroid-stimulating hormone (TSH) Modulates prolactin secretion
Gonadotropin-releasing hormone (GnRH)	Anterior pituitary	Stimulates release of follicle-stimulating hormone (FSH) and luteinizing hormone (LH)
Somatostatin	Anterior pituitary Gastrointestinal tract	Inhibits release of growth hormone (GH) Decreases gastric motility, intestinal secretion, and secretion of TSH, parathyroid hormone, renin, glucagon, and insulin
Growth hormone–releasing factor (GRF)	Anterior pituitary	Stimulates release of GH
Corticotropin-releasing hormone (CRH)	Anterior pituitary	Stimulates release of adrenocorticotropic hormone (ACTH) and beta-endorphin
Substance P	Anterior pituitary	Inhibits synthesis and release of ACTH Stimulates secretion of GH, FSH, LH, and prolactin
Prolactin-inhibiting factor (PIF; possibly dopamine)	Anterior pituitary	Inhibits secretion of prolactin
Prolactin-releasing hormone (PRH)	Anterior pituitary	Stimulates secretion of prolactin

termedia lies between the two lobes of the pituitary gland. In the adult the distinct intermediate lobe disappears and the individual cells are distributed diffusely throughout the pars distalis and pars nervosa (neural lobe) (Reichlin, 1985).

The pituitary gland receives its blood supply primarily from a special portal system (illustrated in Fig. 17-7). This system of blood flow facilitates communication among the hypothalamus, median eminence, and adenohypophysis.

The hormones—neurotransmitters and releasing factors—secreted by the hypothalamus serve as major regulators of anterior pituitary function. The neurosecretory products released into the portal system are known technically as *releasing hormones* if their chemical structures have been identified and as **releasing factors** if there is evidence of their presence but no definitive chemical identification.

When hypothalamic neurons are stimulated and neurosecretory cells respond by releasing hormones, the neurosecretory products are released into the portal circulation and travel to the anterior pituitary. The neurosecretory products apparently bind to plasma membrane receptors in the anterior pituitary, where their action is mediated by cyclic AMP.

The hypothalamus synthesizes and releases hormones that regulate secretion by other glands. These hormones include **prolactin-inhibiting factor (PIF), thyrotropin-releasing hormone (TRH), gonadotropin-releasing hormone (GnRH), somatostatin, growth hormone–releasing factor (GRF), corticotropin-releasing hormone (CRH),** and **substance P.** These hormones are summarized in Table 17-5.

Hormones of the Posterior Pituitary

The posterior pituitary secretes two polypeptide hormones: (1) **antidiuretic hormone (ADH),** also called vasopressin, and (2) **oxytocin.** These peptide hormones are similar in structure, differing by only two amino acids. They are synthesized, along with their binding proteins, the neurophysins, in the supraoptic and paraventricular nuclei of the hypothalamus (Fig. 17-8). Once synthesized, the hormones and their carrier proteins are packaged in secretory vesicles. They are moved down the axons of the infundibular stem to the infundibular process for storage. The posterior pituitary thus can be seen as a storage and releasing site for hormones synthesized in the hypothalamus.

The release of ADH and oxytocin is mediated by cholinergic and adrenergic neurotransmitters. Stimulation of the cholinergic receptors by acetylcholine, angiotensin II, and β-endorphins stimulates the release of ADH and oxytocin, whereas activation of β-adrenergic receptors inhibits hormone secretion. Before release into the

circulatory system, ADH and oxytocin are split from the neurophysins and are secreted in unbound form.

Antidiuretic hormone

The major homeostatic function of the posterior pituitary is the control of plasma osmolality as regulated by ADH, or vasopressin (see Chapter 3). At physiologic levels, ADH acts to increase the permeability of the distal renal tubules and collecting ducts (see Chapter 32). This increased permeability leads to an increase in water reabsorption and the production of more concentrated urine. These effects may be inhibited by hypercalcemia, prostaglandin E, and hypokalemia. ADH has no direct effect on electrolyte levels.

ADH originally was named *vasopressin* because in extremely high doses it does cause vasoconstriction and a resulting increase in arterial blood pressure. These levels are not reached physiologically, but this effect may be achieved pharmacologically. For example, high doses of ADH (as the drug vasopressin) may be administered to achieve hemostasis during hemorrhage.

The secretion of ADH is regulated primarily by the osmoreceptors of the hypothalamus, located near or in the supraoptic nuclei (osmoreceptors are stimulated by increased osmolality). The plasma osmolality is maintained at the mean set point of approximately 280 mOsm/kg. As plasma osmolality increases, the rate of ADH secretion increases.

Other mechanisms affect ADH secretion. ADH secretion is increased by changes in intravascular volume. Intravascular volume changes are monitored by baroreceptors in the left atrium and in the carotid and aortic arches. A volume loss of 7% to 25% acts through these receptors to stimulate ADH secretion. This mechanism for regulating ADH secretion is much less sensitive than that of the osmoreceptors. Stress, trauma, pain, exercise, nausea, nicotine, exposure to heat, and drugs such as chloroform and morphine also increase ADH secretion, apparently by activating cholinergic neurotransmitters in the hypothalamus. ADH secretion decreases with a decrease in plasma osmolality, an increase in intravascular volume, hypertension, and alcohol ingestion.

Oxytocin

Oxytocin is responsible for contraction of the uterus and milk ejection in lactating women and may have a role in sperm motility in men, although this effect has not yet been clearly elucidated. In both sexes, oxytocin has an antidiuretic effect similar to that of ADH. The mechanisms by which this effect is achieved appear similar to those of ADH, but the physiologic significance is not clear. (The function of this hormone is discussed in Chapter 19.)

The release of oxytocin has been studied more exten-

FIG. 17-8 **Nerve tracts from hypothalamus to posterior lobe of pituitary gland.** (From Thompson, McFarland, Hirsch, & Tucker, 1993.)

sively in women. In the woman, oxytocin is secreted in response to suckling and mechanical distention of the female reproductive tract. Oxytocin is required for the milk "let-down" reflex. Stimulated by sucking, oxytocin binds to its receptors on myoepithelial cells in the mammary tissues and causes contraction of those cells. This results in increased intramammary pressure and milk expression.

Oxytocin also acts on the uterus to stimulate contractions. Its role in initiating labor has been debated because levels of oxytocin do not increase until near the end of labor. At this stage, oxytocin functions to enhance effectiveness of contractions, to promote delivery of the placenta, and to stimulate postpartum contractions to prevent excessive bleeding (Martin, 1985).

Hormones of the Anterior Pituitary

The anterior pituitary is composed of two main cell types: (1) the **chromophobes,** which appear to be nonsecretory, and (2) the **chromophils,** which are consid-

ered the secretory cells of the adenohypophysis. The chromophils are subdivided into six secretory cell types, and each cell type secretes specific hormone(s) (Table 17-6).

In general, the regulation of the anterior pituitary hormones is achieved by the following mechanisms: (1) secretion of hypothalamic peptide hormones or releasing factors, (2) feedback effects of the hormones secreted by target glands, and (3) direct effects of other mediating neurotransmitters. (These mechanisms are summarized in Fig. 17-3.)

The hormones secreted by the anterior pituitary include adrenocorticotropic hormone (ACTH), melanocyte-stimulating hormone (MSH), somatotropic hormones (growth hormone and prolactin), and the glycoprotein hormones (follicle-stimulating hormone, luteinizing hormone including the male analogue of LH [interstitial cell-stimulating hormone—ICSH], and thyroid-stimulating hormone). Each of these hormones affects the physiologic function of specific target organs (see Fig. 17-3 and Table 17-6).

TABLE 17-6

Hormones of the Anterior Pituitary and Their Functions

Hormone	Secretory cell type	Target organs	Functions
Adrenocorticotropic hormone (ACTH)	Corticotropic	Adrenal gland	Increased steroidogenesis Synthesis of adrenal proteins contributing to maintenance of the adrenal gland
Melanocyte-stimulating hormone (MSH)	Melanotropic	Anterior pituitary	Promotes secretion of melanin and lipotropin by anterior pituitary; makes skin darker
Somatotropic hormones: Growth hormone (GH)	Somatotropic	Muscle, bone, liver	Regulates metabolic processes related to growth and adaptation to physical and emotional stressors, including skeletal growth, muscle growth, increased protein synthesis, increased liver glycogenolysis, increased fat mobilization
		Liver	Induces formation of somatomedins, or insulin-like growth factors (IGF) that have actions similar to insulin
Prolactin	Lactotropic	Breast	Milk production
Glycoprotein hormones: Thyroid-stimulating hormone (TSH)	Thyrotropic	Thyroid gland	Increased production and secretion of thyroid hormone Increased iodine uptake
Luteinizing hormone (LH)	Gonadotropic	In women: ovarian follicle	Ovulation, progesterone production
		In men: Leydig's cells	Regulates spermatogenesis, testosterone production
Follicle-stimulating hormone (FSH)	Gonadotropic	In women: ovarian follicle	Follicle maturation, estrogen production
		In men: Leydig's cell	Spermatogenesis
β-Lipotropin	Corticotropic	Adipose cells	Fat breakdown and release of fatty acids
β-Endorphins	Corticotropic	Adipose cells	Analgesia; may regulate body temperature, food and water intake

Thyroid and Parathyroid Glands

The thyroid gland, located in the neck just below the larynx, produces hormones that control the rates of metabolic processes throughout the body. The parathyroid glands are located near the thyroid. The four parathyroid glands function to control serum calcium levels.

Thyroid Gland

The **thyroid gland** is composed of two lobes that lie on either side of the trachea, inferior to the thyroid cartilage (Fig. 17-9). The lobes are joined by a small band of tissue, the **isthmus,** which crosses the anterior surface of the trachea and larynx at the cricoid cartilage. The normal thyroid gland is not visible on inspection, but it may be palpated on swallowing, which causes upward displacement of the gland.

The thyroid gland is composed of **follicles.** The follicles are composed of follicular cells that surround a viscous substance called *colloid.* The follicular cells synthesize and secrete some of the thyroid hormones. Neurons terminate on blood vessels within the thyroid gland and on the follicular cells themselves. This anatomic finding suggests that neurotransmitters may directly af-

TABLE 17-7

Thyroid Gland Hormones and Their Regulation and Function

Hormone	Regulation	Functions

Thyroxine (T_4) and triiodothyronine (T_3)	T_4 and T_3 levels are controlled by TSH
	Hormones show diurnal variation with a peak during late evening
	Influences on amount secreted
	  Gender
	  Pregnancy
	  Gonadal- and adrenal cortical–increased steroids = ↑ levels
	  Exposure to extreme cold = ↑ levels
	  Nutritional state
	  Chemicals
	    GHIH = ↓ levels
	    Dopamine = ↓ levels
	    Catecholamines = ↑ levels
		Regulates protein, fat, and carbohydrate catabolism in all cells
		Regulates metabolic rate of all cells
		Regulates body heat production
		Insulin antagonist
		Maintains growth hormone secretion, skeletal maturation
		Affects CNS development
		Necessary for muscle tone and vigor
		Maintains cardiac rate, force, and output
		Maintains secretion of GI tract
		Affects respiratory rate and oxygen utilization
		Maintains calcium mobilization
		Affects RBC production
		Stimulates lipid turnover, free fatty acid release, and cholesterol synthesis

Calcitonin	Elevated serum calcium—major stimulant for calcitonin
	Other stimulants
	  Gastrin
	  Calcium-rich foods (regardless of serum Ca^{++} levels)
	  Pregnancy
	Lowered serum calcium—suppresses calcitonin release
		Major function:
		  Lowers serum calcium by opposing bone-resorbing effects of PTH, prostaglandins, and calciferols by inhibiting osteoclastic activity
		Also lowers serum phosphate levels
		May also decrease calcium and phosphorus absorption in GI tract

From Long, Phipps, & Cassmeyer, 1992.

fect secretory activity of the follicular cells (Ahren, 1986).

Also found in the tissue of the thyroid are parafollicular cells, or **C cells.** The C cells secrete various polypeptides, including calcitonin and somatostatin (Ahren, 1986). **Calcitonin,** also called *thyrocalcitonin,* acts to lower serum calcium levels by direct, rapid, and significant inhibition of bone-resorbing osteoclasts and promotion of osteoblasts that result in bone formation. (Bone resorption is explained in Chapter 21.) The metabolic consequences of calcitonin deficiency or excess, however, have not yet been identified in human beings (see Table 17-7).

Regulation of thyroid hormone secretion

Thyroid hormone (TH) is regulated through a negative feedback loop involving the hypothalamus, the anterior pituitary, and the thyroid gland (see Fig. 17-3). (Fig. 17-9 illustrates the thyroid and parathyroid glands.) The initiating hormone is termed thyrotropin-releasing hor-

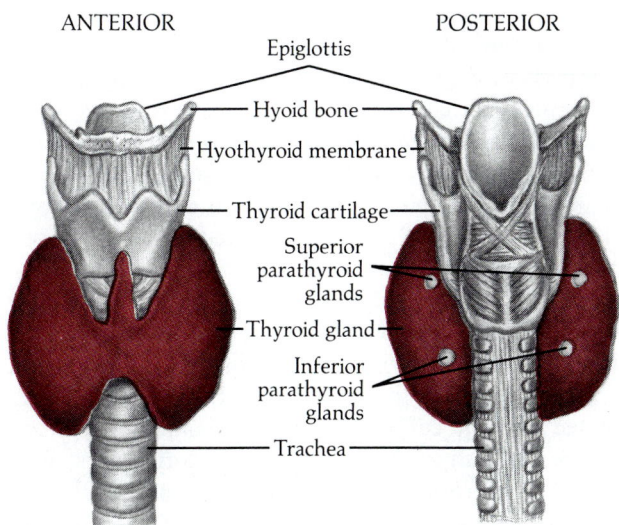

FIG. 17-9 Thyroid and parathyroid glands. Note their location to each other and to the larynx and trachea. (From Thompson, McFarland, Hirsch, & Tucker, 1993.)

mone (TRH) and it is synthesized and stored within the hypothalamus. TRH is released into the hypothalamic-pituitary portal system and circulates to the anterior pituitary, where it stimulates the release of thyroid-stimulating hormone (TSH). TRH is increased with exposure to cold, stress, and decreased levels of thyroxine (T_4).

Thyroid-stimulating hormone (TSH) is a glycoprotein hormone synthesized and stored within the anterior pituitary. Once TSH is secreted by the anterior pituitary, it circulates to bind with TSH receptor sites located on the outer side of the thyroid cell's plasma membrane. The effects of TSH on the thyroid include (1) an immediate increase in the release of stored thyroid hormones, (2) an increase in iodine uptake and oxidation, (3) an increase in thyroid hormone synthesis, and (4) an increase in the synthesis and secretion of prostaglandins by the thyroid. Thyroid gland hormones and their regulation and function are summarized in Table 17-7.

When TH is secreted by the thyroid gland, it acts on the thyroid gland, the anterior pituitary, and the median eminence to regulate further TH production. Thyroid hormones have a negative feedback effect and inhibit TRH and TSH, which decreases TH synthesis and secretion.

Synthesis of thyroid hormone

The thyroid gland is stimulated to produce thyroid hormone by TSH, by low serum iodide levels, or by drugs interfering with the thyroid gland's uptake of iodide in the blood. The first step in the synthesis of TH is the concentration of iodide (an iodine compound) by the thyroid gland. Because there is a iodine concentration gradient of about 30 to 40:1 between the thyroid gland and the blood, iodine is moved by active transport from the extracellular fluid to the thyroid follicular cells. (Mechanisms of active transport are discussed in Chapter 1.) Before being used to form TH, however, the iodide must be oxidized to iodine. This reaction is facilitated by the enzyme peroxidase inside the follicular cells. The major naturally occurring source of iodine is seafood; in the United States iodine is added to salt and flour. Approximately 25% of ingested iodine is trapped by the thyroid gland.

For the synthesis of TH to occur, another molecule, thyroglobulin, also must be present. **Thyroglobulin** is a large glycoprotein synthesized within the follicular cell. After its synthesis the uniodinated thyroglobulin is released into the colloid. Iodine then combines with tyrosine in the thyroglobulin to form iodotyrosines. Two major iodotyrosines are monoiodotyrosine (MIT) with one iodine molecule and diiodotyrosine (DIT) with two iodine molecules. Several hours after the iodotyrosines are formed, coupling of the iodotyrosines takes place to form iodothyronines, two of which are active thyroid

hormones. The exact mechanism for this coupling is not clearly understood. The most commonly held view is that two DIT molecules are coupled to form **thyroxine** (T_4), and one DIT and one MIT molecule are joined to form **triiodothyronine** (T_3). The thyroid gland normally produces 90% T_4 and 10% T_3. In the body tissues, however, T_4 is converted to T_3, and T_3 probably has the greatest metabolic effects. Once released into the circulation, about 99% of T_3 and T_4 is bound to thyroxine-binding globulin for transport to body tissues.

Action of thyroid hormones

Thyroid hormone affects most body tissues by increasing the rate of protein, fat, and glucose metabolism and as a result increases body temperature. Normal growth and development also require thyroid hormone, as does the effectiveness of growth hormone.

Parathyroid Glands

Two pairs of parathyroid glands are normally present. They are small and located behind the upper pole of the thyroid gland and behind the lower pole (see Fig. 17-9). The number of parathyroid glands, however, may range from two to six.

The parathyroid glands produce **parathyroid hormone** (PTH), a regulator of serum calcium. PTH is regulated primarily by the level of ionized plasma calcium, although these regulatory mechanisms are not precisely clear. Calcium also increases intraparathyroid destruction of PTH but apparently does not affect the rate of PTH synthesis.

Magnesium and phosphate levels also affect PTH secretion. Hypomagnesemia in persons with normal calcium levels acts as a mild stimulant to PTH secretion. In hypocalcemic persons, hypomagnesemia decreases PTH secretion. Hyperphosphatemia leads to hypocalcemia, probably because of calcium-phosphate precipitation in soft tissue and bone. Alterations in serum phosphate levels therefore may indirectly influence PTH secretion by affecting serum calcium levels (Fig. 17-10). The overall effect of PTH is to decrease serum phosphate concentration.

Once the parathyroid gland is stimulated, PTH is secreted. On release, PTH enters the circulation in unbound form. The hormone attaches to plasma membrane receptors in target tissues, where the biologic effects of PTH are mediated primarily by activation of the adenylate cyclase system (see Chapter 1).

PTH is the single most important factor in the regulation of serum calcium levels (Fig. 17-11). To achieve regulation of serum calcium, PTH acts directly on bone and on the kidneys. In bone, PTH has at least two effects. The effect of intense acute stimulation involves the breakdown and resorption of bone (see Chapter 21).

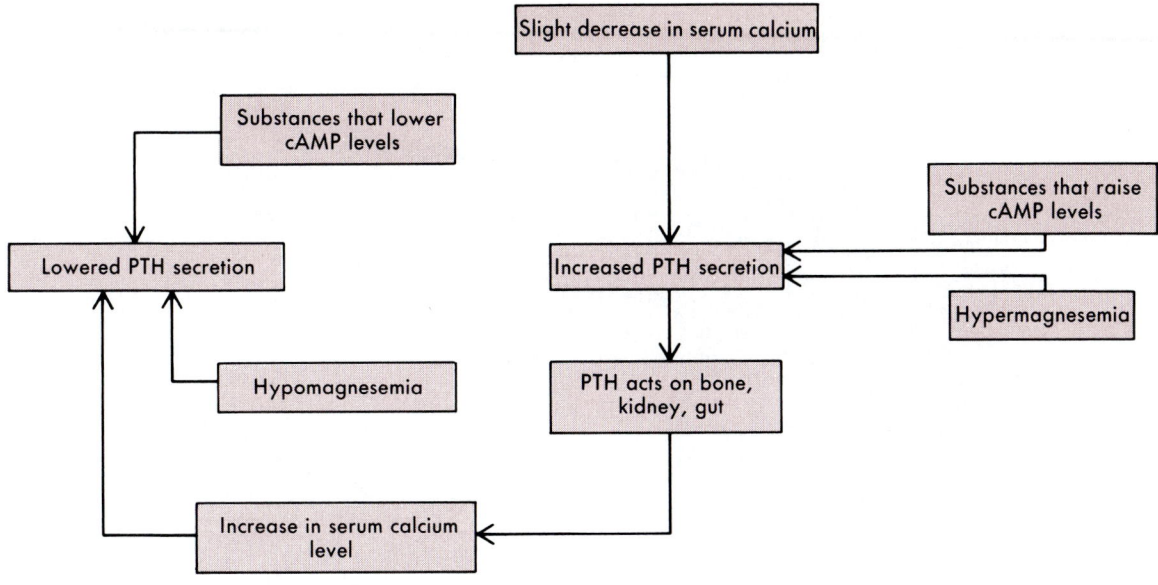

FIG. 17-10 Variables affecting PTH secretion.

FIG. 17-11 Normal calcium metabolism regulated by PTH. (Adapted from Ezrin, Godden, & Volpe, 1979.)

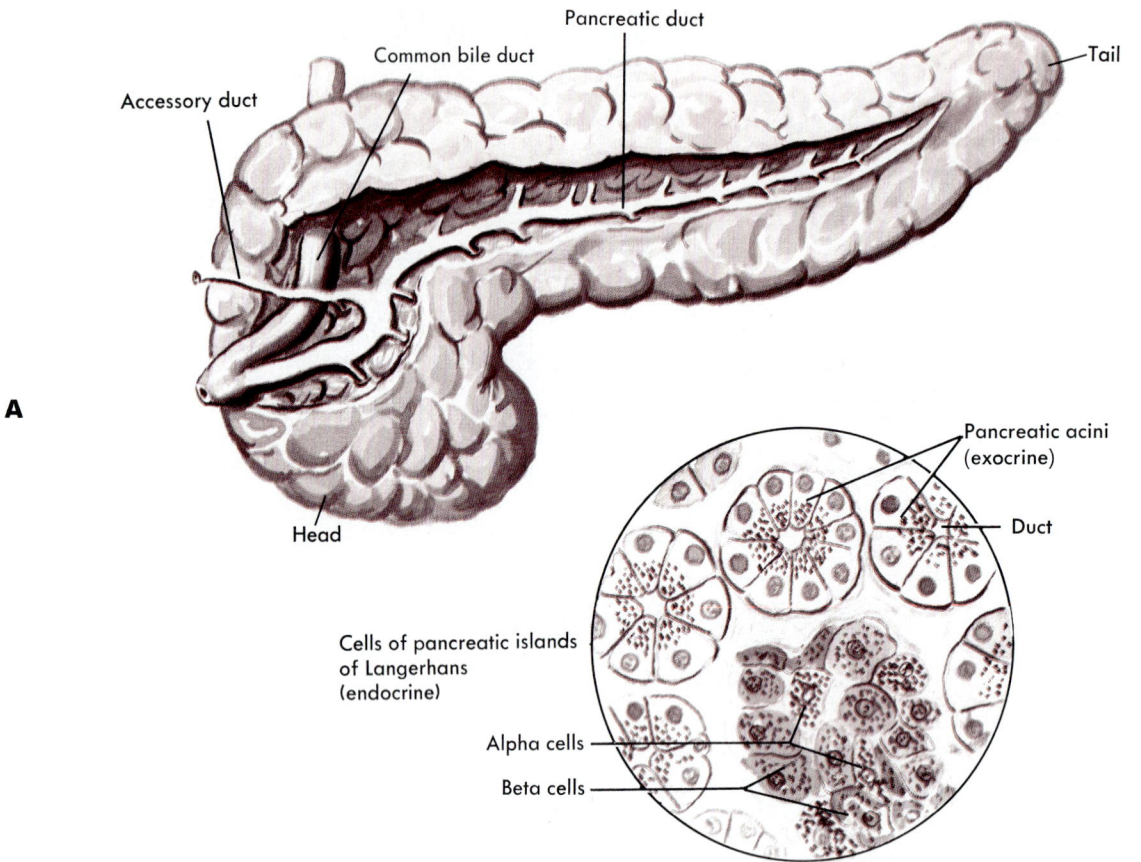

Accessory duct

Common bile duct

Pancreatic duct

Tail

A

B

Head

Pancreatic acini
(exocrine)

Duct

Cells of pancreatic islands
of Langerhans
(endocrine)

Alpha cells

Beta cells

Exocrine cells

C

Island of Langerhans

FIG. 17-12 The pancreas. A, Pancreas dissected to show main and accessory ducts. **B,** Exocrine and endocrine glandular cells. Alpha endocrine cells secrete glucagon, and beta cells secrete insulin. **C,** Photomicrograph of pancreas showing pancreatic islands and adjacent exocrine cells (×150). (From Thibodeau, 1987.)

Chronic stimulation by PTH results in bone remodeling, a process in which bone is broken down and reformed.

In the kidneys, PTH acts on its plasma membrane receptor in the proximal tubule of the nephron to increase reabsorption of calcium and to decrease reabsorption of phosphorus. PTH also decreases proximal tubule reabsorption of bicarbonate. In the kidney, PTH stimulates the synthesis of a biologically active form of vitamin D, a potent stimulator of calcium and phosphate transport in the intestine. In this way PTH apparently increases gastrointestinal absorption of calcium.

Endocrine Pancreas

The **pancreas** is both an endocrine gland that produces hormones and an exocrine gland that produces digestive enzymes. (The exocrine pancreas is discussed in Chapter 35.) The pancreas therefore is responsible for much metabolism within the body. A major disorder of the endocrine pancreas is diabetes mellitus.

The pancreas is located behind the stomach, between the spleen and the duodenum. It houses the **islets of Langerhans,** which secrete **glucagon** and **insulin,** hormones that help to regulate much of the carbohydrate, fat, and protein metabolism within the body. The islets of Langerhans have three types of hormone-secreting cells: **alpha cells,** which secrete glucagon; **beta cells,** which secrete insulin; and **delta cells,** which secrete gastrin or somatostatin, or both. The alpha and delta cells are located at the periphery of the islet, and beta cells are located in the middle. F cells, a fourth type of pancreatic cell, secrete pancreatic polypeptide. (The pancreas is illustrated in Fig. 17-12.) Nerves from both divisions of the autonomic nervous system innervate the pancreatic islets.

Insulin

The beta cells of the pancreas synthesize insulin from the precursor, proinsulin. Proinsulin is formed from a larger and earlier precursor molecule, preproinsulin. Proinsulin is composed of an A peptide and a B peptide connected by a C peptide and two disulfide bonds. C peptide is cleaved by proteolytic enzymes, leaving the A and B peptide chain connected by the disulfide bonds.

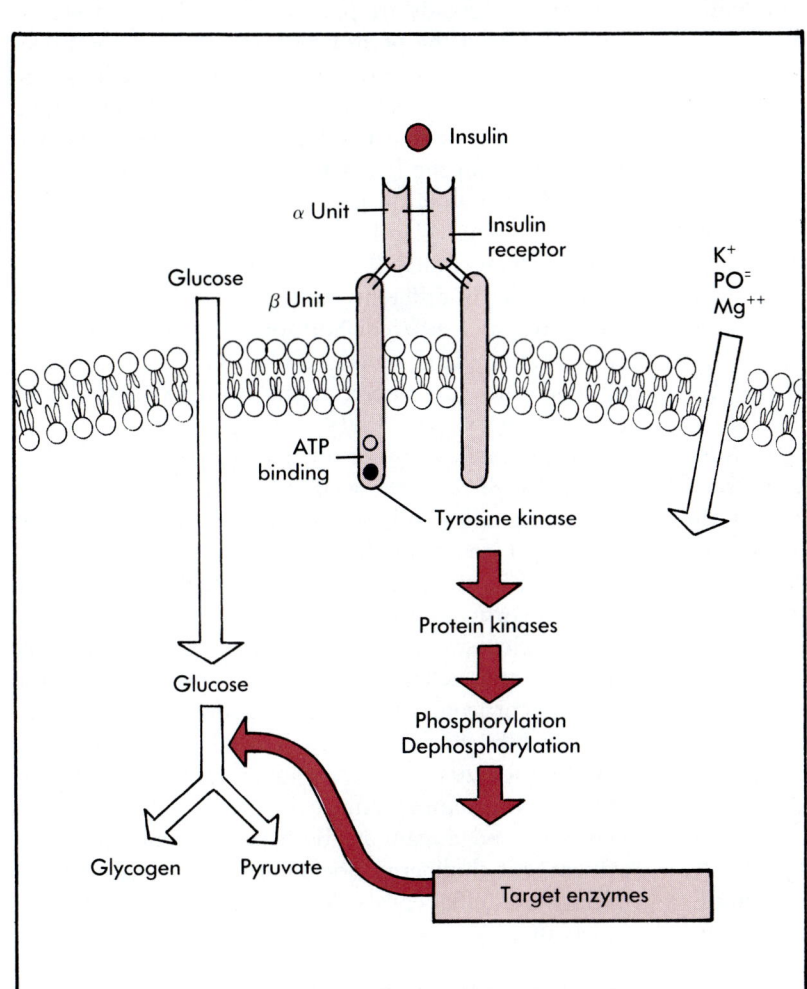

FIG. 17-13 Insulin action on target cell.
See text for explanation.
(Adapted from Berne & Levy, 1993.)

The bonded A and B chains become insulin. Insulin circulates freely in the plasma and is not bound to a carrier.

Secretion of insulin is regulated by chemical, hormonal, and neural control. Insulin secretion is promoted by increased blood levels of glucose, amino acids (arginine and glucagon), and gastrointestinal hormones and by parasympathetic stimulation of the beta cells. Insulin secretion diminishes in response to low blood levels of glucose (hypoglycemia), high levels of insulin (through negative feedback to the beta cells), and sympathetic stimulation of the alpha cells in the islets. Prostaglandins also may inhibit insulin secretion (Felig, 1985).

At the target cell, insulin combines with a plasma membrane receptor composed of alpha and beta subunits that span the plasma membrane. Tyrosine kinase activity in the beta subunit provides a signal for activating glucose transporters and a signal transduction for the phosphorylation of protein kinase with ATP as the substrate. Protein kinase then activates or deactivates target enzymes for glucose metabolism (Fig. 17-13). Potassium, phosphate, and magnesium are independently facilitated to enter the cell.

Insulin is an anabolic hormone that promotes the synthesis of proteins, carbohydrates, lipids, and nucleic acids. The major sites of insulin-promoted synthesis are the liver, muscle, and adipose tissue. The brain and red blood cells do not require insulin for glucose transport. In the liver, insulin increases glucose uptake; stimulates synthesis of glycogen and fatty acids; and inhibits gluconeogenesis (glucose formation), glycogenolysis (the splitting of glycogen to form glucose), and ketogenesis (formation of ketones from fats). In muscle, insulin increases uptake of glucose and amino acids, increases glycogen synthesis, stimulates protein synthesis, and inhibits protein breakdown (proteolysis). In adipose tissue, insulin increases glucose uptake, stimulates fat synthesis, and inhibits fat breakdown (lipolysis). The net effect of insulin in these tissues is to stimulate cellular metabolism. Overall, however, the major consequence of insulin release is to decrease blood glucose. Insulin also facilitates the intracellular transport of potassium.

Insulin is metabolized in the liver and kidney by enzymes that split disulfide bonds. Very little insulin is excreted unchanged in the urine.

Glucagon

Glucagon is produced by the alpha cells of the pancreas and by a number of cells lining the gastrointestinal tract. High glucose levels cause glucagon release to be inhibited; low glucose levels and sympathetic stimulation promote glucagon release, particularly in the liver. Amino acids, such as alanine, glycine, and asparagine, serve to stimulate glucagon secretion. A protein-rich meal has the same effect.

Glucagon acts primarily in the liver and increases blood glucose by stimulating glycogenolysis and gluconeogenesis. Glucagon acts as an antagonist to insulin. Much controversy exists regarding the role of glucagon in carbohydrate regulation, both normally and in diabetes mellitus. Glucagon also stimulates lipolysis, which has a ketogenic effect from the metabolism of free fatty acids by the liver.

Somatostatin

The somatostatin produced by delta cells is a hormone essential in carbohydrate, fat, and protein metabolism (i.e., homeostasis of ingested nutrients). It is different from hypothalamic somatostatin, which inhibits release of growth hormone. Little is known about pancreatic somatostatin, but it probably is involved in the regulation of alpha-cell and beta-cell function within the islets. Presumably, somatostatin inhibits both glucagon and insulin secretion, and it may prevent excess secretion of insulin.

Adrenal Glands

The **adrenal glands** are paired, pyramid-shaped organs located behind the peritoneum and close to the upper pole of each kidney. Each gland is surrounded by a capsule, embedded in fat, and well supplied with blood from the phrenic and renal arteries and the aorta. Venous return on the left is to the renal vein and on the right is to the inferior vena cava.

Each adrenal gland consists of two separate portions—an inner medulla and an outer cortex. These two portions have different embryonic origins, different structures, and different hormonal functions. In effect, each adrenal gland functions like two separate glands, although there are interrelationships between functions of each portion (Fig. 17-14).

The **adrenal cortex,** or outer region of the gland, accounts for 80% of the weight of the adult gland. The cortex is histologically subdivided into three zones. The outer layer, the **zona glomerulosa,** constitutes approximately 15% of the cortex and primarily produces the mineralocorticoid aldosterone. The middle layer, the **zona fasciculata** (78% of the cortex), and the inner layer, the **zona reticularis** (7% of the cortex), secrete the mineralocorticoids, the adrenal androgens and estrogens, and the glucocorticoids. The **adrenal medulla,** accounting for 20% of the gland's total weight, secretes the catecholamines epinephrine (adrenaline), norepinephrine, and dopamine. Both sympathetic and parasympathetic cholinergic fibers innervate the adrenal medulla; the adrenal cortex does not appear to be directly innervated.

Adrenal Cortex

The adrenal cortex secretes several steroid hormones, including the glucocorticoids, the mineralocorticoids,

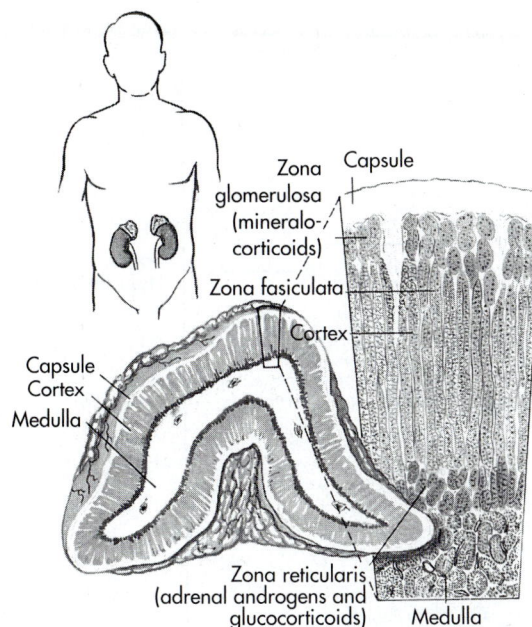

FIG. 17-14 Structure of the adrenal gland showing cell layers (zonae) of the cortex. Zona glomerulosa secretes aldosterone. Zona fasciculata secretes abundant amounts of glucocorticoids, chiefly cortisol. Zona reticularis secretes minute amounts of sex hormones and glucocorticoids. (Line drawings from Thibodeau & Patton, 1993. Photomicrograph from Thibodeau, 1987.)

and the adrenal androgens and estrogens. These hormones are all synthesized from cholesterol. The cells of the adrenal cortex must be stimulated by the extraadrenal regulator, **adrenocorticotropic hormone (ACTH)**, for cholesterol to be used in steroidogenesis. Steroidogenesis is not totally dependent on ACTH, but there appears to be an ACTH-independent baseline glucocorticoid secretion of 3% to 10% (Neville & O'Hare, 1982). The best known pathway of steroidogenesis involves the conversion of cholesterol to pregnenolone, which is then converted to the major corticosteroids.

Little storage of the steroid hormones occurs in the adrenal gland. The adrenal cortex also contains a high concentration of ascorbic acid and vitamin A; the functional roles within the adrenal glands are not known at present.

Glucocorticoids

Functions of the glucocorticoids. The glucocorticoids have metabolic, antiinflammatory, and growth-suppressing effects. They also influence levels of awareness and sleep patterns (Born, deKloet, Kern, & Fehm, 1991). The term **glucocorticoid** is applied to those steroid hormones that have direct effects on carbohydrate metabolism. These hormones increase blood glucose concentration by promoting gluconeogenesis in the liver and by decreasing use of glucose in muscle, adipose tis-

sue, and lymphatic tissue. In extrahepatic tissues the glucocorticoids stimulate protein catabolism and inhibit amino acid uptake and protein synthesis. In hepatic tissue, however, glucocorticoids act primarily to stimulate glucose formation and synthesis of enzymes that mediate glucocorticoid effects. The ultimate effect on the body is protein breakdown (catabolism).

The glucocorticoids act at several sites to inhibit immune and inflammatory reactions (described in Unit III). These include depressing proliferation of T lymphocytes, including those that produce the antiviral protein interferon; decreasing natural killer cell activity; reversing macrophage activity; and suppressing the synthesis, secretion, and actions of chemical mediators involved in inflammatory and immune responses. These chemical mediators include interleukins, prostaglandins, leukotrienes, bradykinin, serotonin, and histamine (Eskay, Grino, & Chen, 1990).

Other actions of the glucocorticoids include increasing circulating erythrocytes, leading to polycythemia; increasing the appetite; promoting fat deposits in the face and cervical areas; increasing uric acid excretion; decreasing serum calcium levels, possibly by inhibiting gastrointestinal absorption of calcium; suppressing the secretion and synthesis of ACTH; and suppressing growth hormone secretion so that somatic growth is inhibited. The glucocorticoids also have important "permissive" effects, sensitizing arterioles to the vasoconstrictive effects of norepinephrine.

Glucocorticoids appear to potentiate the effects of catecholamines, thyroid hormone, and growth hormone on adipose tissue. It also has been speculated that a metabolite of cortisol may act like a barbiturate and depress nerve cell function in the brain. This may account for the noted effects on mood associated with steroid fluctuation in disease or stress (Tepperman, 1987).

Cortisol. The most potent of the naturally occurring glucocorticoids is **cortisol.** It is the main secretory product of the adrenal cortex and is necessary for the maintenance of life and for protection from stress (see p. 649 and Fig. 9-1). Cortisol has a biologic half-life of approximately 90 minutes, with the liver primarily responsible for its deactivation.

The secretion of cortisol is regulated primarily by the hypothalamus and the anterior pituitary gland (Fig. 17-15). In the hypothalamus, corticotropin-releasing hormone (CRH) is produced in several nuclei and stored in the median eminence. Once released, CRH travels through the portal vessels to stimulate the production of ACTH, β-lipotropin, γ-lipotropin, endorphins, and enkephalins by the anterior pituitary. ACTH is the main regulator of cortisol secretion and adrenocortical growth.

Three factors appear to be primarily involved in regulating the secretion of ACTH: (1) high circulating levels of cortisol and synthetic glucocorticoids suppress

FIG. 17-15 Feedback control of glucocorticoid synthesis and secretion.

both CRH and ACTH, whereas low cortisol levels stimulate their secretion; (2) diurnal rhythms affect ACTH and cortisol levels (in persons with regular sleep-wake patterns, ACTH peaks 3 to 5 hours after sleep begins and declines throughout the day), and cortisol levels follow a similar pattern; and (3) stress has been shown to increase ACTH secretion, leading to increased cortisol levels. (Neurologic mechanisms regulating sleep are discussed in Chapter 13.) A form of ACTH (i.e., ir ACTH) also is produced by the cells of the immune system. It is detectable through laboratory techniques, and physiologically it appears to exert the usual feedback effects (see Chapter 9). This mechanism may account, in part, for integration of the immune and endocrine systems.

Once ACTH is secreted, it binds to specific plasma membrane receptors on the cells of the adrenal cortex and on other extraadrenal tissues. Because both adrenal and extraadrenal tissues have ACTH receptors, a number of effects result from stimulation by ACTH. (These are summarized in the box at right.) Both adrenal and extraadrenal effects appear to be mediated through the activation of the adenylate cyclase system. The most well-known extraadrenal effect is melanocyte stimulation, which causes increased pigmentation (Franco-Saenz, Atarashi, Takagi, & Mulrow, 1986).

Once ACTH stimulates the cells of the adrenal cortex, cortisol synthesis and secretion immediately occur. In the normal person the secretory patterns of ACTH and cortisol are nearly identical. After secretion, most cortisol circulates in bound form. Fifteen percent to 30% is bound to albumin, and 55% to 75% is tightly but reversibly bound to a plasma glycoprotein, called *transcortin*, or corticosteroid-binding globulin. Trans-

EFFECTS OF ADRENOCORTICOTROPIC HORMONE

Adrenal

Maintenance of gland size
Depletion of ascorbic acid
Activation of adenylate cyclase
Conversion of cholesterol to pregnenolone
Maintenance of enzymes active in converting pregnenolone to other steroids
Accumulation of cholesterol
Secretion of cortisol and adrenal androgens

Extraadrenal

Melanocyte stimulation
Activation of tissue lipase

cortin levels are significantly elevated by increased estrogen levels that occur with pregnancy and hormone therapy. Ten percent to 15% of the cortisol secreted circulates unbound. The unbound portion is free to diffuse into cells, but only those cells with specific intracellular glucocorticoid receptors respond to cortisol stimulation. ACTH is rapidly inactivated in the circulation, and the liver and kidneys remove the deactivated hormone.

Mineralocorticoids: aldosterone

Mineralocorticoid is the term applied to those steroids that directly affect ion transport by epithelial cells, causing sodium retention and potassium and hydrogen loss.

Aldosterone is the most potent of the naturally occurring mineralocorticoids. The primary role of aldosterone is to conserve sodium. This is accomplished by increasing the activity of the sodium pump of the epithelial cells. (The sodium pump is described in Chapter 1.)

The initial stages of aldosterone synthesis occur in the zona fasciculata and zona reticularis. The final conversion of corticosterone to aldosterone, however, apparently is confined to the zona glomerulosa. Aldosterone synthesis and secretion are regulated primarily by the renin-angiotensin system (described in Chapter 32), although other factors also may be involved. Sodium and potassium levels may directly affect aldosterone secretion; however, the mechanisms involved are not understood. ACTH may transiently stimulate aldosterone synthesis but does not appear to be a major regulator of aldosterone secretion.

Aldosterone secretion is stimulated by angiotensin, which is converted by renin to angiotensin I and then to angiotensin II and III (see Chapter 32). Once angiotensin II and III are formed, they appear to stimulate aldosterone synthesis (Fig. 17-16). The renin-angiotensin system is activated primarily by sodium and

water depletion and a diminished effective blood volume. (The postulated relationships among these factors are summarized in Fig. 17-17.)

When sodium and potassium levels are within normal limits, approximately 50 to 250 mg of aldosterone is secreted daily. Fifty percent to 75% of the secreted aldosterone binds to plasma proteins, including albumin, transcortin, and an α_1-acid glycoprotein (AAG). The relatively large proportion of unbound aldosterone contributes to its rapid metabolic turnover in the liver, its low plasma concentration, and its short half-life of approximately 15 minutes. The main site of aldosterone degradation is the liver, with the metabolic end products excreted by the kidney.

The mechanism for aldosterone action, like that of other steroid hormones, involves binding to a nuclear binding site and acting to alter protein production in the target cell. In the kidney, aldosterone acts on the ascending portion of the loop of Henle, the distal, predominantly convoluted tubule, and the collecting ducts to increase sodium ion reabsorption and increase potassium and hydrogen ion excretion. High levels of aldosterone may result in alkalosis and hypokalemia (see Chapter

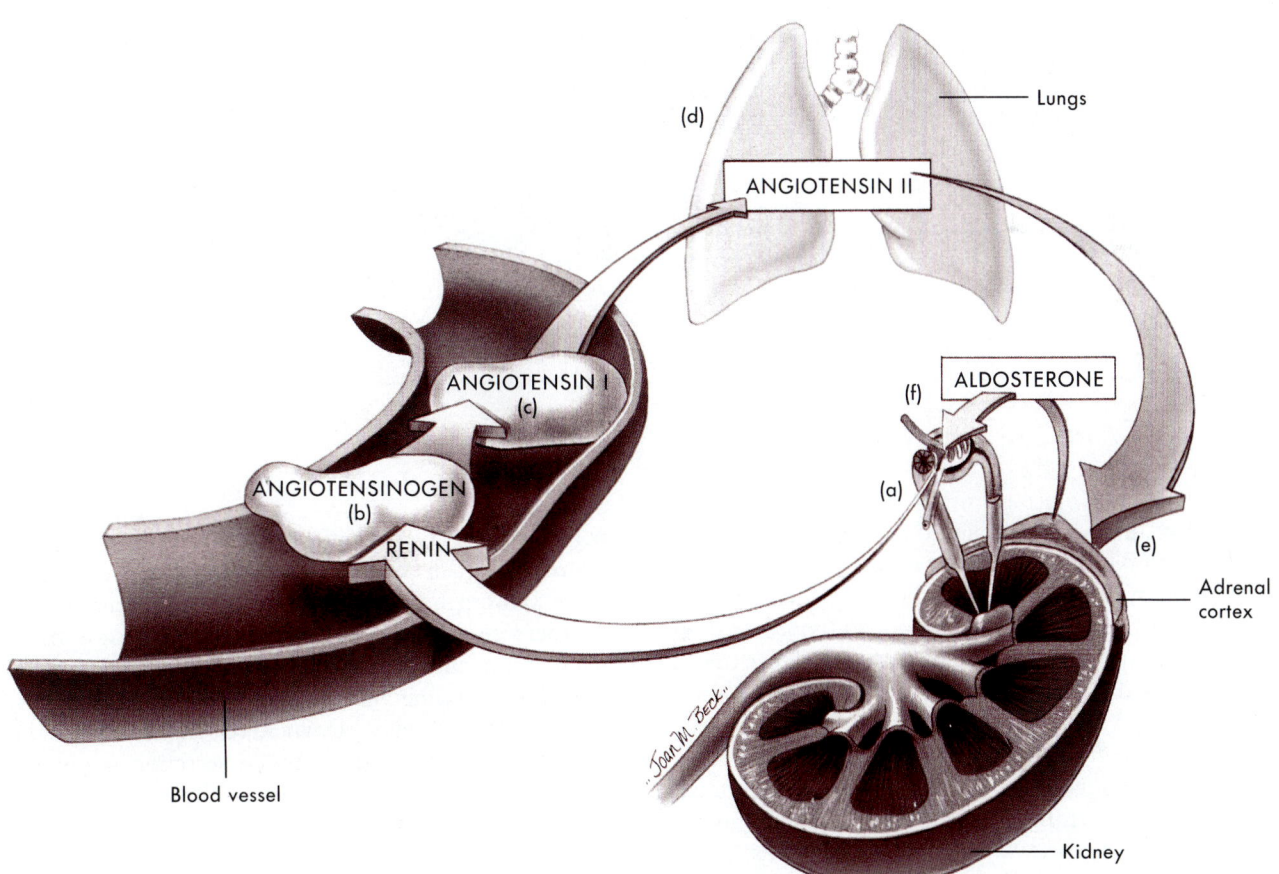

FIG. 17-16 Renin-angiotensin mechanisms for regulating aldosterone secretion. (From Thibodeau & Patton, 1993.)

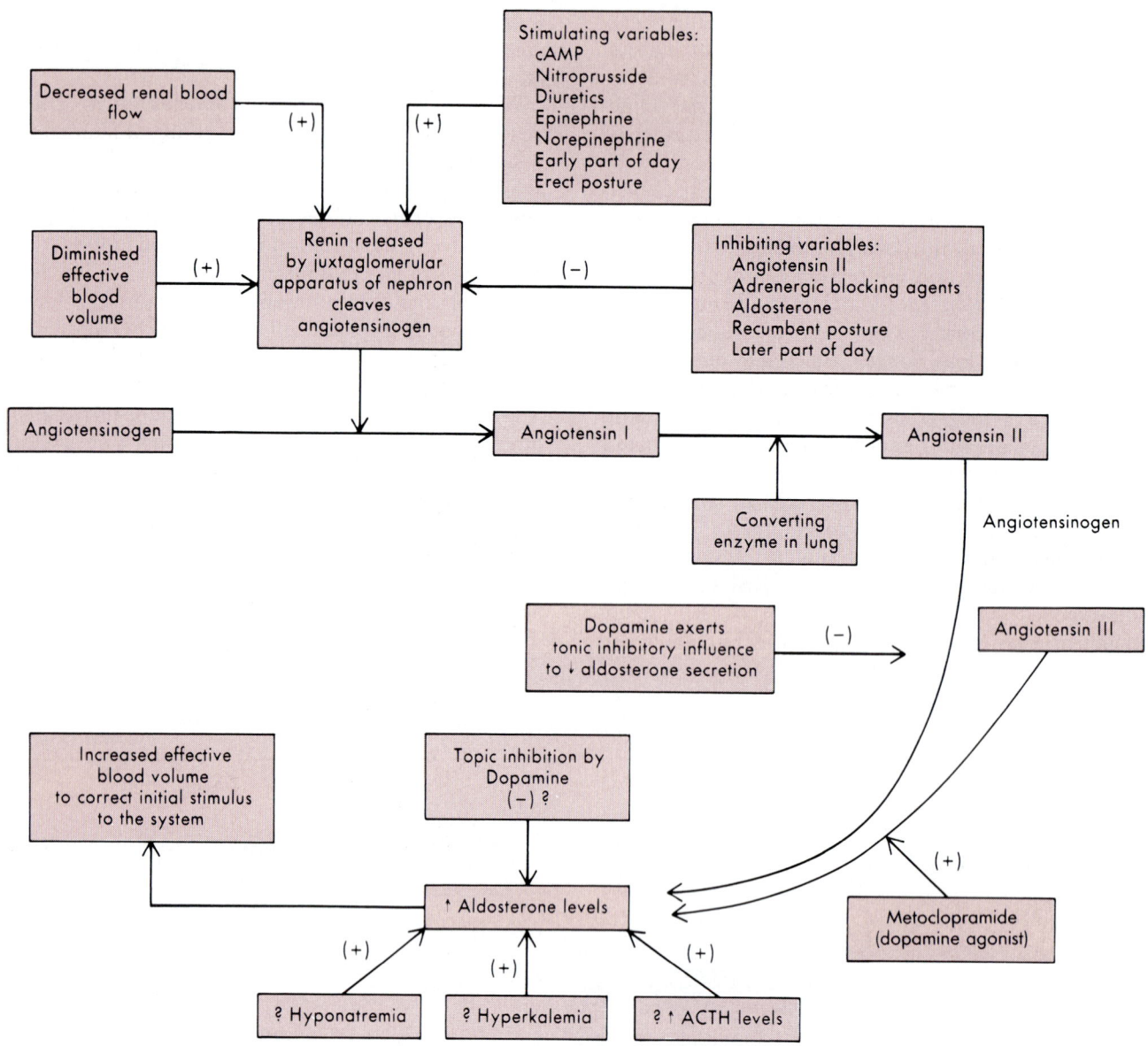

FIG. 17-17 The feedback mechanisms regulating aldosterone secretion.

3). (Kidney function is discussed in Chapter 32.) This renal effect takes 90 minutes to 6 hours to occur after stimulation by aldosterone. Other effects of aldosterone include enhancement of cardiac muscle concentration and possible stimulation of ectopic ventricular activity, secondary cardiac pacemakers in the ventricles.

Adrenal estrogens and androgens

Estrogen secretion by the normal adrenal cortex is so minimal as to be considered physiologically unimportant. The adrenal cortex also secretes androgens. Some of the weakly androgenic substances secreted by the cor-tex are then converted by peripheral tissues to stronger androgens, such as testosterone, thus accounting for some androgenic effect initiated by the adrenal cortex. An increased capacity for peripheral conversion of adrenal androgens to estrogens occurs in particular cases, however, including aging, obesity, liver disease, and hyperthyroidism (Meikle, Daynes, & Araneo, 1991). The modulation of adrenal androgen secretion is not well understood. ACTH appears to be the major regulator rather than the gonadotropins. The biologic effects and metabolism of the adrenal sex steroids do not vary from those produced by the gonads (see Unit VII).

Adrenal Medulla

The adrenal medulla, together with the sympathetic divisions of the autonomic nervous system, is embryonically derived from neural crest cells. The major products secreted by the adrenal medulla are the catecholamines epinephrine (adrenaline) and norepinephrine, although the medulla is only a minor source of norepinephrine.

Catecholamine production in the adrenal medulla consists of approximately 75% to 85% epinephrine and approximately 15% to 25% norepinephrine. Epinephrine is about 10 times more potent than norepinephrine in producing direct metabolic effects. The adrenal medulla synthesizes the catecholamines from the amino acid phenylalanine (Fig. 17-18).

The regulation of adrenal catecholamine release is complex. Secretion is increased by ACTH and the glucocorticoids. The catecholamines apparently exert a direct inhibiting influence on their own secretion by decreasing the formation of the rate-limiting enzyme tyrosine hydroxylase. Other stimuli to adrenal medullary secretion include hypoglycemia, hypoxia, hypercapnia, acidosis, hemorrhage, glucagon, nicotine, pilocarpine, histamine, and angiotensin II. On stimulation of the adrenal medullary cell, cytoplasmic storage granules that contain the catecholamines migrate to the cell surface and undergo exocytosis. The control of exocytosis probably involves calcium, although this mechanism is not fully understood.

Once released, the catecholamines may bind to various target cells, may be taken up by neurons for storage in new cytoplasmic granules, or may be metabolically inactivated and excreted in the urine. The catecholamines exert their biologic effects after binding to a plasma membrane receptor in target cells. This binding activates the adenylate cyclase system.

Catecholamines have diverse effects on the entire body. Their release and the body's response have been characterized as the "fight or flight" response (see Fig. 9-1 and Table 9-2). In general, the metabolic effects of catecholamines promote hyperglycemia through a variety of mechanisms and through interfering with usual glucose regulatory feedback mechanisms.

Neuroendocrine Response to Stressors

The endocrine system acts together with the nervous system to respond to stressors. The integrated response to stressors also includes the immune system. Hormones of the neuroendocrine system affect components of the immune system, and mediators produced by immune components regulate the neuroendocrine response.

Perception that an event is stressful may be essential to the emotional arousal and initiation of the stress response (discussed in Chapter 9). Some events, such as bacterial invasion, can activate the stress response without emotional arousal. The hypothalamus receives input from a variety of areas within the brain and ultimately directs the neuroendocrine response to stress through the actions of corticotropin-releasing factor, the locus ceruleus–norepinephrine autonomic (sympathetic) nervous system, and the pituitary-adrenal axis. In addition to the neuroendocrine components of the stress response, the gamma motor neuron system is activated to increase skeletal motor tone. Central nervous system and peripheral responses promote redirection of energy to the central nervous system and stressed sites. Enhanced availability of vital substrates occurs, and growth and reproduction are restrained to preserve energy for protective responses (Chrousos & Gold, 1992). Details of the stress response are presented in Chapter 9.

FIG. 17-18 Synthesis of catecholamines.

Tests of Endocrine Function

Tests of the endocrine system involve several general types of clinical evaluation. Measurement of hormone level is accomplished by radioimmunoassay, by enzyme-linked immunosorbent assay, and less commonly by bioassay. **Radioimmunoassay (RIA)** is an immunologic technique in which known amounts of antibody and radiolabeled hormone are placed in an assay tube with the unlabeled hormone. The radiolabeled hormone competes chemically with the nonlabeled hormone molecules for binding sites on the antibodies. When increasing amounts of unlabeled hormones are added to the assay, the limited binding sites of the antibody can bind less of the radiolabeled hormone. Therefore the higher the concentration of unlabeled hormone, the fewer the number of radioactive "counts," or labeled hormone, that bind to the fixed concentration of antibody. A quantitative value is established by use of standard reference curves.

Enzyme-linked immunosorbent assays (ELISA) also are used to determine circulating hormone levels. The method is similar to that of RIA but is less expensive and easier to conduct. Instead of radiolabeled hormones, an enzyme-labeled hormone is used. The enzyme activity in either the bound or unbound fraction is determined and related to the concentration of the unlabeled hormone.

A **bioassay** involves the use of graded doses of hormone in a reference preparation and then comparison of the results with an unknown sample. Bioassays are used more commonly in investigative endocrinology than in clinical laboratories.

The concentration of hormones in serum can be measured to assess endocrine function in health and disease. If the serum level is greater or less than the reference values, more definitive tests are required to determine the source of the problem. Measurement of individual hormones does not always permit differentiation between normal and abnormal. For an accurate interpretation the broad normal range of some hormones requires a knowledge of previous hormonal levels (Griffen, 1992).

The major problems in evaluating the endocrine system include these: (1) the complexity of the clinical presentation because of multiple organ system involvement, (2) the nonspecific nature of complaints frequently associated with endocrine dysfunction, and (3) the inappropriate use of laboratory test interpretations.

❑ AGING and the Endocrine System

The precise relationship between aging and the endocrine system is not clear. Perhaps most important, the question of whether changes in endocrine function are

a consequence or a cause of aging has yet to be resolved. These relationships have been difficult to identify, in part because of a number of age-related variables that may coexist, such as acute and chronic nonendocrine disease, use of medications, alterations in diet, body composition and weight, and changes in sleep-wake cycles (Born et al., 1991).

Theories about the Effects of Aging

Investigation into the role of the endocrine glands and their interactions in the aging process has generated much data, although the evidence is contradictory. Altered biologic activity of hormones, altered circulating levels of hormones, altered secretory response of the endocrine glands, altered metabolism of hormones, and loss of circadian control of hormone secretion are among the findings.

Theories of cellular damage deal with adverse cellular conditions that produce the biologic effects associated with aging. (These theories are discussed in Chapter 2.) The endocrine system has not been specifically implicated in any of these theories, particularly as a causative variable. The cellular changes or consequences described by these theories, however, do affect endocrine glands and might contribute to endocrine gland dysfunction or alterations in responsiveness of target organs. For example, the loss of self-regulatory patterns of the immune system leads to an autoimmune phenomenon characterized by either autoimmunity or immunodeficiencies. These mechanisms may account for the onset of type II diabetes mellitus (see Chapter 18).

Theories of stress and adaptation suggest that body structures wear out from overuse or are no longer able to adapt to the cumulative effects of physiologic stress. One such endocrine function that may be affected is the sympathoadrenal axis. Exhaustion of this axis may be associated with an inability of the body to respond effectively to stressors.

Theories of programmed change are concerned with genetic control of cell function. Certain secretory cells may be programmed genetically to secrete hormones for a prescribed length of time. Changes seen with female reproductive function may represent the phenomenon of programmed change.

All changes in cellular activity—as a result of damage, programmed change, or wear and tear—may affect neuroendocrine regulation. Impaired secretion of hypothalamic regulatory factors and hormones or impaired hypothalamic feedback sensitivity may contribute to impaired control of an optimal internal environment. The dynamic equilibrium of the endocrine system also may be affected by altered secretion of neurotransmitters within certain areas of the brain, affecting hypothalamic and pituitary function. Such alterations may include an excess or deficit in secretion of pituitary hormones and loss of appropriate secretory pattern of those hormones. Loss of endocrine steady states may be associated with or contribute to aging.

Effects of Aging on Specific Glands
Thyroid Gland

Changes in thyroid structure and function occur with aging. Structurally, some glandular atrophy and fibrosis occur with nodularity and increasing inflammatory infiltrates. These infiltrative changes may reflect age-related autoimmune damage (Spaulding, 1987).

Changes relative to TH and its function are more difficult to assess. One difficulty is finding older adults who are free of all systemic and thyroid-related illness, so that the resulting changes can be attributed to aging. Much of the available data is contradictory. Most evidence, however, supports the following age-related changes: (1) T_4 secretion and turnover are decreased; (2) plasma levels of T_3 decline, especially in men; (3) hypothyroidism is seen with increasing frequency as age advances; (4) overall TSH secretion is diminished; and (5) responsiveness of plasma TSH concentration to TRH administration is reduced, especially in men (Van Coevorden, Laurent, & Decoster, 1989). In addition, the average dose for TH replacement appears to be lower in elderly persons because the peripheral metabolism of TH decreases with age (Spaulding, 1987). TH must be replaced slowly in elderly individuals with coronary artery disease to prevent angina and myocardial infarction (Urban, 1992).

Parathyroid Gland

An age-related alteration in PTH secretion has been proposed to explain alterations in calcium homeostasis that have been noted in older adults. Such an alteration, however, has not been consistently documented. Calcium intake, especially in women, tends to decrease with aging. The average daily intake of 450 to 500 mg/day causes a negative calcium balance greater than 40 mg/day and may be related to the absolute bone loss of approximately 1.5% per year. Older adults show decreased intestinal adaptation to variations in calcium intake. Many older adults also have a mild, persistent hypercalciuria, which indicates a defective renal mechanism for responding to decreased calcium intake. Decreased circulating levels of vitamin D also have been documented.

The decrease in calcium intake, an age-related decrease in circulating vitamin D, and a blunted response of older persons to PTH may explain these changes seen

in aging (Korenman, 1982). Additional investigation into mechanisms of altered calcium metabolism is required before the age-associated alterations can be explained.

Adrenal Glands

The adrenal cortex loses some weight and has more fibrous tissue after the age of 50. Age does not appear to affect the feedback mechanisms involved in maintaining glucocorticoid levels, but the decrease in the metabolic clearance rate of the glucocorticoids is age related.

The metabolic clearance of cortisol decreases with an age-related decline in liver and kidney function. Furthermore, less cortisol appears to be used by the body when aging is accompanied by a loss of lean body mass. Both decreased clearance and reduced use of cortisol contribute to higher circulating cortisol levels. Because feedback mechanisms are intact, the higher cortisol levels cause a decrease in cortisol secretion. Plasma levels of the adrenal androgens, as well as urinary excretion of the metabolic end products, decrease gradually but dramatically with age, to as much as 50% to 70% of the young adult level. This change appears to reflect a decline in the function of the zona reticularis. The effects of decreased secretion are obscured, however, by the effects of aging on gonadal androgen secretion (see Unit VII). Because cortisol secretion does not vary significantly with aging, the decrease in secretion of adrenal androgens probably is independent of ACTH. Change in both the testis and hypothalamic-pituitary axis may be responsible for decreased testosterone levels (Vermeulin, 1991). Circadian patterns of ACTH and cortisol secretion do not change with aging (Roberts, Barton, & Horan, 1990).

Posterior Pituitary

Although hyponatremia is a common finding in older persons, it appears related to changes in renal function rather than to ADH-related mechanisms. Morphologic studies have not shown significant age-related degenerative changes in the neuroendocrine pathways that regulate the synthesis and secretion of ADH. It appears that ADH secretion is augmented when stimulated by changes in osmotic concentration, whereas baroreceptor-mediated ADH secretion is reduced (Born et al., 1991).

Anterior Pituitary

The anterior pituitary in older persons is characterized by a number of morphologic changes, including increases in fibrosis, focal necrosis, iron deposits, and microadenoma formation and a moderate decrease in size (Lurie, Doraiswamy, & Husain, 1990).

SUMMARY REVIEW

Mechanisms of Hormonal Regulation

1 The endocrine system has diverse functions, including sexual differentiation, growth and development, and continuous maintenance of the body's internal environment.

2 Hormones are chemical messengers synthesized by endocrine glands and released into the circulation.

3 Hormones have specific negative and positive feedback mechanisms. Most hormone levels are regulated by negative feedback, in which hormone secretion raises the level of a specific hormone, ultimately causing secretion to subside.

4 Endocrine feedback is described in terms of short, long, and ultra-short feedback loops.

5 Water-soluble hormones circulate throughout the body in unbound form, whereas lipid-soluble hormones (i.e., steroid and thyroid hormones) circulate throughout the body bound to carrier proteins.

6 Hormones affect only target cells with appropriate receptors and then act on these cells to initiate specific cell functions or activities.

7 Hormones have two general types of effects on cells: (1) direct effects, or obvious changes in cell function, and (2) permissive effects, or less obvious changes that facilitate cell function.

8 Receptors for hormones may be located on the plasma membrane or in the intracellular compartment of a target cell.

9 Water-soluble hormones act as first messengers, binding to receptors on the cell's plasma membrane. The signals initiated by hormone-receptor binding are then transmitted into the cell by the action of second messengers.

10 Second messengers that have been identified include cyclic adenosine monophosphate (AMP), cyclic guanosine monophosphate (GMP), calcium, and prostaglandins.

11 For cells that have cyclic AMP as their second messenger, a series of interactions within the plasma membrane must activate the intracellular cyclic nucleotides, converting intracellular substances to active enzymes.

12 For cells that have calcium as their second messenger, a rise in intracellular calcium causes calcium to bind with calmodulin, a regulatory protein. This step then initiates other intracellular processes.

13 Lipid-soluble hormones (including steroid and thyroid hormones) may cross the plasma membrane through diffusion. These hormones either bind to cytoplasmic proteins or diffuse directly into the cell nucleus and bind to nuclear receptors.

Structure and Function of the Endocrine Glands

1 The pituitary gland, consisting of anterior and posterior portions, is connected to the central nervous system through the hypothalamus.

2 The hypothalamus regulates anterior pituitary function by secreting releasing hormones and releasing factors into the portal circulation. Releasing hormones have identified chemical structures; releasing factors have hormonal properties but no definitive chemical identification.

3 Hypothalamic hormones include prolactin-inhibiting factor (PIF), which inhibits prolactin secretion; thyrotropin-releasing factor (TRF), which affects release of thyroid hormones; gonadotropin-releasing hormone (GRH), which facilitates release of adrenocorticotropic hormone (ACTH) and endorphins; and substance P, which inhibits ACTH release and stimulates release of a variety of other hormones.

4 The posterior pituitary secretes antidiuretic hormone (ADH), which also is called vasopressin, and oxytocin.

5 ADH controls serum osmolality, increases permeability of the renal tubules to water, and causes vasoconstriction when administered pharmacologically in high doses. ADH also may regulate some central nervous system functions.

6 Oxytocin causes uterine contraction and lactation in women and may have a role in sperm motility in men. In both men and women, oxytocin has an antidiuretic effect similar to that of ADH.

7 Hormones of the anterior pituitary are regulated by (1) secretion of hypothalamic-releasing hormones or factors, (2) negative feedback from hormones secreted by target organs, and (3) mediating effects of neurotransmitters.

8 Hormones of the anterior pituitary include ACTH, melanocyte-stimulating hormone (MSH), somatotropic hormones (growth hormone [GH] and prolactin), and glycoprotein hormones—follicle-stimulating hormone (FSH), luteinizing hormone (LH), and thyroid-stimulating hormone (TSH).

9 The two-lobed thyroid gland contains follicles, which secrete some of the thyroid hormones, and C cells, which secrete calcitonin and somatostatin.

10 Regulation of thyroid hormone (TH) levels is complex and involves the hypothalamus, anterior pituitary, thyroid gland, and numerous biochemical variables.

11 Thyroid hormone (TH) secretion is regulated by thyroid-releasing hormone through a negative feedback loop that involves the anterior pituitary and hypothalamus.

12 Thyroid-stimulating hormone (TSH), which is synthesized and stored in the anterior pituitary, stimulates secretion of TH by activating intracellular processes, including uptake of iodine necessary for the synthesis of TH.

13 Once secreted, TH acts on the thyroid gland, the anterior pituitary, and the median eminence to regulate further TH production.

14 Synthesis of TH depends on the glycoprotein thyroglobulin, which contains a precursor of TH, tyrosine. Tyrosine then combines with iodine to form precursor molecules of the thyroid hormones thyroxine (T_4) and triiodothyronine (T_3).

15 When released into the circulation, T_3 and T_4 are bound by carrier proteins in the plasma, which store these hormones and provide a buffer for rapid changes in hormone levels.

16 Thyroid hormones alter protein synthesis and have a wide range of metabolic effects on proteins, carbohydrates, lipids, and vitamins. TH also affects heat production and cardiac function.

17 The paired parathyroid glands normally are located behind the upper and lower poles of the thyroid. These glands secrete parathyroid hormone (PTH), an important regulator of serum calcium levels.

18 PTH secretion is regulated by levels of ionized calcium in the plasma and by cyclic AMP within the cell. Some other substances—hormones, neurotransmitters, and ions—affect PTH secretion by inhibiting cyclic AMP or by changing calcium levels.

19 In bone, PTH causes bone breakdown and resorption. In the kidney, PTH increases reabsorption of calcium and decreases reabsorption of phosphorus and bicarbonate.

20 The endocrine pancreas contains the islets of Langerhans, which secrete hormones responsible for much of the carbohydrate metabolism in the body.

21 The islets of Langerhans consist of alpha cells, beta cells, and delta cells.

22 Delta cells secrete somatostatin, which inhibits glucagon and insulin secretion.

23 Beta cells secrete preproinsulin, which is ultimately converted to insulin.

24 Insulin is a hormone that regulates blood glucose concentrations and overall body metabolism of fat, protein, and carbohydrates.

25 Alpha cells produce glucagon, which is secreted inversely to blood glucose concentrations.

26 The paired adrenal glands are situated in the kidneys. Each gland consists of an adrenal medulla, which secretes catecholamines, and an adrenal cortex, which secretes steroid hormones.

27 The steroid hormones secreted by the adrenal cortex are all synthesized from cholesterol. These hormones include glucocorticoids, mineralocorticoids, and adrenal androgens and estrogens.

28 Glucocorticoids directly affect carbohydrate metabolism by increasing blood glucose concentration through gluconeogenesis in the liver and by decreasing use of glucose. Glucocorticoids also inhibit immune and inflammatory responses.

29 The most potent naturally occurring glucocorticoid is cortisol, which is necessary for the maintenance of life and for protection from stress. Secretion of cortisol is regulated by the hypothalamus and anterior pituitary.

30 Cortisol secretion is related to secretion of adrenocorticotropic hormone (ACTH), which is stimulated by corticotropin-releasing hormone (CRH). ACTH binds with receptors of the adrenal cortex, which activates intracellular mechanisms (specifically cyclic AMP) and leads to cortisol release.

31 Mineralocorticoids are steroid hormones that directly affect ion transport by epithelial cells, causing sodium retention and potassium and hydrogen loss.

32 Aldosterone is the most potent of the naturally occurring mineralocorticoids. Its primary role is to conserve sodium.

33 Aldosterone secretion is regulated primarily by the renin-angiotensin system.

34 Aldosterone acts by binding to a site on the cell nucleus and altering protein production within the cell. Its principal site of action is the kidney, where it causes sodium reabsorption and potassium and hydrogen excretion.

35 Androgens and estrogens secreted by the adrenal cortex act in the same way as those secreted by the gonads.

36 The adrenal medulla secretes the catecholamines epinephrine and norepinephrine. Catecholamines are synthesized from the amino acid phenylalanine. Their release is stimulated by sympathetic nervous system stimulation, ACTH, and glucocorticoids.

37 Catecholamines bind with various target cells and are taken up by neurons or excreted in the urine. They cause a range of metabolic effects that generally are characterized as the "flight or fight" response.

38 The endocrine system acts together with the nervous system to respond to stressors.

39 The response to stressors involves (a) activation of the sympathetic division of the autonomic nervous system and (b) activation of the endocrine system.

40 The adrenal glands and the sympathetic neurons that innervate these glands form the sympathoadrenal axis.

41 Activation of the sympathetic neurons causes the activation of an enzymatic pathway that increases catecholamine synthesis, leading to manifestations of the "fight or flight" response, hyperglycemia, and immune suppression.

42 Both hyperglycemia and immune suppression appear to be adaptive responses that are essential in the body's ability to react to stressors.

43 Other hormones that are secreted in response to stress include growth hormone, prolactin, testosterone, ADH, and insulin.

Aging and the Endocrine System

1 Endocrine changes that may be associated with aging include altered biologic activity of hormones, altered circulating levels of hormones, altered secretory responses of endocrine glands, altered metabolism of hormones, and loss of circadian control of hormone release.

2 Cellular damage associated with aging, genetically programmed cell change, and chronic wear and tear may contribute to endocrine gland dysfunction or alterations in responsiveness of target organs.

3 Aging apparently causes atrophy of the thyroid gland and is associated with infiltrative glandular changes. Secretion of thyroid hormones may diminish with age.

4 Aging is associated with alterations in calcium steady states, which may be related to alterations in PTH secretion from the parathyroid glands.

5 Age-related changes in adrenal function include decreased clearance of glucocorticoids and a decrease in levels of adrenal androgens. The effects of these changes, however, are offset by feedback mechanisms that maintain glucocorticoid levels and by gonadal secretion of androgens.

KEY TERMS

Adrenal cortex, 644
Adrenal gland, 644
Adrenal medulla, 644
Adrenocorticotropic hormone (ACTH), 645
Aldosterone, 647
Alpha cell, 643
Antidiuretic hormone (ADH), 636
Beta cell, 643
Bioassay, 650
C cell, 639
Calcitonin, 639
Chromophil, 637
Chromophobe, 637
Corticotropin-releasing hormone (CRH), 636
Cortisol, 645
Delta cell, 643
Direct effect, 630
Enzyme-linked immunosorbent assay (ELISA), 650
First messenger, 630
Follicle, 638

Glucagon, 643
Glucocorticoid, 645
Gonadotropin-releasing hormone (GnRH), 636
Growth hormone–releasing factor (GRF), 636
Guanylate cyclase, 632
Hormone, 626
Hormone receptor, 630
Infundibular process, 633
Infundibular stem, 633
Insulin, 643
Islet of Langerhans, 643
Isthmus, 638
Median eminence, 633
Mineralocorticoid, 646
Negative feedback, 627
Oxytocin, 636
Pancreas, 643
Parathyroid hormone (PTH), 640
Pars distalis, 633
Pars intermedia, 633
Pars tuberalis, 633

Permissive effect, 630
Pharmacologic effect, 630
Pituitary gland, 633
Positive feedback, 629
Prolactin-inhibiting factor (PIF), 636
Radioimmunoassay (RIA), 650
Releasing factor, 636
Second messenger, 631
Somatostatin, 636
Substance P, 636
Target cell, 630
Thyroglobulin, 640
Thyroid gland, 638
Thyroid hormone (TH), 639
Thyroid-stimulating hormone (TSH), 640
Thyrotropin-releasing hormone (TRH), 636
Thyroxine (T_4), 640
Triiodothyronine (T_3), 640
Zona fasciculata, 644
Zona glomerulosa, 644
Zona reticularis, 644

REFERENCES

Ahren, B. (1986). Thyroid neuroendocrinology: Neural regulation of thyroid hormone secretion. *Endocrine Reviews, 7*(2), 149-155.

Berne, R. M., & Levy, M. N. (1993). *Physiology*. (3rd ed.). St. Louis: Mosby–Year Book.

Born, J., deKloet, E. R., Kern, W., & Fehm, H. L. (1991). Gluco- and antimineralocorticoid effects on human sleep: A role of central corticosteroid receptors. *American Journal of Physiology, 260*, E183-E188.

Chrousos, G. P., & Gold, P. W. (1992). The concepts of stress and stress system disorders: Overview of physical and behavioral homeostasis. *Journal of the American Medical Association, 267*(9), 1244-1252.

Eskay, R. L., Grino, M., & Chen, H. T. (1990). Interleukins, signal transduction and the immune mediated stress response. In J. C. Porter & B. D. Jezava (Eds.), *Advances in experimental medicine and biology: Circulatory regulatory factors and neuroendocrine function* (pp. 331-334). New York: Plenum Press.

Ezrin, C., Godden, J. D., & Volpe, R. (1979). *Systematic endocrinology*. (2nd ed.). New York: Harper & Row.

Felig, P. (1985). Diabetic control: Is it worth it? *Transactions of the Association of Life Insurance Medical Directions of America, 68*, 61-65.

Franco-Saenz, R., Atarashi, K., Takagi, M., & Mulrow, P. J. (1986). Effects of atrial natriuretic factor on the renin-angiotensin aldosterone axis. *Journal of Hypertension, 4* (Suppl. 6), 523-525.

Griffen, J. E. (1992). Dynamic tests of endocrine function. In J. D. Wilson & D. W. Foster (Eds.), *Williams textbook of endocrinology* (8th ed., p. 1663). Philadelphia: W. B. Saunders.

Korenman, S. G. (Ed.). (1982). *Endocrine aspects of aging*. New York: Elsevier.

Lefkowitz, R. J. (1982, August). Biochemical mechanisms of hormone receptor-effector coupling. *Federation Proceedings, 41*(10), 2662-2663.

Long, B. C., Phipps, W. J., & Cassmeyer, V. L. (1992). *Medical-surgical nursing: A nursing process approach.* (3rd ed.). St. Louis: Mosby–Year Book.

Lurie, S. N., Doraiswamy, P. M., & Husain, M. M. (1990). In vivo assessment of pituitary gland volume with magnetic resonance imaging: The effect of age. *Journal of Clinical Endocrinology and Metabolism, 71*, 505.

Martin, C. R. (1985). *Endocrine physiology*. New York: Oxford Press.

Meikle, W. A., Daynes, R. A., & Araneo, B. A. (1991). Adrenal androgen secretion and biologic effects. *Endocrinology and Metabolism Clinics of North America, 20*(2), 381-400.

Neville, A. M., & O'Hare, M. J. (1982). *The human adrenal cortex*. New York: Springer Verlag.

Reichlin, S. (1992). Neuroendocrinology. In J. D. Wilson & D. W. Foster (Eds.), *Williams textbook of endocrinology* (8th ed.). Philadelphia: W. B. Saunders.

Roberts, N. A., Barton, R. N., & Horan, M. A. (1990). Aging and the sensitivity of the adrenal gland to physiologic doses of ACTH in man. *Journal of Endocrinology, 126*, 507.

Seeley, R. R., Stevens, T. D., & Tate, P. (1992). *Anatomy and physiology* (2nd ed.). St. Louis: Mosby–Year Book.

Spaulding, S. (1987). Age and the thyroid. *Endocrinology and Metabolism Clinics of North America, 16*(4).

Tepperman, J. (1987). *Metabolic and endocrine physiology: An introductory text* (5th ed.). St. Louis: Mosby–Year Book.

Thibodeau, G. A., & Patton, K. (1993). *Anatomy and physiology*. (2nd ed.). St. Louis: Mosby–Year Book.

Thompson, J. M., McFarland, G. K., Hirsch, J. E., & Tucker, S. M. (1993). *Mosby's manual of clinical nursing* (3rd ed.). St. Louis: Mosby–Year Book.

Urban, J. R. (1992). Neuroendocrinology of aging in the male and female. *Endocrinology and Metabolism Clinics of North America, 21*(4), 921-931.

Van Coevorden, A., Laurent, E., & Decoster, C. (1989). Decreased basal and stimulated thyrotropin secretion in healthy elderly men. *Journal of Clinical Endocrinology and Metabolism, 69*, 177.

Vermeulin, A. (1991). Clinical review: Androgens in the aging male. *Journal of Clinical Endocrinology and Metabolism, 73*, 221.

SUGGESTED READINGS

Adelman, R., & Roth, G. (1982). *Endocrine and neuroendocrine mechanisms of aging*. Boca Raton, FL: CRC Press.

Barnes, D. M. (1986). Steroids may influence changes in mood. *Science, 232*, 1344-1345.

Berridge, M. J. (1976). The interaction of cyclic nucleotides and calcium in control of cellular activity. *Advances in Cyclic Nucleotide Research, 6*, 1-98.

Berridge, M. J. (1985, October). The molecular basis of communication within the cell. *Scientific American, 253*(4), 142.

Brown, M. R., Koob, G., & Rivier, C. (Eds.). (1990). *Stress: neurobiology and neuroendocrinology*. New York: Dekker.

Burchfield, S. R. (1979). The stress response: A new perspective. *Psychosomatic Medicine, 41*(8), 661-669.

Catt, K. J., & Dufau, M. L. (1977). Peptide hormone receptors. *Annual Review of Physiology, 39*, 529.

Ebersole, P., & Hess, P. (1990). *Toward healthy aging: Human needs and nursing response* (3rd ed.). St. Louis: Mosby–Year Book.

Greer, M. A. (Ed.). (1990). *The thyroid gland*. New York: Raven.

Griffin, J. E., & Sergio, O. R. (Eds.). (1992). *Textbook of endocrine physiology*. New York: Oxford.

Hadley, M. E. (1992). *Endocrinology* (3rd ed.). Englewood Cliffs, NJ: Prentice-Hall.

King, R. J. B. (1984). Enlightenment and confusion over steroid hormone receptors. *Nature, 312*, 20.

Mazzaferri, E. L., Barr, R. S., & Kreisberg, R. A. (1993). *Advances in endocrinology and metabolism, Volume 3*. St. Louis: Mosby–Year Book.

McClain, D. A. (1992). The mechanism and role of insulin receptor endocytosis. *American Journal of Medical Science 304*(3), 192-201.

Munck, A., & Foley, R. (1979). Activation of steroid hormone-receptor complexes in intact target cells in physiological conditions. *Nature, 278*, 752.

O'Mally, B. W., Schwartz, R. J., & Schrader, W. T. (1976). A review of regulation of gene expression by steroid hormone receptors. *Journal of Steroid Biochemistry, 7*, 1151.

Rasmussen, H., Jensen, P., Lake, W., Friedmann, N., & Goodman, D. B. P. (1975). Cyclic nucleotides and cellular calcium metabolism. In G. L. Drummond et al. (Eds.), *Advances in cyclic nucleotide research: Vol. 5*. New York: Raven Press.

Rose, R. M. (1980). Endocrine responses to stressful events. *Psychiatric Clinics of North America, 3*, 251-276.

Ross, E. M., & Gilman, A. G. (1980). Biochemical properties of hormone sensitive adenylate cyclase. *Annual Review of Biochemistry, 49*, 533.

Stanley, J. C. (1981). Mechanisms of hormone action. *British Journal of Anaesthesia, 53*, 147.

Streeten, D. H. P., Anderson, G. H., Dalakos, T. G., Seeley, D., Mallov, J. S., Eusebio, R., Sunderlin, F. S., Badawy, S. Z., & King, R. B. (1984). Normal and abnormal function of the hypothalamic-pituitary-adrenocortical system in man. *Endocrine Reviews, 5*(3), 371-394.

Vinik, A. I. (Ed.). (1992). *Pancreatic islet cell regeneration and growth*. New York: Plenum.

Alterations of Hormonal Regulation

Patti Ludwig-Beymer
Sue E. Huether
D. Patricia Gray*

Chapter Outline

*Contributing author to first edition.

F*unction of the endocrine system involves complex interrelationships and interactions that maintain dynamic steady states and provide growth and reproductive capabilities. Dysfunction of the endocrine system was initially described in terms of excessive or insufficient function of the endocrine gland with alterations in hormone levels. Alterations in function were thought to be caused by either hypersecretion or hyposecretion of the various hormones, leading to abnormal hormone concentrations in the blood. Techniques for studying the various components of the endocrine system have improved, and evidence has shown that dysfunction may result from abnormal receptor function or from altered intracellular response to the hormone-receptor complex.*

MECHANISMS OF HORMONAL ALTERATIONS

Significantly elevated or depressed hormone levels may result from a variety of causes (Fig. 18-1). Feedback systems that recognize the need for a particular hormone may fail to function properly or may respond to inappropriate signals (see Chapter 17). Dysfunction of an endocrine gland may involve the gland's failure to produce adequate amounts of biologically free or active hormone forms. This failure may occur when the secretory cells are unable to produce or obtain an adequate quantity of required hormone precursors, or are unable to convert the precursors to the appropriate form. A gland also may synthesize or release excessive amounts of hormone. Once hormones are released into the circulation, they may be degraded at an altered rate, or they may be inactivated by antibodies before reaching

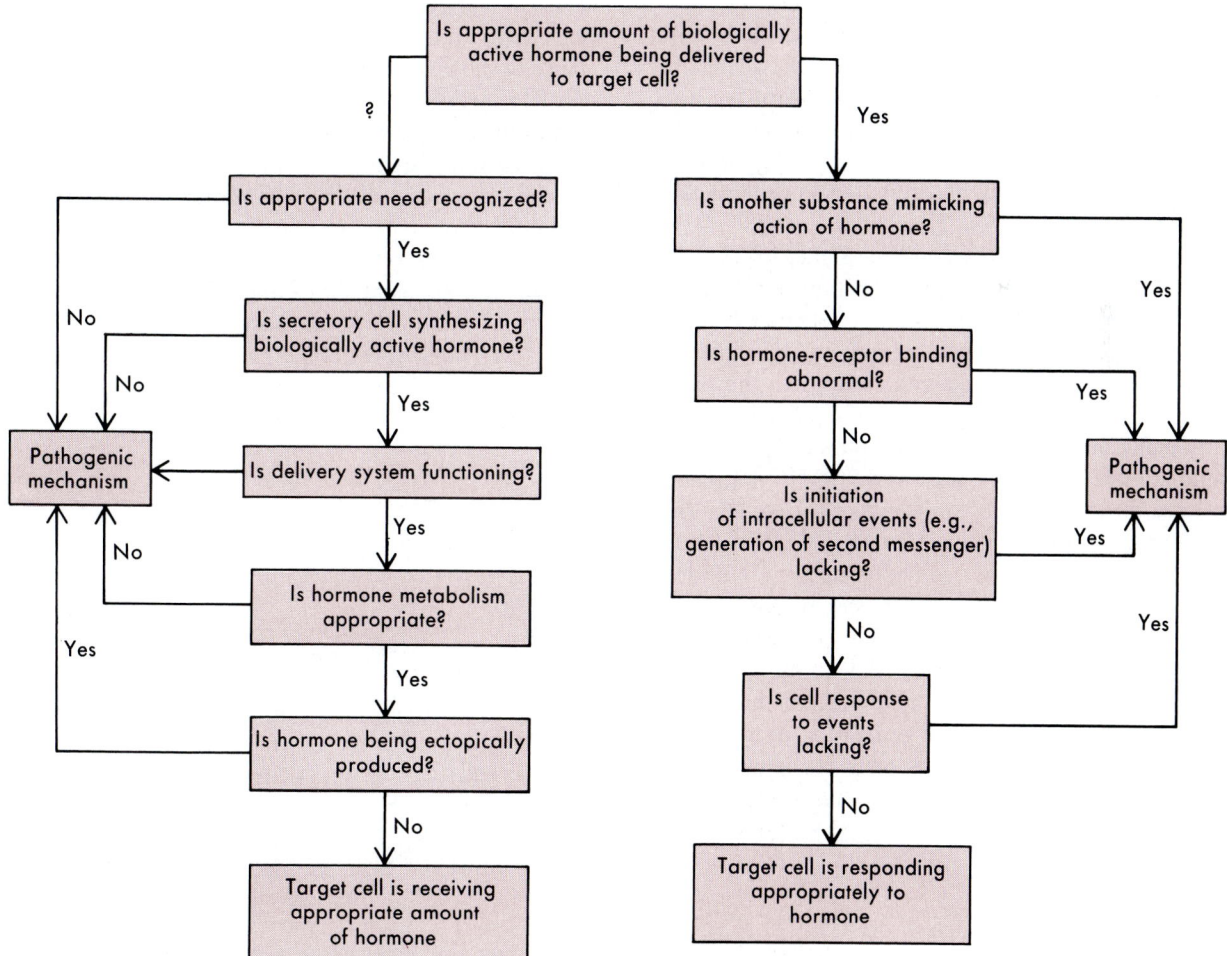

FIG. 18-1 Hormone delivery to cells. Phases at which pathogenic mechanisms may develop in delivering appropriate amounts of hormone to the cells.

the target cell. Ectopic sources of hormones (hormones produced by nonendocrine tissues) may result also in abnormally elevated hormone levels. This mechanism operates without benefit of the normal feedback system for hormone control. In these cases, the ectopic hormone production is said to be autonomous.

Recently, research has been directed toward understanding causes for the failure of the target cell to respond to its hormone. The general types of abnormal target cell responses currently recognized are (1) receptor-associated disorders and (2) intracellular disorders. Receptor-associated disorders have been primarily identified in water-soluble hormones, such as insulin. These types of disorders are usually one of the following: (1) a decrease in the number of receptors, leading to decreased or defective hormone-receptor binding, (2) impaired receptor function resulting in insensitivity to the hormone, (3) presence of antibodies against specific receptors that either reduce available binding sites or mimic hormone action, exaggerating target cell response, or (4) unusual expression of receptor function, as occurs in some tumor cells with abnormal receptor activity.

Intracellular disorders may involve inadequate synthesis of the second messenger, such as cyclic adenosine monophosphate (cAMP), needed to transduce the hormonal signal into intracellular events. The target cell for water-soluble hormones may have a faulty response to hormone-receptor binding and thus fail to generate the required second messenger. The cell also may have an abnormal response to the second messenger if levels of intracellular enzymes or proteins are altered. (Second messengers for various hormones are listed in Chapter 17, Table 17-4). Both of these pathogenic mechanisms result in failure of the target cell to express the usual hormonal effect.

Pathogenic mechanisms affecting target cell response for lipid-soluble hormones, such as thyroid hormone, either occur less frequently or are recognized less frequently than those affecting the water-soluble hormones. These mechanisms are not yet precisely understood, although some theories have been proposed. The number of intracellular receptors may be decreased, or those receptors may have an altered affinity for hormones. Both mechanisms would affect hormone-receptor binding. Alterations in generation of new messenger RNA or absence of substrates for new protein synthesis also may occur, resulting in altered target cell response.

ALTERATIONS OF THE HYPOTHALAMIC-PITUITARY SYSTEM

Because of the relative inaccessibility of the hypothalamic-pituitary unit in the brain and the short half-life and small concentrations of the hypothalamic hormones, documenting abnormal release of hypothalamic-releasing hormones has been difficult. The most common hypothalamic diseases probably result from interruption in the infundibular stem caused by destructive lesions of the stem, rupture of the stem after head injury, surgical transection of the stem, or stem tumor. In these cases, interruption of the physical connections between the hypothalamus and the pituitary causes hypothalamic disease. For example, diabetes insipidus (antidiuretic hormone insufficiency) may result, depending on the location at which the infundibular stem is interrupted. If the lesion is close to the hypothalamus, diabetes insipidus is likely; the farther away the lesion is from the hypothalamus, the less likely is the occurrence of diabetes insipidus.

The absence of hypothalamic hormones (Fig. 18-2) causes a variety of manifestations. In women, the menses cease, and in men spermatogenesis is impaired because of the absence of gonadotropin-releasing hormone (GnRH) stimulation of the gonadotropin follicle-stimulating hormone (FSH) and luteinizing hormone (LH). Adrenocorticotropic hormone (ACTH) response to low serum cortisol levels is decreased because of the absence of corticotropin-releasing hormone (CRH). Hypothalamic hypothyroidism is caused by the absence of thyrotropin-releasing hormone (TRH). Low levels of growth hormone cause the absence of growth hormone regulatory hormones. Hyperprolactinemia is caused by an absence of usual inhibitory controls of prolactin secretion.

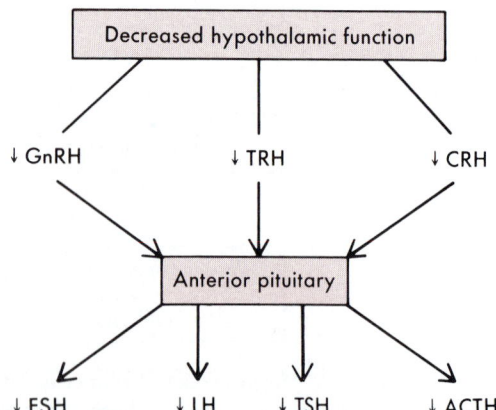

FIG. 18-2 Loss of hypothalamic hormones.

Diseases of the Posterior Pituitary
Syndrome of Inappropriate Antidiuretic Hormone Secretion

Diseases of the posterior pituitary that cause clinically observable symptoms are rare. If they do occur, they are usually related to abnormal antidiuretic hormone (ADH/vasopressin) secretion. **Syndrome of inappropriate ADH secretion** (SIADH) is characterized by high levels of ADH in the absence of normal physiologic stimuli for its release (Kovacs & Robertson, 1992).

The most common cause of elevated levels of ADH is ectopically produced ADH. Syndrome of inappropriate antidiuretic hormone secretion is associated with some forms of cancer, apparently because of the ectopic secretion of ADH by tumor cells. Tumors that have been reported in association with SIADH include oat cell adenocarcinoma of the lung, carcinoma of the duodenum and pancreas, leukemia, lymphoma, Hodgkin disease, sarcoma, and squamous cell carcinoma of the tongue.

Transient SIADH may follow pituitary surgery, because stored ADH is released in an unregulated fashion. When postoperative fluid volume shifts occur after any type of surgery, ADH secretion is increased for 5 to 7 days. The exact mechanism is unknown, but apparently is related to volume changes within the body and may be considered a normal response to surgery. Syndrome of inappropriate antidiuretic hormone secretion may be seen in individuals with a variety of infectious pulmonary diseases. This may be caused by the ectopic production of ADH by infected lung tissue (Kovacs & Lichardus, 1989) or by increased posterior pituitary secretion of ADH in response to a hypoxia-induced decrease in pulmonary perfusion (Labhart, 1986).

Syndrome of inappropriate antidiuretic hormone secretion may be associated with psychiatric disease and also may occur after treatment with a variety of drugs. These include hypoglycemic medications (thioridazine), barbiturates, general anesthesia, vincristine, nicotine, morphine, diuretics, and synthetic hormones. These drugs serve either to simulate ADH release or to potentiate circulating ADH (Labhart, 1986).

Pathophysiology

The main features of SIADH are water retention or increases in total body H_2O; solute loss, particularly Na; and osmotic inactivation of cellular solutes. These features lead to hyponatremia and hypoosmolality. In SIADH, ADH is released continually. Water retention results from the normal action of ADH on the renal tubules and collecting ducts, increasing their permeability to water and increasing water reabsorption by the kidneys. (Renal function is discussed in Chapter 34.)

An expansion of extracellular fluid volume results, and a dilutional hyponatremia develops. Hyponatremia acts to suppress renin and therefore aldosterone secretion, decreasing proximal tubule reabsorption of sodium. This effect explains renal sodium loss during a hyponatremic state.

Clinical Manifestations

A diagnosis of SIADH requires the following signs: (1) serum hypoosmolality and hyponatremia, (2) urine hypersomolarity (that is, the osmolality of the urine is greater than expected for the concomitant serum osmolality), (3) urine sodium excretion that matches sodium intake, (4) improvement in hyponatremia with water restriction, and (5) absence of other causes of decreased diluting ability.

The symptoms of SIADH are primarily the result of hyponatremia. The severity and the sudden onset of the hyponatremia determine the extent of the symptoms. Even if hyponatremia develops slowly, serum sodium levels below 110 to 115 mEq/L are likely to cause severe and sometimes irreversible neurologic damage. Thirst, impaired taste, anorexia, dyspnea on exertion, fatigue, and dulled sensorium occur when the serum sodium decreases rapidly from 140 to 130 mEq/L. Severe gastrointestinal symptoms, including vomiting and abdominal cramps, occur with a drop in sodium from 130 to 120 mEq/L. With a serum sodium level below 115 mEq/L, confusion, lethargy, muscle twitching, and convulsions may occur. Symptoms usually resolve with correction of hyponatremia.

Evaluation and Treatment

Serum electrolyte levels, serum osmolality and urine volume, urine electrolyte levels, and urine osmolality are adequate measures of the presence of SIADH. The treatment of SIADH involves the correction of any underlying causal problems, emergency correction of severe hyponatremia by administration of hypertonic saline, and, most important, fluid restriction to 600 to 800 ml/day. Careful monitoring is important. Resolution usually occurs within 3 days, with a 2- to 3-kg weight loss and correction of hyponatremia and salt wasting. Phenytoin may be administered, particularly for excessive ADH release by the posterior pituitary. No drug therapy is available to suppress ectopically produced ADH.

Diabetes Insipidus

Diabetes insipidus is related to an insufficiency of ADH, leading to polyuria and polydipsia. There are three forms of diabetes insipidus: (1) a neurogenic or central form, (2) a nephrogenic form, and (3) a psychogenic form (Culpepper, Heber, & Andreoli, 1985). The neurogenic form is caused by insufficient amounts of ADH; the nephrogenic form is caused by an inadequate response to ADH. The psychogenic form is caused by extremely large volumes of fluid intake, producing a decreased ADH level.

The neurogenic form of diabetes insipidus occurs when any organic lesion of the hypothalamus, infundibular stem, or posterior pituitary interferes with ADH synthesis, transport, or release. These lesions include primary brain tumors, hypophysectomy, aneurysms, thrombosis, infections, and immunologic disorders. Diabetes insipidus is a well-recognized complication of closed-head trauma.

The nephrogenic form of diabetes insipidus is usually an acquired disorder. An idiopathic form has been documented and is usually genetic. Nephrogenic diabetes insipidus represents end organ failure, with an insensitivity of the renal tubule to ADH, particularly the collecting tubules. Nephrogenic diabetes insipidus is generally related to disorders and drugs that damage the renal tubules or inhibit the generation of cAMP in the tubules. These disorders include pyelonephritis, amyloidosis, destructive uropathies, polycystic disease, and intrinsic renal disease, all of which lead to irreversible diabetes insipidus. Drugs that may induce a generally reversible form of nephrogenic diabetes insipidus include lithium carbonate, general anesthetics, methoxyflurane, and demeclocycline.

Pathophysiology

Individuals with diabetes insipidus may have partial to total inability to concentrate urine. This inability apparently results from chronic polyuria, causing washout of the renal medullary concentration gradient (see Chapter 32).

Insufficient ADH secretion causes immediate excretion of large volumes of dilute urine, leading to an increase in plasma osmolality. In conscious individuals, the thirst mechanism is stimulated and induces polydipsia. For unknown reasons, the person usually craves cold drinks. The urine output is varied. In about one half of cases, urine volume is 4 to 8 L/day, whereas in one fourth of the cases it is 8 to 12 L/day. With profound ADH deficiency, output may be greater than 12 L/day. The urine specific gravity is low, from 1.00 to 1.005. Serum electrolytes are generally not affected. Dehydration develops rapidly without ongoing fluid replacement.

In nephrogenic diabetes insipidus, ADH levels are normal or high but the collecting ducts do not increase their permeability to water in response to ADH. There is a familial form of the disorder or it may be associated with the drugs lithium, demeclocycline, or the anesthetic methoxyflurane.

Diabetes insipidus usually has an acute onset. With neurogenic diabetes insipidus, a classic, three-phase syndrome has been observed. Initially, significant diuresis occurs, apparently as a result of acute damage to the hypothalamic centers involving ADH secretion. The second phase is one of antidiuresis, which may represent necrosis of denervated tissue of the posterior pituitary with release of ADH into the circulation. The final phase is one of polyuria and polydipsia reflecting a permanent loss of the ability to secrete adequate amounts of ADH. Antidiuretic hormone does not have to be completely absent for polyuria and polydipsia to occur.

Clinical Manifestations

The clinical manifestations of diabetes insipidus are caused by the absence of ADH. These signs and symptoms include polyuria, nocturia, continuous thirst, polydipsia, low urine specific gravity, low urine osmolality (Cecil, Wyngaarden, & Smith, 1992), and high-normal plasma osmolality (300 mOsm/kg H_2O or more) (Labhart, 1986). Plasma osmolality is always higher than urine osmolality in diabetes insipidus after 8 hours of water deprivation. Individuals with long-standing diabetes insipidus develop a large bladder capacity and hydronephrosis (see Chapter 33).

Evaluation and Treatment

Diabetes insipidus must be distinguished from other polyuric states, including diabetes mellitus, osmotically induced diuresis, and primary polydipsia. Water restriction is a useful test because people without diabetes insipidus respond with a rapid decrease in urine volume (800 mOsm/kg), whereas persons with diabetes insipidus have no decrease in urine volume and maintain a urine osmolarity of approximately 100 mOsm/kg. Water deprivation tests, or dehydration testing, should be done with careful monitoring because depriving an individual with diabetes insipidus of water can lead to circulatory collapse or hypertonic encephalopathy. During dehydration tests, if the patient has nothing by mouth for 4 to 18 hours, maintains urine osmolarity, and specific gravity taken hourly is greater than 3% of body weight, the test should be terminated to avoid hypotension. The psychogenic form, compulsive water drinking, of diabetes insipidus is diagnosed when 24-hour urine volume is greater than 18 L/24 hours, random plasma osmolarity is less than 285 mOsm/kg of H_2O, and there is episodic polyuria (Cecil et al., 1992).

Treatment of neurogenic diabetes insipidus is based on the extent of the ADH deficiency and on individual variables such as age, endocrine and cardiovascular status, and life-style. Individuals who have a urine output in excess of 9 L/day and a urine osmolality of less than 100 mOsm/kg after a dehydration or water restriction test generally require ADH replacement (Reichlin, 1984).

Oral hydration is often adequate. Replacement therapy for symptomatic central or neurogenic diabetes insipidus includes administration of the synthetic vasopressin analog DDAVP (desmopressin) applied intravascularly. Drugs that potentiate the action of otherwise insufficient amounts of endogenous ADH, such as chlorpropamide, may be used in individuals with incomplete ADH deficiency. Clofibrate and carbamazepine are used in a limited fashion with mildly to moderately affected individuals (Camargo & Kolb, 1988). They stimulate ADH release from the hypothalamus.

Diseases of the Anterior Pituitary

Disorders of the anterior pituitary may involve either hypofunction or hyperfunction of the gland. **Hypopituitarism** is defined as a range of dysfunction, from the absence of selective pituitary hormones to complete failure of hormonal functions of the anterior pituitary. Pituitary hypofunction may be classified as primary (caused by intrinsic pituitary disease), secondary (caused by hypothalamic disorders), or functional (related to anorexia nervosa or chronic starvation). **Hyperpituitarism** is generally caused by a pituitary adenoma.

Anterior pituitary hypofunction may result from infarction of the gland, removal or destruction of the gland, or space-occupying lesions such as pituitary adenomas or aneurysms that compress otherwise-normal secreting pituitary cells and lead to compromised hormonal output. Growth hormone–secreting cells are most sensitive to pressure. Hyperfunction of the anterior pituitary generally implies an adenoma composed of secretory pituitary cells. Compression of a portion of the gland by an adenoma may lead to hypersecretion of one hormone produced by the adenoma, and hyposecretion of another caused by the compression effects of the tumor.

Hypopituitarism

Primary and secondary hypopituitarism are not usually distinguished. Secondary hypopituitarism (resulting from dysfunction of the hypothalamus) is difficult to document because the neurohormonal output of the hypothalamus does not lend itself to measurement.

A cause of hypopituitarism is pituitary infarction. Infarction may be seen in conjunction with Sheehan syndrome (postpartum pituitary necrosis), pituitary apoplexy, shock, sickle cell disease, and diabetes mellitus. Other causes of hypopituitarism are head trauma; infections (such as meningitis, syphilis, and tuberculosis); vascular malformations; surgical ablation related to tumor removal; and, rarely, granulomatous lesions. Hypopituitarism has been studied most frequently in cases of Sheehan syndrome, but it is occurring less frequently because of improved obstetric care.

Pathophysiology

The pituitary gland is extremely vascular and is therefore extremely vulnerable to infarction. The likelihood of infarction is increased with the increased size and vasculature of the gland, which occurs during pregnancy.

Sheehan and Stanfield proposed in 1961 that the primary pathologic mechanism in postpartum pituitary infarction is vasospasm of the artery supplying the anterior pituitary. A frequently identified cause is some event that leads to circulatory collapse and compensatory vasospasm. If vasospasm is sustained for more than several hours, tissue necrosis occurs. The pituitary gland may be particularly susceptible to necrosis because its blood supply, through the portal system, is already partially deoxygenated and, especially in the hyperplastic pituitary of pregnancy, oxygen demands are increased.

After tissue necrosis, edema occurs. Expansion of the pituitary within the fixed confines of the sella turcica further impedes blood supply to the pituitary. A second mechanism, which may be involved in pituitary infarction in the postpartum woman (Sheehan syndrome), is an increased risk for intravascular coagulation. In such individuals, excessive fibrin is deposited in the pituitary vessels, predisposing the woman to decreased blood supply and infarction of the pituitary (Reid, Quigley, & Yen, 1985).

FIG. 18-3 Hypopituitary dwarfism. A 4-year-old boy whose height is 25 inches. Girl is also 4 years old and has a normal height of 39 inches. Dwarf has a normal face, as well as head, trunk, and limbs of approximately normal proportions. (From Brasher & Raney, 1986.)

Clinical Manifestations

The signs and symptoms of hypofunction of the anterior pituitary are highly variable and depend on the affected hormones. If all hormones are absent (a condition termed **panhypopituitarism**), the individual suffers from cortisol deficiency from lack of ACTH, thyroid deficiency from lack of thyroid-stimulating hormone (TSH), diabetes insipidus from lack of ADH, and gonadal failure and loss of secondary sex characteristics from absence of FSH and LH. Growth hormone and, consequently, somatomedin levels are low, which may affect children, but these deficiencies do not generally develop into a symptom complex in adults (Fig. 18-3). Additionally, postpartum women are unable to lactate, because of the absence of prolactin.

Adrenocorticotropic hormone deficiency is a potentially life-threatening disorder, because cortisol is required for functional maintenance. Adrenocorticotropic hormone deficiency is usually encountered with generalized pituitary hypofunction; it rarely occurs as an isolated event. Within 2 weeks of the complete absence of ACTH, symptoms of cortisol insufficiency develop. These include nausea, vomiting, anorexia, fatigue, and weakness. The resulting hypoglycemia is caused by increased insulin sensitivity, decreased glycogen reserves, and decreased gluconeogenesis associated with hypocortisolism. In women, loss of body hair and decreased libido may be caused by decreased adrenal androgen production.

Adrenocorticotropic hormone deficiency also limits maximum aldosterone secretion, although the renin-angiotensin system is capable of stimulating some aldosterone secretion. Glomerular filtration rate is decreased with ACTH deficiency and may explain the decreased urine output. (Renal function is described in Chapter 32.) This may be of some benefit in the individual who has diabetes insipidus, but the polyuria associated with diabetes insipidus worsens after correction of cortisol levels. Frequently, individuals maintain some low level of ACTH secretion, so that cortisol replacement is not necessary. If ACTH is completely absent, however, cortisol replacement is required to maintain life.

Thyroid-stimulating hormone deficiency is rarely seen in isolation but frequently occurs in conjunction with other pituitary hormone deficiencies. The effects of decreased TSH levels may become apparent 4 to 8 weeks after the onset of hypothyrotropinemia. Cold intolerance, dryness of skin, mild myxedema, lethargy, and decreased metabolic rate occur as a result of hypothyroidism induced by decreased TSH levels. The symptoms are usually less severe than those associated with primary hypothyroidism.

The onset of FSH and LH deficiencies in women of reproductive age is associated with amenorrhea and an atrophic vagina, uterus, and breasts. In postpubertal males, atrophy of the testicles and decreased beard growth occur. Both men and women experience a decrease in body hair and diminished libido. Follicle-stimulating hormone and LH deficiencies frequently occur as a result of pressure on the gonadotropes from other sources, such as tumors. If there is enlargement caused by tumor, symptoms may include headache and visual disturbances with blurring and field defects.

Evaluation and Treatment

The diagnostic tests evaluating hypopituitarism are not definitive but must be interpreted together with the individual's signs and symptoms. Radioimmunoassay is used to measure hormone levels, and radiology shows an enlarged sella turcica. In cases of hypopituitarism, the underlying disorder should be corrected as quickly as possible. Frequently, cerebral edema is corrected by the administration of dexamethasone, which also corrects hypocortisolism. Thyroid and cortisol replacement therapy must be maintained. Sex steroid replacement therapy may be initiated, depending on the needs and desires of the individual.

Hyperpituitarism: Primary Adenoma

Pituitary adenomas are usually benign, slow-growing tumors that frequently arise from cells of the anterior pituitary. The incidence of pituitary adenomas may be as high as 22%, but most of these adenomas are microscopic and asymptomatic. Most are found only on postmortem examinations. The cause of pituitary adenomas is not known. The mortality associated with pituitary tumors is usually attributable to alterations in hormone secretion or tissue changes caused by expanding adenomas.

Pathophysiology

Local expansion of pituitary adenomas causes both neurologic and secretory effects. Neurologically, the tumor may impinge on the optic chiasma, particularly if it extends upward from the sella turcica. This causes a variety of visual disturbances, depending on the portion of the nerve that is compressed. If the tumor is malignant, invasion of the oculomotor and trigeminal nerves occurs, evoking symptoms relative to their function. Extension also may involve the hypothalamus, disturbing hypothalamic control of wakefulness, thirst, appetite, and temperature.

The adenomatous tissue secretes the hormone of the cell type from which it arose, without regard to the needs of the body and without benefit of regulatory feedback mechanisms. Because of the pressure exerted by a tumor growing in the unexpandable skull, those secreting cells of the anterior pituitary that are most sensitive to pressure also may be affected (growth hormone–secreting cells, FSH- and LH-secreting cells). The result of such pressure is hyposecretion of these hormones.

Clinical Manifestations

The clinical manifestations of pituitary adenomas are related to tumor growth and hormone hypersecretion and hyposecretion. Effects from an increase in tumor size include such nonspecific complaints as headache, fatigue, neck pain or stiffness, and seizures. Visual changes produced by pressure on the optic chiasma include visual field impairments (frequently beginning in one eye and progressing to the other) and temporary blindness. If the tumor infiltrates other cranial nerves, neuromuscular function is affected.

The hyposecretion of the pituitary hormones caused by pressure changes results in impaired pituitary function. Hyposecretion of growth hormone almost always occurs, but in adults this is clinically asymptomatic. Gonadotropic hyposecretion frequently results in menstrual irregularity in women, decreased libido, and receding secondary sex characteristics in both men and women. If the tumor exerts sufficient pressure, thyroid and adrenal hypofunction may occur because of lack of TSH and ACTH. These result in the symptoms of hypothyroidism and hypocortisolism. Hypersecretion of hormones secreted by the adenoma itself leads to symptoms associated with the particular hormone that is affected.

Evaluation and Treatment

Diagnosis of pituitary adenoma involves physical and laboratory evaluations, including pertinent hormone assays and radiographic examination of the skull. This may be accomplished by computed tomographic scanning used in conjunction with contrast material.

The goal of treatment is to protect the individual from the effects of tumor growth and to control hormone hypersecretion while minimizing damage to appropriately secreting portions of the pituitary. Surgery and radiation therapy are used, depending on the extent of tumor growth and the suitability of the individual for surgery.

Hypersecretion of Growth Hormone: Acromegaly

Acromegaly occurs in adults who are exposed to continuously excessive levels of growth hormone (GH). In children and adolescents whose epiphyseal plates have not yet closed, the effect of increased GH levels is termed **giantism** (Fig. 18-4).

Acromegaly is a relatively uncommon disease, estimated to occur in about 40 cases per million (Melmed, 1990). Approximately 15% of all pituitary tumors release excessive GH. The most common cause of acro-

FIG. 18-4 Giantism. A pituitary giant and dwarf contrasted with normal-sized men. Excessive secretion of growth hormone by the anterior lobe of the pituitary gland during the early years of life produces giants of this type, whereas deficient secretion of this substance produces well-formed dwarfs. (From Thibodeau & Patton, 1993.)

FIG. 18-5 **Acromegaly.** Note thickening of skin on scalp. (From Thibodeau, G. A. [1987]. *Anatomy and physiology*. St. Louis: Mosby–Year Book.)

FIG. 18-6 **Acromegaly.** Note large head, forward projection of jaw, and protrusion of frontal bone. (From Thibodeau, G. A. [1987]. *Anatomy and physiology*. St. Louis: Mosby–Year Book.)

megaly is a primary autonomous GH-secreting pituitary adenoma. Acromegaly occurs more frequently in women than men and is diagnosed most frequently in adults in their 40s and 50s, although the disease was usually present for years preceding the diagnosis.

Acromegaly is a slowly progressive disease that, if untreated, is associated with a decreased life expectancy. The increased number of deaths associated with acromegaly are apparently caused by an increased occurrence of hypertension and diabetes mellitus.

Pathophysiology

With a GH-secreting adenoma, the usual GH baseline secretion pattern is lost, as are sleep-related GH peaks. A totally unpredictable secretory pattern ensues. With only slight elevations of GH, somatomedin levels increase, stimulating growth. In the adult, epiphyseal closure has occurred, and increased amounts of GH and somatomedins cannot stimulate further long bone growth. Instead these elevations cause connective tissue proliferation and an increase in the cytoplasmic matrix, as well as bony proliferation that results in the characteristic appearance of acromegaly.

Growth hormone acts on the renal tubules to increase phosphate reabsorption, leading to mild hyperphosphatemia. The metabolic effects of GH hypersecretion include impaired carbohydrate tolerance and increased metabolic rate. Hyperglycemia may be seen as a result of GH's inhibition of peripheral glucose uptake and increased hepatic glucose production, followed by compensatory hyperinsulinism, and finally, insulin resistance. Diabetes mellitus occurs when the pancreas is unable to secrete enough insulin to offset the effects of GH. Somatotropic tumors are frequently associated with decreased gonadotropin secretion, leading to oligomenorrhea in women and impotence in men.

Clinical Manifestations

As a result of connective tissue proliferation, individuals with acromegaly have enlarged tongues, interstitial edema, increase in the size and function of sebaceous and sweat glands (leading to increased body odor), and coarse skin and body hair. The coarse skin condition becomes very apparent when procedures such as inserting an intravenous needle are performed; the skin is very thick and difficult to penetrate (Fig. 18-5). Bony proliferation involves periosteal vertebral growth and enlargement of the facial bones and the bones of the hands and feet (Fig. 18-6). The associated growth results in protrusion of the lower jaw and forehead and a need for increasingly larger sizes of shoes, hats, rings, and gloves.

Because somatomedins stimulate cartilaginous growth, the increased somatomedin levels cause elongation of ribs at the bone-cartilage junction, leading to a barrel-chested appearance and increased proliferation of cartilage in joints. This in turn causes backache, arthralgia, and arthritis. These are early manifestations of acromegaly. When shaking hands with an individual with acromegaly, one can palpate the large soft tissues. With bony and soft-tissue overgrowth, entrapment of nerves may occur, leading to peripheral nerve damage as manifested by weakness, muscular atrophy, foot drop, and sensory changes in the hands.

Hypertension and left heart failure are seen in one third to one half of individuals with acromegaly, although the associated pathophysiology is not understood at present (Bengtsson, Eden, & Ernst, 1988). Headache occurs in 50% to 87% of cases and does not appear related to GH levels, size, or extension of the tumor or presence of hypertension. Because of a space-occupying lesion, central nervous system symptoms of headache, seizure activity, visual disturbances (such as bitemporal hemianopia from compression of the optic chiasma), papilledema, and compression hypopituitarism may occur (Molitich, 1992).

If compression hypopituitarism does occur, the secretion of the gonadotropins may be affected. This causes amenorrhea in women and impotence in men. The secretion of prolactin-inhibiting factor is impaired in 30% to 40% of individuals with acromegaly. Approximately one third of people with acromegaly have impaired glucose tolerance, and one half of these are diabetic (Ezrin, Horvath, Kaufman, Kovacs, & Weiss, 1980).

Evaluation and Treatment

Diagnosis of GH hypersecretion involves measurement of serum GH by radioreceptor assay or radioimmunoassay at basal conditions and in response to glucose administration. The goals of treatment are to normalize or reduce GH secretion, if possible, allowing normal pituitary function and relieving or preventing complications related to tumor expansion. The treatment of choice in acromegaly is surgical removal of the GH-secreting adenoma. Treatment by radiation therapy may be effective when rapid control of GH levels is not essential, when the individual is not a good surgical candidate, or when hyperfunction persists after subtotal resection.

ALTERATIONS OF THYROID FUNCTION

Thyrotoxicosis
Course of Thyrotoxicosis

Thyrotoxicosis is a condition in which thyroid hormones (TH) from any source exert greater-than-normal responses (Braverman & Utiger, 1991). Thyrotoxicosis has a variety of causes. Identifying the cause is important because the treatment and expected outcome vary accordingly. Hyperthyroidism is a form of thyrotoxicosis in which excess thyroid hormones are secreted by the thyroid gland. Specific diseases that can cause hyperthyroidism include Graves disease, toxic multinodular goiter, thyroid cancer, and increased TSH secretion. Thyrotoxicosis not associated with hyperthyroidism includes subacute thyroiditis, ectopic thyroid tissue, and ingestion of excessive TH. Each of these conditions is associated with specific pathophysiology and manifestations, and the most commonly occurring ones are described in the following pages. All forms of thyrotoxicosis share some common characteristics.

Clinical Manifestations

The clinical features of thyrotoxicosis are attributable to the metabolic effects of increased circulating levels of thyroid hormones. This usually results in an increased metabolic rate with heat intolerance and an increased tissue sensitivity to stimulation by the sympathetic division of the autonomic nervous system. The major manifestations are summarized in Table 18-1. Goiter is almost always present.

Evaluation and Treatment

The diagnosis of thyrotoxicosis is related to the symptoms accompanying specific diseases that cause excessive thyroid hormone and associated laboratory findings. Elevated serum T_4, T_3, and radioactive iodine uptake (RAIU) are common in hyperthyroid states.

Treatment is directed at controlling excessive TH production, secretion, or action. The major types of therapy currently used to achieve these goals include drug therapy, radioactive iodine therapy, and surgery.

Hyperthyroid Conditions
Graves disease

Graves disease is the most common cause of hyperthyroidism. Although the exact cause of Graves disease is currently unknown, the most accepted theory is that the disease is associated with autoimmune abnormalities (see Chapter 8). Graves disease is a familial disorder, characterized as a multisystem syndrome consisting of one or more of the following: (1) hyperthyroidism, (2) diffuse thyroid enlargement, (3) ophthalmopathy, (4) dermopathy, and (5) effects on the extremities (Farid & Stenzky, 1988). The incidence is less than 1% in the U.S. population (McDougall, 1991).

The pathology of Graves disease indicates that normal regulatory mechanisms are overridden by some abnormal thyroid-stimulating mechanism. Substances termed thyroid receptor antibody (or thyroid-stimulating immunoglobulins) of the IgG class are found in more than 95% of subjects with Graves disease. The

TABLE 18-1

Systemic Effects of Hyperthyroidism

System	Manifestations	Mechanisms
Endocrine	Enlarged thyroid gland (97%-99% of cases); systolic or continuous bruit over thyroid; increased cortisol degradation; hypercalcemia and decreased PTH secretion; diminished sensitivity to exogenous insulin	Hyperactivity of the thyroid gland; excess bone resorption leading to hypercalcemia and a disruption of PTH-regulating mechanisms; increased insulin degradation
Reproductive	Oligomenorrhea or amenorrhea in women, impotence and decreased libido in men; increased serum estradiol and estrone but lower than normal levels of free estradiol and estrone	Menstrual cycle alterations that may be related to hypothalamic or pituitary disturbances; increase in sex hormone–binding globulin
Gastrointestinal	Weight loss and an associated increase in appetite; increased peristalsis leading to less formed and more frequent stools; nausea, vomiting, anorexia, abdominal pain; increased use of hepatic glycogen stores and of adipose and protein stores; decrease in serum lipid levels (including triglycerides, phospholipids, and cholesterol); changes in vitamin metabolism leading to decrease in tissue stores of vitamins	Increased catabolism leading to the body's inability to meet its metabolic needs; malabsorption of fat; increased glucose absorption; increase in cholesterol excretion in feces and cholesterol conversion to bile salts; impaired conversion of B vitamins to their coenzymes, causing increased need for water-soluble and fat-soluble vitamins
Integumentary	Excessive sweating, flushing, and warm skin; heat intolerance; hair fine, soft, and straight; temporary hair loss; nails that grow away from nail beds, palmar erythema	Hyperdynamic circulatory state
Sensory (eyes)	Ocular manifestations including elevated upper eyelid leading to decreased blinking and a staring quality; fine tremor of lid; infiltrative ocular changes associated with Graves disease	Overactivity of Müller's muscle
Cardiovascular	Increased cardiac output and decreased peripheral resistance; tachycardia at rest; loud heart sounds; supraventricular arrhythmias	Hypermetabolism and need to dissipate heat
Nervous	Restlessness; short attention span; compulsive movement; fatigue; tremor; insomnia; emotionally labile	Not clearly defined: alterations in cerebral metabolism resulting from excess thyroid hormone
Pulmonary	Dyspnea; reduced vital capacity	Weakness of respiratory muscles

immunoglobulins bind to the plasma membrane and initiate thyroid growth, vascularity, and hypersecretion of hormone. The hyperfunction of the thyroid gland leads to suppression of TSH and TRH, although these usual feedback mechanisms are ineffective in lowering TH levels. The hyperfunction of the thyroid gland is reflected in a dramatically increased iodine uptake and increased rate of thyroid gland metabolism, which may in turn contribute to the hypervascularity and enlargement of the gland. The disproportionate increase in T_3 production reflects chronic hyperstimulation of the thyroid

gland. A decrease in the concentration of thyroid-binding globulin, combined with the increased production of thyroid hormone, causes increased circulating levels of thyroid hormone responsible for many of the thyrotoxic symptoms.

A small number of individuals with Graves disease experience **pretibial myxedema (Graves dermopathy)**, characterized by subcutaneous swelling on the anterior portions of the legs, and by indurated and erythematous skin. These manifestations occasionally appear on the hands as well. Because pretibial myxedema is a widespread alteration in a number of disorders, Graves dermopathy has been proposed as a term to replace pretibial myxedema (Ezrin, 1979).

Many individuals with Graves disease experience ocular manifestations (Fig. 18-7). Two categories of ocular manifestations are associated with Graves disease: (1) functional abnormalities resulting from hyperactivity of the sympathetic division of the autonomic nervous system and (2) infiltrative changes involving the orbital contents with enlargement of the ocular muscles. Functional abnormalities occur in most individuals with Graves disease. These abnormalities include a lag of the globe on upward gaze or a lag of the upper lid on downward gaze. This manifestation does not appear to affect ocular function and appears to resolve with treatment for hyperthyroidism.

Infiltrative ophthalmopathy may occur with Graves disease, although the ophthalmopathy appears to be a separate disorder. It appears in 50% to 70% of individuals with Graves disease (Volpe, 1991), and it is characterized by edema of the orbital contents, protrusion of the globe, paralysis of the extraocular muscles, and damage to the retina and optic nerve, which may lead to blindness. These changes result in exophthalmos, periorbital edema, and extraocular muscle weakness leading to diplopia. The individual may experience irritation, pain, lacrimation, photophobia, and blurred vision. Occasionally, decreased visual acuity, papilledema, visual field impairment, exposure keratosis, and corneal ulceration may occur.

Unfortunately, current treatment for Graves disease does not reverse the infiltrative ophthalmopathy or the pretibial myxedema. Therapy for these problems is palliative, although skin lesions rarely require treatment.

Diffuse toxic goiter

The thyroid gland normally enlarges in response to an increased demand for TH that occurs in puberty, pregnancy, iodine deficiency, and immunologic, viral, or genetic disorders. The increased number of follicles is a compensatory mechanism in response to increased TSH levels. When the condition requiring increased TH resolves, TSH secretion normally subsides and the thyroid gland returns to its original size.

Irreversible changes may have occurred in some follicular cells, however, so that such cells now function autonomously. Hyperthyroidism may or may not result from these irreversible changes. Autonomously functioning cells may produce less TH than the body requires. The remainder of the gland then functions to supply the remainder of the body's need, and a euthyroid state is achieved and maintained. If the autonomously functioning cells produce sufficient or excessive TH for the usual body requirement, the remainder of the gland undergoes involution, becoming normal but

FIG. 18-7 Graves disease. Note large and protruding eyeballs. (From Thibodeau, G. A. [1987]. *Anatomy and physiology*. St. Louis: Mosby–Year Book.)

inactive tissue. This condition may result in euthyroidism or hyperthyroidism, depending on the amount of TH produced.

Once thyrotoxicosis results, the condition is generally termed **toxic multinodular goiter.** The manifestations of hyperthyroidism resulting from toxic nodular goiter are similar to those of Graves disease, although infiltrative ophthalmopathy and myxedema do not occur. The symptoms usually develop slowly and appear over time (Gavin, 1991).

Thyrotoxic crisis

Thyrotoxic crisis (thyroid storm) is a rare but dangerous worsening of the thyrotoxic state, in which death occurs within 48 hours without treatment. The condition may develop spontaneously, but it occurs most frequently in individuals who have undiagnosed or partially treated severe hyperthyroidism and who are subjected to excessive stress from other causes. These causes may include infection, pulmonary or cardiovascular disorders, emotional distress, dialysis, plasmapheresis, or inadequate preparation for thyroid surgery.

The systemic symptoms of thyrotoxic crisis include hyperthermia; tachycardia, especially atrial tachydysrhythmias; high-output heart failure; agitation or delirium; and nausea, vomiting, or diarrhea contributing to fluid volume depletion. The symptoms may be attributed to increased beta-adrenergic receptors and catecholamines (Gavin, 1991). The treatment is designed to reduce both circulating TH levels by inducing a block of thyroid hormone synthesis (i.e., prophylthiouracil) and thereby reducing their effects to eliminate the precipitating disorder; and to provide symptomatic and supportive care.

Hypothyroidism

Deficient production of TH by the thyroid gland results in the clinical state termed **hypothyroidism.** Hypothyroidism may be either primary or secondary. Primary causes include (1) congenital defects or loss of thyroid tissue after treatment for hyperthyroidism and (2) defective hormone synthesis resulting from autoimmune (circulating antithyroid antibodies) thyroiditis, endemic iodine deficiency, or antithyroid drugs (goitrous hypothyroidism). Causes of secondary hypothyroidism that are less common include (1) insufficient stimulation of the normal gland, causing TSH deficiency from hypothyroidism of the pituitary or hypothalamus, and (2) peripheral resistance to TH (Wilson & Foster, 1992). Hypothyroidism is the most common disorder of thyroid function.

Pathophysiology

In primary hypothyroidism, the loss of thyroid tissue leads to a decreased production of TH. The response is an increased secretion of TSH that leads to goiter. Secondary hypothyroidism is most commonly caused by failure of the pituitary to synthesize adequate amounts of TSH. Postpartum pituitary necrosis and a pituitary tumor are the most frequent causes of secondary hypothyroidism.

Clinical Manifestations

Hypothyroidism generally affects all body systems, with the extent of the symptoms closely related to the degree of TH deficiency. The onset is usually insidious over months or years. The lowered levels of TH result in decreased energy metabolism and heat production. The individual develops a low basal metabolic rate, cold intolerance, lethargy, tiredness, and slightly lowered basal body temperature (Table 18-2). A decrease in TH may lead to excessive TSH production and goiter.

The characteristic sign of severe or long-standing hypothyroidism is **myxedema,** which is histologically similar to the pretibial myxedema deposits that often occur with Graves disease. Myxedema is a result of an alteration in the composition of the dermis and other tissues. The connective fibers are separated by an increased amount of protein and mucopolysaccharides.

This protein-mucopolysaccharide complex binds water, producing nonpitting, boggy edema, especially around the eyes, hands, and feet and in the supraclavicular fossae (Fig. 18-8). Binding with water is also responsible for thickening of the tongue and the laryngeal and pharyngeal mucous membranes. This results in thick slurred speech and hoarseness, both common in hypothyroidism.

Evaluation and Treatment

In addition to the clinical symptoms of hypothyroidism, a decrease in serum T_4 and free T_4 is nearly always present. Thyroid-stimulating hormone concentration increases from loss of negative feedback from thyroid hor-

---

TABLE 18-2

Systemic Manifestations of Hypothyroidism

System	Manifestations	Mechanisms
Neurologic	Confusion, syncope, slowed speech and thinking, memory loss; lethargy, headaches, hearing loss, night blindness; slow, clumsy movements; cerebellar ataxia; slow alpha wave activity and loss of amplitude in EEG; reduced cAMP response to epinephrine, glucagon, and PTH	Decreased cerebral blood flow leading to cerebral hypoxia; reduced intracellular processes caused by decreased beta-adrenergic activity that may be related to a decrease in the number of beta-adrenergic receptor sites
Endocrine	Increased TSH production in primary hypothyroidism; enlarged pituitary thyrotropes, increase in serum prolactin levels with galactorrhea; decreased rate of cortisol turnover but with normal serum cortisol levels	Impaired TH synthesis or defects in iodide trapping leading to compensatory TSH production; chronic overstimulation of thyrotropes by TRH and by TSH synthesis; stimulation of lactotropes by TRH related to increased prolactin levels; decreased deactivation of cortisol

TABLE 18-2

Systemic Manifestations of Hypothyroidism—cont'd

System	Manifestations	Mechanisms
Reproductive	Decreased androgen secretion in men, increased estriol formation in women; low total hormone values but with increased amounts of unbound hormone; anovulation, decreased libido, and a high incidence of spontaneous abortion in women; impotence, decreased libido, and oligospermia in men	Altered metabolism of estrogens and androgens; decreased sex hormone–binding globulin
Hematologic	Decrease in red cell mass leading to normocytic, normochromic anemia; macrocytic anemia associated with vitamin B_{12} deficiency and inadequate folate or iron absorption in the GI tract	Decreased basal metabolic rate and reduced oxygen requirements, decreased production of erythropoietin, possible relationship between TH and optimal hematologic response to vitamin B_{12}
Cardiovascular	Reduction in stroke volume and heart rate causing lowered cardiac output; increased peripheral vascular resistance to maintain systolic blood pressure; normal response to exercise but with alterations in circulatory system at rest (prolonged circulation time and decreased blood flow to tissues); cool skin and cold tolerance; enlarged heart; decreased intensity of heart sounds and variety of ECG changes (sinus bradycardia, prolonged PR interval, depressed P waves, flattened or inverted T waves, and low-amplitude QRS complexes); cardiac tamponade (although rare)	Decreased metabolic demands and loss of regulatory and rate-setting effects of TH; protein-mucopolysaccharide-rich fluid in the pericardial sac associated with enlarged heart; pericardial effusions associated with heart sounds and ECG changes
Pulmonary	Dyspnea; myxedematous changes in respiratory muscles leading to hypoventilation and carbon dioxide retention, which contribute to myxedema coma	Pleural effusions associated with dyspnea, although effusions may be asymptomatic
Renal	Reduced renal blood flow and glomerular filtration rate leading to decreased renal excretion of water; increase in total body water and dilutional hyponatremia; reduced production of erythropoietin	Hemodynamic alterations associated with reduced blood flow and filtration; increased total body water related to decreased excretion and mucinous deposits in tissue
Gastrointestinal	Decreased appetite; constipation, weight gain, and fluid retention; decreased absorption of most nutrients; decreased protein metabolism leading to retarded skeletal and soft-tissue growth and slightly positive nitrogen balance; edema; decreased glucose absorption and delayed glucose uptake; increased sensitivity to exogenous insulin; elevated serum lipid values	Reduced intake and reduced peristaltic activity that may progress to fecal impaction; water absorption related to prolonged transit time; fluid retention associated with myxedematous changes; edema associated with high concentrations of exchangeable albumin in the extravascular space caused by increased capillary permeability to proteins; depressed insulin degradation; depressed lipid synthesis and degradation
Musculoskeletal	Muscle aching and stiffness; slow movement and slow tendon jerk reflexes; decreased bone formation and resorption, increased bone density; aching and stiffness in joints	Decreased rate of muscle contraction and relaxation contributing to slow movement and reflexes
Integumentary	Dry, flaky skin; dry, brittle head and body hair; reduced growth of nails and hair, slow wound healing	Reduced sweat and sebaceous gland secretion
	Myxedema	Accumulation of hyaluronic acid, which binds water and causes a puffy appearance
	Cool skin	Decreased circulation to skin

FIG. 18-8 Myxedema. Note the edema around eyes and facial puffiness. (From Thibodeau, G. A. [1987]. *Anatomy and physiology.* St. Louis: Mosby–Year Book.)

mone. When hypothyroidism is caused by pituitary deficiencies, serum TSH levels are decreased; the basal metabolic rate (BMR) is decreased. Hormone replacement therapy is the treatment of choice for hypothyroidism. Thyroid hormone is currently available as a synthetic hormone (levothyroxine or liothyronine) and is generally preferred over the crude extract from animal thyroid glands (desiccated thyroid).

The restoration of normal TH levels should be timed appropriately; a regimen of hormonal therapy depends on the individual's age, the duration and severity of the hypothyroidism, and the presence of other disorders, particularly cardiovascular disorders. The goal is maximal metabolic restoration consistent with the individual's overall well-being.

Hypothyroid Conditions

Hypothyroidism results from three relatively rare disorders, none of which is related to any of the others by cause, symptoms, management, or outcome. These three conditions are acute thyroiditis, subacute thyroiditis, and autoimmune thyroiditis. **Acute thyroiditis** is caused by a bacterial infection of the thyroid gland and is a rare disorder. **Subacute thyroiditis** is a nonbacterial inflammation of the thyroid often preceded by a viral infection. Both conditions are accompanied by fever, tenderness, and enlargement of the thyroid. The inflammatory process results in hypothyroidism caused by tissue infil-

tration of lymphocytes and leukocytes. Symptoms may last for 2 to 4 months, and corticosteroids usually resolve symptoms. **Autoimmune thyroiditis** (Hashimoto disease or chronic lymphocytic thyroiditis) results in destruction of thyroid tissue by circulating thyroid antibodies and infiltration of lymphocytes. Autoimmune thyroiditis also may be caused by an inherited immune defect. Goiter formation is commonly observed.

Myxedema coma

A medical emergency, **myxedema coma** is a diminished level of consciousness associated with severe hypothyroidism. Symptoms include hypothermia without shivering, hypoventilation, hypotension, hypoglycemia, and lactic acidosis. Older patients with severe vascular disease and with moderate or untreated hypothyroidism are particularly at risk for developing myxedema coma. It also may occur after overuse of narcotics or sedatives or after an acute illness in hypothyroid individuals.

Congenital hypothyroidism

Hypothyroidism in infants occurs as a result of absent thyroid tissue (thyroid dysgenesis) and hereditary defects in thyroid hormone synthesis. Thyroid dysgenesis occurs more frequently in female infants, with permanent abnormalities in 1 of every 400 live births (Jubiz, 1985).

Thyroid hormone is essential for embryonic growth, particularly of brain tissue. The infant will be mentally retarded if there is no thyroxine during fetal life, but this can be partially reversed with administration of thyroxine immediately after birth.

Clinical manifestations of hypothyroidism may not be evident until after 4 months of age. Symptoms include difficulty eating, hoarse cry, and protruding tongue caused by myxedema of oral tissues and vocal cords; hypotonic muscles of the abdomen with constipation, abdominal protrusion, and umbilical hernia; subnormal temperature; lethargy; excessive sleeping; slow pulse; and cold mottled skin. Skeletal growth is stunted because of impaired protein synthesis, poor absorption of nutrients, and lack of bone mineralization. The child will be dwarfed, with short limbs, if not treated (cretinism) (Fig. 18-9). Dentition is often delayed. Mental retardation is a function of the severity of hypothyroidism and the delay before initiation of treatment.

Hypothyroidism is difficult to identify at birth, but high birth weight, hypothermia, delay in passing meconium, and neonatal jaundice are suggestive signs. Cord blood can be examined in the first days of life for thyroxine and TSH levels. Treatment is administration of thyroxine. There is a high probability of normal growth and intellectual function if treatment is started before the child is 3 or 4 months old.

FIG. 18-9 Adult cretin. Note characteristic facial features, dwarfism (44 inches), absent axillary and scant pubic hair, poorly developed breasts, potbelly, and small umbilical hernia. (From Schneeberg, 1970.)

Thyroid Carcinoma

Thyroid carcinoma is the most common endocrine malignancy but is relatively rare, accounting for 11,000 new cases annually and approximately 0.5% of all cancer deaths per year (American Cancer Society [ACS], 1993). Iodine deficiency, chronic long-term use of goitrogenic drugs, exposure to ionizing radiation, or a combination of these causal factors has been shown to produce thyroid hyperplasia and, ultimately, malignancy in animals. In approximately 10% of cases, hyperplasia of the thyroid gland leads to thyroid carcinoma in humans. The most consistent causal risk factor in the development of thyroid cancer appears to be exposure to ionizing radiation, especially exposure during childhood.

Most individuals with thyroid carcinoma have normal T_3 and T_4 levels and are therefore euthyroid. Thyroid cancer is typically discovered as a small thyroid nodule or as a metastatic tumor most commonly occurring in the lungs, brain, or bone. Changes in voice and swallowing and difficulty in breathing are related to tumor growth impinging on the trachea or esophagus. Di-

agnosing a thyroid cancer involves (1) measurement of serum thyroid levels, (2) radioisotope scanning, (3) ultrasonography, or (4) small-needle aspiration biopsy.

Treatment for thyroid carcinoma remains controversial, primarily because of the rarity of the disease, its protracted nature, and the relatively low mortality rate regardless of the method of treatment. Treatment may include partial or total thyroidectomy, TSH suppression therapy (levothyroxine), radioactive iodine therapy (in iodine-concentrating tumors), postoperative radiation therapy, and chemotherapy (especially in anaplastic carcinoma) (Camargo & Kolb, 1988).

ALTERATIONS OF PARATHYROID FUNCTION

Hyperparathyroidism

Hyperparathyroidism is characterized by greater than normal secretion of parathyroid hormone (PTH). Hyperparathyroidism is classified as one of three types: primary, secondary, or tertiary.

Pathophysiology

Estimates suggest that **primary hyperparathyroidism** occurs in 0.2% to 0.3% of the adult population and occurs twice as often in women. It is generally found in older adults (Braunwald et al., 1987). Because postmenopausal women are a group already at risk for developing osteoporosis, the effects of increased levels of PTH on bone disease can be significant. Most cases of hyperparathyroidism (approximately 80%) are the result of a chief cell adenoma with an increased secretion of parathyroid hormone.

Primary hyperparathyroidism

In primary hyperparathyroidism (Conn disease, primary aldosteronism) the normal regulatory relationship between serum calcium levels and PTH secretion is interrupted so that PTH secretion is autonomous and not under the usual feedback control mechanisms. The increase in gastrointestinal absorption of calcium is presumed to reflect the kidney's increased generation of biologically active vitamin D in response to increased PTH levels (see Fig. 3-7).

Secondary hyperparathyroidism

Secondary hyperparathyroidism is a compensatory, although not inevitable, response of the parathyroid glands to chronic hypocalcemia. Chronic hypercalcemia can be associated with decreased renal activation of vitamin D as occurs in renal failure (see Chapters 3 and 35). In secondary hyperparathyroidism, secretion of PTH is elevated but PTH is unable to achieve normal calcium levels because of failure of a target organ, the kidney.

Tertiary hyperparathyroidism

Hyperplasia of the parathyroid glands and a loss of sensitivity to circulating calcium levels can cause autonomous secretion of PTH, even with normal calcium levels. The condition is then termed **tertiary hyperthyroidism.** Tertiary hyperthyroidism frequently occurs in individuals with chronic renal failure. Signs and symptoms of this syndrome are similar to those of primary hyperparathyroidism.

Clinical Manifestations

Hypersecretion of PTH causes excessive osteoclastic and osteocytic activity, resulting in bone resorption. (Bone resorption is discussed in Chapter 38.) Pathologic bone changes include pathologic fractures, kyphosis of the dorsal spine, and compression fractures of the vertebral bodies. Parathyroid hormone hypersecretion and its resulting hypercalcemia increase the renal filtration load of calcium, leading to hypercalcuria.

Hypercalcemia also affects proximal renal tubular function, causing metabolic acidosis and production of an abnormally alkaline urine. Because calcium and phosphate levels are inversely related, hypercalcemia results in hypophosphatemia (see Chapter 3). Hyperparathyroidism directly results in hyperphosphaturia. The combination of these three variables—hypercalcuria, alkaline urine, and hyperphosphaturia—predisposes the individual to the formation of calcium stones. Kidney stones are frequently formed in the renal pelvis or in the renal collecting ducts and may be associated with infections. Both kidney stones and renal infection may

---

TABLE 18-3

Manifestations of Primary Hyperparathyroidism

Symptoms	Responsible derangements	Mechanisms
Renal colic, nephrolithiasis, recurrent urinary tract infections, renal failure	Hypercalcemia, hyperphosphaturia, proximal renal tubular bicarbonate leak, urine pH>6	Calcium phosphate salts precipitate in alkaline urine, renal pelvis, and collecting ducts; calcium oxalate stones also formed
Abdominal pain, peptic ulcer disease	Hypercalcemia-stimulated hypergastrinemia	Elevated hydrochloric acid secretion
Pancreatitis	Hypercalcemia	Etiology of relationship unknown
Bone disease, osteitis fibrosa and cystica, osteoporosis	PTH-stimulated bone resorption, metabolic acidosis	Osteoporosis now more commonly encountered, but other disorders more specific for hyperparathyroidism
Muscle weakness, myalgia	PTH excess, possible direct effect on striated muscle and on nerves	Characteristic myopathic changes in muscle histology, nerve conduction rate suppressed
Neurologic and psychiatric problems	Hypercalcemia	Neuropathy; electroencephalographic changes present
Polyuria, polydipsia	Hypercalcemia	Direct effect on renal tubule to decrease responsiveness to antidiuretic hormone
Constipation	Hypercalcemia	Decreased peristalsis of gastrointestinal tract
Anorexia, nausea, and vomiting	Hypercalcemia	Central stimulation of vomiting center
Hypertension	Renal disease, direct effect of calcium on arterial smooth muscle, pheochromocytoma	Plasma renin activity elevated or normal
Arthralgia and arthritis	Gout, pseudogout, periarticular classification	Hyperuricemia, chronic renal failure with high calcium X phosphate product

From Rabin, D., & McKenna, T.J. (1982). *Clinical endocrinology and metabolism: Principles and practice.* New York: Grune & Stratton.

lead to impaired renal function. Hypercalcemia also impairs the concentrating ability of the renal tubule by decreasing its response to ADH.

Chronic hypercalcemia of hyperparathyroidism is associated with insulin resistance, necessitating increased insulin secretion to maintain normal glucose levels. Hypercalcemia also affects the muscular, nervous, and gastrointestinal systems. (The clinical symptoms of primary hyperparathyroidism are summarized in Table 18-3.)

Evaluation and Treatment

The diagnosis of hyperparathyroidism is generally accomplished by excluding all the other possible causes of hypercalcemia. A definitive diagnosis then must be supported by at least a 6-month history of symptoms associated with hypercalcemia, including kidney stones, hypophosphatemia, hyperchloremia, and increased urinary calcium levels. Tests used to document hyperparathyroidism include measurement of serum calcium, phosphorus, magnesium, bicarbonate, chloride, and pH (urinary pH, calcium, and hydroxyproline); bone x-ray films and densitometry; catheterization of the thyroid veins to document the source of PTH secretion; and radioimmunoassays. Radioimmunoassays for PTH are not generally required for the diagnosis of hyperparathyroidism, and this test currently poses many problems in providing clear-cut evidence of hyperparathyroidism.

The treatment of hyperparathyroidism includes lowering of severely elevated calcium levels, increasing urinary calcium excretion with diuretics, and long-term management of hypercalcemia by use of drugs that decrease resorption of calcium from bone. Definitive treatment for hyperparathyroidism involves the surgical removal of the hyperplastic parathyroid glands.

Hypoparathyroidism

Hypoparathyroidism (abnormally low PTH levels) is most commonly caused by damage to the parathyroid glands during thyroid surgery. Overt postoperative parathyroid failure occurs in approximately 1% of all individuals undergoing thyroid surgery, with the incidence increasing to 10% after repeated neck explorations.

In hypoparathyroidism, a lack of circulating PTH causes a depressed serum calcium level and an increased serum phosphate level. In the absence of PTH, the abilities to resorb calcium from bone and to regulate calcium reabsorption from the renal tubules are impaired. Phosphate reabsorption by the renal tubules is therefore increased, causing hyperphosphatemia.

Hypoparathyroidism appears to result from hypomagnesemia, although the effects of hypomagnesemia on the peripheral metabolism and clearance of PTH are not clearly understood. Once serum magnesium levels are returned to normal, however, PTH secretion returns to normal. Hypomagnesemia may be related to chronic alcoholism, malnutrition, malabsorption, increased renal clearance of magnesium caused by the use of aminoglycoside antibiotics or certain chemotherapeutic agents, or prolonged magnesium-deficient parenteral nutritional therapy.

Clinical Manifestations

Symptoms associated with hypoparathyroidism are primarily those of hypocalcemia. Hypocalcemia causes a lowering of the threshold for nerve and muscle excitation so that a nerve impulse may be initiated by a slight stimulus anywhere along the length of a nerve or muscle fiber. This is manifested as muscle spasms, hyperreflexia, clonic-tonic convulsions, laryngeal spasms, and, in severe cases, death of asphyxiation.

Other symptoms of hypocalcemia are caused by mechanisms that are not yet understood. These symptoms include dry skin, loss of body and scalp hair, hypoplasia of developing teeth, horizontal ridges on the nails, cataracts, basal ganglia calcifications (which may be associated with a parkinsonian syndrome), and bone deformities, including brachydactyly and bowing of the long bones.

Phosphate retention caused by increased renal reabsorption of phosphate is associated also with hypoparathyroidism. Hyperphosphatemia is associated with inhibition of the renal enzyme necessary for the conversion of vitamin D to its most active form. This tends to depress serum calcium levels further by reducing gastrointestinal absorption of calcium.

Evaluation and Treatment

A low serum calcium and high phosphorus level in the absence of renal failure, intestinal disorders, or nutritional deficiencies is diagnostic of hypoparathyroidism. Parathyroid hormone levels are usually normal in primary hypoparathyroidism.

The treatment of hypoparathyroidism is directed toward the alleviation of hypocalcemia. In acute states, this involves parenteral administration of calcium, which allows correction of serum calcium within minutes. Maintenance of serum calcium is achieved with pharmacologic doses of an active form of vitamin D and oral calcium. The recommended daily dose of calcium is 1 to 3 g.

Hypoplastic dentition, cataracts, bone deformities, and basal ganglia calcifications do not respond to the correction of hypocalcemia, but the other symptoms of hypocalcemia are reversible. As serum calcium levels return to normal, phosphaturia is usually stimulated. This leads to a return to normal of serum phosphate levels. In some individuals, however, the absence of the phosphaturic effect of PTH causes a persistent hyperphosphatemia.

Significant elevations of phosphorus should be treated with drugs that inhibit gastrointestinal absorption of phosphate and thus prevent ectopic calcifications. Such calcifications are likely to occur if the mathematical product of the serum calcium and serum phosphate levels exceeds 70 (i.e., $Ca^{++} \times PO_4 = 70$). In such instances, calcifications can be expected.

DYSFUNCTION OF THE ENDOCRINE PANCREAS: DIABETES MELLITUS

Diabetes mellitus is not a single disease but a group of disorders with glucose intolerance in common. It encompasses many causally unrelated diseases and includes many different causes of disturbed glucose tolerance (Palmer & Lernmark, 1990). Historically, diabetes was described as a disease distinguished by weight loss and excessive urination, thirst, and hunger. The disease was recognized in at least two forms, one form that primarily affected the obese and another that was more common among younger, thin individuals.

The term *diabetes mellitus* is now used to describe a syndrome characterized by chronic hyperglycemia and other disturbances of carbohydrate, fat, and protein metabolism. The World Health Organization (WHO) (1985) has identified four major classes of diabetes mellitus: insulin-dependent diabetes mellitus (IDDM or type I diabetes mellitus), non-insulin-dependent diabetes mellitus (NIDDM or type II diabetes mellitus), malnutrition-related diabetes mellitus (MRDM), and other types of diabetes mellitus. (Table 18-4 describes terminology and characteristics related to both types.) Types I and II are the most common and are discussed in greatest detail in this text.

The diagnosis of diabetes is based on (1) more than one fasting plasma glucose level greater than 140 mg/dl, (2) elevated plasma glucose levels in response to an oral glucose tolerance test, and (3) random plasma glucose levels above 200 mg/dl combined with classic symptoms of polydipsia, polyphagia, and polyuria (Bennett, 1990). Because numerous epidemiologic studies have shown severe cardiovascular disease in individuals with only impaired glucose tolerance, early screening and detection are important and may be accomplished with plasma or urine testing. Urine glucose tests should never be used exclusively for diagnosis. Although urine tests are still used by some for self-monitoring, glucose testing of capillary blood obtained through finger stick provides a more sensitive indication of glucose status.

An oral glucose tolerance test consists of the administration of a glucose load after a 12-hour fast followed by measurement of serum glucose levels at specified intervals. Impaired glucose tolerance results primarily from reduced suppression of hepatic glucose output

caused by abnormal pancreatic islet-cell function (Mitrakau et al., 1992). Intravenous glucose tolerance tests are rarely used because they are generally less sensitive than oral glucose tolerance tests and may cause painful venous thrombosis. Another mechanism, used primarily to identify the plasma glucose concentration over time, is the measurement of **glycosylated hemoglobin.** In the normal 120-day lifespan of the red blood cell, glucose molecules join hemoglobin, forming glycosylated hemoglobin. In individuals with poorly controlled diabetes, increases in the quantities of three glycosylated hemoglobins, A1A, A1B, and A1C, are noted. Once a hemoglobin molecule is glycosylated, it remains that way. A buildup of glycosylated hemoglobin within the red cell reflects the average level of glucose to which the cell has been exposed during its life cycle. Measuring glycosylated hemoglobin assesses the effectiveness of therapy by monitoring long-term serum glucose regulation (Fajans, 1990).

Types of Diabetes Mellitus
Type I Diabetes Mellitus

Although the cause is unknown (Palmer & Lernmark, 1990), **type I diabetes mellitus (IDDM)** accounts for approximately 10% of all diabetes mellitus in the Western world. The incidence of the condition is increasing in some areas, with other areas showing no change in incidence (Bennett, 1990). Several studies suggest that the incidence and prevalence are higher for whites than for nonwhites, with the highest rate found in Finland and the lowest rate in Japan. Variations occur, however, even within individual countries. (Table 18-5 summarizes the epidemiology of diabetes mellitus.)

Type I diabetes mellitus is thought to be the result of a genetic-environmental interaction. Between 10% and 13% of individuals with newly diagnosed type I diabetes have a first-degree relative (parent or sibling) with type I diabetes. Diagnosis has a seasonal distribution, with more cases reported during autumn and winter in the northern hemisphere. Diagnosis is rare during the first 9 months of life and peaks at age 12 years.

Pathophysiology

Two distinct types of type I diabetes have been identified. In type IA, environmental factors combined with genetic factors are thought to result in cell-mediated destruction of β-cells. Human leukocyte antigen (HLA)-DR4 is strongly associated with this phenomenon. Type IB is an uncommon primary autoimmune condition that occurs in individuals with other autoimmune conditions, such as Hashimoto disease, Graves disease, pernicious anemia, and myasthenia gravis. This condition is associated with histocompatibility antigen HLA-DR3 and occurs later in life, typically between the ages of 30 and 50.

TABLE 18-4

Classification and Characteristics of Diabetes Mellitus

Name	Previous synonyms	Characteristics
Type I		
Insulin-dependent diabetes mellitus (IDDM)	Juvenile diabetes Juvenile onset diabetes Ketosis-prone diabetes Brittle diabetes Idiopathic diabetes	Long preclinical period with abrupt onset of clinical symptoms Individual prone to ketoacidosis Insulin dependent Several syndromes, both primary autoimmune and genetic-environment Often affects young around age of puberty Decrease in size and number of islet cells
Type II		
Non-insulin-dependent diabetes mellitus (NIDDM)	Adult onset diabetes Maturity onset diabetes Stable diabetes Ketosis-resistant diabetes	Usually not insulin dependent Individual not ketosis prone (but may form ketones under stress) Multiple syndromes: obese, nonobese, and maturity onset in the young (MODY) Generally occurs in those over age 40 Strong familial pattern being investigated
Malnutrition-related diabetes (MRDM)	Tropical diabetes Pancreatic diabetes Pancreatogenic diabetes Endocrine pancreatic syndrome	Seen in tropical, developing countries Seen in young persons with severe protein malnutrition and emaciation Develop severe hyperglycemia without ketosis Uncertain etiology and pathophysiology
Other types	Secondary diabetes	Associated with other conditions/syndromes such as pancreatic disease, hormonal disease, drugs, and chemical agents
Other related conditions		
Impaired glucose tolerance (IGT)	Asymptomatic diabetes Chemical diabetes Borderline diabetes Subclinical diabetes Latent diabetes	Show abnormal response to oral glucose tolerance test 10% to 15% will convert to type II diabetes within 10 years Many with IGT are obese
Gestational diabetes mellitus (GDM)	Same as above	Glucose intolerance first recognized during pregnancy, most likely in the third trimester Following pregnancy, glucose may normalize, remain impaired, or progress to diabetes mellitus Occurs in 2% of all pregnancies; 60% will develop diabetes mellitus within 15 years of gestation
Statistical risk class		
Previously abnormal glucose level	Latent diabetes Prediabetes	Previous abnormality of oral glucose tolerance test or increased risk of developing diabetes because of genetic relationship with a diabetic
Potential abnormal glucose tolerance	Potential diabetes	Family history of diabetes mellitus

TABLE 18-5

Epidemiology and Etiology of Diabetes Mellitus

	Type I (IDDM)	Type II (NIDDM)
Incidence		
Frequency	Relatively rare (10% of all DM) Range from 29.5/100,000 (Finland) to 1.6/ 100,000 (Japan)	Accounts for most cases Prevalence rate in United States (for age 18 and over) is 6.6% Prevalence for Pima Indian (western American Indian group) is 39.9%
Change in frequency	Increased frequency in British Isles, Finland, Norway, Denmark, Israel, Germany, and Poland; stable elsewhere	Incidence has risen in United States since 1940
Characteristics		
Age at onset	Peak onset at age 11 to 13 (slightly earlier for girls and later for boys) Rare in children under age 1 and adults over 30	Risk of developing diabetes increases after age 40; in general, incidence increases with age into the 70s; among Pima Indians, incidence peaks betwen ages 40 and 50, then falls
Gender	Conflicting data	In the United States, more females than males
Racial distribution	Rates for whites 1.5 to 2 times higher than for nonwhites Higher rates for those of Scandinavian descent than for those of central or southern European descent	Certain racial groups may be more likely to develop type II diabetes when exposed to a particular environment Common in migrant groups encountering a different environment (e.g., Polynesians moving from traditional to western lifestyle) In the United States, risk is highest for American Indians, rates are higher for Pacific Islanders, Japanese, Puerto Ricans, and blacks than for whites
Socioeconomic status	Conflicting data	A disease of the affluent in developing nations, but more common among those with lower incomes and less education in the United States
Seasonal distribution	More new cases documented during fall and winter in the northern hemisphere	No known association
Childbirth association	No association documented	Effect of parity on subsequent development of type II diabetes varies among different populations
Obesity	Generally normal or underweight	Frequent precipitant of type II diabetes among those susceptible; a major factor in populations recently exposed to westernized environment Increased risk related to duration, degree, and distribution of obesity

TABLE 18-5

Epidemiology and Etiology of Diabetes Mellitus—cont'd

	Type I (IDDM)	Type II (NIDDM)
Etiology		
Common theory	Genetic and environmental factors, resulting in gradual process of autoimmune destruction in genetically susceptible individuals	Disease results from genetic susceptibility (although the precise gene/genes have not yet been determined) combined with environmental determinants and other risk factors
		MODY follows dominant pattern of inheritance
	Strong association with HLA-DR3 and HLA-DR4	Associated with long-duration obesity
Heredity	Risk to sibling is 5% to 10%; risk to offspring is 2% to 5%	Risk to first degree relative (child or sibling) is 10%-15%
		For MODY, risk to siblings and offspring is 50%
Presence of antibody	Islet cell antibodies (ICA) reported in newly diagnosed individuals but tend to disappear with time after diagnosis	Islet cell antibodies rare
Insulin resistance	Insulin resistance is rare	Increased insulin resistance caused by a decrease in number of cell receptor sites and altered cellular metabolism

Historically, type I diabetes mellitus has been thought to have an abrupt onset. More recently, however, prospective studies show a distinctive natural history involving genetic susceptibility, a long preclinical period, immunologically mediated destruction of β-cells, and hyperglycemia.

Genetic susceptibility. Although the exact nature of genetic susceptibility is not yet understood, research findings support an HLA link. (HLA loci and associated histocompatibility antigens are discussed in Chapter 6.) The strongest association with type I diabetes is with alleles HLA-DR4 and HLA-DR3. The risk of developing type I diabetes increases 5 to 8 times when one of those specific loci is present. When the individual is a heterogenous HLA-DR3/4, the risk is 20 to 40 times higher than that of the general population. Specific human antigens also are thought to decrease the risk of developing type I diabetes, with HLA-DR2 associated with an unusually low risk. Current theories of causation hold that islet-cell destruction occurs predominantly in genetically susceptible people.

Long preclinical period. Research has demonstrated the presence of islet cell antibodies (ICA) for years before the occurrence of symptoms. These immune markers precede evidence of β-cell deficiency, and have been found in 70% to 80% of type I diabetes cases at the time

SPECIFIC ENVIRONMENTAL FACTORS LINKED TO TYPE I DIABETES MELLITUS

1. Drugs and chemicals

Alloxan
Streptozocin
Pentamidine
Vacor (a rodenticide)

2. Nutritional intake

Demonstrated in rats; significance in humans unknown

3. Viruses

Mumps and Coxsackie—type I diabetes does occur rarely as a complication of viral infections, but there is no evidence of a substantial relationship

Rubella—40% of individuals with congenital rubella infection develop type I diabetes later

Cytomegalovirus—persistent CMV⁻infections appear to be relevant to pathogenesis of some cases of Type I diabetes of clinical onset (Palmer & Lernmark, 1990). Auto-antibodies against insulin (IAA) also have been noted. Researchers speculate that IAA may form during the process of active islet cell and β-cell destruction. Islet cell antibodies and IAA are probably the result of the autoimmune process rather than the cause (Fajans, 1990). They tend to disappear with time.

Immunologically mediated destruction of β-cells. The presence of islet cell antibodies provides strong evidence for an autoimmune origin and pathogenesis of type I diabetes. Research suggests that a local or organ-specific suppressor deficit may induce the autoimmune phenomenon (Kahn, LeFloch, & Charreire, 1990). The precise sequence of events that trigger migration or attachment of immune cells to the pancreatic islets has not yet been determined. Environmental mechanisms are thought to play a role in the destruction by direct toxicity, increasing the susceptibility of the β-cells to another mechanism or triggering an autoimmune response to β-cells. Specific environmental factors linked to type I diabetes are presented in the box on p. 677. Controversy remains over whether β-cell destruction always progresses to type I diabetes or if it can remit.

Hyperglycemia and other symptoms. Before hyperglycemia occurs, 80% to 90% of the insulin-secreting β-cells of the islet of Langerhans must be destroyed. β-cell abnormalities are present long before the acute clinical onset of type I diabetes. The initiating events of β-cell destruction may be different from the final event that precipitates clinical symptoms.

Regardless of the cause, a disequilibrium of hormones produced by the islets of Langerhans occurs in diabetes mellitus. Considerable evidence suggests that both α-cell and β-cell functions are abnormal and that both a lack of insulin and a relative excess of glucagon (produced by α-cells) exist in type I diabetes.

Hyperglycemia and hyperketonemia are not possible as a result of insulin deficiency alone; glucagon must be present in relative excess. Thus the full metabolic syndrome is caused by both hormones, a finding that ultimately may provide an entirely new therapeutic approach to the management of diabetes mellitus (Palmer & Lernmark, 1990). Relative hyperglucagonemia occurs in every form of diabetes mellitus. The concentration of glucagon therefore is relatively high in comparison with the relative or absolute deficiency of insulin, and elevated blood glucose levels fail to suppress the production of glucagon. Overproduction of glucose and ketones, as occurs in uncontrolled diabetes mellitus, results from excessive glucagon relative to the amount of effective insulin. The ratio of insulin to glucagon in the portal vein—and not the concentration of each hormone—controls hepatic glucose and fat metabolism.

Clinical Manifestations

Type I diabetes mellitus affects the metabolism of fat, protein, and carbohydrates. Glucose accumulates in the blood and spills into the urine as the renal threshold for glucose is exceeded. In addition, protein and fat breakdown occurs because of the lack of insulin, resulting in weight loss.

Initial clinical manifestations of type I diabetes are generally acute. The individual often has the classic symptoms of polyuria, polydipsia, and polyphagia (Table 18-6). Weight loss and wide fluctuations in blood glucose levels occur.

Ketoacidosis, caused by increased levels of circulating ketones without the inhibiting effects of insulin, is also common. Accumulation of ketone acids causes a drop in pH and triggers the buffering system associated with metabolic acidosis (see Chapter 3). Acetone then is blown off, giving the breath a sweet or "fruity" odor. Occasionally, diabetic coma is the initial symptom of the disease.

TABLE 18-6

Clinical Manifestations and Rationale for Type I Diabetes Mellitus

Manifestations	Rationale
Polydipsia	Because of elevated blood sugar levels, water is osmotically attracted from body cells, resulting in intracellular dehydration and stimulation of thirst in the hypothalamus
Polyuria	Hyperglycemia acts as an osmotic diuretic; the amount of glucose filtered by the glomeruli of the kidney exceeds that which can be reabsorbed by the renal tubules; glycosuria results, accompanied by large amounts of water lost in the urine
Polyphagia	Depletion of cellular stores of carbohydrates, fats, and protein results in cellular starvation and a corresponding increase in hunger
Weight loss	Weight loss occurs because of fluid loss in osmotic diuresis and the loss of body tissue as fats and proteins are used for energy
Fatigue	Metabolic changes result in poor use of food products, contributing to lethargy and fatigue

Evaluation and Treatment

The diagnosis of diabetes is not difficult when the symptoms of polydipsia, polyuria, polyphagia, weight loss, and hyperglycemia are present in fasting and postprandial states. The diagnosis may be made also using the oral glucose tolerance test (OGTT). Age, diet, drugs, activity, and presence of disease must be considered when performing and interpreting the OGTT.

Currently, treatment regimens are designed to avoid high and low levels of glucose and insulin. The Diabetes Control and Complications Trial (DCCT), a 10-year, $165 million study that monitored 1441 individuals with type I diabetes mellitus, was designed to evaluate treatment regimens (DDCT Research Group, 1987). In June 1993, the National Institutes of Health announced research results, which have not yet been published. The research compared individuals whose blood sugars were tightly controlled (with blood glucose checks 4 times a day, three or more insulin injections daily, and meal planning) to those who received standard treatment. While long-term complications were decreased in the tightly controlled group (DCCT, 1993), achieving near-normal glucose levels was accompanied by risks, such as hypoglycemia and weight gain (DCCT Research Group, 1988). Management of diabetes mellitus requires individual planning according to type of disease, age, and activity level, but all individuals require some combination of insulin, meal planning, and exercise.

Insulin. Insulin administration is used to normalize blood glucose levels and to avoid or reduce the complications of diabetes. Exogenous insulin has been used only since 1922. Using recombinant DNA techniques, insulin recently has been derived from beef or pork or from synthetic production. The structure of human, porcine, and bovine insulin is fairly similar.

Beef insulin is the least expensive and most readily available of the insulins; however, it is the most immunogenic. Pork insulin more closely resembles human insulin and is therefore less immunogenic. Human insulin is also available. Most types of insulin are available in various strengths and may be treated with zinc or protamine to render the insulin longer lasting.

Insulin is broken down by gastric enzymes and thus may not be given orally. In the management of type I diabetes, insulin is most commonly given subcutaneously one to four times daily. Glucose and insulin levels may fluctuate widely, and self-monitoring though plasma glucose and urine testing is essential (Strowig & Raskin, 1990). Continuous subcutaneous infusion is an alternative treatment using a small battery-powered infusion pump. Although insulin is essential in the treatment of type I diabetes mellitus, it is associated with a variety of complications, including insulin hypertrophy, antibodies, allergy, resistance, and edema (Galloway & deShazo, 1990).

Meal planning. The individual with type I diabetes mellitus must consume sufficient calories to achieve and maintain normal weight for height and age. Caloric intake should be regulated with consideration of age, activity, and severity of the diabetes. In general, approximately 55% to 60% of the total calories should be derived from carbohydrates, with less than 30% derived from fats, and 15% to 20% from proteins. Cholesterol and saturated fats are also restricted (American Diabetes Association, 1989). Meals and snacks should be planned according to the peak action times of insulin.

Exercise. Exercise by individuals with type I diabetes may result in an inability to regulate blood glucose levels (Vranic, Wasserman, & Bukowiecki, 1990). Most commonly, hypoglycemia occurs because of excess insulin. Reducing the insulin dosage before exercise reduces the incidence of hypoglycemia. Further research is needed to formulate exercise programs beneficial for individuals with type I diabetes mellitus.

Transplantation. Transplantation is designed to establish a normoglycemic, insulin-independent state. Pancreas transplants have been performed since 1966 (Sutherland, Moudry-Munns, & Elick, 1990). Research suggests that normal glucose may be maintained for longer than 5 years after pancreatic transplant (Morel, Goetz, Moudry-Munns, Freier, & Sutherland, 1991). Clinical trials on islet transplantation have also begun (Lacy & Shart, 1990). As with any transplant, rejection remains a problem, and lifelong immunosuppression is necessary.

Experimental treatments. New pharmacologic approaches are being tested. Because most cases of type I diabetes appear to be a manifestation of autoimmunity, several clinical trials of general immunosuppressive agents are under way (National Institutes of Health [NIH], 1992).

Type II Diabetes Mellitus

Type II diabetes mellitus (NIDDM) is much more common than type I. The incidence of the disease has risen in the United States since 1940. Current U.S. disease prevalence in those older than age 18 is 6.6%. In addition, one case is undiagnosed for each known case in the United States. Prevalence varies by ethnic group, with the condition more common in native Americans, Hispanics, and blacks in the United States. Prevalence also varies by environment. For example, prevalence among Polynesians living traditionally is 2.9% compared with 12% among migrants (Bennett, 1990). A genetic-environment interaction appears to be responsible for the condition.

Pathophysiology

The cause of type II diabetes mellitus is unknown, although it is thought to be autosomal recessive. It affects people primarily after the age of 40, many of whom are obese (Rotter, Vadheim, & Rimoin, 1990). Individuals with maturity onset diabetes of youth (MODY), a subset of type II diabetes, are normal to underweight. Maturity onset diabetes of youth is thought to be autosomal dominant because it affects 50% of first-degree relatives (Fajans, 1990).

Obesity and subsequent insulin resistance is a factor for 60% to 80% of individuals with type II diabetes in the Western world. Decreased β-cell responsiveness to plasma glucose levels is noted, with abnormal glucagon secretion also demonstrated (Kahn & Porte, 1990). The islet dysfunction may be caused by a decrease in β-cell mass, abnormal function of the β-cells, or some combination.

Pancreatic changes in individuals with type II diabetes mellitus are nonspecific and have been observed to a lesser degree in nondiabetics. Amyloid of the islets occurs in 10% to 40% of the pancreases from individuals with type II diabetes. The extent of amyloid deposits is positively correlated with the age of the individual and the duration and severity of the disease (Volk, 1990). Amyloid formation is associated with islet cell destruction (Clark, Yon, deKorning, & Holman, 1991).

Liver changes are related to elevated serum lipid levels. Fatty pancreatic and hepatic atrophy, although affecting both those with and those without diabetes, occurs with much greater frequency in the individual with type II diabetes. These fatty infiltrates may play a role in the development of amyloid deposits in the islets. Although tissue atrophies, fat infiltration may increase the overall size of the liver and pancreas, and glycogen vacuoles may be found in the cell nuclei. Ischemia caused by vascular sclerosis may cause the fatty atrophy. Pancreatic fibrosis, occurring in 33% to 66% of individuals with type II diabetes, also contributes to pancreatic atrophy.

A decrease in the weight and number of β-cells generally occurs in type II diabetes, but the cause is unclear. The decrease in β-cells may be the result of progressive deterioration over time. To confuse the issue further, the ratio of α-cells to β-cells may be completely normal in the individual with type II diabetes, and most individuals with type II diabetes have plasma and pancreatic insulin levels that are not decreased. This latter finding supports the hypothesis that diabetes is a disorder caused by both insulin and glucagon, so that a deficiency of insulin and an excess of glucagon may be either relative or absolute. An inherited secretory deficiency of the β-cells also may play a role (Kahn & Porte, 1990).

Type II diabetes is usually caused by some combination of gene-environmental interaction, although the contribution of each component varies under different circumstances. The most powerful risk factor for type II diabetes, identified by the World Health Organization Expert Committee (1985), is obesity. (Risk factor analysis is discussed in Chapter 5.) The risk for developing type II diabetes mellitus increases 10 times with severe obesity (Horton & Jeanrenaud, 1990). Excessive caloric intake predisposes an individual to type II diabetes by contributing to obesity.

In the obese, insulin has a decreased ability to influence glucose uptake and metabolism in the liver, skeletal muscles, and adipose tissue. Multiple theories have been presented to explain this phenomenon. One theory postulates that a decreased number of insulin receptors in the plasma membrane causes decreased insulin binding. Another theory holds that postreceptor events in insulin-sensitive cells are responsible for insulin resistance in the obese. A third theory states that hyperinsulinemia, which often occurs in the early stages of type II diabetes, is a compensatory adaptation to insu-

TABLE 18-7

Clinical Manifestations and Rationale for Type II Diabetes Mellitus

Manifestations	Rationale
Recurrent infections (e.g., boils and carbuncles; skin infections) and prolonged wound healing	Growth of microorganisms is stimulated by increased glucose levels; impaired blood supply hinders healing
Genital pruritus	Hyperglycemia and glyucosuria favor fungal growth; candidal infections, resulting in pruritus, are a common presenting symptom in women
Visual changes	Blurred vision occurs as water balance in the eye fluctuates because of elevated blood glucose levels; diabetic retinopathy may ensue
Paresthesias	Paresthesias are common manifestations of diabetic neuropathies
Fatigue	Metabolic changes result in poor use of food products, contributing to lethargy and fatigue

lin resistance in tissues. This theory suggests that elevated levels of circulating insulin are induced by obesity until the pancreas cannot continue to overproduce insulin. Still another theory holds that overeating leads to hyperinsulinemia, which necessitates the development of peripheral insulin resistance to protect against hypoglycemia (Bennett, 1990). In any event, the mechanism responsible for insulin receptor binding or postreceptor activity may be reversed through weight loss.

Clinical Manifestations

Clinical manifestations of type II diabetes are often nonspecific. Although younger people may develop the condition, it generally affects those older than age 40. The individual often is overweight and hyperlipidemic. The onset is frequently slow and insidious. The individual with type II diabetes may show some classic symptoms of diabetes but more often will have nonspecific symptoms such as pruritus, recurrent infections, visual changes, and paresthesias (Table 18-7).

Evaluation and Treatment

The diagnosis of type II diabetes is similar to that of type I (see p. 679). As with type I diabetes, the goal of treatment for individuals with type II diabetes is the restoration of euglycemia (a normal blood glucose level) and correction of related metabolic disorders. Dietary measures, including the restriction of the total caloric intake, are of primary importance in the overweight individual. As the obese individual loses weight, the body's resistance to insulin often diminishes so that weight loss results in improved glucose tolerance. Nonobese individuals with type II diabetes should consume calories consistent with their ideal weight and pattern of activity. As in type I diabetes, the ratio of fats, carbohydrates, and protein is important, and both cholesterol and saturated fats are restricted. Some research suggests that high-fiber diets (Vinik & Wing, 1990) also improve diabetic control.

Although the first approach to treatment of the individual with type II diabetes is appropriate meal planning, medication may be needed for optimal management. Sulfonylurea drugs are useful in treating some individuals with type II diabetes and are the only oral hypoglycemic agents approved for clinical use in the United States (Lebovitz, 1990). Use of sulfonylureas requires a pancreas capable of synthesizing insulin. Insulin may be used also in the treatment of some individuals with type II diabetes.

Exercise is an important aspect of treatment for the individual with type II diabetes. Physical training improves glucose control (Vranic et al., 1990). Exercise not only reduces postprandial blood glucose levels and diminishes insulin requirement, it also lowers triglyceride and cholesterol levels while increasing the level of high-density lipoprotein (HDL) cholesterol. In addition, exercise is a valuable adjunct to weight loss for the overweight individual. Hypoglycemia may result, however, when the exercising individual receives oral hypoglycemic agents. Modification of dose may be needed. In addition, research suggests that regular, vigorous exercise is associated with a decreased incidence of type II diabetes, thus helping prevent the condition (Manson et al., 1992).

Acute Complications of Diabetes Mellitus
Hypoglycemia

Hypoglycemia is a lowered plasma glucose level. It may be caused by exogenous, endogenous, or functional causes (see Tables 18-8, 18-9, and 18-10 for a summary of causes). In general, hypoglycemia occurs when blood glucose levels are below 35 mg/dl in newborns for the first 48 hours of life and 45 to 60 mg/dl in children and adults. Evidence also indicates that some individuals may become symptomatic before glucose levels decrease to 50 mg/dl if the decrease is relatively rapid (Lefebvre, 1990). Hypoglycemia occurs most frequently in individuals with diabetes mellitus (Table 18-11 lists predisposing factors). It occurs in more than 90% of those with type I diabetes and limits the management of the disease (Cryer & Gerich, 1990). Hypoglycemia in diabetes is sometimes called insulin shock, or insulin reaction.

Symptoms result from a neurogenic reaction and from cellular malnutrition. Symptoms frequently vary among individuals but tend to be consistent for each person. Neurogenic reactions occur when the decrease in blood glucose is rapid with tachycardia, palpitations, diaphoresis, tremors, pallor, and arousal anxiety. The response is probably generated when the hypothalamus senses decreased glucose levels. The neuron receives inadequate supplies of carbohydrates to metabolize and is thus unable to maintain normal function. Cellular malnutrition produces further symptoms, including headache, dizziness, irritability, fatigue, poor judgment, confusion, visual changes, hunger, seizures, and coma. If an individual is receiving a beta-blocking medication, the anatomic symptoms may be absent.

When hypoglycemic symptoms are nonspecific, the safest treatment is to provide some form of glucose, because failure to provide glucose may precipitate convulsions, coma, and death. If the hypoglycemic individual is conscious, ingestion of fast-acting carbohydrate is preferred; if the individual is unconscious, intravenous glucose or subcutaneous glucagon administration will reverse the hypoglycemia. After the crisis, the individual should be observed for a subsequent relapse, and an additional, longer-lasting source of carbohydrates should be provided. Prevention of hypoglycemia episodes through alternate therapeutic regimens and proper education should be the goal.

TABLE 18-8

Exogenous Causes of Hypoglycemia

Exogenous cause	Predisposing factor	Occurrence
Insulin	Intentional or accidental overdose; may be combined with inadequate food intake, unusually increased exercise, decrease in insulin requirement, or potentiating medications	Most frequent cause of hypoglycemia
Oral hypoglycemic agents	Intentional or accidental overdose; may be combined with inadequate food intake, increased exercise, or potentiating medications	Frequent cause of hypoglycemia
Alcohol	Particularly likely in chronically malnourished or acutely food-deprived individuals	Occurs within 6-36 hours of ingesting moderate to large amounts of alcohol
Other agents	Salicylates, hypoglycines, pentamidine, perhexiline	Common in children under the age of 2
Exercise	Increased duration and intensity of exercise increase glucose uptake and normally decrease insulin secretion	Occurs with both insulin and sulfonylurea administration and intense exercise, but may be unpredictable in onset

TABLE 18-9

Endogenous Causes of Hypoglycemia

Endogenous cause	Predisposing factors	Occurrence
Organic hypoglycemia	Insulinoma	Uncommon neoplasm of beta cells of islets of Langerhans
	Nesidioblastosis and beta cell hyperplasia	Rare disease causing persistent hypoglycemia of infancy
Extrapancreatic neoplasms	May be mesenchymal tumors, hepatomas, adrenocortical carcinomas, gastrointestinal tumors, lymphomas, or leukemias	Rare; most common in adults 40-70 years of age
Inborn errors of metabolism	Hereditary fructose intolerance	Rare autosomal recessively inherited inborn error of metabolism
	Fructose-1,6-disphosphatase deficiency	Rare autosomal recessive disease
	Galactosemia	Autosomal recessive disease; hypoglycemia less common than in fructose intolerance
	Phosphoenolpyruvate carboxykinase deficiency	Reported in a few infant cases
	Inborn errors in glycogen metabolism, leucine sensitivity	Reported in von Gierke disease, Hers disease, and type IXb glycogen storage disease

TABLE 18-10

Functional Causes of Hypoglycemia

Dysfunction	Precipitating factors	Occurrence
Alimentary hypoglycemia	Rapid dumping of carbohydrates into the upper small intestine	Postgastrectomy
Spontaneous reactive hypoglycemia	Syndrome of unknown cause with symptoms such as diaphoresis, tachycardia, tremulousness, headache, fatigue, drowsiness, and irritability	Rarely diagnosed throughout the world; widely diagnosed in United States, prompting American Diabetes Association and Endocrine Society to issue statement that entity is probably overdiagnosed
Alcohol-promoted reactive hypoglycemia	Drinking on an empty stomach	More common with drinks containing both alcohol and glucose or saccharin (e.g., beer, gin and tonic, rum and cola, whisky and ginger ale, etc.)
Posthyperalimentation hypoglycemia	Rapid discontinuation of total parenteral alimentation	Easily prevented by gradually reducing parenteral administration (alimentation)
Endocrine-deficiency states	Glucocorticoid deficiency	A danger for any person with adrenal insufficiency
	Growth hormone deficiency	Particularly during a prolonged fast
	Catecholamine deficiency	Possible cause in children
Severe liver deficiency	Insufficient glucose output by the liver	Fasting hypoglycemia
Lack of body stores for protein, fat, and carbohydrates	Profound malnutrition	Frequent; also found with relative frequency in kwashiorkor
Prolonged muscular exercise	Metabolism of energy-producing substances	Occurs if exercise is too prolonged or severe or if nutritional intake and carbohydrate stores are insufficient
Functional or transient hypoglycemia in infancy	Transient neonatal hypoglycemia	Occurs in 10% of live births, during first 3 days of life
	Maternal diabetes	Caused by β-cell hyperplasia and possibly relative hypoglucagonemia
	Erythroblastosis fetalis	Frequently associated with erythroblastosis fetalis
	Leucine-induced hypoglycemia	Generally in infants under 6 months of age; severe hypoglycemia attacks may occur postprandially or after short periods of fasting
	Ketotic or ketogenic hypoglycemia	One of the most common forms of hypoglycemia in childhood, occurs after food deprivation in children 1-8 years old; generally, spontaneous recovery before age 10
	Maple sugar urine disease	Frequent in those with maple sugar urine disease
	Adrenal hyporesponsiveness	Found in children born small for dates, after complicated pregnancy

TABLE 18-11

Common Acute Complications of Diabetes Mellitus

Hypoglycemia in those with DM	Diabetic ketoacidosis	Hyperosmolar nonacidotic diabetes
Synonyms		
Insulin shock, insulin reaction	Diabetic coma syndrome	Hyperosmolar hyperglycemia nonketotic coma
Those at risk		
Individuals with type I diabetes Individuals with rapidly fluctuating blood sugar Individuals with type II diabetes taking oral agents, especially chlorpropamide	Individuals with type I diabetes Individuals with nondiagnosed diabetes	Elderly or very young individuals with type II diabetes, nondiabetics with predisposing factors, those with renal insufficiency, individuals with undiagnosed diabetes
Predisposing factors		
Excessive insulin or hypoglycemic agent intake, lack of sufficient food intake, excessive physical exercise, abrupt decline in insulin needs (e.g., renal failure, immediately postpartum; some cases of insulin reaction), simultaneous use of insulin-potentiating agents	Stressful situation such as infection, accident, trauma, emotional stress; omission of insulin; medications that antagonize insulin	High-carbohydrate diets (e.g., tube feedings; total parenteral nutrition), prolonged mannitol diuresis, peritoneal or hemodialysis with hyperosmolar dialysate, medications antagonizing insulin
Typical onset		
Rapid	Slow	Slowest
Presenting symptoms		
Neurogenic reaction: pallor, sweating, tachycardia, palpitations, hunger, restlessness, anxiety, tremors Cellular malnutrition: fatigue, irritablity, headache, loss of concentration, visual disturbances, dizziness, hunger, confusion, transient sensory or motor defects, convulsions, coma, death	Malaise, dry mouth, headache, polyuria, polydipsia, weight loss, nausea, vomiting, pruritus, abdominal pain, lethargy, shortness of breath, Kussmaul respirations, "fruity" or acetone odor to breath	Polyuria, polydipsia, hypovolemia, dehydration (parched lips, poor skin turgor), hypotension, tachycardia, hypoperfusion, weight loss, weakness, nausea, vomiting, abdominal pain, hypothermia, stupor, coma, seizures
Laboratory analysis		
Serum glucose below 30 mg/dl in newborn (first 2-3 days) and below 55-60 mg/dl in adults	Glucose levels 300-750 mg/dl, reduction in bicarbonate concentration, increased anion gap, increased plasma levels of beta-hydroxybutyrate, acetoacetate, and acetone	Glucose levels 600-4800 mg/dl, lack of ketosis, serum osmolarity above 350 mOsm/L, elevated blood urea nitrogen and creatinine

Diabetic Ketoacidosis

Ketoacidosis, a serious complication of diabetes mellitus, is a common cause for hospital admissions, and average mortality rates throughout the United States are 7% to 9%. **Diabetic ketoacidosis (DKA)** develops when there is an absolute or relative deficiency of insulin and an increase in insulin counterregulatory hormones: catecholamines, cortisol, glucagon, and growth hormone. Under these conditions, hepatic glucose production increases, peripheral glucose usage decreases, fat mobilization increases, and ketogenesis is stimulated (Fig. 18-10). The most common precipitating factor is intercur-

rent illness, such as infection, trauma, surgery, or myocardial infection. Interruption of insulin administration also may result in DKA. In 20% to 30% of the cases, no precipitating factors are noted. Emotional factors and stress, particularly in children, are thought to contribute to the development of DKA (Kriesberg, 1990).

Catecholamines, cortisol, glucagon, and growth hormone antagonize insulin by increasing glucose production. In addition, catecholamines, cortisol, and growth hormones decrease use of glucose. Insulin deficiency results in decreased glucose usage, an increased release of fatty acids, and accelerated gluconeogenesis and keto-

Diabetic ketoacidosis

FIG. 18-10 Diabetic ketoacidosis.

genesis. Relatively increased glucagon levels are simultaneously responsible for activation of the gluconeogenic (glucose-forming) and ketogenic (ketone-forming) pathways in the liver. Because of the insulin deficiency, hepatic overproduction of beta-hydroxybutyrate and acetoacetic acids causes increased ketone concentrations. Ordinarily, ketones used by the brain or skeletal muscle as an energy source regenerate bicarbonate. This balances the loss of bicarbonate, which occurs when the ketone is formed. Hyperketonemia (increased blood ketone levels) may be a result of impairment in the use of ketones by peripheral tissue, which permits strong organic acids to circulate freely (Kreisberg, 1990). Bicarbonate buffering then does not occur, and the individual develops a metabolic acidosis.

Clinical Manifestations

The signs and symptoms of diabetic ketoacidosis are fairly nonspecific, and an individual rarely progresses to complete coma without intervention. Polyuria and dehydration result from the osmotic diuresis associated with hyperglycemia. Here the plasma glucose level is higher than the individual's renal threshold, allowing much glucose to be lost in the urine. Although water deficits may reach 100 ml/kg body weight, they are generally not as severe as those experienced by the individual with hyperosmolar nonacidotic diabetes. Sodium, phosphorus, and magnesium deficits are common. The most important electrolyte disturbance, however, is a marked deficiency in total body potassium. Although the serum potassium may appear normal or elevated because of volume contraction and a shift of potassium from the cell caused by metabolic acidosis, total deficiencies reach 3 to 5 mEq/kg. Symptoms of diabetic ketoacidosis include Kussmaul respirations (hyperventilation in an attempt to compensate for the acidosis), postural dizziness, central nervous system depression, ketonuria, anorexia, nausea, abdominal pain, thirst, and polyuria.

Evaluation and Treatment

The diagnosis of ketoacidosis is suggested when individuals have symptoms of vomiting, abdominal pain, dehydration, and an acetone odor on the breath. Laboratory findings include serum glucose greater than 300 mg/dl, arterial pH less than 7.30, and positive urine and serum ketones.

Treatment of diabetic ketoacidosis involves continual administration of low-dose insulin to decrease glucose levels. Fluids are administered to replace lost fluid volume, and electrolytes—particularly sodium, potassium, and phosphorus—are administered as needed. Fluid and electrolytes should be closely monitored. Electrolyte deficits become apparent as fluid volume is replaced. After the administration of insulin, the concentration of

beta-hydroxybutyrate promptly begins to decrease and after a slight increase, acetoacetate also begins to decrease. A persistent ketonuria may be observed for several days after treatment. As with hypoglycemia, prevention is the long-term goal. Health teaching emphasizes predisposing factors and strategies for avoiding diabetic ketoacidosis.

Hyperosmolar Nonacidotic Diabetes

Hyperosmolar nonacidotic diabetes (HNAD), also called hyperosmolar hyperglycemia nonketotic coma, was first described in 1886, but even today no satisfactory evidence has explained how HNAD differs pathophysiologically from diabetic ketoacidosis. Levels of free fatty acids in HNAD are consistently lower than those found in diabetic ketoacidosis. HNAD is characterized also by a lack of ketosis. Because the amount of insulin required to inhibit fat breakdown is less than that needed for effective glucose transport, insulin levels are sufficient to prevent excessive lipolysis but not to use glucose properly. Glucose levels are considerably higher in HNAD than in diabetic ketoacidosis. One hypothesis is that the lack of ketonemia in HNAD permits greater synthesis of glucose and thus more severe hyperglycemia.

Clinical Manifestations

Glycosuria and polyuria in HNAD result from the extreme serum glucose elevation. As much as 19 g of glucose per hour may be lost in diuresis, which also causes severe volume depletion and intracellular dehydration. Water losses are generally between 4.8 and 12.6 L, and although some electrolytes are lost with the fluid, the urine is hypotonic. This, along with increased glucose levels, contributes to the increased serum osmolarity. Neurologic changes, such as stupor, correlate with the degree of hyperosmolarity. Glomerular filtration also decreases with the hyperosmolarity, resulting in further serum glucose increases.

Evaluation and Treatment

The serum ketone concentration is normal or only mildly elevated in HNAD. In addition to the depressed mental state, laboratory findings include serum glucose levels greater than 600 mg/dl, serum osmolarity greater than 310 mOsm/L, and BUN of 70 to 90 mg/dl. Diabetic ketoacidosis and HNAD show considerable overlap in symptoms and treatment. An important distinction, however, is that the dehydration experienced in HNAD is far more severe than that in diabetic ketoacidosis. Thus fluid replacement, with both crystalloids and colloids, is more rapid. As much as 2000 ml may be given the first hour, together with monitoring of the response to therapy. Potassium deficits may be so extreme in HNAD that more than a week may be needed to correct the total body deficits. Phosphorus and sodium also may be needed. The mortality rate is also high in HNAD, currently 14% to 17% (Matz, 1990). Thus, although the exact mechanisms are unknown at this time, real differences exist between diabetic ketoacidosis and HNAD. (Table 18-11 compares and contrasts the three acute complications described thus far.)

Somogyi Effect

The **Somogyi effect** is a unique combination of hypoglycemia during the night with rebound hyperglycemia in the morning. The problem is more common in individuals with type I diabetes mellitus, particularly in children, and should be investigated whenever fluctuations in blood sugar levels are serious. The Somogyi effect occurs when hypoglycemia stimulates glucose counterregulation, including epinephrine, growth hormone, cortisol, and glucagon release (Cryer & Gerich, 1990). These hormones serve to increase blood glucose by gluconeogenesis (formation of glucose from nonglucose sources) and glycogenolysis (breakdown of glycogen into glucose). They mobilize fatty acids and proteins while inhibiting peripheral glucose use (Fig. 18-11).

Clinical Manifestations

In addition to fluctuating glucose levels, subtle symptoms of hypoglycemia occur. The individual often complains of nightmares and early morning headaches. Both symptoms probably reflect a hypoglycemic state. Ketonuria may occur if the mobilization of energy sources overshoots the body's need for glucose and exogenous insulin is depleted.

Evaluation and Treatment

Diagnosis involves the documentation of nighttime hypoglycemia by several plasma glucose analyses at 2:00 A.M., 4:00 A.M., and 7:00 A.M. Treatment consists of decreasing insulin dosage or changing the time of administration.

Dawn Phenomenon

The **dawn phenomenon** is an early morning rise in blood glucose concentration with no hypoglycemia during the night. It appears to be related to nocturnal elevations of growth hormone, which decrease metabolism of glucose by muscle and fat. Increased clearance of plasma insulin also may be involved (Galloway & deShazo,

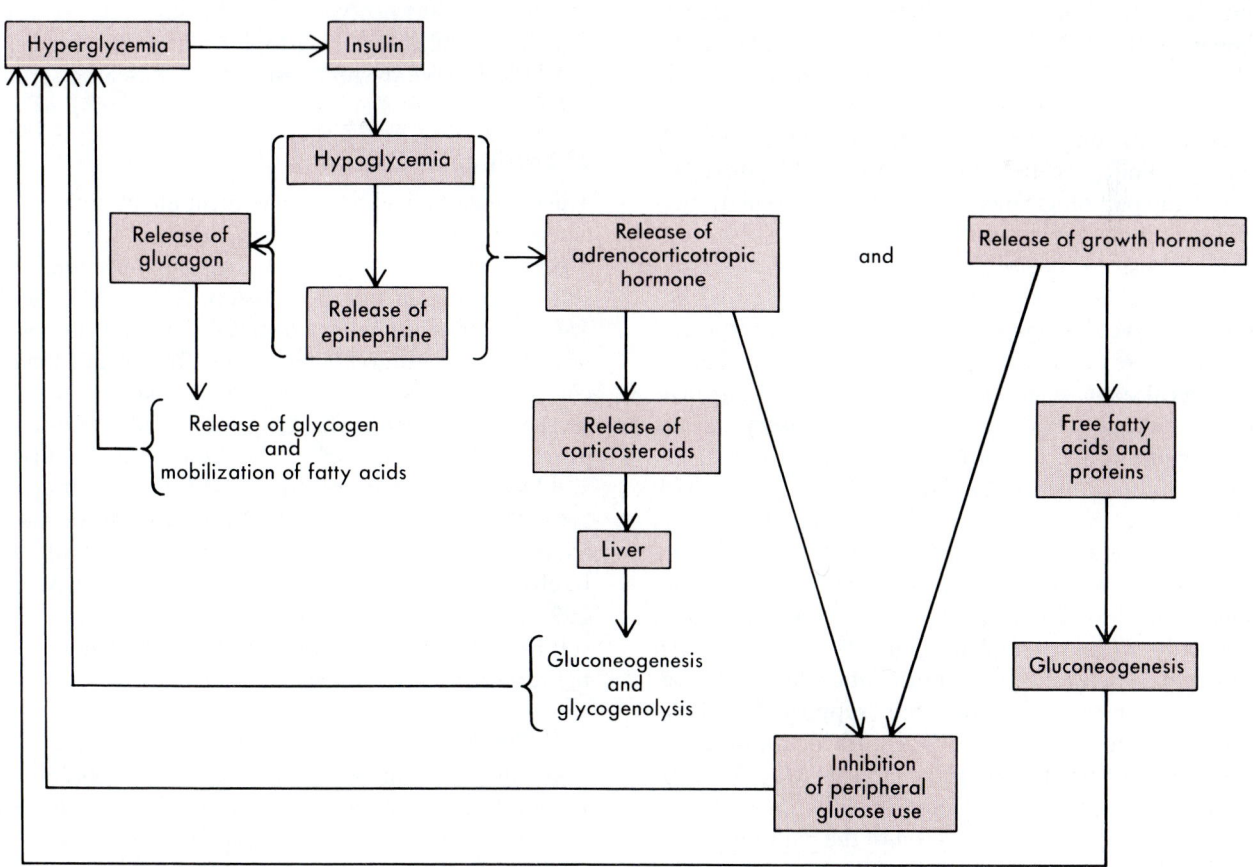

FIG. 18-11 The Somogyi effect.

1990). Periodic monitoring of plasma glucose values in the morning ascertains the need for additional morning insulin. Altering the time and dose of insulin manages the problem. Treating dawn phenomenon may result in the Somogyi effect and vice versa.

Chronic Complications of Diabetes Mellitus

Before the discovery of long-term insulin, complications in individuals with diabetes had little significance because the survival time was short, especially for individuals with type I diabetes. Today, long-term survival is the rule. As a result, the problems of neuropathy, vascular disease, and infection have become important in clinical management. Vascular changes include microvascular disease, such as retinopathy and nephropathy, and macrovascular disease, such as coronary artery disease, stroke, and peripheral vascular disease (Levin & Sicard, 1990). The degree of metabolic control influences the development of complications. Other factors, however, also affect the onset, severity, and progression of complications (Skyler, 1990).

Diabetic Neuropathies

Diabetic neuropathy is the most common cause of neuropathy in the Western world and is probably the most common complication of diabetes. The prevalence is similar for both IDDM and NIDDM (Greene, Sima, Albers, & Pfeifer, 1990). Yet, the disease remains poorly understood. Neuropathy and other long-term complications are thought to result from the interaction of multiple metabolic, genetic, and environmental factors. The underlying pathologic mechanism may be vascular, metabolic, or a combination of both mechanisms. Neuropathy is classified into two stages: subclinical and clinical. In the subclinical stage, there is evidence that peripheral nerve dysfunctions such as slowed motor and sensory nerve conduction exist without clinical sign. In the clinical stage, symptoms or clinically detectable neurologic deficits are present. Generally, sensory deficits and symptoms are greater than motor involvement.

Diabetic neuropathy is considered to be a form of a "dying back" neuropathy, in which the distal portions of the neurons are initially and eventually more severely affected. The earliest morphologic change in both peripheral nerves and the central nervous system is axonal degeneration that preferentially involves unmyelinated nerve fibers. Schwann cell abnormalities then occur because of changes in the axons they support. Metabolic activity of the Schwann cell is disturbed, causing segmental loss of myelin and the characteristic pattern of demyelination and remyelination observed in long-term diabetic neuropathy. The location of the pathology may include the spinal cord, the posterior root ganglia, or the peripheral nerves. These changes may occur alone or in combination.

Motor nerve conduction velocity, electromyography, and sensory perception have shown abnormalities at the onset of diabetes. Sensory nerve conduction also may be impaired at this stage and is probably the most sensitive index of peripheral neuropathy. These abnormalities have sometimes been restored to normal by good glucose control. Although these changes suggest early involvement of the nervous system in individuals with diabetes, they are not generally accompanied by clinical symptomatology.

A number of different diabetic neuropathies occur with varying causes, pathogeneses, and clinical backgrounds (Table 18-12). Some of the diabetic neuropathic syndromes are progressive, but many, such as painful peripheral neuropathy, mononeuropathy (wrist drop, foot drop), diabetic amyotrophy, diabetic neuropathic cachexia, and visceral manifestations associated with autonomic neuropathy, such as diabetic diarrhea and orthostatic hypotension, are reversible. This suggests that metabolic changes are not completely responsible for the neuropathies. In fact, any neuropathy may occur during periods of good glucose control and may be the initial clinical manifestation of diabetes, even without overt glucose intolerance. Obviously, much investigation regarding diabetic neuropathies remains to be done. The Diabetes Control and Complications Trial has not yet released results related to the appearance of clinical neuropathy and parameters of subclinical nerve dysfunction (DCCT Research Group, 1987).

Microvascular Disease

Thickening of the capillary basement membrane is characteristic of diabetic microangiopathy and emerges over a period of 1 to 2 years. The thickening eventually results in decreased tissue perfusion. Although some degree of hyperglycemia is a necessary prerequisite for the vascular changes, no conclusive evidence is available to correlate the basement membrane thickening with the severity of diabetes. The frequency of the lesions appears to be proportional to the duration of the disease and blood glucose levels. In the DCCT study, individuals with tightly controlled blood glucose were half as likely to have renal and eye complications as those who received standard treatment (DCCT Research Group, 1993). Hypoxia and ischemia of various organs may result from microangiopathy. Two areas often affected are the retina and the kidney.

Retinopathy

The retina is the most metabolically active structure per weight of tissue in the body. Thus, the retina is a vulnerable target for microvascular occlusion in diabetes mellitus. **Diabetic retinopathy** appears to be a response to retinal ischemia resulting from blood vessel changes and red blood cell aggregation. The roles of growth hor-

TABLE 18-12

Classification of Diabetic Neuropathies

Location	Characteristics
Somatic (peripheral) neuropathies	
Lower extremities	Most commonly bilateral, symmetric, and sensory
Asymptomatic	Paresthesias, progressive and irreversible, underlie the development of neuropathic ulcers and Charcot joints
Painful	Pain and paresthesias, particularly nocturnally; anorexia, depression, and irritability; absence of knee and ankle jerk reflexes; the greater the pain, the better the prognosis
Upper extremities	Involves muscle atrophy, asthenia, sensory impairment, and radiculitis
Asymmetric neuropathies	Predominantly motor involvement, absent sensory involvement, sudden onset, severe pain, good prognosis
Diabetic neuropathic cachexia	Profound weight loss with severe pain, spontaneous recovery
Visceral neuropathies (generally occur with peripheral neuropathy)	
Cranial nerves	Involves cranial nerve III, leading to pain, diplopia, and ptosis
Gastrointestinal tract	Involves decreased esophageal motility, delayed gastric emptying, and diabetic constipation and diarrhea
Genitourinary tract	Insidious and progressive bladder paralysis with urinary retention; sexual dysfunction in males, including retrograde ejaculation and impotence
Autonomic nervous system	Includes cardiovascular reflexes, anhidrosis, and vasomotor instability

TABLE 18-13

Findings in Diabetic Retinopathy

Type of retinopathy	Pathologic findings
Nonproliferative retinopathy	
Venous abnormalities	Increased tortuosity, dilation with irregular constriction; frequency increases with increased severity of retinopathy
Microaneurysms	Mostly thin-walled, 15-50 μm in diameter, pathogenesis controversial
Interretinal hemorrhage	Circular and small; may take several months to resorb
Macular edema	Caused by serum leakage through incompetent vessel walls, may resorb in several weeks
Hard exudates	Characteristically "hard," exudates with pattern of exudation, irregular in shape, and sharply defined, may appear and disappear over months to years; common with hypertension; "soft" exudates may appear and disappear more frequently; related to increased retinal capillary permeability
Preproliferative diabetic retinopathy	
"Cottonwool" patches	Infarcts of the nerve fiber layer caused by retinal ischemia
Intraretinal microvascular shunts	Tortuous shunts between patent and occluded retinal vessels
Proliferative diabetic retinopathy	
Neovascularization	New vessels surrounded by connective tissue; five distinct groups representing different hazards to the eye
Glial proliferation	Often produced to reinforce neovascularization; may occur on optic disc and along vascular arcades
Vitreoretinal traction hemorrhage; retinal detachment	Traction occurring from the vitreous jelly; eventually causes small blood vessels to hemorrhage and retinal detachment to occur

mone and metabolic control are being explored. The prevalence and severity of the retinopathy are strongly related to the age of the individual and duration of the diabetes. Retinopathy develops more rapidly in individuals with type II than with type I diabetes (L'Esperance, James, & Judson, 1990). The vast majority of individuals with diabetes mellitus have some degree of retinopathy (Nathan, 1993).

There are three stages of retinopathy (Table 18-13). Nonproliferative retinopathy (stage I) is characterized by an increase in retinal capillary permeability, vein dilation, microaneurysm formation, and superficial (flame-shaped) and deep (blot) hemorrhages. Preproliferative retinopathy (stage II) is a progression of retinal ischemia with areas of poor perfusion that culminate in infarcts. Proliferative diabetic retinopathy (stage III) is the result of neovascularization and fibrous tissue formation within the retina or optic disc. Traction of the new vessels on the vitreous humor may cause retinal detachment or hemorrhage into the vitreous humor.

Maculopathy is a progressive process that may accompany the increased retinal capillary permeability, vessel occlusion, and ischemia. If formation of exudates, edema, or ischemia occurs near the fovea, serious loss of vision may result. Although a variety of drugs have been used to treat diabetic retinopathy, proper clinical trials are lacking. Laser treatments are used to handle vision loss.

Diabetic nephropathy

Diabetes is the most common cause of end-stage renal disease in the Western world. Approximately 30% of individuals with type I and 5% to 10% of those with type II diabetes become uremic. The individual typically experiences no clinical signs or symptoms for 10 years (in type I diabetes) or 5 to 8 years (in type II).

The exact process responsible for destruction of kidneys in diabetes is unknown. Mechanisms such as hyperglycemia, hyperfiltration, increased blood viscosity, and increased glomerular pressure are being investigated (Friedman, 1990). The glomeruli are injured by at least two mechanisms: protein denaturation by high glucose levels and adverse effects of intraglomerular hypertension. Renal glomerular changes can occur early in diabetes mellitus and occasionally may precede the overt manifestation of the disease. Glomerular enlargement and glomerular basement membrane thickening, resulting in diffuse intercapillary glomerulosclerosis, develop during the first few years of diabetes. The Kimmelstiel-Wilson nodule, thickening at the center of the glomerular lobules with thickening of the peripheral basement membrane, is distinctive in individuals with diabetes (Harris, Steffes, Bilous, Sutherland, & Mauer, 1991).

Proteinuria, a reliable and consistent sign of renal damage, is the first manifestation of renal dysfunction. Continuous proteinuria generally heralds a life expectancy of less than 10 years. Scanty information is available to explain the determinants of proteinuria in diabetic nephropathy. Leakage of albumin into glomerular filtrate results from factors other than increased membrane pore size, although these other factors are not yet defined. As renal failure progresses, extensive vascular and extravascular changes occur.

Before the development of proteinuria, no clinical signs or symptoms of progressive glomerulosclerosis are likely to be evident. Later, hypoproteinemia, reduction in plasma oncotic pressure, fluid overload, anasarca (generalized body edema), and hypertension may occur (Steffes & Mauer, 1990). As renal function continues to deteriorate, individuals with type I diabetes may experience hypoglycemia, which necessitates a decrease in insulin therapy. The hypoglycemia occurs because the kidney's ability to metabolize insulin is lost along with other renal functions. As the glomerular filtration rate drops below 10 ml/min, uremic signs such as nausea, lethargy, acidosis, anemia, and uncontrolled hypertension occur (see Chapter 33 for a discussion of renal failure). Impaired kidney function also accelerates retinopathy. Death from renal failure is much more common in individuals with type I diabetes mellitus than in those with type II.

Macrovascular Disease

Macrovascular disease is a prominent cause of morbidity and mortality among individuals with type II diabetes mellitus. Unlike microangiopathy, atherosclerotic disease is unrelated to the severity of diabetes and is often present in those with merely an impaired glucose tolerance. (Atherosclerosis is discussed in Chapter 27.) The current theory of the pathogenesis of atherosclerosis is related to the theory of response to injury (McMillan, 1990). The fibrous plaques of atherosclerosis result from the proliferation of subendothelial smooth muscle in the arterial wall. Other factors in the serum of individuals with diabetes also stimulate this proliferation (Fig. 18-12).

In addition, deposition of lipids in the lesions may be facilitated in individuals with diabetes. Triglyceride and serum cholesterol elevations are very common. High-density lipoproteins (HDL), which tend to protect vessels, are present in only low concentrations in individuals with diabetes. As in the nondiabetic, the presence of other risk factors increases vulnerability to atherosclerosis. Further work is needed to clarify the complexities of macrovascular complications.

Coronary artery disease

Coronary artery disease (CAD or coronary heart disease) affects 9.5% to 75% of individuals with diabetes. The risk for those with diabetes is higher than for the

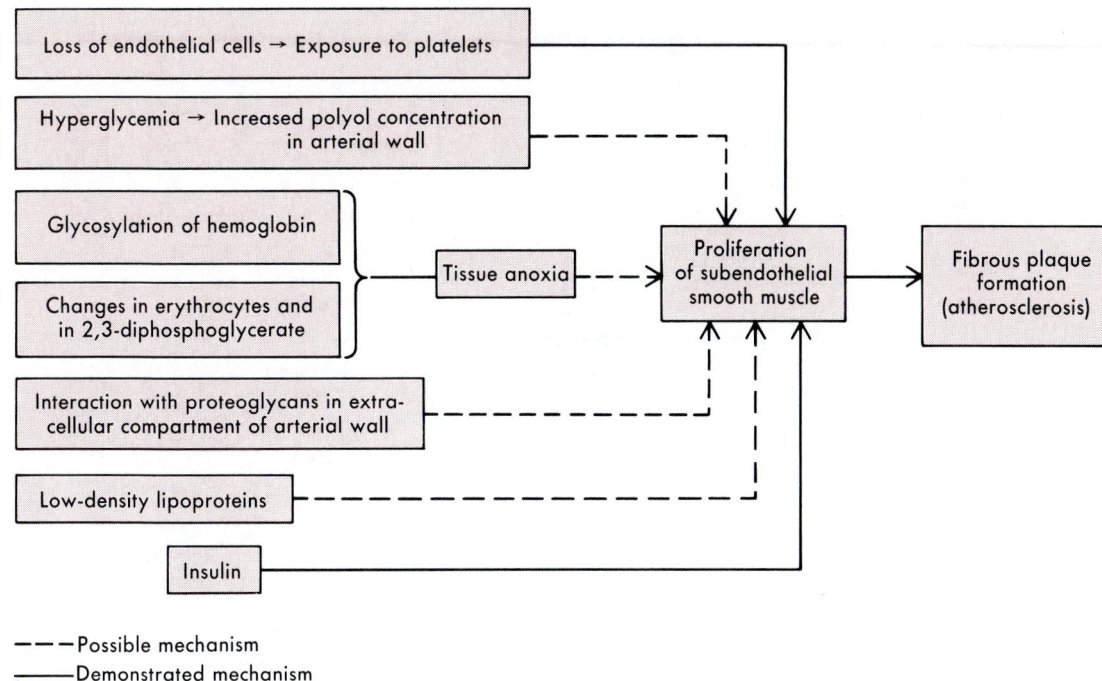

FIG. 18-12 Diabetes mellitus and atherosclerosis. Contributing causes of proliferation of subendothelial smooth muscle in arterial wall, resulting in atherosclerosis.

general population even when hypertension and hyperlipidemia are taken into account. Coronary artery disease is the most common cause of death in individuals with type II diabetes, but is also common in those with type I (Fein & Scheuer, 1990). Whereas the cardiovascular mortality is increased in all age groups, mortality is most marked at or before middle age, particularly in women. In general, the prevalence of coronary artery disease increases with the duration but not the severity of diabetes.

Myocardial infarction (death of heart muscle due to coronary artery occlusion) is the cause of death in 20% of those with diabetes, and individuals with diabetes mellitus have a higher mortality rate during the acute phase of myocardial infarctions than do nondiabetics. In addition, the incidence of congestive heart failure is higher in the individual with diabetes, even without myocardial infarction. The reason is unclear, but may be related to the presence of increased amounts of collagen in the ventricular wall, which reduces the mechanical compliance of the heart during filling. (Heart disease is described in Chapter 27.)

Stroke

Stroke is twice as common in those with diabetes than in the nondiabetic population (McMillan, 1990). The survival rate for an individual with diabetes after a massive stroke is typically shorter than for a nondiabetic.

Hypertension is a definite risk factor (see Chapter 15). No data are available to evaluate the effects of blood glucose control on the incidence of stroke.

Peripheral vascular disease

The increased incidence of peripheral vascular disease (PVD), gangrene, and amputation in the individual with diabetes has been documented in many studies, particularly in individuals with type II diabetes (Levin & Sicard, 1990). To see how foot lesions of diabetes can lead to amputation, see Fig. 18-13. Many individuals with type II diabetes have evidence of peripheral vascular disease at the time of their initial diagnosis. The atherosclerotic process in the individual with diabetes is more common, appears at a younger age, and advances more rapidly than vascular changes in nondiabetics. The prevalence of PVD is nearly equal in males and females with diabetes. Age, duration of diabetes, genetics, and additional risk factors influence the development of PVD.

Because of occlusions of the small arteries and arterioles, most of the gangrenous changes of the lower extremities occur in patchy areas of the feet and toes. Smaller vessels often have more advanced disease than larger vessels in the same individuals. Fifty percent of nontraumatic amputations in the United States are performed on individuals with diabetes. Hospital mortality for individuals with diabetes who undergo major amputation is between 10% and 23%. The survival rate

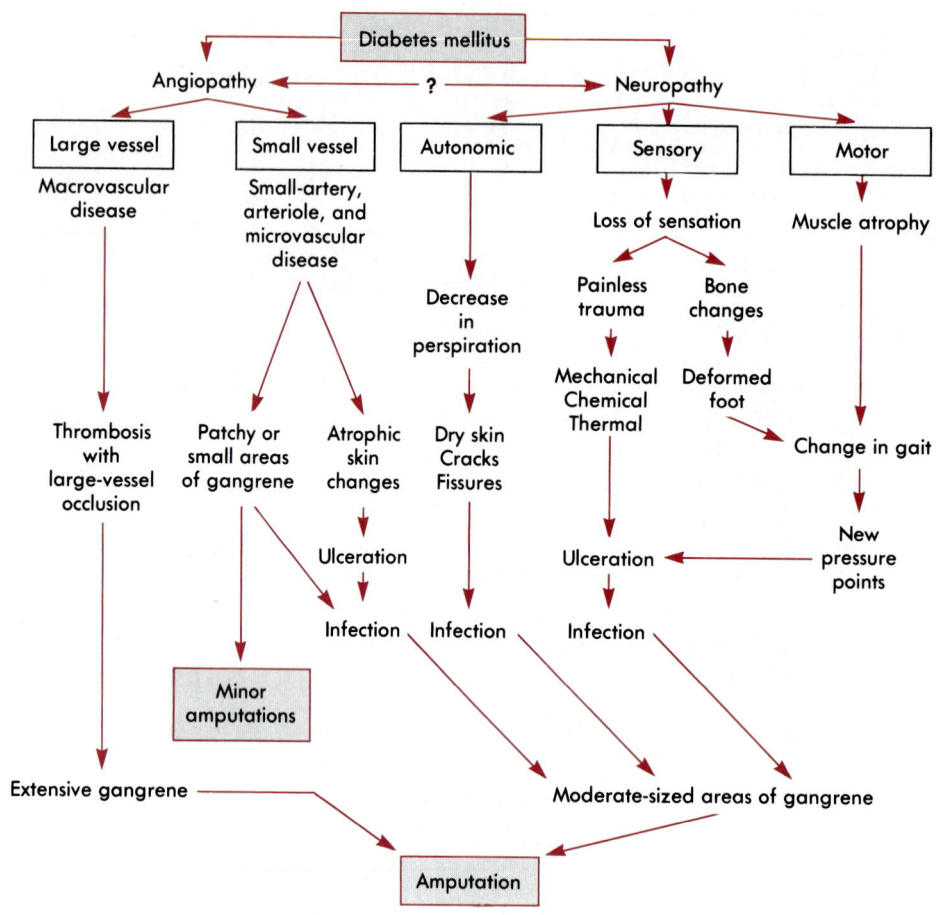

FIG. 18-13 How foot lesions of diabetes can lead to amputation. (From Phipps, Long, Woods, & Cassmeyer, 1991.)

after surgery is only 40% at the end of 5 years (Levin & Sicard, 1990).

Infection

Increased morbidity and mortality from infectious agents have been documented in those with diabetes (Casey, 1990). The individual with diabetes is at increased risk for infection throughout the body for at least five reasons. One major reason involves the senses. Impaired vision caused by retinal changes and impaired touch caused by neuropathy diminish the prevention of breaks in the skin by decreasing the early warning systems. Once breaks in skin integrity occur, tissues may have increased susceptibility to infection because of hypoxia, a second reason for susceptibility to infection. Microvascular and macrovascular complications cause decreased oxygen supply to tissues. In addition, the increased content of glycosylated hemoglobin in the red blood cell impedes the release of oxygen to tissues.

The third general reason for infection in individuals with diabetes is that pathogens are able to multiply rapidly once they have gained access to the tissues. Some

pathogens proliferate rapidly because the increased glucose in body fluids provides an excellent source of energy. Fourth, the decreased blood supply resulting from vascular changes decreases the supply of white blood cells to the affected area. Fifth, the function of the white cells is impaired. Chemotaxis is abnormal, and phagocytosis is defective. The causes for these mechanisms have not been identified, but the end result is an individual at considerable risk for the development of infections. (Factors that promote healing are described in Chapter 7.) The risk of infection is especially high for individuals undergoing surgery and for those taking immunosuppressant medications.

ALTERATIONS OF ADRENAL FUNCTION

Disorders of the Adrenal Cortex

Disorders of the adrenal cortex are related either to hyperfunction or to hypofunction. Hyperfunction that causes increased levels of circulating cortisol leads to

Cushing disease, or Cushing syndrome; that which causes increased secretion of adrenal androgens and estrogens leads to virilization or feminization; and that which causes increased levels of aldosterone leads to hyperaldosteronism, which may be primary or secondary. Hypofunction of the adrenal cortex leads to Addison disease, which has a variety of causal factors.

Hypercortical Function (Cushing Disease, Cushing Syndrome)

Cushing syndrome refers to chronic **hypercortisolism** (excessive levels of circulating cortisol) caused by hyperfunction of the adrenal cortex, with or without pituitary involvement. **Cushing disease** refers specifically to pituitary-dependent hypercortisolism. Additionally, a Cushing-like syndrome may develop as a result of the exogenous administration of cortisone (McNicol, 1992).

Adrenocorticotropic hormone–induced Cushing disease is more common in adults and is two to three times more common in women than in men. Cushing syndrome resulting from ectopic ACTH secretion is more common in older adults, particularly men. Adrenal tumors, rather than pituitary tumors, are more common in children, especially girls. Cushing syndrome can be found in any age, but usually occurs between 30 and 50 years of age.

Pathophysiology

Causes of hypercortisolism often involve excessive circulating ACTH, which may result from a variety of pathophysiologic alterations. Dysregulation of hypothalamic or anterior pituitary hormones may lead to increased levels of ACTH. Autonomous, ectopic ACTH secretion by a tumor outside the pituitary, usually a malignant tumor, and frequently an oat cell carcinoma of the lung, also may cause the development of Cushing syndrome.

Elevated levels of ACTH account for approximately 75% to 80% of all cases of Cushing syndrome. Autonomous secretion of cortisol by an adrenal neoplasm, which may be either benign or malignant, accounts for approximately 10% of the cases of hypercorticoadrenalism.

Whatever the cause, two observations consistently apply to individuals with Cushing syndrome: (1) they do not have diurnal or circadian secretion patterns of ACTH and cortisol, and (2) they do not increase ACTH and cortisol secretion in response to a stressor. In individuals with ACTH-stimulated hypercorticoadrenalism, secretion of both cortisol and adrenal androgens is increased. Hormone-secreting tumors of the adrenal cortex, however, generally only secrete cortisol. When the secretion of cortisol by the tumor exceeds normal cortisol levels, symptoms of hypercortisolism develop.

The elevated cortisol levels suppress CRH and ACTH secretion by the hypothalamus and anterior pituitary, respectively, because normal feedback mechanisms still function. The low circulating levels of ACTH cause atrophy of the remaining normal portions of the adrenal cortex. This atrophy is not considered irreversible if the hypercortisolism is resolved, although recovery of cortisol-secreting activity of such cells may take several months.

Clinical Manifestations

Most of the clinical signs and symptoms of Cushing syndrome are caused by hypercortisolism (see Chapter 9). Weight gain is the most common feature and results from the accumulation of adipose tissue in the trunk, facial, and cervical areas. These characteristic patterns of fat deposition have been described as "truncal obesity," "moon face," and "buffalo hump" (Figs. 18-14 and 18-15). Transient weight gain from sodium and water retention may be present because of the mineralocorticoid effects of cortisol, exhibited when cortisol is present in high levels.

Glucose intolerance occurs because of cortisol-induced insulin resistance and increased gluconeogenesis and glycogen storage by the liver. Overt diabetes mellitus develops in approximately 20% of individuals with hypercortisolism. Polyuria, which is sometimes seen in hypercortisolism, is a manifestation of hyperglycemia and resultant glycosuria.

Protein wasting is commonly observed in hypercortisolism and is caused by the catabolic effects of cortisol on peripheral tissues. Muscle wasting, especially obvious in the muscles of the extremities, leads to muscle weakness. In bone, loss of the protein matrix leads to osteoporosis, with pathologic fractures, vertebral compression fractures, bone and back pain, kyphosis, and reduced height. Bone disease may contribute to hypercalcinuria and resulting renal stones, which are experienced by approximately 20% of individuals with disease. Loss of collagen also leads to thin, weakened integumentary tissues through which capillaries are more visible and which are easily stretched by adipose deposits. Together, these changes account for the characteristic purple striae most frequently observed in the trunk area. Loss of collagenous support around small vessels makes them susceptible to rupture, leading to easy bruising, even with minor trauma. Thin, atrophied skin is also easily damaged, leading to skin breaks and ulcerations.

Hyperpigmentation in Cushing syndrome is associated with very high serum levels of ACTH. The precise hormonal basis for this hyperpigmentation is still undetermined; however, current speculation focuses on the melanotropic activity of ACTH (Franco-Saenz, 1986). The pigmentation involves the mucous membranes,

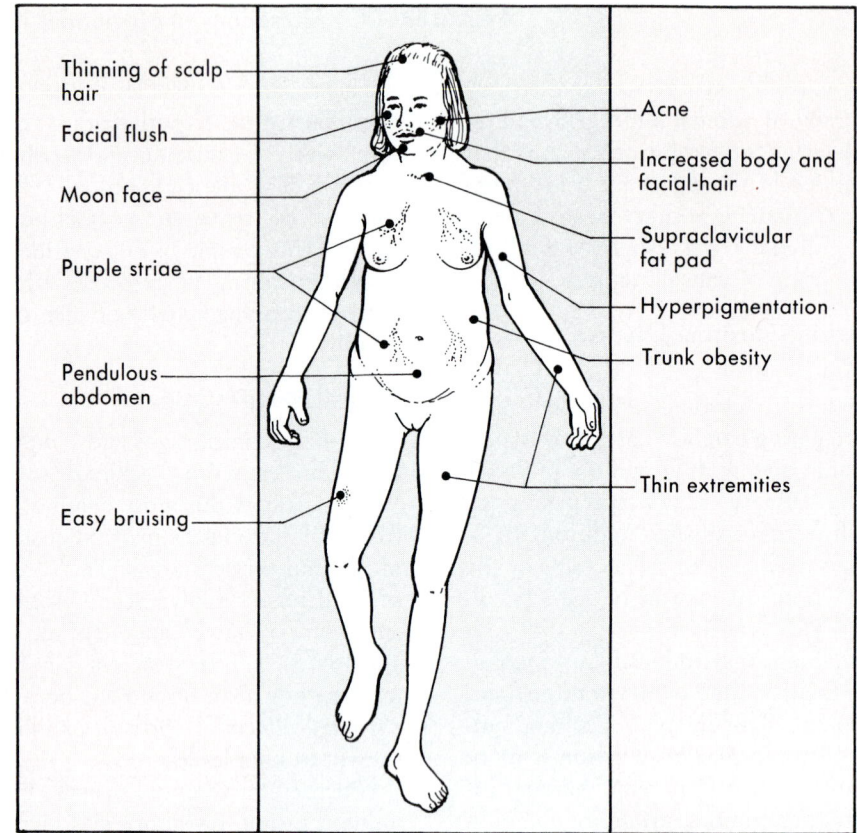

FIG. 18-14 Symptoms of Cushing disease.

FIG. 18-15 Cushing syndrome. A, Preoperatively. B, Six months postoperatively. (From Thibodeau, G. A. [1987]. *Anatomy and physiology*. St. Louis: Mosby–Year Book.)

hair, and skin, all of which acquire a characteristic brownish or bronze color.

Cortisol has a permissive effect on the actions of the catecholamines. With elevated cortisol levels, vascular sensitivity to catecholamines is significantly increased, leading to vasoconstriction and hypertension. Elevated blood pressure occurs in most individuals with Cushing syndrome. Chronically elevated cortisol levels also cause suppression of the immune system and increased susceptibility to infections.

Approximately 50% of individuals with Cushing syndrome experience alterations in their mental status. These may range from irritability and depression to severe psychiatric disturbances such as schizophrenia. The effects of glucocorticoids on mood are complex and are just beginning to be examined (Majewska, 1986).

Females may experience symptoms of increased adrenal androgen levels, increased hair growth (especially facial hair), acne, and oligomenorrhea. Rarely do androgen levels become high enough to cause changes of the voice, recession of the hairline, and clitoral hypertrophy unless an adrenal carcinoma is involved. Routine laboratory examinations may reveal hyperglycemia, glycosuria, hypokalemia, and metabolic alkalosis.

Evaluation and Treatment

A variety of laboratory tests must be used to diagnose Cushing syndrome. These include urinary free cortisol (17-hydroxycorticosterol) greater than 100 µg/24 hours and plasma cortisol obtained late in the evening greater than 20 mg/dl. A dexamethasone suppression test is simple and inexpensive and may be used to confirm the diagnosis and determine the cause.

Without treatment, approximately 50% of individuals with Cushing syndrome die within 5 years of onset. Major causes of death are overwhelming infection, suicide, complications from generalized arteriosclerosis, and hypertensive disease. Treatment is specific for the cause of hypercorticoadrenalism and includes medication, radiation, and surgery. Therefore differentiation among pituitary, adrenal, and ectopic causes of the hypercortisolism is essential for effective treatment.

Hyperaldosteronism

Hyperaldosteronism is characterized by excessive aldosterone secretion by the adrenal glands. The excessive secretion can result from a primary adrenal disorder, such as an aldosterone-secreting adenoma, or from excessive stimulation of the normal adrenal cortex by substances such as angiotensin, ACTH, or elevated potassium. Hyperaldosteronism may be primary or secondary. **Primary hyperaldosteronism** refers to an excessive secretion of aldosterone caused by an abnormality of the adrenal cortex. **Secondary hyperaldosteronism** involves excessive aldosterone secretion from an extraadrenal stimulus, most frequently angiotensin.

Primary hyperaldosteronism (Conn disease, primary aldosteronism) presents a clinical picture of hypertension, hypokalemia, renal potassium wasting, and neuromuscular manifestations. The most common cause of primary aldosteronism is the benign, single adrenal adenoma (80% to 90% of cases), followed by multiple tumors or idiopathic hyperplasia of the adrenals (10% to 15% of cases). Adrenal carcinomas and unknown causes account for the remainder of cases. The incidence of primary hyperaldosteronism is not known, but it is estimated to be 1% to 2% of all hypertensives (Melby, 1991).

Because aldosterone secretion is normally stimulated by the renin-angiotensin system, secondary hyperaldosteronism can be expected to result from sustained elevated renin release and activation of angiotensin. (Factors that affect renin and aldosterone secretion are summarized in Table 18-14.) Increased renin-angiotensin secretion occurs in a variety of situations. In general, these include decreased circulating blood volume (e.g., in de-

TABLE 18-14

Physiologic Factors Affecting Renin and Aldosterone Secretion

Factors	Renin secretion	Aldosterone secretion
Age	Highest in infants; lowest in the aged	Highest in infants
Menstrual cycle	Highest in luteal phase (see Chapter 19)	Highest in luteal phase
Sodium intake	Increased by salt restriction	Increased by salt restriction
	Decreased by salt loading	Decreased by salt loading
Potassium status	Increased by K$^+$ depletion	Decreased by K$^+$ depletion
Posture	Increased with erect posture	Increased with erect posture
Sympathetic nervous stimulation	Increased by catecholamines	Increased through renin secretion
Time of sampling	Highest before noon; lowest in evening	Diurnal rhythm (as for ACTH)

hydration, shock, or hypoalbuminemia) and decreased delivery of blood to the kidneys (e.g., renal artery stenosis, heart failure, or hepatic cirrhosis). In many of these instances, the activation of the renin-angiotensin system and subsequent aldosterone secretion may be seen as compensatory, although in some instances (e.g., congestive heart failure), the increased circulating volume may further worsen the condition.

Increased estrogen levels associated with pregnancy and use of oral contraceptives also increase renin-angiotensin levels, apparently by stimulating renin substrate production by the liver. These pregnancy-induced changes, however, may represent adaptation to pregnancy and are therefore not representative pathophysiologic alterations.

Other causes of secondary hyperaldosteronism are Bartter syndrome, in which the underlying disorder is a renal tubular defect leading to hypokalemia, and renin-

secreting tumors of the kidney. Such tumors, however, cause secondary hyperaldosteronism. (Renal disorders are discussed in Chapter 33.)

Pathophysiology

In primary hyperaldosteronism, pathophysiologic alterations are caused by excessive aldosterone secretion and the fluid and electrolyte imbalances that ensue. Hyperaldosteronism promotes increased sodium reabsorption with corresponding hypervolemia (see Chapter 3). The extracellular fluid volume overload and suppression of normal feedback mechanisms of renin secretion are characteristic of primary disorders.

Edema usually does not occur with primary aldosteronism, possibly because of the renal tubular "escape" phenomenon that is activated in chronic hyperaldosteronism. The escape phenomenon changes or resets the rate of sodium excretion and prevents more severe so-

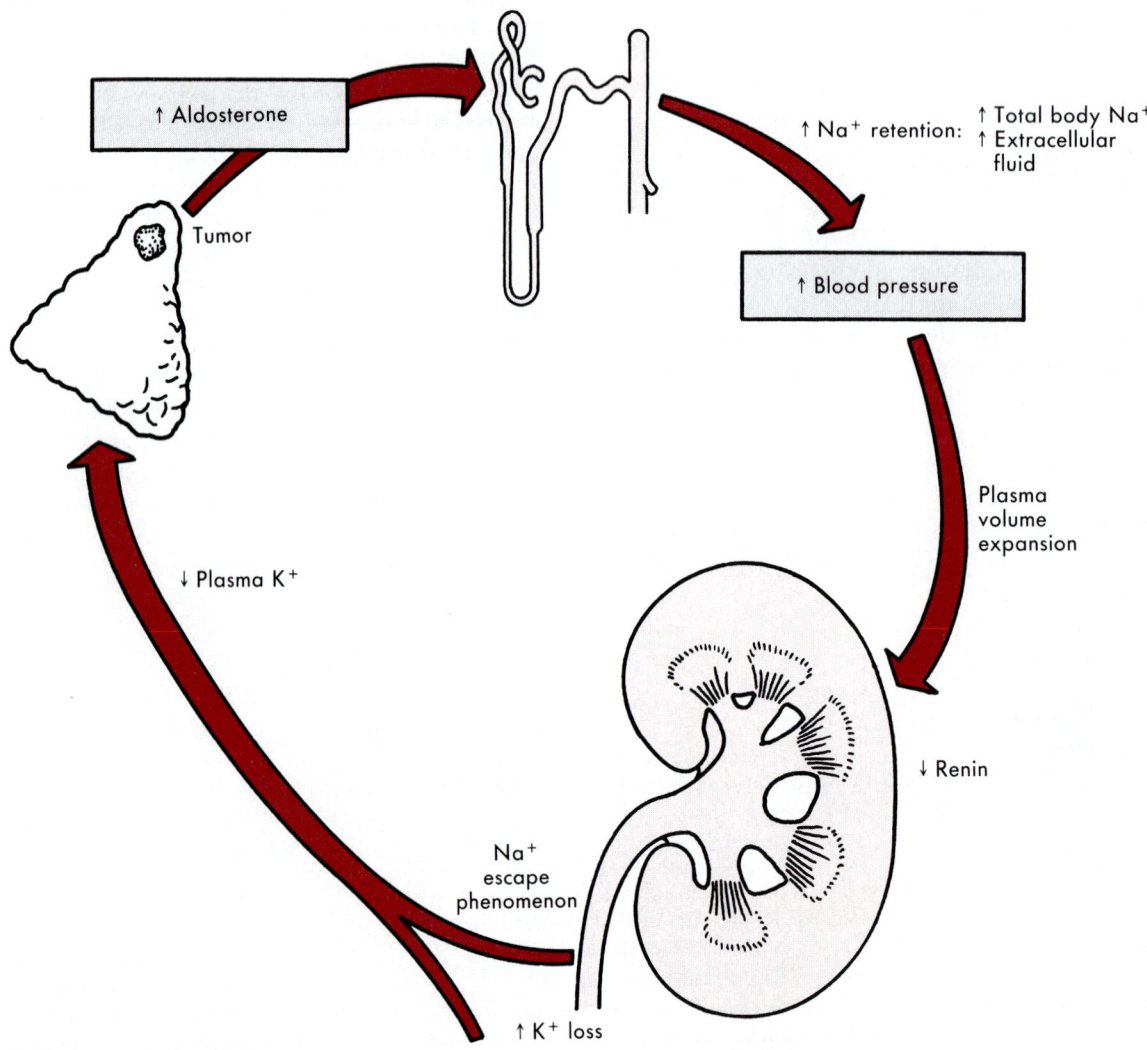

FIG. 18-16 Primary hyperaldosteronism. Pathophysiology of mineralocorticoid excess syndromes in primary hyperaldosteronism.

dium retention. The escape phenomenon operates in the proximal tubules and causes additional sodium to pass to the distal tubules, where the sodium is, to some extent, reabsorbed in exchange for potassium. This mechanism, while protecting from excessive sodium reabsorption and edema, increases urinary losses of potassium (Fig. 18-16).

In secondary hyperaldosteronism, the effect of increased extracellular volume on renin secretion may vary. If renin secretion is being stimulated by variables other than pressure-initiated cellular changes at the juxtaglomerular apparatus (see Chapter 32), then increased circulating blood volume may not decrease renin secretion through feedback mechanisms. This process occurs, for instance, in states of increased estrogen levels.

In Bartter syndrome, a state of hypokalemia develops because of defective renal tubular reabsorptive mechanisms. The hypokalemic state may induce the formation of prostaglandins (especially PGE_2) by the renal cells, which stimulates renin and hence aldosterone secretion. The stimulatory effect on aldosterone secretion is offset somewhat by the aldosterone-suppressing effects of hypokalemia.

Potassium secretion also is promoted by aldosterone, so that with excessive circulating levels of aldosterone, hypokalemia occurs (see Chapter 3). In hyperaldosteronism, hypokalemic alkalosis, changes in myocardial conduction, and skeletal muscle alterations may be seen, particularly with severe potassium depletion (i.e., the renal tubules may become insensitive to ADH, thus promoting excessive loss of free water). In this situation, hypernatremia also may occur because water is not able to follow the sodium that is reabsorbed.

Clinical Manifestations

Hypertension and hypokalemia are the hallmarks of hyperaldosteronism. Hypertension may result from increased intravascular volume, from altered sodium concentrations in vessel walls, or from a state of aldosterone-mediated vasoconstriction, although this requires very high levels of aldosterone. If hypertension is sustained, the chronic effects of elevated arterial pressure become evident. These effects include left ventricular hypertrophy and progressive arteriosclerosis. Because of the increased arterial pressure, renin secretion is typically suppressed, although it may be increased in secondary aldosteronism.

Aldosterone-stimulated potassium loss can be substantial. Serum potassium levels of less than 3.0 mEq/L result in the typical manifestations of hypokalemia: hypokalemic alkalosis caused by the movement of potassium from the intercellular to extracellular space in exchange for hydrogen ions as well as renal loss of hydrogen ions to facilitate sodium reabsorption (see Chapter 3). Individuals with hypokalemic alkalosis may

experience (1) tetany and paresthesia caused by an alkalosis-induced lowering of ionized calcium levels, (2) skeletal muscle weakness that can be so severe as to mimic flaccid paralysis, (3) cardiovascular alterations, including depressed T waves and ST segment, appearance of U waves on the electrocardiogram, and ventricular ectopy, which may or may not be associated with syncopy, and (4) loss of urine-concentrating mechanisms leading to polyuria or nocturia.

Evaluation and Treatment

A variety of clinical and laboratory measurements are useful in the assessment of hyperaldosteronism. These include blood pressure, serum and urinary electrolyte levels, serum and urinary levels of aldosterone and renin, and aldosterone suppression testing. Blood pressure is elevated; serum sodium may be normal or elevated; and serum potassium is depressed, whereas urinary potassium is elevated (i.e., >30 mmol/day). Serum aldosterone, as measured by radioimmunoassay, is usually greater than 20 ng/dl. Plasma renin activity is generally less than 1 ng/ml/hr for individuals with primary aldosteronism. Serum aldosterone and plasma renin activity both must be measured under controlled situations and after careful dietary regulation of sodium and potassium intake (Table 18-14). Aldosterone-suppression testing is commonly accomplished with Florinef. Imaging techniques, such as CT scans or nuclear magnetic resonance (NMR), may be used to localize an aldosterone-secreting adenoma.

Treatment includes management of hypertension and hypokalemia, as well as correction of any underlying causal abnormalities. If an aldosterone-secreting adenoma is present, it must be surgically removed.

Hypersecretion of Adrenal Androgens and Estrogens

Hypersecretion of adrenal androgens and estrogens may be caused by adrenal tumors, either adenomas or carcinomas, Cushing syndrome, or defects in steroid synthesis. The clinical syndrome that results depends on the hormone secreted, the sex of the individual, and the ages at which the hypersecretion was initiated. Hypersecretion of estrogens causes **feminization,** the development of female sex characteristics. Hypersecretion of androgens causes **virilization,** the development of male sex characteristics (Fig. 18-17).

The effects of an estrogen-secreting tumor are most evident in males and result in gynecomastia (98% of cases), testicular atrophy, and decreased libido. In female children, such tumors may lead to early development of secondary sex characteristics. An androgen-secreting tumor indicates changes more easily observed in females, including excessive face and body hair growth, hirsutism, clitoral enlargement, deepening of

FIG. 18-17 Virilization. Virilization of a young girl by a virilizing tumor of the adrenal cortex. The tumor secretes excess androgens, thereby producing masculinizing adrenogenital syndrome. (From Thibodeau, G. A. [1987]. *Anatomy and physiology*. St. Louis: Mosby–Year Book.)

the voice, amenorrhea, acne, and breast atrophy. In children, virilizing tumors promote precocious sexual development and bone aging. Treatment of androgen-secreting tumors usually involves surgical excision.

Hypocortical Functioning

Hypocortisolism (low levels of cortisol secretion) develops either because of inadequate stimulation of the adrenal glands by ACTH or because of a primary inability of the adrenals to produce and secrete the adrenal cortical hormones. In some syndromes, however, there is partial dysfunction of the adrenal cortex so that only synthesis of aldosterone or the adrenal androgens is affected. Hypofunction of the adrenal cortex may affect glucocorticoid or mineralocorticoid secretion or a combination of both.

Primary adrenal insufficiency is termed **Addison disease.** Addison disease is a relatively rare disease, occurring most often in adults ages 30 to 60, although it may

appear at any time throughout the lifespan. Addison disease, caused by autoimmune mechanisms, is more common in women.

In the United States and Europe, tuberculosis (TB) is a rare cause of Addison disease. In Japan, however, TB continues to account for most cases. Once the adrenals are attacked by TB, the destructive process is irreversible and leads to progressive loss of the gland. Amyloidosis, another rare cause of Addison disease, also destroys the tissue of the adrenal cortex. Adrenoleukodystrophy and adrenomyeloneuropathy are two rare types of familial adrenal deficiency that lead to symptoms of hypocortisolism.

Pathophysiology

Addison disease is characterized by elevated serum ACTH levels with inadequate corticosteroid synthesis and output. The most common cause is idiopathic organ-specific autoimmune disease. Other causes include familial adrenal insufficiency, amyloidosis, metastatic destruction of the adrenal glands, adrenal hemorrhage, and infections. Before clinical manifestations of hypocortisolism are evident, more than 90% of total adrenocortical tissue must be destroyed.

Idiopathic Addison disease. Idiopathic Addison disease (**organ-specific autoimmune adrenalitis**), which causes adrenal atrophy and hypofunction, is generally recognized as an organ-specific autoimmune disease. (Autoimmunity is discussed in Chapter 8.) Autoantibodies are present in 50% to 70% of individuals with idiopathic Addison disease, and this percentage increases in younger persons and in those with other autoimmune diseases. The autoantibodies appear to be specific for the cells of the adrenal cortex. A combination of cell membrane and cytoplasmic antibodies and cell-mediated immune mechanisms contributes to the pathology of the disease. Apparently, a genetic defect in immune surveillance mechanisms causes a deficiency of immune suppressor cells. This deficiency allows the proliferation of immunocytes directed against specific antigens within the adrenocortical cells (Wulffraat, Drexhage, & Bottazzo, 1992).

Idiopathic Addison disease is frequently associated with other autoimmune diseases, especially Hashimoto thyroiditis, pernicious anemia, and idiopathic hypoparathyroidism. In these cases, Addison disease may be inherited as an autosomal recessive trait (McGregor, 1990). (Mechanisms of inheritance are described in Chapter 4.)

The adrenal glands in idiopathic Addison disease are smaller than normal and may be misshapen. Microscopically, gland atrophy is evident throughout the cortex, although the medulla appears intact. Extensive diffuse cortical lymphocytic infiltrate supports the immune component of the disease process.

TABLE 18-15

Clinical Manifestations and Pathophysiologic Mechanisms of Addison Disease

Clinical manifestation	Pathophysiologic mechanism
Weakness and easy fatigability that worsens as the day progresses, seen especially after exposure to stressors	Not known, may be related to hypoglycemia, decreased metabolism of proteins
Gastrointestinal disturbances; anorexia, nausea, vomiting, diarrhea, abdominal pain	Not known
Hypoglycemia, manifested by fatigue, mental confusion, apathy, psychosis	Absence of cortisol leads to decreased gluconeogenesis, decreased glycogen storage by liver, decreased metabolism of proteins, increased insulin sensitivity
Hyperpigmentation (only seen in cases of Addison disease with increased ACTH)	Increased secretion of ACTH is accompanied by increased secretion of beta-lipotropin and melanocyte-stimulating hormone; both hormones induce pigment changes in epithelial cells
Vitiligo, white patchy areas of depigmented skin	Autoimmune destruction of melanocytes
Hypotension	Decreased blood volume resulting from hypoaldosteronism causing increased renal sodium losses
Addisonian crisis: severe hypotension and vascular collapse	Combined effects of hypocortisolism, hypoaldosteronism, extracellular volume depletion, and some precipitating stressor (such as infection, vomiting, diarrhea)

Secondary hypocortisolism. Secondary hypocortisolism is characterized by low-to-absent ACTH levels, which cause inadequate adrenal stimulation, adrenal atrophy, and ultimately decreased corticosteroidogenesis. The exogenous administration of glucocorticoids for nonendocrine disease results in this form of hypocortisolism. Cortisol-producing endocrine tumors also cause secondary hypocortisolism. In these cases, increased glucocorticoid levels suppress ACTH production through normal feedback mechanisms. With decreased ACTH levels, corticosteroid synthesis by the adrenal gland is suppressed. This mechanism is ineffective in reducing corticosteroid levels, however, because the alteration in cortisol secretion lies outside the regulation of the normal feedback loop. Pituitary hypofunction, as occurs in postpartum pituitary infarction (Sheehan syndrome) and panhypopituitarism, hypophysectomy, or isolated ACTH deficiency causes inadequate ACTH production and secretion and absence of pituitary responsiveness to normal feedback mechanisms. In all instances of low ACTH levels, adrenal atrophy occurs, and endogenous adrenal steroidogenesis is depressed.

Clinical manifestations of secondary hypocortisolism are similar to those of Addison disease. One difference is that with the typically low levels of ACTH seen in secondary hypocortisolism, hyperpigmentation does not usually occur. Second, the renin-angiotensin system is usually normal in these individuals; therefore aldosterone and potassium levels also tend to be normal.

Clinical Manifestations

The symptoms of Addison disease are primarily a result of hypocortisolism and hypoaldosteronism. Decreased adrenal androgen secretion is usually not clinically obvious in males because the adrenals are not a major source of male androgens. Females may experience a loss of some secondary sex characteristics, such as pubic and axillary hair, normally maintained by the adrenal androgens. The symptoms of Addison disease are summarized in Table 18-15.

Evaluation and Treatment

Serum and urine levels of cortisol, aldosterone, and 17-ketosteroids are all depressed with hypocortisolism. Adrenocorticotropic hormone levels may be increased if there is adrenocortical insufficiency. Because of dehydration, blood urea nitrogen levels and hematocrit levels are increased. Serum glucose is low. Eosinophil and lymphocyte counts are frequently elevated. Hyperkalemia may cause mild alkalosis (see Chapter 3). The ACTH stimulation test may be used to evaluate adrenal cortical function. This is achieved by administering ACTH and monitoring the adrenal steroid levels.

The treatment of Addison disease involves glucocorticoid and possibly mineralocorticoid replacement therapy, together with dietary modifications. All individuals with hypocortisolism require long-term daily glucocorticoid replacement therapy. In the event of acute stressors, additional cortisol must be administered to approximate the amount of cortisol that might be expected to be secreted if normal adrenal function were present (approximately 100 to 300 µg/day).

The individual's diet should include at least 150 mEq sodium per day, with sodium intake increased in the event of excessive sweating or diarrhea. Treatment also must include correction of any underlying disorders such as tuberculosis.

Disorders of the Adrenal Medulla
Adrenal Medulla Hypofunction

No known physiologic alterations are associated with hypofunction of the adrenal medulla. Bilateral adrenalectomy, for example, is followed by a rapid decrease in urinary excretion of epinephrine, but that of norepinephrine remains relatively stable. Pathophysiologic alterations are instead associated with hyperfunctioning of the adrenal medulla.

Adrenal Medulla Hyperfunction

The most prominent cause of adrenal medulla hypersecretion is pheochromocytoma. A **pheochromocytoma** is a catecholamine-producing tumor, usually derived from the adrenal medullary cells (Fig. 18-18). Fewer

FIG. 18-18 Pheochromocytoma. Large pheochromocytoma replacing entire adrenal gland and displacing kidney. (From Rosai, 1989.)

than 10% of these tumors metastasize; if they do, they are usually found in the lungs, liver, bones, or para-aortic lymph glands. Most pheochromocytomas produce norepinephrine, although large tumors secrete both epinephrine and norepinephrine.

The true incidence of pheochromocytoma in the general population is not known. One tenth of one percent of the hypertensive population have a pheochromocytoma (Braunwald et al., 1987). The tumors are most common in people in their 40s and 50s, with men and women equally affected.

Pathophysiology

Pheochromocytomas cause excessive production of catecholamines attributable to autonomous functioning of the tumor. Other causes of elevated levels of catecholamines include defects in the normal inhibition of tyrosine hydroxylate or defects in the control mechanisms responsible for the regulation of catecholamine synthesis and release. Approximately 5% of people with pheochromocytomas have no symptoms, apparently because the tumor is nonfunctioning. Such tumors can, however, release catecholamines, especially in response to a stressor.

Clinical Manifestations

The clinical manifestations of a pheochromocytoma are related to the chronic effects of catecholamine secretion and include persistent hypertension associated with flushing, diaphoresis, tachycardia, and palpitations. Hypertension is a result of increased peripheral vascular resistance and may be sustained or paroxysmal. Headaches appear because of sudden changes in catecholamine levels in the blood, affecting cerebral blood flow. Hypermetabolism may be related to increased thyroid hormone levels resulting from stimulation of the thyroid gland by the catecholamines. Glucose intolerance may occur because of catecholamine-induced inhibition of insulin release by the pancreas. Complaints of warmth, heat intolerance, and weight loss are common despite a normal-to-increased appetite. Other symptoms of catecholamine excess include excessive sweating, palpitations and tachycardia, and gastrointestinal alterations, especially constipation.

An acute episode of hypertension related to hypersecretion of catecholamines may follow specific events. Exercise, excessive ingestion of tyrosine-containing foods (aged cheese, red wine, beer, yogurt), ingestion of caffeine-containing foods, external pressure on the tumor, and induction of anesthesia all can increase secretion of catecholamines by the tumor.

These tumors tend to be extremely vascular and can rupture. Such an event can cause massive and potentially fatal hemorrhage. Rupture of a pheochromocytoma is characterized by a sudden unexplained decrease in blood pressure, sudden severe abdominal pain, and a rigid abdomen.

Evaluation and Treatment

A diagnosis of pheochromocytoma is made when increased catecholamine production is demonstrated in the blood or urine. Individuals with this disorder can have total catecholamines greater than 250 µg/day. After elevation of urinary or plasma catecholamines is documented, the site of the tumor is determined by using radiographic techniques and surgical exploration of the abdomen. Because of the possibility of metastasis, whole-body scanning may be done.

The usual treatment of pheochromocytoma is surgical excision of the tumor. Medical therapy is used to stabilize blood pressure before surgery. Drugs used include alpha-adrenergic blocking agents and, possibly later, beta-adrenergic blocking agents (Cryer, 1992).

SUMMARY REVIEW

Mechanisms of Hormonal Alterations

1 Abnormalities in endocrine function may be caused by hypersecretion or hyposecretion of hormones, causing alterations in normal hormone levels.

2 Endocrine abnormalities also may be caused by alterations in receptor function through a variety of mechanisms: (1) a decrease in number of receptors, (2) receptor insensitivity to the hormone, (3) antibodies against specific receptors, and (4) general receptor dysfunction.

3 Abnormally high levels of circulating hormones are sometimes caused by hormone release from tissues outside the endocrine system (ectopic foci), which may not respond to normal feedback mechanisms, in which case they are said to function autonomously.

Alterations of the Hypothalamic-Pituitary System

1 Dysfunction in the release of hypothalamic hormones is probably related to interruption of the connection between the hypothalamus and pituitary, the infundibular stem.

2 Disorders of the posterior pituitary include syndrome of inappropriate ADH secretion (SIADH) and diabetes insipidus. Syndrome of inappropriate ADH secretion is characterized by abnormally high ADH secretion; diabetes insipidus is characterized by abnormally low ADH secretion.

3 In SIADH, high ADH levels interfere with renal function, leading to hyponatremia and hypoosmolality. Syndrome of inappropriate ADH secretion is associated with certain forms of cancer, apparently because of ectopic secretion of ADH by tumor cells.

4 Diabetes insipidus may be neurogenic, caused by insufficient amounts of ADH, or nephrogenic, caused by an inadequate response to ADH. Its principal clinical features are polyuria and polydipsia.

5 Hypopituitarism is dysfunction of the anterior pituitary that causes failure of hormonal functions. Symptoms may be mild to severe.

6 The most common cause of hypopituitarism is pituitary infarction, in which an initiating event leads to circulatory collapse and compensatory vasospasm. Pregnant and postpartum women are most at risk for pituitary infarction.

7 Hyperpituitarism is caused by pituitary adenomas. These are usually benign, slow-growing tumors that arise from cells of the anterior pituitary.

8 Expansion of a pituitary adenoma causes both neurologic and secretory effects. Pressure from the expanding tumor causes hyposecretion of cells, dysfunction of the optic chiasma (leading to visual disturbances), and dysfunction of the hypothalamus and some cranial nerves.

9 Hypersecretion of GH causes acromegaly, in which GH secretion becomes high and unpredictable. Pituitary adenoma is the most common cause of acromegaly.

10 Prolonged, abnormally high levels of GH lead to proliferation of body and connective tissue and in the cytoplasmic matrix. Renal, thyroid, and reproductive dysfunction develop slowly, together with a change in body proportions.

Alterations of Thyroid Function

1 Thyrotoxicosis is a general condition in which TH levels cause greater-than-normal physiologic responses. The condition can be caused by a variety of specific diseases, each of which has its own pathophysiology and course of treatment.

2 In general, hyperthyroidism has a range of endocrine, reproductive, gastrointestinal, integumentary, and ocular manifestations. These are caused by increased circulating levels of TH and by stimulation of the sympathetic division of the autonomic nervous system.

3 Graves disease, the most common form of hyperthyroidism, is probably caused by an autoimmune mechanism that overrides normal mechanisms for control of TH secretion.

4 Manifestations of Graves disease can include symptoms of hyperthyroidism, diffuse thyroid enlargement, disorders of the skin, and effects on the extremities.

5 Effects on the extremities cause pretibial myxedema, a condition characterized by subcutaneous swelling of the legs and, occasionally, the hands.

6 Ocular manifestations of Graves disease are caused by hyperactivity of the sympathetic division of the autonomic nervous system and by unknown mechanisms that cause infiltrative changes.

7 Toxic nodular goiter and toxic multinodular goiter occur when TH-regulating mechanisms and abnormal hypertrophy of the thyroid gland cause hyperthyroidism.

8 Toxic nodular goiters are follicular cell adenomas that produce symptoms similar to those of Graves disease.

9 Toxic multinodular goiter is caused by independently functioning follicular cells diffused throughout the thyroid gland.

10 Thyrotoxic crisis is a severe form of hyperthyroidism that is often associated with physiologic or psychologic stress. Without treatment, death occurs quickly.

11 Hypothyroidism is caused by deficient production of TH by the thyroid gland. The condition may be primary or secondary.

12 Hypothyroid conditions include a variety of specific disease processes. Hypothyroidism also can be caused by hypothalamic-pituitary dysfunction in which TRH and TSH are not produced in sufficient amounts.

13 Hypothyroidism affects all body systems. Symptoms depend on the degree of TH deficiency. Common manifestations include decreased energy metabolism and heat production.

14 Myxedema is the characteristic sign of hypothyroidism. Myxedema is caused by alterations in connective tissue with water-binding proteins. The excess water leads to edema and thickened mucous membranes.

15 Acute thyroiditis, a form of hypothyroidism, is caused by a bacterial infection.

16 Subacute thyroiditis, a form of hypothyroidism, is a self-limiting nonbacterial inflammation of the thyroid gland. The inflammatory process damages follicular cells, causing leakage of T_3 and T_4. Hyperthyroidism then is followed by transient hypothyroidism, which is corrected by cellular repair and a return to normal levels in the thyroid.

17 Autoimmune thyroiditis is associated with infiltration or fibrosis of the thyroid, circulating thyroid antibodies, and gradual loss of thyroid function. Autoimmune thyroiditis occurs in those individuals with genetic susceptibility to an autoimmune mechanism that causes thyroid damage and eventual hypothyroidism.

18 Myxedema coma is a severe form of hypothyroidism, which may be life-threatening without emergency medical treatment.

19 Thyroid carcinoma is a relatively rare cancer. The most consistent causal risk factor associated with thyroid carcinoma is exposure to ionizing radiation, especially in childhood.

Alterations of Parathyroid Function

1 Hyperparathyroidism, which may be primary, secondary, or tertiary, is characterized by greater than normal secretion of PTH.

2 Primary hyperparathyroidism is caused by an interruption of the normal mechanisms that regulate calcium and PTH levels. Manifestations include chronic hypercalcemia, increased bone resorption, and hypercalcuria.

3 Secondary hyperparathyroidism is a compensatory response to hypocalcemia and often occurs with chronic renal failure.

4 Tertiary hyperparathyroidism is associated with hyperplasia of the parathyroid glands and a loss of the regulatory mechanism that governs PTH and calcium levels.

5 Hypoparathyroidism, defined by abnormally low PTH levels, is caused by thyroid surgery or by hereditary mechanisms.

6 The lack of circulating PTH in hypoparathyroidism causes depressed serum calcium levels, increased serum phosphate levels, decreased bone resorption, and eventual hypocalcuria.

Dysfunction of the Endocrine Pancreas: Diabetes Mellitus

1 Diabetes mellitus is a complex syndrome that causes a number of physiologic changes, some of which are metabolic processes and others of which are vascular.

2 A diagnosis of diabetes mellitus is based on elevated plasma glucose concentrations. Classic signs and symptoms are often present as well.

3 Two most common types of diabetes mellitus are type I and type II, also called insulin-dependent diabetes mellitus (IDDM) and non-insulin-dependent diabetes mellitus (NIDDM).

4 Type I diabetes mellitus is characterized by a lack of insulin and a relative excess of glucagon, which causes improper metabolism of fat, protein, and carbohydrates.

5 Type I diabetes mellitus is most commonly diagnosed among whites younger than 30 years of age.

6 In type I diabetes mellitus, β-cells are destroyed, and islet cell antibodies (ICA) appear. The function of these antibodies is unknown, and they tend to disappear with time.

7 Type I diabetes mellitus seems to be caused by a gradual process of autoimmune destruction in genetically susceptible individuals.

8 In type I diabetes mellitus, decreased use of glucose causes glucose accumulation in the blood and sub-

sequent loss in the urine. This in turn causes polyuria and polydipsia resulting from osmotic diuresis.

9 Ketoacidosis, caused by increased levels of circulating ketones without the inhibiting effects of insulin; increased levels of circulating fatty acids; and weight loss are all manifestations of type I diabetes mellitus.

10 Type II diabetes mellitus is probably caused by genetic susceptibility that is triggered by environmental factors. The most compelling environmental risk factor is obesity.

11 In the obese, insulin has a diminished ability to influence glucose uptake and metabolism.

12 In type II diabetes, amyloid deposits in the islets, fatty atrophy of the pancreas and liver, and vascular sclerosis (causing ischemia) are generally present.

13 Some insulin production continues in type II diabetes mellitus, but the weight and number of β-cells decrease.

14 Because the ratio of α-cells to β-cells may be normal in the individual with type II diabetes, hypotheses suggest that the disease is caused by dysfunctional levels of both insulin and glucagon.

15 Acute complications of diabetes mellitus include hypoglycemia, diabetic ketoacidosis, hyperosmolar nonacidotic diabetes, the Somogyi effect, and the dawn phenomenon.

16 Hypoglycemia is a lowered blood glucose level, which may be related to exogenous, endogenous, or functional causes.

17 Symptoms of hypoglycemia are caused by a neurogenic reaction, which occurs when the neuron receives inadequate amounts of carbohydrates to metabolize, and cellular malnutrition, which causes further symptoms.

18 Diabetic ketoacidosis develops when there is an absolute or relative deficiency of insulin and an increase in the insulin counterregulatory hormones of catecholamines, cortisol, glucagon, and growth hormone.

19 Hyperosmolar nonacidotic diabetes (HNAD) is pathophysiologically similar to diabetic ketoacidosis, although levels of free fatty acids are lower in HNAD and lack of ketosis indicates that some level of insulin is present.

20 The Somogyi effect is a combination of hypoglycemia and ketosis. It is most common in those with type I diabetes mellitus and in children.

21 The dawn phenomenon is an early morning rise in glucose levels caused by nocturnal elevations of growth hormone.

22 Chronic sequelae of diabetes mellitus include diabetic neuropathies, microvascular disease (e.g., retinopathy, nephropathy), macrovascular disease (e.g., coronary artery disease, stroke, and peripheral vascular disease), and infection.

23 Diabetic neuropathies may be caused by vascular or metabolic mechanisms or a combination of both.

24 In diabetic neuropathy, axonal and Schwann cell degeneration and metabolic aberrations are related to abnormalities in motor nerve conduction velocity, electromyography, and sensory perception.

25 Microangiopathy is caused by thickening of the capillary basement membrane and eventual decreased tissue perfusion affecting the microcirculation.

26 Diabetic retinopathy is caused by retinal ischemia related to microvascular occlusion associated with diabetes mellitus.

27 Diabetic nephropathy is related to glomerular enlargement and glomerular basement membrane thickening, which in turn cause diffuse intercapillary glomerulosclerosis.

28 Macrovascular disease associated with diabetes mellitus is probably related to the proliferation of fibrous plaques in the arterial wall and to elevated lipid levels.

29 Incidence of coronary heart disease, peripheral vascular disease, and stroke is greater in those with diabetes than in nondiabetics.

30 Individuals with diabetes are at risk for a variety of infections.

31 Infection may be related to sensory impairment and resulting injury, hypoxia, increased proliferation of pathogens in elevated concentrations of glucose, decreased blood supply associated with vascular damage, and impaired white cell function.

Alterations of Adrenal Function

1 Disorders of the adrenal cortex are related to hyperfunction or hypofunction. No known disorders are associated with hypofunction of the adrenal medulla, but medullary hyperfunction causes clinically defined syndromes.

2 Cortical hyperfunction, or hypercortisolism, causes Cushing syndrome, which may or may not involve the pituitary gland, and Cushing disease, which is hypercortisolism with pituitary involvement.

3 Cushing syndrome may be caused by excessive circulating ACTH related to CRH secretion, a pituitary adenoma, autonomous secretion by a tumor outside the pituitary, or autonomous secretion by an adrenal neoplasm and its metastases.

4 Individuals with Cushing disease lose diurnal and circadian patterns of ACTH and cortisol secretion, and they lack the ability to increase secretion of these hormones in response to a stressor. Individuals experience weight gain, glucose intolerance, protein wasting, bone disease, hyperpigmentation, and immune suppression.

5 Excessive aldosterone secretion causes hyperaldosteronism, which may be primary or secondary. Primary hyperaldosteronism is caused by an abnormal-

ity of the adrenal cortex. Secondary hyperaldosteronism involves an extraadrenal stimulus, often angiotensin.

6 Primary hyperaldosteronism is usually caused by an adrenal adenoma or carcinoma. The condition is characterized by hypertension, hypokalemia, renal potassium wasting, and neuromuscular manifestations.

7 Secondary hyperaldosterone secretion is related to a variety of conditions associated with elevated renin release and activation of angiotensin. These include decreased circulating blood volume and decreased renal blood supply, elevated estrogen levels, Bartter syndrome, and renin-secreting tumors.

8 Hyperaldosteronism promotes increased sodium reabsorption, corresponding hypervolemia, increased extracellular volume (which is variable), and hypokalemia related to renal reabsorption of sodium.

9 Hypersecretion of adrenal androgens and estrogens causes adrenal tumors, either adenomas or carcinomas. Hypersecretion of estrogens causes feminization, the development of female sex characteristics. Hypersecretion of androgens causes virilization, the development of male sex characteristics.

10 Hypofunction of the adrenal cortex can affect glucocorticoid or mineralocorticoid secretion, or both. Hypofunction can be caused by a deficiency of adrenal-stimulating substance or by a primary deficiency in the gland itself.

11 Hypocortisolism, or low levels of cortisol, is caused by inadequate adrenal stimulation by ACTH or by primary cortisol hyposecretion. Primary adrenal insufficiency is termed Addison disease.

12 Addison disease is characterized by elevated ACTH levels with inadequate corticosteroid synthesis and output.

13 Causes of Addison disease include idiopathic autoimmune disease, tuberculosis of the adrenal gland, familial adrenal insufficiency, amyloidosis, metastatic destruction of the adrenal glands, and adrenal hemorrhage.

14 Secondary hypercortisolism is characterized by low to absent ACTH levels, leading to inadequate adrenal stimulation, adrenal atrophy, and decreased corticosteroidogenesis. The most common cause is exogenous administration of glucocorticoids.

15 Manifestations of Addison disease are related to hypocortisolism and hypoaldosteronism. Symptoms include weakness, fatigability, hypoglycemia and related metabolic problems, lowered response to stressors, vitiligo, and manifestations of hypovolemia and hyperkalemia.

16 Hyperfunction of the adrenal medulla is usually caused by a pheochromocytoma, a catecholamine-producing tumor. Symptoms of catecholamine excess are related to their sympathetic nervous system effects and include hypertension, palpitations, tachycardia, glucose intolerance, excessive sweating, and constipation.

KEY TERMS

Acromegaly, 663

Acute thyroiditis, 670

Addison disease (primary adrenal insufficiency), 698

Autoimmune thyroiditis (Hashimoto disease, chronic lymphocyte thyroiditis), 670

Cushing disease (pituitary-dependent hypercortisolism), 693

Cushing syndrome (chronic hypercortisolism), 693

Dawn phenomenon, 687

Diabetes insipidus, 659

Diabetes mellitus, 674

Diabetic ketoacidosis (DKA) 685

Diabetic nephropathy, 690

Diabetic neuropathy, 688

Diabetic retinopathy, 688

Feminization, 697

Giantism, 663

Glycosylated hemoglobin, 674

Graves disease, 665

Hyperaldosteronism, 695

Hypercortisolism, 693

Hyperosmolar nonacidotic diabetes (HNAD), 686

Hyperparathyroidism, 671

Hyperpituitarism, 661

Hypocortisolism, 698

Hypoglycemia (insulin shock/reaction), 681

Hypoparathyroidism, 673

Hypopituitarism, 661

Hypothyroidism, 668

Idiopathic Addison disease (organ-specific autoimmune adrenalitis), 698

Myxedema, 668

Myxedema coma, 670

Panhypopituitarism, 662

Pheochromocytoma, 700

Pituitary adenoma, 662

Pretibial myxedema (Graves dermopathy), 666

Primary hyperaldosteronism (Conn disease, primary aldosteronism), 695

Primary hyperparathyroidism, 671

Secondary hyperaldosteronism, 695

Secondary hypercortisolism, 699

Secondary hyperparathyroidism, 671

Somogyi effect, 687

Subacute thyroiditis, 670

Syndrome of inappropriate ADH secretion (SIADH), 659

Tertiary hyperparathyroidism, 672

Thyrotoxic crisis (thyroid storm), 667

Thyrotoxicosis, 665

Toxic multinodular goiter, 667

Type I diabetes mellitus (insulin-dependent diabetes mellitus [IDDM]), 674

Type II diabetes mellitus (non-insulin-dependent diabetes mellitus [NIDDM]), 679

Virilization, 697

REFERENCES

American Cancer Society (ACS). (1993). *Cancer facts & figures 1993.* New York: Author.

American Diabetes Association. (1989). *Exchange lists for meal planning.* McLean, VA: Author.

Bengtsson, B. A., Eden, S., & Ernst, I. (1988). Epidemiology and long-term survival in acromegaly. A study of 166 cases diagnosed between 1955 and 1984. *Acta Medica Scandinavia, 223,* 327-335.

Bennett, P. H. (1990). Epidemiology of diabetes mellitus. In H. Rifkin & D. Porte (Eds.), *Diabetes mellitus theory and practice* (4th ed.). New York: Elsevier.

Brasher, H. R., & Raney, R. B. (1986). *Shand's handbook of orthopaedic surgery* (10th ed.). St. Louis: Mosby–Year Book.

Braunwald, E., Isselbacher, K. J., Petersdorf, R. G., Wilson, J., Martin, J. B., & Fauci, A. S. (1987). *Harrison's principles of internal medicine* (11th ed.). New York: McGraw-Hill.

Braverman, L. E., & Utiger, R. D. (1991). Introduction to thyrotoxicosis. In S. L. Werner & S. H. Ingbar (Eds.), *The thyroid: A fundamental and clinical text* (p. 645). Philadelphia: Lippincott.

Camargo, C. A., & Kolb, K. O. (1988). Endocrine disorders. In S. A. Schroeder, M. E. Krupp, & L. W. Tierney (Eds.), *Current medical diagnosis and treatment.* Norwalk, CT: Langer.

Casey, J. I. (1990). Host defense and infections in diabetes mellitus. In H. Rifkin & D. Porte (Eds.), *Diabetes mellitus theory and practice* (4th ed.). New York: Elsevier.

Cecil, R. L., Wyngaarden, J. B., & Smith, L. H. (1992). *Cecil's textbook of medicine* (9th ed.). Philadelphia: Saunders.

Clark, A., Yon, S. M., deKoning, D. J., & Holman, R. R. (1991). Autoantibodies to islet amyloid polypeptide in diabetes. *Diabetic Medicine, 8*(7), 668-673.

Cryer, P. E. (1992). Pheochromocytoma. *Western Journal of Medicine 156:*399-407.

Cryer, P. E., & Gerich, J. E. (1990). Hypoglycemia in insulin-dependent diabetes mellitus: Insulin excess and defective glucose counter-regulation. In H. Rifkin & D. Porte (Eds.), *Diabetes mellitus theory and practice* (4th ed.). New York: Elsevier.

Culpepper, R. M., Heber, S. C., & Andreoli, T. E. (1985). The posterior pituitary and water metabolism. In J. D. Wilson & D. W. Foster (Eds.), Williams textbook of endocrinology (9th ed.). Philadelphia: Saunders.

Diabetes Control and Complications Trial (DCCT) Research Group (1987). Diabetes control and complications trial (DCCT): Results of a feasibility study. *Diabetes Care, 10*(1), 1-19.

Diabetes Control and Complications Trial (DCCT) Research Group (1988). Weight gain associated with intensive therapy in the diabetes control and complications trial. *Diabetes Care, 11*(7), 567-573.

Diabetes Control and Complications Trial (DCCT) Research Group (1993). Results presented at June, 1993, American Diabetes Association Conference in Las Vegas. *New England Journal of Medicine* (in press).

Ezrin, C. (1979). *Systemic endocrinology.* Hagerstown, MD: Harper & Row.

Ezrin, C., Horvath, C., Kaufman, B., Kovacs, K., & Weiss, M. (1980). *Pituitary disease.* Boca Raton, FL: CRC Press.

Fajans, S. S. (1990). Classification and diagnosis of diabetes. In H. Rifkin & D. Porte (Eds.), *Diabetes mellitus theory and practice* (4th ed.). New York: Elsevier.

Farid, N. R., & Stenszky, V. (1988). Graves' disease. In N. Fand (Ed.), *Immunogenetics of endocrine disorders.* New York: Alan R. Liss.

Fein, F. S., & Scheuer, J. (1990). Heart disease in diabetes. In H. Rifkin & D. Porte (Eds.), *Diabetes mellitus theory and practice* (4th ed.). New York: Elsevier.

Franco-Saenz, R. (1986). Diseases of the adrenal cortex. In P. J. Mulrow (Ed.), *The adrenal gland.* New York: Elsevier.

Friedman, E. A. (1990). Diabetes renal disease. In H. Rifkin & D. Porte (Eds.), *Diabetes mellitus theory and practice* (4th ed.). New York: Elsevier.

Galloway, J. A., & deShazo, R. D. (1990). Insulin chemistry, pharmacology, dosage algorithms, and complications of insulin treatment. In H. Rifkin & D. Porte (Eds.), *Diabetes mellitus theory and practice* (4th ed.). New York: Elsevier.

Gavin, L. A. (1991). Thyroid crises. *Medical Clinics of North America, 75*(1), 179-193.

Greene, D. A., Sima, A. A. F., Albers, J. W., & Pfeifer, M. A. (1990). Diabetes neuropathy. In H. Rifkin & D. Porte (Eds.), *Diabetes mellitus theory and practice* (4th ed.). New York: Elsevier.

Harris, R. D., Steffes, M. W., Bilous, R. W., Sutherland, D. E., & Mauer, S. M. (1991). Global glomerular sclerosis and glomerular arteriolar hyalinosis in insulin dependent diabetes. *Kidney International, 40*(1), 107-114.

Horton, E. S., & Jeanrenaud, B. (1990). Obesity and diabetes mellitus. In H. Rifkin & D. Porte (Eds.), *Diabetes mellitus theory and practice* (4th ed.). New York: Elsevier.

Jubiz, W. (1985). *Endocrinology* (2nd ed.). New York: McGraw-Hill.

Kahan, A., LeFloch, J. P., & Charreire, J. (1990). Normal suppressive T-cell function of Epstein-Barr virus induced B-cell activation in type I (insulin dependent) diabetes mellitus. *Autoimmunity, 5*(4), 257-264.

Kahn, S. E., & Porte, D. (1990). Pathophysiology of type II (noninsulin-dependent) diabetes mellitus: Implications for treatment. In H. Rifkin & D. Porte (Eds.), *Diabetes mellitus theory and practice* (4th ed.). New York: Elsevier.

Kovacs, L., & Lichardus, B. (1989). Vasopressin: Disturbed secretion and its effects (p. 294). Boston: Dordrecht.

Kovacs, L., & Robertson, G. L. (1992). Syndrome of inappropriate antidiuresis. *Endocrinology and Metabolism Clinics of North America, 21*(4), 859-875.

Kriesberg, R. A. (1990). Diabetic ketoacidosis. In H. Rifkin & D. Porte (Eds.), *Diabetes mellitus theory and practice* (4th ed.). New York: Elsevier.

Labhart, A. (1986). *Clinical endocrinology: Theory and practice.* Berlin: Springer-Verlag.

Lacy, P. E., & Sharp, D. W. (1990). Islet cell transplantation. In H. Rifkin & D. Porte (Eds.), *Diabetes mellitus theory and practice* (4th ed.). New York: Elsevier.

Lebovitz, H. E. (1990). Oral hypoglycemic agents. In H. Rifkin & D. Porte (Eds.), *Diabetes mellitus theory and practice* (4th ed.). New York: Elsevier.

Lefebvre, P. J. (1990). Hypoglycemia. In H. Rifkin & D. Porte (Eds.), *Diabetes mellitus theory and practice* (4th ed.). New York: Elsevier.

L'Esperance, F. A., James, W. A., & Judson, P. H. (1990). The eye and diabetes mellitus. In H. Rifkin & D. Porte (Eds.), *Diabetes mellitus theory and practice* (4th ed.). New York: Elsevier.

Levin, M. E., & Sicard, G. A. (1990). Peripheral vascular disease in the person with diabetes. In H. Rifkin & D. Porte (Eds.), *Diabetes mellitus theory and practice* (4th ed.). New York: Elsevier.

Majewska, M. D. (1986). Steroid hormone metabolites are barbiturate-like modulators of the GABA receptor. *Science, 232,* 1004.

Manson, J. E., Nathan, D. M., Krolewski, A. S., Stampfer, M. J., Willett, W. C., & Hennekins, C. H. (1992). A prospective study of exercise and incidence of diabetes among US male physicians. *Journal of the American Medical Association, 268*(1), 63-67.

Matz, R. (1990). Hyperosmolar nonacidotic diabetes. In H. Rifkin & D. Porte (Eds.), *Diabetes mellitus theory and practice* (4th ed.). New York: Elsevier.

McDougall, I. R. (1991). Graves disease. *Medical Clinics of North America, 75*(1), 79-96.

McGregor, A. M. (1990). Immunoendocrine interactions and autoimmunity. *New England Journal of Medicine, 322,* 1739-1741.

McMillan, D. E. (1990). The role of blood flow in diabetic vascular disease. In H. Rifkin & D. Porte (Eds.), *Diabetes mellitus theory and practice* (4th ed.). New York: Elsevier.

McNicol, A. M. (1992). The human adrenal gland: Aspects of structure, function, and pathology. In V. H. James (Ed.), *The adrenal gland* (2nd ed., p. 12). New York: Raven Press.

Melby, J. C. (1991). Diagnosis of hyperaldosteronism. *Endocrinology and Metabolism Clinics of North America, 20*(2), 247-255.

Melmed, S. (1990). Acromegaly. *New England Journal of Medicine, 322*, 966-977.

Mitrakou, A., Kelley, D., Mokan, M., Veneman, T., Pangburn, T., Reilly, J., & Gerich, J. (1992). Role of reduced suppression of glucose production and diminished early insulin release in impaired glucose tolerance. *New England Journal of Medicine, 326*(1), 22-29.

Molitich, M. E. (1992). Clinical manifestations of acromegaly. *Endocrinology and Metabolism Clinics of North America, 21*(3), 597-614.

Morel, P., Goetz, F. C., Moudry-Munns, K., Freier, E., & Sutherland, D. E. (1991). Long-term glucose control in patients with pancreatic transplants. *Annals of Internal Medicine, 115*(9), 694-699.

Nathan, D. M. (1993). Long-term complications of diabetes mellitus. *New England Journal of Medicine, 328*(23), 1676-1685.

National Institute of Health (NIH). (1992). Prevention of insulin dependent diabetes mellitus by immunomodulation. *NIH Guide for Grants and Contracts, 21*(12, part 2), 9-11.

Palmer, J. P., & Lernmark, A. (1990). Pathophysiology of type I (insulin-dependent) diabetes. In H. Rifkin & D. Porte (Eds.), *Diabetes mellitus theory and practice* (4th ed.). New York: Elsevier.

Phipps, W. J., Long, B. C., & Woods, N. F. (1987). *Medical surgical nursing: Concepts and clinical practice* (3rd ed.). St. Louis: Mosby–Year Book.

Reichlin, S. (Ed.). (1984). *The neurohypophysis*. New York: Plenum.

Reid, R. L., Quigley, M. E., & Yen, S. S. C. (1985). Pituitary apoplexy. *Archives of Neurology, 42*, 712-719.

Rosai, J. (1989). *Akerman's surgical pathology* (p. 806). St. Louis: Mosby–Year Book.

Rotter, J. I., Vadheim, C. M., & Rimoin, D. L. (1990). Genetics of diabetes mellitus. In H. Rifkin & D. Porte (Eds.), *Diabetes mellitus theory and practice* (4th ed.). New York: Elsevier.

Schneeberg, N. G. (1970). *Essentials of clinical endocrinology*. St. Louis: Mosby–Year Book.

Sheehan, H. L., & Stanfield, J. P. (1961). The pathogenesis and postpartum necrosis of the anterior lobe of the pituitary gland. *Acta Endocrinol (Copenh), 37*, 479-510.

Skyler, J. S. (1990). Relation of metabolic control of diabetes mellitus to chronic complications. In H. Rifkin & D. Porte (Eds.), *Diabetes mellitus theory and practice* (4th ed.). New York: Elsevier.

Steffes, M. W., & Mauer, S. M. (1991). Diabetic nephropathy: A disease causing and complicated by hypertension. *Clinical Chemistry, 37*(10, part 2), 1838-1842.

Strowig, S., & Raskin, P. (1990). Insulin treatment and patient management. In H. Rifkin & D. Porte (Eds.), *Diabetes mellitus theory and practice* (4th ed.). New York: Elsevier.

Sutherland, D. E. R., Moudry-Munns, K. C., & Elick, B. A. (1990). Pancreas transplantation. In H. Rifkin & D. Porte (Eds.), *Diabetes mellitus theory and practice* (4th ed.). New York: Elsevier.

Thibodeau, G. A. (1987). *Anatomy and physiology*. St. Louis: Times Mirror/Mosby–Year Book.

Vinik, A., & Wing, R. R. (1990). Nutritional management of the person with diabetes. In H. Rifkin & D. Porte (Eds.), *Diabetes mellitus theory and practice* (4th ed.). New York: Elsevier.

Volk, B. W. (1990). Pathology of the diabetic pancreas. In H. Rifkin & D. Porte (Eds.), *Diabetes mellitus theory and practice* (4th ed.). New York: Elsevier.

Volpe, R. (1991). Graves disease. In S. H. Werner & S. H. Ingbar (Eds.), *The thyroid: A fundamental and clinical text* (6th ed., p. 654). Philadelphia: Saunders.

Vranic, M., Wasserman, D., & Bukowiecki, L. (1990). Metabolic implications of exercise and physical fitness in physiology and diabetes. In H. Rifkin & D. Porte (Eds.), *Diabetes mellitus theory and practice* (4th ed.). New York: Elsevier.

Wilson, J. D., & Foster, D. W. (1992). *Williams textbook of endocrinology* (8th ed.). Philadelphia: Saunders.

World Health Organization (WHO) Expert Committee. (1985). Geneva: World Health Organization.

World Heath Organization (WHO) Study Group. (1985). *Diabetes mellitus report of a WHO study group.* Technical Report Series 727:1-113. Geneva: World Health Organization.

Wulffraat, N. M., Drexhage, H. A., & Bottazzo, G. F. (1992). Autoimmune aspects of Addison's disease. In V. H. T. James (Ed.), *The adrenal gland* (2nd ed., pp. 263-288). New York: Raven Press.

SUGGESTED READINGS

Ahren, B. (1986). Thyroid neuroendocrinology: Neural regulation of thyroid hormone secretion. *Endocrine Reviews, 7*(2), 149-155.

Barnes, D. M. (1986, June). Steroids may influence changes in mood. *Science, 232,* 1344-1345.

Bautter, F. C., & Schwartz, W. B. (1967). The syndrome of inappropriate secretion of antidiuretic hormone. *American Journal of Medicine, 42,* 790-806.

Burchfield, S. R. (1979, December). The stress response: A new perspective. *Psychomotor Medicine, 41*(8), 661-670.

Burry, M., & Martens, L. (1980, February). ADH and its inappropriate secretion. *Canadian Nurse,* 41-43.

Cobb, W. E. (1984). Management of neurogenic DI. In S. Reichlin (Ed.), *The neurohypophysis.* New York: Plenum.

DeQuattro, V., Myers, M., & Campese, V. M. (1989). Pheochromocytoma: Diagnosis and therapy. In L. J. DeGroot (Ed.), *Endocrinology* (2nd ed.). Philadelphia: Saunders.

Fitzgerald, M. G., & Kilveat, A. (1985). The endocrine system—Diabetes. In J. C. Brocklehurst (Ed.), *Textbook of geriatric medicine and gerontology.* London: Churchill Livingstone.

Groop, L. C., & Eriksson, J. G. (1992). The etiology and pathogenesis of non-insulin dependent diabetes. *Annals of Medicine 24*(6):483-489.

Jaffe, R. B. (1984). Stress and health. *Annual Review of Public Health, 5,* 319-341.

Kubo, W. M., & Grant, M. M. (1978). The syndrome of inappropriate secretion of antidiuretic hormone. *Heart & Lung, 7*(3), 469-476.

Moses, A., & Notman, D. D. (1982). Diabetes insipidus and syndrome of inappropriate antidiuretic hormone secretion (SIADH). In G. J. Stollerman (Ed.), *Advances in internal medicine* (vol. 27, pp. 73-100). Chicago: Mosby–Year Book.

Williams, G., & Ginsberg, J. (1993). *Illustrated text of diabetes and endocrinology.* St. Louis: Mosby–Year Book.

Yao, Y. (1981). Current review of thyroid function tests. *Hospital Practice, 16*(9), 149-164.

UNIT VII

The Reproductive System

MOST RECORDED HISTORY about the female and male reproductive systems has focused on issues of fertility, the female reproductive cycle, and venereal diseases. In ancient times the female reproductive cycle and birth were viewed as divine mysteries. As civilizations evolved, reproduction and birth were sometimes viewed as dirty or sinful. This perspective was slow to change, even with the development of modern medicine. The idea that health problems peculiar to women deserved separate attention was not conceived before the middle of the nineteenth century. The first women's hospital in the United States was opened in 1855 by a physician in New York City.

In 1809 in Kentucky the first ovariotomy was performed. Physicians thought that removal of the ovaries might be a successful treatment for "female hysteria." Between 1846 and 1849, Dr. Marion Sims developed expertise in the surgical correction of vesicovaginal fistula by performing 30 operations on a female slave. Also in 1846, practitioners began to associate postpartum infections with the lack of hand washing. In 1871 the first hysterectomy was performed in the United States, and between 1878 and 1882, Poro and Saenger improved techniques of cesarean section, thereby establishing it as a routine procedure. Over the past 20 years, the cesarean rate in the United States has increased steadily from

VENEREAL DISEASE

Spectre of venereal disease shrinks before a large hand with a stick—
"Venereal disease must go."
(Courtesy National Library of Medicine.)

5% in 1970 to approximately 30% today, whereas the current rate for European countries remains between 5% and 15%. This routine performance of cesarean section is receiving intense scrutiny.

Control of fertility was not available until the early 1900s, except through methods developed by lay healers and midwives. Spermatozoa had been known about since the seventeenth century, and the ovum was described in early 1800s. Medically the first means of fertility control was the intrauterine device, initially described in 1909 by Richard Richter. It was not until the 1930s that physicians knew enough about the menstrual cycle to predict the timing of ovulation and fertilization. This knowledge led to development of the rhythm method of birth control, which was proposed independently by Ogino in Japan and Knaus in Austria. Penile protectors were known to the ancient Egyptians, and the first description of

the condom was written in 1854, primarily for protection against syphilis. By the middle of the nineteenth century, sheaths of animal intestine were widely sold in France and England for safety and for prevention of conception.

Knowledge about the specific hormones involved in male and female reproductive function has increased dramatically since the development of techniques to isolate hormones and their derivatives. One of the first sex hormones to be isolated was progesterone; it was discovered by G. W. Corner and W. M. Allen in 1929. This was followed by the isolation of estrogen. This knowledge, together with information regarding the events of the menstrual cycle, led to the development of female birth control pills, which were introduced in the United States in the 1950s. Information about central nervous system control of the reproductive cycle became available in the 1960s with the isolation of follicle-stimulating hormone and luteinizing hormone. These hormones initially were thought to affect only the female reproductive cycle, but in the 1970s they were found to affect the male reproductive system as well.

Testosterone was first isolated in 1935, although evidence for male sex hormones was described in 1849 when testes were transplanted into castrated male chicks and the secondary characteristics of roosters appeared. The most recently discovered reproductive hormone is inhibin, a hormone that influences sperm production.

The recorded history of venereal diseases began in the fifteenth century. The first major epidemic of syphilis occurred among sailors returning to the Old World on Columbus's first voyage. The disease spread to Spanish soldiers who were fighting for the king of Naples and then to the French troops of Charles VIII, after which it became known as the "French disease." Girolamo Fracastoro of Verona (1483-1553), a poet, physician, geologist, classicist, and pathologist, wrote *Syphilis sive Morbus Gallicus* (1530), in which he named the French disease syphilis and noted its sexual means of spread. Jean Fernel (1497-1588), a physician trained in Paris, was the first to suggest that gonorrhea and syphilis were quite separate illnesses that merely shared a common mode of transmission. Syphilis was treated with mercury or guaiac. In the sixteenth century, gonorrhea and syphilis became very common. Fear of these two venereal diseases

prompted the closing of communal baths. This was a great loss, as adequate water for bathing was not generally available.

Not until the 1970s, as medical practitioners realized the complexity of sexually transmitted conditions, did thinking about venereal diseases undergo a major shift. Health care workers and policymakers became increasingly aware of the great number of infections spread from person to person during sexual contact. This category of infections was expanded to include not only the classic venereal diseases, such as syphilis and gonorrhea, but also any disease that could be transmitted through sexual contact, such as amebiasis, tuberculosis, and hepatitis. This new understanding caused the term *sexually transmitted diseases* to replace *venereal diseases* gradually.

CHAPTER 19

Structure and Function of the Reproductive Systems

Kristynia M. Robinson

Kathryn L. McCance

D. Patricia Gray*

Chapter Outline

*Contributing author to first edition.

The male and female reproductive systems have several anatomic and physiologic features in common. Most obvious is their major function, reproduction, through which a 23-chromosome female gamete, the **ovum,** and a 23-chromosome male gamete, the **spermatozoon** (**sperm cell**) unite to form a 46-chromosome zygote that is capable of developing into a new individual. The male reproductive system produces sperm and delivers them to the female reproductive tract. The female reproductive system produces the ovum and, if it is fertilized, can nurture and protect it (now called the embryo and developing fetus), and expel it at birth. These functions are determined not only by anatomic structures but also by complex hormonal, neurologic, and psychogenic factors.

DEVELOPMENT OF THE REPRODUCTIVE SYSTEMS

The structure and function of both male and female reproductive systems depend on steroid hormones called **sex hormones.** Hormonal effects on the reproductive systems begin well before birth and continue for life.

Sexual Differentiation in Utero

During embryonic development, the most important sex hormone is the primary male sex hormone, **testosterone.** Until the eighth week of gestation, the initial reproductive structures of male and female embryos are homologous (the same), consisting of one pair of primary sex organs, or **gonads,** and two pairs of ducts, the mesonephric ducts (wolffian ducts) and the paramesonephric ducts (mullerian ducts) (Fig. 19-1). Both pairs of ducts empty into an opening called the urogenital sinus.

At about 8 weeks' gestation, the gonads of genetically male embryos begin to produce testosterone. Under the influence of testosterone, the male gonads develop into the two testes, which produce sperm. The paramesonephric ducts degenerate, and the mesonephric ducts develop into the vasa deferentia, the two tubes that carry sperm from the testes to the urethra.

In female embryos, the gonads do not produce testosterone. Lack of testosterone causes the two female gonads to develop into ovaries, which will produce ova.

UNDIFFERENTIATED

FIG. 19-1 Internal genitalia development. Embryonic and fetal development of the internal genitalia. (From Bobak, Jensen, & Zalar, 1989.)

In females the mesonephric ducts deteriorate, and the lower ends of the paramesonephric ducts join to become the uterus. The upper portions of the paramesonephric ducts develop into the fallopian (uterine) tubes. These two ducts carry ova from the ovaries to the uterus.

Like the internal reproductive structures the external structures develop from homologous embryonic tissues.

During the first 8 weeks of gestation, both male and female embryos develop an elevated structure called the genital tubercle. Fig. 19-2 shows how the undifferentiated genital tubercle develops into the external reproductive organs. In male embryos, testosterone causes the genital tubercle to form the male external genitalia. Absence of testosterone causes development of the exter-

FIG. 19-2 External genitalia development. Embryonic and fetal development of the external genitalia. (From Bobak & Jensen, 1993.)

nal female genitalia. By 9 months' gestation the internal and external genital structures are all present, and the male gonads (the testes) have descended into the scrotum.

Puberty

From fetal life through childhood the testes secrete low levels of testosterone, and the ovaries secrete low levels of the primary female sex hormone, estrogen. Between the ages of 9 and 12 the gonads begin to produce more of the sex hormones. This triggers sexual maturation, or puberty. In girls puberty begins at about age 10. In boys it begins later, at about age 11. Puberty lasts 2 or 3 years and is complete when the individual is capable of reproduction. *Puberty* is not the same as adolescence. Puberty refers solely to sexual maturation; *adolescence* refers to all aspects of development that occur between the ages of 11 and 19.

Hormonal stimulation of the reproductive systems involves the central nervous system, the endocrine system, and the gonads themselves. As can be seen in Fig. 19-3, specific structures involved are the hypothalamus, the anterior pituitary, and the gonads (ovaries and testes). At the time of puberty the hypothalamus of the brain begins to produce greater amounts of **gonadotropin-releasing hormone (GnRH)**. Increased levels of GnRH stimulate the anterior pituitary to increase its production of the **gonadotropins: luteinizing hormone (LH)** and **follicle-stimulating hormone (FSH)**. The gonadotropins then stimulate the gonads to produce more of the sex hormones. (The sex hormones are discussed in sections on the female and male systems.)

Increased sex hormone production causes the genitalia to grow into their adult proportions. It also stimulates the development of male and female secondary sex characteristics (beard, voice changes, breast develop-

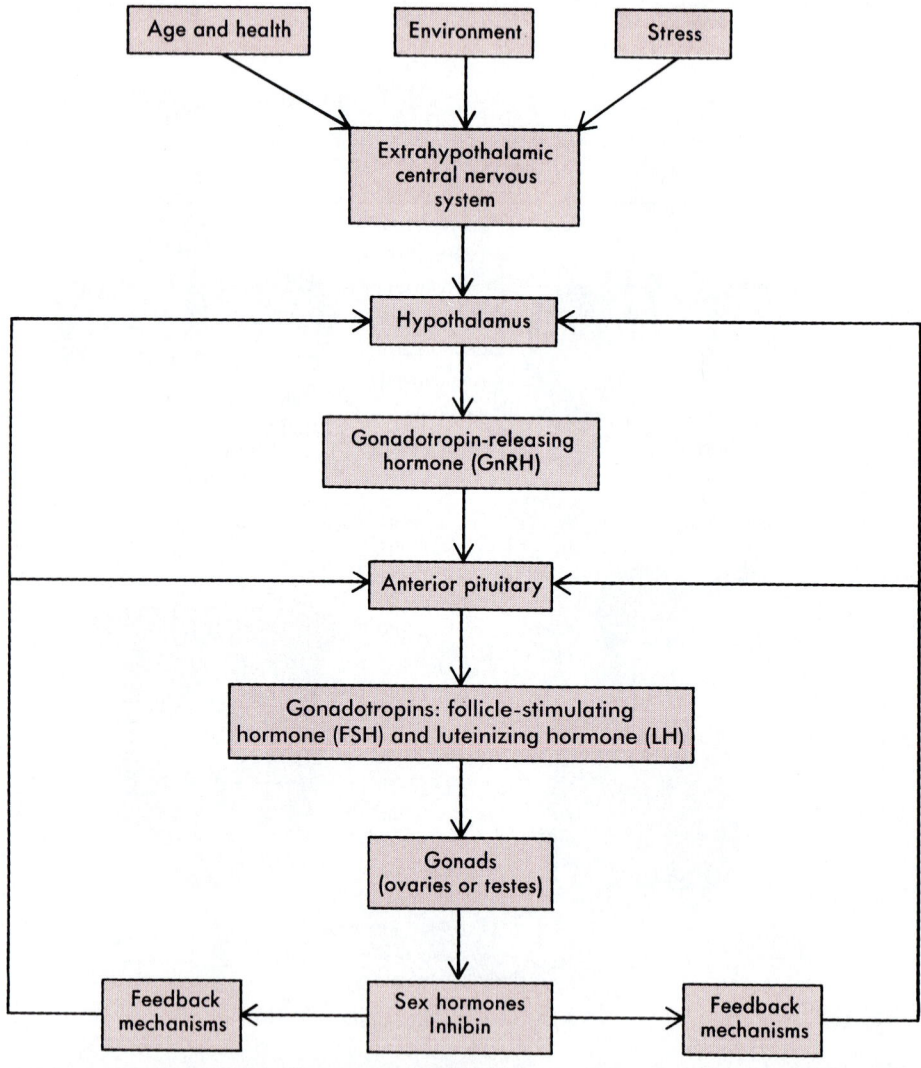

FIG. 19-3 Hormonal stimulation of the gonads. The hypothalamic-pituitary-gonadal axis.

ment, and pubic and axillary hair). The most important hormonal effects occur in the gonads, however. In males the testes begin to produce mature sperm that are capable of fertilizing an ovum. Male puberty is complete with the first ejaculation that contains mature sperm. In females the ovaries begin to release mature ova. Female puberty is complete at the time of the first menstrual period.

THE FEMALE REPRODUCTIVE SYSTEM

In females the most important reproductive organs, or genitalia, are internal. They are the ovaries, fallopian tubes, uterus, and vagina. These organs are essential to reproduction. The external genitalia have accessory functions. They protect body openings and play an important role in sexual functioning.

External Genitalia

Fig. 19-4 shows the external female genitalia, which are known collectively as the **vulva,** or pudendum. The **mons pubis** (veneris) is a fatty layer of tissue over the pubic symphysis (joint of the pubic bones). During puberty the mons pubis becomes covered with pubic hair,

and its sebaceous and sweat glands become more active. Estrogen causes fat to be deposited under the skin, giving the mons pubis a moundlike shape. This cushion of tissue protects the pubic symphysis during sexual intercourse.

SECONDARY SEX CHARACTERISTICS THAT DEVELOP AT PUBERTY

Female	Male
Growth of long bones; widening of pelvis	Growth of long bones; widening of shoulders
Increase of subcutaneous fat, particularly at hips, thighs	Decrease of subcutaneous fat and increase of muscle mass
Growth of pubic and axillary hair	Growth of pubic and axillary hair
Activation of sebaceous and sweat glands in skin	Activation of sebaceous and sweat glands in skin
Some change of voice	Deepening of voice
Development of breasts	Growth of facial hair

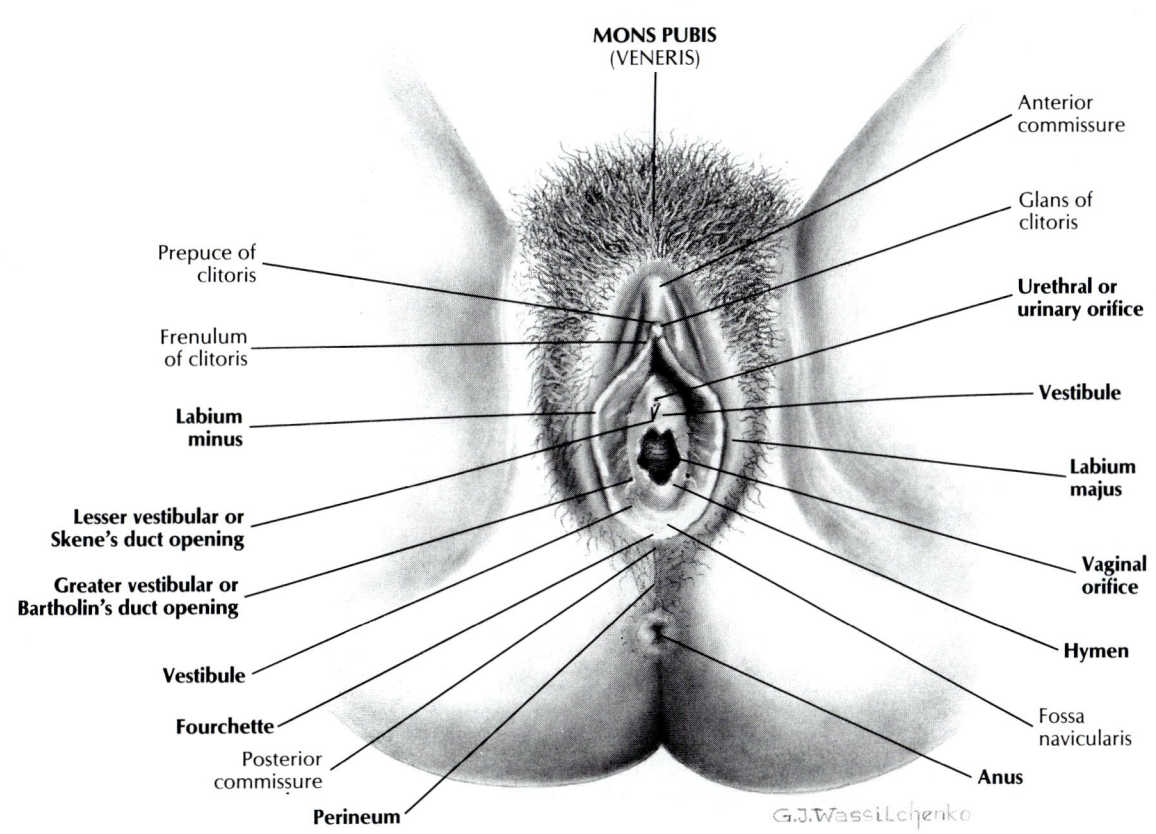

FIG. 19-4 External female genitalia. (From Bobak & Jensen, 1993.)

The **labia majora** (singular, **labium majus**) are two folds of skin that arise at the mons pubis and extend back to the fourchette, forming a cleft. Like the mons pubis, the labia majora undergo changes at puberty: the amount of fatty tissue increases, pubic hair grows on the lateral surfaces, and sebaceous glands on the hairless medial surfaces begin to secrete lubricants. Because of an extensive network of nerve endings, the labia majora are highly sensitive to temperature, touch, pressure, and pain and are homologous to the male scrotum (see Fig. 19-2). The principal function of the labia majora is to protect the inner structures of the vulva.

Within the labia majora lie two smaller, thinner folds of skin, the **labia minora** (singular, **labium minus**). Anteriorly, they form the clitoral hood or prepuce and frenulum, then split to enclose the vestibule, and converge near the anus forming the fourchette. The labia minora are hairless, pink, and moist and are well supplied with nerves, blood vessels, and sebaceous glands. These glands secrete a bactericidal fluid that has a distinctive odor and that lubricates and waterproofs the vulvar skin. During sexual arousal the labia minora become swollen with blood.

The **clitoris** is a richly innervated, erectile organ that lies between the labia minora. It is a small, cylindrical structure having a glans that is visible and a shaft that lies beneath the skin (Fig. 19-4). The clitoris is homologous to the male penis. Like the penis, the clitoris is a major site of sexual stimulation and orgasm. With sexual arousal, erectile tissues in the clitoris fill with blood, causing it to enlarge somewhat. Similar to other vulvar glands, the clitoris secretes a fluid, called smegma, that has a unique odor and may be erotically stimulating to the male.

The area protected by the labia minora is called the **vestibule.** The vestibule contains the external opening of the vagina, which is called the **introitus** or vaginal orifice. The introitus may be covered by a thin, perforated membrane called the hymen. The vestibule also contains the opening of the urethra, or **urinary meatus** (orifice). These structures are lubricated by two pairs of glands: Skene glands and Bartholin glands. The ducts of **Skene glands** (also called the lesser vestibular or paraurethral glands) open on both sides of the urinary meatus. The ducts of **Bartholin glands** (greater vestibular or vulvovaginal glands) open on either side of the introitus. In response to sexual stimulation, Bartholin glands secrete mucus that lubricates the inner labial surfaces, as well as enhances the viability and motility of sperm. Skene glands help to lubricate the urinary meatus and the vestibule. Secretions from both sets of glands facilitate coitus. Also, in response to sexual excitement, the highly vascular tissue just beneath the vestibule fills with blood and becomes engorged.

The less hairy skin and the subcutaneous tissue that lie between the vaginal orifice and the anus are referred to as the **perineum.** Unlike the rest of the vulva, this area has little subcutaneous fat so that the skin is close to the underlying muscles. The perineum covers the muscular **perineal body,** a fibrous structure comprised of elastic fiber, connective tissue, and the common attachment of the bulbocavernosus (not shown), the external anal sphincter, and the levator ani muscles (Fig. 19-5). This area is much larger in the female, and the characteristic median raphe seen in the male is generally absent. The perineum varies in length from 2 to 5 cm or more and stretches remarkably. The length of the perineum and the elasticity of the perineal body influence tissue resistance and injury during childbirth.

Internal Genitalia
Vagina

The **vagina** is an elastic, fibromuscular canal, 9 to 10 cm in length, that extends up and back from the introitus to the lower portion of the uterus. As Fig. 19-5 shows, it lies between the urethra (and part of the bladder) and the rectum. Mucosal secretions from the upper genital organs, menstrual fluids, and products of conception leave the body through the vagina, which also receives the penis during coitus. During sexual excitement, the vagina lengthens and widens and the anterior third becomes congested with blood.

The vaginal wall is composed of four layers. Its lining is a mucous membrane of squamous epithelial cells. (Types of epithelium are described and illustrated in Chapter 1, Table 1-3.) This layer thickens and thins in response to hormones, particularly estrogen. The squamous epithelial membrane is continuous with the membrane that covers the lower part of the uterus. In women of reproductive age, the mucosal layer is arranged in transverse wrinkles, or folds, called **rugae** (singular, **ruga**). The rugae permit the mucosal layer to stretch during coitus and childbirth. The second layer consists of fibrous connective tissue containing numerous blood and lymphatic vessels. Smooth muscle constitutes the third layer. The outermost layer consists of connective tissue and a rich network of blood vessels.

The upper part of the vagina surrounds the cervix, the lower end of the uterus (Fig. 19-5). The recessed space around the cervix is called the **fornix** of the vagina. The posterior fornix is "deeper" than the anterior fornix because of the angle at which the cervix meets the vaginal canal. In most women this angle is about 90 degrees. A pouch called the **cul-de-sac** separates the posterior fornix and the rectum.

Its elasticity and relatively sparse nerve supply enhance the vagina's function as the birth canal. During sexual arousal the vaginal wall becomes engorged with

FIG. 19-5 Internal female genitalia and other pelvic organs. Midsagittal view, with woman lying supine. (From Bobak & Jensen, 1993.)

blood, like the labia minora and clitoris. Engorgement pushes some fluid to the surface of the mucosa, enhancing lubrication. The vaginal wall does not contain mucus-secreting glands; rather, secretions drain into the vagina from the endocervical glands or enter from the vestibule.

Two factors help to maintain the self-cleansing action of the vagina and to defend it from infection, particularly during the reproductive years. They are (1) an acid-base balance that discourages the proliferation of most pathogenic bacteria and (2) the thickness of the vaginal epithelium. Before puberty, vaginal pH is about 7.0 (neutral), and the vaginal epithelium is thin. At puberty the pH becomes more acidic (4.0 to 5.0), and the squamous epithelial lining thickens. These changes are maintained until menopause (cessation of menstruation), at which time the pH rises again to more alkaline levels, and the epithelium thins out. Therefore, protection from infection is greatest during the years when a woman is most likely to be sexually active. Between puberty and menopause, vulnerability to infection varies somewhat with cyclic changes in pH and epithelial thickness. Both defenses are greatest when estrogen levels are high and

the vagina contains a normal population of *Lactobacillus acidophilus*, a harmless resident bacterium that helps to maintain pH at acidic levels. Any condition that causes vaginal pH to rise, such as douching or use of vaginal sprays or deodorants, low estrogen levels, or destruction of *L. acidophilus* by antibiotics, lowers vaginal defenses against infection.

Uterus

The **uterus** is a hollow, pear-shaped organ whose lower end opens into the vagina. The functions of the uterus are to anchor and protect a fertilized ovum, provide an optimal environment while it develops, and push the fetus out at birth. In addition, the uterus plays an important role in sexual response and conception. During sexual excitement, the opening of the uterus (the cervix) dilates slightly. At the same time, the uterus increases in size and moves upward and backward creating a tenting effect in the midvagina that results in the cervix "sitting" in a pool of semen. During orgasm, rhythmic contractions facilitate movement of sperm through the cervical os while enhancing physical pleasure.

At puberty the uterus attains its adult size and proportions and descends from the abdomen to the lower pelvis, between the bladder and the rectum (Fig. 19-5). The uterus of a mature, nonpregnant female is approximately 9 cm long and 6.5 cm wide, with muscular walls 3.5 cm thick. It is held loosely in position by ligaments, peritoneal tissue folds, and pressure of adjacent organs, especially the urinary bladder, sigmoid colon, and rectum. In most women the uterus is anteverted: that is, it is tipped forward so that it rests on the urinary bladder. But it may be retroverted, or tipped backward. Various degrees of flexion are normal (Fig. 19-6).

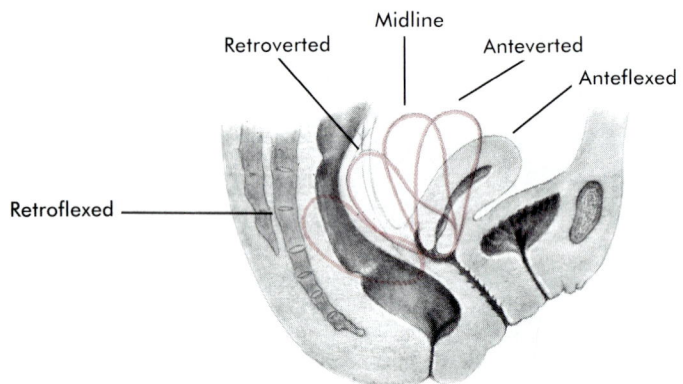

FIG. 19-6 Variations in uterine position.

Fig. 19-7 shows a cross section of the uterus. The uterus has two major parts: the body, or **corpus,** and the cervix. The top of the corpus, above the insertion of the fallopian tubes, is called the **fundus.** The diameter of the uterine cavity is widest at the fundus and narrowest at the **isthmus,** which is the narrowed part of the corpus just above the cervix. The **cervix,** or "neck of the uterus," extends from the isthmus to the vagina. The passageway between the cervix's upper opening (the internal os) and its lower opening (the external os) is called the **endocervical canal.** The entire uterus, like the upper vagina, is innervated exclusively by motor and sensory fibers of the autonomic nervous system.

The uterine wall is composed of three layers: the perimetrium, the myometrium, and the endometrium (Fig. 19-7). The **perimetrium (parietal peritoneum)** is the outer serous membrane that covers the uterus. The **myometrium** is the thick, muscular middle layer. The myometrium is thickest at the fundus, apparently to facilitate birth. The **endometrium,** or uterine lining, is composed of a functional layer (superficial compact layer and spongy middle layer) and a basal layer. The functional layer of the endometrium is responsive to sex hormones. Between puberty and menopause this layer proliferates and sloughs off monthly. The basal layer, which is attached to the myometrium, regenerates the functional layer after the sloughing off (menstruation).

The endocervical canal does not have an endometrial

FIG. 19-7 Cross section of uterus, fallopian tube, and ovary. (From Bobak & Jensen, 1991.)

layer. Rather, it is lined with columnar epithelial cells (see Table 1-3). The endocervical lining is continuous with that of the outer cervix and vagina, but it is not made up of the same type of epithelial cells. The point at which the columnar epithelium of the cervix meets the squamous epithelium of the vagina is called the transformation zone, or the **squamous-columnar junction** (Fig. 19-7). The transformation zone is the usual site of cervical dysplasia or carcinoma in situ.

The cervix acts as a mechanical barrier to infectious microorganisms that may be present in the vagina. The external cervical os is a very small opening that contains thick, sticky mucus (the mucous "plug") during most of the menstrual cycle and all of pregnancy. In addition the downward flow of cervical secretions moves microorganisms away from the cervix and uterus. In women of reproductive age, the pH of these secretions is inhospitable to most bacteria. Furthermore, mucosal secretions contain enzymes and antibodies (mostly immunoglobulin A) of the secretory immune system. (The secretory immune system is discussed in Chapter 6.) These defenses do not always prevent infection, even if they are intact. Besides infection, uterine pathophysiology includes displacement of the uterus within the pelvis, benign growths of the uterine wall, and cancer.

Fallopian Tubes

The two **fallopian tubes** (oviducts, uterine tubes) enter the uterus bilaterally just beneath the fundus (Fig. 19-7). Their function is to conduct the ova from the spaces around the ovaries to the uterus. From the uterus the fallopian tubes curve up and over the two ovaries. Each tube is 8 to 12 cm long and about 1 cm in diameter, except at its ovarian end, which flares out like the bell of a trumpet. This widened end, called the **infundibulum,** is fringed or fimbriated. The **fimbriae** (fringes) move, creating a current that draws the ovum into the infundibulum. Once the ovum has entered the fallopian tube, cilia and peristalsis (muscle contractions) keep it moving toward the uterus.

The ampulla, or distal third, of the fallopian tube is the usual site of fertilization (see Fig. 19-7). Sperm released into the vagina travel upward through the endocervical canal and uterine cavity and enter the fallopian tubes. If an ovum is present in either tube, fertilization can occur. Whether or not the ovum encounters sperm, it continues to travel through the fallopian tube to the uterus. If fertilized, the ovum (now called a blastocyst) implants itself in the endometrial layer of the uterine wall. If not fertilized, the ovum breaks down and leaves the uterus with menstrual fluids.

Disorders that affect the fallopian tubes can block the path of both sperm and ovum and cause infertility. Such disorders include congenital malformations, infection, and inflammation.

Ovaries

The **ovaries,** the female gonads, are the primary female reproductive organs. They have two main functions: secretion of female sex hormones and development and release of female gametes, or ova.

The almond-shaped ovaries are located on both sides of the uterus and are suspended and supported by the mesovarian portions of the broad ligament, ovarian ligaments, and suspensory ligaments (see Fig. 19-7). The ovaries are smaller than their male homologs, the testes. In women of reproductive age, each ovary is 3 to 5 cm long, 2.5 cm wide, and 2 cm thick and weighs 4 to 8 g. Size and weight vary somewhat from phase to phase of the menstrual cycle (see p. 723).

Fig. 19-8 shows a cross section of an ovary. The central part, or medulla, is composed of connective tissue and contains a large number of small arteries, veins, and lymphatics, which enter at the hilum. Surrounding the medulla is the cortex. At birth, the cortex of each ovary contains 200,000 to 400,000 ova within immature **ovarian follicles.** During puberty some of the follicles and the ova within them begin to mature. Between puberty and menopause the ovarian cortex always contains follicles and ova in various stages of development. Once every menstrual cycle (about every 28 days), one of the follicles reaches maturation and discharges its ovum through the ovary's outer covering, the germinal epithelium. During the reproductive years, 300 to 400 ovarian follicles mature completely and release an ovum, an event termed **ovulation.** The rest either fail to develop at all or degenerate without maturing completely.

Having ejected a mature ovum, the follicle develops into another structure, the **corpus luteum** (Fig. 19-8). The immediate fate of the corpus luteum depends on whether the ejected ovum is fertilized. If fertilization occurs, the corpus luteum enlarges and begins to secrete hormones that maintain and support pregnancy. If fertilization does not occur, the corpus luteum secretes these hormones for approximately 14 days and then degenerates, which triggers the maturation of another follicle. The **ovarian cycle**—the process of follicular maturation, ovulation, corpus luteum development, and corpus luteum degeneration—is continuous from puberty to menopause, except during pregnancy. At menopause this process ceases, and the ovaries may shrink to the point that they cannot be felt on palpation.

Sex hormones are secreted by four types of cells present within the ovarian cortex: cells of the stroma, or tissue matrix; two types of cells in the ovarian follicle, **granulosa cells** and **theca cells;** and cells of the corpus luteum (Fig. 19-9). These cells all contain receptors for the gonadotropins (LH and FSH) or for the sex hormones, which are discussed in the next section.

Because ovarian function is regulated by hormones,

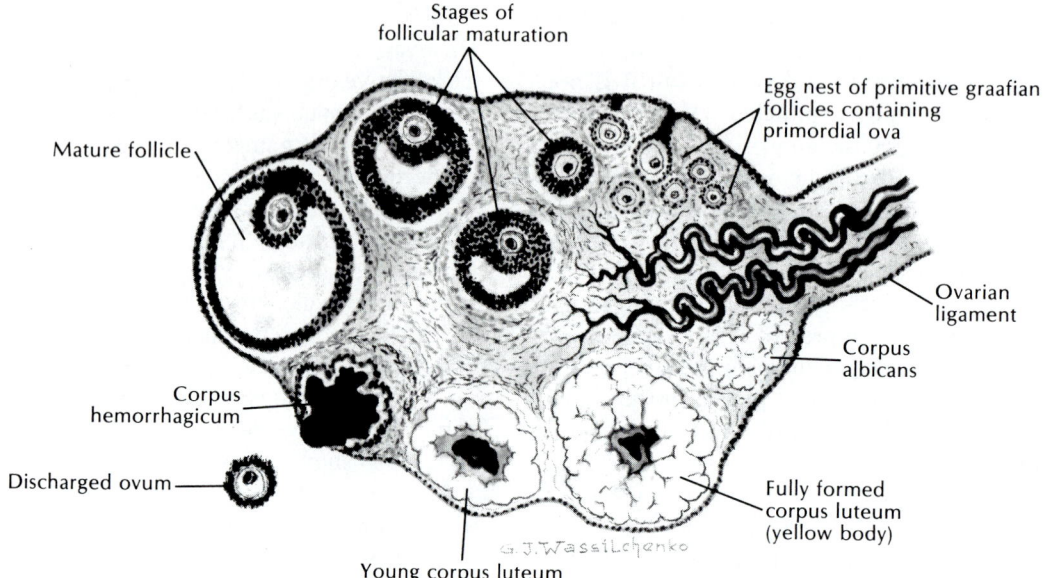

FIG. 19-8 **Cross section of ovary during reproductive years.** (From Bobak & Jensen, 1991.)

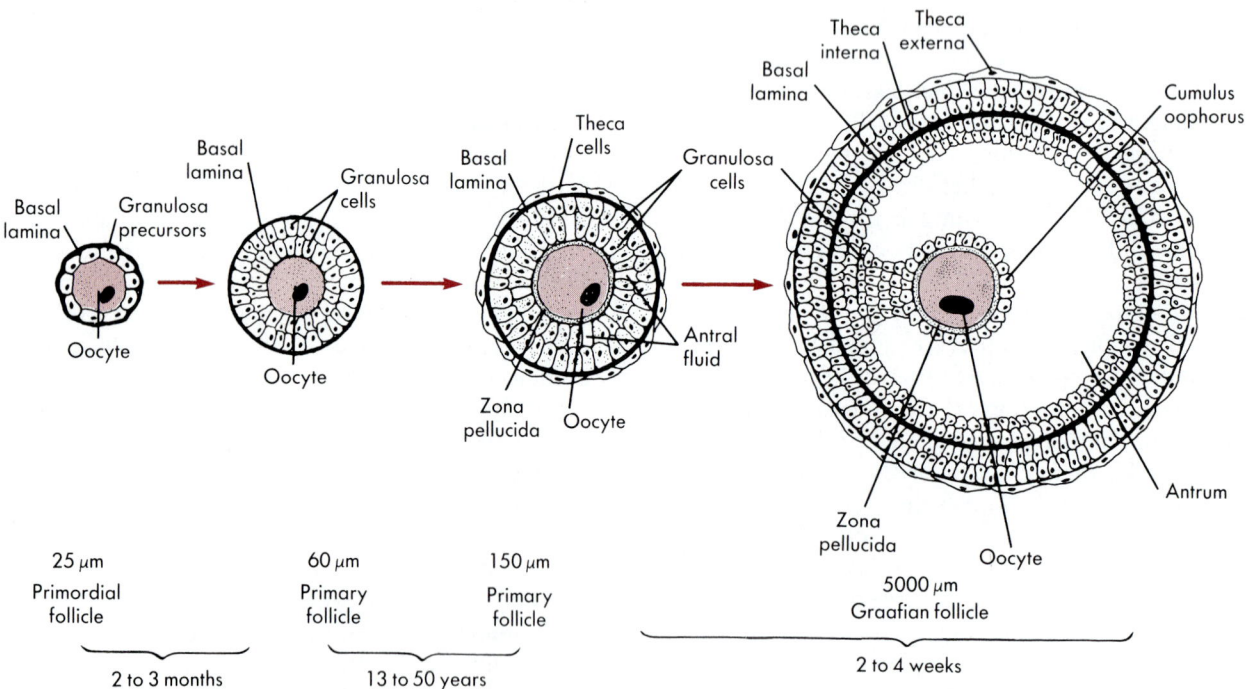

FIG. 19-9 **Development of an ovarian follicle** (not to scale). The graafian follicle has more layers of granulosa and theca cells than shown here. (From Berne & Levy, 1993.)

any disorder that disrupts hormone secretion or reception by target cells can cause ovarian dysfunction and infertility. Ovarian pathology also can be caused by benign or malignant growths, cysts, infection, or inflammation.

Female Sex Hormones

The sex hormones are all steroid hormones; that is, they are synthesized from cholesterol (Chapter 17). Most of the sex hormones, both male and female, are present in adults of both sexes all the time. The female body contains low levels of testosterone, for example, and the male body contains low levels of estrogen. The effects of the sex hormones depend on their amount and concentration in the blood.

Steroid hormones produced by the ovaries maintain female characteristics throughout life. During fetal development, infancy, and childhood, sex hormone production is low. At puberty, hormone production surges, causing sexual maturation and development of secondary sex characteristics. From puberty to menopause, the sex hormones control the ovarian-menstrual cycle, pregnancy, and lactation. The dominant female sex hormones are estrogen and progesterone. These two hormones are not produced steadily. Rather, their production surges and diminishes monthly, creating the ovarian-menstrual cycle. The androgens, which are actually male sex hormones, also have important functions in women. The female body normally produces small amounts of androgens and other male sex hormones.

Estrogens

Estrogen is a generic term for any of three similar hormones: estradiol, estrone, and estriol. **Estradiol** is the most potent and plentiful of the three. The main site of estrogen production is the ovaries (ovarian follicle and corpus luteum), but limited amounts of estrogen are secreted by the cortices of the adrenal glands and the placenta during pregnancy. Androgens are converted to estrogen in peripheral adipose tissue; this process is the major source of estrogen in postmenopausal women and in men.

Estrogen has numerous biologic effects, many of

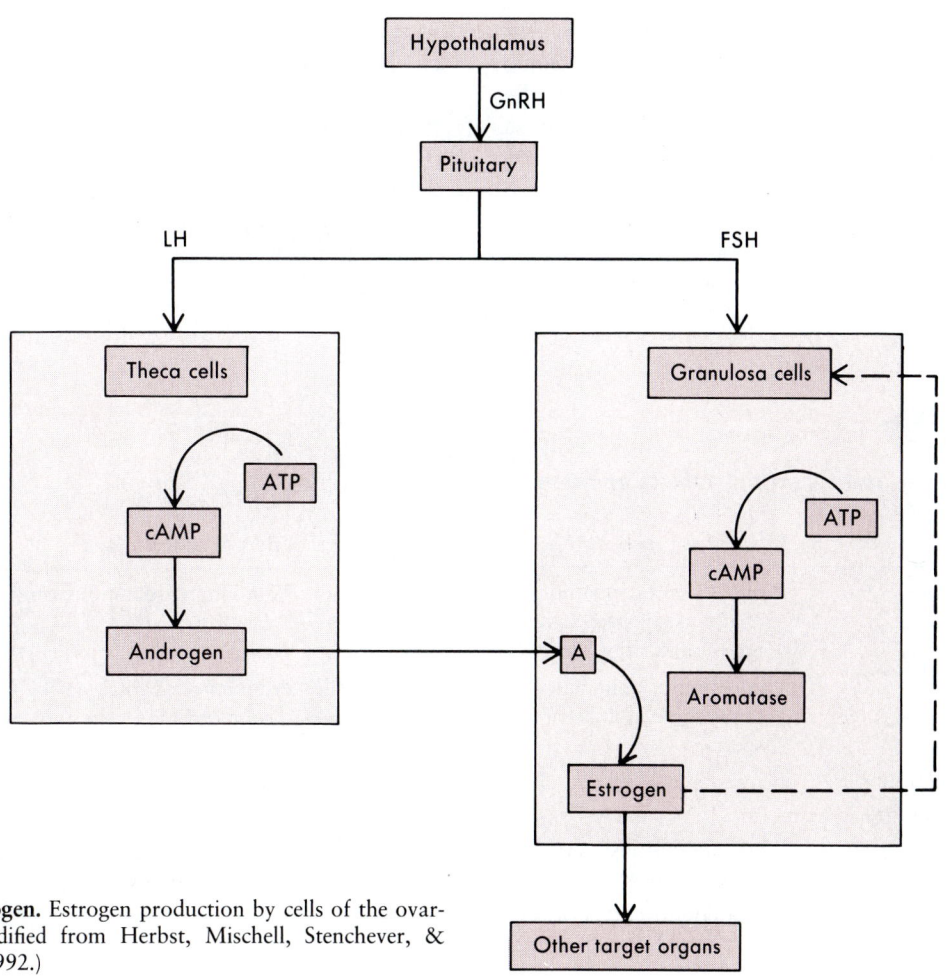

FIG. 19-10 Estrogen. Estrogen production by cells of the ovarian follicle. (Modified from Herbst, Mischell, Stenchever, & Droegemueller, 1992.)

which involve interactions with other hormones. Estrogen is needed for maturation of reproductive organs, development of secondary sex characteristics, closure of long bones after the pubertal growth spurt, regulation of the ovarian-menstrual cycle, endometrial regeneration after menstruation, endometrial maintenance during pregnancy, and lactation. Estrogen also has metabolic effects on the bones, liver, blood vessels, blood, central nervous system, kidneys, and skin. During the reproductive years estrogen helps to maintain the density of bone. The ovaries stop producing estrogen at menopause; for this reason postmenopausal women are susceptible to osteoporosis, a condition in which bone density is reduced.

Like the other steroid hormones, estrogens are derived from cholesterol in a complex, enzyme-mediated series of reactions. (Mechanisms of hormone synthesis and action are described in Chapter 17.) Stimulated by GnRH from the hypothalamus, the anterior pituitary gland secretes gonadotropins (LH and FSH), as shown in Fig. 19-3.

Luteinizing hormone induces estradiol synthesis by the corpus luteum. It also stimulates the ovarian follicle to synthesize estradiol, but not directly. Apparently LH stimulates theca cells of the ovarian follicle to produce androgens. (Androgens are discussed further on p. 731 and in the section on male reproductive function.) Some of these androgens are converted to estradiol by the theca cells themselves; others diffuse into the granulosa cells, where they are converted (aromatized) to estradiol. Conversion within the granulosa cells is made possible by FSH (Fig. 19-10).

Disturbances of estrogen production can be caused by abnormalities that affect (1) secretion of GnRH by the hypothalamus, (2) secretion of LH or FSH by the anterior pituitary, (3) hormonal feedback mechanisms, or (4) structural integrity of the ovaries. Estrogen's role in the menstrual cycle is described on p. 723.

Progesterone

Luteinizing hormone from the anterior pituitary stimulates the corpus luteum to secrete **progesterone,** the second major female sex hormone. Progesterone is an early product in the enzymatic conversion pathway of estrogen. With estrogen, progesterone controls the ovarian-menstrual cycle. Large amounts of progesterone are secreted while the corpus luteum is active, for about 9 to 13 days after ovulation. Small amounts of progesterone are secreted by the adrenal cortices. Adrenal secretion is not cyclic, however.

Progesterone secreted by the corpus luteum stimulates the thickened endometrium to become more complex in preparation for implantation of a blastocyte. If conception and implantation do occur, the corpus luteum persists and secretes progesterone (and estrogen) throughout pregnancy.

Progesterone is sometimes called "the hormone of pregnancy." During pregnancy, it is produced not only by the corpus luteum but also by the placenta. Its effects in pregnancy include (1) maintenance of the thickened endometrium; (2) relaxation of smooth muscle in the myometrium, which prevents premature contractions and helps the uterus to expand; (3) thickening of the myometrium, which prepares it for the muscular work of labor; and (4) prevention of lactation until the fetus is born. Progesterone and estrogen have some opposing and complementary effects, which are summarized in Table 19-1.

TABLE 19-1

Complementary and Opposing Effects of Estrogen and Progesterone

Structure	Effect of estrogen	Effect of progesterone
Vaginal mucosa	Proliferation of squamous epithelium; increase in glycogen content of cells; layering (cornification) of cells	Thinning of squamous epithelium; decornification
Cervical mucosa	Production of abundant fluid secretions that favor survival and enhance motility of sperm	Production of thick, sticky secretions that tend to "plug" the cervical os
Smooth muscle of uterus and fallopian tubes	Increased motility and ciliary action	Decreased motility and ciliary action; relaxes myometrium
Endometrium	Stimulation of growth; increase in number of receptors for progesterone	Activation of glands and blood vessels; accumulation of glucogen and enzymes
Breasts	Promotion of effects of prolactin (hormone that stimulates milk production)	Inhibition of effects of prolactin

Androgens

Although **androgens** are primarily male sex hormones, small amounts of them are produced in the ovaries and adrenal cortices of females. Some androgens are precursors of female sex hormones, notably estrogen and androstenedione. At puberty, androgens contribute to the skeletal growth spurt and cause growth of pubic and axillary hair. The androgens also activate sebaceous glands, accounting for some cases of acne during puberty.

The Menstrual Cycle

Besides pregnancy, the obvious manifestation of female reproductive functioning is menstrual bleeding (the menses), which starts with the **menarche** (first menstruation) and ends with **menopause.** In the United States, the average age of first menstruation is 12.5 years, with a range from 9 to 17 years. Menarche appears to be related to body weight, especially percentage of body fat (ratio of fat to lean tissue), which may trigger a change in the metabolic rate and lead to hormonal changes associated with ovulation. At first, cycles are anovulatory and may vary in length from 10 to 60 days or more. As adolescence proceeds, regular patterns of menstruation and ovulation are established at intervals ranging between 30 and 35 days. During adulthood, menstruation continues to recur in a recognizable and characteristic pattern, with the length of the menstrual cycle varying considerably among women. The commonly accepted cycle average is 28 (27 to 30) days, with rhythmic intervals of 21 to 45 days considered normal. If a woman is to experience regular and predictable menstruation, it usually happens by the third decade. Presumably this strict control of menses is related to sequential ovarian secretion of estrogen and progesterone that are delivered to the endometrium during an ovulatory cycle.

Phases of the Menstrual Cycle

The menstrual cycle consists of three phases of one event. The event is ovulation: the release of an ovum from a mature ovarian follicle. The three phases are the follicular/proliferative phase, the luteal/secretory phase, and menstruation (Fig. 19-11).

During **menstruation,** the functional layer of the endometrium disintegrates and is discharged through the vagina. Menstruation is followed by the **follicular/proliferative phase.** This phase is named for two simultaneous processes: maturation of an ovarian follicle and proliferation of the endometrium (Fig. 19-11). During the follicular/proliferative phase, the anterior pituitary gland secretes FSH, which causes an ovarian follicle to develop. While the follicle is developing, its granulosa cells secrete estrogen, and the estrogen causes cells of the endometrium to proliferate. By the time the ovarian follicle is mature, the endometrial lining is restored. At this point ovulation occurs.

Ovulation marks the beginning of the **luteal/secretory phase** of the menstrual cycle. The ovarian follicle begins its transformation into a corpus luteum (Fig. 19-8), hence the name *luteal phase.* Luteinizing hormone from the anterior pituitary stimulates the corpus luteum to secrete progesterone, which in turn initiates the secretory phase of endometrial development. Glands and blood vessels in the endometrium branch and curl throughout the functional layer, and the glands begin to secrete a thin, glycogen-containing fluid, hence the name *secretory phase.* If conception should occur, the nutrient-laden endometrium is ready for implantation. If conception and implantation do not occur, the corpus luteum degenerates and ceases its production of progesterone and estrogen (which it has been producing in lesser amounts). Without progesterone or estrogen to maintain it, the endometrium enters the ischemic ("blood-starved") phase and disintegrates. Then menstruation occurs, marking the beginning of another cycle.

Ovarian cycles appear to have a minimum length of 25 to 26 days: the ovarian follicle requires 10 to 12.5 days to develop, and the luteal phase appears fixed at 14 days. Menstrual blood flow usually lasts from 3 to 7 days, but may last as long as 8 days or stop after 2 days and still be considered within normal limits. Bleeding is consistently scant to heavy and varies from 30 ml to 100 ml, with most blood loss occurring during the first 3 days of menses. Menstrual discharge consists of blood, mucus, and desquamated endometrial tissue and fails to clot under normal circumstances. It is usually dark and produces a characteristic musty odor on oxidation. Environmental factors (e.g., severe emotional stress, illness, malnutrition, and seasonal variation) may affect the length of the menstrual cycle.

Hormonal Controls

Hormonal control of the menstrual cycle depends on complex interactions among the hypothalamus, the anterior pituitary, and the ovaries. Gonadotropin-releasing hormone is secreted by the hypothalamus into the hypophyseal portal system and travels to the anterior pituitary, where it stimulates the secretion of LH and FSH. Follicle-stimulating hormone and LH are released from the anterior pituitary in pulses that correspond to the secretion of GnRH.

Blood levels of estrogen and progesterone exert a feedback effect on the anterior pituitary, thereby determining how much FSH and LH are secreted (Table 19-2). Follicle-stimulating hormone and LH secretion are not completely parallel: that is, FSH and LH are not secreted simultaneously in equal amounts throughout the menstrual cycle. Nonparallel secretion is caused by cyclic changes in feedback mechanisms. During the early follicular phase, low levels of estrogen inhibit the FSH-secreting cells of the anterior pituitary. In addition, the developing ovarian follicle secretes **inhibin,** a protein

FIG. 19-11 The menstrual cycle. (Modified from Bobak, Jensen, & Zalar. [1989]. *Maternity and gynecologic care.* [4th ed.]. St. Louis: Mosby–Year Book.)

TABLE 19-2

Hormonal Feedback Mechanisms in the Menstrual Cycle

Phase of cycle and ovarian hormone levels	Feedback to hypothalamus and anterior pituitary	Resultant GnRH, FSH, and LH levels	Ovarian and menstrual events
Early follicular phase: estrogen levels low; no progesterone secreted	Negative and inhibitory	All low	Ovarian follicle develops; endometrium proliferates
Late follicular (preovulatory) phase: estrogen levels high; minute amount of progesterone secreted	Positive and stimulatory	All surge; LH dominates	Process of ovulation begins; endometrial proliferation complete
Ovulatory phase: estrogen levels dip; progesterone levels begin to rise	Negative and inhibitory	All fall sharply	Corpus luteum begins to develop; endometrium enters secretory phase
Early luteal phase: estrogen and progesterone levels high; progesterone dominates	Negative and inhibitory	All continue to decline, but gradually	Corpus luteum fully developed; endometrium ready for implantation
Late luteal phase: estrogen and progesterone levels fall sharply	Negative and inhibitory; feedback lessens slightly	All rise slightly	Corpus luteum regresses; endometrium breaks down; menstruation begins
Menstrual phase: estrogen levels low; no progesterone secreted	Negative and inhibitory	All low	More ovarian follicles begin to develop; functional layer of endometrium is shed

hormone that inhibits both GnRH and FSH secretion. As the ovarian follicle grows, it produces more and more estrogen. During the late follicular phase, the preovulatory rise in progesterone facilitates the positive feedback of estrogen; estrogen levels begin to increase, stimulating a surge of FSH and LH secretion from the anterior pituitary. (Progesterone may be necessary also to induce the midcycle FSH peak.) The midcycle surge of LH causes ovulation. Rising estrogen and progesterone levels during the luteal phase may have some inhibitory effect on the anterior pituitary, thereby inhibiting LH and FSH secretion. Just before the onset of menstruation, FSH and LH levels begin to increase slightly, probably because of declining estrogen and progesterone levels.

Ovarian Cycle

To grow and mature, ovarian follicles require FSH, LH, and estradiol. At the end of a cycle in which pregnancy does not occur, FSH and LH levels increase slightly (Fig. 19-11). At this time, a group of ovarian follicles begin

to mature; the exact number is dependent on the remaining pool of inactive follicles. It is not understood why these particular follicles respond to the increase in FSH and LH. As the follicles mature, granulosa cells multiply, increasing the secretion of estradiol. At this time, one follicle becomes dominant, and the others atrophy. It is not clear why one follicle becomes dominant, but it may be because this follicle has more FSH receptors, or better blood supply, or greater ability to convert androgens to estradiol. The dominant follicle begins to secrete progressively larger amounts of estradiol, which exerts a positive-feedback effect, causing the LH surge. Ovulation generally occurs an average of 16 hours after the LH surge, with a range of 8 to 40 hours; specific timing may reflect seasonal variations. Progesterone, proteolytic enzymes, and prostaglandins (E and F series) trigger mechanisms controlling follicular rupture and release of the ovum. Possible mechanisms include thinning, stretching, degradation, and digestion of the follicular wall and contraction of smooth muscle cells of the follicle. Prostaglandins play such a significant role in ovulation that women with fertility problems should avoid all use of antiprostaglandin medication (Speroff, Glass, & Kase, 1989).

The LH surge also transforms the granulosa cells of the ovulatory follicle into the corpus luteum. The corpus luteum secretes both estrogen and progesterone in amounts that depend, in part, on adequate development of the follicle before ovulation. If pregnancy does not occur, the corpus luteum persists for 14 days, then regresses and eventually disappears.

Uterine Phases

Uterine phases of the menstrual cycle—the proliferative phase, the secretory phase, and menstruation—involve the cyclic changes that occur in the endometrium. During the midfollicular phase, increasing levels of estrogen contribute to endometrial repair and proliferation, thus increasing endometrial thickness. Once ovulation occurs and serum progesterone levels increase, the endometrial tissue develops secretory characteristics. If implantation of a fertilized ovum does not take place, endometrial tissue begins to break down approximately 11 days after ovulation. The period of breakdown is sometimes called the ischemic phase (Fig. 19-11). Sloughing of tissue (menstrual bleeding) begins about 14 days after ovulation.

Cervical mucus also undergoes cyclic changes. During the proliferative phase, the cervical mucus is thin and watery. With the preovulatory surge of LH and estradiol, the mucus becomes thicker and more elastic (spinnbarkeit). Increasing progesterone levels apparently contribute to the development of tiny channels in the mucus of the cervical os, providing access for sperm. Changes in the consistency of cervical mucus can be used to identify fertile intervals.

Vaginal Response

The vaginal endothelium also responds to the cyclic hormonal changes of the menstrual cycle. Under the influence of estrogen, cells of the vaginal epithelium grow maximally during the follicular/proliferative phase. After ovulation, layers of keratinized cells overgrow the basal epithelium, a process known as **cornification.** Near the end of the luteal phase, leukocytes invade vaginal epithelium, removing the outer layers in a process termed **decornification.**

Body Temperature

Basal body temperature (BBT) undergoes characteristic biphasic changes during menstrual cycles in which ovulation occurs. During the follicular phase, the BBT fluctuates around 98° F (37° C). During the luteal phase, the average temperature increases by 0.4° to 1.0° F (0.2° to 0.5° C). At the end of the luteal phase, 1 to 3 days before the onset of menstruation, BBT declines to follicular-phase levels. The shift in temperature is related to ovulation, corpus luteum formation, and increased serum progesterone levels. Progesterone probably acts on the thermoregulatory center of the hypothalamus to increase body temperature. Changes in BBT are used to document ovulatory cycles but are not useful to predict the exact timing of ovulation.

THE MALE REPRODUCTIVE SYSTEM

In men, the external genitalia perform the major functions of reproduction, which are to produce sperm and deliver them to the female reproductive tract. Sperm are produced in the male gonads, the testes, and delivered to the female vagina by the penis. The internal male genitalia have a more accessory function. They consist of conducting tubes and fluid-producing glands, all of which aid in the transport of sperm from the testes to the urethral opening of the penis. The male reproductive and urinary structures are shown in Fig. 19-12.

External Genitalia
Testes

In men, the testes are the essential organs of reproduction. Like the ovaries, the testes have two functions: (1) production of gametes (in this case, sperm) and (2) production of sex hormones (in this case, androgens and testosterone). The testes are suspended outside the pelvic cavity because sperm production requires an environment that is 1 or 2 degrees cooler than body temperature.

During embryonic and fetal life, the testes develop within the abdomen (see Fig. 19-1). Then, about 3 months before birth, the testes start to descend toward the developing scrotum. About 1 month before birth, they enter twin passageways called **inguinal canals.** The inguinal canals are vaginal processes created by outpouchings of the peritoneum (lining of the abdominal cavity). The descent of a **testis** is shown in Fig. 19-13. Each testis moves down outside the peritoneum until it is suspended in the scrotal sac by its supply lines: the ducts, blood vessels, lymphatic vessels, and nerves of the **spermatic cord.** When descent is complete, the abdominal end of each vaginal process closes up and the inguinal canal disappears. If peritoneal closure at the site of the inguinal canal is incomplete or weak, an inguinal hernia may occur later in life. Failure of the testes to descend through the inguinal canal is known as cryptorchidism. The scrotal end of each vaginal process becomes the outer covering of the testis, the **tunica vaginalis.** A hydrocele is the accumulation of fluid within the tunica vaginalis.

Fig. 19-14 shows a sagittal section of a mature testis. The adult testis is ovoid and varies considerably in

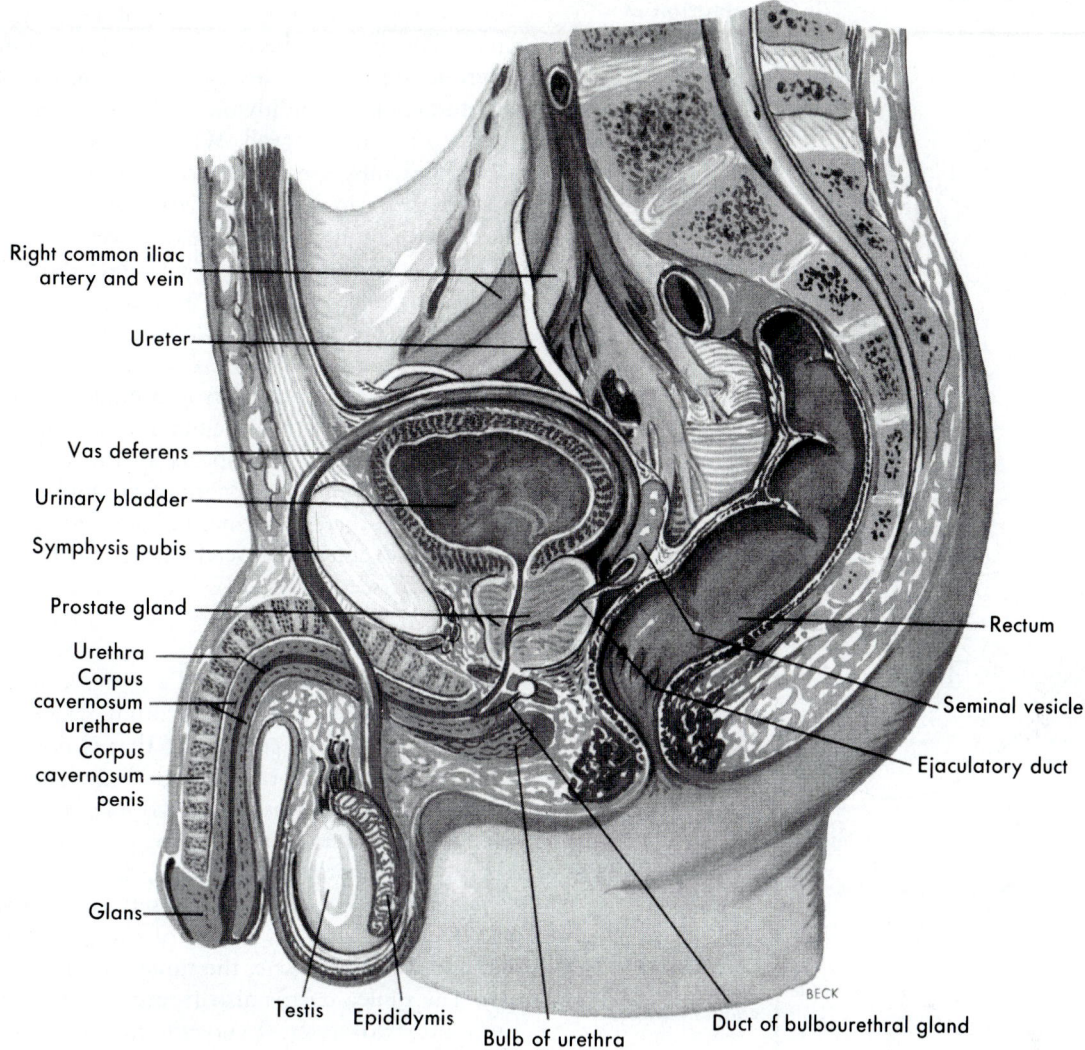

Right common iliac
artery and vein

Ureter

Vas deferens

Urinary bladder

Symphysis pubis

Prostate gland

Urethra
Corpus
cavernosum
urethrae
Corpus
cavernosum
penis

Glans

Rectum

Seminal vesicle

Ejaculatory duct

BECK

Testis   Epididymis   Bulb of urethra   Duct of bulbourethral gland

FIG. 19-12 Sagittal section of the penis. Sagittal section of the male penis showing the location of the reproductive organs. (From Thibodeau, G. A. [1987]. *Anatomy and physiology*. St. Louis: Mosby–Year Book.)

length (3 to 6 cm), width (2 to 3.5 cm), depth (3 to 4 cm), and weight (10 to 40 g). The testis is almost entirely surrounded by an outer covering, the tunica vaginalis, which separates the testis from the scrotal wall, and an inner covering, the **tunica albuginea.** Inward extensions of the tunica albuginea form septa that separate the testis into about 250 compartments, or lobules, each of which contains several tortuously coiled ducts called **seminiferous tubules.** The seminiferous tubules constitute the bulk (80%) of testicular volume and are the site of sperm production. (Sperm production, termed **spermatogenesis,** is described on p. 731.) Tissue surrounding these ducts contains blood and lymphatic vessels, fibroblastic support cells, macrophages, mast cells, and Leydig cells. **Leydig cells,** which occur in clusters and account for about 1% to 5% of testicular volume,

produce androgens, chiefly testosterone. Abnormal dilation of the veins in the testes is referred to as varicocele. Inflammation of the testes is known as orchitis and may be a complication of the mumps virus.

The two ends of each seminiferous tubule join and leave the lobule through a short, straight section called the **tubulus rectus.** Sperm travel from the seminiferous tubules into these straight sections, which lead to the central portion of the testis, the **rete testis.** From the rete testis, sperm move through the **efferent tubules,** or vasa efferentia, to the epididymis, where they mature.

The testes are innervated by adrenergic fibers, whose sole function apparently is to regulate blood flow to the Leydig cells. The testes receive arterial blood from the internal spermatic and differential arteries. Arterial blood flows over the surface of the testes before enter-

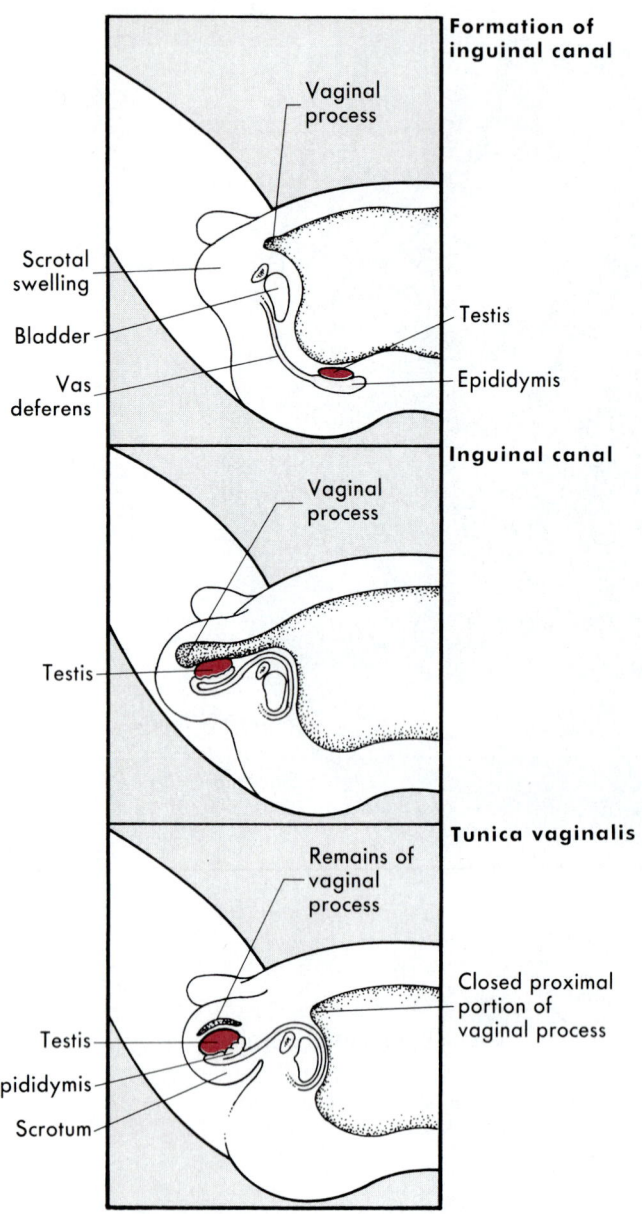

Formation of inguinal canal

Vaginal process

Scrotal swelling

Bladder

Vas deferens

Testis

Epididymis

Inguinal canal

Vaginal process

Testis

Tunica vaginalis

Remains of vaginal process

Testis

Epididymis

Scrotum

Closed proximal portion of vaginal process

FIG. 19-13 **Descent of a testis.** The testes descend from the abdominal cavity to the scrotum during the last 3 months of fetal development.

ing the parenchyma (functional tissues). Surface flow cools the blood to temperatures that promote spermatogenesis, approximately 1° to 2° C below body core temperature.

Epididymis

The **epididymis** (plural, *epididymides*) is a comma-shaped structure that curves over the posterior portion of each testis (see Fig. 19-14). It consists of a single, 60- to 70-cm highly packed and markedly coiled duct measuring 5 cm in length, whose structural function is to

conduct sperm from the efferent tubules to the vas deferens. The duct can become inflamed from infection by microorganisms that ascend the urethra or from the prostate, causing epididymitis. The epididymis has physiologic functions as well. When they enter the head of the epididymis, sperm are not fully mature or motile, nor are they capable of fertilizing an ovum. During the 12 days (or more) sperm take to travel the length of the epididymis, they receive nutrients and testosterone from the epididymal epithelium, and some biochemical or physiologic mechanism enhances their capacity for fertilization.

The tail of the epididymis is continuous with the **vas deferens,** a duct with muscular layers capable of powerful peristalsis that transports sperm toward the urethra. After traveling the length of the epididymis, sperm are stored in the epididymal tail and vas deferens. The vas deferens enters the pelvic cavity through the spermatic cord (see Fig. 19-14).

Scrotum

The testes, epididymides, and spermatic cord are enclosed and protected by the scrotum. The **scrotum** is a skin-covered, fibromuscular sac that is homologous to the female labia majora (see Fig. 19-2). The skin of the scrotum is thin and has rugae (wrinkles or folds), which enable it to enlarge or relax away from the body. At puberty the scrotal skin darkens, develops active sebaceous glands, and becomes sparsely covered with hair. Just under the skin lies a layer of connective tissue (fascia) and smooth muscle, the **tunica dartos** (see Fig. 19-14). The tunica dartos also forms a septum that separates the two testes. Exposure to cold temperatures causes the tunica dartos to contract, pulling the testes close to the warm body. In warm temperatures the tunica dartos relaxes, suspending the testes away from body heat. These mechanisms promote optimal temperatures for spermatogenesis. In addition, scrotal sensitivity to touch, pressure, temperature, and pain protects the testes against potential harm. During sexual excitement, the scrotal skin and tunica thicken, the scrotum tightens and lifts, and the spermatic cords shorten, partially elevating the testes toward the body. As excitement plateaus, the engorged testes increase 50% in size, rotate anteriorly, and flatten against the body, signaling impending ejaculation.

Penis

The **penis** has two main functions: delivery of sperm to the female vagina and elimination of urine. (Urine formation and excretion are the subjects of Chapter 32.) Embryonically, the penis is homologous to the female clitoris (see Fig. 19-2).

Fig. 19-12 shows a sagittal section of the adult penis and its anatomic relation to other urogenital structures.

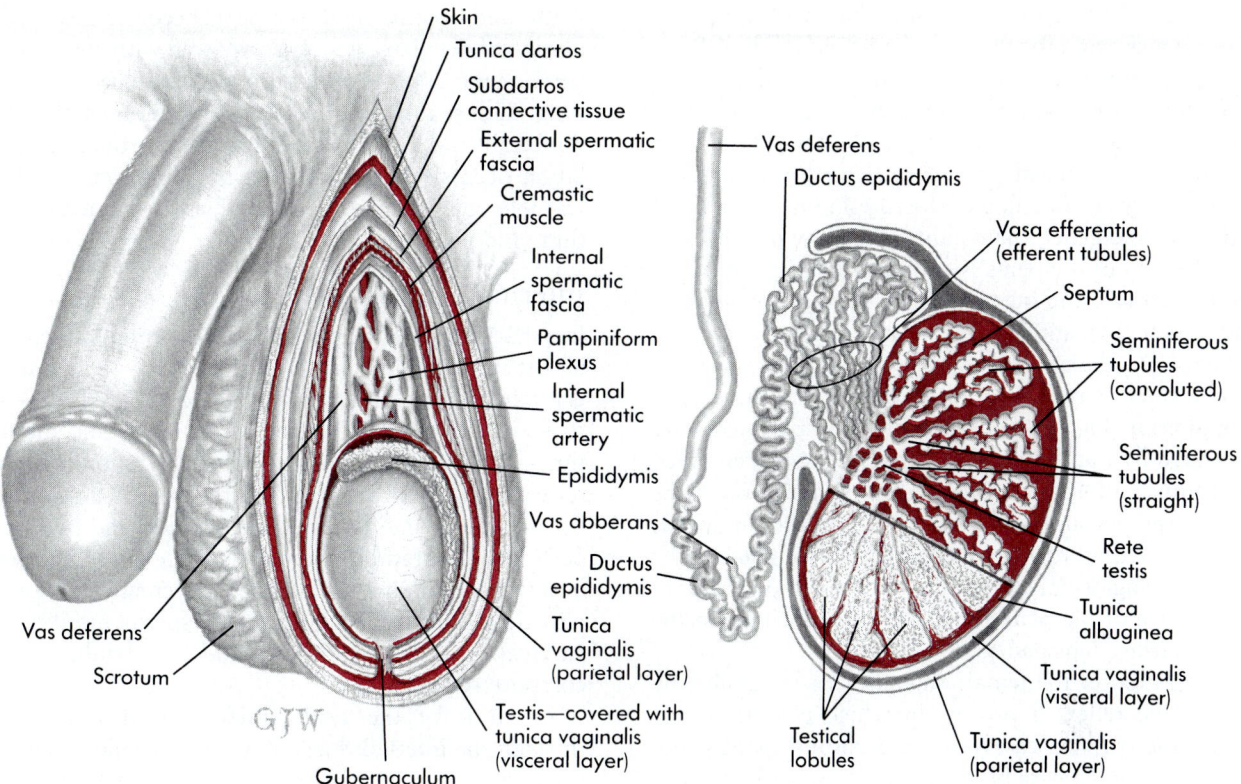

FIG. 19-14 **The testes.** External and sagittal views showing interior anatomy. (From Tanagho & McAninch, 1992.)

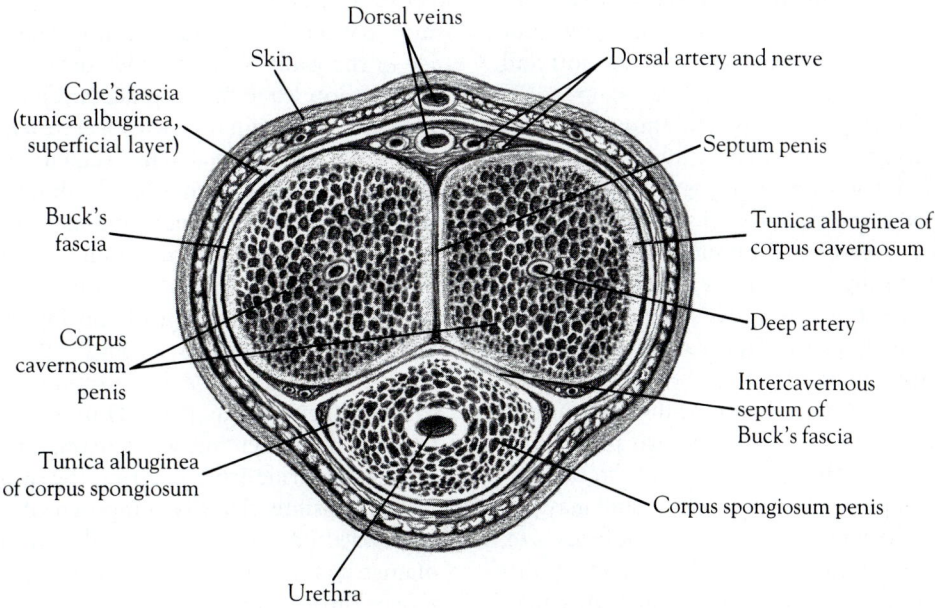

FIG. 19-15 **Cross section of the penis.** (From Thompson, McFarland, Hirsch, & Tucker, 1993.)

Externally the penis consists of a shaft with a tip, the **glans,** which contains the opening of the urethra. Balanitis is an inflammation of the glans. The skin of the glans folds over the tip of the penis, forming the prepuce, or **foreskin.** Soon after birth, the foreskin may be removed in a surgical procedure termed circumcision. If the prepuce or opening of the foreskin is too small to slide over the glans, the condition is known as phimosis. The skin of the penis is continuous with that of the groin, scrotum, and inner thighs. It is hairless, movable, and darker than surrounding skin.

Internally, the penis consists of the urethra and three compartments: two **corpora cavernosa** and the **corpus spongiosum** (Fig. 19-15). The three compartments are separated by Buck's fascia and, like the testes, enclosed by a tunica albuginea. The **urethra** passes through the corpus spongiosum and ends at a sagittal slit in the glans. If the urethra is not completely surrounded by the corpus spongiosum, the meatus may open on the ventral surface of the penile shaft (hypospadias) or on the dorsal surface (epispadias).

Penetration of the female vagina is made possible by the **erectile reflex,** a process in which erectile tissues within the corpora cavernosa and corpus spongiosum become engorged with blood, generally 20 to 50 ml. The erectile tissues consist of vascular spaces, or chambers, which are supplied with blood by arterioles (small arteries). Most of the time, the arterioles are constricted, so that not much blood flows through the erectile tissues. Sexual stimulation, however, causes the arterioles to dilate and fill with blood. Their rapid expansion fills the erectile tissues, causing an erection. Erection apparently is maintained by compression or constriction of veins that drain the corpora cavernosa and corpus spongiosum. When sexual stimulation ceases or orgasm and ejaculation occur, these veins open up, blood flows out of the arterioles, and the penis becomes flaccid (soft and pendulous).

Erection is under the control of the autonomic nervous system but can be stimulated or inhibited by central nervous system input. Stimulation of mechanoreceptors of the penis, particularly of the glans, causes parasympathetic nerves of the autonomic nervous system to relax smooth muscle in the walls of penile arterioles. At the same time the effects of sympathetic nerves, which normally cause arteriolar smooth muscle to constrict, are inhibited.

Erections begin in utero and continue throughout life, but ejaculation does not occur until sperm production begins at puberty. Growth of the penis and scrotal contents continues well past puberty, however, and may not be complete until the late teens or early 20s. Penis size, when flaccid, varies considerably; with an erection, difference in penis size diminishes. Sexual excitement causes the corpora cavernosa to increase in length and width and become rigid; the penis becomes erect. Stimulation of the glans, which is endowed with copious sensitive nerve endings, provides maximum erotic sensation. With sexual arousal, skin color deepens, the glans doubles in size, and the urethral meatus dilates. Ejaculation occurs with frequent, strong contractions of the vas deferens, epididymis, seminal vesicles, prostate, urethra, and penis.

Internal Genitalia

Fig. 19-12 shows the anatomy of the internal genitalia and their relation to other pelvic organs. The internal genitalia consist of ducts and glands. The ducts—the two vasa deferentia, the ejaculatory duct, and the urethra—conduct sperm and glandular secretions from the testes to the urethral opening of the penis. The glands—the prostate gland, two seminal vesicles, and two Cowper (or bulbourethral) glands—secrete fluids that serve as a vehicle for sperm transport and create an alkaline, nutritious medium that promotes sperm motility and survival. Together, the sperm and the glandular fluids compose **semen.**

Sperm leave the epididymides and travel rapidly through the internal ducts in a process called **emission.** Emission occurs just seconds before ejaculation, at the moment when sexual arousal peaks. Emission always leads to ejaculation.

Emission occurs as smooth muscle in the walls of the epididymides and vasa deferentia begins to contract rhythmically, pushing sperm and epididymal secretions through the vasa deferentia. Each vas deferens is a firm, elastic, fibromuscular tube that begins at the tail of the epididymis, enters the pelvic cavity within the spermatic cord, loops up and over the bladder, and ends in the prostate gland (Figs. 19-12 and 19-16). Sperm are moved along by peristaltic contractions of smooth muscle in the walls of the vas deferens.

As sperm leave the ampulla (wide portion) of the vas deferens, the seminal vesicles secrete a nutritive, glucose-rich fluid into the ejaculate (semen). The **seminal vesicles** are a pair of glands, each about 4 to 6 cm long, that lie behind the urinary bladder and in front of the rectum. The ducts of the seminal vesicles join the ampulla of the vas deferens to become the **ejaculatory duct,** which contracts rhythmically during emission and ejaculation. As can be seen in Figs. 19-12 and 19-16, the ejaculatory duct joins the urethra, where both pass through the prostate gland. During emission and ejaculation a sphincter (muscle surrounding a duct) closes, preventing urine from entering the prostatic urethra.

The **prostate gland** is composed of alveoli and ducts embedded in fibromuscular tissue. It measures 4 cm in diameter and weighs approximately 20 g. While semen moves through the prostatic portion of the urethra, the prostate gland contracts rhythmically and secretes pros-

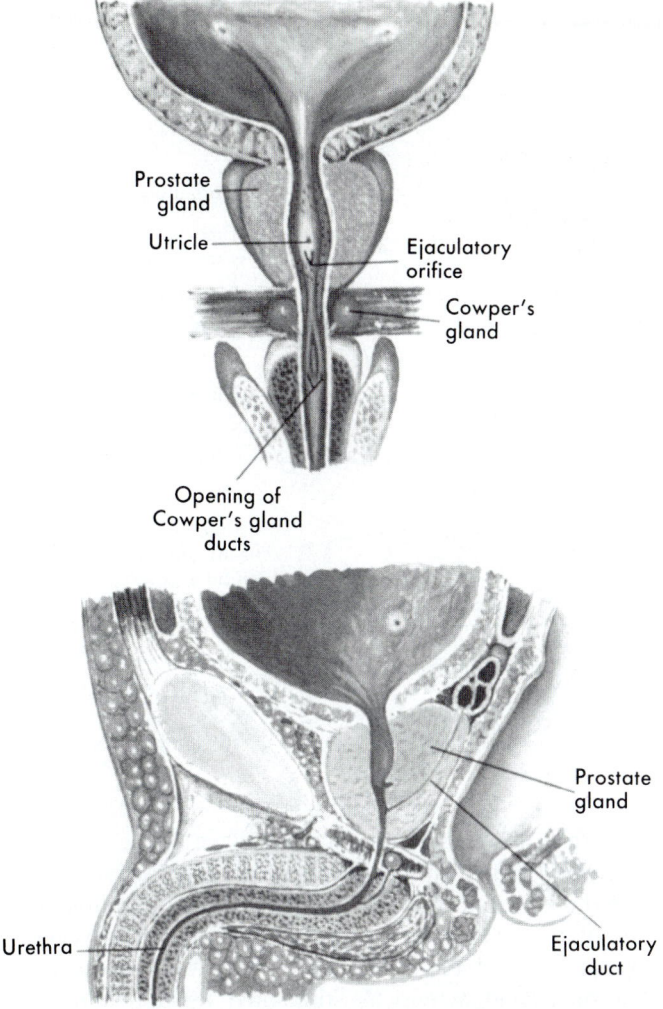

FIG. 19-16 Anatomy of the prostate gland and seminal vesicles. (From Seidel, Ball, Dains, & Benedict, 1991.)

tatic fluid into the mixture. Prostatic fluid is a thin, milky substance with an alkaline pH that helps sperm to survive in the acid environment of the female reproductive tract. In addition, substances in seminal and prostatic fluids help to mobilize sperm after ejaculation. Prostatitis is an inflammation of the prostate often caused by infecting microorganisms from the urinary tract. Enlargement of the prostate is common after 50 years of age and is known as benign prostatic hypertrophy (BPH).

The last pair of glands to add fluid to the ejaculate are **Cowper's glands** (bulbourethral glands), whose ducts secrete mucus into the urethra near the base of the penis. Ejaculation occurs as semen reaches the base of the penis and muscles there begin the rhythmic contractions that push semen out. Normally a man ejaculates between 2 and 6 ml of semen, containing 75 million to 400 million sperm. About 98% of the ejaculate

consists of glandular fluids; 60% to 70% of volume comes from the seminal vesicles and 20% from the prostate. Therefore the ejaculate of a man who has undergone vasectomy (a surgical procedure that prevents sperm from entering the vas deferens) is not reduced by much: about 2%.

Spermatogenesis

Spermatogenesis begins at puberty and continues for life. In this respect, spermatogenesis differs markedly from oogenesis (production of primordial ova), which occurs during fetal life only.

Spermatogenesis takes place within the seminiferous tubules of the testes (see Fig. 19-14). The basement membrane of each seminiferous tubule is lined with diploid (46-chromosome) germ cells called **spermatogonia** (singular, *spermatogonium*). These cells undergo continuous mitotic division. (Mitotic division, in which a cell divides into two identical cells, is described in Chapter 1.) Some of the spermatogonia move away from the basement membrane and mature, becoming **primary spermatocytes** (Fig. 19-17). The primary spermatocytes undergo meiosis, a type of cell division that results in two haploid (23-chromosome) cells called **secondary spermatocytes.** (Meiosis is described and illustrated in Chapter 4.) The two secondary spermatocytes then undergo meiosis, resulting in four **spermatids.** It is the spermatids that differentiate into spermatozoa, or sperm, each of which contains 23 chromosomes (Fig. 19-18).

The development of spermatids into sperm depends on the presence of **Sertoli cells** (nondividing support cells) within the seminiferous tubules. The spermatids attach themselves to Sertoli cells, from which they receive the nutrients and the hormonal signals they need to develop into sperm.

The process of spermatogenesis, from mitotic division of a spermatogonium to maturation of the spermatids, takes about 70 to 80 days. Mature sperm migrate from the seminiferous tubules to the epididymides, where their capacity for fertilization continues to develop. Although they are completely mature by the time they are ejaculated, the sperm do not become motile (capable of movement) until they are activated by biochemicals in semen and in the female reproductive tract.

Male Sex Hormones

The male sex hormones are androgens. Testosterone, the primary male sex hormone, is an androgen. Testosterone and other androgens are produced mainly by Leydig cells of the testes, but they are also produced by the adrenal glands. In men, sex hormone production is relatively constant and does not occur in a cyclic pattern, as it does in women.

The androgens have a number of physiologic actions related to the growth and development of male tissues

A

B

FIG. 19-17 Spermatogenesis. A, Cell division; **B,** sperm developing within seminiferous tubule. (From Bobak & Jensen, 1993.)

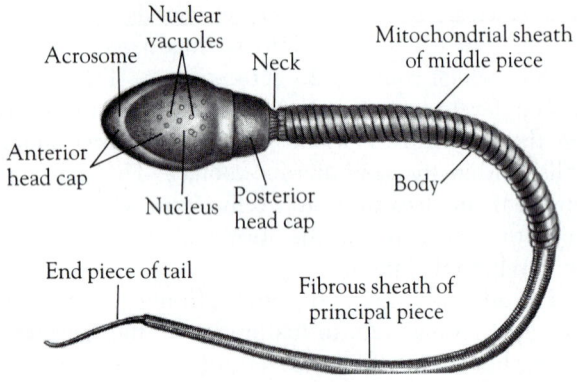

FIG. 19-18 Mature sperm cell (spermatozoon). (From Thompson, McFarland, Hirsch, & Tucker, 1993.)

and organs. The androgens are responsible for the fetal differentiation and development of the male urogenital system and have some effects on the fetal brain. After birth, the Leydig cells become quiescent until activated by the gonadotropins during puberty. At puberty, androgens cause the sex organs to grow and secondary sex characteristics to develop.

Testosterone affects nervous and skeletal tissues, bone marrow, skin and hair, and sex organs. It has an anabolic effect on skeletal muscle tissue, thereby contributing to the difference in body weight and composition between men and women. Testosterone also stimulates

growth of the musculature and cartilage of the larynx, causing a permanent deepening of the voice. Testosterone directly stimulates the bone marrow and indirectly stimulates renal erythropoietin production to achieve increased hemoglobin and hematocrit levels. Because sebaceous gland activity is stimulated by testosterone, acne may develop. Hair becomes coarser in texture, and facial, axillary, and pubic hair grows in male patterns. Later in life, testosterone causes baldness in genetically susceptible individuals. Testosterone is required for spermatogenesis and for secretion of fluid by the prostate gland, seminal vesicles, and Cowper glands. Testosterone is also associated with an increase in libido (sex drive). Other, less well understood effects of testosterone include alterations in fatty acid and cholesterol metabolism.

The regulation of androgen production and spermatogenesis is achieved by a complex feedback system involving the extrahypothalamic central nervous system, the hypothalamus, the anterior pituitary, the testes, and the androgen-sensitive end organs. These relationships, which are essentially the same in women, are summarized in Fig. 19-3. Extrahypothalamic influences include such variables as physiologic and psychologic stress. These factors may inhibit or augment hypothalamic activity. Gonadotropin-releasing hormone secretion by the hypothalamus is stimulated by norepinephrine and inhibited by both serotonin and dopamine. Gonadotropin-releasing hormone is transported by por-

FIG. 19-19 **The female breast.** (From Thompson, McFarland, Hirsch, & Tucker, 1993.)

tal flow to the median eminence of the pituitary gland, where it stimulates the secretion of LH and FSH. Luteinizing hormone and FSH, which are named for their effects in the female reproductive system, have important effects on the male system as well. Luteinizing hormone acts on the Leydig cells to stimulate testosterone secretion, which in turn is enhanced by FSH; FSH binds to Leydig cells and increases the number of LH receptors on the cells. In addition, both FSH and LH are important in the initiation and maintenance of spermatogenesis. Luteinizing hormone and FSH secretion are inhibited by testosterone, other androgens, and estradiol. Follicle-stimulating hormone also is regulated by inhibin secreted by the Sertoli cells. Inhibin appears to act in conjunction with the gonadal steroids to regulate FSH levels.

STRUCTURE AND FUNCTION OF THE BREAST

The **breasts** are modified sebaceous glands that lie on the ventral surface of the thorax, within the superficial fascia of the chest wall. They extend vertically from the second rib to the sixth or seventh intercostal space, and laterally from the side of the sternum to the midaxillary line. Breast tissue also may extend into the axilla; this tissue is known as the tail of Spence.

The Female Breast

The female breast is composed of 15 to 20 pyramid-shaped lobes that are separated and supported by Cooper ligaments (Fig. 19-19). Each lobe contains 20 to 40 lobules (alveoli), which subdivide further into many functional units called **acini** (singular, *acinus*). Each acinus is lined with a layer of epithelial cells capable of secreting milk and a layer of subepithelial cells capable of contracting to squeeze milk from the acinus. The acini empty into a network of lobular collecting ducts, which empty into interlobular collecting and ejecting ducts. These ducts reach the skin through openings (pores) in the nipple. The lobes and lobules are surrounded and separated by muscle strands and fatty connective tissue. The amount of fatty connective tissue varies from individual to individual, depending on weight and genetic and endocrine factors, and contributes to the diversity of breast size and shape.

An extensive capillary network surrounds the acini and is supplied by the internal and lateral thoracic arteries and the intercostal arteries. Venous return follows

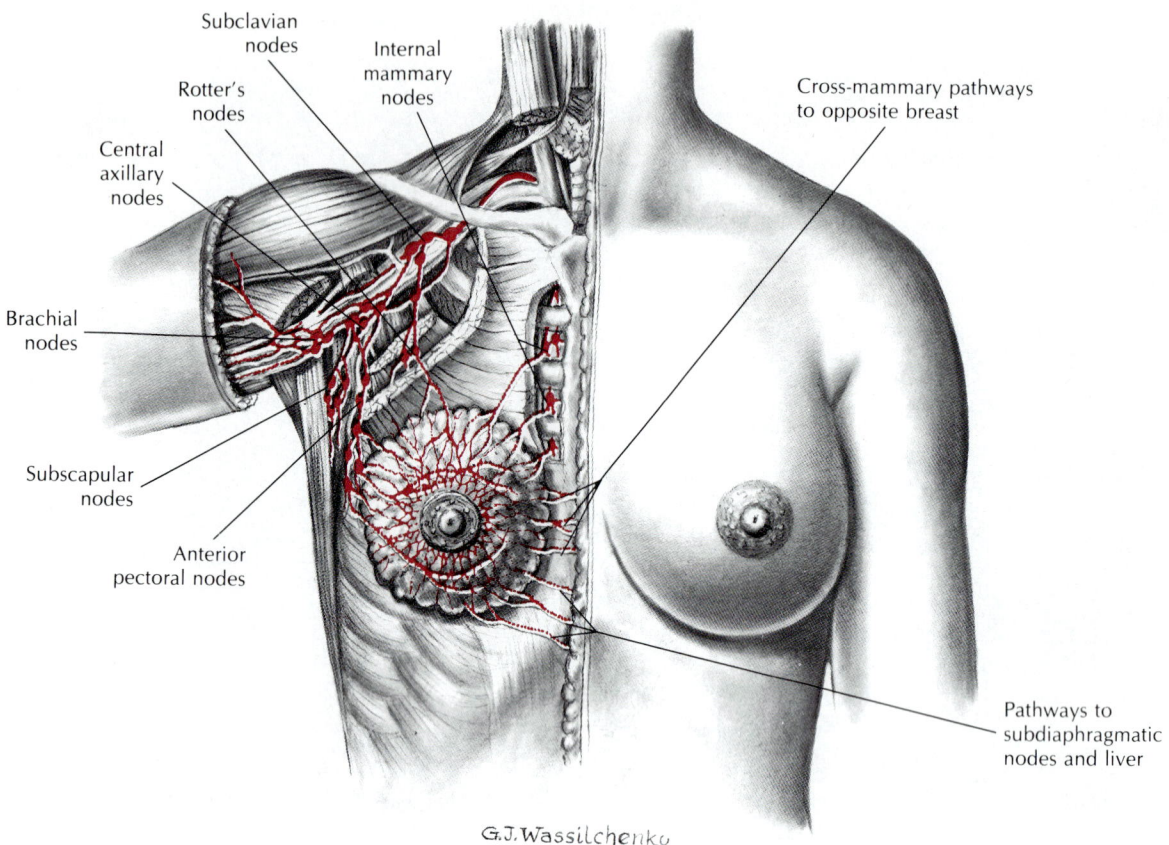

G.J.Wassilchenko

FIG. 19-20 **Lymphatic drainage of the female breast.** (From Bobak, Jensen, & Zalar. [1989]. *Maternity and gynecologic care.* [4th ed.]. St. Louis: Mosby–Year Book.)

arterial supply, with relatively rapid emptying into the superior vena cava. The breasts receive sensory innervation from branches of the second and sixth intercostal nerves and the cervical plexus. This accounts for the fact that breast pain may be referred to the chest, back, scapula, medial arm, and neck. Lymphatic drainage of the breast occurs largely through axillary nodes, but approximately 25% occurs through transpectoral and internal mammary routes (Fig. 19-20).

The **nipple** is a pigmented, cylindrical structure that is usually located at the fourth or fifth intercostal space. It measures 0.05 to 1.3 cm in diameter and is approximately 10 to 12 mm in height when erect. On its surface lie multiple openings, one from each lobe. The **areola** is the pigmented, circular area around the nipple. It may be 15 to 60 mm in diameter. A number of sebaceous glands, the **glands of Montgomery,** are located within the areola and aid in lubrication of the nipple during lactation. The nipple and areola contain smooth muscles, which receive motor innervation from the sympathetic nervous system. Sexual stimulation and exposure to cold cause the nipple to become erect.

The fetal and early postnatal development of breast tissue does not depend on hormones, although fetal breast tissue does become progressively responsive to hormonal stimulation. During childhood, breast growth is latent, and growth of the nipple and areola keeps pace with body surface growth. (Male breast development does not normally progress any further.) At the onset of puberty in the female, estrogen secretion stimulates mammary growth. Breast development, or **thelarche,** is usually the first sign of puberty in the female. Full differentiation and development of breast tissue are mediated by a variety of hormones, including estrogen, progesterone, prolactin, growth hormone, thyroid hormone, insulin, and cortisol. Estrogen promotes development of the lobular ducts; progesterone stimulates development of cells lining the acini. Lactation (milk production) occurs after childbirth in response to increased levels of prolactin; prolactin secretion, in turn, is stimulated by breast feeding. Oxytocin, another hormone released after delivery, controls milk ejection from acini cells.

During the reproductive years, the breast undergoes cyclic changes in response to changes in the levels of estrogen and progesterone associated with the menstrual cycle. During the follicular/proliferative phase of the menstrual cycle, high estradiol levels increase the vascularity of breast tissue and stimulate proliferation of ductal and acinar tissue. This effect is sustained into the luteal/secretory phase of the cycle. During this phase, progesterone levels increase and contribute to the breast changes induced by estradiol. Specific effects of progesterone include dilatation of the ducts and conversion of the acinar cells into secretory cells. Most women experience some degree of premenstrual breast fullness, tenderness, and increased breast nodularity. Breast volume may increase as much as 10 to 30 ml. Because the length of the menstrual cycle does not allow for complete regression of new cell growth, breast growth continues at a slow rate until approximately age 35. Because of the cyclic changes that occur in breast tissue, breast examination should be conducted at the conclusion of or a few days after the menstrual cycle, when hormonal effects are minimal and breasts are at their smallest.

The function of the female breast is primarily to provide a source of nourishment for the newborn. Physiologically, breast milk is the most appropriate nourishment for newborns. Not only does its composition change over time to meet the changing digestive capabilities and nutritional requirements of the infant, but breast milk also contains specific immunoglobulins, especially IgA, and nonspecific antimicrobial factors, such as lysosomes and lactoferrin, which protect the infant against infection. During lactation, high prolactin levels interfere with hypothalamic-pituitary hormones that stimulate ovulation. This mechanism suppresses the menstrual cycle and prevents ovulation. In many parts of the world (underdeveloped or Third World countries), breast feeding is the major means of contraception. Breasts are also a source of pleasurable sexual sensation and in Western cultures have become a sexual symbol.

The Male Breast

Until puberty, development of the male breast is similar to that of the female breast. In the absence of sufficiently high levels of estrogen and progesterone, the male breast does not develop any further. The normal male breast consists of a small, underdeveloped nipple; some fatty and fibrous tissue; and a few ductlike structures in the subareolar area. The male breast may appear enlarged in obese men because of accumulation of fatty tissue. During puberty some males experience gynecomastia, a condition in which the breasts enlarge temporarily as a result of hormonal fluctuations.

TESTS OF REPRODUCTIVE FUNCTION

Diagnostic tests of the male and female reproductive systems are performed to determine the cause of infertility, to detect the presence of cancerous lesions, or to identify the presence of sexually transmitted diseases. (Alterations of the reproductive systems are discussed in Chapter 20; sexually transmitted diseases are discussed in Chapter 21.) Procedures include laboratory tests, such as cultures, smears, stains, biopsies, serologic testing, and hormonal assays. Radiographic procedures are performed to identify abnormal growths or structures. Direct observation of reproductive organs is completed by laparoscopy or culdoscopy.

Infection and Cancer Tests

Smears, stains, cultures, and serologic testing are commonly used to detect infectious diseases. Smears are prepared by spreading a thick layer of specimen material on a glass slide. The specimen may be evaluated microscopically as a wet mount or dried and stained with different dyes. Gram staining is a technique that allows the differential identification of two categories of bacteria according to the tendency of the microorganism to selectively absorb different components of the stain.

A **culture** is the growth of microorganism in a nutrient medium selectively prepared to support the growth of particular microorganisms that are obtained from body secretions or tissues. Both bacteria and viruses, such as cytomegalovirus, can be cultured.

Serologic testing identifies whether an antigen-antibody reaction has occurred in response to an infectious microorganism. Several different techniques can be used to identify the formation of antigen-antibody complexes. With immunofluorescent testing, fluorescein-labeled antibodies react with specific antigen, such as the spirochetes of syphilis. The fluorescent pattern of the reaction can be microscopically observed under ultraviolet light. The flocculation (agglutination) test is the precipitation of clumped cells caused by the reaction of antigen with homologous antiserum. The Venereal Disease Research Laboratory (VDRL) test for syphilis is a type of flocculation test. Certain viral diseases can be diagnosed by using specific serologic antibody markers, for example, the diagnosis of hepatitis A and hepatitis B viruses. Radioimmunoassay (RIA) and enzyme-linked immunoabsorbent assay (ELISA) are more specific tests used to document viral infections. A summary of tests used for the diagnosis of sexually transmitted diseases is presented in Table 19-3.

Tissue biopsy is the surgical resection of a tissue specimen from a suspect site. The biopsy provides cells and tissues to identify infectious processes and to differentiate benign from malignant conditions, and primary from metastatic lesions. In the reproductive tract, tissue may be obtained from the vagina, cervix (by cone or brush biopsy), endometrium of the uterus (by curettage), ovary, testes, prostate, or penis.

Needle biopsy is a technique of aspirating small amounts of tissue by positioning a needle in the tissue

TABLE 19-3

Diagnosis of Sexually Transmitted Diseases

Test	Description	Normal value
Serologic test for syphilis	Detection of antibodies to *Treponema pallidum*	Negative or nonreactive
VDRL	Venereal Disease Research Laboratory (nonspecific)	
RPR	Rapid plasma reagin (more specific)	
FTA	Fluorescent treponemal antibody absorption test (more specific; confirmatory test)	
Other test for syphilis		
Darkfield examination	Direct smear of serous exudate from moist lesions to detect *Treponema pallidum* with corkscrew appearance	Negative
Tests for gonorrhea		
Culture	Isolation and detection of *Neisseria gonorrhoeae* in urethral, anal, and/or pharyngeal secretions	No growth
Gram stain	Direct smear and staining of cervical or urethral discharge to identify gram-negative intracellular diplococci with polymorphonuclear (PMN) leukocytes	Negative
Tests for *Chlamydia*		
Tissue culture	Isolation and detection of *Chlamydia trachomatis* from epithelial cells of endocervix and urethra (expensive, time extensive)	No growth
Antigen detection	Direct immunofluorescence staining of cervical and/or urethral specimens to detect monoclonal antibodies (inexpensive, quick)	Negative
Tests for HIV infection		
ELISA (enzyme-linked immunosorbent assay)	Detects the presence of antibodies to human immunodeficiency virus (HIV)	Nonreactive
IFA (indirect fluorescent antibody)	A more specific test for HIV	Nonreactive
WB (Western blot)	A more specific test for HIV	Nonreactive
Tests for viral infections		
TORCH test	Detects elevations of IgA or IgM caused by *Toxoplasma*, rubella, cytomegalovirus, syphilis, and herpes simplex in mother and newborn infant; herpes requires more specific testing when result is positive	No elevation in antibodies
Cytomegalovirus (herpes virus 5)	Can be grown in cell culture with samples from urine, cervix, semen, saliva, blood	No growth

TABLE 19-4

Tests and Normal Values of Reproductive Function/Fertility

Test	Description	Normal value
I. Basic assessment		
Semen analysis (2 samples at least 2 weeks apart)	Determines number, motility, and structure of sperm cells	Volume = 2-6 ml Number = >20 million/ml Motility = >50%-60% with forward progression quality = >2 (scale 0-4) Morphology = >60% normal shape <10^6 WBC/ml
	Determines presence of bacteria/leukocytes	
Antisperm antibody	Detects antibody to sperm	No sperm agglutinins present
II. Intermediate assessment		
Basal body temperature	Determines whether ovulation has occurred	Decrease in basal body temperature before ovulation followed by a rise in temperature at the time of ovulation
Cervical mucus	Evaluates presence of ovulation from estrogenic effects at ovulation; mucus may also be examined for pH, glucose, or proteins or cultured for presence of infection	Fern pattern appears when cervical mucus dries on a clean slide; mucus is clear, watery, and elastic (spinnbarkeit ≥8-10 cm) with no inflammatory cells
Postcoital cervical mucus (Sims-Huhner test)	Tests ability of sperm to penetrate and maintain motility in cervical mucus 2-4 hours after coitus approximately 1 day before ovulation	≥10 motile sperm in each high-power field; motility in one direction; previous sperm analysis normal
III. More specialized tests		
Endometrial biopsy	Determines whether ovulation has occurred by obtaining endometrial tissue on day 26 of 28-day menstrual cycle (or postovulatory day 12)	Finding is "secretory-type" endometrium if ovulation has occurred; read in conjunction with day of cycle and serum progesterone levels
Hysterosalpingogram	Assessment of uterus and fallopian tubes for obstructions using transuterine injection of contrast material and radiography; performed 1-2 days after cessation of menses	No obstruction evident
Uterotubal insufflation (Rubin test)	Assesses patency of fallopian tubes using transuterine tubal insufflation with carbon dioxide and pressure measurement	Pressure <180-200 mm Hg, no obstruction; pressure >200 mm Hg indicates tubal obstruction; repeated studies differentiate obstruction from tubal spasm
Laparoscopy (pelvic endoscopy)	Visualization of reproductive organs using a laparoscope inserted within the pelvic cavity through the abdomen to assess structure or determine presence of adhesions, endometriosis, tumors, or infection	Normal structure and position of organs
Hysteroscopy	Visualization of uterine cavity using modified cystoscope inserted through cervical os; best done during first 14 days of cycle	Absence of intrauterine lesions

TABLE 19-5

Serum Hormone Values

Hormone	Value
Serum progesterone	Normal = >10 ng/dl, presumptive evidence of ovulation; draw level between days 20-25 of 28-day cycle or 6-10 days postovulation <10 ng/ml = inadequate luteal function <3 ng/ml suggests anovulation
Serum testosterone Resulting from diurnal and pulsatile pattern, need serial blood draws	Normal = 300-1200 ng/dl; must be interpreted with serum LH and FSH levels Low values in male hypogonadism
Serum FSH and LH Resulting from diurnal and pulsatile pattern, need serial blood draws	FSH = <22 IU/L LH = 4-24 IU/L High levels in males indicate primary testicular disease; low levels in males indicate hypogonadism caused by hypothalamic-pituitary dysfunction

and applying negative pressure by pulling back on the plunger of the attached syringe as the needle is moved back and forth at the biopsy site. There is relatively less discomfort with this procedure than with a tissue biopsy that requires opening the surface of the skin to localize the tissue site. Normal findings indicate no abnormal cells or tissues on histologic examination.

The **Papanicolaou smear** is a procedure commonly used for the cytologic examination of the female reproductive tract. Cells from body tissues and fluids (from the vagina or cervix) are stained and examined for the number and types of cells and abnormalities in their morphology. Specimens also may be obtained from the mouth, nipple discharge, or amniotic, pleural, or spinal fluid aspirations. The Papanicolaou smear is particularly useful for diagnosis of premalignant (dysplastic), malignant, atypical, and inflammatory cells.

Evaluations of the breast are commonly performed to detect tumors. Mammography, thermography, and biopsy are specific examination techniques. **Mammography** is a low-dose radiographic examination used to identify nonpalpable (less than 1 cm) or unrecognized lesions. Breast cancer can be detected by radiography 2 to 3 years before its clinical presentation, providing an excellent prognosis for cure. The American Cancer Society (ACS) (1992) recommends a baseline mammogram of all women at 40 years of age, annual or biannual mammogram between 40 and 49 years, and yearly mammogram after age 50.

Thermography is a method of measuring patterns of temperature distribution by using an infrared camera for photography. The pictorial representation of the normal breast has an even distribution of temperature patterns. With increased or decreased blood supply these areas are represented as hot spots (black areas) or cold spots (white areas) on a thermogram. Infection, tumor, and fibrocystic tissue are associated with hot spots, making the test nonspecific. False negatives are also possible because not all breast cancers are associated with increased blood supply. However, because the test is easy and inexpensive, it may be used for screening and followed by other diagnostic procedures.

Fertility Tests

Tests of reproductive function are performed most commonly when infertility exists. Both the male and female partners are examined, and several diagnostic evaluations may be completed. The types of tests and their normal values are summarized in Tables 19-4 and 19-5. The man must have normal number, amount, structure, and motility of sperm, with no obstruction along the reproductive tract. Tests for women determine whether (1) the reproductive tract (cervix, uterus, fallopian tubes) is adequately patent to allow for passage of ovum and sperm, (2) ovulation occurs normally, (3) the endometrium is responding normally to hormones, and (4) reproductive tissues are free of tumors or infections. Hormonal assays evaluate the adequacy of pituitary function and target organ response. The position and size of organs or the presence of tumors can be detected by direct observation procedures using a laparoscope or by radiographic studies, such as plain films, computerized scans, or tomography.

❏ AGING and Reproductive Function
Aging and the Female Reproductive System

Menopause is a normal developmental event that is universally experienced by middle-aged women. The average age at which menopause occurs is 50 to 51 years and does not appear to be affected by age at menarche, childbearing, weight, socioeconomic factors, or race. Because life expectancy has increased significantly, women can now expect to spend one third of their lives after their last menstrual period.

The physiologic changes of menopause are primarily caused by declining ovarian function and a resulting decrease in ovarian hormone secretion. During the 5 to 10 years before menopause, approximately 90% of women note extreme variability in the frequency of menstruation and in the quality of menstrual flow. This transitional interval begins with the onset of changes in ovarian function, including decreased frequency of ovulation, reduced estrogen production by the ovaries, and, finally, menopause. Primordial follicles are present in the ovaries, but they apparently resist gonadotropin stimulation. It is not clear exactly what mechanisms cause this resistance.

Hormonal findings during the years surrounding menopause include significantly elevated FSH and LH levels and maintenance of pulsatile secretion by the pituitary. In the ovary, however, the follicle and corpus luteum no longer develop and thus do not secrete estradiol and progesterone. Therefore, serum levels of both these hormones decline. The stroma of the ovaries does continue to secrete androstenedione, which is converted peripherally to estrone (a form of estrogen). The conversion takes place in adipose tissue; therefore, obese women tend to have higher serum levels of estrone. The physiologic role of estrone is not clearly understood, but increased estrone levels (unopposed by progesterone) are associated with an increased incidence of endometrial cancer. This may account for the higher incidence of endometrial cancer in obese women.

As ovarian function diminishes, breast tissue begins to become involuted. Two phases of involution have been described: (1) the premenopausal phase and (2) the menopausal phase. The premenopausal phase occurs between 35 and 45 years of age. During this phase, there is a moderate decrease in mammary tissue. During the menopausal phase, glandular breast tissue is significantly reduced, and there is some increase of fat deposits and connective tissue. These changes contribute to the reduction in size and firmness of breast tissue.

Several systemic changes are associated with declining ovarian function. They include changes in vasomotor tone, urogenital structures, bone density, and artery walls. The severity of these changes may depend on such variables as the rate at which tissue levels of estradiol decline. Vasomotor changes can cause a hot flash, or **vasomotor flush.** This event is characterized by a rise in skin temperature, dilation of peripheral blood vessels, changes of electrical resistance in the skin, and transient increase in heart rate. Vasomotor flush usually occurs in the face and neck initially and may progress to the chest. The flush may be accompanied by dizziness, nausea, headaches, palpitations, diaphoresis (sweating), or night sweats. Vasomotor flushes vary in intensity and in duration, lasting from 1 to 4 minutes. Approximately 75% to 85% of all menopausal women experience vasomotor flushes. Most have symptoms for more than 1 year, and 25% have symptoms for more than 5 years. Vasomotor flushes apparently are triggered by estrogen withdrawal rather than estrogen lack. They can be triggered also by emotional stress, excitement, fear, or anxiety. The exact causal mechanisms are not known.

The urogenital tract undergoes a number of changes. The ovaries begin to decrease in size around the age of 30 years, and shrinkage accelerates after the age of 60. During the years surrounding menopause, the uterus atrophies and decreases in size. The vagina shortens, narrows, and loses some of its elasticity. Vaginal walls lose their ability to lubricate quickly. When sexually aroused, menopausal women may take 1 to 3 minutes to lubricate compared to premenopausal women, who take 6 to 30 seconds. Intercourse before adequate lubrication may be painful. The vaginal pH, usually maintained at 4.0 to 6.0 as a result of estrogen stimulation, increases to between 6.5 and 8.0 and contributes to a higher incidence of vaginitis. The cervix atrophies, and the cervical os decreases in size. The vaginal epithelium also atrophies; this atrophy can cause vaginal irritation, burning, itching (pruritus), white discharge (leukorrhea), painful intercourse (dyspareunia), and vaginal bleeding. The labia majora and minora become less prominent, and some pubic hair is lost. Urethral tone declines, as does muscle tone throughout the pelvic area. Urinary frequency or urgency, urinary tract infections, and incontinence are thought to be associated with menopausal changes because these symptoms diminish with estrogen therapy (Droegemueller, Herbst, Mischell, & Stenchever, 1987). For unknown reasons, sexually active women have less vaginal atrophy. Regular intercourse, once or twice a week, and masturbation are associated with continued rapid lubrication when sexually aroused, vaginal pliability, and function. Women approaching menopause who have weekly intercourse tend to have higher estrogen levels and milder, if any, hot flashes (Golub, 1992).

Loss of bone mass is also associated with menopause. Bone mass reaches a peak in the early 30s and then begins to decline. The decline amounts to 1% to 2% per year after menopause. Insufficient bone mass leads to increased brittleness and porosity of bone (osteoporosis), predisposing some women to pathologic bone fractures, usually after the age of 60. It is not understood how diminished estrogen production causes loss of bone mass. Bone loss appears to be prevented by estrogen therapy, however, and can be minimized with weight-bearing exercise, proper nutrition, and adequate calcium intake. Smoking doubles a woman's risk for the development of osteoporosis, as does intake of more than two alcoholic drinks per day. Calcium intake in childhood and adolescence determines peak bone mass in adulthood. Those with greater bone mass are less likely to develop osteoporosis after menopause. Increased calcium intake during the postmenopausal years does not appear to prevent osteoporosis.

Premenopausal women have significantly lower risk of developing coronary heart disease than do age-matched men, but immediately after menopause, women are at increased risk of coronary disease. This increase is significant after the age of 55. Levels of serum cholesterol, triglycerides, and iron increase after menopause, whether the menopause is spontaneous or surgically induced, increasing the risk of coronary disease.

The assumption that menopause is a distressing and depressing time is prevalent, but systematic investigations have failed to identify a psychologic syndrome associated with menopause. It may be that responses to the physiologic changes of menopause are influenced by other life changes that tend to occur in the 50s. During these years a woman may be coping with increased responsibility for aging parents, loss of parents, changes in the dependent status of children, daily care of grandchildren, or illness of significant others.

Aging and the Male Reproductive System

Men maintain reproductive capacity longer than women, despite the popular perception that men over the age of 50 are somehow sexually impaired. There is no known discrete event, comparable to menopause, that characterizes aging of the male reproductive system. Changes do occur, however, in male sexual behavior and in testicular structure and function, including hormonal secretion and spermatogenesis.

Components of male sexual behavior include both sexual drive and erectile/ejaculatory capacity. **Libido,** or sexual drive, is a complex phenomenon that requires a baseline hormonal milieu but is influenced significantly by health status and environmental, social, and psychologic factors. Aging causes specific physical changes that influence erectile and ejaculatory capabilities. Alterations in sexual response include the need for longer stimulation to achieve full erection, slower and less forceful ejaculation, with less pelvic muscle involvement; decreased vasocongestive re-

sponse; and longer refractory period (time during which erection and ejaculation are not possible), up to 24 hours in some males.

The testes undergo several age-related structural changes, including decreased weight, atrophy, and softening. Degenerative changes in the seminiferous tubules may include thickening of the basement membrane; increase in lumen size; germ cell (spermatogonium) arrest and a decrease in spermatogenic activity; and collapse of tubules, followed by complete obstruction caused by sclerosis and fibrosis. Areas of mild to severe degenerative change may be interspersed with areas having intact tubules. These morphologic changes may result from atherosclerosis (arterial clogging) in the testicular vascular bed (Mastroianni & Coutifaris, 1990). Alterations of the seminiferous tubules do not appear to diminish sperm counts, but they do reduce fertility because a greater percentage of the sperm lack motility or have structural abnormalities.

Aging probably causes changes in the production of male sex hormones and responsiveness of target tissues. Hormone synthesis by the testes, testicular responsiveness to the gonadotropins (FSH and LH), and pituitary secretion of these gonadotropins are altered. Most studies of testosterone levels in aging men show that their serum testosterone levels are lower than levels in younger men (Brenner, Vitiello, & Primz, 1983; Royer, Seckman, Schwartz, Bennett, & Hendrix, 1984; Vermeulen, Rubens, & Verdonck, 1972).

The reduced levels of testosterone may be related to alterations in the Leydig cells, the testosterone producers of the testes. The number of Leydig cells decreases as age increases, perhaps because of atherosclerotic changes in arteries that supply blood to the testes. Even if testosterone levels are not decreased, older men may have less unbound testosterone in their blood, decreasing the amount of unbound hormone available to stimulate target tissues. Decreased testosterone levels have several effects, including functional deterioration of the accessory sex organs (the prostate gland, seminal vesicles, epididymis, and ductus deferens); loss of muscle mass, strength, and endurance; and, in many men, decrease in libido. This last effect may also be caused by alterations in other variables that affect libido.

Serum levels of the gonadotropins, particularly FSH, increase with age. The change in gonadotropin secretion may result from primary testicular failure or from some hypothalamic-pituitary dysregulation of the gonadotropins.

Androgen replacement therapy is problematic because androgens have adverse systemic effects. Androgens are associated with coronary atherosclerosis, exacerbations of benign prostatic hypertrophy, and induction of prostatic carcinoma (Mastroianni & Coutifaris, 1990).

SUMMARY REVIEW

Development of the Reproductive Systems

1 Differentiation of female and male genitalia begins in the eighth week of embryonic development, when the gonads of genetically male embryos begin to secrete male sex hormones, primarily testosterone. Until that time, the primitive reproductive organs of males and females are homologous (the same).

2 The structure and function of both male and female reproductive systems are controlled by the hypothalamic-pituitary-ovarian axis, a set of complex neurologic and hormonal interactions that accelerate at puberty, causing sexual maturation and making reproduction possible.

3 Extrahypothalamic factors cause the hypothalamus to secrete gonadotropin-releasing hormone (GnRH), which stimulates the anterior pituitary to secrete gonadotropins—follicle-stimulating hormone (FSH) and luteinizing hormone (LH)—which stimulate the gonads (ovaries or testes) to secrete female or male sex hormones.

4 Production of primitive female gametes (ova) occurs solely during fetal life. From puberty to menopause, one female gamete matures per menstrual cycle. Production of the male gametes (sperm) begins at puberty; after that, millions are produced daily, normally for life.

The Female Reproductive System

1 The function of the reproductive system is to produce mature ova and, when they are fertilized, to protect and nourish them through embryonic and fetal life and expel them at birth.

2 The external female genitalia are the mons pubis, labia majora, labia minora, clitoris, vestibule (urinary and vaginal openings), Bartholin glands, and Skene glands.

3 The internal female genitalia are the vagina, uterus, fallopian tubes, and ovaries. Although all of these organs are needed for reproduction, the ovaries are the most essential because they produce the female gametes and female sex hormones.

4 The vagina is a fibromuscular canal that receives the penis during sexual intercourse and is the exit route for menstrual fluids and products of conception. The vagina leads from the introitus (its external opening) to the cervical portion of the uterus.

5 The uterus is the hollow, muscular organ in which a fertilized ovum develops until birth. The uterine walls have three layers: the endometrium (lining), myometrium (muscular layer), and perimetrium (outer covering, which is continuous with the pelvic peritoneum). The endometrium proliferates (thickens) and sloughs off in response to cyclic changes in levels of female sex hormones. The cervix is the narrow, lower portion of the uterus that opens into the vagina.

6 The two fallopian tubes extend from the uterus to the ovaries. Their function is to conduct ova from the spaces around the ovaries to the uterus. Fertilization normally occurs in the fallopian tubes.

7 From puberty to menopause, the ovaries are the site of (a) ovum maturation and release and (b) production of female sex hormones (estrogen and progesterone) and androgens. The female sex hormones are involved in sexual differentiation and development, the menstrual cycle, pregnancy, and lactation. Although they are primarily male sex hormones, androgens in women contribute to the prepubertal growth spurt, pubic and axillary hair growth, and activation of sebaceous glands.

8 Estrogen (primarily estradiol) is produced by cells in the developing ovarian follicle (structure that encloses the ovum). Progesterone is produced by cells of the corpus luteum, the structure that develops from the ruptured ovarian follicle after ovulation (ovum release). Androgens are produced within the ovarian follicle, adrenal glands, and adipose tissue.

9 The average menstrual cycle takes 27 to 30 days and consists of four phases, which are named for ovarian and endometrial changes: the follicular/proliferative phase, ovulation, the luteal/secretory phase, and menstruation.

10 Ovarian events of the menstrual cycle are controlled by gonadotropins. High FSH levels stimulate follicle and ovum maturation (follicular phase); then a surge of LH causes ovulation, which is followed by development of the corpus luteum (luteal phase).

11 Uterine (endometrial) events of the menstrual cycle are caused by ovarian hormones. During the follicular phase of the ovarian cycle, estrogen produced by the follicle causes the endometrium to proliferate (proliferative phase). During the luteal phase, estrogen maintains the thickened endometrium while progesterone causes it to develop blood vessels and secretory glands (secretory phase). As the corpus luteum degenerates, production of both hormones drops sharply, and the "starved" endometrium degenerates and sloughs off, causing menstruation.

12 Cyclic changes in hormone levels also cause thinning and thickening of the vaginal epithelium, thinning and thickening of cervical secretions, and changes in basal body temperature.

The Male Reproductive System

1 The function of the male reproductive system is to produce male gametes (sperm) and deliver them to the female reproductive tract.

2 The external male genitalia are the testes, epididymides, scrotum, and penis. The internal genitalia are the vas deferens, ejaculatory duct, prostatic and membranous sections of the urethra, seminal vesicles, prostate gland, and Cowper glands.

3 The testes (male gonads) are paired glands suspended within the scrotum. The testes have two functions: spermatogenesis (sperm production) and production of male sex hormones (androgens, chiefly testosterone).

4 The epididymis is a long, coiled tube arranged in a comma-shaped compartment that curves over the top and rear of the testis. The epididymis receives sperm from the testis and stores them while they develop further. Sperm travel the length of the epididymis and then are ejaculated into the vas deferens.

5 The scrotum is a skin-covered, fibromuscular sac that encloses the testes and epididymides, which are suspended within the scrotum by the spermatic cord. The scrotum keeps these organs at optimal temperatures for sperm survival (about 1 to 2 degrees lower than body temperature) by contracting in cold environments and relaxing in warm environments.

6 The penis is a cylindrical organ consisting of three longitudinal compartments (two corpora cavernosa and one corpus spongiosum) and the urethra. The urethra runs through the corpus spongiosum. The corpora cavernosa and corpus spongiosum consist of erectile tissue. Externally the penis consists of a shaft and a tip, which is called the glans. The glans contains sebaceous glands and the opening of the urethra. It is covered by a flap of skin (the foreskin), which may be removed in a procedure called circumcision.

7 The penis has two functions: delivery of sperm to the female vagina and elimination of urine. Semen (sperm and glandular secretions) and urine both leave the penis through the urethra, but these two fluids are never in the urethra at the same time.

8 Sexual intercourse is made possible by the erectile reflex, in which tactile or psychogenic stimulation of the parasympathetic nerves causes arterioles in the corpora cavernosa and corpus spongiosum to dilate and fill with blood, causing the penis to enlarge and become firm.

9 Emission, which occurs at the peak of sexual arousal, is the movement of semen from the epididymides to the penis. Ejaculation, which is a continuation of emission, is the pulsatile ejection of semen from the penis. Both emission and ejaculation involve rhythmic contractions of smooth muscle within the internal glands and ducts.

10 Spermatogenesis is a continuous process because spermatogonia, the primitive male gametes, undergo continuous mitosis within the seminiferous tubules of the testes. Some of the spermatogonia develop into primary spermatocytes, which divide meiotically into secondary spermatocytes, then spermatids. The spermatids develop into sperm with the help of nutrients and hormonal signals from Sertoli cells.

11 Production of the male sex hormones is controlled (like production of the female sex hormones) by the hypothalamic-pituitary-gonadal axis and by complex feedback mechanisms. The male hormones are produced steadily rather than cyclically, however.

Structure and Function of the Breast

1 Until puberty the female and male breasts are similar, consisting of a small, underdeveloped nipple, some fatty and fibrous tissue, and a few ductlike structures under the areola. At puberty, however, a variety of hormones (estrogen, progesterone, prolactin, growth hormone, insulin, and cortisol) cause the female breast to develop into a system of glands and ducts that is capable of producing and ejecting milk.

2 The basic functional unit of the female breast is the lobe, a system of ducts that branches from the nipple to milk-producing units called lobules. The lobules contain acini, which are convoluted spaces lined with epithelial cells that secrete milk and subepithelial cells that contract, moving the milk into the system of ducts that leads to the nipple.

3 Each breast contains 15 to 20 lobes, which are separated and supported by Cooper ligaments.

4 Milk production occurs in response to prolactin, a hormone that is secreted in larger amounts after childbirth. Milk ejection is under the control of oxytocin, another hormone of pregnancy and parturition.

5 During the reproductive years, breast tissue undergoes cyclic changes in response to hormonal changes of the menstrual cycle.

Tests of Reproductive Function

1 Diagnostic tests are performed to evaluate fertility or presence of tumors, infection, or sexually transmitted diseases.

2 Smears, stains, cultures, and serologic tests are used to diagnose infections. These tests specifically identify microorganisms or types of infections.

3 Tissue biopsy can be performed by resection or needle aspiration. Specimen analysis permits identification of abnormal cells.

4 The Papanicolaou smear is a cytologic examination of cells taken from body fluids and tissues. Although cells can be obtained from many sites, the smear is most commonly used (with endocervical cells) for diagnosis of cervical carcinoma.

5 Mammography is a low-dose radiographic examination of the breast for cancer detection.

6 Thermography measures patterns of temperature variation. The test is useful for identifying sites of infection or tumor growth, which frequently have an increased blood supply and show as "hot spots."

7 Evaluation of fertility includes reproductive hormone assays and assessment of structural alteration or infections and the determination of normal ovulation or adequate sperm motility and count.

Aging and Reproductive Function

1 In women, the reproductive years end with menopause, which occurs at the average age of 51. At menopause, the menstrual cycle ceases and levels of sex hormones decrease.
2 Reduced levels of female sex hormones cause all the reproductive organs to atrophy. In addition, the vaginal epithelium thins, and glandular secretions diminish and become more alkaline. Continued sexual activity and orgasm reduce vaginal changes.
3 Nonreproductive effects of reduced estrogen levels include increased risk of osteoporosis and coronary artery disease.

4 Male reproductive function diminishes with age, but it does not cease in healthy men.
5 The testes atrophy and produce less testosterone, and some seminiferous tubules may degenerate and become fibrotic. These changes affect sex drive (libido) and sperm morphology. Although sperm count remains normal, the semen tends to contain more defective and nonmotile sperm.
6 The erectile reflex is somewhat diminished and occurs more slowly as age advances.
7 Reduced testosterone levels cause some loss of function in the internal genitalia and enlargement (hypertrophy) of the prostate gland.

KEY TERMS

Acinus of breast, 733
Androgen, 723
Areola, 734
Bartholin gland (greater vestibular gland), 716
Breast, 733
Cervix, 718
Clitoris, 716
Cornification, 726
Corpus cavernosum, 730
Corpus luteum, 719
Corpus spongiosum, 730
Corpus of uterus (body of uterus), 718
Cowper's gland (bulbourethral gland), 731
Cul-de-sac, 716
Culture, 735
Decornification, 726
Efferent tubule, 727
Ejaculatory duct, 730
Emission, 730
Endocervical canal, 718
Endometrium, 718
Epididymis, 728
Erectile reflex, 730
Estradiol, 721
Estrogen, 721
Fallopian tube (oviduct, uterine tube), 719
Fimbriae, 719
Follicle-stimulating hormone (FSH), 714
Follicular/proliferative phase, 723
Foreskin (prepuce), 730
Fornix, 716
Fundus of uterus, 718
Glands of Montgomery, 734

Glans, 730
Gonad, 712
Gonadotropin, 714
Gonadotropin-releasing hormone (GnRH), 714
Granulosa cell, 719
Infundibulum, 719
Inguinal canal, 726
Inhibin, 723
Introitus, 716
Isthmus, 718
Labium majus (labia majora), 716
Labium minus (labia minora), 716
Leydig cell, 727
Libido, 740
Luteal/secretory phase, 723
Luteinizing hormone (LH), 714
Mammography, 738
Menarche, 723
Menopause, 723
Menstruation (menses), 723
Mons pubis, 715
Myometrium, 718
Needle biopsy, 735
Nipple, 734
Ovarian cycle, 719
Ovarian follicle, 719
Ovary, 719
Ovulation, 719
Ovum, 711
Papanicolaou smear, 738
Penis, 728
Perimetrium (parietal peritoneum), 718
Perineal body, 716
Perineum, 716
Primary spermatocyte, 731
Progesterone, 722
Prostate gland, 730

Rete testis, 727
Ruga (rugae; pertains to vagina and testes), 716
Scrotum, 728
Secondary spermatocyte, 731
Semen, 730
Seminal vesicle, 730
Seminiferous tubule, 727
Serologic test, 735
Sertoli cell (nondividing support cell), 731
Sex hormone, 712
Skene gland (lesser vestibular gland), 716
Spermatic cord, 726
Spermatid, 731
Spermatogenesis, 727
Spermatogonia, 731
Spermatozoon (sperm cell), 711
Squamous-columnar junction, 719
Testis, 726
Testosterone, 712
Theca cell, 719
Thelarche, 734
Thermography, 738
Tissue biopsy, 735
Tubulus rectus, 727
Tunica albuginea, 727
Tunica dartos, 728
Tunica vaginalis, 726
Urethra, 730
Urinary meatus, 716
Uterus, 717
Vagina, 716
Vas deferens (ductus deferens), 728
Vasomotor flush, 739
Vestibule, 716
Vulva, 715

REFERENCES

American Cancer Society (ACS). (1992). *Cancer facts and figures 1992*. Atlanta: Author.

Berne, R. M., & Levy, M. N. (Eds.). (1992). *Physiology* (3rd ed.). St. Louis: Mosby–Year Book.

Bobak, I. M., Jensen, M. D., & Zalar, M. K. (1992). *Maternity and gynecologic care: The nurse and the family* (5th ed.). St. Louis: Mosby–Year Book.

Brenner, W. J., Vitiello, M. V., & Primz, P. N. (1983). A loss of circadian rhythmicity in blood testosterone levels with aging in normal men. *Journal of Clinical Endocrine Metabolism, 56*, 1278-1281.

Golub, S. (1992). *Periods: From menarche to menopause*. Newbury Park: Sage.

Herbst, A. L., Mischell, D. R., Stenchever, M. A., & Droegemueller, W. D. (1992). *Comprehensive gynecology* (2nd ed.). St. Louis: Mosby–Year Book.

Mastroianni, L., & Coutifaris, C. (1990). *Reproductive physiology* (vol. 1). New Jersey: Parthenon Publishing.

Royer, G. L., Seckman, C. E., Schwartz, J. H., Bennett, K. P., & Hendrix, J. W. (1984). Relationship between age and levels of total, free, and bound testosterone in healthy subjects. *Current Therapeutic Research, 35*, 345-353.

Seidel, H. M., Ball, J. W., & Benedict, G. W. (1991). *Mosby's guide to physical examination* (2nd ed.). St. Louis: Mosby–Year Book.

Speroff, L., Glass, R. H., & Kase, N. G. (1989). *Clinical gynecology, endocrinology, and infertility* (4th ed.). Baltimore: Williams & Wilkins.

Tanagho, E. A., & McAninch (Eds.). (1992). *Smith's general urology* (13th ed.). Norwalk, CT: Appleton-Lange.

Thibodeau, G. A. (1992). *Structure and function of the body*. St. Louis: Mosby–Year Book.

Thompson, J. M., McFarland, G., Hirsch, J., & Tucker, S. (1993). *Mosby's clinical nursing* (3rd ed.). St. Louis: Mosby–Year Book.

Vermeulen, A., Rubens, R., & Verdonck, L. (1972). Testosterone secretion and metabolism in male senescence. *Journal of Clinical Endocrine Metabolism, 34*, 730-735.

SUGGESTED READINGS

Beard, M., & Curtis, L. (1991). *Menopause and the years ahead* (rev. ed.). Tucson, AZ: Fisher Books.

Davies, T. F., & Kase, N. G. (1990). Male reproduction. In N. Kase, A. B. Weingold, & D. M. Gershenson (Eds.), *Principles and practice of clinical gynecology* (2nd ed.). New York: Churchill Livingstone.

Gordon, T., Castelli, W. P., Hjortland, M. C., & McNamara, P. M. (1978). Menopause and coronary heart disease: The Framingham study. *Annals of Internal Medicine, 89*, 157-161.

Hammond, K. R., & Steinkampf, M. P. (1992, September). Assessing ovulatory function. *Contemporary OB/GYN*, 29-42.

Hatcher, R. A., Stewart, F., Trussell, J., Kowal, D., Guest, F., Stewart, G. K., & Cates, W. (1990). *Contraceptive technology 1990-1992* (15th rev. ed.). New York: Irvington Publishers.

Kase, N. G., Weingold, A. B., & Gershenson, D. M. (Eds.). (1990). *Principles and practice of clinical gynecology* (2nd ed.). New York: Churchill Livingstone.

Lichtman, R., & Papera, S. (1990). *Gynecology: well woman care*. Norwalk, CT: Appleton-Lange.

Swerdloff, R. S., & Heber, D. (1982). Effects of aging on male reproductive function. In S. G. Korenman (Ed.), *Endocrine aspects of aging*. New York: Elsevier.

Valenta, L. H., & Elias, A. N. (1983). Pituitary-gonadal function in the aging male: The male climacteric. *Geriatrics, 38*(12), 67-72.

Yen, S. S. C., & Jaffe, R. B. (1991). *Reproductive endocrinology: Physiology, pathophysiology, and clinical management*. Philadelphia: Saunders.

CHAPTER 20

Alterations of the Reproductive System

Kristynia M. Robinson

Kathryn L. McCance

D. Patricia Gray*

Chapter Outline

*Contributing author to first edition.

lterations of the reproductive system span a wide range of concerns from delayed sexual development and suboptimal sexual performance to structural and functional difficulties. Many common reproductive disorders carry potentially serious physiologic or psychologic consequences. For example, sexual or reproductive dysfunction, such as impotence or infertility, can dramatically affect self-concept, relationships, and overall quality of life. Prostate cancer is the second most common cause of cancer deaths in men, and breast cancer, the number one cancer in women, is the second most frequent cause of death in women. Conversely, organic and psychosocial problems, such as alcoholism, depression, situational stressors, chronic illness, and medications, can affect ovulation and menstruation, sexual performance, and fertility and may be risk factors for the development of some types of reproductive tract cancers. Diagnosis and treatment of reproductive system disorders, however, are often complicated because of the stigma and symbolism associated with the reproductive organs and the emotion-laden beliefs and behaviors related to reproductive health. Treatment and diagnosis for any problem may be delayed because of embarrassment, guilt, fear, or denial.

ALTERATIONS OF SEXUAL MATURATION

A variety of congenital and endocrine disorders can disrupt the timing of puberty, or sexual maturation. These disorders may cause puberty to occur too late (delayed puberty) or too early (precocious puberty). Both types of disorders involve the inappropriate onset of sex hormone production by the gonads.

Delayed Puberty

The first sign of puberty in girls is thelarche, or breast development. Thelarche should begin by the time a girl is 13. In boys the first sign is enlargement of testes and thinning of the scrotal skin; this should happen by age

---

CAUSES OF DELAYED PUBERTY

I. Deficiency of GnRH secretion by hypothalamus
   A. Genetic
      1. Familial
      2. Kallman syndrome
      3. Laurence-Moon-Biedl syndrome
      4. Prader-Willi syndrome
   B. Acquired
      1. Infections
         a. Encephalitis
         b. Granuloma
      2. Neoplasms
         a. Hypothalamus
         b. Pineal region
II. Deficiency of gonadotropic secretion by pituitary
   A. Genetic
      1. Panhypopituitarism
      2. Isolated gonadotropin deficiency
      3. Fertile eunuch (normal FSH, low LH)
   B. Acquired
      1. Infections
      2. Neoplasms
      3. After trauma
III. Gonadal disorders
   A. Genetic
      1. Turner syndrome (45, X or structural X abnormalities or mosaicism)
      2. Klinefelter syndrome (47, XXY)

      3. Noonan syndrome
      4. Syndromes of complete androgen insensitivity (no pubic hair)
      5. Del Castillo syndrome (Sertoli cells only)
      6. Pure gonadal dysgenesis
      7. Myotonic dystrophy
   B. Acquired
      1. Infections
         a. Gonorrhea (male)
         b. Virus (usually mumps—male)
         c. Tuberculosis (male)
      2. Radiotherapy or chemotherapy
      3. Mechanical causes
         a. After torsion
         b. After surgery
IV. Adrenal and gonadal steroid enzyme deficiencies
V. Chronic systemic diseases
   A. Congenital heart disease
   B. Chronic pulmonary disease
   C. Inflammatory bowel disease
   D. Chronic renal failure and renal tubular acidosis
   E. Hypothyroidism
   F. Poorly controlled diabetes mellitus
   G. Sickle cell anemia
   H. Collagen-vascular disease
   I. Anorexia nervosa

From Hoekelman, Friedman, Nelson, & Seidel, 1992.

14. In **delayed puberty,** these secondary sex characteristics show no sign of appearing in a girl of 13 or a boy of 14.

In 90% to 95% of cases, the delayed puberty is a constitutional delay; that is, hormonal levels are normal and the hypothalamic-pituitary-ovarian axis is intact, but maturation is happening slowly. Constitutional delay is much more common in boys than in girls.

The other 5% of cases are caused by some disruption of the hypothalamic-pituitary-gonadal axis or by a systemic disease. The disruption can consist of deficient secretion of gonadotropin-releasing hormone (GnRH) by the hypothalamus, deficient gonadotropin secretion by the pituitary, or gonadal disorders. Treatment of pathophysiologic delayed puberty depends on the cause. Insufficient sex hormone secretion can be corrected by hormone replacement therapy.

Constitutional delay seldom requires treatment, unless the delayed puberty is causing psychosocial problems. The well-being of a boy with constitutional delay sometimes is improved by a short course of testosterone replacement, which accelerates development.

Precocious Puberty

Precocious puberty is the onset of sexual maturation before the age of 8 in girls and 9 in boys. Precocity is 5 times more common in girls than boys, with 75% of precocity in girls being idiopathic. Although boys are affected less often, the cause is more likely to be organic.

Precocious puberty occurs in three forms: isosexual, heterosexual, and incomplete. **Isosexual precocious puberty** is premature development of appropriate characteristics for the child's sex. In true isosexual precocious puberty, the hypothalamic-pituitary-ovarian axis is working normally but prematurely. In pseudoprecocious puberty, the sex hormones are being produced by some mechanism other than stimulation by the gonadotropins.

Heterosexual precocious puberty causes the child to develop some secondary sex characteristics of the opposite sex. This condition is usually evident at birth and is rare in older children.

Incomplete precocious puberty is the partial development of appropriate secondary sex characteristics. A girl with incomplete precocious puberty might undergo only thelarche or adrenarche (growth of pubic hair). Premature thelarche is seen in girls between 6 months and 2 years of age. It does not progress to complete puberty (ovulation and menstruation). Premature adrenarche tends to occur between the ages of 5 and 8. This condition can progress to complete precocious puberty.

All forms of precocious puberty are treated by identifying and removing the underlying cause or administering appropriate hormones. In many cases, precocious puberty can be reversed. The most common form, idiopathic isosexual precocity, is difficult to treat. Besides the premature development of secondary sex characteristics, it can cause long bones to stop growing before the child has reached normal height.

CAUSES OF ISOSEXUAL PRECOCIOUS PUBERTY

I. True puberty (with gonadotropin secretion)
  A. Idiopathic (constitutional predisposition)
  B. CNS abnormalities
    1. Congenital anomalies (hydrocephalus)
    2. Tumors (hypothalamic, pineal, other)
    3. Hamartoma
    4. Postinflammatory condition
    5. Trauma
    6. Syndromes
      a. McCune-Albright (polyostotic fibrous dysplasia)
      b. Neurofibromatosis
      c. Tuberous sclerosis
  C. Hypothyroidism (severe)
  D. Ectopic gonadotropin-secreting tumors (chorioepithelioma, hepatoblastoma, teratoma)
II. Pseudopuberty
  A. Exogenous sex steroids
  B. Gonadal tumors
    1. Ovarian
    2. Testicular

From Hoekelman, Friedman, Nelson, & Seidel, 1992.

CAUSES OF HETEROSEXUAL PRECOCIOUS PUBERTY

I. Female
  A. Congenital adrenal hyperplasia
  B. Androgen-secreting tumors
    1. Adrenal
    2. Ovarian
    3. Teratoma
II. Male
  A. Estrogen-producing tumors
    1. Adrenal
    2. Teratoma
  B. Exogenous estrogens

From Hoekelman, Friedman, Nelson, & Seidel, 1992.

DISORDERS OF THE FEMALE REPRODUCTIVE SYSTEM

Hormonal and Menstrual Alterations

Primary Dysmenorrhea

Primary dysmenorrhea is painful menstruation associated with ovulation but not associated with pelvic disease. More than 50% of women between the ages of 15 and 25 are affected, some (5% to 10%) severely enough to miss work or school. Dysmenorrhea usually begins with the onset of ovulatory cycles, around the age of 15 or 16 years. The incidence steadily rises, peaks in women in their mid-20s, and decreases slowly thereafter.

Pathophysiology

Dysmenorrhea is the result of excessive endometrial prostaglandin production and effect. Women with painful periods produce 10 times as much prostaglandin F ($PGF_{2\alpha}$) as asymptomatic women (Pickles, Hall, & Best, 1965). Likewise, compared with proliferative endometrium, secretory endometrium produces higher levels of prostaglandins. These lipid hormones increase myometrial contractions and constrict endometrial blood vessels, causing ischemia, endometrial bleeding, and pain.

Women who are anovulatory because they use oral contraceptives do not have primary dysmenorrhea. In these women, the progestin (synthetic progesterone) and estrogen in the pill decrease prostaglandin synthesis and myometrial contractility.

Clinical Manifestations

The chief symptom of dysmenorrhea is pelvic pain associated with the onset of menses. The pain frequently radiates into the groin and may be accompanied by backache, anorexia, vomiting, diarrhea, syncope, and headache. The latter symptoms are caused by entry of prostaglandins and prostaglandin metabolites into the systemic circulation. Usually, the discomfort associated with primary dysmenorrhea begins shortly before the onset of menstruation and rarely persists beyond the second day.

Evaluation and Treatment

Primary dysmenorrhea must be differentiated from secondary dysmenorrhea caused by disorders such as endometriosis, pelvic adhesions, inflammatory disease, or uterine fibroid. A thorough medical history and pelvic examination are completed to exclude pelvic pathology.

In women who desire contraception, primary dysmenorrhea can be relieved with oral contraceptives. Prostaglandin inhibitors work in 80% of cases and are most effective if started at the first sign of bleeding or cramping. A diet low in fat and regular exercise seem to prevent or reduce symptoms, and local application of heat, massage, relaxation techniques, and orgasm are common comfort measures.

Primary Amenorrhea

Amenorrhea means lack of menstruation. **Primary amenorrhea** is the failure of menarche and the absence of menstruation by the age of 14 without the development of secondary sex characteristics, or by age 16 regardless of the presence of secondary sex characteristics. The cause of primary amenorrhea includes a diverse group of abnormalities, such as congenital defects of gonadotropin production (Prader-Willi, Kallmann, and Laurence-Moon-Biedl syndromes); genetic disorders (Turner syndrome); congenital central nervous system defects, such as hydrocephalus; congenital anatomic malformations of the reproductive system (e.g., absence of vagina or uterus); and acquired central nervous system (CNS) lesions, including trauma, infection, and tumors.

Pathophysiology

In some of the congenital syndromes that cause primary amenorrhea, the hypothalamic-pituitary-ovarian axis is dysfunctional. The hypothalamus is unable to synthesize GnRH, so the pituitary fails to secrete luteinizing hormone (LH) and follicle-stimulating hormone (FSH). Therefore, the ovary does not receive the hormonal signals that normally initiate the ovarian and endometrial changes of the menstrual cycle, and ovulation and menstruation do not occur. Because the ovarian hormones are absent, secondary sex characteristics do not develop.

Some anatomic defects of the CNS, whether congenital or acquired, impinge on the hypothalamic-pituitary unit so as to interfere with or interrupt the secretion of GnRH or FSH and LH. Examples of such defects include hydrocephalus, craniopharyngiomas, and other space-occupying lesions of the central nervous system. Again the target organ, the ovary, does not receive the necessary signals, and ovulation and menstruation do not occur. In some cases these lesions develop between the onset and conclusion of puberty. Therefore skeletal growth may occur and secondary sex characteristics may develop, but sexual maturation is interrupted before menarche, which normally concludes puberty.

Anatomic defects of the genitalia also are associated with primary amenorrhea. They include congenital absence of the vagina and uterus and congenital uterine hypoplasia (infantile uterus). Females without a uterus or vagina usually have normal ovarian function. Therefore, skeletal growth occurs, and secondary sex characteristics develop in the proper sequence, but menstruation does not occur. In cases of uterine hypoplasia, the uterus does not respond to hormonal stimulation during puberty.

Several genetic disorders are associated with primary

amenorrhea. These include gonadal dysgenesis (Turner syndrome); testicular feminizing syndrome (male pseudohermaphroditism); and poly-X, or superfemale syndrome. With the chromosomal abnormalities of Turner syndrome (XO), the ovaries lack gametes, and ovarian failure is complete. Without primitive gametes and follicles, follicular development and estrogen secretion cannot occur. Lack of estrogen accounts for failure of secondary sex characteristic development, amenorrhea, and high levels of circulating FSH and LH. In male pseudohermaphroditism, the individual is male genetically but female morphologically. The individual does not develop male genitalia because androgen receptors are absent in undifferentiated target organs. The gonads are found either in the abdomen or in the inguinal canal, and they produce both androgens and estrogens. Because target tissues lack androgen receptors but have estrogen receptors, most individuals with male pseudohermaphroditism acquire female external genitalia and female secondary sex characteristics. With the exception of a small vagina, internal female genitalia are absent, accounting for amenorrhea and infertility.

Clinical Manifestations

The major clinical manifestation of primary amenorrhea is the absence of the menses. The cause of the amenorrhea determines whether secondary sex characteristics and height are affected.

Evaluation and Treatment

Diagnosis of primary amenorrhea is based on history and physical examination. If ovarian steroid hormone levels are low, the individual has the appearance of an immature female. Physical examination may show structural or physiologic alterations. Laboratory studies may be required to document abnormal levels of gonadotropins and ovarian hormones. Diagnostic imaging is used to document structural abnormalities.

Treatment involves correction of any underlying disorders and hormone replacement therapy to induce the development of secondary sex characteristics. Surgical alteration of the genitals may be undertaken to correct structural abnormalities. Hormonal manipulation or embryo transplantation may make pregnancy possible for women with primary amenorrhea.

Secondary Amenorrhea

Secondary amenorrhea is the absence of menstruation for a time equivalent to 3 or more cycles or 6 months in women who have previously menstruated. A wide variety of disorders and physiologic conditions are associated with secondary amenorrhea. Besides disease, secondary amenorrhea can be triggered by dramatic weight loss, whether the loss results from malnutrition or excessive exercise. Secondary amenorrhea is normal during early adolescence, pregnancy, and lactation and when approaching menopause.

FIG. 20-1 Cause of secondary amenorrhea.

Pathophysiology

The pathophysiology of secondary amenorrhea is summarized in Fig. 20-1. In women with normal ovarian steroid hormone levels, secondary amenorrhea is caused by structural abnormalities or removal of the uterus. In women with elevated ovarian steroid hormone levels, inhibited ovulation leads to amenorrhea. An excess of ovarian hormones apparently disrupts feedback relationships between the various hormones of the hypothalamic-pituitary-ovarian axis, preventing ovulation. Depressed ovarian hormone levels, which are associated with a variety of clinical disorders, also cause amenorrhea by preventing ovulation. Lack of ovulation, termed **anovulation**, may result from increased levels of prolactin, decreased levels of gonadotropins, irregular secretion of gonadotropins, or abnormally low levels of CNS neurotransmitters. Any of these variables alters the feedback effects that the ovarian hormones have on the hypothalamus and pituitary.

Hyperprolactinemia (overproduction of prolactin by the pituitary) may have short-loop feedback effects that lead to decreased secretion of GnRH by the hypothalamus. The result is a loss of pulsatile LH secretion and an overall reduction in LH levels. Anovulation and secondary amenorrhea may result. In the ovary, elevated prolactin levels appear to inhibit the secretion of progesterone by the granulosa cells of the follicle. This leads to anovulation caused by follicular atresia. These abnormalities may act singly or in combination to cause other alterations in the menstrual cycle.

Clinical Manifestations

The major manifestation of secondary amenorrhea is the absence of menses. Infertility, vasomotor flushes, vaginal atrophy, acne, and **hirsutism** (abnormal hairiness) also may be present, depending on the underlying cause of the amenorrhea.

Evaluation and Treatment

Diagnosis of secondary amenorrhea involves the identification of underlying hormonal or anatomic alterations. A woman with secondary amenorrhea and normal secondary sex characteristics should have a complete history and physical examination. Pregnancy is ruled out before any further workup is undertaken. Initial evaluation begins with a measurement of thyroid-stimulating hormone, a prolactin level, and a progesterone challenge to induce withdrawal bleeding. Further uterine challenge with estrogen and progesterone, radioimmunoassay levels of gonadotropins, x-rays, and computed tomography (CT) scans may be necessary to determine the cause of amenorrhea. Depending on the cause of the amenorrhea, treatment may involve hormone replacement therapy (e.g., estrogens, thyroid hormone, glucocorticoids, clomiphene citrate, gonadotropins, bromocriptine) or a corrective procedure, such as surgical removal of pituitary tumors.

Dysfunctional Uterine Bleeding

Menstrual concerns or abnormal bleeding patterns (Table 20-1) are common complaints. Approximately 33% of all gynecologic visits are for irregular genital bleeding. This proportion increases to 69% in the perimenopausal and postmenopausal age groups (Mencaglia, Perino, & Hamou, 1987). Failure to ovulate as an expression of age, stress, or endocrinopathy is the most common cause of cycle irregularity. Other causes include intrinsic uterine pathology, pregnancy and its complications, and hematologic disorders. A breakdown of common causes of abnormal bleeding based on age group and frequency is listed in Table 20-2.

Dysfunctional uterine bleeding (DUB) is abnormal uterine bleeding resulting from a disturbance of the menstrual cycle. It is not associated with other causes of abnormal uterine bleeding, such as tumor, infection,

---

TABLE 20-1

Abnormal Menstrual Bleeding

Term	Definition
Polymenorrhea	Cycles shorter than 3 weeks; may indicate disturbance in endocrine control of ovulation
Oligomenorrhea	Cycles longer than 6-7 weeks; may indicate disturbance in endocrine control of ovulation
Metrorrhagia	Intermenstrual bleeding or bleeding of light character occurring irregularly between cycles; may be a sign of organic disease
Hypermenorrhea	Excessive flow; may be a sign of organic disease
Menorrhea	Prolonged duration of flow
Menorrhagia	Increased amount and duration of flow
Menometrorrhagia	Prolonged flow associated with irregular and intermittent spotting between bleeding episodes

or systemic disease. Dysfunctional uterine bleeding affects 15% to 20% of all gynecologic women at some time during their menstrual life and accounts for 25% of gynecologic surgery (Weingold, 1990).

Pathophysiology

Dysfunctional uterine bleeding is most commonly associated with anovulatory menstrual cycles. Although it may occur at any time during the reproductive years, more than 50% of DUB occurs in premenopausal women aged 40 to 50 years. Symptoms of hypomenorrhea, followed by missed periods or prolonged intervals between menses, could mark the onset of physiologic ovarian exhaustion and menopause or may be an early sign of pathologically premature ovulatory failure and secondary amenorrhea. Other conditions associated with chronic anovulation include polycystic ovarian syndrome, immaturity of the hypothalamic-pituitary-ovarian axis, obesity, hyperthyroidism and hypothyroidism, and estrogen-secreting ovarian neoplasms.

Dysfunctional uterine bleeding secondary to ovarian dysfunction is a result of either progesterone deficiency or relative estrogen excess. In premenopausal women in their 40s and 50s, progesterone secretion is absent, but variable quantities of estrogen continue to be secreted by the granulosa–theca cell complex. Estrogen stimulates proliferation and hyperplasia of the endometrial glands. Without the usual stromal support induced by progesterone, irregular bleeding occurs.

Usually, with anovulation involving women in their late 30s and 40s, relative estrogen excess results in heavy bleeding. In this case, unopposed estrogen induces a progression of endometrial responses beginning with proliferation, hyperplasia, adenomatous hyperplasia, and, over a course of many years, may end with atypia and carcinoma. In the absence of growth-limiting progesterone and periodic desquamation, the endometrium attains an abnormal height with increasing hypervascularity and back-to-back glandularity, but without an intervening stromal support matrix.

Regardless of whether DUB is caused by progesterone deficiency or relative estrogen excess, the usual endometrial control mechanisms are missing. Menstrual flow is prolonged and excessive because of the large quantity of tissue available for bleeding and the random breakdown of tissue that results in exposure of vascular channels. Vasoconstrictive rhythmicity, tight coiling of spiral vessels, and orderly collapse are absent and stasis does not occur.

Dysfunctional uterine bleeding in ovulatory cycles is less common, and mechanisms underlying the bleeding are unclear. Excessive fibrinolytic activity and changes in prostaglandin production may be implicated.

Clinical Manifestations

Dysfunctional uterine bleeding is characterized by irregular or heavy bleeding or both. Dysfunctional bleeding may also involve the passage of large clots, which often indicate excessive blood loss. It is difficult to estimate the severity of blood loss in otherwise healthy women because such women do not become anemic until blood loss exceeds 1.6 L over a short interval.

Evaluation and Treatment

Dysfunctional uterine bleeding is diagnosed after other organic conditions that could cause abnormal bleeding are ruled out. Usual therapy is hormonal and may consist of intense progestin-estrogen therapy, cyclic low-dose contraceptives, or medroxyprogesterone acetate. For the woman with idiopathic menorrhagia not associated with anovulatory cycles, prostaglandin synthetase inhibitors may be effective in decreasing blood loss. Treatment for DUB with dilation and curettage (D & C) or hysterectomy is not recommended (Lee, Dicker, Rubin, & Ory, 1984; Lichtman & Papera, 1990). The major purpose of a D & C is diagnostic, and it can be a curative procedure in the removal of products of conception, polyps, or focal endometrial hyperplasia.

TABLE 20-2

Common Causes of Abnormal (Vaginal/Genital) Bleeding in Descending Order of Frequency

Age group	Cause
Prepubescence	Sexual assault
	Trauma
	Foreign bodies
	Precocious puberty
Adolescence	Anovulation (immature hypothalamic-pituitary-ovarian axis)
	Trauma and sexual abuse
	Pregnancy
	Pelvic inflammatory disease
	Coagulation disorder
Reproductive years	Pregnancy
	Pelvic inflammatory disease
	Complication of contraceptives
	Endometriosis
	Anovulation
Premenopause	Anovulation
	Malignancy
	Pregnancy
	Endometriosis
	Benign neoplasms (myomas, adenomyosis)
Postmenopause	Malignancy

Polycystic Ovarian Syndrome

Polycystic ovarian syndrome (PCO) includes a variety of symptoms and physiologic abnormalities. In women with PCO, the hypothalamic-pituitary-ovarian axis is intact and the ovary is intrinsically without defects. Rather the ovary is affected by the production of excessive amounts of androgens and conversion of these androgens to estrogen in the peripheral tissues. This hormonal imbalance prevents ovulation. There is no known cause of PCO. For a subgroup of women, PCO is inherited, seemingly through transmission of an X-linked dominant disorder. Also, enlarged polycystic ovaries may be associated with Cushing syndrome, congenital adrenal hyperplasia, thyroid disease, androgen-producing adrenal or ovarian tumors, and syndromes with hyperprolactinemia.

Pathophysiology

The biochemical basis of PCO is complex. The most common biochemical abnormality is inappropriate gonadotropin secretion. Levels of FSH are typically low or below normal, and the midcycle peak is absent. Levels of LH are elevated, and LH does not surge correctly at midcycle. The persistent LH elevation causes both adrenal and ovarian androgen secretion to increase. The androgen is converted to estrogen in peripheral tissues. Thus PCO is characterized by excessive production of both androgen and estrogen.

Increased androgen secretion by the ovaries contributes to premature follicular atresia and persistent anovulation. In turn, persistent anovulation causes enlarged polycystic ovaries. Because estrogen promotes endometrial proliferation, women with PCO are at risk for endometrial polyps and breast cancer.

Clinical Manifestations

Clinical manifestations of PCO usually appear at puberty but may appear after a variable period of normal menstrual function and, possibly, pregnancy. The symptoms are related to anovulation and include dysfunctional bleeding or amenorrhea, hirsutism, and infertility. Approximately 15% of women with PCO are obese.

Evaluation and Treatment

Diagnosis of PCO is based on evidence of androgen excess, chronic anovulation, and inappropriate gonadotropin secretion. Treatment of PCO includes progesterone therapy to oppose estrogen's effects and medication to stimulate ovulation. Most often, clomiphene citrate, an antiestrogen, is used, with resultant decrease in estrogen, increase in FSH, then ovulation. If ovulation induction fails with clomiphene, a bilateral surgical wedge resection of the ovaries may be successful but with a limited effect. A regimen of GnRH agonist combined with menotropins creates a revers-

ible medial wedge resection and may prove to be more effective. For women who do not desire pregnancy, low-dose oral contraceptives may be used to suppress androgen production and hirsutism. Approximately 40% of women with PCO can become pregnant with the proper medical management.

Premenstrual Syndrome

Premenstrual syndrome (PMS) is the cyclic recurrence (in the luteal phase of the menstrual cycle) of physical, psychologic, or behavioral changes distressing enough to impair interpersonal relationships or interfere with usual activities (Reid, 1985). The prevalence of PMS is difficult to determine. It has been estimated that 5% to 10% of menstruating women have severe to disabling premenstrual symptoms, and 50% or more have moderately distressing symptoms. To confuse matters, it seems that (1) symptoms are experienced to some degree by all adolescent and adult women and are more likely to occur throughout all menstrual phases, (2) the presence and severity of symptoms in any one woman may be inconsistent from month to month, and (3) menstrual phase for peak symptom severity may differ depending on the population studied (Woods, Lenz, Mitchell, Lee, & Taylor, 1989; York, Freeman, Lowery, & Strauss, 1989).

Past theories of PMS causes have focused on ovarian, pituitary, and adrenal hormones, as well as insulin, endogenous opioids, prostaglandins, yeast, and bacteria. Support for these varying theories is nonexistent or inconclusive. It is thought that PMS is the end result of abnormal tissue response, for example, nervous, immunologic, vascular, and gastrointestinal, among others, to the normal changes of the menstrual cycle. This biologic response may be triggered by fluctuating estrogen and progesterone levels and is important but not sufficient to produce PMS. Other mediating factors must exist.

A predisposition to PMS runs in families, perhaps because of genetics or environment. A woman's menstrual experience tends to be similar to her mother's or her sister's experience. Although research is limited, further evidence supports a relationship between the severity and frequency of premenstrual symptoms and reports of low general well-being; history of major affective disorder and personality characteristics, such as perfectionism; increased stress; poor nutrition; lack of exercise; low self-esteem; history of sexual abuse; and family conflict. In turn, when premenstrual symptoms are perceived as distressing, the quality of interpersonal relationships and self-image are negatively affected.

Clinical Manifestations

The pattern of symptom frequency and severity is more important than specific complaints. More than 200 physical, emotional, and behavioral symptoms have been attributed to PMS. Emotional symptoms, particularly depression, anger, irritability, and fatigue, have been reported as the most prominent and the most distressing, whereas physical symptoms seem to be the least prevalent and problematic. Approximately 6% of women present with classic PMS, as defined earlier, and 7% report premenstrual magnification of symptoms that are present during the entire cycle. A typical premenstrual symptom pattern may appear after the treatment of a systemic disease. Likewise, underlying physical or psychologic disease may be aggravated premenstrually.

Evaluation and Treatment

Diagnosis of PMS is based on health history and symptoms. Research and diagnostic criteria for PMS are presented in the boxes below. Because the cause of PMS is complex and cannot be reduced to a single biologic explanation and because the occurrence and severity of PMS are mediated by lifestyle, social, and psychologic factors, current treatment for PMS is symptomatic. Nonpharmacologic therapies, with or without medication, tend to be more effective in controlling symptoms than medication alone.

Initial treatment focuses on validation of the premenstrual experience, education on PMS and self-help techniques, and elimination of contributing factors or treatment of coexisting disorders. Individual, marriage, or family counseling, anger management and conflict resolution, and stress-reduction techniques, including biofeedback, relaxation and imagery, regular exercise, adequate rest, and time management, are all recommended. Dietary changes, such as eating six small meals a day; increasing intake of complex carbohydrates, fiber, and water; and decreasing caffeine, alcohol, sugar, and animal fat consumption, are beneficial.

After a trial of nonpharmacologic therapies, medications may be added to the treatment regimen. Drugs frequently prescribed include vitamin and mineral supplements, antidepressants, antiprostaglandins, and alprazolam. Progesterone may be used for its muscle relaxant and sedative properties, even though its efficacy in the treatment of PMS is not documented. Because the edema associated with PMS is a result of local fluid shifts rather than fluid retention, diuretics are not recommended.

GENERAL CRITERIA FOR PREMENSTRUAL DYSPHORIC DISORDER* (PMDD)

"The criteria for PMDD describe those women for whom a rigorous prospective assessment confirms a pattern of severe depressive symptoms that occurs regularly during the last week of the menstrual cycle and markedly interferes with daily living."

From A. Francis, Chair DSM-IV Task Force, personal communication, April 12, 1993.
*PMDD will be included as an example of a nonspecific depressive disorder in the American Psychiatric Association's next edition of *Diagnostic and Statistical Manual of Mental Disorders (DSM-IV)*

NATIONAL INSTITUTES OF HEALTH GUIDELINES

The diagnosis of PMS requires the documentation of at least a 30% increase in symptom severity in the 5 days before menses compared with the 5 days after menses in at least 2 of 3 menstrual cycles.

From National Institutes of Health. (1983). *NIMH premenstrual syndrome workshop guidelines, April 14-15, 1983.* Rockville, MD: Author.

DIAGNOSTIC AND RESEARCH CRITERIA FOR PMS

1. The pretense by self-report of at least one of the following somatic and effective symptoms during the 5 days before menses in each of the three prior menstrual cycles:

AFFECTIVE	SOMATIC
Depression	Breast tenderness
Angry outbursts	Abdominal bloating
Irritability	Headache
Social withdrawal	Swollen extremities
Fatigue	

2. Relief of the above symptoms within 4 days of the onset of menses, without recurrence until at least cycle day 12.
3. The symptoms are present in the absence of any pharmacologic therapy, hormone ingestion, drug, or alcohol.
4. The symptoms occur reproducibly during two cycles of prospective recording.
5. Identifiable dysfunction in social or economic performance by one of the following criteria:
   Marital or relationship discord confirmed by partner
   Difficulties in parenting
   Poor work or school performance, attendance/tardiness
   Increased social isolation
   Legal difficulties
   Suicidal ideation
   Seeking medical attention for somatic symptom(s)

From Mortola, 1992.

In severe cases, menses is abolished, which eliminates cyclic ovarian hormones and, thus, the biologic trigger for PMS. Elimination of menses can be accomplished with the use of oral contraceptives, medroxyprogesterone acetate, or GnRH agonists.

Infection and Inflammation

Infections of the genital tract may result from exogenous or endogenous microorganisms. Exogenous pathogens are most frequently sexually transmitted (see Chapter 21). Endogenous causes of infection include microorganisms that are normally resident in the vagina, bowel, or vulva. Infection occurs if these microorganisms migrate to a new location or overproliferate or if the immune system and other defense mechanisms are impaired.

A number of skin disorders can affect the vulva. They include reactive dermatitis, contact dermatitis, psoriasis, and impetigo. (For a discussion of skin disorders, see Chapter 41.) Most infectious disorders that affect the vulva and vagina are sexually transmitted, however. These disorders are described in Chapter 21.

Pelvic Inflammatory Disease

Pelvic inflammatory disease (PID) is an acute inflammatory process caused by infection (Fig. 20-2). Pelvic inflammatory disease may involve any organ, or combination of organs, of the upper genital tract—the uterus, fallopian tubes, or ovaries—and, in its most severe form, the entire peritoneal cavity. (Infection of the fallopian tubes is termed **salpingitis** [Fig. 20-3]; infection of the ovaries is called **oophoritis**.) Most cases of PID are caused by sexually transmitted microorganisms that migrate from the vagina to the uterus, fallopian tubes, and ovaries.

Pathophysiology

The development of upper genital tract infections is mediated by a number of defense mechanisms that are usually very effective in preventing PID (see Chapter 19). Virulence of the organism, size of the inoculum, and defense status of the individual all determine whether an infectious process results.

Pelvic inflammatory disease is usually considered a polymicrobial infection. Most cases (up to 84%) are caused by mixed nongonococcal-nonchlamydial bacteria, including anaerobes (*Bacteroides* species and peptostreptococci) and facultative organisms (*Gardnerella vaginalis, Haemophilus influenzae,* and streptococci). *Escherichia coli* has been overemphasized as a causal agent, but may contribute to pelvic infections in older women. Recovery of *N. gonorrhoeae, C. trachomatis,* or both, has been reported in 50% to 60% of women with acute PID. Although recovery of gonorrhea and chlamydia is absent in some cases, these organisms may

induce a response from the body that will cause tubonecrosis with repeated infections and may predispose a woman to PID. After one episode of pelvic infection, 15% to 25% of women develop long-term sequelae, such as infertility, ectopic pregnancy, chronic pelvic pain, dyspareunia, pelvic adhesions, perihepatitis, and tuboovarian abscess. The incidence of complications increases markedly with repeated infections. The mortality rate associated with PID is 8% to 9% of cases. Most deaths resulting from PID are caused by septic shock (see Chapter 29).

Clinical Manifestations

The clinical manifestations of PID vary from sudden, severe abdominal pain with fever to no symptoms at all. An asymptomatic cervicitis may be present for some time before PID develops. Of women with salpingitis, 67% to 75% may have a subclinical infection. The first sign of the ascending infection may be the onset of low bilateral abdominal pain, most often characterized as dull and steady with a gradual onset. Symptoms are more likely to develop during or immediately after menstruation. The pain of PID may worsen with walking, jumping, or intercourse. Other manifestations of PID include dysuria (difficult or painful urination) and irregular bleeding.

Evaluation and Treatment

The diagnosis of PID is based on history, abdominal tenderness with or without rebound, presence of uterine and cervical movement tenderness on bimanual pelvic examination, mucopurulent discharge at the cervical os, white blood cells on Gram stain or wet mount of cervical discharge, leukocytosis, and increased erythrocyte sedimentation rate. To support the diagnosis, a chlamydia smear for fluorescent antibody testing or DNA testing and a gonorrhea culture are done; sonography, laparoscopy, and culdocentesis are indicated when a woman has recurrent or unresponsive symptoms to outpatient treatment regimen, fever greater than 38° C, or an adnexal mass. Other conditions that cause pelvic pain must be excluded, including ectopic pregnancy, threatened abortion, or appendicitis.

Treatment involves bed rest, avoidance of intercourse, and combined antibiotic therapy (Table 20-3). Twenty-five percent to 40% of women require hospitalization for intravenous administration of antibiotics and treatment of peritonitis or a tuboovarian abscess. To prevent recurrence, sexual partners are also treated with antibiotic combinations.

Vaginitis

Vaginitis is infection of the vagina. The major causes of vaginitis are sexually transmitted pathogens (see Chapter 21) and *Candida albicans*. The incidence of sexually

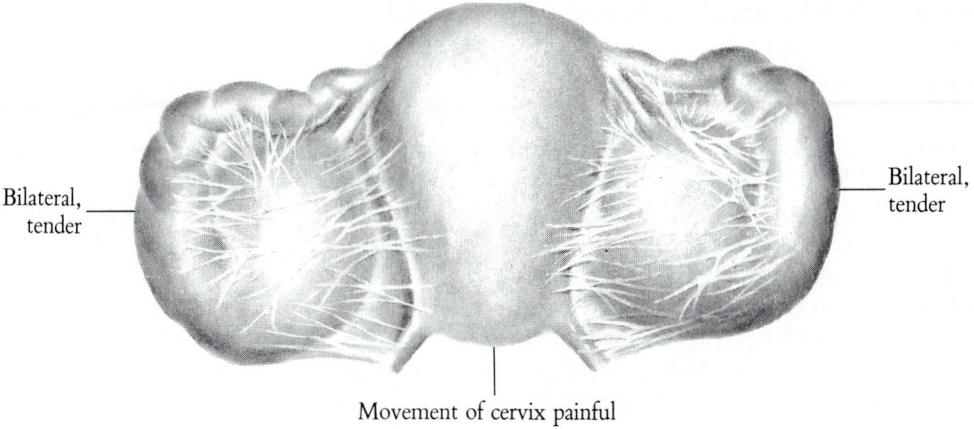

Bilateral, tender

Bilateral, tender

Movement of cervix painful

FIG. 20-2 Pelvic inflammatory disease. (From Seidel, Ball, Dains, & Benedict, 1991.)

Advanced

Pyosalpinx

FIG. 20-3 Salpingitis. (From Seidel, Ball, Dains, & Benedict, 1991.)

TABLE 20-3

CDC Recommended Treatment for Acute PID (1989)

Ambulatory management	Hospital management	
Cefoxitin (2 g IM plus 1 g probenecid orally) or Ceftriaxone (250 mg IM) plus Doxycycline (100 mg orally twice daily for 10-14 days) or Tetracycline (500 mg orally 4 times daily for 10-14 days) For patients who cannot tolerate doxycycline, substitute erythromycin (500 mg orally 4 times daily for 10-14 days)	1. Cefoxitin (2 g IV every 6 hours) or Cefotetan* (2 g IV every 12 hours) or Equivalent cephalosporin plus Doxycycline (100 mg every 12 hours orally or IV) Regimen given for at least 48 hours after patient clinically improves; after discharge from hospital, continue doxycycline (100 mg orally twice daily for 10-14 days)	2. Clindamycin (900 mg IV every 8 hours) plus Gentamicin (2 mg/kg loading dose IV or IM followed by 1.5 mg/kg maintenance dose every 8 hours) Regimen given for at least 48 hours after the patient improves; after discharge from hospital, continue doxycycline (100 mg orally twice daily for 10-14 days) or clindamycin (450 mg orally 5 times daily for 10-14 days)

*Other cephalosporins, such as ceftizoxime, cefotaxime, and ceftriaxone, which provide adequate gonococcal, other facultative growth-negative aerobic, and anaerobic coverage, may be used in appropriate doses.

transmitted vaginitis is highest in young women 15 to 25 years of age.

The development of vaginitis is related to the overall health of a woman and local defense mechanisms, particularly vaginal pH. The pH of the vagina is dependent on cervical secretions and the presence of normal flora that help to maintain an acidic environment. A neutral or alkaline pH normally occurs before puberty, after menopause, and during pregnancy. The acidic nature of vaginal secretions during the reproductive years provides protection against a variety of sexually transmitted pathogens. Therefore, variables that alter the vaginal pH or the bactericidal nature of secretions (see Chapter 19) may predispose a woman to infection. These variables include douching, use of soaps, feminine hygiene sprays, deodorant menstrual pads or tampons, and conditions associated with increased glycogen content of vaginal secretions, such as pregnancy or diabetes.

The use of antibiotics may destroy *Lactobacillus acidophilus*, an anaerobic, gram-positive rod normally found in the vagina that helps maintain an acidic pH. In its absence, alkalinity increases and the vagina is more susceptible to trichomoniasis and bacterial vaginosis; moreover, there may be an overgrowth of *C. albicans*, causing a yeast vaginitis.

Normally, vaginal discharge is a clear, milky, or cloudy secretion with a slippery or clumpy texture. It is nonirritating, has a mild inoffensive odor, and turns yellow after drying. Throughout the menstrual cycle, the amount and texture of a woman's discharge will change in response to hormonal fluctuation. Vaginal secretions increase at the time of ovulation, during pregnancy, and with sexual arousal; just before menstruation, vaginal discharge becomes thick and sticky. Although the amount of vaginal discharge alone is not an indication of infection, any other change in discharge may indicate a problem. Infection is suggested with a marked change in color or if the discharge becomes malodorous or irritating.

Diagnosis is based on history, physical examination, and examination of the discharge by wet mount. Treatment involves developing and maintaining an acidic environment, relieving symptoms (usually pruritus), and administering antimicrobial or antifungal medications to eradicate the infectious organism. If the infection can be sexually transmitted, a woman's partner will also be treated.

Cervicitis

Cervicitis is an inflammation of the cervix. **Mucopurulent cervicitis** (MPC) is usually caused by one or more sexually transmitted pathogens, such as *Trichomonas*, gonorrhea, *Chlamydia*, *Mycoplasma*, or *Ureaplasma*. Infection causes the cervix to become red and edematous. A mucopurulent (mucus- and pus-containing) ex-

udate drains from the external cervical os, and the individual may report vague pelvic pain, bleeding, or dysuria. The infectious organisms are cultured or identified by immunoassay. Definitive diagnosis is followed by oral antibiotic therapy. Sexual partners are usually treated.

Vulvitis

Inflammation of the vulva is termed **vulvitis**. Acute vulvitis is an inflammation of the skin (dermatitis) of the vulva and often of the perianal area. Vulvitis can be caused by contact with soaps, detergents, lotions, hygienic sprays, menstrual pads, or perfumed toilet paper or to nonabsorbent or tight-fitting clothes. Vulvitis is also caused by vaginal infections (e.g., candidiasis or trichomoniasis) that spread to the labia, where they cause inflammation and edema. Other skin diseases, such as tinea cruris, psoriasis, and inflammation of the apocrine (sweat) glands, can involve the vulva (see Chapter 41).

Avoidance of irritants; wearing of loose, cotton clothing; and appropriate antimicrobial/antifungal treatment for recurrent vaginitis are usually effective cures for acute vulvitis. Chronic vulvitis is usually treated with fluorinated hydrocortisone. Biopsy specimens of persistent lesions are examined for the presence of malignancy.

Bartholinitis

Bartholinitis, or Bartholin cyst, is an inflammation of one or both of the ducts that lead from the introitus (vaginal opening) to Bartholin glands (Fig. 20-4). The usual causes of bartholinitis are microorganisms that in-

FIG. 20-4 Inflammation of Bartholin glands. (From Gardner & Kaufman, 1969.)

fect the lower female reproductive tract, such as streptococci, staphylococci, and sexually transmitted pathogens. Acute bartholinitis is usually preceded by an infection, such as cervicitis, vaginitis, or urethritis.

Infection or trauma causes inflammatory changes that narrow the distal portion of the duct, leading to obstruction and stasis of glandular secretions. The obstruction, or cyst, varies from 1 to 8 cm in diameter and is located in the posterolateral portion of the vulva. The cyst is usually reddened and painful, and pus may be visible at the opening of the duct. The individual may have symptoms of the initiating infection, fever, and malaise.

Most Bartholin cysts are asymptomatic and require no treatment. Chronic bartholinitis is characterized by the presence of a small cyst that is slightly tender but otherwise is asymptomatic. Symptoms occur if an exacerbation of infection causes an abscess to form in the gland itself.

Diagnosis of bartholinitis is based on the clinical manifestations and the identification of infectious microorganisms. Antibiotics are given to treat infection, and pain is relieved with analgesics and warm sitz baths. If an abscess forms, it is surgically drained.

Pelvic Relaxation Disorders

The bladder, urethra, and rectum are supported by the endopelvic fascia and the perineal muscles. This muscular and fascial tissue loses tone and strength with aging and may fail to maintain the pelvic organs in the proper position. Progressive relaxation of the pelvic support structures may cause uterine displacement. Uterine displacement can also result if trauma, such as childbirth or pelvic surgery, damages or weakens the supporting structures. Pelvic relaxation is progressive and is related to the inherent strength or weakness of the woman's musculofascial tissue. Malpositioning of the bladder, urethra, or rectum (and hence the uterus) may occur many years after an initial injury to the supporting structure. A strong familial tendency and, perhaps, a multifactorial genetic component place some women at risk for the development of prolapse. Genital prolapse is 80 times more prevalent in whites than in blacks and, despite grand multiparity, pelvic relaxation is rare in Canadian Indians.

Fig. 20-5 shows vaginal prolapse caused by cystocele, rectocele, and enterocele. **Cystocele** is descent of the bladder and the anterior vaginal wall into the vaginal

FIG. 20-5 Cystocele and rectocele. **A,** Cystocele. **B,** Rectocele. (From Seidel, Ball, Dains, & Benedict, 1991.)

TABLE 20-4

Cystocele, Urethrocele, and Rectocele

Condition	Etiology	Symptoms	Treatment
Cystocele	Laceration, stretching, or weakening of supporting fascial tissue; usually caused by prolonged labor, multiple births, or birth of a large baby	Urinary frequency, urgency, and occasional incontinence Difficulty in complete emptying of the bladder Low backache Symptoms become problematic pre- or postmenopausally	Depending on age of woman and severity of the condition, includes: Isometric exercise to strengthen the pubococcygeal muscle Oral or topical estrogen to improve tone and vascularity of fascial support Pessary, a removable device that holds the bladder in position Surgical correction
Urethrocele	Pressure of fetal head on urethra and attachments beneath the symphysis pubis Familial or genetic predisposition	Asymptomatic, unless it occurs in conjunction with cystocele	Isometric exercises (see Cystocele)
Rectocele	Trauma to the fascia and levator muscles; usually caused by childbirth Familial or genetic predisposition	Constipation or feeling of rectal fullness Difficult defecation Pressure and sensation of fullness in the vagina	Isometric exercises Diet counseling to prevent constipation Stool softeners or laxatives Surgery

canal. In severe cases, the bladder and anterior vaginal wall bulge outside the introitus. A cystocele may cause the woman to lose urine when she laughs, sneezes, coughs, or does anything that strains the abdominal muscles. Cystocele is usually accompanied by **urethrocele,** or sagging of the urethra. Urethrocele is usually caused by the shearing effect of the fetal head on the urethra during childbirth. A **rectocele** is the bulging of the rectum and posterior vaginal wall into the vaginal canal. If this condition is severe, defecation is difficult and can only be accomplished by applying manual pressure to the posterior vaginal wall. An enterocele is herniation of the rectouterine pouch into the rectovaginal septum (between the rectum and posterior vaginal wall). It is usually associated with other pelvic relaxation disorders such as uterine prolapse, cystocele, and rectocele. Table 20-4 summarizes the causes, symptoms, and treatment of cystocele, urethrocele, and rectocele.

Uterine prolapse is descent of the cervix or entire uterus into the vaginal canal (Fig. 20-6). In severe cases, the uterus falls completely through the vagina and protrudes from the introitus. First-degree uterine prolapse is not treated unless it causes discomfort. Second- and third-degree prolapse causes feelings of fullness, heaviness, and collapse through the vagina. Symptoms of other pelvic relaxation disorders also may be present. Treatment in these cases is the insertion of a **pessary,**

which is a removable mechanical device that holds the uterus in position. The pelvic fascia may be strengthened through Kegel exercises, a repetitive, isometric tightening and relaxing of the pubococcygeal muscles; or by a course of estrogen therapy, particularly if the woman is past menopause. Surgical repair is the treatment of last resort.

Benign Growths and Proliferative Conditions
Benign Ovarian Cysts

Benign cysts of the ovary may occur at any time during the lifespan, but are most common between puberty and menopause (Fig. 20-7). Two common causes of benign ovarian enlargement in ovulating women are follicular cysts and corpus luteum cysts. These cysts are called functional cysts because they are caused by variations of normal physiologic events. Follicular and corpus luteum cysts are unilateral. They are typically 5 to 6 cm in diameter but can grow as large as 8 to 10 cm.

A **follicular cyst** develops from a dominant ovarian follicle that does not release its ovum but remains active or from a degenerating follicle whose fluid is not reabsorbed. Most follicular cysts are not symptomatic, require no treatment, and either regress or rupture spontaneously within 60 days. A large follicular cyst may cause low back pain, painful intercourse (dyspareunia),

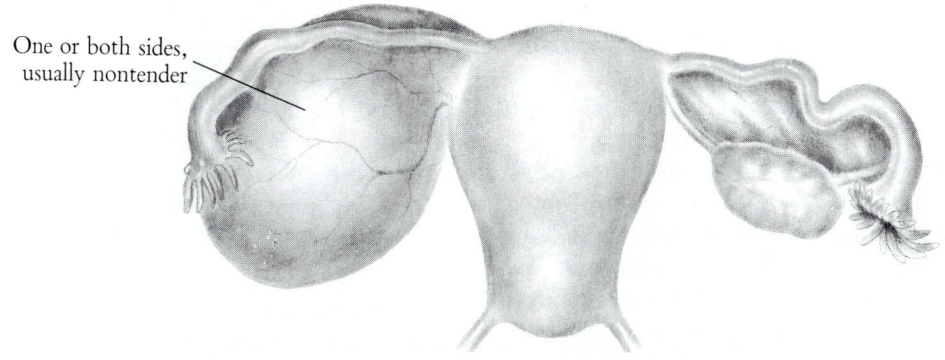

FIG. 20-6 **Degrees of uterine prolapse. A,** Normal uterus. **B,** First-degree prolapse: descent within the vagina. **C,** Second-degree prolapse: the cervix protrudes through the introitus. **D,** Third-degree prolapse: the vagina is completely everted. (From Seidel, Ball, Dains, & Benedict, 1991.)

One or both sides, usually nontender

FIG. 20-7 **Ovarian cyst.** (From Seidel, Ball, Dains, & Benedict, 1991.)

chronic lower abdominal pain, and menstrual irregularities.

A **corpus luteum cyst** develops if a mature corpus luteum persists abnormally and continues to secrete progesterone. The cyst consists of blood or fluid that accumulates in the cavity of the corpus luteum. Corpus luteum cysts are less common than follicular cysts, but luteal cysts typically cause more symptoms, particularly if they rupture. Manifestations include dull pelvic pain and amenorrhea or delayed menstruation, followed by irregular or heavier-than-normal bleeding. Rupture can cause massive bleeding with excruciating pain and require immediate surgery. Corpus luteum cysts usually regress spontaneously, however, within 2 months in nonpregnant women. Oral contraceptives may be used to prevent cysts from forming in the future.

Endometrial Polyps

An **endometrial polyp** is a benign mass of endometrial tissue attached to the inner uterine lining by a pedicle. Polyps usually arise from the uterine fundus in response to estrogen stimulation and often coexist with endometrial hyperplasia. Polyps may be single or multiple with a narrow or broad pedicle and may vary from 0.5 to 3 cm in diameter. Although polyps most often develop in women between the ages of 40 and 49, they can occur at all ages.

Endometrial polyps are a frequent cause of premenstrual spotting or intermenstrual bleeding in the premenopausal woman. These polyps consist of stromal tissue covered by either proliferative or hyperplastic mucosa. In response to subtle hormonal changes, irregular bleeding occurs that is nonsynchronous with the normal endometrial lining. Occasionally, for reasons not understood, significant bleeding occurs.

Diagnosis is made by hysteroscopy, hysterosalpingography, or direct examination of tissue obtained by curettage. The lesions are removed with small curved polyp forceps. Malignancy is extremely rare; coexistence of a separate endometrial atypical hyperplasia or adenocarcinoma is common.

Leiomyomas

Leiomyomas, commonly called uterine fibroids, are benign tumors that develop from smooth muscle cells in the myometrium. Leiomyomas are the most common benign tumors of the uterus and most remain small and asymptomatic. Prevalence increases in women aged 30 to 50 but decreases with menopause. In the United States, it is estimated that myomas develop in 30% of white and 50% of black women by the age of 50. The incidence of leiomyomas in black and Asian women is two to five times higher than that in white women.

The cause of uterine leiomyomas is unknown, although their size appears to be related to hormonal fluc-

tuations. Uterine leiomyomas are not seen before menarche, and those that develop during the reproductive years generally decrease in size after menopause. Tumors in pregnant women enlarge rapidly but often decrease in size after termination of the pregnancy.

Pathophysiology

Most leiomyomas occur in multiples in the fundus of the uterus, although they may occur singly and throughout the uterus. Leiomyomas are classified as subserous, submucous, or intramural, according to their location within the various layers of the uterine wall (Fig. 20-8). Uterine leiomyomas are usually firm and surrounded by a pseudocapsule composed of compressed but otherwise normal uterine myometrium. Degenerative changes, such as ulceration and necrosis, may occur when the leiomyoma outgrows its blood supply and therefore are more common in larger tumors.

Clinical Manifestations

The major clinical manifestations of leiomyomas are abnormal uterine bleeding, pain, and symptoms related to pressure on nearby structures. The leiomyoma tends to make the uterine cavity larger, thereby increasing the en-

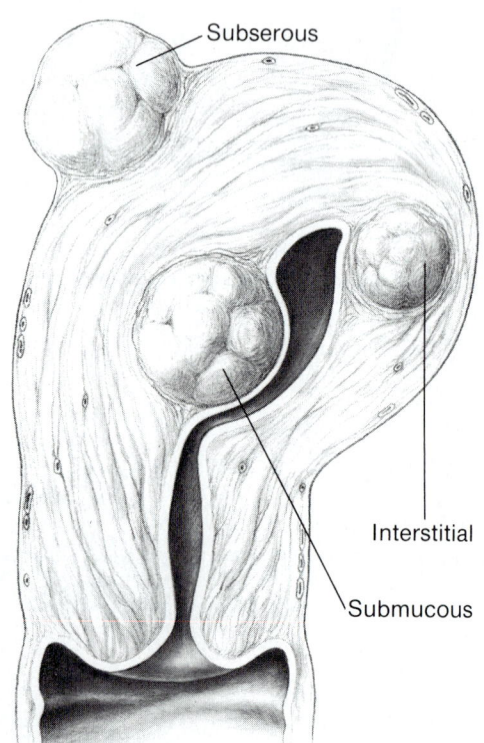

FIG. 20-8 Leiomyomas. Uterine section showing whorl-like appearance and locations of leiomyomas, which are also called uterine fibroids. (From Herbst, Mischell, Stenchever, & Droegemueller, 1992.)

dometrial surface area. This increase may account for the increased menstrual bleeding that is associated with leiomyomas. Pain is not an early symptom, but tends to occur with the devascularization of larger leiomyomas. It is also associated with blood vessel compression that limits blood supply to adjacent structures. Symptoms of abdominal pressure are slow to develop, apparently because the tumor is relatively slow-growing, enabling adjacent structures to adapt to pressure. Pressure on the bladder may contribute to urinary frequency, urgency, and dysuria. Pressure on the ureter may cause it to become distended "upstream" from the pressure point; rectosigmoid pressure may lead to constipation. A sensation of abdominal or genital heaviness may be felt with larger tumors.

Evaluation and Treatment

Uterine leiomyomas are diagnosed by physical examination. The bimanual examination discloses irregular, nontender nodularity of the uterus. Treatment depends on the symptoms, tumor size, age, reproductive status, and overall health of the individual. Most myomas can be treated conservatively. Medical treatment is aimed at shrinking the myoma with either progesterone or GnRH. Myomectomy may be undertaken and is the surgical treatment of choice.

Adenomyosis

Adenomyosis is the presence of endometrial glands and stroma within the uterine myometrium. It commonly develops during the late reproductive years, with the highest incidence among women in their 40s. Adenomyosis may be asymptomatic or may be associated with abnormal menstrual bleeding, dysmenorrhea, uterine enlargement, and uterine tenderness during menstruation.

Treatment, when necessary, is surgical and includes resection of localized areas of adenomyosis or, if severe, hysterectomy.

Endometriosis

Endometriosis is the presence of functioning endometrial tissue or implants outside the uterus. Like normal endometrial tissue, the ectopic (out-of-place) endometrium responds to the hormonal fluctuations of the menstrual cycle.

The incidence of endometriosis is difficult to determine, particularly in asymptomatic fertile women and adolescents. Up to 50% of women evaluated for pelvic pain, infertility, or a pelvic mass are diagnosed as having endometriosis.

The cause of endometriosis is not known, but several theories have been proposed. In 1927, J. A. Sampson proposed that endometriosis is caused by the implantation of endometrial cells during **retrograde menstrua-**

tion, in which menstrual fluids move through the fallopian tubes and empty into the pelvic cavity. It is now known that retrograde menstruation occurs in almost all women; however, not all women develop endometriosis.

Another theory is that women with endometriosis have a slightly depressed cytotoxic T-cell response to endometrial cells or some other defect of the immune response. These alterations may cause the body to tolerate ectopic implantation of endometrial cells. Researchers also have proposed that endometrial cells spread through the lymphatic system or that multipotential cells in the epithelial coverings of reproductive organs are stimulated somehow to develop into endometrial cells. A genetic predisposition to endometriosis has been documented. Studies show that incidence and severity of disease are greatest among women with female relatives who also have endometriosis.

Pathophysiology

Endometrial implants can occur throughout the body. The most common sites of implantation are the ovaries, uterine ligaments, rectovaginal septum, and pelvic peritoneum (Fig. 20-9). Other sites of implantation are the sigmoid colon, small intestine, rectum, appendix, blad-

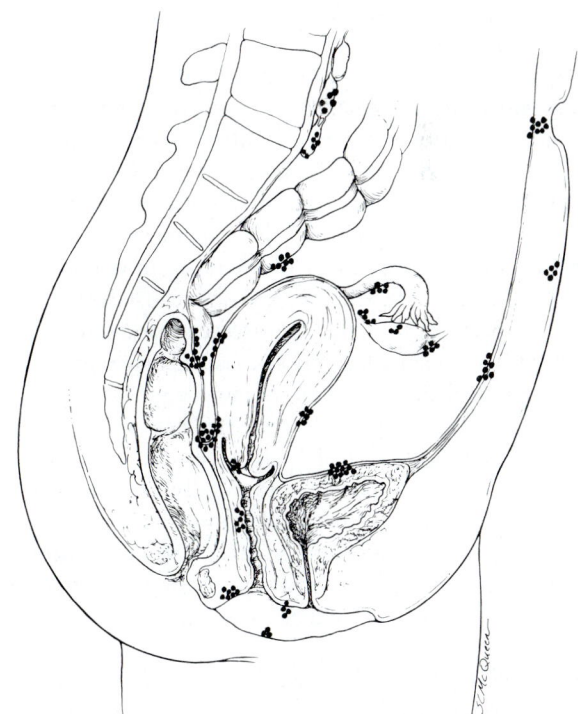

FIG. 20-9 Pelvic sites of endometrial implantation. Endometrial cells may enter the pelvic cavity during retrograde menstruation. (From Herbst, Mischell, Stenchever, & Droegemueller, 1992.)

der, uterus, vulva, vagina, cervix, lymph nodes, extremities, pleural cavity, lungs, laparotomy scars, and hernial sacs.

Cyclic changes depend on the blood supply of the implants. Given that blood supply is sufficient, the ectopic endometrium proliferates, breaks down, and bleeds in conjunction with the normal menstrual cycle. The bleeding causes inflammation and pain in surrounding tissues. The inflammation may lead to fibrosis, scarring, and adhesions.

Clinical Manifestations

The clinical manifestations of endometriosis are variable in frequency and severity and include infertility; abnormal vaginal bleeding; dysmenorrhea; dyschezia (pain on defecation); constipation; dyspareunia (pain on intercourse); and, if implants are located within the pelvis, asymptomatic pelvic mass having irregular, movable nodules and a fixed, retroverted uterus. Most symptoms of endometriosis can be explained by the proliferation, breakdown, and bleeding of the ectopic endometrial tissue, with subsequent formation of adhesions. In many instances, however, the degree of endometriosis is not related to the frequency or severity of symptoms. Dysmenorrhea, for example, does not appear to be related to the degree of endometriosis. With involvement of the rectovaginal septum or the uterosacral ligaments, dyspareunia develops. Dyschezia occurs with bleeding of ectopic endometrium in the rectosigmoid musculature and subsequent fibrosis.

Approximately 30% to 40% of individuals with endometriosis are infertile. The link between endometriosis and infertility is not clear, but it does not appear to involve severity of disease. Infertility may result from mechanical interference with ovulation or ovum transport through the fallopian tube, but mechanical interference is an unlikely cause of infertility in women with mild endometriosis. Another possible cause is phagocytosis of sperm by macrophages in the reproductive tract. It is known that endometriosis causes macrophages in the peritoneal fluid to become more aggressive phagocytes ("eater cells"; see Chapter 7). These macrophages have been found in the fallopian tubes and may account for some cases of infertility, especially in women with mild endometriosis. Other explanations include changes in prostaglandin secretion, luteal phase defect, unruptured luteinizing follicle syndrome, hyperprolactinemia, and autoimmune and genetic factors.

Evaluation and Treatment

Evaluation of the pelvis through laparoscopy is required for definitive diagnosis of endometriosis and should be completed before therapy is begun. On the basis of the extent of the disease, the American Fertility Society has proposed that endometriosis be classified as stage I,

mild; stage II, moderate; stage III, severe; and stage IV, extensive. All treatment is based on the stage of the disease and aimed toward prevention of disease progression, alleviation of pain, and establishment or restoration of fertility. Medical therapies include suppression of ovulation with noncyclic estrogen-progestin oral contraceptives, danazol, or GnRH agonists. Conservative surgical treatment includes laparoscopic removal of endometrial implants with conventional or laser techniques and presacral neurectomy for severe dysmenorrhea. Effectiveness of therapy may be increased when medical regimens are combined with surgical techniques. The overall results of conservative surgery are excellent except in cases of severe endometriosis associated with bilateral large endometriomas. In these instances, radical surgery, total abdominal hysterectomy with bilateral salpingo-oophorectomy (TAH-BSO), may be warranted if the woman's family is complete.

Cancer

Malignant tumors of the female reproductive system are common. Endometrial carcinoma accounts for approximately 5% of all cancers in women; ovarian tumors, 4%; cervical tumors, 2%; and other malignant tumors, 1% to 3% (American Cancer Society [ACS], 1993). The malignant neoplasms of the female reproductive tract account for about 1 of 8 diagnosed cancers and 1 of 11 cancer deaths in women in the United States (ACS, 1992).

Cervical Cancer

Invasive cancer of the cervix is the third most prevalent gynecologic cancer and accounts for approximately 20% of all female cancers. Average age for detection and diagnosis of dysplasia, or precancerous lesions, is 33 to 38 years, and 43 to 48 years for invasive cancer. Invasive carcinoma is most likely to affect women in their 50s and 60s. Whereas the overall incidence of invasive cervical cancer has decreased over the years, rates of abnormal cervical cytology have markedly increased in women under 25, presumably because of increased infection with human papillomavirus (HPV). By age 20, one in eight young women will have cervical dysplasia. Incidence rates tend to be higher in women of low socioeconomic status, perhaps because of the inability to access health care.

Cervical cancer is generally considered a sexually transmitted disease. Infection of the cervix with HPV, intercourse before age 16, and multiple sexual partners or a male partner with multiple partners place a woman at risk. Smoking is a considered a cofactor in the development of cervical carcinoma. Diet and vitamin deficiencies, primarily vitamins A, C, and folic acid, may also be factors, but further investigation is needed.

TABLE 20-5

Clinical Staging for Cancer of the Cervix

Stage	Characteristics
0	Cancer in situ, intraepithelial carcinoma; earliest stage of cancer; means that the cancer is confined to its original site
I	Carcinoma confined to cervix (extension to corpus disregarded)
IA	Microinvasive carcinomas (those diagnosed by microscopy)
IA1	Minimal microscopically evident stromal invasion
IA2	Lesions detected microscopically within specific measurement limits
IB	Lesions of greater dimension than stage IA2 that should be specifically recorded to determine whether it should affect treatment decisions in the future
II	Carcinoma extends beyond cervix but has not extended to the pelvic wall; carcinoma involves the vagina but not as far as the lower third
IIA	No obvious parametrial involvement
IIB	Obvious parametrial involvement
III	Carcinoma extended to the pelvic wall; no cancer-free space between the tumor and pelvic wall on rectal examination; tumor involves lower third of the vagina; all cases with a nonfunctioning kidney are included
IIIA	No extension to the pelvic wall; tumor involves lower third of the vagina
IIIB	Extension to the pelvic wall and/or nonfunctioning kidney
IV	Carcinoma has extended beyond the true pelvis or has clinically involved the mucosa of the bladder or rectum; bullous edema as such does not permit a case to be allotted to stage IV
IVA	Spread of growth to adjacent organs
IVB	Spread to distant organs

From American Cancer Society, 1991.

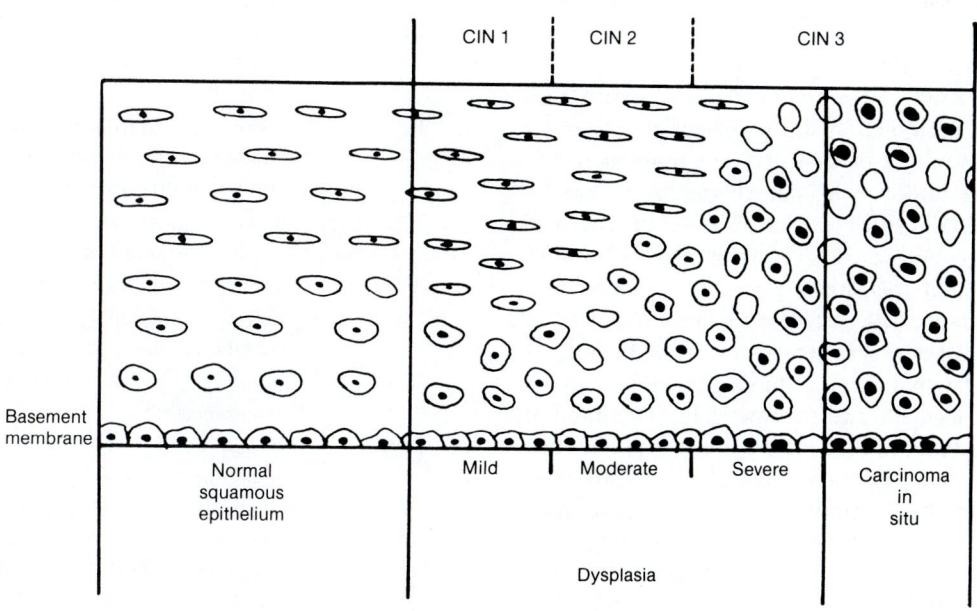

FIG. 20-10 Cervical intraepithelial neoplasia (CIN). Diagram of cervical endothelium showing progressive degrees of CIN. (From Herbst, Mischell, Stenchever, & Droegemueller, 1992.)

Pathogenesis

Cervical cancer is a progressive disease that is staged according to histology (Table 20-5). Premalignant lesions occur 10 to 12 years before the development of invasive carcinoma.

The progressive changes of cervical cells are classified as (1) cervical intraepithelial neoplasia, (2) cervical carcinoma in situ, and (3) invasive carcinoma. **Cervical intraepithelial neoplasia (CIN)**, commonly called cervical dysplasia, is replacement of some epithelial cells by atypical, neoplastic cells. Cervical intraepithelial neoplasia is graded as mild dysplasia (CIN 1), moderate dysplasia (CIN 2), or severe dysplasia and carcinoma in situ (CIN 3), depending on the depth of epithelial involvement (Fig. 20-10).

In **cervical carcinoma in situ,** all or most of the cervical epithelium shows cellular features of carcinoma, but underlying tissue is not affected. Risk of progression to invasive carcinoma steadily rises with the severity of dysplasia. Women with CIN 1 have a 15% chance of developing malignant lesions. This rate increases to 75% in women with CIN 3.

Carcinoma in situ is most likely to develop in the squamous-columnar junction—the so-called transformation zone—where the columnar epithelium of the cervical lining meets the squamous epithelium of the outer cervix and vagina (Fig. 20-11). In this zone, columnar epithelium is constantly being replaced by squamous epithelium in a process known as metaplasia. Metaplasia seems to be affected by hormonal levels; change in cervical epithelium is not understood as well as endometrial tissue change in response to fluctuating hormones. Because metaplastic cells are at increased risk of incorporating foreign or abnormal genetic material, neoplastic changes are most common in the transformation zone.

The spontaneous regression of carcinoma in situ is extremely rare. Carcinoma in situ is generally a precursor of invasive carcinoma of the cervix. A number of factors, including tumor type, contribute to the rate at which carcinoma in situ becomes invasive. **Invasive carcinoma of the cervix** consists of direct invasion into adjacent tissues and metastasis (spread of cancer cells) through the lymphatics. Adjacent tissues most often involved are the ureters and structures of the lateral pelvic wall, the vaginal stroma and epithelium, and the lower uterine segment and myometrium. The internal, external, and common iliac lymph nodes and the obturator nodes are common sites of lymphatic involvement. A staging system for carcinoma of the cervix is set forth in Table 20-5.

Clinical Manifestations

Because cervical neoplasms are asymptomatic, regular cytologic screening (Papanicolaou smear) is necessary. Vaginal bleeding and discharge are common symptoms.

Bleeding is variable and may occur after intercourse or between menstrual periods. At times, women will complain of abnormal menses or postmenopausal bleeding. Vaginal discharge is a less common presenting symptom and may be serosanguineous or yellowish in color. A new or foul odor also may be present. Bleeding and discharge are subtle and are likely to be disregarded by premenopausal women, who mistake these signs for variations of normal processes. Postmenopausal women are more likely to seek medical attention if these signs appear. With severe bleeding, symptoms of anemia may occur. Pelvic or epigastric pain is experienced only with large lesions. Advanced disease may cause urinary or rectal symptoms.

Evaluation and Treatment

Cervical cytology is most accurate if cells obtained by endocervical swabbing and ectocervical scraping are examined. When dysplasia is detected, cervical biopsy and curettage are required. Colposcopy is used to identify suggestive sites for biopsy. The transformation zone moves higher into the cervix as age increases, making biopsy more difficult. If invasive carcinoma is found, lymphangiography, CT scan, ultrasonography, or radio-

TABLE 20-6

Cervical Cancer Treatment Options

Stage	Treatment
0	Conization, cryosurgery, laser surgery, surgery (hysterectomy)
IA	Surgery (total abdominal hysterectomy, may include oophorectomy), radiation therapy
IB	Surgery (radical hysterectomy with lymph node dissection), internal and external radiation therapy combined
IIA	Surgery (radical hysterectomy with lymph node dissection), internal and external radiation therapy combined
IIB	Internal and external radiation therapy combined
III	Internal and external radiation therapy combined
IVA	Internal and external radiation therapy combined; surgery (exenteration) for removal of uterus, vagina, cervix; could include bladder, colon or rectum depending on the area of malignant spread
IVB	Radiation therapy for pain symptoms

From American Cancer Society, 1991.

FIG. 20-11 Cervical carcinoma in situ. Typical transformation zone, where the columnar (grapelike) epithelium is replaced by metaplastic epithelium. At its outer edge, the metaplastic epithelium adjoins the squamous epithelium, which extends into the vagina. (From Coppleson, Pixley, & Reed, 1971; Herbst, Mischell, Stenchever, & Droegemueller, 1992.)

immunodetection methods are used to assess lymphatic involvement.

The treatment depends on the degree of neoplastic change, the size and location of the lesion, and the extent of metastatic spread. For premalignant or early cancer (stage 0), cryosurgery or carbon dioxide laser therapy is commonly used; laser treatment may produce better results in the multiparous cervix. Conization is an alternate treatment. The amount of tissue removed depends on the location of the lesion. None of these measures affects fertility or childbearing. If fertility is not desired, a hysterectomy may be performed.

For invasive cervical carcinoma, treatment depends on the stage of the tumor (Table 20-6). Surgical inter-

vention may include a hysterectomy, pelvic lymphadenectomy, and pelvic exenteration. Radiation therapy is used most frequently in cases of small cell cancer with lymphatic involvement. External radiation is usually combined with use of one or two intracavity implants. Multidrug chemotherapy regimens also have been used. Smokers tend to have a higher stage of disease at diagnosis, and their cancer is more resistant to radiation treatment.

With early detection and treatment, prognosis is excellent. Overall, the 5-year survival rate is 66% and increases to 88% with early diagnosis. A cure rate of 100% is possible for women with dysplasia or carcinoma in situ.

Vaginal Cancer

Cancer of the vagina is the rarest of the female genital cancers. It can occur at any age, but is found predominantly in women 60 years of age and older. More than 90% of women with vaginal cancer have squamous cell carcinoma, although melanomas, sarcomas, and adenocarcinomas are also seen. (Types of tumors are described in Chapter 10.) Metastatic cancers are more common than primary lesions in older women.

Vaginal and cervical cancers seem to have similar epidemiology. Both start as intraepithelial lesions and occur in sexually active women. Prior carcinoma of the cervix places a woman at higher risk for developing vaginal cancer. In utero exposure to nonsteroidal estrogens has also been considered a risk factor. It has been estimated that 100,000 to 160,000 women were exposed in utero to such nonsteroidal estrogens as diethylstilbestrol (DES), dienestrol, or hexestrol from 1960 to 1970. Apparently exposure to such hormones during the first 3 months of gestation inhibits the normal replacement of columnar epithelium by squamous epithelium in the vagina of the fetus. The columnar epithelium, which is not normally found in the vagina, then may undergo malignant transformation. Not all women exposed to DES in utero develop neoplastic changes in the vagina, however. Between 0.14 and 1.4 cases of vaginal cancer develop per 1000 women at risk. Nineteen is the average age at which clear cell carcinoma develops as a result of DES exposure.

Like cervical neoplasms, vaginal cancers are classified as intraepithelial neoplasia (dysplasia), carcinoma in situ, or invasive carcinoma. The lesion is usually not invasive, and it most frequently occurs in the upper third of the vagina.

Vaginal cancer is generally asymptomatic. Therefore, regular pelvic examinations, particularly for those exposed to DES in utero, are extremely important. Clinical manifestations that do occur include abnormal vaginal bleeding or discharge and urinary symptoms. Pain is a symptom of advanced disease or an infected lesion.

Biopsy techniques confirm the tumor type and determine its size, location, and extent. Treatment depends on these findings and on the age of the individual. Vaginal dysplasia or carcinoma in situ is excised by using standard surgical techniques, cryotherapy, or laser surgery. Topical 5-fluorouracil (5-FU) also may be used. If the lesion is invasive, surgery may include hysterectomy, vaginectomy, and pelvic bilateral inguinal lymphadenectomy. Radiation and chemotherapy may follow surgery. Approximately 40% of individuals with invasive vaginal cancer develop recurrent cancer, which is usually confined to the pelvic area.

Endometrial Cancer

Adenocarcinoma of the endometrium is the most prevalent gynecologic malignancy. It accounts for more than 40% of female cancers and usually affects postmenopausal women with higher socioeconomic status (ACS, 1992). Peak incidence occurs at 58 to 60 years of age. Estimates include 44,500 new cases in 1993, with approximately 10,100 deaths. Although the cause of endometrial cancer is not clear, a number of risk factors have been identified, including obesity, a diet high in fat, infertility or never experiencing pregnancy, late menopause (after 52 years), and, possibly, diabetes and hypertension. Postmenopausal women who have endometrial hyperplasia secondary to estrogen replacement therapy are particularly at risk.

The use of oral contraceptives containing synthetic estrogen and progesterone has a protective effect. After 12 months of use, the risk of endometrial cancer is half that of women who have never used oral contraceptives; this effect seems to persist long after the pills are discontinued.

More than 90% of endometrial cancers are adenocarcinomas. Abnormal vaginal bleeding is the only clinical manifestation of endometrial cancer. The bleeding is caused by disruption of the endometrial surface by neoplastic processes.

Screening methods for early detection of endometrial cancer are as effective as those for cervical cancer. Pap smears can show endometrial cancer in up to 50% of cases, but direct cytologic sampling of the endometrium is required for diagnosis. This may be accomplished by endometrial biopsy or fractional curettage that includes biopsies of all sectors of the uterus. Hysteroscopy and hysterography may also be used to examine the endometrium, but these methods may result in uterine perforation or enhancement of tumor cell migration if disease is advanced. Evaluation for metastasis includes routine blood work, metabolic studies, chest x-ray films, intravenous pyelography (IVP), barium enema, ultrasonography, and lymphangiography.

Treatment is based on the extent of the disease and includes surgical removal of the obvious tumor and radiation for control of residual microscopic disease. Surgical interventions may include curettage for carcinoma in situ, total abdominal hysterectomy with bilateral salpingo-oophorectomy, and lymphadenectomy. Chemotherapy also may be used. Progesterone may benefit individuals with advanced or recurrent disease. Multidrug protocols are currently under investigation because the results of single-drug therapy for endometrial cancer have been disappointing. Survival rates range from 75% to 95%.

Ovarian Cancer

Cancer of the ovaries is the sixth most frequent cancer in women. Ovarian cancer accounts for 5% of all female cancer deaths and causes more deaths than any other cancer of the female reproductive system (ACS, 1993). The incidence of ovarian cancer is highest in industrialized countries. Approximately 1 of every 70 (1.4%) women in the United States will develop ovarian cancer during her lifetime. Incidence rates increase with age and peak between the ages of 40 and 80.

Pathogenesis

The cause of ovarian cancer is unknown at present. The risk of the disease is greatest for women with one or more first-degree relatives affected by ovarian cancer. Other risk factors include a personal history of breast, endometrial, or colorectal cancer; infertility; early menopause; obesity; a high-fat diet; and, possibly, exposure to asbestos or talc. Pregnancy and childbirth decrease the risk. Oral contraceptive use provides the same protection from ovarian cancer as it does from endometrial cancer (see p. 766).

There are two major types of ovarian cancer: epithelial ovarian neoplasms and germ cell neoplasms. Most ovarian malignancies are epithelial ovarian neoplasms, which usually develop from the surface epithelium of the ovary. Epithelial ovarian tumors may be serous, mucinous, endometrial, or undifferentiated. These tumors are classified as (1) benign, (2) borderline malignant, or (3) frankly malignant. The malignant forms are collectively classed as ovarian adenocarcinomas, which account for 85% to 90% of all ovarian malignancies. Of the ovarian adenocarcinomas, 40% to 50% are serous epithelial malignancies, which usually involve both ovaries and tend to be bulky. Serous tumors generally affect women from 50 to 55 years of age and are extremely rare in prepubertal girls. The 5-year survival rate is 25% to 30%.

Germ cell tumors are derived from the primitive germ cells (gametes) of the embryonic gonad and may be either malignant or benign. The benign cystic teratoma accounts for approximately 10% of all ovarian tumors. If the germ cell tumor is malignant, it tends to be a highly aggressive and rapidly growing tumor with a poor prognosis. Germ cell tumors almost always occur in children or adolescents.

Clinical Manifestations

The intrapelvic location of the ovaries and the range of tumor activity (from slow to rapid and relentless growth) cause diverse signs and symptoms. Ovarian cancer is generally considered a silent disease, meaning that by the time the individual experiences symptoms and seeks treatment, the disease has spread beyond the primary site.

The most obvious symptoms are pain and abdominal swelling that arise from the primary ovarian mass, epigastricomental plaques, or ascites. Gastrointestinal manifestations may include dyspepsia, vomiting, and alterations in bowel habits caused by the mechanical obstruction by the tumor. Abnormal vaginal bleeding may occur if the postmenopausal endometrium is stimulated

by a hormone-secreting tumor. The tumor also may cause ulcerations through the vaginal wall that result in bleeding.

Systemic manifestations of nonmetastatic malignant disease include connective tissue inflammation (dermatomyositis), abnormal pigmentation (acanthosis nigricans), and subacute cerebellar degeneration. Tumor obstruction of vascular channels can cause venous and, occasionally, arterial thrombosis. Alterations in coagulability also occur, contributing to clot formation. Metastasis frequently causes pleural effusion.

Evaluation and Treatment

Because ovarian cancer has no early symptoms and there are no effective screening techniques to detect it, disease is usually advanced by the time treatment is sought. Diagnosis is made after ultrasound, CT scan, magnetic resonance imaging (MRI), or other imaging techniques that enable clinicians to localize the tumor mass. Staging of disease requires exploratory surgery. The International Federation of Gynecologists and Obstetricians (FIGO) staging system is described in Table 20-7. Other preoperative studies may be used to determine the extent of metastasis. These include an upper gastrointestinal series, barium enema, intravenous pyelogram, mammography, and lymphography.

The search for a tumor marker that could be used as a screen for ovarian cancer is ongoing. Some types of germ cells and, rarely, adenocarcinoma, may be associated with increased levels of alpha-fetoprotein (AFP), human chorionic gonadotropin (HCG), or carcinoembryonic antigen (CEA-125). Increased CEA-125 levels are found in about 78% to 80% of nonmucinous ovarian cancers; however, elevated levels are produced in 29% of nongynecologic tumors and in a variety of noncancerous conditions, for example, endometriosis, PID, benign ovarian cysts, myomas, and pregnancy. Carcinoembryonic antigen is a nonspecific, nonsensitive test for ovarian cancer, but may be more reliable as a screening tool in postmenopausal women. Further research is needed.

The initial approach to treatment is surgery, which is performed to determine the stage of disease and remove as much of the tumor as possible. Radiation therapy may follow if the tumor is smaller than 2 cm in size and is confined to the abdominopelvic area without involvement of the kidneys or liver. Radiation therapy may be administered externally, intraperitoneally, or in both ways. The success of chemotherapy depends on whether the tumor is a discrete mass, the extent of disease, and whether there has been prior exposure to chemotherapeutic agents. Alkylating agents are given alone or in combination with antimetabolites. At this time, chemotherapy can reduce tumor size, but it does not reduce mortality. In 1991, the Food and Drug Administration (FDA) approved al-

TABLE 20-7

FIGO* Staging of Carcinoma of the Ovary

Stage	Characteristics
I	Growth limited to the ovaries
IA	Growth limited to one ovary; no ascites
i.	No tumor on the external surface; capsule intact (90% 5-year survival, with treatment)
ii.	Tumor present on the external surface, or capsule(s) ruptured, or both
IB	Growth limited to both ovaries; no ascites
i.	No tumor on the external surface; capsule intact
ii.	Tumor present on the external surface, or capsule(s) ruptured, or both
IC	Tumor either stage IA or stage IB, with ascites present or with positive peritoneal washings
II	Growth involving one or both ovaries with pelvic extension
IIA	Extension and/or metastases to the uterus and/or tubes
IIB	Extension to other pelvic tissues
IIC	Tumor either stage IIA or stage IIB, but with ascites present or with positive peritoneal washings
III	Growth involving one or both ovaries with intraperitoneal metastases outside the pelvis, or positive retroperitoneal nodes, or both. Tumor limited to the true pelvis with histologically proven malignant extension to small bowel or omentum
IV	Growth involving one or both ovaries with distant metastases. If pleural effusion is present, there must be positive cytology to allot a case to stage IV. Parenchymal liver metastases indicate stage IV
Special category	Unexplored cases that are thought to be ovarian carcinoma

From American Cancer Society, 1992.
*The International Federation of Gynecologists and Obstetricians.

TABLE 20-8

Possible Effects of Chronic Disease on Sexual Functioning in Women

Disease	Sexual function
Cerebral palsy	Intact genital sensations, decreased lubrication; difficulty with sexual activity/positioning because of muscle spasticity, rigidity, and/or weakness; pain with positioning caused by contracture of knees and hips or because of increased spasms with arousal
Cerebrovascular accident (CVA)	Difficulties in sexual positioning and sensitivity because of impaired motor strength, coordination or paralysis; decreased sex drive with stroke on the dominant side of the brain
Diabetes	Diminished intensity of orgasm and gradual decline in ability to achieve orgasm; decreased lubrication and/or recurrent vaginal infections with resultant dyspareunia
Chronic renal failure	Decreased arousal; increasingly rare and less intense orgasms; decreased lubrication
Rheumatoid arthritis (RA)	Painful sexual activity/positions because of swollen, painful joints, muscular atrophy and joint contracture; decreased sex drive because of pain, fatigue, and/or medication; genital sensations remain intact
Systemic lupus erythematosus (SLE)	Similar to RA; decreased lubrication and vaginal lesions result in painful penetration
Myocardial infarction (MI)	Most literature male-oriented; problems related to medications
Multiple sclerosis (MS)	Diminished genital sensitivity; decreased lubrication; declining orgasmic ability; difficulty with sexual activity because of muscle weakness, pain, or incontinence
Spinal cord injury	Reflex sexual response with injury above sacral area; disrupted response with lesion at or below sacrum; loss of sensation, decreased lubrication; spasticity, incontinence, or pain with arousal; continued orgasmic sensations or sensations diffused in general or to specific body parts, such as breast or lips

tretamine as a single agent to treat persistent or recurrent ovarian cancer. Altretamine is used after an initial combination regimen containing an alkylating agent or cisplatin and seems to have the potential to decrease morbidity and, possibly, mortality.

The mortality rate associated with ovarian cancer has not changed significantly over the past 20 years, mostly because disease is already advanced at the time of diagnosis. Five-year mortality rates for epithelial neoplasms range from 15% to 30% for women with early disease (stage IA) to 80% for women with advanced disease (stage IV). The overall survival rate is 39% (ACS, 1993).

Sexual Dysfunction

Increased awareness of female sexual dysfunction is relatively new and most of what is known comes from clinical observations and anecdotal reports from women. Adequate research is needed. Both organic and psychosocial disorders can be implicated in sexual dysfunction. Organic problems may be the underlying cause in 10% to 20% of cases and can contribute to another 15%. The exact cause may not always be identified.

As in men, chronic illness can affect sexual functioning and response in women. For example, neuropathy in the pelvic region may increase the threshold for orgasm in diabetic women. Diminished intensity and gradual decline in orgasm may be analogous to the development of impotence in diabetic men. For women with heart disease, problems in sexual functioning more often are related to drug therapy than the disease itself. Table 20-8 outlines possible effects of specified chronic diseases on female sexual functioning.

Sexual anorexia or inhibited sexual desire (decreased libido) may be a biologic manifestation of depression, alcohol or other substance abuse, prolactin-secreting pituitary tumors, or testosterone deficiency. β-Adrenergic blockers used for heart disease also may inhibit sexual desire.

Vaginismus is an involuntary muscle spasm in response to attempted penetration. Common causes include prior sexual trauma or fear of sex; organic causes are less common and are similar to those that cause dyspareunia. Even after the underlying organic problem is detected and successfully treated, vaginismus may persist.

Anorgasmia or orgasmic dysfunction is the inability of the woman to reach or achieve orgasm. Dysfunction follows a continuum from difficulty in arousal to lack of orgasm. Any chronic illness may affect arousal. Orgasmic dysfunction is linked to organic causes in less than 5% of cases. Diabetes; alcoholism; neurologic disturbances; hormonal deficiencies; and pelvic disorders, such as infections, trauma, and surgical scarring, are specific disorders that may block orgasm. Drugs, such as narcotics, tranquilizers, antidepressants, and antihypertensive medications, also can inhibit orgasm.

Rapid orgasm is a relatively new diagnosis and seems to be rare. In this instance, once orgasm occurs there is little interest in further sexual activity. Rapid orgasm has no known organic cause.

Dyspareunia or painful intercourse is common. Women may experience pain during arousal or at the time of orgasm, at the initiation of intercourse, midway, or after intercourse. The pain may have a burning, sharp, searing, or cramping quality and may be described as external, vaginal, deep abdominal, or pelvic. A variety of psychosocial and organic causes have been identified. Inadequate lubrication may make penetration or intercourse difficult or painful. Drugs with a drying effect, such as antihistamines, certain tranquilizers, and marijuana, and disorders such as diabetes, vaginal infections, and estrogen deficiency, can decrease lubrication. Other causes of dyspareunia include skin problems around the introitus or affecting the vulva; irritation or infection of the clitoris; disorders of the vaginal opening, such as scarring from episiotomy, intact hymen, or chronically infected hymenal remnants; bartholinitis; disorders of the urethra or anus; disorders of the vagina, such as infections, thinning of the walls due to aging or decreased estrogen, irritation due to spermicides or douches; and pelvic disorders, such as infection, tumors, cervical or uterine abnormalities, and torn uterine ligaments.

Sexual dysfunction may develop as a coping mechanism. Women with a history of sexual trauma—rape, incest, or molestation—frequently have problems of desire, arousal, orgasm, or experience pain with sexual activity. In extreme cases, total sexual aversion may develop. At other times, sexual dysfunction may be a symptom of marital or relationship problems. Often unresolved anger may manifest as inhibited desire or diminished arousal.

Impaired Fertility

Infertility affects approximately 15% of all couples and is defined as the inability to conceive after 1 year of unprotected intercourse. Fertility can be impaired by factors in the man or the woman or in both partners. Male factors include diminished quality and production of sperm, and important causes of infertility in the female are associated with malfunctions of the fallopian tubes, the ovaries, or the reproductive hormones. Adhesions from pelvic infection may cause blockage of one or both fallopian tubes preventing access of the sperm to the ovum. Hormonal or local factors may disrupt ovulation or prevent a fertilized egg from implantation. For unclear reasons, endometriosis also may contribute to infertility. These factors have been discussed previously. A number of diagnostic procedures are required in the routine investigation of the infertile couple (Table 19-4). In many instances no cause may be identified.

Treatment of infertility is aimed toward correcting

problems identified during the diagnostic workup. The best treatment for infertility is prevention, specifically prevention of sexually transmitted infection that can result in scarring and adhesion formation in the reproductive tract of either the man or the woman.

DISORDERS OF THE MALE REPRODUCTIVE SYSTEM

Disorders of the Urethra

Urethritis and urethral strictures are common disorders of the male urethra. Urethral carcinoma occurs in men older than 60 years of age, but it is an extremely rare form of cancer.

Urethritis

Urethritis is an inflammatory process that is usually, but not always, caused by a sexually transmitted microorganism. Biologic agents associated with infectious urethritis in males include *Neisseria gonorrhoeae* and *Chlamydia trachomatis*, and, less commonly, *Ureaplasma urealyticum*. Infectious urethritis caused by *N. gonorrhoeae* is often called gonococcal urethritis (GU); that caused by other microorganisms is called nongonococcal urethritis (NGU). (Sexually transmitted urethritis is described in Chapter 21.) Nonsexual origins of urethritis include inflammation or infection as a result of urologic procedures, insertion of foreign bodies into the urethra, anatomic abnormalities, or trauma.

Noninfectious urethritis is rare and is associated with the ingestion of wood or ethyl alcohol or turpentine. It is also seen with Reiter syndrome, which involves a number of mucocutaneous lesions.

Symptoms of urethritis include urethral tingling or itching or a burning sensation on urinating, frequency, and urgency. The individual may notice a purulent or clear mucus-like discharge from the urethra. Treatment consists of appropriate antibiotic therapy for infectious urethritis and avoidance of future exposure or mechanical irritation.

Urethral Strictures

A **urethral stricture** is a narrowing of the urethra caused by scarring. The scars may be congenital but are more likely to result from trauma (e.g., injury or urologic instrumentation) or untreated or severe urethral infections. Prostatitis and infection secondary to urinary stasis are common complications. Severe and prolonged obstruction can result in hydronephrosis and renal failure.

The clinical manifestations of urethral stricture are caused by bladder outlet obstruction. Symptoms include urinary frequency and hesitancy, diminished force and caliber of the urinary stream, dribbling after voiding, and nocturia.

Urethral stricture is diagnosed on the basis of history, physical examination, and cytoscopy. Treatment is usually surgical and may involve urethral dilation, urethrotomy, or a variety of open surgical techniques. The choice of surgical intervention depends on the age of the individual and the severity of the problem.

Disorders of the Penis
Phimosis and Paraphimosis

Phimosis and paraphimosis are both disorders in which the foreskin (prepuce) is "too tight" to be moved easily over the glans penis. **Phimosis** is a condition in which the foreskin cannot be retracted back over the glans, whereas **paraphimosis** is the opposite: the foreskin is retracted and cannot be moved forward (reduced) to cover the glans (Fig. 20-12). Both conditions can cause penile pathology.

The inability to retract the foreskin is normal in infancy and is caused by congenital adhesions. During the first 3 years of life, these adhesions separate naturally with penile erections and are not an indication for circumcision. Phimosis can occur at any age and is most commonly caused by poor hygiene and chronic infection. It rarely occurs with normal foreskin.

Edema, erythema, and tenderness of the prepuce and purulent discharge are usually the reasons for seeking treatment; inability to retract the foreskin is a less common complaint. Circumcision, if needed, is performed after infection has been eradicated. Complications of phimosis include inflammation of the glans (balanitis) or prepuce (posthitis) and paraphimosis. There is a higher incidence of penile carcinoma in uncircumcised males, but chronic infection and poor hygiene are usually the underlying factors in such cases.

Paraphimosis, in which the foreskin is retracted, can constrict the penis, causing edema of the glans. If edema is such that the foreskin cannot be reduced manually, surgery must be performed to prevent necrosis of the glans caused by constricted blood vessels. Severe paraphimosis is a surgical emergency.

Peyronie Disease

Peyronie disease, the "bent nail syndrome," is a fibrotic condition that causes lateral curvature of the penis during erection (Fig. 20-13). Peyronie disease develops slowly and is characterized by tough fibrous thickening of the fascia in the erectile tissue of the corpora cavernosa. A dense, fibrous plaque is usually palpable on the dorsum of the penile shaft. The problem usually affects middle-aged men and is associated with painful erection, painful intercourse (for both partners), and poor erection distal to the involved area. In some cases, impotence or unsatisfactory penetration occurs. There is no pain when the penis is flaccid.

Although the exact cause is unknown, a local vasculitis-like inflammatory reaction occurs and de-

FIG. 20-12 **Phimosis and paraphimosis. A,** Phimosis: the foreskin has a pinpoint opening that is not large enough to permit retraction over the glans. **B,** Paraphimosis: the foreskin is retracted over the glans but cannot be reduced to its normal position. Here it has formed a constricting band around the penis. (From Phipps, Long, Woods, & Cassmeyer, 1991.)

FIG. 20-13 **Peyronie disease.** (Courtesy Patrick C. Walsh, MD. The Johns Hopkins University School of Medicine, Baltimore.) (From Seidel, Ball, Dains, & Benedict, 1991.)

FIG. 20-14 **Priapism.** (From Lloyd-Davies, Gow, & Davies, 1983.)

creased tissue oxygenation results in fibrosis and calcification. Peyronie disease is associated with Dupuytren contracture (a flexion deformity of the fingers or toes caused by shortening or fibrosis of the palmar or plantar fascia), diabetes, and the tendency to develop keloids.

There is no definitive treatment for Peyronie disease. Spontaneous remissions occur up to 50% of the time. Pharmacologic therapies, such as vitamin E and Potaba, that increase oxygenation may hasten self-resolution if used several times a day for prolonged periods. Plication, as well as surgical resection of the fibrous plaque followed by grafting, have been successful (Tanagho & McAninch, 1992).

Priapism

Priapism is an uncommon condition of prolonged penile erection. It is usually painful and is not associated with sexual arousal (Fig. 20-14). Priapism is idiopathic in 60% of cases, whereas the remaining 40% of cases can be associated with spinal cord trauma, sickle cell disease, leukemia, pelvic tumors, or intracavernous injection therapy for impotence. The two corpora cavernosa within the erect penis are filled with blood and tender to palpation; the corpus spongiosum is not engorged. The vascular congestion is thought to be associated with venous obstruction. If the erection remains over a period of days, edema and fibrosis develop, leading to erectile dysfunction (impotence).

Priapism must be considered a urologic emergency. Treatment within hours is effective and prevents impotence. Conservative approaches include iced saline enemas, ketamine administration, and spinal anesthesia. Needle aspiration of blood from the corpus through the dorsal glans is often effective and is followed by catheterization and pressure dressings to maintain decom-

pression. More aggressive surgical treatments include the creation of vascular shunts to maintain blood flow. Erectile dysfunction results in up to 50% of cases.

Balanitis

Balanitis is an inflammation of the glans penis (Fig. 20-15) and usually occurs in conjunction with posthitis, an inflammation of the prepuce. (Inflammation of the glans and the prepuce is called balanoposthitis.) It is associated with poor hygiene and phimosis. The accumulation under the foreskin of glandular secretions (smegma),

FIG. 20-15 Balanitis. (From Lloyd-Davies, Gow, & Davies, 1983.)

TABLE 20-9

Classifications of Carcinoma of the Penis

Stage	Definition
I	Tumor limited to the glans or foreskin
II	Tumor extends to shaft of penis
III	Inguinal lymph nodes involved but operable
IV	Inguinal nodes inoperable or distant metastasis has occurred

sloughed epithelial cells, and *Mycobacterium smegmatis* can irritate the glans directly or lead to infection. Skin disorders (e.g., psoriasis, lichen planus, eczema) and candidiasis must be differentiated from inflammation resulting from poor hygienic practices. Balanitis is most commonly seen in men with poorly controlled diabetes mellitus and candidiasis. Antimicrobials are used to treat infection. Circumcision can prevent recurrences and can be considered after the inflammation has subsided.

Penile Cancer

Carcinoma of the penis is rare in the United States, constituting only 0.3% to 0.6% of all malignancies in men. Although it is considered a disease of the elderly, penile cancer can affect men 40 to 80 years of age, with 40% of diagnosed men younger than age 60. The disease occurs almost twice as frequently in blacks as compared with whites in the United States and tends to be more common in lower socioeconomic groups. Although the exact cause is unknown, cancer of the penis is thought to develop as a result of chronic irritation caused by smegma beneath a phimotic foreskin. The incidence of penile carcinoma is highest in populations where infantile circumcision and adequate genital hygiene are not routinely practiced. In these areas, penile cancer remains a significant health problem and accounts for 10% to 20% of all malignancies in men.

Squamous cell carcinoma accounts for 95% of invasive penile cancers. Other premalignant lesions, in situ forms of epidermal carcinoma, can occur on the penis. These include leukoplakia (white plaque), Paget disease (red, inflamed areas), erythroplasia of Queyrat (raised red areas), and Busche Lowerstein patches (large venous areas). Condylomata (genital warts) caused by the HPV may be involved in the development of precancerous lesions. At times, the penis might be the site of metastatic spread of solid tumors from the bladder, prostate, rectum, or kidney. Early squamous cell carcinoma and premalignant epidermal lesions are easily treated but are often ignored. Delays in seeking treatment are attributed to denial, embarrassment, failure to detect lesions under a phimotic foreskin, fear, guilt, and ignorance.

Squamous cell carcinoma usually begins as a small, fat ulcerative or papillary lesion on the glans or foreskin that grows to involve the entire penile shaft. Extensive lesions are associated with metastases and a poor prognosis. These lesions are not as painful as the amount of tissue involvement would seem to indicate. The regional femoral and iliac nodes are common metastatic sites. Rarely the urethra and bladder are involved. Weight loss, fatigue, and malaise accompany chronic suppurative lesions. Untreated, progressive disease causes death within 2 years.

The specific diagnosis is made by biopsy after examination to document the location, size, and fixation of the lesion and the absence or presence of regional adenopathy. Distant metastases are uncommon. Classifications of carcinoma of the penis are presented in Table 20-9.

For invasive penile carcinoma, complete excision leaving adequate tumor-free margins is the goal. A simple circumcision may be sufficient for localized lesions of the prepuce. If the glans and distal shaft are the primary site, the penis is amputated, leaving a 2-cm margin proximal to the tumor. Inguinal lymph nodes also are removed if metastasis to these structures is known or suspected. Palliative treatment with radiation or chemotherapy may be used when the disease is inoperable and bulky inguinal metastases have occurred. Options for individuals with carcinoma in situ include local excision, radiation, laser surgery, cryosurgery, chemosurgery, or chemotherapy with topical (5%) 5-fluorouracil. The 5-year survival rate for stage I disease is over 80%.

Disorders of the Scrotum, Testis, and Epididymis
Disorders of the Scrotum

Varicocele, hydrocele, and spermatocele are common intrascrotal disorders. A **varicocele** is an abnormal dilatation of a vein within the spermatic cord and is classically described as a "bag of worms" (Fig. 20-16). Most (95%) occur on the left side and may be painful or tender. Varicocele occurs in 10% to 15% of males and is seen most frequently after puberty. Sudden development of a varicocele in an older man is a late sign of renal tumor. Unilateral right-sided varicoceles are rare and result from compression or obstruction of the inferior vena cava by a tumor or thrombus.

The cause of varicocele is incompetent or congenitally absent valves in the spermatic veins. The valves that normally prevent backflow are absent or do not close adequately, permitting blood to pool in the veins rather than flow into the venous system. Varicocele decreases blood flow through the testis. This interferes with spermatogenesis and is a cause of infertility. If infertility is a problem, treatment consists of ligation of the spermatic vein. If varicocele is mild and fertility is not an issue, a scrotal support is usually sufficient to relieve symptoms of scrotal heaviness or "dragging."

A **hydrocele** is a collection of fluid within the tunica vaginalis (Fig. 20-17). It is the most common cause of scrotal swelling. Hydroceles in infants are congenital

FIG. 20-16 **Varicocele.** Dilation of veins within the spermatic cord. (From Seidel, Ball, Dains, & Benedict, 1991.)

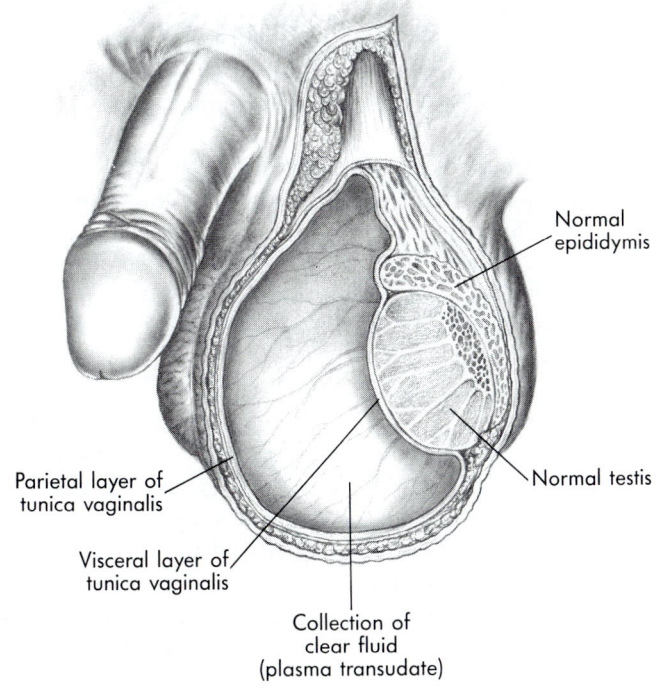

Normal epididymis

Normal testis

Parietal layer of tunica vaginalis

Visceral layer of tunica vaginalis

Collection of clear fluid (plasma transudate)

FIG. 20-17 **Hydrocele.** Accumulation of clear fluid between the visceral and parietal layers of the tunica vaginalis.

FIG. 20-18 Spermatocele. Retention cyst of the head of the epididymis or of an aberrant tubule or tubules of the rete testis. The spermatocele lies outside the tunica vaginalis; therefore, on palpation it can be readily distinguished and separated from the testis. (From Lloyd-Davies, Gow, & Davies, 1983.)

malformations that frequently resolve spontaneously by 1 year of age. Hydroceles in adults may be caused by an imbalance between the secreting and absorptive capacities of scrotal tissues. Hydroceles range in size from slightly larger than the testes to the size of a grapefruit or larger and may be flaccid or tense. Compression of testicular blood supply may lead to atrophy.

The exact mechanism of idiopathic hydrocele is unknown. Secondary hydrocele may result from trauma or infection of the testis or epididymis or from a testicular tumor. Treatment for uncomplicated hydrocele is aspiration of the fluid and injection of a sclerosing drug into the scrotal sac. The goal of treatment is to remove the hydrocele and prevent recurrence by causing sclerosis of the tunica vaginalis. Treatment for recurrent hydroceles is excision of the tunica vaginalis.

A **spermatocele** is a cyst located between the head of the epididymis and the testis that is filled with milky fluid that contains sperm (Fig. 20-18). Spermatoceles that cause pain or discomfort are excised. Usually, however, spermatoceles are asymptomatic or produce mild discomfort that is relieved by scrotal support. Neither hydroceles nor spermatoceles are associated with infertility.

Cryptorchidism

Cryptorchidism is a condition in which one or both testes fail to descend into the scrotum. It is the most common congenital condition involving the testes. Three percent of all full-term males and 20% of all premature males have undescended testes at birth. The testes may remain in the abdomen, or descent may be arrested in the inguinal canal or the puboscrotal junction. In approximately 75% to 90% of infants with cryptorchidism, the testes descend into the scrotum by 1 year of

age, leaving a true incidence of 0.8% of the male population.

The cause of testicular maldescent is not clear. Cryptorchidism may result from a developmental delay, a defect of the testis, deficient maternal gonadotropin stimulation, or some mechanical factor that prevents descent through the inguinal canal. Mechanical possibilities include a short spermatic cord, fibrous bands or adhesions in the normal path of the testes, or a narrowed inguinal canal. Chromosomal studies do not support a genetic component.

Untreated cryptorchidism is associated with a lowered sperm count and, therefore, impaired fertility. Impaired spermatogenesis is caused by higher temperatures within the abdomen. Cryptorchidism does not prevent puberty or maintenance of secondary sex characteristics if the testis is otherwise normal. Undescended testes are susceptible to neoplastic processes: the risk of testicular cancer is 35 to 50 times greater for men with cryptorchidism or a history of cryptorchidism than for the general male population.

Physical examination discloses the absence of one or both testes in the scrotum. Ultrasonography or a CT scan can help clinicians to locate a testis that has migrated intraabdominally. Treatment often begins with administration of HCG, a hormone that may initiate descent, making surgery unnecessary. If hormonal therapy is not successful, the testis is located and moved surgically (orchiopexy). To preserve fertility, surgical correction of cryptorchidism should be attempted when the child is about 2 years of age. Orchiopexy is recommended no later than age 5 or 6. Placement of the cryptorchid testis into the scrotal sac does not decrease the potential for malignancy; it does facilitate examination and tumor detection.

Torsion of the Testis

Torsion of the testis is a condition in which the testis rotates on its vascular pedicle, interrupting its blood supply. This event can occur at any age but is most common among neonates and adolescents, with highest incidence at the time of puberty. Onset may be spontaneous or follow physical exertion or trauma. Torsion twists the arteries and veins in the spermatic cord, reducing or stopping circulation to the testis. Vascular engorgement and ischemia develop, causing scrotal swelling. These manifestations are not relieved by rest or scrotal support. Torsion of the testis is a surgical emergency. If the torsion cannot be reduced manually, surgery must be performed within 6 hours after the onset of symptoms to preserve normal testicular function. Surgery includes untwisting the spermatic cord and anchoring both testicles in correct position within the scrotum to prevent recurrences. With successful manual detorsion, surgical fixation should be done within a few days.

FIG. 20-19 Orchitis. (From Seidel, Ball, Dains, & Benedict, 1991.)

FIG. 20-20 Testicular tumor. (From *400 Self-assessment picture tests*, 1984.)

Orchitis

Orchitis is an acute inflammation of the testes (Fig. 20-19), and is uncommon except as a complication of systemic infection or as an extension of an associated epididymitis (see p. 778). Infectious organisms may reach the testes through the blood or the lymphatics, or, most commonly, by ascent through the urethra, vas deferens, and epididymis. Most cases of orchitis are actually cases of epididymoorchitis. Occasionally in middle-aged men, a nonspecific, apparently noninfectious, inflammatory process (called granulomatis orchitis) can occur. It seems to be an autoimmune disease that triggers a granulomatous response to spermatozoa.

Mumps is the most common infectious cause of orchitis and usually affects postpubertal males. The onset is sudden, occurring 3 to 4 days after the onset of parotitis. Signs and symptoms include high fever, reaching 40° C (104° F), marked prostration, bilateral or unilateral erythema, edema and tenderness of the scrotum, and leukocytosis. An acute hydrocele may develop. Urinary signs and symptoms, which accompany epididymitis, are absent. Atrophy with irreversible damage to the spermatogenesis may result in 30% of affected testes. Bilateral orchitis does not affect androgenic function but may cause permanent sterility.

Treatment is supportive and includes bed rest, scrotal support, elevation of the scrotum, hot or cold compresses, and analgesic agents for relief of pain. If an acute hydrocele develops, it is aspirated. Testicular abscess usually requires orchiectomy (removal of the tes-

tis). Appropriate antimicrobial drugs should be used for bacterial orchitis, and corticosteroids are indicated in proved cases of nonspecific granulomatous orchitis.

Cancer of the Testis

Testicular cancer is among the most curable of cancers; for nearly all common types, cure rates are greater than 95%. Overall, testicular cancers are rare, accounting for approximately 1% of all male cancers; yet, they are the most common solid tumor of young adult men. Approximately 6600 cases are predicted for 1993 (ACS, 1993), with an estimated 350 deaths. Cancer of the testis occurs most commonly in men between the ages of 15 and 34 years. Of interest, within a given race, cancer rates in higher socioeconomic groups are twice the rate of those in the lower levels. In the United States, the lifetime probability of developing testicular cancer is 0.2% for white men, an incidence that is 4.5 times higher than in blacks. Testicular tumors are slightly more common on the right side than on the left, a pattern that parallels the occurrence of cryptorchidism, and are bilateral in 1% to 3% of cases (Fig. 20-20).

Pathogenesis

Most testicular cancers are germ cell tumors: that is, they arise from the male gametes. Germ cell tumors include seminomas, embryonal carcinomas, teratomas, and choriosarcomas. Of these tumors, seminomas are the least and choriosarcomas are the most aggressive. Testicular tumors also can arise from specialized cells of the gonadal stroma. These tumors, which are named for their cellular origins, are the Leydig cell, Sertoli cell, granulosa cell, and theca cell tumors.

The cause of testicular neoplasms is unknown. Because young men are affected most frequently, it is thought that high levels of androgens may contribute to tumorigenesis. A genetic predisposition is suggested by the fact that the incidence is higher among brothers, identical twins, and other close male relatives. Genetic predisposition is supported further by statistics showing that the disease is relatively rare among black Africans, black Americans, Asians, and native New Zealanders. Cryptorchidism is statistically associated with the development of testicular cancer. Apparently the undescended testis has a developmental defect or undergoes gradual involution and degeneration over time, which may contribute to neoplastic changes. A history of trauma or infection also is associated with the development of testicular neoplasms, but it may be that coexisting testicular tumors are discovered by "accident" in men who undergo examination because of trauma or infections. Research regarding the role prenatal exposure to DES, exogenous hormones, or pesticides may play in the development of testicular cancer has been inconclusive.

Clinical Manifestations

Painless testicular enlargement commonly is the first sign of testicular cancer. Enlargement is usually gradual and may be accompanied by a sensation of testicular heaviness or dull ache in the lower abdomen. Occasionally acute pain occurs because of rapid growth resulting in hemorrhage and necrosis. Ten percent of affected men have epididymitis. The testicular mass is usually discovered by the individual or by his sexual partner. Gynecomastia is noted or a hydrocele is present in about 5% of all cases of testicular cancer. Approximately 10% of individuals already have symptoms related to metastases at the time of initial diagnosis. Lumbar pain also may be present and is usually caused by retroperitoneal node metastasis. Signs of metastasis to the lungs include cough, dyspnea, and bloody sputum (hemoptysis). Supraclavicular node involvement may cause difficulty swallowing (dysphagia) and neck swelling. Alterations in vision or mental status, papilledema, and seizures may be experienced with metastasis to the central nervous system.

Evaluation and Treatment

Evaluation begins with careful physical examination, including palpation of the scrotal contents with the individual in the erect and supine positions. Signs of testicular cancer include abnormal consistency, induration, nodularity, or irregularity of the testis. Transillumination may be helpful in identifying scrotal contents. The abdomen and lymph nodes are palpated to seek evidence of metastasis. Tumor type is identified after or-

chiectomy. Testicular biopsy is not recommended because it may cause dissemination of the tumor and increase the risk of local recurrence. Chest x-ray films, lymphangiograms, intravenous pyelograms, abdominal ultrasound or CT scan, and measurement of serum markers (α-fetoprotein and β-subunit gonadotropin) are used in clinical staging of disease. Besides surgery, treatment involves radiation and chemotherapy singly or in combination. A number of factors influence the prognosis (Table 20-10). They include histology of the tumor stage of the disease, and selection of appropriate treatment. Serum markers are useful for detecting metastases and assessing responses to therapy. Most patients treated for cancer of the testis can expect a normal lifespan; some have persistent paresthesias, Raynaud phenomenon, or infertility. Almost 90% of disease-related deaths occur in the first 2 years after cessation of therapy; disease-free survival of 3 years is considered a cure. Orchiectomy does not affect sexual function.

Impairment of Sperm Production and Quality

Spermatogenesis requires adequate secretion of FSH and LH by the pituitary and sufficient secretion of testosterone by the testes. Inadequate secretion of gonadotropins may be caused by hypothyroidism, hyperadrenocortisolism, hyperprolactinemia, or hypogonadotropic hypogonadism. In these situations, gonadotropin levels are low because of feedback inhibition or idiopathic hyposecretion. In the absence of adequate gonadotropin levels, the Leydig cells are not stimulated to secrete testosterone, and sperm maturation is not promoted in the Sertoli cells. Spermatogenesis depends not only on appropriate stimulation by the gonadotropins, but also on an appropriate response by the testes. Defects in testicular response to the gonadotropins result in decreased secretion of testosterone and, as a result of normal feedback mechanisms, high levels of circulating gonadotropins. In the absence of adequate testosterone levels, spermatogenesis is impaired.

Impaired spermatogenesis also can be caused by testicular trauma, infection, or atrophy of the testes from any cause. Other conditions associated with impaired spermatogenesis include systemic illness involving high fever, ingestion of various drugs, exposure to environmental toxins, and cryptorchidism.

Fertility is adversely affected if spermatogenesis is normal but the sperm are chromosomally or morphologically abnormal or are produced in insufficient quantities. Chromosomal abnormalities are caused by genetic factors and by external variables, such as exposure to radiation or toxic substances. A sperm count of 10 to 20 million sperm per milliliter of semen has been suggested as the minimum concentration required for fertility. Average fertile men have 50 to 100 million sperm per milliliter.

Sperm motility is another important variable affect-

TABLE 20-10

Testicular Tumors of Germ Cell Origin

Cell types	Occurrence	Metastatic pattern	Prognosis/remission rate
Single-cell tumors			
Seminoma (germinoma)	35%-40% of all testicular tumors	Rarely to retroperitoneal lymph nodes	Excellent; tumor usually remains localized and is responsive to radiation; cure rate stage I and II >95%; stage II and IV >80%
Embryonal carcinoma	20%-25% of all testicular tumors	Earlier to regional lymphatics, also lung, liver, bone	Good; complete remission rate stage I and II >95%; stage II and IV >70-80%
Teratoma	5%-10% of all testicular tumors (occurs primarily in infants and young children)	Through lymphatics and bloodstream; affects same organ systems as embryonal type	Fair
Choriocarcinoma	1%-3% of all testicular tumors	Earliest and widest, initially through bloodstream	Poor; early metastasis
Mixed tumors			
Teratocarcinoma	20%-25% of all testicular tumors	Mixed pattern; depends on cell types	Variable; prognosis becomes that of the most malignant element
Other Teratocarcinoma with seminoma Embryonal cancer with seminoma Teratoma with seminoma Any combination with choriocarcinoma	10%-15% of all testicular tumors	Mixed pattern; depends on cell types	Variable; prognosis becomes that of the most malignant element

From American Cancer Society, 1991; Tanagho & McAninch, 1992.

TABLE 20-11

Volume and Characteristics of Semen

	Normal semen quality	Marginal semen quality	Abnormal semen quality
Semen volume (ml)	≥2	1-1.9	< 1
Sperm concentration ($\times 10^6$ ml [million/ml])	≥20	10-19.9	<10
Sperm motility (% motility)	≥50 with forward progression; ≥25 with rapid linear progression within 60 min after collection	40-40.9	<40
Morphology (% with normal morphology)	≥50	40-40.9	<40

From Davies & Kase, 1990; Fathalla, Rosenfield, Indriso, Sen, & Ratnam, 1990.

ing fertility. Motility appears to be affected by the sperm's chemical environment, that is, the characteristics of semen (Table 20-11). Prostatic dysfunction, excessive semen viscosity, presence of drugs or toxins in the semen, and presence of antisperm antibodies are associated with impaired sperm motility. Approximately 17% of infertile males have antisperm antibodies in their semen. Antisperm antibodies may develop as a result of trauma to or obstruction of the reproductive organs or genetic defect in self-recognition or may be stimulated by cross-reactive microbial antigens present in urinary tract infections. Antisperm antibodies may be (1) cytotoxic antibodies, which attack sperm and reduce their number in the semen, or (2) sperm-immobilizing antibodies, which impair sperm motility and reduce their ability to transverse the endocervical canal.

Treatment for impaired spermatogenesis involves correction of any underlying disorders and avoidance of radiation or toxins. Androgens, human gonadotropins, and antiestrogens (such as clomiphene citrate or tamoxifen citrate) may enhance spermatogenesis. Semen can be modified to improve sperm motility. If conception is desired, the semen is obtained by masturbation, after which it can be diluted, concentrated, or washed to remove antisperm antibodies. These alterations are followed by artificial insemination.

Epididymitis

Epididymitis, or inflammation of the epididymis, generally occurs in sexually active young males (younger than 35 years of age) and is rare before puberty (Fig. 20-21). In young men the usual cause is a sexually transmitted microorganism, such as *Neisseria gonorrhoeae* or *Chlamydia trachomatis*. In men older than 35 years of age, Enterobacteriaceae (intestinal bacteria) and *P. aeruginosa* associated with urinary tract infections and prostatitis also may cause epididymitis. Rarely epididymitis occurs after strenuous lifting or straining, or after scrotal trauma.

Pathophysiology

The pathogenic microorganism usually reaches the epididymis by ascending the vasa deferentia from an already infected urethra or bladder. The presence of bacteria initiates the inflammatory response, causing symptoms of bacterial epididymitis. Epididymitis caused by heavy lifting or straining results from reflux of urine from the bladder into the vas deferens and epididymis. Urine is extremely irritating to the epididymis and initiates an inflammatory response called chemical epididymitis.

Clinical Manifestations

Pain is the main symptom of epididymitis. Scrotal or inguinal pain is caused by inflammation of the epididymis and surrounding tissues. The pain is usually acute and severe. Flank pain may occur if, as the urethra passes over the spermatic cord, edematous swelling of the cord obstructs the urethra. The individual may have pyuria and bacteriuria and a history of urinary symptoms, including urethral discharge. The scrotum on the involved side is red and edematous as a result of inflammatory changes. The tail of the epididymis near the lower pole of the testis usually swells first; then swelling ascends to the head of the epididymis. The spermatic cord also may be swollen and tender.

Complications of epididymitis include abscess formation, infarction of the testis, recurrent infection, and infertility. Infarction is probably caused by thrombosis (obstruction by blood clots) of the prostatic vessels secondary to severe inflammation. Recurrent epididymitis may result from inadequate initial treatment or failure to identify or treat predisposing factors. Chronic epididymitis can cause scarring of the epididymal endothelium. Once scarring has occurred, treatment with antibiotics is ineffective because adequate antibiotic levels cannot be achieved within the epididymis.

Evaluation and Treatment

A history of recent urinary tract infection or urethral discharge suggests the diagnosis of epididymitis. The relief of pain when the inflamed testis and epididymis are elevated (Phren sign) is also diagnostic. Definitive diagnosis is based on culture or Gram stain of a urethral swab. Epididymal aspiration may be necessary to obtain a specimen, especially if the individual has been taking antibiotics and has sterile urine.

Treatment includes antibiotic therapy for the infection itself and various measures to provide sympto-

FIG. 20-21 Epididymitis. (From Lloyd-Davis, Gow, & Davies, 1983.)

matic relief. Bed rest and scrotal elevation are recommended until the scrotum is no longer tender. Scrotal elevation facilitates maximal lymphatic and venous drainage. Abscess formation is rare with antibiotic therapy. If an abscess occurs and persists, it is drained surgically and an orchiectomy may be indicated. Complete resolution of swelling and pain may take several weeks to months. The individual's sexual partner should be treated with antibiotics if the causative microorganism is a sexually transmitted pathogen.

Disorders of the Prostate Gland
Benign Prostatic Hyperplasia

Benign prostatic hyperplasia (BPH), also called benign prostatic hypertrophy, is the enlargement of the prostate gland (Fig. 20-22). This condition becomes problematic as prostatic tissue compresses the urethra, where it passes through the prostate. Approximately 51% of men between 60 and 69 years of age have prostatic enlargement. Although BPH is common, its cause remains obscure. Its relationship to aging is well-documented, however. At birth, the prostate is pea-sized and growth of the gland is gradual until puberty. There is a period of rapid development that continues until the third decade of life when the prostate reaches adult size (see Chapter 19). Around 40 to 45 years of age, benign hyperplasia begins and continues slowly until death. Although androgenic stimulation is necessary for normal prostatic development, its role in BPH remains unclear. Current causative theories of BPH focus on estrogen/androgen synergism or undefined prostatic growth factors with possible hormonal involvement.

Benign prostatic hyperplasia begins in the periurethral glands, which are the inner glands or layers of the pros-

FIG. 20-22 Benign prostatic hypertrophy. (From Seidel, Ball, Dains, & Benedict, 1991.)

tate. The prostate enlarges as nodules form and grow (nodular hyperplasia) and glandular cells enlarge (hypertrophy). As nodular hyperplasia and cellular hypertrophy progress, tissues that surround the prostatic urethra compress it, usually but not always causing bladder outflow obstruction.

During the early stages of urethral obstruction, the detrusor muscle hypertrophies to help the bladder force urine out against increasing resistance. Symptoms include the urge to urinate frequently, some delay in starting urination, and decreased force of the urinary stream. As the obstruction progresses, often over a period of several years, the bladder is unable to empty all of the urine. Increasing volumes of urine are retained until urine retention is chronic. The volume of urine retained may be great enough to produce uncontrolled "overflow incontinence" with any increase in intraabdominal pressure. At this stage, the force of the urinary stream is significantly reduced, and it takes much more time to initiate and complete voiding.

Progressive bladder distention causes sacculations or diverticular outpouchings of the bladder wall. The ureters may be obstructed where they pass through the hypertrophied detrusor muscle. Hydroureter, hydronephrosis, and bladder or kidney infection then develop.

There is no way to reverse progressive BPH, but the hyperplasia is not always progressive. Annual digital rectal examinations (DRE) are used to screen men over 40 for BPH. When necessary, the hyperplastic tissue may be removed surgically to prevent the serious consequences of urethral obstruction. A permanent indwelling catheter is inserted if the individual cannot tolerate surgery. Recently, BPH has been successfully treated with drugs. α-Adrenergic blockers (prazosin and terazosin) are used to relax the smooth muscle of the bladder and prostate. In the fall of 1992, the FDA approved the use of finasteride (Proscar) for BPH. This drug shrinks the prostate gland by interrupting the action of hormones and offers an alternative to surgery for up to 75% of men with mild prostate enlargement (Gilbaugh, 1992). Neither the α-blockers nor finasteride seems to affect sexual desire or potency; finasteride may cause bone loss and lower levels of prostate-specific antigen (PSA). Prostate-specific antigen is used as a screen for prostate cancer.

Prostatitis

Prostatitis is an inflammation of the prostate. Some degree of prostatic inflammation is present in 4% to 36% of the male population. This percentage increases to 50% in older men. Inflammation is usually limited to a few of the gland's excretory ducts (Fig. 20-23).

Prostatitis is characterized as (1) acute bacterial prostatitis, (2) chronic bacterial prostatitis, or (3) nonbacterial prostatitis. **Prostatodynia** (pain in the prostate) is

FIG. 20-23 Prostatitis. (From Seidel, Ball, Dains, & Benedict, 1991.)

sometimes considered a form of prostatitis. Men with prostatodynia have the same clinical manifestations as those with nonbacterial prostatitis, but physical and laboratory examinations do not show prostatic pathology. Prostatodynia may not be caused by a pathologic condition of the prostate but rather by spasms in the genitourinary tract or tension in the muscles of the pelvic floor.

A number of defense mechanisms normally protect the lower urogenital tract from infection. Mechanical defenses include urethral length, micturition (urination), and ejaculation. Structural malformations and instrumentation of the genitourinary tract may weaken these defense mechanisms. Chemical defenses include antimicrobial substances in the prostatic fluid. The most important of these is a zinc-containing polypeptide known as prostatic antibacterial factor.

Bacterial prostatitis

Acute bacterial prostatitis is an ascending infection of the urinary tract that tends to occur in men between the ages of 30 and 50 but is also associated with BPH in older men. Coliform bacteria, particularly *Escherichia coli, Pseudomonas,* and *Streptococcus faecalis,* are common causes of acute bacterial prostatis. Mycoplasmas, ureaplasmas, and chlamydiae are infrequent causes of prostate infection. Infection stimulates an inflammatory response in which the prostate becomes enlarged, tender, and firm. The onset of prostatitis may be acute and unrelated to previous illnesses, or it may follow catheterization or cystoscopy.

Clinical manifestations of acute bacterial prostatitis are those of urinary tract infection. Symptoms include dysuria and urinary frequency, which result from bacterial contamination and inflammation of the bladder, and lower abdominal and suprapubic discomfort. The individual also may have symptoms of lower urinary tract obstruction, such as slow, small urinary stream, inability to empty the bladder, and nocturia (need to urinate frequently during the night). Acute inflammatory prostatic edema can compress the urethra, causing urinary obstruction. Systemic signs of infection include sudden onset of a high fever (up to 40° C [104° F]), fatigue, arthralgia, and myalgia. Prostatic pain may occur, especially when the individual is in an upright position, because the pelvic floor muscles tighten with standing and compression of the prostate gland occurs. Some individuals experience low back pain, painful ejaculation, and rectal or perineal pain. Palpation discloses an extremely tender and enlarged prostate.

Because acute bacterial prostatitis is usually associated with a bladder infection caused by the same microorganism, urine cultures disclose its identity. Prostatic massage may express enough secretions from the urethra for direct bacterial examination, but massage may be painful and increases the risk that the infection will ascend to adjacent structures or enter the bloodstream.

Long-term, broad-spectrum-antibiotic therapy (up to 6 weeks) may be required to resolve the infection and control its spread. In severe cases the individual is hospitalized and treated with an aminoglyoside, such as gentamicin sulfate, kanamycin sulfate, or tobramycin sulfate. Pain relievers, antipyretics, bed rest, and adequate hydration are also therapeutic. Complications include urinary retention that resolves with antibiotic therapy; prostatic abscess that may rupture into the urethra, rectum, or perineum; epididymitis; bacteremia; and septic shock. Urinary retention requiring drainage is best managed with a suprapubic catheter; Foley catheterization is contraindicated during acute infection.

Chronic bacterial prostatitis is characterized by recurrent urinary tract infections and persistence of pathogenic bacteria. This form of prostatitis is the most common recurrent urinary tract infection in men. Symptoms are variable and may be similar to those of an acute bladder infection: frequency, urgency, dysuria, perineal discomfort, low back pain, myalgia, and arthralgia. The prostate may be only slightly enlarged, but fibrosis can cause it to be firm and irregular in shape.

When the initial urine sample is bacteria free, prostatic massage is used to express secretions. Subsequently, the first 10 ml of voided urine is collected and examined microscopically. Prostatic secretions showing greater than 10 white blood cells (WBC)/high-power field (hpf) and macrophages containing fat are indicative of bacterial infection; diagnosis is confirmed by culture. Prostatic calculi may be seen on pelvic x-ray.

Treatment of chronic bacterial prostatitis is difficult,

mainly because damage caused by chronic inflammation blocks passage of antibiotics into prostatic tissues. Therefore, therapeutic levels are hard to achieve. The usual treatment is a 12-week course of trimethoprim-sulfamethoxazole. Alternative antibiotics include doxycycline hyclate, minocycline, carbenicillin, and erythromycin. Men whose chronic bacterial prostatitis is not cured may require continuous, low-dose suppressive therapy or may benefit from a radical transurethral prostatectomy.

Nonbacterial prostatitis

Nonbacterial prostatitis is the most common prostatitis syndrome and consists of prostatic inflammation without evidence of bacterial infection. The cause of nonbacterial prostatitis is not clear. Microbiologic, urodynamic, and psychologic factors have been studied, but results are inconclusive.

Men with nonbacterial prostatitis may complain of pain or a dull ache that is continuous or spasmodic in the suprapubic, infrapubic, scrotal, penile, or inguinal area. Other symptoms are pain on ejaculation and urinary symptoms, such as frequency of urination. The prostate gland generally feels normal on palpation.

Digital examination of the prostate, bacterial cultures of the urogenital tract, microscopic examination of expressed prostatic fluid, urethroscopy, and urodynamic studies are used to verify the diagnosis of nonbacterial prostatitis. Nonbacterial prostatitis is a diagnosis by exclusion.

There is no generally accepted treatment for nonbacterial prostatitis. Some clinicians prescribe a 1- to 3-week course of antibiotics for both affected individuals and sexual partners. This approach sometimes reduces symptoms. Symptoms can be relieved by hot sitz baths, bed rest, anticholinergics, and antiinflammatory drugs.

Cancer of the Prostate

Cancer of the prostate accounts for more than 13% of all cancer deaths and more than 28% of all cancers in men in the United States; only lung cancer accounts for more (ACS, 1993). Prostatic cancer rarely occurs in men younger than age 40. Incidence increases with advancing age, with more than 80% of all prostate cancers diagnosed in men older than age 65.

Prostatic cancer is more common in North America and Northern Europe and is relatively rare in Eastern Europe and the Far East. Migration from low-incidence to high-incidence areas increases the risk of developing this cancer, indicating that an environmental risk factor is involved. In the United States, the incidence and mortality among blacks are approximately 50% higher than those among whites.

The cause of prostatic cancer is poorly understood.

FIG. 20-24 **Carcinoma of prostate.** (From Seidel, Ball, Dains, & Benedict, 1991.)

Four possible causes studied thus far are genetic predisposition, endogenous hormones, environmental and dietary factors, and sexually transmitted infectious pathogens. Evidence from most of these studies is inconclusive or conflicting. It is believed that both genetic and environmental influences play a role in the cause of prostate cancer, with male hormones playing an essential additional role as tumor-promoter. There is no clear evidence of a causal link between BPH and prostate cancer even though they may frequently occur together.

Pathogenesis

More than 95% of prostatic neoplasms are adenocarcinomas, and most occur in the periphery of the prostate. Several histologic grading systems have been developed on the basis of the glandular pattern, the degree of differentiation (anaplasia) of the cancer cells, or both. The biologic aggressiveness of the neoplasm appears to be related to the degree of differentiation rather than the size of the tumor.

Prostatic cancer is thought to metastasize by local extension and through lymphatic and blood vessels. The most frequent sites of distant metastasis are the lymph nodes, bones, lungs, liver, and adrenals. The pelvis, lumbar spine, femur, thoracic spine, and ribs are the most common sites of bone metastasis. Local extension is usually posterior, although late in the disease the tumor may invade the rectum or encroach on the prostatic urethra and cause bladder outlet obstruction (Fig. 20-24).

Clinical Manifestations

Prostatic cancer often causes no symptoms until it is far advanced. The first manifestations of disease are those of bladder outlet obstruction: slow urinary stream, hesitancy, incomplete emptying, frequency, nocturia, and dysuria. Unlike the symptoms of obstruction caused by BPH, the symptoms of obstruction caused by prostatic cancer are progressive and do not remit. Local extension of prostatic cancer can obstruct the upper urinary tract ureters as well. If rectal obstruction occurs, the individual may experience a large bowel obstruction or difficulty in defecation. Symptoms of late disease include bone pain at sites of bone metastasis, edema of the lower extremities, enlargement of lymph nodes, liver enlargement, pathologic bone fractures, and mental confusion associated with brain metastases.

Evaluation and Treatment

Rectal examination is extremely important in the diagnosis of prostatic cancer; however, abnormalities may not be palpable in the early stages of disease. The tumor is typically palpated as an area of induration. Biopsy and microscopic examination of tissue are required to establish the diagnosis. Computed tomography scans, bone scans, intravenous urograms, MRI, arteriography, lymphangiography, and ultrasound can be used to assess the extent of spread. New procedures for early diagnosis are transrectal ultrasound (TRUS) and PSA blood tests. It seems that the ability to predict cancer rises significantly (from 41% to 71%) when TRUS and PSA tests are combined with a digital rectal examination.

Treatment of prostatic cancer depends on the age of the individual and the stage of the neoplasm. Options include no treatment, hormonal therapy, orchiectomy, chemotherapy, radiation therapy, surgery (radical prostatectomy, extended radical prostatectomy, or pelvic exenteration), or any combination of these. Treatments aimed at relieving symptoms of urinary obstruction, bladder outlet obstruction, colon obstruction, and spinal cord compression may be undertaken. Pain, especially that of bony metastases, may be relieved by narcotics.

Sexual Dysfunction

In males, the normal sexual response involves three processes: erection, emission, and ejaculation. **Sexual dysfunction** is the impairment of any or all of these processes. Impairment can be caused by a number of physiologic, psychologic, and emotional factors.

Until the late 1970s, most cases of male sexual dysfunction were thought to be psychogenic. Recent studies of this problem indicate that, in men older than 40 years of age, organic factors are involved in more than 50% of cases. The causes of organic sexual dysfunction include (1) vascular, endocrine, and neurologic disorders; (2) chronic disease, including renal failure and diabetes mellitus; (3) penile diseases and penile trauma;

and (4) iatrogenic factors, such as surgery and pharmacologic therapies. Most of these disorders cause erectile dysfunction.

Pathophysiology

Vascular disorders can prevent erection. Some arterial diseases diminish or interrupt circulation to the penis. This prevents engorgement of erectile tissues in the corpora cavernosa and corpus spongiosum. Rarely, excessive venous drainage of the corpora cavernosa prevents erection.

Endocrine disorders that reduce testosterone production affect sexual function and libido. The reduction may be caused by inadequate secretion of the gonadotropins caused by pituitary dysfunction or hyperprolactinemia. Feminizing tumors and estrogen therapy reduce relative levels of testosterone. Testicular atrophy from any cause also decreases testosterone levels and contributes to sexual dysfunction.

Neurologic disorders can interfere with the important sympathetic, parasympathetic, and central nervous system mechanisms required for erection, emission, and ejaculation. They include spinal cord injury or tumor, multiple sclerosis, and disorders that cause peripheral neuropathies, for example, diabetes mellitus and chronic renal failure. Spinal cord injuries or tumors can alter one or more components of the sexual response, depending on the location of the lesion. For example, in most men with upper motor neuron lesions, reflexogenic erection is possible, but emission and ejaculation (i.e., orgasm) are not possible. Lesions affecting the lower motor neurons usually prevent erection. In approximately 40% of such cases, emission and ejaculation are prevented.

Many chronic diseases are associated with sexual dysfunction. In some conditions the sexual dysfunction has a specific physiologic cause. Diabetes mellitus, for example, causes both peripheral vascular and neurologic pathology that can lead to erectile dysfunction. In other chronic conditions, sexual dysfunction is associated with low energy levels and loss of libido. The pathophysiologic mechanisms responsible for such changes are not known.

Priapism causes fibrosis of trabeculae (erectile tissues) within the corpora cavernosa, making erection difficult. The penile curvature caused by Peyronie disease does not make erection impossible but may make it extremely painful and intercourse impossible. Penile trauma can damage the erectile tissue, disrupt the posterior urethra, and disrupt the pudendal arteries or nerves.

Iatrogenic factors, including drugs and surgery, have a significant impact on erectile function. The following surgical procedures all carry the risk of erectile dysfunction: radical pelvic surgery; radical prostatectomy; transurethral, suprapubic, or simple retropubic prostatectomy; and aortoiliac surgery. Erectile dysfunction is caused by the severing of small nerve branches that are essential for erection. Aortoiliac surgery, retroperitoneal lymphadenectomy, and sympathectomy cause the loss of ejaculation capacity in some individuals.

A few pharmacologic agents enhance the sexual response, but most have the opposite effect. Men who are taking antihypertensives, antidepressants, antihistamines, antispasmodics, sedatives or tranquilizers, barbiturates, diuretics, sex hormone preparations, narcotics, or psychoactive drugs may experience some degree of sexual dysfunction. Ethyl alcohol also has a negative effect on sexual function. Drug-induced sexual dysfunction consists of decreased desire, decreased erectile ability, or decreased ejaculatory ability. A number of pharmacologic agents also diminish the quality or quantity of sperm. A few may cause priapism.

Evaluation and Treatment

Evaluation of sexual dysfunction includes a physical examination, with particular attention to the genitalia, prostate, and nervous system, and basic laboratory tests to identify the presence of endocrinopathies or other underlying disorders that can cause the dysfunction. If no physiologic cause is found and the condition does not improve with psychotherapy, the man is referred for further investigation of organic causes. Psychologic evaluation is indicated for younger men with a sudden onset of sexual dysfunction or men of any age who are able to achieve but not maintain an erection.

Sophisticated diagnostic techniques can be used to assess penile blood flow, erectile tissue anatomy, nervous system function, and occurrence of erection or emission during sleep (nocturnal emission). Penile blood flow is measured by Doppler techniques and penile arteriography. Corpus cavernosography, in which contrast material is injected into the corpora cavernosa, provides anatomic information about the erectile tissue of the penis. Neuropathic causes of sexual dysfunction are evaluated by measuring the speed of the bulbocavernous reflex. Nocturnal penile tumescence monitoring measures the frequency of nocturnal erections. Depending on the equipment used, this information may be correlated to rapid-eye-movement (REM) or non-REM sleep.

Treatments for organic sexual dysfunction include both medical and surgical interventions. Nonsurgical interventions include correction of underlying disorders, particularly drug-induced dysfunction and endocrinopathy-related (e.g., reduced testosterone associated with chronic renal failure) dysfunction. Vasodilators and cessation of smoking can benefit individuals with vasculogenic erectile dysfunction. Surgical interventions include penile implants, penile revascularization, and correction of other anatomic defects contributing to sexual dysfunction.

DISORDERS OF THE BREAST
Disorders of the Female Breast
Galactorrhea

Galactorrhea (inappropriate lactation) is the persistent and sometimes excessive secretion of a milky fluid from the breasts of a woman who is not pregnant or nursing an infant. Galactorrhea, which also can occur in men, may involve one or both breasts and is not associated with breast cancer.

The incidence of galactorrhea is difficult to estimate because of differences among definitions of the condition, examination techniques, and populations of women who have been studied. Prevalence has been documented as 0.1% to 32% of all women.

Pathophysiology

Galactorrhea is not a breast disorder per se. Rather it is a manifestation of pathophysiologic processes elsewhere in the body. These processes are chiefly hormone imbalances caused by hypothalamic-pituitary disturbances, pituitary tumors, or neurologic damage. Exogenous causes include drugs, estrogen (e.g., in oral contraceptives), and manipulation of the nipples.

The most common cause of galactorrhea is **nonpuerperal hyperprolactinemia,** or excessive amounts of prolactin in the blood not related to pregnancy or childbirth. Prolactin is a pituitary hormone that stimulates milk production. Elevated prolactin levels are found in 49% to 77% of cases of galactorrhea. Nonpuerperal hyperprolactinemia can be caused by any factor that (1) stimulates or overstimulates the prolactin-secreting units of the pituitary gland; (2) interferes with production of **prolactin-inhibiting factor** (PIF), a neurotransmitter (probably dopamine) that inhibits prolactin secretion; or (3) interferes with pituitary receptors for PIF. A variety of exogenous agents and disorders can trigger one of these three mechanisms, thereby causing hyperprolactinemia.

Several drugs can cause nonpuerperal hyperprolactinemia. They include the phenothiazines, reserpine, and methyldopa; exogenous estrogens, particularly in oral contraceptives; morphine; and the tricyclic antidepressants.

Hypothyroidism causes increased secretion of hypothalamic thyroid-releasing hormone (TRH), which stimulates prolactin release from the pituitary. Hypothyroidism also is associated with reduced metabolic clearance of prolactin, which prolongs its effects.

Many types of pituitary tumors cause hyperprolactinemia. Approximately 20% of cases of galactorrhea are caused by a prolactin-secreting pituitary adenoma or prolactinoma. Prolactinomas cause hyperprolactinemia by secreting prolactin, decreasing production of PIF, or putting pressure on the pituitary stalk such that delivery of PIF to the anterior pituitary is prevented. Growth hormone–secreting pituitary tumors may cause galactorrhea through the intrinsic lactogenic effect that growth hormone appears to have on mammary tissue. Prolactin-secreting lung and kidney tumors also cause hyperprolactinemia.

Chronic stress may cause hyperprolactinemia by inhibiting PIF release. Cervical spinal injuries, head trauma, encephalitis, meningitis, herpes zoster, or thoracotomy scars may stimulate the afferent portion of the suckling reflex arc, which is carried in the second to sixth thoracic nerves. The suckling reflex increases prolactin secretion.

Galactorrhea can be induced by persistent and repeated sucking or squeezing of the nipples and has been documented in women who manipulate their breasts and nipples daily (Haagensen, 1986). Monthly examination of the breasts for nipple discharge is usually not associated with the development of galactorrhea.

Clinical Manifestations

Inappropriate lactation is manifested by the appearance of a milky breast secretion, usually from both breasts. Most women with galactorrhea have some menstrual abnormality. In fact, the most common complaint for which evaluation is sought is infertility, not galactorrhea.

If a hypothalamic or pituitary process is involved, the individual may report CNS symptoms. These include intractable headache, visual field abnormalities, and abnormal temperature, thirst, or appetite.

Evaluation and Treatment

The evaluation of galactorrhea includes a variety of diagnostic tests. Breast secretions are examined for fat globules and neoplastic cells to verify their source. Serum prolactin levels are measured. Because such variables as eating, sleeping, stress, and breast examinations all increase prolactin levels, at least two positive results are needed for diagnosis of hyperprolactinemia. Prolactin levels greater than 25 to 30 ng/ml (by radioimmunoassay) are considered elevated. Those in the range of 75 to 100 ng/ml are considered to be caused by a pituitary tumor until proved otherwise. Serum T_4 and TSH levels are measured to rule out hypothyroidism, and LH and FSH levels are obtained if the individual is amenorrheic. Computed tomography scans, MRI evaluations, and carotid angiography may assist in the localization of adenomas.

Treatment for galactorrhea consists of identification and treatment of the cause. Medical and surgical therapies may be involved. If a pituitary microadenoma is found, it may be surgically removed, particularly if there has been progressive tumor growth, loss of visual field or acuity, cranial nerve dysfunction, increased intracra-

nial pressure, cerebrospinal fluid leak or obstruction, or infertility. A microadenoma may be treated medically with bromocriptine (Parlodel). This drug controls the tumor, but does not cure it, and must be taken indefinitely. A pituitary macroadenoma is usually treated medically because surgical and radiologic therapies seldom succeed.

Benign Breast Disease (Fibrocystic Disease)

A great many terms have been used to describe benign breast lesions of epithelial origin. **Fibrocystic disease** (physiologic nodularity) is perhaps most descriptive of the clinical manifestations: palpable lumps in the breast that fluctuate with the menstrual cycle and may become progressively worse until menopause. Fibrocystic disease is not, however, an accurate term for the wide range of breast lesions it has been used to describe. Microcysts, macrocysts, adenosis, apocrine change, fibrosis, fibroadenomas, and ductal hyperplasia are all termed *fibrocystic disease*. This is unfortunate for two reasons. First, physiologic nodularity is present in approximately 50% of all menstruating women, and at least some of these pathophysiologic changes are seen in up to 90% of all women. It is probably a misnomer to term so widespread a process a "disease" (Hutter, 1985). Second, some of the lesions called fibrocystic disease are associated with an increased risk of breast cancer, particularly when such variables as age and family history are considered. Having all these epithelial processes grouped together under one name generates significant confusion regarding potential outcomes, particularly the development of breast cancer.

On the basis of a study of 3303 women and at least a 15-year follow-up, Dupont and Page (1985) devised a three-category classification system for benign breast lesions and a risk index for the development of breast cancer. The three classifications are (1) lesions with no proliferative activity (nonproliferative lesions), including mild hyperplasia, microcysts, epithelium-related calcification, and fibroadenomas; (2) proliferative lesions without atypia, including moderate to florid hyperplasia, papillomas, ductal involvement with atypical lobular hyperplasia, and sclerosing adenosis; and (3) atypical hyperplasia, including the so-called borderline lesion (a lesion with some of the morphologic characteristics of carcinoma in situ). The risk index for classifications 2 and 3 is shown in Table 20-12.

Pathophysiology

The histologic changes associated with fibrocystic breast disease, fibrosis, cyst formation, an increase in acini, and hyperplasia appear to be responses to hormonal stimulation; however, the exact causative mechanisms are not known. The hormone involved appears to be estrogen, but it is not known whether estrogen level alone or the

COLUMBIA CLASSIFICATION OF BENIGN BREAST LESIONS COMMONLY DIAGNOSED AS FIBROCYSTIC DISEASE*

A. Microscopic features normally seen in the breasts of women. They do not form a palpable tumor and are not predisposing factors for carcinoma.
  1. Blunt ducts
  2. Microcysts: cysts less than 3 mm in diameter that evolve from blunt ducts
  3. Apocrine gland epithelium
B. Microscopic lesions frequently seen in the breasts of modern women, but not often enough to be regarded as normal components of breast tissue. They do not form a palpable tumor and are not predisposing factors for carcinoma.
  4. Adenosis: When very extensive, it may form a palpable tumor and therefore constitute a separate category
  5. Papillomatosis
C. Clinically evident lesions that often form a palpable tumor but are not predisposing factors for carcinoma
  6. Fibrous disease
  7. Solitary intraductal papilloma in a subareolar terminal duct
D. A microscopic lesion that does not form a palpable tumor but is a predisposing factor for carcinoma
  8. Lobular neoplasia (misnamed lobular carcinoma in situ)
E. Clinically evident breast lesions that form a palpable tumor and are predisposing factors for carcinoma
  9. Multiple intraductal papilloma. A number of ducts, usually peripheral, are involved.
  10. Gross cysts that are 3 mm and more in diameter and are visible to the naked eye. When they reach 10 mm in diameter, they are usually palpable.

Modified from Haagensen, 1986.
*Also called chronic cystic mastitis, cystic mastitis, mammary dysplasia, and, in Sweden, fibroadenomatosis.

TABLE 20-12

Relative Risk of Breast Cancer in Women With Proliferative Breast Disease

Lesion	Risk
Proliferative lesion without atypia	
Age 46-55	1.1
Without calcifications	1.5
Without family history	1.5
Age greater than 55	1.7
Age 20-45	1.8
With calcifications	1.9
With family history	2.1
Atypical hyperplasia	
Without family history	3.5
Without calcifications	4.0
With calcifications	6.5
With family history	8.9
Overall risk, all women	1.5

From Dupont & Page, 1985.

size, and presence of multiple lesions distinguish benign fibrocystic lesions from carcinoma.

Evaluation and Treatment

Breast biopsy is used to make a definitive diagnosis and assess an individual's risk for the development of breast cancer. Mammography may be helpful, but the very dense breast tissue frequently seen in young women can make interpretation extremely difficult. Sonography can be used to differentiate a solid mass from a cystic (fluid-filled) mass.

Treatment consists largely of relieving symptoms. The individual can minimize breast pain by wearing a brassiere that provides good support. Cystic pain is reduced by draining the cysts under local anesthesia. Many women find that the elimination or reduction of caffeine in their diet reduces both the pain and the nodularity. Women with breast pain also may benefit from a diet low in fat and high in complex carbohydrates.

Danazol, a synthetic androgen, has been used to treat individuals with severe pain caused by proliferative breast disease. Danazol is thought to minimize the hormonal fluctuations to which breast tissue is exposed.

Benign breast tumors include fibroadenomas, mammary duct ectasia, solitary intraductal papilloma, multiple papilloma, and fat necrosis. These benign conditions are summarized in Table 20-13.

estrogen-to-progesterone ratio is more important. Histologic changes may result from inappropriate responses by breast tissue to hormones rather than inappropriate hormone levels (Table 20-13).

Clinical Manifestations

Pain or tenderness is the most common complaint associated with fibrocystic disease. Discomfort increases as menstruation approaches. Pain, fluctuation in lesion

TABLE 20-13

Benign Breast Disorders

Benign breast disease	Period of greatest risk	Pathophysiology	Clinical manifestations of lesion	Treatment
Fibroadenoma	Puberty, early adulthood, rare after menopause	Unknown, but thought to be associated with exposure to increased estrogen levels	Painless, firm, solitary, well-circumscribed mobile mass; usually in upper outer quadrant of breast	Surgical excision of mass
Mammary duct ectasia (comedomastitis)	Menopausal, post-menopause, during lactation and nursing	Subareolar ducts become dilated and fill with cellular debris, initiating inflammatory reaction; rupture of ducts may occur	Blood-stained, sticky, thick, spontaneous, multiple-duct discharge; ductal rupture creates palpable mass; burning pain, swelling of areolar area may occur	Condition usually resolves 7-10 days after onset with or without antibiotic therapy
Solitary intraductal papilloma	Age 40-50	Unknown	Lesion is slow-growing, cauliflowerlike, and extends length of involved duct, nipple discharge from one or two ductal openings may be watery, serous, serosanguineous, or sanguineous	Surgical excision of involved duct
Multiple papilloma	Age 35-40	Unknown	Similar to solitary intraductal papilloma, except that discharge is from multiple ductal openings	Depends on extent of involvement; if lesion is small, excision of that breast segment; total mastectomy if disease is widespread
Fat necrosis	Age 14-80, average age 50	Breast trauma, including silicone injections and breast biopsy, cause hemorrhage and induration, leading to formation of a palpable mass	Unilateral, fairly immobile breast mass, located close to the surface; mass is usually tender and painful	Mass may be reabsorbed spontaneously; biopsy, excision may be required if no resorption occurs

Breast Cancer

Breast cancer is the most common cancer in American women and the second biggest killer after lung cancer. Breast cancer (*lifetime* risk; Table 20-14) afflicts approximately one in every eight women (Elliott, 1993). Generally, incidence is much higher among North American and Northern European women than among South American and Asian women. The risk of breast cancer increases as age advances, reaching a peak in women aged 45 to 64 (Table 20-14). The incidence rate increased by 21% between 1973 and 1989; however, this increase is reportedly attributable to earlier detection of cancer while the tumor is in situ (before invasion) (Eliott, 1993). Breast cancer is the leading cause of death in women between 40 and 44 years of age, and deaths have remained steady at 27 per 100,000 women for decades (Eliott, 1993). The risk factors and possible causes of breast cancer can be classified as reproductive, hormonal, environmental, and familial (Table 20-15).

Reproductive factors

A woman's age when her first child is born affects her risk for developing breast cancer (ACS, 1993). The younger she is, the lower the risk. Pregnancies that do not proceed to term apparently have no protective effect. Women who have never given birth are at greater risk than those who have. The duration of a woman's reproductive life also affects her risk of developing breast cancer. Late menarche and early menopause (i.e., a short reproductive life) reduce risk (see Pathogenesis).

Hormonal factors

The link between breast cancer and hormones is based on three factors that affect risk: (1) the protective effect of an early first pregnancy; (2) the protective effect of removal of the ovaries and pituitary gland; and (3) the increased risk associated with early menarche, late menopause, and nulliparity. Oral contraceptive use and estrogen replacement therapy may be risk factors for breast cancer. Study results to date are conflicting and inconclusive (Henrich, 1992; McPherson & Doll, 1991). Yet, a renewed interest is emerging in an old suspect: hormones, especially estrogen. Increasing exposure to hormones may be partly the result of declining age of first menstruation—presumably reflecting improved nutrition—and a trend toward later childbirth and menopause (Eliott, 1993). Hormones are discussed further in the pathogenesis section.

TABLE 20-14

Risk of Developing Breast Cancer

By age	By ratio
25	1 in 19,608
30	1 in 2525
35	1 in 622
40	1 in 217
45	1 in 93
50	1 in 50
55	1 in 33
60	1 in 24
65	1 in 17
70	1 in 14
75	1 in 11
80	1 in 10
85	1 in 9
Ever*	1 in 8

Modified from Eliott, 1993.
*Lifetime risk.

SUMMARY: FAMILIAL BREAST CANCER

PREVALENCE: Approximately 12.5% of women will develop breast cancer during their lifetime. About 7% of these women have the familial form of breast cancer discussed here (i.e., about 1/150 women in the general population).

SURVIVAL: For all cases of breast cancer diagnosed in the U.S. from 1983 to 1988, the 5-year survival rates are 79% (whites) and 62% (blacks).

PRESENTATION: The *familial* form of breast cancer is more often bilateral and early onset (premenopausal) than nonfamilial breast cancer.

GENETICS: The mode of inheritance is autosomal dominant. Penetrance for females is 90% by age 50. Males also can be affected, but the penetrance is much lower. The gene has been mapped to chromosome 17q.

OTHER: It is important to keep in mind that, *in general,* having one first-degree female relative (i.e., mother or a sister) affected with breast cancer *doubles* a female's risk of developing a breast tumor. If two first-degree relatives develop breast tumors before age 55, the risk increases to 54%.

From Jorde, L.B. (1993). *Human genetics syllabus,* University of Utah, Salt Lake City.
Data from Hall, J.M., 1992.

TABLE 20-15

Risk Factors for Breast Cancer in Women

Factor	High risk	Low risk	Magnitude of risk
Age	Old	Young	***
Country of birth	North America Northern Europe	Asia Africa	**
Socioeconomic status	Upper	Lower	**
Marital status	Never married	Ever married	*
Place of residence	Urban	Rural	*
Place of residence	Northern United States	Southern United States	*
Race	White	Black	*
Age at first pregnancy	Older than 30	Younger than 20	**
Oophorectomy	No	Yes	**
Body build, postmeno- pausal	Obese	Thin	**
Age at menarche	Early	Late	*
Family history of pre- menopausal bilateral breast cancer	Yes	No	***
History of cancer in one breast	Yes	No	***
History of fibrocystic dis- ease (atypia hyperpla- sia)	Yes	No	**
Any first-degree relative with breast cancer	Yes	No	**
History of primary can- cer in ovary or endo- metrium	Yes	No	**
Radiation to chest	Large doses	Minimal exposure	**

Modified from Eliott, 1993.

***, Relative risk greater than 4.0; **, relative risk between 2.0 and 4.0; *, relative risk between 1.1 and 1.9. (Relative risk is defined and discussed in Chapter 5.)

Environmental factors

High doses of ionizing radiation are associated with an increased risk of breast cancer, especially if exposure occurs during adolescence or pregnancy. These are periods when breast cells are proliferating rapidly.

A high-fat diet may increase the risk of breast cancer. The incidence of breast cancer is significantly higher in populations with high fat intake than in those with low fat intake. Breast cancer is rare in Japan, but not in Japanese immigrants in the United States who adopt Western eating habits. In 1980 a group of 89,538 registered nurses in the United States participated in a study to measure individual fat consumption and incidence of breast cancer (Stampfer, Bechtel, & Hunter, 1992). Although the study period was limited (4 years), results suggested that total fat intake or consumption of specific types of fat among women did not increase the risk of breast cancer (Eliott, 1993). One diet hypothesis that has not been examined carefully is the possibility that *very* low-fat diets (20% or less) could have a beneficial effect not provided by low-fat diets (Eliott, 1993).

Several studies have shown some correlation between breast cancer and alcohol ingestion (ACS, 1993; Stampfer et al., 1992). The relationship between alcohol and breast cancer risk appears to be present for all forms of alcoholic beverages. Differences in alcohol intake, however, explain only a small fraction of breast cancer rates (Stampfer et al., 1992).

The mechanisms by which alcohol increases the risk of breast cancer are unknown. Alcohol may hinder the liver's ability to rid the body of cancer-causing agents, impair the body's immune system, or make breast tissue more susceptible to cancer cells. It is not known whether decreasing or stopping alcohol consumption in midlife lessens the risk of breast cancer.

Familial factors

A history of breast cancer in first-degree relatives (mother or sister) increases a woman's risk 2 to 3 times. Risk increases even more if two first-degree relatives are involved, especially if the disease occurred before menopause and was bilateral. In some families, breast cancer occurs at an earlier age and the frequency of bilateral tumors is greater.

Pathogenesis

Table 20-16 lists the different types of breast carcinomas and summarizes their major characteristics. Most breast cancers arise from the ductal epithelium. Tumors of the infiltrating ductal type do not grow to a large size, but they metastasize early. This type accounts for 70% of breast cancers.

Breast cancer is a disease of the glandular epithelium and is thought to result from a mutation during the differentiation of stem cells into mature epithelial cells (Russo, Tay, & Russo, 1982). Unlike most human organs that are differentiated at the end of fetal life, development and differentiation of the mammary gland occur after puberty. The mammary gland at birth is formed by primary mammary ducts that branch during childhood. At premenarche, the duct epithelium proliferates. At menarche, under the influence of progesterone and, presumably, estrogen, terminal duct tubular units (acini) are formed. Acini are the dynamic structure of the mammary gland (Fig. 19-19). The number of these acini increases at each menstruation with new budding of structures until approximately age 35 years (Morabia & Wynder, 1990; Russo & Russo, 1987).

With pregnancy, there is an increase in the number of acini, resulting in full differentiation of their structure and function. When pregnancy does not happen, full differentiation of the breast may never be attained. At menopause, acini, as well as interlobular fibrous tissues, undergo atrophy but the large and intermediate duct system persists (Morabia & Wynder, 1990). Involution of the glandular epithelium continues and the breast becomes composed mainly of large ducts, increased connective tissue, and fat.

Mammary epithelial cells achieve rapid renewal by a small number of mitotic divisions of immortal stem cells. (Cell renewal is discussed in Chapters 1 and 10.) Because the number of mutations is proportional to the rate and number of stem cell divisions, factors that accelerate cell division can have a carcinogenic effect. Hormones may act as accelerators and influence the susceptibility of the breast epithelium to environmental carcinogens because hormones control the differentiation of the mammary gland epithelium and, thereby, regulate the rate of stem cell division. Current knowledge of the mechanisms of differentiation of the mammary gland suggests that both estrogens and progestins may be involved in breast carcinogenesis. This hypothesis is supported by two facts: (1) the increased incidence of breast cancer in women (e.g., 100 times more frequent in women than in men), and (2) the association of breast cancer with the events of reproductive life.

The period of highest proliferative activity of mammary epithelium stem cells is during each ovulatory cycle between puberty and either the first full-term pregnancy or menopause among nulliparous women. Thus, it is important to know whether the proliferation occurs mostly in the first part of the menstrual cycle (the follicular phase), which is under the influence of estrogen, or in the second part (the luteal phase), which is under the influence of both estrogen and progesterone. The answer to this critical question is controversial. Vogel and co-workers (1981) reported that mitotic activity was highest during the follicular phase, suggesting that estrogen has a proliferative effect on the mammary gland epithelium, whereas progesterone acted as an antiestrogen in inhibiting proliferation. These reports were consistent with Korenman's (1980) "open window theory" stating that breast cancer is related to an abnormal luteal phase with low or absent progesterone secretion. Thus, women with anovulatory cycles were predicted to be at higher risk because the proliferative effect of estrogens was unopposed or uninhibited by progesterone.

Vogel and co-workers based their conclusions on structural changes identified in the mammary epithelium during the phases of the menstrual cycle. Their approach has been criticized because it does not allow quantitation (e.g., counting of the number of mitoses) during the follicular and luteal phases. Other researchers have actually compared the differences in mitoses between the two phases (Longacre & Bartow, 1986; Potten et al., 1988). Most of these quantitative studies show that human and animal mammary glands proliferate mostly during the luteal phase. During the estrogen follicular phase, terminal ductules are few and there is no mitotic activity. During the luteal phase, because of the increased progesterone levels, perhaps on the background of estrogen priming or as a result of cooperation between the two hormones, there is increased mi-

TABLE 20-16

Types of Breast Carcinomas and Major Distinguishing Features

Histologic type	Distinguishing features
Carcinoma of mammary ducts	
Papillary	Well-delineated cystic masses in multiple areas; hemorrhage often present; majority appear in 40-60 age group; often involves skin
Intraductal (comedo)	Often accompanied by evidence of infection; well-circumscribed tumors within the duct; well-differentiated tumor cells; rarely ulcerates the skin
Infiltrating carcinoma	
Ductal	Fibrous, firm, glistening, gray-tan mass with chalky streaks, mixture of patterns; causes discharge from the nipple; represents about 70% of all breast cancer
Mucinous	Usually large, >3 cm in diameter, circumscribed and encapsulated, glistening appearance, varies in color; two types: pure and mixed; pure tumor is surrounded by mucin; infrequent; found in the lateral half of the breast; tends to occur in women over 70
Medullary	Encapsulated and grows to be very large (7-8 cm in diameter); commonly infiltrates lymphoid tissue; occurs after age 50
Tubular	Well-differentiated with orderly tubules in center (stroma) of mass; associated with noninfiltrating ductal carcinoma; occurs in women about 50 years of age; nodal metastasis infrequent; occurrence rare
Adenoid cystic	Very rare; well-circumscribed, painless mass arising from the nipple and areola
Metaplastic	Involves cartilage or bone, mixed tumors or osteogenic sarcomas
Squamous cell	Frequent in blacks; originates in ductal epithelium
Carcinoma of mammary lobules	
Lobular carcinoma in situ	Found in individuals with fibrocystic disease; localized to upper breast quadrants; risk of 10%-35% becoming invasive; occurs frequently in mid-40s; infiltrating variety occurs in early 50s
Infiltrating lobular	Infiltrates from duct; firm mass with chalky streaks
Paget disease	Eczema of the nipple that extends to the areola; cancer usually found underneath the nipple; poorly circumscribed; large Paget's cells arise from the duct and directly invade nipple; history of scaly, red rash spreading from the nipple; lesion palpable beneath the nipple, often bilateral; occurs in middle age
Inflammatory carcinomas	Not a histologic type; fairly diffuse within the breast tissue, diffuse edema of the overlying skin; extremely undifferentiated, very rare, most metastasize to axilla
Sarcoma of the breast	
Cytosarcoma phyllodes	Usually large (>17 cm in diameter); mostly localized, but can rupture through the skin; rarely metastasizes to lymph nodes; history of painless nodule present for years before it forms a large mass; ulceration and bleeding of skin often present; occurs in wide age range (13-77 years)
Fibrosarcoma	Well-circumscribed, firm, and usually does not involve the skin or nipple; well-differentiated to extremely undifferentiated; arises from connective tissue; extremely rare (e.g., liposarcoma, angiosarcoma)

totic activity (Morabia & Wynder, 1990). These studies contradict the "open window theory," because if progesterone were acting as an antiestrogen, proliferation of the mammary epithelium would be less extensive during the luteal than during the follicular phase (Morabia & Wynder, 1990).

Thus it can be suggested that the risk of carcinogenic mutations is proportional to the *time* required for all stem cells to undergo differentiation. The risk then would be proportional to the duration of the interval separating menarche from the first full-term birth and to the number of ovulatory cycles during this period of time (Morabia & Wynder, 1990). In human studies, an increased risk of breast cancer is associated with young age at menarche, later age at menopause, or longer duration of ovulatory activity. Likewise, a protective effect or decreased risk of breast cancer is associated with young age at first live birth; full-term birth shifts the mammary gland from a proliferative state with high susceptibility to carcinogens to a low-proliferative, low-risk state (Morabia & Wynder, 1990).

Approximately 60% of carcinomas of the breast occur in the upper outer quadrant because most of the glandular tissue of the breast is there (Fig. 20-25). The lymphatic spread of cancer to the opposite breast, to lymph nodes in the base of the neck, and to the abdominal cavity is caused by obstruction of the normal lymphatic pathways or destruction of lymphatic vessels by surgery or radiotherapy. The less common inner-quadrant tumors may spread to mediastinal nodes or Rotter nodes, which are located between the pectoral muscles. Internal mammary chain nodes are frequent sites of metastasis.

Metastases from the vertebral veins can involve the vertebrae, pelvic bones, ribs, and skull. The lungs, kidneys, liver, adrenal glands, ovaries, and pituitary gland are also sites of metastasis.

Approximately one third of breast cancers are hormone dependent and regress in response to surgical removal of the ovaries. Estrogen and progesterone are of primary significance in maintaining some breast cancer growths. Not all breast tumors, however, are estrogen-receptor− (ER-) or progesterone-receptor− (PR-) positive. It is now known that estrogens, like other steroid hormones, modulate gene expression in target (e.g., breast) cells through their interaction with specific nuclear proteins (receptors). Current research, however, identifies two levels of control of cell growth: (1) paracrine signaling by estrogen and progesterone steroids; and (2) autocrine signaling by locally secreted growth factors, such as transforming growth factor (TGF) (Fig. 20-26). (Paracrine and autocrine signaling are discussed in Chapters 1 and 17. Transforming growth factor is also discussed in Chapter 10.) Current evidence indicates that estrogen-dependent breast cancer growth may

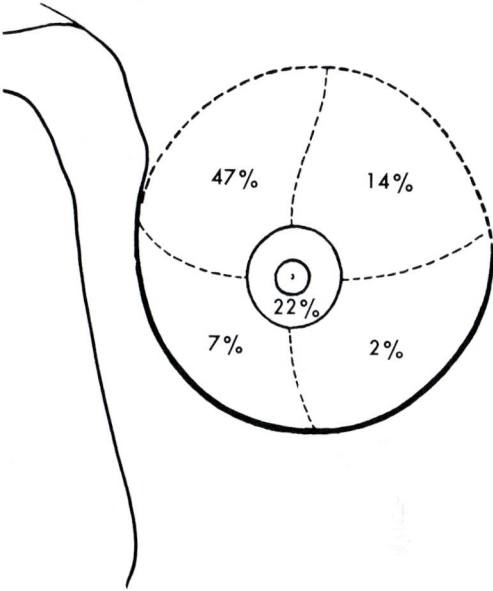

FIG. 20-25 Distribution of carcinomas in different areas of the breast. (From del Regato, Spjut, & Cox, 1985.)

be regulated by positive growth stimulators like TGF-α and negative (inhibiting) growth stimulators like TGF-β (Knabbe et al., 1987; Waxman, 1991).

Clinical Manifestations

The first sign of breast cancer is usually a painless lump. Lumps caused by breast tumors do not have any classic characteristics. Other presenting signs include palpable nodes in the axilla, retraction of tissue (dimpling) (Fig. 20-27), or bone pain caused by metastasis to the vertebrae. Table 20-17 summarizes the clinical manifestations of breast cancers. Manifestations vary according to the type of tumor and stage of disease.

Evaluation and Treatment

Mammography, percutaneous needle aspiration, biopsy, and hormone receptor assays are generally used in evaluating breast cancer. Biopsy is the definitive diagnostic test.

Treatment is based on the extent or stage of the cancer (Table 20-18). The extent of the tumor at the primary site, the presence and extent of lymph node metastasis, and the presence of distant metastases are all evaluated to determine the stage of disease.

Surgery, radiation, chemotherapy, hormone therapy, biologic therapy, and bone marrow transplantation may

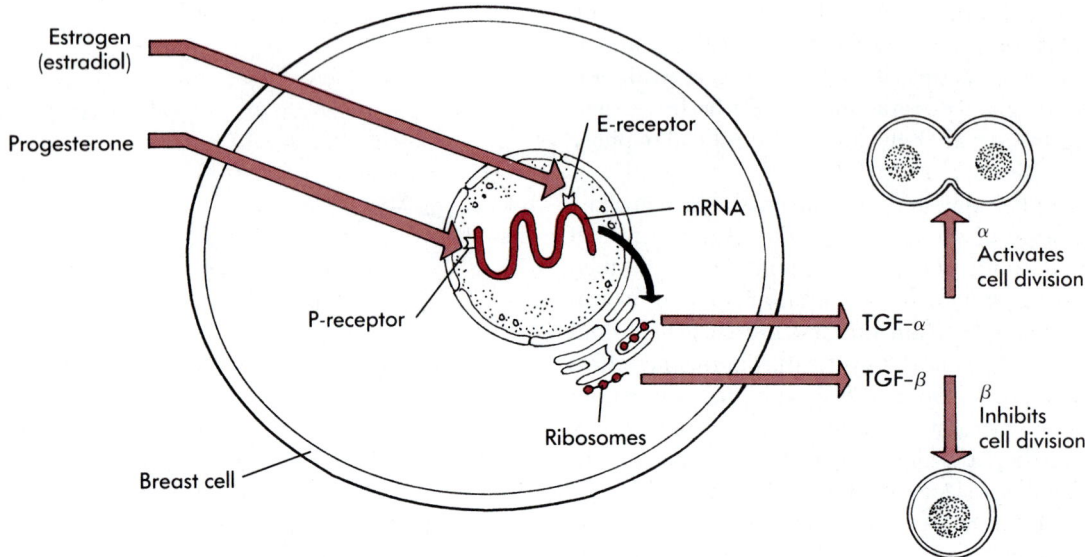

FIG. 20-26 **Control of breast cell growth.** Two levels of control of breast cell growth: (1) paracrine signaling by estrogen and progesterone steroids and (2) autocrine signaling by locally secreted growth factors, such as transforming growth factor: TGF (α and β).

TABLE 20-17

Clinical Manifestations of Breast Cancer

Clinical manifestation	Pathophysiology
Local pain	Local obstruction caused by the tumor
Dimpling of the skin	Can occur with invasion of the dermal lymphatics because of retraction of Cooper's ligament, or involvement of the pectoralis fascia
Nipple retraction	Shortening of the mammary ducts
Skin retraction	Involvement of the suspensory ligaments
Edema	Local inflammation or lymphatic obstruction
Nipple/areolar eczema	Paget disease
Pitting of the skin (similar to the surface of an orange [peau d'orange])	Obstruction of the subcutaneous lymphatics, resulting in the accumulation of fluid
Reddened skin, local tenderness, and warmth	Inflammation
Dilated blood vessels	Obstruction of venous return by a fast-growing tumor; obstruction dilates superficial veins
Nipple discharge in a non-lactating woman	Spontaneous and intermittent discharge caused by tumor obstruction
Ulceration	Tumor necrosis
Hemorrhage	Erosion of blood vessels
Edema of the arm	Obstruction of lymphatic drainage in the axilla
Chest pain	Metastasis to the lung

Modified from Griffiths, Murray, & Russo, 1984.

FIG. 20-27 Retraction of nipple caused by carcinoma. (From del Regato, Spjut, & Cox, 1985.)

TABLE 20-18

Staging and TMN Classification of Breast Cancer

Stage	TNM Classification
Stage 1	T_1 (tumor 2 cm or less) N_0 (no palpable axillary nodes) M_0 (no evident metastasis)
Stage 2	T_0 (no palpable tumor) T_1 (tumor 2 cm or less) T_2 (tumor less than 5 cm) N_1 (palpable axillary nodes with histologic evidence of breast malignancy)
Stage 3	T_3 (tumor more than 5 cm; may be fixed to muscle or fascia) N_1 or N_2 (fixed nodes) M_0 (no evident metastasis)
Stage 4	T_4 (tumor any size with fixation to chest wall or skin; presence of edema, including *peau d'orange;* ulceration; skin nodules; inflammatory carcinoma) N_3 (supraclavicular or intraclavicular nodes or arm edema) M_1 (distant metastasis present or suspected)

From Phipps, Long, Woods, & Cassmeyer, 1991.

be used to treat breast cancer. The extent of the surgery depends on the tumor's histology, predictability, and stage and the individual's age and medical and psychologic history. Beginning with the most conservative, the surgical procedures commonly used are (1) tylectomy or lumpectomy, in which the tumor and a small amount of surrounding tissue are removed; (2) quadrant excision, in which a quadrant of the breast is removed; (3) partial mastectomy, in which a larger amount of tissue is removed; (4) total or simple mastectomy, in which the tumor and all breast tissue are removed (the nipple may or may not be removed); (5) modified radical mastectomy, in which the breast, pectoralis minor, and axillary contents are removed; and (6) radical mastectomy, in which the breast, axillary contents, and pectoralis major and minor are removed. Radiation therapy is infrequently used except to prevent metastasis of a small tumor (<2 cm) that has been surgically excised. Chemotherapy and hormone therapy are most successful as an adjunct to surgery in premenopausal women with hormone-dependent tumors. They are also used in individuals with advanced disease. Endocrine therapy (androgens, estrogens, progesterones, and steroids) may be used to prolong survival time and appears most effective in women with ER- and PR-positive tumors. ER- and PR-negative tumors are unlikely to respond to hormonal therapy. Newer treatments that include biologic response modifiers (see Chapter 11) and bone marrow transplantation are being used in clinical research trials.

Disorders of the Male Breast
Gynecomastia

Gynecomastia is the overdevelopment of breast tissue in a male. Gynecomastia accounts for approximately 85% of all masses that develop in the male breast and affects 32% to 40% of the male population. If only one breast is involved, it is typically the left. Incidence is greatest among adolescents and men older than age 50.

Gynecomastia results from hormonal alterations, which may be idiopathic or caused by systemic disorders, drugs, or neoplasms. Gynecomastia usually involves an imbalance of the estrogen/testosterone ratio. The normal estrogen/testosterone ratio can be altered in one of two ways. First, estrogen levels may be excessively high, although testosterone levels are normal. This is the case in drug-induced and tumor-induced cases of hyperestrogenism. Second, testosterone levels may be extremely low, although estrogen levels are normal, as is the case in hypergonadism. Gynecomastia also can be caused by alterations in breast-tissue responsiveness to hormonal stimulation. Breast tissue may have increased responsiveness to estrogen or decreased responsiveness to androgen. Alterations of responsiveness may cause many cases of idiopathic gynecomastia.

Besides puberty and aging, estrogen-testosterone imbalances are associated with hypogonadism, Klinefelter syndrome, and testicular neoplasms. Hormone-induced gynecomastia is usually bilateral. Pubertal gynecomastia is a self-limiting phenomenon that usually disappears within 4 to 6 months. Senescent gynecomastia usually regresses spontaneously within 6 to 12 months.

Systemic disorders associated with gynecomastia include cirrhosis of the liver, infectious hepatitis, chronic renal failure, chronic obstructive lung disease, hyperthyroidism, tuberculosis, and chronic malnutrition. It may be that these disorders ultimately alter the estrogen/testosterone ratio, initiating the gynecomastia.

Gynecomastia is frequently seen in males receiving estrogen therapy, either in preparation for a sex-change operation or for prostatic carcinoma. Other drugs that can cause gynecomastia include digitalis, cimetidine, spironolactone, reserpine, thiazide, isoniazid, ergotamine, tricyclic antidepressants, amphetamines, vincristine, and busulfan. Gynecomastia is usually unilateral in these instances.

Malignancies of the testes, adrenals, or liver can cause gynecomastia if they alter the estrogen/testosterone ratio. Pituitary adenomas and lung cancer are also associated with gynecomastia.

Pathophysiology

The enlargement consists of hyperplastic stroma and ductal tissue. Hyperplasia results in a firm, palpable mass, at least 2 cm in diameter and located beneath the areola.

Evaluation and Treatment

The diagnosis of gynecomastia is based on physical examination. Identification and treatment of the cause are likely to be followed by resolution of the gynecomastia. The man should be taught to perform breast self-examination and is examined at 6- and 12-month intervals if the gynecomastia persists.

Carcinoma

Breast cancer in males accounts for 0.2% of all male cancers and 1% of all breast cancers. Breast cancer in men is seen most commonly after the age of 60, with the peak incidence between 60 and 69 years. It has, however, been reported in males as young as 6 and in adolescents. Possible risk factors include gynecomastia, radiation of the chest wall, and family history of breast cancer. The relationship between these factors and risk of disease is not clearly defined.

Male breast tumors frequently resemble carcinoma of the breast in women. Estrogen receptors have been found in up to 84% of biopsy specimens from men (deVita, Hellman, & Rosenberg, 1985). The malignant male breast lesion is usually a unilateral solid mass located near the nipple. Because the nipple is commonly involved, crusting and nipple discharge are typical clinical manifestations. Other findings include skin retraction, ulceration of the skin over the tumor, and axillary node involvement. Patterns of metastasis are similar to those in females.

The diagnosis of cancer is confirmed by biopsy. Because of delays in seeking treatment, male breast cancer tends to be advanced at the time of diagnosis and therefore to have a poor prognosis. Treatment protocols are similar to those for female breast cancer, but endocrine therapy is used more frequently for males because a higher percentage of male tumors are hormone-dependent. Orchiectomy is performed to treat metastatic disease.

SUMMARY REVIEW

Alterations of Sexual Maturation

1 Sexual maturation, or puberty, should begin in girls between the ages of 8 and 13, and in boys between the ages of 9 and 14. Delayed puberty is the onset of sexual maturation after these ages; precocious puberty is onset before these ages.

2 Alterations of sexual maturation can be idiopathic or caused by a disease or congenital anomaly. In most cases of delayed puberty the hypothalamic-pituitary-gonadal axis is intact, but the surge of activity that stimulates puberty is delayed. This situation is common in boys. Precocious puberty, more common in girls, can also be caused by mistiming of the stimulatory surge in a child whose hypothalamic-pituitary-ovarian system is otherwise normal.

3 Precocious puberty can be isosexual (sex-appropriate), heterosexual (not sex-appropriate), or partial (development of one secondary sex characteristic only).

Disorders of the Female Reproductive System

1 The female reproductive system can be altered by hormonal imbalances, infectious microorganisms, inflammation, structural abnormalities, and benign or malignant proliferative conditions.

2 Menstrual disorders usually involve some disruption of the hypothalamic-pituitary-ovarian axis and subsequent alteration of hormone production, reception by target organs, or feedback mechanisms.

3 Primary dysmenorrhea is painful menstruation not associated with pelvic disease. It results from excessive synthesis of prostaglandins, which cause the myometrium to contract and constrict blood vessels, resulting in ischemic pain.

4 Primary amenorrhea is the continued absence of menarche and menstrual function by age 14 without the development of secondary sex characteristics or by age 16 if these changes have occurred.

5 Primary amenorrhea may be caused by decreased or absent secretion of GnRH, FSH, or LH; ovarian resistance to FSH or LH; anatomic defects, such as congenital absence of the uterus; or genetic disorders, including Turner syndrome.

6 Secondary amenorrhea is the absence of menstruation for a time equivalent to more than 3 cycles or 6 months in women who have previously menstruated. Secondary amenorrhea is associated with anovulation.

7 Secondary amenorrhea can be physiologic (e.g., during adolescence, premenopause, during pregnancy) or pathophysiologic. This condition develops if the uterus is removed or if levels of regulatory hormones are altered so as to inhibit ovulation.

8 Dysfunctional uterine bleeding (DUB) is heavy or irregular bleeding caused by a disturbance of the menstrual cycle.

9 Polycystic ovarian syndrome (PCO) is a condition in which excessive androgen production is triggered by inappropriate secretion of gonadotropins. Depressed FSH and elevated LH levels perpetuate adrenal and ovarian secretion of androgens, which are converted to estrogen in peripheral tissues. This hormonal imbalance prevents ovulation and causes enlargement and cyst formation in the ovaries, excessive endometrial proliferation in the uterus, and, occasionally, hirsutism.

10 Premenstrual syndrome (PMS) is the cyclic recurrence of physical, psychologic, or behavioral changes distressing enough to disrupt normal activities or interpersonal relationships. More than 200 emotional, physical, and behavioral symptoms have been attributed to PMS. Emotional symptoms, particularly depression, anger, irritability, and fatigue, are reported as the most distressing symptoms; physical symptoms tend to be less problematic. Treatment is symptomatic and includes self-help techniques, lifestyle changes, counseling, and medication.

11 Infection and inflammation of the female genitalia can result from microorganisms from the environment or overproliferation of microorganisms that normally populate the genital tract.

12 Pelvic inflammatory disease (PID) is an acute ascending infection of the upper genital tract. Its usual cause is a sexually transmitted pathogen.

13 Vaginitis, or vaginal infection, is usually caused by sexually transmitted pathogens or *Candida albicans*, which causes candidiasis. Susceptibility to infection is highest when estrogen levels are lowest (e.g., before puberty or after menopause). Risk factors associated with low estrogen levels are alkaline pH, relatively thin epithelium, and decreased populations of lactobacilli.

14 Cervicitis, which is infection of the cervix, can be acute (mucopurulent cervicitis) or chronic. Its most common cause is a sexually transmitted pathogen.

15 Vulvitis is an inflammation of the skin of the vulva. It can be caused by chemical irritants, allergens, skin disorders, irritation from tight-fitting clothing, or spread of vaginal infections, such as candidiasis.

16 Bartholinitis, also called Bartholin cyst, is an infection of the ducts that lead from the Bartholin glands to the surface of the vulva. Infection blocks the glands, preventing the outflow of glandular secretions.

17 The pelvic relaxation disorders—uterine displacement, uterine prolapse, cystocele, rectocele, and urethrocele—are caused by the relaxation of muscles and fascial supports, usually with age or after childbirth or other trauma, and are more likely to occur in women with a familial or genetic predisposition.

18 Benign growths and proliferative conditions of the female reproductive tract tend to affect the ovaries (benign ovarian cysts) or uterine tissues (endometrial polyps, leiomyomas, and endometriosis).

19 Benign ovarian cysts develop from mature ovarian follicles that do not release their ova (follicular cysts) or from a corpus luteum that persists abnormally instead of degenerating (corpus luteum cyst). Cysts usually regress spontaneously.

20 Endometrial polyps consist of overgrowths of endometrial tissue and frequently cause abnormal bleeding in the premenopausal woman.

21 Leiomyomas, also called uterine fibroids, are tumors arising from the muscle layer of the uterus, the myometrium. Incidence increases in women between the ages of 30 and 50; most myomas remain small and asymptomatic. Adenomyosis is the presence of endometrial glands and stroma within the uterine myometrium.

22 Endometriosis is the presence of functional endometrial tissue (i.e., tissue that responds to hormonal stimulation) at sites outside the uterus. Endometriosis causes an inflammatory reaction at the site of implantation and is a cause of infertility.

23 Most cancers of the female genitalia involve the uterus (particularly the cervix) and the ovaries. Cancer of the vagina is rare.

24 Risk factors for cervical cancer are young age at first coitus, multiple sexual partners, exposure to sexually transmitted infections, and exposure to cigarette smoke. Incidence is greatest among women in their 40s; however, it is increasing in younger women.

25 Cervical cancer arises from the cervical epithelium and is considered a sexually transmitted disease. The progressively serious neoplastic alterations are (a) cervical intraepithelial neoplasia (cervical dysplasia),

cervical carcinoma in situ, and invasive cervical carcinoma. Smoking is a cofactor.

26 Risk factors for cancer of the vagina are exposure in utero to nonsteroidal estrogens (e.g., DES), exposure to sexually transmitted infection, and prior cervical cancer. Incidence is greatest in women older than 60 years of age.

27 Most vaginal cancers are not invasive. Like cervical cancers, they arise from the epithelium and are identified as intraepithelial neoplasia (dysplasia), carcinoma in situ, or invasive carcinoma.

28 Risk factors for endometrial cancer include exposure to unopposed estrogen, obesity, high-fat diet, infertility or no pregnancies, late menopause, diabetes, and hypertension. Oral contraceptive use protects against endometrial and ovarian cancers. Incidence of endometrial cancer is greatest among women in their 50s and early 60s.

29 Risk factors for ovarian cancer include family history, residence in an industrialized country, prior breast or endometrial cancer, infertility, early menopause, obesity, a high-fat diet, and exposure to asbestos or talc. Ovarian cancer causes more deaths than any other genital cancer in women.

30 Ovarian tumors can arise from the ovarian epithelium or from the female germ cells (developing ova). Epithelial neoplasms account for 85% to 90% of all ovarian malignancies.

31 Infertility, or the inability to conceive after 1 year of unprotected intercourse, affects approximately 15% of all couples. Fertility can be impaired by factors in the male, female, or both partners.

32 Awareness of sexual dysfunction is relatively new. Chronic illness, medications, infection, sexual trauma, and a variety of psychosocial concerns have been implicated as causes.

Disorders of the Male Reproductive System

1 Disorders of the urethra include urethritis (infection of the urethra) and urethral strictures (narrowing or obstruction of the urethral lumen caused by scarring).

2 Most cases of urethritis result from sexually transmitted pathogens. Urologic instrumentation, foreign body insertion, trauma, or an anatomic abnormality can cause urethral inflammation with or without infection. Noninfectious urethritis can also be caused by drinking a toxic fluid (wood or ethyl alcohol, turpentine) and by Reiter syndrome.

3 Urethritis causes urinary symptoms (dysuria), including a burning sensation during urination, frequency, urgency, urethral tingling or itching, and clear or purulent discharge.

4 The scarring that causes urethral stricture can be caused by trauma or by severe untreated urethritis.

5 Manifestations of urethral stricture include those of bladder outlet obstruction: urinary frequency and hesitancy, diminished force and caliber of the urinary stream, dribbling after voiding, and nocturia.

6 Phimosis and paraphimosis are penile disorders involving the foreskin (prepuce). In phimosis, the foreskin cannot be retracted over the glans. In paraphimosis, the foreskin is retracted and cannot be reduced (returned to its normal anatomic position over the glans). Phimosis is caused by poor hygiene and chronic infection and can lead to paraphimosis. Paraphimosis can constrict the penile blood vessels, preventing circulation to the glans.

7 Peyronie disease consists of fibrosis, affecting the corpora cavernosa, which causes penile curvature during erection. Fibrosis prevents engorgement on the affected side, causing a lateral curvature that can prevent intercourse.

8 Priapism is a prolonged, painful erection that is not stimulated by sexual arousal. The corpora cavernosa (but not the corpus spongiosum) fill with blood that does not drain out, probably because of venous obstruction. Priapism is associated with spinal cord trauma, sickle cell disease, leukemia, and pelvic tumors. It can also be idiopathic.

9 Balanitis is an inflammation of the glans penis. It is associated with phimosis, inadequate cleansing under the foreskin, skin disorders, and pathogens (e.g., *Candida albicans*).

10 Cancer of the penis is rare and tends to occur in uncircumcised men with phimosis who practice poor hygiene. Penile carcinoma in situ tends to involve the glans; invasive carcinoma of the penis involves the shaft as well.

11 A varicocele is an abnormal dilation of the veins within the spermatic cord caused by either congenital absence of valves in the internal spermatic vein or acquired valvular incompetence.

12 A hydrocele is a collection of fluid between the testicular and scrotal layers of the tunica vaginalis. Hydroceles can be idiopathic or caused by trauma or infection of the testes.

13 A spermatocele is a cyst located between the testis and epididymis that is filled with fluid and sperm.

14 Cryptorchidism is a congenital condition in which one or both testes fail to descend into the scrotum. It may be caused by a developmental delay of descent, presence of a defective testicle, or a mechanical factor preventing descent, such as a short spermatic cord or a narrowed inguinal canal. Uncorrected cryptorchidism is associated with infertility and significantly increased risk of testicular cancer.

15 Testicular torsion is the rotation of a testis, which twists blood vessels in the spermatic cord. This interrupts blood supply to the testis, resulting in edema and, if not corrected within 6 hours, necrosis and atrophy of testicular tissues.

16 Orchitis is an acute infection of the testes. Pathogenic organisms may reach the testes through the blood or the lymphatics; most commonly, they reach the testes by ascending through the vas deferens and epididymis. Complications of orchitis include hydrocele and abscess formation.

17 Testicular cancer is the most common malignancy in males from 15 to 34 years of age. Although its cause is unknown, high androgen levels, genetic predisposition, and history of cryptorchidism, trauma, or infection may contribute to tumorigenesis. Most testicular neoplasms are germ cell tumors.

18 Spermatogenesis (sperm production by the testes) can be impaired by disruptions of the hypothalamic-pituitary-testicular axis that reduce testosterone secretion and by testicular trauma, infection, or atrophy from any cause. Sperm production is also impaired by neoplastic disease, cryptorchidism, or any factor (e.g., circulatory impairment, wearing of tight clothing) that causes testicular temperature to rise.

19 Sperm quality is impaired by chromosomal abnormalities resulting from genetic factors, irradiation, or toxins. Sperm motility can be impaired by unfavorable constituents or characteristics of semen. Reductions in quality, motility, or number (per milliliter of semen) all impair fertility.

20 Epididymitis, an inflammation of the epididymis, is usually caused by a sexually transmitted pathogen that ascends through the vasa deferentia from an already infected urethra or bladder.

21 Benign prostatic hyperplasia (BPH), also called benign prostatic hypertrophy, is the enlargement of the prostate gland. This condition becomes symptomatic as the enlarging prostate compresses the urethra, causing symptoms of bladder outlet obstruction and urine retention.

22 Bacterial prostatitis is an infection of the prostate. Acute bacterial prostatitis causes an inflammatory response in which the prostate becomes enlarged, tender, and firm. Infection may spread to the bladder. Chronic bacterial prostatitis is recurrent prostatic infection that eventually causes fibrosis.

23 Nonbacterial prostatitis is prostatic inflammation without evidence of bacterial infection.

24 Prostate cancer is the second leading cause of cancer deaths in men (after lung cancer). Possible causes involve genetic predisposition, environmental and dietary factors, and sexually transmitted pathogens. Incidence is greatest among Northern European and North American men (particularly blacks) older than 65 years of age.

25 Most cancers of the prostate are adenocarcinomas that develop at the periphery of the gland. Because there are no early symptoms, disease is often advanced at the time of diagnosis.

26 Sexual dysfunction in males can be caused by any physical or psychologic factor that impairs erection, emission, or ejaculation.

27 Vascular disorders can prevent initiation or maintenance of an erection; endocrine disorders that reduce testosterone levels can decrease libido; neurologic disorders can interfere with erection, emission, and ejaculation; chronic diseases can cause physiologic or psychologic dysfunction; priapism and Peyronie disease can impair erectile function; and surgical procedures and many drugs can disrupt processes necessary for sexual function.

Disorders of the Breast

1 Most disorders of the breast are disorders of the mammary gland, that is, the female breast.

2 Galactorrhea, or inappropriate lactation, is the persistent secretion of a milky substance by the breasts of a woman who is not in the postpartum state or nursing an infant. Its most common cause is nonpuerperal hyperprolactinemia, a rise in serum prolactin levels that is not associated with pregnancy and childbirth.

3 Fibrocystic breast disease is a catch-all term used to describe a variety of benign epithelial breast lesions, including microcysts, macrocysts, adenosis, apocrine gland change, fibroadenomas, and ductal hyperplasia. Many of these lesions are risk factors for breast cancer, and most appear to represent a response of breast tissue to estrogen stimulation.

4 The lesions of fibrocystic disease (physiologic nodularity) are nodular, are multiple, and become tender and large as menstruation approaches. They are palpable and may worsen until menopause. Symptoms tend to lessen with a diet low in fat and caffeine. Physiologic nodularity is present in about 50% of menstruating women.

5 Other benign breast lesions are fibroadenomas, mammary duct ectasia (an inflammatory condition), intraductal papillomas, and fat necrosis.

6 Breast cancer is the most common form of cancer in women and second to lung cancer as the most frequent cause of cancer death.

7 The major risk factors for breast cancer are environmental factors, such as a high-fat diet; reproductive factors, such as nulliparity; and familial factors, such as a family history of breast cancer.

8 Approximately one third of breast cancers are hormone-dependent, or progesterone- or estrogen-receptor–positive. Treatment protocols are often based on whether the tumor is receptor-positive or -negative.

9 Most breast cancers arise from the ductal epithelium and then may metastasize to the lymphatics, opposite breast, abdominal cavity, lungs, bones, kidneys, liver, adrenal glands, ovaries, and pituitary glands.

10 The first clinical manifestation of breast cancer is usually a small, painless lump in the breast. Other manifestations include palpable lymph nodes in the axilla, dimpling of the skin, nipple and skin retraction, nipple discharge, ulcerations, reddened skin, and bone pain associated with bony metastases.

11 Gynecomastia is the overdevelopment (hyperplasia) of breast tissue in a male. It is first seen as a firm, palpable mass at least 2 cm in diameter and is located in the subareolar area.

12 Gynecomastia affects 32% to 40% of the male population. Incidence is greatest among adolescents and men older than 50 years of age.

13 Gynecomastia is caused by hormonal or breast tissue alterations that cause estrogen to dominate. These alterations can result from systemic disorders, drugs, neoplasms, or idiopathic causes.

14 Breast cancer is relatively uncommon in males, but it has a poor prognosis because men tend to delay seeking treatment until the disease is advanced. Incidence is greatest in men in their 60s.

15 Most breast cancers in men are estrogen-receptor–positive.

KEY TERMS

Acute bacterial prostatitis, 780
Adenomyosis, 761
Amenorrhea, 748
Anorgasmia (orgasmic dysfunction), 769
Anovulation, 750
Balanitis, 771
Bartholinitis (Bartholin cyst), 756
Benign prostatic hyperplasia (BPH) (benign prostatic hypertrophy), 779
Cervical carcinoma in situ, 764
Cervical intraepithelial neoplasm (CIN) (cervical dysplasia), 764
Cervicitis, 756
Chronic bacterial prostatitis, 780
Corpus luteum cyst, 760
Cryptorchidism, 774
Cystocele, 757
Delayed puberty, 747
Dysfunctional uterine bleeding (DUB), 750
Dyspareunia (painful intercourse), 769
Endometrial polyp, 760
Endometriosis, 761
Epididymitis, 778
Fibrocystic disease (physiologic nodularity), 784

Follicular cyst, 758
Galactorrhea (inappropriate lactation), 783
Gynecomastia, 793
Heterosexual precocious puberty, 747
Hirsutism, 750
Hydrocele, 773
Hyperprolactinemia, 750
Incomplete precocious puberty, 747
Infertility, 769
Invasive carcinoma of the cervix, 764
Isosexual precocious puberty, 747
Leiomyoma (uterine fibroid), 760
Mucopurulent cervicitis (MPC) (acute cervicitis), 756
Nonbacterial prostatitis, 781
Nonpuerperal hyperprolactinemia, 783
Oophoritis, 754
Orchitis, 775
Paraphimosis, 770
Pelvic inflammatory disease (PID), 754
Pessary, 758
Peyronie disease (bent nail syndrome), 770

Phimosis, 770
Polycystic ovarian syndrome (PCO), 752
Precocious puberty, 747
Premenstrual syndrome (PMS), 752
Priapism, 771
Primary amenorrhea, 748
Primary dysmenorrhea, 748
Prolactin-inhibiting factor (PIF), 783
Prostatitis, 779
Prostatodynia, 779
Rapid orgasm, 769
Rectocele, 758
Retrograde menstruation, 761
Salpingitis, 754
Secondary amenorrhea, 749
Sexual anorexia (inhibited sexual desire, decreased libido), 769
Sexual dysfunction, 782
Spermatocele, 774
Torsion of the testis, 774
Urethral stricture, 770
Urethritis, 770
Urethrocele, 758
Uterine prolapse, 758
Vaginismus, 769
Vaginitis, 754
Varicocele, 773
Vulvitis, 756

REFERENCES

400 Self-assessment picture tests in clinical medicine. (1984). London: Wolfe Medical Publications, Ltd.

American Cancer Society (ACS). (1991). CA cancer source book for nurses (6th ed.). New York: Author.

American Cancer Society (ACS). (1991, July). Cervical cancer: Risk factors, detection, diagnosis, staging, treatment. Cancer Response System Report #408574. New York: Author

American Cancer Society (ACS). (1992). Cancer facts & figures—1992. New York: Author.

American Cancer Society (ACS). (1993). Cancer statistics 1993. CA—A Cancer Journal for Clinicians, 43(1).

Coppleson, M., Pixley, E., & Reed, B. (1971). Colposcopy: A scientific approach to the cervix in health and disease. Springfield, IL: Charles C Thomas.

Davies, T. F., & Kase, N. G. (1990). Male reproduction. In N. Kase, A. B. Weingold, & D. M. Gershenson (Eds.), Principles and practice of clinical gynecology (2nd ed.). New York: Churchill Livingstone.

del Regato, J. A., Spjut, H. J., & Cox, J. D. (1985). Ackerman and del Regato's cancer: Diagnosis, treatment, and prognosis (6th ed.). St. Louis: Mosby–Year Book.

deVita, V. T., Hellman, S., & Rosenberg, S. A. (1985). Cancer principles and practice of oncology (2nd ed.). Philadelphia: Lippincott.

Drugs that cause sexual dysfunction. (1983). Medical Letter, 25 (641), 73-76.

Dupont, W., & Page, D. (1985). Risk factors for breast cancer in women with proliferative breast disease. New England Journal of Medicine, 312(2), 146-151.

Eliott, M. (1993). Special report. Search for a killer: Focus shifts from fats to hormones. Science, 259, 616-618.

Fathalla, M. F., Rosenfield, A., Indriso, C., Sen, D. K., & Ratnam, S. S. (Eds.). (1990). The FIGO manual of human physiology: Reproductive health global issues (Vol. 3). New Jersey: Parthenon Publishing.

Gardner, H. L., & Kaufman, R. H. (1969). Benign diseases of the vulva and vagina. St. Louis: Mosby–Year Book.

Gilbaugh, J. H. (1992). A doctor's guide to men's private parts. Glendale, CA: Crown Publishers.

Griffiths, M. J., Murray, K. H., & Russo, P. C. (1984). *Oncology nursing: Pathophysiology, assessment, and intervention.* New York: Macmillan.

Haagensen, C. D. (1986). *Diseases of the breast.* Philadelphia: Saunders.

Hall, J.G. (1990). Genomic imprinting: Review and relevance to human diseases. *American Journal of Human Genetics, 46,* 857-873.

Hall, J. M., Friedman, L., Guenther, C., Lee, M. K., Weber, J.L., Black, D. M., & King, M. (1992). Closing in on a breast cancer gene on chromosome 17q. *American Journal of Human Genetics, 15*(6), 1235–1242.

Henrick, J. B. (1992). The post-menopausal estrogen/breast cancer controversy. *Journal of the American Medical Association, 268*(14), 1900-1902.

Herbst, A.L., Mischell, D.R., Stenchever, M.A., & Droegemueller, W. D. (1992). *Comprehensive gynecology* (2nd ed.). St. Louis: Mosby–Year Book.

Hoekelman, R. A., Friedman, S. B., Nelson, N. M., & Seidel, H. M. (1992). *Primary pediatric care* (2nd ed.). St. Louis: Mosby–Year Book.

Hutter, R. V. P. (1985). Goodbye to fibrocystic disease. *New England Journal of Medicine, 312*(3), 179-181.

Knabbe, C., Lippman, M. E., Wakefield, L. M., Flanders, K. C., Kasid, A., Derynck, R., & Dickson, R. B. (1987). Evidence that transforming growth factor-B is a hormonally regulated negative growth factor in human breast cancer cells. *Cell, 48,* 417-428.

Korenman, S. G. (1980). Estrogen window hypothesis of the etiology of breast cancer. *Lancet, 8,* 700-701.

Lee, N. C., Dicker, R. C., Rubin, G. L., & Ory, H. W. (1984). Confirmation of the preoperative diagnosis for hysterectomy. *American Journal of Obstetrics and Gynecology Clinics of North America, 150*(3), 283-287.

Lichtman, R., & Papera, S. (1990). *Gynecology well woman care.* Norwalk, CT: Appleton-Lange.

Lloyd-Davies, R. W., Gow, J. G., & Davies, D. R. (1983). *Color atlas of urology.* London: Wolfe Medical Publications, Ltd.

Longacre, T. A., & Bartow, S. A. (1986). A correlative morphologic study of human breast and endometrium in the menstrual cycle. *American Journal of Surgical Pathology, 10,* 382-393.

McPherson, K., & Doll, H. (1991). Oestrogens and breast cancer: Exogenous hormones. *British Medical Bulletin, 47*(2), 484-492.

Mencaglia, L., Perino, A., & Hamou, J. (1987). Hysteroscopy in perimenopausal and postmenopausal women with abnormal uterine bleeding. *The Journal of Reproductive Medicine, 32*(8), 577-582.

Morabia, A., & Wynder, E. L. (1990). Epidemiology and natural history of breast cancer. *Surgical Clinics of North America, 70*(4), 739-752.

Pfau, A. (1986). Prostatitis. *Urologic Clinics of North America, 13*(4), 695-714.

Phipps, W. P., Long, B. C., Woods, N. F., & Cassmeyer, V.L. (1991). *Medical-surgical nursing: Concepts and clinical practice.* (4th ed.). St. Louis: Mosby–Year Book.

Pickles, V. R., Hall, W. S., & Best, F. A. (1965). Prostaglandins in endometrium and menstrual fluid from normal and dysmenorrheic subjects. *British Journal of Obstetrics and Gynecology, 72,* 185.

Potten, C. S., Watson, R. J., Williams, G. T., Tickle, S., Roberts, S. A., Harris, M., & Howell, A. (1988). The effect of age and menstrual cycle upon proliferative activity of the normal human breast. *British Journal of Cancer, 58*(2), 163-170.

Reid, R. (1985). *Premenstrual syndrome: Current problems in obstetrics, gynecology, and fertility* (Vol. VIII, No. 2). St. Louis: Mosby–Year Book.

Russo, J., & Russo, I. H. (1987). Development of the human mammary gland. In M. C. Neville & C. W. Daniel (Eds.), *The mammary gland development, regulation, and function* (pp. 67-96). New York: Plenum Press.

Russo, J., Tay, L. K., & Russo, I. H. (1982). Differentiation of the mammary glands and susceptibility to breast cancer. *Breast Cancer Research Treatment, 2,* 5-73.

Sampson, J. A. (1927). Peritoneal endometriosis due to the menstrual dissemination of endometrial tissue into the peritoneal cavity. *American Journal of Obstetrics & Gynecology, 14,* 422.

Seidel, H., Ball, J., Dains, J., & Benedict, G. W. (1991). *Mosby's guide to physical examination* (2nd ed.). St. Louis: Mosby–Year Book.

Stampfer, M. J., Bechtel, S. D., & Hunter, D. (1992). Fat, alcohol, selenium, and breast cancer risk. *Contemporary OB/GYN, 37,* 42-47.

Sweet, R. L. (1991, December). Infection protocols: Acute salpingitis treatment—An update. *Contemporary OB/GYN, 36,* 43-52.

Tanagho, E. A., & McAninch, J. W. (Eds.). (1992). *Smith's general urology* (13th ed.). Norwalk, CT: Appleton-Lange.

Vogel, P.M., Georgiade, N. G., Fetter, B. F., McCarty, K. S. (1981). The correlation of histologic changes in the human breast with the menstrual cycle. *American Journal of Pathology, 104,* 23-34.

Waxman, J. (1991). A new understanding of the hormonal regulation of endocrine dependent cancer. *British Medical Bulletin, 47*(1), 197-208.

Weingold, A. B. (1990). Abnormal bleeding. In N. Kase, A. B. Weingold, & D. M. Gershenson (Eds.), *Principles and practice of clinical gynecology* (2nd ed.). New York: Churchill Livingston.

Woods, N. F., Lentz, M. J., Mitchell, E. S., Lee, K. A., & Taylor, D. (1989). *Prevalence of perimenstrual symptoms: Final report.* Seattle: University of Washington.

York, R., Freeman, E., Lowery, B., & Strauss, J. F. (1989). Characteristics of premenstrual syndrome. *Obstetrics & Gynecology, 73*(4), 601-605.

SUGGESTED READINGS

American Cancer Society (ACS). (1992, January). Testicular cancer: Organ/site description, incidence/statistics, cause/prevention. *Cancer Response System Report #476657.*

American Cancer Society (ACS). (1992, June). Prostate cancer: Detection/diagnosis. *Cancer Response System Report #462514, #462515.*

Bain, J. (1991). Disorders of the testes. *Comprehensive Therapy, 17*(7), 19-24.

Beard, M., & Curtis, L. (1991). *Menopause and the years ahead* (revised edition). Tucson, Arizona: Fisher Books.

Burgers, J. K., Badalament, R. A., & Drago, J. R. (1992). Penile cancer: Clinical presentation, diagnosis, and staging. *Urologic Clinics of North America, 19*(2), 247-256.

Doody, K. M., & Carr, B. R. (1990). Amenorrhea. *Obstetrics and Gynecology Clinics of North America, 17*(2), 361-388.

Faro, S. (1990). Pelvic pain and infections. *Obstetrics and Gynecology Clinics of North America, 17*(2), 441-455.

Hammond, K. R., & Steinkampf, M. P. (1992, September). Assessing ovulatory function. *Contemporary OB/GYN, 37,* 29-42.

Hatcher, R. A., Stewart, F., Trussell, J., Kowal, D., Guest, F., Stewart, G. K., & Cates, W. (1990). *Contraceptive technology 1990-1992* (15th revised ed.). New York: Irvington Publishers.

Kaplan, H. S. (1987). *The illustrated manual of sex therapy* (2nd ed.). New York: Brunner/Mazel.

Kase, N. G., Weingold, A. B., & Gershenson, D. M. (Eds.). (1990). *Principles and practice of clinical gynecology* (2nd ed.). New York: Churchill Livingstone.

Masters, W. H., Johnson, V. E., & Kolodny, R. C. (1992). *Human sexuality* (4th ed.). New York: Harper Collins.

Rous, S. M. (1992). *The prostate book: Sound advice on symptoms and treatment.* New York: W. W. Norton.

Rubinow, D. R. (1992). The premenstrual syndrome: New views. *Journal of the American Medical Association, 268*(14), 1908-1912.

Scottish Cancer Trials Breast Group and ICRS Breast Unit, Guy's Hospital London. (1993). Adjuvant ovarian ablation versus CMS chemotherapy in premenopausal women with pathological stage II breast carcinoma: The Scottish trial. *Lancet, 341,* 1293-1298.

Van Wijngaarden, W. J., & Duncan, I.D. (1993). Rationale for stopping cervical screening in women over 50. *British Medical Journal, 306,* 967-971.

Wein, A. J., & Van Arsdalen, K. N. (1988). Drug-induced male sexual dysfunction. *Urologic Clinics of North America, 15*(1), 23-31.

Woods, N. F., Taylor, D., Mitchell, E. S., & Lentz, M. J. (1992). Perimenstrual symptoms and health seeking behavior. *Western Journal of Nursing Research, 14*(40), 418-443.

Sexually Transmitted Diseases

Thom J. Mansen
Deborah L. Greener*

Chapter Outline

*Contributing author to first edition.

Throughout recorded history humans have been threatened by infectious diseases. Even into this century epidemics of diphtheria, smallpox, tuberculosis, typhoid, and other catastrophic infections could decimate entire communities almost overnight. Today, however, many of these diseases are virtually unknown, or at least under control, in North America. Unfortunately, despite medical advances, improved living standards, and better nutrition, new epidemics are now considered major public health problems, and some pose lethal threats to individuals and communities. These epidemics are the venereal or sexually transmitted diseases (STDs).

Within the past decade, the study and categorization of STDs have broadened to include both bacterial and viral, as well as other, agents as causes of STDs and other syndromes (Table 21-1) (Quinn & Cates, 1992). The more recent viral-induced STDs are generally considered incurable. The overall impact on the world is staggering when one considers the statistics related to these diseases.

It is estimated by the World Health Organization (WHO) that 250 million cases of STD occur each year in the world, and in many countries they have reached epidemic proportions (Quinn & Cates, 1992). The magnitude of the occurrence of STDs has

FIG. 21-1 Sexually transmitted diseases. A young couple, blindfolded, approach the edge of a cliff. (Courtesy National Library of Medicine.)

TABLE 21-1

Currently Recognized Sexually Transmitted Infections

Causal microorganism	Disease
Bacteria	
Campylobacter	Campylobacter enteritis
Calymmatobacterium granulomatis	Granuloma inguinale
Chlamydia trachomatis	Urogenital infections; lymphogranuloma venereum
Gardnerella vaginalis	Bacterial vaginosis
Haemophilus ducreyi	Chancroid
Mycoplasma	Mycoplasmosis
Neisseria gonorrhoeae	Gonorrhea
Shigella	Shigellosis
Treponema pallidum	Syphilis
Viruses	
Cytomegalovirus	Cytomegalic inclusion disease
Hepatitis B virus (HBV)	Hepatitis
Herpes simplex virus (HSV)	Genital herpes
Human immunodeficiency virus (HIV)	Acquired immune deficiency syndrome (AIDS)
Human papillomavirus	Condylomata acuminata
Molluscum contagiosum virus	Molluscum contagiosum
Protozoa	
Entamoeba histolytica	Amebiasis; amebic dysentery
Giardia lamblia	Giardiasis
Trichomonas vaginalis	Trichomoniasis
Ectoparasites	
Phthirus pubis	Pediculosis pubis
Sarcoptes scabiei	Scabies
Fungus	
Candida albicans	Candidiasis

a significant impact on the mortality and morbidity of adults and exposed infants. This is particularly true in developing countries, where STDs were not recognized until recently as a major cause of acute and chronic illnesses in women (Ronald et al., 1991).

The incidence and increase in STDs are attributable to changes in demographic and sociocultural factors. Such changes include increased premarital sex (especially among teens), an increase in the divorce rate, nonmonogamy among married people, and bisexuality. All of these contribute to the increase in numbers of sexual partners and an increased exposure to STDs. Concern also is expressed about the numbers of individuals who fail to take protective measures when engaging in sexual activities (Fig. 21-1). This is especially prevalent among teenagers (Schwartz & Gilmore, 1990).

Sexually transmitted diseases are stereotyped as occurring only among the urban poor and minority populations. Because the Centers for Disease Control (CDC) does not require that all STDs be reported, private physicians often do not report them. Thus, reported STDs often come from public health clinics, giving the impression that a greater number of the urban poor and minority populations are inflicted with STDs. The fact is that STDs are prevalent among all individuals in all socioeconomic groups.

SEXUALLY TRANSMITTED UROGENITAL INFECTIONS

Bacterial Infections
Gonorrhea

Gonorrhea is caused by **gonococci** (singular, *gonococcus*), which are microorganisms of the species *Neisseria gonorrhoeae*. Gonococci were first identified by Neisser in stained smears of vaginal, urethral, and conjunctival exudate in 1879. Gonorrhea is the most commonly reported communicable disease in the United States. In 1991, 620,478 cases (not including military cases) were reported (Centers for Disease Control [CDC], 1992).

The incidence of gonorrhea appears to be declining in men, possibly because of safer sex practices among sexually active homosexuals and bisexuals. Sexually active adolescents and young adults between 15 and 29 years of age have the highest incidence of gonorrhea, with females between the ages of 15 and 19 being in the highest risk category. Other demographic risk factors include nonwhite race, early onset of sexual activity, single marital status, and previous gonorrhea (Hook & Handsfield, 1990). The risk of developing gonorrhea from intercourse with an infected partner is between 50% and 90% for females and 20% for males. The risk increases threefold to fourfold for males after four exposures to an infected partner (Hook & Handsfield, 1990).

Transmission of gonococcal infection generally requires contact of epithelial surfaces, such as occurs during sexual intercourse. Gonorrhea also can be transmitted by a pregnant woman to her fetus. The infection passes from mother to child across the amniotic membranes, by direct inoculation with a fetal scalp electrode during labor monitoring, during passage through the birth canal, or through mother-infant contact after birth. **Fomites** (contaminated objects) are rarely involved in the transmission of *N. gonorrhoeae*, primarily because the gonococcus requires a rich medium (such as bodily fluids) and an environment high in carbon dioxide (5% to 10%) for growth.

Pathophysiology

Humans are the only natural hosts for *N. gonorrhoeae*, which is an aerobic, non–spore-forming, oxidase-positive, gram-negative coccal (round) microorganism that usually appears in pairs (diplococci), with the adjacent sites slightly flattened. Hairlike filaments, called pili, appear to help the microorganisms attach themselves to host cells: the epithelial cells of mucous membranes. Columnar, transitional, and stratified squamous epithelial cells are most frequently infected. First the microorganisms become attached to the plasma membranes (cell walls) of these cells, then they invade the cells and begin to damage the mucosa. Generally a quick leukocytic (inflammatory) response and exudation at the site of infection occur.

In females, the endocervical canal (inner portion of the cervix) is the usual site of original gonococcal infection, although urethral colonization is also common, as is the infection of Skene and Bartholin glands. Several factors can facilitate ascent of gonococci into the uterus and the fallopian tubes, where they cause pelvic inflammatory disease (PID). Among these factors are (1) hor-

monal and cervical mucous changes associated with menstruation that lower natural bacteriostatic and mechanical protection; (2) the presence of an intrauterine contraceptive device (IUD); (3) retrograde menstruation; and (4) individual organisms associated with chlamydia and gonococcal PID that may possess virulent potentiating factors (CDC, 1991b). Bacteria (*N. gonorrhoeae, Chlamydia trachomatis*) also may adhere to sperm and be transported to the fallopian tubes (Westrom & Mardh, 1990). In the fallopian tubes, progressive mucosal and submucosal invasion and sloughing of normal, ciliated tubal epithelium are accompanied by marked inflammatory response, causing the fallopian tubes to fill with exudate. In males, the gonococci typically infect the urethra. Infection of the epididymis and other complications in men are rare and if present are the result of chlamydia infection (Zenilman, 1992).

Clinical Manifestations

The clinical manifestations of gonorrhea can be categorized as local or systemic and uncomplicated or complicated. Uncomplicated local infections are seen as urethral infections in males and urogenital infections in females. Urethral infection in males has an incubation period of 2 to 5 days, but may be as long as 3 weeks. Approximately 60% of those infected suddenly experience marked dysuria (painful or difficult urination), and a profuse, mucopurulent discharge spontaneously appears at the urethral meatus. Some individuals have little discharge, however, and some may have no symptoms at all. Most cases of untreated gonococcal urethritis resolve spontaneously after several weeks, and more than 95% of individuals are asymptomatic by 6 months after infection (Pelouze, 1941).

In females, the incubation period varies, but those who develop symptoms generally do so within 10 days of exposure. The clinical manifestations of uncomplicated gonorrhea in women may be slight or very severe; they include a vaginal discharge that is often yellowish, dysuria, bleeding or spotting between menstrual periods, and heavy menses. Physical examination may disclose cervical friability and erythema (redness) and purulent or mucopurulent discharge from the os. There may be a discharge from the Skene or Bartholin glands if these sites are involved (Fig. 21-2).

Gonococcal infection of the anus and rectum is found in 35% to 50% of women who are diagnosed with urogenital gonorrhea. Anorectal infection probably is caused by the spread of infected exudate from the cervix and vagina, because few such individuals report having had anogenital sexual contact. Among homosexual men, the infection results from rectal intercourse.

Symptoms of anorectal gonorrhea range from mild anal pruritus (itching), mucopurulent rectal discharge, and slight rectal bleeding, to severe rectal pain, tenes-

FIG. 21-2 Gonorrhea. Gonorrhea that has caused bartholinitis with purulent exudate. (From Handsfield, 1990.)

mus (painful and ineffectual straining at stool), and constipation. Physical examination may disclose anal erythema and discharge and evidence of mucosal damage to the anus and rectum, such as friability, edema, and purulent exudate. The frequency of such signs and symptoms is not well known.

Gonococcal infection can be transmitted to the pharynx by orogenital sexual contact, particularly fellatio. Pharyngeal infection occurs in 3% to 25% of cases of gonorrhea, primarily in heterosexual women and homosexual men. Most of these infections are asymptomatic, but acute pharyngitis or tonsillitis with lymphadenopathy and fever occasionally may occur.

Other sites of uncomplicated local infections include the eye, leading to conjunctivitis; however, this is rare in adults. Primary cutaneous infection has also been reported and is usually manifested as a localized ulcer of the genitals, perineum, proximal lower extremities, or fingers. It is important to determine if such infections are the result of *N. gonorrhoeae* or secondary colonization by a preexisting lesion (Hook & Handsfield, 1990).

Local complicated gonorrhea infections include epididymitis and lymphangitis in males and salpingitis (PID) in females. Before the advent of antimicrobial therapy, approximately 20% of infected males developed acute epididymitis. Men with this condition report unilateral testicular pain and swelling and commonly have overt urethritis at the same time.

Penile lymphangitis is a rare complication with an unclear pathogenesis (Hook & Handsfield, 1990). Before modern antibiotics, individuals with this condition were

at risk for developing urethral strictures; however, this complication is now uncommon if treatment is sought and therapy instituted properly.

Acute salpingitis, or pelvic inflammatory disease (PID), is the most common local complication in females. Approximately 10% to 20% of those with acute gonococcal infection develop this condition. Salpingitis is significant in its development because of the potential long-term sequelae associated with it—infertility and ectopic pregnancy.

The onset of symptoms may be very rapid and includes chills, fever, nausea, vomiting, and lower abdominal pain that worsens with coughing, sneezing, or intercourse. Abdominal palpation often discloses bilateral lower quadrant tenderness and rebound tenderness resulting from peritoneal irritation caused by tubal exudate. Marked tenderness of the internal genitalia is frequently noted during pelvic examination. Enlargement or masses also may be palpable in the upper genital tract. Abscess of Bartholin's gland is also a local complication associated with gonococcal infection in females. Apart from PID, abscess formation of Bartholin's gland is the most common complication in females.

Disseminated gonococcal infection (DGI) is a rare systemic complication brought about by the spread of infection through the bloodstream. Approximately 1% of individuals with untreated gonococcal infection develop this type of complication (Elkins & Sparling, 1992).

Spread of *N. gonorrhoeae* to the liver causes a condition known as **perihepatitis** or Fitz-Hugh-Curtis syndrome. *C. trachomatis* also has been identified as a causative agent. Inflammation of the capsule of the liver is the primary pathology and produces sudden and intense upper right quadrant pain (Sperling, 1992).

Gonococcal infection of the newborn is usually manifested as an eye infection (**ophthalmia neonatorum**). Onset generally occurs 1 to 12 days after birth, with a mean of 4 to 6 days. Affected newborns are usually born to mothers who have had prolonged ruptured membranes. In these cases immediate treatment with a topical antibiotic or chemical eyedrop (e.g., silver nitrate) is not effective, because the infection is already established. Established infection causes bilateral corneal ulceration, with a profuse yellow or gray purulent exudate, and is followed by necrosis, scarring, and compromised vision. Signs of systemic disease are seldom apparent.

Evaluation and Treatment

Clinical signs and symptoms are not sufficient for the differential diagnosis of gonococcal infections. Microscopic evaluation of Gram-stained slides of clinical specimens are deemed positive for *N. gonorrhoeae* if gramnegative diplococci with typical "kidney bean" morphology are seen inside polymorphonuclear leukocytes.

Such a finding is considered adequate for the diagnosis of gonococcal urethritis in a symptomatic male. For screening purposes or diagnosis of pharyngeal or anorectal gonorrhea, cultures are recommended. For females, the Gram stain technique is less accurate and reliable and is replaced with a single culture of endocervical secretions. Because the pharynx or anus and rectum are rarely the only sites of infection for females, routine cultures of these sites are optional.

The many different strains of *N. gonorrhoeae* vary with respect to pathogenicity, virulence, and susceptibility to antibiotics. The development of resistance to antibiotics by *N. gonorrhoeae* has become a major concern in the treatment of gonococcal infections. Since 1980 and especially in the last 4 years, the incidence of both plasmid and chromosomal resistance of *N. gonorrhoeae* has increased dramatically (Quinn & Cates, 1992). It is estimated that 11% of the gonococci in the United States have plasmid-mediated penicillin resistance and 5% have plasmid-mediated tetracycline resistance; an additional 11% have chromosomally mediated resistance (Zenilman, 1992).

Another major concern is the coexistence of chlamydial infection with gonorrhea (Leu, 1991). (Chlamydial infections are discussed on pp. 811-814.) Approximately 20% to 30% of males and a higher proportion of females have coexistent chlamydia infections. Symptoms of chlamydia often go undetected until complications such as PID or urethritis manifest themselves.

Treatment for gonorrhea is influenced by four factors: (1) the spread of infection caused by penicillinase-producing *N. gonorrhoeae* (PPNG) and tetracycline resistant *N. gonorrhoeae* (TRNG); (2) the high frequency of chlamydia infection accompanying gonorrhea; (3) recognition of the serious complications of chlamydia and gonorrhea infections; and (4) the recent development of fast, inexpensive, and highly accurate tests for chlamydial infections (CDC, 1989). A single dose of intramuscular ceftriaxone followed by doxycycline is the most recent recommended treatment. Fluoroquinolone antibiotics are offering promising results in treating PPNG and non-PPNG strains of gonorrhea, as well as chromosomally mediated resistant *N. gonorrhoeae* and TRNG (Mogabgab, 1991).

Sexual partners are also assessed and treated according to these protocols, and sexual contact is avoided by all until treatment is completed. Condoms are strongly recommended to prevent future infection.

Syphilis

Syphilis, a disease having local and systemic manifestations, has been well known throughout history. Many famous figures from biblical and Roman times and the royal families of the Old World were thought or known to have had syphilis (Brandt, 1987). In the early half of the 1900s, it was estimated that the prevalence of syphilis in the United States was between 5% and 25% (Sparling, 1990).

There were 128,569 new cases of syphilis (excluding military cases) reported in the United States during 1991 (CDC, 1992). Since 1985, the incidence of syphilis has been increasing, and since 1986 it has been considered to be an epidemic (CDC, 1991c). The greatest increase in incidence has been in black heterosexuals, accounting for approximately 85% of all cases reported in 1991. Other factors contributing to the epidemic include changes in the geographic distribution and the relationship between syphilis and crack-cocaine use (CDC, 1991c).

The highest incidence of syphilis is associated with urban areas, with cities in the Midwest that had not been previously involved reporting substantial increases in the incidence. Cocaine use and the environment in which it is used apparently promote high-risk sexual encounters (sex with multiple anonymous partners in exchange for drugs) (CDC, 1991c).

As with gonorrhea, the incidence of syphilis is declining in the white male population. This, again, is attributed to safer sex practices among the homosexual community related to the spread of the acquired immunodeficiency syndrome (AIDS) virus.

Pathophysiology

Treponema pallidum, the cause of syphilis, is an anaerobic bacterium. The treponemata (individual microorganisms) look like corkscrews, with regular, tight spirals and a rotary motion (Fig. 21-3). *T. pallidum* has never been cultured in vitro.

The bacterium is present in exudate from the moist mucosal or cutaneous lesions of early syphilis and is transmitted through macroscopically invisible abrasions produced during sexual intercourse. Individuals are able to transmit the virus only during the first few years of infection. Approximately one half of individuals who have sexual intercourse with a partner who has early-stage syphilis develop the disease (Wooldridge, 1991). Syphilis becomes a systemic disease shortly after infec-

FIG. 21-3 **Syphilis.** *Treponema pallidum* as seen with dark-field microscope. (From Habif, 1990.)

tion and can be transmitted from a pregnant women to her fetus as early as the ninth week of gestation. The risk of transmission to the fetus gradually declines with each subsequent pregnancy; therefore, a mother who has had several children with severe congenital syphilis may go on to bear a healthy child. After about 8 years, even without treatment, the mother's infection is not transmitted to her fetus (Sparling, 1990).

The course of untreated syphilis consists of four stages: primary, secondary, latent, and tertiary. **Primary syphilis** begins at the site of bacterial invasion. There *T. pallidum* multiplies in the epithelium, producing a granulomatous tissue reaction called a **chancre**. Some microorganisms drain with lymph into adjacent lymph nodes. Within the nodes and at the site of the chancre, the cell-mediated and humoral immune responses are stimulated.

Secondary syphilis is systemic. During this stage blood-borne bacteria spread to all major organ systems. The secondary stage is followed by a period during which the immune system is able to suppress the infection. Even without treatment, spontaneous resolution of the skin lesions occurs and the individual enters the latent stage of infection. **Latent syphilis** may be subdivided into early and late; however, there are no specific criteria established that delineate one from the other (Hook & Marra, 1992). Medical history and serologic studies show that syphilis is present, but the individual has no clinical manifestations. Transmission is possible during the late and early latent stages.

Tertiary syphilis is the most severe stage, involving significant morbidity and mortality. The pathogenesis of syphilitic manifestations at this stage remains unclear. The destructive skin, bone, and soft tissue lesions (called **gummas**) of tertiary syphilis are probably caused by a severe hypersensitivity reaction to the microorganism. Within the cardiovascular system, infection with *T. pallidum* may cause aneurysms, heart valve insufficiencies, and heart failure. Within the central nervous system (CNS), the presence of *T. pallidum* in cerebrospinal fluid may cause the manifestations of **neurosyphilis** (Sparling, 1990).

Congenital syphilis is characterized by vasculitis, necrosis, fibrosis, and distribution of *T. pallidum* throughout the tissues. As would be expected with the increased incidence of syphilis, the incidence of congenital syphilis also has risen. In the last half of 1987, congenital syphilis has increased by 21% over 1986 (Wooldridge, 1991). Dental malformations and extensive, destructive bone lesions are found in the affected infant. Pathophysiology depends on gestational age at the time of infection. The placenta itself may be infected, causing it to become pale and diffusely fibrotic. The longer the maternal infection, the less likely that the fetus will be infected (Wooldridge, 1991).

Clinical Manifestations

Primary stage. In adults the incubation period of syphilis ranges from 12 days to 12 weeks after exposure and averages 3 weeks. At the site of treponemal entry a sore, or "hard chancre," develops. Typically the chancre is an eroded, painless, firm, and indurated (hard) ulcer that may be from a few millimeters to 2 cm in diameter. Chancres are accompanied by firm, enlarged, and nontender regional lymph nodes. Fig. 21-4 shows typical chancres of the penis and vulva. Syphilitic chancres are not always typical, however. Secondary infection can cause chancres to become necrotic and painful, and lesions on the fingers may be dry, scaly, and papular or moist and vegetative. If left untreated, the chancre of primary syphilis heals in 2 to 8 weeks and then spontaneously disappears, usually without leaving a scar.

Secondary stage. Clinical manifestations of secondary syphilis may overlap with those of the primary stage or may not appear for several weeks. Generally about 6 weeks after the appearance of the chancre the individ-

FIG. 21-4 Primary syphilis. A, Chancre of the penis. **B,** Chancre of the vulva. (From Wehrle & Top, 1981.)

FIG. 21-5 **Secondary syphilis in an infant.** Papulosquamous lesions of an infant with secondary syphilis. (From Wehrle & Top, 1981.)

FIG. 21-6 **Secondary syphilis.** Condylomata lata of the vulva. (From Wehrle & Top, 1981.)

ual develops cutaneous (skin) lesions of any type, from macular to pustular. These lesions are usually widespread, bilateral, and almost always present on the palms and soles (Fig. 21-5). Some moist papules may become elevated and bumpy, or vegetative; these are known as **condylomata lata.** The condylomata lata are usually whitish and flattened and appear most frequently in women, in the labial folds and on the skin of the groin and inner thighs (Fig. 21-6). Men and women may also develop these highly infectious lesions in the anal area.

Mild to severe systemic signs and symptoms, such as malaise, fever, sore throat, headache, hoarseness, anorexia, and joint pain, may occur with secondary syphilis. Lymphadenopathy, pruritus, and alopecia are commonly present. Some individuals develop anemia, leukocytosis, increased sedimentation rate, hepatitis, transitory proteinuria, arthritis, electrocardiographic abnormalities, and CNS symptoms. Regardless of whether treatment is given, the cutaneous lesions generally heal in 2 to 10 weeks, but relapses may occur for several years (Wooldridge, 1991).

Latent and tertiary stages. The asymptomatic, latent stage of syphilis may be as long as the life of the individual or as short as 1 year. The clinical manifestations of tertiary syphilis then may appear. These include gummas, cardiovascular lesions, and neurosyphilis. Because antibiotics can cure syphilis, manifestations of tertiary syphilis are quite rare.

Congenital syphilis. Congenital syphilis is usually divided into two clinical syndromes: early (manifested in the first 2 years of life) and late (manifested later, often near puberty). Newborns with congenital syphilis are often premature and show evidence of intrauterine growth retardation, hepatosplenomegaly, nasal discharge, varied cutaneous lesions, osteochondritis, anemia, leukocytosis or leukopenia, thrombocytopenia, nephrotic syndrome, varying degrees of CNS involvement, retinal inflammation, and glaucoma (Shultz, Murphy,

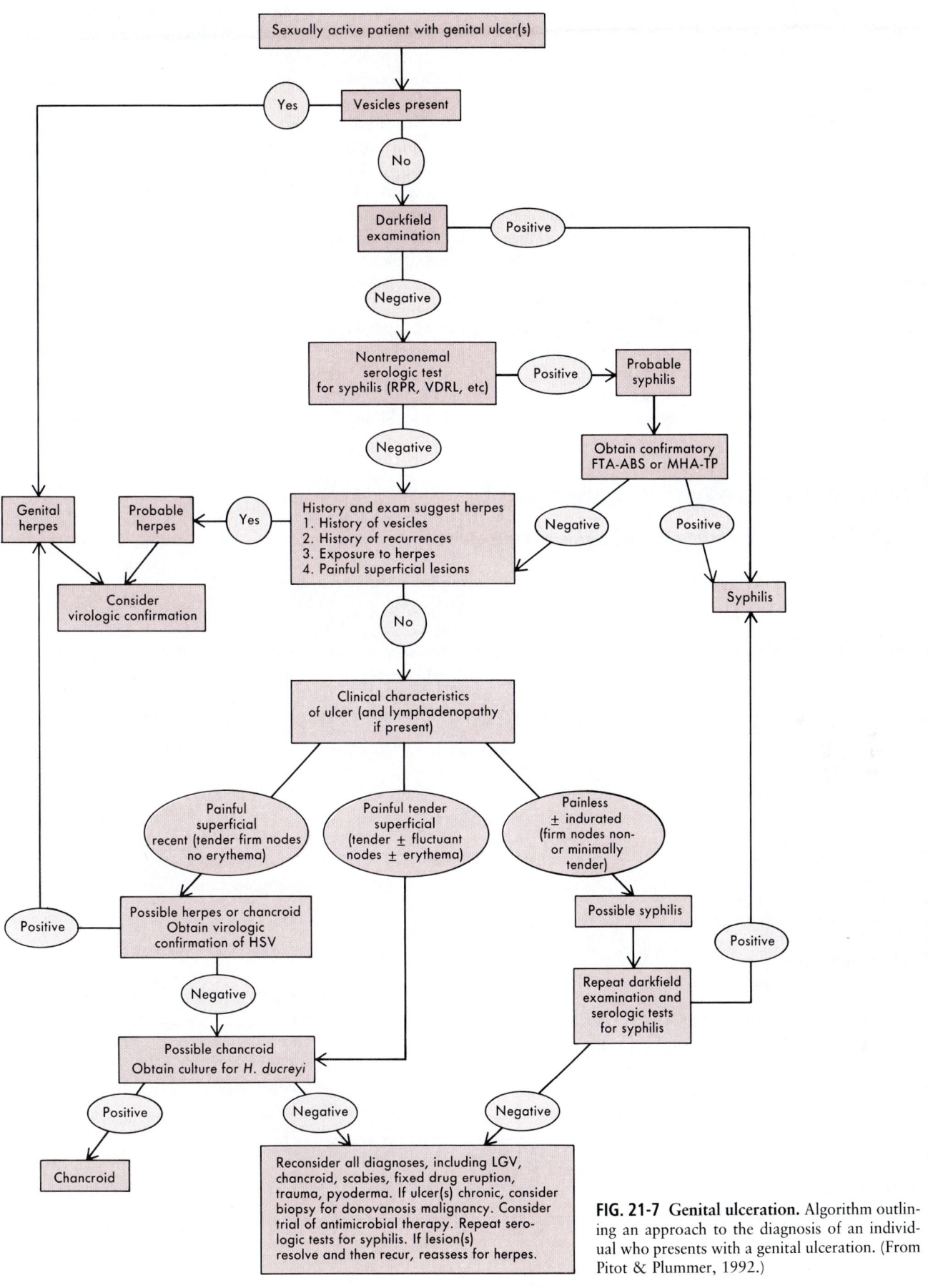

FIG. 21-7 Genital ulceration. Algorithm outlining an approach to the diagnosis of an individual who presents with a genital ulceration. (From Pitot & Plummer, 1992.)

Patamasucon, & Mehaus, 1990). The late clinical manifestations of classic congenital syphilis correspond to those of tertiary syphilis in the adult and are now rare.

Evaluation and Treatment

Because *T. pallidum* cannot be cultured in vitro, definitive diagnosis of early syphilis depends upon dark-field microscopy of a specimen taken from the chancre. The examination is repeated on 2 successive days if the result is initially negative (Thin, 1990). Genital ulcers are sometimes difficult to diagnose; an algorithm outlining an approach to the diagnosis of the individual presenting with a genital ulcer is given in Fig. 21-7.

Serologic tests for primary syphilis provide indirect evidence of infection. The Venereal Disease Research Laboratory (VDRL) antigen or rapid plasma reagin (RPR) test yields a positive result in more than half of infected individuals. The nonspecific serologic tests are based on a nonspecific antibody that is produced within an individual with syphilis. This antibody reacts against the negatively charged phospholipids found mainly in the inner membrane of mitochondria of all cells. A reaction would be considered positive for a diagnosis of syphilis (Farnes & Setness, 1990). Serologic-specific tests are used to assess antibody response to *T. pallidum* and include the fluorescent treponomal antibody absorption (FTA-ABS) and the microhemagglutination test (MHA-TP).

Numerous dermatologic disorders can mimic the skin lesions of secondary syphilis, making differential diagnosis difficult. Again laboratory confirmation is important; dark-field microscopy of scrapings from the condylomata lata or other skin lesions discloses the treponemata. Serologic tests are almost always strongly positive in this stage.

During the latent stage, individuals continue to have serologic evidence of untreated disease, but it is difficult to obtain confirmation through dark-field micros-

FALSE-POSITIVE SEROLOGIC TESTS FOR SYPHILIS

Reasons for false-positive, nontreponemal reactions (VDRL, RPR):

Transient reactions (<6 months)	Chronic reactions (>6 months)
Technical error (low titer)	Malaria
Smallpox vaccination	Leprosy
Mycoplasma pneumonia	Systemic lupus erythematosus
Enterovirus infections	Narcotic abuse
Infectious mononucleosis	Other connective tissue diseases
Pregnancy	Elderly population
Narcotic abuse	Hashimoto thyroiditis
Advanced tuberculosis	Rheumatoid arthritis
Scarlet fever	Reticuloendothelial malignancy
Viral and atypical pneumonia	Familial false-positives
Brucellosis	Idiopathic
Ratbite fever	
Leptospirosis	
Measles	
Mumps	
Lymphogranuloma venereum	
Malaria	
Trypanosomiasis	
Varicella	

Reasons for false-positive, *Treponema*-specific reactions (FTA-ABS)

Technical error
Inefficient sorbents
Healthy individuals without syphilis
Genital herpes simplex
Pregnancy
Lupus erythematosus (skin only or systemic)
Alcoholic cirrhosis
Scleroderma
Mixed connective tissue disease

copy. Examination of cerebrospinal fluid may confirm that the treponemata are present and the insidious onset of neurosyphilis has begun.

Treatment for all stages of syphilis is parenteral injection of benzathine penicillin G. If the individual has had signs of disease for less than 1 year, a single dose is appropriate. If signs have been present for more than 1 year, the treatment is three weekly injections. This therapy is also appropriate in pregnancy. There is no evidence to date that *T. pallidum* has developed resistance to penicillin (Thin, 1990). Individuals who are allergic to penicillin receive tetracycline, or if pregnant, erythromycin (CDC, 1989). Because treatment failures do occur, all individuals should have follow-up evaluation. Sexual partners are also examined and treated, and the use of condoms is recommended.

Definitive diagnosis of congenital syphilis is made by microscopic identification of *T. pallidum* in material from skin lesions or nasal discharge. Probable diagnosis is assumed on the basis of a rising or persistently reactive FTA-ABS value and clinical manifestations. In all cases of maternal syphilis, the goal is to treat the mother to prevent congenital syphilis. Maternal treatment with penicillin before delivery usually prevents congenital syphilis. If the infant requires treatment, penicillin is the drug of choice, because allergy does not pose a problem in the neonatal period. Such infants are then followed with serologic tests for syphilis at 3, 6, and 12 months. Nearly all of the tests become nonreactive (negative) by the time the infant is 6 months of age (Shultz et al., 1990).

Chancroid

Chancroid, or soft chancre, is an acute infectious disease that was first differentiated from syphilis in 1852. It is caused by the bacterium *Haemophilus ducreyi*.

Chancroid is most common in heterosexual males (more than 90% of reported cases), particularly those who are not circumcised. Chancroid lesions in women tend to be asymptomatic and internal (in the vagina and cervix); this may account for the low incidence of reported cases among women. There is no evidence that chancroid is transmitted from mother to fetus, either before or during delivery.

The incidence of chancroid in the United States has been decreasing since 1987, when reported cases peaked at 5035. The CDC reported 3476 cases in 1991 (CDC, 1992). Despite the decreasing incidence of chancroid, there continue to be sporadic outbreaks and a concern that the actual numbers reported are not a true representation of the prevalence. Underreporting of chancroid is suspected and is attributable to two factors: (1) the availability of culture media for *H. ducreyi* is limited and (2) no uniform reporting definition of probable cases existed until recently (Schulte & Martich, 1992).

Pathophysiology

H. ducreyi is a gram-negative bacillus with rounded ends. Under a microscope it is commonly observed in small clusters along strands of mucus. The only known route of transmission from person to person is through sexual contact. Fomites have not been identified as playing any role in transmission of *H. ducreyi*. Like other pathogens, *H. ducreyi* does not easily penetrate intact skin or mucous membranes. Therefore, it is thought that these surfaces must be abraded or traumatized to permit entry of the organism (Ronald & Albritton, 1990). Chancroid lesions are usually found on the internal surface of the foreskin or its point of attachment to the penis (the frenulum) in men, and on the labia, clitoris, or fourchette in women. Initially the papule enlarges, then erodes into a soft, circumscribed ulcer containing a superficial exudate. Beneath the ulcer is a lesion characterized by edema, endothelial proliferation, and a base of granulation tissue that is full of lymphocytes and plasma cells. Adjacent lymph nodes are acutely inflamed and full of polymorphonuclear leukocytes and necrotic cells (Para & Baird, 1985).

Clinical Manifestations

Chancroid has an incubation period of 4 to 7 days, after which the chancre appears. The chancre of chancroid, in contrast to the chancre of syphilis, is inflamed and painful. It erodes to an irregular ulcer that is 3 to 20 mm in diameter (Fig. 21-8). Occasionally more than one lesion is present. Lymphadenopathy, when present, is unilateral and painful. An inguinal **bubo** (fluid-filled lymph node) develops 7 to 10 days after the initial chancre in approximately 50% of individuals—primarily men. The bubo may fill with exudate and rupture spontaneously.

Evaluation and Treatment

Chancroid is easily confused with other types of genital ulcers, particularly those of syphilis, genital herpes, and granuloma inguinale (Fig. 21-8). Microscopic analysis of a Gram-stained smear from the chancroid helps identify the microorganism. Definitive diagnosis depends on recovery of *H. ducreyi* from cultured specimens. All individuals with ulcers are tested for syphilis. There are no serologic tests specific for *H. ducreyi*.

Recommended treatment for chancroid includes erythromycin or trimethoprim-sulfamethoxazole; however, resistance has emerged worldwide in isolated instances. Recent recommendations are a single intramuscular injection of ceftriaxone (Cazchor & Gleckman, 1989). Sexual partners are treated simultaneously. Buboes and inflamed nodes are not excised and drained, because these procedures would delay healing. Rather, fluctuant (fluid-filled) lymph nodes or buboes are generally aspirated through adjacent, healthy skin. Relapses

A   B

FIG. 21-8 **Chancroid. A,** Typical chancroid ulcer in a male. **B,** Ruptured inguinal bubo in an individual with chancroid from STD. (From Ronald & Albritton, 1990.)

at the site of original ulcer have occurred after complete healing in approximately 5% of cases (Ronald & Albritton, 1990). The use of condoms is recommended to prevent future infections.

Granuloma Inguinale

Granuloma inguinale is a chronic, progressively destructive bacterial infection caused by the microorganism *Calymmatobacterium granulomatis*, formerly known as *Donovania granulomatis*. The infection is also known by other names, the most common of which is *donovanosis*.

Granuloma inguinale is among the most prevalent sexually transmitted diseases in some parts of the world, predominantly in tropical climates. It appears to be concentrated in parts of southeast India, New Guinea, the Caribbean, and neighboring parts of South America, particularly the Guianas and Brazil. Additionally, it is found among the aborigines of Australia and New Zealand, and cases are also documented in Vietnam, Japan, and Zambia, South Africa (Richens, 1991). It is quite rare in the United States, with most cases being confined to the southern and southeastern regions. In 1991, there were only 29 cases reported in the United States (CDC, 1992), and it does not appear to be increasing in incidence. Although it is sexually transmissible, granuloma inguinale is only mildly contagious. Repeated exposure is necessary to cause disease. Syphilis is often reported in conjunction with granuloma inguinale (Richens, 1991).

Pathophysiology

C. granulomatis is a gram-negative, nonsporing, nonmotile encapsulated rod that is not easily isolated in the laboratory. After exposure, the bacteria survive and multiply within vacuoles of large histocytic cells or polymorphonuclear leukocytes. The bacteria reproduce within these cells until a vacuole may contain 20 to 30

microorganisms. These bacteria-filled vacuoles were identified by Donovan in 1905 and are termed **Donovan bodies** (Hart, 1990). The presence of Donovan bodies in tissue smears of material from the lesions is considered the "gold standard" for diagnosis of lymphogranuloma inguinale (Richens, 1991).

The initial lesion is an indurated subcutaneous nodule that is often preceded and accompanied by itching. The primary sites for development of the lesions are the distal penis in males and the introitus in females (Richens, 1991). Single lesions often coalesce with nearby lesions or form new lesions by autoinoculation of nearby skin surfaces. The progression from the initial nodule to a large, granulomatous heaped ulcer occurs slowly. Secondary infection may occur, increasing tissue damage and residual scarring. The disease may spread to the bones, joints, and liver.

Clinical Manifestations

The incubation period of granuloma inguinale is between 8 and 80 days. The first signs of disease are the indurated nodules, which are sharply defined and usually painless. They bleed easily; contain abundant, red, beefy-looking granulation tissue; and enlarge slowly. Systemic symptoms are quite rare; however, in some cases the infection spreads to the inguinal area, producing **pseudobuboes**. In these instances, the affected lymph nodes are not directly affected, but the surrounding area may be infected and abscessed.

Evaluation and Treatment

Although the clinical manifestations of this disease are important for diagnosis, confirmation involves microscopic examination in which Donovan bodies are seen in a smear or biopsy specimen. Cultures and serologic tests for granuloma inguinale are not available.

Many antibiotics have been used successfully against *C. granulomatis*. They include tetracycline, streptomycin, chloramphenicol, gentamicin, and trimethoprim with sulfamethoxasole. If an antibiotic is effective, the lesions begin to heal within 7 days. Treatment is continued for 21 days or until all lesions are healed. Relapses can occur, so prolonged follow-up is necessary, as is treatment of sexual partners (Richens, 1991).

Bacterial Vaginosis

Bacterial vaginosis (BV) is a condition in which the normal flora of the vagina is altered and is characterized by a noninflammatory response. *Gardnerella vaginalis* is considered to be the primary causative agent of BV; however, the presence of other anaerobic bacteria is necessary to produce the clinical manifestations. Epidemiologic studies of bacterial vaginosis are scarce, and the evidence for sexual transmission is circumstantial. Although 50% or more of sexually active women may be infected with *G. vaginalis* at any time, 50% of these individuals are asymptomatic (Sparks, 1991). Active disease occurs almost exclusively in sexually active women of reproductive age. There may be a correlation between *G. vaginalis*–associated infection and race, promiscuity, marital instability, previous pregnancy, other sexually transmitted infections, and presence of an intrauterine device (Hiller & Holmes, 1990). Although most male sexual partners of infected women harbor the microorganism in their urethra, *G. vaginalis* does not cause disease in men.

Pathophysiology

G. vaginalis is a nonmotile, gram-negative or gram-variable rod. Its exact role in the development of bacterial vaginosis is unclear, primarily because *G. vaginalis* is part of the normal flora of the vagina. Apparently the microorganism acts in concert with anaerobic bacteria to produce some of the clinical manifestations of vaginosis. These anaerobic bacteria have been identified as *Bacteroides,* peptococci, *Mycoplasma,* and the newly identified *Mobiluncus* species (Mardh, 1991) that produce various aromatic amines, including abundant amounts of foul-smelling putrescine and cadaverine. These amines raise the pH of vaginal secretions, further promoting the growth of *G. vaginalis. G. vaginalis* adheres readily to vaginal epithelial cells and mucosal surfaces but is not invasive and produces a minimal inflammatory response. Recent evidence suggests that the microorganism may be associated with ascending infections or pelvic inflammatory disease (Hiller & Holmes, 1990). There is increasing evidence that BV is associated with prematurity based on gestational age, premature rupture of membranes, and postpartum infection (Mead, Eschenbach, Ledger, & Thomason, 1989).

Clinical Manifestations

Bacterial vaginosis associated with *G. vaginalis* is characterized by a thin, gray, homogenous, and malodorous discharge, which adheres to the vaginal walls but is often copious enough to drain into the vulva. Occasionally the discharge is bubbly or frothy. Usually the vaginal pH is 5.0 to 5.5 and there are no signs of vaginal or cervical inflammation. Individuals often complain of a strong, fishy vaginal odor, particularly after intercourse. Odor is caused by the release of aromatic amines after bacterial contact with alkaline semen.

Evaluation and Treatment

Diagnosis is made by microscopic analysis of a wet mount (a specimen of vaginal secretions placed on a slide and mixed with normal saline). The wet mount shows "clue cells," which are considered to be almost pathognomonic for *Gardnerella*-associated bacterial vaginosis. The clue cells are vaginal epithelial cells that are covered with bacteria and look as if pepper has been shaken on them. Few leukocytes are visible on the wet mount, and lactobacilli are also absent. If a drop of potassium hydroxide (KOH) solution is added to vaginal secretions, a characteristic foul, fishy odor is immediately released. Cultures are rarely required or performed.

The most effective and commonly used treatment for *Gardnerella*-associated bacterial vaginosis is a week-long course of oral metronidazole (Flagyl) or gel. Secondary choices for treatment include clindamycin gel applied topically or oral tablets. Ampicillin and amoxicillin also may be used, but are only 50% effective. Some clinicians routinely treat sexual partners; others treat partners only if infection recurs after at least one successful course of treatment. The use of condoms helps to prevent future infections.

Chlamydial Infections
Urogenital Infections

Chlamydia trachomatis is a sexually transmitted urogenital pathogen responsible for many clinical manifestations in both men and women. Transmission from mother to fetus can result in substantial newborn morbidity.

Infection with *C. trachomatis* is a reportable disease in most states, is often not microbiologically confirmed, and often may be asymptomatic. Therefore, it is difficult to assess the incidence of infections in men or women. *Chlamydia* infections are estimated to be the most prevalent STD in the United States, with approximately 4 million individuals affected annually (Perlman & McNeeley, 1992; Potts, 1992).

Evidence of chlamydial infection is rare in the sexually inexperienced. It is most common among young (younger than age 25) heterosexuals who have had multiple partners, have a gonococcal infection, and are of lower socioeconomic status. Other factors include gender and ethnicity, being more common in females who are black. Pregnancy and oral contraceptives also increase the risk of contracting *Chlamydia*, probably as a result of the hormone-induced increase in cervical ectopy, which exposes more columnar epithelial cells to the microorganism. The incidence of *Chlamydia* infection in pregnancy is between 2% and 30%, and the estimated rate of transmission from infected mother to neonate ranges from 60% to 70% (Sargent, 1992). Like gonorrhea, *Chlamydia* infection is transmitted from mother to infant during passage through the infected birth canal.

Pathophysiology

C. trachomatis is an obligate, gram-negative, intracellular bacterium that lacks the ability to reproduce independently. Like viruses, *Chlamydia* can reproduce only within host cells. It is differentiated from other bacteria by its unique two-part growth cycle. The first part consists of an elementary body that is small, resilient, metabolically inert, and able to survive extracellularly. Once this elementary body attaches itself to a receptor host cell, it is able to enter by endocytosis. Once inside the cell, the second part begins and becomes a metabolically active parasite, reproducing within the cell until the cell is destroyed and ruptures, disseminating up to 1000 new elementary bodies. Rarely does this cause a secondary infection. Infection with *C. trachomatis* produces a mononuclear inflammatory reaction rather than a polymorphonuclear inflammatory reaction. The former reaction produces permanent scarring of tissues (Potts, 1992).

Chlamydia organisms are always pathogens; they are not part of the normal flora of the urogenital tract, despite the fact that infection is often asymptomatic. There are numerous different serotypes, or strains, of *C. trachomatis*. Some cause urogenital infection, some ocular trachoma, and others lymphogranuloma venereum, which is discussed in the next section.

The strains of *C. trachomatis* that cause urogenital infection apparently require squamous-columnar and columnar epithelial cells as hosts. *C. trachomatis* infects and disrupts epithelial tissues but does not seem to invade or destroy deeper tissues or organs. Urogenital chlamydial infections may have a fairly self-limited acute course, which is followed by a chronic, low-grade, persistent infection that lasts for years (Schachter, 1990).

In newborns, several sites may be inoculated with *Chlamydia* during passage through the infected maternal cervix. These include the eye, nasopharynx, rectum, and vagina. The infant also may aspirate infected secretions with its first breath.

Clinical Manifestations

Asymptomatic chlamydial infection is very common. Urogenital infections caused by *Chlamydia* closely parallel those caused by gonorrhea. Both microorganisms infect superficial genital tract tissues, such as mucosa of the urethra and cervix, and both can invade the epididymides, fallopian tubes, and hepatic capsule. Table 21-2 lists the pathophysiologic similarities of chlamydial and gonococcal infections.

Chlamydial infection accounts for 50% to 60% of cases of **nongonococcal urethritis** (**NGU**) in men. Clinically, urethritis caused by gonorrhea and chlamydia cannot be differentiated, because both have a 7- to 21-day incubation period, and individuals with either infection have dysuria and a whitish urethral discharge. Chlamydial urethritis is generally milder and more likely to be asymptomatic. Gram-stained smears of the urethral discharge show numerous polymorphonuclear leukocytes, which indicates ongoing inflammation.

Chlamydial epididymitis can accompany chlamydial urethritis and is characterized by fever and a unilaterally painful, swollen scrotum. Chlamydial infection also causes proctitis (rectal inflammation) in homosexual men and occasionally in heterosexual women and is linked to the practice of passive anal intercourse. Chlamydial proctitis is generally mild, although it may, like gonorrheal proctitis, cause rectal bleeding, mucous discharge, and diarrhea. Reiter syndrome (urethritis, conjunctivitis, arthritis, and characteristic mucocutaneous lesions) is also associated with untreated chlamydial infections of the urogenital tract.

In young, sexually active women, *C. trachomatis* is a cause of **acute urethral syndrome** (dysuria, urinary frequency, and presence of sterile pus in the urine). *C. trachomatis* also causes asymptomatic urethral infection in women. Chlamydial infection of Bartholin glands can cause purulent discharge and formation of a Bartholin cyst. Women with chlamydial cervicitis may be asymptomatic or may have a yellow mucopurulent discharge from the os and a hypertrophic, edematous, and friable area of cervical ectopy. The woman also may report intermenstrual or postcoital spotting. Although ectopy alone is not indicative of pathology, a raised, erythematous, raw, and friable ectopy is abnormal and strongly suggestive of chlamydial cervicitis. Chlamydial cervicitis is also often associated with cytologic atypia suggestive of cervical dysplasia (Stamm & Holmes, 1990) and is a leading cause of PID.

The most common clinical manifestations of chlamydial infections in the newborn are conjunctivitis and pneumonia. Chlamydial conjunctivitis begins between 5 and 14 days after delivery, when the infant's eyes begin to water. This discharge may become purulent, and both eyes become red and swollen. Scarring of the conjunctivae may result, but this infection does not cause blindness, as does the ophthalmia neonatorum caused by *N. gonorrhoeae*. *C. trachomatis* accounts for 20% to 60% of all cases of pneumonia in infants up to 6 months of age (Maurice, 1983). The pneumonia is mild or severe and may accompany the conjunctivitis. Infants with

TABLE 21-2

Similarity of Clinical Syndromes Caused by
C. trachomatis and *N. gonorrhoeae*

	Clinical syndrome	
Site of infection	*N. gonorrhoeae*	*C. trachomatis*
Men		
Urethra	Urethritis	Nongonococcal urethritis; post-gonococcal urethritis
Epididymis	Epididymitis	Epididymitis
Rectum	Proctitis	Proctitis
Conjunctiva	Conjunctivitis	Conjunctivitis
Systemic	Disseminated gonococcal	Reiter syndrome
Women		
Urethra	Acute urethral syndrome	Acute urethral syndrome
Bartholin's gland	Bartholinitis	Bartholinitis
Cervix	Cervicitis	Cervicitis; cervical atypia
Fallopian tube	Salpingitis	Salpingitis
Conjunctiva	Conjunctivitis	Conjunctivitis
Liver capsule	Perihepatitis	Perihepatitis
Systemic	Disseminated gonococcal infection	Arthritis-dermatitis syndrome

Modified from Stamm & Holmes, 1990.

FIG. 21-9 **Lymphogranuloma venereum.** Bilateral inguinal buboes that discharge purulent material. (From Habif, 1990.)

chlamydial pneumonia are seen at 3 to 11 weeks of age with staccato coughing spells, nasal congestion, dyspnea, and minimal fever. Other signs include otitis media, tachypnea, wheezing, bronchospasm, crepitant inspiratory rales, and apneic spells.

Evaluation and Treatment

Methods for diagnosing chlamydial infections include tissue culture techniques, direct chlamydia enzyme immunoassay, and fluorescein-labeled monoclonal antibody tests, such as Microtrak. The last two techniques are the least expensive and time consuming. Papanicolaou smears may suggest the presence of chlamydial cervicitis, but they cannot confirm the diagnosis. Cultures for *N. gonorrhoeae* also must be performed, because chlamydial infection and gonorrhea frequently coexist and have similar clinical manifestations.

Treatment for urogenital infections with *C. trachomatis* include a week of tetracycline or doxycycline for men and nonpregnant women and erythromycin for pregnant women and newborns (CDC, 1989). Treat-

ment for those who cannot tolerate this regimen includes erythromycin and sulfasoxazole. There is no known antimicrobial resistance (Potts, 1992). A tetracycline-resistant *C. trachomatis* has been reported (Mogabgab, 1991), however. Sexual partners should be identified, examined, and treated, and all individuals should avoid sex until the chlamydial infection is cured. Condoms should be used to prevent future infections.

Lymphogranuloma Venereum

C. trachomatis also can cause a chronic sexually transmitted disease known as **lymphogranuloma venereum** (**LGV**), which is often confused with other STDs, particularly syphilis, genital herpes, and chancroid (Fig. 21-9). Lymphogranuloma venereum is uncommon in the United States: during 1991, only 471 cases were reported to the CDC (1992). In contrast, LGV is endemic in many other areas, including Africa, India, Southeast Asia, South America, and the Caribbean. Like other STDs, it is more common in urban areas, among those with multiple sexual partners, and in men.

Pathophysiology

The strain of *C. trachomatis* that causes LGV probably penetrates skin and mucous membranes through tiny abrasions. Lymphogranuloma venereum begins as a skin lesion and spreads to lymphatic tissue, where it causes marked inflammation, necrosis, buboes, abscesses of inguinal lymph nodes, and infection of surrounding tissues. Healing occurs by fibrosis after several weeks or months and results in scarring, which damages the lymph nodes and disrupts nodal function. Affected nodes become chronically swollen, hardened, and enlarged. *C. trachomatis* also spreads systematically through the bloodstream and can enter the CNS (Perine & Osoba, 1990).

Clinical Manifestations

The primary lesion of LGV appears after an incubation period of 3 to 12 days or more. The lesion is most commonly a herpetiform (multivesicular) ulcer, but it can take various forms. The ulcer generally is asymptomatic and inconspicuous and heals rapidly, leaving no scar. In men the lesion is most commonly found on the penis or scrotum; in women it is found on the vaginal wall, cervix, or labia. Other signs of primary LGV include a large, tender lymphatic nodule or bubo, urethritis, and cervicitis.

The secondary stage of untreated LGV in men is characterized by inflammation and swelling of the lymph nodes. At first the inguinal bubo is a firm, somewhat painful mass. As the bubo gradually enlarges, it becomes very painful, thereby restricting mobility, and takes on a deep blue color (see Fig. 21-9). This color change signals impending rupture of the bubo through the skin. Thick yellow pus may drain from the site for weeks or months. Healing is very slow and results in scar formation. Systemic manifestations of secondary LGV can include meningitis, pneumonitis, and other major infections. In some cases the bubo does not rupture, but rather involutes and becomes firm. Bubo formation is most common in men. In women the inguinal lymph nodes are involved in fewer than one third of cases.

Anorectal LGV may be caused by direct inoculation during anal intercourse, or it may be a chronic or late manifestation of lymphatic spread from the inguinal area. Most individuals with anorectal LGV are women and homosexual men. Clinical symptoms include multiple ulcerations of the rectal mucosa, chronic inflammation, mucopurulent rectal discharge, and rectovaginal fistulas in women. Individuals may have fever, rectal pain, and tenesmus. Rectal strictures, perirectal abscesses, and anal fissures may develop and are the cause of most of the severe morbidity associated with LGV.

Evaluation and Treatment

Clinical manifestations and laboratory tests are used to diagnose LGV. Tests include the LGV complement-fixation tests, isolation of the microorganism in tissue culture, and monoclonal antibody tests. Lymphogranuloma venereum is treated with a 2-week course of tetracycline. Sex partners also should be treated (CDC, 1989).

Viral Infections
Genital Herpes

Genital herpes, which causes blisterlike lesions, is the most common infectious genital ulceration in the United

States. In fact, genital infection with the herpes simplex virus (HSV) is an epidemic in the United States. Genital herpes can be caused by either of the two serotypes of HSV, type 1 (HSV-1) or type 2 (HSV-2). Although infections caused by the serotypes are clinically indistinguishable, serologic studies show that more than 80% of initial and 98% of recurrent genital HSV infections are caused by HSV-2 (Ashley & Koelle, 1992).

Herpes simplex virus is not a reportable disease, and any reporting that is done is nonstandardized so that national statistics are not available; however, primary HSV infections are estimated to affect 700,000 individuals each year. Recurrent infections are even more common, with an estimated 20 million episodes occurring yearly (Sargent, 1992). The seroprevalence of HSV-2 is estimated to range from 16% to 20% of the total adult population to 35% to 60% for subgroups, for example, STD clinic clients and black women (Ashley & Koelle, 1992). The incidence of HSV infection tends to be highest in the teen to young adult age group (15 to 29) and in nonwhite lower socioeconomic status groups. Infection with HSV is not commonly associated with other types of STDs, for example, gonorrhea (Corey, 1990).

Herpes simplex virus infection is transmitted through intimate contact with a person who is shedding the virus in a secretion or from a peripheral lesion or mucosal surface. Transmission from an infected individual can take place even when the infected individual is asymptomatic. Transmission rates are not well identified; however, it is estimated that a woman has an 80% to 90% risk of developing genital herpes after being exposed to an infected male. The likelihood of nonsexual transmission of genital herpes, through aerosolized secretions of other fomites, is quite rare and unlikely (Peaceman & Gonik, 1991; Sargent, 1992).

Neonatal infections can occur in utero, intrapartum, and postpartum. Of the three, the latter two are the most common. The incidence of neonatal infections has been estimated to be 1 in 2500 to 1 in 20,000 births (Ball & Murph, 1992). Genital herpes causes extensive perinatal morbidity and mortality.

Intrauterine transmission may occur through transplacental or ascending infection. The risk factors for this type of transmission are well identified (Stagno & Whitley, 1990). Intrauterine HSV may cause spontaneous abortion or premature delivery (Corey, 1990).

Intrapartum infection is the most common mode of transmission. Infants are at greatest risk if the mother has a primary infection rather than a recurrent infection. Infants delivered vaginally to mothers with primary HSV have a 20% to 50% risk of contracting HSV, whereas infants delivered vaginally to mothers with recurrent infections only have a 0% to 8% risk of contracting HSV infection. Ruptured membranes have a role in the development of HSV. Membranes that have been ruptured for greater than 6 hours increase the risk for the contracting of HSV. Fetal monitoring devices also increase the risk of the infant contracting HSV (Stagno & Whitley, 1990).

Pathophysiology

After initial exposure and entry of the virus at mucocutaneous sites or abraded skin, the virus undergoes replication locally in the dermis and epidermis. This leads to cell destruction, transudation, and vesicle formation. There is spread of the virus to contiguous cells and eventually into sensory nerves. Eventually, the virus is transported intraaxonally to the dorsal root, where it remains in a latent stage until it becomes reactivated. During the latent period, the genome for the virus is maintained in the host cell nucleus without causing the death of the cell (Smith & Singer, 1992). After oral infection, the latent virus resides in the trigeminal ganglion; after genital infection it resides in the dorsal sacral nerve roots.

Latent infections can become reactivated and cause a recurrent infection with similar manifestations. Reactivation of the HSV-2 is twice as common as HSV-1 infections, and the likelihood of HSV-2 recurrent infections is 8 to 10 times (Smith & Singer, 1992). Reacti-

vation of the HSV is not well understood but may be attributable to physical, hormonal, and immunologic stimuli (Peaceman & Gonik, 1991). Other triggering events may be menstruation, stress, and sun exposure (Sargent, 1992). During reactivation, the viral genomes are transported through the peripheral sensory nerves back to the dermal surface.

Clinical Manifestations

There are three distinct syndromes associated with HSV infection: (1) first-episode primary genital infection, (2) first-episode nonprimary HSV, and (3) recurrent infections. The manifestations of each one depend on the individual's previous immune state. First-episode primary genital infection occurs when an individual has no antibodies to HSV-1 or HSV-2. The individual has small—1 to 2 mm—multiple, vesicular lesions, which are generally located on the labia minora, fourchette, or penis (Fig. 21-10). They also may appear on the cervix, buttocks, and thighs and are often painful and pruritic. These lesions usually last about 10 to 20 days. The lesions of HSV-1 and HSV-2 are indistinguishable to the naked eye. These wet lesions actively shed virus for about 10 to 14 days, after which they heal by reepithelialization. Small lesions may coalesce into larger ulcers and become secondarily infected.

FIG. 21-10 Recurrent herpes genitalis. Ulcers are noted following rupture of vesicles. (From Kaufman & Faro, 1985.)

FIG. 21-11 Clinical course of primary genital herpes. (From Corey, 1990.)

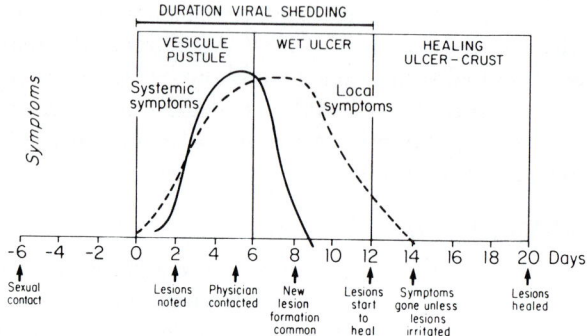

Systemic manifestations often accompany HSV infection, and an individual may suffer from fever, malaise, myalgias, and lymphadenopathy. An individual also may complain of urinary retention. Pharyngitis, aseptic meningitis, and hepatitis also may accompany primary HSV infection. Fig. 21-11 illustrates the clinical course of primary genital HSV.

First-episode nonprimary HSV occurs in individuals who have preexisting antibodies. In some individuals, the primary infection may not have any clinical manifestations. The HSV becomes latent within the nerve root and becomes reactivated at a later date. This first episode with clinical manifestations is often a milder case with fewer lesions that are less painful and heal faster. There are also fewer systemic manifestations, and viral shedding is of shorter duration.

Recurrent infections produce mild local symptoms. The number of lesions is greatly reduced and are less painful. Lesions are often unilateral, with crusting occurring within 4 to 5 days. Complete recovery and healing are usually complete within 10 days.

Recurrent infections may occur on an average of 5 to 8 times per year; individuals infected with HSV-2 are more likely to experience recurrent infections. Individuals may experience prodromal symptoms, for example, pruritus, tingling, or dysesthesias, from a few hours up to 2 days before the eruption of lesions. Women may experience a vaginal discharge and dysuria.

Symptomatic HSV infection of the newborn may occur any time in the first month of life. Manifestations range from a local infection of the eyes, skin, or mucous membranes to a severe, disseminated infection with CNS involvement. About 70% of affected infants present with skin lesions. Central nervous system involvement includes seizures and is associated with a mortality rate of more than 50% and extensive neurologic sequelae in survivors.

Evaluation and Treatment

Genital HSV infection is suggested if typical genital lesions are present. A presumptive diagnosis of HSV-associated infection is supported by the identification in a Papanicolaou smear of multinucleated giant cells with intranuclear inclusions. Definitive diagnosis is made after viral tissue culture. Herpes simplex virus 1 and HSV-2 are distinguished by fluorescent antibody, neutralization, or other serologic techniques.

There is currently no curative treatment for HSV in-

fection. Acyclovir may be used orally and topically for primary HSV and orally to prevent recurrences. Intravenous acyclovir is reserved for severely immunocompromised individuals (Rose & Camp, 1988). Acyclovir-resistant strains of HSV have been identified periodically; no specific definitive resistant strains are known to exist. Although condoms offer some protection, individuals with HSV should refrain from all sexual contact in areas of lesions and understand that an undetermined risk of transmission exists even during asymptomatic periods.

Condylomata Acuminata

Condylomata acuminata, or genital warts, is caused by the human papillomavirus (HPV), of which there are about 60 types. Of these, only about 20 infect mucosal surfaces. The genital tract is the reservoir for 18 HPV types, and the oral cavity is the reservoir for two types (Shah, 1992).

Although condylomata acuminata is not a reportable disease, more than 2 million cases are diagnosed yearly, and the incidence of HPV infection is considered to be of epidemic proportions. Often HPV infection is subclinical so that the actual number of cases is greater than estimated.

Human papillomavirus infection is closely linked to multiple sexual partners and early onset of sexual activity and is most common among males and females aged 16 to 25. Previous thought regarding HPV infection was that it was a relatively harmless condition rather than a serious threat to health. The seriousness of the infection may be related to the type of HPV causing the infection. Serotypes 6 and 11 are identified with most of the cases of benign condylomata acuminata (Peterson & Rao, 1989). There is a growing body of knowledge that links HPV infection with cervical and vulvar cancer in females and anorectal and squamous cell carcinoma of the penis in males (Handsfield, 1992). The increased incidence of genital dysplasias that may lead to cancers has been associated with serotypes 16 and 18, and occasionally 31, 33, 35, and 39 (Peterson & Rao, 1989).

Genital warts are quite contagious, with transmission rates between individuals estimated to be between 38% and 95%. Such a wide range is attributable to the subclinical nature of some infections and various influencing factors that include number of exposures, HPV type, location of lesions, and cellular immunity response (Peaceman & Gonik, 1991). Infants and children also have been identified as being infected with HPV. Infants can be infected in utero and by passage through an infected birth canal. Human papillomavirus infection in children has been traced to child sexual abuse; however, reports vary in making this connection (Derksen, 1992).

Pathophysiology

Human papillomavirus is a nonenveloped, circular, double-stranded DNA virus and belongs to the Papovaviridae family (Peterson & Rao, 1989). Information about HPV was not readily available until the late 1970s when it became possible to clone the viral genomes directly from infected tissues by recombinant DNA technology (Shah, 1992).

Transmission of the virus is believed to occur through sexual contact; however, the exact transmissibility of the virus is unknown. Human papillomavirus is transmissible by fomites and may account for nonsexually transmitted genital warts (Goldsmith, 1990). The initial infection follows trauma to the epithelium that allows the virus to reach and infect the basal cells of the epithelium, which appear to be supportive of viral propagation. Such minor trauma may occur during sexual intercourse. Epithelial cells that are infected with HPV undergo transformation, proliferate, and form a warty growth. Human papillomavirus appears in about 2 to 3 months.

Clinical Manifestations

Condylomata acuminata warts are soft, skin-colored, whitish pink to reddish brown, discrete growths. They may occur singly or in clusters and may be broad-based or pedunculated, feathery, or smooth (Fig. 21-12). Sometimes the warts enlarge to form cauliflowerlike masses on the male frenulum, glans, foreskin, urinary meatus, shaft, scrotum, or anus and on the female labia, clitoris, perineum, vagina, or anus (Fig. 21-13). Although the lesions are usually not painful, they may cause dyspareunia (painful intercourse) and may be friable and bleed easily. Some individuals complain of pruritus. Cervical lesions are generally flattened and may not be seen easily without colposcopy (Camisa, 1985).

Laryngeal papillomas can occur in infants whose mothers had genital warts at the time of delivery. Clinical manifestations of laryngeal warts include stridor, hoarseness, abnormal cry, cough, and respiratory distress (Camisa, 1985).

FIG. 21-12 **Small warts of condylomata acuminata.** Multiple, small warts under the foreskin, the type of moist area where autoinoculations tend to occur. (From Habif, 1990.)

FIG. 21-13 **Large warts of condylomata acuminata.** Massive, cauliflowerlike inoculation of warts on the vulva. (From Habif, T. P. [1985]. *Clinical dermatology: a color guide to diagnosis and therapy.* St. Louis: Mosby–Year Book.)

Evaluation and Treatment

Generally, diagnosis of condylomata acuminata is made on the basis of clinical manifestations. Koilocytosis (typical cellular changes of HPV infection) seen on the Papanicolaou smear aid in the diagnosis of cervical HPV infection. Pointy, fleshy pink lesions caused by HPV must be differentiated from condylomata lata (the whitish-gray, flat lesions) of secondary syphilis. Because HPV infection often accompanies other STDs, gonorrhea culture, chlamydia culture, serology test for syphilis, and wet mount for other vaginal microorganisms also should be performed. Human papillomavirus infection also is associated with the development of squamous cell carcinoma; therefore, all atypical or persistent lesions should have biopsy examination (CDC, 1989). Some clinicians recommend that Papanicolaou smears be repeated every 6 months for women with a history of HPV infection.

Treatments for genital warts include application of topical agents, such as podophyllin, trichloroacetic acid, and 5-fluorouracil cream, cryosurgery, CO_2 laser surgery, electrosurgery, and surgical excision. Podophyllin is quite toxic and must be used with extreme care; it should never be used in pregnancy. Surgery and CO_2 laser surgery require local or regional anesthesia, but these therapies are precise and sterile and cause minimal bleeding (Bourcier & Seidler, 1987; CDC, 1989). Interferons that have general antiviral, antiproliferative, and immunomodulating effects have been successfully used in treating stubborn genital warts. Approximately one third of individuals experience a cure and another one third experience a decrease in wart size (Shah, 1992). Surgical excision is the treatment for laryngeal warts in infants.

Molluscum Contagiosum

Molluscum contagiosum is a benign viral infection of the skin in children and adults. It adults it tends to occur on the genitals and to be transmitted by sexual contact.

Molluscum contagiosum occurs throughout the world and is a very common childhood disease in Papua New Guinea and Fiji. It is much less common in the United States, where incidence is highest among young adults. The childhood disease is transmitted by skin-to-skin contact and fomites (swimming pools, towels, gym equipment) and affects the face, trunk, and limbs. Adult disease is more commonly sexually transmitted and affects the lower abdomen, genitals, and perianal area (Smith & Singer, 1992). Molluscum contagiosum is most common in males 20 to 29 years of age and in those with multiple sexual partners (Smith & Singer, 1992).

The molluscum contagiosum virus is taken into epi-

FIG. 21-14 Papules typical of molluscum contagiosum. (From Habif, T. P. [1985]. *Clinical dermatology: a color guide to diagnosis and therapy.* St. Louis: Mosby–Year Book.)

thelial cells by phagocytosis and replicates within the cytoplasm, where it produces cytoplasmic inclusions (**molluscous bodies**) and cellular hyperplasia. The underlying skin usually is not affected (Lambert & Yoder, 1985).

After an incubation period of 2 to 7 weeks, white or flesh-colored, round or oval, dome-shaped papules appear. The lesions are relatively small (3 to 5 mm) but occasionally may coalesce to form larger lesions up to 15 mm. The surface has a characteristic central umbilication, from which a thick, creamy core material can be expressed (Fig. 21-14). Generally the lesions are not painful or pruritic unless secondarily infected. The papules may last several months or several years and spread by autoinoculation.

The appearance of the lesions is generally all that is needed to make the diagnosis, although direct microscopic examination of stained material from the core of the papule discloses molluscous bodies within the swollen and rounded epithelial cells. The lesions often heal spontaneously after several months. Other effective means of removing the lesions include curettage and application of liquid nitrogen (cryotherapy) or silver nitrate.

Epstein-Barr Virus

Recent investigations have indicated that the **Epstein-Barr virus** (EBV), which is transmitted orally, is also capable of being harbored within the male and female genital tract and transmitted sexually. Further research is needed to specifically identify the role that EBV plays in STDs; however, the significance of EBV infection of the genital tract relates to its ability to transform cells and potentially contribute to the development of cancers in the genital tract (Naher, Grissman, Freese, Petzoldt, & Helfrich, 1992).

Parasitic Infections
Trichomoniasis

Originally discovered in 1836, *Trichomonas vaginalis* was at first thought to be a harmless commensal microorganism. *T. vaginalis* is now known to be one of the most common causes of sexually transmitted lower genital tract infection.

Because **trichomoniasis** (infection by *T. vaginalis*) is not a reportable disease, its prevalence can only be estimated. Between 2.5 and 3 million American women are infected with trichomoniasis every year, and *T. vaginalis* accounts for one of four cases of infectious vaginitis (Herbst, Mischell, Stenchever, & Droegemueller, 1992). Trichomoniasis is usually found in both sexual partners and often coexists with gonorrhea. Although sexual transmission is clearly the most common means of disease spread, transmission through fomites is theoretically possible. To cause infection, the fomite would have to introduce an inoculum of about 10,000 microorganisms directly into the vagina (Rein & Holmes, 1983).

Pathophysiology

T. vaginalis is an anaerobic, unicellular, flagellated, parasitic protozoan that adheres to and damages squamous epithelial cells. Because this protozoan selectively affects squamous epithelium, vaginal and urethral tissue is often infected, as are Skene and Bartholin glands. The endocervical canal is not affected because it is lined with columnar epithelium. In men the urethra is the most common site of infection, although the protozoa, called **trichomonads,** also can infect the epididymis and (rarely) the prostate. Zinc, which has potent antibacterial properties, is found in high concentrations in the prostate. Hence many trichomonads are cleared from the male urethra during ejaculation. This action makes urethral trichomoniasis a fairly self-limiting infection in men. Most infections of the male urethra clear up within 2 weeks.

Trichomoniasis is most common in women of reproductive age, and it is primarily an infection of the vagina. *T. vaginalis* can induce a marked inflammatory response in the vagina, causing a copious discharge that contains large numbers of polymorphonuclear neutrophils. Trichomonads adhere to, but do not invade, the squamous epithelial cells.

Clinical Manifestations

Manifestations of vaginal trichomoniasis range from none to severe, with some women reporting an increase in distressing symptoms immediately after menses. Vaginal discharge and internal pruritus are the most common complaints. Dyspareunia and dysuria are also fairly common. Secretions are usually copious, some-

times frothy or bubbly, and gray-green. The vaginal walls may appear erythematous and sore. Rarely small, punctate red marks, the so-called strawberry spots, are visible. Vaginal pH is usually greater than 5.0.

Most men with trichomoniasis remain asymptomatic. Possible clinical manifestations include scant intermittent discharge, slight pruritus, and mild dysuria.

Evaluation and Treatment

History and symptoms are inadequate for diagnosis of trichomoniasis. Microscopic confirmation of the presence of the trichomonads in vaginal secretions or urine provides a definitive diagnosis. In a fresh wet mount preparation that has been warmed slightly, the epithelial cells have relatively clean and sharp edges, the ratio of polymorphonuclear leukocytes to epithelial cells exceeds 1:1, and the trichomonads are visible. The ovoid microorganism is slightly larger than a polymorphonuclear leukocyte and has one rounded, flagellated end and one slightly pointed, flagellated end. The flagella give the trichomonads their characteristic twisting motility. In an acidic environment, such as urine, the trichomonads assume a "balled-up" or spherical shape and become less motile.

The treatment of choice for trichomoniasis is a single dose of metronidazole (Flagyl). The single-dose therapy is effective, has few side effects, and obviates the need for individual compliance with longer regimens. Sexual partners, even if asymptomatic, are also treated and examined for coexisting STDs. Metronidazole is contraindicated in pregnancy, during which topical clotrimazole is the treatment of choice (Moldwin, 1992).

Scabies

Scabies is a rather benign, common parasitic infection that can be spread by skin-to-skin and sexual contact. Discovered by Bonomo in 1687, it is considered to be the first human disease with a known cause (Orkin & Maibach, 1990).

Scabies has a worldwide distribution and accounts for approximately 2% to 3% of visits to dermatologists in the United States (Shaw & Juranek, 1976). Traditionally the disease was attributed to conditions of poverty, overcrowding, uncleanliness, and sexual promiscuity. Today it is recognized that scabies occurs in individuals with good personal hygiene and is not limited to any social class. Outbreaks of scabies occur every 30 years or so and last about 15 years. The most recent outbreak in the United States began in 1971 and subsided in the 1980s (Fitzpatrick, Polano, & Suurmond, 1983).

Transmission of scabies requires close skin-to-skin contact, which typically occurs within families or between sexual partners. Transmission through fomites is possible but not likely (Lambert & Yoder, 1985).

FIG. 21-15 Scabies distribution. Typical distribution of lesions. (From Habif, 1990.)

FIG. 21-16 Scabies burrow. An S-shaped burrow with a tiny vesicle at one end. (From Habif, T. P. [1985]. *Clinical dermatology: A color guide to diagnosis and therapy*. St. Louis: Mosby–Year Book.)

Pathophysiology

The adult female itch mite, *Sarcoptes scabiei*, is 0.3 to 0.4 mm long and has a lifespan of about 30 days. Once deposited on human skin, it burrows through the horny layer of the stratum granulosum. Within hours of burrowing the female begins laying two to three large eggs per day, each of which progresses through larval and nymphal stages to become an adult itch mite in about 10 days. The most common places for scabies to burrow are on the hands (between the fingers) and on the flexor surfaces of the wrists and the extensor surfaces of the elbows. Genital burrowing occurs on the penis and buttocks and in the crease of skin where the buttock meets the thigh (Orkin & Maibach, 1990). Fig. 21-15 shows the typical sites of scabies burrows.

Clinical Manifestations

The classic symptom of scabies is intense pruritus, which may be pronounced at night. The typical burrow of the *S. scabiei* is a short, wavy line (Fig. 21-16). There may be small, erythematous, excoriated larval papules near the burrows. Secondary infections are common and are caused by scratching. In some individuals, a hypersensitivity reaction occurs 1 or more months after the infestation and causes multiple reddish-brown, pruritic

nodules to develop on the covered portions of the body, most commonly the upper thighs, buttocks, male genitalia, and axillary regions. These nodules may persist for more than a year, despite treatment with a scabicide.

Evaluation and Treatment

Although the diagnosis is often made on clinical grounds, microscopic identification of the mite or its eggs, larvae, or feces is recommended because the symptoms of scabies can imitate those of many other dermatologic conditions. Superficial scrapings from a recently developed, unexcoriated papule or burrow can easily be observed under the microscope; the addition of potassium hydroxide allows easier visualization of the mite.

Treatment consists of topical application of lindane 1% cream or lotion (Kwell, Gammexane, Scabene). Close household and sexual contacts should also be treated. For very young children and pregnant or lactating women, crotamiton 10% cream (Eurax) or sulfur 6% in petrolatum is substituted. To prevent reinfestation, clothing and bed linen should be machine washed and dried at high temperatures (CDC, 1989; Orkin & Maibach, 1990).

Pediculosis Pubis

Phthirus pubis, the crab louse, is one of three species of lice that infest humans. *P. pubis* is commonly transmitted sexually and causes **pediculosis pubis**, or "crabs."

The prevalence of pubic lice infestation is difficult to estimate. Pediculosis pubis is common among individuals being treated for other STDs. Statistics show that incidence is somewhat higher in women than in men (Hatcher et al., 1988) and that the disease is most common in single persons aged 15 to 25 (Billstein, 1990). *P. pubis* is transmitted primarily by intimate sexual contact, although fomites (toilet seats and beds) do play a role in some cases.

FIG. 21-17 Pubic louse and crab lice. A, Pubic louse. B, Crab lice and nits of pediculosis pubis (*arrows*). (**A,** from Billstein, 1990; **B,** from Herbst, Mischell, Stenchever, & Droegemueller, 1992.)

Pathophysiology

The crab louse has a five-stage life cycle: an egg (or nit) stage, three nymphal stages, and an adult stage, all of which occur in the host. The nits of crab lice are found "glued" to hairs; they are oval, 0.8 by 0.3 mm, and whitish and hatch in 5 to 10 days (Fig. 21-17). In the adult stage, pubic lice are grayish, are approximately 1 mm in length, and have a segmented body and claws particularly designed for clinging to pubic hairs. Dependent on blood for nutrition, the lice bite into the skin to obtain food.

Clinical Manifestations

Symptoms range from mild pruritus to severe, intolerable itching, depending on the individual's sensitivity to louse bites. Allergic sensitization occurs in about 5 days, when itching, erythema, and inflammation may worsen. Excessive scratching may lead to secondary infection.

Evaluation and Treatment

The individual's history usually discloses a recent exposure and the typical symptoms of infestation. Because both the lice and nits are visible to the naked eye, a thorough clinical examination permits definitive diagnosis. Pediculosis pubis is treated with lindane 1% lotion, cream, or shampoo (by prescription) or by pyrethrin and piperonyl butoxide (Rid, Triple X, or A-200 Pyrinate, available without a prescription). Sexual contacts and any other intimate household contacts should also be examined and treated, and clothing and bed linen should be machine washed and dried at high temperatures (Billstein, 1990).

SEXUALLY TRANSMITTED INFECTIONS OF OTHER BODY SYSTEMS

Gastrointestinal Infections
Shigellosis and *Campylobacter* Enteritis

A variety of enteric bacterial pathogens are now recognized as sexually transmitted, particularly among homosexual men. The bacteria most frequently implicated in the so-called gay bowel syndrome are species of *Shigella* and *Campylobacter*. *Shigella* infection, termed **shigellosis,** is transmitted by contact with infected feces. Very few microorganisms are needed to cause infection. Anal-oral spread occurs very easily through household contact and anal-oral sexual practices. *Campylobacter jejuni,* which causes ***campylobacter*** enteritis, is primarily an animal pathogen but also may be transmitted among humans through anal-oral sexual practices. Again very few microorganisms are necessary for inoculation and infection.

Pathophysiology

Shigella are nonmotile, gram-negative rods that are related to *Escherichia coli.* They invade and kill intestinal epithelial cells, thereby inducing a marked inflammatory response and diarrhea. *Campylobacter* are highly motile, curved, gram-negative rods that also invade and kill intestinal cells and cause bloody, inflammatory exudate and diarrhea.

Clinical Manifestations

Either microorganism may cause a mild, self-limited gastroenteritis or severe dysentery. After a 24- to 48-hour incubation period, shigellosis begins with fever, abdominal distress, and diarrhea. It may resolve completely or progress to dysentery with severe cramping, abdominal pain, tenesmus, and bloody mucoid discharge from the rectum. Campylobacter enteritis typically begins, after a 1- to 7-day incubation period, with sudden fever and abdominal pain followed by diarrhea.

Malaise, anorexia, headache, arthralgia, and myalgia are common (Caldwell, 1985).

Evaluation and Treatment

Clinical manifestations and cultures of fresh stool samples are used to diagnose shigellosis. Culturing *Campylobacter* is expensive; therefore, microscopic analysis of a Gram-stained smear of rectal exudate may be used as a diagnostic aid.

Treatment for mild illness includes correction of fluid and electrolyte imbalance. Antidiarrheals are avoided because they may delay clearance of the microorganism. Because *Shigella* and *Campylobacter* are both highly contagious, antibiotic treatment may be advisable even for mild cases. The usual treatment for shigellosis is 1 week of trimethoprim and sulfamethoxazole. Erythromycin is used to treat campylobacter enteritis (Caldwell, 1985; CDC, 1989). Sexual partners are examined and treated, and individuals are instructed to avoid oral-anal contact until the infection is cured.

Giardiasis and Amebiasis

Two enteric protozoa that are sexually transmitted, primarily among homosexual men, are *Giardia lamblia,* the cause of **giardiasis,** and *Entamoeba histolytica,* the cause of **amebiasis.** The incidence of these infections in the male homosexual population has decreased over the past years, presumably because of safer sex practices (Quinn & Stamm, 1990). Although the principal route of transmission is contaminated drinking water, giardiasis and amebiasis are also transmitted by anal-oral or genital-anal contact.

Pathophysiology

G. lamblia and *E. histolytica* are both parasites having two forms, cysts and **trophozoites** (uncysted protozoa). The cysts are the infective form because they can survive in moist environments outside the host. Giardiasis commonly begins with ingestion of a small number of *G. lamblia* cysts. Once in the upper small bowel, each cyst becomes a trophozoite, which multiplies and attaches to the bowel mucosa. Enzyme deficiencies, inflammation, and immunologic damage then apparently occur, resulting in intestinal malabsorption. Amebiasis begins similarly: the ingested cysts pass to the small or large bowel, where each returns to the trophozoite state, multiplies quickly, and begins to invade the mucosa through cytotoxic activity. Mucosal invasion results in the development of ulcers and an inflammatory response (Guerrant, Werkel & Raydin, 1990). Individuals infected with *E. histolytica* may excrete up to 45 million cysts per day.

Clinical Manifestations

Giardiasis begins with sudden, explosive diarrhea, distention, and flatulence. Upper gastrointestinal symp-

toms are also prominent and may include epigastric pain; vomiting; foul, sulfuric burping; and nausea. After the acute illness, which usually lasts several days, milder symptoms may persist for months, with evidence of malabsorption and weight loss. Amebiasis is often asymptomatic. Symptoms that do occur range from mild diarrhea to severe dysentery. Amebiasis may spread from the intestine to other organs, such as the liver.

Evaluation and Treatment

Diagnosis of both entities is usually made by history and microscopic examination of fresh stool specimens for either trophozoites or cysts. Small bowel biopsy may aid in the diagnosis of giardiasis; rectal biopsy may aid in the diagnosis of amebiasis. Serologic testing is useful in the differential diagnosis of symptomatic individuals with amebiasis. Metronidazole (Flagyl) is the usual treatment for both conditions (Quinn & Stamm, 1990).

Hepatitis B

Hepatitis is a liver infection that can be caused by three types of viruses: hepatitis A, hepatitis B, and hepatitis non-A, non-B. All cause a syndrome of acute, icteric (jaundice-producing) liver inflammation. Of the three types, the **hepatitis B virus** (**HBV**) is known to be sexually transmitted. (Hepatitis A, like most other predominantly enteric infections, may be considered an STD because of oral-anal transmission.) Additional information about hepatitis is found in Chapter 36.

The prevalence of HBV infection varies dramatically worldwide. In Southeast Asia and Africa, 60% to 80% of the population may harbor serologic evidence of past or current infection. In the United States, approximately 5% to 20% of the general population have evidence of HBV infection. Seropositivity generally increases with age. At risk for HBV infection are those with low socioeconomic status, blacks, Indochinese refugees, health care workers, and male homosexuals. In groups of male homosexuals, the seropositivity rates may be as high as 80%. Other groups at risk are intravenous drug users, institutionalized mentally retarded persons, hemodialysis patients, and heterosexual partners of HBV carriers (Lemon & Newbold, 1990).

Transmission of HBV can occur through needle puncture, blood transfusion, cuts or abrasions in the skin, and absorption by mucosal surfaces. Direct contact with infected body fluids, such as tears, cerebrospinal fluid, synovial fluid, gastric juices, pleural fluid, semen, and urine, may pass the infection. Fomites also can transmit hepatitis: HBV can survive on inanimate objects for up to 1 week (Klein, 1988).

Perinatal transmission of HBV is relatively common. Neonates whose mothers are infectious have a 70% to 90% chance of becoming infected with HBV during labor or delivery and a 90% chance of becoming chronic carriers. Hepatitis B virus can be found in maternal vaginal secretions, blood, amniotic fluid, saliva, and breast milk (Klein, 1988).

Hepatitis delta agent is a defective virus that is similar to HBV antigen but is unable to cause hepatitis B by itself, requiring the presence of HBV to cause hepatitis. Hepatitis delta infection is rare in the United States, but cases have been documented in intravenous drug users and their sexual contacts, and also in recipients of contaminated blood. It is commonly found in homosexuals, persons requiring kidney dialysis, or health care workers (Smith & Singer, 1992).

Pathophysiology

After exposure, HBV passes through the bloodstream to the liver, where it infects liver cells and multiplies. The infection is usually self-limiting, with most patients mounting an effective immune response. Approximately 6% to 10% of infected individuals are unable to eradicate the virus and become chronic carriers of HBV.

Clinical Manifestations

Most HBV infections are clinically inapparent and result in solid and permanent immunity. Symptoms of hepatitis usually develop only after a certain HBV antigen has been circulating in the blood for 3 to 6 weeks. Approximately 15% to 20% of individuals develop a prodromal syndrome that is similar to serum sickness. This syndrome is characterized by an erythematous rash, urticaria, polyarthralgias, and arthritis. Symptoms of infection also may include lassitude, anorexia, nausea, vomiting, headache, fever, dark urine, jaundice, and moderate liver enlargement with tenderness. Long-term sequelae include chronic persistent and chronic active hepatitis, cirrhosis, hepatocellular carcinoma, hepatic failure, and death. In neonates who contract HBV, the disease may be manifested in many ways, from mild illness to a severe, fulminant infection with a mortality rate of 75%.

Evaluation and Treatment

Hepatitis B virus infection is clinically indistinguishable from other types of hepatitis. Diagnosis can be made only through serologic testing.

No specific therapy exists for HBV infection in adults. Treatment consists of supportive care and relief of symptoms. Vaccination is urged for members of high-risk groups.

The infant who is born to a mother with infectious HBV is given HBV immune globulin and Hepatavax-B vaccine within 12 hours of birth. The HBV vaccine is administered again at 1 and 6 months, provided that serologic tests show that a chronic carrier state has not developed (CDC, 1991a).

Systemic Diseases
Acquired Immune Deficiency Syndrome

Epidemiology, modes of transmission, pathophysiology, clinical manifestations, and evaluation and treatment of AIDS are discussed in detail in Chapter 8.

Cytomegalovirus Infection

Cytomegalovirus (CMV) is a sexually transmissible herpes virus. It is associated with a number of clinical syndromes in newborns, otherwise healthy adults, and immunosuppressed individuals.

Cytomegalovirus infection causes no specific genital disease, but its incidence is high in individuals being treated for other STDs. Cytomegalovirus infection is prevalent worldwide, especially in developing countries and lower socioeconomic groups. The virus is found in semen, cervical secretions, urine, blood, saliva, breast milk, and stool, and transmission is associated with close (although not always genital) interpersonal contact or direct transfer of cells or body fluids (Smith & Singer, 1992). It is more common in homosexual men and in young women with multiple sexual partners. Perinatal transmission of CMV may occur across the placenta, by contamination with infected secretions during passage through the birth canal, or during breast-feeding. Approximately 1% (0.4%-2.2%) of infants born in the United States are infected with CMV (Smiley & Huang, 1990).

Pathophysiology

After CMV infects a human cell, it may replicate and destroy the infected cell or become incorporated into the host cell's DNA. Local CMV infections can persist despite the presence of large quantities of systemic antibody to CMV. Cell-mediated immunity seems to have a particular role in protecting against CMV infections. Depression of CMV-specific cell-mediated immunity has been noted in otherwise normal hosts with CMV infection. This may be caused by injury of T cells or macrophages by the cytomegalovirus (Wilson, 1990).

Clinical Manifestations

In healthy individuals, CMV infection can cause a number of mild subclinical or nonspecific illnesses, including mononucleosis, pneumonitis, hemolytic anemia, and thrombocytopenia purpura. In contrast, a CMV infection in an immunocompromised individual, such as a transplant recipient or an individual with AIDS, can cause a devastating, life-threatening illness.

Congenital CMV infection is the most common serious viral infection among infants. Approximately 1% of all infants (40,000) are born with congenital CMV. Of these, 10% (4000) demonstrate typical manifestations of the infection, for example, hepatosplenomegaly, intracranial calcifications, microcephaly, small for gestational age, and hearing impairments. An additional

10% to 15% of these are asymptomatic at birth; however, they begin to develop manifestations of the infection within the first few months of life. Recent evidence suggests that symptomatic infection of infants is caused by a primary infection of the mother during her pregnancy and not necessarily by reinfection or reactivation of a prior infection (Dobbins, Stewart, & Demmler, 1992).

Evaluation and Treatment

The most definitive diagnostic test for CMV is isolation of the virus, usually through growth in human fibroblast cell culture. Several methods for measuring antibodies to CMV are available, including complement fixation (CF) tests and indirect immunofluorescent antibody (IFA) tests. These methods are frequently used in clinical situations.

With the increased incidence of CMV infection among immunocompromised individuals (AIDS and persons with transplants), various treatment modalities have been investigated. Ganciclovir is similar to acyclovir and inhibits viral DNA polymerase (see Chapter 4). Relapses of CMV infection are frequent after therapy ceases; thus, lifelong therapy is particularly indicated in individuals with AIDS (Smith & Singer, 1992). Acyclovir has been used, but optimum therapeutic benefits have not been established. Future therapies still under investigation include ganciclovir plus cytomegalovirus immunoglobulin and vaccine (Smith & Singer, 1992).

Experimental antiviral drugs may prove helpful in the treatment of severe CMV infection, and preliminary studies to develop a vaccine appear promising. No treatment is indicated, however, in most cases of CMV infection.

SUMMARY REVIEW

Sexually Transmitted Urogenital Infections

1 Gonorrhea is a communicable disease that can be local or systemic and is usually transmitted sexually. Complications, such as pelvic inflammatory disease in women and disseminated infections, spread through the bloodstream to the skin, joints, and heart.

2 Gonorrhea passed to the fetus from the mother is usually manifest as an eye infection and develops 1 to 12 days after birth.

3 Penicillin is the drug of choice for treatment of gonorrheal infections.

4 Syphilis is a sexually transmitted disease that becomes systemic shortly after infection. The four stages of the disease are: (1) primary syphilis with a chancre at the site of infection, (2) secondary syphilis with systemic spread to all body systems, (3) **latent syphilis** with minimal symptoms or the development of skin lesions, and (4) tertiary syphilis, the most severe stage, with destruction of bone, skin, and soft tissues.

5 Congenital syphilis contributes to prematurity of the newborn with bone marrow depression, CNS involvement, renal failure, and eye disorders. Late clinical manifestations are those of tertiary syphilis and are rare.

6 Serologic testing is used to diagnose syphilis, and penicillin is the drug of choice.

7 Chancroid is a soft genital chancre most common among uncircumcised men. The lesion appears 1 to 14 days after exposure and is painful and inflamed. The infected person and sexual partner are treated with erythromycin.

8 Granuloma inguinale (donovanosis) is rare in the United States. The bacteria are gram-negative and survive within macrophages. Localized nodules coalesce to form granulomas and ulcers on the penis in men and labia in women. Antibiotics provide effective treatment.

9 Bacterial vaginosis (Gardnerella vaginalis) is caused by anaerobic bacteria that produce aromatic amines that raise the pH of the vagina, promoting further bacterial growth with an inflammatory response and a fishy-smelling odor. "Clue cells" are found on the wet mount. Flagyl provides effective treatment.

10 Infections of Chlamydia trachomatis are probably the most common STD in the United States. Cervicitis associated with pregnancy and use of oral contraceptives is common in women, and urethritis is common in men. C. trachomatis localizes to epithelial tissue and can spread throughout the urogenital system. Microorganisms also may pass from the mother to the eyes and respiratory tract of the infant during birth. Tetracycline or doxycycline is used for treatment in men and nonpregnant women, and erythromycin in infants and pregnant women.

11 Lymphogranuloma venereum is a chronic STD that is uncommon in the United States. The lesion begins as a skin infection and spreads to the lymph tissue, causing inflammation, necrosis, buboes, and abscesses of the inguinal lymph nodes. Primary lesions appear on the penis and scrotum in men, and on the cervix, vaginal wall, and labia in women. Secondary lesions involve inflammation and swelling of the lymph nodes with formation of large blue buboes that rupture and form draining ulcerative lesions. Tetracycline provides effective treatment.

12 Genital herpes is the most common genital ulceration in the United States and is caused by either type 1 (HSV-1) or type 2 (HSV-2) herpes virus. HSV-1 often presents as a "cold sore" of the oral mucosa, and HSV-2 is commonly a genital lesion. Lesions initially appear as groups of vesicles that

progress to ulceration with pain, lymphadenopathy, and fever. Herpes simplex virus passed from mother to fetus can cause spontaneous abortion or prematurity. Acyclovir reduces symptoms but does not cure the disease.

13 Three distinct syndromes are associated with HSV infection: (1) first-episode primary, (2) first-episode nonprimary, and (3) recurrent infections. Recurrent infections are most often attributable to HSV-2 and are generally milder and of shorter duration.

14 Condylomata acuminata (genital warts) is associated with multiple sexual partners and is highly contagious. The velvety cauliflowerlike lesions occur in the genital and anal areas, vagina, and cervix and are painless. They can be transmitted to the infant at birth. Surgical excision with laser or cryosurgery is most effective.

15 Epstein-Barr virus may be harbored in the genital tract and passed on through sexual encounters.

16 Trichomoniasis (*T. vaginalis*) is a common cause of genital infection, vaginitis in women, and urethritis. Both partners are usually infected. Women usually have a copious gray-green discharge with pruritus. Men are usually asymptomatic. Metronidazole is the treatment for both partners.

17 Scabies is a common parasitic infection that can be spread by skin-to-skin contact and sexual contact. The scabies mite burrows through the skin, depositing two or three large eggs per day. Intense pruritus is the most pronounced clinical manifestation. Treatment consists of topical application of lindane 1% cream or lotion.

18 Pediculosis pubis (crabs) is commonly transmitted sexually and is caused by the crab louse, *Phthirus pubis*. The lice bite into the skin for nutrition. Symptoms include mild and severe pruritus. Treatment consists of lindane 1% cream, lotion, or shampoo, or pyrethrins and piperonyl butoxide.

Sexually Transmitted Infections of Other Body Systems

1 A variety of enteric bacterial pathogens are now recognized as sexually transmitted, particularly among homosexual men. The infections include shigellosis, campylobacter enteritis, giardiasis, amebiasis, and hepatitis B.

2 Shigellosis is transmitted by contact with infected feces. Campylobacter enteritis can be transmitted through anal-oral sexual practices.

3 Giardiasis and amebiasis are primarily transmitted through contaminated drinking water, but are also transmitted by anal-oral and genital-anal contact.

4 Transmission of hepatitis B virus (HBV) can occur through needle puncture, blood transfusion, cuts in the skin, and contact with infected body fluids.

5 Perinatal transmission of HBV is relatively common.

6 Systemic diseases known to be sexually transmitted include AIDS (see Chapter 8) and cytomegalovirus infection.

7 Cytomegalovirus (CMV) is a sexually transmissible herpesvirus. The infection causes no specific genital disease, but its incidence is high in individuals being treated for other STDs. The virus is found in semen, cervical secretions, urine, blood, saliva, breast milk, and stool.

8 Cytomegalovirus infection is more common in homosexual men and in young women with multiple sexual partners.

9 Cytomegalovirus infection can cause mononucleosis, pneumonitis, hemolytic anemia, and thrombocytopenia purpura. A CMV infection in an immunosuppressed individual can cause a life-threatening illness. No treatment is indicated in most cases of CMV infection.

KEY TERMS

REFERENCES

Ashley, R., & Koelle, D. M. (1992). Immune responses to genital herpes infection. *Sexually Transmitted Diseases, 8*, 201-238 [T. C. Quinn, Guest Ed.].

Ball, J. F., & Murph, J. R. (1992). Congenital infections and the nervous system. *Pediatric Clinics of North America, 39*, 669-690.

Billstein, S. (1990). Human lice. In K. K. Holmes, P. A. Mardh, P. F. Sparling, & P. J. Weisner (Eds.), *Sexually transmitted diseases* (pp. 467-472). New York: McGraw-Hill.

Bourcier, K. M., & Seidler, A. J. (1987). Chlamydia and condylomata acuminata: An update for the nurse practitioner. *Journal of Obstetric, Gynecologic, and Neonatal Nursing, 16*(1), 17-22.

Brandt, A. M. (1987). *No magic bullet: A social history of venereal disease in the United States since 1880, expanded edition.* New York: Oxford University Press.

Caldwell, J. H. (1985). The "gay bowel" syndrome. In V. A. Spagna & R. B. Prior (Eds.), *Sexually transmitted disease: A clinical syndrome approach* (pp. 255-274). New York: Marcel Dekker.

Camisa, C. (1985). Condyloma acuminatum and other human papillomavirus-induced diseases. In V. A. Spagna & R. B. Prior (Eds.), *Sexually transmitted disease: A clinical syndrome* (pp. 309-332). New York: Marcel Dekker.

Cazchor, J. S., & Gleckman, R. A. (1989). Third generation cephalosporins: A plea to save them for specific infections. *Postgraduate Medicine, 85*, 169-176.

Centers for Disease Control (CDC). (1989). 1989 sexually transmitted diseases treatment guidelines. *Morbidity and Mortality Weekly Report, 38*, 1-43.

Centers for Disease Control (CDC). (1991a). Hepatitis B virus: A comprehensive strategy for eliminating transmission in the United States through universal childhood vaccination. *Mortality and Morbidity Weekly Report Summary, 40*.

Centers for Disease Control (CDC). (1991b). Pelvic inflammatory disease: Guidelines for prevention and management. *Mortality and Morbidity Weekly Report, 40*, 1-24.

Centers for Disease Control (CDC). (1991c). Primary and secondary syphilis—United States, 1981-1990. *Morbidity and Mortality Weekly Report, 40*, 314-323.

Centers for Disease Control (CDC). (1992). Summary of notifiable diseases. United States 1991. *Morbidity and Mortality Weekly Report, 40*, 1-12.

Corey, L. (1990). Genital herpes. In K. K. Holmes, P. A. Mardh, P. F. Sparling, & P. J. Weisner (Eds.), *Sexually transmitted diseases* (2nd ed.). New York: McGraw-Hill.

Derksen, D. J. (1992). Children with condylomata acuminata. *The Journal of Family Practice, 34*, 419-423.

Dobbins, J. G., Stewart, J. A., & Demmler, G. J. (1992). Surveillance of congenital cytomegalovirus disease, 1990-91. *Mortality and Morbidity Weekly Report, 41*, 35-44.

Elkins, C., & Sparling, P. F. (1992). Immunobiology of *Neisseria gonorrhoeae*. *Sexually Transmitted Diseases, 8*, 113-140 [T. C. Quinn, Guest Ed.].

Farnes, S. W., & Setness, P. A. (1990). Serologic tests for syphilis. *Postgraduate Medicine, 87*, 37-46.

Fitzpatrick, T. B., Polano, M. K., & Suurmond, D. (1983). *Color atlas and synopsis of clinical dermatology.* New York: McGraw-Hill.

Goldsmith, L. A. (1990). Bridging the gap: Notes of a wart watcher. *Archives in Dermatology, 125*, 1432-1435.

Guerrant, R. L., Werkel, C. S., & Raydin, J. I. (1990). Intestinal protozoa: *Giardia lamblia, Entamoeba histolytica,* and *Cryptosporidium.* In K. K. Holmes, P. A. Mardh, P. F. Sparling, & P. J. Weisner (Eds.), *Sexually transmitted diseases* (2nd ed., pp. 493-514). New York: McGraw-Hill.

Habif, T. P. (1985). *Clinical dermatology: A color guide to diagnosis and therapy.* St. Louis: Mosby–Year Book.

Handsfield, H. H. (1992). Recent development in STDs: Viral and other syndromes. *Hospital Practice,* January 15, 175-200.

Hart, G. (1990). Donovanosis. In K. K. Holmes, P. A. Mardh, P. F. Sparling, & P. J. Weisner (Eds.), *Sexually transmitted diseases* (2nd ed., pp. 273-277). New York: McGraw-Hill.

Hatcher, R. A., Guest, F., Stewart, F., Stewart, G. K., Trussell, J., Bowen, S. C., & Cates, W. (1988). *Contraceptive technology 1988-1989* (14th revised ed.). Atlanta, GA: Irvington.

Herbst, A. L., Mischell, D. R., Stenchever, M. A., & Droegemueller, W. D. (1992). *Comprehensive gynecology* (2nd ed.). St. Louis: Mosby–Year Book.

Hiller, S., & Holmes, K. K. (1990). Bacterial vaginitis. In K. K. Holmes, P. A. Mardh, P. F. Sparling, & P. J. Weisner (Eds.), *Sexually transmitted diseases* (2nd ed., pp. 547-559). New York: McGraw-Hill.

Hook, E. W. III, & Handsfield, H. H. (1990). Gonococcal infections in the adult. In K. K. Holmes, P. A. Mardh, P. F. Sparling, & P. J. Weisner (Eds.), *Sexually transmitted diseases* (2nd ed., pp. 149-165). New York: McGraw-Hill.

Hook, E. W., & Marra, C. M. (1992). Medical progress: Acquired syphilis in adults. *New England Journal of Medicine, 326*(16), 1060-1068.

Kaufman, R. N., & Faro, S. (1985). Herpes genitalis: Clinical features and treatment. *Clinical Obstetrics & Gynecology, 28*, 156.

Klein, M. B. (1988). Hepatitis B virus: Perinatal management. *Journal of Perinatal and Neonatal Nursing, 1*(4), 12-23.

Lambert, D. R., & Yoder, F. W. (1985). Ectoparasites and molluscum contagiosum. In V. A. Spagna, & R. B. Prior (Eds.), *Sexually transmitted diseases: A clinical syndrome approach* (pp. 333-356). New York: Marcel Dekker.

Lemon S. M., & Newbold, J. E. (1990). Viral hepatitis. In K. K. Holmes, P. A. Mardh, P. F. Sparling, & P. J. Weisner (Eds.), *Sexually transmitted diseases* (2nd ed., pp. 449-466). New York: McGraw-Hill.

Leu, R. H. (1991). Complications of coexisting chlamydial and gonococcal infections. *Postgraduate Medicine, 89*, 56-60.

Mardh, P-A. (1991). The vaginal ecosystem. *American Journal of Obstetrics and Gynecology, 165*(40), 1163-1167.

Maurice, J. (1983). Ubiquitous parasites: Chlamydia infections now commonest sexually transmitted disease. *International Health, 3*, 19-20.

Mead, P. B., Eschenbach, D. A., Ledger, W. J., & Thomason, J. L. (1989, December). Symposium—cover story: Reconsidering bacterial vaginosis. *Contemporary OB/GYN,* 76-89.

Mogabgab, W. J. (1991). Recent developments in the treatment of sexually transmitted diseases. *American Journal of Medicine 91* (suppl 6A), 142-144.

Moldwin, R. M. (1992). Sexually transmitted protozoal infections. *STDs and Other Lesions of the External Genitalia, 19*(1), 93-101.

Naher, H., Grissman, L., Freese, U. K., Petzoldt, D., & Helfrich, S. (1992). Subclinical Epstein-Barr virus infection of both the male and female genital tract: Indication for sexual transmission. *Journal of Investigative Dermatology, 98*, 791-793.

Orkin, M., & Maibach, H. I. (1990). Scabies. In K. K. Holmes, P. A. Mardh, P. F. Sparling, & P. J. Weisner (Eds.), *Sexually transmitted diseases* (2nd ed., pp. 473-480). New York: McGraw-Hill.

Para, M. F., & Baird, I. M. (1985). Genital ulcer syndromes. In V. A. Spagna, & R. B. Prior (Eds.), *Sexually transmitted diseases: A clinical syndrome approach* (pp. 161-186). New York: Marcel Dekker.

Peaceman, A. M., & Gonik, B. (1991). Sexually transmitted viral disease in women. *Postgraduate Medicine, 89*, 133-140.

Pelouze, P. S. (1941). *Gonorrhea in the male and female.* Philadelphia: Saunders.

Perine, P. I., & Osoba, A. O. (1990). Lymphogranuloma venereum. In K. K. Holmes, P. A. Mardh, P. F. Sparling, & P. J. Weisner (Eds.), *Sexually transmitted diseases* (2nd ed., pp. 195-204). New York: McGraw-Hill.

Perlman, M. D., & McNeeley, S. G. (1992). A review of the microbiology, immunology, and clinical implications of *Chlamydia trachomatis* infections. *Obstetrical and Gynecological Survey, 47*, 448-461.

Peterson, I. M., & Rao, R. (1989). Genital warts: Newly discovered consequences of an ancient disease. *Postgraduate Medicine, 86*, 197-204.

Pitot, P., & Plummer, F. A. (1990). Genital ulcer adenopathy syndrome. In K. K. Holmes, P. A. Mardh, P. F. Sparling, & P. J. Weisner (Eds.), *Sexually transmitted diseases* (2nd ed., pp. 711-716). New York: McGraw-Hill.

Potts, J. E. (1992). Chlamydial infection: Screening and management update, 1991. *Postgraduate Medicine, 91,* 120-126.

Quinn, T. C., & Cates, W. (1992). Epidemiology of sexually transmitted diseases in the 1990s. *Sexually Transmitted Diseases, 8* [T. C. Quinn, Guest Ed.].

Quinn, T. C., & Stamm, W. E. (1990). Proctocolitis, enteritis, and esophagitis in homosexual men. In K. K. Holmes, P. A. Mardh, P. F. Sparling, & P. J. Weisner (Eds.), *Sexually transmitted diseases* (2nd ed., pp. 663-683). New York: McGraw-Hill.

Rein, M. R., & Holmes, K. K. (1983). Nonspecific vaginitis, vulvovaginal candidiasis, and trichomoniasis: Clinical features, diagnosis, and management. In J. Remington & M. N. Schwartz (Eds.), *Current clinical topics in infectious diseases* (pp. 281-315). New York: McGraw-Hill.

Richens, J. (1991). The diagnosis of treatment of donovanosis (granuloma inguinale). *Genitourinary Medicine, 67,* 441-452.

Ronald, A. R., & Albritton, W. (1990). Chancroid and *Haemophilus ducreyi.* In K. K. Holmes, P. A. Mardh, P. F. Sparling, & P. J. Weisner (Eds.), *Sexually transmitted diseases* (2nd ed., pp. 263-269). New York: McGraw-Hill.

Ronald, A., Plummer, F., Ngugi, E., Ndinya-Achola, J. O., Pitot, P., Kreiss, J., & Brunham, R. (1991). The Nairobi STD program. *Infectious Disease Clinics of North America, 5,* 337-353.

Rose, F. B., & Camp, C. J. (1988). Genital herpes: How to relieve patients' physical and psychological symptoms. *Postgraduate Medicine, 84,* 81-86.

Sargent, S. J. (1992). The "other" sexually transmitted diseases: Chlamydial, herpes simplex virus, and human papillomavirus infections. *Postgraduate Medicine, 9,* 359-372.

Schachter, J. (1990). Biology of *Chlamydia trachomatis.* In K. K. Holmes, P. A. Mardh, P. F. Sparling, & P. J. Weisner (Eds.). *Sexually transmitted diseases* (2nd ed., pp. 161-180). New York: McGraw-Hill.

Schulte, J. M., & Martich, F. A. (1992). Chancroid in the United States, 1921-1990: Evidence for underreporting of cases. *Morbidity and Mortality Weekly Report, 41,* 57-61.

Schultz, K. F., Murphy, F. K., Patamasucon, P., & Mehaus, A. Z. (1990). Congenital syphilis. In K. K. Holmes, P. A. Mardh, P. F. Sparling, & P. J. Weisner (Eds.), *Sexually transmitted diseases* (2nd ed., pp. 821-842). New York: McGraw-Hill.

Schwartz, P., & Gilmore, M. R. (1990). Sociological perspectives on human sexuality. In K. K. Holmes, P. A. Mardh, P. F. Sparling, & P. J. Weisner (Eds.), *Sexually transmitted diseases* (2nd ed., pp. 45-53). New York: McGraw-Hill.

Shah, K. V. (1992). Biology of genital tract human papillomaviruses. *Urologic Clinics of North America, 19,* 63-69.

Shaw, P., & Juranek, D. (1976). Recent trends in scabies in the United States. *Journal of Infectious Disease, 134,* 414-416.

Smiley, L., & Huang, E. S. (1990). Cytomegalovirus as a sexually transmitted disease. In K. K. Holmes, P. A. Mardh, P. F. Sparling, & P. J. Weisner (Eds.), *Sexually transmitted diseases* (2nd ed., pp. 415-424). New York: McGraw-Hill.

Smith, M. A., & Singer, C. (1992). Sexually transmitted viruses other than HIV and papillomavirus. *Urologic Clinics of North America, 19,* 47-62.

Sparks, J. M. (1991). Vaginitis. *Journal of Reproductive Medicine, 36*(10), 745-752

Sparling, P. F. (1990). Natural history of syphilis. In K. K. Holmes, P. A. Mardh, P. F. Sparling, & P. J. Weisner (Eds.), *Sexually transmitted diseases* (2nd ed., pp. 213-219). New York: McGraw-Hill.

Sperling, R. S. (1992, June). Infection protocols: Perihepatitis. *Contemporary OB/GYN, 51-52.*

Stagno, S., & Whitley, R. J. (1990). Herpesvirus infection in the neonate and children. In K. K. Holmes, P. A. Mardh, P. F. Sparling, & P. J. Weisner (Eds.), *Sexually transmitted diseases* (2nd ed., pp. 863-888). New York: McGraw-Hill.

Stamm, W. E., & Holmes, K. K. (1990). *Chlamydia trachomatis* infections of the adult. In K. K. Holmes, P. A. Mardh, P. F. Sparling, & P. J. Weisner (Eds.), *Sexually transmitted diseases* (2nd ed., pp. 181-194). New York: McGraw-Hill.

Thin, R. N. (1990). Early syphilis in the adult. In K. K. Holmes, P. A. Mardh, P. F. Sparling, & P. J. Weisner (Eds.), *Sexually transmitted diseases* (2nd ed., pp. 221-229). New York: McGraw-Hill.

Wehrle, P. F., & Top, F. H. (1981). *Communicable and infectious diseases* (9th ed.). St. Louis: Mosby–Year Book.

Westrom, L., & Mardh, P-A. (1990). Acute pelvic inflammatory disease (PID). In K. K. Holmes, P. A. Mardh, P. F. Sparling, & P. J. Weisner (Eds.), *Sexually transmitted diseases* (2nd ed., pp. 493-514). New York: McGraw-Hill.

Wilson, C. B. (1990). The cellular immune system and its role in host defense. In G. Mandell, R. G. Douglas, & J. E. Bennett (Eds.), *Principles and practice of infectious diseases* (3rd ed., pp. 101-138). New York: Churchill Livingstone.

Wooldridge, W. E. (1991). Syphilis: A new visit from an old enemy. *Postgraduate Medicine, 89,* 193-202.

Zenilman, J. M. (1992). Update on bacterial sexually transmitted disease. *Urologic Clinics of North America, 19,* 25-34.

SUGGESTED READINGS

Cates, W., & Holmes, K. K. (1986). Sexually transmitted diseases. In J. M. Last, J. Chin, J. E. Fielding, A. L. Frank, J. C. Lashof, & R. B. Wallace (Eds.), *Maxcy-Rosenau public health and preventive medicine* (12th ed.) (pp. 257-295). East Norwalk, CT: Appleton-Century-Crofts.

Centers for Disease Control. (1987). Summary of notifiable diseases—United States 1987. *Morbidity and Mortality Weekly Report, 36*(54).

Centers for Disease Control. (1988). Continuing increase in infectious syphilis—United States. *Morbidity and Mortality Weekly Report, 37*(3), 35-38.

Darrow, W. W., & Siegel, K. (1990). Preventive health behavior and STD. In K. K. Holmes, P. A. Mardh, P. F. Sparling, & P. J. Weisner (Eds.), *Sexually transmitted diseases* (2nd ed., pp. 85-92). New York: McGraw-Hill.

UNIT VIII

The Hematologic System

THE IDEA that blood is a life force has intrigued people since ancient times. Healers in primitive cultures apparently recognized that blood is connected to the heart and without blood life ceases. The ancient Greeks referred to the life-giving role of blood. In Greek mythology, Aesculapius, the son of Apollo and god of medicine, was given Gorgon's blood from the goddess of wisdom, Athena. Aesculapius supposedly used this blood to raise the dead (Hart, 1980).

Anthony van Leeuwenhoek (1632-1723), a janitor from Holland, is given credit for first describing erythrocytes (red blood cells). Van Leeuwenhoek may have seen the white blood cells, but William Hewson (1739-1774), often called the "father of hematology," first described them.

Leukemia was simultaneously discovered by Rudolph Virchow in Berlin (leukamie) and by John Bennett in Edinburgh in 1845 (Wintrobe, 1980). Both investigators used autopsy findings to report their patient's symptoms and two important features: an enlarged spleen and a peculiar appearance of the blood with changes in both color and consistency. The question that was pursued for many years was why the colorless corpuscles were almost as numerous as the red corpuscles. Virchow made an important distinction that leukemia could be subdivided into two forms: one characterized by swelling of the spleen (splenic leukemia) and the other by swelling of the lymph nodes (lymphatic leukemia). Each form had its own dominant type of corpuscle. Although still observed, this distinction was further qualified in 1870 by Ernst Neumann, who suggested that in splenic leukemia the marrow, rather than the spleen, is the source of the excess corpuscles. This observation lead to the term *my-*

For pure blood, take Hood's sarsaparilla. (Courtesy National Library of Medicine.)

covered that Hodgkin had already described the condition, he named it Hodgkin disease and gave a more complete account of the condition.

Paul Ehrlich's (1854-1915) development of a triacid stain, one of the most significant advances for hematology, enabled researchers to distinguish the cell's nucleus, cytoplasm, and other details. Leukocytes were discovered after the red corpuscles, probably because they are fewer in number and colorless, thus easily overlooked (Wintrobe, 1980).

The modern era of hematology commenced in the 1920s, with the investigations of George Whipple, George Minot, and William Castle. These investigators promoted understanding of the pathogenesis of pernicious anemia and the role of certain foods, particularly liver, in promoting production of hemoglobin, the oxygen-carrying molecules of the blood (Wintrobe, 1980). It was during this time that hematology evolved into a quantitative science based on intricate observation and measurement.

Understanding of the humoral mechanism of blood cell regulation began in

eloid, or marrow derived. The classifications of leukemia started in 1889 when A. Epstein introduced the term *acute*.

The first case of Hodgkin disease was reported by Thomas Hodgkin of Gay's Hospital in London in 1832. He had seven patients who were admitted to the hospital shortly before they died. They all had enlarged lymph nodes and some had an enlarged spleen. Hodgkin's observations were apparently ignored, because the condition was rediscovered in 1856 by Samuel Wilks, also of Gay's Hospital (Wintrobe, 1980). When Wilks dis-

the early 1900s. The development of hormones that constitute the hematopoietic growth factors includes work begun by Carnot and Deflandre. Eventually it became clear that specific hematopoietic growth factors, or colony-stimulating factors (CSFs), are necessary for the adequate growth of myeloid, erythroid, lymphoid, and megakaryocytic lineages. In 1977, the first CSF, macrophage-CSF, was purified. Today, many other CSFs have been purified and their clinical utility is the subject of current cytotoxic therapy.

CHAPTER 22

Structure and Function of the Hematologic System

Kathryn L. McCance
Pamela F. Cipriano

Chapter Outline

B lood cells travel long distances and, thus, must be flexible or blood would hardly flow at all. Blood cells act as vehicles—cells and chemicals—that travel along the tens of thousands of miles of blood vessels packed into the human body. Most cells are red blood cells that, like tanker trucks, function as carriers. Yet, red blood cells maneuver more like sports cars, flexing and deforming to squeeze through capillaries smaller than their own diameters. White blood cells are larger than red blood cells and less flexible. Spherical and stiffer, white cells create more resistance and are much more likely to create "traffic jams." White blood cells travel the main highways, avoiding the small capillaries that red blood cells so expertly squeeze through. But disease can make the white cells "sticky" and create traffic jams and cause the red cells to lose their cargo. These alterations can lead to difficulties in oxygenation, acid-base balance, and immune function and, like a major thoroughfare at rush hour, may alter streamline flow.

COMPONENTS OF THE HEMATOLOGIC SYSTEM

Composition of the Blood

Blood consists of a variety of formed elements (cells and proteins) that circulate in the cardiovascular system suspended in plasma, which is approximately 90% water and 10% dissolved substances (solutes). All of these elements constitute blood volume, which in adults amounts to about 6 quarts (5.5 L). Approximately 45% to 50% of blood volume consists of formed elements, and the remainder is plasma. The continuous movement of blood keeps the formed elements dispersed throughout the plasma, where they are available to carry out their chief functions: (1) delivery of substances needed for cellular metabolism in the tissues, (2) defense against invading microorganisms and injury, and (3) acid-base balance.

Plasma and Plasma Proteins

In adults, plasma accounts for 55% to 60% of blood volume. **Plasma** is a complex aqueous liquid containing a number of organic and inorganic elements (Table 22-1). The concentration of these elements varies depending on diet, metabolic demand, hormones, and vitamins. Plasma differs from serum in that **serum** is plasma that has been altered in the laboratory so as to remove fibrinogen (a clotting factor) or some other element that is unwanted or unneeded in the sample.

In circulating plasma, the dominant elements by weight are the plasma proteins, which constitute about 7% of the total plasma weight. The **plasma proteins** vary in structure and function but can be classified into three major groups: the **albumins, globulins,** and **clotting factors.** The albumins are the most numerous, followed by the various globulins (immunoglobulins or gamma globulins) and the clotting factors, chiefly fibrinogen. The plasma proteins are synthesized in the liver, with the exception of the immunoglobulins, which are synthesized by lymphocytes in the lymph nodes and other lymphoid tissues (see Chapter 6 and p. 216).

Albumin is present at a concentration of about 4 g/dl and is essential for regulating the passage of water and solutes through the capillaries. Because albumin molecules are large and do not diffuse freely through the vascular endothelium, they provide the critical colloid osmotic or oncotic pressure that regulates the passage of water and solutes through the microcirculation (arterioles, capillaries, and venules) (Berne & Levy, 1992) (see Chapters 1 and 3). Water and solute particles diffuse out of the arterial portions of the capillaries because blood pressure is greater in arterial than in venous blood vessels (see Chapter 29). Water and solutes move from tissue cells into the venous portions of the capillaries, where the pressures are reversed, oncotic pressure being greater than intravascular pressure. Albumin also serves as a carrier molecule for both normal components of blood and exogenous agents, such as drugs.

The immunoglobulins, or antibodies, are synthesized by mature lymphocytes called plasma cells in the lymphoid organs, chiefly lymph nodes. The immunoglobulins include IgA, IgG, IgM, IgD, and IgE. Most of them are critical for defense against infectious microorganisms. (Lymphocyte and antibody function is described in Chapter 6.)

The third important class of plasma proteins is the clotting factors, which promote coagulation and stop bleeding from damaged blood vessels. Fibrinogen is the most plentiful of the clotting factors and is the precursor of the fibrin clot (see p. 849). Other plasma proteins include complement proteins, a group of proteins involved in the immune response, a variety of enzymes and their inhibitors, and specific carriers of such elements as iron and copper. The plasma lipids, triglycerides, phospholipids, cholesterol, and fatty acids are carried through the blood as complexes with plasma proteins; they are known as **lipoproteins** (see Chapters 1 and 27).

The electrolytes (electrically charged solutes) of the plasma maintain the osmolarity and pH of blood within a physiologic range (Table 22-1). (Electrolytes are described in Chapters 1 and 3.)

Cellular Components of the Blood

The cellular elements of the blood are broadly classified as **erythrocytes** (red blood cells), **leukocytes** (white blood cells), and **platelets** (thrombocytes). The components of the blood are listed in Table 22-2.

Erythrocytes

In 1628, Robert Burton described blood as a "hot, temperate red humor whose office is to nourish the whole body, to give it strength and color being dispersed by the veins through every part of it" (Babior & Stossel, 1984). A few years later, with the invention of the microscope, researchers learned that erythrocytes give blood its red color.

Erythrocytes are the most abundant cells of the blood, occupying approximately 48% of the blood volume in men and about 42% in women. Erythrocytes are primarily responsible for tissue oxygenation. Their shape, size, and structure reflect their unique function as deliverers of gases throughout the body. The erythrocyte's cytoplasm consists of a solution containing protein (mostly **hemoglobin [Hb]**, which carries the gases) and electrolytes, which regulate diffusion through the cell's plasma membrane. The mature erythrocyte lacks the cytoplasmic organelles—a nucleus, mitochondria, and ribosomes—that would enable it to divide or carry out metabolic functions. Therefore it cannot synthesize pro-

TABLE 22-1

Organic and Inorganic Components of Arterial Plasma

Constituent	Amount/concentration	Major functions
Water	93% of plasma weight	Medium for carrying all other constituents
Electrolytes	Total <1% of plasma weight	Maintain H_2O in extracellular compartment; act as buffers; function in membrane excitability
Na^+	142 mEq/L (142 mM)	
K^+	4 mEq/L (4 mM)	
Ca^{++}	5 mEq/L (2.5 mM)	
Mg^{++}	3 mEq/L (1.5 mM)	
Cl^-	103 mEq/L (103 mM)	
HCO_3^-	27 mEq/L (27 mM)	
Phosphate (mostly HPO_4^{2-})	2 mEq/L (1 mM)	
SO_4^{2-}	1 mEq/L (0.5 mM)	
Proteins	7.3 g/dl (2.5 mM)	Provide colloid osmotic pressure of plasma; act as buffers; bind other plasma constituents (lipids, hormones, vitamins, minerals, etc.); clotting factors; enzymes; enzyme precursors; antibodies (immune globulins); hormones
Albumins	4.5 g/dl	
Globulins	2.5 g/dl	
Fibrinogen	0.3 g/dl	
Gases		
CO_2 content	22-20 mmol/L plasma	By-product of oxygenation, most CO_2 content is from HCO_3 and acts as a buffer
O_2	Pao_2 80 torr or greater (arterial); Pvo_2 30-40 torr (venous)	Oxygenation
N_2	0.9 ml/dl	By-product of protein catabolism
Nutrients		Provide nutrition and substances for tissue repair
Glucose and other carbohydrates	100 mg/dl (5.6 mM)	
Total amino acids	40 mg/dl (2 mM)	
Total lipids	500 mg/dl (7.5 mM)	
Cholesterol	150-250 mg/dl (4-7 mM)	
Individual vitamins	0.0001-2.5 mg/dl	
Individual trace elements	0.001-0.3 mg/dl	
Waste products		
Urea (BUN)	7-18 mg/dl (5.7 mM)	End product of protein catabolism
Creatinine (from creatine)	1 mg/dl (0.09 mM)	End product from energy metabolism
Uric acid (from nucleic acids)	5 mg/dl (0.3 mM)	End product from protein metabolism
Bilirubin (from heme)	0.2-1.2 mg/dl (0.003-0.018 mM)	End product of red blood cell destruction
Individual hormones	0.000001-0.05 mg/dl	Functions specific to target tissue

From Vander, Sherman & Luciano, 1990.

tein or carry out oxidative reactions. Because it cannot undergo mitotic division, it lives out its lifespan (approximately 120 days) in the circulation, dies, and is replaced by a new erythrocyte.

The erythrocyte's size and shape are ideally suited to its function as a gas carrier. It is a small disk with two unique properties: (1) **biconcavity** and (2) **reversible**

deformability (Fig. 22-1). The flattened, biconcave shape provides a surface area/volume ratio that is optimal for gas diffusion into and out of the cell. Reversible deformity enables the erythrocyte to alter its shape to squeeze through the microcirculation and then return to normal. During its 120-day lifespan, the erythrocyte, which is 8 μm in diameter, must repeatedly circulate

TABLE 22-2

Cellular Components of the Blood

Cell	Structural characteristics	Normal amounts of circulating blood	Function	Lifespan
Erythrocyte (red blood cell)	Nonnucleated cytoplasmic disk containing hemoglobin	4.2-6.2 million/mm³	Gas transport to and from tissue cells and lungs	80-120 days
Leukocyte (white blood cell)	Nucleated cell	5000-10,000/mm³	Bodily defense mechanisms	See below
Lymphocyte	Mononuclear immunocyte	25% to 33% of leukocyte count (leukocyte differential)	Humoral and cell-mediated immunity (see Chapter 6)	Days or years depending on type
Monocyte and macrophage	Large mononuclear phagocyte	3% to 7% of leukocyte differential	Phagocytosis; mononuclear phagocyte system	Months or years
Eosinophil	Segmented polymorphonuclear granulocyte	1% to 4% of leukocyte differential	Phagocytosis, antibody-mediated defense against parasites, allergic reactions, associated with Hodgkin disease, recovery phase of infection	Unknown
Neutrophil	Segmented polymorphonuclear granulocyte	57% to 67% of leukocyte differential	Phagocytosis, particularly during early phase of inflammation	4 days
Basophil	Segmented polymorphonuclear granulocyte	0% to 0.75% of leukocyte differential	Unknown, but associated with allergic reactions and mechanical irritation	Unknown
Platelet	Irregularly shaped cytoplasmic fragment (not a cell)	140,000 to 340,000/mm³	Hemostasis following vascular injury; normal coagulation and clot formation/retraction	8-11 days

FIG. 22-1 Mature erythrocytes.
Scanning electron micrograph of mature
erythrocytes (×3000). (From Thibodeau, 1993.)

through splenic sinusoids (see p. 836) and capillaries that are only 2 μm in diameter. To do this, the erythrocyte assumes the torpedo-like conformation.

Several hypotheses attempt to explain how the erythrocyte's resting biconcave shape is maintained. Sakagami, Minari, and Orii (1965) proposed that the convex portion of the cell's plasma membrane may have a higher concentration of cholesterol than the concave portion and that the cholesterol molecules may serve as a wedge, bending the membrane into the biconcave shape. (See Chapter 1 for a discussion of plasma membrane structure.) Other investigators have suggested that biconcavity is maintained by the interaction of elastic or electrical forces, surface tension, and colloid osmotic pressure (Lopez, Duck, & Hung, 1968). Whatever the mechanism, maintenance of erythrocyte shape apparently depends on both internal and external factors.

Leukocytes

Leukocytes are white blood cells that defend the body against organisms that cause infection and remove debris, including dead or injured host cells of all kinds (Fig. 22-2). The leukocytes act primarily in the tissues but are transported in the circulation. They are fewer in number than erythrocytes; the average adult has approximately 5000 to 10,000 leukocytes/mm³ of blood.

Leukocytes are classified according to structure as either **granulocytes** or **agranulocytes** and according to function as either **phagocytes** or **immunocytes**. The

FIG. 22-2 Blood cells. Leukocytes are spherical and have irregular surfaces with numerous extending pili. Erythrocytes are flattened spheres with a depressed center. (From Raven & Johnson, 1992.)

granulocytes, which include neutrophils, basophils, and eosinophils, are all phagocytes. (Phagocytic action is described in Chapter 7.) Of the agranulocytes, the monocytes and macrophages are phagocytes, whereas the lymphocytes are immunocytes (cells that create immunity; see Chapter 6).

Granulocytes. The granulocytes are so called because of the many membrane-bounded granules in their cytoplasm. The granules contain enzymes capable of killing microorganisms and catabolizing debris ingested by the process of phagocytosis. The granules also contain powerful biochemical mediators with a variety of inflammatory and immune functions. These mediators, along with the digestive enzymes, are released from some granulocytes in response to specific stimuli and from all granulocytes as they reach the end of their natural lifespan and die. The biochemical mediators have various vascular and intercellular effects, and the enzymes participate in the breakdown of free-floating debris from sites of infection or injury.

Granulocytes are capable of ameboid movement, by which they migrate through vessel walls and then to sites where their action is needed. Migration through vessel walls, called diapedesis, and movement through the tissues, which occurs in response to chemotactic factors, are described and illustrated in Chapter 7.

The **neutrophil** (polymorphonuclear neutrophil, or PMN) is the most numerous and best understood of the granulocytes (Fig. 22-3). Neutrophils constitute about 55% of the total leukocyte count in adults. The cytoplasm of neutrophils contains small lysosomal granules and a central nucleus with two to five distinct lobes. Immature neutrophils are called bands or stabs. Mature neutrophils are called segmented neutrophils because of the characteristic appearance of their nucleus.

Neutrophils are the chief phagocytes of early inflammation. Soon after bacterial invasion or tissue injury, neutrophils migrate out of the capillaries and into the inflamed site, where they ingest and destroy microorganisms and debris, then die in a day or two. The dissolution of dead neutrophils releases digestive enzymes from their cytoplasmic granules. These enzymes dissolve cellular debris and prepare the site for healing. (This final function, called debridement, is described in Chapter 7.)

Eosinophils, which have large, coarse granules, constitute only 1% to 4% of the normal leukocyte count in adults. Like neutrophils, eosinophils are capable of ameboid movement and phagocytosis. Unlike neutrophils, which ingest cellular debris, eosinophils ingest antigen-antibody complexes and are induced by immunoglobulin E (IgE)-mediated hypersensitivity reactions to attack parasites. Eosinophils also help to control inflammatory processes. (Their function in inflammation and defense against parasites is described in Chapter 7.)

High eosinophil counts in atopic (allergy-prone) individuals experiencing type I allergic reactions, such as asthma or allergic rhinitis, have led researchers to think that eosinophils participate in hypersensitivity reactions to allergens besides parasites (see Chapter 8).

Basophils, which make up less than 1% of the leukocytes, are structurally similar to the mast cells found throughout extravascular tissue (see Fig. 22-3). Like the mast cells, whose role in stimulating the inflammatory response is described in Chapter 7, the basophils have cytoplasmic granules that contain vasoactive amines (histamine, bradykinin, and serotonin) and an anticoagulant (heparin). The precise function of basophils is poorly understood.

Agranulocytes. The agranulocytes—monocytes, macrophages, and lymphocytes—differ from the granulocytes in that they do not contain lysosomal granules in their cytoplasm. The lymphocytes do not contain *any* enzyme-filled digestive vacuoles, and the digestive vacuoles of the monocytes and macrophages are larger and fewer than those of the granulocytes.

The **monocytes** and **macrophages** make up the **mononuclear phagocyte system (MPS)**, formerly called the reticuloendothelial system (RES). (The MPS is described on p. 837.) Both monocytes and macrophages participate in the immune and inflammatory response, being powerful phagocytes. They also ingest dead or defective host cells, particularly blood cells.

Monocytes are immature macrophages (see Fig. 22-3). After monocytes are formed and released by the bone marrow, they enter the bloodstream and circulate for about 36 hours while maturing into macrophages. Some of the circulating macrophages migrate out of the vessels in response to infection or inflammation anywhere in the body. Other macrophages migrate to fixed sites in lymphoid tissues of the liver, spleen, lymph nodes, peritoneum, or gastrointestinal tract, where they are active for months or years.

Lymphocytes, which constitute approximately 36% of the total leukocyte count, are the primary cells of the immune response (see Fig. 22-3). Most lymphocytes are located in lymphoid tissues; only a small percentage circulate in the blood. There are many types of lymphocytes, the most important of which are T cells, B cells, and mature B cells (plasma cells). The lifespan of the lymphocyte can be days, months, or years, depending on its type and subtype. (Lymphocyte function and dysfunction are described in detail in Unit III.)

FIG. 22-3 Leukocytes. An example of leukocytes in human blood smear: **A,** Neutrophil; **B,** lymphocyte; **C,** basophil; **D,** monocyte. (From Thibodeau, G. A. [1987]. *Anatomy and physiology.* St. Louis: Mosby–Year Book.)

Platelets

Platelets are not cells, but disk-shaped cytoplasmic fragments. Platelets are essential for blood coagulation and control of bleeding. They lack a nucleus; therefore they have no DNA and are incapable of mitotic division. They do, however, contain cytoplasmic granules capable of releasing biochemical mediators when stimulated to do so by injury to a blood vessel.

There are approximately 140,000 to 340,000 platelets/mm^3 of circulating blood. An additional one third of the body's available platelets are in a reserve pool in the spleen. A platelet lives approximately 10 days, after which it dies and is removed by macrophages of the MPS, mostly in the spleen.

Lymphoid Organs

The lymphoid organs, some of which are merely aggregations of lymphoid tissue, are classified as primary or secondary. The **primary lymphoid organs** are the thymus and the bone marrow. The **secondary lymphoid organs** consist of the spleen, lymph nodes, tonsils, and Peyer's patches of the small intestine (see Fig. 6-4). All of the lymphoid organs link the hematologic and immune systems in that they are sites of residence, proliferation, differentiation, or function of lymphocytes and mononuclear phagocytes (monocytes and macrophages). (The liver, which also has hematologic functions, is primarily a digestive organ and is described in Chapter 35.)

Spleen

The **spleen** is the largest of the secondary lymphoid organs. It is a site of fetal hematopoiesis, its mononuclear phagocytes filter and cleanse the blood, its lymphocytes mount an immune response to blood-borne microorganisms, and it serves as a blood reservoir (see Chapter 24).

The spleen is a concave, encapsulated organ that weighs about 150 g and is about the size of a fist (see Chapter 6; Fig. 6-4). It is located in the left upper abdominal cavity, curved around a portion of the stomach. Strands of connective tissue (trabeculae) extend throughout the spleen from the splenic capsule, dividing the spleen into compartments. The compartments contain masses of lymphoid tissue called splenic pulp. The spleen is interlaced with many blood vessels, some of which are capable of distending to store blood.

Blood that circulates through the spleen comes from the splenic artery, which branches from the descending aorta and reenters the circulatory system through the splenic vein, which feeds into the portal vein. The portion of arterial blood that enters the spleen first encounters the white splenic pulp, which consists of masses of lymphoid tissue containing lymphocytes and macrophages. The white pulp forms clumps around the splenic arterioles and is the chief site of immune and phago-

cytic function within the spleen. Here blood-borne antigens encounter lymphocytes, initiating the immune response (see Chapter 6).

Some of the blood that enters the terminal capillaries of the spleen continues through the microcirculation and enters highly distensible storage areas called venous sinuses. Most of the blood, however, oozes through the extremely permeable capillary walls into the principal site of splenic filtration, the red pulp. Here the resident macrophages of the MPS phagocytose old, damaged, or dead blood cells of all kinds (but chiefly erythrocytes), microorganisms, and particles of debris. Hemoglobin from phagocytosed erythrocytes is catabolized, and heme (iron) is stored in the cytoplasm of the macrophages or released back into the blood plasma (see p. 843 and Fig. 22-9). The macrophages also can remove certain particulate inclusions from erythrocytes without harming the cells themselves. Blood that filters through the red pulp also finds its way into the venous sinuses and hence into the portal circulation.

The venous sinuses (and the red pulp) are capable of storing more than 300 ml of blood. Passive dilation of the venous sinuses enables the spleen to increase its storage capacity as needed by the body. Sudden reductions in blood pressure cause the sympathetic nervous system to stimulate constriction of the sinuses. Constriction, which can expel as much as 200 ml of blood into the venous circulation, helps to restore blood volume or pressure in the circulation and also can increase the hematocrit by as much as 4% (Guyton, 1992).

The spleen is not necessary for life or for adequate hematologic function. Splenic absence from any cause, however, whether it be atrophy, traumatic injury, or removal because of disease, has several effects that indicate its function. For example, leukocytosis (high levels of circulating leukocytes) often occurs after splenectomy. This suggests that the spleen exerts some control over the rate of proliferation of leukocyte stem cells in the bone marrow or their release into the bloodstream. Splenic absence is associated also with decreased levels of iron in the circulation, reflecting the spleen's role in the iron cycle (see p. 844). Immune function decreases in the absence of the spleen. Antibody production in response to small doses of soluble (i.e., blood-borne) antigen diminishes. Finally, the splenic function of removing old and defective blood cells seems to be confirmed by the fact that the blood of individuals lacking spleens contains more morphologically defective blood cells than normal.

Lymph Nodes

Structurally, **lymph nodes** are part of the lymphatic system. Thousands of them are clustered around the lymphatic veins, the vessels that collect interstitial fluid from the tissues and transport it, as lymph, back into the circulatory system near the heart. Functionally, however, lymph nodes are part of the hematologic and immune systems because they are the site of development or activity of large numbers of lymphocytes, monocytes, and macrophages. As the lymph filters through the bean-shaped lymph nodes clustered in the inguinal, axillary, and cervical regions of the body, it is cleansed of foreign particles and microorganisms by the monocytes and macrophages. The microorganisms in lymph stimulate the resident lymphocytes to develop into antibody-producing plasma cells (see Chapter 6). Lymphocytes, monocytes, and macrophages proliferate in the lymph nodes and are released into the lymphatic stream. During an infection, the rate of proliferation of macrophages within the nodes is so great that the nodes enlarge and become tender.

Each lymph node is enclosed in a fibrous capsule (Fig. 22-4). Strands of connective tissue (trabeculae) extend inward from the capsule, dividing the node into several compartments. Reticular fibers that extend between the trabeculae divide the compartments into smaller sections. The reticular fibers trap and store large numbers of lymphocytes, monocytes, and macrophages. The node is composed of an outer cortex area and an inner medullary area. Within the cortex of each node are germinal centers, or separate masses of lymphoid tissue. Lymph enters the node through several afferent lymphatic vessels, filters through the sinuses in the node, and leaves by way of efferent lymphatic vessels. Lymph flows slowly through the nodes, which facilitates the phagocytosis of foreign substances within the node and prevents them from reentering the bloodstream.

The Mononuclear Phagocyte System (MPS)

The MPS consists of a line of cells that originate in the bone marrow, are transported by the bloodstream, and, after differentiation to blood monocytes, finally settle in the tissues as mature macrophages. It is composed of monoblasts, promonocytes, and monocytes in bone marrow, monocytes in peripheral blood, and macrophages in tissue. Table 22-3 lists the various names given to macrophages localized in specific tissues.

The cells of the MPS ingest and destroy (by phagocytosis) unwanted materials in the blood and in organs. During inflammation, they engulf and digest foreign protein particles, microorganisms, debris from dead or injured cells, defective or injured erythrocytes, and dead neutrophils (see Fig. 7-15). The MPS (mostly in the liver and spleen) also is the main line of defense against bacteria in the bloodstream. In addition, the MPS cleanses the blood by removing old, injured, or dead erythrocytes, leukocytes, platelets, coagulation products, antigen-antibody complexes, and macromolecules, such as lipids and carbohydrates synthesized by the body as the result of faulty metabolism (as in storage diseases).

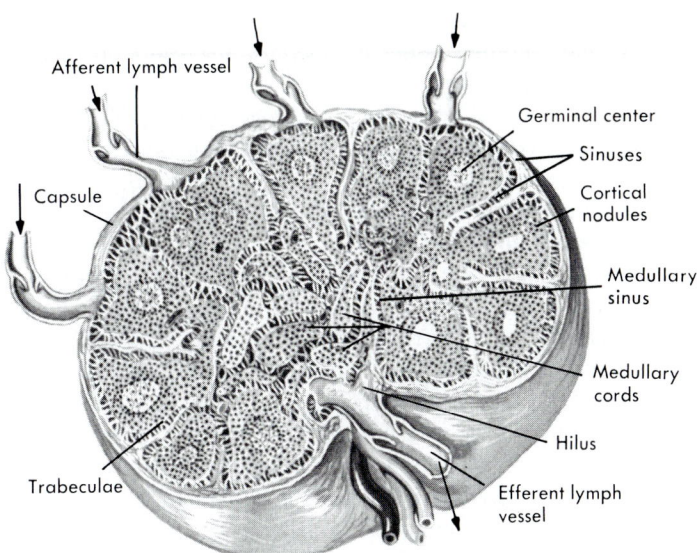

FIG. 22-4 Cross-section of lymph node. Several afferent valved lymphatics bring lymph to node. Efferent lymphatics leave node at the hilus. Blood vessels enter and leave at the hilus. (From Thibodeau, 1993.)

TABLE 22-3

Mononuclear Phagocyte System (Formerly Called the Reticuloendothelial System)

Name of cell	Location
Committed stem cells*	Bone marrow
Monoblasts	Bone marrow
Promonoblasts	Bone marrow
Monocytes	Bone marrow and peripheral blood
Macrophages	Tissue
Kupffer's cells (inflammatory macrophages)	Liver
Alveolar macrophages	Lung
Histiocytes	Connective tissue
Macrophages	Bone marrow
Fixed and free macrophages	Spleen and lymph nodes
Pleural and peritoneal macrophages	Serous cavities
Microglial cells	Nervous system
Mesangial cells	Kidney
Osteoclasts	Bone
Langerhan's cells	Skin
Dendritic cells	Lymphoid tissue

From Robbins, Cotran, & Kumar, 1989; Halma, Daha, & van-Es-La, 1992.

*Development of blood cells from stem cells in the marrow is described on p. 839, and illustrated in Fig. 22-5.

Macrophages also play a role in blood coagulation, wound healing, tissue remodeling, and the control of blood production.

Multiple cell types, including endothelial cells, fibroblasts, and lymphocytes, produce substances called colony-stimulating factors (CSFs) (Metcalf, 1991). Colony-stimulating factors control the production, maturation, and function of granulocytes and monocyte-macrophages (see Fig. 22-6), and the development of blood cells.

The origin and turnover of all the tissue macrophages named in Table 22-3 are not precisely known. It seems clear that once monocytes leave the circulation, they do not return. In the tissues, monocytes differentiate into macrophages without dividing. They can survive many months or perhaps even years (Shand & Bell, 1972). Under normal circumstances, macrophages show little evidence of mitotic division, probably because the levels of CSF production are normally low, but production can be rapidly elevated in response to need, such as the occurrence of an infection (Metcalf, 1991).

DEVELOPMENT OF BLOOD CELLS

Hematopoiesis

Blood cell production, termed **hematopoiesis,** occurs in the liver and spleen of the fetus, but after birth it normally occurs only in bone marrow (see Chapter 28). Blood cell production in bone marrow is known as medullary hematopoiesis. It is still a mystery why hematopoiesis is restricted to bone marrow after birth.

Hematopoiesis is a two-stage process that involves mitotic division, or **proliferation,** and maturation, or **differentiation.** Each type of blood cell has parent cells, called **stem cells,** that undergo mitosis when they receive specific biochemical signals indicating that populations of circulating blood cells have diminished to a certain point. The stem cells continue to proliferate until the requisite number of mature daughter cells has entered the circulation. The stem cells of lymphocytes and possibly monocytes are stimulated to proliferate and differentiate by other mechanisms, particularly activation of the immune response, but they, too, originate in bone marrow.

Certain blood cells proliferate and differentiate simultaneously for a period. Proliferation usually ceases after a number of doubling divisions, but differentiation continues. Erythrocytes and neutrophils are usually mature before entering the blood. Monocytes and other leukocytes are not. They enter the bloodstream and continue to mature as they travel to the spleen, peritoneal cavity, and lung.

Hematopoiesis continues throughout life to replace blood cells that grow old and die, are killed by disease,

or are lost through bleeding. Medullary hematopoiesis increases in response to proliferative disease, hemorrhage, hemolytic anemia (in which erythrocytes are destroyed), chronic infection, idiopathic thrombocytopenic purpura (bleeding caused by platelet insufficiency; see Chapter 28), and other disorders that deplete blood cells. In general, long-term stimuli, such as chronic diseases, cause a greater increase in hematopoiesis than acute conditions, such as hemorrhage. Abnormal proliferation of erythrocytes occurs in polycythemia vera, a myeloproliferative disease.

Medullary hematopoiesis can be accelerated by any or all of three mechanisms: (1) conversion of yellow bone marrow, which does not produce blood cells, to red marrow, which does; (2) faster differentiation of daughter cells; and presumably (3) faster proliferation of stem cells. Marrow conversion is stimulated by erythropoietin, the hormone that stimulates erythrocyte production (Maniatis, Tavassoli, & Crosby, 1971). An increase in blood cell production occurs in response to emergencies, such as infection (see the next section).

In adults, extramedullary hematopoiesis—blood cell production in tissues other than bone marrow—is usually a sign of disease. Extramedullary production of one or more types occurs in disease states that affect erythrocytes (e.g., pernicious anemia, sickle cell anemia, thalassemia, hemolytic disease of the newborn [erythroblastosis fetalis], hereditary spherocytosis) and leukocytes (certain leukemias). Extramedullary hematopoiesis of apparently normal blood cells has been reported also to occur in the spleen and liver and, less frequently, in lymph nodes, adrenal glands, cartilage, adipose tissue, intrathoracic areas, and kidneys (Wintrobe et al., 1981).

Stem Cell System

The processes by which blood cells develop from a common ancestor, or stem cell, are known collectively as the **stem cell system.** This system is a hierarchy in which the earliest, most primitive ancestor is the **totipotential hematopoietic stem cell (THSC)** (Fig. 22-5). Because these cells have the potential to develop into many types of blood cells, they are also called multipotential stem cells. One pathway of development leads to various lymphoid tissues, where T and B lymphocytes mature. The other pathway leads to myeloid tissue—the bone marrow. The stem cell of the myeloid pathway is called the pluripotential myeloid stem cell (PMSC), or simply the **pluripotential stem cell.** The pluripotential stem cell triggers differentiation of (1) neutrophils and monocytes, (2) eosinophils, (3) erythrocytes, and (4) platelets (Fig. 22-5).

Blood cell production in any one pathway requires numerous amplifying cell divisions coupled with complex maturation changes to produce the mature cells

FIG. 22-5 **Bone marrow and stem cell systems.** Probable pathways of differentiation, from the toti-potential stem cell to mature blood cells.

that are released into the blood. Regulation of hemato-poiesis is achieved by two interacting control systems (Metcalf, 1991). The first is specialized stromal cells in the marrow that control some of the cellular events in hematopoiesis by "cell contact processes" or by the production of short-range regulatory molecules (Metcalf, 1991). A second control system involves the interaction of a group of regulatory molecules or cytokines called **hematopoietic growth factors** or **colony-stimulating factors** (CSFs), which stimulate the proliferation of progenitor cells and their progeny and initiate the maturation events necessary to produce fully mature cells (Metcalf, 1991). Specific humoral CSFs are necessary for the adequate growth of myeloid, erythroid, lymphoid, and megakaryocytic pathways (Table 22-4 and Fig. 22-6).

Clinical Uses of CSFs

Blood granulocyte numbers (e.g., eosinophils, neutrophils, basophils/mast cells) are normally in the range of 4000 to 6000 cells per microliter, and susceptibility to

infection develops below 1000 cells per microliter. During a natural response to a bacterial infection, granulocytes usually rise to 10,000 to 20,000 cells per microliter. The CSFs can raise white cell numbers even higher. No advantage, however, is gained from extreme numbers because of the formation of toxic products and tissue damage (Metcalf, 1991). Colony-stimulating factors have been studied in individuals with subnormal hematopoiesis either as a result of diseases such as acquired immune deficiency syndrome (AIDS), aplastic anemia, or congenital neutropenia or as a consequence of cytotoxic therapy for cancer, including lymphoma and leukemia. The CSFs can stimulate increases in granulocyte-macrocyte populations in such individuals, but responses are quantitatively restricted if the available numbers of stem and progenitor cells have been drastically depleted by chemotherapy or disease (Metcalf, 1991). Responses to CSF treatment are evident from the corrections of a preexisting disorder, for example, in congenital neutropenia or hematopoietic response after

FIG. 22-6 Physiologic effects of some CSFs.

TABLE 22-4

Human CSFs

CSF	Cell origin	Cell stimulated
M-CSF	Macrophage, fibroblast	Macrophage
GM-CSF	T cell, macrophage, fibroblast	Neutrophil, macrophage, eosinophil
G-CSF	Macrophage, fibroblast	Neutrophil, eosinophil, basophil
IL-3	T cell	Neutrophil, macrophage
Erythropoietin	Kupffer and peritubular kidney cells	Erythrocyte

Data from Metcalf, 1991; Rowe & Rapoport, 1992.
M-CSF, macrophage; *GM-CSF*, granulocyte-macrophage; *G-CSF*, granulocyte; *IL-3*, interleukin-3.

cytotoxic therapy (e.g., after bone marrow transplantation). Colony-stimulating factor treatment can result in shorter periods of intensive nursing and hospitalization (Metcalf, 1991).

Bone Marrow

Bone marrow, also called myeloid tissue (*myelos* = marrow), is confined to the cavities of bone. Bone marrow consists of blood vessels, nerves, mononuclear phagocytes, stem cells, blood cells in various stages of differentiation, and fatty tissue. Adults have two kinds of bone marrow: red, or active (hematopoietic), marrow

and yellow, or inactive, marrow. The large quantities of fat in inactive marrow make it yellow. Not all bones contain active marrow. In adults there is active marrow in the pelvic bones (34%), vertebrae (28%), cranium and mandible (13%), sternum and ribs (10%), and extreme proximal portions of the humerus and femur (4% to 8%) (Russell, Yoshinaga, Shigetoshi, & Mizuno, 1966). Inactive marrow predominates in cavities of other bones. (Bones are discussed further in Chapter 38.)

Stem cells in hematopoietic marrow receive the oxygen and nutrients they need for mitosis and maturation from the primary or nutrient arteries of the bones. Branches of these arteries terminate in a capillary network that coalesces into large venous sinuses, which eventually drain into a central vein. Hematopoietic marrow and fat fill the spaces surrounding the network of venous sinuses. Some mechanism of transport enables the newly produced blood cells to traverse narrow openings in venous sinus walls and thus enter the circulation. It is not known whether the movement of the new blood cells forces an opening or whether certain sites open in response to the presence of the newly formed cells. Normally, cells do not enter the circulation until they have differentiated to a certain extent, but premature release is known to occur in certain diseases.

Development of Erythrocytes

For almost 100 years, it was believed that erythrocytes developed from lymphocytes that were transformed in the spleen. It was not until the 1850s that the bone marrow was accepted as the site of **erythropoiesis** (Wintrobe et al., 1981). It is now known that erythrocytes are derived from precursor cells called **erythroblasts** (Fig. 22-7). Normal erythroblasts are also called **normoblasts,** whereas abnormal ones are called **megaloblasts.**

Erythrocyte development is shown in detail in Fig. 22-7. The proerythroblast (pronormoblast) possesses a huge nucleus, is rich in ribosomes, and can synthesize protein. The signal that causes an increase in circulating erythrocytes is the glycoprotein erythropoietin. Erythropoietin stimulates uncommitted stem cells to differentiate into proerythroblasts (Quesenberry, 1992; Rowe & Rapoport, 1992; Wintrobe et al., 1981). Whether hemoglobin has been synthesized at this stage is controversial. Hemoglobin is, however, readily apparent and increases in quantity as nuclear size shrinks throughout the basophilic and polychromatophilic stages. The orthochromatic erythroblast (normoblast) is the smallest of the nucleated erythrocyte precursors. Once the nucleus is lost, the cell that remains is called a **reticulocyte.** Although it lacks a nucleus, the reticulocyte contains polyribosomes (for globin synthesis) and mitochondria (for oxidative metabolism and heme synthesis). The reticulocyte matures to an erythrocyte

FIG. 22-7 Erythrocyte differentiation. Erythrocyte differentiation from large, nucleated stem cell to small, nonnucleated erythrocyte.

within 24 to 48 hours. During this period, mitochondria and ribosomes disappear, and the cell becomes smaller and more disklike. With these final changes, the erythrocyte loses its capacity for hemoglobin synthesis and oxidative metabolism.

Reticulocytes remain in the marrow approximately 1 day and then are released into the venous sinuses before maturation is complete. Reticulocytes continue to mature in the bloodstream and may travel to the spleen for several days of additional maturation. The normal reticulocyte count is 1% of the total red blood cell count. Approximately 1% of the body's circulating erythrocyte mass normally is generated every 24 hours. Therefore the reticulocyte count is a useful clinical index of erythropoietic activity and indicates whether new red cells are being produced. The concept "erythron" has been used to describe all the tissues that produce erythrocytes and their precursors. Thus included in this term are stem cells, all stages of developing erythrocytes, and mature red blood cells.

One of the most significant advances in the hematopoietic growth factors has been the development of erythropoietin for use in individuals with chronic renal failure. In 1986, large amounts of recombinant human erythropoietin (rhEpo) became widely available for clinical research (Rowe & Rapoport, 1992). Erythropoietin has been used to correct the anemia of chronic renal failure. Several researchers at present are evaluating the use of rhEpo in individuals with AIDS as well as enhancing the ability of individuals to donate blood for blood transfusions (Rowe & Rapoport, 1992).

Hemoglobin Synthesis

Hemoglobin, the oxygen-carrying protein of the erythrocyte, constitutes approximately 90% of the cell's dry weight. The cytoplasm of a single erythrocyte can contain as much as 300 hemoglobin molecules. Hemoglobin enables the blood to transport 100 times more oxygen than could be transported dissolved in plasma alone. Hemoglobin is not one but a family of molecules whose members differ slightly in primary structure.

FIG. 22-8 Molecular structure of hemoglobin. Molecule is spherical tetramer weighing approximately 64,500 daltons. It contains a pair of α polypeptide and a pair of β polypeptide chains and several heme groups.

Nonetheless, each member is composed of two pairs of polypeptide chains (the **globins**) and four colorful complexes of iron plus protoporphyrin (the **hemes**) (Fig. 22-8).

Hemoglobin synthesis is precisely coordinated by mechanisms not completely understood. Three requisites for hemoglobin synthesis are (1) formation of protoporphyrin, (2) availability of iron (heme), and (3) generation of the proteinaceous globin. Several genes dictate the synthesis of globin in maturing human erythroblasts, each gene resulting in the formation of a structurally different polypeptide chain (alpha, beta, gamma, delta, epsilon, or zeta). Each polypeptide chain contains approximately 150 amino acids and is arranged in the knotted-sausage configuration shown in Fig. 22-8. The chains assemble to form a tetrahedron containing two pairs of identical chains. Hemoglobin A, the most common type of hemoglobin in adults, is com-

TABLE 22-5

Structure of Normal Hemoglobin Molecules

Type of hemoglobin (Hb)	Identity of polypeptide chain	Significance
Hb A	$\alpha_2\beta_2$	92% of adult Hb
Hb A$_{1c}$	$\alpha_2(\beta$-NH-glucose)	5% of adult Hb; increased in diabetes (see Chapter 19)
Hb A$_2$	$\alpha_2\delta_2$	2% of adult Hb; increased in β-thalassemia (see Chapter 23)
Hb F	$\alpha_2\gamma_2$	Major fetal Hb from the third through ninth month of gestation; promotes oxygen transfer across platelets; increase in β-thalassemia
Hb Gower I	ϵ_4 or $\zeta_2\epsilon_2$	Present in early embryo; function unknown
Hb Gower 2	$\alpha_2\epsilon_2$	Present in early embryo; function unknown
Hb Portland	$\zeta_2\gamma_2$	Present in early embryo; function unknown

Modified from Bunn, H.F. (1977). Hemoglobin I structure and function. In W.S. Beck (Ed.), *Hematology* (2nd ed.). Cambridge, MA: MIT Press.

TABLE 22-6

Nutritional Requirements for Erythropoiesis

Nutrient	Role in erythropoiesis	Consequence of deficiency
Protein (amino acids)	Structural component of plasma membrane	Decreased strength, elasticity, and flexibility of membrane; hemolytic anemia
	Synthesis of hemoglobin	Decreased erythropoiesis and lifespan of erythrocytes
Cobalamin (vitamin B$_{12}$)	Synthesis of DNA, maturation of erythrocytes, facilitator of folate metabolism	Macrocytic (megaloblastic) anemia
Folate (folic acid)	Synthesis of DNA and RNA, maturation of erythrocytes	Macrocytic (megaloblastic) anemia
Vitamin B$_6$ (pyridoxine)	Heme synthesis	Hypochromic-microcytic anemia
Vitamin B$_2$ (riboflavin)	Oxidative reactions	Normochromic-normocytic anemia
Vitamin C (ascorbic acid)	Iron metabolism, acts as a reducing agent to maintain iron in its ferrous (Fe^{++}) form	Normochromic-normocytic anemia
Pantothenic acid	Heme synthesis	Unknown in humans*
Niacin	None, but needed for respiration in mature erythrocytes	Unknown in humans
Vitamin E	Heme synthesis (?); protection against oxidative damage in mature erythrocytes	Hemolytic anemia with increased cell membrane fragility; shortens lifespan of erythrocytes in individual with cystic fibrosis
Iron	Hemoglobin synthesis	Iron deficiency anemia
Copper	Required for optimal mobilization of iron from tissues to plasma	Hypochromic-microcytic anemia

From Wintrobe, 1981; Williams, Beutler, Erslev, & Lichtman, 1990.
*Although pantothenic acid is important for optimal synthesis of heme, experimentally induced deficiency *failed* to produce anemia or other hematopoietic disturbances.

posed of two alpha and two beta polypeptide chains. Seven different types of hemoglobin have been identified in healthy human blood at all stages, from fetal life to adulthood, testimony to the heterogeneity of the molecule (Table 22-5). The timing of synthesis and relative amount of each type of hemoglobin are determined by complex developmental processes.

Heme is a large, flat, iron-protoporphyrin disk that is capable of carrying one molecule of oxygen (O_2). Recall that hemoglobin contains four heme groups; thus it is capable of carrying four oxygen molecules. Through a series of complex biochemical reactions, protoporphyrin, a complex four-ringed molecule, is produced and abounds with ferrous iron. The biochemical reactions of heme synthesis include condensation, oxidation, and reduction, all of which are powered by catalytic enzymes. It is crucial that the iron be correctly charged. Presence of the reduced ferrous iron (Fe_2^{++}) allows the formation of normal hemoglobin, which is capable of binding oxygen where it is plentiful (in the lungs) and releasing it where it is less plentiful (in the tissues). Oxidized ferric iron (Fe_3^{+++}) carries an extra positive charge and results in the formation of **methemoglobin,** an unstable type of hemoglobin that is not capable of binding oxygen. An excess of ferric iron occurs in the presence of certain drugs and chemicals, such as nitrates and sulfonamides.

Hemoglobin that is carrying oxygen is called **oxyhemoglobin.** If all four oxygen-binding sites on the oxyhemoglobin's hemes are occupied by oxygen, the molecule is said to be saturated. Oxyhemoglobin that has released its oxygen or is not bound to oxygen for some other reason is called reduced hemoglobin, or **deoxyhemoglobin.**

Nutritional Requirements for Erythropoiesis

Normal development of erythrocytes and synthesis of hemoglobin depend on an optimal biochemical milieu and adequate supplies of the necessary building blocks, including protein, vitamins, and minerals (Table 22-6). If these components are lacking, it is usually the result of a nutritional deficiency or a metabolic imbalance in which other organs or tissues use up a disproportionate share of these nutrients or are unable to absorb the needed nutrients (Wintrobe et al., 1981). If abnormal distribution of nutrients is prolonged, erythrocyte production slows, and anemia (insufficient numbers of functional erythrocytes) may result (see Chapter 23).

Protein is an important structural component of the erythrocyte's plasma membrane, contributing to its strength, flexibility, and elasticity. Amino acid chains form hemoglobin. Without proteins and amino acids, erythrocyte production decreases, and the lifespan of cells that are produced may be shortened because of structural defects (Delmonte, Aschkenasy, & Eyquem,

1964). One of the most important proteins is **intrinsic factor (IF)**, a glycoprotein necessary for gastrointestinal absorption of vitamin B_{12}. Lack of vitamin B_{12} causes pernicious anemia. Intrinsic factor is secreted by the parietal cells in the gastric mucosa and facilitates vitamin B_{12} uptake at its absorptive site, the ileum.

Erythropoiesis cannot proceed in the absence of vitamins, especially B_{12}, folate (folic acid), B_6, riboflavin, pantothenic acid, niacin, ascorbic acid, and vitamin E. Vitamin B_{12} is a large molecule; therefore it requires assistance from IF to penetrate the gastrointestinal mucosa. Once absorbed, vitamin B_{12} is stored in the liver and used as needed in erythropoiesis.

Folate is the second most important vitamin for erythrocyte production and maturation. Folate is necessary for deoxyribonucleic acid (DNA) synthesis, being a component of three of the four DNA bases (thymine, adenine, and guanine). Folate is also needed for ribonucleic acid (RNA) synthesis. Intrinsic factor is not required for folate absorption, which occurs principally in the upper small intestine. Folate is stored in and circulates through the liver. Folate deficiency is more common than vitamin B_{12} deficiency and occurs more rapidly. Folate stores can be depleted within a few months, whereas vitamin B_{12} depletion can take years. Folate supplements are prescribed for pregnant women because pregnancy increases the demand for folate and deficiency can cause anemia.

Iron Cycle

Approximately 67% of total body iron is bound to heme in erythrocytes and muscle cells, and approximately 30% is stored bound to ferritin or hemosiderin mononuclear phagocytes (i.e., macrophages) and hepatic parenchymal cells. The remaining 3% (less than 1 mg) is lost daily in urine, sweat, bile, and epithelial cells shed from the gut. Iron not lost is continuously recycled as shown in Fig. 22-9. Recycling is made possible by **transferrin,** a glycoprotein synthesized primarily by the liver but also by tissue macrophages, submaxillary and mammary glands, and ovaries or testes.

Dietary iron is absorbed primarily in the duodenum and proximal jejunum. Some of it passes into the bloodstream, and the rest is sequestered in intestinal epithelial cells as ferritin. This iron is lost when epithelial cells are sloughed off in the intestinal lumen. Iron that is released to the bloodstream is picked up by transferrin, which is the body's major iron-transport molecule. Iron for hemoglobin production is delivered to erythroblasts in erythropoietic bone marrow. Under normal conditions, only one third of the iron-binding sites on transferrin molecules are occupied.

It is postulated that iron is transferred from transferrin to erythroblasts in the marrow as follows: (1) the transferrin–iron complex binds to a receptor on the

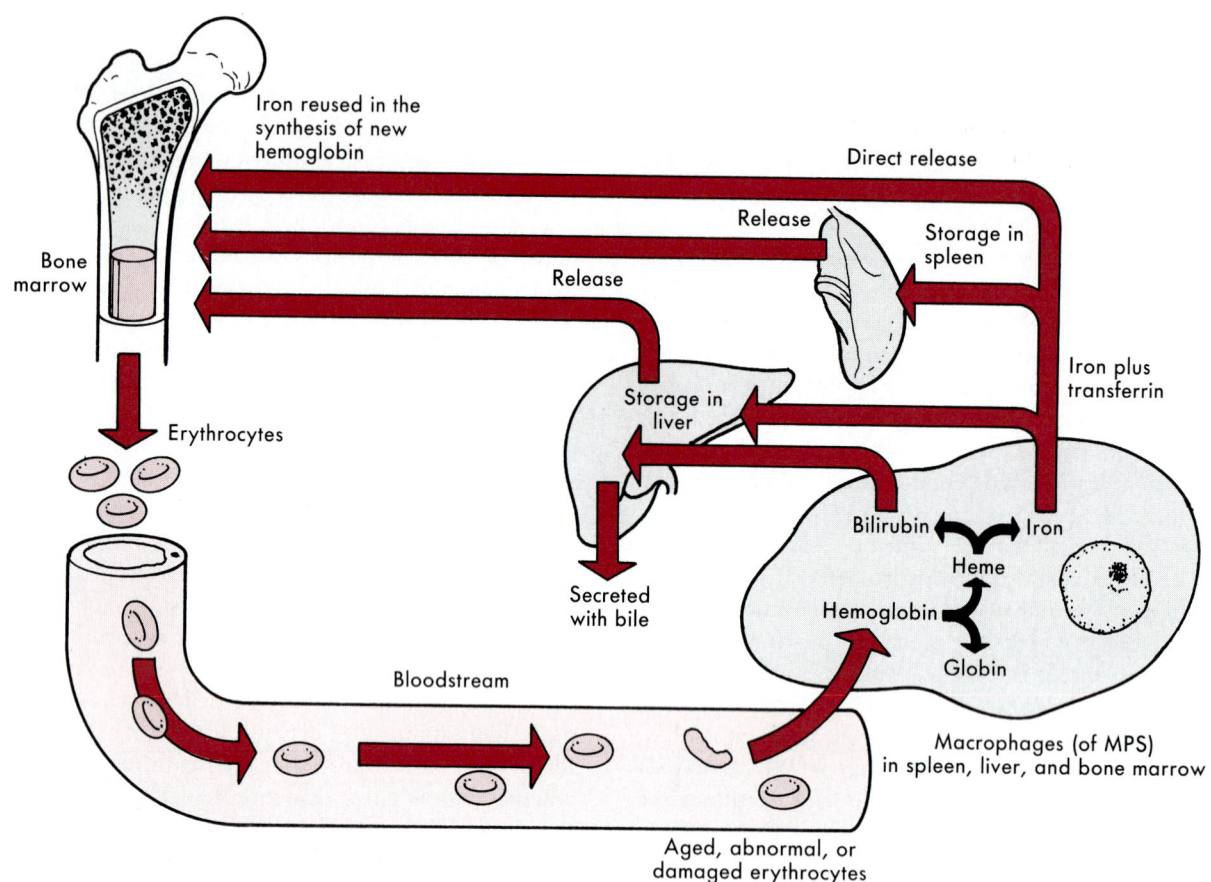

FIG. 22-9 Iron cycle. Iron *(Fe)* released from gastrointestinal epithelial cells circulates in bloodstream associated with its plasma carrier, transferrin. It is delivered to erythroblasts in bone marrow, where most of it is incorporated into hemoglobin. Mature erythrocytes circulate for approximately 120 days, after which they become senescent and are removed by MPS. Macrophages of MPS (mostly in spleen) break down ingested erythrocytes and return iron to bloodstream directly or after storing it as ferritin or hemosiderin.

erythroblast's plasma membrane; (2) the complex moves into the cell, possibly by active transport; (3) iron is released (dissociated) from transferrin; and (4) the dissociated transferrin is returned to the bloodstream (Fig. 22-9) (Guyton, 1992; Wintrobe et al., 1981). Another source of iron for erythropoiesis is the iron stored by ferritin and hemosiderin in the cytoplasm of mononuclear phagocytes (macrophages) resident in the marrow. Once the iron is released into the marrow and incorporated into the erythroblast's mitochondria, the enzyme heme synthetase inserts ferrous iron into protoporphyrin to form heme. Heme then is bound to globin to form hemoglobin. Iron not used in erythropoiesis is stored temporarily as ferritin or hemosiderin and later excreted.

After mature erythrocytes have circulated for 120 days, they are removed from the bloodstream by macrophages of the MPS—chiefly in the spleen. Within the phagolysosomes (digestive vacuole) of the macrophage, the erythrocyte is catabolized and the iron in hemoglo-

bin is oxidized, forming Fe_3^{+++} (methemoglobin). The heme and globin of methemoglobin dissociate easily, and globin may be reduced to its component amino acids. The iron released by methemoglobin dissociation is stored in the macrophage's cytoplasm as ferritin or hemosiderin or released into the bloodstream, where it is free to bind again to transferrin (Fig. 22-9). A minute amount of iron is stored in muscle cells by the heme-containing protein myoglobin. Unavailable stores of iron are present in cytochromes, catalases, and peroxidase enzymes.

Iron balance is achieved through mechanisms controlling its absorption rather than its excretion. Regulation of iron transport across the plasma membrane of gastrointestinal epithelial cells is related to the cell's iron content and the overall rate of erythropoiesis. If the body's iron stores are low or the demand for erythropoiesis is increased, iron passes rapidly through the epithelial cell and into the plasma, probably by mechanisms of active transport. (Transport mechanisms are described in Chapter 1.) If body stores are high and erythropoiesis is not increased, iron crosses the epithelial cell's plasma membrane passively and is stored there bound to ferritin. Excretion of iron occurs when the epithelial cells of the intestinal mucosa slough off.

Regulation of Erythropoiesis

In healthy humans, the total volume of circulating erythrocytes remains surprisingly constant. The feedback mechanism that maintains an optimal population of erythrocytes is mediated by erythropoietin. Erythropoietin induces the selective proliferation and differentiation of proerythroblasts (see Fig. 22-7). Its earliest effects are to stimulate RNA synthesis, after either binding to receptors on the erythroblast's plasma membrane or entrance into the cell. Hemoglobin synthesis begins hours after initial stimulation by erythropoietin.

Erythropoietin is secreted by the kidney in response to tissue hypoxia (Fig. 22-10). Erythropoietin causes a compensatory increase in erythrocyte production if the oxygen content of blood decreases because of anemia, high altitude, or pulmonary disease. The normal steady-state rate of production of approximately 2.5 million erythrocytes per second in humans can increase up to about 17 million per second under anemic or low-oxygen states (Goldwasser, 1990). The receptors that detect hypoxia are within the kidney because production of erythropoietin is known to increase after renal artery constriction, which reduces oxygen supply to renal cells (Fisher, Samuels, & Langston, 1967; Goldwasser, 1990). Unlike the peripheral chemoreceptors of the carotid body and aortic arch that send messengers to the brain to increase respiration in individuals with hypoxia, receptors in the kidney are on cells that synthesize and secrete erythropoietin. Thus the body responds to reduced oxygenation of blood in two ways: (1) by increasing intake of oxygen through increased respiration and (2) by increasing the oxygen-carrying capacity of the blood through increased erythropoiesis. Erythropoietin not only stimulates proliferation of committed stem cells in the marrow but also accelerates maturation of existing erythroblasts. (Erythropoiesis is also discussed in the hematopoiesis section.)

Normal Destruction of Senescent Erythrocytes

Although mature erythrocytes lack nuclei, mitochondria, and endoplasmic reticulum, they do have cytoplasmic enzymes capable of glycolysis (anaerobic glucose metabolism) and production of small quantities of adenosine triphosphate (ATP). The ATP provides the energy necessary to keep the cell alive and its plasma membrane pliable (see Fig. 22-1). Metabolic processes diminish as the erythrocyte ages. Consequently, less ATP is available to maintain the functions essential for life. The senescent red cell becomes increasingly fragile and loses

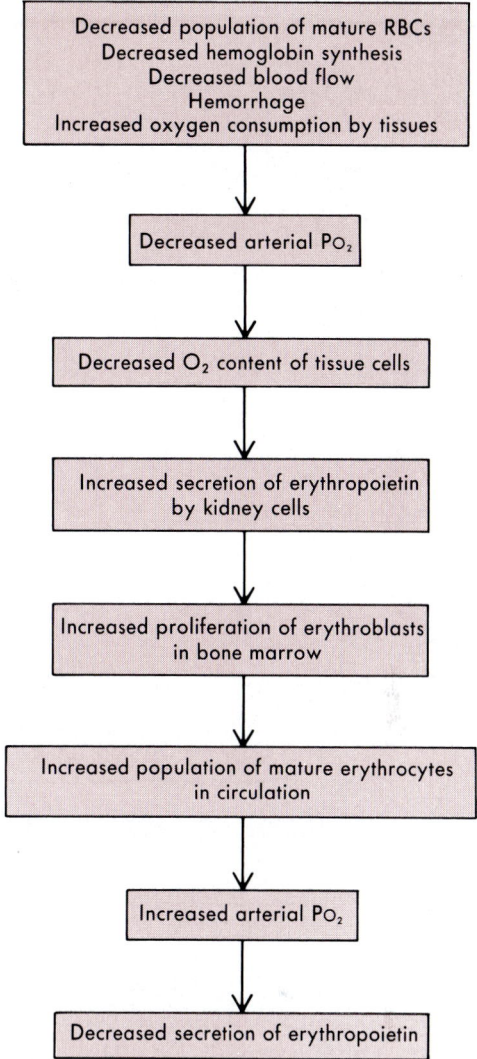

Decreased arterial oxygen levels stimulate production of erythropoietin, which in turn stimulates red cell production and expansion of the erythron. The increase in red cells frequently corrects the problem of low oxygen levels (hypoxia). This restoration to normal oxygen levels alerts the kidney to stop producing erythropoietin (negative feedback). Further erythrocyte production is not needed.

FIG. 22-10 Role of erythropoietin in regulation of erythropoiesis. P_{O_2}, Partial pressure of oxygen in the blood (see Chapter 29).

its property of reversible deformability. Its membrane therefore is susceptible to rupture during passage through narrowed regions of the microcirculation.

Aged red cells are selectively sequestered and destroyed by macrophages of the MPS, primarily in the spleen. If the spleen is dysfunctional or absent, macrophages in the liver (Kupffer cells) take over. The signal that identifies an erythrocyte as senescent and ready for disposal by the MPS is not known. Alterations in the erythrocyte's plasma membrane, including altered ionic

FIG. 22-11 Metabolism of bilirubin released by heme breakdown.

and osmotic gradients across it and a decrease in its electrical charge, and an increase in methemoglobin within the erythrocyte all accompany cellular aging. These factors may contribute to sluggish erythrocyte movement through the spleen and other lymphoid tissues, increasing opportunities for phagocytosis by resident macrophages.

Phagocytosis of the erythrocyte is followed by its digestion by proteolytic and lipolytic enzymes within the phagolysosome of the macrophage. Globin is broken down into amino acids, and iron is recycled (see Fig. 22-9). Porphyrin is reduced to bilirubin, which is transported to the liver, conjugated, and finally excreted in the bile as glucuronide (Fig. 22-11). Approximately 6 g of hemoglobin is catabolized daily, producing 200 mg of bilirubin. (Liver function is described in Chapter 35.) Bacteria in the intestinal lumen transform conjugated bilirubin into urobilinogen. A small portion of this urobilinogen is reabsorbed, to be either metabolized further by the liver or excreted by the kidney into the urine. Most of the urobilinogen is excreted in feces.

Conditions causing accelerated erythrocyte destruc-tion increase the load of bilirubin for hepatic clearance, leading to increased serum levels of unconjugated bilirubin and increased urinary excretion of urobilinogen. Gallstones (cholelithiasis) can result from a chronically elevated rate of bilirubin excretion.

Development of Leukocytes

All of the leukocytes arise from stem cells in the bone marrow (their pathways of differentiation are shown in Fig. 22-5). The granulocytes (neutrophils, eosinophils, and basophils/mast cells) normally mature fully in the marrow and then are released into the bloodstream. The agranulocytes (monocytes and lymphocytes), however, are released into the bloodstream before they undergo their final phase of maturation. The monocytes mature into macrophages within a day or two of release, and the lymphocytes travel to lymphoid tissues, where they are stimulated to differentiate into T cells or B cells (see Chapter 6).

The bone marrow exhibits selective retention of immature granulocytes. Hematopoietic growth factors, granulocyte-macrophage colony–stimulating factor

(GM-CSF), and granulocyte colony–stimulating factor (G-CSF) are required for granulocyte growth and differentiation. Although the biologic effects of GM-CSF and G-CSF depend on binding to specific progenitor cell surfaces, the signaling pathway remains poorly understood (Rowe & Rapoport, 1992). Because elevated blood levels of G-CSF, but not GM-CSF, are seen with infections, G-CSF may be more important as a signal for neutrophils. (Remember neutrophils are always increased with infection.)

Maintenance of optimal levels of granulocytes and monocytes in the blood depends on the availability of pluripotential stem cells in the marrow, induction of these into committed stem cells, and timely release of new cells from the marrow. The marrow contains a reserve pool that can be rapidly mobilized in response to the body's needs. Once cells are released from the marrow, they join the marginating pool or the circulating pool. The cells in the marginating pool lie along the capillary walls and can move into tissues and mucous membranes. Cells from the circulating pool join the marginating pool to replace the cells that have migrated out of the capillaries. Leukocyte production increases in response to infection, to the presence of steroids, and to reduction or depletion of reserves in the marrow. It is also associated with strenuous exercise, convulsive seizures, heat, intense radiation, paroxysmal tachycardias, pain, nausea and vomiting, and anxiety (Wintrobe, 1986).

Normally, some leukocytes are lost in saliva, urine, the lungs, liver, spleen, and gastrointestinal tract. Most exist in the body from days to years, depending on type (Table 22-2).

Development of Platelets

Platelets (thrombocytes) develop from megakaryocytes by a unique process of proliferation termed endomitosis (see Fig. 22-5). In endomitosis, the megakaryocyte undergoes the nuclear phase of cellular division (mitosis) but fails to undergo the cytoplasmic phase (cytokinesis) (see Chapter 1). Without cytokinesis, the cell does not divide into two daughter cells. Rather, the megakaryocyte expands to accommodate the doubling of its DNA (nuclear) content, and breaks up into fragments known as platelets.

An optimal number of platelets and committed platelet precursors (megakaryoblasts) in the bone marrow are maintained in part by the actions of GM-CSF and interleukin-3 (IL-3) that presumably bind to plasma membranes of pluripotential stem cells in the bone marrow, causing them to become committed megakaryoblasts. Granulocyte-macrophage colony–stimulating factor and IL-3 stimulate committed cells at further stages of differentiation to differentiate faster. Rates of the processes of megakaryocyte development, endomi-

tosis, and platelet release are increased (Rowe & Rapoport, 1992).

Platelets, once released, circulate for 10 days before they begin to lose their capacity to carry out biochemical reactions. The initial alteration of function is possibly attributable to proteolytic enzymes present at sites of chronic vascular inflammation. (See Chapter 7 for a discussion of biochemicals involved in inflammation.) Senescent platelets are phagocytosed by neutrophils and monocytes if they are circulating freely or by neutrophils and macrophages if they are part of a clot, or thrombus. Senescent platelets may be removed also by tissue macrophages of the MPS in the liver or spleen.

MECHANISMS OF HEMOSTASIS

Hemostasis means arrest of bleeding. Mechanisms of hemostasis maintain a relatively steady state of blood volume, pressure, and flow through injured blood vessels. Hemostasis after vascular damage and bleeding involves a complex sequence of events: (1) vasoconstriction (vasospasm), (2) formation of a platelet plug, (3) activation of the coagulation (or clotting) cascade, and (4) formation of a blood clot. All four of these events are necessary for hemostasis, and all four involve platelets or clotting factors or both in some way.

Function of Platelets

Mechanisms of platelet participation include adherence of platelets to injured vessel walls; platelet degranulation, which releases biochemical mediators; and platelet aggregation into clumps, or plugs. Normally, platelets circulate freely, suspended in plasma, and do not adhere to endothelial cells that line the vessels. When a vessel is damaged, however, collagen-containing subendothelial tissue is exposed. Collagen attracts platelets out of the plasma within 15 to 20 seconds after injury. The platelets adhere rapidly to this "foreign" surface, after which they undergo dynamic changes in shape, develop protrusions (pseudopods), and degranulate, releasing a variety of potent biochemicals (Fig. 22-12).

Several factors affect platelet adherence to exposed subendothelial tissues. The platelets must contain sufficient concentrations of calcium to change shape, aggregate, degranulate, and activate arachidonic pathways. Evidence suggests that calcium within platelets activates degranulation. Erythrocytes apparently increase the rate of platelet adherence by facilitating migration of circulating platelets toward vascular surfaces and by liberating adenosine diphosphate (ADP), which enables platelets to stick to exposed collagen.

Two of the biochemical mediators released by adhered platelets have immediate effects on smooth muscle in the vascular endothelium. These mediators, sero-

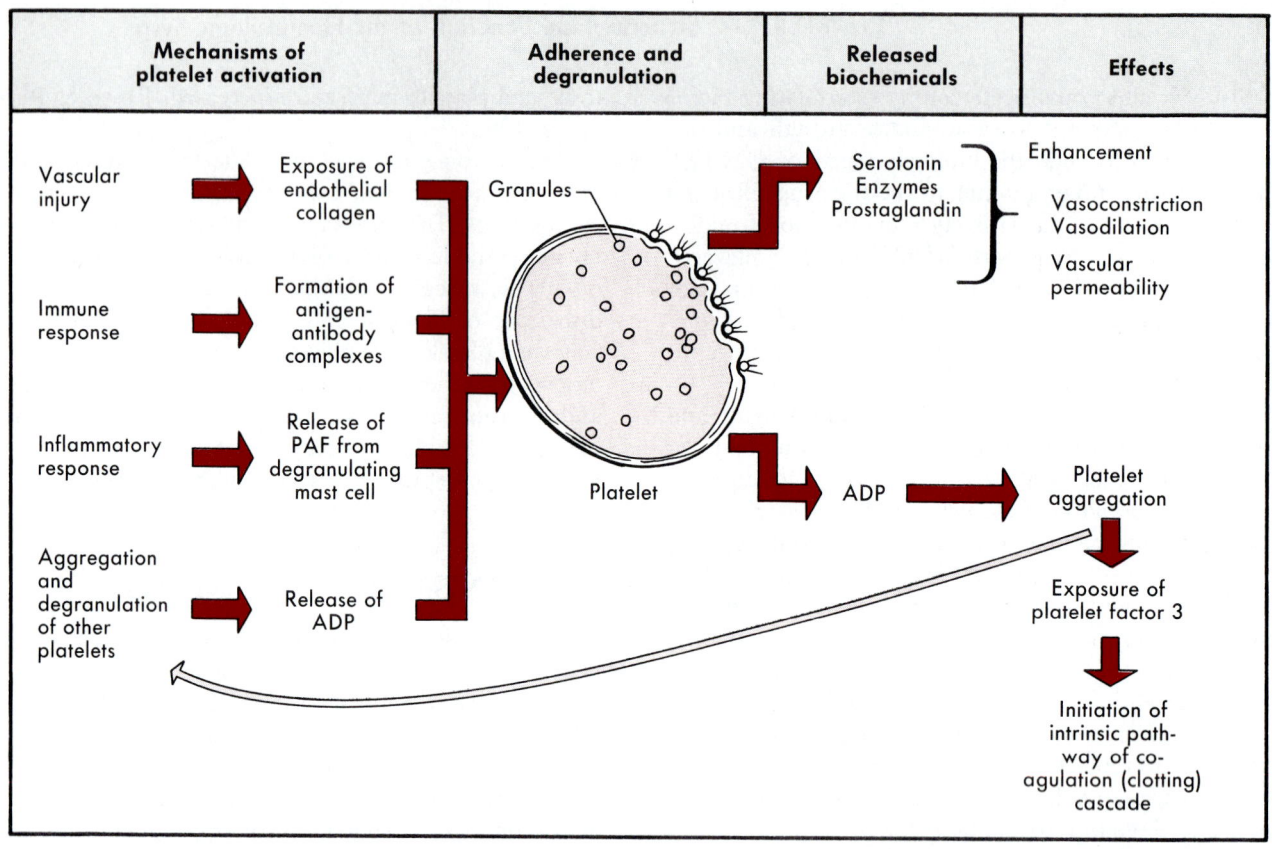

Mechanisms of platelet activation	Adherence and degranulation	Released biochemicals	Effects

FIG. 22-12 Platelet degranulation. *PAF,* platelet-activating factor.

FIG. 22-13 Main steps in blood clotting. A, Platelet aggregation at site of injury, formation of thrombin from prothrombin, and fibrin clot with trapped red cells. **B,** Mesh of fibrin forming a clot. (**A,** from Thibodeau, 1987; **B,** from Raven, P. H., & Johnson, G. B. [1989]. *Biology.* [2nd ed.]. St. Louis: Mosby–Year Book.)

tonin and histamine, cause an immediate temporary constriction of the injured vessel. Vasoconstriction reduces blood flow and thereby diminishes bleeding. (Vasoconstriction is also produced by local reflexes of the nervous system.) Vasodilation soon follows, permitting the inflammatory response to proceed. (The inflammatory response is necessary for healing; see Chapter 7.)

Other biochemical mediators released by degranulation (also called the platelet-release reaction) either promote or inhibit platelet activity and the eventual process of clot formation (see Fig. 7-8). Adenosine diphosphate promotes the adherence and subsequent degranulation of nearby platelets by causing their plasma membranes to become ruffly and sticky. The new activated platelets also adhere to the exposed collagen, causing a platelet plug to seal the injured endothelium. If the effects of ADP were not counteracted and laminar flow were not sufficient, platelet aggregation could continue indefinitely. This eventuality is prevented by two mutually antagonistic prostaglandin derivatives, thromboxane A_2 (TxA_2) and prostacyclin I_2 (PGI_2). Thromboxane A_2 is synthesized and released by degranulating platelets. It causes vasoconstriction and promotes the degranulation of other platelets, which then release more ADP. Prostacyclin I_2 is synthesized and released by uninjured endothelial cells in vessel walls. It is a thromboxane antagonist: it inhibits the effects of TxA_2 by promoting vasodilation and inhibiting platelet degranulation. The net effect of TxA_2 and PGI_2 is to permit platelet aggregation to proceed at the site of injury while preventing adherence to normal vascular endothelium (Fischbach & Fogdall, 1981). Heparin-neutralizing factor (platelet factor 4), which is also released by degranulating platelets, enhances clot formation at the site of injury.

If blood vessel injury is minor, hemostasis is achieved temporarily by the platelet plug, which usually forms within 3 to 5 minutes of injury. Platelet plugs seal the many minute ruptures that occur daily in the microcirculation, particularly in capillaries. In the absence of sufficient numbers of platelets, numerous small hemorrhagic areas called purpuras develop under the skin and throughout the tissues (see Chapters 24 and 25). The plug becomes stable during the process of clot formation.

Function of Clotting Factors

Clot formation is the third major event of hemostasis, following vasoconstriction and formation of the platelet plug. A **blood clot** is a meshwork of protein strands that stabilizes the platelet plug and traps other cells, such as erythrocytes, phagocytes, and microorganisms (Fig. 22-13). The strands are made of fibrin. Unlike platelets, which are formed elements of the blood, fibrin is not normally present in the circulation. Rather,

it is the end product of the **coagulation cascade,** a series of enzymatic reactions among the clotting factors (Fig. 22-14). During the coagulation cascade, clotting factors in the blood are activated and transformed, in turn, until fibrin is produced. (Characteristics of the clotting factors are listed in Table 22-7.) In effect, soluble clotting factors become insoluble fibrin.

The coagulation cascade is initiated through two mechanisms. The intrinsic pathway is activated when Hageman factor (factor XII) in plasma comes into contact with subendothelial substances exposed by vascular injury. The extrinsic pathway is activated when tissue thromboplastin, a substance released by damaged endothelial cells, comes into contact with one of the clotting factors, serum prothrombin conversion factor (factor VII). Both pathways lead to a final common pathway when each has activated factor X (Stuart-Prower factor). The common pathway proceeds to clot formation.

Control of Hemostatic Mechanisms

The major regulatory events in the clotting processes, including the activation of the clotting factors, the inhibition of these active clotting factors, and the production of circulating anticoagulant proteins, takes place on membrane surfaces. The endothelium is a major site of hemostasis. Despite the continual presence of clotting factors and platelets in the circulation, blood normally remains fluid. Two properties of normal vascular endothelium prevent clotting. The first is the smooth texture of the endothelial lining, which prevents adherence of platelets. The second is the negative charge of protein in the endothelial cells, which repels some negatively charged platelets and clotting factors. Damage to the vascular endothelium destroys both of these properties, enabling platelets to adhere and initiating the intrinsic pathway of coagulation.

Once activated, the processes of coagulation are controlled by anticoagulants, some of which are products of the coagulation cascade itself. For example, once a clot has formed, its fibrin strands absorb 85% to 90% of the thrombin subsequently produced at the site. The remaining thrombin is inactivated rapidly by antithrombin III, another plasma protein. Other anticoagulants, most notably heparin, are produced and secreted locally by tissue mast cells and basophils that have been activated by the injury (see Chapter 7). Heparin not only halts the coagulation cascade but also enhances thrombin absorption by fibrin in the clot.

Retraction and Lysis of Blood Clots

After a clot is formed, it retracts, or "solidifies." Clot retraction is the final stage of hemostasis. Fibrin strands shorten, becoming denser and stronger. This helps to approximate the edges of the injured vessel wall and seal

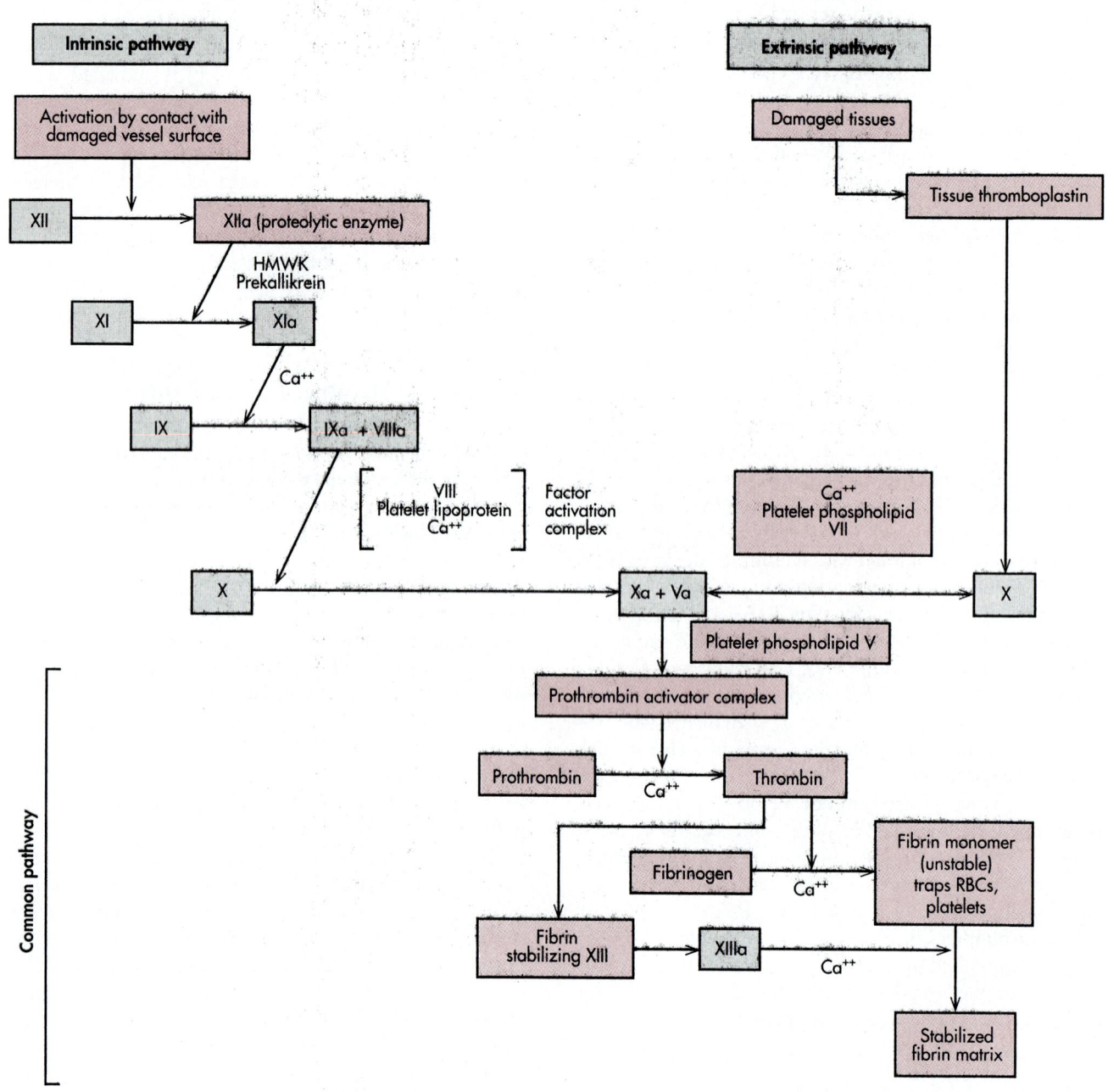

FIG. 22-14 The coagulation cascade.

TABLE 22-7

Clotting Factors

International nomenclature	Synonyms	Substance	Source	Enzymatic function	Pathway of activation
I	Fibrinogen	Plasma protein	Liver	Precursor of fibrin	Final common pathway
II	Prothrombin	Plasma protein	Liver	Precursor of thrombin	Final common pathway
III	Tissue thromboplastin Tissue factor Thrombokinase	Lipoprotein and phospholipid	Released from damaged tissues	Activates prothrombin	Extrinsic pathway
IV	Calcium ion	Ion in plasma	Diet and bones	Activates prothrombin and fibrin formation	All
V	Labile factor Proaccelerin accelerator globulin (AcG) Thrombogen	Plasma protein	Liver	Accelerates conversion of prothrombin to thrombin	Final common pathway
VI	Obsolete; same as V				
VII	Serum prothrombin conversion factor Proconvertin Stable factor	Plasma protein	Liver	Accelerates conversion of prothrombin to thrombin; part of enzyme complex	Extrinsic pathway
VIII	Antihemophilic globulin (AGH) Antihemophilic factor (AHF) Thromboplastinogen Platelet cofactor 1	Plasma protein (three subunits)	Large molecular weight Subunit by endothelium	Associated with platelet factor 3 and Christmas factor (IX); activates prothrombin (II)	Intrinsic pathway
IX	Plasma thromboplastin component (PTC) Christmas factor Antihemophilic factor B Autoprothrombin II (protein C) Platelet cofactor 2	Plasma protein	Liver	Associated with platelet factors 3 and 6; activates prothrombin	Intrinsic pathway
X	Stuart-Prower factor Stuart factor Autoprothrombin III	Plasma protein	Liver and plasma	Activated by Hageman factor	Extrinsic and intrinsic pathway

NOTE: The factors are numbered in the order of their discovery. Numerals do not denote their sequence of activation in the coagulation cascade.

Continued.

TABLE 22-7

Clotting Factors—cont'd

International nomenclature	Synonyms	Substance	Source	Enzymatic function	Pathway of activation
XI	Plasma thrombo-plastin antecedent (PTA) Antihemophilic factor C	Plasma protein	Possibly liver	Activated by Hageman factor; accelerates thrombin formation; substrate for activator enzymatic complex	Intrinsic pathway
XII	Hageman factor Contact factor Glass factor Antihemophilic factor D	Plasma protein	Liver (and plasma?)	Involved in first step of activation of intrinsic pathway; activates XI	Intrinsic pathway
XIII	Fibrin stabilizing factor (FSF) Fibrinase Fibrinoligase Laki-Lorand factor (LLF) Plasma transglutaminase	Plasma protein	Present in plasma and platelets Liver	Produces stronger fibrin clot; stabilizes clot formation	Common
High molecular weight kininogen	HMWK Fitzgerald factor Williams factor Fluajeac factor Reid factor Washington factor	α-Globulin	Tissues	Activates contraction of clot	Intrinsic kinin cascade
Prekallikrein	Fletcher factor	γ-Globulin	Tissues	Activates contraction of clot	Intrinsic kinin cascade

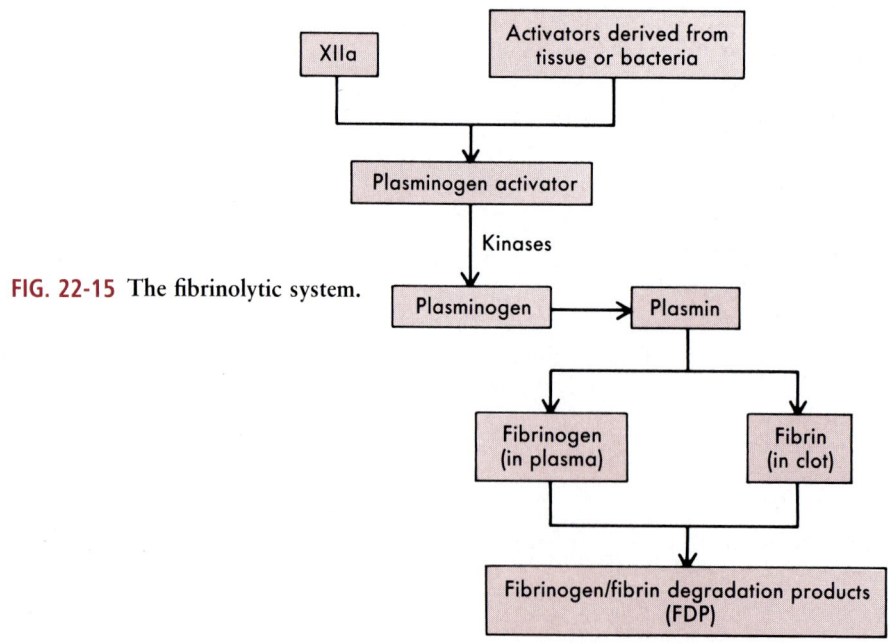

FIG. 22-15 The fibrinolytic system.

the site of injury. Retraction is facilitated by the large numbers of platelets trapped within the fibrin meshwork. The platelets, which contain actinomyosin-like contractile protein, contract and "pull" the fibrin threads closer together while releasing a factor that stabilizes the fibrin. Contraction expels protein-free serum from the fibrin meshwork. This process usually begins within a few minutes after a clot has formed, and most of the serum is expressed within 20 to 60 minutes (Guyton, 1992).

Lysis (breakdown) of blood clots is carried out by the **fibrinolytic system** (Fig. 22-15). Lysis is mediated by plasmin (fibrinolysin), a proteolytic enzyme that is activated by substances present during coagulation and inflammation, such as factor XII, thrombin, and lysosomal enzymes. Plasmin splits fibrin and fibrinogen into **fibrin degradation products (FDP),** which dissolve the clot. The fibrinolytic system removes clotted blood from tissues and dissolves small clots (thrombi) in blood vessels. A balance between amounts of thrombin and plasmin in the circulation maintains normal coagulation and lysis.

CLINICAL EVALUATION OF THE HEMATOLOGIC SYSTEM

Tests of Bone Marrow Function

In tests of marrow function, or hematopoiesis, small amounts of myeloid tissue are removed from the bone cavity and examined under a microscope. Cells contained in the marrow specimen are assessed with respect to (1) relative numbers of stem cells and their developing daughter cells and (2) morphologic structure.

Bone marrow aspiration, in which marrow is withdrawn using a hollow needle, provides information on gross cellular structure, estimation of iron stores in reticulocytes, determination of the ratio of erythrocyte precursor cells to myeloid cells (the normal ratio is 3:3), and the presence or absence of abnormal cells, such as tumor cells. A marrow aspirate that is richly cellular implies normal or increased hematopoiesis but does not indicate whether marrow activity is effective.

Bone aspiration is an important diagnostic test for several anemias (see Chapter 23) and is also performed to diagnose suggested acute leukemia (see Chapters 24 and 25). (Chronic leukemias can be diagnosed from blood samples alone.) Other disorders requiring marrow aspiration for diagnosis or monitoring of disease progression include platelet disorders (to determine whether platelet counts are increased, decreased, or normal; see Chapter 24) and immunoglobulin disorders (to gauge populations of plasma cells and lymphocytes; see Chapter 8).

Bone marrow biopsy, a surgical procedure in which

TABLE 22-8

Differential Cell Counts in Bone Marrow with Age

Developing cells in marrow	Birth	1 mo-1 yr	1-4 yr	4-12 yr	Adult
Erythrocytic series	14	8	19	21	20
Lymphocytic series	14	47	22	18	17
Eosinophilic series	3	3	6	3	3
Neutrophilic series	60	33	50	52	57
Myeloid/erythroid ratio	4:3	4:0	1:3	2:5	1:3

NOTE: Values are percentages of cell types counted during examination of a marrow specimen containing approximately 400 nucleated cells.

a "slice" of marrow is removed, is performed if aspiration is not diagnostic, tumors are suggested (tumors are more easily detected in biopsy sections), marrow is fibrotic, or populations of more than one type of blood cell are reduced. Because marrow aspiration disturbs marrow structure, only general cellularity (numbers of constituent cells) of the marrow can be gauged. Biopsy specimens provide the most reliable and specific information about marrow cellularity. Marrow biopsy is, however, usually more painful and expensive than marrow aspiration. Therefore biopsy is not performed unless insufficient information is obtained from aspiration.

A direct measure of iron stores can be obtained only from liver or marrow biopsy specimens. The bone marrow technique is preferred, not only because it is safer than liver biopsy but also because the red cell is the immediate source of plasma iron destined for erythrocyte production.

Examination of biopsy specimens and aspirate routinely includes a differential cell count (Table 22-8). The differential cell count involves examining approximately 400 nucleated cells under oil-immersion magnification and counting populations of different stem cells. The relative number of each type of stem cell is expressed as a percentage of 400.

Blood Tests

Blood tests provide information about the absolute and relative numbers of blood cells in a specimen of blood, as well as various structural and functional characteristics of the cells. Deviations from normal can reflect disease, physiologic states (e.g., pregnancy, infancy, old age), injury, or dysfunction in almost any part of the body. Blood tests that reflect chiefly hematologic disorders are listed in Table 22-9.

TABLE 22-9

Blood Tests for Hematologic Disorders

Cell type and test	Property evaluated by test	Possible hematologic cause of abnormal findings
Erythrocyte		
Red cell count	Number (in millions) of erythrocytes/μl of blood	Altered erythropoiesis, anemias, hemorrhage, Hodgkin disease, leukemia
Mean corpuscular volume	Size of erythrocytes	Anemias, thalassemias
Mean corpuscular hemoglobin (MCH)	Amount of hemoglobin in each erythrocyte (by weight)	Anemias, hemoglobinopathy
Mean corpuscular hemoglobin concentration (MCHC)	Concentration of hemoglobin in each erythrocyte (percentage of erythrocyte occupied by hemoglobin)	Anemias, hereditary spherocytosis
Hemoglobin determination	Amount of hemoglobin (by weight)/dl of blood	Anemias
Hematocrit determination	Percentage of a given volume of blood that is occupied by erythrocytes	Hemorrhage, polycythemia, erythrocytosis, anemias, leukemia
Reticulocyte count	Number of reticulocytes/μl of blood (also expressed as percentage of reticulocytes in total red cell count)	Hyperactive or hypoactive bone marrow function
Erythrocyte osmotic fragility test	Cellular shape (biconcavity), structure of plasma membrane	Anemias, hemolytic disease caused by ABO or Rh incompatibility, Hodgkin disease, polycythemia vera, thalassemia major
Hemoglobin electrophoresis	Relative percentage of different types of hemoglobin in erythrocytes	Sickle cell disease, sickle cell trait, hemoglobin C disease, hemoglobin C trait, thalassemias
Sickle cell test	Presence of hemoglobin S in erythrocytes	Sickle cell trait, sickle cell anemia
Glucose-6-phosphate dehydrogenase (G-6-PD) deficiency test	Deficiency of G-6-PD in erythrocytes	Hemolytic anemia
Hemoglobin metabolism		
Serum ferritin determination	Depletion of body iron (potential deficiency of heme synthesis)	Iron deficiency anemias
Total iron-binding capacity (TICB)	Amount of iron in serum plus amount of transferrin available in serum (μg/dl)	Hemorrhage, iron deficiency anemia, hemochromatosis, hemosiderosis, iron overload, anemias, thalassemia
Transferrin saturation	Percentage of transferrin that is saturated with iron	Acute hemorrhage, hemochromatosis, hemosiderosis, sideroblastic anemia, iron deficiency anemia, iron overload, thalassemia
Porphyrin analysis (protoporphyrin analysis)	Concentration of protoporphyrin in erythrocytes (μg/dl); an indicator of iron-deficient erythropoiesis	Megaloblastic anemia, congenital erythropoietic porphyria
Direct antiglobulin test (DAT)	Antibody binding to erythrocytes	Hemolytic disease of the newborn, autoimmune hemolytic anemia, drug-induced hemolytic anemia, transfusion reaction
Antibody screen (indirect Coombs' test)	Detection of antibodies to erythrocyte antigens (other than the ABO antigens)	Same as for DAT

From Byrne, C. J., et al. (1986). *Laboratory tests: Implications for nursing care.* Menlo Park, CA: Addison-Wesley.
NOTE: See Fig. 22-13 and Table 22-7 for information about clotting factors and their sequence of activation in the coagulation cascade.

TABLE 22-9

Blood Tests for Hematologic Disorders—cont'd

Cell type and test	Property evaluated by test	Possible hematologic cause of abnormal findings
Leukocytes: differential white cell count (absolute number of a type of leukocyte/µl of blood)	See below	See below
Neutrophil count	Neutrophils/µl	Myeloproliferative disorders, hematopoietic disorders, hemolysis, infection
Lymphocyte count	Lymphocytes/µl	Infectious lymphocytosis, infectious mononucleosis, hematopoietic disorders, anemias, leukemia, lymphosarcoma, Hodgkin disease
Plasma cell count	Plasma cells/µl	Infectious mononucleosis, lymphocytosis, plasma cell leukemia
Monocyte count	Monocytes/µl	Hodgkin disease, infectious mononucleosis, monocytic leukemia, non-Hodgkin lymphoma, polycythemia vera
Eosinophil count	Eosinophils/µl	Hematopoietic disorders
Basophil count	Basophils/µl	Chronic myelogenous leukemia, hemolytic anemias, Hodgkin disease, polycythemia vera
Platelets and clotting factors		
Platelet count	Number of circulating platelets (in thousands)/µl of blood	Anemias, multiple myeloma, myelofibrosis, polycythemia vera, leukemia, disseminated intravascular coagulation (DIC), hemolytic disease of the newborn, idiopathic thrombocytopenic purpura, transfusion reaction, lymphoproliferative disorders
Bleeding time	Duration of bleeding following a standardized superficial puncture wound of the skin, integrity of the platelet plug, measured in minutes following puncture	Leukemia, anemias, DIC, fibrinolytic activity, purpuras, hemorrhagic disease of the newborn, infectious mononucleosis, multiple myeloma, clotting factor deficiencies, thrombasthenia, thrombocytopenia, von Willebrand disease
Clot retraction test	Platelet number and function, fibrinogen quantity and use, measured in hours required for expression of serum from a clot incubated in a test tube	Acute leukemia, aplastic anemia, factor XIII deficiency, increased fibrinolytic activity, Hodgkin disease, hyperfibrinogenemia or hypofibrinogenemia, idiopathic thrombocytopenic purpura, multiple myeloma, polycythemia vera, secondary thrombocytopenia, thrombasthenia
Platelet adhesion studies	Ability of platelets to adhere to foreign surfaces	Anemia, macroglobulinemia, Barnard-Soulier syndrome, multiple myeloma, myeloid metaplasia, plasma cell dyscrasias, thrombasthenia, thrombocytopathy, von Willebrand disease

Continued.

TABLE 22-9

Blood Tests for Hematologic Disorders—cont'd

Cell type and test	Property evaluated by test	Possible hematologic cause of abnormal findings
Platelets and clotting factors—cont'd		
Platelet aggregation tests	Ability of platelets to adhere to one another	Afibrinogenemia, Bernard-Soulier syndrome, thrombasthenia, hemorrhagic thrombocythemia, myeloid metaplasia, plasma cell dyscrasias, platelet release defects, polycythemia vera, preleukemia, sideroblastic anemia, von Willebrand disease, Waldenström macroglobulinemia, hypercoagulability
Whole blood clotting time (Lee-White coagulation time)	Overall ability of blood to clot, as measured in minutes in a test tube	Afibrinogenemia, clotting factor deficiencies, excessive fibrinolysis, hemorrhagic disease of the newborn, hypofibrinogenemia, hypoprothrombinemia, leukemia
Circulating anticoagulants (IgG antibodies that inhibit coagulation)	Presence of antibodies that neutralize clotting factors and inhibit coagulation, as indicated by prolonged clotting time, prothrombin time, or partial thromboplastin time	Afibrinogenemia, presence of fibrin-fibrinogen degradation products, macroglobulinemia, multiple myeloma, DIC, plasma cell dyscrasias
Partial thromboplastin time (PTT)	Effectiveness of clotting factors (except factor VII and VIII), effectiveness of intrinsic pathway of coagulation cascade, as measured by a test tube (in seconds)	Presence of circulating anticoagulants, DIC, clotting factor deficiencies, excessive fibrinolysis, hemorrhagic disease of the newborn, hypofibrinogenemia and afibrinogenemia, prothrombin deficiency, von Willebrand disease, acute hemorrhage
Prothrombin time	Effectiveness of activity of prothrombin, fibrinogen, and factors V, VII, and X; effectiveness of vitamin K–dependent coagulation factors of the extrinsic and common pathways of the coagulation cascade as measured in a test tube (in seconds)	Hypofibrinogenemia, dysfibrinogenemia, and afibrinogenemia; presence of circulating anticoagulants; DIC; deficiency of factors V, VII, or X; presence of fibrin degradation products, increased fibrinolytic activity, hemolytic jaundice, hemorrhagic disease of the newborn; acute leukemia, polycythemia vera, prothrombin deficiency, multiple myeloma
Thrombin time	Quantity and activity of fibrinogen as measured in a test tube (in seconds)	Hypofibrinogenemia, dysfibrinogenemia, and afibrinogenemia; presence of circulating anticoagulants; hemorrhagic disease of the newborn, polycythemia vera; increase in fibrinogen-fibrin degradation products; increased fibrinolytic activity
Fibrinogen assay	Amount of fibrinogen available for fibrin formation	Acute leukemia, congenital hypofibrinogenemia or afibrinogenemia, DIC, increased fibrinolytic activity, severe hemorrhage
Fibrin-fibrinogen degradation products (fibrin-fibrinogen split products)	Fibrinogenic activity as measured by levels of fibrin-fibrinogen degradation products (in μg/ml of blood)	Transfusion reactions, DIC, internal hemorrhage in the newborn, deep vein thrombosis, pulmonary embolism

☐ AGING and the Hematologic System

Blood composition changes little with age. Although anemia is frequent in the elderly population, it is usually a result of other conditions. Erythrocyte lifespan is normal in the elderly, although a delay in erythrocyte replenishment may occur after bleeding, probably because of iron depletion. Total serum iron, total iron-binding capacity, and intestinal iron absorption are all decreased in the elderly (Bothwell & Finch, 1962). Iron deficiency is often responsible for the low hemoglobin levels noted in elderly people (Williams, Beutler, Erslev, & Lichtman, 1990). The plasma membranes of erythrocytes become increasingly fragile because they contain fewer and fewer proteins and membrane-associated enzymes (Kadlubowski, 1978; Kadlubowski & Agutter, 1977). Increased fragility causes portions of the membrane to be lost, presumably because of physical trauma inflicted during circulation.

Although it is unclear whether aging alters the numbers of lymphocytes, their function does decrease with age (see Chapters 6 and 7). The most significant changes are with cellular immunity with some decline in T cell function. The humoral immune system has a decreased ability to respond to antigenic challenge (Williams et al., 1990).

No changes in platelet numbers or structure have been observed in the elderly, yet evidence shows that platelet adhesiveness probably increases (Adams & Mayet, 1966). There is disagreement about whether hemostasis and coagulation are altered with age. Although fibrinogen levels and factors V, VII, and IX tend to be increased in the elderly, evidence about hypercoagulability is inconclusive.

SUMMARY REVIEW

Components of the Hematologic System

1 Blood consists of a variety of formed elements: about 90% water and 10% solutes. In adults the total blood volume is approximately 5.5 L.

2 Plasma, a complex aqueous liquid, contains three major groups of plasma proteins: (1) albumins, (2) globulins, and (3) clotting factors.

3 The cellular elements of blood are the erythrocytes, leukocytes, lymphocytes, and platelets.

4 Erythrocytes are the most abundant cells of the blood, occupying approximately 48% of the blood volume in men and approximately 42% in women. Erythrocytes are responsible for tissue oxygenation.

5 Leukocytes are fewer in number than erythrocytes and constitute approximately 5000 to 10,000 cells/mm^3 of blood. Leukocytes defend the body against infection and remove dead or injured host cells.

6 Leukocytes are classified as either granulocytes (neutrophils, basophils, and eosinophils) or agranulocytes (monocytes, macrophages).

7 Platelets are not cells, but disk-shaped cytoplasmic fragments. Platelets are essential for blood coagulation and control of bleeding.

8 The lymphoid organs are classified as primary (thymus and bone marrow) or secondary (spleen, lymph nodes, tonsils, and Peyer's patches of the small intestine).

9 The lymphoid organs are sites of residence, proliferation, differentiation, or function of lymphocytes and mononuclear phagocytes.

10 The spleen is the largest of the secondary lymphoid organs and functions as the site of fetal hematopoiesis, filters and cleanses the blood, and is a reservoir for lymphocytes and other blood cells.

11 The lymph nodes are the site of development or activity of large numbers of lymphocytes, monocytes, and macrophages.

12 The mononuclear phagocyte system (MPS), previously called the reticuloendothelial system (RES), is composed of monoblasts, promonocytes, and monocytes in bone marrow, monocytes in peripheral blood, and macrophages in tissue.

13 The MPS is the main line of defense against bacteria in the bloodstream and cleanses the blood by removing old, injured, or dead blood cells; antigen-antibody complexes; and macromolecules.

Development of Blood Cells

1 Hematopoiesis, or blood cell production, occurs in the liver and spleen of the fetus and in the bone marrow after birth.

2 Hematopoiesis involves two stages: (1) proliferation and (2) differentiation, or maturation. Each type of blood cell has parent cells called stem cells.

3 Hematopoiesis continues throughout life to replace blood cells that grow old and die, are killed by disease, or are lost through bleeding.

4 Bone marrow consists of blood vessels, nerves, mononuclear phagocytes, stem cells, blood cells in various stages of differentiation, and fatty tissue.

5 Hemoglobin, the oxygen-carrying protein of the erythrocyte, enables the blood to transport 100 times more oxygen than could be transported dissolved in plasma alone.

6 Erythropoiesis depends on the presence of vitamins (especially vitamin B$_{12}$, folate, B$_6$, riboflavin, pantothenic acid, niacin, ascorbic acid, and vitamin E).

7 Regulation of erythropoiesis is mediated by erythropoietin. Erythropoietin is secreted by the kidneys in response to tissue hypoxia and causes a compensatory increase in erythrocyte production if the oxygen content of the blood decreases because of anemia, high altitude, or pulmonary disease.

8 Maintenance of optimal levels of granulocytes and monocytes in the blood depends on the availability of pluripotential stem cells in the marrow, induction of these into committed stem cells, and timely release of new cells from the marrow.

9 Specific humoral CSFs are necessary for the adequate growth of myeloid, erythroid, lymphoid, and megakaryocytic lineages.

10 Platelets develop from megakaryocytes by a process called endomitosis. In endomitosis, the megakaryocytes undergo mitosis but not cytokinesis; thus, the cell does not divide into two daughter cells.

Mechanisms of Hemostasis

1 Hemostasis, or arrest of bleeding, involves (1) vasoconstriction (vasospasm), (2) formation of a platelet plug, (3) activation of the clotting cascade, and (4) formation of a blood clot.

2 Two properties of normal vascular endothelium prevent clotting: (1) the smooth texture of the endothelial lining that prevents adherence of platelets and (2) the negative charge of protein in the endothelial cells that repels some negatively charged platelets and clotting factors.

3 Lysis of blood clots is the function of the fibrinolytic system. Plasmin, a proteolytic enzyme, splits fibrin and fibrinogen into fibrin degradation products that dissolve the clot.

Clinical Evaluation of the Hematologic System

1 Tests of bone marrow function include bone marrow aspiration and bone marrow biopsy.

Aging and the Hematologic System

1 Blood composition changes little with age. A delay in erythrocyte replenishment may occur after bleeding, presumably because of iron deficiency.

2 Lymphocyte function appears to decrease with age. Particularly affected is a decrease in cellular immunity.

3 Platelet adhesiveness probably increases with age.

KEY TERMS

Agranulocyte, 834
Albumin, 831
Basophil, 835
Biconcavity, 832
Blood clot, 849
Bone marrow (myeloid tissue), 840
Clotting factor, 831
Coagulation cascade, 849
Colony-stimulating factor (CSF), 839
Deoxyhemoglobin (reduced hemoglobin), 843
Differentiation (maturation), 838
Eosinophil, 834
Erythroblast, 840
Erythrocyte (red blood cell [RBC]), 831
Erythropoiesis, 840
Fibrin degradation product (FDP), 853
Fibrinolytic system, 853
Globin, 841
Globulin (immunoglobulin), 831

Granulocyte, 834
Hematopoiesis, 838
Hematopoietic growth factor, 839
Heme, 841
Hemoglobin (Hb), 831
Hemostasis, 847
Immunocyte, 834
Intrinsic factor (IF), 843
Leukocyte (white blood cell), 831
Lipoprotein, 831
Lymph node, 836
Lymphocyte, 835
Macrophage, 835
Megaloblast, 840
Methemoglobin, 843
Monocyte, 835
Mononuclear phagocyte system (MPS) (reticuloendothelial system [RES]), 835
Neutrophil (polymorphonuclear neutrophil [PMN]), 834

Normoblast, 840
Oxyhemoglobin, 843
Phagocyte, 834
Plasma, 831
Plasma protein, 831
Platelet (thrombocyte), 831
Pluripotential stem cell (pluripotential myeloid stem cell [PMSC], 838
Primary lymphoid organ, 836
Proliferation (mitotic division), 838
Reticulocyte, 840
Reversible deformability, 832
Secondary lymphoid organ, 836
Serum, 831
Spleen, 836
Stem cell, 838
Stem cell system, 838
Totipotential hematopoietic stem cell (THSC) (multipotential stem cell), 838
Transferrin, 843

REFERENCES

Adams, E. B., & Meyet, F. G. (1966). Hypochromic anaemia in chronic infections. *South African Medical Journal, 40,* 738-740.

Babior, B. M., & Stossel, T. P. (1984). *Hematology: A pathophysiological approach.* New York: Churchill-Livingstone.

Berne, R. M., & Levy, M. N. (1992). *Physiology* (3rd ed.). St. Louis: Mosby–Year Book.

Bothwell, T. H., & Finch, C. A. (1962). *Iron metabolism.* Boston: Little, Brown & Co.

Breuil, J., & Obermaier, H. (1935). The case of altumira at Santillana del Mar (Madrid, Spain, Tip. de Archivos, Plate XIX). In M. W. Wintrobe (Ed.), (1980). *Blood, pure and eloquent: A story of discovery, of people, and of ideas.* New York: McGraw-Hill.

Byrne, C. J., et al. (1986). *Laboratory tests: Implications for nursing care.* Menlo Park, CA: Addison-Wesley.

Cotran, R. S., Kumar, V., & Robbins, S. L. (1989). *Pathologic basis of disease* (4th ed.). Philadelphia: Saunders.

Delmonte, L., Aschkenasy, A., & Eyquem, A. (1964). Studies of the hemolytic nature of protein deficiency anemia in the rat. *Blood, 24,* 49.

Fischbach, D., & Fogdall, R. (1981). *Coagulation, the essentials.* Baltimore: Williams & Wilkins.

Fisher, J. W., Samuels, A. I., & Langston, J. W. (1967). Effects of angiotensin and renal artery constriction on erythropoietin production. *Journal of Pharmacological and Experimental Therapeutics, 157*(3), 618.

Goldwasser, E. (1990). Erythropoietin: Molecular and cellular biology. In J. Spivak, W. Drohan, & D. Dooley (Eds.), *Hematopoietic growth factors in transfusion medicine.* New York: Wiley-Liss.

Guyton, A. C. (1992). *Human physiology and mechanisms of disease* (5th ed.). Philadelphia: Saunders.

Halma, C., Daha, M. R., & van-Es-La. (1992). In vivo clearance by the mononuclear phagocyte system in humans: An overview of methods and their interpretation. *Clinical Experimental Immunology, 89*(10), 1-7.

Hart, G. (1980). Ancient diseases of the blood. In M. W. Wintrobe (Ed.), *Blood pure and eloquent: A story of discovery, of people, and of ideas.* New York: McGraw-Hill.

Kadlubowski, M. (1978). The effect of in vivo aging of the human erythrocyte on the protein of the plasma membrane: A characterization. *International Journal of Biochemistry, 9*(2), 67-78.

Kadlubowski, M., & Agutter, P. S. (1977). Changes in the activities of some membrane associated enzymes during in vivo aging of the normal human erythrocyte. *British Journal of Haematology, 37*(1), 111-125.

Lee, G.R., Bithell, T.C., Foerster, J., Athens, J.W., & Lukens, J.N. (Eds.). (1993). *Wintrobe's clinical hematology* (9th ed.). Philadelphia: Lea & Febiger.

Lopez, L., Duck, I. M., & Hung, W. A. (1968). On the shape of the erythrocyte. *Biophysical Journal, 8,* 1228.

Maniatis, A., Tavassoli, M., & Crosby, W. H. (1971). Factors affecting the conversion of yellow to red marrow. *Blood, 37,* 581.

Metcalf, D. (1991). Control of granulocytes and macrophages: Molecular, cellular, and clinical aspects. *Science, 254*(5031), 529-533.

Purtilo, D. T. (1978). *A survey of human diseases.* Menlo Park, CA: Addison-Wesley.

Quesenberry, P. J. (1992). Biomodulation of chemotherapy-induced myelosuppression. *Seminars in Oncology, 19*(3) [Suppl. 8], 8-13.

Raven, P. H., & Johnson, G. B. (1989). *Biology.* (2nd ed.). St. Louis: Times Mirror/Mosby.

Robbins, S., Cotran, R. S., & Kumar, V. (1989). *Pathophysiologic basis of disease.* (4th ed.). Philadelphia: Saunders.

Rowe, J. M., & Rapaport, A. P. (1992). Hemopoietic growth factors: A review. *Journal of Clinical Pharmacology, 32,* 486-501.

Russell, W. J., Yoshinaga, H., Shigetoshi, A., & Mizuno, M. (1966). Active bone marrow distribution in the adult. *British Journal of Radiology, 39,* 735.

Sakagami, T., Minari, D., & Orii, T. (1965). Interaction of individual phospholipids between rat plasma and erythrocytes in vitro. *Biochimica et Biophysica Acta, 98,* 356-364.

Shand, F. L., & Bell, E. B. (1972). Studies on the distribution of macrophages derived from rat bone marrow cells in xenogenic radiation chimaeras. *Immunology, 22,* 549.

Thibodeau, G. A. (1987). *Anatomy and physiology.* St. Louis: Times Mirror/Mosby.

Vander, A. J., Sherman, J. H., & Luchiano, D. S. (1990). *Human physiology: The mechanisms of body function.* New York: McGraw-Hill.

Williams, W., Beutler, E., Erslev, A., & Lichtman, M. (1990). *Hematology* (4th ed.). New York: McGraw-Hill.

Wintrobe, M. M. (1986). *Hematology, the blossoming of a science: A story of inspiration and effort.* Philadelphia: Lea & Febiger.

Wintrobe, M. M. (Ed.). (1980). *Blood pure and eloquent: A story of discovery, of people, and of ideas.* New York: McGraw-Hill.

SUGGESTED READINGS

Cunningham, A. S. (1975). Eosinophil counts: Age and sex differences. *Journal of Pediatrics, 87,* 426.

Dallman, P. R. (1981, June). Iron deficiency: Diagnosis and treatment. *The Western Journal of Medicine, 134,* 496-505.

DeGabriele, G., & Penington, D. G. (1967). Physiology of the regulation of platelet production. *British Journal of Haematology, 13,* 202.

Diesselhoff-den Dulk, M. M. C., Crofton, R. W., & Van Furth, R. (1979). Origin and kinetics of Kupffer cells during an acute inflammatory response. *Immunology, 37,* 7.

Alterations of Erythrocyte Function

Thom J. Mansen
Kathryn L. McCance
Pamela D. Parker-Cohen*

Chapter Outline

*Contributing author to first edition.

A lterations of erythrocyte function involve either insufficient or excessive numbers of
erythrocytes in the circulation or normal numbers of
cells with abnormal components. Anemias are conditions in which there are too few erythrocytes or an
insufficient volume of erythrocytes in the blood. Polycythemias are conditions in which erythrocyte numbers or volume is excessive. Each of these two conditions has many causes, which is why each has so
many names. Anemia and polycythemia are not diseases per se, but rather they are pathophysiologic
manifestations of a variety of disease states.

ANEMIA

Strictly speaking, **anemia** is a reduction in the total number of circulating erythrocytes or a decrease in the quality or quantity of hemoglobin. Anemic conditions are usually a result of (1) impaired erythrocyte production, (2) blood loss, (3) increased erythrocyte destruction, or (4) a combination of the three.

Classification of Anemias

Anemias are classified according to their etiologic or morphologic basis (see box). The most common classification of anemias is based on cellular morphology or structure. Descriptions of anemias based on erythrocyte morphology refer to the cell's size and hemoglobin content. Because all anemias can be described with respect to these two cellular features, the morphologic classification is widely used (Table 23-1). Terms that refer to cellular size end with "cytic," whereas terms that describe hemoglobin content end with "chromic." An erythrocyte can be **macrocytic** (abnormally large) or **microcytic** (abnormally small); **hyperchromic** (containing an unusually high concentration of hemoglobin within its cytoplasm) or **hypochromic** (containing an abnormally low concentration of hemoglobin). For comparison, cells of normal size are termed **normocytic,** and cells with normal amounts of hemoglobin are termed **normochromic.** In some anemias, the erythrocytes take on various sizes (**anisocytosis**) or they have various shapes (**poikilocytosis**) (Fig. 23-1).

Clinical Manifestations of Anemias

The number and severity of symptoms caused by anemia depend on the body's ability to compensate for the reduced oxygen-carrying capacity of the blood. If the anemia is mild and its onset is gradual, compensation may be so successful that the individual is asymptomatic except during periods of physical exertion. Although anemia may manifest itself in many organs and systems, compensation generally involves the cardiovascular, respiratory, and hematologic systems. Hematologic findings in various anemias are listed in Table 23-2.

A reduction in the number of circulating erythrocytes, such as is seen after hemorrhage, affects the consistency and volume of the blood. To compensate for reduced blood volume, fluids from the interstitium move into the blood vessels, and plasma volume expands. Although this compensatory mechanism maintains adequate blood volume, it decreases the viscosity (thickness) of the blood. The "diluted" blood flows faster and more turbulently than normal blood. Increased blood flow within the heart can cause ventricular dysfunction, cardiac dilation, and heart valve insufficiency. Some cardiovascular manifestations of anemia are caused by hypoxia, which causes arterioles, capillaries, and venules to

ETIOLOGIC (PATHOPHYSIOLOGIC) CLASSIFICATION OF ANEMIAS

Decreased/defective production of erythrocytes

Altered hemoglobin synthesis
  Iron deficiency
  Thalassemia
  Anemia of chronic inflammation

Altered DNA synthesis resulting from deficient nutrients
  Pernicious anemia (decreased B_{12} folate)

Stem cell dysfunction
  Aplastic anemia
  Myeloproliferative leukemia

Bone marrow infiltration
  Carcinoma
  Lymphoma

Pure red cell aplasia

Increased erythrocyte destruction

Blood loss
  Acute—hemorrhage, trauma
  Chronic—GI bleed, menorrhagia

Hemolysis (intracorpuscular defect)
  Membrane—hereditary spherocytosis
  Hemoglobin—sickle cell trait/disease
  Glycolysis—pyruvate kinase
  Oxidation—G6PD deficiency

Hemolysis (extracorpuscular defect)
  Immune mechanisms—warm antibody/cold antibody
  Infection—claustridial, malarial
  Trauma to erythrocyte—hemolytic uremic syndrome
  Splenic sequestration—hypersplenism

dilate, speeding blood flow even further. As venous return to the heart increases, the heart must pump harder and faster to meet normal oxygen demand and to prevent cardiopulmonary congestion. All of these mechanisms of cardiovascular compensation can cause congestive heart failure. (Mechanisms of congestive heart failure are described in Chapter 27.)

Tissue hypoxia has other effects on the heart and lungs. The rate and depth of breathing increase in an attempt to make more oxygen available to the remaining erythrocytes. Cardiac output increases to handle the increased venous return and speed the remaining oxygen-carrying erythrocytes to and from hypoxic tissue cells. Hemoglobin in the erythrocytes releases its oxygen more readily than usual at the tissue level. (Mechanisms of oxygen transport and release by hemoglobin are described in Chapter 29.)

TABLE 23-1

Morphologic Classification of Anemias

Morphology and cause of reduced oxygen-carrying capacity of the blood	Name and mechanism of anemic condition	Primary cause of associated disorder
Macrocytic-normochromic anemia: large, abnormally shaped erythrocytes but normal hemoglobin concentrations	Pernicious anemia: lack of vitamin B_{12} (cobalamin) for erythropoiesis; abnormal DNA and RNA synthesis in the erythroblast; premature cell death	Congenital or acquired deficiency of intrinsic factor (IF); genetic disorder of DNA synthesis
	Folate-deficiency anemia: lack of folate for erythropoiesis; premature cell death	Dietary folate deficiency
Microcytic-hypochromic anemia: small, abnormally shaped erythrocytes and reduced hemoglobin concentration	Iron-deficiency anemia: lack of iron for hemoglobin production; insufficient hemoglobin	Chronic blood loss; dietary iron deficiency, disruption of iron metabolism or iron cycle (see Chapter 22)
	Sideroblastic anemia: dysfunctional iron uptake by erythroblasts and defective porphyrin and heme synthesis	Congenital dysfunction of iron metabolism in erythroblasts, acquired dysfunction of iron metabolism as a result of drugs or toxins
	Thalassemia: impaired synthesis of α or β chain of hemoglobin A; phagocytosis of abnormal erythroblasts in the marrow	Congenital genetic defect of globin synthesis
Normocytic-normochromic anemia: destruction or depletion of normal erythroblasts or mature erythrocytes	Aplastic anemia: insufficient erythropoiesis	Depressed stem cell proliferation resulting in bone marrow aplasia
	Posthemorrhagic anemia: blood loss	Acute or chronic hemorrhage that stimulates increased erythropoiesis, which eventually depletes body iron
	Hemolytic anemia: premature destruction (lysis) of mature erythrocytes in the circulation	Any condition that increases fragility of erythrocytes
	Sickle cell anemia: abnormal hemoglobin synthesis, abnormal cell shape with susceptibility to damage, lysis, and phagocytosis	Congenital dysfunction of hemoglobin synthesis
	Anemia of chronic disease: abnormally increased demand for new erythrocytes	Chronic infection or inflammation; malignancy

If anemia is severe enough to overcome the usual compensatory mechanisms, the individual experiences shortness of breath (dyspnea), a rapid pounding heartbeat, dizziness, and fatigue, even at rest.

When anemia is severe or sudden in onset, peripheral blood vessels constrict so as to direct available blood flow chiefly to the vital organs. A number of systemic symptoms result from this lifesaving maneuver. Decreased blood flow is sensed by the kidneys, and in an effort to improve kidney perfusion, the renal renin-angiotensin response is activated, resulting in salt and water retention. The skin, mucous membranes, lips, nailbeds, and conjunctivae become pale because of re-

duced hemoglobin concentration or yellowish because of accumulation in the skin of products of red blood cell breakdown (hemolysis). Decreased oxygen delivery to the skin results in impaired healing and loss of elasticity, as well as thinning and early graying of the hair. If the anemia is caused by vitamin B_{12} deficiency, the nervous system is affected. Myelin degeneration may occur with loss of nerve fibers in the spinal cord. Paresthesias (numbness), gait disturbances, extreme weakness, spasticity, and reflex abnormalities can result. Decreased oxygen supply to the gastrointestinal tract often produces abdominal pain, nausea, vomiting, and anorexia. Low-grade fever (less than 101° F) occurs in

FIG. 23-1 **Appearance of red blood cells in various disorders. A,** Normal blood smear. **B,** Hypochromic microcytic anemia (iron deficiency). **C,** Macrocytic anemia (pernicious anemia). **D,** Macrocytic anemia in pregnancy. **E,** Hereditary elliptocytosis. **F,** Myelofibrosis (teardrop). **G,** Hemolytic anemia associated with prosthetic heart valve. **H,** Microangiopathic anemia. **I,** Stomatocytes. **J,** Spherocytes (hereditary spherocytosis). **K,** Sideroblastic anemia; note the double population of red blood cells. **L,** Sickle cell anemia. **M,** Target cells (after splenectomy). **N,** Basophil strippling in case of unexplained anemia. **O,** Howell-Jolly bodies (after splenectomy). (From Wintrobe et al., 1981.)

TABLE 23-2

Laboratory Findings for Various Anemias

Test	Pernicious anemia	Folate deficiency anemia	Iron deficiency anemia	Sideroblastic anemia	Aplastic anemia	Posthemorrhagic anemia	Hemolytic anemia	Anemia of chronic inflammation
Hemoglobin	Low	Low	Low	Low	Low/normal	Normal/low	Low	Low
Hematocrit	Low	Low	Low	Low	Low/normal	Normal/low	Low	Low
Reticulocyte count	Low	Low	Normal or slightly high or low	Normal or slightly high	Low	Increased	High	Normal
Mean corpuscular volume	High	High	Low	Low	Normal or slightly high	Slightly low	Normal or high	Normal or low
Plasma iron	High	High	Low	High	High	Normal	Normal or high	Low
Total iron-binding capacity	Normal	Normal	High	Normal	Normal	Normal	Normal	Low
Ferritin	High	High	Low	High	Normal	Normal	Normal	Normal
Serum B_{12}	Low	Normal	Normal	Normal	Normal	Normal	Normal	Normal
Folate	Normal	Low	Normal	Normal	Normal	Normal	Normal	Normal
Bilirubin	Slightly high	Slightly high	Normal	High	Normal	Normal	Slightly high	Normal
Free erythrocyte protoporphyrin	Normal	Normal	High	Increased or normal	High	Normal	Normal	Normal or slightly high
Transferrin	Slightly high	Slightly high	Low	High	Normal	Normal	Normal	Slightly low

some anemic individuals and may be the result of leukocyte pyrogens being released from ischemic tissues.

Therapeutic intervention for any anemic condition calls for treatment of the underlying disorder and palliation of symptoms. Therapies for anemia include transfusions, dietary corrections, and administration of supplemental vitamins or iron.

Macrocytic-Normochromic Anemias

The **macrocytic anemias,** also termed megaloblastic anemias, are characterized by unusually large stem cells (megaloblasts) in the marrow that mature into unusually large erythrocytes (macrocytes) in the circulation. Megaloblastic stem cells are larger at all maturational stages than normal stem cells (normoblasts). In addition, the nucleus of the megaloblast is disproportionately small in relation to the size of the cell. As the cell matures and begins to synthesize hemoglobin, chroma-

tin in the nucleus fails to clump normally. Hemoglobin content is normal, however. The macrocytic anemias are morphologically classified as macrocytic-normochromic anemias (see Table 23-1).

Defective DNA synthesis, usually caused by deficiencies of vitamin B_{12} (cobalamin) or folate, produces a pattern of ineffective erythropoiesis in the macrocytic anemias. As a result of ineffective erythropoiesis, erythrocytes experience premature cell death, resulting in a reduced number of circulating mature erythrocytes.

Defective DNA synthesis in megaloblastic anemias causes cell growth to proceed at unequal rates. DNA replication and cell division, both nuclear functions, are blocked or delayed. However, RNA replication and protein (hemoglobin) synthesis continue at their normal rates. The end result is an overproduction of hemoglobin that occurs during delayed cellular division, creating a larger than normal erythrocyte (Lee, 1993).

Pernicious Anemia

Pernicious anemia, the most common type of megaloblastic anemia, is a chronic condition caused by malabsorption of vitamin B_{12} (Fig. 23-1, *C*). The term *pernicious* means highly injurious or destructive and reflects the fact that this condition was once fatal. Pernicious anemia is most common in late adult life and rare in individuals younger than 30, except in the congenital type that usually occurs before 2 years of age. Pernicious anemia is most common among Scandinavian, English, and Irish peoples. In Great Britain and Scandinavia, women are more commonly affected than men. In the United States, both sexes appear to be equally affected.

Pathophysiology

The underlying disorder in pernicious anemia is defective gastric secretion of intrinsic factor (IF), which is necessary for absorption of vitamin B_{12}. Vitamin B_{12} is in turn necessary for nuclear maturation and DNA synthesis in red blood cells. Pernicious anemias can be caused by a congenital deficiency of IF alone or by adult-onset atrophy of the gastric mucosa that causes deficiencies of all gastric secretions, including IF. Partial or complete surgical excision of the stomach (gastrectomy) also produces a deficiency of IF.

The specific cause of the gastric atrophy that results in IF deficiency in adult-onset pernicious anemia is unknown. An autoimmune, genetic predisposition is highly probable because of the familial occurrence of pernicious anemia. More than 90% of individuals with pernicious anemia demonstrate parietal cell autoantibodies in their serum; 20% to 30% of their relatives also demonstrate the presence of these antibodies along with the presence of type A chronic atrophic gastritis. Additionally, these relatives have a higher than normal frequency of autoantibodies to antigens of the other organ-specific autoimmune diseases of the endocrine glands that cluster with pernicious anemia (Gleeson & Toh, 1991).

Other causes of pernicious anemia include chronic atrophic gastritis and gastrectomy. Chronic atrophic gastritis may be precipitated by heavy alcohol ingestion, hot tea, and smoking. It is also more common in the elderly. Chronic gastritis destroys the gastric gland with concomitant decreased gastric secretion of IF, hydrochloric acid, and pepsin. Impaired vitamin B_{12} absorption parallels the progress of gastric atrophy and glandular destruction.

Pernicious anemia affects both erythrocyte and leukocyte precursors in the marrow. Platelet precursors are less affected. The number and size of all developing erythroid cells increase, and enormous leukocytes with large and unusually shaped nuclei are found. Hematopoietic alterations vary, depending on the degree of vitamin B_{12} deficiency and metabolic causes leading to the anemia.

Clinical Manifestations

Pernicious anemia develops slowly. By the time it is diagnosed, it is usually severe. Vague early symptoms often are ignored by the individual, including infections, mood swings, and gastrointestinal, cardiac, or kidney ailments. When the hemoglobin has decreased significantly (7 to 8 g/dl), the individual experiences the classic symptoms of anemia: weakness, fatigue, paresthesias of feet and fingers, and difficulty walking. The individual also may complain of loss of appetite, abdominal pain, weight loss, and a sore tongue that is smooth and beefy red. The skin may become "lemon yellow," caused by a combination of pallor and icterus.

Evaluation and Treatment

Evaluation is based on blood tests (Table 23-2), bone marrow aspiration, clinical manifestations, and the Schilling test. In the Schilling test, cobalamin absorption is measured indirectly by administering radioactive cobalamin and measuring its excretion in the urine.

Untreated pernicious anemia is fatal, usually because of heart failure. Death occurs after a course of remissions and exacerbations lasting from 1 to 3 years. Since the advent in 1926 of replacement therapy with vitamin B_{12}, mortality has decreased significantly. Today, death caused by pernicious anemia is rare, and relapses are caused primarily by the individual's noncompliance with therapy.

Treatment for pernicious anemia and other anemias caused by cobalamin deficiency is the administration of cobalamin. Cyanocobalamin or hydroxocobalamin is administered intramuscularly or subcutaneously approximately once a month (weekly until the deficiency is corrected). Oral preparations are not effective because of lack of IF. The effectiveness of cobalamin replacement therapy is manifested by a rising reticulocyte count. Within 5 to 6 weeks, blood counts can return to normal. Pernicious anemia cannot be cured, so maintenance therapy must continue for life. Blood transfusions are given if the individual shows signs of circulatory collapse, heart failure, or severe angina pectoris.

Folate Deficiency Anemias

Folate (folic acid) is a vitamin essential to erythrocyte production and maturation. Folate is necessary for DNA synthesis, being a component of three of the four DNA bases (that is, thymine, adenine, and guanine). Folic acid is also required for RNA synthesis. Absorption of folate occurs primarily in the upper small intestine and does not depend on IF. Folate circulates through and is stored in the liver. Deficiency of folate is more common than cobalamin deficiency, especially in alcoholics and other chronically malnourished individuals. Folate stores are depleted more rapidly than cobalamin stores. Without proper dietary intake of folate, megaloblastic anemia develops.

Clinical manifestations are similar to those of pernicious anemia, except for the lack of neurologic symptoms associated with folate deficiency. Evaluation is based on blood tests, measurement of serum folate levels, and clinical manifestations.

Treatment of folate deficiency anemia requires administration of oral folate preparations daily. One milligram per day is sufficient for most individuals, although alcoholics may require 5 mg. Alcohol interferes with folate metabolism in the liver and results in profound depletion of folate stores (Lee, 1993). Prophylactic doses of 0.1 to 0.4 mg/day are sometimes given in pregnancy. Parenteral administration of folic acid can relieve acute symptoms within 48 hours. Blood transfusions are given to treat severe cardiac or respiratory distress.

Microcytic-Hypochromic Anemias

The microcytic-hypochromic anemias are characterized by erythrocytes that are abnormally small and contain abnormally reduced amounts of hemoglobin (Fig. 23-1, B). Hypochromia occurs even in cells of normal size.

Microcytic-hypochromic anemia can result from a variety of conditions that are caused by (1) disorders of iron metabolism, (2) disorders of porphyrin and heme synthesis, or (3) disorders of globin synthesis. Specific disorders include iron deficiency anemia, sideroblastic anemia, and thalassemia.

Iron Deficiency Anemia

There are several interesting historical tales about iron deficiency anemia (Lee, 1993). The Greek mythologic character, Iphiclus, supposedly drank iron rust dissolved in wine and thereby was cured of impotence. From the sixteenth through the early nineteenth centuries, adolescent girls suffered a malady called chlorosis ("green sickness") that caused a greenish pallor associated with palpitations, breathlessness, ankle edema, thrombophlebitis, and diffuse gastrointestinal complaints. Around 1830, scientists defined chlorosis as a disease of the blood characterized by anemia and lack of iron. Pierre Blaud became famous by successfully treating affected individuals with a combination of ferrous sulfate and potassium carbonate (Haden, 1938). Between 1890 and 1920, the incidence of chlorosis decreased dramatically, not because of iron therapy but because women stopped wearing tight-fitting corsets. Apparently, tight-fitting garments compressed the liver and other abdominal organs or induced reflux of stomach contents, causing blood loss resulting from esophageal inflammation. Women who wore corsets also may have had restricted dietary intake in pursuit of fashionably small waists.

Pathophysiology

Bleeding is the usual cause of **iron deficiency anemia,** although inadequate dietary intake is also a problem in impoverished populations. Recently, investigators have reevaluated the significance of a reduced dietary intake of iron in certain populations as contributing to the development of iron deficiency anemia. Iron plays an important role in the body's defense system and **hypoferremia** has been hypothesized to be an adaptive response to an increased exposure to pathogens. Pathogens require iron to survive; thus, with a reduced amount of iron available, they perish (Stuart-Macadam, 1992).

A daily blood loss of 2 to 4 ml/day (1 to 2 mg of iron) is sufficient to cause this anemia (Lee, 1993). In men, gastrointestinal bleeding is most common and may be caused by gastric or duodenal ulcers, hiatal hernia, esophageal varices, cirrhosis, hemorrhoids, ulcerative colitis, or carcinoma. In women, menorrhagia (profuse menstruation) and pregnancy are reasons for primary iron deficiency anemia. Other causes in both sexes are (1) use of medications that cause gastrointestinal bleeding; (2) surgical procedures that decrease stomach acidity, intestinal transit time, and absorption; (3) insufficient dietary intake of iron; and (4) eating disorders such as pica, the craving and eating of nonnutritional substances. Iron deficiency is common in children younger than 2 years of age because of greatly increased iron requirements associated with growth.

Iron deficiency anemia develops slowly through three overlapping stages. In stage I, the body's iron stores for erythropoiesis are depleted. At this stage, erythropoiesis remains normal, as does the hemoglobin content of the maturing erythrocytes. In stage II, however, not enough iron is transported to the marrow, and iron-deficient erythropoiesis begins. Stage III begins when the small, hemoglobin-deficient cells enter the circulation in sufficient numbers, replacing normal erythrocytes that have grown old and have been removed from the circulation. The development of iron deficiency anemia occurs in stage III and is associated with depleted transport of iron stores and diminished hemoglobin production.

Clinical Manifestations

Iron deficiency anemia is the most common type of anemia throughout the world. The onset of symptoms is gradual, and individuals usually do not seek medical attention until hemoglobin levels drop to a certain point (about 7 to 8 g/dl). Early symptoms include fatigue, weakness, and shortness of breath. Pale ear lobes, palms, and conjunctivae are also common signs.

As the condition progresses and becomes more severe, structural and functional changes in epithelial tissue become apparent. The nails become brittle, thin, and "spoon-shaped" or concave as a result of impaired capillary circulation. The tongue may be sore, with redness and burning caused by atrophy of the papillae. These changes can be reversed after 1 to 2 weeks of iron replacement. Changes also occur in the epithelium at the corners of the mouth, causing soreness and dryness. This defect is called angular stomatitis. Difficulty swallowing is often associated with a "web" of mucus and inflammatory cells at the juncture between the hypopharynx and esophagus. These lesions may become malignant. The pathophysiology of the epithelial changes is unclear.

Because iron is a component of compounds other than hemoglobin (e.g., cytochromes, myoglobin, catalase), deficiencies probably alter several tissue enzymes. Deficient iron enzymes may cause many of the clinical manifestations. Individuals with iron deficiency anemia also exhibit gastritis, neuromuscular changes, irritability, headache, numbness, tingling, and vasomotor disturbances. The pathogenesis of neurologic symptoms is unknown but may be caused by hypoxia in already compromised cerebral vessels. Gait disturbances are rare. Mental confusion, memory loss, and disorientation are frequently associated with anemia in the elderly and may be overlooked as "normal" changes caused by aging.

Evaluation and Treatment

Evaluation is based on clinical manifestations and laboratory tests (Table 23-2). Iron stores are measured directly, by bone marrow biopsy, or indirectly, by tests that measure serum ferritin, transferrin saturation, or total iron-binding capacity. A sensitive indicator of heme synthesis is the amount of free erythrocyte protoporphyrin (FEP) within erythrocytes.

The first step in treatment of iron deficiency anemia is to find and eliminate, or rule out, sources of blood loss. Without this strategy, any pharmacologic therapy is simply palliative. Iron replacement is very effective in the treatment of iron deficiency anemia. In fact, the most conclusive evidence for the diagnosis of iron deficiency anemia is an increase in hemoglobin of 1 to 2 g/dl after iron therapy is initiated. Iron preparations can be administered orally, intramuscularly, or intravenously. Oral administration of ferrous sulfate, gluconate, or fumarate, 6 mg/kg/day up to approximately 200 mg of elemental iron daily, is effective.

Once iron therapy has been instituted, individuals often show a rapid decrease in fatigue, lethargy, and other symptoms. Two thirds of the hemoglobin deficit is generally corrected within the first month of therapy, regardless of the severity of the anemia (Dallman, 1981). Therapy is usually continued for 6 to 12 months after bleeding has been contained. For menstruating women, daily therapy may be needed until menopause. An increase in reticulocyte count is a good measure of response to iron therapy.

Sideroblastic Anemia

Sideroblastic anemias are a heterogenous group of disorders characterized by (1) ineffective erythropoiesis caused by altered hemoglobin, (2) large numbers of sideroblasts in the bone marrow, (3) increased levels of tissue iron, and (4) varying proportions of hypochromic erythrocytes in the blood. Sideroblasts are erythroblasts that contain iron complexes that have been deposited in the mitochondria (Fig. 23-1, *K*).

Pathophysiology

Sideroblastic anemia may be acquired or hereditary. The inherited form of sideroblastic anemia is quite rare, with almost all the reported cases occurring in males, supporting a recessive X-linked transmission; however, autosomal transmission affecting females has been documented. Primary acquired sideroblastic anemia is less rare and usually affects elderly individuals. Secondary acquired sideroblastic anemia is caused by drugs or toxins, such as ethanol, isoniazid, chloramphenicol, phenylbutazone, antineoplastic medications, and lead.

The exact cause of the anemia is not clearly understood; however, evidence exists for lack of or decreased activity of some enzymes that control heme synthesis. Formation of small, hypochromic erythrocytes of various sizes and shapes (anisocytosis and poikilocytosis) occurs, and destruction of defective erythroblasts by phagocytes residing in the marrow is seen. Low hemoglobin levels stimulate erythropoiesis, which causes the marrow to become grossly hyperplastic and perpetuates the anemia.

Clinical Manifestations

In addition to the cardiovascular and respiratory manifestations common to all anemias, individuals with hereditary sideroblastic anemia may show signs of iron overload. Signs include mild to moderate enlargement of the liver (hepatomegaly) and spleen (splenomegaly); however, liver function remains normal or only mildly affected. Occasionally abnormal skin pigmentation (bronze-tinted) may occur. Neurologic and epithelial manifestations often associated with anemias are absent. A major complication of iron overload is heart rhythm disturbances, which, fortunately, are rare and occur late in the disease process. Individuals with acquired sideroblastic anemia generally display mild symptoms.

Evaluation and Treatment

At first, sideroblastic anemia may be mistaken for deficiency of stem cells in the marrow (**hypoplastic anemia**) or iron deficiency anemia. (Laboratory findings are listed in Table 23-2.) Bone marrow examination establishes the diagnosis of sideroblastic anemia. The marrow is packed with erythrocyte stem cells, and mononuclear phagocytes in the marrow are loaded with iron in the form of hemosiderin. Presence of sideroblasts confirms the diagnosis of sideroblastic anemia.

Treatment and management of sideroblastic anemia are straightforward. If the anemia results from a drug or noxious substance, the offending treatment is discontinued or the substance is avoided. Pyridoxine therapy is sometimes beneficial in the hereditary form. Iron is not given. Blood transfusions are limited to prevent hemochromatosis (an accumulation of iron in tissues), which would result in cellular damage. Deferoxamine, an iron chelating agent, may be used; however, it is time-consuming (12-hour infusions) and may require treatment over a period of years. The course and prognosis of sideroblastic anemia are variable. Death may occur because of infection, bone marrow failure, liver failure, or cardiac dysrhythmias. Sideroblastic anemia also has the potential to convert to **myelodysplastic syndrome** with the possibility of developing acute myeloblastic leukemia.

Normocytic-Normochromic Anemias

Normocytic-normochromic anemias are anemias in which erythrocytes are relatively normal in size and hemoglobin content but insufficient in number. The normocytic-normochromic anemias do not share any common cause, pathologic mechanism, or morphologic characteristics. These anemias are less common than the macrocytic-normochromic and microcytic-hypochromic anemias. Five distinct anemic conditions—aplastic anemia, posthemorrhagic anemia, hemolytic anemia, anemia of chronic inflammation, and sickle cell anemia—exemplify the diversity of the normocytic-normochromic classification.

Aplastic Anemia

Aplastic anemia is caused either by **bone marrow hypoplasia** or **bone marrow aplasia,** conditions in which hematopoietic marrow or erythrocyte stem cells are underdeveloped, defective, or absent. Many disease processes interfere temporarily or permanently with the viability of the pluripotential stem cell. Reduction in numbers of pluripotential stem cells or their ability to become committed stem cells causes reduced hematopoiesis. If all the cell lines are affected and all cellular components of circulating blood are reduced, a life-threatening condition known as **pancytopenia** results. If only the erythrocyte stem cells are affected, the condition in the marrow is termed **pure red cell aplasia,** and in the circulation is called aplastic anemia.

Pathophysiology

Pure red cell aplasia in an adult is rare and may result from infiltrative disorders of the bone marrow (myelofibrosis, leukemia, myeloma, or carcinoma); autoimmune diseases; renal failure; splenic dysfunction; cobalamin or folate deficiency; parvovirus infection; and exposure to radiation, drugs, and toxins. Drugs known to cause aplastic anemia are identified in Table 23-3. A thymoma is often found in association with red cell aplasia. A congenital condition (Diamond-Blackfan syndrome) also has been identified.

The exact mechanism that halts erythropoiesis is not known, but two theories have been proposed. The first, called the seed or stem-cell–deficiency theory, proposes that a common stem cell population is irreversibly altered, rendering it incapable of proliferation and differentiation. The second theory, the microenvironmental

---

TABLE 23-3

Anemias Secondary to Drug Effects

Drug	Hemolytic	Megaloblastic	Sideroblastic	Aplastic
Antibiotics				
Amphotericin B				X
Bactrim (trimethoprim-sulfamethoxazole)		X		
Chloramphenicol (chloromycetin)			XX	XXXX
Erythromycin	X			X
Gantrisin (Sulfisoxazole)				X
Penicillin	XXX			X
Sulfanilamide/sulfonamides	XX			X,X*
Streptomycin	X			X

X, rare number of reported cases; *XXXX*, substantial number of reported cases; *XX, XXX*, intermediate number of reported cases; *X**, "pure red cell" aplasia.

TABLE 23-3

Anemias Secondary to Drug Effects—cont'd

Drug	Hemolytic	Megaloblastic	Sideroblastic	Aplastic
Anticonvulsants				
Diphenylhydantoin (Dilantin)		XXX		XXX,X*
Mephenytoin		XXX		XXX
Mysoline (primidone)		XX		
Phenobarbitol		XX		
Tridione (trimethadione)				XXX
Antiinflammatory				
ASA (aspirin)				X*
Colchicine		X?		X*
Gold compounds				XX
Ibuprofen (Motrin)	X			X
Indomethacin (Indocin)				X
Phenacetin	XXX			
Phenylbutazone				XX,X*
Antihypertensive/diuretics				
Aldomet	XXX			
Diamox				X
Thiazides	X			
Tranquilizers				
Chlordiazepoxide (Librium)				X
Chlorpromazine (Thorazine)	XX			X
Meprobamate				X
Oral hypoglycemics				
Chlorpropamide (Diabinese)	X			
Tolbutamide (Orinase)				X,X*
Immunosuppressants				
Azathioprine (Imuran)			X	X*
Cyclosporine	X			
Miscellaneous agents				
Benzene	XX			XX
Tagamet (cimetidine)				X
Heparin				X*
INH (isoniazid) ⎱ Anti-TB agents	XX			
PASA (paraamino- salicylic acid) ⎰	XX	X		
Pyridium (phenazopyridine HCl)				XX
Potassium perchlorate				XX
Quinine/quinidine	XX			

deficiency theory, proposes that the stem cell environment (i.e., the marrow) is altered so as to inhibit erythropoiesis (Williams, 1993). An immune response is implicated in aplastic anemia regardless of the precipitating agent or cause (Nissen, 1991).

If the erythrocyte stem cells or the marrow is unable to recover from the insult within months, bone marrow aplasia leads to death from anemia, infection, or hemorrhage. If the insult is mild, causing bone marrow hypoplasia, anemia is less severe and the individual may live for years.

Clinical Manifestations

Aplastic anemia causes the classic cardiovascular and respiratory manifestations of anemia. If the stem cells of platelets and leukocytes also are damaged or deficient, anemia is accompanied by platelet deficiency (thrombocytopenia), which results in hemorrhage into the tissues and leukocyte deficiency (leukopenia), and infection.

Evaluation and Treatment

Bone marrow biopsy is necessary to determine whether the anemia is caused by pure red cell aplasia or hypoplasia (Table 23-2).

The most important aspect of treatment for aplastic anemia is to treat the underlying disorder or prevent further exposure to the causal agent. Hemoglobin levels can be improved temporarily with blood transfusions. Definitive treatment is marrow transplant or pharmacologic stimulation of the marrow function. Hemorrhage or infection is treated as needed. Splenectomy is considered if transfused erythrocytes are being destroyed in the spleen. Immunosuppression therapy is also recommended (Nissen, 1991).

Posthemorrhagic Anemia

Posthemorrhagic anemia is a normocytic-normochromic anemia caused by sudden blood loss in an individual with normal iron stores. Hemorrhage may be obvious (after surgery or trauma) or occult, such as that caused by malignancy or gastrointestinal disorders. Minor prolonged hemorrhage does not result in classic posthemorrhagic anemia, but rather in iron deficiency anemia—a microcytic-hypochromic anemia.

Within 24 hours of blood loss, the body begins to replace lost plasma and blood cells. Water and electrolytes from tissues and interstitial spaces are mobilized to expand plasma volume and accelerate hematopoiesis. Clinical manifestations of anemia are likely to be obscured by the cardiovascular manifestations of acute hemorrhage. Severe shock, lactic acidosis, and death can occur if blood loss exceeds 40% to 50% of plasma volume.

Treatment entails restoring blood volume by intravenous administration of saline, dextran, albumin, or plasma. For large blood losses, transfusion of fresh whole blood is the treatment of choice. The anemia itself does not require specific therapy unless it is associated with iron, folate, or cobalamin deficiency. A normal erythrocyte count is usually evident in 4 to 6 weeks, but hemoglobin restoration can take 6 to 8 weeks.

Hemolytic Anemia

Premature, accelerated destruction of erythrocytes, either episodically or continuously, is a clinical manifestation of many disease states and is the predominant pathogenic event in **hemolytic anemias**. Erythropoiesis is normal and production of erythrocytes may accelerate to 8 times normal; eventually production is not able to compensate for destruction, and anemia results.

Pathophysiology

Hemolytic anemias may be acquired or hereditary. Acquired hemolytic anemias generally are caused by extrinsic (extracellular) defects, such as infection, systemic disease, drugs or toxins, liver disease, kidney disease, or abnormal immune responses. Hereditary forms are caused by intrinsic (cellular) abnormalities, typically of the erythrocyte's plasma membrane or cytoplasmic contents (enzymes of hemoglobin). Congenital hemolytic anemias are present at birth and may or may not be inherited. Causes of acquired and inherited hemolytic anemias are listed in Table 23-4.

Hemolysis occurs within blood vessels or in lymphoid tissues that filter blood, i.e., spleen and liver. Hemolysis that occurs within the vessels tends to be caused by chemicals (drugs or toxins), antibodies, or erythrocyte fragility. Hemolysis within lymphoid tissues is mostly caused by destruction and digestion by macrophages of the mononuclear phagocyte system (MPS). Erythrocytes become more rigid, thus slowing their passage through the spleen, making them vulnerable to phagocytosis. Erythrocytes coated with IgG are particularly vulnerable (Delamaire et al., 1992).

Most hemolytic anemias are acquired and are caused by immune mechanisms. The two most common types are **autoimmune hemolytic anemias (AIHA)** and **drug-induced hemolytic anemias**. The autoimmune hemolytic anemias may be of two types: **warm antibody disease** and **cold antibody disease**.

Warm antibody disease is mediated by immunoglobulin (IgG) antibody that is specific for erythrocyte antigens and binds to the surface of the erythrocyte at normal body temperature (37° C). Immunoglobulin A also has been implicated in this immune process.

Cold antibody disease is mediated by a different immunoglobulin (IgM) specific for erythrocyte antigens. The IgM binds to erythrocytes only at colder temperatures (below 31° C), which may occur in the fingers and toes during cold weather. Agglutination of IgM-bound

TABLE 23-4

Causes of Hemolytic Anemias

Type of hemolytic disorder	Primary cause or associated disorder	Mechanisms of erythrocyte destruction
Acquired forms		
Immune system—mediated hemolysis	Transfusion reaction Hemolytic disease of the newborn (see Chapter 25) Autoimmune hemolytic anemia (see text)	Antibody-mediated erythrocytes by enzymes of the complement system (see Chapter 7)
Traumatic hemolysis	Presence of prosthetic heart valves Structural abnormalities of the heart Hemolytic uremic syndrome Disseminated intravascular coagulation Hemodialysis	Physical destruction of erythrocytes by "mechanical" means (trauma)
Infectious hemolysis	Bacterial infection (clostridia, cholera, typhoid fever) Protozoal infection (malaria, toxoplasmosis)	Infection of erythrocytes
Toxic (chemical) hemolysis	Exposure to toxic chemical agents Hemodialysis or uremia Venoms	Chemical injury of erythrocytes (see Chapter 2)
Physical hemolysis	Burns Radiation	Heat or radiation injury (see Chapter 2)
Hypophosphatemic hemolysis	Hypophosphatemia (phosphate deficiency in plasma; see Chapter 3)	Diminished cellular production of substances required for erythrocyte life and function
Hereditary forms		
Structural defects	Plasma membrane defects	Fragility of the erythrocyte
Enzyme deficiencies	Deficiency of glycolytic enzymes Deficiency of metabolic enzymes (i.e., glucose-6-phosphate dehydrogenase deficiency)	Diminished cellular function
Defects of globin synthesis or structure	Sickle cell anemia	Increased membrane fragility and deformation during sickle crises
	Thalassemia	Defective hemoglobin structure and function
	Miscellaneous hemoglobin defects	Defective hemoglobin structure and function

From Lee, G. R., Bithell, T. C., Foerster, J., Athens, J. W., & Lukens, J. N. (1993). *Wintrobe's clinical hematology* (9th ed.). Philadelphia: Lea & Febiger.

erythrocytes in the extremities produces pain and tissue destruction. In addition, when the antibody-coated cells are warmed on reentering the general circulation, the antibody may dissociate from the erythrocyte. If it does not, hemolysis of the cell may occur. Thus, cold antibody disease is more a problem of vascular obstruction than hemolysis. Cold antibody disease is often a complication of infectious mononucleosis, mycoplasma pneumonia, and lymphoid malignancies. It has also been identified with the Epstein-Barr virus, cytomegalovirus infection, mumps, and Legionnaire disease.

Drug-induced immune hemolytic anemia is initiated by three mechanisms of actions (Fig. 23-2). The first mechanism induces a disorder much like the warm antibody immunohemolytic anemia described previously. The second mechanism—the drug-adsorption mechanism—induces hemolysis by the binding of the drug with the erythrocyte surface and the formation of antibodies directed against this erythrocyte-drug complex. The final mechanism—the immune complex "innocent bystander" mechanism—induces hemolysis through a drug—plasma protein complex to which an antibody

1. Warm antibody mechanism

Binds to erythrocytes at
normal body temperature 37° C

Hemolysis

2. Drug absorption mechanism

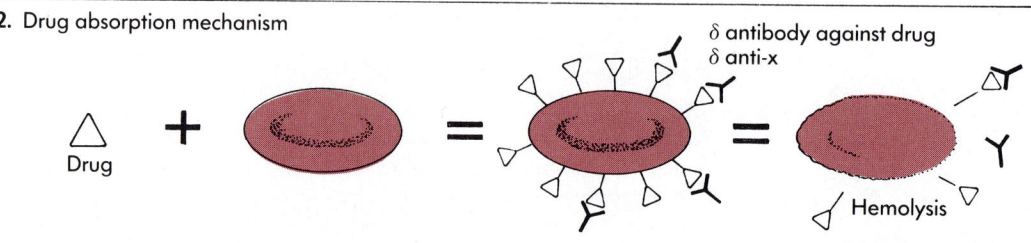

δ antibody against drug
δ anti-x

Drug

Hemolysis

3. Immune complex "innocent bystander" mechanism

Blood vessel

RBC

Activates
complement

Xp = Drug plasma protein complex

FIG. 23-2 **Drug-induced immune hemolytic anemia.** (Discussion in text.)

TABLE 23-5

Types of Polycythemia

Type of polycythemia	Mechanism of increased erythropoiesis	Cause or associated disorder
Primary polycythemia (polycythemia vera)	Excessive proliferation of erythroid precursors in marrow; increased sensitivity of pluripotential stem cell to erythropoietin	Unknown
Secondary polycythemia	Physiologic increase in erythropoietin secretion by the kidneys in response to underlying systemic disorder	Tissue hypoxia caused by cardiopulmonary disorders (chronic obstruction pulmonary disease, congestive heart failure), decreased barometric pressure, cardiovascular malformations causing mixing of arterial and venous blood, methemoglobinemia, carboxyhemoglobinemia, smoking, obesity
	"Nonphysiologic"* increase in erythropoietin secretion	Renal disorders, cerebellar hemangioblastomas, hepatoma (liver tumor), ovarian carcinoma, uterine leiomyoma, pheochromocytoma, adrenocortical hypersecretion
Familial polycythemia	Genetically induced increase in erythroid precursors of the marrow Abnormal Hb with increased oxygen affinity Decreased 2,3-DPG Increased sensitivity of stem cells to erythropoietin Increased erythropoietin in secretion	Genetic defect

*Nonphysiologic means that there is no obvious physiologic explanation for hypersecretion of erythropoietin.

forms. This drug–plasma protein complex attaches itself to the erythrocyte. Complement becomes fixed as a result of the antigen-antibody interaction, resulting in the complete lysis of the red cell. Drugs that have been known to cause hemolytic anemia are identified in Table 23-3.

Clinical Manifestations

The presence and severity of signs and symptoms of hemolytic anemia depend on the degree of hemolysis and the success of compensatory erythropoiesis. The spleen enlarges as it removes more and more dead or defective erythrocytes from the circulation. Jaundice (icterus) occurs if heme breakdown exceeds the liver's ability to conjugate and excrete bilirubin.

Acute conditions—aplastic, hemolytic, or megaloblastic crises—frequently develop if other diseases, particularly viral infections, are also present. Crises are associated with further declines in levels of hemoglobin in the peripheral blood and occasionally bone marrow hypoplasia or aplasia.

In severe hemolytic anemia, the bones become deformed as a result of expansion of hematopoietic bone marrow, and pathologic fractures often occur. Cardiovascular and respiratory manifestations vary with the degree of anemia.

Evaluation and Treatment

Evaluation is based on clinical manifestations, bone marrow studies, and blood tests (Table 23-2). Abnormally increased numbers of erythrocyte stem cells are found in the marrow, a finding termed *erythroid hyperplasia*. Acceleration of erythropoiesis causes large numbers of fragile and immature erythrocytes (stem cells and reticulocytes) to be released prematurely into the circulation. These cells are seen in blood smears.

Acquired hemolytic anemias can be treated by removing the cause or treating the underlying disorder. Acute, fulminating hemolytic anemia (hemolytic crisis) is treated with fluid and electrolyte replacement to prevent shock and renal damage from clogging the kidney tubules by red cell debris. Transfusions of blood products are sometimes given. Splenectomy is performed if the spleen is the major site of hemolysis and splenomegaly is significant.

Steroids are often used to treat autoimmune hemolytic anemias. Folate is given for chronic hemolytic disease because long-term erythrocyte turnover increases folate requirements.

Anemia of Chronic Inflammation (Disease)

Anemia of chronic inflammation is a mild to moderate anemia associated with chronic infections, including acquired immune deficiency syndrome (AIDS); chronic noninfectious inflammatory diseases, including rheumatoid arthritis and other autoimmune conditions (systemic lupus erythematosus [SLE], inflammatory bowel conditions); and malignancies. The anemia develops after 1 to 2 months of active disease. The severity of anemia is related to that of the underlying disorder and may be an asymptomatic or coincidental clinical finding. Morphologically, anemia of chronic inflammation is usually normocytic-normochromic, but it may also be normocytic-hypochromic or microcytic-hypochromic. The exact incidence of anemia of chronic inflammation is unknown. Because it is associated with so many pathologic conditions, it is probably second only to iron deficiency anemia in overall incidence.

Pathophysiology

Three pathogenic mechanisms cause anemia of chronic inflammation: (1) decreased erythrocyte lifespan, (2) failure of mechanisms of compensatory erythropoiesis, and (3) disturbances of the iron cycle (Fig. 23-3).

The decreased erythrocyte lifespan appears to be attributable to red cell destruction mediated by some extrinsic factor that renders the erythrocyte more vulnerable to phagocytosis. Macrophages activated during infection, inflammation, and malignancy have been suggested as the agents that act on the erythrocytes (Erslev, 1990). Red cell destruction in the presence of cancer also may be caused by (1) release of hemolytic agents from the tumor (Sheets, Hamilton, DeGowin, & Janney, 1954) and (2) destruction of the erythrocytes as they enter the tumor (Price & Greenfield, 1958). Anemia associated with chronic infections is thought to be the result of the hemolytic action of bacterial toxins. Coating of the erythrocytes with a small amount of antibody, as seen in infections, also initiates destruction of the red cell (Atkinson & Frank, 1974).

The erythropoietic defect in anemia of chronic inflammation is a failure to increase erythropoiesis in response to hemolysis. Erythropoiesis does not accelerate, but rather continues at the normal rate. This failure is the result of suppression of erythroid progenitor cells by cytokines that have been released from activated macrophages and lymphocytes. The cytokines include prostaglandins, acidic isoferritin, interferons, and tumor necrosis factor. Synergistic effects of these cytokines have been demonstrated (Fuchs et al., 1991). Concomitant with suppression of bone marrow function, there is a reduction in the amount of iron in the blood that impairs the ability of bone marrow to respond to erythropoietin and hemoglobin synthesis.

Impaired iron stores are a major contributing factor to the anemia of chronic inflammation (Fig. 23-3). It is hypothesized that this is caused by iron binding with **lactoferrin** in the plasma. Lactoferrin is a compound that closely resembles transferrin, the protein that normally binds with iron in the plasma and transports it to

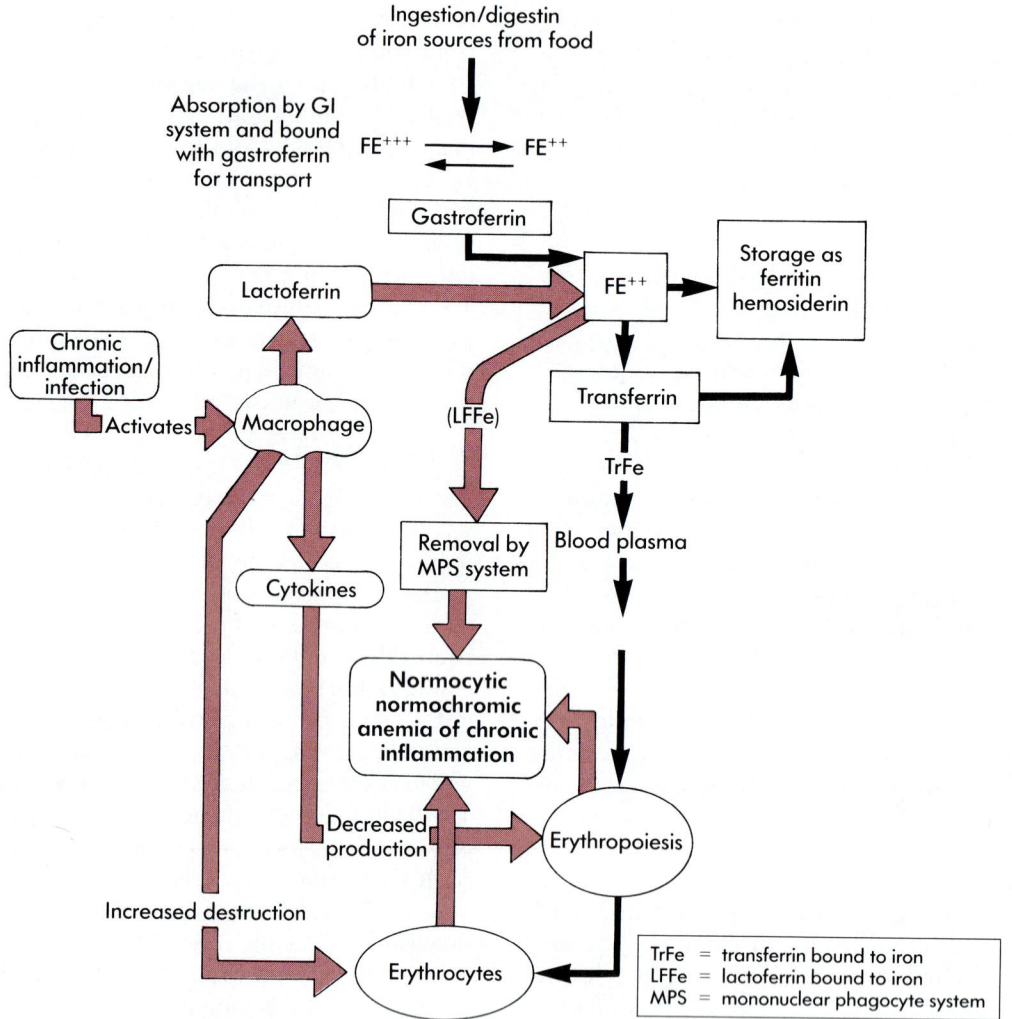

FIG. 23-3 Pathophysiology of anemia of chronic inflammation. Normal iron metabolism is indicated by the narrow arrows. Abnormal mechanisms that are instrumental in the development of anemia of chronic inflammation are indicated by thick arrows. (Discussion in text.)

the bone marrow for erythropoiesis. Under normal conditions, lactoferrin is only present in the blood in minute amounts. During periods of inflammation and infection, however, neutrophils release lactoferrin, making it available to bind with iron competing with transferrin for the available iron. The affinity of iron for lactoferrin is 260 times greater than for transferrin. Iron that is bound to lactoferrin is removed by the MPS instead of being transported to the marrow. Lactoferrin also has significant antibacterial effects because of its ability to bind with iron, thus depriving bacteria of an essential nutritional supplement (Birgens, 1991).

Clinical Manifestations

Anemia of chronic inflammation has fewer and milder clinical manifestations than most other anemias. Manifestations depend on the degree of anemia. As a rule,

disability caused by chronic disease limits physical activity, so that hemoglobin levels are adequate. If hemoglobin levels drop significantly, however, the clinical manifestations of iron deficiency anemia appear.

Evaluation and Treatment

The significant finding in anemia of chronic inflammation is iron deficiency in the marrow despite normal or increased iron stores elsewhere in the body. (Blood test findings are listed in Table 23-2.) Individuals with anemia of chronic inflammation but no evidence of inflammation or infection are screened for the presence of neoplasms.

Anemia of chronic inflammation does not respond to iron replacement therapy because iron is unable to reach the bone marrow. Use of erythropoietin in treatment of anemias associated with arthritis, malignancies, and

AIDS has met with limited success (Drueke, 1991). The mainstay of treatment, therefore, is alleviation of the underlying disorder. The anemia itself does not require treatment unless it becomes symptomatic.

MYELOPROLIFERATIVE RED CELL DISORDERS (POLYCYTHEMIA VERA)

Hematologic dysfunction may result from an overproduction of cells, as well as a deficiency. One or more marrow elements may be produced in excess, responding to exogenous (radiation, drugs) or endogenous (physiologic compensatory response, immune disorder) signals. An overabundance of white cells results in leukemia (see Chapters 24 and 25). An excess of red cells produces a group of disorders classified as polycythemia (Table 23-5).

Polycythemia vera is an unusual myeloproliferative disease that causes **erythrocytosis**—excessively large numbers of erythrocytes in the blood. It was first described in 1892 by a French physician, M. H. Vaquez. In the early 1900s, William Osler undertook an extensive investigation of the disease. Not much more was learned about polycythemia vera until the 1960s, at which time researchers began to investigate a link between polycythemias of all kinds and neoplasia affecting stem cells.

Pathophysiology

Polycythemia vera is caused by excessive proliferation of erythrocyte precursors in the marrow. The fact that it typically is accompanied by increases of circulating platelets and granulocytes suggests that polycythemia vera is caused by an abnormality of the pluripotential stem cell. Controversy exists as to whether polycythemia vera should be classified as a leukemia (see Chapter 24) or a problem of marrow hyperplasia (i.e., myeloproliferative disorder).

There are essentially two types of polycythemia vera: primary (absolute) and secondary (relative). The primary form of polycythemia vera is relatively rare and tends to occur in men between the ages of 40 and 60. It is more common in whites, particularly Jews of European ancestry, than in blacks. Rarely is polycythemia vera found in children or multiple members of a single family. The cause of secondary polycythemia, the more common form, is an essentially physiologic response to hypoxia. Therefore it is not uncommon to find an increased red cell count in individuals living at high altitudes (10,000 feet) and in smokers and individuals with congestive heart failure and chronic obstructive pulmonary disease.

Erythrocytosis causes blood volume and blood viscosity to increase because of an increased erythrocyte count. The liver and spleen become increasingly con- gested with erythrocytes as viscosity causes blood flow to slow. Eventually, the thick, sticky, slow-flowing blood becomes an ideal environment for clotting and acidosis. If thrombi obstruct vessels, tissue or organ infarction (blood deprivation) results.

Clinical Manifestations

The clinical manifestations of polycythemia vera are caused by increased blood volume and viscosity and clogging of microcirculatory blood vessels. They include (1) plethora (ruddy, red color of the face, hands, feet, ears, and mucous membranes), (2) engorgement of retinal and sublingual veins, (3) splenomegaly, and (4) hepatomegaly. Symptoms include headache, a feeling of fullness in the head, dizziness, weakness, elevated blood pressure, itching, sweating, weight loss, epigastric distress, fatigue on exertion, backache, and visual disturbances. The eyes may be bloodshot, and intense pruritus (itching) after bathing may be so troublesome that the individual avoids bathing with warm water. The cause of the pruritus is unknown, and the symptoms do not respond to antihistamines.

Clinical manifestations of vascular disease may predominate, including angina pectoris, calf pain associated with walking-induced vasospasm (intermittent claudication), thrombotic disease, and cerebral insufficiency. Thrombosis of gastric vessels can cause ulcers and mesenteric pain. Respiratory infections are common, as is hoarseness. Some individuals with polycythemia vera tend to bleed, especially from the gastrointestinal and genitourinary tracts. Microvascular clots interfere with normal coagulation mechanisms, and a disseminated intravascular coagulation—like syndrome can occur.

Evaluation and Treatment

Blood and laboratory findings establish the diagnosis. Diagnosis is characterized by an absolute increase in red blood cells and in the total blood volume, although it is not unusual to also have moderate increases in white blood cells and platelets. A bone marrow examination may be done; however, it is incapable of definitively establishing the diagnosis. Treatment for polycythemia vera consists of reducing erythrocytosis and blood volume, controlling symptoms, and preventing thrombosis. Erythrocytosis and blood volume are reduced by phlebotomy, a procedure in which a vein is opened and blood is removed. Three hundred to 500 ml may be removed 2 to 3 times per week until hematocrit drops sufficiently. After that, phlebotomy may be done every 3 to 4 months. Frequent phlebotomies also reduce the amount of iron available; thus, the individual may become iron deficient. Iron deficiency impedes erythropoiesis so that phlebotomies are not needed as frequently. Smokers should be urged to quit, and patients with congestive heart failure and chronic obstructive pulmonary disease require appropriate pharmaceutical intervention.

Radioactive phosphorus is sometimes given orally or intravenously to suppress erythropoiesis. Unfortunately, a side effect of this therapy can be the general suppression of hematopoiesis, resulting in anemia, leukopenia, or thrombocytopenia. Radioactive phosphorus is not given at frequent intervals—as much as 18 months may elapse between treatments. Myelosuppressive drugs (marrow suppressants) are also used, but their effects can be more unpleasant than the disease.

Without proper treatment, 50% of individuals with polycythemia vera die within 18 months of the onset of initial symptoms. The major cause of death is thrombosis or hemorrhage. A significant potential outcome of polycythemia vera is the conversion to acute myeloid leukemia (AML), occurring in approximately 10% of individuals, which is generally resistant to conventional therapy. Conversion to AML is probably related to treatment methods associated with cytotoxic agents. Although polycythemia vera is a chronic disorder, appropriate therapy results in remissions and prevention of significant morbidity and mortality.

SUMMARY REVIEW

Anemia

1 Anemia is generally defined as a reduction in the number or volume of circulating red cells or an alteration in hemoglobin.

2 Anemias can be classified according to erythrocyte size or concentration of hemoglobin, cause of low blood count, or according to the kinetics of why constant and adequate numbers of mature erythrocytes are not maintained in the circulation.

3 Clinical manifestations of anemia can be found in all organs and tissues throughout the body. Decreased oxygen delivery to tissues can cause fatigue, dyspnea, syncope, angina, compensatory tachycardia, and organ dysfunction.

4 Macrocytic/megaloblastic anemias are most commonly caused by deficiency of vitamin B_{12}. Pernicious anemia can be fatal unless vitamin B_{12} replacement is given.

5 Microcytic-hypochromic anemias are characterized by abnormally small red cells with insufficient hemoglobin content. The most common cause is iron deficiency.

6 Iron deficiency anemia usually develops slowly, with gradual insidious onset of symptoms. Fatigue, weakness, dyspnea, alteration of various epithelial tissues, and vague neuromuscular complaints result.

7 Iron deficiency anemia is usually a result of blood loss or poor nutritional intake. Once the source of blood loss is defined and corrected, iron replacement therapy can be initiated. Elevated reticulocyte count is a good index of response to iron therapy.

8 Sideroblastic anemia results from impaired iron metabolism and abnormal sequestration of iron. Treatment varies depending on the cause.

9 Normocytic-normochromic anemias are characterized by insufficient numbers of normal erythrocytes. Included in this category are aplastic, posthemorrhagic, and hemolytic anemia, and anemia of chronic disease.

10 In aplastic anemia erythrocyte stem cells are underdeveloped, defective, or absent. Unless the cause is determined, bone marrow aplasia results in death.

11 Sudden blood loss after hemorrhage results in a normocytic-normochromic anemia. Restoration of blood volume by plasma expanders or transfusions may diminish subjective symptoms of anemia. Hemoglobin restoration may take 6 to 8 weeks.

12 Premature destruction of erythrocytes (hemolytic anemia) may be acquired or hereditary. Of the acquired forms, autoimmune reaction and drug-induced hemolysis are the most common.

13 Failure of erythropoiesis in anemia of chronic inflammation may result in release of cytokines and lactoferrin by phagocytic cells. Lactoferrin has been shown to cause abrupt decreases in plasma iron levels and interferes with the normal iron cycle.

Myeloproliferative Red Cell Disorders (Polycythemia Vera)

1 Polycythemia vera is characterized by excessive proliferation of erythrocyte precursors in the bone marrow. Signs and symptoms result directly from increased blood volume and viscosity. Therapeutic phlebotomy to remove excessive blood volume and use of radioactive phosphorus have been helpful in decreasing the excessive red cell pool.

KEY TERMS

Anemia, 861
Anemia of chronic inflammation, 873
Anisocytosis, 861
Aplastic anemia, 868
Autoimmune hemolytic anemia (AIHA), 870
Bone marrow aplasia, 868
Bone marrow hypoplasia, 868
Cold antibody disease, 870
Drug-induced hemolytic anemia, 870
Erythrocytosis, 875

Hemolysis, 862
Hemolytic anemia, 870
Hyperchromic erythrocyte, 861
Hypochromic erythrocyte, 861
Hypoferremia, 866
Hypoplastic anemia, 867
Iron deficiency anemia, 866
Lactoferrin, 873
Macrocytic anemia (megaloblastic anemia), 864
Macrocytic erythrocyte, 861
Microcytic erythrocyte, 861

Myelodysplastic syndrome, 868
Normochromic cell, 861
Normocytic cell, 861
Pancytopenia, 868
Pernicious anemia, 865
Poikilocytosis, 861
Polycythemia vera, 875
Posthemorrhagic anemia, 870
Pure red cell aplasia, 868
Sideroblastic anemia, 867
Warm antibody disease, 870

REFERENCES

Atkinson, J. P., & Frank, M. M. (1974). The effect of bacillus Calmette-Guerin-induced macrophage activation on the in vivo clearance of sensitized erythrocytes. *Journal of Clinical Investigation, 53,* 1742.

Birgens, H. S. (1991). The interaction of lactoferrin with human monocytes. *Danish Medical Bulletin, 38,* 244-252.

Dallman, P. R. (1981). Anemia of prematurity. *Annual Review of Medicine, 32,* 143-160.

Delamaire, M., Durand, F., Grosbois, B., LeDantec, G., LeGoff, M. C., LeBlay, R., & Gentetet, B. (1992). Is there a mechanical factor of haemolysis in patients with positive IgG type direct antiglobulin test? *British Journal of Haematology, 80,* 91-96.

Drueke, T. B. (1991). Modulating factors in the hematopoietic response to erythropoietin. *American Journal of Kidney Disease, 18,* 87-92.

Erslev, A. J. (1990). Anemia of chronic disorders. In W. J. Williams, E. Beutler, A. J. Erslev, & M. A. Lichtman (Eds.), *Hematology* (4th ed., pp. 540-545). New York: McGraw-Hill.

Fuchs, D., Hausen, A., Gilbert, R., Werner, E. R., Werner-Felmayer, G., Dierich, M. P., & Wachter, H. (1991). Immune activation and the anaemia associated with chronic inflammatory disorders. *European Journal of Haematology, 46,* 65-70.

Gleeson, P. A., & Toh, B. (1991). Molecular targets in pernicious anemia. *Immunology Today, 12,* 233-238.

Haden, R. L. (1938). Historical aspects of iron therapy in anemia. *Journal of the American Medical Association, 111,* 1059.

Lee, G. R. (1993). Megaloblastic and nonmegaloblastic macrocytic anemias. In G. R. Lee, T. C. Bithell, J. Foerster, J. W. Athens, & J. N. Lukens (Eds.), *Wintrobe's clinical hematology* (9th ed.). Philadelphia: Lea & Febiger.

Lee, G. R., (1993). Nutritional factors in the production and function of erythrocytes. In G. R. Lee, T. C. Bithell, J. Foerster, J. W. Athens, & J. N. Lukens (Eds.), *Wintrobe's clinical hematology* (9th ed.). Philadelphia: Lea & Febiger.

Lee, G. R., (1993). Iron deficiency and iron deficiency anemia. In G. R. Lee, T. C. Bithell, J. Foerster, J. W. Athens, & J. N. Lukens (Eds.), *Wintrobe's clinical hematology* (9th ed.). Philadelphia: Lea & Febiger.

Nissen, C. (1991). The pathophysiology of aplastic anemia. *Seminars in Hematology, 28,* 313-318.

Price, V. E., & Greenfield, R. E. (1958). Anemia in cancer. In J. P.

Greenstein & A. Haddow (Eds.), *Advances in cancer research* (Vol. 5). New York: Academic Press.

Sheets, R. F., Hamilton, H. E., DeGowin, E. L., & Janney, C. D. (1954). Spontaneous x-ray induced hemolysis in malignancy. *Journal of Clinical Investigations, 33,* 179.

Stuart-Macadam, P. (1992). Porotic hyperostosis: A new perspective. *American Journal of Physical Anthropology, 87,* 39-47.

Wintrobe, M. M., Lee, G. R., Boggs, D. R., Bithell, T. C., Foerster, J., Athens, J. W., & Lukens, J. N. (1981). *Clinical hematology* (8th ed.). Philadelphia: Lea & Febiger.

Williams, D. M. (1993). Pancytopenia, aplastic anemia, and pure red cell aplasia. In G. R. Lee, T. C. Bithell, J. Foerster, J. W. Athens, & J. N. Lukens (Eds.), *Wintrobe's clinical hematology* (9th ed.). Philadelphia: Lea & Febiger.

SUGGESTED READINGS

Berkowitz, F. E. (1991). Hemolysis and infection: Categories and mechanisms of their interrelationship. *Review of Infectious Diseases, 13,* 1151-1162.

Brown, R. G. (1991). Determining the cause of anemia. *Postgraduate Medicine, 89,* 161-170.

Brown, R. G. (1991). Normocytic and macrocytic anemias. *Postgraduate Medicine, 89,* 125-136.

Erslev, A. J. (1991). Erythropoietin. *New England Journal of Medicine, 324,* 1339-1344.

Isbister, J. P., & Pittiglio, D. H. (1988). *Clinical hematology: A problem oriented approach.* Baltimore: Williams & Wilkins.

Murphy, W. G., & Kelton, J. G. (1991). Immune haemolytic anaemia and thrombocytopenia: Drugs and autoantibodies. *Biochemical Society Transactions, 19,* 183-186.

Nusbaum, N. J. (1991). Concise review: Genetic bases for sideroblastic anemia. *American Journal of Hematology, 41,* 37-41.

Simmons, A. (1989). *Hematology: A combined theoretical and technical approach.* Philadelphia: Saunders.

Treleaven, J., & Barrett, J. (1990). Drugs and the bone marrow. *British Journal of Hospital Medicine, 44,* 245-250.

Williams, W. J., Beutler, E., Erslev, A. J., & Lichtman, M. A. (1990). *Hematology* (4th ed.). New York: McGraw-Hill.

Alterations of Leukocyte, Lymphoid, and Hemostatic Function

Thom J. Mansen

Kathryn L. McCance

Rosemary Field

Pamela F. Cipriano*

Chapter Outline

Many of the disorders involving leukocytes range from purely reactive alterations, such as leukocytosis, to proliferative disorders, such as leukemia. An event of importance to hematology has been its increasing relationship with oncology. Many hematologic disorders are malignancies, and many nonhematologic malignancies metastasize to bone marrow. Thus, a large portion of this chapter is devoted to malignant disease.

Because the only role of clotting (hemostasis) is to stop bleeding, this interesting self-regulatory system is obviously essential to survival. Remarkable is the fact that blood clots when shed and does not normally clot within blood vessels. Platelets—through a renaissance of research interest—are known to have roles in clotting, wound healing, inflammation, and phagocytosis of foreign matter. They also play deleterious roles, however, in the pathogenesis of many diseases. This chapter also covers various clotting factors and their control systems.

ALTERATIONS OF LEUKOCYTE FUNCTION

Leukocyte function is affected if too many or too few cells are present in the blood or if the cells that are present are structurally or functionally defective. The presence of too many or too few cells, the so-called quantitative disorders, can be the result of bone marrow dysfunction or premature destruction of cells in the circulation. Many quantitative alterations, however, originate in the circulation or lymphoid organs in response to invasion by infectious microorganisms.

Most qualitative disorders consist of disruptions of leukocyte function in mechanisms of self-defense. The phagocytic cells (granulocytes, monocytes, and macrophages) may lose their capacity to function as effective phagocytes. The lymphocytes may lose their capacity to respond to antigens. (Disruptions of inflammatory and immune processes caused by leukocyte disorders are described in Chapter 8.) Other leukocyte alterations are not primarily immune or inflammatory defects, but rather are hematologic defects. These disorders include infectious mononucleosis and cancers of the blood—leukemia and multiple myeloma.

Quantitative Alterations of Leukocytes

Quantitative alterations are increases and decreases in numbers of leukocytes in the blood. **Leukocytosis** is a condition in which the leukocyte count is higher than normal; **leukopenia** is a condition in which the count is lower than normal. Usually leukocytosis or leukopenia affects a specific type of leukocyte.

Leukocytosis and leukopenia can result from a variety of bodily conditions and alterations. Leukocytosis is a normal protective response to physiologic stressors, such as invading microorganisms, strenuous exercise, emotional changes, temperature changes, anesthesia, surgery, pregnancy, and some drugs, hormones, and toxins. It also is caused by pathologic conditions, such as malignancies and hematologic disorders. Unlike leukocytosis, leukopenia is never beneficial. As the leukocyte count decreases to below 1000 per cubic millimeter, the individual is at risk for infection. With counts below 500 per cubic millimeter, the risk for very serious life-threatening infections is high. Leukopenia can be caused by radiation, anaphylactic shock, systemic lupus erythematosus, and certain chemotherapeutic agents.

Granulocytes and Monocytes

Increased levels of circulating granulocytes (neutrophils, eosinophils, and basophils) and monocytes are chiefly a physiologic response to infection. Elevations can occur also as a result of myeloproliferative disorders (polycythemia vera, chronic myelocytic leukemia [CML]) that increase stem cell proliferation in the bone marrow.

Decreases occur when infectious processes "use up" the circulating granulocytes and monocytes, drawing them out of the circulation and into infected tissues faster than they can be replaced. Decreases can be caused also by disorders that suppress marrow function.

Granulocytosis begins with the release of blood cells that have been stored in the venous sinuses of the marrow. Because the neutrophil is the most numerous of the granulocytes, the term granulocytosis is often used to describe **neutrophilia** (see Table 22-2). Neutrophilia is prevalent in the early stages of infection or inflammation, when stored neutrophils from the venous sinuses are released into the circulating blood. Stored neutrophils account for approximately 20 to 40 times more neutrophils than are normally present in the blood. Emptying of the venous sinuses stimulates granulopoiesis to replenish stores in the marrow. Specific conditions associated with neutrophilia are identified in Table 24-2.

When the demand for neutrophils exceeds the supply in the circulation, the marrow begins to release immature neutrophils (and other leukocytes) into the blood. Premature release of the immature cells is responsible for the phenomenon that hematologists call the shift to the left. The **shift to the left** refers to the microscopic detection of disproportionate numbers of immature leukocytes in smears of peripheral blood. The term can be understood if one visualizes cellular differentiation and maturation as occurring from left to right, as is shown in Chapter 22, Fig. 22-5. (The shift to the left is sometimes called a leukemoid reaction because it is similar to morphologic findings in blood smears of individuals with leukemia.) As infection or inflammation diminishes and granulopoiesis replenishes circulating granulocytes, a **shift to the right,** or back to normal, occurs.

Neutropenia is the condition associated with a reduction in circulating neutrophils. Clinically, neutropenia exists when the neutrophil count is less than 2000 per milliliter. A reduction in neutrophils occurs in severe prolonged infections when production of granulocytes cannot keep up with demand.

Other causes of neutropenia in the absence of overwhelming infection may be (1) decreased neutrophil production or ineffective granulopoiesis, (2) reduced neutrophil survival, and (3) abnormal neutrophil distribution and sequestration (Russin, Fillipo, & Alder, 1990). Ineffective or defective neutrophil production may be caused by hematologic disorders, for example, hypoplastic anemia or aplastic anemia, leukemia, or drug- or toxin-induced neutropenia. Reduced neutrophil survival is seen in autoimmune disorders, particularly systemic lupus erythematosus and rheumatoid arthritis. Abnormal neutrophil distribution and sequestration are associated with hypersplenism and pseudoneutropenia, which can be caused by starvation and anorexia nervosa.

If neutrophils are drastically reduced (less than 500/ml) and the entire granulocyte count is extremely low, a very serious condition called **granulocytopenia** or **agranulocytosis** results. The usual cause is interference with hematopoiesis in the bone marrow or increased cell destruction in the circulation. Chemotherapeutic agents commonly used in the treatment of hematologic and other malignancies cause bone marrow suppression. Other drugs that have been known to cause agranulocytosis are listed in Table 24-1. Although drug-induced agranulocytosis is rare, it does carry a mortality rate of 10% to 48% (Julia et al., 1991). Clinical manifestations of agranulocytosis include infection (particularly of the respiratory system), general malaise, septicemia, fever, tachycardia, and ulcers in the mouth and colon. If untreated, sepsis caused by agranulocytosis results in death within 3 to 6 days. Other conditions associated with neutropenia are identified in Table 24-2.

Eosinophilia, an absolute increase in the total numbers of circulating eosinophils, has a variety of causes. Allergic disorders associated with asthma, hay fever, and drug reactions are frequently the cause of eosinophilia. During the hypersensitivity reaction, eosinophilic chemotaxic factor of anaphylaxis (CTF-A) and histamine are released from mast cells, attracting eosinophils to the area. Areas abundant in mast cells, such as the respiratory and gastrointestinal tracts, are particularly common sites for eosinophil invasion. Other causes of eosinophilia are associated with dermatologic disorders, such as atopic dermatitis, eczema, and pemphigus. Most recently, increased levels of eosinophils have been identified with eosinophilia-myalgia syndrome, which is associated with ingestion of tryptophan (Ashinsky, 1990).

Parasitic invasion also is associated with eosinophilia, particularly those parasites that invade tissues. Eosinophils are attracted out of the circulation to the site of infestation, where they degranulate powerful enzymes onto the parasites. (This process is described and illustrated in Chapter 7.) Other conditions that cause eosinophilia are detailed in Table 24-2.

Eosinopenia, a decrease in circulating eosinophils, is generally caused by migration of eosinophils into inflammatory sites. It also may be seen in Cushing syndrome and as a result of stress caused by surgery, shock, trauma, burns, or mental distress. Other conditions that cause eosinopenia are detailed in Table 24-2.

Basophilia is quite rare and when present is generally seen as a response to inflammation and hypersensitivity reactions of the immediate type. Basophils contain histamine that is released during an allergic reaction (Wintrobe et al., 1981). An increase in basophils is seen also in myeloproliferative disorders, such as chronic myeloid leukemia and myeloid metaplasia. Other conditions that are associated with basophilia are listed in Table 24-2.

Basopenia is seen in hyperthyroidism, in acute infection, and in long-term therapy with steroids. A decrease in basophils is seen also during ovulation and pregnancy. Other conditions associated with basopenia are listed in Table 24-2.

Monocytosis, an increase in monocytes, is often transient and correlates poorly with disease states. When present, it is most commonly associated with neutropenia associated with bacterial infections, particularly in the late stages or recovery stage, when they are needed to phagocytize surviving microorganisms and debris. An increased level of monocytes also may indicate marrow recovery from agranulocytosis. Monocytosis often is seen in chronic infections such as tuberculosis (TB) and subacute bacterial endocarditis. Other conditions associated with monocytosis are identified in Table 24-2.

Monocytopenia, a decrease in monocytes, is rare and not much is known about this condition because of the

TABLE 24-1

Drugs Associated with Neutropenia and Agranulocytosis

Drug group	Neutropenia	Agranulocytosis
Analgesics, sedatives, antiinflammatory agents	Gold compounds; phenylbutazone; indomethacin	Phenacetin; barbiturates; aminopyrine; dipyrone
Antibiotics	Cephalosporins; semisynthetic penicillins	Sulfonamides; chloramphenicol; methicillin
Antithyroid agents	Methimazole	Propylthiouracil
Psychotropic agents	Tricyclic antidepressants	Phenothiazines
Anticonvulsant agents	Trimethadione	Phenytoin
Antiarrhythmic agents	Procainamide; quinidine	

TABLE 24-2

Other Conditions Associated with Neutrophils, Eosinophils, Basophils, Monocytes, and Lymphocytes

Condition	Cause	Example
Neutrophil		
Neutrophilia	Inflammation or tissue necrosis	Surgery, burns, MI, pneumonitis, rheumatic fever, rheumatoid arthritis
	Infection	Gram-positive (staphylococci, streptococci, pneumococci), gram-negative (*E. coli, Pseudomonas* species)
	Physiologic	Exercise, extreme heat/cold, third trimester pregnancy, emotional distress
	Hematologic	Acute hemorrhage, hemolysis, myeloproliferative disorder, CGL
	Drugs/chemicals	Epinephrine, steroids, heparin, histamine, endotoxin
	Metabolic	Diabetes (acidosis), eclampsia, gout, thyroid storm
	Neoplasms	Liver, GI tract, bone marrow
Neutropenia	Decreased marrow production	Radiation, chemotherapy, leukemia, aplastic anemia, abnormal granulopoiesis
	Increased destruction	Splenomegaly, hemodialysis, immune reaction
	Infection	Gram-negative (typhoid), viral (influenza, hepatitis B, measles, mumps, rubella), severe infections, protozoal infections (malaria)
Eosinophil		
Eosinophilia	Allergy	Asthma, hay fever, drug sensitivity
	Infection	Parasites (trichinosis, hookworm), chronic (fungal, leprosy, TB)
	Malignancies	CML, lung, stomach, ovary, Hodgkin disease
	Dermatoses	Pemphigus, exfoliative dermatitis (drug-induced)
	Drug	Digitalis, heparin, streptomycin, tryptophan (eosinophilia-myalgia syndrome), penicillins, propranolol
Eosinopenia	Stress response	Trauma, shock, burns, surgery, mental distress
	Drugs	Steroids (Cushing syndrome)
Basophil		
Basophilia	Inflammation	Infection (measles, chicken pox), hypersensitivity reaction (immediate)
	Hematologic	Myeloproliferative disorders (CGL, polycythemia vera, Hodgkin disease, hemolytic anemia)
	Endocrine	Myxedema, antithyroid therapy
Basopenia	Physiologic	Pregnancy, ovulation, stress
	Endocrine	Graves disease
Monocyte		
Monocytosis	Infection	Bacterial (SBE, TB), recovery phase of infection
	Hematologic	Myeloproliferative disorders, Hodgkin disease, agranulocytosis
	Physiologic	Normal newborn
Monocytopenia	Rare	
Lymphocyte		
Lymphocytosis	Physiologic	4 months to 4 years
	Acute infections	Infectious mononucleosis, CMV infection, pertussis, hepatitis, mycoplasma pneumonia, typhoid
	Chronic infections	Congenital syphilis, tertiary syphilis
	Endocrine	Thyrotoxicosis, adrenal insufficiency
	Malignancies	ALL, CLL, lymphosarcoma cell leukemia
Lymphocytopenia	Immunodeficiency syndromes	AIDS, agammaglobulinemia
	Lymphocyte destruction	Steroids (Cushing syndrome), radiation, chemotherapy
	Malignancies	Hodgkin disease
	Debilitating illness	CHF, renal failure, TB, SLE, aplastic anemia

small numbers of monocytes generally present in the blood. Monocytopenia, however, has been identified with hairy cell leukemia and prednisone therapy.

Lymphocytes

Quantitative alteration of lymphocytes occurs when lymphocytes are activated by antigenic stimuli, usually microorganisms (see Chapter 6). A **lymphocytosis** is rare in acute bacterial infections and occurs most commonly in acute viral infections, particularly those caused by the Epstein-Barr virus (EBV) (a causative agent in infectious mononucleosis). Other specific disorders associated with lymphocytosis are listed in Table 24-2.

Lymphocytopenia may be attributable to abnormalities of lymphocyte production associated with neoplasias and immune deficiencies, and destruction by drugs, viruses, or radiation. It also is known to occur in individuals for no apparent reason. Other conditions associated with lymphocytopenia are identified in Table 24-2. It has been hypothesized that the lymphocytopenia associated with heart failure and other acute illnesses may be caused by elevated levels of cortisol. The mechanisms in other disease states are not well understood (Athens, 1993).

The most recent condition in which lymphocytopenia is a major problem is in AIDS. The lymphocytopenia associated with this condition is caused by the HIV virus, which is cytopathic for T-helper lymphocytes. (For a more detailed discussion of AIDS, see Chapter 8.)

Infectious Mononucleosis

Infectious mononucleosis is an acute infection of B lymphocytes (B cells). The most common virus is the Epstein-Barr virus (EBV); however, CMV and other viruses, as well as the bacterium *Toxoplasma gondii*, have been identified as causative agents for the disease (Betts, 1990). Although CMV mononucleosis is benign and self-limiting, it does carry significant morbidity (Yarrish et al., 1989).

Infectious mononucleosis usually affects young adults between the ages of 15 and 30. It has been called "kissing disease" because the EBV begins with widespread invasion of B lymphocytes, all of which possess an EBV receptor site.

Unaffected B cells produce antibodies against the virus, and T lymphocytes (T cells) assist the B cell response of attacking the virus directly (see Chapter 6). The proliferation of clones of B and T cells and removal of dead and damaged leukocytes are largely responsible for the swelling of lymphoid tissues (lymph nodes, spleen, tonsils, and occasionally, liver). Sore throat and fever, two of the earliest manifestations of infectious mononucleosis, are caused by inflammation at the site of viral entry (and initial infection), the mouth and throat.

The incubation period for infectious mononucleosis is approximately 30 to 50 days. Mild symptoms, such as headache, malaise, and fatigue, appear during the first 3 to 5 days, with symptoms varying in severity for the next 7 to 20 days. Most cases include fever with temperature elevation lasting 7 to 10 days, sore throat, and enlargement and tenderness of the cervical lymph nodes. Sore throat is the most common symptom. It appears in the first week and is usually accompanied by hyperplasia of the pharyngeal lymphoid tissue with inflammation and edema, as well as exudative tonsillitis.

Lymph node enlargement is the predominant clinical manifestation of infectious mononucleosis. Enlargement occurs gradually, most commonly in the anterior and posterior cervical chains, and generalized lymph node enlargement also may develop. Splenomegaly occurs in about one half of affected individuals.

On rare occasions, other manifestations may occur, including hepatitis, erythematous maculopapular rash on the trunk and extremities, and edema around the eyes. Neurologic involvement can include aseptic meningitis, encephalitis, blurred vision, coma, acute cerebellar syndrome, and Guillain-Barré syndrome (inflammation of the nerves).

Infectious mononucleosis is usually self-limiting, and recovery occurs in a few weeks. Treatment consists of rest and alleviation of symptoms with analgesics.

Laboratory findings include an increase in relative and absolute lymphocyte and monocyte counts, with 10% to 20% atypical forms. In early phases of infectious mononucleosis, this is caused by an increase in both B and T cells. Atypical T cells predominate later. The atypical lymphocytes are large, with oval, horseshoe-shaped, or indented nuclei and vacuolated, spongy cytoplasm, similar to that of basophils. During the first week of infection, the leukocyte count may be normal or slightly low, secondary to mild neutropenia. After the first week, the leukocyte count (predominantly lymphocytes and monocytes) increases to 10,000 to 20,000 per microliter and persists at this level from 4 to 8 weeks. Platelet counts are low (less than 140,000 per cubic millimeter).

Serologic tests are necessary to diagnose infection by Epstein-Barr virus. A Monospot agglutination test is performed to show the presence of heterophilic antibodies associated with infection by Epstein-Barr virus. (Heterophilic antibodies are a heterogeneous group of antibodies that are agglutinins against sheep red blood cells.) Specificity can be increased by differential agglutination tests. Other serologic tests that detect antibodies specific for the virus are used in children.

Leukemias

Leukemia is a malignant disorder of the blood and blood-forming organs causing an accumulation of dysfunctional cells and a loss of cell division regulation. The common pathologic feature of all forms of leukemia is an uncontrolled proliferation of leukocytes. The excessive proliferation of the leukemia cells results in an overcrowding of bone marrow, which causes decreased production and function of normal hematopoietic cells.

The first description of a "leukemic" individual was by Velpeau in 1827 (Gunz, 1980). His patient, a florist and seller of lemonade, aged 63 years, "who had abandoned himself to the abuse of spiritus liquor and of women, without, however, becoming syphilitic," became ill in 1825. This patient had great swelling of the abdomen, fever, weakness, and symptoms related to urinary stones. On autopsy, he was found to have a very large liver and spleen, and blood and pus resembling the

color of yeast and red wine (Gunz, 1980). Not until 1945, however, did the physiologist Bennet and pathologist Virchow separately describe leukemia. Virchow coined the term "white blood" (weissus blut) and later the term "leukemia." He is largely credited with discoveries that have led to current knowledge of the pathology of leukemia.

Since Virchow's time, the classification of leukemia has become increasingly complex. Leukemias are classified as either chronic or acute and as either myeloid or lymphoid. The classification system for leukemia is based on the type of cell that predominates; the type of leukemia is named according to the point at which cell maturation is arrested (Fig. 24-1). In 1976, the French-American-British Cooperative Group developed criteria

FIG. 24-1 Cell-specific leukemias. Differentiation pathways of blood-forming cells and reported sites of block resulting in cell-specific leukemias.

for the classification of acute leukemias. This classification system is based on structure, number of cells, genetics, identification of surface markers, and histochemical staining. These findings produce important therapeutic and prognostic information.

The two major forms of leukemia, acute and chronic, are classified by predominant cell type and the rate at which the affected individual develops clinical symptoms. Acute leukemia is characterized by undifferentiated or immature cells, usually a blast cell. The onset of disease is abrupt and rapid. Disease progression results in a short survival time. In chronic leukemia, the predominant cell is mature in appearance but does not function normally. The onset of disease is gradual and the prolonged clinical course results in a relatively longer survival time. The past two decades have shown advances in remission induction rates, as well as survival. Thus, progress has occurred as a result of more effective chemotherapeutic agents, improved blood product and antimicrobial support, and specialized nursing care (Mayer, 1987). Chemotherapy and bone marrow transplants have significantly increased the survival time for individuals with acute leukemia.

Leukemia occurs with varying frequencies at different ages and is more frequent in adults (about 29,300 cases/year) than in children (2500 cases/year) (American Cancer Society [ACS], 1993). Acute lymphoblastic leukemia is the most common type in children and accounts for more than two thirds of all cases. Acute nonlymphoblastic leukemia (approximately 6500 cases/year) and chronic lymphocytic leukemia (approximately 8200 cases/year) are the most common types in adults (ACS, 1992). The sites of highest overall incidence are the United States, Canada, Sweden, and New Zealand.

Pathogenesis

Leukemias are considered clonal disorders, in that a single cell undergoes transformation and leukemic cells then proliferate. An interesting paradox is that leukemic cells apparently divide more *slowly* and take longer to synthesize DNA than other blood precursors. Acute leukemia therefore is not caused by rapid cellular proliferation, but is instead caused by the blocking of blood cell precursors. Leukemic cells do accumulate relentlessly in most affected individuals, and they compete with normal cellular proliferation. Thus, acute leukemia has also been termed an accumulation disorder, as well as a proliferation disorder.

Although the exact cause of leukemia is unknown, it is clear that causal risk factors acting together with a genetic predisposition can alter nuclear DNA. The leukemic cell is then unable to mature and respond to normal regulatory mechanisms. Abnormal chromosomes are reported in 40% to 50% of patients with acute leukemia, and certain chromosomes are repeatedly more involved than others. It thus appears that a mutation in a single cell gives rise to some leukemias.

Although the genetic mechanism remains unknown, studies indicate a statistically significant tendency for leukemia to recur in families. This tendency to cluster is seen among twins and siblings in certain families. Hereditary abnormalities are also associated with an increased incidence of leukemia, Down syndrome, Fanconi aplastic anemia, Bloom syndrome, ataxia telangiectasia, trisomy 13 (Patau syndrome), Wiskott-Aldrich syndrome, and congenital X-linked agammaglobulinemia.

Acquired disorders that progress to acute leukemia include chronic myelocytic leukemia (CML), polycythemia vera, myelofibrosis, Hodgkin disease, multiple myeloma, ovarian cancer, chronic lymphocytic leukemia (CLL), and sideroblastic anemia. Large doses of ionizing radiation are associated with an increased incidence of myelogenous leukemia. Viruses are known to cause leukemia in certain animals, but have not yet been proved to cause leukemia in human beings. Drugs that cause bone marrow depression (e.g., chloramphenicol, phenylbutazone, and certain alkylating agents, such as cytoxan) also can predispose an individual to leukemia. Acute myelogenous leukemia (AML) is the most frequently reported secondary cancer after high doses of chemotherapy for Hodgkin disease, multiple myeloma, ovarian cancer, non-Hodgkin lymphoma, and breast cancer (Fraser & Tucker, 1988).

In some cases, the development of leukemia occurs in the most primitive blood precursors—pluripotential stem cells—which give rise to all other blood cells (Fig. 24-1). The leukemia blasts, or precursor cells, literally "crowd out" the marrow and cause cellular proliferation of the other cell lines to cease. Normal granulocytic-monocytic, lymphocytic, erythrocytic, and megakaryocytic stem cells cease to function, causing **pancytopenia** (a reduction in all cellular components of the blood). Transformation also may occur specifically in the granulocyte-monocyte series and not in the erythrocyte series.

Much research in acute leukemia has concerned the depression of granulopoietic precursors and the subsequent granulocytopenia. Granulocytes fail to proliferate if cultured in vitro with leukemic cells. The process created in vitro is termed **leukemia-associated inhibitory activity (LIA)**. Leukemia-associated inhibitory activity is produced by lymphoidlike cells from patients with acute nonlymphoblastic leukemia (ANLL), acute lymphoblastic leukemia (ALL), acute erythroleukemia (AEL), chronic myelocytic leukemia (CML), and acute transformation of CML. Individuals in remission exhibit LIA, but the process is usually not detectable because of an inhibitor produced by rapid sedimenting of bone marrow cells (Broxmeyer, Mendelsohn, Moore, & Alcolm,

1977). During remission, leukemic granulopoietic precursors are thus resistant to LIA.

Acute Leukemias

For all types of acute leukemia, the mortality rate for the United States is about 7 per 100,000 individuals. North America and the Scandinavian countries have the highest mortality; Eastern European countries, Asia (except Japan), and Central America have the lowest mortality. The higher mortality in Japan is the result of the atomic bombs. Black Americans have consistently shown a lower mortality than whites.

Leukemia strikes both sexes and all ages. Incidence rises steeply, however, beyond age 50 (Clarkson, Elles, & Little, 1985). The 5-year survival rate for individuals with leukemia is 35%, partly because of the poor survival of those with ANLL. Over the last 30 years, however, there has been a dramatic improvement in survival of individuals with ALL: from a 4-year survival rate of 4% for people diagnosed in the 1960s to 73% in the 1990s (ACS, 1992). The decrease in mortality for ALL appears to be the result of chemotherapy.

Clinical Manifestations

The clinical manifestations of all the varieties of acute leukemia are generally similar. (Mechanisms associated with common manifestations are summarized in Table 24-3.) Signs and symptoms related to bone marrow depression include fatigue caused by anemia, bleeding resulting from **thrombocytopenia** (reduced numbers of circulating platelets), and fever caused by infection. Bleeding can occur in skin, gums, mucous membranes, and gastrointestinal and genitourinary tracts. Signs of bleeding include petechiae and ecchymosis visible in dependent areas, discoloration visible through the skin, gingival bleeding, hematuria, and midcycle menstrual bleeding or heavy bleeding associated with menstruation.

Sites of infection include the oral cavity, throat, respiratory tract, lower colon, urinary tract, and skin. Common organisms include the gram-negative bacilli *Escherichia coli*, *Pseudomonas aeruginosa*, and *Klebsiella pneumoniae*. Fever is an early sign. Chills and tissue infiltration are common.

Anorexia is associated with weight loss, diminished

TABLE 24-3

Clinical Manifestations and Related Pathophysiology in Leukemia

Clinical manifestations	Laboratory abnormalities	Cause	Comments
Anemia	Either a decrease or normal number of erythroblasts; key is the relative *proportion* of erythroblasts to total count; decreased iron in mature RBC	Decreased RBC production may be caused by decreased stem cell input or ineffective erythropoiesis or both; proposed reasons are: 1. Replacement of erythropoietic stem cells (ESCs) by leukemic clone 2. Inhibition of ESCs by leukemic cells 3. Inhibition of pluripotent stem cell 4. Decreased erythropoietin responsiveness from impaired interaction of ESCs with T-lymphocytes (in leukemia there is an increase in T-lymphocytes) 5. Hemorrhage 6. Splenic pooling of RBC 7. Drug therapy	In acute leukemia, anemia is usually present from beginning, often the first symptom noticed, and severe; mild form without symptoms is common in CML and CLL; hemorrhage is common in acute forms, occasional in CML, but rare in CLL

Continued.

TABLE 24-3

Clinical Manifestations and Related Pathophysiology in Leukemia—cont'd

Clinical manifestations	Laboratory abnormalities	Cause	Comments
Bleeding, purpura, petechiae, ecchymosis, thrombosis, or hemorrhage	Decreased and possibly abnormal platelets; abnormal clotting	Reduction in megakaryocytes leading to thrombocytopenia	Bleeding occurs more commonly in acute than in chronic leukemia
Disseminated intravascular coagulation (DIC)	Abnormal promyelocytes; hypofibrinogenemia; prolonged prothrombin, thrombin, and reptilase times; elevated fibrin degranulation products; and decreased levels of factor V, fibrinogen, and platelets	Proliferation of promyelocytic granulocytes with an excessive release of procoagulants from granules within the leukemic promyelocyte	Correction of coagulopathy in DIC is dependent on the successful treatment of leukemia
Infection	Infection is likely with an absolute granulocyte count below 500/mm^3 (Absolute granulocyte count [AGC] is the proportion of neutrophils and bands to the total white blood cell count)	Infections are caused by organisms endogenous to the host or present in the environment; granulocytopenic persons have an impaired inflammatory response; immunodeficiency resulting from chemotherapy, corticosteroids, and the disease process contribute to the infection	Major sites of infection are the alimentary tract sinuses, lungs, and skin; prevention of infection focuses on the restoration of host defenses, decreasing invasive procedures, and reducing colonization of organisms
Weight loss	Decreased 24-hour urinary creatinine excretion; hypoalbuminemia	Condition can be attributed to pain, depression, chemotherapy, radiotherapy, some unknown circulating inhibitor, and alterations in taste	Causes of weight loss are poorly understood; severe alterations in taste; highly seasoned foods seem bland, aggravate condition; patients with liver involvement often detest red meat; some patients have good appetites in the morning, but become satiated later; increased metabolism also aggravates the condition
Bone pain	Frequently no radiographic evidence of bone problems	Result of bone infiltration by leukemic cells or intramedullary infarction	If combination drug regimens are ineffective, radiotherapy is used
Elevated uric acid	Normal excretion of uric acid is 300 to 500 mg daily; the leukemic patient can excrete 50 times more; uric acid precipitates (urates) are commonly found in the proximal collecting tubules and pelvises of the kidney; oliguria and concentrated urine are sometimes found	Uric acid is a normal byproduct of protein catabolism; nucleic acid catabolism is accelerated in the leukemic patient; uric acid precipitation occurs at an acidic, or low, pH; urate precipitation in the leukemic patient is increased from dehydration caused by anorexia or fever and drug therapy	Hyperuricemia is present in both acute leukemia and CML; kidney pathology can be prevented by ensuring increased urine flow, increasing urine pH by administering sodium bicarbonate, or decreasing acid production through allopurinol, which inhibits the enzyme xanthine oxidase
Liver, spleen, and lymph node enlargement	Biopsy is abnormal for liver and spleen	Leukemic cell infiltration causes splenic, hepatic, and lymph node enlargement; lymph nodes also undergo leukemic proliferation as in CLL	

sensitivity to sour and sweet tastes, wasting away of muscle, and difficulty swallowing. Liver, spleen, and lymph node enlargement are more common in ALL than in ANLL. Splenomegaly and hepatomegaly usually occur together. The leukemic individual often experiences abdominal pain and tenderness and breast tenderness.

Neurologic manifestations are frequent and may be due to either leukemic infiltration or cerebral bleeding. Headache, vomiting, papilledema, facial palsy, blurred vision, auditory disturbances, and meningeal irritation can occur if leukemic cells infiltrate the cerebral or spinal meninges. Because chemotherapeutic agents do not pass the blood-brain barrier, leukemia cells can grow easily.

Evaluation and Treatment

Because leukemia is frequently confused with other conditions, early detection is difficult. Persistent symptoms need intensive medical investigation. The diagnosis is made through blood tests and examination of bone marrow.

Chemotherapy is the treatment of choice for leukemia. Controversial are immunotherapy agents that induce differentiation of immature granulocytes (i.e. cisretinoic acid), and marrow transplants. Drugs are used in various combinations. Supportive measures include blood transfusions, antibiotics, antifungals, and antivirals. Allopurinol is used for preventing production of uric acid (which is elevated from cellular death because of treatment). Marrow transplantation using both allogeneic (other than from twins) and autologous (the individual's own) marrow is being investigated as a treatment option for individuals younger than 50 years of age. Although there has not been a marked improvement in response or survival of ANLL, dramatic improvements in survival and response of people with ALL has occurred. Future studies will define the role of biotherapy in the treatment of leukemia and perhaps improve survival rates.

Improved survival rates in individuals with acute leukemia have occurred in the past three decades. Factors influencing increased survival rate include the use of combined and multimodality treatment regimens, improved supportive services, such as blood banking and nutritional support, and microbial treatment.

Chronic Leukemias

The two main types of chronic leukemia are (1) myelocytic (CML) and (2) lymphocytic (CLL). Unlike cells in acute leukemia, chronic leukemic cells are well differ-

FIG. 24-2 Philadelphia chromosome. Metaphase spread of marrow cell in chronic myelocytic leukemia. Ph[1] chromosome is G21 *(arrow and enlarged inset).* It is recognized by partial deletion of long arm. (Courtesy Dr. A. K. Sinha, Houston, Texas. From del Regato, Spjut, & Cox, 1985.)

entiated and can be readily identified. Individuals with chronic leukemia have a longer life expectancy, usually of several years from the time of diagnosis.

Pathophysiology and Clinical Manifestations

The chronic leukemias have a presentation and progression different from the acute leukemias. Chronic leukemia advances slowly and surreptitiously, without warning. Symptoms—when they do appear—include splenomegaly, extreme fatigue, weight loss, night sweats, and low-grade fever.

The incidence of CML is approximately 1 per 100,000 people. Chronic myelocytic leukemia (CML) is a group of diseases called myeloproliferative disorders, along with polycythemia vera, primary thrombocytosis, and idiopathic myelofibrosis (invasion of bone marrow by fibrous tissue).

The presence of the Philadelphia chromosome is a diagnostic marker of CML (Fig. 24-2). The Philadelphia chromosome results from a reciprocal translocation between the long arms of chromosomes 9 and 22, and is demonstrable in all blood cell precursors, meaning that the disease originates in a progenitor stem cell (Rowley, 1990) (see Chapter 4). The median age for persons with Philadelphia chromosome–positive CML is 40 to 45 years. Identifying the Philadelphia chromosome allows the clinician to follow the transformation process. Transformation is identified in erythroid, megakaryocytic, and macrophage cell lines. With such strong evidence that CML begins in a stem cell, however, it is *not* clear why myeloid cells predominate in the chronic phase of the disease (Buschsbaum & Schwartz, 1990). The chromosome appears not to be genetically transmitted, but to occur because of mitotic error. Evidence thus indicates that CML has a clonal origin. The malignant transformation arises from pluripotential stem cells or lymphoid stem cells (see Fig. 24-1). Structural cellular abnormalities are not readily identified in CML. Absent or low levels of the enzyme neutrophil alkaline phosphatase, with subsequent decreased phagocytic capabilities, do, however, indicate that cells fail to differentiate normally.

Although the Philadelphia chromosome is present in erythrocytes, monocytes, and megakaryocytes, erythrocytes and platelets are produced and function relatively normally. The acute effects of CML resemble those of acute leukemia, but with more prominent and painful splenomegaly. Liver function is rarely altered despite enlargement, and lymphadenopathy is generally found only in the acute phase of the disease. Hyperuricemia is invariably present and produces gouty arthritis. Infections, fever, and weight loss are common findings in patients with CML.

Chronic lymphocytic leukemia predominantly involves malignant transformation of B cells, although T cell CLL occurs less commonly. The major pathophysiologic deficit in CLL of B cells is their failure to mature into plasma cells that synthesize immunoglobulin (antibody; see Chapter 6). A possible mechanism responsible for CLL of B cells is a deficiency of normal helper T cells with an increase in suppressor T cells. Together, the T cell abnormalities might account for the impaired differentiation of B cells in CLL.

Suppression of humoral immunity caused by reduction in normally functioning B cells is the most significant effect of CLL. Individuals are at risk both for infections commonly combated by B cell–produced immunoglobulins and for the development of autoimmune diseases that result in secondary cancers. Anemia, thrombocytopenia, and neutropenia are typically present with overt CLL (Table 24-3). Invasion of most organs is uncommon, but infiltration does occur in lymph nodes, liver, spleen, and salivary glands. Central nervous system involvement is rare. Elevated levels of the enzyme lactic dehydrogenase (LDH) and hyperuricemia are common, whereas hypercalcemia is rarely evident.

Evaluation and Treatment

State-of-the-art treatment for CML does not cure the disease, prevent blastic transformation, or prolong the average survival time. New therapeutic approaches include bone marrow transplantation, biologic response modifiers, and combination chemotherapy (Cunningham, 1990) (see Chapter 11). Marrow transplantation should be considered for individuals with CML who are younger than 50 years of age when appropriate donors are available.

Multiple Myeloma

Multiple myeloma is a B-cell cancer, typically associated with mature plasma cell structure and function (Epstein, Xiao, & He, 1990). Recent studies, however, support involvement of early B lymphocytes, such as hematopoietic stem cells, as the origin of myeloma (Epstein, 1992). These data suggest that myeloma originates in the bone marrow and moves through the circulation to and from extramedullary sites, probably lymph nodes, which are required for their development (Epstein, 1992). Subsequently, the myeloma cells return to the bone marrow or soft-tissue sites, using adhesion molecules (see Chapter 10) for "homing" to sites that can provide the environment for expansion and maturation (Epstein, 1992). Development of myeloma is governed by cytokines, whereby IL-6 is the major myeloma growth factor (cytokine). (Lymphocytes and cytokines are described in Chapter 6.) Multiple myeloma is characterized by multiple malignant tumor masses of plasma cells scattered throughout the skeletal system and sometimes in soft tissue. The reported incidence of multiple myeloma has doubled in the past two decades, possibly because of more sensitive testing used for diagnosis (Cancer in Focus, 1991; Silverburg & Lubera, 1989). It now has an annual incidence rate of approximately 32,000 cases in the United States (ACS, 1993). Malignant myeloma has been reported in all races, but the incidence rate in blacks (7 to 10 per 100,000) is at least twice that in whites (3 to 4 per 100,000) (Cancer in Focus, 1991; Silverburg & Lubera, 1989). It is rare before the age of 40 and then occurs increasingly with age, reaching a peak during the seventh decade. The neoplasm is also more common in men than women.

The exact cause of multiple myeloma remains uncertain, but a few clues have been gleaned from studies of animals and clinical observations of human disease. Genetic factors are suggested as a possible cause because tumors occur in specific strains of mice and in human siblings and other near relatives. Chronic stimulation of the mononuclear phagocyte system by chemicals, bacteria, and viral agents has also been suggested as a possible cause. This suggestion is supported by the increased frequency of plasma cell neoplasms in individuals with long-standing chronic infections, such as tuberculosis, osteomyelitis, and pneumonitis, and by the effects of chemical injections in mice (Cotran, Kumar, & Robbins, 1989).

Pathophysiology

Malignant plasma cells arise from one clone of B cells that produce abnormally large amounts of one class of immunoglobulin (usually IgG, occasionally IgA, and rarely IgM, IgD, or IgE). The abnormal immunoglobulin produced by the malignant transformed plasma cell is called the **M-protein**. The M-protein is responsible for many of the clinical manifestations of the disease. M-protein that is produced in excessive amounts results in ineffective antibody production. **Bence Jones proteins,** the light chains of immunoglobulin molecules, are present in the urine. These proteins may result in damage to renal tubular cells.

Multiple myeloma becomes evident as diffuse destructive bone lesions (Fig. 24-3). The bones most commonly affected are the vertebrae (66%), ribs (44%), skull (41%), pelvis (28%), femur (24%), clavicle (10%), and scapula (10%) (Cotran et al., 1989). The lesions progressively destroy the cortical bone. (Bone structures are described in Chapter 38.)

Clinical Manifestations

Clinical manifestations are the result of (1) infiltration and destruction of organs, particularly bone, by the neoplastic plasma cells and (2) an M-protein consisting of an excess of immunoglobulins with altered physiologic

FIG. 24-3 Multiple (plasma cell) myeloma. A, Roentgenogram of femur showing extensive bone destruction caused by tumor. Note absence of reactive bone formation. **B,** Gross specimen from same individual; myelomatous sections appear as dark granular sections. (From Kissane, 1990.)

properties and immune function. Infiltration of bones by malignant plasma cells causes pain and pathologic fractures. Because of an excessive accumulation of neoplastic plasma cells, the most common presenting symptom is bone pain. The production of osteoclast activating factors by the myeloma cells results in extensive osteolysis (breakdown of bone), bone pain, and pathologic fractures. Hypercalcemia resulting from bone resorption can cause neurologic disturbances, such as confusion, lethargy, and weakness, and can contribute to renal disease.

A major clinical manifestation is recurrent infections resulting from suppression of the humoral (antibody-mediated) immune response. Cell-mediated immune function (i.e., T cell function) is relatively normal (Cotran et al., 1989). Humoral immune function is thought to be suppressed by unknown factors secreted from malignant plasma cells. These factors activate macrophages that inhibit maturation of B cells into plasma cells that would be capable of producing immunoglobulins normally (Ullrich & Zolla-Pazner, 1982; Lee, 1993). Renal disease, a complication of multiple myeloma, is thought to be the result of Bence Jones proteinuria. The excreted Bence Jones proteins may be toxic to the tubular epithelial cells of the kidney (Defonzo, Cooke, Wright, & Humphrey, 1978).

Evaluation and Treatment

Diagnosis of multiple myeloma is made by radiographic and laboratory studies and biopsy of a lesion. Chemotherapy, radiation therapy, plasmapheresis (exchange), and marrow transplant have been used for treatment. Individuals with multiple bony lesions, if untreated, rarely survive for more than 6 to 12 months. With chemotherapy and aggressive management of complications, the prognosis can improve significantly with a median survival of 24 to 30 months and a 10-year survival rate of 3%.

ALTERATIONS OF LYMPHOID FUNCTION

Lymphadenopathy

Normally, lymph nodes are not palpable or only barely palpable. Nodes are generally classified as tender or nontender, and movable or fixed. **Lymphadenopathy** is characterized by enlarged lymph nodes (Fig. 24-4). Localized lymphadenopathy usually indicates drainage of an inflammatory lesion. Generalized lymphadenopathy occurs less frequently as a result of infection and is, therefore, usually associated with a malignant or nonmalignant disease. Lymphadenopathy reflects significant diseases more often in adults than in children.

Enlargement of the lymph node is often caused by an increase in size and number of the germinal centers within the node caused by proliferation of lymphocytes or monocytes (immature macrophages). Enlargement also may be caused by invasion of the node by malignant cells or cells not normally present within the node. Palpable nodes, however, do not always indicate serious disease and may only indicate a reaction to minor trauma or infection of a specific structure. The location and size of the enlarged node are important factors in diagnosing the cause of the lymphadenopathy, as are the individual's age, gender, and geographic location. Generalized lymphadenopathy occurs with non-Hodgkin lymphomas, chronic lymphocytic leukemia, histiocytoses, and disorders that produce lymphocytosis. In general, lymphadenopathy results from four types of conditions: (1) neoplastic disease, (2) immunologic or inflammatory conditions, (3) endocrine disorders, or (4) lipid storage diseases. Diseases of unknown cause, including autoimmune diseases and reactions to drugs, also may lead to generalized lymphadenopathy.

FIG. 24-4 Lymphadenopathy. Individual with lymphocyte leukemia with extreme but symmetrical lymphadenopathy. (Courtesy Dr. A. R. Kagan, Los Angeles. From del Regato, Spjut, & Cox, 1985.)

Malignant Lymphomas

Lymphomas are tumors of primary lymphoid tissue (thymus and bone marrow) or secondary tissue (lymph nodes, spleen, tonsils, and intestinal lymphoid tissue). Most lymphomas are neoplasms of secondary lymphoid tissue and involve mostly lymph nodes or spleen. Malignant lymphoid cells are sometimes found in circulating blood, indicating bone marrow involvement. The major subdivisions of malignant lymphomas are **Hodgkin disease** and **non-Hodgkin lymphoma.** Bone marrow involvement occurs more often in non-Hodgkin lymphoma than in Hodgkin disease.

Histopathologic classifications for Hodgkin disease have grown and changed since the first attempt by Ewing in 1928. The current classification for Hodgkin disease is the Rye modification of the Lukes, Butler, and Hicks classification, as shown in the box. Non-Hodgkin lymphoma also has several classifications. Rappaport's widely used classification distinguishes two major histopathologic patterns: nodular and diffuse. The diffuse pattern does not show the cell aggregates that are evident in the nodular pattern. Rappaport's system correlates well with clinical observations, but it gives little insight into the pathophysiology involved. Lukes and Collins proposed an immunologic classification system that produces important correlations with the pathophysiology of the immune system. Other classifications for non-Hodgkin lymphoma have been developed by Lennert (the Kiel classification), the World Health Organization, and Dorfman. It has only been recently that an international working group has developed what may be the standard histologic classification, currently referred to as the "Working Formulation" (Table 24-4).

These two patterns in non-Hodgkin lymphoma illustrate two different pathologic states. The nodular (and diffuse, well-differentiated lymphocytic) pattern involves nodal and extranodal sites. Initially, the disease is slow-growing with few symptoms. After a time, rapid growth can cause the disease to become diffuse. With the diffuse pattern, disease is rapidly growing with early extranodal invasion.

Incidence rates differ with respect to age, gender, geographic location, and socioeconomic class. Approximately 7900 new cases of Hodgkin disease and 41,000 new cases of non-Hodgkin lymphoma are diagnosed annually in the United States (ACS, 1993). The incidence rate of Hodgkin disease is approximately 2.6 per 100,000 in men and 2.2 per 100,000 in women (Skarin, Canellos, Maych, & Nieman, 1986). The incidence rate of non-Hodgkin lymphoma is approximately 8.1 per 100,000 in men and 5.7 per 100,000 in women (Newell, Cabanillas, & Hagemeister, 1987). Both diseases occur more frequently in men than in women. Hodgkin

MAJOR CLASSIFICATIONS OF HODGKIN DISEASE

Lymphocytic predominant
Nodular sclerosing
    Most common in developing countries
Mixed cellularity
    Together with modular sclerosing accounts for 80% of cases in the United States; predominant type in individuals with AIDS
Lymphocytic depletion
    Least common
Unclassified
Data from Lukes, Carver, & Hall, 1966.

disease peaks at two different ages. The first peak occurs early in life during the second and third decades, and the second peak occurs late in life during the sixth and seventh decades. Non-Hodgkin lymphoma is a disease of the middle years, usually in persons older than 50 years of age. The Netherlands, Denmark, and the United States have the highest incidence of Hodgkin disease; Japan and Australia have the lowest rates. High socioeconomic status is also associated with the disease.

Hodgkin Disease
Pathogenesis

Distinctive abnormal chromosomes are present in multiple cells from the lymph nodes of an individual with Hodgkin disease. Hodgkin disease is therefore a clonal disorder. The classically abnormal cell is the Reed-Sternberg cell, which is large and often confused with giant cells found in tuberculosis (Fig. 24-5). Reed-Sternberg cells are polyploid with large nuclei and are derived from the monocyte-macrophage series. Hodgkin disease is unusual because the bulk of the disease is composed of normal cells within which the malignant Reed-Sternberg cells are found (Urba & Longo, 1992). The origin of the Reed-Sternberg cell may differ for various subtypes of disease—some T cell, some B cell, and some monocyte lineage (Urba & Longo, 1992).

Cancerous transformation occurs from a particular site in the lymph node. With continuing growth, the entire node becomes replaced, with zones of necrosis obscuring the normal nodular pattern. The cause of Hodgkin disease remains unknown.

Current evidence indicates that an inhibitor in the serum and spleen of individuals with Hodgkin disease selectively binds to T cells and interferes with their function. Another reported mechanism is suppressor activity by monocytes. Individuals in sustained long remission after total lymphoid radiation continue to exhibit

TABLE 24-4

Classification of Non-Hodgkin Lymphoma: Comparison of Rappaport and Luke-Collins Systems of Nomenclature with Working Formulation

Working formulation	Rappaport system	Luke-Collins system
Low grade		
Small lymphocytic	Lymphocyte lymphocytic well-differentiated	Small lymphocytic B cell or T cell
Follicular, small cleaved	Nodular, lymphocytic, poorly differentiated	Follicular, small cleaved follicular center cell (FCC)
Follicular, mixed small cleaved and large cell	Nodular mixed lymphocytic and histiocytic	Follicular, mixed small cleaved and large follicular center cell
Intermediate grade		
Follicular, large cell	Nodular histiocytic	Follicular, large cleaved and/or noncleaved FCC
Diffuse, small cleaved	Diffuse lymphocytic, poorly differentiated	Diffuse small cleaved FCC
Diffuse, mixed small and large	Diffuse mixed, lymphocytic and histiocytic	Diffuse mixed small and large cleaved or noncleaved FCC
Diffuse, large cell	Diffuse histiocytic	Diffuse large cleaved or noncleaved FCC
High grade		
Immunoblastic, large cell	Diffuse histiocytic	Immunoblastic sarcoma, B or T cell
Lymphoblastic	Diffuse, lymphoblastic	Convoluted T cell
Small, noncleaved	Diffuse undifferentiated (Burkitt/non-Burkitt)	Small noncleaved FCC

deficient cell-mediated immunity, which is associated with a T-lymphocytopenia and a B-lymphocytosis (Kaplan, 1980). Impaired cell-mediated immunity causes delayed responsiveness to natural antigens (hypersensitivity) and delayed homograft rejection.

Two theories are proposed for the mechanism of spread of Hodgkin disease: (1) the contiguity theory and (2) the susceptibility theory. The contiguity theory suggests that Hodgkin disease spreads by the movement of existing tumor cells through lymphatic routes. This theory is based on the notion that spread occurs through immediate connections between pairs of lymph node chains connected by one or more lymphatic channels. Thus transmission is orderly, from one chain to another.

The susceptibility theory suggests that Hodgkin disease is a disorder of the whole lymphatic system, involving certain susceptible multiple sites of origin. Thus the spread occurs because of a traveling causative agent rather than spread of preexisting tumor cells. This theory also suggests that Hodgkin cells may travel to different lymph nodes through the bloodstream, much as normal lymphocytes do. Because Hodgkin disease is currently more accepted as a clonal disorder and con-

tiguous lymph nodes have been described, the contiguity theory is better supported.

Clusters of cases in high schools and certain geographic locations suggest that transmissible agents, such as a virus, might be involved in the pathogenesis of Hodgkin disease. The isolation of herpes virus in individuals with Hodgkin disease (i.e., the presence of Reed-Sternberg cells in lymph nodes of individuals with infectious mononucleosis) further substantiates the viral theory. Higher-than-normal antibody titers to the Epstein-Barr virus also are reported in individuals with Hodgkin disease. Some familial clustering of Hodgkin disease suggests an unknown genetic mechanism.

Clinical Manifestations

An enlarged painless mass, lump, or swelling, most commonly in the neck, is frequently an initial sign of Hodgkin disease (Fig. 24-6). Fever, especially in the evening for several days, may occur intermittently. Older persons more readily experience weakness, malaise, weight loss, and anemia. Back and neck pain with hyperreflexia can be present in both Hodgkin disease and non-Hodgkin lymphoma, suggesting epidural in-

FIG. 24-5 **Lymph node. A,** Hodgkin disease, lymphocytic predominance type (125×). **B,** Note large darker cell. Reed-Sternberg cell, characteristic of Hodgkin disease with lymphocytic predominance (250×). (From Kissane, J. M. [1985]. *Anderson's pathology.* [8th ed.]. St. Louis: Mosby—Year Book.)

FIG. 24-6 **Hodgkin disease and enlarged cervical lymph node.** Typical enlarged cervical lymph node in the neck of a 35-year-old woman with Hodgkin disease. (From del Regato, Spjut, & Cox, 1985.)

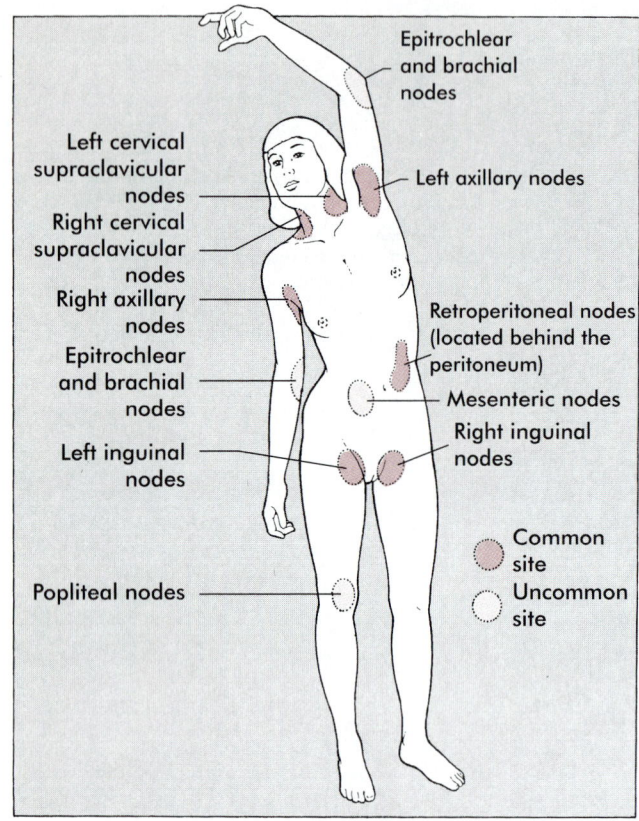

Left cervical supraclavicular nodes

Right cervical supraclavicular nodes

Right axillary nodes

Epitrochlear and brachial nodes

Left inguinal nodes

Popliteal nodes

Epitrochlear and brachial nodes

Left axillary nodes

Retroperitoneal nodes (located behind the peritoneum)

Mesenteric nodes

Right inguinal nodes

Common site

Uncommon site

FIG. 24-7 Common and uncommon involved lymph node sites for Hodgkin disease.

volvement. Pain to the enlarged nodes is reported after ingestion of alcohol.

The cervical, axillary, inguinal, and retroperitoneal lymph nodes are most commonly affected in Hodgkin disease, whereas the mesenteric epitrochlear, bronchial, and popliteal nodes are rarely involved (Fig. 24-7). Local symptoms are produced by lymphadenopathy, usually caused by pressure or obstruction. Extremity involvement can manifest itself by pain, nerve irritation, and obliteration of the pulse.

Although Hodgkin disease rarely arises in the lung, mediastinal, and hilar node, adenopathy can cause secondary involvement of the trachea, bronchi, pleura, or lungs. Determination that pulmonary involvement is because of Hodgkin disease is complicated by infections that can occur together with Hodgkin disease in the same lung. Retroperitoneal nodes can involve vertebral bodies and nerves and can cause displacement of ureters. In the spinal cord, involvement is more common in the dorsal and lumbar regions than in the cervical region. Although infrequent, skin manifestations can include psoriasis and eczematoid lesions, causing itching and scratching.

Pericardial involvement can occur by direct invasion from mediastinal lymph nodes. This involvement can

cause pericardial friction rub, pericardial effusion, and engorgement of neck veins. The gastrointestinal tract and urinary tract are rarely sites of involvement. Anemia is frequently found in individuals with a low serum iron and iron-binding capacity. Hemolytic anemia is rare. Other laboratory findings include elevated sedimentation rate, leukocytosis, and eosinophilia. With advanced stages of Hodgkin disease, leukopenia occurs.

Splenic involvement in Hodgkin disease depends on histopathologic type (Table 24-3). The spleen is involved in 60% of cases of mixed-cellularity and lymphocyte depletion types. Only 34% of cases reveal splenic involvement with lymphocyte predominance and nodular sclerosis types.

Mixed-cellularity and lymphocyte depletion patterns are usually widespread at time of diagnosis. In the lymphocyte depletion type of Hodgkin, an abundance of Reed-Sternberg cells with few lymphocytes is evident. This type has a higher incidence of spleen, liver, and bone marrow involvement. (Initially, the lymphocytic predominance pattern tends to involve a single peripheral node or chain of nodes.) At diagnosis, nodular sclerosing Hodgkin disease can include groups of nodes in the cervical regions as well as mediastinal involvement. (See Table 24-5 for clinical staging classification.)

Evaluation and Treatment

Because of the variability in symptoms, early definitive detection may be difficult. Asymptomatic lymphadenopathy can progress undetected for several years. Careful evaluation, including chest x-ray films, lymphangiography, and biopsy, should be carried out for individuals with fever of unknown origin and peripheral lymphadenopathy. Biopsy establishes the diagnosis for both Hodgkin disease and non-Hodgkin lymphoma. Both are treated with radiotherapy and chemotherapy (Fig. 24-8). Localized gastrointestinal lymphoma occasionally is cured by surgery.

More than 75% of all newly diagnosed individuals with non-Hodgkin disease are cured with radiation therapy or combination chemotherapy regimens. The prognosis for a given person depends on several factors, presence or absence of systemic symptoms, the stage of the disease, and suitability of treatment administered. Individuals whose disease recurs after combination chemotherapy may be helped when retreated with the same or another regimen, depending on the duration of the remission after the drug treatment was stopped.

Non-Hodgkin Lymphoma
Pathogenesis

The cause of lymph node enlargement and cancerous transformation in non-Hodgkin lymphoma is unknown. The diffuse form is characterized by more systemic symptoms (Table 24-4).

FIG. 24-8 Cervical Hodgkin disease. **A,** Young boy with extensive cervical Hodgkin disease. **B,** Appearance several years later, when axillary manifestation developed. **C,** Appearance 23 years after initial treatment with radiation. (From del Regato, Spjut, & Cox, 1985.)

TABLE 24-5

Ann Arbor Modification of the Rye Staging System for Lymphoma

Stage	Extent of involvement
Stage I	Involvement of a single lymph node region (I) or localized involvement of a single extralymphatic organ of site (I E)
Stage II	Involvement of 2 or more lymph node regions on the same side of the diaphragm (II) or localized involvement of a single associated extralymphatic organ or site and its lymph node(s) with or without involvement of other lymph node regions on the same side of the diaphragm (II E)
Stage III	Involvement of lymph node regions of both sides of the diaphragm (III), which may be accompanied by localized involvement of an associated extralymphatic organ or site (III E), by involvement of the spleen (III S), or both (III E & III S)
Stage IV	Disseminated (multifocal) involvement of one or more extralymphatic organs with or without associated lymph node involvement

For Hodgkin disease the presence or absence of systemic manifestations should be indicated by adding either a letter A or B (*A*, asystemic; *B*, fever, sweat, 10% weight loss).

Immunosuppressed persons have a greater incidence of non-Hodgkin lymphoma, suggesting an immune mechanism. In contrast to Hodgkin disease, T cell function is minimally affected. B cell abnormalities, such as impaired and decreased antibody production, are more common in non-Hodgkin lymphoma than in Hodgkin disease. Disorders of mononuclear phagocytes, particular macrophages fixed in tissues, occur more often in individuals with non-Hodgkin lymphoma. A greater-than-expected incidence of non-Hodgkin lymphoma is reported in individuals with ataxia-telangiectasia, Wiskott-Aldrich syndrome, and Chediak-Higashi syndrome.

Clinical Manifestations

The cervical, axillary, inguinal, and femoral chains are the most frequent sites of lymph node enlargement.

Generally, the swelling is painless and the nodes have enlarged and transformed over a period of months or years. Extranodal sites of involvement are the nasopharynx, gastrointestinal tract, bone, thyroid, testes, and soft tissue. Some individuals have retroperitoneal and abdominal masses with symptoms of abdominal fullness, back pain, ascites (fluid in the peritoneal cavity), and leg swelling. Several sites of involvement for non-Hodgkin lymphoma are not common for Hodgkin disease. These sites include the Waldeyer ring (lymphoid tissue that encircles the tonsils), stomach, small and large bowel, mesenteric lymph nodes, thyroid, skin, pancreas, kidney, and central nervous system. With diffuse non-Hodgkin lymphoma, symptoms are variable and generally involve more systemic findings.

Initially, the blood count at diagnosis for non-Hodgkin lymphoma is normal. Blood abnormalities are not seen until the disease is advanced, although the bone marrow is involved earlier than in Hodgkin disease. Pancytopenia, when present, indicates hypersplenism or extensive replacement of bone marrow by lymphoma.

Evaluation and Treatment

Individuals with non-Hodgkin lymphoma can survive for long periods. Survival with nodular lymphoma ranges up to 15 years. Individuals with diffuse disease generally do not survive as long. Many investigators believe that more aggressive treatment increases the cure rate. Autologous marrow transplantation has recently been proposed for recurrent disease when no curative regimen exists and those with poor-risk lymphomas. High-grade non-Hodgkin lymphoma is seen with increasing frequency in persons with acquired immune deficiency syndrome (AIDS) with extremely poor prognosis.

Burkitt Lymphoma

Burkitt lymphoma is a tumor with unique clinical and epidemiologic features. It occurs in children from Eastern Central Africa and New Guinea and primarily involves the jaw and facial bones (Fig. 24-9). The Epstein-Barr virus is associated with Burkitt lymphoma in African children. The virus is found in nasopharyngeal secretions (Borden, Steeves, & Hogan, 1983).

The American type of Burkitt lymphoma usually involves the abdomen and is characterized by extensive marrow replacement. The cancerous cell is a B cell that undergoes cancerous transformation and progression. The African variety has been successfully treated with radiotherapy and cyclophosphamide. The American type is more resistant to treatment.

Conditions That Mimic Lymphomas

Certain other clinical conditions mimic the malignant lymphomas. These conditions include tuberculosis, syphilis, systemic lupus erythematosus, lung cancer, and bone cancer. An important distinction between lymphomas and other conditions is that lymphomas usually involve localized lymphadenopathy. Infectious precursors of malignant lymphomas are characterized by more generalized lymphadenopathy with systemic signs and symptoms.

ALTERATIONS OF SPLENIC FUNCTION

Most alterations of splenic function, particularly those caused by **splenomegaly** (splenic enlargement), result from disorders elsewhere in the body. Sometimes, however, primary physiologic or anatomic alterations do occur. Primary anatomic alterations include splenic rupture (usually caused by trauma), tumors, cysts, and vas-

FIG. 24-9 Burkitt lymphoma. Burkitt lymphoma involving the jaw in young African boy. (Courtesy Dr. J. N. P. Davies, Albany, NY. From del Regato, Spjut, & Cox, 1985.)

cular anomalies, particularly infarction (blockage) or aneurysm (a sac or outpouching in a vessel wall). **Hypersplenism** (hyperactivity of the spleen) is the most common primary physiologic alteration.

Splenomegaly

Splenic enlargement can be caused by proliferation of lymphocytes or macrophages of the white pulp, invasion of neoplastic cells, or chronic congestion with blood. These mechanisms of splenomegaly have several different causes. Proliferation of lymphocytes is caused by infection and is almost always associated with lymphadenopathy. Proliferation of macrophages, however, is usually the result of a blood disorder, such as hemolytic anemia, in which macrophages increase in number so as to phagocytose the defective or dead erythrocytes. Infiltration of neoplastic cells causes splenomegaly resulting from tumor growth. Congestive splenomegaly, or congestion with blood, is caused by hypertension in the portal vein (the vein that receives blood from the spleen), causing blood to leave the spleen more slowly and with more turbulence than it enters. Other causes of splenomegaly include metabolic-infiltrative disorders and splenic abnormalities.

Infiltrative splenomegaly is caused by engorgement of macrophages within the spleen. These macrophages contain indigestible materials associated with specific rare diseases, such as Gaucher disease, Niemann-Pick disease, amyloidosis, diabetic lipemia, and gargoylism

(Wintrobe et al., 1981). The spleen also may develop cysts that cause enlargement. Cysts are benign tumors.

The spleen is usually not palpable in the adult. Splenomegaly without lymphadenopathy is associated with such conditions as hemolytic anemia and portal hypertension. Splenomegaly with lymphadenopathy is very common and is likely to be associated with any condition involving inflammation or infection. Increased activity of the spleen may be appropriate, as in idiopathic thrombocytopenic purpura, or inappropriate, as in portal hypertension (Erslev, 1990).

Hypersplenism

Hypersplenism is a primary or secondary syndrome of accelerated splenic function, particularly the function of blood cell filtration and removal. Compensation for hypersplenism results in bone marrow hyperplasia. Hypersplenism is therefore associated with splenomegaly and pancytopenia. Symptoms depend on the extent of the pancytopenia. Neutropenia causes frequent bacterial infections, whereas thrombocytopenia (platelet counts less than 50,000 per cubic millimeter) cause easy bruising and hemorrhage from mucous membranes of the gastrointestinal and genitourinary tracts or from cerebral blood vessels.

Treatment for hypersplenism is splenectomy, which is performed if granulocytopenia (granulocyte count less than 5000 cells per cubic millimeter) or thrombocytopenia is severe. Improvement after splenectomy is fairly rapid and dramatic. Long-term effects of splenectomy are not entirely beneficial, however, and include leukocytosis, decreased levels of serum iron, and slight decreases in immune function. A mild thrombocytosis also may be evident.

ALTERATIONS OF PLATELETS AND COAGULATION

Alterations of platelets and coagulation all affect hemostasis, either by preventing hemostasis or by causing hemostasis to occur when it is not needed. (Hemostasis is described in Chapter 22.) Platelet and coagulation disorders can prevent hemostasis to varying degrees, causing (or failing to cause) internal or external hemorrhage. Diffuse internal hemorrhage that is visible through the skin causes a discoloration identified as a **purpura.** Purpuric disorders occur when there are not enough normal platelets to plug damaged vessels or prevent leakage from the many minute tears that occur daily in normal capillaries. Coagulation disorders tend to result in more serious bleeding and are usually caused by a deficiency of one or several clotting factors.

Disorders in which coagulation proceeds unnecessarily tend to result from vascular abnormalities that stimulate clotting. These disorders are known collectively as thromboembolic disease.

Disorders of Platelets

Quantitative or qualitative abnormalities of platelets can interrupt normal blood coagulation and prevent hemostasis. The quantitative abnormalities are **thrombocytopenia,** a decrease in the number of circulating platelets, and **thrombocytosis,** an increase in the number of platelets. Qualitative disorders affect the structure or function of individual platelets and can coexist with the quantitative disorders. Qualitative disorders usually prevent platelet adherence and aggregation, preventing formation of a platelet plug.

Thrombocytopenia

Thrombocytopenia is defined as a platelet count below 100,000 platelets per cubic millimeter of blood. A count of 50,000 or less increases the potential for hemorrhage associated with minor trauma. Spontaneous bleeding can occur with counts between 20,000 and 10,000, resulting in petechiae, ecchymoses, larger purpuric spots, or frank bleeding from mucous membranes. Severe bleeding results if the count is below 10,000 and can be fatal if it occurs in the gastrointestinal tract, respiratory system, or central nervous system.

Thrombocytopenia may be classified as either primary or secondary. Primary idiopathic thrombocytopenic purpura (ITP) exists in two forms—acute and chronic—and is thought to be an autoimmune disorder in which an IgG autoantibody is formed that binds to the platelets. Thus, the platelets are destroyed by the individual's immune system.

The acute form is most common in children and young adults (see Chapter 25) and is generally preceded by a viral infection. Chronic ITP is more common in females between the ages of 10 and 50, and generally is not preceded by a viral infection. The individual most commonly presents with mucosal or skin bleeding. Common types of bleeding are epistaxis, menorrhagia, purpura, and petechiae (Tierney, McPhee, Papadakis, & Schroeder, 1993). Enlargement of the spleen is uncommon.

Thrombocytopenia has been identified also as a complication of heparin therapy. Approximately 5% of all individuals treated with heparin develop thrombocytopenia (Chang, 1990). Some individuals have been known to develop paradoxical thrombosis. These thrombi consist of white platelet aggregates; thus, the condition is known as **"white clot syndrome."** The exact mechanism is unknown; however, an antibody of the IgG class has been implicated. If this condition is not recognized and treated, intravascular aggregation of platelets causes rapid development of multiple thrombotic disease in some individuals that can lead to arterial, venous, cerebral, and pulmonary thrombosis, and acute myocardial infarction (Chang, 1990). The individual may have gangrene in an upper or lower extremity or signs and symptoms of pulmonary emboli and stroke.

Secondary thrombocytopenia is caused by conditions associated with drug hypersensitivities that produce antibodies, viral and bacterial infections, and some autoimmune conditions. Viruses produce thrombocytopenia by (1) involving the megakaryocyte and inhibiting platelet production, (2) destroying circulating platelets, or (3) forming viral antigen-antibody complexes. Bacterial infections may increase consumption of platelets in the setting of septicemia associated with disseminated intravascular coagulation (DIC).

Thrombocytosis

Thrombocytosis is defined as a platelet count greater than 400,000 per cubic millimeter of blood. Thrombocytosis may be primary or secondary and is usually asymptomatic until the count exceeds 1 million/mm^3. At that point, intravascular clot formation (thrombosis), hemorrhage, or other abnormalities can occur.

Transient thrombocytosis is a normal, physiologic response to stress, infection, trauma, exercise, and ovulation. Abnormal thrombocytosis is caused by accelerated platelet production in the bone marrow.

Primary thrombocytosis (also called hemorrhagic thrombocythemia) is a myeloproliferative disorder in which megakaryocytes in the marrow overproliferate. It is associated with other myeloproliferative disorders, such as chronic nonlymphoblastic leukemia, polycythemia vera, and myelofibrosis (replacement of hematopoietic bone marrow with fibrous tissue).

Clinical manifestations of primary thrombocytosis typically include thrombosis of peripheral blood vessels (particularly in the digits) or, in severe episodes, thrombosis of hepatic, mesenteric, or pulmonary vessels. The other clinical hallmarks are splenomegaly and easy bruising.

Bleeding time may be prolonged or normal. If the course is benign, treatment is not necessary. In those with thrombotic and hemorrhagic complications, the goal of therapy is to lower the platelet count by use of chemotherapy agents or phlebotomy. Splenectomy is usually contraindicated because it causes a transient rise in the platelet count.

Secondary thrombocytosis occurs after splenectomy because platelets that normally would be stored in the spleen remain in circulating blood. The increase in platelets may be gradual, so that thrombocytosis does not occur for up to 3 weeks after splenectomy. Other forms of secondary thrombocytosis (reactive thrombocytosis) usually consist of a moderate rise in the platelet count that resolves with treatment of the underlying condition, such as rheumatoid arthritis and cancers. Secondary

thrombocytosis also can be caused by the accelerated thrombopoiesis that commonly accompanies accelerated erythropoiesis. This form of secondary thrombocytosis may be seen in conjunction with hemolytic anemias and some polycythemias, or as compensatory thrombocytosis after thrombocytopenia.

Alterations of Platelet Function

Alterations in platelet adherence (or adhesion) can result in prolonged bleeding times despite a normal platelet count. These qualitative disorders may be inherited or acquired. Inherited disorders may be the result of: (1) a lack of cell membrane glycoprotein; (2) reduced or absent cytoplasmic storage granules; (3) a platelet enzyme deficiency; or (4) a plasma factor deficiency, also known as von Willebrand disease (see Chapter 25).

Acquired disorders of platelet function result in membrane abnormalities, intracellular abnormalities, deficiencies in cellular contents, or defects in thromboxane synthesis. These disorders of platelet function are commonly caused by drugs, such as antiinflammatory agents, antimicrobials, antidepressants, and adrenergic blocking agents. Drugs interrupt and inhibit the synthesis of thromboxane A$_2$, as well as alter normal platelet adherence to endothelium. Uremia and a variety of other disorders that affect the hematopoietic system also can result in acquired disorders of platelet function.

Disorders of Coagulation

Disorders of coagulation are usually caused by defects or deficiencies of one or more of the clotting factors. (The characteristics of normal function of the clotting factors are described in Chapter 22.) Qualitative or quantitative abnormalities of clotting factors prevent the enzymatic reactions by which these factors are normally transformed from circulating plasma proteins to a stable fibrin clot (see Fig. 22-14).

Some clotting factor defects are inherited and usually involve a single factor. Two of the most common inherited disorders, the hemophilias and von Willebrand disease, are caused by deficiencies of clotting factors (see Chapter 25). Other coagulation defects are acquired and tend to result from deficient synthesis of clotting factors by the liver. Liver disease is one cause of acquired coagulation deficiency. Another is a dietary deficiency of vitamin K, which is necessary for normal synthesis of the clotting factors.

Other coagulation disorders that are not caused by quantitative or qualitative clotting factor defects are attributed to pathologic conditions that trigger coagulation inappropriately, engaging the clotting factors and causing detrimental clotting within blood vessels. For example, any cardiovascular abnormality that alters normal blood flow by speeding it up, slowing it down, or obstructing it can create conditions in which coagulation proceeds within the vessels. This is a cause of **thromboembolic disease,** in which blood clots obstruct blood vessels. Coagulation is also stimulated by the presence of tissue thromboplastin, which is released by damaged or dead tissues. Therefore, any condition in which tissue decay or damage releases a great deal of tissue thromboplastin, such as occurs in complications of pregnancy, including death of the fetus and placental decay within the mother, can cause widespread and possibly fatal intravascular coagulation. Another cause of detrimental coagulation processes is vasculitis, or inflammation of the blood vessels. Damage to inflamed vessels causes platelet activation, which in turn activates the coagulation cascade. In extensive or prolonged vasculitis, blood clot formation can overcome mechanisms that normally control clot formation and breakdown, leading to clogging of the vessels. In each of these acquired conditions, normal hemostatic function proves detrimental to the body by consuming coagulation factors excessively or by overwhelming normal control of clot formation and breakdown (fibrinolysis).

Vitamin K Deficiency

Vitamin K, a fat-soluble vitamin, is necessary for synthesis of normal prothrombin; clotting factors II, VII, IX, and X; and proteins C and S. Vitamin K is usually taken into the body in green, leafy vegetables. Resident intestinal bacteria also are a source of vitamin K. Deficiencies occur because of insufficient dietary intake, the absence of bile salts necessary for vitamin K absorption, intestinal malabsorption syndromes, and oral antibiotics that kill resident intestinal bacteria. Bleeding caused by vitamin K deficiency resembles that of other coagulation defects and may be moderate to fatal. Laboratory tests disclose an elevated prothrombin time.

Parenteral administration of vitamin K and transfusion of fresh frozen plasma are appropriate ways to replace vitamin K as well as factors II, VII, IX, and X. Resolution of the condition that caused vitamin K deficiency is also necessary. Neonates are deficient in vitamin K because of the immaturity of their livers and lack of normal intestinal flora, so some clinicians administer vitamin K routinely at birth to eliminate the risk of hemorrhagic disease of the newborn.

Liver Disease

A pattern of hemostatic derangements resulting from disruption of synthesis of vitamin K–dependent clotting factors is present with advanced liver disease. Factor VII levels are the first to decline because of its rapid turnover. Fibrinogen, however, seems to be well conserved, and synthesis does not decrease until liver insufficiency is well advanced.

The hemostatic system is affected in other ways by liver disease. Fibrinolysis occurs because of inadequate hepatic synthesis of alpha$_2$ antiplasmin, which is the main inhibitor of fibrinolysis by clearing plasminogen factor from the blood. Concurrent splenomegaly may produce a mild thrombocytopenia and biliary tract congestion may result in inadequate absorption of vitamin K. Treatment is administration of vitamin K and replacement of plasma and blood volume as indicated.

Disseminated Intravascular Coagulation (DIC)

Disseminated intravascular coagulation (DIC) is an acquired coagulopathy that results from a variety of predisposing conditions. It has been described as "a dynamic pathologic process triggered by activation of the clotting cascade with the resultant activation of excess thrombin within the vascular system. Excess thrombin leads to further activation of the coagulation system, shortened survival of certain hemostatic elements, deposition of fibrin in the microcirculation, and activation of the fibrinolytic system" (Feinstein, 1988). In short, DIC is a paradoxical condition in which clotting and hemorrhage occur within the vascular system simultaneously.

The incidence of DIC is estimated to occur in 1 of every 900 to 2400 adult admissions in large urban hospitals, with a mortality rate of 50% to 80% (Bell, 1992). The mortality rate can reach 90% if shock and infection are the precipitating event (Logan, 1988).

Disseminated intravascular coagulation is caused by a wide variety of clinical conditions, specifically those that activate the clotting mechanisms. Significant clinical conditions include (1) arterial hypotension, often associated with shock; (2) hypoxemia; (3) acidemia; and (4) stasis of capillary blood flow (Bell, 1992).

The development of DIC is generally associated with three pathologic processes, including (1) endothelial damage, (2) release of tissue thromboplastin (TTP), and (3) direct activation of factor X. There are also unclassified processes that may precipitate the development of DIC. Specific clinical disorders associated with these processes are shown in the box on p. 900.

Damage to the endothelium exposes the negatively charged basement membrane, which becomes a hemostatically active vascular surface. Sepsis—particularly gram-negative and septic shock—hypoxia, and low-flow states associated with cardiopulmonary arrest can damage the endothelium and precipitate DIC by activating the intrinsic clotting pathway. Endotoxins of gram-negative sepsis cause activation of both intrinsic and extrinsic clotting pathways (Bell, 1992).

Release of TTP is associated with numerous conditions, most commonly those associated with various types of trauma (burns, brain injury, myocardial infarctions, surgeries, obstetric accidents, and malignancies). Endothelial cells and monocytes, however, also have been reported to express TTP on their cell surfaces when

PRECIPITATING MECHANISMS IN THE DEVELOPMENT OF DIC

Endothelial damage

Sepsis (gram-negative)
Hypoxia
Cardiac/pulmonary arrest
Shock (hemorrhagic, septic, cardiogenic, traumatic)
ARDS
Aortic aneurysms (dissecting)

Release of TTP

Trauma (burns, head injury, fat emboli, surgery [extensive procedures])
Myocardial infarction
Dissecting aortic aneurysms
Malignancies (acute leukemia, adenocarcinomas, carcinomas, sarcomas, pheochromocytoma)
Obstetric conditions (abruptio placentae, eclampsia, retained dead fetus, retained placenta, missed/septic abortion, amniotic fluid embolism, hydatidiform mole)

Factor X activation

Acute pancreatitis
Snake venom
Liver disease

Miscellaneous

Hematologic conditions (massive blood transfusion, hemolytic anemia, sickle cell crisis)
Anaphylaxis
Fresh water near-drowning
Hypothermia
Malignant hyperthermia
Pulmonary embolism
Aspirin poisoning
Extracorporeal membrane oxygenation
Necrotizing enterocolitis

stimulated with interleukin-1 and endotoxins (Bailes, 1992). Excessive amounts of TTP in the circulation cause activation of the extrinsic clotting pathway through the activation of factor VII.

Direct proteolytic activation is the activation of the clotting mechanism at factor X. Activation of factor X is stimulated by various substances released into the bloodstream from a variety of sources. Pancreatic and hepatic enzymes act in this way, as well as venom from snake bites.

Disseminated intravascular coagulation also can be precipitated by miscellaneous conditions, most notably blood transfusion. Transfused blood dilutes the clotting factors, as well as the circulating naturally occurring antithrombins. In hemolytic transfusion reactions, procoagulant material is released from disrupted platelets and red blood cells (RBCs) as a result of antigen-antibody reactions. The release of procoagulant material contributes to the diffuse hemorrhaging and hypotension in these individuals. Antigen-antibody reactions are also responsible for the development of DIC after anaphylaxis (Bell, 1992).

The pathophysiology of DIC is shown in Fig. 24-10. Disseminated intravascular coagulation is initiated by one of the above-described mechanisms activating either the intrinsic or extrinsic clotting cascade, although it appears that the extrinsic system is predominant. Once either system is activated, widespread coagulation occurs throughout the body, leading to thrombiotic events within the vasculature. The normal inhibitory mechanisms become overwhelmed so that clotting can occur unrestricted. As a result of the widespread clotting that occurs, the clotting factors become used up and hemorrhage ensues. This leads to the two primary pathophysiologic alterations of DIC—thrombosis in the presence of hemorrhage.

Once clotting occurs, the fibrinolytic pathway is activated, which promotes the degradation of the clot that has formed. After the coagulation and fibrinolytic systems have been activated, large amounts of circulating prothrombin and plasminogen are converted to thrombin and plasmin (Bailes, 1992). In addition, the kallikrein-kinin and complement systems are activated. All of these activated systems further contribute to the thrombosis and hemorrhage characteristics of DIC.

The amount of thrombin that enters the systemic circulation during DIC greatly exceeds the ability of the body's naturally occurring antithrombins (protein C and AT III) to regulate it. Initially, thrombin is released during activation of the clotting cascade and facilitates platelet aggregation and clotting factor consumption. Thrombin also divides fibrinogen into fibrin monomers that polymerize into fibrin clots and become deposited in the microcirculation.

The obstruction that results from circulatory deposition of thrombin interferes with blood flow and causes widespread organ hypoperfusion that can lead to ischemia, infarction, and necrosis. The aggregated platelets contribute to thrombus formation by becoming entrapped within the microvascular fibrin deposits. These events are potentiated when a low blood flow state exists, as in shock (see Chapter 27). Because organ perfusion is drastically impaired, manifestations of multisystem organ dysfunction or failure ultimately result (Bell, 1992). Multisystem organ failure is discussed further in Chapter 27.

Excessive amounts of thrombin, which contributes to the coagulation, also contribute to the hemorrhage associated with DIC. The aggregation of platelets causes a thrombocytopenia that increases the risk of bleeding.

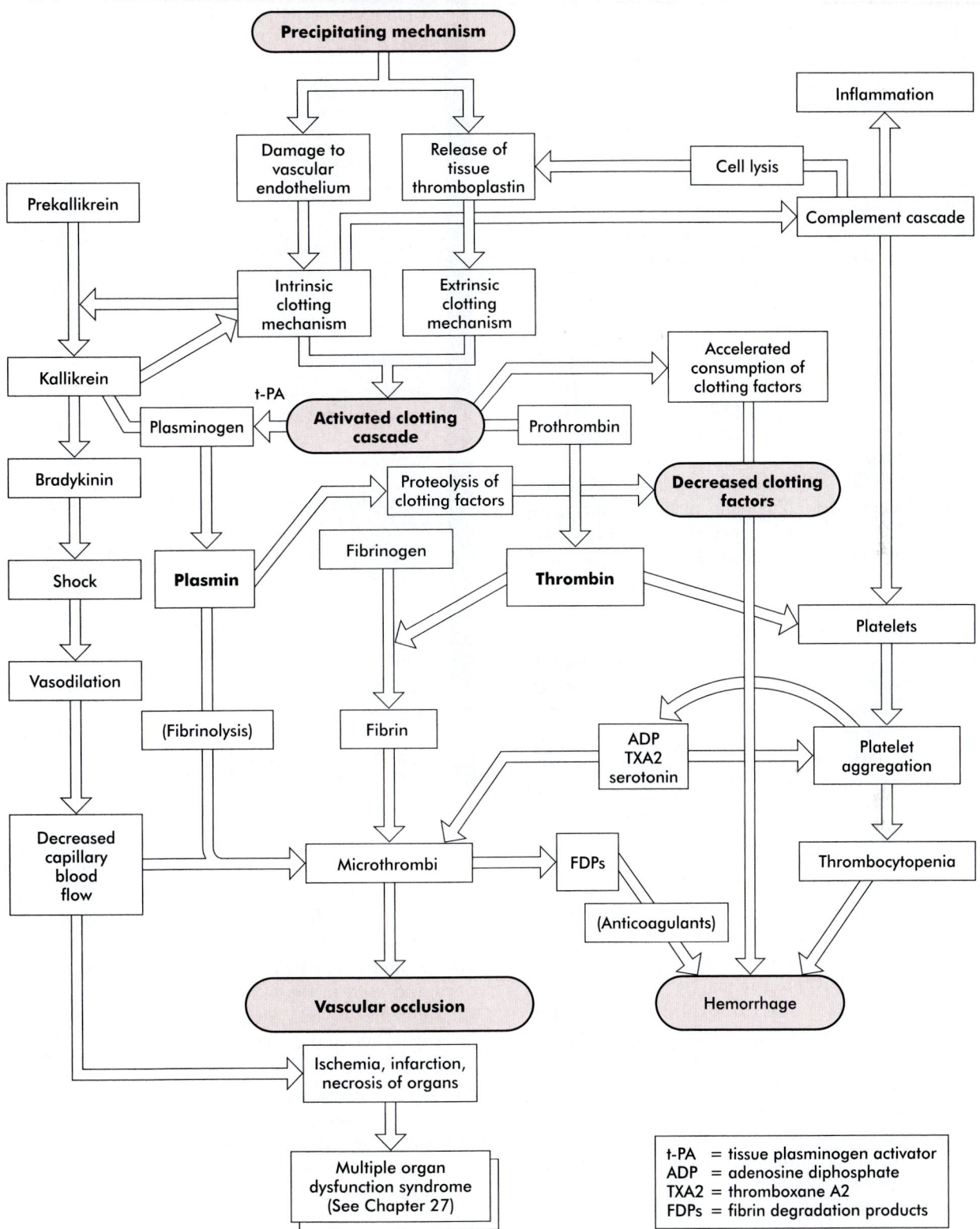

FIG. 24-10 Pathophysiology of DIC. The coagulation cascade is activated if sufficient amounts of specific substances are released into the blood. If the linings of the blood vessels are damaged, the substance released by the injured endothelium initiates the intrinsic pathway for coagulation (see Chapter 22). If tissues anywhere in the body are dead, their decay releases tissue thromboplastin into the blood, initiating the extrinsic pathway of coagulation. (Adapted from Lee et al., 1993.)

Thrombin also activates the fibrinolytic system, causing bleeding.

Plasmin, also present because of overstimulation of the clotting cascade, begins to degrade fibrin before a stable clot has developed. As fibrin is broken down by plasmin, fibrin degradation products (FDPs) are released into the circulation. High concentrations of FDPs, which are potent anticoagulants, further contribute to the bleeding of DIC. Normally, FDPs are cleared from the blood by the macrophage system. The inability of the macrophage system to clear the blood of FDPs is thought to be the result of a lack of fibronectin, a glycoprotein with adhesive properties that mediates clearance of particulate matter (e.g., fibrin clumps). Low levels of fibronectin in individuals with DIC carry a poor prognosis (Bell, 1992). The positive feedback loop that perpetuates the cycle of thrombosis and hemorrhage persists until the underlying mechanism that precipitated DIC is removed or appropriate therapeutic interventions are used.

The onset of DIC can be an acute process, as seen in obstetric situations, for example, placenta previa, abruptio placentae, missed abortion, and hypertonic saline-induced abortion. Chronic DIC can occur with many types of malignancies. Bleeding from numerous sites becomes the predominant problem. Oozing or frank bleeding occurs from mucous membranes, deep tissue, injured tissues, sites of venipuncture or injection, and every natural orifice. Petechiae and ecchymoses are common. Although major organ dysfunction is sometimes caused by underlying disorders, DIC is often the cause, particularly of pulmonary, renal, hepatic, and central nervous system dysfunction. Clinical manifestations of these organ disruptions are summarized in the following box.

The diagnosis of DIC is primarily based on a high index of suspicion and laboratory results. Although no one laboratory test exists to confirm the diagnosis of DIC, multiple tests are performed to establish the existence of DIC. These tests are identified and the results of the presence of DIC are summarized in Table 24-6.

Treatment of DIC is directed toward (1) removal of the underlying pathology, (2) restoration of an appropriate balance between coagulation and fibrinolysis, and (3) maintaining organ viability (Bell, 1992). Removal of the underlying pathology is the initial intervention in the treatment phase. Once the underlying pathology has been removed, coagulation factors can be restored by the liver within 24 to 48 hours, assuming that liver functions are intact (Bell, 1992). Heparin therapy as a way of restoring balance between coagulation and fibrinolysis is controversial and appears to be more therapeutic in certain types of DIC. Heparin is indicated when organ function is compromised by microthrombi or when there is evidence of loss of life or limb. Heparin

---

CLINICAL MANIFESTATIONS ASSOCIATED WITH DIC

Integumentary system

Widespread hemorrhage/vascular lesions
Oozing from puncture sites, incisions, mucous membranes
Acrocyanosis (irregular-shaped cyanotic patches)
Gangrene

Central nervous system

Subarachnoid hemorrhage
Altered state of consciousness (slight confusion to convulsions and coma)

Gastrointestinal system

Occult bleeding to massive GI bleeding
Abdominal distention
Malaise
Weakness

Pulmonary system

Pulmonary infarctions
ARDS
Cyanosis
Tachypnea
Hypoxemia

Renal system

Hematuria
Oliguria
Renal failure

Modified from Bailes, 1992.

---

also appears to be effective in conditions in which DIC is precipitated by retained dead fetus and acute promyelocytic leukemia. In DIC that is precipitated by septic shock or where there is postoperative bleeding, peptic ulcer bleeding, or central nervous system bleeding, heparin is contraindicated. Newer drugs are being developed and used in the treatment of DIC (Antithrombin III and Gabexate mesylate); however, their use remains investigational and controversial (Bell, 1992).

Maintenance of organ viability is treated primarily by adequate fluid replacement to ensure adequate circulating blood volume so that optimal tissue perfusion can be maintained. Fluid resuscitation also may be required to restore blood pressure, cardiac output, and urine output to normal limits.

Thromboembolic Disease

Abnormal clots may occur occasionally within the vascular system. If the clot is stationary or adheres to the vessel wall, it is called a **thrombus** (Fig. 24-11). A thrombus may block blood flow within a vessel that

FIG. 24-11 Thrombus. Thrombus arising in valve pocket at upper end of superficial femoral vein. Postmortem clot on the right is shown for comparison. (From McLachlin & Paterson, J. C. [1951]. Some basic observations on venous thrombosis and pulmonary embolism. *Surgery, Gynecology, & Obstetrics, 93,*1-8, by permission of *Surgery, Gynecology, & Obstetrics.*)

TABLE 24-6

Tests Used to Identify DIC

Test	Result*
Bleeding time	>7 min
Platelet count	<130,000†
Plasma fibrinogen levels	<195 mg/dl
Fibrin degradation products (FDP)	>10 μg/ml
Activated partial thromboplastin time (APTT)	>36 seconds
Prothrombin time (PT)	>12 seconds
One-stage factor assays‡ (extrinsic coagulation system)	
Factor II	<25 μg/ml
Factor V	<50%
Factor VII	<65%
Factor X	<45%

Data from Bailes, 1992; Coffin, 1989.
*Results may vary depending on the laboratory and measurements used.
†In endotoxin-induced DIC, platelets decrease earlier than fibrinogen level; in other causes of DIC, fibrinogen levels fall earlier.
‡One-stage factor assay may be used when APTT and PT are done to determine deficiencies of specific factors.

supplies nutrients to tissue critical to survival, such as the heart, brain, or lungs. It is not completely known why the endothelial lining of these vessels changes, but many causes are under investigation.

An intravascular clot that floats within the blood is called an **embolus.** The mobile embolus travels within the bloodstream until it comes to rest in a very small vessel, where it usually blocks circulation to distal structures. This has dangerous effects in vessels that supply vital organs.

Prethrombotic conditions predispose an individual to the development of thrombi. The prethrombotic state, in general, is caused by **hypercoagulability** within the vasculature. Hypercoagulability may be attributable to hereditary or acquired causes. Hereditary hypercoagulability may result from a deficiency of protein C, protein S, or antithrombin III, or from a variety of inheritable disorders (Bower & Vukelja, 1992).

Both proteins C and S are vitamin K–dependent inhibitors of coagulation and are synthesized in the liver. Decreased levels of either of these proteins interfere with the normal homeostatic balance of procoagulant and anticoagulant activity at the endothelial level.

Inheritance of protein C deficiency is autosomal dominant. Heterozygotes have protein C levels 50% to 60% of normal and may develop superficial thrombophlebitis, deep venous thrombosis, or pulmonary embolism in

their 20s. Homozygotes have less than 1% of normal levels of protein C and tend to develop thrombosis of the cutaneous vessels with large areas of skin necrosis. Infants with this condition rarely survive. Individuals with protein C deficiency require lifelong therapy with coumadin.

Protein S deficiency is inherited as a codominant autosomal recessive disorder (Bower & Vukelja, 1992). Affected individuals experience recurrent thrombosis and thrombophlebitis, often before the age of 35. The homozygous state is not as common; however, when present, thrombosis may be evident as early as the teen years.

Antithrombin III (AT-III) deficiency is inherited as an autosomal dominant condition. Heterozygotes have AT-III levels that are 40% to 60% of normal and may experience thrombotic problems in early adulthood, primarily lower extremity deep venous thrombosis, and pulmonary embolism. These individuals also are placed on long-term anticoagulant therapy.

Other inherited conditions that may predispose an individual to hypercoagulability include (1) decreased fibrinolysis and (2) presence of antiphospholipid antibodies (Freed, 1990). Decreased fibrinolysis results from decreased levels of tissue plasminogen activator (TPA); antiphospholipid antibodies appear to damage the phospholipid surfaces of platelets on which coagulation factors assemble.

The acquired hypercoagulable states are mostly

caused by conditions that promote venous stasis. The most common clinical states that predispose to thromboembolic phenomena are major surgery (orthopedic), acute myocardial infarction, congestive heart failure, limb paralysis, spinal injury, malignancy, advanced age, the postpartum period, and bed rest greater than 1 week (Freed, 1990). In these conditions, it is imperative that one is familiar with factors that promote thrombus formation. These three factors are referred to as the **triad of Virchow** and are (1) loss of integrity of the vessel wall, (2) abnormalities of blood flow, and (3) alterations in the blood constituents.

The vessel wall can be injured, for example, by atherosclerosis (plaque deposits on arterial walls). Atherosclerosis initiates platelet adhesion, aggregation, and formation of a thrombus that resembles a platelet plug. It is not known why atherosclerosis causes arterial thrombosis. Venous thrombosis is apparently caused by alterations of the integrity and tone of the veins by extrinsic factors.

Several abnormalities of blood flow can cause thrombus formation. In arterial vessels, thrombosis occurs in conditions of rapid flow. Changes that create turbulence or change the rate of blood flow promote thrombus enlargement that can ultimately occlude the vessel. In veins, slow blood flow contributes to thrombosis, which becomes more severe with further slowing or stagnation. The slower the flow, the greater the quantity of activated clotting factors that remain in close proximity in the vessels. This is the mechanism by which thrombosis occurs in conditions of venous stasis.

Quantitative or qualitative alterations of blood constituents (chiefly clotting factors and platelets) also contribute to thrombosis. Thrombocytopenia, thrombocytosis, elevated levels of clotting factors, deficiencies of antithrombin III, and reduced fibrinolytic activity all can increase the risk or presence of thromboembolism. Increased viscosity of the blood and increased platelet activity also can lead to thrombus formation.

Whether episodes of thromboembolism are life-threatening depends on the site of vessel occlusion. Therapy consists of removal or breakdown of the clot and supportive measures. Anticoagulant therapy is effective in treating or preventing venous thrombosis; it is not useful in treating or preventing arterial thrombosis. Parenteral heparin is the major anticoagulant used to treat thromboembolism. Oral coumarin drugs are also widely used, particularly for outpatients.

More aggressive therapy may be indicated for such conditions as pulmonary embolism, coronary thrombosis, or thrombophlebitis. Streptokinase and urokinase activate the fibrinolytic system, and are administered to accelerate the lysis of known thrombus. Thrombolytic therapy has limited uses and is prescribed with a high degree of caution because it can cause hemorrhagic complications.

SUMMARY REVIEW

Alterations of Leukocyte Function

1 Quantitative alterations of leukocytes (too many or too few) can be caused by bone marrow dysfunction or premature destruction of cells in the circulation.
2 Many quantitative changes in leukocytes occur in response to invasion by microorganisms.
3 Leukocytosis is a condition in which the leukocyte count is higher than normal and is usually a response to stress and invasion of microorganisms.
4 Leukopenia is a condition in which the leukocyte count is lower than normal and is caused by pathologic conditions, such as malignancies and hematologic disorders.
5 Granulocytosis (particularly as a result of neutrophilia) occurs in response to infection.
6 When the demand for neutrophils exceeds the supply in the circulation, the marrow releases immature cells, causing a shift to the left.
7 Eosinophilia results most commonly from parasitic invasion and ingestion or inhalation of toxic foreign particles.

8 Basophilia is seen in hypersensitivity reactions because of the high content of histamine and subsequent release.
9 Monocytosis occurs during the late or recuperative phase of infection when macrophages (mature monocytes) phagocytose surviving microorganisms and debris.
10 Granulocytopenia, a condition resulting in a decrease in neutrophils, can be a life-threatening condition if sepsis occurs; it is often caused by chemotherapeutic agents, severe infection, and radiation.
11 The common pathologic feature of all forms of leukemia is an uncontrolled proliferation of leukocytes.
12 All leukemias can be designated as (1) lymphocytic, (2) myelocytic or myelogenous, or (3) monocytic. The acute leukemias are divided into two major types: (1) acute nonlymphoblastic leukemia (ANLL) or acute myelogenous leukemia (AML), and (2) acute lymphoblastic leukemia (ALL).
13 The two principal types of chronic leukemia are (1) chronic granulocytic leukemia (CGL) or chronic myelocytic leukemia (CML), and (2) chronic lymphocytic leukemias (CLL).

14 Although the exact cause of leukemia is unknown, it is considered a clonal disorder. A high incidence of acute leukemias and CLL is reported in certain families, suggesting a genetic predisposition.

15 In leukemia, blasts (precursor cells) "crowd out" the marrow and cause cellular proliferation of the other cell lines to cease.

16 The major clinical manifestations of leukemia include fatigue caused by anemia, bleeding caused by thrombocytopenia, fever secondary to infection, anorexia, and weight loss.

17 Chemotherapy is the treatment of choice for leukemia. Acute leukemias are associated with a 20% to 50% long-term survival. Chronic leukemias are associated with a longer life expectancy.

18 Chronic leukemias progress differently than acute leukemias, advancing slowly and without warning.

19 Multiple myeloma is a neoplasm of B cells (immature plasma cells) and mature plasma cells. It is characterized by multiple malignant tumor masses of plasma cells scattered throughout the skeletal system and sometimes in soft tissue.

20 The exact cause of multiple myeloma is unknown, but genetic factors and chronic stimulation of the mononuclear phagocyte system by bacteria, viral agents, and chemicals have been suggested.

21 The major clinical manifestations for multiple myeloma include recurrent infections caused by suppression of the humoral immune response and renal disease as a result of Bence Jones proteinuria.

22 Chemotherapy is the treatment for multiple myeloma. Survival is still only 2 to 3 years with chemotherapy, however.

Alterations of Lymphoid Function

1 The number of lymphocytes is decreased (lymphocytopenia) in most acute infections and in some immune deficiency syndromes.

2 Lymphocytosis occurs in viral infections, infectious mononucleosis and infectious hepatitis, in particular, leukemia, lymphomas, and some chronic infections.

3 Infectious mononucleosis is an acute infection of B-lymphocytes most commonly associated with the Epstein-Barr virus (EBV) (a type of herpes virus).

4 Two of the earliest manifestations of infectious mononucleosis are sore throat and fever caused by inflammation at the site of viral entry.

5 Most cases of EBV infectious mononucleosis include fever with temperature elevation lasting 7 to 10 days, sore throat, and enlargement and tenderness of the cervical lymph nodes.

6 Lymphomas are tumors of primary lymphoid tissue (thymus and bone marrow) or secondary tissue (lymph nodes, spleen, tonsils, and intestinal lymphoid tissue). The two major types of malignant lymphomas are (1) Hodgkin disease and (2) non-Hodgkin disease.

7 Distinctive abnormal chromosomes are present in multiple cells of the lymph nodes of an individual with Hodgkin disease. The abnormal cell is called the Reed-Sternberg cell.

8 A virus might be involved in the pathogenesis of Hodgkin disease. Some familial clustering suggests an unknown genetic mechanism.

9 An enlarged, painless mass or swelling, most commonly in the neck, is an initial sign of Hodgkin disease. Local symptoms are produced by lymphadenopathy, usually caused by pressure or obstruction.

10 Treatment of Hodgkin disease includes radiation therapy and chemotherapy. A cure is possible regardless of stage of Hodgkin disease; however, individuals treated with chemotherapy who relapse in less than 2 years have a poor prognosis.

11 The cause of lymph node enlargement and cancerous transformation in non-Hodgkin lymphoma is unknown. Immunosuppressed persons have greater incidence of non-Hodgkin lymphoma, suggesting an immune mechanism.

12 Generally, with non-Hodgkin lymphoma, the swelling of lymph nodes is painless and the nodes have enlarged and transformed over a period of months or years.

13 Individuals with non-Hodgkin lymphoma can survive for long periods. Treatment is with chemotherapy.

14 Burkitt lymphoma involves the jaw and facial bones and occurs in children from east-central Africa and New Guinea.

Alterations of Splenic Function

1 Splenomegaly (enlargement of the spleen) is a secondary effect to other disorders in the body.

2 Splenomegaly results from (1) proliferation of lymphocytes or macrophages of the white pulp, (2) invasion of neoplastic cells, or (3) chronic congestion with blood.

3 Hypersplenism is associated with splenomegaly and pancytopenia.

Alterations of Platelets and Coagulation

1 Thrombocytopenia is characterized by a platelet count below 100,000 platelets per cubic millimeter of blood; a count below 50,000 increases the potential for hemorrhage associated with minor trauma.

2 Thrombocytopenia exists in primary or secondary forms.

3 Thrombocytopenia is commonly associated with autoimmune diseases and viral infections; bacterial sepsis with DIC also results in thrombocytopenia.

4 Thrombocytosis is characterized by a platelet count greater than 400,000 platelets per cubic millimeter of blood and is symptomatic when the count exceeds one million when risk for intravascular clotting (thrombosis) is high.

5 Thrombocytosis is caused by accelerated platelet production in the bone marrow.

6 Alterations in normal platelet adherence or aggregation prevent platelet plug formation and may result in prolonged bleeding times.

7 Platelet dysfunction results from changes in the cellular contents and integrity.

8 Disorders of coagulation are usually caused by defects or deficiencies of one or more of the clotting factors.

9 Pathologic conditions can trigger coagulation, inappropriately using up the clotting factors, causing detrimental clotting within blood vessels.

10 Coagulation is impaired when there is a deficiency of vitamin K because of insufficient production of prothrombin and clotting factors II, VII, IX, and X.

11 Liver disease accounts for a pattern of hemostatic derangement caused by a disruption of the synthesis of clotting factors.

12 Disseminated intravascular coagulation (DIC) is a complex syndrome resulting from a variety of chemical conditions that cause clotting through the vascular system.

13 Disseminated intravascular coagulation is characterized by a cycle of intravascular clotting followed by active bleeding because of the consumption of coagulation factors, platelets, and diffuse fibrinolysis.

14 Thromboembolic disease results from a fixed (thrombus) or moving (embolism) clot that blocks flow within a vessel, denying nutrients to tissues distal to the occlusion; death can result when clots are located in the heart, brain, or lungs.

15 Hypercoagulability is the result of deficient anticoagulation proteins. Secondary causes are conditions that promote venous stasis.

16 The term *triad of Virchow* refers to three factors that can cause thrombus formation: (1) loss of integrity of the vessel wall, (2) abnormalities of blood flow, and (3) alterations in the blood constituents.

KEY TERMS

Agranulocytosis, 880
Basopenia, 880
Basophilia, 880
Bence Jones protein, 889
Burkitt lymphoma, 896
Disseminated intravascular coagulation (DIC), 899
Embolus, 903
Eosinopenia, 880
Eosinophilia, 880
Granulocytopenia, 880
Granulocytosis, 879
Hodgkin disease, 891
Hypercoagulability, 903
Hypersplenism, 896
Infectious mononucleosis, 882

Leukemia, 882
Leukemia-associated inhibitory activity (LIA), 884
Leukocytosis, 879
Leukopenia, 879
Lymphadenopathy, 890
Lymphocytopenia, 882
Lymphocytosis, 882
M-protein, 889
Monocytopenia, 880
Monocytosis, 880
Multiple myeloma, 888
Neutropenia, 879
Neutrophilia, 879
Non-Hodgkin lymphoma, 891

Pancytopenia, 884
Primary thrombocytosis (hemorrhagic thrombocythemia), 898
Purpura, 897
Secondary thrombocytosis, 898
Shift to the left (leukemoid reaction), 879
Shift to the right, 879
Splenomegaly, 896
Thrombocytopenia, 885, 897
Thrombocytosis, 897
Thromboembolic disease, 899
Thrombus, 902
Triad of Virchow, 903
White clot syndrome, 897

REFERENCES

American Cancer Society (ACS). (1993). *Cancer facts & figures 1993.* New York: Author.

American Cancer Society (ACS). (1992). *Cancer facts & figures 1992.* New York: Author.

American Joint Committee on Cancer. (1988). *Manual for staging cancer* (3rd ed., pp. 25-282). Philadelphia: Lippincott.

Ashinsky, D. (1990). Eosinophilia-myalgia syndrome linked to tryptophan. *Postgraduate Medicine, 88,* 193-195.

Athens, J. W. (1993). Variations of leukocytes in disease. In G. R. Lee, T. C. Bithell, J. Foerster, J. W. Athens, & J. N. Lukens (Eds.), *Wintrobe's clinical hematology* (9th ed.). Philadelphia: Lea & Febiger.

Bailes, B. K. (1992). Disseminated intravascular coagulation. *AORN Journal, 55*(2), 517-529.

Bell, T. N. (1992). Coagulation and disseminated intravascular coagulation. In V. B. Huddleston (Ed.), *Multisystem organ failure: Pathophysiology and clinical implications* (pp. 57-81). St. Louis: Mosby—Year Book.

Betts, R. F. (1990). Mononucleosis syndromes. In W. J. Williams, E. Beutler, A. J. Erslav, & M. A. Lichtman (Eds.), *Hematology* (4th ed., pp. 955-962). New York: McGraw-Hill.

Borden, E. C., Steeves, R. A., & Hogan, J. F. (1983). Infectious carcinogenesis: Viruses and human neoplasia. In S. B. Kahn, R. R. Lone, C. Sherman, & R. Chakravorty (Eds.), *Concepts in cancer medicine.* New York: Grune & Stratton.

Bower, K. J., & Vukelja, S. J. (1992). Hypercoagulable states: Their causes and management. *Postgraduate Medicine, 91*, 117-125, 128-132.

Broxmeyer, H. E., Mendelsohn, N., Moore, M., & Alcolm, A. S. (1977). Abnormal granulocyte feedback regulation of colony forming and colony stimulating activity—Producing cells from patients with chronic myelogenous leukemia. *Leukemia Research, 1*, 3.

Buchsbaum, R. J., & Schwartz, R. S. (1990). Cellular origins of hematologic neoplasms. *New England Journal of Medicine, 233*(10), 694-695.

Cancer in Focus. (1991). The war on cancer: Giant leaps at the bench, small steps in the trench. *The Journal of NIH Research, 3*, 41-72.

Chang, J. C. (1990). White clot syndrome: A serious complication of heparin therapy. *Postgraduate Medicine, 87*, 293, 296-297.

Clarkson, B., Elles, S., & Little, C. (1985). Acute lymphoblastic leukemia in adults. *Seminars in Oncology, 12*, 160-179.

Coffin, C. M. (1989). Potentially catastrophic bleeding disorders: Approaches to diagnosis and management. *Bleeding Disorders, 85*(3), 217-225.

Cotran, R. S., Kumar, V., & Robbins, S. L. (1989). *Robbins pathologic basis of disease* (4th ed.). Philadelphia: Saunders.

Cunningham, I. (1990). Bone marrow transplantation for chronic myelogenous leukemia. *Oncology, 4*(11), 101-108.

Defonzo, R., Cooke, C. R., Wright, J. R., & Humphrey, R. L. (1978). Renal function in patients with multiple myeloma. *Medicine, 57*, 151.

DelRegato, J. A., Spjut, H. J., & Cox, J. D. (1985). *Cancer: Diagnosis, treatment, and prognosis* (6th ed.). St. Louis: Mosby—Year Book.

Epstein, J. (1992). Myeloma phenotype: Clues to disease origin and manifestation. *Hematology Oncology Clinics of North America, 6*(2), 249-256.

Epstein, J., Xiao, H., & He, X. (1990). Markers of multiple hematopoietic cell linages in multiple myeloma. *New England Journal of Medicine, 322*(10), 664-668.

Erslev, A. J. (1990). Erythrocyte disorders: Anemias and red cell changes related to altered splenic function. In W. J. Williams, E. Beutler, A. J. Erslev, & Lichman, M. A. (Eds.), *Hematology* (4th ed., pp. 694-698). New York: McGraw-Hill.

Feinstein, D. I. (1988). Treatment of disseminated intravascular coagulation. *Seminars in Thrombosis and Hemostasis, 14*(4), 351-361.

Fraser, M. C., & Tucker, M. A. (1988). Late effects of cancer therapy: Chemotherapy related malignancy. *Oncology Forum, 15*, 67-77.

Freed, J. (1990). Hypercoagulability: Should every patient with venous thrombosis be tested? *Postgraduate Medicine, 90*, 157-160, 165-167.

Gunz, F. W. (1980). The dread leukemias and the lymphomas: Their nature and their prospects. In M. M. Wintrope (Ed.), *Blood, pure and eloquent: A story of discovery, of people, and of ideas*. New York: McGraw-Hill.

Julia, A., Olona, M., Revilla, E., Rossello, J., Morey, M., Flores, A., Font, L., & Macia, J. (1991). Drug induced agranulocytosis: Prognostic factors in a series of 168 episodes. *British Journal of Haematology, 70*, 366-371.

Kaplan, H. S. (1980). *Hodgkin's disease* (2nd ed.). Cambridge, MA: Harvard University Press.

Kissane, J. M. (Ed.). (1990). *Anderson's pathology* (9th ed.). St. Louis: Mosby—Year Book.

Lee, G. R., Bithell, T. C. Foerster, J., Athens, J. W., & Lukens, J. N. (Eds.). (1993). *Wintrobe's clinical hematology* (9th ed.). Philadelphia: Lea & Febiger.

Lukes, R. J., Carver, L. F., & Hall, T. C. (1966). Report of the Nomenclature Committee from Symposium on Obstacles to the Control of Hodgkin's Disease. *Cancer Research, 26*, 1311.

Logan, J. J. (1988). Hemostasis and bleeding disorders. In J. J. Mazza (Ed.), *Manual of intensive care medicine*. Boston: Little Brown.

Martin, S. E., Zhang, H. Z., & Magyarosy, E. (1984). Immunologic methods in cytology: Definitive diagnosis of NHL using immunologic markers for T- and B-cells. *American Journal of Clinical Pathology, 82*(6), 666-673.

Mayer, R. (1987). Current chemotherapeutic treatment approaches to the management of previously untreated adults with de novo AML. *Seminars in Oncology, 14*, 384-396.

National Cancer Institute. (1982). The NHL pathologic classification project: National Cancer Institute sponsored study of classification of non-Hodgkin lymphoma. *Cancer, 49*(10), 2112-2135.

Newell, G. R., Cabanillas, F. G., & Hagemeister, F. J. (1987). Incidence of lymphoma in the US classified by the working formulation. *Cancer, 59*, 857-861.

Rowley, D. (1990). Molecular cytogenetics. *Cancer Research, 50*(13), 3816-3825.

Russin, S. J., Fillipo, B. H., & Alder, A. G. (1990). Neutropenia in adults: What is its clinical significance. *Postgraduate Medicine, 88*, 209-216.

Silberburg, E., & Lubera, J. (1989). Cancer statistics 1989. *Cancer, 39*, 3-20.

Skarin, A. T., Canellos, G. P., Maych, P. M., & Nieman, R. S. (1986). Lymphoma. In *Cancer manual*. Boston, MA: American Cancer Society.

Tierney, L. M., McPhee, S. J., Papadakis, M. A., & Schroeder, S. A. (Eds.). (1993). *Current medical diagnosis and treatment*. Norwalk, CT: Appleton & Lange.

Ullrich, S., & Zolla-Pazner, S. (1982). Immunoregulatory circuits in myeloma. *Clinical Hematology, 11*, 87.

Urba, W. J., & Longo, D. L. (1992). Hodgkin's disease. *New England Journal of Medicine, 326*(10), 678-687.

Yarrish, R. L., Wromser, G. P., Bittker, S. J., Aron-Hott, L., Cabello, F., & Huang, E. (1989). The febrile father with a cytomegalovirus infection. *Postgraduate Medicine, 58*, 251-254.

SUGGESTED READINGS

Bell, T. N. (1990). Disseminated intravascular coagulation and shock: Multisystem crisis in the critically ill. *Critical Care Nursing Clinics of North America, 2*, 255-268.

Coffin, A. M. (1989). Potentially catastrophic bleeding disorders. *Postgraduate Medicine, 86*, 217-221, 224-225.

Isbister, J. P., & Pittiglio, D. H. (1988). *Clinical hematology: A problem oriented approach*. Baltimore: Williams & Wilkins.

Kjeldsberg, C., Beutler, E., Bell, C., Hougie, C., Foucar, K., & Savage, R. (1989). *Practical diagnosis of hematologic disorders*. Chicago: ASCP Press.

Lukes, R. J. & Butler, J. J. (1966). The pathology and nomenclature of Hodgkin's disease, *Cancer Research, 26*, 1063-1081.

Simmons, A. (1989). *Hematology: A combined theoretical and technical approach*. Philadelphia: Saunders.

Alterations in Hematologic Function in Children

Margaret M. Andrews

Kathleen Hardin Mooney

Chapter Outline

In this chapter a brief explanation of fetal and neonatal hematopoiesis and postnatal changes in blood is presented as a foundation for understanding the pathophysiology of specific blood disorders in childhood. Among the diseases that affect erythrocytes are acquired disorders such as iron deficiency anemia, hemolytic disease of the newborn, and anemia of infectious disease, and inherited disorders, such as glucose-6-phosphate dehydrogenase deficiency, hereditary spherocytosis, sickle cell disease, and the thalassemias. Disorders of coagulation and platelets include inherited hemorrhagic diseases, such as the hemophilias, and antibody-mediated hemorrhagic diseases, which include idiopathic thrombocytopenic purpura, transient neonatal thrombocytopenias, and autoimmune vascular purpuras. Finally, leukocyte disorders, such as leukemia and the lymphomas (both non-Hodgkin lymphoma and Hodgkin disease) are discussed.

FETAL AND NEONATAL HEMATOPOIESIS

As the developing embryo becomes too large for oxygenation of tissues by simple diffusion, the production of erythrocytes begins within the vessels of the yolk sac. Shortly after 2 weeks' gestation, circulating erythrocytes play a major role in delivering oxygen to the tissues. At approximately the eighth week of gestation, the site of erythrocyte production shifts from the vessels to the liver sinusoids, and the production of leukocytes and platelets begins in the liver and spleen. Erythropoiesis in the liver and, to a lesser extent, in the spleen and lymph nodes reaches a peak at approximately 4 months.

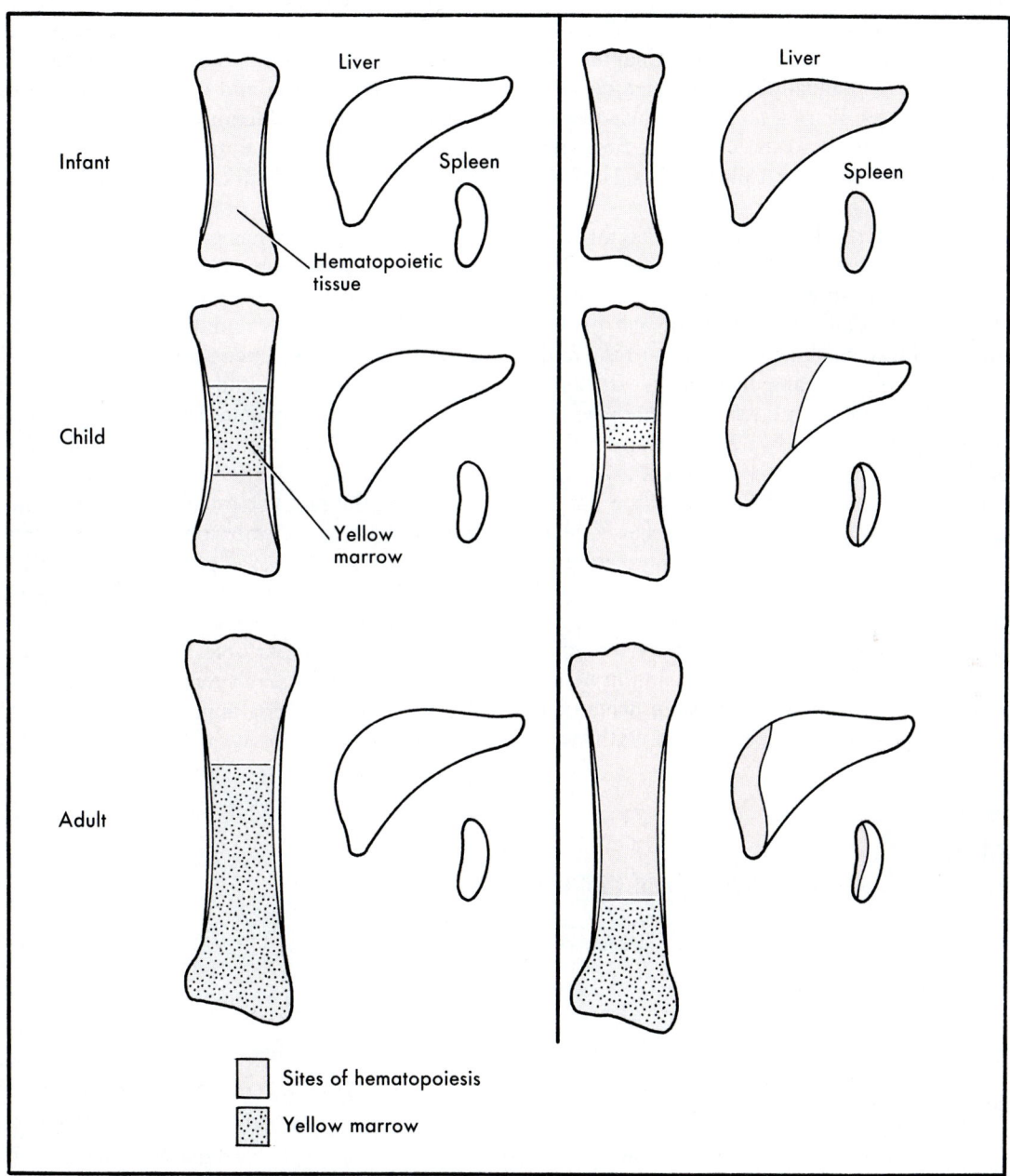

FIG. 25-1 Sites of hematopoiesis in health and illness. With normal maturation, red marrow is partly replaced by yellow marrow in the shafts of the long bones. In adults, red marrow is largely restricted to the proximal ends of the femur and humerus. In response to hemolysis, red marrow replaces yellow marrow in the long bones. In infants, whose long bones are already filled with red marrow, additional hematopoiesis takes place in the liver and spleen. In children and adults, red marrow can replace yellow marrow in response to hemolysis, necessitating less hematopoiesis in the liver and spleen.

Hepatic blood formation declines steadily thereafter but does not disappear entirely during the remainder of gestation. By the fifth month of gestation, hematopoiesis begins to occur in the bone marrow and increases rapidly until hematopoietic (red) marrow fills the entire bone marrow space. By the time of delivery the marrow is the only significant site of hematopoiesis.

In neonates and young infants, hematopoietic marrow progressively fills the bony cavities of the entire axial skeleton (skull, vertebrae, ribs, and sternum), the long bones of the limbs, and many intramembranous bones. (These structures are described in Chapter 38.) Fatty (yellow) marrow gradually replaces hematopoietic marrow in some bones. During childhood, hematopoietic tissue retreats centrally to the vertebrae, ribs, sternum, pelvis, scapulae, skull, and proximal ends of the femur and humerus.

In diseases characterized by hemolysis, erythrocyte production can increase as much as eight times normal because erythropoietin causes hematopoietic marrow to increase in volume. Initially, hematopoietic marrow expands from the ends of the long bones toward the middle of the shafts, replacing fatty marrow. Next, blood cell production begins to occur outside the marrow cavities, especially in the liver and spleen. Extramedullary hematopoiesis is more likely to occur in children than in adults because the bony cavities of children are already filled with red marrow (Fig. 25-1). This is why hemolytic disease causes especially pronounced enlargement of the spleen and liver in children.

The erythrocytes undergo striking changes during gestation, particularly during the first two trimesters, during which they nearly double in numbers and in hemoglobin content. A proportionate increase in hematocrit also occurs. By the end of gestation the erythrocyte count has more than tripled, but the size of each erythrocyte has decreased.

A biochemically distinct type of hemoglobin is synthesized during fetal life. The three **embryonic hemoglobins (Gower 1, Gower 2, and Portland)** and the **fetal hemoglobin (Hb F)** are composed of two alpha and two gamma chains of polypeptides, whereas the adult hemoglobins (Hb A and Hb A$_2$) are composed of two alpha and two beta chains. (The structure of an adult hemoglobin molecule is illustrated in Fig. 22-8, and types of hemoglobin are defined in Table 22-5.) Some unknown regulatory mechanism promotes gamma chain synthesis and inhibits beta and delta chain synthesis in utero. This results in production of embryonic or fetal hemoglobin. After birth, gamma chain synthesis is inhibited, whereas beta and delta chain synthesis is facilitated, resulting in production of adult hemoglobins.

Fetal hemoglobin has greater affinity for oxygen than does adult hemoglobin because it interacts less readily with an enzyme (2,3-diphosphoglycerate) that inhibits hemoglobin-oxygen binding. The decreased inhibitory effects of 2,3-diphosphoglycerate enable fetal blood to transport oxygen despite the relative lack of oxygen in the uterine environment. The increased affinity for oxygen enables Hb F to bind with maternal oxygen in the placental circulation.

During the first trimester, nearly all of the hemoglobin in the fetus is embryonic, but some Hb A can be detected. Therefore it is possible to identify as early as 16 to 20 weeks' gestation some disorders of adult hemoglobin, such as sickle cell anemia and thalassemia major. In the 6-month-old fetus, Hb F constitutes 90% of the total. This percentage then begins to decline. At birth, neonatal hemoglobin consists of 70% Hb F, 29% Hb A, and 1% Hb A$_2$. Between 6 and 12 months of

---

TABLE 25-1

Hematologic Values During Infancy and Childhood

Age	Hemoglobin (g/dl)		Hematocrit (%)		Reticulocytes (%)	Leukocytes (WBC/mm^3)	
	Mean	Range	Mean	Range	Mean	Mean	Range
Cord blood	16.8	13.7-20.1	55	45-65	5.0	18,000	(9-30,000)
2 wk	16.5	13.0-20.0	50	42-66	1.0	12,000	(5-21,000)
3 mo	12.0	9.5-14.5	36	31-41	1.0	12,000	(6-18,000)
6 mo-6 yr	12.0	10.5-14.0	37	33-42	1.0	10,000	(6-15,000)
7-12 yr	13.0	11.0-16.0	38	34-40	1.0	8000	(4500-13,500)
Adult							
Female	14	12.0-16.0	42	37-47	1.6	7500	(5-10,000)
Male	16	14.0-18.0	47	42-52			

Modified from Behrman & Vaughan, 1992.
*Relatively wide range.

age, normal adult hemoglobin percentages are established (see Chapter 22).

POSTNATAL CHANGES IN THE BLOOD

Blood cell counts tend to rise above adult levels at birth, then decline gradually throughout childhood. Table 25-1 lists normal ranges during infancy and childhood. The immediate rise in values is the result of accelerated hematopoiesis during fetal life, increased numbers of cells that result from the trauma of birth, and cutting of the umbilical cord. These events surrounding the birth also are accompanied by a "shift to the left," that is, the presence of large numbers of immature erythrocytes and leukocytes (particularly granulocytes) in peripheral blood (see Chapter 24). The shift to the left disappears as the infant develops, usually within the first 2 to 3 months of life. Other unique postnatal characteristics, particularly of lymphocytes, may be caused by exogenous factors, such as viral infections.

Average blood volume in the full-term neonate is 85 ml/kg of body weight. The premature infant has a slightly larger average blood volume of 90 ml/kg of body weight, with the mean increasing to 150 mg/kg during the first few days after birth. In both full-term and premature infants, blood volume decreases during the first few months. Thereafter the average blood volume is 75 to 77 ml/kg, which is similar to that of older children and adults.

Erythrocytes

The hypoxic intrauterine environment stimulates erythropoietin production in the fetus. This accelerates fetal erythropoiesis, producing polycythemia (excessive proliferation of erythrocyte precursers) of the newborn. After birth the oxygen from the lungs saturates arterial blood, and the amount of oxygen delivered to the tissues increases. In response to the change from a placental to a pulmonary oxygen supply during the first few days of life, levels of erythropoietin and the rate of blood cell formation decrease. The very active rate of fetal erythropoiesis is reflected by the large numbers of immature erythrocytes (reticulocytes) in the peripheral blood of full-term neonates. After birth the number of reticulocytes decreases about 50% every 12 hours so that it is rare to find an elevated reticulocyte count after the first week of life. A decrease in extramedullary hematopoiesis also occurs at this time. In the peripheral blood the erythrocyte count drops for 6 to 8 weeks after birth. During this period of rapid growth the rate of erythrocyte destruction is greater than that in later childhood and adulthood. In full-term infants, normal erythrocyte life span is 60 to 80 days; in premature infants it may be as short as 20 to 30 days; and in children and adolescents it is the same as that in adults— 120 days. (Mechanisms of hemolysis are described in Chapter 22.)

In the premature infant the postnatal fall in hemoglobin and hematocrit values is more marked than in the full-term infant. In the preschool and school-age child, there is a gradual rise in hemoglobin, hematocrit, and red blood cell count. Values in males and females first begin to diverge in adolescence. In the female the gradual hemoglobin increase continues into early puberty, at which time it stabilizes. In the male the hemoglobin increase keeps pace with growth and maturation and eventually surpasses that of the female. This higher value in the mature male is related to androgen secretion.

| Neutrophils (%) | | Differential counts | | | | Platelets |
Mean	Range	Lymphocytes (%) Mean*	Eosinophils (%) Mean	Monocytes (%) Mean	Nucleated red cells (100 WBC)	(/mm³)
					7.0	84-478 × 10³
61	(40-80)	31	2	6	(3-10)	
40		48	3	9	0	
30		63	2	5	0	
45		48	2	5	0	
55		38	2	5	0	
55	(35-70)	35	3	7	0	150-400 × 10⁶
						150-400 × 10⁶

Metabolic processes within the erythrocytes of neonates differ significantly from those of erythrocytes in the normal adult. The relatively young population of erythrocytes in the newborn consumes greater quantities of glucose than do erythrocytes in adults. Several enzymes that regulate glucose consumption are increased in the erythrocytes of neonates, with a subsequent increase in the rate of glycolysis.

Leukocytes and Platelets

The lymphocytes of children tend to have more cytoplasm and less compact nuclear chromatin than do the lymphocytes of adults. The significance of these differences is unknown. One possible explanation is that children tend to have more frequent viral infections, which are associated with atypical lymphocytes. Even minor infections, in which the child fails to exhibit clinical manifestations of illness, and administration of immunizations may result in lymphocyte changes (Mauer, 1969).

The lymphocyte count is high at birth and continues to rise in some healthy infants during the first year of life. Then a steady decline occurs throughout childhood and adolescence until lower adult values are reached. It is unknown whether these developmental variations are physiologic or are a pathologic response to frequent viral infections and immunizations in children.

At birth, the neutrophil count is very high and rises during the early days of life (Manroe, Weinberg, Roenfeld, & Browne, 1979). After 2 weeks, neutrophil counts fall to within or below normal adult ranges. By approximately 4 years of age the neutrophil count is the same as that of an adult. White children have slightly higher counts than black children (Caramihai, Karayaclin, Aballi, & Lanzkowsky, 1975).

Eosinophil count is high in the first year of life and is higher in children than in teen-agers or adults (Cunningham, 1975). Monocyte counts are high in the first year of life and then decrease to adult levels. No relationship between age and basophil count has been found.

Platelet counts in full-term neonates are comparable to platelet counts in adults and remain so throughout infancy and childhood (Albin, Kushner, Murphy, & Zippin, 1961). Controversy exists as to whether premature infants tend to have thrombocytopenia.

DISORDERS OF ERYTHROCYTES

Anemia is the most common blood disorder in children. Like the anemias of adulthood the anemias of childhood are caused by ineffective erythropoiesis or premature destruction of erythrocytes. The most common cause of insufficient erythropoiesis is iron deficiency, which may result from insufficient dietary intake or chronic loss of iron caused by bleeding. The hemolytic anemias of childhood may be divided into two large categories. The first consists of disorders that result from premature destruction caused by intrinsic abnormalities of the erythrocytes, whereas the second consists of disorders that result from damaging extraerythrocytic factors. The hemolytic anemias tend to be inherited (because of a genetic anomaly) or congenital (acquired or manifested before birth), or both.

The most dramatic form of acquired congenital hemolytic anemia is **hemolytic disease in the newborn (HDN),** also termed **erythroblastosis fetalis**. HDN is an isoimmune disease in which maternal blood and fetal blood are antigenically incompatible, causing the mother's immune system to produce antibodies against fetal erythrocytes. Fetal erythrocytes that have been attacked by (i.e., bound to) maternal antibodies are recognized as foreign or defective by the fetal mononuclear phagocyte system and are removed from the circulation by phagocytosis, usually in the fetal spleen. (For a complete discussion on HDN, see p. 914.) Other acquired hemolytic anemias—some of which begin in utero—include those caused by infections or the presence of toxic chemicals.

The inherited forms of hemolytic anemia result from intrinsic defects of the child's erythrocytes, any of which can lead to erythrocyte removal by the mononuclear phagocyte system. Structural defects include abnormal cellular size or shape and abnormalities of plasma membrane structure (spherocytosis). Intracellular defects include enzyme deficiencies, the most common of which is **glucose-6-phosphate dehydrogenase (G6PD) deficiency,** and defects of hemoglobin synthesis, which manifest as sickle cell disease or thalassemia, depending on which component of hemoglobin is defective. These and other causes of childhood anemia, some more common than others, are listed in Table 25-2.

Acquired Disorders
Iron Deficiency Anemia

Iron deficiency anemia is the most frequent blood disorder of infancy and childhood, with the highest incidence occurring between 6 months and 2 years of age. Incidence is not related to sex or race, but socioeconomic factors are important because they affect nutrition. Recent studies document the risk of iron deficiency anemia in children of single, homeless women (Drake, 1992). Iron deficiency anemia is a common disorder in children because of their extremely high need for normal growth to occur.

Between 4 years of age and the onset of puberty, dietary iron deficiency is uncommon. During adolescence, however, it is relatively common, especially in menstruating females. Rapid growth, together with the average teen-ager's dietary habits, causes iron depletion to oc-

TABLE 25-2

Anemias of Childhood

Cause	Anemic condition
Deficient erythropoiesis or hemoglobin synthesis	
Decreased stem cell population in marrow (congenital or acquired pure red cell aplasia)	Normocytic-normochromic anemia
Decreased erythropoiesis despite normal stem cell population in marrow (infection, inflammation, cancer, chronic renal disease, congenital dyserythropoiesis)	Normocytic-normochromic anemia
Deficiency of a factor or nutrient needed for erythropoiesis	
Cobalamin (vitamin B_{12}), folate	Megaloblastic anemia
Iron	Microcytic-hypochromic anemia
Increased or premature hemolysis	
Isoimmune disease (maternal-fetal Rh, ABO, or minor blood group incompatibility)	Hemolytic disease of the newborn (HDN)
Autoimmune disease (idiopathic autoimmune hemolytic anemia, symptomatic systemic lupus erythematosus, lymphoma, drug-induced autoimmune processes)	Autoimmune hemolytic anemia
Inherited defects of plasma membrane structure (spherocytosis, elliptocytosis, stomatocytosis) or cellular size, or both (pyknocytosis)	Hemolytic anemia
Infection (bacterial sepsis, congenital syphilis, malaria, cytomegalovirus infection, rubella, toxoplasmosis, disseminated herpes)	Hemolytic anemia
Intrinsic and inherited enzymatic defects (deficiencies of glucose-6-phosphate dehydrogenase [G-6-PD], pyruvate kinase, 5′-nucleotidase, glucose phosphate isomerase)	Hemolytic anemia
Inherited defects of hemoglobin synthesis	Sickle cell anemia; Thalassemia
Disseminated intravascular coagulation (see Chapter 24)	Hemolytic anemia
Galactosemia	Hemolytic anemia
Prolonged or recurrent respiratory or metabolic acidosis	Hemolytic anemia
Blood vessel disorders (cavernous hemangioma, large vessel thrombus, renal artery stenosis, severe coarctation of the aorta) (see Chapter 28)	Hemolytic anemia

cur readily. (Mechanisms of iron depletion are described in Chapter 22.)

Pathophysiology

Although inadequate intake of iron is the most common cause of iron deficiency anemia during the first few years of life and during adolescence, blood loss is the most frequent cause in childhood. Chronic iron deficiency anemia from occult ("hidden") blood loss may be caused by a gastrointestinal lesion, parasitic infestation, or hemorrhagic disease. As many as one third of infants with severe iron deficiency anemia have chronic intestinal blood loss induced by exposure to a heat-labile protein in cow's milk. Such exposure causes an inflamma-

tory gastrointestinal reaction that damages the mucosa and results in diffuse hemorrhage.

The amount of iron available for hemoglobin synthesis in the infant depends on iron stores present at birth, rate of growth, the amount of dietary iron absorbed, and physiologic or pathologic loss of iron. During the period of inactive erythropoiesis immediately after birth, iron from erythrocytes that die at the end of their normal life span is stored, as hemosiderin, in bone marrow and liver tissue. This creates an iron reserve that can be used in lieu of dietary intake. The greatest stores are present 4 to 8 weeks after birth. Until erythropoiesis resumes, these iron stores are mobilized. In the premature infant, resumption of erythropoiesis depletes iron stores within 6 to 12 weeks; in the full-term infant, depletion takes longer— about 16 to 20 weeks. Once iron stores have been used, the infant depends on dietary iron.

The amount of dietary iron available for erythropoiesis depends on which foods are consumed. Iron-fortified cereals, green and yellow vegetables, fruits, and milk are common in the average 6-month-old infant's diet and provide iron in the amount of 0.9 to 1.5 mg/kg/day, amounts that satisfy the normal average daily requirement. Iron-fortified formulas are commercially available and are being used with increasing frequency.

Clinical Manifestations

The symptoms of mild anemia—lethargy and lassitude—are usually not present or detectable in infants and young children, who are unable to describe these symptoms. Therefore parents usually do not notice any change in the child's behavior or appearance until moderate anemia has developed. General irritability, decreased activity tolerance, weakness, and lack of interest in play are nonspecific indications of anemia. In mild to moderate iron deficiency anemia (Hb 6 to 10 g/dl), compensatory mechanisms of tissue oxygenation, such as increased amounts of 2,3-DPG within erythrocytes and a shift of the oxyhemoglobin dissociation curve, may be so effective that few clinical manifestations are apparent. When the hemoglobin determination falls below 5 g/dl, however, pallor, anorexia, tachycardia, and systolic murmurs may occur.

Splenomegaly is evident in 10% to 15% of children with iron deficiency anemia and, if the condition is long-standing, the sutures of the skull may be widened. Chronic anemia also may result in decreased physical growth and developmental delays. Some children exhibit pica, a behavior in which nonfood substances are eaten. Because children with iron deficiency anemia may be obese, underweight, or of normal weight, other manifestations of undernutrition must be identified.

Iron deficiency anemia may affect neurologic and intellectual function. Some research findings indicate that low iron in the blood affects attention span, alertness, and learning ability, even when anemia is not severe (Prasad & Prasad, 1991).

Evaluation and Treatment

The most definitive test for differentiating iron deficiency from other microcytic states is the absence of iron stores in the bone marrow. However, measurement of serum ferritin iron concentration, transferrin saturation, iron-binding capacity, and, more recently, serum transferrin receptors may prevent proceeding to actual bone marrow evaluation (Massey, 1992). Evaluation and treatment of iron deficiency anemia in children are sim-

ilar to those in adults (see Chapter 23). Oral administration of simple ferrous salts usually is satisfactory, but additional vitamin C may be needed to promote absorption because vitamin C must be present in adequate amounts. Administration of supplementary trace metals or other vitamins is not necessary. If malabsorption is the cause of the anemia (or if oral administration has not been successful), iron dextran (Inferon) is given intravenously. Iron therapy continues for 4 to 6 weeks after erythrocyte indexes have returned to normal.

Dietary modification is required to prevent recurrences of iron deficiency anemia. The child's intake of iron-rich foods is increased, and the intake of cow's milk may be restricted, with the exact amount depending on the child's age (from 1 pint to 32 ounces). Limiting milk intake makes the child hungrier for other iron-rich foods and prevents gastrointestinal blood loss in children whose anemia is aggravated or caused by inflammatory reactions to proteins in cow's milk.

Hemolytic Disease in the Newborn

HDN can occur only if antigens on fetal erythrocytes differ from antigens on maternal erythrocytes. The antigenic properties of erythrocytes are determined genetically: they may be type A, B, or O and may or may not include Rh antigen D. Erythrocytes that express Rh antigen D are Rh-positive; those that do not are Rh-negative. Maternal-fetal incompatibility exists if mother and fetus differ in ABO blood type or if the fetus is Rh-positive and the mother is Rh-negative. (The antigenic properties of erythrocytes are described in Chapter 6.)

ABO incompatibility occurs in about 20% to 25% of all pregnancies, but only one in 10 cases of ABO incompatibility results in HDN. Rh incompatibility occurs in fewer than 10% of pregnancies and rarely causes HDN in the first incompatible fetus. Even after five or more pregnancies, only 5% of women have babies with hemolytic disease. Usually erythrocytes from the first incompatible fetus cause the mother's immune system to produce antibodies that affect the fetuses of subsequent incompatible pregnancies. Only one in three cases of HDN is due to Rh incompatibility; most cases are caused by ABO incompatibility.

Pathophysiology

Given that the mother and fetus have antigenically incompatible erythrocytes, HDN will result (1) if the mother's blood contains preformed antibodies against fetal erythrocytes or produces them on exposure to fetal erythrocytes, (2) if sufficient amounts of antibody (usually IgG) cross the placenta and enter fetal blood, and (3) if IgG binds with sufficient numbers of fetal erythrocytes to cause widespread antibody-mediated hemolysis or splenic removal. (Antibody-mediated cellular destruction is described in Chapter 6.)

Maternal antibodies may be formed against type B erythrocytes if the mother is type A or against type A if the mother is type B. Usually, however, the mother is type O and the fetus is A or B. ABO incompatibility can cause HDN even if fetal erythrocytes do not escape into the maternal circulation during pregnancy. This occurs because the blood of most adults already contains anti-A or anti-B antibodies, which are produced on exposure to certain foods or infection by gram-negative bacteria. (Anti-O antibodies do not exist because type O erythrocytes are not antigenic.) Therefore IgG against type A or B erythrocytes usually is preformed in maternal blood and can enter the fetal circulation throughout the first incompatible pregnancy.

Anti-Rh antibodies, on the other hand, are *only* formed in response to the presence of incompatible (Rh-positive) erythrocytes in the blood of an Rh-negative mother. Sources of exposure include fetal blood that is mixed with the mother's blood at the time of delivery, transfused blood, and, rarely, previous sensitization of the mother by her own mother's incompatible blood.

The first Rh-incompatible pregnancy usually presents no difficulties because very few fetal erythrocytes cross the placental barrier during gestation. When the placenta detaches at birth, however, a large number of fetal erythrocytes usually enter the mother's bloodstream. If the mother is Rh-negative and the fetus is Rh-positive, the mother produces anti-Rh antibodies. The capacity of the mother's immune system to produce anti-Rh antibodies depends on many factors, including her genetic capacity to make antibodies against the Rh antigen D, the amount of fetal-to-maternal bleeding, and the occurrence of any bleeding earlier in the pregnancy. Anti-Rh antibodies persist in the bloodstream for a very long time, and if the next offspring is Rh-positive, the mother's anti-Rh antibodies can enter the fetus's bloodstream and destroy the erythrocytes. Antibodies against Rh antigen D are of the IgG class and easily cross the placenta.

IgG-coated fetal erythrocytes are destroyed extravascularly, primarily by mononuclear phagocytoses in the spleen. As hemolysis proceeds, the fetus becomes anemic. Erythropoiesis accelerates, particularly in the liver and spleen, and immature nucleated cells (erythroblasts) are released into the bloodstream. (This phenomenon is responsible for the other name of HDN, erythroblastosis fetalis). The degree of anemia depends on the length of time the antibody has been in the fetal circulation, antibody concentration, and the ability of the fetus to compensate for increased hemolysis. Unconjugated (indirect) bilirubin, which is formed during catabolism (breakdown) of hemoglobin, is transported across the placental barrier into the maternal circulation and is ex-

creted by the mother. **Hyperbilirubinemia** occurs in the neonate after birth because excretion of lipid-soluble unconjugated bilirubin through the placenta no longer is possible.

The pathophysiologic effects of HDN are more severe in Rh incompatibility than in ABO incompatibility. ABO incompatibility may resolve after birth without life-threatening complications. Maternal-fetal incompatibility in which a mother with type O blood has a child with type A or B blood usually is so mild that it does not require treatment.

Rh incompatibility is more likely than ABO incompatibility to cause severe or even life-threatening anemia, death in utero, or damage to the central nervous system. Severe anemia alone can cause death as a result of cardiovascular complications (see Chapter 23). Extensive hemolysis also results in increased levels of unconjugated bilirubin in the neonate's circulation. If bilirubin levels exceed the liver's ability to conjugate and excrete bilirubin, some of it is deposited in the brain, causing cellular damage and eventually, if the neonate does not receive exchange transfusions, death.

Fetuses that do not survive anemia in utero usually are stillborn, with gross edema in the entire body, a condition called **hydrops fetalis**. Death can occur as early as 17 weeks' gestation and results in spontaneous abortion.

Clinical Manifestations

A wide spectrum of hemolytic disease occurs in affected infants born to sensitized mothers. Neonates with mild HDN may appear healthy or slightly pale, with slight enlargement of the liver or spleen. Pronounced pallor, splenomegaly, and hepatomegaly indicate severe anemia, which predisposes the neonate to cardiovascular failure and shock.

Because the maternal antibodies remain in the neonate's circulatory system after birth, erythrocyte destruction can continue. This causes hyperbilirubinemia and **icterus neonatorum (neonatal jaundice)** shortly after birth. Without replacement transfusions, in which the child receives Rh-negative erythrocytes, the bilirubin is deposited in the brain, a condition termed **kernicterus**. Kernicterus produces cerebral damage and usually causes death (**icterus gravis neonatorum**). Infants who do not die may have mental retardation, cerebral palsy, or high-frequency deafness.

Evaluation and Treatment

Routine evaluation of fetuses at risk for HDN (i.e., fetuses resulting from Rh- or ABO-incompatible matings) includes the Coombs' test. The indirect Coombs' test measures antibody in the mother's circulation and indicates if the fetus is at risk for HDN. The direct Coombs'

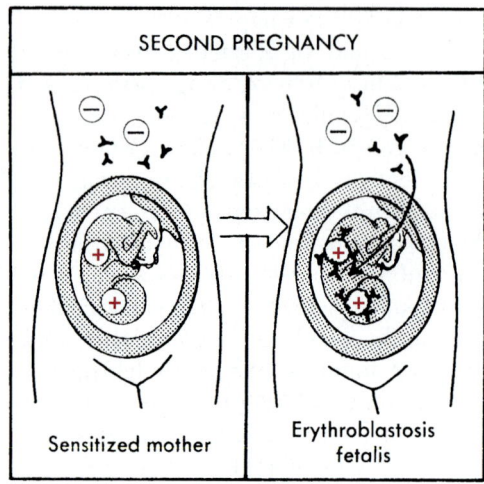

FIG. 25-2 Occurrence and prevention of hemolytic disease in the newborn caused by Rh incompatibility. (See text for explanation.)

test measures antibody already bound to the surfaces of fetal erythrocytes and is used primarily to confirm the diagnosis of antibody-mediated HDN. A recent advancement in the early diagnosis of HDN is the access to the fetal circulation directly through intravenous umbilical cord sampling.

The key to treatment of HDN resulting from Rh-incompatibility lies in prevention (immunoprophylaxis). One of the success stories of immunology has been the spectacular results obtained through the use of Rh immune globulin (RhoGAM), a preparation of antibody against Rh antigen D. If an Rh-negative woman is given Rh immune globulin within 72 hours of exposure to Rh-positive erythrocytes, she will not produce antibody against the D antigen, and the next Rh-positive baby will be protected (Fig. 25-2). Apparently the injected antibodies remain in the mother's bloodstream long enough to prevent her immune system from producing its own anti-Rh antibodies, but not long enough to affect subsequent offspring. The mother must be given Rh immune globulin injections after the birth of each Rh-positive baby and with any abortion. Also, the mother must be especially careful not to receive a transfusion containing Rh-positive blood, because this also would stimulate production of anti-Rh antibodies. In many hospitals, Rh immune globulin is given prophylactically at 28 weeks to all pregnant Rh-negative women with Rh-positive partners. Immunoprophylaxis with Rh immune globulin, unfortunately, appears to be underutilized in the United States. Failure to use immunoprophylaxis, such as in cases of unrecognized abortion, has led to a small increase in mothers who will require comprehensive treatment during subsequent pregnancies (Gibble & Ness, 1992).

If antigenic incompatibility of the parents' erythrocytes is not discovered in time to administer prophylac-

tic immune globulin (RhoGAM) and a child is born with HDN, treatment consists of exchange transfusions in which the neonate's blood is replaced with new Rh-positive blood that is not contaminated with anti-Rh antibodies. This treatment is instituted during the first 24 hours of extrauterine life to prevent kernicterus. Phototherapy also is used to reduce the toxic effects of unconjugated bilirubin.

Jaundice and indirect hyperbilirubinemia are reduced when the infant is exposed to a high intensity of light in the visible spectrum, the most effective being the blue range (from 420 to 470 nm). Bilirubin in the skin absorbs light energy which, by photoisomerization, converts the toxic unconjugated bilirubin into conjugated isomers that are excreted in the bile. Phototherapy also causes autosensitization that results in oxidation reactions. Breakdown products from the oxidation reactions are excreted by the liver and kidney without need for conjugation. The therapeutic effect of phototherapy depends on the light energy emitted in the effective wavelengths, the distance between the infant and the light source, and the amount of skin exposed; the rate of hemolysis and the infant's ability to excrete bilirubin also are factors in determining the effectiveness of phototherapy in lowering serum bilirubin levels.

Anemia of Infectious Disease

Infections of the newborn, often initially acquired by the mother and transmitted to the fetus, may result in a hemolytic anemia with clinical manifestations similar to those of HDN. Congenital syphilis, toxoplasmosis, cytomegalic inclusion disease, rubella, coxsackievirus B infection, herpes virus infection, and bacterial sepsis can all cause hemolytic anemia in the neonate.

The exact mechanism of anemia caused by congenital infections is unclear. In some instances it is related to direct injury of erythrocyte membranes or erythrocyte precursors by the infectious organism. In other instances it results from traumatic destruction of erythrocytes during their passage through inflamed capillaries.

Inherited Disorders

A number of inherited and intrinsic erythrocyte defects are known to cause increased hemolysis (see Table 25-2). These defects may be associated with enzymatic abnormalities that disrupt metabolic processes and prevent normal biochemical balance within the cell, with alterations of hemoglobin structure or synthesis, or with plasma membrane defects accompanied by changes in erythrocyte size or shape.

Glucose-6-Phosphate Dehydrogenase Deficiency

G6PD deficiency is an inherited, X-linked, recessive disorder, most fully expressed in homozygous males, although partial expression (and a carrier state) is possible in heterozygous females. (X-linked inheritance is discussed in Chapter 5.) The deficiency is present in 10% of African Americans and also tends to occur in Sephardic Jews, Greeks, Iranians, Chinese, Filipinos, and Indonesians, with a frequency ranging from 5% to 40%.

Pathophysiology

G6PD is an enzyme that normally enables erythrocytes to maintain metabolic processes despite injurious conditions, such as the presence of certain drugs (sulfonamides, antimalarial agents, salicylates, or naphthaquinolones); ingestion of fava beans (a dietary staple in some Mediterranean areas); hypoxemia; or acidosis. Therefore G6PD deficiency is usually asymptomatic unless one of these stressors is present. Erythrocyte damage in affected children begins after intense or prolonged exposure to one of these substances or conditions, and it ceases when they are removed. In African-American males the G6PD defect becomes more pronounced as the erythrocyte ages; in other populations the defect is profound even in young erythrocytes. By ingesting a substance with oxidant properties, such as a salicylate (aspirin), a pregnant woman may precipitate an episode of hemolysis in a fetus with G6PD deficiency.

In the absence of G6PD, oxidative stressors damage hemoglobin and the plasma membranes of erythrocytes, and they possibly interfere with the activities of other enzymes within the cell. Hemoglobin is oxidized progressively to methemoglobin, sulfmethemoglobin, and denatured globin-glutathione complexes. Eventually, exposure to oxidizing substances results in the precipitation of insoluble hemoglobin inclusions, called *Heinz bodies,* within the cell. Plasma damage and the presence of Heinz bodies cause hemolysis, chiefly in the spleen.

Clinical Manifestations

In Oriental and Mediterranean infants, G6PD deficiency is likely to be associated with icterus neonatorum. The most common clinical manifestation of G6PD deficiency is acute hemolytic anemia, usually after infections or the ingestion of certain oxidative drugs. The fava bean produces a severe hemolytic reaction called *favism* in infants with G6PD deficiency.

Hemolytic episodes are characterized by pallor, icterus, dark urine, back pain, and, in severe cases, shock, cardiovascular collapse, and death. Between hemolytic episodes, anemia is absent and erythrocyte survival is normal.

Evaluation and Treatment

Direct or indirect demonstration of reduced G6PD activity in erythrocytes is required for evaluation. Satisfactory screening test results are based on discoloration of methylene blue and on reduction of methemoglobin. Immediately after a hemolytic episode, reticulocytes and young erythrocytes predominate. Because young erythrocytes have significantly higher enzyme activity than do older cells, testing should be performed a few weeks after a crisis so that a low level of enzyme activity can be demonstrated. G6PD activity that is within the low normal range in the presence of a high reticulocyte count suggests G6PD deficiency. The disorder G6PD also can be detected by electrophoretic analysis.

Prevention of hemolysis is the most important therapeutic measure. Males belonging to high-risk groups (Greeks, Southern Italians, Sephardic Jews, Filipinos, Chinese, Africans, and Thais) should be tested for the defect before being given drugs known to be oxidant. When hemolysis has occurred, supportive treatment may include blood transfusions and oral iron therapy. Spontaneous recovery generally follows treatment.

Hereditary Spherocytosis

Hereditary spherocytosis, also known as congenital hemolytic anemia or congenital acholuric jaundice, is the most common of the hemolytic disorders in which there is no abnormality of hemoglobin.

Pathophysiology

Transmitted as an autosomal dominant trait, hereditary spherocytosis is presumed to represent new mutations in about 25% of cases. The defect is believed to be caused by an undefined abnormality of proteins or spectrins of the erythrocyte membrane. Affected cells are unduly permeable to sodium and acquire a particular characteristic structure (Fig. 25-3). An increased concentration of intracellular sodium is believed to lead to increased use of adenosine triphosphate (ATP) to drive the so-called cation pump. Early aging and destruction of erythrocytes are believed to result from metabolic over-

FIG. 25-3 **The microspherocyte.** **A,** Blood smear from patient with hereditary spherocytosis. (Wright's stain.) **B,** Scanning electron microscope photograph. (Courtesy Dr. M. Bessis; from Miale, 1982.)

Normal

| Valine | Histidine | Leucine | Threonine | Proline | Glutamic acid | Glutamic acid |

Sickle cell anemia

| Valine | Histidine | Leucine | Threonine | Proline | Valine | Glutamic acid |

First seven amino acids in normal and sickle cell hemoglobin

Valine

Valine

Structure of sickle-cell hemoglobin

Sickle fibers

Normal red blood cell   Formation of sickled red blood cell   Sickled red blood cell

FIG. 25-4 **Sickle cell hemoglobin.** Sickle cell hemoglobin is produced by a recessive allele of the gene encoding the beta chain of hemoglobin. It represents a single amino acid change from glutamic acid to valine at the sixth position in the chain. In the folded beta chain molecule the sixth position contacts the alpha chain, and the amino acid change causes the hemoglobins to aggregate into long chains, altering the shape of the cell. (From Raven & Johnson, 1992.)

work and loss of erythrocyte membrane (Delauney, Aloisio, Morle, & Baklouti, 1991).

Circulation of blood to the spleen creates a metabolic environment that is stressful to spherocyte cells, and repeated passages through this stressful environment result in their sequestration and destruction. The spherocyte is relatively rigid and passes with difficulty through the small openings between the splenic cords and sinuses. Thus the spleen is intimately involved in the hemolytic process.

Clinical Manifestations

With onset in the neonatal period or in early infancy, anemia and hyperbilirubinemia are severe enough to require phototherapy or exchange transfusions. During infancy and childhood, severity of the anemia varies widely but tends to be similar within families. Slight jaundice usually is present. Moderate expansion of the marrow cavity of the skull may occur because of compensatory mechanisms to overproduce cells. After infancy, the spleen almost always is enlarged. Although gallstones have been reported to occur as early as 4 to 5 years of age, they usually do not develop until late childhood or early adolescence. If the spleen is not surgically removed, gallstones will form in approximately one half of cases. Aplastic crises are the most serious complication occurring during childhood (Behrman, Kliegmann, Nelson, & Vaughan, 1992).

Evaluation and Treatment

It is important to evaluate the family history, blood smear, and studies of osmotic fragility and autohemolysis. As yet, however, there is no single test specific for the diagnosis of hereditary spherocytosis (Armbrust,

Eber, & Schroter, 1992). Surgical removal of the spleen invariably produces a clinical cure and should be performed when the child is 5 to 6 years of age or older.

Sickle Cell Disease

Sickle cell disease is a group of disorders characterized by the presence of an abnormal form of hemoglobin—**hemoglobin S (Hb S)** within the erythrocytes. Hb S is formed by a genetic mutation in which one amino acid (valine) replaces another (glutamic acid) (Fig. 25-4). Hb S, the so-called sickle hemoglobin, reacts to deoxygenation and dehydration by solidifying and stretching the erythrocyte into an elongated sickle shape. This change has a variety of pathologic consequences, including hemolytic anemia.

Sickle cell disease is an inherited, autosomal recessive disorder that is expressed as sickle cell anemia, sickle cell–thalassemia disease, or sickle cell–hemoglobin C disease, depending on mode of inheritance (Table 25-3). (See Chapter 4 for a discussion of genetic inheritance of disease.) **Sickle cell anemia,** a homozygous form, is the most severe. **Sickle cell–thalassemia** and **sickle cell–Hb C disease** are heterozygous forms in which the child simultaneously inherits another type of abnormal hemoglobin from one parent. **Sickle cell trait,** in which the child inherits Hb S from one parent and normal hemoglobin (Hb A) from the other, is a heterozygous carrier state that rarely has clinical manifestations. Because the child has more than 50% Hb S, clinical manifestations occur only with extreme stress. All forms of sickle cell disease are lifelong conditions and have no known cure.

Sickle cell disease tends to occur in persons with origins in equatorial countries, particularly central Africa,

---

TABLE 25-3

Inheritance of Sickle Cell Disease

Hemoglobin inherited from first parent	Hemoglobin inherited from second parent	Form of sickle cell disease in child
Hb S (an abnormal hemoglobin)	Hb S	Sickle cell anemia: homozygous inheritance in which the child's hemoglobin is mostly Hb S, with the remainder Hb F (fetal hemoglobin)
Hb S	Defective or insufficient alpha or beta chains of Hb A (alpha- or beta-thalassemia)	Sickle cell: thalassemia disease (heterozygous inheritance of Hb S and alpha- or beta-thalassemia)
Hb S	Hb C or D (both abnormal hemoglobins)	Sickle cell: hemoglobin C (or D) disease (heterozygous inheritance of hemoglobin S and either C or D)
Hb S	Normal hemoglobins (mostly Hb A)	Sickle cell trait, the carrier state (heterozygous inheritance of Hb S and normal hemoglobin)

NOTE: See Chapter 22 for a description of normal fetal and adult hemoglobins.

FIG. 25-5 **Sickle cell anemia.** A, A sickled cell. B, Peripheral blood smear in sickle cell anemia. (Courtesy Dr. M. Bessis. From Miale, 1982.)

FIG. 25-6 **Normal and sickle-shaped blood cells.** Scanning electron micrograph of normal and sickle-shaped red blood cells. The irregularly shaped cells are the sickle cells; the circular cells are the normal blood cells. (From Raven & Johnson, 1992.)

the Near East, the Mediterranean area, and parts of India. In the United States, sickle cell disease is most common in African Americans, with a reported incidence ranging from 1:400 to 1:500 live births. In the general population the risk of two African-American parents having a child with sickle cell anemia is 0.7%. Sickle cell hemoglobin C disease is less common (1 in 800 births), and sickle cell–thalassemia occurs in 1 in 1700 births.

Sickle cell trait occurs in 7% to 13% of African Americans, whereas its incidence among East Africans may be as high as 45%. The sickle cell trait may provide protection against lethal forms of malaria. This would be a genetic advantage to carriers who reside in endemic regions for malaria (Mediterranean and African zones) but is of no advantage to carriers living in the United States.

Pathophysiology

Deoxygenation is probably the most important variable in determining the occurrence of sickling (Steingart, 1992). The degree of deoxygenation required to produce sickling varies with the percentage of Hb S in the cells. Sickle-trait cells will sickle at oxygen tensions of about 15 mm Hg, whereas those from an individual with sickle cell disease will begin to sickle at about 40 mm Hg. Hb S that is not bound with oxygen forms aggregates of semisolid gel that become stacked within the erythrocyte, stretching it into an elongated crescent (Figs. 25-5 and 25-6). Sickled erythrocytes are stiff and cannot change shape as easily as normal cells when they pass through the microcirculation. (The reversible deformability of erythrocytes is described in Chapter 22.) As a result, sickled erythrocytes tend to plug the blood vessels, causing vascular occlusion, pain, and organ infarction. Sickled cells undergo hemolysis in the spleen or become sequestered there, causing blood pooling and infarction of splenic vessels. The anemia that follows triggers erythropoiesis in the marrow and, in extreme cases, in the liver.

Sickling usually is not permanent; most sickled erythrocytes regain a normal shape after reoxygenation and rehydration. Some cells, however, do become irreversibly sickled despite treatment. Irreversible sickling is not caused by irreversible hemoglobin changes but rather by irreversible plasma membrane damage caused by sickling. The precise nature of the permanent membrane injury is not known, but it is known that, while in tne sickled state, the plasma membrane loses some of its capacity for active transport, permitting an influx of calcium ions. (Membrane transport and the effects of calcium influx are described in Unit I.) In persons with sickle cell anemia, in which the erythrocytes contain a high percentage of Hb S (75% to 95%), up to 30% of the erythrocytes can become irreversibly sickled. Occasionally, irreversible sickling occurs in sickle cell disease but never in the carrier state (sickle cell trait).

Sickling is an occasional, intermittent phenomenon that can be triggered or sustained by one or more of the following stressors: decreased oxygen tension (PO_2) of the blood (i.e., hypoxemia), increased hydrogen ion concentration in the blood (decreased pH), increased plasma osmolality, decreased plasma volume, and low temperature. The same decrease in PO_2 will cause the most sickling in persons with sickle cell anemia (high concentrations of Hb S), the second most in children with sickle cell–thalassemia, the third most in those with sickle cell–hemoglobin C disease, and the least or none in those with sickle cell trait. The duration of the PO_2 disease also is important, because sickling tends to occur only after the inciting stimulus has been present for some time.

The level of PO_2 in the microcirculation also affects sickling because hemoglobin releases whatever oxygen it is carrying to tissues. Thus PO_2 normally is lower in the microcirculation. The added reduction in PO_2 caused by persistent hypoxemia—induced by stressors—eventually results in sickling in the microcirculation of all cells that contain Hb S in that site (not throughout the body). Sickling within the microcirculation decreases blood flow as sickled cells clog the vessels. Slow blood flow promotes hypoxemia and perpetuates sickling. Finally, decreased blood pH decreases hemoglobin's affinity for oxygen. As less oxygen is taken up by hemoglobin in the lungs, PO_2 drops, promoting sickling further.

Increased osmolality of the plasma (increased concentration of solutes; see Chapters 1 and 3) draws water out of the erythrocytes. This promotes sickling by raising the relative Hb S content in erythrocytes. Decreased plasma volume, which occurs in states of dehydration, causes the blood to become viscous (thick and sticky). Increased viscosity of the blood is the final common pathway leading to many pathologic effects of sickle cell disease. Viscous blood flows slowly and promotes vascular obstruction by increasing opportunities for sickling while decreasing opportunities for reoxygenation in the lungs. This is an example of positive feedback in a vicious cycle of events. Low temperatures precipitate sickle crisis, presumably because of vasoconstriction (Steingart, 1992).

Once sickling begins, it tends to perpetuate itself until PO_2 returns to normal; then it ceases spontaneously. The extent, severity, and clinical manifestations of sickling depend to a great extent on the percentage of hemoglobin that is Hb S. That is why homozygous inheritance of Hb S produces the severest form of sickle cell disease, sickle cell anemia. Heterozygous inheritance of sickle cell disease results in less sickling because the individual's erythrocytes contain other forms of abnormal hemoglobin that, although defective, do not participate

in sickling to any great degree. Heterozygous inheritance (sickle cell trait), in which abnormal hemoglobin is inherited from one parent and normal hemoglobin from the other, rarely results in sickling because normal fetal hemoglobin (Hb F) and adult hemoglobin (Hb A) do not participate in sickling at all. Anemia persists because Hb F does not live 120 days.

Clinical Manifestations

When sickling occurs, the general manifestations of hemolytic anemia—pallor, fatigue, jaundice, and irritability—sometimes are accompanied by acute manifestations called *crises*. Extensive sickling can precipitate four types of crises: (1) vasoocclusive (or thrombotic) crisis, (2) aplastic crisis, (3) sequestration crisis, or, rarely, (4) hyperhemolytic crisis. Sites of specific dysfunction are shown in Fig. 25-7.

Vasoocclusive crisis (thrombotic crisis) begins with sickling in the microcirculation. As blood flow is obstructed by tangled masses of rigid, sickled cells, some degree of vasospasm occurs and a "log-jam" effect brings all blood flow through the vessel to a halt. Unless the process is reversed, thrombosis and infarction (death caused by lack of oxygen) of local tissue follow. Vasoocclusive crisis is extremely painful and may last for days or even weeks, with an average duration of 4 to 6 days. The frequency of this type of crisis is variable and unpredictable.

Vasoocclusive crises may develop spontaneously or be precipitated by infection, exposure to cold, dehydration, low PO_2, acidosis (low pH), or localized hypoxemia. Symmetric, painful swelling of the hands and feet (hand-foot syndrome) caused by infarction in the small vessels of the extremities, often is the initial manifestation of sickle cell disease in infancy. In older children and adults the large joints and surrounding tissue become painful and swollen. Priapism (persistent erection of the penis) may occur if penile veins become obstructed. Severe abdominal pains often are caused by infarction in abdominal structures. Strokes resulting from cerebral occlusion may leave the child with paralysis (usually hemiplegia) or other central nervous system deficits.

In **sequestration crisis,** large amounts of blood become acutely pooled in the liver and spleen. This type of crisis is seen only in the young child. Because the spleen can hold as much as one fifth of the body's blood supply at one time, up to 50% mortality rate has been reported, with death caused by cardiovascular collapse. If blood volume and pressure are maintained by hydration and blood transfusion, much of the sequestered blood eventually is remobilized. Removal of the spleen (splenectomy) is the treatment for recurrent sequestration crises.

Aplastic crisis consists of profound anemia caused by diminished erythropoiesis, despite increased need for

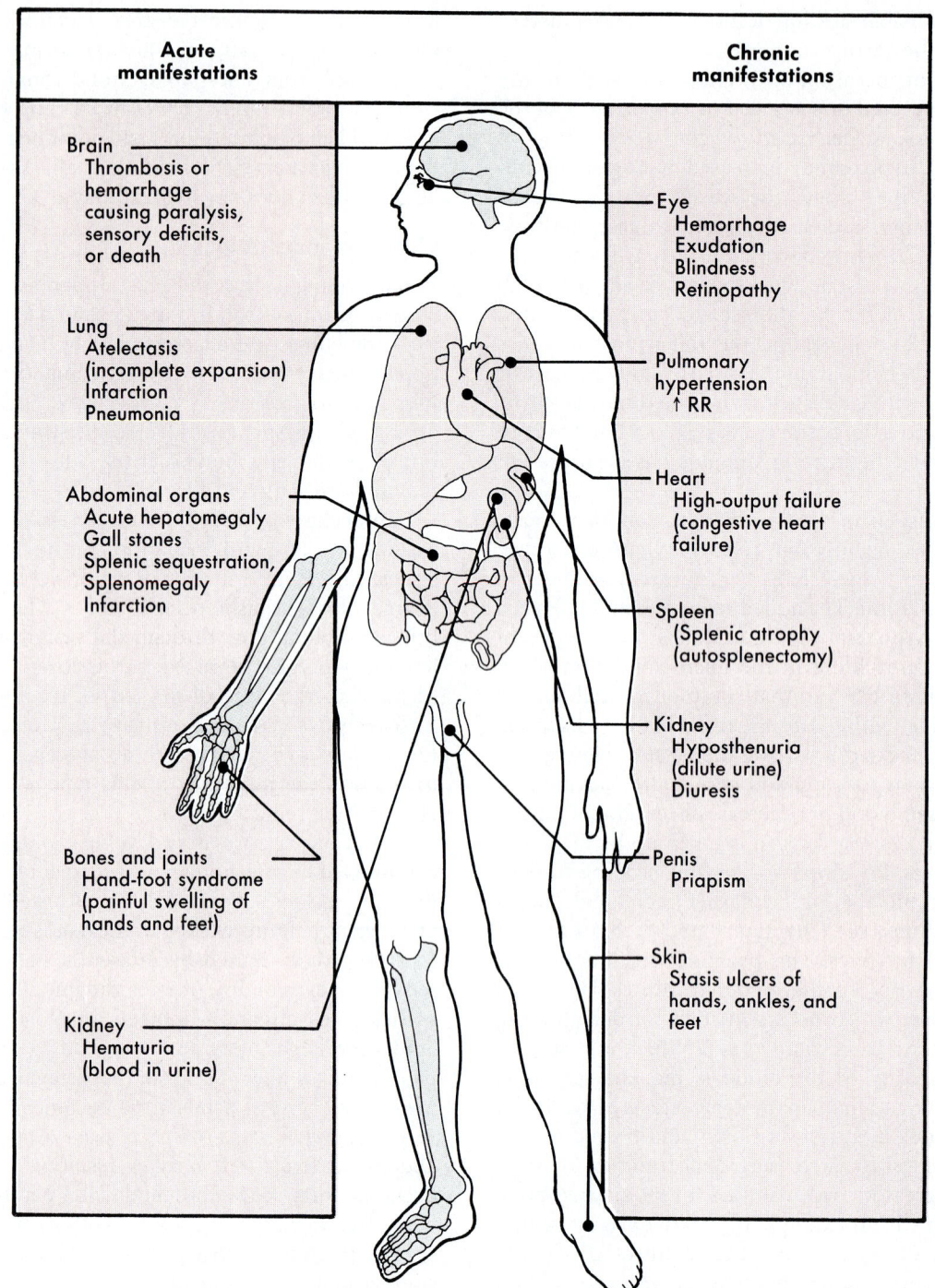

Acute manifestations	Chronic manifestations

Brain
    Thrombosis or
    hemorrhage
    causing paralysis,
    sensory deficits,
    or death
	Eye
	    Hemorrhage
	    Exudation
	    Blindness
	    Retinopathy

Lung
    Atelectasis
    (incomplete expansion)
    Infarction
    Pneumonia
	Pulmonary
	    hypertension
	    ↑RR

Abdominal organs
    Acute hepatomegaly
    Gall stones
    Splenic sequestration,
    Splenomegaly
    Infarction
	Heart
	    High-output failure
	    (congestive heart
	    failure)

	Spleen
	    (Splenic atrophy
	    (autosplenectomy)

	Kidney
	    Hyposthenuria
	    (dilute urine)
	    Diuresis

Bones and joints
    Hand-foot syndrome
    (painful swelling of
    hands and feet)
	Penis
	    Priapism

Kidney
    Hematuria
    (blood in urine)
	Skin
	    Stasis ulcers of
	    hands, ankles, and
	    feet

FIG. 25-7 Clinical manifestations of sickle cell disease.

new erythrocytes. In sickle cell anemia, erythrocyte survival is only 10 to 20 days. Normally a compensatory increase in erythropoiesis (five to eight times normal) replaces the cells lost through premature hemolysis. If this compensatory response is compromised, aplastic crisis develops in a very short time.

Hyperhemolytic crisis is unusual but may occur in association with certain drugs or infections. The concomitant presence of G6PD deficiency (see p. 917) contributes to hyperhemolytic episodes, especially when combined with infections.

Although intravascular sickling and hemolysis can begin by 6 to 8 weeks of age, clinical manifestations are not yet present. Clinical manifestations of sickle cell disease usually do not appear until the infant is at least 6 months old, at which time the postnatal decrease in Hb F causes concentrations of Hb S to rise.

Infection is the most frequent cause of death because of sickle cell disease. Sepsis and meningitis develop in as many as 10% of children with sickle cell anemia during the first 5 years of life, with a mortality rate of 25%. Survival time is unpredictable but averages in the twenties.

Sickle cell–Hb C disease, in which about half the hemoglobin is Hb S and half is Hb C, usually is milder than sickle cell anemia. The peripheral blood contains many target cells resulting from the presence of Hb C. The main clinical problems are related to vasoocclusive crises and are believed to result from higher hematocrit values and viscosity. In older children, sickle cell retinopathy, renal necrosis, and aseptic necrosis of the femoral heads occur along with obstructive crises.

Sickle cell–thalassemia has the mildest clinical manifestations of all the sickle cell diseases. Even though most of the child's hemoglobin is Hb S (60% to 90%), normal hemoglobins (Hb A and Hb F) also are present. The normal hemoglobins, particularly Hb F, inhibit sickling. In addition, the erythrocytes tend to be small (microcytic) and to contain relatively little hemoglobin (hypochromic). Their small size makes them less likely than normal-sized cells to clog the microcirculation, even when in a sickled state.

The sickle cell trait does not affect life expectancy or interfere with daily activities. Yet on rare occasions, *severe* hypoxia caused by shock, vigorous exercising at high altitudes, flying at high altitudes in unpressurized aircraft, or undergoing anesthesia is associated with vasoocclusive episodes in persons with sickle cell trait. These cells form an ivy shape instead of a sickle shape.

Evaluation and Treatment

The parents' hematologic history and clinical manifestations may suggest that a child has sickle cell disease, but hematologic tests are necessary for diagnosis. If the sickle solubility test confirms the presence of Hb S in peripheral blood, hemoglobin electrophoresis provides information about the amount of Hb S in erythrocytes. Prenatal diagnosis can be made after chorionic villus sampling as early as 8 to 10 weeks' gestation or amniotic fluid analysis at 15 weeks' gestation.

Treatment of sickle cell disease consists of supportive care aimed at preventing consequences of anemia and avoiding crises. Crises can be prevented by avoiding fever, infection, acidosis, dehydration, constricting clothes, and exposure to cold. Immediate correction of acidosis and dehydration with appropriate intravenous fluids is imperative. Therapeutic use of antisickling agents (urea, cyanate, carbamoyl phosphate) currently are regarded as unsafe and ineffective. The most definitive approach to the treatment of sickle cell disease involves a permanent alteration in the hemoglobin phenotype. Bone marrow transplantation has been successful in persons with both homozygous sickle cell disease and acute leukemia (Steingart, 1992). In order to avoid increased acidosis, acetaminophen is preferable to salicylates for antipyretic therapy. Immunization against influenza and pneumococcal organisms should be seriously considered. Blood transfusion, including hypertransfusion therapy (e.g., packed red blood cells to raise the hematocrit to a level of 35% for a period of time), can be very effective but must be weighed against the risks of hepatitis, human immunodeficiency virus (HIV), hemosiderosis, and splenic overload. Oral maintenance therapy with folic acid or iron, or both, is needed to meet the increased demands of chronic hemolytic anemia. Splenectomy may be performed if sequestration crises recur.

Genetic counseling and psychologic support are important for the child and family. Genetic counseling enables persons with sickle cell disease or trait to make informed decisions about transmitting this genetic disorder to their offspring, inasmuch as there is a 25% chance with each pregnancy that a child born to two parents with sickle cell trait will have sickle cell disease.

Thalassemias

The alpha- and beta-thalassemias are inherited autosomal recessive disorders that cause an impaired *rate* of synthesis of one of the two chains—alpha or beta—of adult hemoglobin (Hb A). The disorder was named **thalassemia**, which is derived from the Greek word for "sea," because it was defined initially in persons with origins near the Mediterranean Sea. Beta-thalassemia, in which synthesis of the beta globin chain is slowed or defective, is prevalent among Greeks, Italians, and some Arabs and Sephardic Jews. Alpha-thalassemia, in which the alpha chain is affected, is most common among Chinese, Vietnamese, Cambodians, and Laotians. Both alpha- and beta-thalassemia are common among African Americans.

Alpha- and beta-thalassemia can be major or minor, depending on (1) how many of the genes that control alpha or beta chain synthesis are defective and (2) whether the defects are inherited homozygously (thalassemia major) or heterozygously (thalassemia minor). Pathophysiologic effects range from mild microcytosis to death in utero, depending on the number of defective genes and mode of inheritance. The anemic manifestation of thalassemia is microcytic-hypochromic hemolytic anemia.

Pathophysiology

Normally two genes control beta chain synthesis, and four genes control alpha chain synthesis. The number of genetic defects in the controlling genes determines the severity of the disorder. As in sickle cell disease the hemoglobin abnormality usually consists of the substitution of a single amino acid for another. Other molecular abnormalities that cause thalassemia are two amino acid substitutions, amino acid deletions or fusions, and synthesis of elongated chains.

The fundamental defect in beta-thalassemia is the uncoupling of alpha and beta chain synthesis. Beta chain production is depressed—moderately in the heterozygous form, **beta-thalassemia minor,** and severely in the homozygous form, **beta-thalassemia major** (also called **Cooley anemia**). Depression of beta chain synthesis results in erythrocytes having a reduced amount of hemoglobin and accumulations of free alpha chains. The free alpha chains are unstable and easily precipitate in the cell. Most erythroblasts that contain precipitates are destroyed by mononuclear phagocytes in the marrow, resulting in ineffective erythropoiesis and anemia. Some of the precipitate-carrying cells do mature and enter the bloodstream but they are destroyed prematurely in the spleen, resulting in mild hemolytic anemia.

There are four forms of alpha-thalassemia: (1) **alpha trait** (the carrier state), in which a single alpha chain—forming gene is defective, (2) **alpha-thalassemia minor,** in which two genes are defective, (3) **hemoglobin H disease,** in which three genes are defective, and (4) **alpha-thalassemia major,** a fatal condition in which all four alpha-forming genes are defective. Death is inevitable because alpha chains are absent and oxygen cannot be released to the tissues.

Beta-thalassemia occurs more commonly than does alpha-thalassemia. Occasionally synthesis of gamma or delta polypeptide chains is defective, resulting in gamma- or delta-thalassemia. (Hemoglobin chains are described in Chapter 22.)

Clinical Manifestations

Beta-thalassemia minor causes mild to moderate microcytic-hypochromic anemia, mild splenomegaly, bronze coloring of the skin, and hyperplasia of the bone marrow. The degree of reticulocytosis depends on the severity of the anemia, resulting in skeletal changes. Hemolysis of immature (and therefore fragile) erythrocytes may cause a slight elevation in serum iron and indirect bilirubin levels. Persons with beta-thalassemia minor are usually asymptomatic.

Persons with beta-thalassemia major may become quite ill. Anemia is severe and results in a significant cardiovascular burden, with high-output congestive heart failure. In the past, death resulted from cardiac failure.

Today, blood transfusions can increase life span by a decade or two, and death usually is caused by hemochromatosis (from transfusions). (Hemosiderosis and hematochromatosis are described in Chapter 23.) Liver enlargement occurs as a result of progressive hemosiderosis, whereas enlargement of the spleen is caused by extramedullary hemopoiesis and increased destruction of red blood cells. Growth and maturation are retarded, and a characteristic deformity (chipmunk deformity) develops on the face, caused by expansion of bones to accommodate hyperplastic marrow.

Persons who inherit the mildest form of alpha-thalassemia, the alpha trait, usually are symptom-free, having at most, mild microcytosis. Alpha-thalassemia minor has clinical manifestations that are virtually identical to those of beta-thalassemia minor: mild microcytic-hypochromic reticulocytosis, bone marrow hyperplasia, increased serum iron concentrations, and moderate splenomegaly.

Signs and symptoms of alpha-thalassemia are similar to those of beta-thalassemia major, but milder. Moderate microcytic-hypochromic anemia, enlargement of the liver and spleen, and bone marrow hyperplasia are evident.

Alpha-thalassemia major causes hydrops fetalis and fulminant intrauterine congestive heart failure. In addition to edema and massive ascites, the fetus has a grossly enlarged heart and liver. Diagnosis usually is made post mortem. Prenatal screening for this disorder can be performed by use of chorionic villus sampling. These cells can be analyzed and a DNA genetic map can be constructed and evaluated for the abnormalities characteristic of hydrops fetalis.

Both alpha- and beta-thalassemia major are life-threatening. Children with thalassemia major generally are weak, fail to thrive, show poor development, and experience cardiovascular compromise with high-output failure secondary to anemia. Untreated, they will die by 5 to 6 years of age.

Evaluation and Treatment

Evaluation of thalassemia is based on familial disease history, clinical manifestations, and blood tests. Peripheral blood smears that show microcytosis and hemoglobin electrophoresis that demonstrates diminished amounts of alpha or beta chains are used to make the diagnosis. Analysis of fetal DNA from withdrawn amniotic fluid is used as a screening test to detect hydrops fetalis (alpha-thalassemia major).

Persons who are "silent" carriers or have thalassemia minor generally have few if any symptoms and require no specific treatment. Therapies to support and prolong life are necessary, however, for thalassemia major. There is no cure for either condition.

At present, thalassemia major is treated with the following therapies:

1. Blood transfusions, which can return hemoglobin and hematocrit levels to normal, thus alleviating the anemia-induced cardiac failure. Iron overload and hemochromatosis are complications of transfusion therapy.

2. Iron chelation therapy in combination with hypertransfusion (transfusion to a hematocrit of 35 ml/dl to correct all manifestations of thalassemia). This therapy currently is under investigation. If it is proved effective, what once was a fatal disease may in the future be merely an expensive nuisance.

3. Splenectomy, which can reduce the need for transfusions by eliminating a site of hemolysis, thus prolonging erythrocyte survival.

4. Neocyte transfusion, in which young erythrocytes (neocytes) in a unit of blood are separated by centrifugation from old erythrocytes (gerocytes). Neocytes may last longer in the circulation and thus reduce the problem of hemolysis and premature cell destruction. This therapy is being investigated.

For both symptom-free carriers and those with the disease, prenatal diagnosis and genetic counseling may be the most important therapeutic measures that can be offered.

DISORDERS OF COAGULATION AND PLATELETS

Inherited Hemorrhagic Disease
Hemophilias

Awareness of a serious bleeding disorder in males was documented nearly 2000 years ago in the Babylonian Talmud, which exempted from the rite of circumcision those boys having male relatives prone to excessive bleeding. In 1803 the first description of this disorder appeared in the medical literature, where it was noted to be X-linked in nature and associated with joint bleeding and crippling.

Table 25-4 lists the coagulation factors that are associated with clinical bleeding. Until 1952 the term *hemophilia* was reserved for deficiency of factor VIII (antihemophilic factor). Since that time two additional coagulation proteins, factor IX (plasma thromboplastin component [PTC]) and factor XI (plasma thromboplastin antecedent [PTA]), have been identified and their deficiency associated with similar clinical manifestations. Congenital deficiencies of these three plasma clotting factors—VIII, IX, and XI—account for 90% to 95% of the hemorrhagic bleeding disorders collectively called hemophilia. (Table 25-5 lists coagulation disorders in children.)

TABLE 25-4

Phase, Factor, and Disease Name for Coagulation Disorders in Children

Phase/factor	Synonyms
Phase I disorders	
Factor VIII deficiencies	Classic hemophilia; hemophilia A; antihemophilic factor (AHF) deficiency
Factor IX deficiency	Christmas disease; hemophilia B
Factor XI deficiency	Plasma thromboplastin antecedent (PTA) deficiency; hemophilia C
Factor XII deficiency	Hageman factor deficiency
von Willebrand disease	Vascular hemophilia
Phase II disorders	
Congenital deficiency of factors II, V, and VII	Hemorrhagic disease of the newborn; parahemophilia, Owren disease (factor V)
Phase III disorders	
Congenital afibrinogenemia	Congenital fibrinogen deficiency
Congenital dysfibrinogenemia	Congenital fibrinogen deficiency
Factor XIII deficiency	Fibrin-stabilizing factor deficiency

TABLE 25-5

Coagulation Disorders in Children

Factor/deficient	Genetics	Frequency in population (per 10^6)	Disorder
I (fibrinogen)	AR	0.1	Afibrinogenemia, hypofibrinogenemia
II (prothrombin)	AR	0.1	Hypoprothrombinemia
III (thromboplastin)			
IV (Ca^{++})			
V	AR	0.1	Parahemophilia, factor V deficiency
VII	AR	0.1	Factor VII deficiency
VIII (AHP)	X-R	30-40	Hemophilia A, classic hemophilia; von Willebrand disease
IX (PTC)	X-R	3-4	Hemophilia B, Christmas disease
X	AR	0.1	Factor X deficiency
XI (PTA)	AR	1	Hemophilia C, PTA deficiency
XII	AR	0.1	Hageman trait
XIII	AR	0.1	Factor XIII deficiency

Modified from Kelley, 1983. *AR*, autosomal recessive; *X-R*, sex-linked recessive.

Types of hemophilia

Hemophilia A (classic hemophilia) is caused by factor VIII deficiency. It is the most common of the hemophilias. Inherited as an X-linked recessive disorder that affects males and is transmitted by females, its estimated incidence rate is 1 per 10,000 male births.

Hemophilia B (Christmas disease), caused by factor IX deficiency, also is transmitted as an X-linked recessive trait and is clinically indistinguishable from factor VIII deficiency. Approximately 15% of cases, or 1 in every 25,000 to 30,000 males born with hemophilia, are caused by factor IX (Guy, Baxi, Hurlet-Jensen, & Chao, 1992).

Hemophilia A and B occur with varying degrees of clinical severity, depending on concentrations of clotting factor VIII or IX in the blood. Severe hemophilia (concentration of clotting factors less than 1% of normal) is associated with spontaneous bleeding. In moderate hemophilia (1% to 5% of normal), bleeding usually occurs only after trauma; in the mild form (5% to 35% of normal), bleeding occurs only after severe trauma or surgery. The severity of hemophilia is similar in all affected members of a family.

Hemophilia C (factor XI deficiency) occurs as an autosomal recessive disease and occurs equally in males and females. Bleeding usually is less severe than in hemophilia A or B.

Von Willebrand disease results from an inherited autosomal dominant trait with variable clinical manifestations and hematologic findings. The factor VIII deficiency differs from that of hemophilia A in mode of inheritance and response to treatment. In hemophilia A the deficiency is inherited as an X-linked recessive trait, whereas in von Willebrand disease it is inherited as an autosomal dominant trait. The most important difference, however, manifests by the responses to the infusion of plasma. In von Willebrand disease, infusion of plasma causes factor VIII activity to increase for several days because infusion of factor VIII temporarily induces endogenous synthesis of factor VIII.

Pathophysiology

Two types of defects dominate the hereditary defects of hemophilia to date, gene deletions and point mutations. Gene deletions are associated with severe hemophilia A, in which no factor VIII circulates in the blood. To date, about 50 deletion mutations in the gene for factor VIII have been identified at the molecular level, and about 34 independent deletion mutations in the factor IX gene have been found to be the cause of hemophilia B (Furie & Furie, 1992; White & Shoemaker, 1989). The molecular defect that leads to hemophilia is identical among members of a given family; however, the deletional mutation has been unique in each family studied (Furie & Furie, 1992).

Point mutations, in which a single base in the DNA is mutated to another base, represent a second type of mutation that causes hemophilia. When a point mutation gives rise to a "de novo stop codon" (nonsense mutation), translation of the protein ceases and a shortened version of the protein is synthesized. Usually the protein is destroyed intracellularly and never reaches the plasma. This type of defect is associated with severe hemophilia, that is, with coagulant activity levels below 1% (Furie & Furie, 1992). Point mutations in which one amino acid is substituted for another can cause phenotypes of varying severity. The mutation of an important amino acid can destroy protein function, activation, or folding; inhibit intracellular processing; or cause protein clearance (Furie & Furie, 1992). Unlike deletional mutations, point mutations at the same site have been recorded in different families with hemophilia.

Table 25-4 summarizes the types of coagulation disorders according to the phase of coagulation affected. Not all the disorders are discussed in this chapter because some are extremely rare (congenital dysfibrinogenemias), whereas others have no clinical significance (e.g., Hageman factor deficiency, a condition in which profound laboratory deficiency of factor XII has absolutely no clinical effects on the child).

Clinical Manifestations

Although abnormal bleeding may occur in the newborn period, particularly after circumcision, spontaneous bleeding as a result of hemophilia is infrequent during the first year of life. Although there is no transfer of maternal clotting factor to the fetus, many boys with hemophilia are circumcised without excessive bleeding. Normal hemostasis is achieved in these infants because clotting is activated through the extrinsic coagulation cascade, which does not involve factors VII, IX, or XI.

During the first year, spontaneous bleeding often is minimal, but hematoma formation may result from injections and from firm holding (such as under the arms). Easy bruising or hemarthrosis (bleeding into joints), or both, occurs with ambulation. By age 3 to 4 years, 90% of children with hemophilia have had episodes of persistent bleeding from relatively minor traumatic lacerations (e.g., to the lip or tongue). This usually is the first clinical manifestation of hemophilia. Hemorrhage into the elbows, knees, and ankles causes pain, limits joint movement, and predisposes the child to degenerative joint changes. Spontaneous hematuria and epistaxis are troublesome but minor complications.

Recurrent bleeding, both spontaneous and after minor trauma, is a lifelong problem. Many affected persons experience phases or cycles of spontaneous bleeding episodes. Mechanisms that cause this phenomenon are unknown. Intracranial hemorrhage and bleeding into the neck constitute life-threatening emergencies.

Evaluation and Treatment

Although laboratory tests are of primary value in the evaluation of hemorrhagic disorders, the history and physical assessment also should be given careful consideration. The three phases of coagulation can be individually assessed by simple, reliable tests. In any hemorrhagic condition, the adequacy of phase III should be determined first. Unless adequate fibrinogen is present, the blood is incapable of coagulation; thus other laboratory tests that require formation of a visible clot will be invalid. Phase III can be evaluated by the **thrombin time,** the time required for plasma to clot after the addition of bovine thrombin. Fibrinogen can be measured by chemical or immunologic methods.

Phase II is assessed by the **prothrombin time (PT),** the time required for plasma to clot after the addition of thromboplastin and calcium. If phase III is intact, a prolonged prothrombin time indicates a deficiency involving factors II, V, VII, or X, alone or in combination. Specific assays for each of the factors are available.

Phase I, the most complex part of coagulation, can be evaluated by several tests. The **activated partial thromboplastin time (PTT)** is the time required for clotting of plasma that has been activated by incubation with kaolin when calcium and platelets, or partial thromboplastin, are added. PTT assesses the adequacy of factors XII, XI, IX, and VII. The **prothrombin consumption time** is a standard prothrombin test of serum instead of plasma. Because prothrombin is used up during coagulation, the serum normally contains little prothrombin and the serum prothrombin time is prolonged. Deficiencies of the phase I factors are associated with poor use of prothrombin. If the serum and plasma prothrombin times are similar, deficiency of a phase I factor is likely. The **thromboplastin generation** test is the most sensitive of all phase I tests. The test can precisely identify deficiencies of factors VIII and IX. If the PTT, prothrombin consumption, or thromboplastin generation test results are abnormal, the way in which they can be corrected identifies the specific deficiency.

The treatment of hemophilia has advanced during the last 50 years. Plasma first was used in the 1920s, and by the 1940s it was used routinely to treat persons with hemophilia. The disadvantages of fresh frozen plasma (FFP), which is low in factor VIII per volume of plasma, led to the development of cryoprecipitate. In 1964, cryoprecipitate (quick-frozen precipitate), which is rich in factor VIII per volume, was used to treat persons with hemophilia. Although cryoprecipitate advanced the treatment of hemophilia A, there are several disadvantages to its use. The most notable complication is the possibility of transmission of viral diseases. Mild immune suppression and hemolysis, the result of exposure to anti-A antibodies or anti-B antibodies, also have been reported (Roberts, 1991). Factor VIII concentrates were first introduced in 1965. In addition to the predictable factor VIII content, other advantages of the early factor VIII concentrates included greater purity than cryoprecipitate and less contamination with other plasma proteins (Roberts, 1991). The recent cloning of the factor VIII gene and the purification of the recombinant factor VIII have resulted in new factor VIII products that minimize the risk of transmission of viral infection (e.g., HIV and hepatitis) and are potentially less expensive than plasma-derived factor VIII.

The prognosis for children with hemophilia is far more promising now than in the past. Programs of comprehensive care and home treatment have improved the quality of life for those with hemophilia and enhanced their general physical capabilities.

Antibody-Mediated Hemorrhagic Disease

The antibody-mediated hemorrhagic diseases are a group of disorders caused by the immune response. Antibody-mediated destruction of platelets or antibody-mediated inflammatory reactions to allergens damage blood vessels and cause seepage into tissues. The thrombocytopenic purpuras may be intrinsic or idiopathic, or they may be transient phenomena transmitted from mother to fetus. The inflammatory, or "allergic," purpuras occur in response to allergens in the blood. All these disorders first appear during infancy or childhood.

Idiopathic Thrombocytopenic Purpura

Acute **idiopathic thrombocytopenic purpura (ITP)** (**autoimmune** or **primary thrombocytopenic purpura**) is the most common of the thrombocytopenic purpuras of childhood. It is a disorder of platelet consumption in which antiplatelet antibodies bind to the plasma membranes of platelets, causing platelet sequestration and destruction by mononuclear phagocytes in the spleen and other lymphoid tissues at a rate that exceeds the ability of the bone marrow to produce them.

Pathophysiology

Platelets have several tissue-specific antigens on their plasma markers that may be targets for antiplatelet antibody. In approximately 70% of cases of ITP, there is an antecedent viral disease (such as rubella, rubeola, or viral respiratory infection), thus suggesting that viral sensitization has occurred. The interval between infection and onset of purpura averages 2 weeks. A comparison with purpura seen in adults has identified an immune mechanism as the basis for ITP. High levels of IgG have been found bound to platelets and may represent immune complexes on the platelet surface (Karpatkin, 1981; Lightsey & Koenig, 1979; Simons, Main, & Yarsh, 1975; Weiss, 1975).

Clinical Manifestations

One to 4 weeks after a viral infection, bruising and a generalized petechial rash often occur with acute onset. Asymmetric bleeding is typical and is found most frequently throughout the legs. Hemorrhagic bullae of the gums, lips, and other mucous membranes may be prominent. Epistaxis (nose bleeding) may be severe and difficult to control. Except for the signs of bleeding, the child appears well. The acute phase of the disease associated with spontaneous hemorrhages lasts 1 to 2 weeks, but thrombocytopenia often persists even longer. Although its incidence is less than 1%, intracranial hemorrhage is the most serious complication of ITP. In some cases the onset is more gradual, and clinical manifestations consist of moderate bruising and a few petechiae.

Evaluation and Treatment

On examination of the blood the platelet count is reduced and the few platelets observed on a smear are large in size, reflecting increased bone marrow production. The tourniquet test and tests of bleeding time and clot reaction give abnormal results. Bone marrow aspiration reveals normal or increased megakaryocytes and normal erythrocytes and granulocytes.

Even without treatment, the prognosis for children with ITP is excellent. Three fourths recover completely within 3 months. After the initial acute phase, spontaneous clinical manifestations subside. By 9 to 12 months after onset, about 90% of affected children have regained normal platelet counts.

Because of the short lifespan of platelets (10 days), fresh blood or platelets are of no value or of transient benefit; however, their use is indicated when life-threatening hemorrhage occurs. For 20% of cases, corticosteroid therapy reduces the severity and shortens the duration of the initial phase by suppressing the immune attack on platelets. Bacterial infections should be treated with antibiotics. Parents should be instructed to protect the child from falls or other trauma that might result in bleeding. Splenectomy should be reserved for chronic cases that fail to respond to nonsurgical intervention.

Transient Neonatal Thrombocytopenias

Antibody-mediated thrombocytopenic purpura occurs in neonates in either autoimmune or isoimmune form. Both forms are characterized by the immunologic destruction of platelets by antibodies (IgG) against tissue-specific antigens expressed by the platelets (i.e., platelet-specific antigens).

Transient neonatal thrombocytopenia was first noted in the early 1950s when it was observed that mothers with ITP frequently delivered infants who were transiently thrombocytopenic. Neonatal thrombocytopenia was observed in approximately 50% of infants at risk and lasted an average of 1 month. As platelet counts returned to normal, there was a concomitant drop in the level of maternal antiplatelet antibody on the child's platelets. The particular platelet-specific antigens that are the targets of antiplatelets have not yet been identified, but they do not appear to be among known platelet-specific antigens. The prognosis generally is favorable, but several fetal complications do occur. Perinatal intracranial hemorrhage, for example, occurs in approximately 6% to 17% of affected infants born by vaginal delivery.

Isoimmune thrombocytopenic purpura (IITP) is less common, occurring in approximately 1 in 5000 births. IITP is suspected in thrombocytopenic infants of mothers with normal platelet counts and no history of purpura. The disorder is caused by the production of a maternal antibody against a fetal platelet-specific antigen inherited from the father and not shared by the mother. Approximately 50% of IITP cases are associated with the presence of the Pl^A1 antigen on neonatal and paternal platelets but not on maternal platelets.

It is not known why IITP occurs in only half of the neonates genetically at risk for IITP. Because 98% of the population show Pl^A1 positivity, approximately 1 in 50 pregnancies would be expected to show maternal-fetal incompatibility, but the incidence of IITP is 100 times less. IITP does not develop in neonates born to some mothers with high antiplatelet antibody levels.

The diagnosis of IITP is confirmed by detection in the maternal serum of antibody that reacts with platelets from the infant and father but not with platelets from the mother. In approximately 75% to 85% of cases, IITP recurs in subsequent pregnancies. Purpura usually develops in the affected infant shortly after delivery, and intracranial, renal, and gastrointestinal hemorrhages are possible. Mortality rates from intracranial hemorrhage have been estimated at 10% to 15%.

Most of the life-threatening clinical manifestations of both transient neonatal thrombocytopenia and IITP can be avoided through delivery by cesarean section. If the mother has antiplatelet disease, however, surgery can result in hemorrhage and serious maternal morbidity. Maternal mortality resulting from IITP during pregnancy is low (less than 5%): the principal maternal risk is bleeding from surgical incisions during cesarean section. This poses a problem for the obstetrician. The incidence of transient thrombocytopenia in infants born to mothers with IITP is about 50%. If all deliveries were performed by cesarean section, half the mothers would undergo cesarean section unnecessarily. Conversely, if all deliveries were vaginal, then half the infants—those with thrombocytopenia—would be at risk for intracranial bleeding. A considerable amount of research has focused on methods of predicting whether the fetus is thrombocytopenic so that the route of delivery can be chosen to minimize the risks for both mother and child. No satisfactory method has been found, despite reports from many laboratories that fetal platelet counts correlate closely with levels of antiplatelet antibody on maternal platelets or in the maternal circulation. Equally unreliable are predictions of neonatal thrombocytope-

nia based on immunosuppression with corticosteroids. Research continues in such areas as the identification of specific subclasses of antiplatelet antibodies.

Autoimmune Vascular Purpura

Autoimmune vascular purpura (allergic purpura) is caused by antibody-mediated injury of blood vessel walls, typically arterioles and capillaries. The inflammatory reaction is to foreign proteins or chemicals in the blood (microorganisms, drugs, or other chemicals).

Autoimmune vascular purpura usually is seen in children, with the incidence decreasing in adolescents and adults and occurring only rarely in elderly persons. The average age at onset is 5 years, with a slightly higher proportion of males affected. Purpura occurs as vessel integrity is disrupted by inflammatory processes, causing effusion of serosanguineous exudate to perivascular tissues.

Clinical manifestations may vary and include headache, anorexia, fever, abdominal pain, arthralgias, and skin lesions (urticaria and erythema). The lesions usually are located symmetrically on the proximal portions of the extremities, particularly on the legs and buttocks, and may be accompanied by itching or paresthesias (Lee et al., 1993). Abdominal pain results from hemorrhage into the bowel, which may lead to colic, nausea, and vomiting. These symptoms may precede the appearance of skin lesions. The pain usually is midabdominal but may radiate to other parts of the abdomen. Constipation may occur.

Some forms of autoimmune vascular purpura may produce joint pain and tenderness. Periarticular swelling and edema of the hands and feet are common, but hemarthrosis does not occur. These symptoms may precede the onset of symptoms associated with abdominal pain and purpura. Subacute glomerulonephritis occurs in some cases but usually is reversible.

The characteristic skin lesions (purpura and cutaneous manifestations of allergy), accompanied by a history of joint and abdominal pain, are clues for diagnosis. Laboratory test results often reveal no major abnormalities. Attacks may last several weeks and may recur at odd intervals and with changing manifestations with each episode. Treatment, if necessary, consists of the alleviation of symptoms.

LEUKEMIA AND LYMPHOMA

Leukemia, the most common malignancy of childhood, represents approximately 33% of all childhood cancers. Childhood lymphoma is the third most common malignant neoplasm of children in the United States, representing approximately 11% of all childhood cancers. (See Chapter 24 for a discussion of leukemia in adults.)

Leukemia

Of the varieties of childhood leukemia, 80% to 85% of leukemias in children are acute lymphoblastic leukemia (ALL) or acute undifferentiated leukemia (AUL). The remaining 15% to 20% are acute nonlymphocytic leukemias (ANLL) (which include myeloblastic, promyelocytic, monocytic, myelomonoblastic) and the very rare red blood cell leukemia, erythroleukemia. Since the vast majority of ANLL involves the myeloblastic cell, many experts refer to the disease as AML (acute myelogenous leukemia). Leukemia accounts for 25% of cases of cancer in black children and 34% of cases of cancer in white children. Approximately 2200 new cases are diagnosed each year in the United States (Bleyer, 1990). Of those 2200 children, 1700 are diagnosed with ALL. Both a juvenile and an adult form of chronic granulocytic leukemia (CGL) in children develop, but this condition is uncommon and accounts for only 2% of all leukemias in childhood. Chronic lymphocytic leukemia (CLL) is virtually nonexistent in children.

The peak incidence for childhood ALL is between 2 and 6 years of age. Although this peak is very evident in white children in the United States, it is not observed in African-American children. The reason for this difference is unknown, but it may be related to genetic susceptibility or to exposure to the environmental influences that might play a role in leukemia. Furthermore, acute leukemia is nearly twice as common in white children as in nonwhite children (4.2/100,000 vs. 2.4/100,000, respectively). For a white child the risk of acute leukemia developing before the age of 10 is 1:2800 (Pendergrass, 1985). Childhood ALL also is more common in boys than in girls (1.3:1.0). The reason for this difference is again unknown, although sex hormones may play a role in the leukemia process.

Types of Leukemia

A number of different classifications are used for the leukemias. First, acute leukemia is differentiated from chronic leukemia. Second, the cell line determines whether lymphoid cells or myeloid cells are involved. In acute leukemia, this difference separates ALL from ANLL and vice versa. Then, within each of these categories, further subdivisions have been developed. (See Chapter 24 for a discussion of leukemias that occur in adults.)

Cytogenic studies of leukemic cells are routinely performed at most major treatment centers during the diagnostic process. Abnormal morphologic characteristics, as well as abnormalities in the number of copies of chromosomes, are found in leukemic cells. Hyperdiploidy (increased number of chromosome copies) is associated with a good prognosis. Other genetic abnormalities include chromosome translocations and fragility (break sites). Translocations are more common in children with a poor prognosis. Some oncogenes have been associated with various types of childhood leukemia, including *src, abl,* N-*ras,* and c-*myb* (Israel, 1993).

Two additional classifications of ALL, morphologic and immunologic, have proved clinically useful because they have prognostic value. Although a number of different morphologic classifications have been developed, the accepted system was developed by a cooperative effort of French, American, and British scientists and is known as the French-American-British Cooperative Group (FAB) classification (Bennett et al., 1981). This system divides lymphoblasts into three categories—L_1, L_2, and L_3—on the basis of histologic appearance of the abnormal lymphoblast. Approximately 85% of ALL is of the L_1 subtype; less than 15% is L_2 and is more common in adults with ALL, and the L_3 subtype, which is rare, occurs in fewer than 1% of children with ALL.

The immunologic classification of ALL currently is evolving as advances are made in immunologic techniques (Poplack, 1993). Because of the new techniques, distinguishing between lymphoblastic and nonlymphoblastic leukemia is much easier than in the past when the degree of immaturity of the cell had sometimes made such distinction difficult. In addition, immunologic classifications have assisted clinicians in determining the degree of aggressive therapy needed.

Immunologic classification has been based on identification of various surface markers. Five categories of ALL have been identified on the basis of their presumed origin from thymic cells (T cells) and bursa-equivalent cells (B cells) of normal lymphocytes:

1. T cell ALL, characterized by the presence of abnormal T lymphoblasts and found more commonly in older boys whose diagnosis includes mediastinal masses, high white blood cell counts, and hepatosplenomegaly (20% of ALL)
2. B cell ALL, characterized by the presence of abnormal B lymphoblasts and associated with a poor prognosis (5% of ALL)
3. Pre–B cell ALL, characterized by the presence of pre-B lymphoblasts (20% of ALL)
4. Unclassified ALL, also known as *null cell,* meaning neither T nor B lymphoblasts, and now classified as early B cell lineage (15% of ALL)
5. Common ALL, characterized by the presence of a specific antigen known as *common ALL antigen,* or common lymphocytic leukemia antigen (CALLA), in which the actual cell usually is considered to be of the B lineage (39% of ALL)

The identification of CALLA is important because this type of ALL has a more favorable prognosis.

Subtypes of ANLL also have been classified by the FAB system according to the morphologic and cytochemical characteristics of the leukemic cell. Seven categories have been established. M1 involves cells that are myeloblastic without differentiation, M2 involves cells that are myeloblastic with differentiation, M3 involves the promyelocyte, M4 involves the myeloblastic and monoblastic cell lines, M5 involves monoblasts, M6 involves precursors of erythrocytes, and M7 involves precursors of megakaryocytes. Nearly half of all childhood ANLL is M1 or M2. Another third is categorized as M4 or M5. ANLL subtypes M3, M6, and M7 are quite rare (Grier & Weinstein, 1993).

Pathogenesis

The exact cause of childhood leukemia is unclear. Investigations have focused on genetic susceptibility, environmental factors, and viral infections (see Chapters 10 and 11). Observations of a familial tendency and links with a number of inherited disorders have implicated genetic factors in the origin of leukemia. For example, if ALL develops in one identical twin, the other twin is at very high risk for development of the disease—particularly during the first year after diagnosis of the leukemic twin. Miller (1963) found the risk of development of leukemia in the co-twin to be 1 in 4. After approximately 7 years the risk to the unaffected twin returns to the same risk as that of the general population. Some evidence suggests that multiple cases of leukemia occur in families. The incidence of leukemia in siblings of leukemic children is reported to be between 1/720 and 1/1000, which represents a fourfold risk over that of the general population (Miller, 1967).

Inherited diseases that predispose a child to leukemia (both ALL and ANLL) include Down syndrome (1:74 before the age of 10), Fanconi anemia (1:12 before the age of 21), Bloom syndrome (1:8 before the age of 26), and ataxia-telangiectasia (1:8 before the age of 25) (Pendergrass, 1985). Leukemia also has been associated with known genetic diseases, such as congenital agammaglobulinemia. ANLL in children sometimes is associated with loss or deletion of chromosome 7 (Grier & Weinstein, 1993). ANLL can develop from preexisting myeloproliferative disorders that also are preleukemia syndromes. When these disorders progress to ANLL, an insidious pattern of leukemic dysfunction usually is revealed.

Most research on environmental factors as etiologic agents has centered on exposure to ionizing radiation. Atomic bomb survivors have been shown to have an increased risk for leukemia. The degree of risk depends on the distance from the epicenter. The peak incidence period is 4 to 8 years after exposure to the radiation. Whereas ANLL most often develops in adults who are exposed to radiation, ALL is more likely to develop in children. The therapeutic use of x-rays for thymic enlargement in children also has been linked to subsequent development of ALL in children (Murray, Heckel, & Hempelmann, 1959). In a more recent study, no increased risk of childhood leukemia was found in children who had received small doses of radiation from di-

agnostic x-rays (Baverstam & Holmberg, 1989). Some doubt remains concerning the relative risk of prenatal exposure to radiation. A study conducted by the National Academy of Sciences (1980), however, found that radiation exposure during the prenatal period was associated with a marked risk of development of a variety of pediatric cancers. During the first trimester the risk was fivefold; the risk dropped to 1.5 times the normal rate during the second and third trimesters. Leukemia accounted for approximately one half of the subsequent cancers. Further evidence of prenatal exposure to radiation and leukemia was found in a study of twins who had received in utero exposure to diagnostic x-rays (Harvey, Boice, & Honeyman, 1985). Although most studies of radiation exposure have focused on manmade radiation sources, there is considerable interest in natural background radiation, particularly the possible role of radon exposure in subsequent childhood and adult cancers. Studies continue in this area (Henshaw, Eatough, & Richardson, 1990).

Electromagnetic field (EMF) exposure from power poles and small appliances is an area of current study for causative factors in acute leukemias. Two studies conducted in Denver, Colorado, have shown an increased risk of leukemia and other childhood cancers for children living in high EMF environments (Savitz, Wachtel, & Barnes, 1987; Wertheimer & Leeper, 1979). Other studies, however, have not supported these findings, and further investigation is ongoing (Pool, 1990; Savitz, John, & Kleckner, 1990).

Although chemicals such as benzene have been associated with the development of ANLL in adults, no evidence suggests a similar chemical or drug association in childhood leukemia. Leukemia (primarily ANLL) has been reported as a secondary malignancy (development of a second cancer after the first) in children treated for Hodgkin disease and Wilms tumor, although such cases are rare. In most cases the children received both chemotherapy (alkylating agents or dactinomycin) and radiation therapy for the primary cancer, perhaps accounting for the subsequent development of another cancer.

Leukemic "clusters" that represent a greater number of leukemia cases occurring in a particular geographic location have raised speculation about environmental factors of infectious patterns of transmission. Careful follow-up, however, has failed to document the abnormal clustering. Explanations for this phenomenon therefore are statistical artifact and coincidence. However, one reported leukemic cluster in the town of Woburn, Massachusetts, has been linked to possible water supply contamination by chemicals from factory waste (Lagakos, Wessen, & Zelen, 1986).

Another area of interest has been the role viruses may play in the development of leukemia. Viruses clearly have been known to cause leukemia in a number of animals, including cats, fowl, and mice. Scientists have linked retroviruses with several adult cancers, including human T-cell leukemia/lymphoma virus (HTLV)-I with an unusual form of adult T-cell leukemia, HTLV-II with hairy-cell leukemia, and HIV with Kaposi sarcoma (Reitz et al., 1984). However, retroviruses have not been linked with childhood leukemia.

Gibson and colleagues (1968) reported findings that indicate the interaction of multiple factors in the cause of childhood leukemia. They investigated risk factors in children in whom leukemia developed between the ages of 1 and 4 years. They found that children exposed to four specific factors had a 4.64 times greater risk for development of leukemia than did children who had not experienced similar exposures. The four factors are (1) radiation of the mother before conception, (2) prenatal radiation of the child, (3) maternal history of miscarriages, and (4) early viral illness in the child. These, along with other evidence, strongly suggest that childhood leukemia is likely to be the result of a multiple interaction between hereditary or genetic predisposition and environmental influences (Mulvihill, 1993). This interaction is called *ecogenetics* and focuses on the genetic variations that occur in relation to environmental factors.

Clinical Manifestations

Few variations appear in the presenting symptoms of the various cell types of acute leukemia. The onset may be abrupt or insidious, but the most common symptoms reflect the consequence of bone marrow failure, which results in decreased red blood cells and platelets and changes in white blood cells. Pallor, fatigue, petechiae, purpura, bleeding, and fever generally are present. Approximately 45% of children have a hemoglobin level below 7 g/ml; in contrast to adults, children seem to demonstrate fewer symptoms. If acute blood loss occurs, however, characteristic symptoms of tachycardia, air hunger, restlessness, and thirst may be present. Epistaxis frequently occurs in children with severe thrombocytopenia. Three fourths of children with ALL have platelet counts below 100,000/mm³ at diagnosis, and 28% have a platelet count below 20,000/mm³. Half of all children newly diagnosed with ANLL have platelet counts below 50,000/mm³. Disseminated intravascular coagulation occurs more commonly with ANLL, particularly with promyelocytic leukemia. The granules in the leukemic promyelocytes may then indicate thromboplastin activity.

Fever is usually present as a result of two causes: (1) infection associated with the decrease in functional neutrophils and (2) hypermetabolism associated with the ongoing rapid growth and destruction of leukemic cells. In most children with ALL, the total white blood count is less than 10,000/mm³, and with ANLL most have

white cell counts below 50,000/mm³. In a few children, however, the peripheral white blood count can go well above 100,000/mm³. White blood cell counts greater than 200,000/mm³ can cause leukostasis, an intravascular clumping of cells that results in infarction and hemorrhage, usually in the brain and lung.

Renal failure as a result of hyperuremia (high uric acid levels) can be associated with ALL, particularly at diagnosis or during active treatment. Cell breakdown results as a natural process in the presence of a high white blood cell count and/or as a result of cellular breakdown caused by chemotherapy. Uric acid levels rise as an end product of purine metabolism from cellular destruction. Because the major excretory pathway is through the kidney, urates can precipitate in renal tubules or ureters and can lead to oliguria and acute renal failure. Renal failure is preventable if uric acid levels are monitored and treatment is aimed at optimal hydration, alkalinization of urine to assist with the excretion of soluble urates, and blockage of further uric acid formation by administration of the drug allopurinol.

Extramedullary invasion with leukemic cells can occur in nearly all body tissue. Most children with ALL have some extramedullary involvement at diagnosis. Leukemic invasion of tissue other than bone marrow is believed to represent metastatic infiltration. Hepatosplenomegaly and lymphadenopathy, resulting from extramedullary hematopoiesis, occur in nearly one half of children with ALL, but they are less common in children with ANLL.

The central nervous system (CNS) is a common site of infiltration of extramedullary leukemias, although fewer than 10% of children with ALL have CNS involvement at diagnosis. CNS infiltration manifests later in the course of the disease. Because successful chemotherapy prolongs the time of remission, the incidence of CNS involvement has increased. The most common symptoms of CNS involvement relate to increased intracranial pressure, causing early morning headaches, nausea, vomiting, irritability, and lethargy. Prophylactic CNS treatment therefore is necessary, because systemic treatment with chemotherapy does not cross the blood-brain barrier.

Gonadal involvement, with testicular and ovarian infiltration, has been demonstrated in postmortem examination in 57% and 35% of children, respectively. Clinical detection of gonadal involvement is much less frequent. The incidence of testicular involvement, like CNS involvement, has increased with lengthened duration of remission. Prophylactic treatment has not been successful and currently is not recommended.

Leukemic infiltration into bones and joints is frequent in children. Reports of bone or joint pain actually lead to the diagnosis of leukemia in some children. In most children, bone pain is characterized as migratory, vague, and without areas of swelling or inflammation. If joint pain is the primary symptom and some swelling is associated with the pain, however, misdiagnoses of rheumatoid arthritis and rheumatic fever have occurred.

Other organs reported to be sites of leukemic invasion include the kidneys, heart, lungs, thymus, eyes, skin, and the gastrointestinal tract. Of these, kidneys, lungs, and the gastrointestinal tract are the most frequently reported sites. Skin involvement is more common in ANLL than in ALL.

Children with leukemia usually have had symptoms for only 1 week before diagnosis. In 1990 a nationwide study was begun to document the symptom profile of children with cancer, including leukemia. The 5-year study is investigating the relationship of demographic and socioeconomic factors.

Evaluation and Treatment

Although blood test results can raise the clinician's suspicion of leukemia, a bone marrow aspiration is required to establish the diagnosis. The **blast cell** is the hallmark of acute leukemia. The blast cell is a relatively undifferentiated cell characterized by diffusely distributed nuclear chromatin, with one or more nucleoli and basophilic cytoplasm. Normal children have fewer than 5% blast cells in the bone marrow and none in the peripheral blood. The bone marrow is categorized on the basis of blast percentage. Normal bone marrow is called M1 marrow; M2 and M3 represent an increased percentage of blasts in the sample. This categorization system should not be confused with the similar terminology used to denote subtypes of ANLL. In ALL the bone marrow often is replaced by 80% to 100% blast cells, with a reduction in normal developing red blood cells and granulocytes. The marrow, which is considered hypercellular, is composed of a homogenous population of cells. Occasionally, however, the marrow appears hypocellular, making the diagnosis difficult to differentiate from aplastic anemia. When this occurs, bone marrow biopsy or biopsy of extramedullary sites is necessary to confirm the diagnosis.

Combination chemotherapy, with or without radiation therapy to localize sites, such as the CNS, is the treatment of choice for acute leukemia. In ALL, identification of various risk groups has led to the development of different intensities of drug protocols. Thus treatment is tailored specifically for a particular risk group. (Table 25-6 outlines the various prognostic factors for ALL that are considered in determining the degree of risk.)

Most ALL treatment programs have four distinct phases: (1) induction of remission, (2) preventive therapy for the CNS, (3) intensification (also called *consolidation),* and (4) maintenance. In remission induction the goal is no clinical evidence of disease and a normal

TABLE 25-6

Prognostic Factors in ALL

Prognostic factor	Better prognosis	Worse prognosis
*Age		
<2 years or >10 years		X
2-7 years	X	
*Sex		
Male		X
Female	X	
*Initial white blood count		
>50,000/mm^3		X
<10,000/mm^3	X	
Race		
Black		X
White	X	
Morphology		
L_2 or L_3		X
L_1	X	
*Immunology		
T or B cell ALL		X
Early pre-B cell or CALLA	X	
Leukemic involvement		
Mediastinal mass		X
Central nervous system involvement at diagnosis		X
Splenic enlargement		X

*The four most reliable prognostic factors. Initial prognostic factors become less effective predictors with increasing length of remission. Age and sex are not significant after 15 months of continuous remission and white blood count after 24 months of continuous remission.

bone marrow biopsy result, which is achieved in 95% of children with ALL. Prophylactic CNS treatment has included both chemotherapy and radiation in the past, but evidence has increasingly shown that this therapy, although effective in preventing CNS leukemia, adversely affects neurologic and intellectual function. A marked incidence of learning disabilities has been identified in children previously treated to prevent CNS disease. New, less toxic treatment protocols are now being studied to deal with this problem (Poplack, 1993). Once remission is achieved, an intensification phase of treatment is begun. This treatment is necessary because leukemic cells will continue to be present despite successful remission. Thus the goal of the intensification phase is to further decrease and eliminate the remaining leukemic cells. Intensification therapy often overlaps prophylactic CNS treatment. The final phase of initial treatment is called *maintenance therapy.* The goal of this phase is to maintain disease control. The optimal duration of maintenance therapy is not well defined, but it usually continues for 2½ to 3 years. During maintenance therapy, intermittent "pulses" of new drugs may be given. Periods of intensified therapy are believed to minimize development of drug-resistant leukemic cells.

ALL is a curable disease. This prognosis is indeed a dramatic reversal of the outlook for a child diagnosed with this disease 30 years ago, when ALL was uniformly fatal, the average survival time being only 2 to 3 months. Today, with prompt and appropriate treatment, 60% to 70% of children with ALL are cured. Those children with the more favorable early pre–B cell or CALLA-positive ALL have a survival rate of 90% (Crist, Boyett, Pullen, Van Eys, & Vietti, 1986).

Prognostic factors in ANLL are not as well defined as they are for ALL because of the small number of affected children and their overall poor prognosis (Grier et al., 1987). The goal of treatment for ANLL is similar to that of ALL except that much more aggressive chemotherapy is administered. With intensive chemotherapy, significant bone marrow suppression both is necessary and predisposes children to infection, bleeding, and anemia. The use of colony-stimulating factor (CSF), which stimulates the rapid proliferation of specific blood cell lines, is a recent advancement that now shortens this period of bone marrow aplasia (CSFs are discussed in Chapter 22). Although initial remission is achieved relatively easily in all cases of ALL, successful lasting remission can be achieved in only 70% to 80% of children with ANLL (Buckley et al., 1989). If remission is achieved, further treatment, called *continuation therapy,* is required. The specific intensity, timing, and length of continuation therapy are controversial. Bone marrow transplantation (BMT) is an important treatment consideration in ANLL. Because long-term remission and cure of ANLL are difficult to achieve with chemotherapy alone, BMT often is recommended after the first remission is achieved. BMT is the treatment of choice after relapse of ANLL. The long-term survival rate for children with ANLL, whether treated with chemotherapy or chemotherapy and BMT, is approximately 40% (Krischer et al., 1989).

Lymphomas

Non-Hodgkin lymphoma (NHL) and Hodgkin disease comprise approximately 11% of all childhood cancer. Approximately 750 cases of childhood lymphoma are diagnosed in the United States annually (Bleyer, 1990). Either group of diseases is rare before the age of 5 years, and the relative incidence increases throughout childhood. NHL is 1.5 times more common than Hodgkin disease in children. Boys are more likely to be diagnosed with a malignant lymphoma than are girls, and high-risk groups have been identified. At particular risk are children with inherited or acquired immunodeficiency syndromes. These children have been found to have increased rates of lymphoreticular cancers that range between 100 and 10,000 times the rate of normal children. The cancers are most commonly NHLs (Link, 1985). Children who are artificially immunosuppressed after organ transplantation, especially if cyclosporine is the immunosuppressive agent, also are at increased risk for lymphomas.

Non-Hodgkin Lymphoma

The classification of NHL has been confusing because of the heterogeneity of this group of diseases. Generally, most classification systems divide NHL into two categories, nodular or diffuse, on the basis of cellular pattern. Whereas one half of all adults with NHL have a nodular form of the disease, children rarely demonstrate this pattern. Nodular disease represents a less aggressive form of lymphoma. Almost without exception, childhood NHL becomes evident as a diffuse disease and can be further subdivided into three groups: (1) large cell (histiocytic), (2) lymphoblastic, and (3) small noncleaved cell (Burkitt or non-Burkitt lymphoma). Large-cell NHL often involves chromosomal translocations. Disease sites commonly involve extranodal sites, such as brain, lung, bone, and skin. Lymphoblastic NHL also shows chromosomal translocations, particularly chromosomes 7 and 14. Disease sites commonly include the mediastinum and peripheral lymph nodes. Small noncleaved cell NHL involves chromosome translocations of 8 and 14. It is believed that this translocation triggers the c-*myc* oncogene. Children with small noncleaved cell NHL commonly have intraabdominal disease at diagnosis.

An area of intensive study concerns the apparent biologic similarities of NHL and ALL in children. These two diseases are cytologically identical, and the histologic distinction between them is indicated by the degree of infiltration in the blood and bone marrow. The more bone marrow involvement and the less nodal and organ infiltration that are present, the more likely the disease is to be classified as ALL. Childhood NHL also is much more like ALL in its clinical manifestations and much less like Hodgkin disease or adult NHL.

As in ALL, immunophenotyping is an important part of the classification of childhood NHL. Almost 45% of the disease in children originates from T cells; an equal number originates from B cells. The remaining group, which represents less than 10% of childhood NHLs, is classified as non-T, non-B.

Pathogenesis

The origin of NHL in childhood is still elusive. Although defective host immunity is implicated in most children in whom NHL develops, an immune deficit cannot be identified. Viral etiology is suggested, but the role in development of human lymphoma is still unclear. The strongest correlation exists between the Epstein-Barr virus and African Burkitt lymphoma. This form of NHL is associated with a break point on chromosome 8 that is located near the c-*myc* oncogene (Magrath, 1987). The relationship between the Epstein-Barr virus infection and Burkitt lymphoma outside Africa is weak, however, even though the tumor is histopathologically and clinically indistinguishable. Chronic immunostimulation also has been suggested as a factor in the development of lymphomas because these diseases are seen more frequently when chronic persistent antigenic stimulation occurs from infection, such as malaria or intestinal parasites. Genetic susceptibility also may play a role in the process of malignant transformation. There is increased evidence of NHL in children with congenital immunodeficiency syndromes, such as Wiskott-Aldrich syndrome, ataxia-telangiectasia, and Bloom syndrome. Children with acquired immunodeficiency syndrome (AIDS) also are at greater risk for NHL (Beral, Peterman, & Berkelman, 1991).

Clinical Manifestations

In children, NHL has been found to arise from any lymphoid tissue. Signs and symptoms therefore are specific for the site involved. Some children have such widespread involvement that no original site can be determined. Because childhood NHL is a rapidly progressive disease, symptoms generally are present only a few weeks before diagnosis is made. Rapidly enlarging lymphoid tissue and painless lymphadenopathy are common in about one third of children with abdominal sites of involvement, usually representing a gastrointestinal origin for the disease. Symptoms often include abdominal pain and vomiting, but a palpable mass is not always present. Most children with abdominal symptoms have diffuse, small noncleaved cell NHL (Burkitt or non-Burkitt) of B cell origin. If the tumor recurs, it appears again in the abdomen before distant spread.

The other frequent site of childhood NHL is the chest region. An anterior mediastinal mass, with or without pleural effusion, often is present. If the mass is large enough, respiratory compromise, tracheal compression, and superior vena cava syndrome may arise, which constitutes a medical emergency. Children with anterior mediastinal involvement often are male adolescents and usually have diffuse lymphoblastic lymphoma of T cell origin. This form of diffuse lymphoblastic lymphoma often evolves into extensive bone marrow involvement and is considered to be an overt leukemic phase, therefore referred to as *leukemic transformation*. CNS involvement and testicular infiltration often then occur.

The bone marrow is less common than other primary sites, whereas CNS involvement is common. A relatively small number (10% to 20%) of children with NHL have lymphoid tissue involvement of the head and neck (Waldeyer's ring, nasopharynx, and sinuses). Signs and symptoms include tonsillitis, sinusitis, and a painless nasopharynx mass. In African Burkitt lymphoma, involvement of facial bones, particularly the jaw, is common, although this occurs infrequently in non-African cases.

Evaluation and Treatment

Diagnosis is made by biopsy of disease sites, usually the involved lymph nodes. Other sites of biopsy include the tonsils, bone marrow, spleen, liver, bowel, or skin. Advances in understanding the disease and progress in treatment strategies have meant that most children with NHL are cured of the disease. Optimal treatment is still being developed, but combination chemotherapy, with or without radiation therapy for prevention of CNS involvement, currently is being used successfully (Magrath, 1993). Treatment programs are based on the same four phases used in ALL. Radiation therapy may be combined with chemotherapy in treatment of lymphomatous masses because lymphoma cells are easily destroyed by radiation.

Children with advanced small noncleaved cell lymphoma of the abdomen have the poorest prognoses. Although remission occurs in more than 90% of these children, most experience subsequent relapses. Even in the presence of advanced lymphoblastic lymphoma, however, 60% to 80% of children can be cured. Children with localized disease in more easily treated sites are very likely to be cured with prompt and appropriate treatment. Overall, children with localized disease have a 90% survival rate, and those with advanced disease have a 60% to 70% survival rate (Leventhal & Kato, 1990).

Hodgkin Disease

Although the etiologic agent for **Hodgkin disease,** a lymphoma, has not been identified in children, an infectious mode of transmission has been implicated. Major interest currently concerns viral activity, particularly in light of the association between the Epstein-Barr virus and African Burkitt lymphoma (Leventhal & Donaldson, 1993). Many persons with Hodgkin disease have high Epstein-Barr virus titers. At this time, however, the evidence is not sufficient to link an Epstein-Barr virus infection to Hodgkin disease.

The interest in a viral cause of Hodgkin disease has been supported by epidemiologic studies (Gutensohn & Cole, 1981; Gutensohn & Shapiro, 1982). Childhood factors that might influence the time of exposure to an infectious agent were studied. A striking similarity between the epidemiology of Hodgkin disease in children and the prevaccine era of poliomyelitis gives support to the theory that Hodgkin disease may be the rare consequence of a common infection. Gutensohn (1982) suggested that the pathogenesis of Hodgkin disease in children may be different from that of adults.

Genetic susceptibility also has been suggested. Observations show that siblings have a sevenfold increase in risk, particularly siblings of the same sex. In general, Hodgkin disease is more common in males—in childhood, 60% of all cases occur in males.

Hodgkin disease is rare in childhood. It occurs only infrequently in children younger than 2 years of age, and few cases are observed before the age of 5. A gradual rise in incidence occurs through the age of 11, with a marked increase through adolescence that continues into the thirties. The annual incidence of Hodgkin disease in the United States is 4/1,000,000 in children younger than 15 years of age.

Painless adenopathy in the lower cervical chain, with or without fever, is the most common symptom in children. Mediastinal involvement can cause pressure on the trachea or bronchi, leading to airway obstruction. Extranodal primary sites in Hodgkin disease are rare. Initial symptoms consist of anorexia, malaise, and lassitude. Intermittent fever is present in 30% of children, and weight loss also may accompany these symptoms. Hodgkin disease has a well-defined staging system that considers extent and location of disease and the presence of fever, weight loss, or night sweats at diagnosis. Treatment for Hodgkin disease includes chemotherapy and radiation therapy. For many years the standard chemotherapy was a regimen of *m*echlorethamine, Oncovin (vincristine), *p*rocarbazine, and *p*rednisone (MOPP). However, these drugs can cause permanent sterility. A new drug combination consisting of *A*driamycin (doxorubicin), *b*leomycin, *v*inblastine, and *d*acarbazine (ABVD) has been shown to be superior to MOPP; it is less toxic and requires 6 to 8 months of treatment rather than the traditional 12 months of MOPP treatment. The survival rate for children with Hodgkin disease is very high. Most children are seen initially with limited disease and have a 90% survival rate. Even children who are first seen with advanced disease have a 70% to 80% survival rate (Kornblith et al., 1992).

SUMMARY REVIEW

Fetal and Neonatal Hematopoiesis

1 After 2 weeks' gestation, circulating erythrocytes play a major role in delivering oxygen to the tissues.
2 Erythropoiesis in the liver and, to a lesser extent, in the spleen and lymph nodes reaches a peak at about 4 months.
3 By the fifth month of gestation, hematopoiesis begins to occur in the bone marrow and by the time of delivery it is the only significant site of hematopoiesis.
4 A biochemically distinct type of hemoglobin is synthesized during fetal life, including Gower 1, Gower 2, and Portland.

Postnatal Changes in the Blood

1 Blood cells tend to rise above adult levels at birth and then decline gradually throughout childhood.
2 The immediate rise in blood cell counts is the result of increased hematopoiesis during fetal life, trauma of birth, and cutting of the umbilical cord.

Disorders of Erythrocytes

1 Iron deficiency anemia is the most frequent blood disorder of infancy and childhood; the highest incidence occurs at 6 months and 2 years of age.
2 Hemolytic disease of the newborn (HDN) results from incompatibility between the maternal and the fetal blood, which may involve differences in Rh factors or blood type (ABO). Maternal antibodies enter the fetal circulation and cause hemolysis of fetal erythrocytes. Because the immature liver is unable to conjugate and excrete the excess bilirubin that results from the hemolysis, icterus neonatorum or kernicterus, or both, can develop. Kernicterus also may result from other causes, which causes increased breakdown of red blood cells or decreased liver output of enzymes.
3 Infections of the newborn, often acquired by the mother and transmitted to the infant, may result in hemolytic anemia.
4 Glucose-6-phosphate dehydrogenase (G6PD) deficiency is an inherited enzyme deficiency in erythrocytes that results in a disruption of a common pathway of glycolysis, shortening erythrocyte lifespan to a pathologic state.
5 Hereditary spherocytosis is the most common of the hereditary hemolytic states in which there is no abnormality of hemoglobin. The basic defect is an undefined abnormality of the proteins or spectrins of the erythrocyte membrane in which affected cells are unduly permeable to sodium and acquire a characteristic structure.
6 Sickle cell disease is a genetically determined defect of hemoglobin synthesis, inherited by an autosomal recessive transmission and causing a change in the shape of a red blood cell that results in decreased oxygen or hydration. It is most common among Africans and those of Mediterranean descent.

7 The thalassemias are a heterogenous group of hereditary hypochromic anemias of varying severity. Basic genetic defects include abnormalities of messenger-RNA processing or deletion of genetic materials, resulting in a decrease in the chains for hemoglobin.

Disorders of Coagulation and Platelets

1 Hemophilia is a condition characterized by impairment of the coagulation of blood and subsequent tendency to bleed. The classic disease is hereditary and limited to males, being transmitted through the female to the second generation. Many similar conditions attributable to the absence of various clotting factors are now recognized.

2 Von Willebrand disease is a dominantly inherited disease characterized by a vascular abnormality that produces a prolongation of bleeding time and by decreased levels of clotting factor VIII. The platelets in von Willebrand disease have decreased adhesiveness because the plasma factor is absent.

3 The acquired antibody-mediated hemorrhagic diseases include idiopathic thrombocytopenic purpura (ITP), transient neonatal thrombocytopenia, and autoimmune vascular purpura.

4 ITP, the most common of the childhood thrombocytopenic purpuras, is a disorder of platelet consumption in which antiplatelet antibodies bind to the plasma membranes of platelets. This results in platelet sequestration and destruction by mononuclear phagocytes at a rate that exceeds the ability of the bone marrow to produce them.

5 Transient neonatal thrombocytopenia is an antibody-mediated disorder that occurs in either autoimmune or isoimmune form.

6 The autoimmune vascular purpuras (allergic purpuras) are caused by the body's responses to allergens in the blood.

Leukemia and Lymphoma

1 The childhood leukemias include, in order of their rate of incidence, acute lymphoblastic, acute nonlymphoblastic, and the very rare chronic granulocytic leukemia.

2 Although the cause of childhood leukemia is not known, it is probably the result of multiple interactions between hereditary or genetic predisposition and environmental influences.

3 Acute lymphoblastic leukemia is a potentially curable disease, with more than 60% to 70% of cases cured.

4 The lymphomas of childhood are non-Hodgkin lymphoma and Hodgkin disease.

5 The origin of non-Hodgkin lymphoma is unknown. Factors that have been implicated include defective host immunity, a viral agent, chronic immunostimulation, and genetic predisposition.

6 Non-Hodgkin lymphoma has a favorable prognosis, with a 60% to 80% rate of cure.

7 Hodgkin disease is thought to be caused by a yet unidentified etiologic agent.

8 Hodgkin disease is a readily curable disease with survival statistics similar to those of adults.

KEY TERMS

Activated partial thromboplastin time (PTT), 927
Alpha-thalassemia major, 924
Alpha-thalassemia minor, 924
Alpha trait, 924
Aplastic crisis, 921
Autoimmune vascular purpura (allergic purpura), 929
Beta-thalassemia major (Cooley anemia), 924
Beta-thalassemia minor, 924
Blast cell, 933
Embryonic hemoglobins (Gower 1, Gower 2, and Portland), 910
Fetal hemoglobin (Hb F), 910
Glucose-6-phosphate dehydrogenase (G6PD) deficiency, 912
Hemoglobin H disease, 924
Hemoglobin S (Hb S), 919
Hemolytic disease in the newborn (HDN) (erythroblastosis fetalis), 912

Hemophilia A (classic hemophilia), 926
Hemophilia B (Christmas disease), 926
Hemophilia C (factor XI deficiency), 926
Hereditary spherocytosis, 917
Hodgkin disease, 935
Hydrops fetalis, 915
Hyperbilirubinemia, 915
Hyperhemolytic crisis, 922
Icterus gravis neonatorum, 915
Icterus neonatorum (neonatal jaundice), 915
Idiopathic thrombocytopenic purpura (ITP) (autoimmune, or primary, thrombocytopenic purpura), 928
Isoimmune thrombocytopenic purpura (IITP), 929
Kernicterus, 915

Non-Hodgkin lymphoma (NHL), 934
Prothrombin consumption time, 927
Prothrombin time, 927
Sequestration crisis, 921
Sickle cell anemia, 919
Sickle cell disease, 919
Sickle cell–Hb C disease, 919
Sickle cell–thalassemia, 919
Sickle cell trait, 919
Thalassemia, 923
Thrombin time, 927
Thromboplastin generation, 927
Transient neonatal thrombocytopenia, 928
Vasoocclusive crisis (thrombotic crisis), 921
von Willebrand disease, 926

REFERENCES

Albin, A. R., Kushner, J. H., Murphy, A., & Zippin, C. (1961). Platelet enumeration in the neonatal period. *Pediatrics, 28,* 822.

American Cancer Society (ACS). (1993). *Cancer facts and figures 1993.* New York: American Cancer Society.

Armbrust, R., Eber, S. W., & Schroter, W. (1992). Absence of phosphorylation-induced gelation of erythrocyte membrane skeletons: A diagnostic tool for hereditary spherocytosis. *Annals of Hematology, 64*(2), 93-96.

Baverstam, U., & Holmberg, M. (1989). Are low doses of radiation leukemogenic in children. *Leukemia Research, 13*(7), 515-517.

Behrman, R., Kliegman, R., Nelson, W., & Vaughan, V., III. (Eds.). (1992). *Nelson textbook of pediatrics.* Philadelphia: W. B. Saunders.

Bennett, J., Catovsky, D., Daniel, M., Flandrin, G., Galton, D. A. G., Gralnick, H. R., Sultan, C., & The French-American-British (FAB) Cooperative Group. (1981). French-American-British (FAB) Cooperative Group: The morphological classification of acute lymphoblastic leukaemia—Concordance among observers and clinical correlations. *British Journal of Haematology, 47,* 553-561.

Beral, B., Peterman, T., & Berkelman, R. (1991). AIDS-associated non-Hodgkin's lymphoma. *Lancet, 337,* 805-809.

Bleyer, W. A. (1990). The impact of childhood cancer on the United States and the world. *CA: A Cancer Journal for Clinicians, 40,* 355-367.

Buckley, J. D., Lampkin, B. C., Nesbit, M. E., Bernstein, I. D., Feig, S. A., Kersey, J. H., Piomelli, S., Kim, T., & Hammond, G. D. (1989). Remission induction in children with acute nonlymphocyte leukemia using cytosine arabinoside and doxorubicin or daunorubicin: A report from the Children's Cancer Study Group. *Medicine and Pediatric Oncology, 17,* 382-390.

Caramihai, E., Karayaclin, G., Aballi, A. J., & Lanzkowsky, P. (1975). Leukocyte count differences in healthy white and black children. *Journal of Pediatrics, 86,* 252.

Crist, W., Boyett, J., Pullen, J., Van Eys, J., & Vietti, T. (1986). Clinical and biological features predict poor prognosis. *Medicine and Pediatric Oncology, 13,* 135-139.

Cunningham, A. S. (1975). Eosinophil counts—Age and sex differences. *Journal of Pediatrics, 87,* 426.

Delauney, J., Alloisio, N., Morle, L., & Baklouti, F. (1991). The genetic disorders of the red cell skeleton. *Nouvelle Revue Francaise D Hematologie (Heidelberg), 33*(2), 63-70.

Drake, M. A. (1992). The nutritional status and dietary adequacy of single homeless women and their children in shelters. *Public Health Reports, 107*(3), 312-319.

Furie, B., & Furie, B. C. (1992). Molecular and cellular biology of blood coagulation. *New England Journal of Medicine, 326*(12), 800-806.

Gibble, J. W., & Ness, P. M. (1992). Maternal immunity to red cell antigens and fetal transfusion. *Clinical Laboratory Medicine, 12*(3), 553-576.

Gibson, R. W., Bross, I., Graham, S., Lilienfield, A. M., Schuman, L. M., Levin, M. L., & Dowd, J. E. (1968). Leukemia in children exposed to multiple risk factors. *New England Journal of Medicine, 279,* 906-909.

Grier, H. E., Gelber, R. D., Camitta, B. M., Delorey, M. J., Link, M. P., Prince, K. N., Leavitt, P. R., & Weinstein, H. G. (1987). Prognostic factors in childhood acute myelogenous leukemia. *Journal of Clinical Oncology, 5,* 1026-1032.

Grier, H., & Weinstein, H. (1985). Acute nonlymphocytic leukemia. *Pediatric Clinics of North America, 32,* 653-668.

Grier, H., & Weinstein, H. (1993). Acute myelogenous leukemia. In P. A. Pizzo & D. G. Poplack (Eds.), *Principles and practices of pediatric oncology* (2nd ed.). Philadelphia: J. B. Lippincott.

Gutensohn, N. (1982). Social class and age at diagnosis of Hodgkin's disease: New epidemiologic evidence for the "two-disease hypothesis." *Cancer Treatment Report, 66,* 689-695.

Gutensohn, N., & Cole, P. (1981). Childhood social environment and Hodgkin's disease. *New England Journal of Medicine, 304,* 135-140.

Gutensohn, N., & Shapiro, D. (1982). Social class risk factors among children with Hodgkin's disease. *Internal Journal of Cancer, 30,* 433-435.

Guy, G. P., Baxi, L. V., Hurlet-Jensen, A., & Chao, C. R. (1992). An unusual complication in a gravida with factor IX deficiency: Case report with review of the literature. *Obstetrics and Gynecology, 80*(3, Pt. 2), 502-505.

Harvey, E. G., Boice, J. D., & Honeyman, M. (1985). Prenatal x-ray exposure and childhood cancer in twins. *New England Journal of Medicine, 312,* 531-545.

Henshaw, D. L., Eatough, J. P., & Richardson, R. B. (1990). Radon as a causative factor in induction of myeloid leukemia and other cancers. *Lancet, 355,* 100-112.

Israel, M. A. (1993). Cancer cell biology. In P. A. Pizzo & D. G. Poplack (Eds.), *Principles and practices of pediatric oncology* (2nd ed.). Philadelphia: J. B. Lippincott.

Karpatkin, S. (1981). Autoimmune thrombocytopenic purpura. *Blood, 56,* 329-333.

Kelley, V. S. (1983). *Practice of pediatrics* (vol. 5). New York: Harper & Row.

Kornblith, A. B., Anderson, J., Cella, D. F., Tross, S., Zuckerman, E., Cherin, E., Henderson, E. S., Canellos, G. P., Kosty, M. P., Cooper, M. R., Weiss, R. B., Gottlieb, A. (deceased), & Holland, J. C. (1992). Comparison of psychosocial adaptation and sexual function of survivors of advanced Hodgkin disease treated by MOPP, ABVD, or MOPP alternating with ABVD. *Cancer, 70*(10), 2508-2516.

Krischer, J. P., Steuber, C. P., Vietti, T. J., Culbert, S. J., Fagab, A. H., Morgan, S. K., Berry, D. H., Hvizdala, E., Thomas, P. J., Land, V. J., & Castleberry, R. P. (1989). Long-term results in the treatment of acute nonlymphocytic leukemia: A Pediatric Oncology Group Study. *Medicine and Pediatric Oncology, 17,* 401-408.

Lagakos, S. W., Wessen, B. J., & Zelen, M. (1986). An analysis of contaminated well water and health effects in Woburn, Massachusetts. *Journal of the American Statistical Association, 81,* 583-596.

Lee, G. R., Bithell, T. C., Foerster, J., Athens, J. W., & Lukens, J. N. (Eds.). *Wintrobe's clinical hematology* (9th ed.). Philadelphia: Lea & Febiger.

Leventhal, B., & Donaldson, S. (1993). Hodgkin's disease. In P.A. Pizzo & D.G. Poplack (Eds.), *Principles and practices of pediatric oncology* (2nd ed.). Philadelphia: Lippincott.

Leventhal, B., & Kato, G. (1990). Childhood Hodgkin and non-Hodgkin lymphoma. *Pediatric Review, 12,* 171-179.

Lightsey, A. L., & Koenig, H. M. (1979). Platelet associated immunoglobulin G in childhood idiopathic thrombocytopenic purpura. *Journal of Pediatrics, 94,* 20-22.

Link, M. (1985). Non-Hodgkin's lymphoma in children. *Pediatric Clinics of North America, 32,* 699-720.

Magrath, I. T. (1987). Malignant non-Hodgkin's lymphoma in children. *Hematology and Oncology Clinics of North America, 1,* 577-603.

Magrath, I. T. (1993). Malignant non-Hodgkin's lymphomas in children. In P. A. Pizzo & D. G. Poplack (Eds.), *Principles and practices of pediatric oncology* (2nd ed.). Philadelphia: Lippincott.

Manroe, B. L., Weinberg, A. G., Rosenfeld, C. R., & Browne, R. (1979). The neonatal blood count in health and disease. Reference values for neutrophilic cells. *Journal of Pediatrics, 95,* 89-98.

Massey, A. C. (1992). Microcytic anemia. Differential diagnosis and management of iron deficiency anemia. *Medical Clinics of North America, 76*(3), 549-566.

Mauer, A. M. (1969). *Pediatric hematology.* New York: McGraw-Hill.

Miale, J. B. (1982). *Laboratory medicine: Hematology* (6th ed.). St. Louis: Mosby—Year Book.

Miller, R. W. (1967). Persons with exceptionally high risk of leukemia. *Cancer Research, 27,* 2420.

Miller, R. W. (1963). Down's syndrome (mongolism), other congenital malformations, and cancers among the siblings of leukemic children. *New England Journal of Medicine, 268*(8), 393-401.

Mulvihill, J. (1993). Childhood cancer, the environment, and heredity. In P. A. Pizzo & D. G. Poplack (Eds.), *Principles and practices of pediatric oncology* (2nd ed.). Philadelphia: Lippincott.

Murray, R., Heckel, P., & Hempelmann, L. (1959). Leukemia in children exposed to ionizing radiation. *New England Journal of Medicine, 261,* 585-589.

National Academy of Sciences. (1980). *Biological effects of atomic radiation.* Washington, DC: National Research Council.

Pendergrass, T. (1985). Epidemiology of ALL. *Seminars in Oncology, 12*(2), 80-91.

Pool, R. (1990). Is there an EMF-cancer connection? *Science, 249,* 1096-1098.

Poplack, D. G. (1993). Acute lymphoblastic leukemia. In P. A. Pizzo & D. G. Poplack (Eds.), *Principles and practices of pediatric oncology* (2nd ed.). Philadelphia: Lippincott.

Prasad, A. N., & Prasad, C. (1991). Iron deficiency; non-hematological manifestations. *Progress in Food and Nutrition Science, 15*(4), 255-283.

Raven, P. H., & Johnson, G. B. (1993). *Biology* (3rd ed.). Boston: Little, Brown.

Reitz, M., Jr., Robert-Guroff, M., Kalyanaraman, V., Sarngadharan, M. G., Sarin, P., Popovic, M., & Gallo, R. C. (1984). A retrovirus associated with human adult T-cell leukemia-lymphoma. In I. Magrath, G. O'Conor, & B. Ramot (Eds.), *Pathogenesis of leukemia and lymphomas: Environmental influences.* New York: Raven Press.

Roberts, H. R. (1991). Factor VIII replacement therapy. Issues and future prospects. *Annals of the New York Academy of Science, 614,* 106-113.

Savitz, D. A., John, E. M., & Kleckner, R. C. (1990). Magnetic field exposure from electrical appliances and childhood cancer. *American Journal of Epidemiology, 131,* 763-772.

Savitz, D. A., Wachtel, H., & Barnes, F. (1987) Case-control study of childhood cancer and electromagnetic field exposure. *American Journal of Epidemiology, 126,* 780-783.

Simons, S. M., Main, C. A., & Yarsh, H. M. (1975). Idiopathic thrombocytopenic purpura in children. *Journal of Pediatrics, 293,* 531-535.

Steingart, R. (1992). Management of patients with sickle cell disease. *Medical Clinics of North America, 76*(3), 669-682.

Weiss, H. J. (1975). Platelet physiology and abnormalities of platelet function. *Journal of Medicine, 293,* 531-535.

Wertheimer, D., & Leeper, E. (1979). Electrical wiring configuration and childhood cancer. *American Journal of Epidemiology, 109,* 270-284.

White, G. C., II, & Shoemaker, C. B. (1989). Factor VIII gene and hemophilia A. *Blood, 73,* 1-12.

SUGGESTED READINGS

Miller, D. R., Baehner, R. L., & Miller, L. P. (Eds.). (1990). *Blood disorders of infancy and childhood* (6th ed.). St. Louis: Mosby—Year Book.

Rote, N. S. (1982). Pathophysiology of Rh isoimmunization. *Clinical Obstetrics and Gynecology, 25,* 243-254.

Whaley, L. F. & Wong, D. L. (1991). *Nursing care of infants and children* (4th ed.). St. Louis: Mosby—Year Book.

UNIT IX

The Cardiovascular and Lymphatic Systems

THE HEART'S ROLE was questioned by ancient societies. For example, the Egyptians attributed breathing to the heart, whereas the ancient Chinese connected the action of the heart to the pulse. The *Nei Ching*, a collection of Chinese medical writings, reported that all the blood was under the control of the heart and that the heart was the seat of happiness. The Greeks thought of the heart as the region in the body in which thinking originated.

The works of the renowned Greek physician, Galen (ca AD 129 to 200), survived for nearly 1500 years as the "unimpeachable authority on medicine." Galen thought blood was pro-duced in the liver, where it received "natural spirit" and from which it was pulled to the periphery of the body by some attractive force. When he first looked at the heart in the second century AD, Galen noted that the sides of the heart did not contract simultaneously, as he thought a pump should. Galen concluded that blood was displaced from the right to the left chambers of the heart through tiny pores in the membrane that separated the chambers. He believed that the arterial and venous circulatory systems were joined by these pores.

Galen's theories finally collapsed when William Harvey (1578-1657), an Englishman,

HEART AND ARTERIES

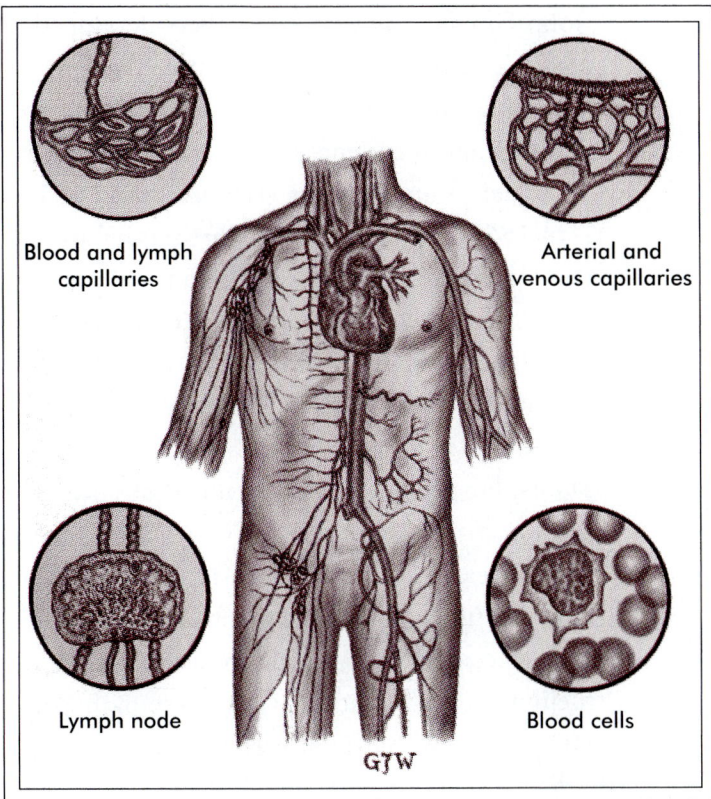

Blood and lymph capillaries

Arterial and venous capillaries

Lymph node

Blood cells

GJW

Atlas of human anatomy and physiology.
(Redrawn from Tuner, William, & Goodsir, 1857; courtesy National Library of Medicine.)

published his studies on circulation. Harvey's writings were based on dissection of cadavers and physiologic experiments performed on animals. He showed that the heart pumped blood continuously and that the veins returned the blood to the heart. Observing that both ventricles of the heart contracted and expanded together, Harvey concluded that there was no pressure difference between these chambers to drive blood through the thick membrane that separated them. He also noted that when the heart was removed from an animal, it continued to contract and expand like a muscle. This demonstrated that the heart was an independent pump and not just an organ that sucked in blood. Harvey's achievement became the foundation of modern cardiovascular physiology.

Thomas Wharton (1614-1673) described the distinguishing characteristics of the lymphatic

glands. He denied the old and persistent idea that the brain was a gland that secreted mucus, yet he continued to believe that tears came from the brain. He recognized that there were ductless glands (now called endocrine glands), whose secretions entered the blood, and ductile glands, whose secretions were discharged into cavities (exocrine glands). In 1661, Niels Steensen made the distinction between the exocrine glands and the lymph nodes. He also disproved the idea that tears originated in the brain.

In 1733, more than 100 years after Harvey's work was published, Stephan Hales (1677-1761), a clergyman, made the first blood pressure measurements. He inserted a hollow tube into the neck artery of a horse and was surprised to see the blood rise 9 feet in a glass column. In the middle of the nineteenth century, Harry Goldblatt, R. Tigerstedt, P. G. Bergman, and others first showed that blood pressure could be affected by a substance thought to be from the kidney. A little later, intensive studies by researchers, including G. W. Pickering, M. Prinzmetal, I. Page, and D. van-Slyke, revealed the existence of a complex enzymatic hormonal mechanism of blood pressure regulation involving the adrenal glands, kidneys, and nervous system.

In the early twentieth century a Dutch physicist, Willem Einthoven, invented the string galvanometer, an instrument to measure electric circuits. This instrument was the forerunner of the electrocardiogram. By the end of World War I, the string galvanometer and its applications had been developed by Englishman Thomas Lewis, establishing the science of electrocardiography.

In 1929, Weiner Forssmann, a young intern in a German hospital, worked out a technique for emergency injection of drugs directly into the heart. While looking into a mirror and standing behind a fluoroscopic screen, he threaded a thin catheter into his own arm vein, through the venous channels, and into his heart. Dangerous as the procedure was, it had been performed 15 years earlier by three other researchers without the aid of x-rays. Forssmann, along with A. Cournand and D. W. Richards, Jr., received the Nobel Prize in 1956 for developing the procedure of intracardiac catheterization.

Until midcentury, surgical repair of congenital heart defects and malarrangements of the large blood vessels was performed entirely by feel, since the heart could not be stopped during surgery. In 1939, Robert Gross reported the first successful cure of a congenital heart anomaly. After 19 years of experimentation, John Gibbon, his wife, and others developed a heart-lung machine that could take over the pumping function of the heart during surgery. This advancement enabled Gibbon to repair a heart defect under direct visualization in 1953.

In 1967, in South Africa, Christiaan Barnard performed the first heart transplantation in a human being. In 1969, Denton Cooley and his colleagues used an artificial heart to keep a person alive for 2½ days to await the transplantation of a living heart. Most heart transplants, however, occurred in the 1980s with 85% occurring since 1985. Today, cardiovascular research includes signalling systems in vascular tissue, metabolism and its interaction with electrophysiology, and injury to the endothelium as the initiating event in the pathogenesis of cardiovascular disease.

CHAPTER 26

Structure and Function of the Cardiovascular and Lymphatic Systems

Kathryn L. McCance
Stephanie J. Richardson

Chapter Outline

943

he function of the circulatory system is quite simple: to deliver oxygen, nutrients, and other substances to all of the body's cells and to remove the waste products of cellular metabolism. Delivery and removal are achieved by a wonderfully complex array of tubing—the blood vessels—connected to a pump—the heart. The heart pumps blood continuously through the blood vessels with cooperation from other systems, particularly the nervous and endocrine systems, which are intrinsic regulators of the heart and blood vessels. Nutrients and oxygen are supplied by the digestive and respiratory systems; gaseous wastes of cellular metabolism are blown off by the lungs; and other wastes are removed by the kidneys.

THE CIRCULATORY SYSTEM

The heart pumps blood through two separate circulatory systems, one to the lungs and one to all other parts of the body. Structures on the right side of the heart, or **right heart,** pump blood through the lungs. (This system, termed the **pulmonary circulation,** is described in Chapter 29.) The left side of the heart, or **left heart,** sends blood throughout the **systemic circulation,** which supplies all of the body except the lungs (Fig. 26-1). These two systems are serially connected; thus the output of one becomes the input of the other.

Arteries carry blood flow from the heart to all parts of the body, where they branch into even smaller vessels until they become a fine meshwork of capillaries. Capillaries allow the closest contact and exchange between the blood and the interstitial space, or interstitium—the environment in which the cells live. Veins channel blood flow from capillaries in all parts of the body back to the heart. The plasma passes through the walls of the capillaries into the interstitial space. This fluid is eventually returned to the cardiovascular system by vessels of the lymphatic system.

THE HEART

The adult heart weighs less than 1 pound and is about the size of a fist. It lies obliquely (diagonally) in the **mediastinum,** an area above the diaphragm and between the lungs.

Heart structures can be described with respect to three general categories of function: (1) structural support of heart tissues and circulation of pulmonary and systemic blood through the heart; (2) maintenance of

heart cells; and (3) stimulation and control of heart action. Included in the first category are the heart wall and fibrous skeleton, which enclose and support the heart and divide it into four heart chambers: the valves that direct flow through the chambers, and the great vessels that conduct blood to and from the heart. The second category comprises vessels of the coronary circulation—the arteries and veins that serve the metabolic needs of all the heart's cells, particularly its muscle cells. Also included in the second category are the lymphatic vessels of the heart. The third category of structures, those responsible for heart action, consists of the nerves and specialized muscle cells that direct the rhythmic contraction and relaxation of the heart muscles, which propel blood throughout the pulmonary and systemic circulatory systems.

Structures That Direct Circulation Through the Heart
The Heart Wall

The heart wall has three layers—the pericardium, myocardium, and endocardium. The **pericardium** is a double-walled membranous sac that encloses the heart (Fig. 26-2). The pericardium has several functions. It (1) prevents displacement of the heart during gravitational acceleration or deceleration, (2) is a physical barrier that protects the heart against infection and inflammation from the lungs and pleural space, and (3) contains pain receptors and mechanoreceptors that can elicit reflex changes in blood pressure and heart rate. The outer layer of the pericardium, the **parietal pericardium,** is composed of a surface layer of mesothelium over a thin layer of connective tissue. The **visceral pericardium,** or epicardium, is the inner layer of the pericardium. At one point, the visceral pericardium folds back and becomes continuous with parietal pericardium, allowing the large vessels to enter and leave the heart without breaching the pericardial layers.

The visceral and parietal pericardia are separated by a fluid-containing space called the **pericardial cavity.** The **pericardial fluid** (10 to 30 ml), which is secreted by cells of the mesothelium, lubricates the membranes that line the pericardial cavity, enabling them to slide over one another with a minimum of friction as the heart beats. The amount and character of the pericardial fluid are altered by inflammation of the pericardium (see Chapter 27).

The thickest layer of the heart wall, the **myocardium,** is composed of cardiac muscle and is anchored to the heart's fibrous skeleton. The thickness of the myocardium varies tremendously from one heart chamber to another. Thickness is related to the amount of resistance the muscle must overcome to pump blood from the different chambers. The internal lining of the myocardium

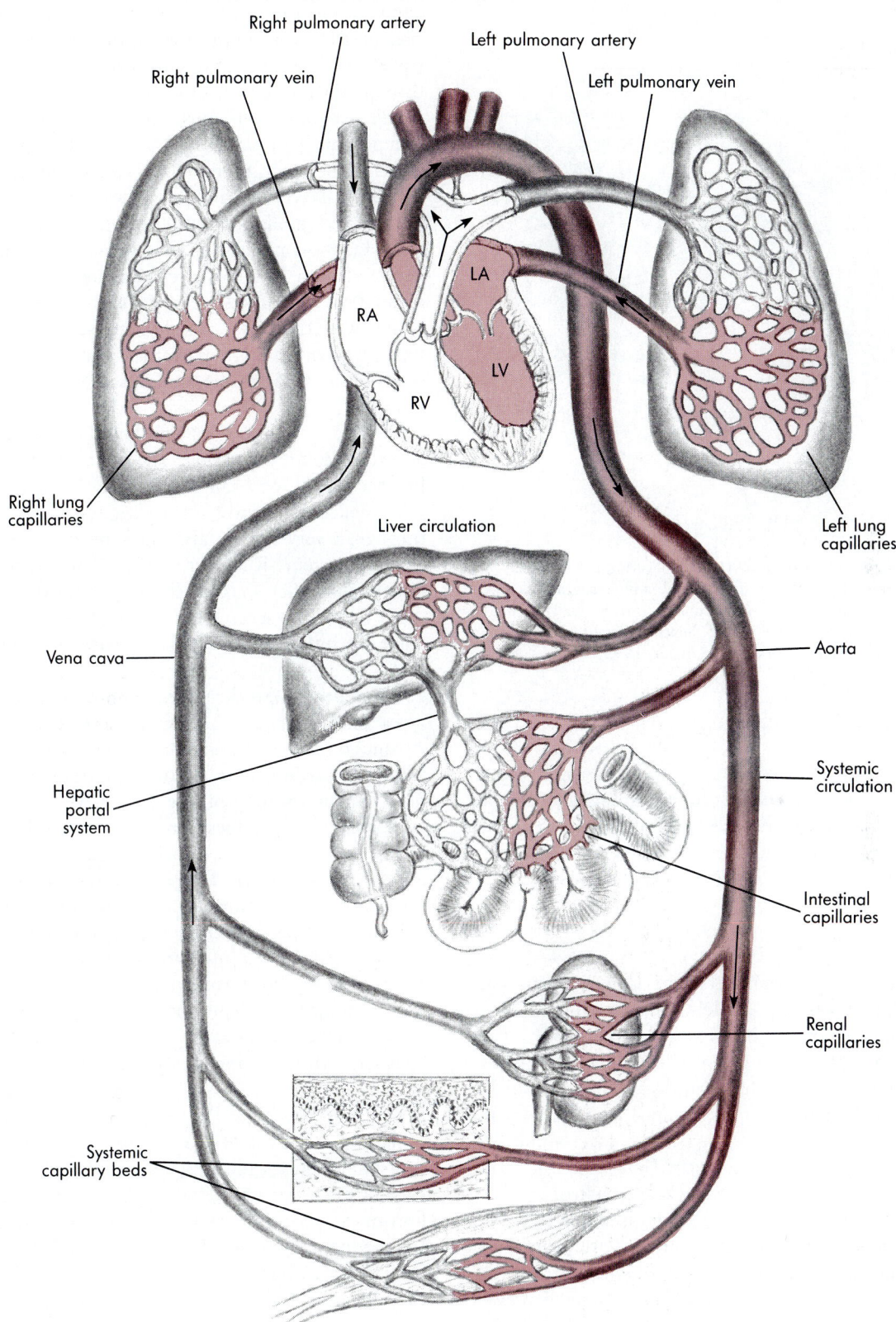

FIG. 26-1 **Diagram showing serially connected pulmonary and systemic circulatory systems.** Right heart chambers propel unoxygenated blood through pulmonary circulation, while left heart propels oxygenated blood through systemic circulation.

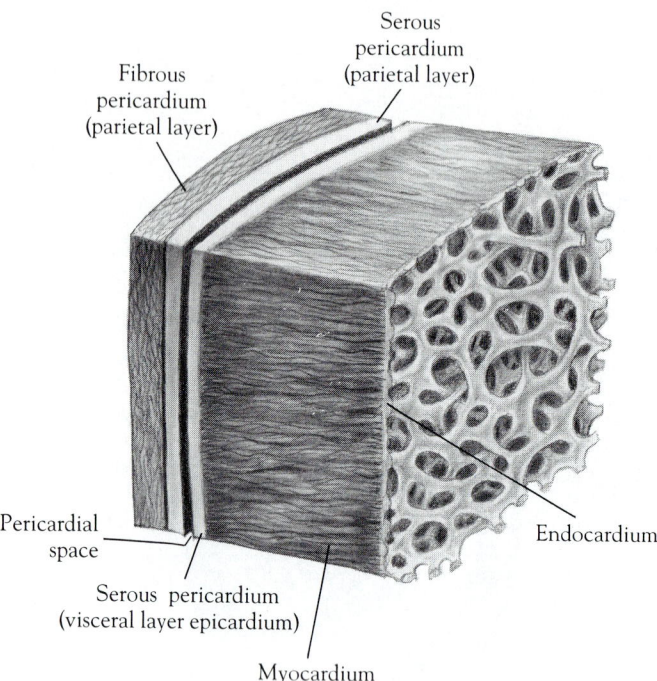

Serous
pericardium
(parietal layer)

Fibrous
pericardium
(parietal layer)

Pericardial
space

Serous pericardium
(visceral layer epicardium)

Myocardium

Endocardium

FIG. 26-2 Cross section of heart walls. Section through wall of heart, showing pericardium (outer sac), myocardium (cardiac muscle), and endocardium (inner lining). Heart wall encloses chambers (atria and ventricle) of left heart and right heart. (From Thompson, McFarland, Hirsch, & Tucker, 1993.)

is composed of connective tissue and a layer of squamous cells called the **endocardium** (see Fig. 26-2). The endocardial lining of the heart is continuous with the endothelium that lines all the arteries, veins, and capillaries of the body, creating a continuous, closed circulatory system.

Chambers of the Heart

The heart has four chambers, the **right atrium, left atrium, right ventricle,** and **left ventricle.** (Blood flow through these chambers is illustrated in Fig. 26-3.) The atria are smaller than the ventricles and have thinner walls. The wall of the right atrium is about 2 mm thick, and that of the left atrium is about 3 to 5 mm thick. The ventricles have a thicker myocardial layer and comprise much of the bulk of the heart. The wall of the right ventricle is about 3 to 5 mm thick and that of the left ventricle, the most muscular chamber, is about 13 to 15 mm. It is now known that the ventricles are formed by a continuum of muscle fibers that take origin from the fibrous skeleton at the base of the heart (Berne & Levy, 1992).

The myocardial thickness of each cardiac chamber depends on the amount of pressure or resistance it must overcome to eject blood. The two atria have the thinnest walls because they are low-pressure chambers that

serve as storage units and conduits for blood that is emptied into the ventricles. Normally, there is little resistance to flow from the atria to the ventricles. The ventricles, on the other hand, must propel blood all the way through the pulmonary or systemic circulation. The ventricular myocardium must also be strong enough to pump against pressures in the pulmonary or systemic vessels. The mean pulmonary capillary pressure that is the major force favoring movement of fluid out of the pulmonary capillaries into the interstitium is only 15 mm Hg. By comparison, the mean arterial pressure is about 92 mm Hg. Pressure is greatest in the systemic circulation, which is driven by the left ventricle. This explains why the left ventricle's myocardium is several times thicker than that of the right ventricle, which sends blood through the low-pressure pulmonary circulation.

The shapes of the right and left ventricles also differ according to their function. The right ventricle is shaped like a crescent, or triangle, enabling its bellowslike action, which efficiently ejects large volumes of blood through a very small valve into the low-pressure pulmonary system (Rushmer, 1976). The left ventricle is larger and bullet shaped. Its shape and thick myocardium help it to eject blood through a relatively large valve opening into the high-pressure systemic circulation.

The ventricles are structurally more complex than the atria. Each ventricle contains muscle fibers that divide it roughly into an **inflow tract,** which receives blood from the atrium, and an **outflow tract,** which sends blood to the circulation (see Fig. 26-3).

Normally, blood does not flow between the chambers of the right side of the heart and the chambers of the left side of the heart. The adult right and left sides of the heart are separated by an intact septal membrane. The atria are separated by the interatrial septum, and the ventricles by the interventricular septum. The interventricular septum is an extension of the fibrous skeleton of the heart. Indentations of the endocardium form valves that separate the atria from the ventricles and the ventricles from the aorta and pulmonary arteries.

Fibrous Skeleton of the Heart

Four rings of dense fibrous connective tissue provide a firm anchorage for the attachments of the atrial and ventricular musculature, as well as the valvular tissue. The fibrous rings are adjacent and form a central, fibrous supporting structure collectively termed the annuli fibrosi cordis. The fibrous rings serve as attachments for the four heart valves (Fig. 26-4).

Valves of the Heart

One-way blood flow through the heart is ensured by the four heart valves. During ventricular relaxation the two **atrioventricular valves** open and blood flows from the

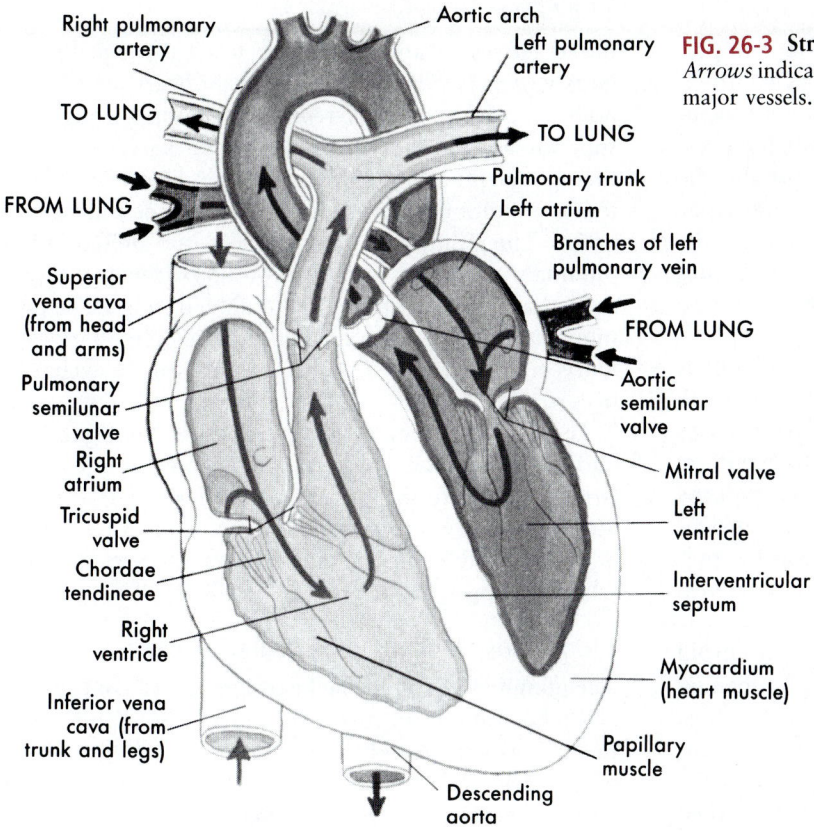

Right pulmonary artery

Aortic arch

Left pulmonary artery

TO LUNG

TO LUNG

FROM LUNG

Pulmonary trunk

Left atrium

Branches of left pulmonary vein

Superior vena cava (from head and arms)

FROM LUNG

Aortic semilunar valve

Pulmonary semilunar valve

Right atrium

Mitral valve

Tricuspid valve

Left ventricle

Chordae tendineae

Interventricular septum

Right ventricle

Myocardium (heart muscle)

Inferior vena cava (from trunk and legs)

Papillary muscle

Descending aorta

FIG. 26-3 **Structures that direct blood flow through the heart.** *Arrows* indicate path of blood flow through chambers, valves, and major vessels. (From Thibodeau, 1987.)

Pulmonary artery

Pulmonary semilunar valve

Aortic semilunar valve

Opening of coronary artery

Coronary artery

Aorta

Left ventricle

Right ventricle

Left fibrous ring

Right fibrous ring

Mitral valve

Tricuspid valve

FIG. 26-4 **Fibrous skeleton and valves of heart.** Fibrous rings serve as attachments for all of the heart's valves. Two atrioventricular valves, mitral and tricuspid, separate atria from ventricles, while pulmonic and aortic semilunar valves separate ventricles from their receiving vessels, pulmonary artery, and aorta, respectively. (From Thibodeau, 1987.)

higher pressure atria to the relaxed ventricles. With in-creasing ventricular pressure these valves close and pre-vent backflow into the atria as the ventricles contract. The **semilunar valves** of the heart open when intraven-tricular pressure exceeds aortic and pulmonary pres-sures and blood flows out of the ventricles and into the pulmonary and systemic circulations. After ventricular contraction and ejection, intraventricular pressure falls and the **pulmonic** and **aortic semilunar valves** close, pre-venting backflow into the right and left ventricle (see Figs. 26-3 and 26-4).

The openings of the heart valves are guarded by flaps of tissue called leaflets or cusps. The cusps of the atrio-ventricular valves are attached to the papillary muscles by the **chordae tendineae** (see Fig. 26-3). The **papillary muscles** are extensions of the myocardium that pull the cusps together and downward at the onset of ventricu-lar contraction, thus preventing their backward expul-sion into the atria. (See p. 949 for a description of pres-sure changes and valvular function.)

The right atrioventricular valve is called the **tricuspid valve** because it has three cusps. The tricuspid opening (orifice) has the largest diameter of all the heart valves. The three cusps are unequal in size. The left atrioven-tricular valve is a bicuspid (two-cusp) valve called the **mitral valve.** The mitral valve resembles a cone-shaped funnel that extends into the cusps, which are connected by a fibrous tissue called the commissure. The anterior cusp of the mitral valve is continuous with supporting tissues of the aortic semilunar valve cusps and the left coronary valve cusps. (The coronary circulation is de-scribed on p. 952). Thus, damage to this continuous tis-sue can alter function of both the aortic and mitral valves.

The tricuspid and mitral valves function as a unit be-cause the atrium, fibrous rings, valvular tissue, chordae tendineae, papillary muscles, and ventricular walls are connected. Collectively, these six structures are known as the **mitral and tricuspid complex.** Damage to any one of the complex's six components can alter function sig-nificantly.

Blood leaves the right ventricle through the pulmonic semilunar valve, and it leaves the left ventricle through the aortic semilunar valve (see Figs. 26-3 and 26-4). Both the pulmonic and aortic semilunar valves have three cup-shaped cusps that arise from the fibrous skel-eton. The pulmonic cusps are slightly thinner than the aortic cusps. The lower edges of each cusp are sus-pended from the root of the pulmonary artery or aorta, with the upper valve edges freely projecting into the ves-sel lumen. When the ventricles contract, the cusps be-have like one-way swinging doors. The force of the blood propels the cusps outward against the vessel wall. When the ventricles relax, blood fills the cusps and causes their free edges to meet in the middle of the ves-sel, closing the valve and preventing any backflow.

The Great Vessels

Blood moves in and out of the heart through several large vessels (see Fig. 26-3). The right heart receives ve-nous blood from the systemic circulation through the **superior** and **inferior venae cavae.** These vessels enter the right atrium. Blood leaves the right ventricle and en-ters the pulmonary circulation through the **pulmonary artery.** The pulmonary artery divides into **right** and **left pulmonary arteries** to transport unoxygenated blood from the right heart to the right and left lungs. The pul-monary arteries branch further into the pulmonary cap-illary bed, where oxygen and carbon dioxide exchange occurs.

The four **pulmonary veins,** two from the right lung and two from the left lung, carry oxygenated blood from the lungs to the left side of the heart. The oxygen-ated blood moves through the left atrium and ventricle and out into the **aorta,** which delivers it to systemic ves-sels that supply the body.

Blood Flow During the Cardiac Cycle

The pumping action of the heart consists of contraction and relaxation of the myocardial layer of the heart wall. Each contraction, and the relaxation that follows it, is one **cardiac cycle.** (Blood flow through the heart during a single cardiac cycle is illustrated in Fig. 26-5.) During relaxation, termed **diastole,** blood fills the ventricles. The contraction that follows, termed **systole,** propels the blood out of the ventricles and into the circulation. Con-traction of the left ventricle is slightly earlier than con-traction of the right ventricle.

During diastole, blood from the veins of the systemic circulation enters the thin-walled right atrium from the superior vena cava and the inferior vena cava (see Figs. 26-3 and 26-5). Venous blood from the coronary circu-lation enters the right atrium through the coronary si-nus. The right atrium fills and distends, pushing open the right atrioventricular (tricuspid) valve. This permits blood to fill the right ventricle. The same sequence of events occurs a split second earlier in the left heart. The four pulmonary veins, two from the right lung and two from the left lung, carry blood from the pulmonary cir-culation to the left atrium. As the left atrium fills, it pushes the cusps of the mitral valve open, and blood flows into the left ventricle. Left atrial contraction, "atrial kick," provides a significant increase of blood to the left ventricle. Filling of the right and left sides of the heart occurs during one period of diastole.

Four phases of the cardiac cycle can be identified on initiation of ventricular myocardial contraction (Fig. 26-6).

Phase 1: Systole begins with "isovolumic contrac-tion," so called because ventricular volume is con-stant, i.e., the lengths of the muscle fibers remain relatively constant. Isovolumic contraction is the first detectable rise in left ventricular pressure. Con-

A

B

FIG. 26-5 **Blood flow through the heart during a single cardiac cycle. A,** During diastole, blood flows into atria, atrioventricular valves are pushed open, and blood begins to fill ventricles. Atrial systole *(center)* squeezes any blood remaining in atria out into ventricles. **B,** During ventricular systole *(right),* ventricles contract, pushing blood out through semilunar valves into pulmonary artery (right ventricle) and aorta (left ventricle).

FIG. 26-6 **Major phases of cardiac cycle.** Schematic at top shows four major phases of cardiac cycle. Left atrial, aortic, and left ventricular pressure pulses correlated in time with aortic flow, ventricular volume, heart sounds, venous pulse, and electrocardiogram for a complete cardiac cycle in the dog. (From Berne & Levy, 1992.)

traction pushes the atrioventricular valves shut. Their cusps bulge backward but are prevented from opening back into the atria by their anchors, the chordae tendineae (see Fig. 26-3).

Phase 2: When left ventricular pressure reaches that of the aorta, the aortic valve opens and ventricular ejection occurs. Intraventricular pressure and ventricular volume decrease rapidly.

Phase 3: With left ventricular relaxation and ventricular pressure decreases, the aortic valve closes and "isovolumic relaxation" occurs.

Phase 4: When sufficient decreases exist in left ventricular pressure, the mitral valve opens and ventricular filling from the atrium occurs.

The ventricle fills rapidly in early diastole and again in late diastole when the atrium contracts. As blood is pushed through the inflow and outflow tracts of the ventricles, it flows around the **crista supraventricularis**— the muscle that separates the inflow from the outflow tracts—and is mixed by passing through the strands of the **trabeculae carneae.** Expulsion of blood from the ventricles marks the end of one cardiac cycle.

Normal Intracardiac Pressures

Normal intracardiac pressures are shown in Table 26-1 and Figs. 26-6 and 26-7. Atrial pressure curves are composed of the **a wave,** which is generated by atrial contraction, and the **v wave,** which is an early diastolic peak

TABLE 26-1

Normal Intracardiac Pressures

	Mean (mm Hg)	Range (mm Hg)
Right atrium	4	0-8
Right ventricle		
Systolic	24	15-28
End-diastolic	4	0-8
Left atrium	7	4-12
Left ventricle		
Systolic	130	90-140
End-diastolic	7	4-12

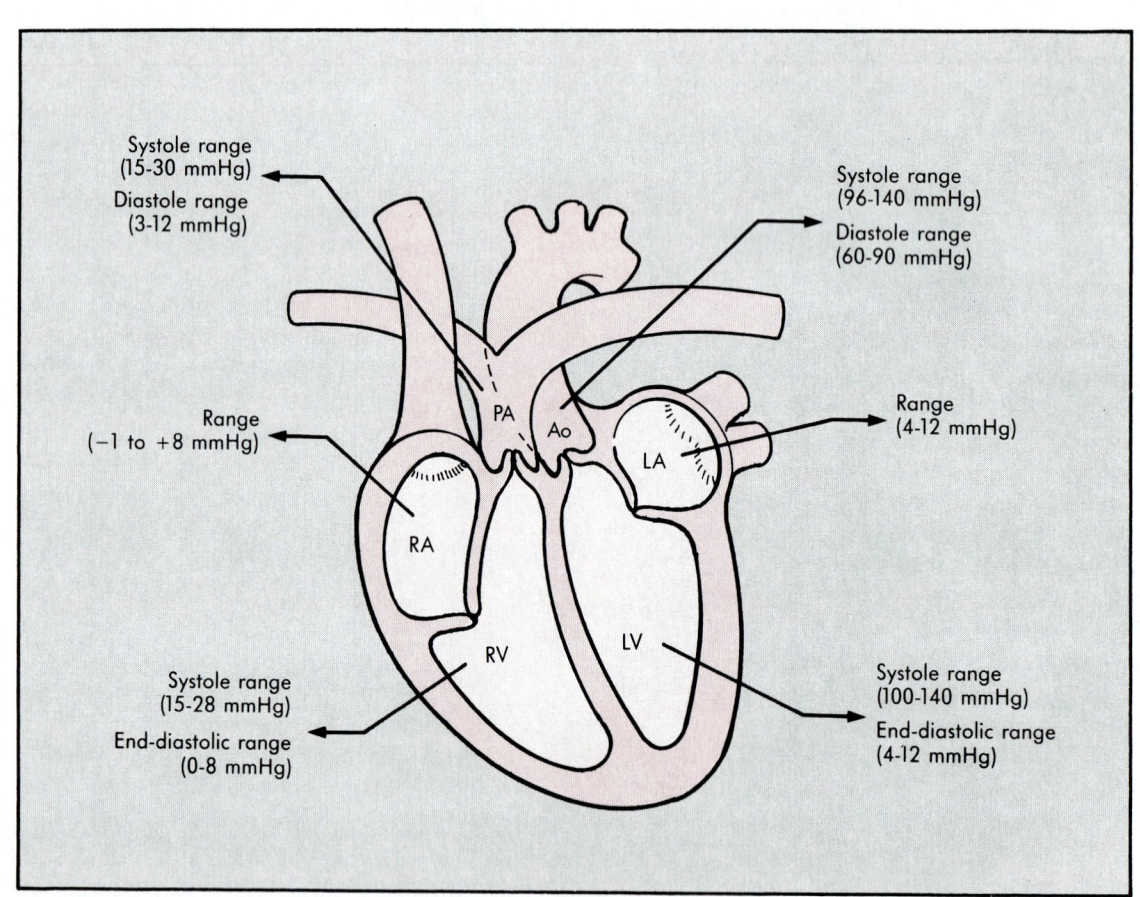

FIG. 26-7 Normal intracardiac pressures. *RA,* Right atrium; *LA,* left atrium; *RV,* right ventricle; *LV,* left ventricle; *PA,* pulmonary artery; *AO,* aorta.

caused by filling of the atrium from the peripheral veins. The **x descent** follows the a wave and is produced because of descent of the tricuspid valve ring and by the ejection of blood from both ventricles. The **y descent** follows the v wave and reflects the rapid flow of blood from the great veins and right atrium into the right ventricle. A small deflection, the **c wave,** occurs after the a wave in early systole and may represent bulging of the mitral valve into the left atrium during early systole. Ventricular pressures are illustrated by a peak systolic pressure and an end-diastolic pressure, which is the ventricular pressure immediately before the onset of systole. The minimal left ventricular pressure occurs in early diastole.

Structures That Support Cardiac Metabolism: The Coronary Vessels

The blood within the heart chambers does not supply oxygen and other nutrients to the cells of the heart. Like all other organs, including the lungs, heart structures are nourished by vessels of the systemic circulation. The branch of the systemic circulation that supplies the heart is termed the **coronary circulation.** The coronary circulation consists of **coronary arteries,** which receive blood through openings in the aorta called the **coronary ostia,** and the **cardiac veins,** which empty into the right atrium through another ostium, the opening of a large vein called the **coronary sinus** (Fig. 26-8). (Regulation of the coronary circulation, which is similar to regula-

ANTERIOR VIEW

FIG. 26-8 Anterior and posterior surfaces of the heart. Location and distribution of the principal coronary vessels are illustrated. (From Berne & Levy, 1992.)

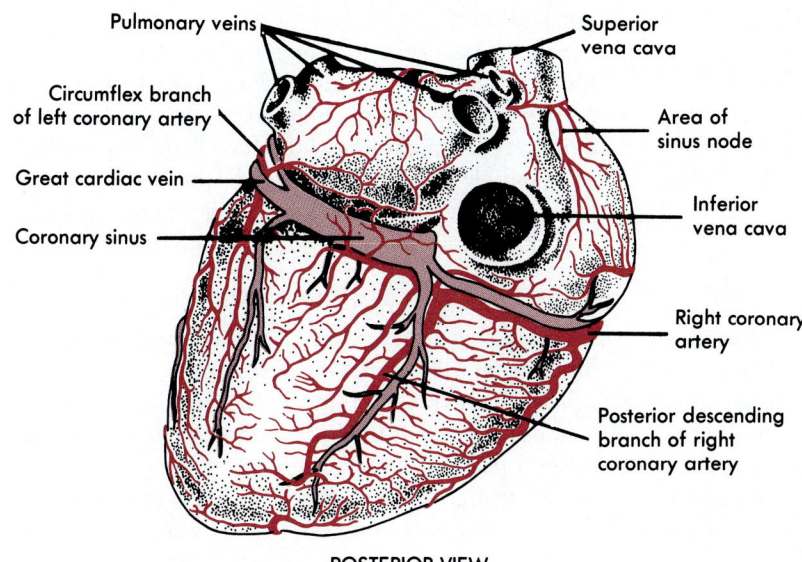

POSTERIOR VIEW

tion of flow through systemic and pulmonary vessels, is described elsewhere.)

Coronary Arteries

The major coronary arteries are the **right coronary artery** and the **left coronary artery** (see Fig. 26-8). These arteries traverse the epicardium and branch several times. The pattern of branching through the visceral pericardium differs from heart to heart. The branches enter the myocardium and endocardium and branch further to become arterioles, then capillaries.

The left coronary artery arises from a single ostium (opening) behind the left cusp of the aortic semilunar valve. This artery ranges from a few millimeters to a few centimeters in length. It passes between the left atrial appendage and the pulmonary artery and generally divides into two branches, the left anterior descending artery and the circumflex artery. Other branches of the left main coronary artery are distributed diagonally across the free wall of the left ventricle.

The **left anterior descending artery,** also called the anterior interventricular artery, delivers blood to portions of the left and right ventricles and much of the interventricular septum. The left anterior descending artery travels down the anterior surface of the interventricular septum toward the apex of the heart.

The **circumflex artery** travels in a groove called the **coronary sulcus,** which separates the left atrium from the left ventricle, to the left border of the heart (see Fig. 26-8). It supplies blood to the left atrium and the lateral wall of the left ventricle. The circumflex artery often branches to the posterior surfaces of the left atrium and left ventricle (see Fig. 26-8).

The right coronary artery originates from an ostium behind the right aortic cusp, travels behind the pulmonary artery, and extends around the right heart to the heart's posterior surface, where it branches to the atrium and the ventricle. The three major branches of the right coronary artery include the conus, which supplies blood to the upper right ventricle; the right marginal branch, which travels the right ventricle to the apex; and the posterior descending branch, which lies in the posterior interventricular sulcus and supplies smaller branches to both ventricles.

Collateral Arteries

The **collateral arteries** are really connections, or anastomoses, between two branches of the same coronary artery or connections of branches of the right coronary artery with branches of the left. They are particularly common within the interventricular and interatrial septa, at the apex of the heart, over the anterior surface of the right ventricle, and around the sinus node (Thomas et al., 1982). The epicardium contains more collateral vessels than the endocardium.

The functional importance of the collateral circulation is debated: does it protect the heart or does it represent more severe ischemia? In some studies individuals with good collateral arteries had a significantly higher prevalence of two- or three-vessel disease than individuals with poor collateral arteries. These same individuals, however, had a lower prevalence of acute myocardial infarction and heart failure (Fuster, Badimon, Badimon, & Chesebro, 1992; Hansen, 1989). Although the collateral circulation apparently contributes to recovery after occlusion of coronary arteries and myocardial tissue death (infarction) caused by occlusion (Thomas et al., 1982), it cannot prevent infarction after the sudden occlusion of a major vessel. A gradual occlusion of a coronary artery may, however, cause collateral vessels to develop and reestablish blood flow to the deprived tissue (Fuster et al., 1992; Gregg, 1974; Schaper, 1971). Overall, investigators concluded that the development of collateral circulation provides some protection against the myocardial effects of coronary occlusion (Fuster et al., 1992; Hansen, 1989; Kirk & Jennings, 1985).

Collateral coronary arteries in normal hearts are generally straight or slightly curved, whereas those in hearts with occluded coronary arteries are severely twisted and tortuous (Baroldi, Manteo, & Scomozoni, 1956). The twisted shapes are possibly caused by the wear and tear caused by higher blood pressures generated by the occlusion.

Coronary Capillaries

The heart has an extensive capillary network, with approximately 3300 capillaries per square millimeter (ca/mm^2) or about one capillary per muscle cell (muscle fiber) (Underhill, Woods, Sivarajan, & Halpenny, 1982). Blood travels from the arteries to the arterioles, then into the capillaries, where exchange of oxygen and other nutrients takes place.

Alterations of the cardiac muscles dramatically affect blood flow in the capillaries. For example, in ventricular hypertrophy (enlargement of the ventricular myocardium), the capillary network does not expand along with muscle fiber size. Therefore the same number of capillaries must now perfuse a larger area. This results in decreased exchange of oxygen and nutrients.

Coronary Veins and Lymphatic Vessels

After passing through the extensive capillary network, blood from the coronary arteries drains into the cardiac veins, which travel alongside the arteries. Most of the venous drainage of the heart occurs through veins in the visceral pericardium.

The cardiac veins feed into the **great cardiac vein** and then into the enlarged vessel cavity called the coronary sinus. The coronary sinus is located on the posterior surface of the heart, between the atria and ventricles, in the coronary sulcus. Venous coronary blood empties into the right atrium from the coronary sinus. Blood from the left ventricular walls is generally drained through the coronary sinus and its tributaries, which together form the largest system of coronary veins. The great cardiac vein primarily drains the anterior surface of the heart. The **posterior vein of the left ventricle** branches from the coronary sinus and accompanies the circumflex artery. This vein is the largest vein on the posterior surface of the heart.

The myocardium has an extensive system of lymphatic vessels. With cardiac contraction, the lymphatic vessels drain fluid to lymph nodes in the anterior mediastinum that eventually empty into the superior vena cava. The lymphatics are important for protecting the myocardium against injury. (The lymphatic vessels are described on p. 983.)

Structures That Control Heart Action

Continuous, rhythmic repetition of the cardiac cycle (systole and diastole) depends on the continuous, rhythmic transmission of electrical impulses, termed **cardiac action potentials,** through the myocardium. (Action potentials are described in Chapters 1 and 3.) As an electrical impulse passes from cell to cell (fiber to fiber) in the myocardium, it stimulates the fibers to shorten. Shortening causes muscular contraction, or systole. After the action potential passes, the fibers relax and return to their resting length, causing diastole. The muscle fibers of the myocardium are uniquely joined so that action potentials pass from cell to cell very rapidly and efficiently. Therefore an action potential generated in one part of the myocardium passes almost simultaneously through all its contiguous fibers, causing rapid contraction.

The myocardium differs from other muscle tissues in that it contains its own **conduction system**—specialized cells that enable it to generate and transmit action potentials without stimulation from the nervous system. These cells are concentrated at certain sites in the myocardium called **nodes.** Although the heart is innervated by the autonomic nervous system (both sympathetic and parasympathetic fibers), neural impulses are not needed to maintain the cardiac cycle. Thus, the heart will beat in the absence of any nervous connection. The cardiac cycle is stimulated by the nodes of specialized cells and "fine tuned" as needed by the autonomic fibers. The sympathetic and parasympathetic nerves have different effects on the speed of the cardiac cycle (**heart rate,** or beats per minute) and on the diameter of the coronary vessels (see Fig. 26-12).

Other factors that influence heart action are substances delivered to the myocardium in coronary blood. Nutrients and oxygen are needed for cellular survival and normal function, whereas hormones and biochemicals affect the strength and duration of myocardial contraction and the degree and duration of myocardial relaxation. Normal or appropriate function depends on the availability of these substances, which is why coronary artery disease can seriously disrupt heart function.

The Conduction System

Normally electrical impulses arise in the **sinoatrial node** (SA node, sinus node), which is often called the pacemaker of the heart. The SA node is located at the junction of the right atrium and superior vena cava, just above the tricuspid valve (Fig. 26-9). The SA node lies only a millimeter or less beneath the visceral pericardium, making it vulnerable to injury and disease, especially pericardial inflammation (James, 1962). The SA node is nourished by the sinus node artery, which passes through the center of the node. There are numerous autonomic nerve endings within the node. The SA node's **P cells,** so called because they are pale and primitive appearing, are assumed to be the site of impulse formation (DeHaan, 1965; Harary, 1962).

In the resting adult the SA node generates about 75 action potentials per minute. Each action potential travels rapidly from cell to cell and through special pathways in the atrial myocardium, causing both atria to contract. Atrial contraction begins systole. Ventricular contraction is delayed because the fibrous skeleton of the heart interrupts cell-to-cell transmission of the electrical impulses. Transmission of the action potential from the atrial to the ventricular myocardium occurs through fibers of the conduction system. The action potential travels first to the **atrioventricular node** (AV node), then to the **bundle of His** (atrioventricular bundle, common bundle), and finally through the **bundle branches** of the interventricular septum to Purkinje fibers in the heart wall (see Fig. 26-9).

The AV node is well situated for mediating conduction between the atria and ventricles. It is located in the right atrial wall above the tricuspid valve and anterior to the ostium of the coronary sinus. There is much variation from one heart to another in the size and length of the AV node fibers. Generally the AV node is thicker and shorter and has fewer P cells than the SA node. Behind the AV node are numerous autonomic ganglia, presumably vagal (parasympathetic) (James, 1968). (The nervous systems are described in Chapter 12.) These ganglia may serve as receptors for the vagus nerve and cause slowing of the cardiac cycle.

Conducting fibers from the AV node converge to form the bundle of His. The bundle of His, which is triangular in shape, lies within the posterior border of the interventricular septum. The two lower ends of the triangle give rise to the right and left bundle branches. The **right bundle branch (RBB)** is thin and travels without

FIG. 26-9 Excitation and conduction system of heart. Arrows indicate stimulatory impulse from sinoatrial node as it travels through myocardium of both atria and stimulates conduction through ventricle. (From Thibodeau, 1987.)

much branching to the right ventricular apex. Because of its thinness and relative lack of branches, the RBB is susceptible to interruption by damage to the endocardium.

The **left bundle branch** (LBB) arises perpendicularly from the bundle of His and, in some hearts, divides into two branches, or fascicles. The left anterior bundle branch (LABB) passes the left anterior papillary muscle and the base of the left ventricle and crosses the aortic outflow tract. Damage to the aortic valve or the left ventricle can interrupt this branch. The left posterior bundle branch (LPBB) travels posteriorly, crossing the left ventricular inflow tract to the base of the left posterior papillary muscle. This branch spreads diffusely through the posterior inferior left ventricular wall. Blood flow through this portion of the left ventricle is relatively nonturbulent, so the LPBB is somewhat protected from injury caused by wear and tear.

Because the LBB divides and crosses the ventricles to the anterior and posterior papillary muscles, action potentials reach the left ventricle before they reach the right ventricle. Therefore the left ventricle contracts slightly ahead of the right.

The **Purkinje fibers** are the terminal branches of the right and left bundle branches. They extend from the ventricular apices to the fibrous rings and penetrate the heart wall to the outer myocardium. P cells are also found among the Purkinje fibers.

Because impulses from the SA node arrive at the AV node extremely quickly, investigators have proposed that these nodes are connected by internodal pathways. In 1916, Bachmann first described a pathway between the right atrium and the left atrium. Although controversy exists as to whether this pathway, termed **Bachmann's bundle,** is made up of conducting fibers, the bundle is well developed and has been extensively demonstrated in autopsy dissections. Purkinje fibers also have been found in Bachmann's bundle (James, Sherf, Schlat, & Silverman, 1985). Two other pathways, the middle internodal pathway and the posterior internodal pathway, apparently connect the SA node and the AV node (Berne & Levy, 1992; Katz, 1977; Soderstrom, 1948; Thorel, 1909; Wenckebach, 1908).

Cardiac excitation

From the SA node, the impulse that begins systole spreads throughout the right atrium at a conduction velocity of about 1 m/sec. Bachmann's bundle conducts

Intracellular and Extracellular Ion Concentrations in the Myocardium

Ion	Intracellular concentration	Extracellular concentration
Sodium (Na$^+$)	15 mM	145 mM
Potassium (K$^+$)	150 mM	4 mM
Chloride (Cl$^-$)	5 mM	120 mM
Calcium (Ca^{++})	10^{-7} M	2 mM

NOTE: *mM*, millimoles per kilogram; *M*, moles.

the impulse from the SA node to the left atrium, and the three internodal pathways conduct the impulse from the SA node to the AV node.

The action potential is delayed in the region of the AV node, possibly because of electrophysiologic differences in the cells comprising the AV region (Berne & Levy, 1992; Halpenny, 1982a). The delay between atrial and ventricular excitation permits an additional boost to ventricular filling by atrial contraction (atrial kick). From the AV node, the impulse travels from the atrioventricular bundle and through the bundle branches to the Purkinje fibers. Conduction velocities in the atrioventricular and Purkinje fibers are 2 to 4 m/sec, the most rapid in the heart.

Ventricular activation occurs sequentially in three phases: (1) septal activation, (2) apical activation, and (3) basal (upper) and posterior activation. The first areas of the ventricles to be excited are portions of the interventricular septum. The septum is activated from both the RBB and the LBB, although the impulse travels from left to right. The extensive network of Purkinje fibers promotes the rapid spread of the impulse to the ventricular apices. Activation traverses the heart wall from the inside outward (from the endocardium to the epicardium; see Fig. 26-2). The basal and posterior portions of the ventricles are the last to be activated. Deactivation, which begins diastole, occurs in the opposite direction, spreading from the outside inward (epicardium to endocardium). All areas of the ventricle recover at about the same time.

Propagation of cardiac action potentials

Electrical activation of the muscle cells, termed **depolarization,** is caused by the movement of electrically charged solutes (ions) across cardiac cell membranes. Deactivation, called **repolarization,** occurs the same way. (Movement of ions across cell membranes is described in Chapter 1; electrical activation of muscle cells is described in Chapter 38.)

Movement of ions into and out of the cell creates an

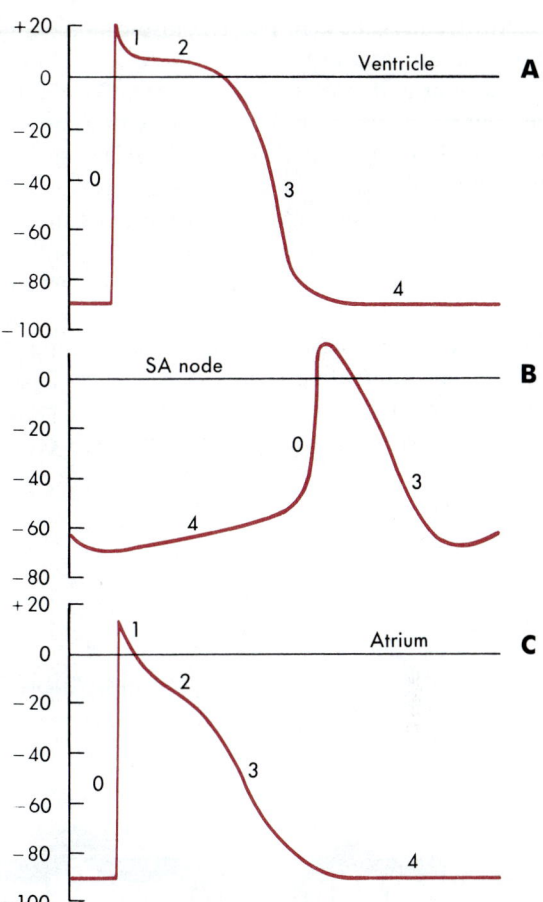

FIG. 26-10 Cardiac action potentials. **A,** Ventricle; **B,** SA node; and **C,** atrium. Sweep velocity in **B** is one half that in **A** or **C.** (From Berne & Levy, 1992.)

electrical (voltage) difference across the cell membrane called the membrane potential. The resting membrane potential of myocardial cells is −80 to −90 millivolts (mV), whereas that of SA and AV node cells is −60 mV. During depolarization, the inside of the cell becomes less negatively charged. In cardiac cells the difference between resting membrane potential (in millivolts) and the decreased negative charge caused by depolarization is the cardiac action potential. Table 26-2 summarizes the intracellular and extracellular ionic concentrations of cardiac muscle. The various phases of the cardiac action potential are related to changes in the permeability of the cell membrane, primarily to sodium and potassium. Threshold is the point at which the cell membrane's selective permeability to sodium and potassium is temporarily disrupted, leading to depolarization.

Normal myocardial cell depolarization and repolarization occur in four phases (Fig. 26-10). Phase 0 consists of depolarization. This phase lasts from 1 to 2 milliseconds (msec) and represents rapid sodium entry into the cell. Phase 1 is early repolarization, in which calcium slowly enters the cell. Phase 2, also called the **pla-teau,** is a continuation of repolarization, with slow entry of calcium and sodium into the cell. Potassium is moved out of the cell during phase 3, with a return to resting membrane potential in phase 4. This time between action potentials corresponds to diastole. If the resting membrane potential becomes more negative, for example with a decrease in extracellular potassium concentration (hypokalemia), it is termed **hyperpolarization.**

The phases of depolarization and repolarization occur somewhat differently in the SA and AV node cells, a difference that enables these cells to generate cardiac action potentials independently. Although the cells of

the Purkinje fibers, atria, and ventricles begin with a negative resting membrane potential and proceed to a rapid upstroke, or depolarization (phase 0), a rapid early repolarization (phase 1), a plateau (phase 2), and a rapid later repolarization (phase 3), cells of the SA and AV nodes begin with a less negative resting membrane potential, proceed to a slow upstroke (phase 0) and usually lack a plateau (phase 2) (see Fig. 26-10, *B*). The fast inward current, mediated by sodium ions flowing through "fast channels" in the cell membrane, causes the rapid upstroke of the action potential in Purkinje fibers, atria, and ventricles (see Fig. 26-10, *A*). The slow inward current, mediated by calcium and sodium ions flowing through "slow channels" of the cell membrane,

FIG. 26-11 ECG and cardiac electrical activity. **A,** Normal ECG. Depolarization and repolarization. **B,** ECG intervals between P, QRS, and T waves. **C,** Schematic representation of ECG and its relationship to cardiac electrical activity. (**A** and **B** from Thibodeau & Patton, 1993. **C** from Thibodeau, 1987.)

is responsible for the action potential of the SA node and the AV node. Hence, drugs that block calcium have profound effects on the slow inward current and can alter heart rate (Wu, 1984). Slow channel-blocking drugs, such as verapamil, are used to treat a variety of cardiovascular disorders.

A **refractory period,** during which no new cardiac action potential can be initiated by a stimulus, follows depolarization. This period, called the effective or absolute refractory period, corresponds to the time needed for the reopening of channels that permit sodium and calcium influx (phase 0 through half of phase 3). A relative refractory period occurs near the end of repolarization, following the effective refractory period. During this time the membrane can be depolarized again but only by a greater-than-normal stimulus. Abnormal refractory periods as a result of disease can cause abnormal heart rhythms or dysrhythmias, including ventricular fibrillation and cardiac arrest (see Chapter 27).

The normal electrocardiogram. The genesis of the normal electrocardiogram is from electrical activity recorded by skin electrodes, that is, the sum of all the cardiac action potentials (Fig. 26-11). The **P wave** represents atrial depolarization. The **PR interval** is a measure of time from the onset of atrial activation to the onset of ventricular activation; it normally ranges from 0.12 to 0.20 second. The PR interval represents the time necessary to travel from the sinus node through the atrium, AV node, and His-Purkinje system to activate ventricular myocardial cells. The **QRS complex** represents the sum of all ventricular muscle cell depolarizations. The configuration and amplitude of the QRS complex vary considerably among individuals. The duration is normally between 0.06 and 0.10 second. During the **ST interval** the entire ventricular myocardium is depolarized. The **QT interval** is sometimes called the "electrical systole" of the ventricles. Its duration is about 0.4 second, but it varies inversely with the heart rate.

Automaticity. Automaticity, or the property of generating spontaneous depolarization to threshold, enables the SA and AV nodes to generate cardiac action potentials without any stimulus. Cells capable of spontaneous depolarization are called **automatic cells.** The automatic cells of the cardiac conduction system can stimulate the heart to beat even when the heart is removed from the body. Spontaneous depolarization is possible in automatic cells because the membrane potential does not "rest" during phase 4. Instead, it slowly creeps toward threshold during the diastolic phase of the cardiac cycle. Because threshold is approached during diastole, phase 4 in automatic cells is called **diastolic depolarization.** The electrical impulse normally begins in the SA node because its cells depolarize more rapidly than other automatic cells.

Rhythmicity. Rhythmicity is the regular generation of an action potential by the heart's conduction system.

The SA node sets the pace because normally it has the fastest rate, which is why it is called the natural pacemaker of the heart. The SA node depolarizes spontaneously 60 to 100 times a minute. If the SA node is damaged, the AV node will become the heart's pacemaker at a rate of about 40 to 60 spontaneous depolarizations per minute. Eventually, however, conduction cells in the atria usually take over from the AV node. Purkinje fibers are capable of spontaneous depolarization, but at a rate of only 30 to 40 beats/min.

Cardiac Innervation

Although the heart's nodes and conduction system generate cardiac action potentials independently, the autonomic nervous system influences the *rate* of impulse generation (firing), depolarization, and repolarization of the myocardium and the strength of atrial and ventricular contraction. Autonomic neural transmission produces changes in the heart and circulatory system faster than metabolic or humoral agents (Fig. 26-12). Speed is important, for example, in stimulating the heart to increase its pumping action during times of stress or fear, the so-called fight or flight response. Although increased delivery of oxygen, glucose, hormones, and other bloodborne factors sustains increased cardiac activity, the rapid initiation of increased activity depends on the sympathetic and parasympathetic fibers of the autonomic nervous system. (The autonomic nervous system is described and illustrated in Chapter 12.)

Sympathetic and parasympathetic nerves

Sympathetic nerve fibers innervate all parts of the atria and ventricles. Parasympathetic fibers from the vagus nerve innervate these structures plus the SA and AV nodes. Strong vagal stimulation can block cardiac action potentials transmitted from the atria. Sympathetic nerves can also shorten the conduction time through the AV node and increase the rhythmicity of the AV pacemaker fibers.

Efferent sympathetic fibers originate in the thoracic spinal cord and branch into the superior middle and inferior cardiac nerves. The efferent parasympathetic fibers originate in the medulla oblongata and travel by way of the vagus nerves to join the sympathetic nerves in the **cardiac plexus,** a neural junction located at the root of the aorta, in front of the trachea.

Sympathetic nervous activity enhances myocardial performance (Berne & Levy, 1992). Neurally released norepinephrine or circulating catecholamines interact with beta-adrenergic receptors on the cardiac cell membranes. The overall effect is an increased influx of Ca^{++} during the action potential plateau. The increased calcium increases the contractile strength of the heart. In addition, sympathetic nervous activity increases heart rate, whereas parasympathetic (vagal) activity decreases heart rate. The vagus nerve releases acetylcholine. In the

FIG. 26-12 Autonomic innervation of cardiovascular system. *ACh,* Acetylcholine; *NE,* norepinephrine; *E,* epinephrine; *SA,* sinoatrial node; *AV,* atrioventricular node.

heart, receptors for these neurotransmitters are found in the myocardium and in the coronary vessels. When the autonomic nervous system is active, the vagal effects usually dominate (Berne & Levy, 1992).

Adrenergic receptor function

Sympathetic neural stimulation of the myocardium and coronary vessels depends on the presence of adrenergic receptors, which bind specifically with neurotransmitters of the sympathetic nervous system. (Receptor physiology is discussed in Chapter 1.) The effects of sympathetic stimulation depend on (1) whether α- or β-adrenergic receptors are most plentiful on cells of the effector tissue and (2) whether the neurotransmitter is norepinephrine or epinephrine.

Overall, cardiovascular structures have more β than α receptors; therefore effects mediated by the β receptors predominate. β_1 receptors are found mostly in the heart, specifically the conduction system (AV and SA

nodes, Purkinje fibers) and the atrial and ventricular myocardium. Norepinephrine binding with β_1 receptors increases the rate of impulse generation (firing) and conduction and also the strength of myocardial contraction during systole. These effects enable the heart to pump more blood. At the same time, epinephrine binds with β_2 receptors, which are most plentiful in the coronary arterioles. This causes the coronary arterioles to dilate, supplying the hard-working myocardium with more oxygen and nutrients (see Table 12-6).

α-Adrenergic receptors are also present in the coronary vessels, but in fewer numbers than the β receptors. Norepinephrine binding with α_1 receptors in the coronary arteries causes vasoconstriction. The α_2 receptors are located mostly on the sympathetic ganglia and nerve terminals. The effect of norepinephrine on the α_2 receptors is to inhibit release of more norepinephrine, which promotes vasodilation.

Epinephrine stimulates all four types of receptors (β_1,

β_2, α_1, α_2) strongly, whereas norepinephrine stimulates α_1, α_2, and β_1 receptors and certain β_2 receptors weakly or not at all. Thus both epinephrine and norepinephrine stimulate the heart (β_1) and constrict certain blood vessels (α_1), but only epinephrine dilates certain blood vessels (β_2) (Vick, 1984).

Myocardial Cells

The cells of cardiac muscle (the myocardium) and of muscle that makes voluntary movement possible (skeletal muscle) are nearly identical in structure, function, and microscopic appearance. (The properties of skeletal muscle are described in detail in Chapter 38.) Both types of muscle tissue are composed of long, narrow cells, called fibers, which contain basically the same structures: bundles of longitudinally arranged myofibrils; a nucleus (cardiac muscle) or many nuclei (skeletal muscle); mitochondria; an internal membrane system (the sarcoplasmic reticulum); cytoplasm (sarcoplasm); and a plasma membrane (the sarcolemma), which encloses the cell. Cardiac and skeletal muscle cells also have an "external" membrane system made up of transverse tubules (t-tubules) formed by invaginations of the sarcolemma. The sarcoplasmic reticulum forms a network of channels that surrounds the muscle fiber.

The microscopic appearance of cardiac and skeletal muscle is somewhat similar as well (see Chapter 1, Table 1-5). Because the myofibrils in both types of fibers are made up of alternating light and dark bands of protein, the fibers appear striped, or striated. The dark and light bands of the myofibrils comprise longitudinal repeating units called sarcomeres. The length of the sarcomeres, normally between 1.6 to 2.2 μm, is important because it determines the limits of myocardial stretch at the end of diastole and subsequently the force of contraction during systole.

Cardiac muscle differs from skeletal muscle in several respects that reflect heart function. Cardiac cells are arranged in branching networks throughout the myocardium, whereas skeletal muscle cells tend to be arranged in parallel throughout the length of the muscle. Cardiac fibers have only one nucleus, whereas skeletal muscle cells have many nuclei. Other differences enable cardiac fibers to (1) transmit action potentials quickly from cell to cell, (2) maintain high levels of energy synthesis, and (3) gain access to more ions, particularly sodium and potassium, in the extracellular environment.

Rapid transmission of electrical impulses from cardiac fiber to cardiac fiber is possible because the network of fibers is connected at specialized intercellular junctions called intercalated disks (see the illustration in Chapter 1, Table 1-7). **Intercalated disks** are thickened portions of the sarcolemma that enable electrical impulses to spread quickly in a continuous cell-to-cell (syncytial) fashion. The intercalated disks contain two junctions: desmosomes, which attach one cell to another;

and gap junctions, which allow the electrical impulse to spread from cell to cell (see Chapter 1). Together, these junctions provide a low-resistance pathway for impulse propagation.

Unlike skeletal muscle, the heart cannot rest and is in constant need of energy compounds, such as adenosine triphosphate (ATP). Therefore the cytoplasm surrounding the bundles of myofibrils in each cardiac muscle cell contains a superabundance of mitochondria (25% of the cellular volume). Cardiac muscle cells have more mitochondria than skeletal muscle cells. The large number of mitochondria provide the necessary respiratory enzymes for aerobic metabolism and supply quantities of ATP sufficient for the constant action of the myocardium. (The role of mitochondria in cellular energy production is described in Chapter 1.)

The third major difference between cardiac and skeletal muscle cells has to do with the transverse tubule (t-tubule) system. Cardiac fibers contain more t-tubules than skeletal muscle fibers. This feature gives each myofibril in the myocardium ready access to molecules it needs for the continuous transmission of action potentials, a process that involves transport of sodium and potassium through the walls of the t-tubules. (The mechanisms by which sodium and potassium transport cause transmission of cardiac action potentials are described in Chapters 1 and 38.)

Because the t-tubule system is continuous with the extracellular space and the interstitial fluid, it facilitates the rapid transmission of the electrical impulses from the surface of the sarcolemma to the myofibrils inside the fiber. This activates all the myofibrils of one fiber simultaneously. The sarcoplasmic reticulum is located around the myofibrils. When an action potential is transmitted through the t-tubules, it induces the sarcoplasmic reticulum to release its stored calcium, which activates the contractile proteins, actin and myosin.

Actin, myosin, and the troponin-tropomyosin complex

The thick filaments of **myosin** constitute the central dark band called the **anisotropic** or **A bands** (Fig. 26-13). The myosin molecule resembles a golf club with two large bulbous heads protruding from one end of a straight shaft (Fig. 26-14). The bilobed heads contain an actin-binding site and a site of ATPase activity. A thick filament is composed of about 200 myosin molecules bundled together with the heads of the molecules (called crossbridges) facing outward (see Fig. 26-14). The actin molecules are part of the thin filaments (Fig. 26-15). The light bands are called **isotropic** or **I bands** (see Fig. 26-13). The thin filaments of actin appear light and extend from the Z line. The dense fibrous **Z line** crosses the center of each I band. A sarcomere is the area from one dark Z line to an adjacent Z line with a length that varies from 1.6 to 2.2 μm. In the center of a sarcomere is the H zone, a somewhat less dense region. A thin, dark **M line** travels the center of the H zone. A single tropomyosin molecule (a relaxing protein) lies alongside seven actin molecules. Troponin, another relaxing protein, associates with the tropomyosin molecule forming the **troponin-tropomyosin complex** (Fig. 26-16). The troponin complex, itself, has three components. **Troponin T** aids in the binding of the troponin complex to actin and tropomyosin; **troponin I** inhibits the ATPase of actomyosin; and **troponin C** contains binding sites for the calcium ions involved in contraction.

Myocardial metabolism

Cardiac muscle, like other muscle tissue in the body, depends on the constant production of ATP for energy. ATP is produced within the mitochondria mainly from glucose, fatty acids, and lactate. If the myocardium is inadequately perfused because of coronary artery dis-

ease, anaerobic metabolism becomes an essential source of energy (see Chapter 1). The energy produced by metabolic processes is used for muscle contraction and relaxation, electrical excitation, membrane transport, and synthesis of large molecules. Normally, the amount of ATP produced supplies sufficient energy to pump blood systemically.

FIG. 26-14 Structure of myosin. A, Each myosin molecule is a coil of two chains wrapped around one another. At the end of each chain is a globular region, much like a golf club, called the "head." **B,** Myosin molecules are usually combined into filaments, which are stalks of myosin from which the heads protrude at regular intervals. (From Raven & Johnson, 1986.)

FIG. 26-13 Sarcomere. A, Electron photomicrograph of sarcomere. **B,** Schematic of location and interaction of actin and myosin. (From Andreoli, Carpenter, Plus, & Smith, 1986.)

FIG. 26-15 Actin filament. (From Raven & Johnson, 1986.)

Cardiac work is often expressed in terms of **myocardial oxygen consumption** (MVO$_2$). Because oxidative metabolism is the main process of cardiac energy generation, the rate of MVO$_2$ correlates closely with total cardiac energy requirements. MVO$_2$ is determined by three major factors. The three major determinants of MVO$_2$ include (1) the amount of wall stress during systole, which can be estimated by measuring the systolic blood pressure; (2) duration of systolic wall tension, which is measured indirectly by the heart rate; and (3) the contractile state of the myocardium. No clinical measurement for the contractile state exists.

The oxygen supply to the myocardium is delivered exclusively by the coronary arteries. Approximately 70% to 75% of the oxygen from the coronary arteries is used immediately by cardiac muscle, leaving little oxygen in reserve. Therefore increased energy needs can only be met by increasing coronary blood flow. When oxygen content decreases, the local concentration of local metabolic factors increases. One of these factors, adenosine, dilates coronary arterioles, increasing coronary blood flow. Oxygen content of the blood cannot be increased under normal atmospheric conditions, nor can the amount of O$_2$ extracted from the blood be appreciably increased from the resting level (see Chapter 29). Myocardial O$_2$ consumption can increase several fold with exercise and decrease moderately under conditions such as hypotension and hypothermia (Berne & Levy, 1992).

FIG. 26-16 Mechanisms of muscle contraction. A, Thin myofilament. **B,** Thick myofilament. **C,** Cross-section of thick and thin myofilaments showing arrangement of myofilaments and crossbridges. **D,** Sliding filament theory of muscle contraction; note changes in banding patterns. (From Thibodeau, 1993.)

FIG. 26-17 Crossbridge theory of muscle contraction (or sliding filament theory). Crossbridges of single myosin fiber are thought to point at 60° angles at six actin filaments. Crossbridges bond to actin filaments and slide them toward center of sarcomere. Sequence of events in muscular contraction: **A,** in preparation for contraction, ATP bonding of myosin head causes conversion to high-energy form of myosin; **B,** Ca⁺⁺ is released from the sarcoplasmic reticulum and is bound to troponin-tropomyosin complex, changing its conformation so that troponin no longer holds tropomyosin in a blocking position between actin and myosin; **C,** as tropomyosin is pulled out of position, myosin head makes contact with actin molecule (bonding process displaces high-energy phosphate group [ADP + Pi]) from myosin head; **D,** loss of energy causes myosin to contract back to its original position, exerting traction on the rest of the myosin bridge, causing thin filaments to slide past the thick filaments. (From Thibodeau, 1993.)

Myocardial Contraction and Relaxation

Myocardial contractility can be defined as a change in developed tension at a given resting fiber length. In functional terms, contractility is the ability of the heart muscle to shorten (Berne & Levy, 1992). The molecular basis of myocardial contraction is the sliding of the thin filaments of actin over thick filaments of myosin, called the **crossbridge theory of muscle contraction.** Anatomically, contraction occurs when the sarcomere shortens with adjacent Z lines moving closer together (Fig. 26-17). The width of the A band, which contains the thick myosin filaments, is unchanged. The movement comes from the long sets of filaments. The degree of shortening of the muscle fibers depends on how much the thin filaments overlap the thick filaments. Maximal contraction occurs when the sarcomere length is 2.2 μm. At 2.2 μm, the number of crossbridge attachments between actin and myosin is maximal.

The crossbridge theory

The globular head-end of the myosin contains a binding site for actin and a separate enzymatic site that catalyzes the breakdown of ATP to ADP and inorganic phosphate (see Fig. 26-17). This reaction releases the chemical energy stored in ATP. Magnesium is required for the binding of ATP to the myosin site. The splitting of ATP occurs on the myosin molecule before it attaches to actin, but the ADP and inorganic phosphate released remain bound to the active site on myosin. The chemical energy released is transferred to myosin (m), producing a high-energy form of myosin (M) (Vander, Sherman, & Luciano, 1990):

$$m \cdot ATP \rightarrow M \cdot ADP + P_i$$

The binding of this high-energy form of myosin to actin through a crossbridge releases the energy stored in myosin (e.g., ADP and P_i), producing the force necessary for movement of the crossbridge. With the attachment of actin to myosin at the crossbridge, the myosin head molecule undergoes a position change exerting traction on the rest of the myosin bridge, causing the thin filaments to slide past the thick filaments (see Fig. 26-17). During contraction, each crossbridge undergoes cycles of attachment, movement, and dissociation from the thin filaments.

Calcium and excitation-contraction coupling

Excitation-contraction coupling is the process by which an action potential in the plasma membrane of the muscle fiber triggers the cycle of events leading to crossbridge activity and contraction. This cycle of events and contraction depends on the availability of calcium. When the extracellular calcium concentration is increased, there is an increase in myocardial contractility, and a reduction in extracellular calcium causes a decrease in myocardial contractility.

Calcium is stored in the tubule system and the sarcoplasmic reticulum. Calcium enters the myocardial cell from the interstitial fluid after electrical excitation, which increases the membrane permeability to calcium. Two types of calcium channels (L-type and T-type) are identified in cardiac tissues. The L-type, or long-lasting, channels are the predominant type of calcium channels and are the channels blocked by **calcium channel-blocking drugs.** These drugs include verapamil, nifedipine, and diltiazem and their major effect is to decrease the strength of cardiac contraction. The T-type, or transient, channels are much less abundant in the heart and are not blocked by calcium channel-blocking drugs (Berne & Levy, 1992). Calcium that enters the cell from the interstitial fluid triggers release of calcium from the storage sites. The storage sites most important for contraction are from the sarcoplasmic reticulum. Calcium from these sites diffuses toward the myofibrils and there it binds with troponin.

The calcium and its interaction with the troponin complex facilitate the contraction process. In the resting state, troponin I is bound to actin and the configuration of the tropomyosin molecule is such that it covers the sites where the myosin heads bind to actin. Thus interaction between actin and myosin is prevented. Calcium binding to troponin inhibits troponin C (which enhances troponin I–actin binding). This, in turn, causes tropomyosin to move away, thus uncovering the binding sites on the myosin heads. Myosin and actin can now form crossbridges and ATP can be dephosphorylated to ADP. Sliding of the thick and thin filaments can now occur and the muscle contracts.

Myocardial relaxation

Adequate relaxation is just as vital to optimal cardiac function as contraction. Studies have shown that various heart diseases affect relaxation long before they result in inadequate contraction (Brutsaert, Rademakers, & Sys, 1984). Calcium also facilitates relaxation. After contraction, free calcium ions are actively pumped out of the cell back into the interstitial fluid or reaccumulated in the sarcoplasmic reticulum and stored. Troponin releases its bound calcium. The tropomyosin complex blocks the active sites on the actin molecule preventing crossbridges with the myosin heads. Each tropomyosin molecule is held in this blocking position by a molecule of troponin. Troponin is bound to both tropomyosin and actin (see Figs. 26-16, *A*, and 26-17).

Adequate relaxation is just as vital to optimal cardiac function as contraction. Studies have shown that various heart diseases affect relaxation long before they result in inadequate contraction (Brutsaert et al., 1984).

Relaxation, or inhibition of contraction, is made possible by the so-called relaxing proteins in the myofibrils, troponin, and tropomyosin. The release of calcium also facilitates relaxation.

Factors Affecting Cardiac Performance

Four factors affect cardiac performance directly: (1) preload, (2) afterload, (3) heart rate, and (4) myocardial contractility. **Preload** (pressure generated at the end of diastole) and **afterload** (resistance to ejection during systole) depend on both the heart and the vascular system. Heart rate and contractility are characteristics of the cardiac tissue, per se, and are influenced by neural and humoral mechanisms (Fig. 26-18). To understand the role of these factors in cardiac performance, it is first necessary to understand two physical laws that explain the mechanisms of heart action: the Frank-Starling law of the heart and Laplace's law.

Frank-Starling Law of the Heart

Cardiac muscle, like other muscle, increases its strength of contraction when it is stretched. This relationship was described in 1914 by a British physiologist, Ernest Starling, who based his studies on the earlier work of a German physiologist, Otto Frank. In 1914, Starling wrote that "the output of any heart can be varied within wide limits by alterations of the venous inflow, and that within these limits it varies directly as the venous inflow. So long as the functional condition of the heart remains constant, the amount put out at each beat depends directly on the diastolic filling" (Fye, 1983).

The **Frank-Starling law of the heart,** or the length-tension relationship of cardiac muscle, relates resting sarcomere length, expressed as the volume of blood in the heart at the end of diastole, or **end-diastolic volume,** to tension generation, described as development of left ventricular pressure. Thus there is a direct relationship between the volume of blood in the heart at the end of diastole (the length of its muscle fibers) and the force of contraction during the next systole. Although the change in pressure is related to volume of the ventricle and, consequently, to the length of the ventricular muscle fibers, it is common to use preload (i.e., filling pressure) as an index of ventricular volume. The length-tension mechanism is the major mechanism by which the normal right and left ventricles maintain equal minute outputs even though their stroke outputs may vary considerably during normal respiration (Schlant & Sonnenblick, 1990). For example, changes in volume occur when an individual assumes a reclining position after being in a standing position; the volume of blood returning to the heart temporarily increases. The right ventricle stretches to accommodate this increase in volume and, thereby, increases its force of contraction. A

```
                              ┌──────────────────┐
        ┌─────────────────────│  Cardiac output  │◀─────────────────────┐
        │                     └──────────────────┘                      │
        │                                                                │
  ┌───────────┐                                              ┌─────────────────┐
  │ Heart rate│                                    ┌─────────│  Stroke volume  │◀────────┐
  └───────────┘                                    │         └─────────────────┘         │
        ▲                                          ▲                                     ▲
        │                                          │                                     │
        │     ┌──────────────┐          ┌────────────────────┐         ┌────────────────────┐
        ├─────│  Autonomic   │          │ End-diastolic volume│        │ End-systolic volume │
        │     │nervous system│          └────────────────────┘        └────────────────────┘
        │     └──────────────┘                     ▲                             ▲
        │                                          │                             │
        │     ┌──────────────┐          ┌────────────────────┐         ┌────────────────────┐
        ├─────│ Temperature  │          │ Ventricular filling│         │ Ventricular emptying│
        │     └──────────────┘          └────────────────────┘         └────────────────────┘
        │                                          ▲                             ▲
        │     ┌──────────────┐                     │                             │
        ├─────│     Ions     │          ┌────────────────────┐         ┌────────────────────┐
        │     └──────────────┘          │  Length of diastole│         │Strength of contraction│
        │                               └────────────────────┘         └────────────────────┘
        │  ┌─────────────────┐                     │                             ▲
        │  │ Epinephrine and │          ┌────────────────────┐                   │
        └──│norepinephrine from│        │   Venous return    │     ┌──────────────────────────┐
           │ adrenal medulla │         └────────────────────┘     │ Degree of stretch of      │
           └─────────────────┘                                    │ cardiac muscle            │
                                                                   ├──────────────────────────┤
                                                                   │ Sympathetic division of   │
                                                                   │ autonomic nervous system  │
                                                                   ├──────────────────────────┤
                                                                   │ Epinephrine and           │
                                                                   │ norepinephrine from       │
                                                                   │ adrenal medulla           │
                                                                   └──────────────────────────┘
```

FIG. 26-18 Factors affecting cardiac performance. Cardiac output, which is amount of blood (in liters) ejected by heart per minute, depends on heart rate (beats per minute) and stroke volume (milliliters of blood ejected during ventricular systole).

FIG. 26-19 Frank-Starling law of the heart. Relationship between length and tension in heart. End-diastolic volume determines end-diastolic length of ventricular muscle fibers and is proportional to tension generated during systole, as well as to cardiac output, stroke volume, and stroke work. A change in myocardial contractility causes the heart to perform on a different length-tension curve. *A*, Increased contractility; *B*, normal contractility; *C*, heart failure or decreased contractility. (See text.)

larger stroke volume (i.e., the amount of blood ejected per beat) is pumped to the lungs, generating higher pressures. Pulmonary vascular pressure increases causing a rise in the left ventricular filling pressure or preload. Left ventricular volume and pressure increases. The left ventricle pumps a larger stroke volume and arterial vascular pressure rises.

The mechanical function of the heart is characterized by a number of length-tension curves (Fig. 26-19). Factors that increase contractility (i.e., positive inotropic), such as sympathetic nerve stimulation, cause the heart to operate on a higher length-tension curve (curve A). A higher tension or increase in ventricular stroke volume is generated without a necessary change in left ventricular end-diastolic volume or fiber length. Heart failure (curve C) is characterized by a lower length-tension curve (Chapter 27). The failing or dilated heart may not be able to use the Frank-Starling law of the heart because its fibers are lengthened maximally already. The failing heart is unable to respond significantly to increased filling or stretch with a greater force (Schlant & Sonnenblick, 1990). Thus at the same left ventricular end-diastolic volume as curves A and B, the force of contraction of stroke volume is decreased. The relationship between stretch and contraction can be compared to that of a rubber band. To a certain point, the more the rubber band is stretched, the farther it will fly when one end is released. Beyond that point, however, the rubber band will break.

The crossbridge theory partially accounts for the length-tension mechanism of cardiac muscle. According to the Frank-Starling law, the longer the initial resting length of the cardiac muscle fiber (optimal length is between 2.2 μm and 2.4 μm), the greater the strength of contraction. At 2.2 μm there is an optimal number of active crossbridges between actin and myosin. If the fibers are stretched beyond 2.2 μm to 2.4 μm, the force of contraction decreases because actin and myosin become partially disengaged, disrupting many of the crossbridges. Excessive stretching, to about 3.65 μm, causes actin and myosin to become completely disengaged and causes developed tension (force of contraction) to drop to zero. Heart failure occurs when it takes higher and higher filling pressures to accomplish normal contractile force.

Laplace's Law

Laplace's law demonstrates the relationship between wall thickness, pressure, and wall tension. Wall tension is related directly to the product of intraventricular pressure and internal radius, and inversely to the wall thickness. Wall tension can be calculated by Laplace's equation:

$$T = \frac{p \times v}{\mu m}$$

where T = wall tension, p = intraventricular pressure, v = internal radius of the sphere, and μm = wall thickness. In other words, the amount of tension generated in the wall of the ventricle (or any chamber or vessel) to produce a given intraventricular pressure depends on the size (radius and wall thickness) of the ventricle.

The law of Laplace is useful for understanding aneurysm formation, distensibility in blood vessels, and the effects of ventricular dilation on myocardial contraction. Dilation is an important factor in heart failure (see Chapter 27). With a dilated ventricle there is a need for the myocardial fibers in the wall to develop greater tension to produce a given pressure within the ventricle. The disadvantage of dilation is that the increased force, or tension, in the myocardial fibers required to develop a given pressure inside a dilated ventricle results in a decrease in the *rate* of fiber shortening, thereby decreasing the ability of the ventricle to eject blood (Schlant & Sonnenblick, 1990).

Preload

Left ventricular preload is the pressure generated in the left ventricle at the end of diastole, or left ventricular **end-diastolic pressure**. Preload is determined by end-diastolic volume. According to the Frank-Starling law, the end-diastolic volume stretches the cardiac muscle fibers, which in turn develop tension, or force, for contraction. Within a physiologic range of muscle stretching (2.2 μm to 2.4 μm), an increase in preload increases cardiac output (volume of blood pumped per minute; see Fig. 26-18). In monitoring preload the clinician measures indexes of left ventricular end-diastolic pressure. Pressure changes are important because increased left ventricular filling pressures "back up" into the pulmonary circulation, where they force plasma out through vessel walls, causing fluid to accumulate in lung tissues. (This condition is called pulmonary edema; see Chapter 30.) Treatment goals are to maintain an end-diastolic volume that will maintain or increase cardiac output.

Afterload

Left ventricular afterload is the resistance or impedance to ejection of blood from the left ventricle. It is the load the muscle must move after it starts to contract. Aortic systolic pressure is a good index of afterload. Low aortic pressures (decreased afterload) enable the heart to contract more rapidly, whereas high aortic pressures (increased afterload) slow contraction. Increased afterload, or high aortic pressures, causes higher work loads against which the heart must function and therefore the less blood it can eject and vice versa. Pressure in the ventricle must exceed aortic pressure before blood can be pumped out during systole. Afterload involves a force-velocity relationship; that is, the lighter the afterload, the faster the contraction, and the heavier the afterload, the slower the contraction.

In addition to influencing the speed of shortening, afterload is related to extent of shortening. Increases in aortic pressure, with a constant preload, result in decreased blood pumped by the left ventricle. Decreased aortic pressure allows the left ventricle to pump a larger volume.

Heart Rate

The average heart rate in normal adults is about 70 beats/min. The average heart rate is significantly greater in children. Heart rate diminishes by 10 to 20 beats/min during sleep and can accelerate to more than 100 beats/min during muscular activity or emotional excitement. In well-conditioned athletes at rest the heart rate is normally about 50 to 60 beats/min. In highly trained or elite athletes the resting heart rate can be below 50 beats/min. Highly trained athletes have a lower resting heart rate, greater stroke volume, and lower peripheral resistance in active muscles than they had before training. The low resting heart rate is due to an increased vagal stimulation and lower sympathetic stimulation (Berne & Levy, 1992). The lowered peripheral resistance is thought to be due to an increase in the number of arterioles in skeletal muscle. The decrease in peripheral resistance increases the venous return, causing the cardiac output to increase (Berne & Levy, 1992). As the resting heart rate falls in individuals during physical training, the end-diastolic fiber length of the ventricles increases; this occurs because the longer duration of diastole results in greater filling. The increased end-diastolic fiber length increases stroke volume, which helps to compensate for the decreased heart rate.

Neural factors, including neural reflexes, and hormonal and chemical factors influence the heart rate. Neural control is exerted by both the central and autonomic nervous systems. Hormonal factors include the catecholamines (norepinephrine and epinephrine), thyroid hormones, growth hormones, and pancreatic hormones. (Hormonal function is described in Unit VI.) Stimulation by the sympathetic nervous system increases the rhythmicity of the cardiac pacemaker (SA node), whereas the parasympathetic stimulation has an inhibiting effect.

Cardiovascular control centers in the brain

The major **cardiovascular control center** is in the brain stem in the medulla. Other areas of central cardiovascular control are in the hypothalamus, the cerebral cortex, the thalamus, and complex networks of exciting or inhibiting interneurons (connecting neurons) throughout the brain. The hypothalamic centers regulate cardiovascular responses to changes in temperature; the cerebral cortex centers adjust cardiac reaction to a vari-

ety of emotional states; and the medullary control center regulates heart rate and blood pressure (see p. 980 for a discussion of blood pressure regulation). The medullary neurons are often classified as cardiac and vasomotor (vasoconstrictor or vasodilator) centers; yet, because these centers are not discrete anatomic areas and actually constitute diffuse networks of interneurons, it is preferable to call the entire area the cardiovascular control center (Vander et al., 1990).

The nerve fibers from the cardiovascular control center synapse with the autonomic neurons (see Chapter 12 and Table 12-7). When the parasympathetic nerves to the heart are stimulated, the sympathetic nerves to the heart, arterioles, and veins are usually inhibited. The opposite is also true: when the sympathetic nerves are stimulated, the parasympathetic nerves are usually inhibited. Because parasympathetic excitation and simultaneous sympathetic inhibition generally depress cardiac function (e.g., decrease the heart rate), these interneurons are often referred to as the **cardioinhibitory center** (Little, 1985). Excitation occurs with parasympathetic inhibition and sympathetic stimulation, and these interneurons are collectively called the **cardioexcitatory center** (Little, 1985). Therefore heart rate can be slowed by two simultaneous events that begin in the cardiovascular control center: (1) inhibition of sympathetic stimulation of the SA node and (2) activation of parasympathetic stimulation of the SA node. Heart rate can be increased by activation of sympathetic nerves and inhibition of parasympathetic nerves.

The resting heart rate in healthy individuals is primarily under the control of parasympathetic stimulation. While the individual is at rest, parasympathetic effects from the vagus nerves override sympathetic effects in the SA node. Interruption of the vagus nerves causes significant tachycardia (abnormally fast heart rate) because the inhibitory parasympathetic influence is lost.

Neural reflexes

Two important neural reflexes that affect heart rate and rhythm are the Bainbridge reflex and the baroreceptor reflex. The **Bainbridge reflex** causes heart rate to increase after intravenous infusions of blood or other fluid. The increased rate is thought to be due to a reflex mediated by volume receptors in the atria that are innervated by the vagus nerves. (Volume receptors are thought to respond to increased plasma volume.) The magnitude of the change in heart rate depends on the initial heart rate. If the initial rate is slow, intravenous infusion usually accelerates it, but if the initial rate is rapid, infusions will usually slow it down (Berne & Levy, 1992). Contractility is usually not affected by the Bainbridge reflex.

The **baroreceptor reflex** is an important facilitator of blood pressure changes, but it also facilitates heart rate changes. The baroreceptor reflex is mediated by tissue pressure receptors (pressoreceptors) in the aortic arch and carotid arteries. (Because the receptors respond to mechanical factors, they are also called aortic and carotid mechanoreceptors.) The pressoreceptors increase their rate of discharge when stretched by blood pressure elevations. Neural impulses are then transmitted over the glossopharyngeal nerve (ninth cranial nerve) from the carotid artery and through the vagus nerve from the aorta to the cardiovascular control centers in the medulla. These centers initiate an increase in parasympathetic activity and a decrease in sympathetic activity, causing blood vessels to dilate and heart rate to decrease. In the heart, the initial response is caused by a decrease in sympathetic stimulation, but most of the decrease in heart rate is probably due to increased parasympathetic activity. Responses to the baroreceptor reflex return the blood pressure to its previous level, which may or may not be normal. The higher the blood pressure, the greater the reflexive decrease in heart rate.

If blood pressure is decreased, the baroreceptor reflex accelerates heart rate and causes vessels to constrict. These responses raise blood pressure back toward normal (see p. 980 and the section about shock in Chapter 27). The pressoreceptors are more effective in compensating for a decrease in arterial blood pressure than a rise in pressure (Kirchheim, 1976).

Neural receptors in the lungs cause heart rate to increase during inspiration and decrease during expiration. The increase in heart rate during inspiration is caused by the stretching (activation) of vagal fibers in the lungs that cause heart rate to speed up by inhibiting the cardioinhibitory center of the medulla. Inhibition of this center allows unopposed sympathetic acceleration of heart rate.

Hormones and biochemicals

Hormones and biochemicals affect the arteries arterioles, venules, capillaries and, both directly and indirectly, contractility of the myocardium. The catecholamines (norepinephrine and epinephrine) and hormones affect both heart rate and myocardial contractility. Norepinephrine increases heart rate, enhances myocardial contractility, and constricts blood vessels. Epinephrine dilates vessels of the liver and skeletal muscle and also causes an increase in myocardial contractility. Some adrenocortical hormones, such as hydrocortisone, potentiate the effects of the catecholamines.

Thyroid hormones enhance sympathetic activity, promoting an increase in cardiac output. The exact mechanism by which this occurs is not known. A decrease in growth hormone, as well as thyroid and adrenal hormones, results in bradycardia (heart rate below 60 beats/min), reduced cardiac output, and low blood pressure (hypotension; see Chapter 27).

Myocardial Contractility

Stroke volume, or the volume of blood ejected during systole, depends on the *force* of contraction, which depends on myocardial contractility, or the degree of myocardial fiber shortening. Two major factors determine the force of contraction: (1) changes in the stretching of the ventricular myocardium caused by changes in ventricular volume (preload) and (2) alterations in the sympathetic activation of the ventricles. An increase in the flow of blood from the veins into the heart distends the ventricle by increasing preload. Greater preload increases the stroke volume and, subsequently, cardiac output. Increased output then causes increased venous return, atrial volume and pressure, and eventually end-diastolic volume and stroke volume.

Myocardial contractility is difficult to measure because measurement requires keeping preload, afterload, and heart rate constant. Only when these factors are held constant can changes in cardiac performance be attributed to changes in the inotropic (contractile) state of the myocardium itself.

Factors affecting contractility are called **inotropic agents.** Positive inotropic agents increase the velocity of myocardial contraction (phase 0) and stroke volume. The positive inotropic agents are excess thyroid hormone, epinephrine, norepinephrine, dopamine or isoproterenol infusion, and calcium salt infusion. The negative inotropic agents decrease the velocity of myocardial contraction and the stroke volume. These agents include alcohol, procainamide, quinidine, and propranolol.

Myocardial contractility is also affected by oxygen and carbon dioxide levels (tensions) in the coronary blood. (Blood gases are discussed in Chapter 29.) Different degrees of arterial oxygen deficiency—termed hypoxemia—affect contractility differently. With severe hypoxemia (arterial oxygen saturation less than 50%) contractility is decreased. With less severe hypoxemia (saturation more than 50%) contractility is stimulated. Moderate degrees of hypoxemia may increase contractility by enhancing the myocardial response to circulating catecholamines (Berne & Levy, 1992).

Factors Determining Cardiac Output

Cardiac output is a measure of the amount of blood flow usually expressed in liters per minute. It is the volume of blood flowing through either the systemic or the pulmonary circuit per minute (Vander, Sherman, & Luciano, 1990). Heart rate and stroke volume determine cardiac output. The volume to which the ventricle fills is determined by the ventricular filling pressure and the compliance of the ventricle. The filling pressure of the right ventricle is the **right atrial pressure,** and the filling pressure of the left ventricle is the **left atrial pressure.** The cardiac output is determined by multiplying the heart rate and the stroke volume. Normal cardiac output is about 5 L/min for a resting adult. A summary of the major factors that determine cardiac output is presented in Fig. 26-20. (Also see heart rate and myocardial contractility [stroke volume], pp. 966-967.)

The ventricle does not eject all of the blood it contains; the amount ejected is called the **ejection fraction,** or the stroke volume divided by the end-diastolic vol-

ume. The end-diastolic volume of the normal ventricle is about 70 to 80 ml/m^2; the normal ejection fraction of the resting heart is about 60% to 75% (Schlant & Sonnenblick, 1990). The ejection fraction is increased by factors that increase contractility (e.g., sympathetic nervous system activity), and a decrease in ejection fraction is a hallmark of ventricular failure (Schlant & Sonnenblick, 1990).

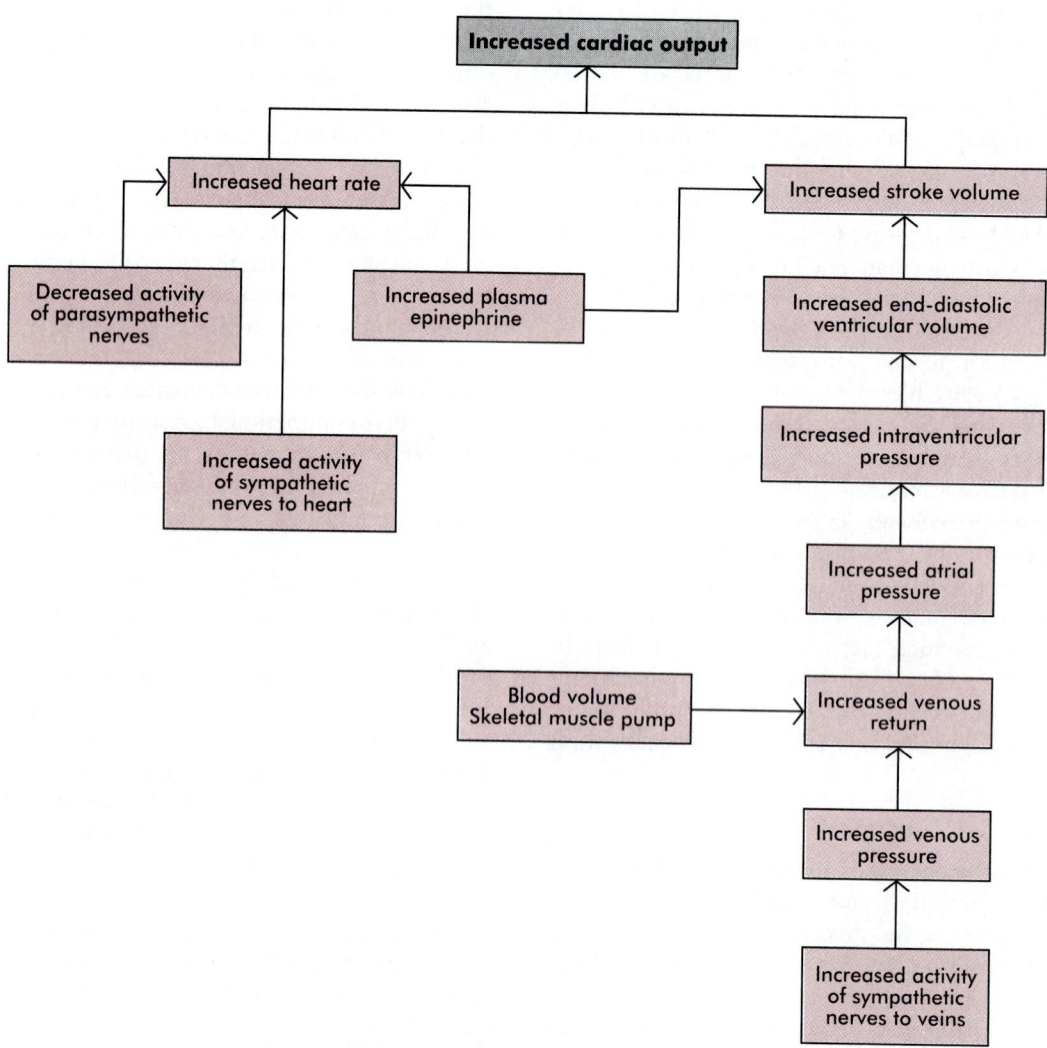

FIG. 26-20 **Major factors determining an increased cardiac output.** (Adapted from Vander, Sherman, & Luciano, 1990, and Halpenny, 1982b.)

THE SYSTEMIC CIRCULATION

The arteries and veins of the systemic circulation are illustrated in Fig. 26-21. Blood from the left side of the heart flows through the aorta and into the systemic arteries. The **arteries** branch into small **arterioles** that branch further into the smallest vessels, the **capillaries,** where nutrient exchange between the blood and tissues occurs. Blood from the capillaries then enters tiny **venules** that join together to form the larger **veins,** which return venous blood to the right heart. **Peripheral vascular system** is an imprecise term used to describe the part of the systemic circulation that supplies the skin and the extremities, particularly the legs and feet.

Structure of Blood Vessels

Blood vessel walls are composed of three layers: (1) the tunica intima (innermost or intimal layer), (2) the tunica media (middle or medial layer), and (3) the tunica externa or adventitia (outermost or external layer). These structures are illustrated in Figs. 26-22 and 26-23. The **tunica intima** is composed of a layer of squamous epithelium or endothelium, a layer of connective tissue, and a basement membrane. (These cellular structures are described in Chapter 1.) The **tunica media** is composed of smooth muscle fibers mixed with elastic fibers. The **tunica externa,** or adventitia, has a thin layer of connective tissue containing elastic and collagenous fibers that run lengthwise in the vessel. Blood vessel walls vary in thickness depending on the thickness or absence of one or more of these three layers. Cells of the larger vessels are nourished by the **vasa vasorum,** small vessels located in the tunica externa. The vasa vasorum arise from the blood vessel itself or from other vessels nearby.

Arterial Vessels

Arterial walls are composed of elastic connective tissue, fibrous connective tissue, and smooth muscle. There are two types of arteries: elastic arteries and muscular arteries. The **elastic arteries** have a very thick tunica media that contains more elastic fibers than smooth muscle fibers. Elastic arteries include the aorta and its major branches and the pulmonary trunk. Elasticity enables the vessel to stretch as blood is ejected from the heart during systole. During diastole, elasticity promotes recoil of the arteries, which is important for maintaining blood pressure within the vessels.

The **muscular arteries** are the medium-sized and small arteries farther from the heart than the elastic arteries. They contain fewer elastic fibers and more muscle fibers than the elastic arteries because, being farther from the heart, they have less need of the properties of stretch and recoil. The function of the muscular arteries is to distribute blood to arterioles throughout the body. They also play a role in controlling blood flow because their smooth muscle can be stimulated to contract or relax. Contraction narrows the vessel **lumen** (the internal cavity of the vessel), which diminishes flow through the vessel. This condition is termed **vasoconstriction.** The smooth muscle layer can also be stimulated to relax, which permits more blood to flow through the vessel lumen. This state is called **vasodilation.**

An artery becomes an arteriole where the diameter of its lumen narrows to less than 0.5 mm. The arterioles are composed almost exclusively of smooth muscle, with little elastic tissue. Arterioles regulate the flow of blood into the capillaries by vasoconstriction, which retards the flow of blood into the capillaries, and vasodilation, which permits blood to enter the capillaries freely (Fig. 26-24). The thick smooth muscle layer of the arterioles is a major determinant of the resistance blood encounters as it flows through the systemic circulation.

The capillary network is composed of connective channels, or thoroughfares, called **metarterioles,** and "true" capillaries (Fig. 26-25). The capillaries branch from the metarterioles, which are the main channels connecting arterioles and venules. The metarteriole and capillary meet at a ring of smooth muscle called the **precapillary sphincter.** As the sphincters contract and relax, they regulate blood flow through the capillaries. Appropriately stimulated, the precapillary sphincters help to maintain arterial pressure and regulate selective flow to vascular beds.

The capillary walls are very thin, making possible the rapid exchange of substrates, metabolites, and special products (such as hormones) between the blood and the interstitial fluid, from which they are taken up by the cells. The capillary wall consists of a single layer of endothelial cells surrounded by the thin basement membrane of the tunica intima. A single endothelial cell may form the entire vessel wall if the capillary has no tunica media or tunica externa. In some capillaries, the endothelial cells contain oval windows or pores termed **fenestrations.** Fenestrations are generally covered by a thin diaphragm.

Substances pass between the capillary lumen and the interstitial fluid in several ways: (1) through junctions between endothelial cells, (2) through fenestrations in endothelial cells, (3) in vesicles moved by active transport across the endothelial cell membrane, or (4) by diffusion through the endothelial cell membrane. (Movement across cell membranes is described in Chapter 1.) A single capillary may be only 0.5 mm to 1 mm in length and 0.01 mm in diameter, but the capillaries are so numerous that their total surface area may be more than 600 m^2 or larger than 100 football fields.

Text continued on p. 974.

A

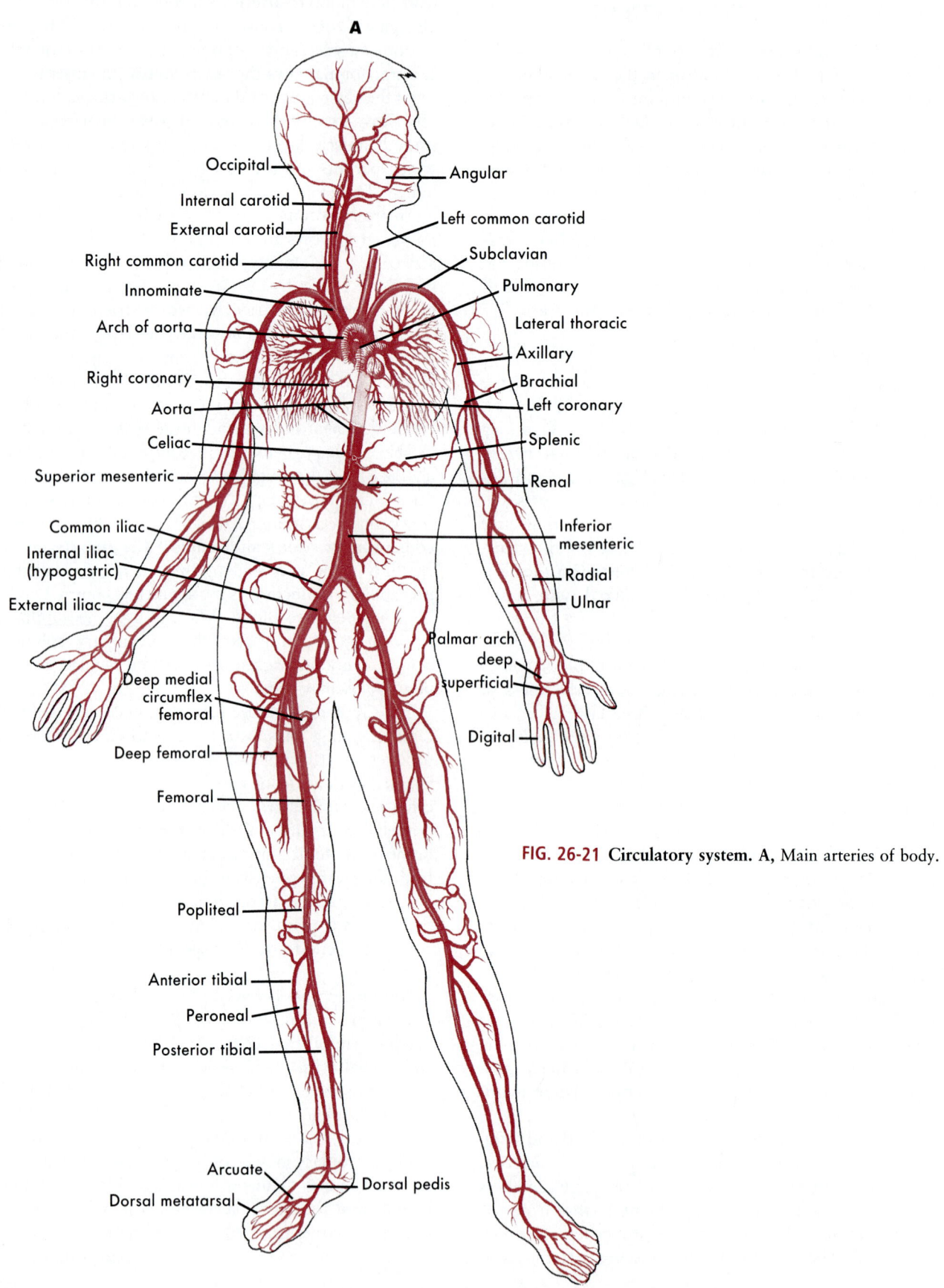

Occipital

Angular

Internal carotid

External carotid

Left common carotid

Right common carotid

Subclavian

Innominate

Pulmonary

Arch of aorta

Lateral thoracic

Axillary

Right coronary

Brachial

Aorta

Left coronary

Celiac

Splenic

Superior mesenteric

Renal

Common iliac

Inferior mesenteric

Internal iliac (hypogastric)

Radial

External iliac

Ulnar

Palmar arch deep

Deep medial circumflex femoral

superficial

Deep femoral

Digital

Femoral

Popliteal

Anterior tibial

Peroneal

Posterior tibial

Arcuate

Dorsal pedis

Dorsal metatarsal

FIG. 26-21 Circulatory system. **A,** Main arteries of body.

B

FIG. 26-21, **cont'd** B, Principal veins of body. Only superficial veins are shown on forearms and hands. (From Thibodeau, 1987.)

ARTERY   VEIN

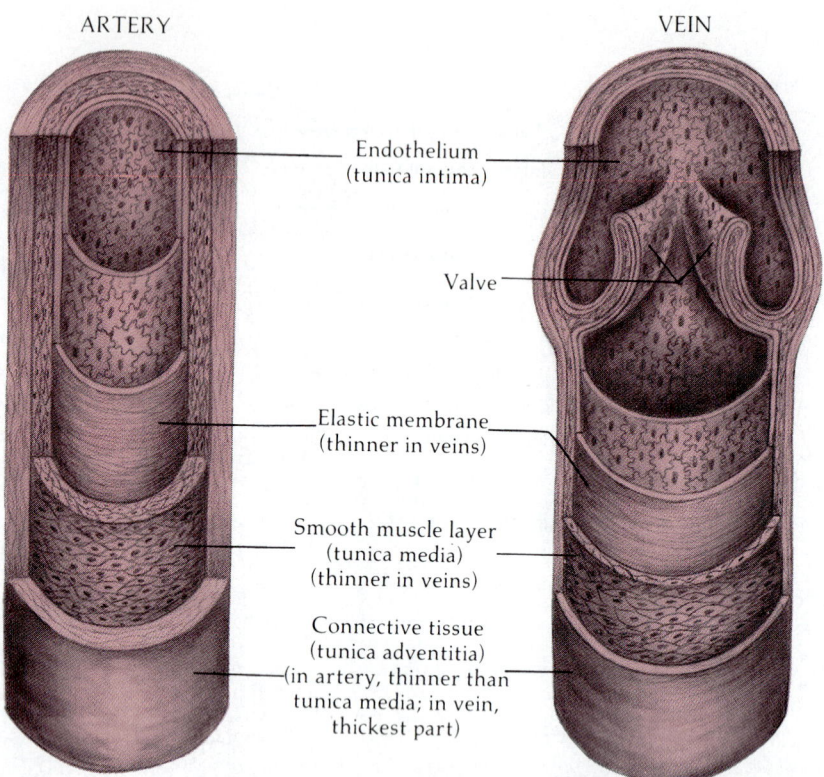

Endothelium
(tunica intima)

Valve

Elastic membrane
(thinner in veins)

Smooth muscle layer
(tunica media)
(thinner in veins)

Connective tissue
(tunica adventitia)
(in artery, thinner than
tunica media; in vein,
thickest part)

FIG. 26-22 Schematic drawings of artery and vein. Shown are the comparative thickness of three coats: outer coat (tunica adventitia), muscle coat (tunica media), and lining of endothelium (tunica intima). Note that muscle and outer coats are much thinner in veins than in arteries and that veins have valves. (From Thompson, McFarland, Hirsch, & Tucker, 1993.)

FIG. 26-23 This ruptured tube is a blood vessel. It is full of red blood cells, which move through these blood vessels transporting oxygen and carbon dioxide from one place to another in the body. (From Raven & Johnson, 1992.)

FIG. 26-24 Capillary wall. Walls of capillaries consist of only a single layer of epithelial cells. These thin, flattened cells permit rapid movement of substances between blood and interstitial fluid. Note thicker walls and presence of precapillary sphincters (smooth muscle cells) on arteriole. (From Thibodeau, 1993.)

FIG. 26-25 Capillary network. Blood enters network as arterial blood and exits as venous blood.

FIG. 26-26 Valves of vein. Pooled blood is moved toward heart as valves are forced open by pressure from volume of blood downstream. (From Thibodeau, 1993.)

FIG. 26-27 Muscle pump.

Control of Vessel Contraction or Relaxation: Vasomotion

Recently it has been demonstrated in vitro that the endothelium is a source of substances that promote contraction or relaxation, **vasomotion,** of the vascular smooth muscle. **Prostacyclin,** a prostaglandin formed in the endothelium from arachidonic acid, can relax vascular smooth muscle through increases in cyclic adenosine monophosphate (cAMP). Mechanisms that cause the *release* of prostacyclin are not known. The primary function of prostacyclin, however, is to inhibit platelet adherence to the endothelium, thereby preventing intravascular clot formation.

More significant to endothelial-mediated vascular dilation is the formation and release of the **endothelial-derived relaxing factor (EDRF).** Stimulation of the endothelial cells in vivo causes the production and release of EDRF (Berne & Levy, 1992). The EDRF activates guanylate cyclase in the vascular smooth muscle to increase cyclic guanosine monophosphate (cGMP) concentration, which produces relaxation. The endothelium can also produce an **endothelial-derived contracting factor (EDCF),** yet little is known about its function. It is apparently not *endotelin,* a small vasoconstrictor protein that has been isolated from endothelial cells (Berne & Levy, 1992).

Veins

The smallest venules closest to the capillaries have an inner lining, which is composed of the endothelium of the tunica intima and surrounded by some fibrous tissue. The largest venules, those farthest from the capillaries, are surrounded by a few smooth muscle fibers that comprise a thin tunica media.

Compared to arteries, veins are thin-walled, fibrous, and have a larger diameter (see Fig. 26-22). A given vein is larger than the artery that lies within the same sheath. Veins are more numerous than arteries. In veins the tunica externa has less elastic tissue than it does in the arteries. Therefore veins do not recoil after distention as quickly as arteries. Like arteries, veins receive nourishment from the tiny vasa vasorum. Some veins, most commonly in the lower limbs, contain valves that regulate the one-way flow of blood toward the heart (Fig. 26-26). These valves are folds of the tunica intima and resemble the semilunar valves of the heart. Backflow in veins of the legs is stopped as the flaps of the valves fill with blood and block the vessel. The position of the valves also facilitates blood flow in the proper direction during venous compression. When a person stands up, contraction of the skeletal muscles of the legs compresses the deep veins of the legs and assists the flow of blood toward the heart. This important mechanism of venous return is called the **muscle pump** (Fig. 26-27).

Factors Affecting Blood Flow

Blood flow is the amount of fluid moved per unit of time and is usually expressed as liters or milliliters per minute (ml/min) or cubic centimeters per second (cm³/sec). Blood flow is regulated by the same physical properties that govern the movement of simple fluids in a closed, rigid system. These properties include pressure, resistance, velocity, turbulent versus laminar flow, and compliance.

Pressure and Resistance

Blood flow is determined primarily by two factors, pressure and resistance. **Pressure** in a liquid system is the force exerted on the liquid per unit area. Pressure is expressed as dynes per square centimeter (dyn/cm²), mm Hg, or torr. Blood flow depends partly on the difference between pressures in the arterial and venous vessels supplying the organ. Fluid moves from the arterial "side" of the capillaries, a region of greater pressure, to the venous side, a region of lesser pressure.

Resistance is the opposition to force. In the cardiovascular system most opposition to blood flow is provided by the diameter and length of the blood vessels themselves. Therefore most of the changes in blood flow through an organ are due to changes in the vascular resistance within the organ. The major mechanisms causing changes in vascular resistance are an increase or decrease in vessel diameter and the opening or closing of vascular channels. Resistance in a vessel is inversely related to blood flow; that is, increased resistance leads to decreased blood flow.

Blood flow (Q) through a vessel can be calculated from measurements of pressure at the inflow end of the vessel (P_1), pressure at the outflow end of the vessel (P_2), and resistance (R). The difference between P_1 and P_2 is often referred to as the change in pressure and is expressed as δP. The following formula, which expresses **Poiseuille's law**, shows the relationship between blood flow, pressure, and resistance:

$$Q = \frac{\delta P}{R}$$

where Q = blood flow, δP = the pressure difference ($P_1 - P_2$), and R = resistance.

Resistance to flow cannot be measured directly, but it can be calculated if the pressure difference and flow volumes are known. To determine resistance, the equation for flow is rearranged as follows:

$$R = \frac{\delta P}{Q}$$

Another factor that influences blood flow is the consistency of the blood. Flow varies inversely with the viscosity of the fluid. Thick fluids move more slowly and cause greater resistance to flow than thin fluids. The viscosity of blood depends on its red cell content. The greater the percentage of red cells in the blood, the more viscous the blood. This relationship is expressed as the hematocrit, the ratio of the volume of red blood cells to the volume of whole blood (see Chapter 22). A high hematocrit reduces flow through the blood vessels, particularly the microcirculation (arterioles, capillaries, and venules). Conditions in which the hematocrit is elevated, for example, dehydration, cyanotic congenital heart disease (see Chapter 28), or polycythemia (see Chapter 23), can lead to increased cardiac work as a result of increased vascular resistance.

The viscosity of blood also increases if blood flow becomes very slow or stagnates. This condition is called **anomalous viscosity**. Anomalous viscosity is generally not significant unless cardiac output is low (Little, 1985). When cardiac output is reduced, as in shock, venous flow may be slowed to the point that anomalous viscosity develops. (Shock is described in Chapter 27.)

Poiseuille's formula for resistance to fluid flow through a tube takes into account the length of the tube, the viscosity of the fluid, and the radius of the tube's lumen. According to Poiseuille's formula, resistance (R) is proportional to a constant $8/\pi$, the viscosity of the blood (η), and the length of the vessel (l), and is inversely proportional to the fourth power of the lumen's radius (v_4) (Berne & Levy, 1992). Thus

$$R = \frac{8\eta l}{\pi v_4}$$

Because this equation was derived using straight, rigid tubes with steady, streamlined flow, it cannot be applied directly to the vascular system. Nevertheless, it is a useful model of vascular resistance.

The most important factor determining resistance *in a single vessel* is the caliber of the vessel's lumen, expressed in Poiseuille's formula as its radius and in Fig. 26-28 as its diameter. Small changes in the lumen's radius lead to large changes in vascular resistance. Because vessel length is relatively constant, length is not as important as lumen size in determining flow through a single vessel.

Generally, resistance to flow is greater in longer tubes because resistance increases with length. That resistance increases with increased length is demonstrated by comparing flow of the same amount of blood under the same pressure through vessels arranged in different configurations. Blood flowing through the distributing arteries, beginning with branches off the aorta and ending at arterioles in the capillary bed, encounters more resistance than blood flowing through the capillary bed itself, where flow is distributed among many short, tiny branches arranged in parallel. This is because the dis-

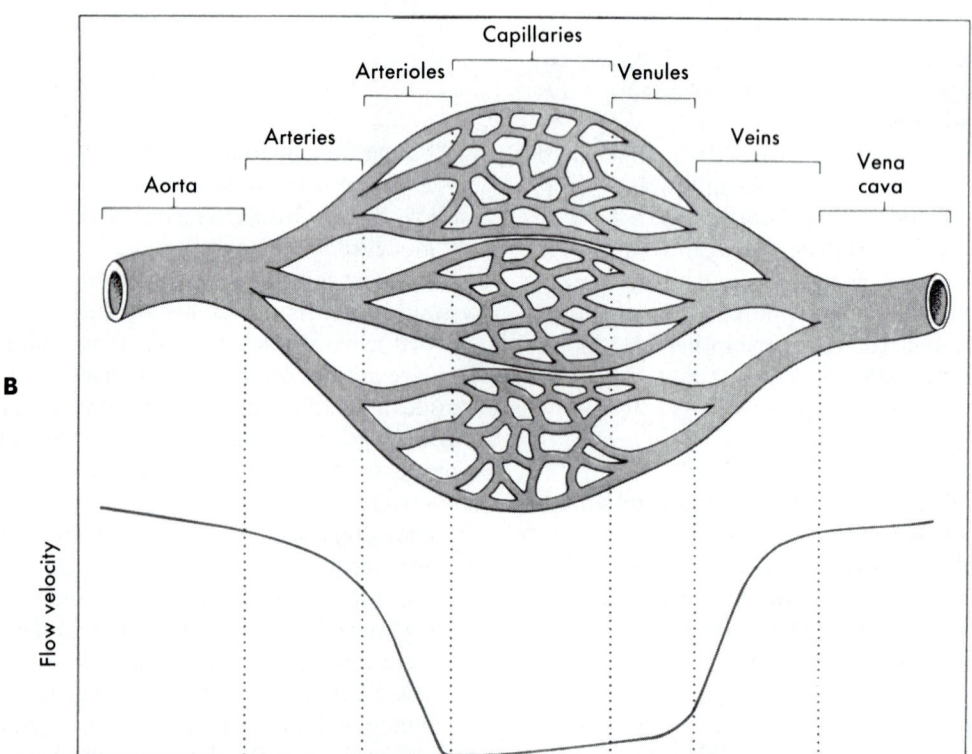

FIG. 26-28 Lumen diameter, blood flow, and resistance. A, Effect of lumen diameter on flow through vessel. **B,** Effect of vessel diameter on resistance and flow velocity. The narrower a tube, the greater the resistance it presents to liquid flowing through it. The resistance is inversely proportional to the fourth power of the radius of the tube. (**B** from Raven & Johnson, 1992.)

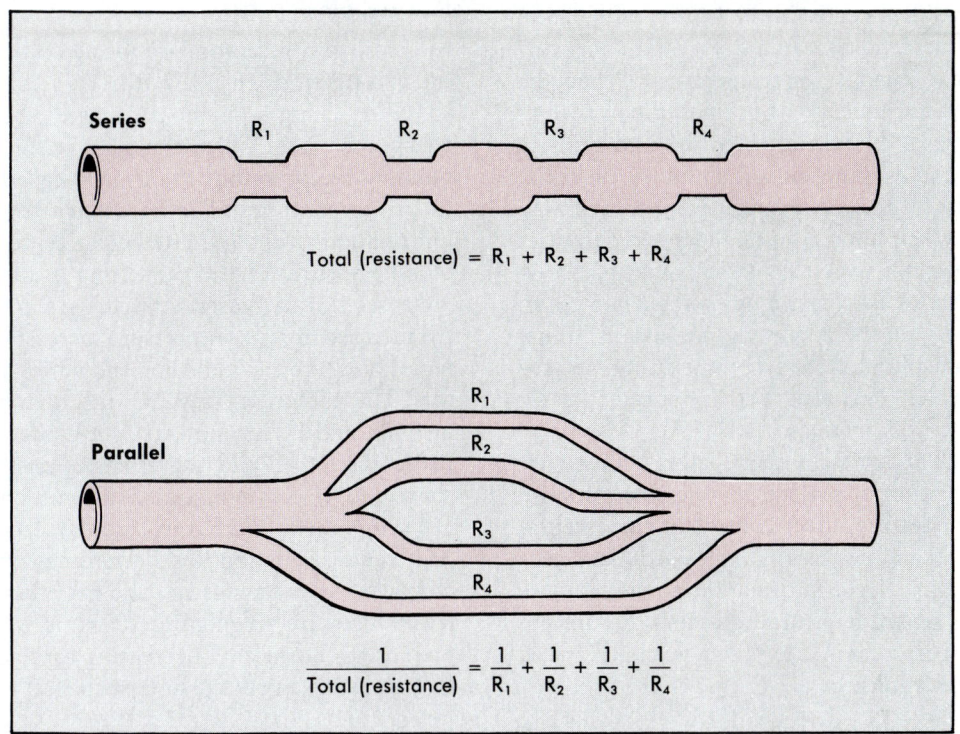

FIG. 26-29 **Resistance in blood vessels arranged in series or parallel.** *R,* Resistance in an individual vessel.

tributing arteries comprise a long system of tubes connected in series (end to end), whereas the arterioles and capillaries comprise a short system of many vessels arranged in parallel (side by side) (Fig. 26-29). Although the arterioles are arranged in series with the distributing arteries and the capillaries, they are arranged in parallel with other arterioles. Similarly, the capillaries are in series with the metarterioles, but they are in parallel with other capillaries.

Resistance to flow through a system of vessels, or **total resistance,** depends not only on characteristics of individual vessels but also on whether the vessels are arranged in series or in parallel. Total resistance is calculated differently for vessels arranged in series and in parallel (see Fig. 26-29). For vessels arranged in series, total resistance equals the sum obtained by adding all the individual resistances calculated using Poiseuille's formula. For vessels arranged in parallel, total resistance equals the sum of the reciprocals *(I/R)* of the individual resistances.

Total resistance is related to the total cross-sectional area of a system of vessels in parallel and to the number of vessels in parallel that make up the total cross-sectional area. The larger the total cross-sectional area, as in the capillary system, the lower the resistance. However, if a cross-sectional area is made up of a very large number of parallel vessels, the overall resistance will be

greater than it would be if the cross-sectional area were made up of only two or three parallel vessels. Therefore, resistance is greater in smaller vessels than in larger vessels. The total cross-sectional area of the arteriolar system is greater than that of the arterial system, yet the greater number of arterioles arranged in parallel leads to great resistance to flow in the arteriolar system. Although the capillary system has a larger number of vessels in parallel than the arteriolar system, the total cross-sectional area is greater, resulting in lower resistance overall through the capillary system. The relationship between flow and cross-sectional area has physiologic significance. Despite the narrow diameter of each vessel (which normally increases resistance), total resistance in any capillary bed is relatively low. This, plus the slow velocity of flow in each vessel, promotes optimal capillary-tissue exchange.

Neural Control of Total Peripheral Resistance

Total resistance in the systemic circulation, sometimes called total peripheral resistance, is determined primarily by change in the diameter of the arterioles. Reflex control of total cardiac output and peripheral resistance includes (1) sympathetic stimulation of heart, arterioles, and veins; and (2) parasympathetic stimulation of the heart only.

The autonomic nervous system is monitored by the

cardiovascular control center in the brain (see p. 966). The hypothalamic centers regulate vascular (and cardiac) responses to changes in temperature. When the body's core temperature exceeds normal, the hypothalamus reflex initiates dilation of arterioles and veins in the skin. This causes shunting of blood to the skin, where heat is lost from sweating, radiation, conduction, or convection. When body core temperature decreases below normal, surface vessels constrict, shunting blood to the vital organs. Vasoconstriction is regulated by an area of the brain stem that maintains a constant (tonic) output of norepinephrine from sympathetic fibers in the peripheral arterioles. This tonic activity is essential for maintenance of blood pressure.

During exercise and stress, the sympathetic fibers that stimulate vasodilation of skeletal muscle arterioles are thought to be under the direct control of the cerebral cortex and hypothalamus, and *not* the medullary centers (Vander et al., 1990). Information about pressure and resistance is sensed by neural receptors (baroreceptors and chemoreceptors) in arterial walls and delivered to the medullary centers.

Baroreceptors

Major stretch receptors are located in the aorta and in the carotid sinus (Fig. 26-30). These baroreceptors respond to changes in smooth muscle fiber length by altering their rate of discharge. (Technically, they are mechanoreceptors but are usually called baroreceptors or pressoreceptors.) The baroreceptors supply sensory information to the cardiovascular center that regulates blood pressure. The rate of firing of the baroreceptors increases and decreases with changes in blood pressure. An increase in arterial pressure increases the rate of firing of both the carotid sinus and aortic arch baroreceptors. These impulses travel up the afferent nerves to the medulla and (1) slow heart rate by decreasing sympathetic discharge and increasing parasympathetic discharge, (2) decrease myocardial contractility by inhibiting sympathetic discharge, and (3) decrease arteriolar and venous dilation by decreasing sympathetic discharge to smooth muscle. The net effect of this major blood pressure–regulating reflex is to reduce blood pressure to normal by decreasing cardiac output (heart rate and stroke volume) and peripheral resistance. (Pos-

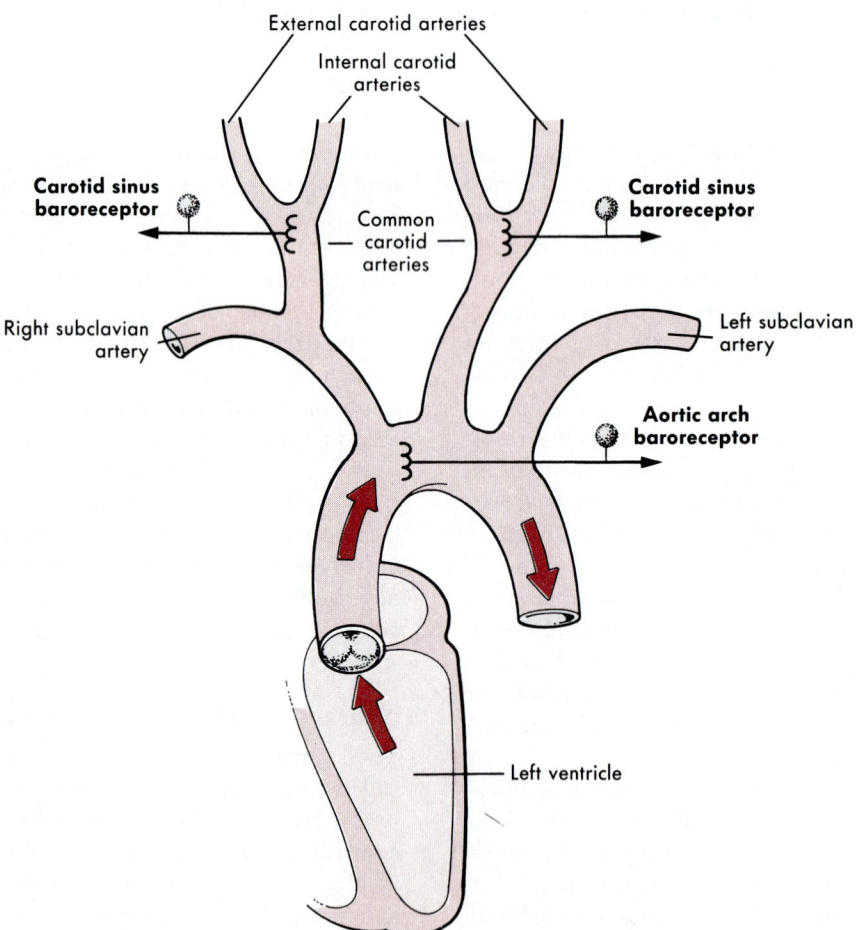

FIG. 26-30 Location of arterial baroreceptors.

tural changes and the baroreceptor reflex are discussed in Chapter 27.)

Arterial chemoreceptors

Specialized areas within the aortic and carotid arteries are sensitive to concentrations of oxygen, carbon dioxide, and hydrogen ions (pH) in the blood. Although these receptors, called chemoreceptors, are more important for the control of respiration, they also transmit impulses to the medullary cardiovascular centers that regulate blood pressure. A decrease in arterial oxygen concentration or pH causes a reflexive increase in blood pressure, whereas an increase in carbon dioxide causes a decrease in blood pressure. Blood pressure changes are carried out by smooth muscle layers in the vessels. Vasoconstriction raises blood pressure and vasodilation lowers it. The major chemoreceptive reflex is due to alterations in arterial oxygen concentration. The effects of altered pH or carbon dioxide levels are minor.

Velocity

Blood velocity is the *distance* blood travels in a unit of time, usually centimeters per second (cm/sec). Blood velocity is directly related to blood flow (*amount* of blood moved per unit of time) and inversely related to the cross-sectional area of the vessel in which the blood is flowing.

The relationship between velocity and flow can be understood by thinking of a river. The volume of water flowing in a river is the same whether the river is narrow or wide. Where the river narrows, the water flows quickly; where it widens out the water flows slowly. The volume of water moving between the riverbanks does not change. In the body, as blood moves from the aorta to the capillaries, the total cross-sectional area of the vessels increases and velocity of flow decreases.

Laminar versus turbulent flow

Flow through any tubular system is either laminar or turbulent. Normally, blood flow through the vessels is laminar. In **laminar flow,** concentric layers of molecules move "straight ahead." Each concentric layer flows at a different velocity (Fig. 26-31). The cohesive attraction between the fluid and the vessel wall prevents the molecules of blood that are in contact with the wall from moving. The next thin layer of blood is able to slide

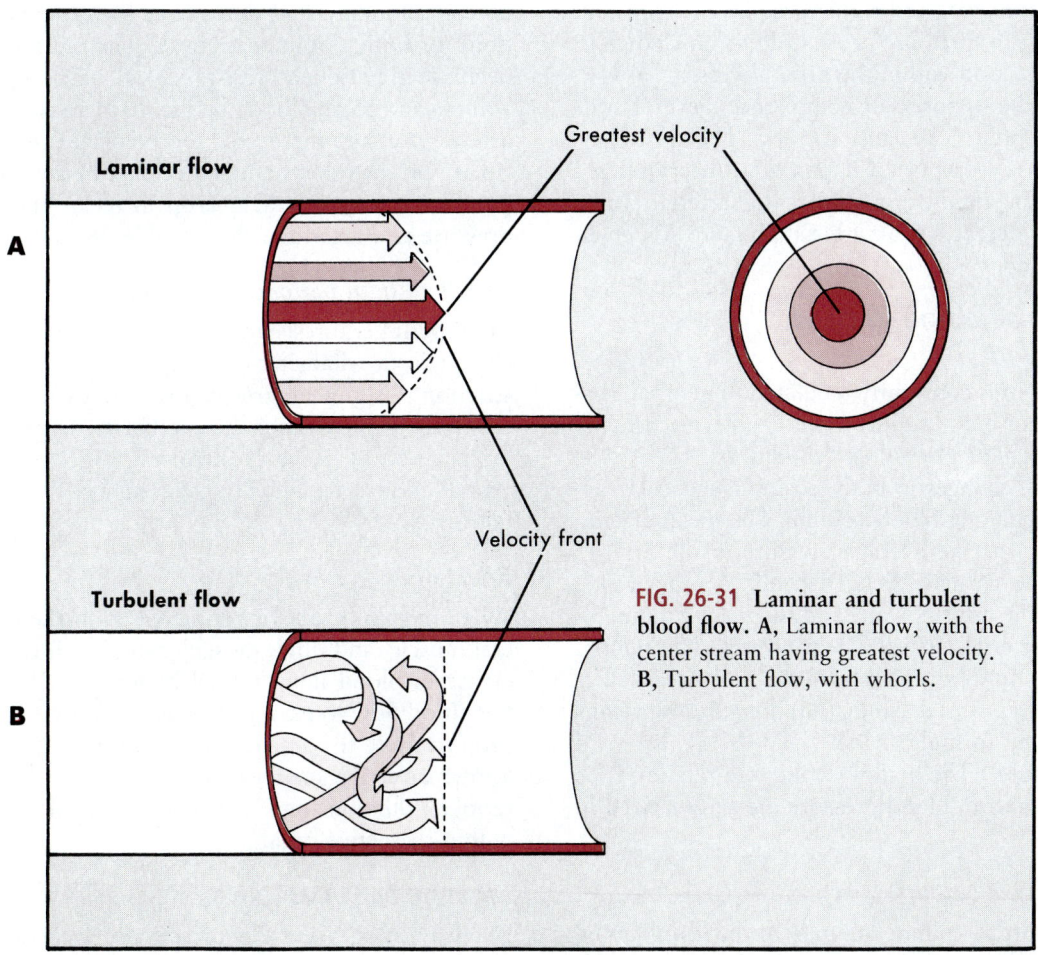

FIG. 26-31 Laminar and turbulent blood flow. **A**, Laminar flow, with the center stream having greatest velocity. **B**, Turbulent flow, with whorls.

slowly past the stationary layer, and so on until, at the center, the blood velocity is greatest. The centermost concentric layer of fluid is not slowed by friction against the vessel wall. Large vessels have room for a large center layer; therefore they have less resistance to flow and greater flow and velocity than smaller vessels.

Where flow is obstructed, or the vessel turns, or blood flows over rough surfaces, it becomes turbulent. **Turbulent flow** consists of whorls or eddy currents and is noisy, causing a murmur to be heard on auscultation. Resistance increases with turbulence.

Vascular Compliance

Vascular compliance is the increase in volume a vessel is able to accommodate for a given increase in pressure (e.g., C = VP). Compliance depends on the ratio of elastic fibers to muscle fibers in the vessel wall. The elastic arteries are more compliant than the muscular arteries, and the veins are more compliant than either type of artery because they serve as storage areas for the circulatory system.

Compliance determines a vessel's response to pressure changes. For example, with a very small increase in pressure, a large volume of blood can be accommodated by the venous system. In the less compliant arterial system, where smaller volumes and higher pressures are normal, small variations in pressure cause little or no change in the volume of blood within the arterial vessels.

Stiffness is the opposite of compliance. Several conditions and disorders can cause stiffness. The most common is arteriosclerosis (see Chapter 27). Arteriosclerosis increases the rigidity or stiffness of arterial walls, which in turn increases peak arterial pressure at a given volume of blood.

Regulation of Blood Pressure
Arterial Pressure

Arterial pressure is constantly regulated to maintain tissue **perfusion,** or blood supply to the capillary beds, during a wide range of physiologic conditions. These conditions include changes in body position, muscular activity, and circulating blood volume. The **mean arterial pressure,** which is the average pressure in the arteries throughout the cardiac cycle, depends on the elastic properties of the arterial walls and the *mean* volume of blood in the arterial system. The mean arterial pressure (MAP) can be approximated from the measured values of the systolic (Ps) and diastolic (Pd) pressures by means of the following formula: MAP = Pd + 1/3 (Ps − Pd or pulse pressure). The major factors and relationships that regulate arterial blood pressure are summarized in Fig. 26-32.

Effects of cardiac output

The cardiac output (minute volume) of the heart can be changed by alterations in heart rate, stroke volume (vol-

TABLE 26-3

Factors That Affect Mean Arterial Pressure and Capillary Flow

	Mean arterial pressure	Capillary flow
Peripheral resistance*		
Increased	Increased	Decreased
Decreased	Decreased	Increased
Heart rate†		
Increased	Increased	Increased
Decreased	Decreased	Decreased
Stroke volume‡		
Increased	Increased	Increased
Decreased	Decreased	Decreased

From Little, R.C. (1985). *Physiology of the heart and circulation* (3rd ed.). St. Louis: Mosby–Year Book.
*Cardiac output maintained constant.
†Peripheral resistance and stroke volume contrast.
‡Peripheral resistance and heart rate constant.

ume of blood ejected during each ventricular contraction), or both. An increase in cardiac output without a decrease in peripheral resistance will cause both arterial volume and mean blood pressure to increase. The higher arterial pressure increases blood flow through the arterioles. On the other hand, a decrease in the cardiac output causes an immediate drop in mean arterial blood pressure and arteriolar flow (Table 26-3).

Effects of total peripheral resistance

Total peripheral resistance is primarily determined by a change in the diameter of the arterioles: arteriolar constriction raises mean arterial pressure by preventing the free flow of blood into the capillaries. Dilation has the opposite effect. Reflex control of vasoconstriction and vasodilation is mediated by the sympathetic nervous system.

Effect of hyperemia

When metabolic activity is increased in the heart, skeletal muscle, and other muscular organs, it causes an increase in blood flow termed **hyperemia.** For example, the blood flow to exercising skeletal muscle increases in proportion to the activity of the muscle. This condition, known as active (exercise) hyperemia, is the result of arteriolar dilation and autoregulation of blood flow within the active organ.

Effects of hormones

Many hormones cause contraction or relaxation of arteriolar smooth muscle. By constricting or dilating arte-

FIG. 26-32 Factors regulating blood pressure.

rioles in specific vascular beds, hormones can (1) increase the blood supply to vital organs requiring more flow in times of stress, (2) redistribute blood volume during hemorrhage or shock, and (3) regulate heat loss.

Epinephrine, the hormone released from the adrenal medulla, causes vasoconstriction in most vascular beds (exceptions are the liver and skeletal muscles). However, the effects of norepinephrine (from the sympathetic nervous system and adrenal medulla) are quantitatively more vasoconstrictive than the effects of epinephrine.

The systemic renin-angiotensin system

Renin is an enzyme synthesized and secreted by the juxtaglomerular cells of the kidney. To date, however, renin has also been found in the adrenal cortex, in the salivary gland, in the prolactin-producing and luteinizing hormone–producing cells of the pituitary, in arterial smooth muscle cells in the vascular endothelial cell, in the brain, and in the myocardium (Re, 1987). Factors that control renin release include (1) a drop in blood pressure (e.g., the renal artery); (2) a decrease in the amount of sodium delivered to the kidney (although recent evidence indicates a role for chloride in regulating renin secretion) (Re, 1987); (3) β-adrenergic stimuli stimulate release, whereas β-adrenergic inhibitors decrease renin release; (4) angiotensin II reduces renin re-

lease; and (5) low potassium concentrations in plasma increase renin release.

Once in the circulation, renin splits off a polypeptide from angiotensinogen to generate **angiotensin I.** Angiotensin I appears to be physiologically inactive (Re, 1987). Angiotensin I, however, is converted by an enzyme (kininase II) to **angiotensin II.** Angiotensin II is a powerful vasoconstrictor and also stimulates the secretion of **aldosterone** from the adrenal gland (Fig. 26-33; also see Fig. 17-6). Aldosterone causes reabsorption of sodium in the kidneys. In addition, angiotensin II causes some sodium retention in the kidneys and suppresses renin secretion from the juxtaglomerular cells (Re, 1987; Re et al., 1978). In some tissues, angiotensin II is converted to angiotensin III, which is also biologically active.

The kidney-based renin-angiotensin system serves as an important regulatory loop. For example, decreases in blood pressure or sodium delivery to the kidneys (macula densa), as might occur after hemorrhage or extracellular volume deficits (dehydration), stimulate secretion of renin, which acts in the blood on angiotensinogen to form angiotensin I. Angiotensin I is converted to angiotensin II and restores blood pressure, as well as sodium retention caused by increased secretion of aldosterone. Overall the renin-angiotensin system is acti-

FIG. 26-33 Renin-angiotensin system.

vated after volume depletion or hypotension, or both, and is suppressed after volume repletion and hypertension.

Venous Pressure

The main determinants of venous blood pressure are (1) the volume of fluid within the veins and (2) the compliance (distensibility) of the vessel walls. Veins have much thinner walls than arteries and are more distensible than arteries. The venous system accommodates approximately 60% of the total blood volume at any given moment, with a venous pressure averaging less than 10 mm Hg. Conversely, the arteries accommodate about 15% of the total blood volume, with an average arterial pressure (blood pressure) of about 100 mm Hg (Vander et al., 1990).

The sympathetic nervous system regulates venous blood pressure by controlling compliance. The walls of the veins are highly innervated by sympathetic fibers that, when stimulated, cause venous smooth muscle to contract. This increases muscle tone (i.e., prevents distention) rather than causing vasoconstriction, as occurs in arterial vessels. The effect of increased muscle tone is to stiffen the wall of the vein, which reduces distensibility and increases blood pressure. The increased venous pressure forces more blood through the veins and into the right heart.

Two other mechanisms that increase venous pressure and venous return to the heart are (1) the skeletal muscle pump and (2) the respiratory pump. During skeletal muscle contraction, the veins within the muscles are par-

tially compressed, causing a decrease in venous capacity and increased return to the heart. The respiratory pump acts during inspiration, when the veins of the abdomen are partially compressed by the downward movement of the diaphragm. Increased abdominal pressure moves blood toward the heart.

Regulation of the Coronary Circulation

Flow of blood (F) in the coronary circulation, as in vascular beds, is directly proportional to the perfusion pressure (P) and inversely proportional to the vascular resistance (R) of the bed (F = P/R). **Coronary perfusion pressure** is the difference between pressure in the aorta and pressure in the coronary vessels of the right atrium. Aortic pressure is the driving pressure that perfuses vessels of the myocardium. Mechanisms of vasodilation and vasoconstriction normally maintain coronary blood flow despite stresses imposed by the constant contraction and relaxation of the heart muscle and despite shifts (within a physiologic range) of coronary perfusion pressure.

Several anatomic factors influence coronary blood flow. Because of their location, the aortic valve cusps obstruct coronary blood flow by pushing against the openings of the coronary arteries during systole. Also during systole, the coronary arteries are compressed by ventricular contraction. These anatomic factors have a **systolic compressive effect,** which is particularly evident in the subendocardial layers of the left ventricular wall and can greatly decrease coronary blood flow. Therefore most coronary blood flow in the left ventricle occurs during diastole. During the period of systolic compression, when flow is slowed or stopped, oxygen is supplied by **myoglobin,** a protein that is present in heart muscle. This protein binds oxygen during diastole and then releases it when blood levels of oxygen fall during systole (Sparks & Rooke, 1987).

Autoregulation

Autoregulation (automatic self-regulation) enables individual vessels to regulate blood flow by altering their own arteriolar resistances. Autoregulation in the coronary circulation maintains constant blood flow at perfusion pressures (mean arterial pressure) between 60 and 180 mm Hg, provided that other influencing factors are held constant (Berne & Levy, 1992). Thus autoregulation ensures constant coronary blood flow despite shifts in the perfusion pressure within the stated range.

The mechanism of autoregulation is not known, but two explanations have been proposed: the myogenic hypothesis and the metabolic hypothesis. The myogenic hypothesis proposes that autoregulation originates in vascular smooth muscle, presumably of the arterioles, as a response to an increase in arterial pressure. According to the myogenic hypothesis of autoregulation, smooth muscle stretches in response to an increase in perfusion pressure. The stretching eventually stimulates contraction of the smooth muscles, which increases vascular resistance. Initially, coronary blood flow increases with the abrupt distention of the blood vessels. The return of more normal flow follows constriction of the arterioles. This mechanism also works in the opposite direction; that is, vasodilation is stimulated by decreased arterial pressure (Sparks & Rooke, 1987).

The myogenic hypothesis illustrates the law of Laplace (tension = pressure × radius). Increased coronary perfusion pressure increases the pressure against the vessel wall, and the stretch increases the vessel's radius, resulting in an increase in wall tension. The increase in tension stimulates constriction of the vessel to a radius less than the original radius, so that the product of pressure (increased) times radius (decreased) is restored to normal.

The metabolic hypothesis of autoregulation, which is better documented, proposes that autoregulation of coronary vessels originates in the myocardium. The stimulus is a drop in coronary perfusion pressure or an increase in the metabolic needs of the myocardium (e.g., because of strenuous exercise). The metabolic hypothesis proposes that with an increased myocardial oxygen requirement, myocardial cells release substances that promote vasodilation. The best known of these substances is adenosine, a potent vasodilator released in response to a decrease in myocardial oxygenation. Low coronary blood flow, hypoxemia, or increased meta-

bolic activity of the heart can all increase the heart muscle's need for oxygen (Berne, 1980; Berne & Levy, 1992). An increased concentration of adenosine in the interstitial fluid decreases the resistance of the coronary arterioles and increases blood flow. Perfusion strongly correlates with the amount of adenosine released (Berne, 1980). When coronary perfusion pressure is increased, the increased flow washes out the vasodilatory substances. As the dilators are washed out, vasoconstriction occurs and returns flow toward normal (Sparks & Rooke, 1987).

Autonomic Regulation

Stimulation of the sympathetic nerves to the heart causes a marked increase in coronary blood flow, even though it also causes vasoconstriction of the coronary vessels. Why? The increase in coronary flow is due to acceleration of heart rate and enhancement of myocardial contractility (more forceful systole). Although the longer, forceful myocardial contraction and the tachycardia (heart rate greater than 100 beats/min) tend to restrict coronary flow, the increase in myocardial metabolism tends to counteract these factors by dilating the coronary arterioles (Berne & Levy, 1992). Therefore the net effect of sympathetic stimulation is to increase coronary blood flow.

Although the coronary vessels themselves contain sympathetic (α- and β-adrenergic) and parasympathetic neural receptors, coronary blood flow is regulated locally through metabolic autoregulation. Metabolic autoregulation overrides neurogenic influences (Berne & Levy, 1992; Schlant & Sonnenblick, 1990).

THE LYMPHATIC SYSTEM

The lymphatic system is a special vascular system that picks up excess tissue fluid and returns it to the bloodstream. Normally, fluid is forced out of the blood at the arterial end of the capillary bed and is reabsorbed into the bloodstream at the venous end. Yet not all of this interstitial fluid returns to the blood at the venous end; capillary outflow exceeds venous reabsorption by about 3 L/day. Thus some fluid lags behind in the interstitium. To maintain sufficient blood volume in the cardiovascular system, this fluid must eventually rejoin the bloodstream. Returning interstitial fluid to the bloodstream is the function of the lymphatic system.

The lymphatic system consists of lymphatic vessels and the lymph nodes (Fig. 26-34). (Lymph nodes are described in Chapter 8.) It is a pumpless system in which a series of valves ensures one-way flow of the excess interstitial fluid (now called lymph) toward the heart. The lymphatic capillaries are closed at the ends as shown in Fig. 26-35.

Superior nodes of
deep cervical chain

Submandibular
nodes

Entry of right lymphatic
trunk into junction
of right subclavian
and internal jugular
veins

Entry of thoracic
duct into left
jugular trunk

Infraclavicular and
supraclavicular nodes

Axillary nodes

Right lymphatic
duct

Thoracic duct

Cisterna chyli

Cubital
nodes

Internal iliac
nodes

Superficial and
deep inguinal
nodes

FIG. 26-34 Schematic representation of lymphatic vessels, larger lymphatic trunks, and lymph nodes. (From Thibodeau, 1987.)

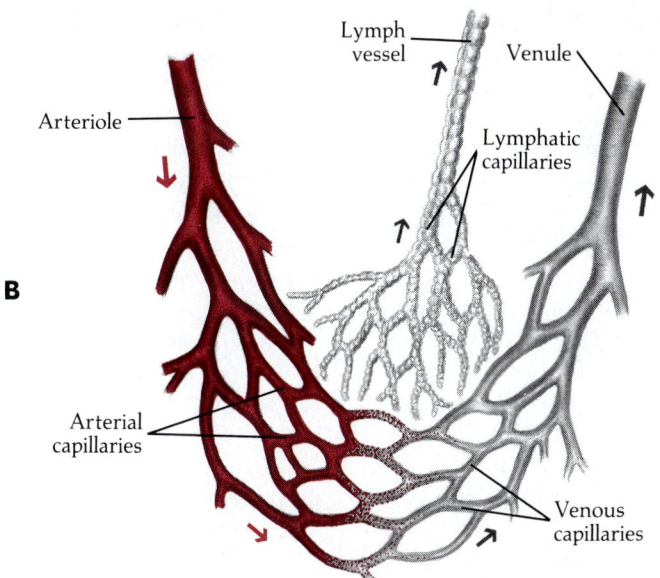

FIG. 26-35 **Lymphatic capillaries. A,** Schematic representation of lymphatic capillaries. **B,** Anatomic components of microcirculation. (From Thompson, McFarland, Hirsch, & Tucker, 1993.)

Lymph consists primarily of water and small amounts of dissolved proteins, mostly albumin, that are too large to be reabsorbed into the less permeable blood capillaries. Once within the lymphatic system, lymph travels successively through larger and larger vessels called **lymphatic venules** and **lymphatic veins.** The lymphatic vessels run in the same sheaths with the arteries and veins and eventually drain into one of two large ducts in the thorax, the right lymphatic duct and the thoracic duct. The **right lymphatic duct** drains lymph from the right arm and the right side of the head and thorax, whereas the larger **thoracic duct** receives lymph from the rest of the body (see Fig. 26-34). The right lymphatic duct and the thoracic duct drain lymph into the right and left subclavian vein, respectively.

The lymphatic veins are thin walled like the veins of the cardiovascular system. In the larger lymphatic veins, endothelial flaps form valves similar to those in the circulatory veins (see Fig. 26-26). The valves permit lymph to flow in only one direction because lymphatic vessels are compressed intermittently by contraction of skeletal muscles, pulsatile expansion of an artery in the same sheath, and contraction of the smooth muscles in the walls of the lymphatic vessel.

As lymph is transported toward the heart, it is filtered through thousands of bean-shaped lymph nodes clustered along the lymphatic vessels (see Fig. 26-34). Lymph enters the node through several **afferent lymphatic vessels,** filters through the sinuses in the node, and leaves by way of **efferent lymphatic vessels.** Lymph flows slowly through the node, which facilitates the phagocytosis of foreign substances within the node and prevents them from reentering the bloodstream. (Phagocytosis is described in Chapter 7.)

TESTS OF CARDIOVASCULAR FUNCTION

Historically, cardiac function was first measured by subjective means and by simple objective observations that included the individual's sensorium, mucous membrane color, and a manually palpated pulse. Currently, there are many sophisticated ways to measure heart function, ranging from no-risk, noninvasive electrocardiography to relatively high-risk, invasive cardiac catheterization.

Noninvasive Assessment of Function
Sensorium of the Individual

Often, the first observation indicating an impairment of cardiac function is a decreased level of consciousness. Should the pumping ability of the heart decrease for whatever reason, the amount and pressure of blood ejected from the heart will decrease. Consequently, the amount and pressure of blood that reaches all body tissues will be insufficient to supply oxygen and nutrients to cells and remove waste products.

Perhaps no other system is more sensitive to a decrease in oxygen and nutrient supply, particularly of glucose, than the central nervous system. A decrease in cardiac pumping ability, if sufficiently severe, will almost immediately be followed by a decrease in neural efficiency, which includes impairment of mentation and such simple motor functions as conjugate gaze, enunciation, and pupillary reflexes (see Chapters 12 and 13).

Mucous Membrane Color

Provided that lung, blood, and vessel structure and function are normal, a darkening or bluing of the mucous membranes, called cyanosis, signifies decreased cardiac function. Mucous membrane color is a reflection of hemoglobin saturation in the capillary blood (see Chapters 22 and 29). Hemoglobin that is well-oxygenated

and well-saturated takes on a bright red color, whereas poorly oxygenated hemoglobin is dark red or purple. These colors are best observed in the mucous membranes of the conjunctivae, gums, nail beds, and genitalia where the capillary network is dense and the epithelium is thin.

Cardiac function indirectly affects the affinity of hemoglobin for oxygen. If cardiac function decreases and blood flow slows in the capillary beds, two changes occur. First, hemoglobin will come in contact with tissues for an extended time, allowing more oxygen to diffuse into the tissues. The capillary blood will darken, as will mucous membranes. Second, a decrease in the amount of oxygen delivered per minute to the tissues will result in a metabolic acidosis, as cells switch from aerobic to anaerobic metabolism and produce lactic acid. Interstitial pH and capillary blood pH will drop. Acidosis causes more oxygen to dissociate from hemoglobin and diffuse out of the capillaries (see Chapter 29). Capillary blood in mucous membranes will darken further.

Manually Palpated Pulse

If cardiac function is impaired, the pulse will be affected. When palpated, changes in the radial, femoral, and carotid pulses offer information regarding heart rate, regularity of heart rhythm, the length and strength of ventricular systole, and peripheral artery patency. A decrease in cardiac function may be detected as a decrease in pulsatile strength. A bilateral comparison of pulses may reveal decreased pulsatile flow unilaterally, in which case arterial narrowing or occlusion would be suspected.

Irregular heartbeats (dysrhythmias) may be reflected in changes in pulse rhythmicity and pulse pressure per beat. Turbulent blood flow caused by valve or septal disease may be reflected in the carotid pulses and felt as a "thrill." A pulsatile thrill elsewhere may indicate the presence of a fistula, or opening, between an artery and a nearby vein.

Auscultation of Heart Sounds

Auscultation (auditory examination) of the heart is done with a stethoscope placed over the valve, chamber, or great vessel being examined. Different sounds are normally heard over different heart structures during systole and diastole. The dominant sounds are made by the four heart valves as they close. The first sound, S_1, is made by atrioventricular valve closure. The second, S_2, is made by closure of the aortic and pulmonic semilunar valves. The first two heart sounds provide information about heart rate, heart rhythm, and the length of ventricular systole.

Abnormal heart sounds indicate abnormalities of the heart valves or chamber walls. In heathy adults, only S_1 and S_2 can be heard. Abnormalities of these sounds or detection of the third and fourth heart sounds (S_3 and S_4) indicates disease. The mechanisms causing the normal heart sounds are listed in Table 26-4. Causes of abnormal heart sounds, or **adventitious sounds,** are listed in Table 26-5.

Cardiography

Electrocardiography, typically the 12-lead electrocardiogram (ECG), gives information about heart rate and rhythm, the effects of electrolytes or drugs on the heart, and the electrical orientation of the cardiac muscle. An ECG gives no direct information about the contractile state or mechanical performance of the heart.

Einthoven's triangle places the heart in the center of a triangle, with angles placed at the right shoulder, left shoulder, and the pubic area. Body fluids conduct electrical potential differences that can be detected by bipolar or unipolar electrical leads placed on the skin. Einthoven's triangle gives a triaxial (three-axis) reference for the detection of cardiac electrical potentials.

Serial 12-lead ECGs are of primary importance in establishing the presence of myocardial infarction. This examination has become part of the routine hospital admission assessment, even when the admitting diagnosis is not cardiac in nature, because it establishes baseline information about the electrical function of the heart.

TABLE 26-4

Normal Heart Sounds

Sound	Event in cardiac style	Cause of sound	Comments
First sound (S_1)	Beginning of ventricular systole	Closure of atrioventricular valves, particularly mitral valve	With S_2, the loudest heart sound normally heard
Second sound (S_2)	End of ventricular systole	Closure of semilunar valves, particularly aortic valves	With S_1, the loudest heart sound normally heard
Third sound (S_3)	Early ventricular diastole (filling)	Vibration of ventricular walls as blood rushes in	Normally heard only in children and young adults
Fourth sound (S_4)	Atrial systole during late ventricular diastole (filling)	Uncertain, but thought to be the result of a sudden change in filling rate (i.e., shudder of the left ventricle)	Rarely heard in the normal heart

TABLE 26-5

Abnormal Heart Sounds

Sound	Cause of sound	Typical underlying abnormality
Accentuated S_1	Forceful closure of mitral valve	Rapid heart rate resulting from exercise, anemia, or hyperthyroidism Mitral valve stenosis (narrowing)
Diminished S_1	Premature partial closure of the mitral valve before systole, so that systole causes only the completion of closure	Prolonged diastole resulting from blockage in conduction system that slows impulse conduction to or within the atrioventricular node
	Failure of the mitral valve to close completely	Mitral valve incompetence (regurgitation)
Accentuated S_2	Forceful closure of the aortic or pulmonic semilunar valve, which closes late and must close quickly	Prolonged systole resulting from high blood pressure in the systemic or pulmonary circulation; systole is slightly prolonged so as to force all the blood out against high pressure
	Valvular stiffness, which increases the impact of closure	Aortic valve syphilis

Continued.

TABLE 26-5

Abnormal Heart Sounds—cont'd

Sound	Cause of sound	Typical underlying abnormality
Diminished S₂	Gentle closure of aortic semilunar valve	Low blood pressure in the systemic arteries, which reduces pressure that pushes valve leaflets shut
	Gentle closure of aortic semilunar valve caused by incomplete opening	Aortic stenosis
Split heart sounds (S₁ and S₂)	Delayed closure of various heart valves, usually caused by late right ventricular systole	Normal increase in venous return to the right heart with inspiration Conduction defects involving the right or left bundle branches Defect of the interatrial septum that raises pressures in the right heart Pulmonic semilunar valve stenosis, which causes delayed closure
Gallop sounds S₃ (in adults)	Possibly the "thud" of blood hitting noncompliant ventricular walls at the start of ventricular filling	Myocardial damage that stiffens muscle and prevents relaxation during systole
S₄ (in children)	Ejection of blood into overfilled ventricle during atrial systole	Incomplete emptying of ventricle during systole of preceding cardiac cycle, causing overfilling and overdistention during next cycle; causes include myocardial damage or disease, aortic stenosis, high blood pressure, fluid overload (see Chapter 3)
Murmurs	Turbulent blood flow at high blood pressure	Irregularity, constriction, or dilation of any structure that blood flows through, such as valvular stenosis or incompetence, perforation of interatrial or interventricular septum Increased rate of flow (blood flow) through normal structures (e.g., during pregnancy)
Rub	Friction within the pericardium, usually caused by disruption of the pericardial fluid; loss of fluid causes the visceral and parietal pericardium to rub against one another	Surgery, infection, inflammation, or adhesion that damages the parietal or visceral pericardium
Click	Sudden, abnormal movement of an aortic or pulmonic semilunar valve leaflet	Valve prolapse, in which valve leaflets open backward as well as forward; usually resulting from increase in valve opening (anulus)
Snap	Opening of stenotic (stiff) atrioventricular valve (mitral or tricuspid)	Atrioventricular valve stenosis
Hum	Vibration of heart walls or vessel walls caused usually by movement during turbulent blood flow at low pressure	Irregularity of any structure that blood flows through; normal in jugular veins of children

Also, recent ECGs can be compared to ECGs obtained from the same individual in the past. Changes in the ECG over time assist in determining the cause, amount, or nature of changes in cardiac anatomy and physiology over time. Fig. 26-11 depicts a normal ECG.

In conjunction with a 12-lead ECG, a vectorcardiogram can assist to (1) precisely locate the site of a myocardial infarction, (2) diagnose conduction defects, and (3) diagnose chamber hypertrophy. Commonly, five electrodes are placed over the precordium, one electrode is placed on the left leg, and one is placed on the back of the neck. Recorded in conjunction with the ECG, the electrodes of the vectorcardiogram provide a series of dots over time that represent the vector of the heart in microseconds.

Pulse Tracing

The pulsation described by the flow of blood through an artery during the cardiac cycle can be drawn as a waveform plotting pressure against time (Fig. 26-36). The waveform can be obtained noninvasively by placing a transducer on the skin over the carotid artery, while the individual's head is turned slightly away from the transducer. In conjunction with phonocardiography and an ECG, the arterial pulse tracing gives a reference for the phonocardiograph and assists in the timing of the events of the cardiac cycle.

Like an arterial pulse tracing, a venous pulse tracing gives a reference for the phonocardiograph and assists

in the timing of the cardiac cycle. A venous pulse tracing is obtained by placing a transducer over the jugular vein at the supraclavicular area near the manubrium. A waveform is produced that reflects pressures in the vein over time during the cardiac cycle.

Vibrations at the apex of the heart during the cardiac cycle are recorded by placing a transducer at the point of maximal impulse. An apexcardiogram is used to assist in the timing of the cardiac cycle and is made along with a phonocardiogram and an ECG.

A phonocardiogram is made by placing microphones over the precordium. An ECG is recorded simultaneously as a reference point. By recording the sounds made during the cardiac cycle, the phonocardiogram can assist to time the events and length of diastole and systole. Abnormal sounds can also be examined more closely for timing, characteristics, and sources of those sounds.

An echocardiogram is an ultrasonic examination. The skin is first prepared by applying a lubricating agent (usually cooking oil), and a piezoelectric crystal is placed against the chest. Ultrasonic sound waves are then generated and directed into the cardiac structures, which reflect the waves at different angles and lengths according to structure and density. The crystal picks up these deflected waves and passes them through a transducer, which transforms the waves into electrical impulses. The impulses are displayed on an oscilloscope and are viewed with a simultaneously recorded ECG.

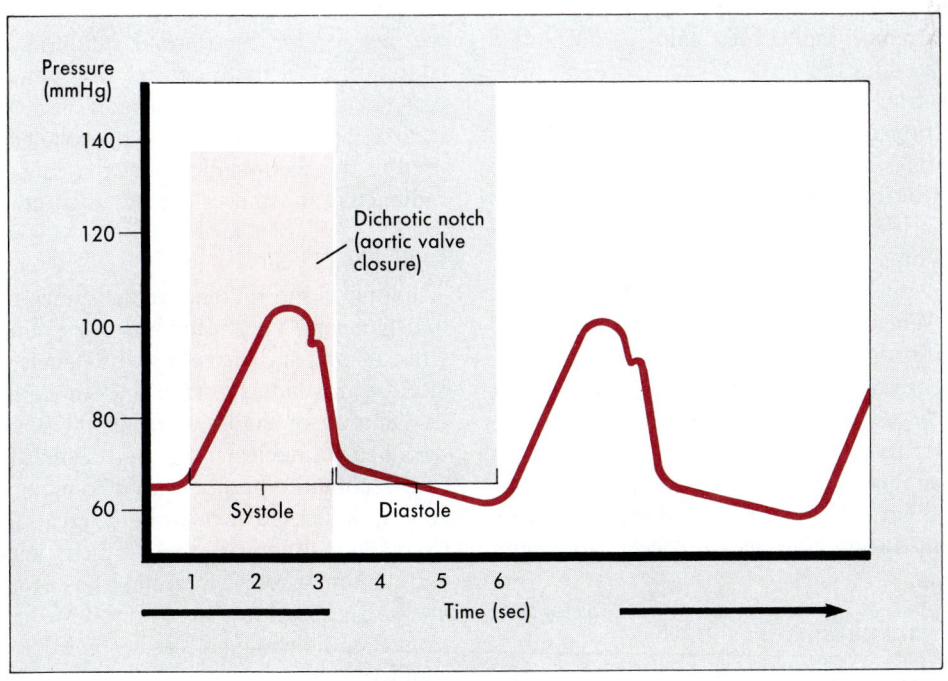

FIG. 26-36 Arterial pulse waveforms.

Like an ECG, an echocardiogram is recorded continuously over time so that changes in the heart during the cardiac cycle (such as valve position, chamber size, and myocardial wall position) can be examined. Information about cardiac anatomy and function, including stroke volume and cardiac output, is gained.

Doppler Studies

A Doppler study is made by using a hand-held microphone placed on the skin over a lubricating gel. The microphone amplifies and can record sounds made by blood flowing in peripheral vessels. The Doppler microphone is placed over the vessel to be studied, and sounds related to obstructions to flow, vessel wall mobility, and heart murmurs are transmitted through the gel to the microphone. The microphone amplifies sound waves so that they are audible to the human ear.

Stress Testing

Cardiac activity during exercise is examined during a stress test. Stress testing elicits signs and symptoms of heart disease and coronary artery disease that may not appear at rest. A 12-lead ECG, blood pressure measurement, and bipolar ECG strip-recording are done before the study and at regular intervals during and after the study. Cardiac stress from exercise is induced by having the individual walk on a treadmill. Other, less frequently used forms of exercise include stair climbing (the Stairmaster's double two-step) and bicycle ergometry. The individual exercises until the maximal heart rate for sex and age is reached or until other subjective or objective indicators of cardiac dysfunction or distress appear. Subjective indicators include chest pain, extreme fatigue, extreme dyspnea, leg pain, or the individual's request to stop the test. Objective criteria are ST segment elevation or depression, SA node or atrial dysrhythmias, atrioventricular node dysrhythmias, ventricular dysrhythmias, elevated or decreased blood pressure, signs of cerebral hypoxia, and signs of circulatory insufficiency.

A stress test is also useful in determining the rate or progress of recovery from a myocardial infarction or cardiac surgery. When a differential diagnosis for chest pain has been difficult to determine, stress testing may help distinguish coronary artery insufficiency from other causes of pain. There is some risk associated with stress testing. The mortality rate is about 1 per 10,000, and the morbidity rate is approximately 24 per 10,000 (Rochmis & Blackburn, 1971). The risk is greater when the test is performed soon after an acute ischemic event (Chaitman, 1992).

Chest X-Ray Examinations

In a chest x-ray examination, the size and contour of the heart and related structures are visualized. A chest

x-ray examination is a routine part of a cardiac examination. The most commonly obtained views are anterior-posterior and lateral, with the individual upright and the lungs fully expanded.

Invasive Assessment of Cardiac Function

Invasive studies generally carry a greater risk to the individual than noninvasive studies, with the possible exception of stress testing. Ingestion of substances is considered invasive.

X-Ray Films with Barium

The cardiac silhouette obtained with routine radiographic studies of the chest can be enhanced by ingestion of barium. The contrast medium causes the esophagus to appear as white on the x-ray film, creating a bright background against which the heart is more distinctly outlined. X-ray films are taken using four different axes.

Nuclear Imaging with Radiolabeled Pharmaceuticals

Hot spot imaging

Technetium pyrophosphate (^{99m}TcPYP) is injected intravenously into a resting individual during a hot spot imaging examination. Two hours after injection, the distribution pattern of the radioactive solution is recorded by nuclear scan. During the 2-hour delay, the injected material will have been taken up by infarcted areas of the myocardium, particularly 1 to 3 days after the onset of symptoms. This study is not definitive during the first 12 hours after an infarct.

Hot spot imaging is used when (1) there is a conflicting history for myocardial infarction, (2) there are equivocal ECG abnormalities, or (3) an individual's cardiac enzymes have been elevated because of surgery or trauma. Such small amounts of the injected material are used in this examination that the risks associated with radioactive substances are not an issue.

Cold spot imaging

Thallium is the radioactive substance injected intravenously during a perfusion imaging examination. During stress testing and at the peak of exercise, thallium is injected intravenously. After a 1- or 2-minute delay, the distribution of thallium within the myocardium is determined by nuclear scan, and again after a period of rest. Thallium typically is not taken up by areas of ischemic or infarcted myocardium, creating "cold spots." Cold spots disappear at rest if the ischemia is reversible and remain at rest if infarction has occurred. Perfusion imaging is useful to differentiate a myocardial infarction from reversible angina (cardiac pain) in the presence of conflicting or equivocal enzymatic and historical data. Risks associated with perfusion imaging are the same as for stress testing. No risk attributable to the small quantity of injected material has been documented.

Atrioventricular Bundle Electrocardiography

Two electrode-tipped catheters are inserted percutaneously into the femoral vein, floated up the inferior vena cava, and positioned in or near the right atrium during atrioventricular bundle (His bundle) electrocardiography. The first electrode is quadripolar and is lodged against the right atrial wall. Two poles of this electrode record the difference in electrical potential between two points, and the other two poles are a pacing electrode and a ground (that allow for pacing of the right atrium). The second electrode is bipolar and is placed across the tricuspid valve, at the location of the bundle of His, and records the electrical potentials across the bundle. These recordings across the bundle divide the P-R interval into two segments: (1) the atrial-His interval (AHI), and (2) the His-ventricular interval. The atrial-His interval is the interval from the onset of atrial electrical activity to the arrival of the impulse at the bundle of His. The His-ventricular interval is the interval between the passage of the impulse through the His bundle and the passage of the impulse through the ventricular conduction system and muscle.

His bundle electrocardiography can detect secondary sites of impulse generation (ectopic foci), as well as accessory pathways of conduction. Other conduction defects and the effects of drugs on conduction can also be illuminated. Risks related to this procedure can be grave and include dysrhythmias, death, vessel or heart perforation, clot or plaque embolization, and kidney failure.

Cardiac Catheterization

One or both sides of the heart can be examined using cardiac catheterization. This procedure requires the use of fluoroscopy and strict sterile techniques and takes place in a specially equipped catheterization laboratory. Local anesthesia is given, and a catheter is introduced percutaneously into the vasculature and passed caudally into the atrium and ventricle. For a right-heart catheterization, the catheter is placed in the brachial or femoral vein. The femoral artery is commonly used for a left-heart study. Once the catheter has been guided into the atrium, pressures are recorded, blood samples are obtained to examine oxygen content, and a contrast medium is injected to visualize chamber function and valve patency. The catheter is then passed into the ventricles and the sequence repeated.

Cardiac catheterization provides a means to visualize the chambers of the heart continuously, although for a short time. A great deal of information can be obtained about heart structure and function. Pressures in each chamber and across heart valves can be precisely measured, along with timing of events in the cardiac cycle.

Of particular value is the ability to compare the oxygen content of blood in each heart chamber.

Risks for this procedure have decreased over time and mortality rates range from 0.1% to 0.3% (Abrams, 1983). Morbidity rates, including serious and relatively minor complications, ranged from 3.1% to 10.1% in 1968 (Braunwald, 1968), but are quoted currently as less than 0.5% (Silverman & Neeld, 1984). One of the most serious complications of cardiac catheterization is the development of dysrhythmias. Death is usually caused by cardiac arrest after ventricular fibrillation.

Coronary Angiography

Fluoroscopic visualization of the coronary arteries and left heart structures using contrast dye is called coronary angiography or arteriography. Like cardiac catheterization, this study takes place in a catheterization laboratory using local anesthesia and a sterile field. A catheter is threaded into the left ventricle through the femoral artery. A ventriculogram is generally performed first. Contrast dye is injected into the apex of the ventricle and the next few cardiac cycles are visualized and filmed. The contrast dye used is 66% diatrizoate meglumine and 10% diatrizoate sodium, an iodine preparation that is not tolerated by individuals who are allergic to iodine. Like cardiac catheterization, coronary angiography is used to gain information about the structure and function of the ventricle and related valves.

After the ventriculogram, catheters are introduced individually into the ostia of the coronary arteries. When the catheter is in position, 5 to 10 ml of contrast dye is mechanically and rapidly injected into the artery, and the results are visualized and filmed. Dye injection is repeated with the individual tilted at various angles to afford views of the artery other than the anterior-posterior view. The catheter is then either moved to the next artery to be studied or withdrawn to conclude the study. Pressures in the left side of the heart are usually obtained, but blood samples are not. The right side of the heart is not studied.

The risks of this procedure are similar to those of cardiac catheterization, but with exceptions. Because the blood supply to the cardiac muscle is briefly interrupted when dye is introduced into the coronary arteries, angina (chest pain) caused by ischemia (lack of oxygen) is much more common. Coronary artery spasms can also occur. Interrupted flow also causes decreased heart rate (bradycardia), as well as some tachydysrhythmias, hypotension, and ST segment depression. In persons at low risk, the need for emergency coronary surgery occurs in at least 7.4 per 1000 individuals (Stewart et al., 1990).

The administration of nitroglycerin sublingually or directly into the coronary artery can dilate the artery sufficiently to alleviate ischemic complications. Persistent bradycardia is corrected by having the individual

TABLE 26-6

Indicators of Cardiac Function

Indicator	Definition*	Common cause of abnormality
Heart rate (HR)	Number of heartbeats (cardiac cycles) per minute Normal adult value: 70 beats/min	Ischemia, electrolyte disturbances, drug toxicity
Cardiac output (CO)	Amount of blood (in liters) moved by the heart in 1 minute Normal range: 4-8 L/min	Decrease indicates heart failure Increase indicates decreased systemic vascular resistance, common in sepsis
Cardiac index (CI)	Relationship between cardiac output and body surface area (BSA, in square meters) Normal range: 2.8-4.2 L/min/m²	Decrease indicates heart failure Increase indicates decreased systemic vascular resistance, common in sepsis
Stroke volume (SV)	Amount of blood (in milliliters) ejected by the left ventricle during systole, i.e., per beat Normal range: 60-100 ml/beat	Decrease indicates heart failure Increase indicates decreased systemic vascular resistance, common in sepsis
Stroke volume index (SVI)	Relationship between stroke volume and body surface area Normal range: 33-47 ml/beat/m²	Decrease indicates heart failure Increase indicates decreased systemic vascular resistance, common in sepsis
Oxygen consumption index (VO₂I)	Amount of oxygen (VO₂ in milliliters) consumed per minute in relation to body surface area	Decrease: sedation, anesthesia, hypothermia Increase: elevated temperature, sepsis, seizures
Stroke work index (SWI)	Amount of work (expressed as done) by the left or right ventricle per systole per square meter of body surface area Normal value: 35 gm-m	Decreases within specific ranges indicate cardiogenic or hypovolemic shock (see Chapter 27) Increase: elevated systemic vascular resistance
Systemic mean arterial pressure (MAP)	Mean blood pressure (in millimeters of mercury) in the systemic arteries Normal range: 70-100 mm Hg	Elevated: epinephrine release, diseases of arteries, primary hypertension Decreased: cardiac failure, decreased vascular resistance of sepsis
Pulmonary vascular resistance (PVR)	Relationship between cardiac output, preload, and afterload, expressed as units of force of resistance per second per centimeter of water Normal value: less than 250 dyn/sec/cm⁻⁵	Increased: ARDS, pneumonia, primary pulmonary hypertension, congestive heart failure Decreased: late shock
Systemic vascular resistance (SVR)	Same definition as for PVR Normal range: 770-1500 dyn/sec/cm⁻⁵	Increased: epinephrine release Decreased: inflammatory response

*Values given are for adults at rest.

cough to stimulate the heart rate or, in severe cases, by the administration of atropine. Bradycardia is such a common complication that a temporary pacer is often introduced into the right ventricle through the femoral vein at the beginning of coronary angiography. Heparin is given to avoid thrombus formation. The effects of heparin may be reversed after the procedure by using protamine.

Combined Indicators of Cardiac Function

Cardiac function can be evaluated using indicators calculated from pressures and flow rates in the heart and vessels. Table 26-6 defines the indicators most frequently used in the clinical setting.

❏ AGING and the Cardiovascular System

Cardiovascular disease is the most common cause of hospitalization and death in the elderly population in Western society. The most common cardiovascular pathologic condition is coronary atherosclerosis. It is difficult to describe normal physiologic changes in cardiac function with aging because many pathologic changes are usually present as well. Studies of the effect of age on cardiovascular function must be rigorous in their distinction between persons who are free of disease and those who have disease that may only be evident during stress testing. A consistent finding is the large variation in the older population for nearly every cardiovascular variable (Weisfeldt, LaKatta, & Gerstenblith, 1992). To obtain an understanding of the effects of age on cardiovascular functioning it is, therefore, necessary to consider cardiac performance at rest and during exercise.

Resting Cardiac Performance

For many years it has been believed that advanced age is associated with a progressive decline in resting cardiovascular function. The physiologic changes were reported to involve most of the major determinants of cardiac performance: heart rate, cardiac output, blood volume, filling rate, filling volume, afterload, and blood pressure. However, recent studies are challenging these findings.

The Baltimore Longitudinal Study on Aging (BLSA) was conducted in a group of 61 participants, ranging from 26 to 79 years of age, who were free of heart disease (Rodeheffer et al., 1984). The volunteers were active but not conditioned athletes. Subjects were studied in the upright position at rest and during progressive bicycle exercise to exhaustion. In contrast to previous studies, there were no age-related changes in cardiac output. Resting heart rate has been reported to be unchanged with age (Strandell, 1964), but there was a trend toward lower heart rates in the BLSA subjects. Resting stroke volume has previously been reported to be decreased or unchanged with age (Julius, Antoon, Whitlock, & Conway, 1967; Strandell, 1964), but there was a slight age-related increase in stroke volume at rest in the BLSA population. Thus, the lack of any change in cardiac output in the BLSA subjects is possibly related to the slight decrease in heart rate and slight increase in stroke volume. Table 26-7 summarizes both the findings of the BLSA study and previous findings of resting cardiac function in the elderly.

In summary, resting healthy/fit subjects show no age-related changes in cardiac output or heart rate, and a small increase in stroke volume. No age-related changes

---

TABLE 26-7

Resting Cardiac Function in the Elderly: A Comparison of New and Old Data

Determinant	Previous studies	Baltimore Longitudinal Study
Cardiac output	Decreased	No change
Heart rate	No change	Slight decrease
Stroke volume	Decreased or unchanged	Slight increase
Ejection fraction	Unchanged	Unchanged
Afterload (systolic blood pressure)	Increased	Increased
End-diastolic volume	Unchanged	Unchanged
End-systolic volume	Unchanged	Unchanged
Contraction	Increased	Increased because of prolonged relaxation

were noted in cardiac volume and the ejection fraction; however, there may be an increase in systolic arterial pressure. There is also evidence of an age-related prolonged and delayed left ventricular relaxation in humans and in animal models (Rodeheffer & Gerstenblith, 1985; Weisfeldt et al., 1992).

Exercise Cardiac Performance

Stress testing is used to uncover changes in functional capacity that are not apparent at rest. In contrast to the subtle age effects on resting cardiac tests, there are more dramatic changes during exercise. Most researchers have reported a decline in maximum oxygen uptake and heart rate with aging, even in athletes (Weisfeldt et al., 1992). Several have reported a decline in exercise cardiac output with increasing age because of a decrease in both heart rate and stroke volume (Weisfeldt et al., 1992). Ejection fraction increases more from rest to exercise in younger than in older people. During exercise,

heart rate increases less in older people, possibly because of a decreased cardiovascular response to catecholamines. The decrease in catecholamine-mediated effects during exercise is probably not caused by decreased amounts of catecholamines, since plasma levels are higher, not lower, in humans during exercise. Finally, the benefit of the Frank-Starling mechanism is unaltered with age and used effectively during exercise to maintain cardiac output through a higher stroke volume at a greater end-diastolic volume (Weisfeldt et al., 1992).

In summary, age does not appear to significantly alter left ventricular performance except in the presence of a superimposed stress like severe exercise or disease, particularly dysrhythmia or hypertension. In these instances, impaired diastolic relaxation and systolic emptying may occur; the latter is probably related to a decreased responsiveness to catecholamine beta-adrenoreceptor stimulation (Weisfeldt et al., 1992).

SUMMARY REVIEW

The Circulatory System

1 The circulatory system is the body's transport system. It delivers oxygen, nutrients, metabolites, hormones, neurochemicals, proteins, and blood cells through the body and carries metabolic wastes to the kidneys and lungs for excretion.

2 The circulatory system consists of the heart and blood vessels and is made up of two separate, serially connected systems: the pulmonary circulation and the systemic circulation.

3 The pulmonary circulation is driven by the right side of the heart. The function of the pulmonary circulation is to deliver blood to the lungs for oxygenation.

4 The systemic circulation is driven by the left side of the heart, and its function is to move oxygenated blood throughout the body.

5 The lymphatic vessels collect fluids from the interstitium and return the fluids to the circulatory system.

The Heart

1 The heart consists of four chambers (two atria and two ventricles), four valves (two atrioventricular valves and two semilunar valves), a muscular wall, a fibrous skeleton, a conduction system, nerve fibers, systemic vessels (the coronary circulation), and openings where the great vessels enter the atria and ventricles.

2 The heart wall, which encloses the heart and divides it into chambers, is made up of three layers: the pericardium (outer layer), the myocardium (muscular layer), and the endocardium (inner lining).

3 The myocardial layer of the two atria, which receive blood entering the heart, is thinner than the myocardial layer of the ventricles, which have to be stronger to squeeze blood out of the heart.

4 The right and left sides of the heart are separated by portions of the heart wall called the interatrial septum and the interventricular septum.

5 Unoxygenated (venous) blood from the systemic circulation enters the right atrium through the superior and inferior venae cavae. From the atrium the blood passes through the right atrioventricular (tricuspid) valve into the right ventricle. In the ventricle the blood flows from the inflow tract to the outflow tract and then through the pulmonic semilunar valve (pulmonary valve) into the pulmonary artery, which delivers it to the lungs for oxygenation.

6 Oxygenated blood from the lungs enters the left atrium through the four pulmonary valves (two from the left lung and two from the right lung). From the left atrium, the blood passes through the left atrioventricular valve (mitral valve) into the left ventricle. In the ventricle the blood flows from the inflow tract to the outflow tract and then through the aortic semilunar valve (aortic valve) into the aorta, which delivers it to systemic arteries of the entire body.

7 The heart valves ensure the one-way flow of blood from atrium to ventricle and from ventricle to artery.

8 Oxygenated blood enters the coronary arteries through an opening in the aorta, and unoxygenated blood from the coronary veins enters the right atrium through the coronary sinus.

9 The pumping action of the heart consists of two phases: diastole, during which the myocardium relaxes and the chambers fill with blood, and systole, during which the myocardium contracts, forcing blood out of the ventricles. A cardiac cycle consists of one systolic contraction and the diastolic relaxation that follows it. Each cardiac cycle comprises one "heartbeat."

10 The conduction system of the heart generates and transmits electrical impulses (cardiac action potentials) that stimulate systolic contractions. The autonomic nerves (sympathetic and parasympathetic fibers) can adjust heart rate and systolic force, but they do not stimulate the heart to beat.

11 The normal electrocardiogram is the sum of all action potentials. The P wave represents atrial depolarization; the QRS complex is the sum of all ventricular cell depolarizations. The ST interval occurs when the entire ventricular myocardium is depolarized.

12 Cardiac action potentials are generated by the sinoatrial node at the rate of about 75 impulses per minute. The impulses can travel through the conduction system of the heart, stimulating myocardial contraction as they go.

13 Cells of the cardiac conduction system possess the properties of automaticity and rhythmicity. Automatic cells return to threshold and depolarize rhythmically without outside stimulus. The cells of the sinoatrial node depolarize faster than other automatic cells, making it the natural pacemaker of the heart. If the sinoatrial node is disabled, the next fastest pacemaker, the atrioventricular node, takes over.

14 Each cardiac action potential travels from the sinoatrial node to the atrioventricular node to the bundle of His (atrioventricular bundle), through the bundle branches, and finally to the Purkinje fibers. There the impulse is stopped. It is prevented from reversing its path by the refractory period of cells that have just been polarized. The refractory period ensures that diastole (relaxation) will occur, thereby completing the cardiac cycle.

15 Adrenergic receptor number, type, and function govern autonomic (sympathetic) regulation of heart rate, contractile force, and the dilation or constriction of coronary arteries. The presence of specific receptors (α-1, α-2; β-1, β-2) in the myocardium and coronary vessels determines the effects of the neurotransmitters norepinephrine and epinephrine.

16 Unique features that distinguish myocardial cells from skeletal cells enable myocardial cells to transmit action potentials faster (through intercalated disks), synthesize more ATP (because of a large number of mitochondria), and have readier access to ions in the interstitium (because of an abundance of transverse tubules). These combined differences enable the myocardium to work constantly, which skeletal muscle is not required to do.

17 Crossbridges between actin and myosin enable contraction. Calcium and its interaction with the troponin complex facilitate the contraction process. With troponin release of calcium, myocardial relaxation begins.

18 Cardiac performance is affected by preload, afterload, heart rate, and myocardial contractility.

19 Preload, or pressure generated in the ventricles at the end of diastole, depends on the amount of blood in the ventricle. Afterload is the resistance to ejection of the blood from the ventricle. Afterload depends on pressure in the aorta.

20 Heart rate is determined by the sinoatrial node and by components of the autonomic nervous system, including cardiovascular control centers in the brain, neuroreceptors in the atria and aorta, hormones, and catecholamines (epinephrine and norepinephrine).

21 Contractility is the potential for myocardial fiber shortening during systole. It is determined by the amount of stretch during diastole (i.e., preload) and by sympathetic stimulation of the ventricles.

22 The Frank-Starling law of the heart states that the myocardial stretch determines the force of myocardial contraction (the greater the stretch, the stronger the contraction).

23 Laplace's law states that the amount of contractile force generated within a chamber depends on the radius of the chamber and the thickness of its wall (the smaller the radius and the thicker the wall, the greater the force of contraction).

The Systemic Circulation

1 Blood flows from the left ventricle into the aorta and from the aorta into arteries that eventually branch into arterioles and capillaries, the smallest of the arterial vessels. Oxygen, nutrients, and other substances needed for cellular metabolism pass from the capillaries into the interstitium, where they are available for uptake by the cells. Capillaries also absorb products of cellular metabolism from the interstitium.

2 Venules, the smallest veins, receive capillary blood. From the venules, the venous blood flows into larger and larger veins until it reaches the venae cavae, through which it enters the right atrium.

3 Vessel walls consists of three layers: the tunica intima (inner layer), the tunica media (middle layer), and the tunica externa (the outer layer).

4 Layers of the vessel wall differ in thickness and composition from vessel to vessel, depending on the vessel's size and location within the circulatory system.

In general, the tunica media of arteries close to the heart contains a greater proportion of elastic fibers because these arteries must be able to distend during systole and recoil during diastole. Distributing arteries farther from the heart contain a greater proportion of smooth muscle fibers because these arteries must be able to constrict and dilate to control blood pressure and volume within specific capillary beds.

5   Blood flow into the capillary beds is controlled by the contraction and relaxation of smooth muscle bands (precapillary sphincters) at junctions between metarterioles and capillaries. *The endothelium is probably a source of prostaglandins that control vasomotion.*

6   Blood flow through the veins is assisted by the contraction of skeletal muscles (the muscle pump), and backflow in the lower body is prevented by one-way valves, particularly in the deep veins of the legs.

7   Blood flow is affected by blood pressure; resistance to flow within the vessels; blood consistency (which affects velocity); anatomic features that may cause turbulent or laminar flow; and compliance (distensibility) of the vessels.

8   Poiseuille's law describes the relationship of blood flow, pressure, and resistance as the difference between pressure at the inflow end of the vessel and pressure at the outflow end divided by resistance within the vessel.

9   According to Poiseuille's formula, resistance depends on the vessel's length and radius and on the viscosity of the blood. The greater the vessel's length and the blood's viscosity and the narrower the radius of the vessel's lumen, the greater the resistance within the vessel.

10 Total peripheral resistance, or the resistance to flow within the entire systemic circulatory system, depends on the combined lengths and radii of all the vessels within the system and on whether the vessels are arranged in series (greater resistance) or in parallel (lesser resistance).

11 Poiseuille's law and Poiseuille's formula are based on physical laws governing the behavior of fluids in a straight tube. In the body blood flow is also influenced by neural stimulation (of vasoconstriction or vasodilation) and by autonomic features that cause turbulence within the vascular lumen (e.g., protrusions from the vessel wall, twists and turns, bifurcations).

12 Arterial blood pressure is influenced and regulated by factors that affect cardiac output (heart rate and stroke volume), total resistance within the system, and blood volume.

13 Venous blood pressure is influenced by blood volume within the venous system and compliance of the venous walls.

14 Blood flow through the coronary circulation is governed not only by the same principles as flow through other vascular beds but also by adaptations dictated by cardiac dynamics. First, blood flows into the coronary arteries during diastole rather than systole because, during systole, the cusps of the aortic semilunar valve block the openings of the coronary arteries. Second, systolic contraction inhibits coronary artery flow by compressing the coronary arteries.

15 Autoregulation enables the coronary vessels to maintain optimal perfusion pressure despite systolic effects, and myoglobulin in heart muscle stores oxygen for use during the systolic phase of the cardiac cycle.

The Lymphatic System

1   The vessels of the lymphatic system run in the same sheaths with the arteries and veins.

2   Lymph (interstitial fluid) is absorbed by lymphatic venules in the capillary beds and travels through ever larger lymphatic veins until it is emptied through the right or left thoracic duct into the right or left subclavian vein.

3   As lymph travels toward the thoracic ducts, it is filtered by thousands of lymph nodes clustered around the lymphatic veins. The lymph nodes are sites of immune function.

Tests of Cardiovascular Function

1   Observable signs of cardiovascular disease include a decreased level of consciousness (caused by insufficient perfusion of brain tissue) and cyanosis, particularly mucous membrane color (caused by insufficient perfusion of vascular beds of the skin).

2   Palpable signs of cardiovascular disease include abnormal pulses of the radial, femoral, and carotid arteries.

3   Abnormal heart sounds, which are detected by auscultation with a stethoscope or by phonocardiography, are auditory signs of cardiovascular disease.

4   Stress tests elicit clinical manifestations of cardiovascular disease that might not be present at rest.

5   Noninvasive diagnostic tests include electrocardiography (ECG) and Holter monitoring, which detect disturbances of impulse generation or conduction; pulse tracings and Doppler studies, which detect abnormalities of blood flow; phonocardiography; ultrasound (echocardiography), which detects the structural and functional abnormalities over time; and chest x-ray films, which detect cardiac enlargement and structural abnormalities.

6   Invasive diagnostic tests involve intravenous injection of radiolabeled substances (barium x-rays, nuclear imaging) or the introduction of a catheter that is threaded through the vascular system to the heart

(atrioventricular bundle ECG, cardiac catheterization, coronary angiography).

7 Cardiac catheterization is used to measure the oxygen content and pressure of blood in the heart's chambers and to inject contrast media for x-ray examination of the size and shape of the chambers and valves. Injection of contrast medium in the coronary arteries (coronary angiography), on the other hand, permits visualization of the coronary circulation and every tissue perfused by the coronary arteries.

Aging and the Cardiovascular System

1 Much controversy exists regarding the effects of normal aging on the cardiovascular system. Separating the physiologic from the pathologic alterations is difficult because of the presence of arteriosclerosis in the majority of the elderly population.

2 Recent studies have documented no change in cardiac output, a slight decrease in heart rate, and a slight increase in stroke volume in healthy (lack of ischemic heart disease) elderly persons at rest. Also no changes were noted at rest in ejection fraction. A slight increase in afterload (e.g., as systolic blood pressure) and prolonged left ventricular relaxation were noted.

3 With exercise, the healthy elderly subjects demonstrated a decrease in maximum oxygen consumption and no age-related changes in cardiac output but did demonstrate significant decreases in heart rate and increases in stroke volume. Thus the healthy elderly subjects maintained a normal cardiac output during exercise by dilating the ventricle and using the Frank-Starling mechanism to increase stroke volume.

4 Contrary to previous studies, recent studies have found no age-related increase with exercise for systolic blood pressure and systemic vascular resistance.

KEY TERMS

A band, 959
Adventitious sound, 987
Afferent lymphatic vessel, 986
Afterload, 963
Aldosterone, 981
Angiotensin I, 981
Angiotensin II, 981
Anisotropic band, 959
Anomalous viscosity, 975
Aorta, 948
Aortic semilunar valve (aortic valve), 948
Arteriole, 969
Artery, 969
Atrioventricular node (AV node), 953
Atrioventricular valve, 946
Automatic cell, 957
Automaticity, 957
Autoregulation, 983
a wave, 950
Bachmann's bundle, 954
Bainbridge reflex, 966
Baroreceptor reflex, 966
Blood flow, 975
Blood velocity, 979

Bundle branch, 953
Bundle of His (atrioventricular bundle, common bundle), 953
Calcium channel-blocking drug, 963
Capillary, 969
Cardiac action potential, 953
Cardiac cycle, 948
Cardiac output, 967
Cardiac plexus, 957
Cardiac vein, 951
Cardioexcitatory center, 966
Cardioinhibitory center, 966
Cardiovascular control center, 966
Chordae tendineae, 948
Circumflex artery, 952
Collateral artery (collateral circulation), 952
Conduction system, 953
Coronary artery, 951
Coronary circulation, 951
Coronary ostium, 951
Coronary perfusion pressure, 982
Coronary sinus, 951
Coronary sulcus, 952
Crista supraventricularis, 950

Crossbridge theory of muscle contraction, 962
c wave, 951
Depolarization, 955
Diastole, 948
Diastolic depolarization, 957
Efferent lymphatic vessel, 986
Ejection fraction, 968
Elastic artery, 969
End-diastolic pressure, 965
End-diastolic volume, 963
Endocardium, 946
Endothelial-derived contracting factor (EDCF), 974
Endothelial-derived relaxing factor (EDRF), 974
Excitation-contraction coupling, 962
Fenestration, 969
Frank-Starling law of the heart, 963
Great cardiac vein, 952
Heart rate, 953
Hyperemia, 980
Hyperpolarization, 956
I band, 959
Inferior vena cava, 948
Inflow tract, 946

REFERENCES

Abrams, H. L. (1983). Complications of coronary arteriography (Chapter 23, pp. 503-518). In H. L. Abrams (Ed.), *Angiography: Vascular and interventional radiology* (3rd ed.). Boston: Little, Brown.

Andreoli, T. E., Carpenter, C. C. J., Plus, F., & Smith, L. H. (1986). *Cecil essentials of medicine.* Philadelphia: W. B. Saunders.

Bachmann, G. (1916). The inter-auricular time interval. *American Journal of Physiology, 41,* 309.

Baroldi, G., Manteo, O., & Scomozoni, G. (1956). The collaterals of the coronary arteries in normal and pathologic heart. *Circulatory Research, 4,* 223.

Berne, R. M. (1980). The role of adenosine in the regulation of coronary blood flow. *Circulation Research, 47,* 807.

Berne, R. M., & Levy, M. N. (1992). *Cardiovascular pathophysiology* (6th ed.). St. Louis: Mosby–Year Book.

Braunwald, E. (1968). Cooperative study on cardiac catheterization. *Circulation, 37* (Suppl. 3).

Brutsaert, D. L., Rademakers, F. E., & Sys, S. U. (1984). Triple control of relaxation: Implications in cardiac disease. *Circulation, 69,* 190-196.

Chaitman, B. (1992). Exercise stress testing. In E. Braunwald (Ed.), *Heart disease: A textbook of cardiovascular medicine* (4th ed.). Philadelphia: W. B. Saunders.

DeHaan, R. L. (1965). Development of pacemaker tissue in the embryonic heart. *Annals of the New York Academy of Sciences, 127,* 7.

Fuster, V., Badimon, L., Badimon, J. J., & Chesebro, J. H. (1992). The pathogenesis of coronary artery disease and the acute coronary syndromes. *New England Journal of Medicine, 326*(4), 242-250.

Fye, W. B. (1983). Ernest Henry Starling: His law and its growing significance in the practice of medicine. *Circulation, 68*(5), 1145-1148.

Gregg, D. E. (1974). The natural history of collateral development. *Circulation Research, 35,* 355.

Halpenny, C. J. (1982a). Cardiac electrophysiology. In S. L. Underhill, S. L. Woods, E. S. Sivarajan, & C. J. Halpenny (Eds.), *Cardiac nursing* (p. 36). Philadelphia: J. B. Lippincott.

Halpenny, C. J. (1982b). Regulation of cardiac output and blood pressure. In S. L. Underhill, S. L. Woods, E. S. Sivarajan, & C. J. Halpenny (Eds.), *Cardiac nursing.* Philadelphia: J. B. Lippincott.

Hansen, J. F. (1989). Coronary collateral circulation: Clinical significance and influence on survival in patients with coronary artery occlusion. *American Heart Journal, 117,* 290-295.

Harary, I. (1962). Heart cells in vitro. *Scientific American, 206,* 141.

James, T. N. (1962). Pericarditis and the sinus nodes. *Archives of Internal Medicine, 110,* 305.

James, T. N. (1968). The coronary circulation and conduction system in acute myocardial infarction. *Progressive Cardiovascular Disease, 10,* 410.

James, T. N., Sherf, L., Schlat, R. C., & Silverman, M. E. (1985). Anatomy of the heart. In J. W. Hurst & C. Rackley (Eds.), *The heart: Arteries and veins* (6th ed.). New York: McGraw-Hill.

Julius, S., Antoon, A., Whitlock, L. S., & Conway, J. (1967). Influence of age on the hemodynamic response to exercise. *Circulation, 36,* 222-230.

Katz, A. M. (1977). *Physiology of the heart* (pp.1-24). New York: Raven Press.

Kirchheim, H. R. (1976). Systemic arterial baroreceptor reflexes. *Physiological Review, 56*(1), 110-176.

Kirk, E. S., & Jennings, R. B. (1985). Pathophysiology of myocardial ischemia. In J. W. Hurst & C. Rackley (Eds.), *The heart: Arteries and veins* (6th ed.). New York: McGraw-Hill.

Little, R. C. (1985). *Physiology of the heart and circulation* (3rd ed.). Chicago: Year Book.

Raven, R. H. & Johnson, G. B. (1986). *Biology.* St. Louis: Mosby–Year Book.

Re, R. N. (1987). The renin-angiotensin systems. In E. D. Frohlich (Ed.), *Essential hypertension. Medical Clinics of North America, 71*(5).

Re, R., Novelline, R., Escourrou, M. T., Atnansouhs, C., Burton, J., & Aarber, E. (1978). Inhibition of angiotensin-converting enzyme for diagnosis of renal artery stenosis. *New England Journal of Medicine, 298*(11), 582-586.

Rochmis, P., & Blackburn, H. (1971, August 23). Exercise tests: A survey of procedures, safety, and litigation experience in approximately 170,000 tests. *JAMA, 217,* 1061-1066.

Rodeheffer, R. J., & Gerstenblith, G. (1985). Effect of age on cardiovascular function. In H. A. Johnson (Ed.), *Relations between normal aging and disease.* New York: Raven Press.

Rodeheffer, R. J., Gerstenblith, G., Becker, L. C., Fleg, J. L., Weisfeldt, M. L., & Lakatta, E. G. (1984). With exercise cardiac output is maintained with advancing age in healthy human subjects: Cardiac dilatation and increased stroke volume compensate for a diminished heart rate. *Circulation, 69,* 203-213.

Rushmer, R. F. (1976). *Cardiovascular dynamics.* Philadelphia: W. B. Saunders.

Schaper, W. (1971). *The collateral circulation of the heart.* New York: American Elsevier.

Schlant, R. C., & Sonnenblick, E. H. (1990) Normal physiology of the cardiovascular system. In J. W. Hurst, R. B. Logue, C. E. Rackley, R. C. Schlant, E. H. Sonnenblick, & N. K. Wenger (Eds.), *The heart: Arteries and veins* (7th ed.). New York: McGraw-Hill.

Silverman, B. D., & Neeld, J. B., Jr. (1984). Evaluation of the cardiac patient for noncardiac surgery. *Journal of the Medical Association of Georgia, 73*(5), 315-318.

Soderstrom, M. (1948). Myocardial infarction and mitral thrombosis in the atria of the heart. *Acta Medica Scandinavian Supplementum, 132*(217), 114.

Sparks, H. V., & Rooke, T. W. (1987). *Essentials of cardiovascular physiology.* Minneapolis: University of Minnesota Press.

Starling, E. H. (1918). *The Linacre lecture on the law of the heart.* London: Longmans, Green & Co.

Stewart, J. T., Gray, H. H., Wars, D. E., Pumphrey, C. W., Redwood, D. R., & Parker, D. J. (1990). Major complication of coronary arteriography: The place of cardiac surgery. *British Medical Journal, 63*(2), 73.

Strandell, T. (1964). Circulation studies on healthy old men. *Acta Medica Scandinavian Supplementum 175* (414), 1-14.

Thibodeau, G. A. (1987). *Anatomy and physiology.* St. Louis: Times Mirror/Mosby.

Thibodeau, G. A., & Patton, K. T. (1993). *Anatomy and physiology* (2nd ed.). St. Louis: Mosby–Year Book.

Thomas, J. L., Dickstein, R. A., Parker, F. B., Jr., Potts, J. L., Poirer, R. A., et al. (1982). Prognostic significance of the development of left bundle conduction defects following aortic valve replacement. *Journal of Thoracic and Cardiovascular Surgery, 84*(3), 382-386.

Thompson, J. M., McFarland, G. K., Hirsch, J. E., Tucker, S. M., & Bowers, A. C. (1989). *Mosby's manual of clinical nursing* (2nd ed.). St. Louis: Mosby–Year Book.

Thorel, C. (1909). Vorlarifig mittelung uber eine beson dere muskel ver bindung zwischen der cava superior und dem hisschen bundel. *Munich Med Wochenschrift, 56,* 2159.

Underhill, S. L., Woods, S. L., Sivarajan, E. S., & Halpenny, C. J. (Eds.). (1982). *Cardiac nursing.* Philadelphia: J. B. Lippincott.

Vander, A. J., Sherman, J. H., & Luciano, D. S. (1990). *Human physiology: The mechanisms of body function* (5th ed.). New York: McGraw-Hill.

Vander, A., Sherman, J.H., & Luciano, D. S. (1980). *Human physiology* (3rd ed.). New York: McGraw-Hill.

Vick, R. L. (1984). *Contemporary medical physiology.* Menlo Park, CA: Addison-Wesley.

Weisfeldt, M. L., LaKatta, E. G., & Gerstenblith, G. (1992). Aging and the heart. In E. Braunwald (Ed.), *Heart disease: A textbook of cardiovascular medicine* (4th ed.). Philadelphia: W. B. Saunders.

Wenckebach, K. F. (1908). Bietrage zur kenntnis der mengchlichen hertztatigkeit. *Archives of Anatomy and Physiology, 3,* 53.

Wu, D. (1984). What is the role of calcium antagonists for ventricular tachycardia. *International Journal of Cardiology, 5,* 543-547.

SUGGESTED READINGS

Braunwald, E. (Ed.). (1992). *Heart disease: A textbook of cardiovascular medicine* (4th ed.). Philadelphia: W. B. Saunders.

Halpenny, C. J. (1982). Systemic and pulmonary circulations. In S. L. Underhill, S. L. Woods, E. S. Sivarajan, & C. J. Halpenny (Eds.), *Cardiac nursing.* Philadelphia: J. B. Lippincott.

James, T. N. (1967). Cardiac innervation: Anatomic and pharmacologic relations. *Bulletin of the New York Academy of Medicine, 43,* 1041.

Schauf, C. L., Moffett, D. F., & Moffett, S. B. (1990). *Human physiology: Foundations and frontiers.* St. Louis: Mosby–Year Book.

Alterations of Cardiovascular Function

Sandra W. Haak

Stephanie J. Richardson

Sheryl S. Davey

Pamela D. Parker-Cohen*

Chapter Outline

*Contributing author to first edition.

I

*n the past, pathophysiology of the heart cen-
tered on coronary artery disease or on congenital heart diseases. Today emphasis is on reperfusion
injury, myocardial hypertrophy, injury to the endothelium as the initiating event in the pathogenesis of
cardiovascular disease, and those diseases requiring
cardiac transplants.*

DISEASES OF THE ARTERIES AND VEINS

Arteriosclerosis

Arteriosclerosis is a chronic disease of the arterial system characterized by abnormal thickening and hardening of the vessel walls. In arteriosclerosis, the tunica intima undergoes a series of changes that decrease the artery's ability to change lumen size. Smooth muscle cells
and collagen fibers migrate into the tunica intima, causing it to stiffen and thicken. This process gradually narrows the arterial lumen (Fig. 27-1). Changes in lipid,
cholesterol, and phospholipid metabolism within the tunica intima also contribute to arteriosclerosis. Although
these structural changes may be part of the normal aging process, they can cause or worsen pathophysiologic
conditions such as high blood pressure, insufficient perfusion of tissues, or weakening and outpouching of arterial walls.

Atherosclerosis

Atherosclerosis is a form of arteriosclerosis in which the
thickening and hardening of the vessel walls are caused
by soft deposits of intraarterial fat and fibrin that
harden over time. Atherosclerosis is not a single disease
entity. It can take several forms, depending on the anatomic location, the age, genetic and physiologic status,
and the risk factors to which each individual may have
been exposed. It is the leading contributor to coronary
artery and cerebrovascular disease. (Atherosclerosis of
the coronary arteries is described on p. 1022; that of
the cerebral arteries in Chapter 15.)

Pathophysiology

It has long been recognized that lipid deposition is an
early event in atherogenesis and occurs when influx and
deposition of cholesterol into the arterial wall exceed efflux (Ross, 1992; Virchow, 1862). The lesions of atherosclerosis occur primarily within the tunica intima (innermost layer) and include the fatty streak, fibrous
plaque, and the advanced or complicated lesion. The
fatty streak, the earliest atherosclerotic lesion, is a flat,
yellow, lipid-filled smooth muscle cell that causes no obstruction of the affected vessel. Fatty streaks are commonly present in the aorta of children older than 1 year
regardless of race, sex, or environmental factors
(Cotran, Kumar, & Robbins, 1989). These lesions are
thought to be reversible.

Fibrous plaque is the characteristic lesion of advancing atherosclerosis and is rarely found in people younger
than 25 years of age. It consists of lipid-laden smooth

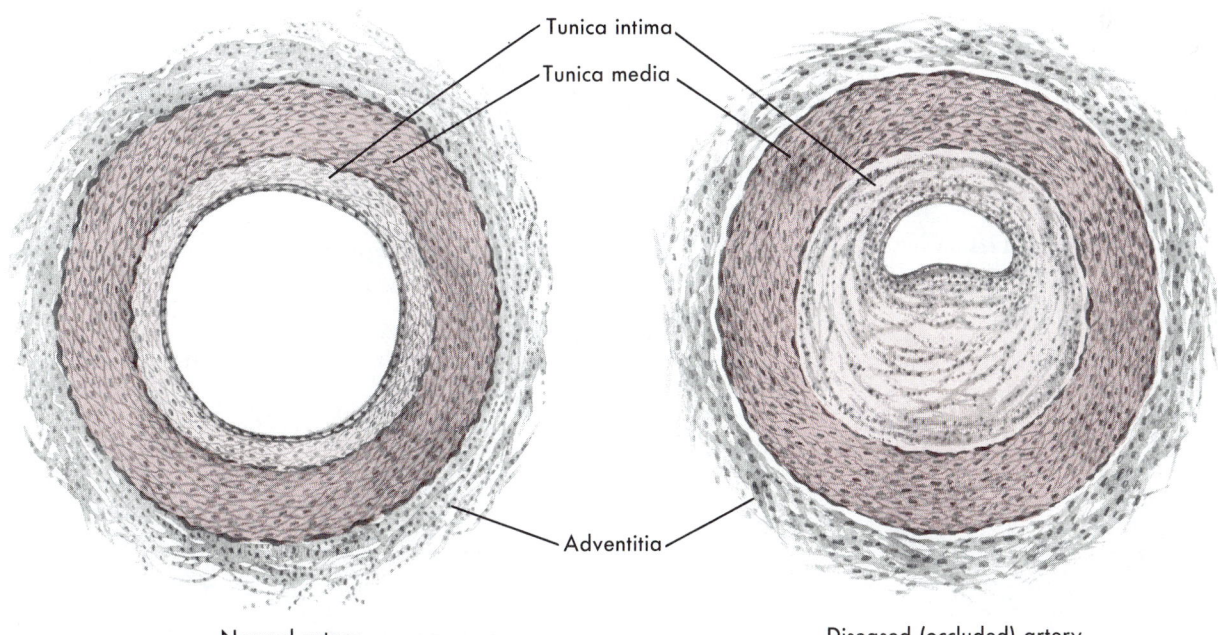

FIG. 27-1 **Arteriosclerosis.** Cross section of a normal artery and an artery altered by disease.

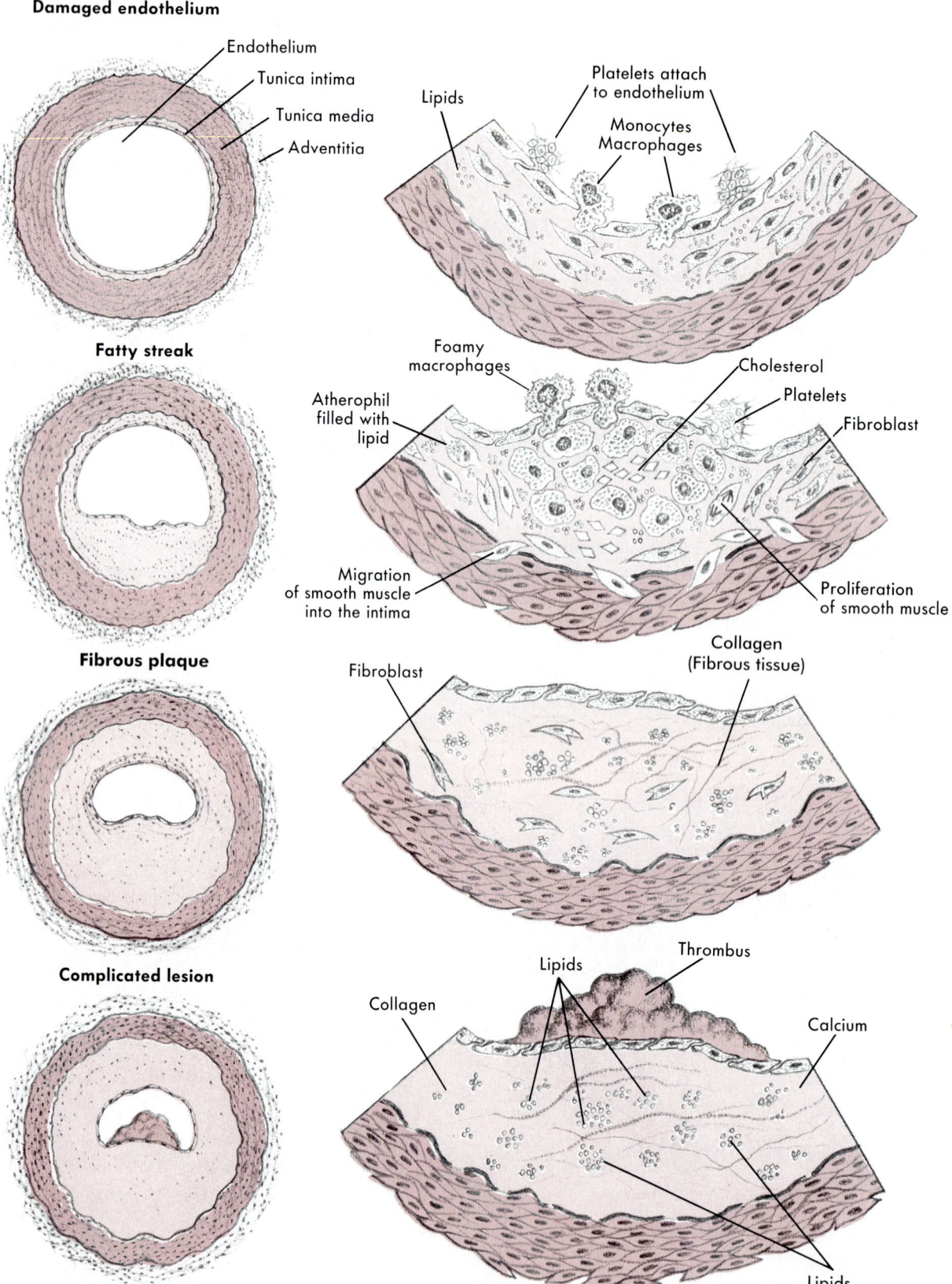

Damaged endothelium

Endothelium
Tunica intima
Tunica media
Adventitia

Lipids

Platelets attach
to endothelium

Monocytes
Macrophages

Fatty streak

Foamy
macrophages

Atherophil
filled with
lipid

Cholesterol

Platelets

Fibroblast

Migration
of smooth muscle
into the intima

Proliferation
of smooth muscle

Fibrous plaque

Collagen
(Fibrous tissue)

Fibroblast

Complicated lesion

Lipids

Thrombus

Collagen

Calcium

Lipids

FIG. 27-2 Progression of atherosclerosis.

muscle cells surrounded by collagen, elastic fibers, and a mucoprotein matrix. The lesion is white and elevated and protrudes into the lumen of the artery (Fig. 27-2). The growing mass fixes to the inner wall of the tunica intima and may invade the muscular tunica media. Fibrous plaques are thought to develop from fatty streaks in which cellular proliferation, lipid accumulation, and connective tissue formation occur. The core of the fibrous plaque may consist of lipids and debris resulting from cellular necrosis caused by insufficient blood supply. If the lesion progresses sufficiently, it can occlude the arterial lumen. This is most likely to occur at arterial bifurcations, curves, or regions in which the arteries taper.

Complicated or advanced lesions occur if the fibrous plaques are altered over time by hemorrhage, calcification, cellular necrosis, and mural thrombosis (occlusion by blood clots throughout the intimal layer). The intimal surface may disintegrate or ulcerate as the lipid-laden lesion enlarges and hardens. This rigid complex structure is often the cause of vascular occlusion.

Atherosclerotic lesions generally cause no symptoms until 60% or more of the tissue's blood supply is occluded. If plaque formation occurs slowly, collateral arteries may develop to supply tissue.

Several hypotheses have been proposed to explain the pathogenesis (atherogenesis) and progression of athero-

sclerosis, but there is disagreement about which is correct. Atherogenesis and atherosclerosis probably occur as a result of several of the hypotheses described in Table 27-1.

Clinical Manifestations

Atherosclerosis may have many different manifestations, again depending on the vessel involved, site of the lesion, and the age, genetic makeup, and physiologic status of the individual. High blood pressure ensues if atherosclerosis elevates systemic vascular resistance. Cerebral or myocardial ischemia is a life-threatening manifestation of atherosclerosis in vessels of the brain or heart.

Evaluation and Treatment

In evaluating individuals for the presence of atherosclerosis, the complete health history, including risk factors, and physical examination, including laboratory data, are considered. Judicious use of x-ray films, electrocardiography, ultrasonography, nuclear scanning, and angiography may be necessary to identify affected vessels, particularly coronary vessels.

Dietary modification is always the first treatment for atherosclerosis. Fat intake should be reduced to less than 30% of daily calorie consumption, with no more than 10% saturated fats, no more than 10% polyun-

---

TABLE 27-1

Hypotheses of Atherogenesis

Hypothesis	Mechanism of atherogenesis
Response to injury	Arterial endothelium is injured by altered hemodynamic forces (hypertension), harmful chemicals (nicotine, catecholamines), bacterial infection, hyperlipidemia, or mechanical trauma; endothelial membrane is disrupted, permeability is altered, and platelets, lipids, and smooth muscle aggregate on the intimal layer.
Monoclonal hypothesis	Phenotypically identical smooth muscle cells are transformed into benign neoplasms by viruses or chemicals.
Lipogenic hypothesis	Elevated levels of low-density lipoproteins (LDLs), decreased levels of high-density lipoproteins (HDLs) result in migration and accumulation of LDLs and cholesterol in the tunica intima and tunica media.
Clonal senescence	Aging interferes with immune function in the tunica intima and tunica media, and smooth muscle cell replication continues unchecked, allowing muscle cells and lipids to accumulate.
Thrombogenic hypothesis	Repeated deposition of blood elements (fibrin, platelets, etc.) on the endothelium results in formation of microthrombi; old deposits degenerate as new material continues to accumulate and platelets release a factor that stimulates smooth muscle proliferation (von Rokitansky, 1852).
Lipid infiltration	Circulating lipids enter arterial endothelium and accumulate around the smooth muscle; endothelial permeability is adversely affected, allowing continued lipid filtration (Virchow, 1862).

saturated fats, and 10% to 15% monounsaturated fats. Monounsaturated fats reduce atherogenesis while avoiding the problems of polyunsaturated fats (see Chapter 10). Daily cholesterol intake must be reduced to 250 to 300 mg.

The NIH Consensus Development Conference has recommended target total blood cholesterol levels of less than 200 mg/dl with low-density lipoproteins (LDL) less than 130 mg/dl (LaRosa, 1990). Drugs that decrease lipidemia are prescribed only if serum lipoproteins are not reduced by a reasonable trial of dietary modification or if lipid levels are dangerously elevated in an individual who will require a considerable time for significant dietary change and weight reduction.

Hypertension

Hypertension is consistent elevation of systemic arterial blood pressure. Approximately 62.8 million Americans, including 2.8 million children aged 6 to 17 years, have hypertension. Individuals are diagnosed as having hypertension when the average of two or more diastolic blood pressure measurements made on two or more consecutive clinical visits is 90 mm Hg or higher, or when the average of systolic blood pressure measurements made on two or more consecutive visits is greater than 140 mm Hg (Joint National Committee, 1988).

Hypertension is caused by increases in cardiac output, total peripheral resistance, or both. (The many factors affecting cardiac output and peripheral resistance are described in Chapter 26. See Figs. 26-18 and 26-28.) Cardiac output is increased by any condition that increases heart rate or stroke volume, whereas peripheral resistance is increased by any factor that increases blood viscosity or reduces vessel diameter, particularly arteriolar diameter.

Individuals with hypertensive disease may have combined systolic and diastolic hypertension or isolated systolic hypertension. Most cases of combined systolic and diastolic hypertension have no known cause and are therefore diagnosed as **primary hypertension.** Primary hypertension, also called essential or idiopathic hypertension, affects 92% to 95% of hypertensive individuals (Danielson & Dammstrom, 1981; Joint National Committee, 1988; Kaplan, 1992; Rudnick, Sackett, Hirst, & Holmes, 1977). **Secondary hypertension** is caused by altered hemodynamics associated with a primary disease, such as arteriosclerosis. Although many diseases can cause secondary hypertension, this form of hypertension accounts for only 5% to 8% of cases. **Isolated systolic hypertension** is elevated systolic blood pressure accompanied by normal diastolic blood pressure (below 90 mm Hg). Isolated systolic hypertension is a manifestation of increased cardiac output, or rigidity of the aorta, or both.

Estimates of the prevalence of hypertension in the United States (American Heart Association, 1991) indicate that the prevalence rate of hypertension in adults is lowest for white women (25%) and highest for black women (39%). The prevalence rate for white men (33%) is lower than that for black men (38%). Among whites, the incidence of hypertension in men is higher than in women.

Factors Associated with Primary Hypertension

A specific cause for primary hypertension has not been identified, and a combination of genetic and environmental factors is thought to be responsible for its development. Genetic predisposition to hypertension is thought to be polygenic. The inherited defects are associated with renal sodium excretion, cell membrane sodium or calcium transport, and sympathetic response to neurogenic hormones (Fackelmann, 1991; Hilbert et al., 1992; Kaplan, 1992; Lifton et al., 1992; Williams et al., 1990). Factors associated with primary hypertension include (1) family history of hypertension, (2) advancing age, (3) gender (man younger than age 50 and woman older than age 50), (4) black race, (5) high dietary sodium intake, (6) glucose intolerance (diabetes mellitus), (7) cigarette smoking, (8) obesity, and (9) heavy alcohol consumption (Kaplan, 1992). Many of these factors are risk factors for other cardiovascular disorders. In fact, hypertension, hyperlipidemia, and glucose intolerance are often found together.

Although populations with high dietary sodium intake have long been shown to have a high incidence of hypertension, recent studies indicate that low dietary potassium, calcium, and magnesium intake are also risk factors (Joint National Committee, 1988; Scrogin, Hatton, & McCarron, 1992). The nicotine in cigarette smoke is a vasoconstrictor that can elevate both systolic and diastolic blood pressure acutely. In habitual smokers, an individual cigarette may not raise blood pressure, yet habitual smoking is associated with a high incidence of severe hypertension and with death resulting from hypertension (Joint National Committee, 1988; Kaplan, 1992). The incidence of hypertension is higher among heavy drinkers of alcohol (more than three drinks per day) than among abstainers, but moderate drinkers (two to four drinks per week) appear to have lower blood pressures, as well as lower cardiovascular mortality, than either abstainers or heavy drinkers (Joint National Committee, 1988; Kaplan, 1992).

Pathophysiology

Chronic hypertension damages the walls of systemic blood vessels. Prolonged vasoconstriction and high pressures within these vessels, particularly the arteries and arterioles, stimulate the vessels to thicken and strengthen to withstand the stress. Arterial smooth muscle undergoes hypertrophy (cellular enlargement) and hyperplasia (cellular proliferation). Eventually, the tunica intima and tunica media undergo fibromuscular thickening sufficient to narrow their lumina. At this point, regardless of stimuli that cause vasoconstriction, the vessels are permanently narrowed.

Hypertensive injury of vessel walls also stimulates the biochemical mediators of inflammation (histamine, leukotrienes, and prostaglandins) to increase the permeability of the vascular endothelium. As permeability increases, sodium, calcium, water, plasma proteins, and other blood-borne (humoral) substances enter vessel walls, causing further thickening and, in the case of calcium, increasing responsiveness to stimuli that cause smooth muscle contraction (i.e., vasoconstriction). (Inflammation is discussed in Chapter 7.)

In the coronary vessels, hypertension causes or aggravates other conditions, such as atherosclerosis, that diminish vessel caliber. Therefore, hypertension combined with coronary artery disease increases the risk of coronary artery occlusion and infarction of myocardial tissue.

Primary hypertension

Despite research by numerous investigators, the exact pathogenesis of primary hypertension has not been established. In view of the multiple, interdependent factors involved in normal blood pressure regulation, it seems likely that no single cause or defect will be identified.

Several hypotheses have been proposed to explain the onset of primary hypertension in individuals at risk. They include (1) increases in blood volume, (2) inappropriate autoregulation, (3) overstimulation of sympathetic neural fibers in the heart and vessels, (4) water and sodium retention by the kidneys, and (5) hormonal inhibition of sodium-potassium transport across cell walls in the kidneys and blood vessels. Any or all of these mechanisms may be at work, but researchers disagree about which is dominant during pathogenesis of primary hypertension.

Fig. 27-3 illustrates the hemodynamic hypothesis of onset. This hypothesis, which is closely related to all but the neural hypothesis, attributes the onset of hypertension to fluid overload. According to the hemodynamic hypothesis, early primary hypertension consists of a series of cardiovascular adjustments to an increase in blood volume. First, cardiac output increases to handle the increased volume of blood circulating through the heart. As the systemic arteries sense the volume increase, their autoregulatory mechanisms try to slow things down by causing vasoconstriction. Because blood volume remains high, the increase in total peripheral resistance caused by vasoconstriction leads to hypertension. At this point, hypertension has not damaged the vessels and, if blood volume is reduced, cardiac output and vascular smooth muscle tone return to normal.

In individuals in whom persistent primary hypertension develops, however, cardiac output returns to nor-

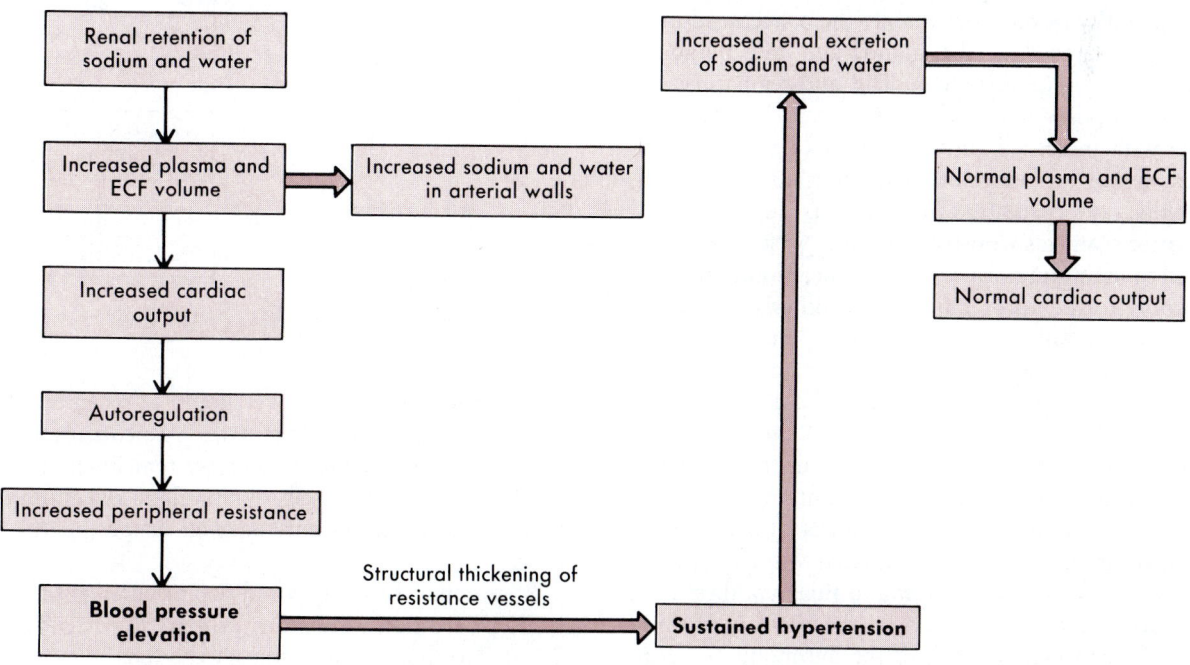

FIG. 27-3 Primary hypertension. Hemodynamic events of early primary hypertension *(thin arrows)* and established primary hypertension *(thick arrows)*. *ECF,* Extracellular fluid volume.

FIG. 27-4   Two related mechanisms of sodium-induced primary hypertension.

mal but vascular smooth muscle tone does not, so peripheral resistance remains high. At this point, hypertension becomes established and vascular damage begins. This simple hypothesis leaves unexplained many mechanisms that might be involved. The amount of increase in extracellular fluid and cardiac output that must occur before hypertension results is unknown (Kaplan, 1992).

Autoregulation in the cardiovascular system chiefly involves the intrinsic capability of the arterioles in the vascular beds to regulate the flow of blood according to the quantity of blood available, the concentration of metabolites carried in the blood, and the metabolic needs of surrounding tissues. The autoregulatory hypothesis proposes that, although primary hypertension begins with increased cardiac output (Fig. 27-3), it is *maintained* by an alteration of vascular autoregulation. Normally, autoregulatory mechanisms adjust arterial and arteriolar vasoconstriction and vasodilation as needed to maintain normal, or baseline, blood pressure. According to the autoregulatory hypothesis, the defect consists of the failure of autoregulatory mechanisms to return vascular tone to normal after cardiac output and blood volume have returned toward baseline (because of water and sodium excretion by the kidneys). Hypertension is established as the new baseline, and autoregulation subsequently functions to maintain it.

The third hypothesis about the onset of primary hypertension is that neurally stimulated vasoconstriction is the initiating event. According to this hypothesis, the cardiovascular control centers in the brain overstimulate the sympathetic branch of the autonomic nervous system, causing vasoconstriction. Overstimulation also could be caused by some abnormality of α-adrenergic

receptor function, or an oversupply of receptors for the neurotransmitter that stimulates vasoconstriction. Because the sympathetic nervous system innervates both the heart and the vessels, sympathetic overstimulation increases cardiac output, as well as peripheral resistance.

Researchers have proposed two mechanisms by which sodium retention can initiate primary hypertension (Fig. 27-4). The first is that primary hypertension begins with an inherited defect of sodium excretion in the kidneys (Kaplan, 1992; Page, 1987). The defect in renal sodium excretion is aggravated by dietary sodium intake of more than 50 mEq/day, which initiates the hemodynamic events of early hypertension (Fig. 27-3).

The second mechanism of sodium retention is thought to be an interruption of the sodium-potassium pump, which normally governs the transport of sodium and potassium across cell membranes (see Chapters 1 and 3). In individuals with this defect, a humoral factor (a hormone) is thought to inhibit sodium excretion from cells. The factor or factors have not been discovered. Elevated levels of the humoral sodium-transport inhibitor not only cause intracellular sodium to accumulate, but also seem to cause increases of intracellular calcium. Because intracellular calcium promotes smooth muscle contractility, the presence of extra calcium in vascular smooth muscle cells increases vascular reactivity. This vascular reactivity produces vasoconstriction with increased peripheral resistance and leads to the final outcome of hypertension. The cellular events related to sodium-induced hypertension are summarized in Fig. 27-4.

Secondary hypertension

Secondary hypertension is caused by a systemic disease process that raises peripheral vascular resistance or cardiac output. If the cause is identified and removed before permanent structural changes occur, blood pressure returns to normal. Table 27-2 summarizes the pathogenesis of major forms of secondary hypertension.

Isolated systolic hypertension

Elevations of systolic pressure alone are usually caused by increases in cardiac output, or total peripheral vascular resistance, or both. Isolated systolic hypertension caused by increased cardiac output can be secondary to dysfunction of the aortic semilunar valve (aortic valve insufficiency), any abnormal opening between heart chambers (arterioventricular fistula, patent ductus arteriosus; see Chapter 28), thyrotoxic crisis (thyroid storm), Paget disease of the bone, and beriberi. Rigidity of the aorta is the chief vascular cause of isolated systolic hypertension.

Isolated systolic hypertension is most common in the

TABLE 27-2

Pathogenesis of Major Forms of Secondary Hypertension by Cause

Primary disease	Pathogenesis of hypertension
Renal disorders	
Renal parenchymal disease	Disturbances in filtration and reabsorption of serum sodium, potassium, and calcium initiate the hemodynamics of early hypertension
Renovascular disease	Impaired blood flow and renal ischemia invoke the compensatory renin-angiotensin-aldosterone mechanism in an effort to raise the renal perfusion pressure
Renin-producing tumors	Elevated blood renin levels invoke elevations in angiotensin and aldosterone, which cause blood pressure to rise
Renal failure	Disturbances in filtration and reabsorption of serum sodium, potassium, and calcium initiate the hemodynamics of early hypertension
Primary sodium retention	Disturbance in filtration and/or reabsorption of serum sodium initiates the hemodynamics of early hypertension
Endocrine disorders	
Acromegaly	Excess human growth hormone causes increased peripheral resistance
Hypothyroidism	Mucopolysaccharide deposits in vascular tissue increase resistance
Hypercalcemia	Calcium ion directly affects vascular tonicity; elevated serum calcium levels increase vascular tone and peripheral resistance
Hyperthyroidism	Increased inotropic effect on the heart elevates systolic pressure; diastolic pressure decreases as a result of decreased peripheral resistance
Adrenal disorders Cortical disturbances Cushing syndrome	Glucocorticoids facilitate sodium and water retention, initiating the hemodynamics of early hypertension

From Kaplan, N.M. (1990). *Clinical hypertension* (5th ed.). Baltimore: Williams & Wilkins.

Continued.

TABLE 27-2

Pathogenesis of Major Forms of Secondary Hypertension by Cause—cont'd

Primary disease	Pathogenesis of hypertension
Endocrine disorders—cont'd	
Primary aldosteronism	Excess aldosterone promotes sodium retention and initiation of the hemodynamics of early hypertension
Congenital adrenal hyper-plasia	Excess production of adrenal cortical hormones promotes sodium and water retention
Medullary disturbance: pheochromocytoma	Excess catecholamines raise vascular tone and increase peripheral resistance
Extraadrenal chromaffin tumors	Excess catecholamines raise vascular tone and increase peripheral resistance
Vascular disorders	
Coarctation of the aorta	Decreased blood flow in distal areas initiates maximum peripheral resistance as an auto-regulatory effort to adjust perfusion pressure
Arteriosclerosis	Loss of elasticity in vessel walls results in increased peripheral resistance
Pregnancy-induced hypertension	Pathogenesis unclear
Neurologic disorders	
Elevated intracranial pressure (brain tumor, encephalitis, respiratory acidosis of pulmonary or CNS origin)	Higher systemic blood pressure required to maintain adequate cerebral perfusion
Quadriplegia, acute porphyria, familial dysautonomia, lead poisoning, Guillain-Barré syndrome	Interface with neural control of blood pressure initiates increased systemic blood pressure
Acute stress	
Surgery, psychogenic hyperventilation, hypoglycemia, burns, pancreatitis, alcohol withdrawal, sickle-cell crisis, resuscitation, increased intravascular volume	Acute stress precipitates release of catecholamines and glucocorticoids
Drugs and other substances	
Oral contraceptives and estrogen	Unknown; possibly caused by sodium retention, plasma retention, weight gain, changes in levels and actions of renin, angiotensin, and aldosterone
Corticosteroids	Same as for Cushing disease
Sympathetic stimulants, appetite suppressants, antihistamines	Raises vascular tone and increases vascular resistance
Licorice	Contains glycerrhizic acid, a mineralocorticoid causing salt and water retention
Monoamine oxidase inhibitors	Hypertension may develop in an individual who routinely takes MAO inhibitor with ingestion of a food containing tyramine

TABLE 27-3

Pathologic Effects of Sustained, Complicated Primary Hypertension

Site of injury	Mechanism of injury	Potential pathologic effect
Heart		
Myocardium	Increased workload combined with diminished blood flow through coronary arteries	Left ventricular hypertrophy, myocardial ischemia, left heart failure
Coronary arteries	Accelerated atherosclerosis (coronary artery disease)	Myocardial ischemia, myocardial infarction, sudden death
Kidneys	Renin and aldosterone secretion stimulated by reduced blood flow	Retention of sodium and water, leading to increased blood volume and perpetuation of hypertension
	Reduced oxygen supply	Tissue damage that compromises filtration
	High pressures in renal arterioles	Nephrosclerosis leading to renal failure
Brain	Reduced blood flow and oxygen supply; weakened vessel walls	Transient ischemic attacks, cerebral thrombosis, aneurysm, hemorrhage
Eyes (retinas)	Reduced blood flow	Retinal vascular sclerosis
	High arteriolar pressure	Exudation, hemorrhage
Aorta	Weakened vessel wall	Dissecting aneurysm (see p. 1013)
Arterial vessels of lower extremities	Reduced blood flow and high pressures in arterioles	Intermittent claudication, gangrene

elderly. Rigidity of the aorta is caused by arteriosclerosis, which increases total peripheral vascular resistance. Changes associated with aging alter the aortic valve so that increased cardiac output is needed to maintain blood flow into the systemic circulation.

Complicated hypertension

Complicated hypertension is sustained primary hypertension that has pathologic effects besides hemodynamic alterations and fluid and electrolyte imbalances. Complicated hypertension commonly compromises the structure and function of the vessels themselves, the heart, aorta, kidneys, eyes, brain, and lower extremities. The two major mechanisms of tissue damage are ischemia and edema. Ischemia deprives tissues of the oxygen and nutrients they need for survival and function. Leakage of fluids into the interstitial space, and even hemorrhage, is caused by high pressures in the vessels. The heart is particularly susceptible to injury because although high cardiac output is stimulating myocardial hypertrophy, vasoconstriction is diminishing blood flow through the coronary arteries. The pathophysiology of complicated hypertension is summarized in Table 27-3.

Cardiovascular complications include left ventricular hypertrophy, angina pectoris, congestive heart failure (left heart failure), coronary artery disease, myocardial infarction, and sudden death. Vascular complications include the formation, dissection, and rupture of aneu-

rysms (outpouchings in vessel walls); intermittent claudication; and gangrene resulting from vessel occlusion. Possible renal complications are parenchymal damage, nephrosclerosis, renal arteriosclerosis, and renal insufficiency or failure.

Changes in the vascular beds can be estimated by viewing the arterioles of the retina. Complications specific to the retina include retinal vascular sclerosis, exudation, and hemorrhage. Cerebrovascular complications are similar to those of other arterial beds and include transient ischemia, stroke, cerebral thrombosis, aneurysm, and hemorrhage.

Malignant hypertension (rapidly progressive hypertension in which diastolic pressure is usually above 140 mm Hg) can cause encephalopathy, a profound cerebral edema that disrupts cerebral function and causes loss of consciousness. Encephalopathy occurs because high arterial pressure renders the cerebral arterioles incapable of regulating blood flow to the cerebral capillary beds. Capillary permeability is increased by high hydrostatic pressures in the capillaries and vascular fluid exudes into the interstitial space. If blood pressure is not reduced, cerebral edema and cerebral dysfunction increase until death occurs. Organ damage resulting from malignant hypertension is life-threatening. Besides encephalopathy, malignant hypertension can cause papilledema, cardiac failure, uremia, retinopathy, and cerebrovascular accident.

Clinical Manifestations

The early stages of hypertension have no clinical manifestations other than elevated blood pressure. Most important, there are no signs and symptoms to cause the individual to seek health care; thus, hypertension is called a lanthanic (silent) disease. Some hypertensive individuals never have signs, symptoms, or complications, whereas others become very ill, in which case hypertension can be a cause of death. Others have anatomic and physiologic damage caused by past hypertensive disease, despite current blood pressures within normal ranges.

The chance of developing primary hypertension increases with age, over and above the natural rise in blood pressure associated with aging. In individuals at risk for primary hypertension, the factors leading to development of hypertension accumulate during the first two or three decades of life. Although hypertension is usually thought to be an adult health problem, it is important to remember that hypertension does occur in children and is being diagnosed with increasing frequency (Liebermann, 1990; Robson & Leung, 1991). Usually, however, increased peripheral resistance and early hypertension develop in the second, third, and fourth decades of life. If elevated blood pressure is not detected and treated, it becomes established and may begin to accelerate atherosclerosis when the individual is 30 to 50 years of age. This sets the stage for the complications of hypertension that begin to appear during the fourth, fifth, and sixth decades of life.

Most of the clinical manifestations of hypertensive disease are caused by complications that damage organs and tissues outside the vascular system. Besides elevated blood pressure, the signs and symptoms, therefore, tend to be specific for the organs or tissues affected. Evidence of heart disease, renal insufficiency, central nervous system dysfunction, impaired vision, impaired mobility, vascular occlusion, or edema can all be caused by sustained hypertension. (See appropriate chapters for specific clinical manifestations of organ dysfunction.)

Evaluation and Treatment

Diagnostic tests for suggested hypertension include repeated blood pressure measurements, complete blood count, urinalysis, biochemical blood profile (plasma glucose, potassium, creatinine, cholesterol, and triglycerides), and an electrocardiogram. Individuals who have elevated blood pressure are assumed to have primary hypertension unless their history, physical examination, or initial diagnostic screening indicates secondary hypertension.

Treatment of primary hypertension depends on its severity. Table 27-4 lists blood pressure levels and categories of severity used as guidelines for treatment.

Hypertension is usually managed with both pharmacologic and nonpharmacologic methods. Treatment begins with reducing or eliminating risk factors. Lifestyle modification can control hypertension and enhance the effects of drug treatment. The usual dietary recommendations are to restrict sodium intake to 2 g/day, to increase potassium intake, to restrict saturated fat intake, and to adjust calorie intake as required to maintain optimum weight. An exercise program that promotes en-

TABLE 27-4

Classification of Hypertension by Category of Severity and Recommended Follow-up

Blood pressure (mm Hg)	Category of severity	Recommended follow-up
Diastolic		
Below 85	Normal blood pressure	Recheck within 2 years
85-89	High normal blood pressure	Recheck within 1 year
90-104	Mild hypertension	Prompt confirmation (2 months or less)
105-114	Moderate hypertension	Prompt care (2 weeks or less)
Above 115	Severe hypertension	Immediate care
Systolic (diastolic below 90 mm Hg)		
Below 140	Normal blood pressure	Recheck within 2 years
140-159	Borderline isolated systolic hypertension	Prompt confirmation (2 months or less)
160-199	Isolated systolic hypertension	Prompt confirmation (2 months or less)
Above 200	Isolated systolic hypertension	Prompt care (2 weeks or less)

From Joint National Committee (1988). The 1988 report of the Joint National Committee on detection, evaluation, and treatment of high blood pressure, *Archives of Internal Medicine 148*(5), 1023-1038.

durance and relaxation is usually recommended. Physical training increases stroke volume, which has the effect of lowering heart rate and hence systolic blood pressure. Relaxation is expected to reduce levels of circulating catecholamines, which has the effect of reducing vascular tone and blood pressure. Individuals are counseled to stop smoking cigarettes to eliminate vasoconstrictor effects of nicotine.

Four groups of drugs are used to manage hypertension in a tailored therapy approach: (1) diuretics, (2) angiotensin inhibitors, (3) vascular smooth muscle relaxants, and (4) adrenergic blockers. Diuretics reduce blood pressure initially by facilitating renal excretion of sodium and water, thereby reducing blood volume and cardiac output. Subsequently, the cardiovascular system adjusts to restore cardiac output, but reduced blood pressure is maintained because peripheral resistance is lower. Angiotensin inhibitors reduce blood pressure by preventing the renin-angiotensin mechanism from acting on the vascular smooth muscle, adrenal cortex, kidney, and brainstem. Captopril, for example, acts by inhibiting the enzyme that converts inactive angiotensin I to the active form, angiotensin II. With less active angiotensin II in the blood, blood pressure decreases. Vascular smooth muscle relaxants lower blood pressure by blocking calcium influx to smooth muscle cells. This decreases vascular reactivity and promotes vasodilation. Adrenergic blockers interfere with the transmission of the neurohumoral facilitators (e.g., norepinephrine) of vasoconstriction and cardiac stimulation. These agents bind with adrenergic receptors, preventing receptor binding with neurohumoral stimulators of increased cardiac output and vasoconstriction.

Orthostatic (Postural) Hypotension

The term **orthostatic (postural) hypotension** means a decrease in both systolic and diastolic arterial blood pressure on standing. When a normal individual stands up, the resultant gravitational changes on the circulation are compensated for by several mechanisms that include reflex arteriolar and venous constriction, increased heart rate, and mechanical factors, such as the closure of valves in the venous system, pumping of the leg muscles, and a decrease in intrathoracic pressure (Hurst et al., 1986). The normally increased sympathetic activity during upright posture is mediated through stretch receptors (baroreceptors) in the carotid sinus and the aortic arch (see Chapter 26). Their reflex response to shifts in volume caused by postural changes leads to a prompt increase in heart rate and constriction of the systemic arterioles. Thus, despite a marked decrease in cardiac output, arterial blood pressure is maintained.

Orthostatic hypotension is often accompanied by dizziness, blurring or loss of vision, and syncope or fainting. Fainting is caused by insufficient vasomotor com-

pensation and reduction of blood flow through the brain. The normal or compensatory vasoconstrictor response to standing is thus replaced by a marked vasodilation and blood pooling in the muscle vasculature, as well as in the splanchnic and renal beds.

Orthostatic hypotension may be acute and temporary or chronic. **Acute orthostatic hypotension,** or temporary type, is caused when the normal regulatory mechanisms are sluggish. This delay may be the result of (1) anatomic variation, (2) altered body chemistry, (3) drug action (e.g., antihypertensives and antidepressants), (4) prolonged immobility caused by illness, (5) starvation, (6) physical exhaustion, (7) any condition that produces volume depletion (e.g., massive diuresis, potassium or sodium depletion), and (8) venous pooling (e.g., pregnancy, extensive varicosities of the lower extremities). The elderly are susceptible to this type of orthostatic hypotension in which postural reflexes are apparently slowed as part of the aging process. This is not a universal finding in the elderly, however.

The two forms of **chronic orthostatic hypotension** are (1) secondary to a specific disease and (2) idiopathic or primary. The diseases that cause secondary orthostatic hypotension are endocrine disorders (e.g., adrenal insufficiency, diabetes mellitus), metabolic disorders (e.g., porphyria), or diseases of the central or peripheral nervous system (e.g., intracranial tumors, cerebral infarcts, Wernicke encephalopathy, and peripheral neuropathies).

Idiopathic, or primary, orthostatic hypotension is the term for the group in which there is no known initial cause (Silber, 1987). There is controversy, however, about this group. Some define the disorder as a separate entity, whereas others suggest it is a part of a generalized degenerative central nervous system disease. Idiopathic orthostatic hypertension affects men more often than women and usually occurs between the ages of 40 and 70. In addition to cardiovascular symptoms, impotence and bowel and bladder dysfunction are often found in this type.

No curative treatment is available for idiopathic orthostatic hypertension. In the secondary form, syncope ceases when the underlying disorder is corrected (Silber, 1987). Several treatments can help acute and chronic orthostatic hypotension.

Aneurysm

An **aneurysm** is a localized dilatation or outpouching of a vessel wall or cardiac chamber. The law of Laplace can provide an understanding of the hemodynamics of an aneurysm (Fig. 27-5). (The law of Laplace is discussed in detail in Chapter 26.) Presumably, formation of a ventricular wall aneurysm occurs when intraventricular tension stretches the noncontracting infarcted muscle (Braunwald, 1988). The stretching produces in-

FIG. 27-5 Pressure-tension and wall thickness relations in blood vessels (Laplace's law). (From Kissane, 1990.)

FIG. 27-6 Infrarenal atherosclerotic aneurysm of abdominal aorta. A, Origins of celiac axis and superior mesenteric artery, as well as the right and left renal arteries, are above aneurysm. Aortic bifurcation and common iliac arteries are below. **B,** Opened atherosclerotic aneurysm of distal abdominal aorta demonstrates laminated fibrin thrombus *(dark material)* in aneurysm. Renal arteries are at top of photograph, and aortic bifurcation with severely atherosclerotic and aneurysmal common iliac arteries is at bottom. (From Kissane, 1990.)

A   B farct expansion, a weak and thin layer of necrotic muscle, and fibrous tissue that bulges with each systole. With time, the aneurysm becomes more fibrotic, but continues to bulge with each systole, thus acting as a "reservoir" for some of the stroke volume.

The aorta is particularly susceptible to aneurysm formation because of constant stress on the vessel wall and the absence of penetrating vasa vasorum in the adventitial layer. Three fourths of all aneurysms occur in the abdominal aorta (Fig. 27-6). Atherosclerosis is the most common cause of aneurysms because plaque formation erodes the vessel wall. Arteriosclerosis and hypertension are found in more than half of all individuals with aneurysms. Syphilis and other infections also can cause aortic aneurysms.

True aneurysms involve all three layers of the arterial wall and are best described as a weakening of the vessel wall. Most are fusiform and circumferential (Fig. 27-7). **False aneurysms** and **saccular aneurysms** are usually the result of trauma. These aneurysms are caused by a dissection of the layers of the arterial wall, so that

blood is contained at the point of aneurysm by the adventitial layer (dissecting saccular aneurysm) or by a clot (false aneurysm).

Clinical manifestations of aneurysm include a variety of symptoms. Aortic aneurysms can be very painful. Symptoms of dysphagia (difficulty swallowing) and dyspnea (breathlessness) are caused by the pressure of a large volume of blood on surrounding organs. An aneurysm that impairs flow to an extremity causes symptoms of ischemia. Cerebral aneurysms, which frequently occur in the circle of Willis, are associated with signs and symptoms of increased intracranial pressure. Signs and symptoms of stroke occur when cerebral aneurysms leak. (Cerebral aneurysms are described in Chapter 15.)

Treatment of aneurysms is nearly always surgical. Saccular aneurysms are repaired more easily than fusiform and circumferential aneurysms. If the weakness or separation of vascular layers spreads, the aneurysm becomes a **dissecting aneurysm** (Fig. 27-8). Dissecting aneurysms and leaking aneurysms require emergency treatment. Leaking cerebral aneurysms, especially those

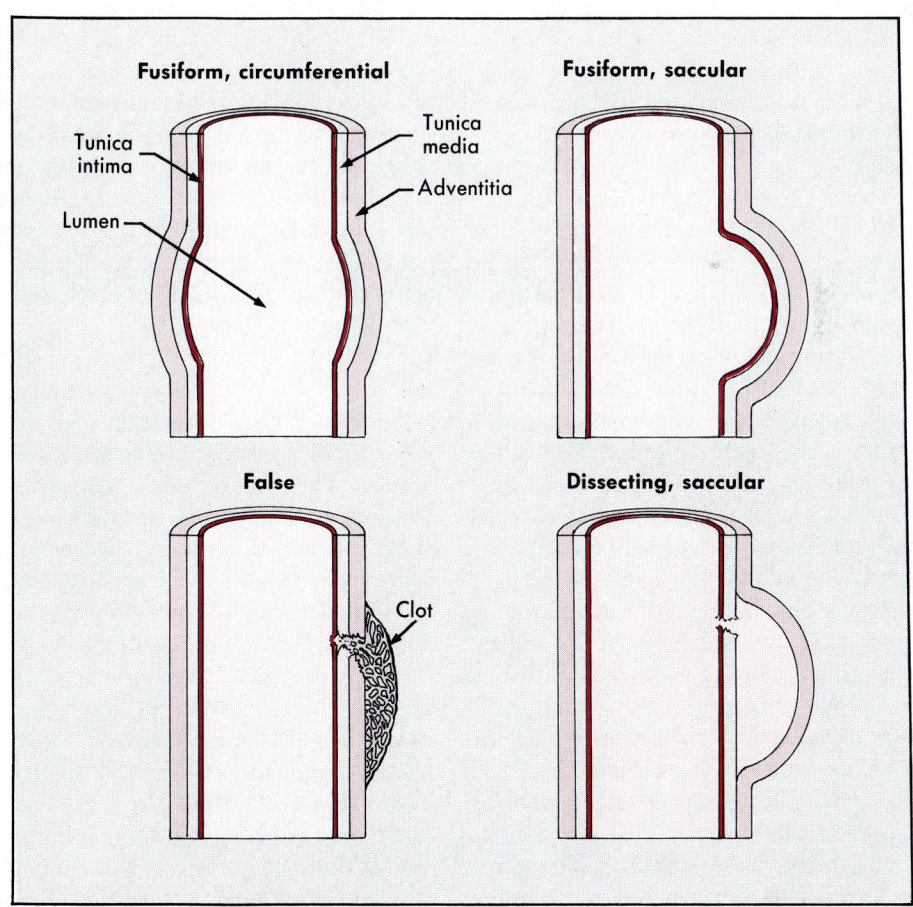

FIG. 27-7 **Longitudinal sections showing types of aneurysms.** The fusiform circumferential and fusiform saccular aneurysms are true aneurysms, caused by weakening of the vessel wall. False and saccular aneurysms involve a break in the vessel wall, usually caused by trauma.

FIG. 27-8 **Dissecting aneurysm.** Cross section of the aorta with dissecting aneurysm showing true aortic lumen *(above and right)* compressed by dissecting column of blood that separates media and creates false lumen. (From Kissane, 1990.)

associated with vascular spasms as a compensatory mechanism, are treated with clot-stabilizing drugs and a number of clinical measures designed to reduce intracranial pressure and induce hemodynamic stability before surgical intervention.

Thrombus Formation

A **thrombus** is a blood clot that remains attached to a vessel wall (see Figure 24-11). A detached thrombus is called **thromboembolus.** Thrombi tend to develop wherever intravascular conditions promote activation of the coagulation, or clotting, cascade. These conditions include intimal irritation, roughening, inflammation, traumatic injury, infection, and low blood pressures or obstructions that cause blood stasis and pooling within the vessels. (Mechanisms of coagulation are described in Chapter 22.) In the arteries, activation of the coagulation cascade is usually caused by roughening of the tunica intima by atherosclerosis. Invasion of the tunica intima by an infectious agent also roughens the normally smooth lining of the artery, causing platelets to adhere readily. Anatomic changes of an artery can stimulate thrombus formation, particularly if the change results in a pooling of arterial blood. This can occur, for example, in blood that is pooled within an aneurysm. In the veins, thrombus formation is more often associated with inflammation (phlebitis), a condition termed thrombophlebitis. Thrombi also form on heart valves altered by calcification or bacterial vegetation. Valvular thrombi are most commonly associated with inflammation of the endocardium (endocarditis) and rheumatic heart disease.

Shock (circulatory failure), particularly shock resulting from septicemia, can activate the intrinsic and extrinsic pathways of coagulation. The impaired cellular metabolism that occurs with all types of shock activates the extrinsic pathway of coagulation, whereas blood stasis caused by very low blood pressures activates the intrinsic pathway (see Chapter 22). Thrombus formation may be confined to one area or may progress to diffuse coagulopathy, such as disseminated intravascular coagulation (see Chapter 24).

A thrombus poses two potential threats to the circulation. First, the thrombus may grow large enough to occlude the artery, causing ischemia in tissue supplied by the artery. Second, the thrombus may dislodge, becoming a thromboembolus that travels through the vascular system until it occludes flow into a distal systemic or pulmonic vascular bed.

Pharmacologic treatment includes the administration of heparin and warfarin derivatives. These derivatives interfere with the clotting cascade by accelerating the activity of antithrombin III, thereby slowing or stopping thrombus growth. Pharmacologic treatment also includes the intravenous or intraarterial administration of streptokinase, which dissolves the thrombus.

A balloon-tipped catheter can be used to remove or compress a thrombus. This type of catheter is inserted into the vessel containing the thrombus at a point proximal to the thrombus and is threaded past the thrombus until the tip of the catheter is past the thrombus. The balloon on the tip of the catheter is then inflated and drawn backward out of the vessel, pulling out the clot by a "dredging" action. Various combinations of drug and catheter therapies are sometimes used concurrently.

Embolism

Embolism is the obstruction of a vessel by an **embolus**—a bolus of matter that is circulating in the bloodstream. The embolus may consist of a dislodged thrombus; an air bubble; an aggregate of amniotic fluid; an aggregate of fat, bacteria, or cancer cells; or a foreign substance. An embolus travels in the bloodstream until it reaches a vessel through which it cannot fit. No matter how tiny it is, an embolus will eventually lodge in a systemic or pulmonary vessel. The source of the embolus determines whether the embolus will lodge in a vessel of the pulmonary or systemic circulation. Pulmonary emboli originate on the venous side (mostly from the deep veins of the legs) of the systemic circulation or in the right heart; systemic emboli (or arterial) most commonly originate in the left heart and are associated with thrombi after myocardial infarction, valvular disease, left heart failure, endocarditis, and dysrhythmias.

Embolism causes ischemia or infarction in tissues distal to the obstruction. A limb that is ischemic because of arterial occlusion is characterized by an almost waxy whiteness of the skin because the vasculature is devoid of erythrocytes, and by numbness and pain resulting from neural ischemia.

Embolism of a central organ causes organic dysfunction and pain. For example, pulmonary artery embolism causes chest pain and dyspnea; renal artery embolism causes abdominal pain and oliguria; and mesenteric artery embolism causes abdominal pain and a paralytic, ischemic bowel. Infarction and subsequent necrosis of a central organ are life-threatening, not only because of organ dysfunction but also because of sepsis. Necrotic tissue is a rich medium for the growth of bacteria from the lungs, bowel, and, occasionally, the bladder. Necrosis of the bladder, in particular, can quickly lead to peritonitis or septicemia.

Embolism of a coronary or cerebral artery is an immediate threat to life if the embolus severely obstructs a major vessel. Occlusion of a coronary artery will cause a myocardial infarction (see p. 1026), whereas occlusion of a cerebral artery causes a stroke (see Chapter 15).

Thromboembolism

Thromboembolism is a vascular obstruction by a dislodged thrombus. The most common source of arterial thromboemboli is the heart. Mitral or aortic valvular disease, especially that associated with abnormal heart rhythms (atrial fibrillation and flutter), causes thrombus formation on roughened vascular surfaces and in atrial blood as a result of stasis. More than half of these thromboemboli lodge in the lower extremities (in the femoral and popliteal arteries). Others lodge in the coronary arteries and the cerebral vasculature.

Air Embolism

Room air that enters the circulation through intravenous lines is probably the most common cause of air embolism. Room air is about 70% nitrogen. Although nitrogen dissolves quickly in blood, large amounts of air cannot be dissolved rapidly enough to prevent the displacement of blood in the arterioles and capillary beds. Ischemia and necrosis occur when air totally blocks a vessel.

Air also can be introduced into the bloodstream if trauma to the chest causes air from the lungs to enter the vascular space. For example, gunshot wounds and puncture wounds of the thorax sometimes introduce air emboli. Treatment for air embolism is supportive, including bed rest and supplemental oxygen, once the connection between the source of air and the vascular system has been eliminated.

Amniotic Fluid Embolism

The great intraabdominal pressures generated during labor and delivery may force amniotic fluid into the bloodstream of the mother through the highly vascular uterine wall. Amniotic fluid not only displaces blood, reducing oxygen, nutrient, and waste exchange, but also introduces antigens, cells, and protein aggregates that trigger inflammation, coagulation, and the immune response within the bloodstream. Capillary beds are usually affected by amniotic fluid emboli, especially the capillary beds of the lungs and kidneys. Treatment is supportive and may include dialysis, particularly after a cesarean section or hysterectomy.

Bacterial Embolism

Isolated bacteria in the bloodstream do not cause embolism, but aggregates of bacteria may be large enough to do so. The most common cause of bacterial embolism is subacute bacterial endocarditis, during which clumps of vegetation are dislodged from infected cardiac valves and ejected into the pulmonary or systemic circulation. A less common cause is erosion of an artery or vein by bacteria at a source of infection, such as an abscess. Treatment for bacterial embolism includes bed rest, supplemental oxygen, and antibiotics to eradicate the source of infection.

Fat Embolism

Trauma to the long bones is associated with fat embolism, particularly in the lungs. Two mechanisms have been proposed to account for the generation of fat emboli after skeletal trauma. The first is that trauma to the bones initiates defective fat metabolism, causing globules of fat to form in the blood. Platelets adhere to these globules until the conglomerate is large enough to lodge in a capillary bed. The second possible explanation is that globules of fat are released from fatty bone marrow exposed by fracture. Again, platelets adhere to the fat globules and embolism occurs.

Treatment for fat embolism consists of prompt immobilization of fractures and supportive measures that include administration of supplemental oxygen, steroids, and glucose. Steroid administration may decrease the inflammation that occurs with vascular occlusion. Inflammation in the pulmonary bed is especially dangerous because it can cause adult respiratory distress syndrome (see Chapter 30). Intravenous administration of glucose is thought to prevent inappropriate fat metabolism.

Foreign Matter

Foreign matter can enter the bloodstream during trauma or through an intravenous or intraarterial line. If the bolus of foreign matter is relatively large, it is usually removed surgically. Small particles, such as drug precipitates, small glass shards, or fibers from linen, are sometimes introduced unintentionally into a vessel through intravenous injections or manipulation of monitoring lines. Once in the blood, these small particles initiate the coagulation cascade. The thromboemboli that form around the particles are large enough to occlude a vessel and result in ischemia. Treatment is aimed at preventing thrombus formation around the particle, dissolution of the particle, and supportive measures to alleviate ischemia.

Peripheral Arterial Disease
Thromboangiitis Obliterans (Buerger Disease)

Thromboangiitis obliterans (Buerger disease), which tends to occur in young men who are heavy cigarette smokers, is an inflammatory disease of the peripheral arteries. The inflammatory lesions are accompanied by thrombi and sometimes by vasospasm of arterial segments. Inflammation, thrombus formation, and vasospasm can eventually occlude and obliterate (render physiologically useless) portions of small and medium-sized arteries in the feet and sometimes in the hands. Typically affected are the digital, tibial, and plantar arteries of the feet and the digital, palmar, and ulnar arteries of the hands. The disease is sometimes associated with inflammation of adjacent veins and nerves. The pathogenesis of thromboangiitis obliterans is not known.

The chief symptom of thromboangiitis obliterans is pain and tenderness of the affected part. Clinical manifestations are caused by sluggish blood flow and include rubor (redness of the skin), which is caused by dilated capillaries under the skin, and cyanosis, which is caused by blood that remains in the capillaries after its oxygen has diffused into the interstitium. Chronic ischemia causes the skin to thin and become shiny, and the nails to become thickened and malformed. In advanced disease, ischemia resulting from vessel obliteration can cause gangrene.

The most important part of treatment is cessation of cigarette smoking. All other measures are aimed at improving circulation to the foot or hand. Vasodilators are prescribed to alleviate vasospasm, and exercises are taught that use gravity to improve blood flow. If vasospasm persists, sympathectomy may be performed. Gangrene necessitates amputation.

Raynaud Phenomenon and Disease

Raynaud phenomenon and **Raynaud disease** are both characterized by attacks of vasospasm in the small arteries and arterioles of the fingers and, less commonly, the toes. Although the clinical manifestations of the phenomenon and the disease are the same, their causes differ.

Raynaud phenomenon is secondary to systemic diseases, particularly collagen vascular disease (scleroderma), pulmonary hypertension, thoracic outlet syndrome, myxedema trauma, serum sickness (see Chapter 8), or long-term exposure to environmental conditions, such as cold or vibrating machinery in the workplace. (The effects of segmental vibration are described in

Chapter 2.) Raynaud disease, however, is a primary vasospastic disorder of unknown origin. Raynaud disease tends to affect young women and to consist of vasospastic attacks triggered by brief exposure to cold or by emotional stress. Genetic predisposition may play a role in its development.

The clinical manifestations of the vasospastic attacks of either disorder are changes in skin color and sensation caused by ischemia. Vasospasm occurs with varying frequency and severity and causes pallor, numbness, and the sensation of cold in the digits. Attacks tend to be bilateral, and manifestations usually begin at the tips of the digits and progress to the proximal phalanges. Sluggish blood flow resulting from ischemia may cause the skin to appear cyanotic. Rubor follows as vasospasm ends and the capillaries become engorged with oxygenated blood. Rubor is often accompanied by throbbing and paresthesias. Skin color returns to normal after the attack, but frequent, prolonged attacks interfere with cellular metabolism, causing the skin of the fingertips to thicken and the nails to become brittle. In severe, chronic Raynaud phenomenon or disease, ischemia can eventually cause ulceration and gangrene. This outcome is rare, however.

Treatment for Raynaud phenomenon consists of removing the stimulus or treating the primary disease process. Attacks of vasospasm sometimes can be alleviated at their onset by an exercise in which the arms are swung forward and backward. This maneuver increases hydrostatic pressure (and perfusion pressure) in the arteries by means of centrifugal force.

Treatment of Raynaud disease is limited to prevention or alleviation of vasospasm itself, because no underlying disorder has been identified. Stimuli that trigger attacks (e.g., cold and emotional stress) are avoided, and cigarette smoking is stopped to eliminate the vasoconstricting effects of nicotine. Exercises that build centrifugal force in the extremities are also helpful in the early stages of vasospasm. If attacks of vasospasm become frequent or prolonged, vasodilators (e.g., the antihypertensive drugs Dibenamine or Roniacal) and rauwolfia alkaloids such as reserpine are administered. Sympathectomy, which is not always effective, is the next line of treatment. If ischemia leads to ulceration and gangrene, amputation is necessary. Calcium blockers also may be tried to decrease vasospasm caused by vascular reactivity from calcium influx.

Diseases of the Veins
Varicose Veins and Chronic Venous Insufficiency

A **varicose vein** is a vein in which blood has pooled. Varicose veins, typically the saphenous veins of the legs, are distended, tortuous, and palpable. Varicose veins are caused by (1) trauma to the saphenous veins that damages one or more valves or (2) gradual venous distention caused by a combination of standing for long periods, which diminishes the action of the muscle pump, and the action of gravity on blood within the legs.

Veins are thin-walled, highly distensible vessels. Normally, valves prevent backflow and pooling of blood. If a valve is damaged, permitting backflow, a section of the vein is subjected to the pressure exerted by a larger volume of blood under the influence of gravity. The vein swells as it becomes engorged and surrounding tissue becomes edematous because increased hydrostatic pressure pushes plasma through the stretched vessel wall.

Valvular incompetence is also caused by venous distention that develops over time in individuals who habitually stand for long periods, wear constricting garments, or cross the legs at the knees. Distention progresses until the pressure in the vein damages venous valves, rendering the valves incompetent. Damaged valves are unable to maintain normal venous pressure, which causes hydrostatic pressure in the vein to increase. As the vein distends further, it becomes tortuous, and edema develops in the extremity.

Varicose veins and valvular incompetence can progress to **chronic venous insufficiency** (CVI). Chronic venous insufficiency is inadequate venous return over a long period. It causes pathologic changes as a result of ischemia in the vasculature, skin, and supporting tissues. Chronic venous insufficiency is marked by chronic pooling of blood in the veins of the lower extremities and leads to hyperpigmentation of the skin over the feet and ankles. Edema of the feet and ankles becomes marked and may progress proximally to the knees.

Circulation to the extremities becomes so sluggish that the metabolic demands of the cells for oxygen, nutrients, and waste removal are barely met. Any trauma or pressure can, therefore, lower the oxygen supply to injurious levels by further reducing blood flow into the area. Cell death occurs and necrotic tissue develops into **venous stasis ulcers.** Persistent ulceration develops because the high metabolic demands of healing tissue, particularly an increased need for oxygen, cannot be met by the existing circulation. Venous stasis ulcers are susceptible to infection because poor circulation impairs the delivery of the cells and biochemicals of the immune and inflammatory responses. (The role of inflammation in processes of healing is described in Chapter 7.)

Treatment of varicose veins and chronic venous insufficiency begins conservatively. The individual wears antiembolism stockings and avoids standing and other factors, such as constrictive clothing, that contribute to venous stasis. If conservative treatment is ineffective, saphenous vein stripping is performed.

Thrombus Formation in Veins

The process of thrombus formation in the veins is the same as that of thrombus formation in the arteries. Ve-

FIG. 27-9 **Multiple venous thrombi.** (From Rosai, 1981.)

nous thrombi are more common than arterial thrombi, however, because flow and pressure are lower in the veins than in the arteries (Fig. 27-9). With aging, in particular, the deep veins in the lower extremities become susceptible to thrombus formation, particularly with long-term bed rest or the wearing of constrictive clothing.

The inflammatory response triggered by the clotting cascade causes extreme tenderness, swelling, and redness in the area of thrombus formation. Deep venous thrombi rarely detach and cause embolism. Thrombi that form in superficial veins are almost always caused by trauma to the venous intima.

The clinical manifestations of venous occlusion differ markedly from those of arterial occlusion. With venous occlusion, the skin is discolored rather than pale (ranging from an angry red to deep blue-purple), edema is prominent, and pain is most marked at the site of occlusion, although extreme edema can render all the skin of the limb quite tender. Neuralgia develops if the edema causes soft tissues to compress local nerves.

Superior Vena Cava Syndrome

Superior vena cava syndrome (SVCS) is a progressive occlusion of the superior vena cava (SVC) that leads to venous distention in the upper extremities and head. The leading cause of SVCS is bronchogenic cancer (75% of cases), followed by lymphomas (15%), and metastasis of other cancers (7%). The right main stem bronchus abuts the SVC so that cancers occurring in this bronchus may press on the SVC. The SVC is also a relatively low-pressure vessel that lies in the closed thoracic compartment; therefore, tissue expansion within the thoracic compartment can easily compress the SVC. Finally, the SVC is surrounded by lymph nodes and lymph chains that commonly become involved in thoracic cancers and compress the SVC during tumor growth. Because onset of SVCS is slow, collateral venous drainage to the azygous vein usually has time to develop.

Clinical manifestations of SVCS include edema and venous distention in the upper extremities and face, including the ocular beds. Cerebral and central nervous system edema may cause headache, visual disturbance, and impaired consciousness. The skin of the face and arms is purple and taut, and capillary refill time is prolonged. Respiratory distress may be present because of edema of bronchial structures or compression of the bronchus by a carcinoma.

Treatment of SVCS is usually delayed for 24 hours to determine its cause. Because of its slow onset and the development of collateral venous drainage, SVCS is generally not a vascular emergency, but rather is an oncologic emergency. Treatment consists of radiation therapy and the administration of diuretics, steroids, and anticoagulants, as necessary (Varricchio, 1985).

Coronary Artery Disease, Myocardial Ischemia, and Myocardial Infarction

Coronary artery disease, myocardial ischemia, and myocardial infarction form a pathophysiologic continuum that impairs the pumping ability of the heart by depriving the heart muscle of blood-borne oxygen and nutrients. The earliest lesions of the continuum are those of **coronary artery disease**—virtually any vascular disorder that narrows or occludes the coronary arteries (Fig. 27-10). Coronary artery disease can diminish the myocardial blood supply until deprivation impairs myocardial metabolism enough to cause **ischemia,** a local state in which the cells are temporarily deprived of blood sup-

FIG. 27-10 Atherosclerosis. Narrowed lumen of small branch of anterior descending coronary artery caused by atherosclerosis. Note thick fibrous and atheromatous plaque on one side, greatly reduced lumen, and reduced media. This woman died of a myocardial infarction. (From Kissane, 1990.)

ply. They remain alive but are unable to function normally. Persistent ischemia or the complete occlusion of a coronary artery causes **infarction,** or death, of the deprived myocardial tissue. Infarction constitutes the often-fatal event known as the "heart attack."

Development of Coronary Artery Disease

In the United States, coronary artery disease (CAD) is responsible for nearly 50% of all deaths and one third of deaths of persons between 35 and 65 years of age (American Heart Association, 1991). In the 1960s, researchers began to identify risk factors that contribute to the onset and escalation of coronary artery disease. The factors were classified as either modifiable or nonmodifiable. The nonmodifiable risk factors refer to variables that cannot be altered by persons wishing to decrease their risk of cardiovascular disease. These include advanced age, male gender (until age 60), black or Oriental race, genetic predisposition (which many consider modifiable if genetic risk includes hypertension and hyperlipidemia, which are treatable), and diabetes mellitus type I. The modifiable risk factors include hyperlipidemia (high levels of circulating lipoproteins), hypertension, cigarette smoking, diabetes mellitus type II, obesity, sedentary lifestyle, psychosocial factors (e.g., stress), hormone therapy, and heavy alcohol consumption. The role that some of the modifiable risk factors play in precipitating or exacerbating cardiovascular disease is controversial. Hyperlipidemia (e.g., hypercholesterolemia), hypertension, and cigarette smoking have, however, been identified objectively as most predictive of CAD (Criqui, 1986).

Hyperlipidemia

The strong link between coronary artery disease and elevated plasma lipoprotein concentrations is well documented (The Expert Panel, 1988, 1991; Titus & Kim, 1990). The term *lipoprotein* refers to lipids, phospholipids, cholesterol, and triglycerides bound to carrier proteins. Lipids (cholesterol in particular) are required by most cells for the manufacture and repair of plasma membranes. Cholesterol is also a necessary component for the manufacture of such essential substances as bile acids and steroid hormones. Although cholesterol can easily be obtained from dietary fat intake, most body cells are also able to manufacture cholesterol.

The cycle of lipid metabolism is complex. Dietary fat is packaged into particles known as **chylomicrons** in the small intestine. Chylomicrons are required for absorption of fat and function by transporting exogenous lipid from the intestine to the liver and peripheral cells. Chylomicrons are the least dense of the lipoproteins, and primarily contain triglyceride. Some of the triglyceride may be removed and either stored by adipose tissue or used by muscle as an energy source. The chylomicron remnants, composed mainly of cholesterol, are taken up by the liver. A series of chemical reactions in the liver results in the production of several lipoproteins that vary in density and function. These include very low-density lipoproteins (VLDL), primarily triglyceride and protein; low-density lipoproteins (LDL), mostly cholesterol and protein; and high-density lipoproteins (HDL), mainly phospholipids and protein. Investigators suggest that high levels of VLDL and LDL are directly related to increased risk of atherosclerosis of the coronary arteries because of their fat content. High serum levels of copper and iron, as well as low levels of selenium, have been implicated in accelerated atherogenesis and increased risk of coronary heart disease (Salonen et al., 1992). Risk is thought to be the result of oxygen free radical production and lipid peroxidation (see Chapter 2).

High-density lipoproteins, however, are thought to prevent or delay atherogenesis and thus are thought to be protective. This may be because of their lower fat content or their possible role in carrying lipids away from body tissues to the liver for degradation, that is, "reverse" cholesterol transport (Hancock, 1991).

Hyperlipidemia may develop in individuals because of high dietary fat intake, systemic disease (pancreatitis, diabetes mellitus, hypothyroidism, nephrosis, systemic lupus erythematosus), and genetic defects (familial dyslipoproteinemias). The most convincing evidence that hyperlipidemia is an important risk factor in the development of atherosclerosis is seen in cases of familial hypercholesterolemia. Individuals who are homozygous for this disorder rarely reach the age of 20; most die of severe atherosclerosis in their teens. Myocardial infarctions have been documented in children as young as 3 to 5 years of age in whom this familial disorder occurs (Assmann, 1987). Causes of the familial dyslipoproteinemias include abnormalities of lipid-metabolizing enzymes and abnormal cellular lipid receptors (Table 27-5) (Goldstein & Brown, 1989).

Hypertension

Elevated blood pressure may precipitate or exacerbate the atherosclerotic process by causing trauma to the arterial walls. A vicious cycle results as atherogenic plaques stiffen and narrow arterial walls, increasing peripheral resistance and myocardial workload. Escalating hypertension and cardiac muscle hypertrophy result.

Cigarette smoking

Studies indicate that 30% of the annual mortality from coronary artery disease is traceable to cigarette smoking (Hancock, 1991). The mechanism by which smoking increases atherosclerosis is uncertain. Nicotine stimulates the release of catecholamines (epinephrine and norepinephrine), which increase heart rate and peripheral vascular constriction. As a result, blood pressure in-

creases, as do cardiac workload and oxygen demand. Elevated catecholamines also stimulate release of free fatty acids. In one study, men and women who smoked more than 15 cigarettes per day were found to have lower HDL levels and higher LDL, cholesterol, and triglyceride levels (Brischetto, Connor, Connor, & Matarazzo, 1983). Cigarette smoking also may increase platelet adhesiveness, thereby increasing the risk of clot formation within the arteries. Furthermore, the carbon monoxide in cigarette smoke reduces the oxygen content of arterial blood. Hypoxemia (insufficient oxygen in arterial blood) may promote atherosclerosis by decreasing the availability of oxygen to the vessel walls and increasing vessel wall permeability. The cadmium in cigarette smoke may be related to elevations in blood pressure. The risk of coronary artery disease increases with heavy smoking and decreases when smoking is stopped. After smoking is discontinued, the risks associated with coronary artery disease may decrease as much as 50% in 1 year (Farmer & Gotto, 1992).

Diabetes mellitus

Diabetes mellitus is often associated with increased lipid levels, obesity, and hypertension. Glucose intolerance doubles the occurrence of coronary disease in men and may quadruple the incidence in women (Hurst, Schlant, Rackley, Sonnenblick, & Wenger, 1990). Control of hyperglycemia alone, however, does not eliminate the coronary risk. The pathophysiologic link to atherosclerosis is unclear, but multifactorial risk reduction is implied (see Chapter 5).

Genetic predisposition

A strong family predisposition to early coronary heart disease occurs in approximately 5% of the general population of families; however, these coronary-prone families account for more than 50% of cases of coronary disease occurring before the age of 55 (Williams, 1984). Serum cholesterol level is one of the most predictive risk factors for coronary heart disease (CHD) (Hjermann, Velve Byrek, Holm, & Leren, 1981; Kannel, Feinleib, McNamara, Garrison, & Castelli, 1979). It is the cholesterol risk factor that clinicians most often refer to as the genetic contribution to CHD (McCance, 1983). Coronary disease usually develops by age 45 in men who have familial hypercholesterolemia (Williams, 1984).

A phenomenon called "tracking" exists in children, whereby the level of serum cholesterol at school age is predictive of the level 4 years later. This suggests an inborn genetic control of cholesterol over time (Schrott, Bucker, Clarke, & Lauer, 1979). The Framingham Offspring Study (Kannel et al., 1979), as well as twin studies (Feinleib & Garrison, 1979), indicate that the cholesterol subfractions LDL, HDL, and VLDL show famil-

TABLE 27-5

Familial Dyslipoproteinemias

Name	Laboratory findings	Clinical features	Therapy
Type I; exogenous hyperlipidemia; fat-induced hypertriglyceridemia	Cholesterol normal Triglycerides increased 3 times Chylomicrons increased	Abdominal pain Hepatosplenomegaly Skin and retinal lipid deposits Usual onset: childhood	Low-fat diet
Type IIa; hypercholesterolemia	Triglycerides normal LDL increased Cholesterol increased	Premature vascular disease Xanthomas of tendons and bony prominences Common Onset: all ages	Low–saturated fat and cholesterol diet Cholestyramine[1] Colestipol[2] Nicotinic acid[3] Neomycin[4] Intestinal bypass
Type IIb; combined hyperlipidemia; carbohydrate-induced hypertriglyceridemia	LDL, VLDL increased Cholesterol increased Triglycerides increased	Same as IIa	Same as IIa; *plus* carbohydrate restriction Clofibrate[5] Gemfibrozil[6]
Type III; dysbetalipoproteinemia	IDL or chylomicron remnants increased Cholesterol increased Triglycerides increased	Premature vascular disease Xanthomas of tendons and bony prominences Uncommon Onset: adulthood	Weight control Low carbohydrate, saturated fat, and cholesterol diet Alcohol restriction Clofibrate Gemfibrozil Nicotinic acid Estrogens[7] Intestinal bypass
Type IV; endogenous hyperlipidemia; carbohydrate-induced hypertriglyceridemia	Glucose intolerance Hyperuricemia Cholesterol normal or increased VLDL increased Triglycerides increased	Premature vascular disease Skin lipid deposits Obesity Hepatomegaly Common onset: adulthood	Weight control Low-carbohydrate diet Alcohol restriction Clofibrate Nicotinic acid Intestinal bypass
Type V; mixed hyperlipidemia; carbohydrate and fat-induced hypertriglyceridemia	Glucose intolerance Hyperuricemia Chylomicrons increased VLDL increased LDL increased Cholesterol increased Triglycerides increased 3 times	Abdominal pain Hepatosplenomegaly Skin lipid deposits Retinal lipid deposits Onset: childhood	Weight control Low–carbohydrate and fat diet Clofibrate Nicotinic acid Progesterone[8] Intestinal bypass

[1]*Cholestyramine* (Questram), anion exchange resin; binds bile acids; enhances cholesterol excretion.
[2]*Colestipol* (Colestid), same as cholestyramine.
[3]*Nicotinic acid* (niacin), decreases release of free fatty acids from adipose tissue; increases lipogenesis in liver; decreases glucagon release; most effective for type V disorder.
[4]*Neomycin*, experimental medication; questionable mode of action; decreases LDLs.
[5]*Clofibrate* (Atromid S), decreases release of free fatty acids from adipose tissue; decreases hepatic secretion of VLDL and increases catabolism of VLDL.
[6]*Gemfibrozil* (Lopid), similar to clofibrate, but increases HDLs more.
[7]*Estrogens*, decrease IDL levels in type III disorders; experimental.
[8]*Progesterone*, decreases plasma triglycerides in type V disorders; experimental.

ial associations and heritability similar to those of total cholesterol levels. Familial hypercholesterolemia (type IIa) has the greatest predictive power in characterizing genetic disorders leading to early CAD.

Hypertension also plays a significant role in approximately one fourth of coronary-prone families. Estimates of heritability for blood pressure indicate that about 50% of the population variability for blood pressure could be attributed to genetic factors (Williams et al., 1991).

Obesity

Obesity is not always shown to be an independent risk factor. When it is classified as to the pattern of fat distribution, however, those persons with upper body obesity are found to have a higher risk of cardiovascular disease than those with lower body obesity (Blackburn & Kanders, 1987). Obesity also affects the risk profile by predisposing individuals to hypertension, hyperlipidemias, and impaired glucose tolerance. Studies have consistently reported a decrease in HDL levels associated with obesity (Criqui, 1986). As obesity progresses, the heart increases in size, resulting in increased oxygen consumption and increased work load.

Sedentary lifestyle

Investigations of physical fitness and coronary heart disease and all-cause mortality have shown that a sedentary lifestyle predisposes to coronary artery disease and that physical exercise may delay or prevent its development (Blair et al., 1989; Powell, Thompson, Caspersen, & Kendrick, 1987). Physical exercise may reduce blood pressure, decrease the urge to smoke and eat, improve carbohydrate metabolism, and improve psychologic outlook. (Increased fibrinolysis with decreased blood clotting has been noted in individuals who exercise regularly [Estok & Rudy, 1986].) In addition, persons who are habitually physically active tend to have higher plasma HDL levels than do sedentary individuals (Criqui, 1986). There is no evidence that exercise increases development of coronary collateral vessels or results in regression of atheromatous plaques. Physical activity does increase heart volume and mass, increase cardiac capillary vascularity, and decrease heart rate, however—all of which may protect from the effects of ischemic damage (Hurst et al., 1990). Studies on sudden death in joggers and runners older than age 30 show that coronary atherosclerosis is most often the cause (Estok & Rudy, 1986; Scragg, Stewart, Jackson, & Beaglehole, 1987).

Hormone therapy

Mortality from coronary artery disease has been reportedly reduced in women who receive estrogen replacement post menopause (Criqui, 1986). It is thus interest-

ing to note that estrogens do not reduce the incidence of coronary artery disease in men. Moreover, use of estrogen-containing oral contraceptives in premenopausal women may increase the risk of myocardial infarction (Hurst et al., 1990). The mechanism involved is enhanced thrombosis rather than accelerated atherogenesis. Presumably, contraceptives affect the coagulation profile, i.e., high platelet counts, short thromboplastin time, elevation of various clotting factors, increased platelet adhesiveness, lowered levels of antithrombin III (complexes with thrombin; a reduction promotes thrombosis), and decreased clearance of activated clotting factors (Farmer & Gotto, 1992). Oral contraceptives have been associated with increases in body weight, blood pressure, and triglyceride levels while decreasing glucose tolerance and HDL concentrations. Women who smoke may be at an even greater risk for untoward effects of estrogen therapy (Farmer & Gotto, 1992). Further research is needed to elucidate the relationship of estrogens and coronary artery disease.

The reason for the male-female differential in susceptibility to coronary artery disease is not understood. Although initial studies lauded estrogen as the reason women younger than age 50 experienced lower incidence of CAD, the previous paragraph disputes this claim. Perhaps androgen levels are responsible. Postmenopausal women experience increased effects from circulating androgens as a result of decreased estrogen opposition. It is possible that male-linked hormones also may be correlated significantly with increased coronary risk.

Alcohol

Moderate alcohol intake (less than three drinks per day) has been associated with increased HDL levels (Rimm et al., 1991). Regardless, the apparent protective nature of alcohol may be more likely the consequence of multiple advantageous characteristics, such as low blood pressure, healthy genetic endowment, and so forth (Shaper, Phillips, Pocock, & Walker, 1987). Alcohol is known to increase body weight, triglyceride levels, and systolic blood pressure and may impair left ventricular function. Some studies have demonstrated a direct cardiotoxic effect of excessive alcohol on myocardial tissue, resulting in collagen accumulation, diminished nucleic acid pools, and loss of membrane transport systems (Hurst et al., 1990). Further research is needed to clarify this issue (Sheehy, 1992).

Women and coronary artery disease

The incidence of coronary artery disease is lower in premenopausal women than in age-matched men. In the early 1980s, this difference was attributed to women's low participation in work outside the home and consequent fewer job-related risk factors (Detre, 1984; Haynes, Eaker, & Feinleib, 1984). Further study has shown both sexes are equally affected by coronary artery disease risk factors, and the process of atherosclerosis does not appear to differ between men and women. The gender differences in prevalence of coronary artery disease are now attributed to differences in circulating estrogen and androgenic hormones (Das & Banka, 1992; Farmer & Gotto, 1992; Hazzard, 1989). In postmenopausal women, the incidence of coronary artery disease increases rapidly and by age 65 approaches the same rate as that for men.

Although HDL cholesterol levels are inversely related to the risk of cardiovascular disease in both men and women, the risk posed by high levels of LDL cholesterol is not as dramatic or clearcut in women as it is in men (Crouse, 1989). Data from two large studies suggest that low HDL levels are riskier for women than high LDL levels (Crouse, 1989). The study of women and cardiovascular disease needs direct investigation rather than extrapolation from studies of men.

Type A personality

Beginning in the 1950s, Friedman and Rosenman (1974) and other investigators argued compellingly that persons with the type A personality are at higher risk for the development of coronary disease. Many epidemiologic studies support that view; however, crucial support came from two other types of studies—a prospective study and a number of angiographic studies (Dimsdale, 1988). Individuals with type A personality are described as hard-driving, aggressive, compulsive, domineering, and deadline conscious (Rose, 1987).

The well-known prospective study was the Western Collaborative Group Study (WCGS), which followed 3154 healthy men for 8½ years. Data demonstrated three significant findings: (1) that persons with type A behavior had about twice the chance of acquiring CAD, (2) that the increased risk associated with type A behavior was not dependent on other known risk factors, and (3) that type A behavior was a predictor of subsequent reinfarction (Jenkins, Zyzanski, & Rosenman, 1976). Three separate research groups found that persons with type A behavior had more extensive CAD at the time of coronary angiography (Blumenthal, Williams, Kong, Schanberg, & Thompson, 1978; Frank, Heller, Kornfield, Sporn, & Weiss, 1978; Jenkins, Zyzanski, & Rosenman, 1976).

As a result of these studies, a review panel recognized type A behavior as a risk factor for CAD in 1981 (The Review Panel on Coronary-Prone Behavior and Coronary Heart Disease, 1981). Since the early 1980s, however, a large number of contradictory findings have been reported regarding the risk status of type A behavior (Dimsdale, 1988). For example, Ragland and Brand

(1988) found that subsequent coronary mortality in patients who had experienced a first coronary event was surprisingly lower among type A than among type B persons (an opposite type of behavior). Thus, type A behavior became a protective factor!

Recent studies now fail to demonstrate an association between type A behavior and the extent of coronary artery disease (Dimsdale, 1988). Perhaps there is a better, tighter, more predictive description of the type A behavior. For example, suppressed hostility has been described as a more predictive core of the "coronary-prone personality" (MacDougall, Dembroski, Dimsdale, & Hackett, 1985). Expressive hostility was positively related to LDL levels (Dujovne & Houston, 1991) and a strong belief in personal control predicted severe coronary atherosclerosis (Seeman, 1991). Emotional stresses are known to precipitate an acute myocardial infarction (Pasternak, Braunwald, & Sobel, 1992). Rahe and colleagues (1974) noted a significant increase in stressful life events in individuals who subsequently experienced myocardial infarction or sudden death.

Myocardial Ischemia
Pathophysiology

The coronary arteries normally supply blood flow sufficient to meet the demands of the myocardium as it labors under varying work loads. Oxygen extraction from these vessels occurs with maximal efficiency. If efficient exchange does not meet myocardial oxygen needs, healthy coronary arteries are able to dilate to increase the flow of oxygenated blood to the myocardium. A variety of pathologic mechanisms can interfere with blood flow through the coronary arteries, giving rise to myocardial ischemia. Narrowing of a major coronary artery by more than 50% impairs blood flow sufficiently to hamper cellular metabolism under conditions of increased myocardial demand (Fig. 27-10).

The most common cause of myocardial ischemia is atherosclerosis. Plaque formation within the arterial system often results in occlusion of vessel lumina, depriving the myocardium of oxygen and nutrients. Thrombus formation in the coronary arteries may result from ulceration of atherosclerotic plaques. The growing mass of plaque, platelets, fibrin, and cellular debris eventually can narrow the lumen enough to impede blood flow (Fig. 27-2). Platelet aggregations are known to release the prostaglandin thromboxane A_2, a potent vasoconstrictor capable of causing spasm of the coronary arteries. Thromboxane A_2 also promotes platelet aggregation, resulting in a vicious positive feedback cycle of vasoconstriction and platelet buildup in the vessel walls.

Myocardial ischemia develops if coronary blood flow or the oxygen content of coronary blood is not sufficient to meet the metabolic demands of myocardial cells. Imbalances between blood supply and myocardial demand can result from a number of conditions. Supply is reduced by (1) hemodynamic factors, such as increased resistance in coronary vessels, hypotension, or decreased blood volume (e.g., due to hemorrhage); (2) cardiac factors, such as decreases of diastolic filling time, increases in heart rate, or valvular incompetence; (3) hematologic factors, such as the oxygen content of the blood; or (4) systemic disorders that reduce blood flow or the availability of oxygen (e.g., shock). Myocardial ischemia is usually caused by increased resistance in coronary vessels, but because the myocardium has little tolerance for hypoxia, it is particularly vulnerable (along with brain tissue) to the hypoxemia caused by respiratory disease (e.g., chronic obstructive pulmonary disease), anemia, or erythrocyte disorders that interfere with oxygen binding (see Chapters 23 and 30).

Demand is increased by (1) high systolic blood pressure; (2) increased ventricular volume; (3) increased thickness of the myocardium (e.g., left ventricular hypertrophy caused by increased systemic resistance, such as occurs with aortic valve stenosis and hypertension); (4) increased heart rate resulting from exercise, stress, hyperthyroidism, anemia, or hyperviscosity of the blood (e.g., polycythemia); or (5) conditions that heighten the myocardium's contractile response. Ischemia occurs if demand exceeds supply. For example, in an individual with coronary artery disease, supply may be adequate for myocardial function while the individual is at rest, provided respiratory and erythrocyte function are normal. Any factor that increases demand, such as strenuous exercise, or decreases supply, such as the develop-

ment of anemia or respiratory disease, places the individual at risk for an episode of myocardial ischemia.

Myocardial cells become ischemic within 10 seconds of coronary occlusion. After several minutes, the heart cells lose the ability to contract, thus hampering pump function and depriving the myocardium of a glucose source necessary for aerobic metabolism. Anaerobic processes take over, and lactic acid accumulates. Cardiac cells remain viable for approximately 20 minutes under ischemic conditions. If blood flow is restored, aerobic metabolism resumes, contractility is restored, and cellular repair begins. If the coronary arteries cannot compensate for lack of oxygen, myocardial infarction occurs (Fig. 27-11).

Clinical Manifestations

Angina pectoris is chest pain caused by myocardial ischemia. The discomfort is usually transient, lasting approximately 3 to 5 minutes. If blood flow is restored, no permanent change or damage results. The effects of temporary ischemia are reversible.

Angina pectoris is typically experienced as substernal chest discomfort, ranging from a sensation of heaviness or pressure to moderately severe pain. Individuals often describe the sensation by clenching a fist over their left chest. Discomfort may radiate to the neck, lower jaw, left arm, and left shoulder. It may occasionally radiate to the back or down the right arm. Discomfort is commonly mistaken for indigestion. The pain is presumably caused by the buildup of lactic acid or abnormal stretching of the ischemic myocardium that irritates myocar-

FIG. 27-11 Cycle of ischemic events.

dial nerve fibers. These afferent sympathetic fibers enter the spinal cord from levels C3 to T4, accounting for the variety of locations and radiation pattern of anginal pain. Pallor, diaphoresis, and dyspnea may be associated with the pain.

There are three types of angina: stable angina, unstable angina, and Prinzmetal angina. **Stable angina** (classic, exertional angina) is caused by luminal narrowing and hardening of the arterial walls, so that the affected vessels cannot dilate in response to increased myocardial demand associated with physical exertion or emotional stress. The discomfort of stable angina is generally predictable. It is brought on by known stimuli and causes the same type of sensation with each ischemic attack. Stable angina is usually relieved by rest and nitrates; if unrelieved by either treatment, the individual may be progressing toward an infarction.

Unstable angina (preinfarction angina, acute coronary insufficiency, crescendo angina) may indicate advanced ischemic heart disease. Unstable angina can seldom be predicted. The onset and course of pain differ with each attack, and attacks tend to increase in frequency and duration with time, often occurring at rest. Ischemia is often caused by a combination of vasospasm and atherosclerotic lesions that cause inadequate oxygen supply at rest. Unstable angina is a manifestation of ischemia that may signify impending infarction.

Prinzmetal angina (variant angina) is chest pain attributable to transmural ischemia of the myocardium (ischemia that involves the entire thickness of the myocardial layer). It occurs unpredictably and almost exclusively at rest. The underlying pathology is vasospasm of one or more of the major coronary arteries, with or without associated atherosclerosis. Variant angina frequently occurs at night, during rapid-eye-movement sleep. It may have a cyclical pattern of occurrence. The cause of vasospasm is postulated to be (1) hyperactivity of the sympathetic nervous system, (2) an increase in calcium flux within arterial smooth muscle, or (3) impaired production or release of prostaglandin I_2 or thromboxane A_2 (Ganz & Alexander, 1985; McFadden et al., 1991).

Evaluation and Treatment

Physical examination may disclose extra, rapid heart sounds (left ventricular gallop or S_3), indicating impaired left ventricular function during the ischemic attack. The presence of xanthelasmas (small fat deposits) around the eyelids or arcus senilis of the eyes (a yellow lipid ring around the cornea) suggests hyperlipidemia and possible atherosclerosis.

Electrocardiography is a critical tool for the diagnosis of myocardial ischemia. Because many individuals have normal electrocardiograms in the absence of pain, diagnosis requires that electrocardiography be per-

formed during an attack of angina. Transient ST segment depression and T wave inversion are characteristic signs of subendocardial ischemia. ST elevation, indicative of transmural ischemia, is seen in individuals with Prinzmetal's angina (Fig. 27-12). The electrocardiogram can also give some indication of which coronary artery is involved. Exercise stress testing is useful in differentiating angina from other types of chest pain, as well as detecting ischemic changes that occur in the absence of anginal pain.

Radioisotope imaging with thallium-201 is another technique used to diagnose coronary artery disease. Active transport mechanisms (the Na-K-ATPase system) cause thallium to enter myocardial cells. An area of myocardial infarction appears as a region of diminished activity or no activity (a "cold spot"). Defects that are absent at rest, but can be induced by exercise, represent ischemia.

Coronary angiography is useful in determining the anatomic extent of coronary artery disease. Although the procedure is expensive and carries some risk, it is considered essential in the diagnostic evaluation of angina.

The primary aim of therapy for myocardial ischemia and angina is to reduce myocardial oxygen consumption by altering its various determinants in a favorable way. The factors most amenable to pharmacologic manipulation are blood pressure, heart rate, contractility, and left ventricular volume.

Nitrates are often the first drug of choice because they increase oxygen supply and reduce demand. Nitrates cause peripheral veins and, to a lesser extent, peripheral arteries to dilate. Dilation reduces both peripheral vascular resistance and venous return to the heart (preload) and thereby reduces left ventricular filling pressure and left ventricular volume. Reduced filling pressure and volume decrease workload (myocardial demand). Nitrates also improve coronary blood flow by reducing coronary artery spasm and thereby increase myocardial blood supply. These drugs cannot enhance vasodilation in coronary vessels altered by atherosclerosis or arteriosclerosis, because these disorders impair the vessels' ability to change lumen size.

β-Adrenergic blocking agents have had great impact on therapy for ischemic heart disease in the past 20 years. By blocking β receptors, these medications can increase oxygen supply and reduce myocardial demand. β-Blockers diminish catecholamine-induced elevations of heart rate, myocardial contractility, and blood pressure. Coronary blood flow also can be augmented by β-blockade. Reduction in heart rate provides additional diastolic filling time for coronary perfusion, leading to enhanced oxygen delivery to the heart.

Calcium plays a key role in the electrical excitation of cardiac cells and in mechanical contraction of the

Normal ECG deflections

A

P
R
Q S
T

Atrial depolarization
Ventricular depolarization
Ventricular repolarization

ST segment depression

P
R
Q
S
T

T wave inversion

P
R
Q S
T

ST segment elevation

P
R
Q
T

B

FIG. 27-12 ECG and ischemia. A, Normal ECG. **B,** Electrocardiographic alterations associated with ischemia.

myocardial and vascular smooth muscle cells (see Chapter 26). By blocking the influx of calcium into myocardial cells and vascular smooth muscle cells, the pacemaker activity of the sinoatrial node and conduction properties of the atrioventricular node can be modified. The three calcium channel blockers available in the United States are verapamil, nifedipine, and diltiazem. Combinations of nitrates, β-blockers, and calcium antagonists may provide dramatic relief from clinical manifestations of ischemic heart disease and make more invasive interventions unnecessary. The effects of these drugs are summarized in Table 27-6.

Experimental evidence linking platelet aggregation with decreased coronary blood flow has led to the use of antiplatelet agents for individuals with ischemic heart disease. Effective antiplatelet agents include aspirin, sulfinpyrazone, dipyridamole, or combinations of these drugs.

Percutaneous transluminal coronary angioplasty (PTCA) is a procedure whereby stenotic (narrowed) cor-

onary vessels are dilated with a balloon dilatation catheter. The lesion most suitable for angioplasty is one that is discrete, concentric, located in a proximal portion of the vessel, noncalcified, and less than 10 mm in size (Baim, 1992). Percutaneous transluminal coronary angioplasty is generally used to treat single-vessel disease, but can be effective with multiple-vessel disease or stenosis of a coronary artery or a venous bypass graft.

Ischemic heart disease can be surgically treated by a coronary artery bypass graft. A saphenous vein from the thigh is most commonly used to bypass the obstructed coronary artery. A more recent technique, using the left internal mammary artery (LIMA) rather than the saphenous vein, has shown promise for significant improvement in long-term graft patency. One of the most common indications for bypass surgery is incapacitating angina in an individual who has good left ventricular function and technically operable coronary arteries, but who has not responded to medical therapy (Baim, 1992). Although surgery has been shown to relieve angina, it does

TABLE 27-6

Effects of Antianginal Agents on Myocardial Supply and Demand

	Nitrates	Beta blockers	Calcium antagonists
Demand			
Wall tension	Decrease	Increase	Increase or no apparent effect
Sysolic blood pressure	Decrease	Decrease	Decrease
Ventricular volume	Decrease	Increase	Decrease or no apparent effect
Heart rate	Increase	Decrease	Increase, decrease, or no apparent effect
Contractility	No apparent effect	Decrease	Decrease
Supply			
Coronary blood flow	Increase	Increase or no apparent effect	Increase
Coronary vascular resistance	Decrease	Increase or no apparent effect	Decrease
Coronary spasm	Decrease	Increase or no apparent effect	Decrease
Diastolic perfusion time	Decrease	Increase	Decrease, increase, or no apparent effect
Collateral blood flow	Increase	No apparent effect	Decrease

From Kafka, Meltzer, & Frishman, 1985.

ιot halt the progress of atherosclerosis or prolong life. A successful coronary artery bypass graft can, however, diminish the probability of lethal insult to the coronary tissues.

Myocardial Infarction

Acute myocardial infarction can be considered the endpoint of the coronary artery disease—myocardial ischemia continuum. Prolonged, unrelieved ischemia that interrupts the blood supply to the myocardium results in an acute coronary event. Unlike the temporary ischemia that causes angina and reversible cellular injury, the prolonged ischemia that causes infarction leads to irreversible hypoxia and cellular death (Fig. 27-13).

The precipitating cause of irreversible hypoxia is controversial. If myocardial infarction is on a continuum with the ischemic attacks of angina, then hypoxia could be the result of long-term obstruction by atherosclerotic plaques, hemorrhage into a plaque, embolism caused by thrombi or atheromatous material, or coronary spasm. Thrombus formation resulting from abnormal platelet aggregation seems to be the most likely cause of eventual arterial occlusion. Evidence indicates that the fissuring and rupturing of atherosclerotic plaques stimulate platelet aggregation, platelet-thrombus formation, and abnormal vasomotor tone on the plaque location (Fuster, Badimon, Badimon, & Chesebro, 1992a,

1992b; Shah & Forrester, 1991). Such substances as serotonin, thromboxane A_2, adenosine diphosphate (ADP), adenosine triphosphate (ATP), plateletactivating factor (PAF), and platelet-activated growth factor contribute to acute myocardial infarction.

Atherosclerotic complicated lesions may be either fibromuscular or fibrolipid. Fibromuscular lesions have more smooth muscle and less lipid incorporated into their cores and are less likely to rupture than fibrolipid lesions. Although fibrolipid lesions tend to be smaller, they are more often associated with acute myocardial infarction, sudden death, and unstable angina because of the rapid development of occluding thrombus after rupture of the lesion (Fuster et al., 1992a, 1992b).

Pathophysiology

Cellular injury. Cardiac cells can withstand ischemic conditions for about 20 minutes before cellular death takes place. After only 30 to 60 seconds of hypoxia, electrocardiographic changes are visible. Yet even if cells are metabolically altered and nonfunctional, they can remain viable if blood flow returns within 20 minutes (Braunwald & Sobel, 1992).

After 8 to 10 seconds of decreased blood flow, the affected myocardium becomes cyanotic and cooler. Myocardial oxygen reserves are used very quickly (within about 8 seconds) after complete cessation of cor-

FIG. 27-13 Recent infarct of myocardium of left ventricle. (From Kissane, 1990.)

onary flow. Glycogen stores decrease as anaerobic metabolism begins. Unfortunately, glycolysis can supply only 65% to 70% of the total myocardial energy requirement and produces much less ATP than aerobic processes. Hydrogen ions and lactic acid accumulate. Because myocardial tissues have poor buffering capabilities and myocardial cells are very sensitive to low cellular pH, accumulation of these products further compromises the myocardium. Acidosis may make the myocardium more vulnerable to the damaging effects of lysosomal enzymes, and may suppress impulse conduction and contractile function, thereby leading to heart failure.

Oxygen deprivation also is accompanied by electrolyte disturbances, specifically, loss of potassium, calcium, and magnesium from cells. Myocardial cells deprived of necessary oxygen and nutrients lose contractility, thereby diminishing the pumping ability of the heart. Normally, the myocardium takes up varying quantities of catecholamines (epinephrine and norepinephrine). Significant arterial occlusion causes the myocardial cells to release catecholamines, predisposing the individual to serious imbalances of sympathetic and parasympathetic function, irregular heartbeats (dys-

rhythmia), and heart failure. Catecholamines mediate the release of glycogen, glucose, and stored fat from body cells. Therefore, plasma concentrations of free fatty acids and glycerol rise within 1 hour after onset of acute myocardial infarction. Excessive levels of free fatty acids can have a harmful detergent effect on cell membranes. Norepinephrine elevates blood sugar levels through stimulation of liver and skeletal muscle cells. It also suppresses pancreatic β-cell activity, which reduces insulin secretion and elevates blood glucose further. Not surprisingly, hyperglycemia is noted approximately 72 hours after an acute myocardial infarction.

Cellular death. After about 20 minutes of myocardial ischemia, irreversible hypoxic injury causes cellular death and tissue necrosis. (Types of necrosis are described in Chapter 2.) Necrosis of myocardial tissue results in the release of certain intracellular enzymes through the damaged cell membranes into the interstitial spaces. The lymphatics pick up the enzymes and transport them into the bloodstream, where they can be detected by serologic tests.

Structural and functional changes. Myocardial infarction results in both structural and functional changes of cardiac tissues. Table 27-7 outlines the tissue changes

TABLE 27-7

Tissue Changes After Myocardial Infarction

Time after myocardial infarction	Tissue changes	Stage of healing process
6-12 hours	No gross changes; subcellular cyanosis with decreased temperature	Not begun
18-24 hours	Pale to gray-brown; slight pallor	Inflammatory response; intercellular enzyme release
2-4 days	Visible necrosis: yellow-brown in center and hyperemic around edges	Proteolytic enzymes remove debris; catecholamines, lipolysis, and glycogenolysis elevate plasma glucose and increase free fatty acids to assist depleted myocardium recovery from anaerobic state
4-10 days	Area soft, with fatty changes in center, regions of hemorrhage in infarcted area	Debris cleared; collagen matrix laid down
10-14 days	Weak, fibrotic scar tissue with beginning revascularization	Healing continues, but area very mushy, vulnerable to stress
6 weeks	Scarring usually complete	Tough inelastic scar replaces necrotic myocardium

NOTE: Processes of tissue healing are described and illustrated in Chapter 7.

that may follow myocardial infarction. Gross tissue changes may not become apparent for several hours, despite almost immediate onset (within 30 to 60 seconds) of electrocardiographic (ECG) changes. Ischemic tissues around the area of necrosis may not be irreversibly damaged at the onset of myocardial infarction. Researchers are seeking ways to salvage these tissues and reduce the size of the infarction.

The severity of functional impairment depends on the size of the lesion and the site of infarction. Functional changes can include (1) decreased cardiac contractility with abnormal wall motion, (2) altered left ventricular compliance, (3) decreased stroke volume, (4) decreased ejection fraction, (5) increased left ventricular end-diastolic pressure, and (6) sinoatrial node malfunction. Life-threatening dysrhythmias and heart failure often follow myocardial infarction.

Repair. Myocardial infarction causes a severe inflammatory response that ends with wound repair (see Chapter 7). Repair consists of degradation of damaged cells, proliferation of fibroblasts, and synthesis of scar tissue. Many cell types, hormones, and nutrient substrates must be available for optimal healing to proceed. Within 24 hours, leukocytes infiltrate the necrotic area, and proteolytic enzymes from scavenger neutrophils degrade necrotic tissue. A pseudodiabetic state often develops as catecholamines released from damaged cells stimulate release of glucose and free fatty acids. By the

second week, insulin secretion increases to mobilize glucose from the repair processes. The collagen matrix that is deposited is initially weak, mushy, and vulnerable to reinjury. Unfortunately it is at this time in the recovery period (10 to 14 days after infarction) that individuals feel more like increasing activities and may stress the newly formed scar tissue. After 6 weeks, the necrotic area is completely replaced by scar tissue, which is strong but is unable to contract and relax like healthy myocardial tissue.

Clinical Manifestations

The first symptom of acute myocardial infarction is usually sudden, severe chest pain. The pain is similar to angina pectoris but is more severe and persistent and is not relieved by nitrates. It may be described as heavy and crushing, such as a "truck sitting on my chest." Radiation to the neck, jaw, back, shoulder, or left arm is common. Some individuals, especially those who are elderly or diabetic, experience no pain, thereby having a "silent" infarction. Infarction often stimulates a sensation of unrelenting indigestion. Nausea and vomiting may occur because of reflex stimulation of vomiting centers by pain fibers. Vasovagal reflexes from the area of the infarcted myocardium may also affect the gastrointestinal tract. Catecholamine release results in sympathetic stimulation, producing diaphoresis and peripheral vasoconstriction that cause the skin to become cool and clammy. Fever may develop in the first 24 hours and persist for a week because of inflammatory activity within the myocardium.

A variety of cardiovascular changes may be found on physical examination. With an acute myocardial infarction, blood pressure may initially decrease. The drop in blood pressure reflexively activates the sympathetic nervous system to compensate and then causes a temporary increase in heart rate and blood pressure. Abnormal extra heart sounds (S_3, S_4) reflect left ventricular dysfunction. Inflammation can cause pericardial friction rub, along with a variety of cardiac murmurs.

Laboratory data reveal leukocytosis and elevated sedimentation rate, both of which indicate inflammation. The individual's blood sugar is usually elevated, and the glucose tolerance level may remain abnormal for several weeks.

A transient rise in plasma enzyme levels can confirm the occurrence of myocardial infarction and indicate its severity. The enzymes released by myocardial cells include creatine kinase (CK), lactic dehydrogenase (LDH), and, to a lesser extent, serum glutamic oxaloacetic transaminase (SGOT; also known as aspartate aminotransferase, or AST). These enzymes exist in several different active molecular forms called isoenzymes, which are present in different amounts within particular tissues. If serologic tests show abnormally high levels of isoenzymes associated with cardiac tissue (CK-MB, LDH-1), acute myocardial infarction has probably oc-

curred. Of the three isoenzymes, CK-MB is most specific for myocardial infarction, although its level may also increase in individuals with certain other conditions (such as muscular dystrophy, hypothermia, chronic obstructive pulmonary disease associated with left heart failure and pulmonary embolism, extensive third-degree burns, or small bowel infarction). A new assay based on monoclonal antibodies against troponin I may be a more specific marker for myocardial injury than CK-MB (Adams et al., 1993). Elevation of CK-MB, LDH-1, and SGOT will be noted at characteristic times. The amount of CK elevation may be correlated with severity of infarction. The higher the serum concentration of CK-MB, the more extensive the tissue damage that has occurred. Blood is drawn for enzyme determinations as soon as possible after the onset of symptoms, and serial enzyme levels are assessed for several days. Three consecutive days of negative enzyme elevations rule out myocardial infarction.

Myocardial infarction can occur in various regions of the heart wall and may be described as anterior, inferior, posterior, lateral, subendocardial, endocardial, subepicardial, epicardial, intramural, or transmural, depending on the anatomic location and extent of tissue damage from infarction. (For descriptions of these locations see Chapter 26.) Twelve-lead ECGs help to localize the affected area through identification of Q waves and changes in ST segments and T waves (Fig. 27-14). The infarcted myocardium is surrounded by a

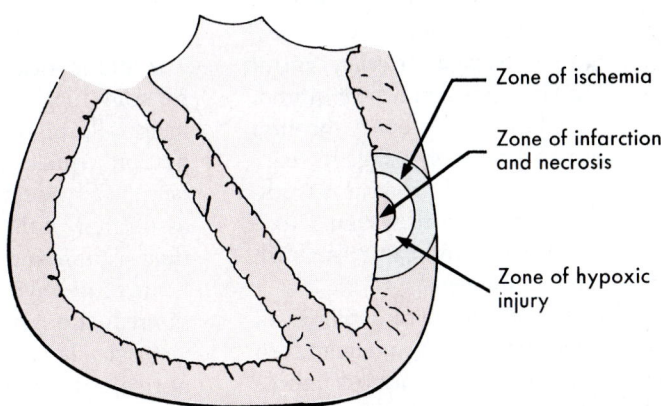

FIG. 27-14 Electrocardiographic alterations associated with the three zones of myocardial infarction.

zone of hypoxic injury, which may progress to necrosis or return to normal. Infarcted tissue is electrically silent and does not contribute to the ECG. Transmural infarcts are large enough to create inscription of a Q wave on the ECG (Q wave infarction). Small infarcts are usually subendocardial and do not create a Q wave (non–Q wave infarction). Adjacent to the zone of hypoxic injury is a zone of reversible ischemia. Ischemic and injured myocardial tissue causes ST and T wave changes. As the myocardium heals, the ST segment and T waves gradually return to normal, but abnormal Q waves generally persist.

Radionucleotide imaging with thallium-201 can provide a diagnostic picture in individuals with acute or healed myocardial infarction. Technetium-99m pyrophosphate is also taken up by areas of myocardial infarction, which appear as "hot spots." Unfortunately, the area of infarction must be large enough to visualize the hot spot, and the scan may remain positive for many months after infarction.

Evaluation and Treatment

The diagnosis of acute myocardial infarction is made on the basis of ECG, serial enzyme alterations, radionucleotide imaging, and physical examination (see Clinical Manifestations). Acute myocardial infarction requires immediate admission to a hospital with a coronary care unit, if possible. Continuous close monitoring of cardiac rhythms and enzymatic changes is especially important. The first 24 hours after onset of symptoms is the time of highest risk for sudden death. In complicated cases, invasive monitoring techniques (such as arterial, central venous pressure, and Swan-Ganz lines) may be required. Myocardial infarction caused by intracoronary thrombi can be relieved by infusion of thrombolytic agents (e.g., streptokinase) that dissolve clots and promote vasodilation. The treatment must be performed within 3 to 4 hours after the onset of infarction, and can reestablish blood flow in approximately 3 minutes.

Bed rest, followed by gradual return to activities of daily living, reduces the myocardial oxygen demands of the compromised heart. Pain relief is of utmost importance. If sublingual nitroglycerin is ineffective, small, carefully titrated doses of morphine sulfate (4 to 6 mg) may be given for sedation and vasodilation. Supplemental oxygen (2 to 4 L/min) is administered to increase arterial oxygen content and deliver more oxygen to the ischemic myocardium. Dietary measures are aimed at preventing nausea and vomiting, and consumption of sodium, saturated fats, sugar, and caffeine is limited.

Besides pain relief, pharmacologic intervention is used to limit infarction size, reduce vasoconstriction, prevent thrombus formation, and augment repair. Emergent utilization of PTCA, thrombolytic therapy (streptokinase, urokinase, tissue plasminogen activators), and judicious

use of β blockers are among the techniques showing promise in reducing infarction size and salvaging ischemic tissues (Tiefenbrunn, 1992; Woo, 1992). Stool softeners are given to eliminate the need for straining, which can precipitate bradycardia and can be followed by increased venous return to the heart, causing possible cardiac overload.

Complications

The number and severity of postinfarction complications depend on the location and extent of necrosis, the individual's physiologic condition before the infarction, and the availability of swift therapeutic intervention (Khan, 1992).

Dysrhythmias (arrhythmias), which are disturbances of cardiac rhythm, are the most common complication of acute myocardial infarction, affecting more than 90% of individuals. Dysrhythmias can be caused by (1) ischemia, (2) hypoxia, (3) autonomic nervous system imbalances, (4) lactic acidosis, (5) electrolyte abnormalities, (6) alterations of impulse conduction pathways or conduction defects, (7) drug toxicity, or (8) hemodynamic abnormalities. Dysrhythmias may originate from the atria, ventricles, nodal regions, or conduction tissues. The seriousness of dysrhythmias depends on the hemodynamic consequences. There is no ventricular contraction in ventricular fibrillation; consequently there is no cardiac output. Atrial fibrillation, however, does not affect ventricular contraction and thus can be tolerated by most individuals. (Dysrhythmias are described on p. 1048.)

Acute myocardial infarction is usually accompanied by some degree of left ventricular failure (congestive heart failure), which is characterized by pulmonary congestion, reduced myocardial contractility, and abnormal heart wall motion (see p. 1056). Anterior infarction is associated with more severe congestive heart failure than is inferior infarction (Cheng, 1990). Mortality from acute myocardial infarction is directly related to the reduction in stroke volume caused by the infarcted ventricle. If cardiac output is insufficient to maintain normal arterial pressure and to perfuse the kidneys and other organs adequately, cardiogenic shock develops. Cardiogenic shock characteristically develops if 40% or more of the left ventricular myocardium is infarcted. (Cardiogenic shock is discussed on p. 1063.)

Inflammation of the pericardium (pericarditis) is a frequent complication of acute myocardial infarction. Pericardial friction rubs are often noted 2 to 3 days later, associated with anterior chest pain that worsens with respiratory effort. Specific treatment is not required, but corticosteroids dramatically relieve symptoms.

Dressler's postinfarction syndrome, which is essentially a delayed form of acute pericarditis, can occur from 1 week to several months after acute myocardial infarction. Although poorly understood, the syndrome is thought to be an immunologic (antigen-antibody) response to the necrotic myocardium. Pain, fever, friction rub, pleural effusion, and arthralgias may accompany this syndrome. Steroids may alleviate symptoms.

Organic brain syndrome may occur in acute or chronic form if blood flow to the brain is impaired secondary to myocardial infarction. Transient ischemic attacks or an outright cerebrovascular accident may result from thromboemboli that have broken loose from coronary arteries or cardiac valves.

Cardiac complications of myocardial infarction include rupture of heart structures. Necrosis of tissue in or around the papillary muscles can cause rupture of these muscles or of the chordae tendineae. Factors that lead to rupture of the free wall of the infarcted ventricle include thinning of the wall, poor collateral flow, shearing effect of muscular contraction against the stiffened necrotic area, marked necrosis at the terminal end of the blood supply, and aging of the myocardium with laceration of the myocardial microstructure (Pasternak, Braunwald, & Sobel, 1992).

Rupture of the wall of the infarcted ventricle may be a consequence of aneurysm formation (Fig. 27-15). According to the law of Laplace, with decreased muscle mass at the infarcted site, the wall is weakened and tension stretches the noncontracting infarcted heart muscle, thus producing infarct expansion or aneurysm formation (see aneurysm, p. 1011). Decreased muscle mass causes an increase in the radius of the ventricle and, because the radius is directly proportional to pressure and tension, both increase with time. The wall of the aneurysm becomes more fibrotic but continues to bulge with systole. The bulge results in impaired pump function. Although rare, rupture may occur when the tension becomes too great. Death in individuals with a left ventricular aneurysm is presumably related to ventricular tachyarrhythmias and not to ventricular rupture (Pasternak et al., 1992). Left ventricular aneurysm is a late complication of myocardial infarction, occurring months or years after the acute event.

Infarctions around septal structures that separate the heart chambers can lead to septal rupture. Ruptures are associated with audible, harsh cardiac murmurs, increased left ventricular end-diastolic pressure, and decreased systemic blood pressure.

Systemic thromboembolism is commonly found during postmortem examinations of individuals who have died of myocardial infarction. Thromboemboli may disseminate from debris and clots that collect inside dilated aneurysmal sacs, or from the infarcted endocardium. Pulmonary emboli are especially common, as are deep venous thrombi of the legs. Early mobilization and prophylactic anticoagulation therapy should reduce the incidence of this complication.

Sudden death resulting from cardiac arrest is often caused by dysrhythmias, particularly ventricular fibrillation. Other dysrhythmias may be equally lethal. Widespread knowledge of cardiopulmonary resuscitation has increased the probability of survival during the first few hours after cardiac insult. Immediate intervention and careful monitoring have also reduced mortality and have improved chances for long-term survival. Several factors, however, contribute to the risk of death during acute infarction or reduce the chances of long-term survival, despite the best possible treatment. They are (1) age greater than 65 years, (2) previous angina pectoris, (3) hypotension or cardiogenic shock, (4) acute systolic hypertension at the time of admission, (5) diabetes mellitus, (6) dysrhythmias or conduction defects, and (7) previous myocardial infarction (Pasternak et al., 1992).

FIG. 27-15 Aneurysm of left ventricle, a result of myocardial infarct. **A,** External view. **B,** Interior view. On right, between forceps, is thin fibrotic wall. On left, aneurysm sac is filled with thrombus. (From Kissane, J. M. [1985]. *Anderson's pathology,* ed. 8. St. Louis: Mosby–Year Book.)

DISORDERS OF THE HEART WALL

Disorders of the Pericardium

Pericardial disease is often a localized manifestation of another disorder, such as infection (bacterial, viral, fungal, rickettsial, or parasitic); trauma or surgery; neoplasm; or a metabolic, immunologic, or vascular disorder (uremia, rheumatoid arthritis, systemic lupus erythematosus, periarteritis nodosa). The pericardial response to injury from these diverse causes may consist of acute pericarditis, pericardial effusion, or constrictive pericarditis (Hancock, 1989).

Acute Pericarditis

Although frequently idiopathic, **acute pericarditis** (acute inflammation of the pericardium) is also commonly caused by infection, connective tissue disease, or radiation therapy (Fig. 27-16). The pericardial membranes become inflamed and roughened, and an exudate may develop.

Symptoms include sudden onset of severe chest pain that worsens with respiratory movements. Although the

pain may radiate to the back, it is generally felt in the anterior chest and may be confused initially with the pain of acute myocardial infarction. Individuals with acute pericarditis may also report dysphagia, restlessness, irritability, anxiety, weakness, and malaise.

Physical examination often discloses low-grade fever and sinus tachycardia. Friction rub, a short, scratchy, grating sensation similar to the sound of sandpaper, may be heard at the cardiac apex and left sternal border and is pathognomonic for pericarditis. The rub is caused by the roughened pericardial membranes rubbing against each other. Friction rubs are not always present, and may be intermittently heard and transient. Electrocardiographic changes may reflect inflammatory processes through diffuse ST segment elevation without Q waves.

Treatment for uncomplicated acute pericarditis consists of relieving symptoms. Analgesics are given to relieve pain, but doses are limited to avoid excessive respiratory depression in individuals who are already limiting respiratory effort because of pain. Salicylates and nonsteroidal antiinflammatory drugs reduce inflammation. Corticosteroids may diminish symptoms, but rebound pain may occur after the steroids are discontinued. Rest is helpful during episodes of acute pain. Exploration of the underlying cause is important. If pericardial effusion develops, aspiration of the excessive fluid may be necessary. Acute pericarditis is usually self-limiting but occasionally may progress to chronic constrictive pericarditis (Shabetai, 1990).

FIG. 27-16 **Acute pericarditis.** Notice shaggy coat of fibers covering surface of heart. (From Anderson & Scotti, 1980.)

FIG. 27-17 **Exudate of blood in the pericardial sac from rupture of aneurysm.** (From Anderson & Scotti, 1980.)

Pericardial Effusion

Pericardial effusion—the accumulation of fluid in the pericardial cavity—can occur in all forms of pericarditis. The fluid may be a transudate, such as the serous effusion that develops with congestive heart failure, overhydration, or hypoproteinemia. More often, however, the fluid is an exudate, which reflects pericardial injury and inflammation (Fig. 27-17). (Types of exudate are described in Chapter 7.) If the fluid is serosanguineous, the underlying cause is likely to be tuberculosis, neoplasm, uremia, or radiation. Idiopathic serosanguineous (cause unknown) effusion is possible, however. Effusions of frank blood are generally related to aneurysms, trauma, or coagulation defects. If chyle leaks from the thoracic duct, it may enter the pericardium and lead to cholesterol pericarditis.

Pericardial effusion, even in large amounts, is not necessarily clinically significant, except that it indicates an underlying disorder. The important consideration is whether the fluid creates sufficient pressure to cause cardiac compression, which is a serious condition known as **tamponade.** If an effusion develops gradually, the pericardium can stretch to accommodate large quantities of fluid without compressing the heart. If the fluid accumulates rapidly, however, even a small amount (50 to 100 ml) may cause serious tamponade. The danger is that pressure exerted by the pericardial fluid eventually will equal diastolic pressure within the heart chambers. The first structures to be affected by tamponade are the right atrium and ventricle, where diastolic pressures are normally lowest. Compression by pericardial fluid interferes with right atrial filling during diastole, resulting in increased venous pressure, systemic venous congestion, and signs and symptoms of right heart failure (distention of the jugular veins, edema, and hepatomegaly). Decreased atrial filling leads to decreased ventricular filling, decreased stroke volume, and reduced cardiac output. Life-threatening circulatory collapse may occur.

The most significant clinical finding is pulsus paradoxus, in which arterial blood pressure during expiration exceeds arterial pressure during inspiration by more than 10 mm Hg. Pulsus paradoxus indicates tamponade. This clinical finding reflects impairment of diastolic filling of the left ventricle plus reduction of blood volume within all four cardiac chambers. Presence of a large pericardial effusion or tamponade magnifies the normally insignificant effect of inspiration on intracardiac flow and volume.

Other clinical manifestations of pericardial effusion are distant or muffled heart sounds, poorly palpable apical pulse, dyspnea on exertion, and dull chest pain. A chest x-ray film may disclose a "water-bottle" configuration of the cardiac silhouette. An echocardiogram can detect an effusion as small as 20 ml.

Treatment of pericardial effusion or tamponade generally consists of pericardiocentesis (aspiration of excessive pericardial fluid). Pericardiocentesis is both diagnostic and therapeutic: the fluid is analyzed to identify the cause of the effusion, and its removal alone may bring dramatic relief from symptoms. Persistent pain may be treated with analgesics, antiinflammatory medications, or steroids. Surgery may be required if the underlying cause of tamponade is trauma or aneurysm.

Individuals with acute pericarditis secondary to certain underlying conditions may have pericardial effusion. This manifestation is common in (1) individuals with uremia who are in need of dialysis and have fluid overload and left ventricular failure; (2) individuals who have lymphoma or breast cancer or who are receiving radiation therapy; (3) individuals who are taking such drugs as procainamide and minoxidil; and (4) individuals who have undergone surgery that involved an incision of the heart wall. If an effusion is neoplasm induced, chemotherapeutic agents may be injected into the pericardial space. Tetracycline also may be injected into the pericardium to induce pericardial sclerosis and prevent further fluid accumulation (Hancock, 1989).

Constrictive Pericarditis

Constrictive pericarditis (chronic pericarditis) was synonymous with tuberculosis years ago (Fig. 27-18). Currently in the United States, this form of pericardial disease is either idiopathic or associated with radiation exposure, rheumatoid arthritis, uremia, or coronary artery bypass graft. In constrictive pericarditis, fibrous scarring with occasional calcification of the pericardium causes the visceral and parietal pericardial layers to adhere, obliterating the pericardial cavity. The fibrotic lesions encase the heart in a rigid shell. Like tamponade, constrictive pericarditis compresses the heart and eventually reduces cardiac output. Unlike tamponade, however, constrictive pericarditis always develops gradually.

Because the onset of constrictive pericarditis is gradual, clinical manifestations seldom include pulsus paradoxus. Symptoms tend to be exercise intolerance, dyspnea on exertion, fatigue, and anorexia. Clinical assessment shows weight loss, edema, distention of the jugular vein, and hepatic congestion. Restricted ventricular filling may cause a pericardial knock (early diastolic sound).

Electrocardiographic findings include T wave inversions and atrial fibrillation. An echocardiogram may suggest evidence of nonspecific pericardial thickening. Computed tomography is best able to detect constrictive processes (Hancock, 1989). Chest x-ray films frequently disclose prominent pulmonary vessels and calcification of the pericardium.

Initial treatment for constrictive pericarditis is pharmacologic and dietary. Digitalis glycosides, diuretics,

FIG. 27-18 **Constrictive pericarditis.** Notice band of calcified tissue that constricts heart. (From Kissane, 1990.)

and sodium restriction are often prescribed. If these modalities are successful, surgical excision of the restrictive pericardium is indicated. Removal of the pericardium (pericardiectomy) results in no noticeable cardiac impairment. For individuals with severe restrictive disease, pericardiectomy may prevent untimely death from heart failure.

Disorders of the Myocardium: the Cardiomyopathies

The **cardiomyopathies** are a diverse group of diseases that primarily affect the myocardium itself and are not secondary to the usual cardiovascular disorders, such as coronary artery disease, hypertension, or valvular dysfunction. They may, however, be secondary to infectious disease, exposure to toxins, systemic connective tissue disease, infiltrative and proliferative disorders, or nutritional deficiencies. Despite this large number of possible causes, most cases of cardiomyopathy are idiopathic; that is, their cause is unknown. The cardiomyopathies are categorized as dilated (formerly, congestive), hypertrophic, or restrictive, depending on their physiologic effects on the heart (Fig. 27-19 and Table 27-8).

Dilated Cardiomyopathy

Dilated cardiomyopathy (congestive cardiomyopathy) is characterized by ventricular dilatation and grossly impaired systolic function, leading to dilated heart failure (Fig. 27-20). The basic problem is diminished myocardial contractility, which is reflected in diminished systolic performance of the heart. Dilated cardiomyopathy causes decreased ejection fractions, increased end-diastolic and residual volumes, decreased ventricular stroke volume, and biventricular failure.

About one half of the cases of dilated cardiomyopathy are idiopathic, and the remainder result from some known disease process. Serious myocardial damage can result from certain drugs used in cancer chemotherapy, especially doxorubicin and daunorubicin. Cardiotoxicity increases with dosage, and the severity of the toxic reaction is directly related to the cumulative dose. It is not known whether ischemia related to coronary artery disease can cause dilated cardiomyopathy. Recurrent and extensive myocardial infarction can, however, cause the same outcome as dilated cardiomyopathy; that is, left heart failure. Dilated cardiomyopathies occur most often in black men between 40 and 60 years of age.

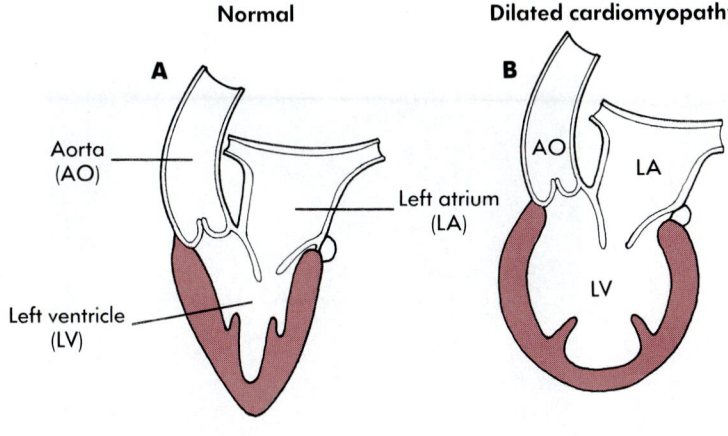

Normal

Dilated cardiomyopathy

Aorta (AO)

Left atrium (LA)

Left ventricle (LV)

Hypertrophic cardiomyopathy

Constrictive cardiomyopathy (amyloid)

FIG. 27-19 Diagram showing major distinguishing pathophysiologic features of the three types of cardiomyopathy. **A,** The normal heart. **B,** In the dilated type of cardiomyopathy, the heart has a globular shape and the largest circumference of the left ventricle is not at its base but midway between apex and base. **C,** In the hypertrophic type, the wall of the left ventricle is greatly thickened; the left ventricular cavity is small but the left atrium may be dilated because of poor diastolic relaxation of the ventricle. **D,** In the restrictive (constrictive) type, the left ventricular cavity is of normal size but, again, the left atrium is dilated because of the reduced diastolic compliance of the ventricle. (From Kissane, 1990.)

TABLE 27-8

Effects of Cardiomyopathies on Circulation Through the Heart

Effect	Type of cardiomyopathy		
	Dilated	Hypertrophic	Restrictive
Hemodynamic			
Cardiac output	Decreased	Normal	Normal or decreased
Stroke volume	Decreased	Normal or increased	Decreased
Ventricular filling pressure	Increased	Normal or increased	Increased
Ejection fraction	Decreased	Increased	Normal or decreased
Inflow resistance	Normal	Increased	Increased
Outflow tract obstruction	None	Increased	None
Formation of intracardiac thrombi	Increased	None	Increased
Structural or functional			
Chamber size	Increased	Normal or decreased	Decreased or normal
Myocardial mass	Increased	Increased	Normal or increased
Endocardial thickness	Normal or increased	Increased	Increased
Contractility	Decreased	Increased or decreased	Normal or decreased
Mitral valve competence	Decreased	Decreased	Decreased

Data from DeSanctis, 1990; Wenger, Abelmann, & Roberts, 1990.

FIG. 27-20 Cross-sectional view of dilated cardiomyopathy. (From Kinney, 1991.)

FIG. 27-21 **Hypertrophied heart.** (From Kinney, 1991.)

A disproportionate number of individuals with idiopathic dilated cardiomyopathy are alcoholics. Heavy consumption of alcohol is thought to cause cardiomyopathy through three mechanisms: (1) a direct toxic effect of alcohol or of its metabolites; (2) effects of nutritional deficits, especially thiamine deficiency; and (3) toxic effects of beverage additives such as cobalt. In contrast to other forms of cardiomyopathy, the progression of myocardial dysfunction may be stopped or reversed if alcohol consumption is reduced or stopped early in the course of the disease (Wynne & Braunwald, 1992).

Peripartum cardiomyopathy is another idiopathic form of dilated cardiomyopathy. The cardiomyopathy usually develops in the first 3 to 4 months after completion of a pregnancy, after the period of maximum physiologic stress is thought to have ended. A few cases have resulted from acute myocardial inflammation (myocarditis).

A third group of dilated cardiomyopathies may be the late consequences of previous viral, bacterial, or parasitic infections or an autoimmune process. Endocardial biopsies have shown that a significant number of these cases also involve active myocarditis. The implications of these findings remain unclear. (Pathophysiologic effects of the cardiomyopathies are summarized in Table 27-9.)

The most common symptoms of dilated cardiomyopathy are dyspnea and fatigue. Pulmonary congestion is expected, but acute pulmonary edema is not. Palpitations are common, and associated dysrhythmias may cause dizziness (syncope). Systemic and pulmonary emboli are common complications. Chest pain may be present, but it is unlike anginal pain.

In the presence of dilated heart failure, blood pressure is often elevated. Extra heart sounds and cardiac murmurs may be present as well. Dilated cardiomyopathy may be difficult to distinguish from acute myocarditis, valvular heart disease, coronary artery disease, and hypertensive heart disease.

Treatment for dilated cardiomyopathy consists of salt restriction and the prescription of digitalis glycosides and diuretics. Anticoagulants are given to prevent pulmonary and systemic embolism. Bed rest for extended periods can be used to reduce the workload of the weakened heart. Corticosteroids and immunosuppressants

TABLE 27-9

Pathophysiologic Effects of the Cardiomyopathies

Pathophysiology	Type of cardiomyopathy		
	Dilated	Hypertrophic	Restrictive
Major symptoms	Fatigue, weakness, palpitations	Dyspnea, angina pectoris, fatigue, dizziness (syncope), palpitations	Dyspnea, fatigue
Cardiomegaly	Moderate to marked	Mild to moderate	Mild
Hypertrophy	Left ventricular myocardium	Left ventricular myocardium and interventricular septum	Left ventricular myocardium
Alterations of chamber volume	Volume increased	Volume decreased, particularly in left ventricle	Volume normal to decreased
Alterations of chamber compliance	Compliance increased	Compliance decreased, particularly in left ventricle	Compliance decreased, particularly in left ventricle
Alterations of systolic function (myocardial contractility)	Contractility decreased in left ventricle	Contractility increased or vigorous	None
Valvular incompetence	Atrioventricular valves, particularly mitral	Mitral valve	Atrioventricular valve
Conduction defects	Intraventricular	Nonspecific	Atrioventricular
Dysrhythmias	Sinoatrial tachycardia; atrial and ventricular dysrhythmias	Atrial and ventricular dysrhythmias	Tachyarrhythmias
Thromboembolism	Systemic or pulmonary	Systemic or pulmonary	Systemic or pulmonary
Associated conditions	Alcoholism, pregnancy, infection, nutritional deficiency, exposed to toxins	Possible inherited defect of muscle growth and development	Infiltrative disease
Eventual cardiovascular event	Left heart failure	Left heart failure	Right heart failure

can benefit individuals with documented inflammatory disease, and vasodilators are administered to combat congestion. Venous dilation reduces preload by promoting peripheral venous pooling, thereby decreasing central blood volume and alleviating pulmonary congestion. Arterial dilation reduces afterload and aortic impedance, making it easier for the failing left ventricle to eject blood. Combinations of these drugs have been effective in improving symptoms, although there is no indication that they prolong life.

The prognosis is poor. About 50% of individuals with dilated cardiomyopathy die within 2 years of the onset of symptoms (Ahumada, 1987). Sudden death from congestive failure or dysrhythmias is most common.

Hypertrophic Cardiomyopathy

This form of cardiomyopathy is also known as asymmetric septal hypertrophy, muscular subaortic stenosis, and idiopathic hypertrophic subaortic stenosis. The name *hypertrophic* is preferable, however, because the cardiac changes are not always obstructive and the hypertrophy is not always subaortic or asymmetric (Cotran, Kumar, & Robbins, 1989). An autosomal dominant inheritance has been linked to this disorder (DeSanctis, 1990). Although its origin is unknown, the basic abnormality appears to reside in the contractile elements of the heart muscle. The hallmark of **hypertrophic cardiomyopathy** is disproportionate thickening of the interventricular septum (Fig. 27-21). There is disorganization of the septal muscle cells and greater hypertrophy of the ventricular septum than of the ventricular chambers. Thus the heart may actually appear to be of normal size. Thickening of the septum results in a hyperdynamic state, with subsequent increased myocardial contractility and ejection fraction. Diastolic relaxation is impaired, however, and ventricular compliance is decreased (increased stiffness). If the septum is asymmetrically enlarged, it actually may obstruct left ventricular outflow and result in decreased cardiac output. Under these circumstances, any condition or medication that increases contractility also increases the degree of obstruction. For example, nitroglycerin aggravates obstruction by increasing the heart rate, decreasing chamber size, and decreasing blood pressure (afterload) (DeSanctis, 1990).

Major clinical manifestations of hypertrophic cardiomyopathy are angina, syncope, palpitations, and congestive heart failure. Myocardial infarction can occur if the hypertrophied myocardium outgrows its blood supply. Dysrhythmias are common, and extra heart sounds and murmurs are not unusual. Electrocardiography discloses left ventricular hypertrophy and dysrhythmias, if any are present. Echocardiograms may prove helpful in recognizing and assessing the severity of this disorder.

Beta-blockers, such as propranolol, are favored for initial therapy because they may decrease left ventricular stiffness and reduce the heart rate enough to permit a longer time for ventricular filling. Calcium antagonists may or may not be beneficial. Surgical resection of the hypertrophic tissue may be done to relieve symptoms in individuals who do not respond to pharmacologic therapy. Although the course and prognosis of hypertrophic cardiomyopathy vary, long-term survival is expected.

Restrictive Cardiomyopathies

Restrictive cardiomyopathy is usually caused by an infiltrative disease of the myocardium, such as amyloidosis, hemochromatosis, or glycogen storage disease. The myocardium becomes rigid and noncompliant, impeding ventricular filling and raising filling pressures during diastole. The overall clinical and hemodynamic picture mimics that of constrictive pericarditis.

The most common clinical manifestation of restrictive cardiomyopathy is congestive heart failure, particularly right heart failure. Cardiomegaly and dysrhythmias are common. In most cases, there is no therapy for restrictive cardiomyopathy other than treating the underlying disease process. Death occurs as a result of congestive failure or dysrhythmias.

Disorders of the Endocardium
Valvular Dysfunction

Disorders of the endocardium, the innermost lining of the heart wall, all damage the heart valves, which are made up of endocardial tissue. Endocardial damage can be either congenital or acquired. The acquired forms cause inflammatory, ischemic, traumatic, degenerative, or infectious alterations of valvular structure and function (Braunwald, 1992).

The usual cause of acquired valvular dysfunction is inflammation of the endocardium secondary to acute rheumatic fever or infectious endocarditis (see pp. 1043-1045). Structural alterations of the heart valves lead to stenosis, incompetence, or both.

In **valvular stenosis,** the valve orifice is constricted and narrowed, impeding the forward flow of blood and increasing the workload of the cardiac chamber "in front" of the diseased valve (Fig. 27-22). Pressure (intraventricular or atrial) increases in the chamber to overcome resistance to flow through the valve. Increased pressure causes the myocardium to work harder, causing myocardial hypertrophy. In **valvular regurgitation** (also called insufficiency or incompetence), the valve leaflets, or cusps, fail to shut completely, permitting blood flow to continue even when the valve is supposed to be closed (Fig. 27-22). During systole, some blood leaks back into the atrial chamber "upstream." Valvular regurgitation increases the volume of blood the heart must pump and increases the workload of both atrium and ventricle. Valvular incompetence causes cardiomegaly. Increased volume leads to chamber dilatation, and increased workload leads to hypertrophy. Although all four heart valves may be affected, those of the left heart (mitral and aortic semilunar valves) are far more commonly affected than those of the right heart (tricuspid and pulmonic semilunar valves).

Valvular dysfunction stimulates chamber dilatation and myocardial hypertrophy, both of which are compensatory mechanisms intended to increase the pumping capability of the heart. Eventually, myocardial contractility is diminished, the ejection fraction is reduced, diastolic pressure increases, and the ventricles fail from overwork. Depending on the severity of the valvular dysfunction and the capacity of the heart to compensate, valvular alterations cause a range of symptoms and some degree of incapacitation (Table 27-10). Valvular dysfunction is treated with cardiac glycosides, diuretics, dietary salt restriction, and antibiotics until prosthetic valve replacement becomes necessary.

Stenosis

Aortic stenosis. Aortic stenosis has three common causes: (1) inflammatory damage caused by rheumatic heart disease, (2) congenital malformation (see Chapter 3), and (3) degeneration resulting from calcification (see Chapter 2). The orifice of the aortic semilunar valve narrows, causing diminished blood flow from the left ventricle into the aorta (see Fig. 27-22). Outflow obstruction increases pressure within the left ventricle as it tries to eject blood through the narrowed opening.

Aortic stenosis tends to develop gradually. Clinical

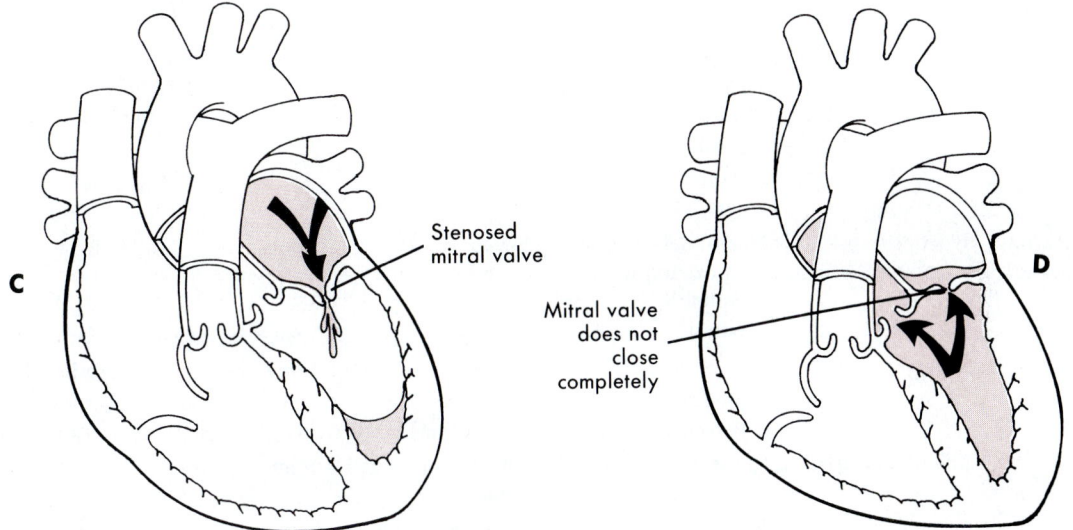

FIG. 27-22 **Valvular stenosis and regurgitation. A,** Normal position of the valve leaflets, or cusps, when the valve is open and closed. **B,** Open position of a stenosed valve *(left)* and open position of a closed regurgitant valve *(right).* **C,** Hemodynamic effect of mitral stenosis. The stenosed valve is unable to open sufficiently during left atrial systole, inhibiting left ventricular filling. **D,** Hemodynamic effect of mitral regurgitation. The mitral valve does not close completely during left ventricular systole, permitting blood to reenter the left atrium.

manifestations include decreased stroke volume, reduced systolic blood pressure, and narrowed pulse pressure (difference between systolic and diastolic pressure). Heart rate is often slow, and pulses are faint. Resistance to flow gives rise to a crescendo-decrescendo systolic heart murmur. Left ventricular hypertrophy develops to compensate for the increased workload. Eventually, hypertrophy increases myocardial oxygen demand, which the coronary arteries may not be able to supply. If this occurs, ischemia may cause attacks of angina. Untreated aortic stenosis can lead to dysrhythmias, myocardial infarction, and heart failure. Most symptoms of aortic stenosis are attributable to diminished stroke volume, which results in diminished tissue perfusion.

Mitral stenosis. **Mitral stenosis** impairs the flow of blood from the left atrium to the left ventricle. Mitral stenosis is most commonly caused by acute rheumatic

fever or bacterial endocarditis, although uncommonly it can be congenital. Narrowing of the orifice occurs as inflammatory lesions in the valvular leaflets heal (Fig. 27-23). Scarring causes the leaflets to become fibrous and fused, and the chordae tendineae to become shortened.

Clinical manifestations depend on the size of the valvular orifice. As in aortic stenosis, impedance to blood flow results in incomplete emptying of the left atrium and elevated atrial pressure, as the chamber tries to force blood through the stenotic valve. Continued increases in left atrial volume and pressure cause chamber dilatation and hypertrophy. The risk of developing atrial dysrhythmias (especially fibrillation) and dysrhythmia-induced thrombi is high. As mitral stenosis progresses, symptoms of decreased cardiac output occur, especially during exertion. Continued elevation

TABLE 27-10

Clinical Manifestations of Valvular Stenosis and Regurgitation

Manifestation	Aortic stenosis	Mitral stenosis	Aortic regurgitation	Mitral regurgitation	Tricuspid regurgitation
Cardiovascular outcome*	Left ventricular failure	Right ventricular failure	Left heart failure	Left heart failure	Right heart failure
General symptoms	Fatigue	Fatigue, weakness		Fatigue, weakness	Peripheral edema (with heart failure)
Respiratory effects	Dyspnea on exertion	Dyspnea on exertion, orthopnea, paroxysmal nocturnal dyspnea, predisposition to respiratory infections, hemoptysis, pulmonary hypertension, and edema	Dyspnea with effort	Dyspnea; occasional hemoptysis	Dyspnea
Central nervous system effects	Syncope, especially on exertion	Neural deficits only associated with emboli (e.g., hemiparesis)	Syncope	None	None
Gastrointestinal effects	None	Ascites; hepatic angina with hepatomegaly	None	None	Ascites, hepatomegaly (with heart failure)
Pain	Angina pectoris	Chest pain	Chest pain (anginal)	None	Palpitations
Heart rate, rhythm	Bradycardia, dysrhythmias (with heart failure)	Palpitations (atrial fibrillation)	Palpitations, water-hammer pulse	Palpitations	Atrial fibrillations
Heart sounds	Systolic murmur	Diastolic murmur, accentuated first heart sound, opening snap	Diastolic and systolic murmurs	Murmur throughout systole	Murmur throughout systole
Most common cause	Congenital, rheumatic fever	Rheumatic fever	Bacterial endocarditis; aortic root disease	Floppy valve; coronary artery disease	Congenital

Data from Braunwald, 1992; Hancock, 1992.
*Untreated disease.

of left atrial pressure and volume causes pressure to rise in the pulmonary circulation. The outcome of untreated chronic mitral stenosis is pulmonary hypertension, edema, and right ventricular failure.

Atrial enlargement is demonstrated by chest x-ray films and electrocardiography. Blood flow through the stenotic valve gives rise to a rumbling decrescendo diastolic murmur. The first heart sound (S_1) is often accentuated and somewhat delayed because of increased left atrial pressure. Other signs and symptoms are generally those of pulmonary congestion and right heart failure.

Regurgitation

Aortic regurgitation. **Aortic regurgitation** is caused by an acute or chronic lesion of rheumatic fever, bacterial endocarditis, syphilis, hypertension, connective tissue disorders (e.g., Marfan syndrome), or atherosclerosis. The hemodynamic repercussions depend on the size of the "leak." During systole, blood is ejected from the left ventricle into the aorta. If the aortic semilunar valve is affected, some of the ejected blood flows back into the left ventricle. Volume overload occurs in the ventricle because it receives blood from the left atrium during di-

FIG. 27-23 Mitral stenosis with classic "fishmouth" orifice. (From Kissane, 1990.)

astole and blood from the aorta during systole. Over time, the end-diastolic volume of the left ventricle increases, and myocardial fibers stretch to accommodate the extra fluid. Compensatory dilatation permits the left ventricle to increase its stroke volume and maintain cardiac output. Ventricular dilation and hypertrophy eventually cease to compensate for aortic incompetence, and heart failure develops.

Clinical manifestations include widened pulse pressure resulting from increased stroke volume and backflow. Turbulence across the aortic valve during diastole produces a characteristic murmur. Large stroke volume and rapid runoff of blood from the aorta result in prominent carotid pulsations and throbbing peripheral pulses (water-hammer pulse). Other symptoms are usually associated with heart failure that occurs when the ventricle can no longer enlarge. Dysrhythmias and endocarditis are common complications of aortic regurgitation.

Mitral regurgitation. **Mitral regurgitation,** unlike mitral stenosis, has a variety of causes. The most common are mitral valve prolapse and rheumatic heart disease. Other causes include infective endocarditis, coronary artery disease, connective tissue diseases (Marfan syndrome), and congestive cardiomyopathy. Mitral regur-

gitation permits backflow of blood from the left ventricle into the left atrium during ventricular systole, giving rise to a loud pansystolic (throughout systole) murmur that radiates into the back and axilla. The left ventricle becomes dilated and hypertrophied to maintain adequate cardiac output, despite increased volume from the left atrium. The volume of backflow reentering the left atrium gradually increases, causing atrial dilatation. As the left atrium enlarges, the valve structures stretch and become deformed, leading to further backflow. As mitral valve regurgitation progresses, left ventricular function may become impaired to the point of failure. Eventually, increased atrial pressure also causes pulmonary hypertension and failure of the right ventricle. Mitral incompetence is usually well tolerated—often for years—until ventricular failure occurs. Most clinical manifestations are caused by heart failure.

Tricuspid regurgitation. **Tricuspid regurgitation** is more common than tricuspid stenosis and is usually associated with failure and dilatation of the right ventricle secondary to high blood pressure in the pulmonary circulation or right ventricle. Rheumatic heart disease and infective endocarditis are less common causes. Tricuspid valve incompetence leads to volume overload in the right ventricle, increased systemic venous blood pressure, and right heart failure. Pulmonic semilunar valve dysfunction can have the same consequences as tricuspid valve dysfunction.

Mitral valve prolapse syndrome (MVPS)

Mitral valve prolapse syndrome is a condition in which the anterior and posterior cusps of the mitral valve billow upward (prolapse) into the atrium during systole (Fig. 27-24). The cusps are enlarged, thickened, and scalloped, possibly secondary to collagenous abnormalities, and the chordae tendineae may be elongated, permitting the valve cusps to stretch upward. Mitral regurgitation occurs if the ballooning valve permits blood to leak into the atrium.

Mitral valve prolapse is the most common valve disorder in the United States (Cheng, 1989). It tends to be most prevalent in young women. Recent studies suggest an autosomal dominant inheritance pattern. Because mitral valve prolapse is often associated with other inherited connective tissue disorders (Marfan syndrome, Ehlers-Danlos syndrome, osteogenesis imperfecta), it may result from a genetic or environmental disruption of valvular development during the fifth or sixth week of gestation (Devereux, Kramer-Fox, & Kligfield, 1989). There also may be a relationship between symptomatic mitral valve prolapse and hyperthyroidism.

Many cases of mitral valve prolapse are completely asymptomatic. Cardiac auscultation on routine physical examination may disclose a regurgitant murmur or midsystolic click in an otherwise healthy individual, or echocardiography may demonstrate the condition in the absence of auscultatory findings. Symptomatic mitral valve prolapse can cause palpitations related to dysrhythmias, tachycardia, light-headedness, syncope, fatigue (especially in the morning), lethargy, weakness, dyspnea, chest tightness, hyperventilation, anxiety, depression, panic attacks, and atypical chest pain (Hancock, 1992). Many symptoms are vague and puzzling and are unrelated to the degree of prolapse. Mitral valve prolapse was once considered a psychiatric malady. Recent research has suggested that individuals with mitral valve prolapse have an autonomic dysfunction in which inordinate quantities of catecholamines are produced, with or without adrenergic stimulation (Boudoulas & Wooley, 1988). This finding could explain why mitral valve prolapse causes such a variety of subjective complaints.

Its high incidence rate suggests that mitral valve prolapse may be a normal variant rather than a pathologic entity. Although severe sequelae, such as chorda rupture, ventricular failure, systemic emboli, and sudden death, are possible, the disorder is actually associated with minimal mortality and morbidity. Most individuals experience no physical limitations. In fact, the psychological effects of chest pain and knowledge of the diagnosis may be more disabling than the disease itself.

Evaluation of mitral valve prolapse includes physical assessment and laboratory evaluation. Echocardiography is the procedure of choice for diagnosing the disor-

FIG. 27-24 **Mitral valve prolapse.** Normal mitral valve *(left)* and prolapsed mitral valve *(inset).* Prolapse permits the valve leaflets to billow back into the atrium during left ventricular systole. The billowing causes the leaflets to part slightly, permitting regurgitation into the atrium.

der (Hershman, Moskowitz, Marton, & Balady, 1989). Cardiac angiography is rarely necessary to confirm the diagnosis.

Management is matched to the degree of mitral regurgitation. If regurgitation is present, antibiotic prophylaxis for infective endocarditis is given before invasive procedures, but physical activities are not restricted. Occasionally beta blockers are needed to alleviate syncope, severe chest pain, or palpitations. Hypovolemia (resulting from diuretics or donating blood) is avoided because it can decrease ventricular volume, thereby increasing stress on the prolapsed mitral valve (Hunt, 1985). Surgical repair or valve replacement may be required.

Acute Rheumatic Fever and Rheumatic Heart Disease

Rheumatic fever is a diffuse, inflammatory disease caused by a delayed immune response to infection by the group A β-hemolytic streptococcus. In its acute form, rheumatic fever is a febrile illness characterized by inflammation of the joints, skin, nervous system, and heart. If untreated, rheumatic fever can cause scarring and deformity of cardiac structures resulting in **rheumatic heart disease.**

The incidence of acute rheumatic fever declined in the United States during the 1960s, '70s, and early '80s because of medical and socioeconomic improvements, as well as changes in the virulence of group A streptococci (Harris, 1991). Recent outbreaks in Utah and Pennsylvania corresponded with the reappearance of highly virulent strains. Because crowding and poor hygiene are environmental risk factors for acute rheumatic fever, the disease continues to be a major cause of death and disability for underprivileged populations.

The acute disease occurs most frequently in children between the ages of 5 and 15 years. Only 3% of those in whom pharyngeal streptococcal infection develops acquire acute rheumatic fever. Because the β-hemolytic streptococcus infection must persist for some time to cause acute rheumatic fever, appropriate antibiotic therapy given within the first 9 days of infection usually prevents rheumatic fever (Harris, 1991; Stollerman, 1975). Initiation of antibiotic therapy 2 weeks after the start of streptococcal infection does not prevent rheumatic fever in susceptible individuals (Fitzmaurice, 1980).

The incidence of rheumatic fever tends to run in families, lending support to the concept of genetic predisposition (Zabriskie & Friedman, 1983), perhaps involving an abnormal immune response to antigens expressed by the bacterial membrane. Individuals who have experienced one attack of acute rheumatic fever are more susceptible than the general population to recurrent attacks.

Pathophysiology

Acute rheumatic fever can develop *only* as a sequel to pharyngeal infection by group A β-hemolytic streptococcus. Streptococcal skin infections do not progress to acute rheumatic fever, although both skin and pharyngeal infections can cause acute glomerulonephritis (Harris, 1991). Acute rheumatic fever probably affects the heart, joints, central nervous system, and skin through an abnormal humoral and cell-mediated immune response to group A streptococcal cell membrane antigens. These antigens can bind to receptors on heart, muscle, and brain cells. They also have an affinity for membrane receptors within synovial joints, where they trigger an autoimmune response.

Diffuse, proliferative, and exudative inflammatory lesions develop in the connective tissues, especially in the heart, joints, and skin. The inflammation may subside before treatment, leaving behind damage to the heart valves and increasing the individual's susceptibility to recurrent acute rheumatic fever after any subsequent streptococcal infections. Repeated attacks of acute rheumatic fever cause chronic proliferative changes in the previously mentioned organs as a result of scarring, granulomas, and thromboses.

Approximately 10% of cases of rheumatic fever develop rheumatic heart disease (Cheng, 1986). Rheumatic heart disease begins as **carditis,** or inflammation of the heart. Even mild cases of rheumatic fever can cause carditis in all three layers of the heart wall (endocardium, myocardium, and pericardium; see Chapter 26, Fig. 26-2). The primary lesion usually involves the endocardium, which lines the heart chambers and includes the heart valves. Endocardial inflammation causes swelling of the valve leaflets, with secondary erosion along the lines of leaflet contact. Small, beadlike

FIG. 27-25 Mitral stenosis. Mitral leaflets are thickened and fused and have clumps of vegetation containing platelets and fibrin. (From Kissane, 1990.)

clumps of vegetation containing platelets and fibrin are deposited on eroded valvular tissue and on the chordae tendineae (Fig. 27-25). (The chordae tendineae anchor the valve leaflets; see Chapter 26, Fig. 26-3.) These lesions can become progressively adherent. Scarring and shortening of the involved structures occur over time. The valves lose their elasticity and the leaflets may adhere to each other.

If inflammation penetrates the myocardium, localized fibrin deposits develop that are surrounded by areas of necrosis. These fibrinoid necrotic deposits are called Aschoff bodies. Pericardial inflammation is usually characterized by serofibrinous effusion within the pericardial cavity. Cardiomegaly and congestive heart failure may occur during episodes of untreated acute or recurrent rheumatic fever. Conduction defects and atrial fibrillation are frequently associated with rheumatic heart disease.

Clinical Manifestations

Many of the common clinical manifestations of acute rheumatic fever—fever, lymphadenopathy, arthralgia, nausea, vomiting, epistaxis, abdominal pain, and tachycardia—are associated with other disorders as well and are by no means diagnostic of the disease. The major specific manifestations of acute rheumatic fever are carditis, acute migratory polyarthritis, chorea, and erythema marginatum, which may occur singly or in combination after a latent period of 1 to 5 weeks after streptococcal infection of the pharynx.

Carditis. The earliest cardiac manifestation of acute rheumatic fever may be a previously undetected murmur caused by mitral or aortic semilunar valve dysfunction. Chest pain is caused by pericardial inflammation. Pericardial effusion produces an audible friction rub. Extra heart sounds, heart block (see p. 1051), atrial fibrillation, and a prolonged PR interval are frequently associated with chronic rheumatic heart disease.

Polyarthritis. The classic presenting manifestation of acute rheumatic fever is acute migratory polyarthritis (inflammation of more than one joint). Although all of the synovial joints may be involved, the large joints of the extremities are most frequently affected. Two or more joints are usually involved simultaneously or in succession. Exudative synovitis causes heat, redness, swelling, severe pain, and tenderness, but no permanent disability. Palpable subcutaneous nodes often develop over bony prominences and along extensor tendons. They do not interfere with joint function and often go unnoticed.

Chorea. Sydenham chorea, or St. Vitus dance, is a disorder of the central nervous system characterized by sudden, aimless, irregular, involuntary movements. (Chorea is described in Chapter 14.) It is more common in girls than in boys and may occur several months af-

ter the streptococcal infection. The chorea is self-limiting. It runs its course within weeks or months and has no permanent neural sequelae (Harris, 1991).

Erythema marginatum. Erythema marginatum is a distinctive truncal rash that often accompanies acute rheumatic fever. It consists of nonpruritic, pink, erythematous macules that never occur on the face or hands. The rash is transitory and may change in appearance within minutes or hours. Heat (e.g., bathing) darkens the rash. The macules may fade in the center and be mistaken for ringworm.

Evaluation and Treatment

When correlated with physical assessment findings, laboratory values lend significant support to the diagnosis of acute rheumatic fever. A positive throat culture for group A β-hemolytic streptococci can be an important finding when associated with certain physical signs. Cultures may be negative when the rheumatic attack begins, however. Documented recent scarlet fever is another potentially strong diagnostic aid to acute rheumatic fever, but diagnosis of scarlet fever may depend on a positive throat culture and may be difficult to distinguish from other disorders associated with a similar rash. A high or rising antistreptolysin O antibody titer (ASO) is a more accurate means of diagnosing the presence of a streptococcal infection. Most strains of group A β-hemolytic streptococcus produce a hemolytic factor called streptolysin O. Antibodies against this hemolytic factor increase as the individual's immune system fights the disease. Antistreptolysin O antibody titers greater than 250 Todd units in adults and 333 Todd units in children are considered elevated. Several other antibody tests are sensitive prognosticators of streptococcal infection. These include antideoxyribonucleotidase (anti-DNase B), antihyaluronidase, and antistreptozyme (ASTZ).

Elevated white blood cell count, erythrocyte sedimentation rate, and C-reactive protein indicate inflammation. All three are usually increased at the time cardiac or joint symptoms begin to appear. They are more useful in identifying an acute inflammatory process and suggesting prognosis than in diagnosing acute rheumatic fever. The levels of these tests decrease as the inflammatory process resolves.

In 1944, the Jones criteria (Table 27-11) were established to assist in the diagnosis of acute rheumatic fever. The criteria have been modified several times by the American Heart Association, most recently in 1965 (Markowitz, 1988). No single laboratory test, sign, or symptom is pathognomonic of acute rheumatic fever, but certain combinations of criteria indicate that acute disease is probably present.

Therapy for acute rheumatic fever is aimed at eradicating the streptococcal infection. This is accomplished

TABLE 27-11

Jones Criteria (revised) Used for Diagnosis of Rheumatic Fever

Criteria	Description
Major manifestations	Carditis, polyarthritis, chorea, erythema marginatum, subcutaneous nodes
Minor manifestations	Clinical: previous rheumatic fever or rheumatic heart disease, arthralgia, fever; laboratory: elevated appearance of C-reactive protein, leukocytosis; electrocardiographic: prolonged PR interval
Supporting evidence of streptococcal infection	Increased titer of streptococcal antibodies: antistreptolysin O (ASO), other; positive throat culture for group A *Streptococcus;* recent scarlet fever

From American Heart Association, 1982.

by a 10-day regimen of oral penicillin or erythromycin administration. Salicylates are used as antiinflammatory agents for both rheumatic carditis and arthritis. Serious carditis may require that cardiac glycosides, corticosteroids, diuretics, and bed rest be added to the regimen. Surgical repair of damaged valves may be necessary in cases of chronic recurrent rheumatic fever/carditis. Active disease is considered resolved when (1) the murmur has disappeared or cardiac status becomes stable, (2) major manifestations are no longer present, (3) the individual is afebrile, and (4) the erythrocyte sedimentation rate is normal or stabilized. This may take anywhere from 1 to 6 months (Harris, 1991; Stollerman, 1992).

Research suggests that a rheumatic recurrence will develop in 50% to 65% of children with known rheumatic fever if they have another group A streptococcal infection. Recurrence rates decline with the length of time elapsed since the last infection. To prevent recurrence of acute rheumatic fever, continuous prophylactic antibiotic therapy is necessary (Stollerman, 1992).

Infective Endocarditis

Infective endocarditis is a general term used to describe inflammation of the endocardium—especially the car-

diac valves. Causal agents include bacteria, viruses, fungi, rickettsiae, and parasites, but bacterial infection, particularly by streptococci or staphylococci, is most common. Infective carditis was once a lethal disease, but morbidity and mortality diminished significantly with the advent of antibiotics and improved diagnostic techniques.

Risk factors for infective carditis include acquired valvular heart disease (especially mitral valve prolapse) and implantation of prosthetic heart valves. Congenital lesions associated with highly turbulent flow, such as ventricular septal defect, are also risk factors. (Congenital lesions are discussed in Chapter 28.) Other risk factors include a previous attack of infective endocarditis, male gender, intravenous drug abuse, long-term indwelling catheterization (e.g., for pressure monitoring, hyperalimentation, or hemodialysis), and recent cardiac surgery.

Pathophysiology

The pathogenesis of infective endocarditis is a complex process that requires at least three critical elements (Fig. 27-26). First, the endocardium (e.g., heart valve) must be "prepared," usually by endothelial damage, for microorganism colonization. Second, blood-borne microorganisms must adhere to the damaged endocardial surface. Third, the adherent microorganisms must proliferate and promote the propagation of infective endocardial vegetation (Friedman, 1987; Sullam, Drake, & Sande, 1985).

The first critical element, endocardial damage, exposes the endothelial basement membrane. The basement membrane contains a type of collagen that attracts platelets and thereby stimulates thrombus formation on the membrane. Platelet activation and thrombus formation can cause an inflammatory reaction termed **nonbacterial thrombotic endocarditis.** Infective endocarditis cannot develop unless microorganisms gain access to the bloodstream. Microorganisms may enter the bloodstream as a result of minor procedures, such as dental cleaning or bladder catheterization, or they may spread from uncomplicated upper respiratory or skin infections. Any time pathogens gain access to the bloodstream, the potential for endocardial infection exists. Bacteremia and adherence constitute the second critical element. Adherence of microorganisms to the endocardial surface is facilitated by the coexistence of nonbacterial thrombotic endocarditis. It should be noted, however, that bacteremia can cause infective endocarditis even on healthy, intact endocardium (Freedman, 1987; Sullam et al., 1985). The third critical element, bacterial proliferation and vegetation formation, is also promoted by coexistent nonbacterial thrombotic endocarditis.

Not all microorganisms are capable of colonization. This capability, which determines the microorganism's

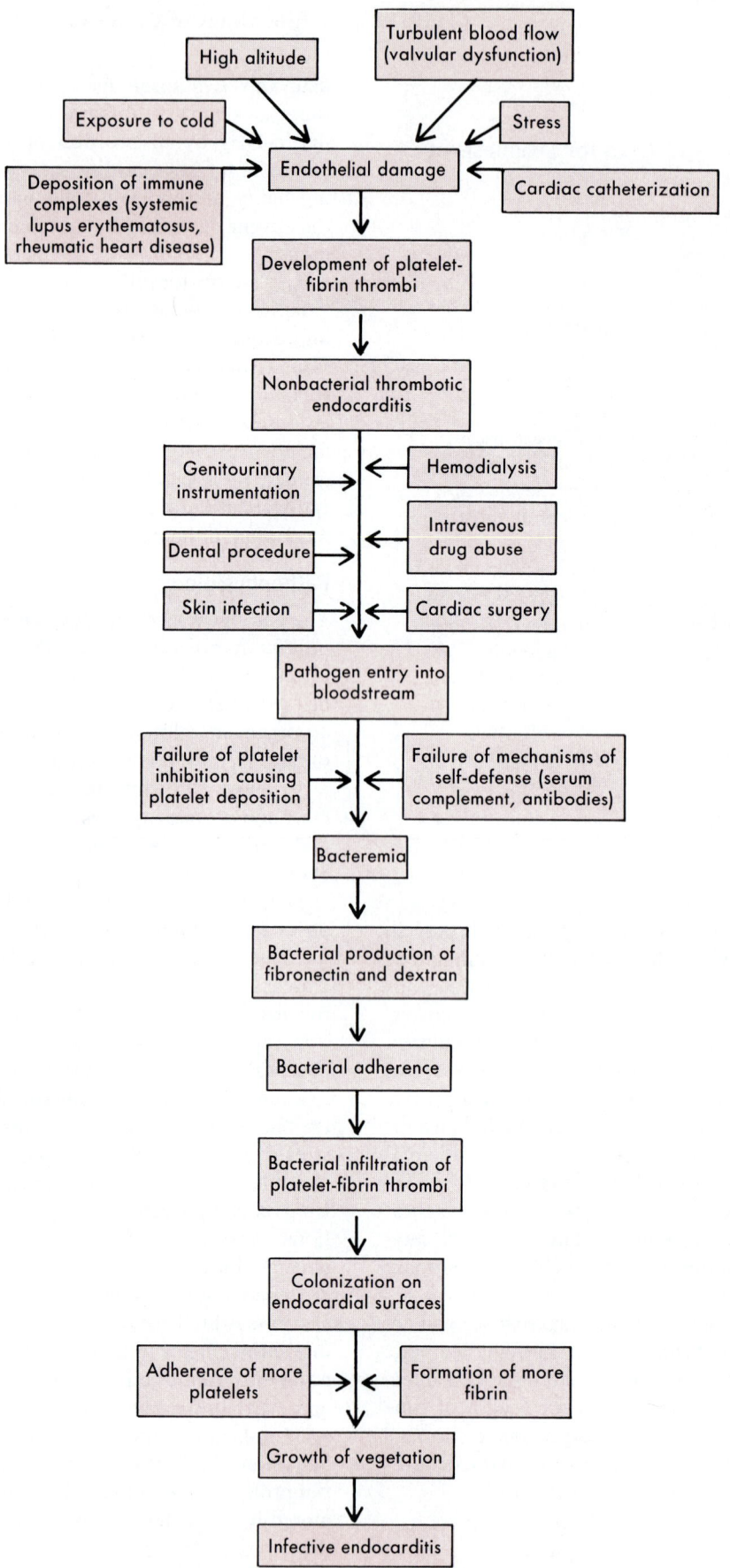

FIG. 27-26 Pathogenesis of infective endocarditis.

FIG. 27-27 Bacterial endocarditis of mitral valve. Lesion in combination with old rheumatic valvulitis. (From Kissane, 1990.)

pathogenicity, depends on the organism's ability to survive interactions with circulating serum complement, antibodies, and platelets aggregated on the endocardial surface. Complement, antibodies, and platelets may serve as effective inhibitors to bacterial colonization.

In addition to circumventing the host's defense mechanisms, the circulating microorganisms must adhere to the endocardial surface to initiate endocardial infection. Studies suggest that bacteria are able to synthesize extracellular polysaccharides, such as dextran or fibronectin, which promote stickiness on endocardial surfaces (Gould, Ramirez-Ronda, Holmes, & Stanford, 1975).

Once the endocardial surface is colonized, formation of infected vegetation proceeds by a series of complex steps (Fig. 27-27). Within 3 to 6 hours after infection, microbial replication occurs and bacterial colonies form within aggregates of fibrin and platelets. Within 24 hours, infected vegetation has increased in size, with colonies of microorganisms sandwiched between layers of fibrin and platelets. Bacteria may accelerate fibrin formation by activating the clotting cascade in some as yet undetermined manner (Sullam et al., 1985). As the growing bacterial colonies become progressively enmeshed in the tight fibrin network, which contains few phagocytic cells, they become less and less susceptible to the host's mechanisms of self-defense (Archer, 1977). Although endocardial tissue is constantly bathed in antibody-containing blood and is surrounded by scavenging monocytes and polymorphonuclear leukocytes,

bacterial colonies are inaccessible to host defenses because they are embedded in the protective fibrin clots (Korzeniowski & Kaye, 1992). The lesions can form anywhere on the endocardium, but usually occur on the endocardial surfaces of heart valves and surrounding structures.

Clinical Manifestations

Infective endocarditis may be acute, subacute, or naggingly chronic. It causes varying degrees of valvular dysfunction and may be associated with manifestations involving any number of organ systems (lungs, eyes, kidneys, bones, joints, central nervous system), making diagnosis exceedingly difficult. The "classic" findings of fever, cardiac murmur, and petechial lesions of the skin, conjunctiva, and oral mucosa are not always present.

Signs and symptoms of infective endocarditis are caused by infection and inflammation, systemic spread of microemboli, and immune complex deposition in various organs. A history of fever, anorexia, weight loss, back pain, and night sweats; a new or significantly changed cardiac murmur; petechiae; positive blood cultures; elevated erythrocyte sedimentation rate; and urine abnormalities make the diagnosis quite clear. Sudden onset of severely debilitating symptoms indicates acute disease.

If infective endocarditis extends farther into the heart wall and invades the conduction system, electrocardiography may show prolonged PR interval, left bundle branch block, or complete heart block (see p. 1052). Emboli may travel to the coronary arteries and cause an acute myocardial infarction.

Evaluation and Treatment

Echocardiography is useful for diagnosing infective endocarditis and predicting the prognosis, especially in cases in which blood cultures are negative. If peripheral emboli are suggested, organ scans can be performed to confirm their presence. Antimicrobial therapy is generally given for 4 to 6 weeks, beginning with intravenous and ending with oral administration. In some cases, two different antibiotics are given simultaneously to eliminate the offending microorganism and prevent the development of drug resistance. Penicillin and streptomycin are commonly used to treat infective endocarditis. Other drugs may be necessary to treat congestive heart failure secondary to valvular dysfunction.

Recurrent infective endocarditis or severe impairment of the heart valves may require implantation of prosthetic valves. Unfortunately, the presence of an artificial valve is itself a significant risk factor for infective endocarditis. Valve failure and valve-induced embolization are known sequelae of prosthetic valve placement.

Individuals who are known to be at risk for infective endocarditis can avoid the disease by taking antibiotics before and after any procedure that carries the risk of transient bacteremia. Such procedures include dental cleaning, genitourinary instrumentation, and open cardiovascular surgery. The Committee on Rheumatic Fever, Endocarditis, and Kawasaki Disease of the Council on Cardiovascular Disease in the Young periodically updates its recommendations concerning prevention of infective endocarditis for individuals at risk (Dajani et al., 1990).

Cardiac Complications in Acquired Immunodeficiency Syndrome (AIDS)

There is growing evidence that 25% to 50% of individuals infected with the human immunodeficiency virus (HIV) have cardiac involvement consisting of myocarditis, endocarditis, pericarditis, or cardiomyopathy (Acierno, 1989; Wynne & Braunwald, 1992). Cardiac involvement can result from the HIV itself, inflammation, other infections, malignancy, or drugs. In addition to HIV infection, the cardiac involvement may be induced by the accompanying inflammatory response. Infection also may be caused by a variety of bacterial, viral, protozoan, mycobacterial, and fungal pathogens. Malignancies, such as lymphoma and Kaposi sarcoma, are frequently seen in individuals with AIDS and can affect the heart. Anti-HIV drugs or drugs used to combat opportunistic infections may produce toxic lesions. Myocarditis is the most common pathologic finding.

Clinical manifestations of cardiac disease are seen in about 10% of those with HIV (Acierno, 1989; Wynne & Braunwald, 1992). Congestive heart failure is the most common and is related to left ventricular dilation and dysfunction. Pericardial effusion, ventricular arrhythmias, electrocardiographic changes, and right ventricular dilation and hypertrophy are other less common findings. Treatment includes antibiotic therapy when appropriate and relief of symptoms.

MANIFESTATIONS OF HEART DISEASE

Dysrhythmias

A dysrhythmia, or arrhythmia, is a disturbance of heart rhythm. Normal heart rhythms are generated by the sinoatrial node (SA node) and travel through the heart's conduction system, causing the atrial and ventricular myocardium to contract and relax at a regular rate that is appropriate to maintain circulation at various levels of physical activity (see Chapter 26). Dysrhythmias range in severity from occasional "missed" or rapid beats to serious disturbances that impair the pumping ability of the heart, contributing to heart failure and death. Dysrhythmias can be caused by either an abnormal rate of impulse generation (Table 27-12) by the SA

node or other pacemaker, or the abnormal conduction of impulses (Table 27-13) through the heart's conduction system, including the myocardial cells themselves.

Heart Failure

Heart failure is the inability of the heart to supply the body and heart muscle itself with adequate circulatory volume and pressure. Failure encompasses a large number of causes and a spectrum of clinical manifestations. Heart failure is occasionally defined as reduced stroke volume with adequate venous return. This definition does not, however, apply to heart failure in which venous return is excessive or cardiac output is high. The causes of heart failure include elevated systemic and pulmonic vascular resistance, myocardial infarction, infection, anemia, and beriberi. These and other causes of heart failure usually involve alterations of (1) contractility, (2) preload, (3) afterload, and (4) the ratio of oxygen supply to oxygen demand. (These factors are described in Chapter 26.)

Mechanisms of Heart Failure
Altered contractility

According to Starling's law of the heart, contractility is optimal within a certain range of myocardial cell lengths. Within this range, the more the myocardium is stretched, the harder it contracts. This increases the force of systole and the amount of blood that is ejected with each ventricular contraction. In other words, an increase of diastolic stretch results in a larger systolic ejection force and a larger stroke volume.

As the sarcomeres of the muscle cell microfilaments are stretched to the upper limits of their length, two things happen: not only do a large number of crossbridges have an opportunity to form, but more room is created within the cell to allow for the sliding of the microfilaments upon contraction. (The crossbridge theory and the Frank-Starling law of the heart are discussed in Chapter 25.) At a cell length of less than 0.5 μm, the microfilaments are overlapped so completely that there is little room for them to slide when the crossbridges are moved (Fig. 27-28). At 0.5 μm, the sarcomere is already nearly as short as it can get and still contract. At lengths less than 0.5 μm, the actin filaments themselves may have begun to overlap. Because actin filaments cannot form crossbridges with each other (i.e., they require the thick filaments of myosin), contractile force is limited. Clinically, 0.5 μm is the minimal length at which the myocardium contracts satisfactorily. Therefore, low blood volume resulting from hemorrhage, for example, can reduce contraction even in the absence of cardiac disease because the nearly empty ventricle is not stretched sufficiently to contract with much force.

At cell lengths greater than 2.2 μm, the amount of contact the filaments have with each other begins to be

Text continued on p. 1054.

TABLE 27-12

Disorders of Impulse Formation

Type	ECG	Effect	Pathophysiology	Treatment
Sinus bradycardia	P rate 60 or less PRI normal QRS for each P	Increased preload Decreased mean arterial pressure	Hyperkalemia: slows depolarization Vagal hyperactivity: unknown Digoxin toxicity common Late hypoxia: lack of ATP	If hypotensive, treat cause and support Follow with sympathomimetics, cardiotonics, and pacer Vagolytics
Simple sinus tachycardia	P rate 100-150 PRI normal QRS for each P	Decreased filling times Decreased mean arterial pressure Increased myocardial demand	Catecholamines: rise in resting potential, calcium influx Fever: unknown Early failure and lung disease: hypoxic cell metabolism Hypercalcemia	Oxygen, bed rest Calcium blockers
Premature atrial contractions or beats*	Early P waves that may have changed morphology PRI normal QRS for each P	Occasional decreased filling time and mean arterial pressure	Electrolyte disturbances: decrease all phases Hypoxia and elevated preload: cell membrane disturbances Hypercalcemia	Treat underlying cause Digoxin
Sinus arrhythmia	Rate varies P-P regularly irregular, short with inspiration, long with exhalation PRI normal QRS for each P	Variable filling times Variable mean arterial pressures Variable oxygen demand	Unknown Common in young and young adults	None
Atrial tachycardia (includes premature atrial tachycardia if onset is abrupt)	P rate 151-250 P morphology may differ from sinus P PRI normal P:QRS ratio variable	Decreased filling time Decreased mean arterial pressure Increased myocardial demand	Same as PACs: leads to increased atrial automaticity, atrial reentry Digoxin toxicity: common	Control ventricular rate Digoxin, calcium blockers, vagus stimulation Pace to override
Atrial flutter*	P rate 251-300, morphology may vary from sinus P PRI usually not observable P:QRS ratio variable	Decreased filling time Decreased mean arterial pressure	Same as atrial tachycardia Aging	Same as atrial tachycardia Synchronous cardioversion
Atrial fibrillation*	P rate >300 and usually not observable No PRI QRS rate variable and rhythm irregular	Same as atrial flutter	Same as atrial tachycardia Aging	Same as atrial tachycardia

*Most common in adults.
†Life-threatening in adults.

Continued.

TABLE 27-12

Disorders of Impulse Formation—cont'd

Type	ECG	Effect	Pathophysiology	Treatment
Idiojunctional rhythm	P absent or independent QRS normal, rate 41-59, regular	Decreased cardiac output from loss of atrial contribution to ventricular preload Decreased mean atrial pressure as a result of bradycardia	Atrial and sinus bradycardia, or standstill, or block	Same as sinus bradycardia
Junctional bradycardia	P absent or independent QRS normal, rate 40 or less	Same as idiojunctional rhythm	Same as idiojunctional rhythm Vagal hyperactivity	Same as sinus bradycardia
Premature junctional contractions or beats	Early beats without P waves QRS morphology normal	Decreased cardiac output from loss of atrial contribution to ventricular preload for that beat	Hyperkalemia (6-5.4 mEq/L) Hypercalcemia, hypoxia, and elevated preload (see PACs)	Same as PAC
Accelerated junctional rhythm	P absent or independent QRS morphology normal, rate 60-99	Decreased cardiac output from loss of atrial contribution to ventricular preload	Same as PJCs	Same as PAC
Junctional tachycardia	P absent or independent QRS morphology normal, rate 100 or more	Decreased cardiac output from loss of atrial contribution to ventricular preload Increased myocardial demand because of tachycardia	Same as PJCs	Same as PAC
Idioventricular rhythm†	P absent or independent QRS >0.11 and rate 20-39	Same as idiojunctional rhythm	Sinus, atrial, and junctional bradycardia, standstill, or block	Same as sinus bradycardia
Ventricular bradycardia†	P absent or independent QRS >0.11 and rate 60-21	Same as idiojunctional rhythm	Same as idiojunctional rhythm	Same as sinus bradycardia
Agonal rhythm/ electromechanical dissociation†	P absent or independent QRS >0.11 and rate 20 or less	Absent or barely present cardiac output and pulse Not compatible with life	Depolarization and contraction not coupled: electrical activity present with little or no mechanical activity Usually caused by profound hypoxia	Vigorous pharmacology aimed at restoring rate and force Usually ineffective May attempt to pace
Ventricular standstill or asystole†	P absent or independent QRS absent	No cardiac output Not compatible with life	Profound ischemia, hyperkalemia, acidosis	Same as agonal rhythm, including electrical defibrillation

*Most common in adults.
†Life-threatening in adults.

TABLE 27-12

Disorders of Impulse Formation—cont'd

Type	ECG	Effect	Pathophysiology	Treatment
Premature ventricular contraction or depolarizations*	Early beats with P waves QRS occasionally opposite in deflection from usual QRS	Same as premature junctional contractions	Same as PJCs, including aging and induction of anesthesia Impulse originates in cell outside normal conduction system and spreads through intercalated disks	Pharmacology to change thresholds, refractory periods, reduce myocardial demand increase supply Removal of cause
Accelerated ventricular rhythm	P absent or independent QRS >0.11 and rate 41-99	Same as accelerated junctional rhythm	Same as PVCs	Same as PVCs
Ventricular tachycardia†	P absent or independent QRS >0.11 and rate 100 or more	Same as junctional tachycardia	Same as PVCs	Same as PVCs, including electrical cardioversion
Ventricular fibrillation†	P absent QRS >300 and usually not observable	Same as ventricular standstill	Same as PVCs Rapid infusion of potassium	Same as PVCs including electrical defibrillation

*Most common in adults.
†Life-threatening in adults.

TABLE 27-13

Disorders of Impulse Conduction

Type	ECG	Effect	Pathophysiology	Treatment
Sinus block	Occasionally absent P, with loss of QRS for that beat	Occasional decrease in cardiac output Increase in preload for the following beat	Local hypoxia, scarring of intraatrial conduction pathways, electrolyte imbalances Increased atrial preload	Conservative Usually do not progress in severity Pharmacologic treatment includes vagolytics, sympathomimetics, pacing
First-degree block*	PRI >0.2	None	Same as sinus block Hyperkalemia (>7 mEq/L) Hypokalemia (>3.5 mEq/L) Formation of myocardial abscesses in endocarditis	Conservative Discovery and correction of cause

*Most common in adults.
†Life-threatening in adults.

Continued.

TABLE 27-13

Disorders of Impulse Conduction—cont'd

Type	ECG	Effect	Pathophysiology	Treatment
Second-degree block, Mobitz I, or Wenckebach*	Progressive prolongation of PRI until one QRS is dropped Pattern of prolongation resumes	Same as sinus block	Hypokalemia (>3.5 mEq/L) Faulty cell metabolism in A-V node Severity increases as heart rate increases Supports theory that A-V node is fatiguing Digoxin toxicity, beta-blockade CAD, MI, hypoxia, increased preload, valvular surgery and disease, diabetes	Same as sinus block
Second-degree block or Mobitz II	Same as sinus block	Same as sinus block	Hypokalemia (>3.5 mEq/L) Faulty cell metabolism below A-V node Antiarrhythmics, cyclic antidepressants CAD, MI, hypoxia, increased preload, valvular surgery and disease, diabetes	More aggressively than Mobitz I, since can progress to type III Pacemaker after pharmacologic treatment
Third-degree block†	P waves present and independent of QRS No observed relationship between P and QRS Always A-V dissociation	Same as idiojunctional rhythm	Hypokalemia (>3.5 mEq/L) Faulty cell metabolism low in bundle of His MI, especially inferior wall, as nodal artery interrupted; results in ischemia of A-V node	Pharmacologic until pacemaker inserted Temporary pacing if caused by inferior MI, since ischemia usually resolves
Atrioventricular dissociation	P waves present and independent of QRS, but not always because of block (e.g., ventricular tachycardia) A-V dissociation not always third-degree block	Decreased cardiac output from loss of atrial contribution to ventricular preload Variable effect on myocardial demand, depending on ventricular rate	May result from third-degree block or accelerated junctional or ventricular rhythm, or be caused by sinus, atrial, and junctional bradycardias	Treat according to cause Pacemaker or reducing rate of A-V or ventricular discharge, or increasing rate of sinus or A-V node discharge

*Most common in adults.
†Life-threatening in adults.

TABLE 27-13

Disorders of Impulse Conduction—cont'd

Type	ECG	Effect	Pathophysiology	Treatment
Ventricular block	QRS > 0.11 R-S-R′ in V1, V2, V5, V6	None	Faulty cell metabolism in right and left bundle branches RBBB more common than LBBB because of dual blood supply to left bundle branch CHR, MR, especially anterior MI, because of infarct of fascicles Left anterior hemiblock more common than left posterior hemiblock, since posterior fascicles have dual blood supply	Isolated RBBB or LBBB or hemiblock not treated If acute and/or associated with acute anterior MI, treated with permanent pacer and vigorous pharmacology
Aberrant conduction	QRS >0.11	None, unless ventricular rate abnormalities present	Conduction of impulse through intercalated disks, since conduction system transiently blocked because of hypoxia, electrolyte imbalances, digoxin toxicity, excessively rapid rates of discharge	Correct underlying cause
Preexcitation syndromes (Wolff-Parkinson-White and Lown-Ganong-Levine)	P present with QRS for each P PRI >0.12 and QRS >0.11 because of presence of delta wave in PRI	None	Congenital presence of accessory pathways (bundle of Kent and fiber of Mahaim) that conduct very rapidly and bypass the A-V node, causing early ventricular depolarization in relation to atrial depolarization Prone (reason unknown) to tachycardias and atrial fibrillation that can result in very rapid ventricular rates	Aimed at lining up refractory periods of accessory pathway and A-V node to prevent reentry May slow rate with pharmacology May surgically cut pathways

*Most common in adults.
†Life-threatening in adults.

FIG. 27-28 Effects of sarcomere overlap on myocardial contractility. **A,** The position of myocardial sarcomeres at lengths from 0.5 to 2.2 μm. **B,** The position of myocardial sarcomeres at a length of less than 0.5 μm. Overlap is excessive, and contractility is diminished. **C,** The position of myocardial sarcomeres at a length greater than 2.3 μm. Overlap is insufficient, and contractility is diminished.

reduced. Contractile force progressively degenerates as length increases (Fig. 27-28). The fewer the number of crossbridges, the less force will be generated, even though the stretched microfilaments have adequate room to move within the sarcomere. At 2.2 μm or more, the force of systole is reduced, causing the heart chamber to supply inadequate blood volume and pressure to the body, even though the chamber is very full and stretched. Consequently, blood pressure drops. If the chamber empties poorly but venous return remains normal, the chamber will "overfill" during diastole. Overfilling increases stretch further, which weakens systole more. This forms a positive feedback loop that can lead to chamber failure.

Preload determines the amount of stretch, usually exerted by blood volume, that occurs before systole. Preload in the right heart depends on venous return to the heart from the systemic circulation. Preload in the left heart depends on venous return from the pulmonary system. Preload is also increased by outflow impedance from any chamber, even when venous return is not increased. If the chamber cannot empty fully, the end-diastolic volume increases, and myocardial stretch increases. Idiopathic hypertrophic subaortic stenosis and aortic stenosis increase left ventricular preload, whereas pulmonary stenosis increases right ventricular preload.

Prolapse of the aortic semilunar valve enables blood to enter the ventricle during diastole from both the left

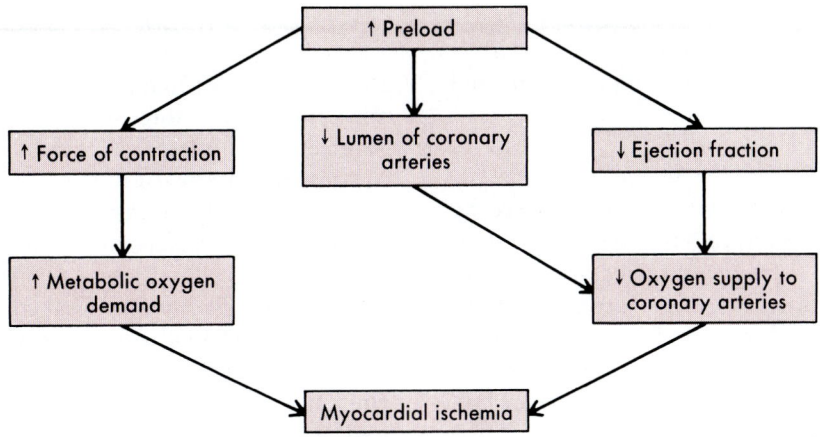

FIG. 27-29 The effect of elevated preload on myocardial oxygen supply and demand.

atrium and the aorta. This increases the end-diastolic volume and increases stretch in the left ventricle. If the mitral valve is prolapsed, blood reenters the left atrium from the left ventricle during systole and from the pulmonary vasculature during diastole. Blood volume and pressures in the left atrium become very high before atrial systole, and atrial stretch occurs.

If preload stretches the sarcomere beyond 2.2 μm, contractile force diminishes, ejection is reduced, and the cardiac chamber contains more blood than usual at the end of systole. Because there is no reduction in the amount of blood entering the chamber during diastole, the chamber is "overfilled" during diastole, preload climbs, and the systolic ejection fraction diminishes further.

Increases of preload also increase myocardial oxygen consumption by necessitating a greater force of contraction to accomplish systole. The increased force of cardiac contraction is accompanied by increased metabolic demand in the myocardium, and more oxygen is required to support myocardial metabolism (Fig. 27-29). Unfortunately, elevated preload can also decrease the amount of oxygen available to the myocardium by two mechanisms. First, increased myocardial stretch decreases myocardial capillary perfusion by mechanically narrowing coronary capillary lumina. Second, if preload increases beyond the ventricle's ability to empty, the coronary artery blood supply decreases as the ejection fraction decreases. Increases of metabolic demand in the face of coronary capillary lumen narrowing and decreased blood flow to the coronary arteries cause the overworked and overstretched myocardium to become hypoxic.

Afterload is the force or pressure against which a cardiac chamber must eject blood during systole. Increased afterload can be caused by and equated with mechanical outflow impedance, as in subaortic and aortic ste-

nosis. Subaortic and aortic stenosis will, through impeding outflow of blood, eventually cause decreased left ventricular emptying, which will lead to elevated left ventricular preload. More commonly, increased afterload is equated with increased systemic vascular resistance (SVR) or pulmonary vascular resistance (PVR), such as occurs in systemic or pulmonary hypertension. To maintain cardiac output, the left ventricle must eject the same amount of blood over the same amount of time into an area of higher resistance. Therefore, the ventricular myocardium must use greater force during ejection and consume more oxygen with each contraction. To maintain blood pressure, the heart rate and stroke volume must rise. To increase stroke volume, the ventricle must contract with more force than usual and raise the ejection fraction. The ventricular myocardium also requires more oxygen as the force of contraction increases.

Altered ratio of oxygen supply and demand

The myocardial need for oxygen is affected by a number of factors—among them heart rate, force of contraction, and metabolic rate. The myocardial oxygen supply is affected by the patency or lumen size of the coronary arteries, oxygen content of the blood, and the oxygen content of ambient air.

Because both oxygen supply and oxygen demand are always in states of flux, they are thought of as a ratio. The optimum ratio of supply to demand is 1.0 or greater. When the ratio decreases to below 1.0 (i.e., demand exceeds supply), the myocardium suffers grave consequences. Two of the most common and devastating sequelae to a ratio of less than 1 are myocardial infarction and impaired myocardial contractility. A decrease in the ratio can precipitate, exacerbate, or follow heart failure.

Types of Heart Failure

The four major types of heart failure are (1) right heart failure, (2) left heart failure, (3) low-output failure, and (4) high-output failure.

Right heart failure (cor pulmonale)

Right heart failure (cor pulmonale) is rarely caused by excessive systemic venous return. High venous return to a right heart that is on the verge of failing as a result of myocarditis or other diseases can be forced "over the line" into frank failure, however. Right heart failure more commonly results from pulmonary disease and elevated PVR. The most common cause of right heart failure is left heart failure.

The pathophysiology of right heart failure is sometimes said to "progress backward," meaning that the disease process moves from the left heart or lungs to the right atrium, contrary or opposite to the flow of blood (Fig. 27-30). Right heart failure begins in the left heart because of left heart disease (e.g., cardiomyopathy) or an event, such as myocardial infarction, that decreases the amount of blood the left heart is able to accept from the pulmonary circulation. The lung capillary beds become engorged with blood, and the lungs become a high-pressure system. Right heart failure can begin also in the lungs as a result of disease or an event, such as pulmonary embolism, that alters the alveolocapillary membrane (the blood-air interface in the lungs). Elevated pressures across affected capillary beds are transferred to the pulmonary arteries, and PVR is increased. Whether it is caused by left heart disease or lung disease, elevated PVR promotes right heart failure because the right ventricle must work harder to maintain its systolic ejection fraction; therefore, more oxygen is required and consumed with each contraction.

The ratio of oxygen supply to oxygen demand is normally quite high in the right ventricular myocardium. The pulmonary vasculature is normally a low-pressure system. Therefore, PVR is normally low, and the coronary arteries supply more than enough blood and oxygen for routine right ventricular activity. Even in the presence of coronary artery disease, right ventricular infarction is less common than left ventricular infarction because of low right ventricular demand. Unless coexistent lung disease reduces the availability of oxygen, pulmonary hypertension may develop and exist for quite some time before the supply-demand ratio is compromised.

As the supply-demand ratio falls, the right ventricle loses its ability to maintain a normal ejection fraction and empties less completely with each beat. In addition, if increasing PVR makes ejection of a normal volume of blood more and more difficult for the right ventricle, right ventricular end-diastolic pressure (RVEDP) increases.

Increases of RVEDP and volume cause increases of right ventricular preload, which stretch the right ventricle. Within the optimum range of stretch, the right ventricle increases its force of contraction as the myofibrils lengthen. The increased force of contraction increases the amount of oxygen required with each systole. This lowers the supply-demand ratio further and contributes to ventricular weakening as myocardial metabolism becomes anaerobic. Preload continues to increase, and the ventricle continues to weaken.

The high RVEDP causes right atrial preload to increase because the right atrium begins to have trouble emptying fully into the engorged right ventricle. The right atrium stretches, and its contractility and oxygen consumption increase until it, too, begins to fail.

Blood volume and pressure rise in the vena cava as the right atrial preload increases because blood cannot empty from the venae into the engorged right atrium. Elevated blood volumes and pressures are transmitted backward from the venae cavae through the veins, venules, and capillaries of the systemic circulation. Elevated central venous pressure (CVP) occurs early in right heart failure. In the absence of central venous pressure monitoring, distention of the jugular vein is used as an indicator of elevated right atrial and ventricular end-diastolic pressures. As pressures in the capillaries increase, hydrostatic pressure exceeds interstitial pressure, and fluid leaks out of the capillaries, causing peripheral edema. Peripheral edema progresses to anasarca (generalized, massive edema) and abdominal organ distention, especially of the liver and spleen.

Treatment for right heart failure begins with treatment of underlying left heart failure (see below), or pulmonary disease. The goal is to reduce pulmonary hypertension and increase arterial oxygen content. Diuretics, in conjunction with restricted water and sodium intake, are used to reduce venous blood volume (preload). Myocardial contractility is enhanced with digoxin or other cardiotonic medications. Bed rest reduces myocardial oxygen demand and promotes diuresis by increasing renal perfusion.

Left heart failure (congestive heart failure)

Left heart failure, commonly called congestive heart failure, is really left ventricular failure. Myocardial infarction resulting from coronary artery disease is a very common cause of left heart failure that can be thought of as intrinsic to the myocardium (Castaner et al., 1984). Causes extrinsic to the myocardium are systemic hypertension, and aortic stenosis and regurgitation.

In left heart failure resulting from systemic hypertension or elevated SVR, the progression of events is similar to that of right heart failure (Fig. 27-31). Elevated SVR increases myocardial oxygen demand until contractile force is decreased. As the ejection fraction falls,

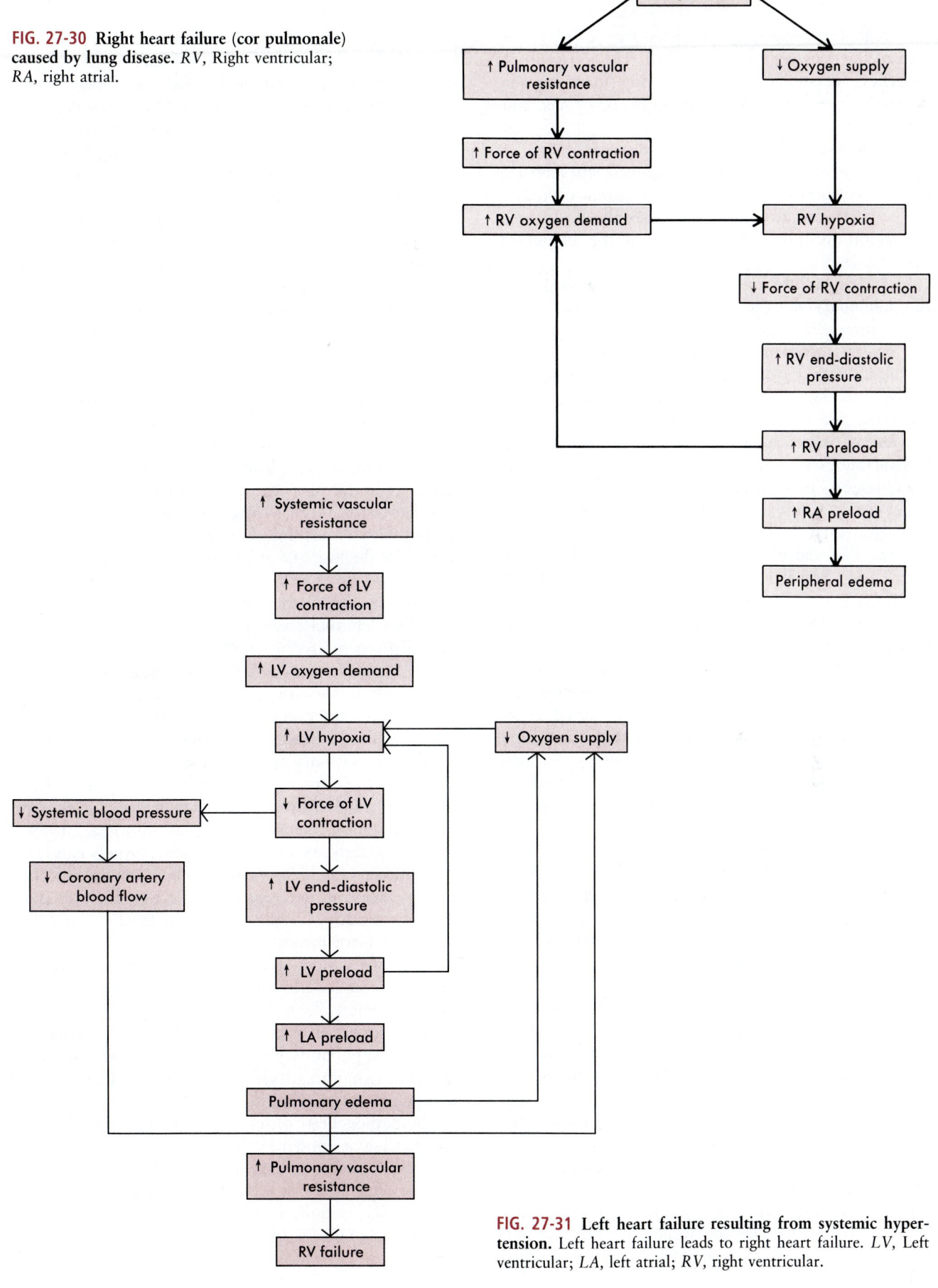

FIG. 27-30 Right heart failure (cor pulmonale) caused by lung disease. *RV,* Right ventricular; *RA,* right atrial.

FIG. 27-31 Left heart failure resulting from systemic hypertension. Left heart failure leads to right heart failure. *LV,* Left ventricular; *LA,* left atrial; *RV,* right ventricular.

left ventricular end-diastolic pressure (LVEDP) increases, as does ventricular preload. The left ventricle stretches, works harder, and requires more oxygen. When the increased demand for oxygen is not met, contractile force decreases further.

The increase in LVEDP makes it difficult for the left atrium to empty fully into the engorged left ventricle, and the ejection fraction of the left atrium decreases. Preload in the left atrium then increases, the atrium fails, and blood pressure and volume rise in the pulmonary veins.

Elevated pressure and volume are transmitted from the pulmonary veins to the pulmonary capillary beds, where increased hydrostatic pressure drives fluid into the low-pressure air sacs (alveoli; see Chapter 30). The alveoli fill with plasma, and pulmonary edema results.

When the lungs become fluid filled, gas exchange is impaired, and the failing left ventricle is faced with a decrease in oxygen supply. This further impairs ventricular metabolism and contractility. Pressures increase in the lungs, and pressures in the systemic circulation fail.

Pulmonary vascular resistance will increase if the pulmonary edema is not treated or if the left heart failure persists. Elevated PVR causes right ventricular failure (Fig. 27-32). **Biventricular heart failure** is failure of both ventricles.

Systemic blood pressure decreases because of decreased contractile force and decreased ejection fraction of the left ventricle (Fig. 27-32). This triggers receptors in the glomerular apparatus of the kidneys to release renin. Renin converts angiotensinogen (produced in the liver and circulating in the blood) to angiotensin. Angiotensin stimulates release of aldosterone by the adrenal cortex. Under the influence of aldosterone, renal tubular reabsorption of sodium increases. As sodium and water are reabsorbed, plasma volume increases.

The extent to which renin and angiotensin contribute to congestive heart failure varies. Cody, Covit, Schaer, and Laragh (1984) demonstrated that occupation of receptor sites for angiotensin II in individuals with heart failure ranges from low (with low SVR) to quite high (with high SVR). This has implications for treatment aimed at manipulation of vascular resistance.

The decrease in systemic blood pressure is also detected by various baroreceptors (Sleight, 1984). Through neuronal pathways, baroreceptors stimulate the hypothalamus to cause the symptom of thirst. The hypothalamus also causes the posterior pituitary to release antidiuretic hormone (ADH). Antidiuretic hormone increases the renal tubular permeability to water. This causes water reabsorption to increase, and plasma volume increases further.

Increased plasma volume increases right ventricular preload. High preload exacerbates right ventricular failure if that chamber has begun to be affected by elevated

PVR. If right ventricular function is intact, a greater volume of blood is delivered to the pulmonary vasculature. If pulmonary edema has not already developed, it will soon do so, causing an increase in PVR and a decrease in oxygen diffusion into the pulmonary capillaries. The right ventricle fails if the PVR increases enough or if the atrial oxygen content decreases enough to affect right ventricular contractility.

As blood pressure decreases, sympathetic activity is stimulated, causing the release of epinephrine and norepinephrine (Sleight, 1984). These neurotransmitters are cardiotonic; that is, they increase the action of the myocardium. This lowers the supply-demand ratio further while contributing to decreased left ventricular contractility.

Epinephrine also constricts arterioles, reducing their radii. Arteriolar constriction increases SVR directly, and may decrease blood flow to the coronary arteries. An increased SVR contributes to failure by increasing oxygen demand, whereas a narrowing of the coronary arteries' radii decreases the oxygen supply.

If left heart failure is caused by ventricular infarction, contractility is not decreased by an elevated SVR, but rather by the loss of functional myofibrils (Fig. 27-33). In this case, heart failure begins with a decrease in contractility, which leads to decreased blood pressure and increased left ventricular preload. Left heart failure resulting from infarction eventually causes the same array of manifestations as failure resulting from elevated SVR. Risk factors for left heart failure as a result of myocardial infarction include triple-vessel coronary artery disease (Castaner et al., 1984), left bundle branch block with coronary artery disease (Hamby, Weissman, Prakash, & Hoffman, 1983), diabetes mellitus (Jaffe et al., 1984), and early atrioventricular node block with anterior myocardial infarction (Sclarovsky et al., 1984).

In the elderly, ventricular diastolic stiffness can lead to pulmonary circulatory congestion without a concomitant decrease in left ventricular ejection fraction (Luchi, Snow, Luchi, Nelson, & Pircher, 1982). Aortic stenosis and aortic insufficiency, which are rather common in individuals older than 75 years of age, elevate left ventricular preload to the point where the left ventricle becomes relatively stiff and noncompliant. Elevated pressures are transmitted to the pulmonary vasculature and lead to pulmonary edema and other manifestations of left heart failure, despite the fact that left ventricular systole remains normal.

The pathogenesis of left atrial failure caused by mitral stenosis is shown in Fig. 27-34. Left atrial failure progresses to the right ventricle without a decrease in cardiac output. If the valvular stenosis is severe, however, cardiac output diminishes because of a decrease in the volume of blood delivered to the ventricle during diastole.

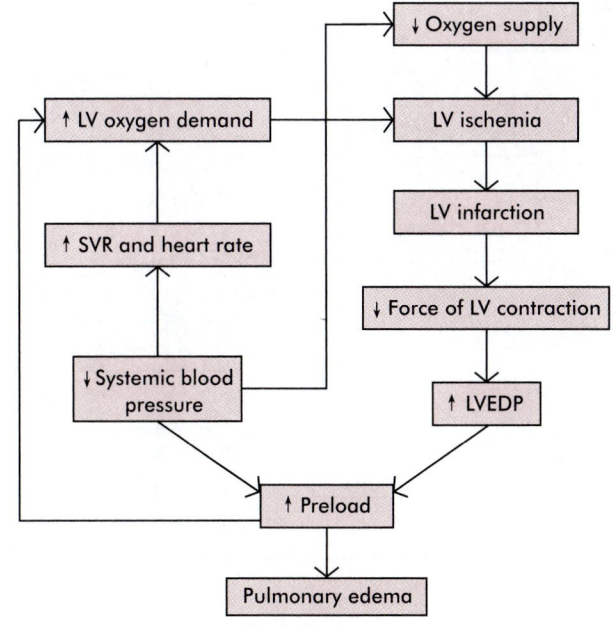

FIG. 27-32 Left heart failure (congestive heart failure) from elevated systemic vascular resistance. Left heart failure leads to right heart failure. Systemic vascular resistance and preload are exacerbated by renal and adrenal mechanisms. *LV,* Left ventricular; *LVEDP,* left ventricular end-diastolic pressure; *LA,* left atrial; *ADH,* antidiuretic hormone.

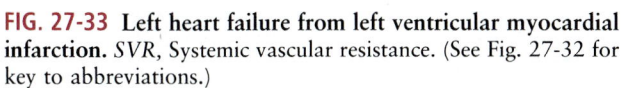

FIG. 27-33 Left heart failure from left ventricular myocardial infarction. *SVR,* Systemic vascular resistance. (See Fig. 27-32 for key to abbreviations.)

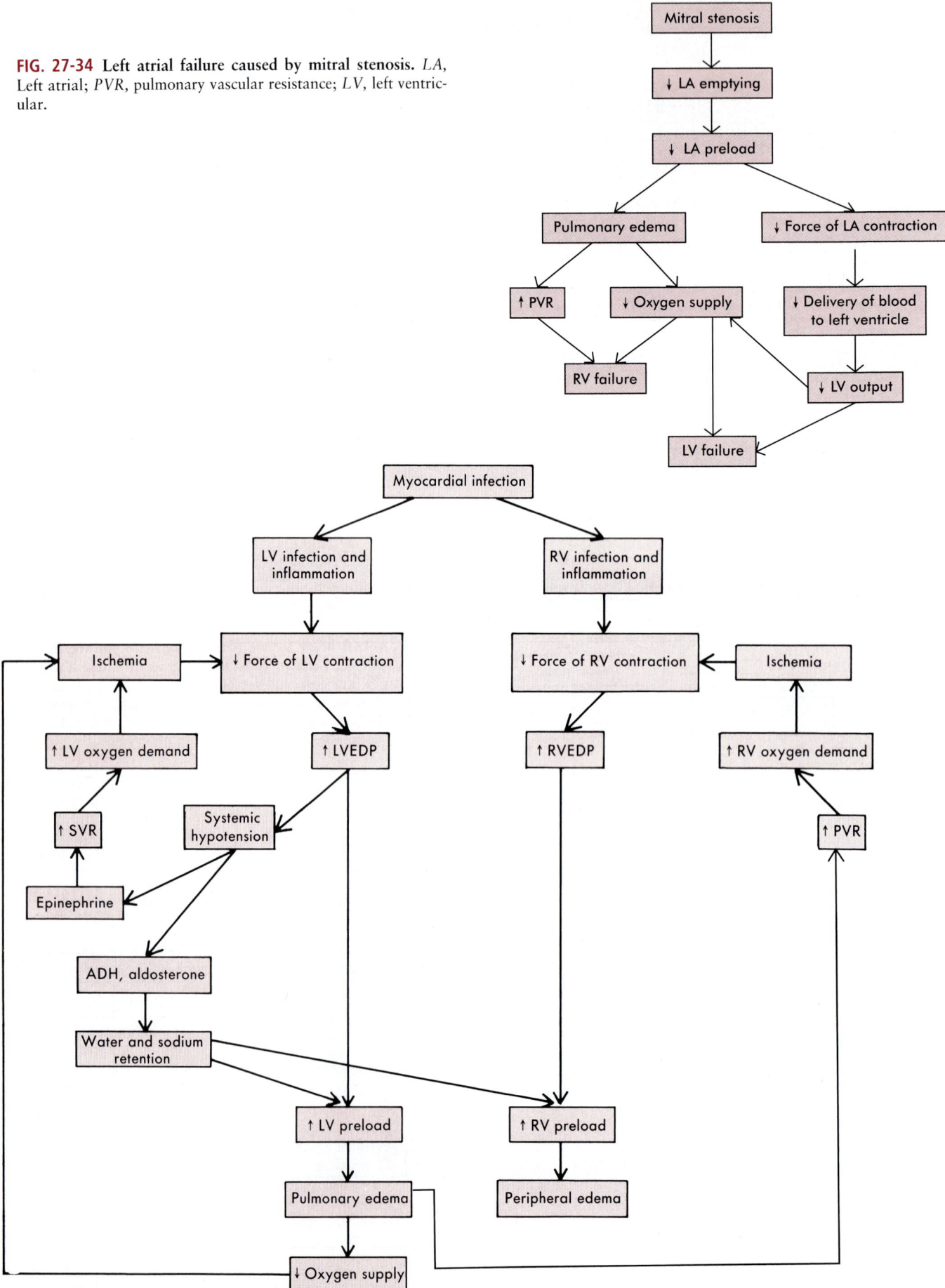

FIG. 27-34 Left atrial failure caused by mitral stenosis. *LA,* Left atrial; *PVR,* pulmonary vascular resistance; *LV,* left ventricular.

FIG. 27-35 Low-output failure. *EDP* End-diastolic pressure. (See legends to preceding figures for key to other abbreviations.)

The earliest clinical manifestation of left ventricular failure is an increase in LVEDP, which corresponds to a rise in the pulmonary capillary wedge pressure as measured by a Swan-Ganz catheter. Because compensatory mechanisms enable the body to maintain systemic blood pressure for a while, a decrease in blood pressure is usually not the first sign of left ventricular failure. Cardiac output may decrease quite early, however. Decreased cardiac output is accompanied by an increase in the SVR. Pulmonary edema, which is manifested by frothy sputum, dyspnea, decreasing oxygen content of the blood, and white fields visible on lung x-ray films, is a later sign of left ventricular failure.

Treatment of left heart failure is aimed at the underlying cause. Valvular dysfunction may require surgery. Elevated SVR is treated with vasodilators, such as nitroprusside and nitroglycerin. Vasodilators also can improve coronary artery perfusion. The **hypotension** associated with left ventricular failure, however, is usually treated with a cardiotonic antihypotensive, such as dopamine or dobutamine, especially if vasodilators also are being given to treat elevated SVR. At low doses, dopamine also increases renal perfusion.

Oxygen is administered continuously to increase the supply of oxygen to the myocardium, and diuretics are given to decrease pulmonary edema and blood volume. Sodium and fluid intake are restricted. Moderate bed rest can reduce oxygen consumption further.

Morphine sulfate is often used to treat left ventricular failure accompanied by pulmonary edema, because morphine dilates the pulmonary and systemic vessels enough to decrease pulmonary and systemic capillary hydrostatic pressure. Morphine sulfate is also an analgesic and an opiate. These properties help to improve the emotional state of the individual and may limit the cerebrally mediated release of epinephrine.

The intraaortic balloon pump (IABP) is sometimes used to treat left heart failure. The IABP is a counterpulsation device that sits in the aorta and decreases afterload, decreases preload, increases coronary artery perfusion, and increases mean systemic arterial blood pressure. The IABP has not been shown to change the mortality rate of left heart failure, however, which is 60% to 80% despite treatment.

Low-output failure

Low-output failure is biventricular. Common causes of low-output failure are cardiomyopathies and myocardial infection (myocarditis). The pathophysiology of low-output failure, like that of failure caused by myocardial infarction, begins with a loss of contractility and a decrease in cardiac output (Fig. 27-35). Because myocardial disease renders the myocardium unable to con-

tract more forcefully no matter what the stimulus, low-output failure may be unresponsive to treatments aimed at elevating preload (Howard, Puri, & Paidipaty, 1984), to cardiotonic drugs, or to sympathetic stimulation.

High-output failure

High-output failure is the inability of the heart to adequately supply the body with blood-borne nutrients, despite adequate blood volume and normal or elevated myocardial contractility. In high-output failure, the heart increases its output, but the body's metabolic needs are still not met. Common causes of high-output failure are anemia, septicemia, hyperthyroidism, and beriberi (Fig. 27-36).

Anemia decreases the oxygen-carrying capacity of the blood (see Chapter 23). Metabolic acidosis occurs as the body's cells switch to anaerobic metabolism (see Chapter 3). In response to metabolic acidosis, heart rate and stroke volume increase in an attempt to circulate blood faster. If anemia is severe, however, even maximum cardiac output does not supply the cells with enough oxygen for metabolism.

In septicemia, disturbed metabolism, bacterial toxins, and the inflammatory process cause systemic vasodilation and fever. Faced with a lowered SVR and an elevated metabolic rate, cardiac output increases to maintain blood pressure and prevent metabolic acidosis. In overwhelming septicemia, however, the heart may not be able to raise its output enough to compensate for vasodilation. Body tissues show signs of inadequate blood supply despite a very high cardiac output.

Hyperthyroidism accelerates cellular metabolism through the actions of elevated levels of thyroxine from the thyroid gland. This may occur chronically (e.g., thyrotoxicosis) or acutely (e.g., thyroid storm). Because the body's demand for oxygen threatens to cause metabolic acidosis, cardiac output increases. If blood levels of thyroxine are high and the metabolic response to thyroxine is quite vigorous, even an abnormally elevated cardiac output may be inadequate.

In the United States, beriberi (thiamine deficiency) is usually caused by malnutrition secondary to chronic alcoholism. Beriberi actually causes a mixed type of heart failure. Thiamine deficiency impairs cellular metabolism in all tissues, including the myocardium. In the heart, impaired cardiac metabolism leads to insufficient contractile strength. In blood vessels, thiamine deficiency leads mainly to peripheral vasodilation, which decreases SVR. Heart failure ensues as decreased SVR triggers increased cardiac output, which the impaired myocardium is unable to deliver. The strain of demands for increased output in the face of impaired metabolism may deplete cardiac reserves until low-output failure begins.

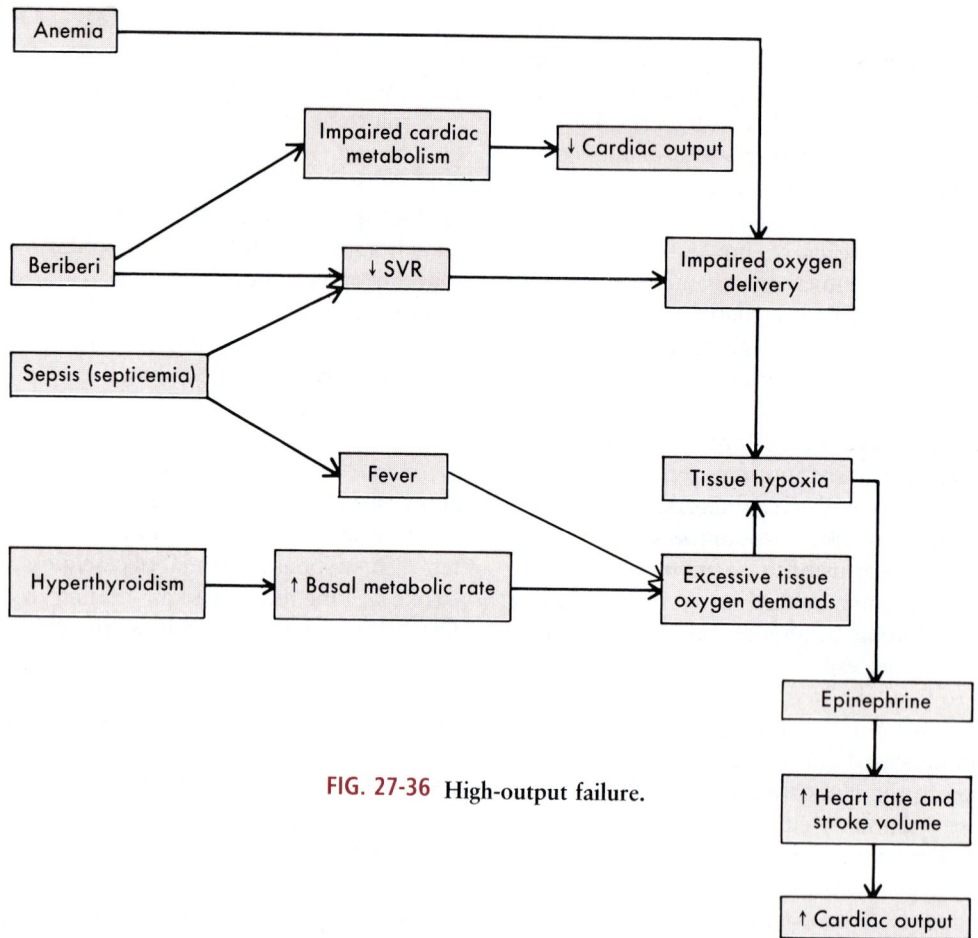

FIG. 27-36 High-output failure.

SHOCK

Shock is a condition in which the cardiovascular system fails to perfuse the tissues adequately, resulting in widespread impairment of cellular metabolism. Because tissue perfusion can be disrupted by any factor that alters heart function, blood volume, or blood pressure, shock has many causes and various clinical manifestations. Ultimately, however, shock from any cause progresses to organ failure and death, unless compensatory mechanisms reverse the process or clinical intervention succeeds. Untreated severe shock overwhelms the body's compensatory mechanisms through positive feedback loops that initiate and maintain a downward physiologic spiral.

Because the body is made up of many cells, which may function or malfunction at different stages of metabolic impairment, shock causes many diverse signs and symptoms. Subjective complaints are usually nonspecific, and may not be particularly helpful to the clinician attempting diagnosis and treatment. The individual may report feeling sick, weak, cold, hot, nauseated, dizzy, confused, afraid, thirsty, and short of breath. Observable and measurable signs and symptoms are often conflicting in nature. Blood pressure, cardiac output, and urinary output are usually—but not always—decreased. Respiratory rate is usually increased. Variable indicators of shock include alterations of heart rate, core body temperature, skin temperature, systemic vascular resistance, and skin color. Dyspnea, diaphoresis, and altered sensorium may be obvious.

Types of Shock

Shock can be classified by cause, by principal pathophysiologic process, or by clinical manifestations. Classification by cause is perhaps the most useful because it suggests the principal pathophysiologic process and focuses on the underlying disorder, which must be treated to prevent the irreversible impairment of cellular metabolism. Shock is classified by cause as cardiogenic (caused by heart failure), hypovolemic (caused by insufficient intravascular fluid volume), neurogenic (caused by neural alterations of vascular smooth muscle tone), anaphylactic (caused by immunologic processes), or septic (caused by infection). Each type of shock involves numerous clinical manifestations that are also characteristic of many other conditions, making diagnosis difficult. In addition, the body's many compensatory mechanisms can mask, for a time, many definitive signs of shock.

Cardiogenic Shock

Cardiogenic shock results from heart failure from any cause. Most cases of cardiogenic shock follow myocardial infarction. Up to 20% of all individuals with myocardial infarction (MI) can develop cardiogenic shock (Ranjadayalan, Umachandran, & Timmis, 1992). Shock also can follow congestive heart failure, myocardial ischemia, myocardial or pericardial infections, and heart failure resulting from drug toxicity. Cardiogenic shock is notoriously unresponsive to treatment, with in-hospital mortality rates of 71% reported. Mortality rates improve with the use of percutaneous coronary angioplasty and thrombolytic/aspirin therapy (Crimi et al., 1988; Hibbard et al., 1992; Ranjadayalan et al., 1992). The pathophysiology of cardiogenic shock is shown in Fig. 27-37. As cardiac output decreases, renal and hypothalamic adaptive responses maintain or increase blood volume. Blood pressure is maintained through vasoconstriction in response to catecholamine release from the adrenals. Catecholamines also increase contractility and heart rate. Increases in blood volume and vascular resistance succeed in normalizing blood pressure and increasing cardiac performance, but at the cost of increasing myocardial demands for oxygen and nutrients. Increasing myocardial requirements further strain the al-

ready failing heart, which can no longer pump an adequate volume of blood with sufficient force to perfuse the tissues. The direct effect of decreased tissue perfusion is impaired cellular metabolism. (Normal cellular metabolism is discussed in Chapter 1.)

The clinical manifestations of cardiogenic shock are caused by widespread impairment of cellular metabolism. They include impaired mentation, elevated preload in the systemic and pulmonary vasculature, systemic and pulmonary edema, dusky skin color, low blood pressure, oliguria, ileus, and dyspnea. Elevated preloads and low cardiac output are manifestations of heart failure (Howard et al., 1984).

Hypovolemic Shock

Hypovolemic shock is caused by loss of whole blood (hemorrhage), plasma (burns), or interstitial fluid (diaphoresis, diabetes mellitus, diabetes insipidus, emesis, or diuresis) in large amounts. Loss of whole blood or plasma causes hypovolemia directly. Loss of interstitial fluid causes it indirectly by promoting diffusion of plasma from the intravascular to the extravascular space. Hypovolemic shock begins to develop when intravascular volume has decreased by about 15%.

Hypovolemia is offset initially by compensatory

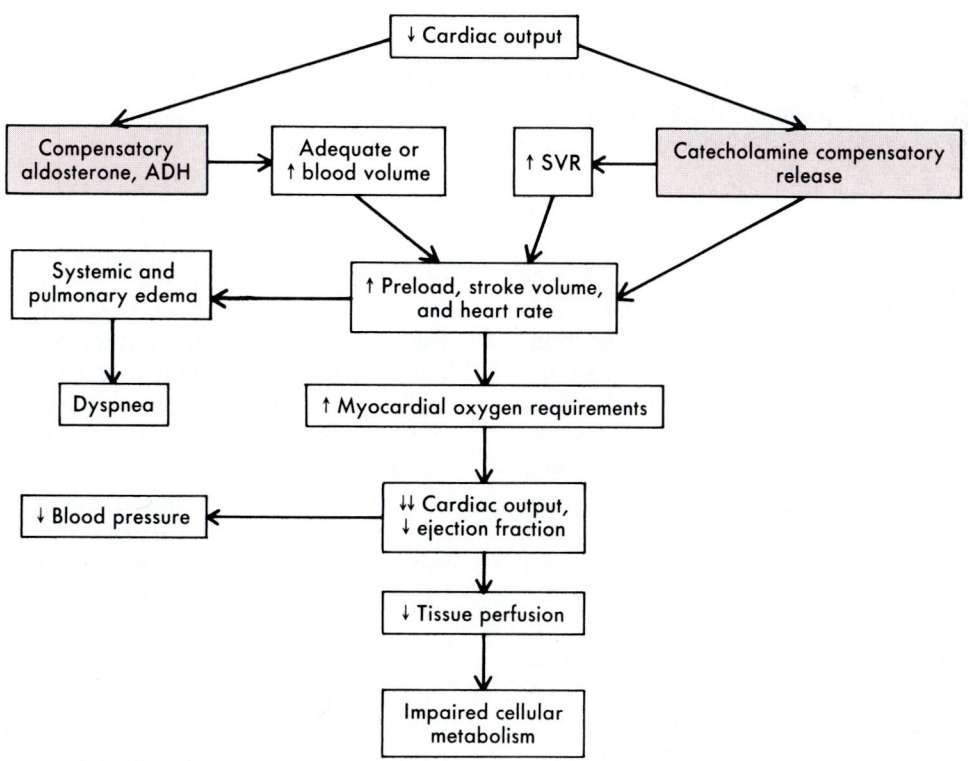

FIG. 27-37 Cardiogenic shock. Shock becomes life threatening when compensatory mechanisms (colored labels) cause increased myocardial oxygen requirements.

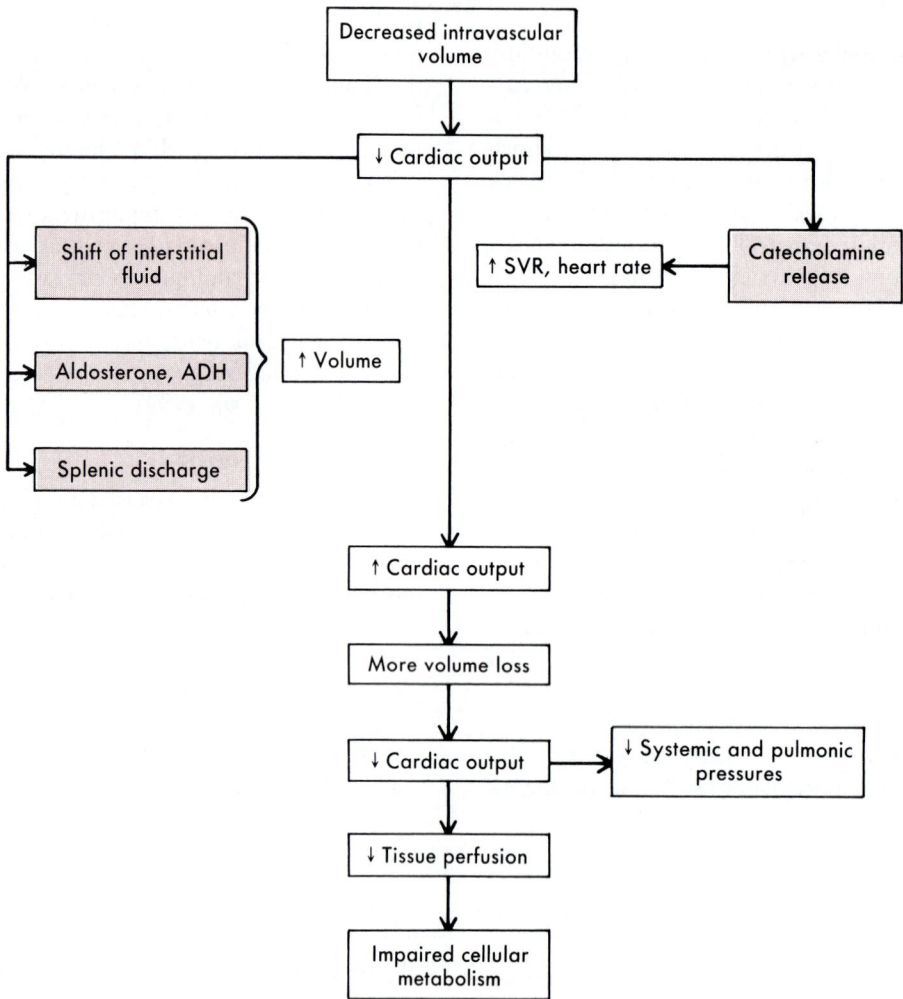

FIG. 27-38 Hypovolemic shock. This type of shock becomes life threatening when compensatory mechanisms (colored labels) are overwhelmed by continued loss of intravascular volume.

mechanisms (Fig. 27-38). Heart rate and SVR increase as a result of catecholamine release by the adrenals. This boosts both cardiac output and tissue perfusion pressures. Compelled by a decrease in capillary hydrostatic pressures, interstitial fluid moves into the vascular compartment. The liver and spleen add to blood volume by disgorging stored red blood cells and plasma. In the kidneys, renin (through several intermediaries) stimulates aldosterone release and the retention of sodium (and hence water), whereas ADH from the posterior pituitary gland increases water retention.

These compensatory mechanisms are finite, however. If the initial fluid or blood loss is great, or if loss continues, compensation fails, resulting in decreased tissue perfusion. As in cardiogenic shock, nutrient delivery to the cells is impaired, and cellular metabolism fails.

Mortality rates for traumatic hemorrhagic shock range from 10% to 31%. Fluid replacement is the treat-

ment of choice and time to normalization of blood volume is critical because delays increase mortality rates (Esposito, Gens, Smith, Scorpio, & Buchman, 1991; Mattox, Bickell, Pepe, Burch, & Feliciano, 1989).

The clinical manifestations of hypovolemic shock include high SVR, poor skin turgor, thirst, oliguria, low systemic and pulmonary preloads, and rapid heart rates. The differences between the signs and symptoms of hypovolemic shock and those of cardiogenic shock are mainly because of differences in fluid volume and cardiac muscle health (Howard et al., 1984).

Neurogenic Shock

Neurogenic shock is sometimes called vasogenic shock. Both terms refer to a widespread and massive vasodilation that results from an imbalance between parasympathetic and sympathetic stimulation of vascular smooth muscle (see Chapter 26). Occasionally, parasympathetic overstimulation or sympathetic understimulation persists, causing vasodilation for an extended period. Extreme, persistent vasodilation leads to neurogenic shock (Fig. 27-39). Neurogenic shock creates "relative hypovolemia." Blood volume has not changed, but the amount of space containing the blood has increased, so that SVR decreases drastically. With a decreased SVR, pressure in the vessels is inadequate to drive nutrients across capillary membranes, and nutrient delivery to the cells is impaired. As with other types of shock, this leads to impaired cellular metabolism.

Neurogenic shock can be caused by any factor that stimulates parasympathetic or inhibits sympathetic stimulation of vascular smooth muscle. (Parasympathetic stimulation automatically inhibits sympathetic activity, and vice versa; see Chapter 26.) Normally, sympathetic stimulation maintains muscle tone. If sympathetic stimulation is interrupted or inhibited, vasodilation occurs. Therefore, trauma to the spinal cord or medulla, conditions that interrupt the supply of oxygen to the medulla, or conditions that deprive the medulla of glucose (e.g., insulin reactions) all can cause neurogenic shock by interrupting sympathetic activity. Depressive drugs, anesthetic agents, and severe emotional stress and pain are other causes of neurogenic shock.

The clinical hallmark of neurogenic shock is a very low SVR, along with other indicators of excessive parasympathetic activity. Bradycardia is the most obvious manifestation, especially in the early stages. Bradycardia may cease when compensatory mechanisms, particularly an increase in sympathetic system activity, have been initiated. The ejection fraction remains high, indicating a healthy myocardium, whereas central venous pressure decreases as the veins dilate. Neurogenic shock causes fainting if blood pressure decreases to the point that cerebral metabolism is not sufficient to support consciousness. Most episodes of fainting are *not* shock, however; for such episodes to progress to shock is rare. By allowing the blood pressure to equalize from head to toe as the individual becomes prone, fainting can actually prevent shock.

Anaphylactic Shock

Anaphylactic shock is the outcome of a widespread hypersensitivity reaction known as anaphylaxis. The basic physiologic alteration in anaphylactic shock is the same as that of neurogenic shock; that is, vasodilation, **peripheral pooling,** and relative hypovolemia, leading to decreased tissue perfusion and impaired cellular metabolism (Fig. 27-40). Anaphylactic shock is often more severe than other types of normovolemic shock because the hypersensitivity reaction that triggers vasodilation has other pathophysiologic effects that rapidly involve the entire body.

Anaphylactic shock begins as an allergic reac-

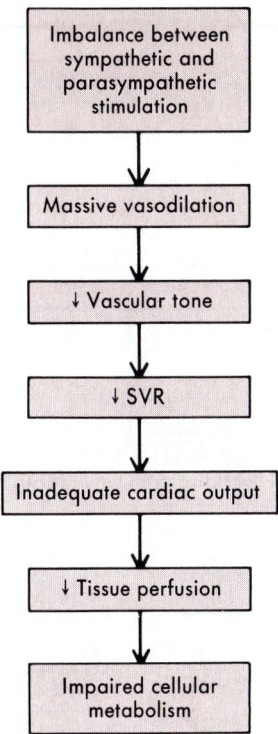

FIG. 27-39 Neurogenic shock.

tion—an immune and inflammatory response—to an allergen. (An allergen is an antigen to which an individual is hypersensitive; see Chapters 6, 7, and 8 for discussion of immunity, inflammation, and hypersensitivity.) Some allergens known to cause hypersensitivity reactions are insect venoms, pollens, shellfish, penicillin, and animal sera. Once in the body, the allergen causes an extensive immune and inflammatory response. The vascular effects of this response include vasodilation and increased vascular permeability, resulting in peripheral pooling and tissue edema. The extravascular effects include constriction of extravascular smooth muscle. Constriction often causes respiratory difficulty because it tends to affect smooth muscle layers in airway walls (e.g., the larynx and bronchioles; see Chapter 29).

The onset of anaphylactic shock is usually sudden, and progression to death can occur within minutes unless emergency treatment is given. The first manifestations of shock may be anxiety, difficulty breathing, gastrointestinal cramps, edema, hives (urticaria), and sensations of burning or itching of the skin. A precipitous decrease in blood pressure occurs and is followed by impaired mentation. Other signs include decreased SVR, with high or normal cardiac output, and oliguria. Treatment begins with removal of the antigen (if possible). Epinephrine is administered to cause vasoconstriction and reverse airway constriction. Volume expanders

FIG. 27-40 Anaphylactic shock.

(such as lactated Ringer's solution) are given intravenously to reverse the relative hypovolemia, and antihistamines and steroids are given to stop the inflammatory reaction.

Septic Shock

Septic shock is complex, and the body of knowledge that explains its genesis and progression is the most rapidly changing of all the types of shock. Gram-negative bacteria account for more than half of all cases of septic shock, gram-positive bacteria for about 10%, and *Candida albicans* for about 2% (Smith, Arregui, Promnitz, & Feldman, 1991). The two most common sources of infection are the respiratory tract and the gastrointestinal tract (Smith et al., 1991). Mortality rates from septic shock vary from 10% (Cunnion & Parrillo, 1989) to 90% (Parker & Parrillo, 1983) in current literature, but the most believable rates range from about 40% to 70% (Bone, Fisher, & Clemmer, 1987; Pilz et al., 1991; Ruokonen, Takala, Kari, & Alhava, 1991).

Septic shock begins with the development of bacteremia (Fig. 27-41) (infection of the blood; see Chapter 2).

Bacteremia may exist for quite some time before shock develops (Table 27-14). In general, individuals who are aged, critically ill, or immune compromised are at an increased risk to develop shock from bacteremia. At a cellular level, the development of sepsis seems dependent on several factors (Bone, 1991a): (1) the response of target cells to the chemicals of inflammation, (2) the presence of multiple mediators of inflammation in the immediate cellular environment, (3) the ability of the target cell to release mediators of inflammation, and (4) the efficacy of the negative feedback mechanisms that the host is able to generate.

Although endotoxin (see Chapters 2 and 7) from the infectious agent can directly cause the hypothalamus to induce fever and can produce the vasodilation characteristic of septic shock (Snell & Parrillo, 1991), the generation of shock from bacteremia is dependent on several inflammatory chemicals other than endotoxin. Four major chemicals among nearly a dozen have been implicated in the genesis of shock: interleukins (IL), tumor necrosis factor (TNF), platelet-activating factor (PAF), and myocardial depressant substance (MDS). Curiously,

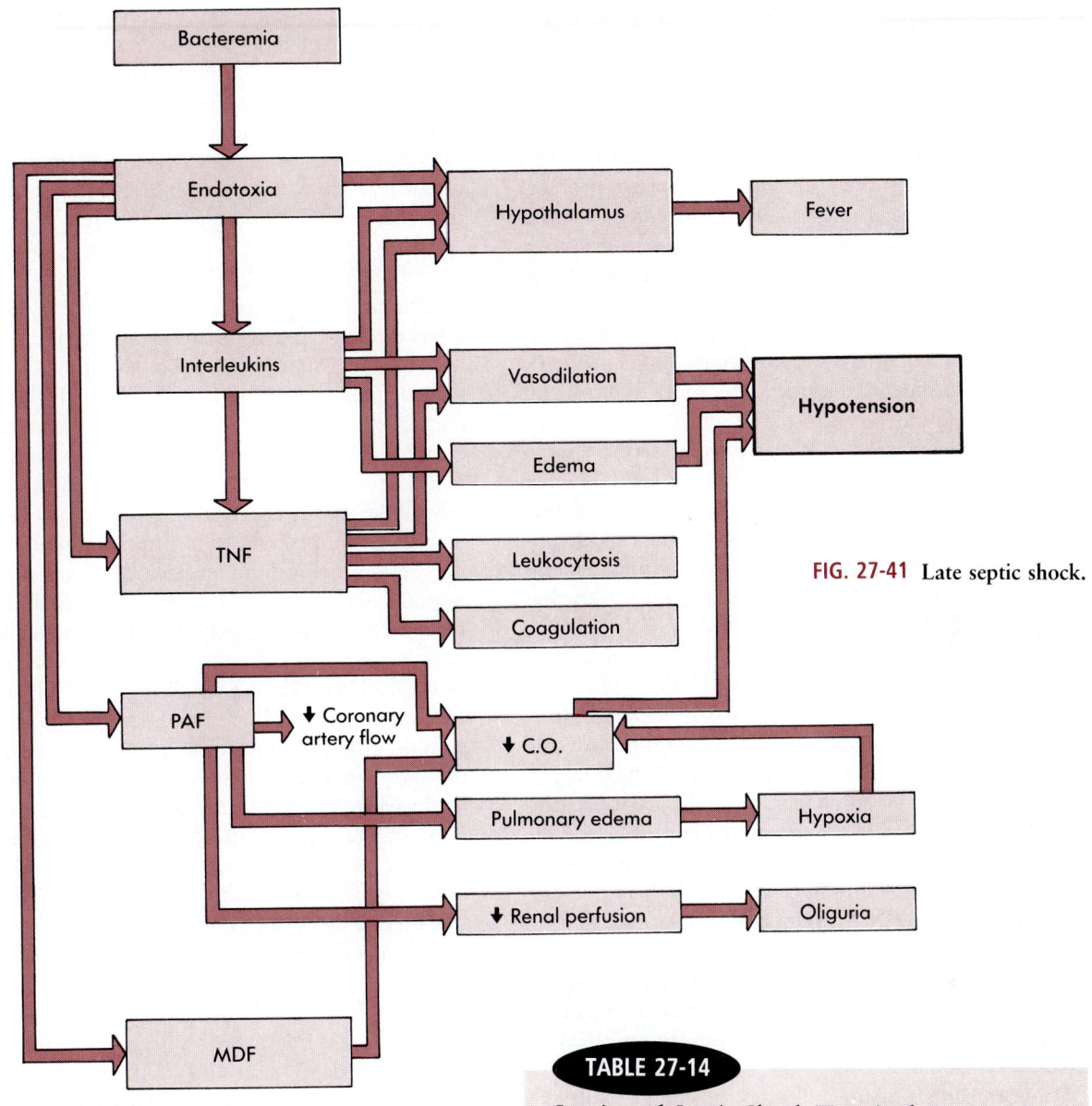

FIG. 27-41 Late septic shock.

it appears that the only chemical of inflammation that is not elevated in septic shock is a potent vasodilator, histamine (Jacobs, Shelhamer, Kaliner, & Parrillo, 1989).

The interleukins

Interleukins (IL) are cytokines with variable, often opposing functions (see Chapter 6). They are released in septic shock in response to endotoxin and TNF. In shock, interleukin-1 (IL-1) causes arteriolar smooth muscle dilation, capillary basement membrane leaks, and changes in carbohydrate production and uptake. Interleukin-1 causes the hypothalamus to induce fever and initiates the complement cascade; stimulates the release of TNF and several other interleukins; enhances tissue cell sensitivity to TNF; and promotes polymor-

TABLE 27-14

Sepsis and Septic Shock Terminology

Term	Definition/comments
Bacteremia	At least one positive blood culture
Septicemia	Too broadly used, confusing; delete from use
Sepsis syndrome	Bacteremia plus evidence of altered organ perfusion
Septic shock	Sepsis syndrome with reversible hypotension
Refractory septic shock	Sepsis syndrome with irreversible, prolonged (>1 hr) hypotension

Modified from Bone, 1991a.

phonuclear cell production and adhesion (Bone, 1991a; Cerami, 1991; Dal Nogare, 1991; Snell & Parrillo, 1991; Zentella, Kanogue, & Cerami, 1991).

Interleukin-3 stimulates mast cells and natural killer cells to produce TNF. Interleukin-6 acts as a helper cell for T- and B-cells and stimulates the release of acute-phase proteins from the liver. One acute-phase protein, C-reactive protein, is released so consistently in acute septic shock that its serum levels are used to establish the diagnosis of septic shock (Bone, 1991a; Zentella et al., 1991).

Interleukin-4 and IL-8 supply negative feedback to the chemical mediators of septic shock (Bone, 1991a). In susceptible individuals, the generation of IL-4 and IL-8 may simply be both too little and too late to prevent the massive cellular alterations of septic shock. Thus, the interleukins have several target cells. The net effect of the interleukins in bacteremia leading to septic shock is the symptoms of fever, vasodilation and hypotension, edema, and elevated white blood count. The interleukins trigger other chemicals of inflammation that ensure and reinforce these symptoms.

Tumor necrosis factor

Like the interleukins, TNF is also a cytokine. It is thought to be the major chemical responsible for the generation of septic shock in bacteremic individuals. It is produced from macrophages, natural killer cells, and mast cells in response to endotoxin and interleukins. Two kinds of TNF are currently known: TNF alpha, or cachectin from macrophages; and TNF beta, or lymphotoxin from T cells. Tumor necrosis factor alpha predominates in septic shock, probably because of the increased activation of macrophages when compared with T-cells during bacteremia (Cerami, 1991; Zentella et al., 1991). (See Chapter 7 for a complete list of all cytokines.)

Tumor necrosis factor infiltrates the complement and coagulation cascades. Tumor necrosis factor induces the production of several interleukins. It stimulates polymorphonuclear cell production and acts directly in the hypothalamus to produce fever. It activates the complement and coagulation cascades and is directly toxic to vascular endothelial cells. Tumor necrosis factor assists with tissue regeneration in healthy individuals, but in the bacteremic individual its overproduction leads to capillary dilation and leak, changes in carbohydrate metabolism, and fever (Bone, 1991a; Dal Nogare, 1991; Snell & Parrillo, 1991; Tracey, 1991; Zentella et al., 1991).

Tumor necrosis factor generates the same symptoms of septic shock in susceptible individuals as do the interleukins. Tumor necrosis factor and interleukins, together, are redundant, which indicates the importance to the body of these initially compensatory and later damaging responses in bacteremia.

Platelet-activating factor (PAF) is released from mononuclear phagocytes, platelets, and some endothelial cells in response to endotoxin. Like endotoxin, interleukins, and TNF, PAF causes vascular dilation and leak and mobilization of white blood cells. Platelet-activating factor induces systemic hypotension, promotes leukocyte and platelet activation, and stimulates the release of TNF.

Platelet-activating factor

Platelet-activating factor is a singular chemical in that it has direct toxic effects on certain organs. In the heart, it causes coronary artery constriction and decreases myocardial contractility. In the lungs, PAF is responsible for the generation of pulmonary edema through increased vascular permeability, margination of leukocytes, and endothelial damage in the alveoli. In the kidneys, PAF decreases renal blood flow and the production of urine through renal arterial vasoconstriction. It decreases urine sodium levels and induces interstitial albumin leakage. In the gastrointestinal tract, PAF causes ulceration in animals. Platelet-activating factor also may be neurotoxic (Anderson, Bensard, & Harken, 1991; Bone, 1991a). Like interleukins and TNF, PAF generates symptoms of shock in susceptible bacteremic individuals. However, PAF differs from these two chemicals of septic shock in that it may initiate multiple organ failure in septic shock. Platelet-activating factor directly impairs other, vital organ systems. This characteristic of PAF becomes critical when it is understood that if the individual with septic shock survives the hypotension of this illness, he or she is at risk to die of multiple organ failure (Ruokonen et al., 1991).

Myocardial depressant substance

Septic shock is characterized by, and confounded by, a myocardial depression and dilation that is resilient to treatment and unrelated to myocardial oxygenation and perfusion (Snell & Parrillo, 1991). In early septic shock, cardiac output ranges from normal to elevated; this cardiac output was thought previously to be related to the ease with which the heart could empty into the dilated vasculature. Later in septic shock, the heart fails even when the myocardium was not previously subjected to hypoxemia or low-flow states. The reason for this initial high cardiac output and later biventricular failure remained obscure until the discovery of **myocardial depressant substance** (MDS). Myocardial depressant substance is secreted from white blood cells in response to endotoxin. It is produced in septic shock regardless of what bacteria served as the nidus of infection. In response to MDS, the myocardium becomes depressed and dilated, with both ventricles involved simultaneously (Demeules, 1984; Parker et al., 1990). The dilation initially may allow the heart to compensate for myofibril depression, according to Starling's law of the heart, with a normal or elevated cardiac output. Later, the ventricular dilation is insufficient to counteract myofibril depression. This biventricular failure does not respond to volume infusion as it often does in individuals with septic shock. Hypotension is the main cause of early death in septic shock (Ruokonen et al., 1991). If the individual survives the shock, however, cardiac failure is reversible (Ognibene, Parker, Nataneon, Shelhamer, & Parrillo, 1988).

The result of these chemical mediators initially is a hyperdynamic state. This hyperdynamic state of early septic shock includes fever, vasodilation, increased cardiac output, interstitial edema, and changes in carbohydrate metabolism. Fever raises cellular metabolic rates so that tissues become oxygen-starved and lactic acidosis develops. Lactic acidosis is a hallmark of septic shock, and changes in lactate levels indicate the relative success of treatment efforts (Howard et al., 1984; Mizock & Falk, 1992). Vasodilation in capillary beds, arterioles, and venules makes the individual appear pink and feel hot, and lowers blood pressure. Vasodilation increases the oxygen deficit in the capillary beds as sluggish blood flow through the capillaries decreases perfusion pressure into the tissues. The raised cardiac output of early septic shock initially can compensate for fever and vasodilation in some individuals, but in many, even very high outputs simply do not meet the metabolic demands of others. Interstitial edema impairs the delivery of oxygen and other nutrients into the cells and further increases the oxygen deficit of tissues. (See multiple organ dysfunction syndrome at right.)

The pathogenesis of the changes in carbohydrate metabolism of septic shock is not yet understood. Serum levels of both glucagon and insulin increase. Serum glucose levels fluctuate, whereas the use of glucose is enhanced. Glycogen degradation increases and glycogen synthesis decreases (Zentella et al., 1991). Later in septic shock, glucose and glycogen stores are depleted and the heart reaches its dilatable limits. The heart, like all other tissues, is oxygen- and glucose-depleted. Cardiac output decreases and tissue oxygenation and function further degenerate. Multiple organ dysfunction syndrome often develops.

The wide range of symptoms in and responses to septic shock can be accounted for when individual physiologies are considered. The strength of the inflammatory response varies among individuals, as does the strength of each person's immune response. The involvement of a varying number of cells, tissues, and organs as the septic shock progresses also accounts for the varying and confusing spectrum of symptoms seen clinically. The type of infective agent involved does not affect the course or outcome of septic shock significantly (Siegel, 1983).

Toxic shock syndrome (TSS), which is most common in menstruating women, is a form of septic shock with a similar set of clinical manifestations. Toxic shock syndrome is characterized by extremely low blood pressure, high fever, cerebral manifestations (confusion, syncope, headache), and skin rash. In toxic shock, bacterial toxins, usually those of *Staphylococcus aureus*, may migrate from the site of infection (e.g., the vagina) into the blood, triggering a widespread inflammatory response that leads to peripheral vasodilation, impaired cellular metabolism, and septic shock.

Toxic shock syndrome can be caused by *S. aureus* invasion from any site, but occurs most frequently from the vagina during menstruation. In approximately 70% of all toxic shock cases, the strain of *S. aureus* cultured from the individual makes TSS toxin-1 (TSST-1). In the remaining 30%, the *S. aureus* recovered excretes enterotoxins B and C (Reingold, 1991; Schlievert, 1989). Toxic shock syndrome toxin-1 and enterotoxins B and C are postulated to trigger an outpouring of the interleukins and TNF (Parsonnet, 1989).

The number of cases of toxic shock syndrome has decreased considerably since it was first recognized 10 years ago. Most cases in the first half of the 1980s were related to tampon use. Current incidence of menstrual toxic shock syndrome ranges from 1 to 3 per 100,000. Current morbidity rates are approximately 2% (Reingold, 1991). The decline in TSS resulted from: (1) lowering of tampon absorbency, (2) change in tampon composition from polyester foam and cross-linked carboxymethylcellulose to entirely cotton or rayon, (3) public education leading to improved recognition by women and their health care providers, and (4) a decrease in tampon use (Schuchat & Broome, 1991).

Multiple Organ Dysfunction Syndrome

Multiple organ dysfunction syndrome (MODS) is the progressive failure of two or more organ systems after a very severe illness or injury. Although sepsis and septic shock are the most common causes, MODS also can be triggered by persistent inflammatory foci, necrotic tissue, severe trauma, major surgery, burns, circulatory shock, acute pancreatitis, acute renal failure, adult respiratory syndrome, and other severe injuries. Multiple organ dysfunction syndrome is a relatively new diagnosis, first described in 1975 (Baue, 1975). Today, MODS is diagnosed in 15% of individuals admitted to critical care units (Bone, 1991b; Knaus & Wagner, 1989). The mortality rate of MODS is 60% to 90%, and approaches 100% if three or more organs are involved, sepsis is present, and the individual is older than 65 years of age (Bone, 1991b; Cerra, 1990; Huddleston, 1992). It is the major cause of death following septic, traumatic, and burn injuries.

Pathophysiology

Although sepsis is a frequent component of MODS, clinical infection is not necessary for its development.

FIG. 27-42 Pathogenesis of multiple organ dysfunction syndrome.

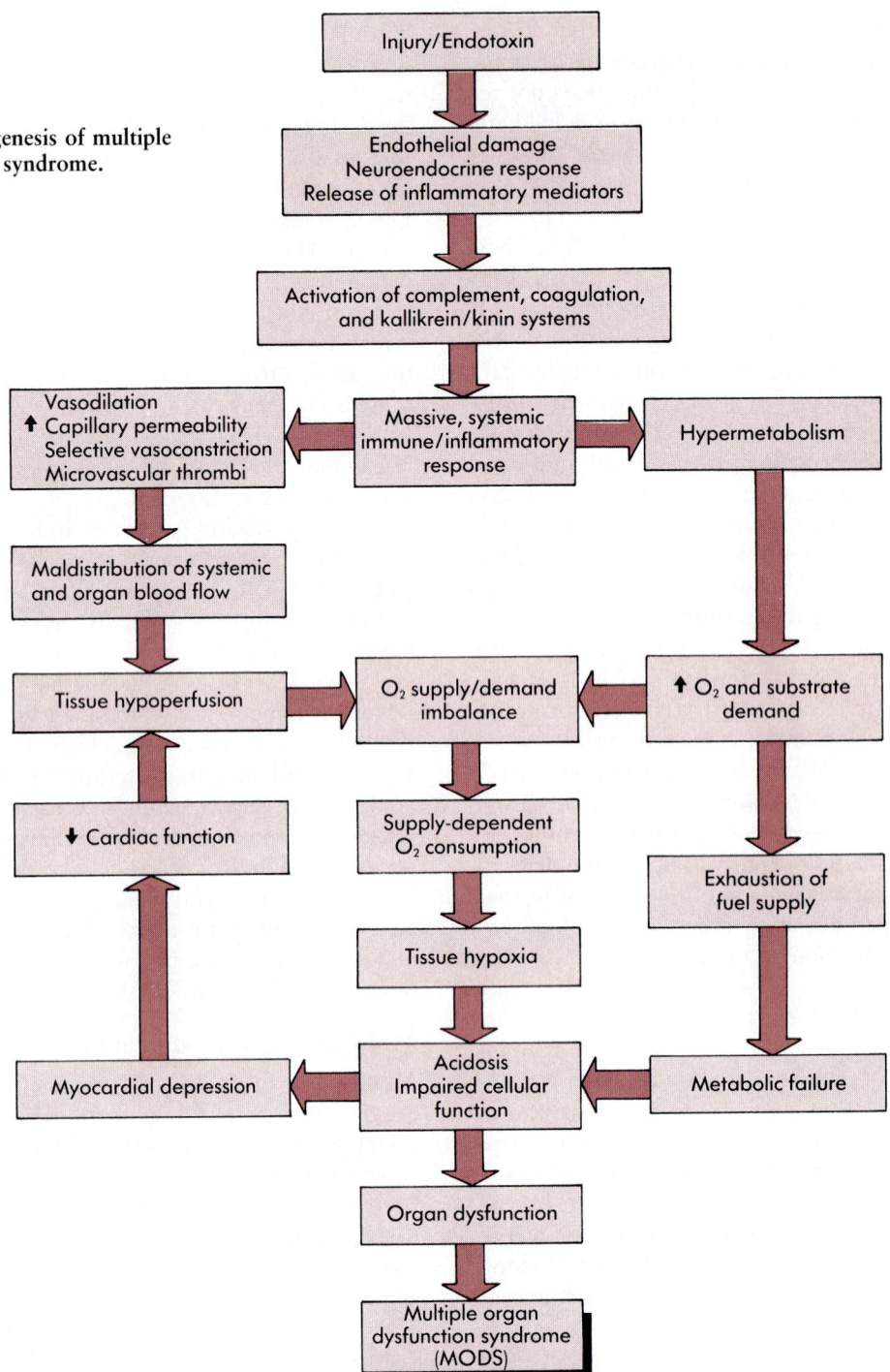

Any process that triggers the body's inflammatory response has the potential to initiate MODS, including direct mechanical, chemical, and thermal injury to tissue or damage by bacterial endotoxin (Fig. 27-42).

After an insult, the neuroendocrine system is activated. The stress hormones cortisol, epinephrine, norepinephrine, and endorphins are released into the circulation (see Chapter 9). The sympathetic nervous system is stimulated to compensate for complications resulting from the injury, such as fluid loss and hypotension. Vascular endothelial damage occurs as a direct result of injury or from damage by endotoxin or inflammatory mediators released into the circulation. The vascular endothelium becomes permeable, allowing fluid and cells to leak into the interstitial spaces, contributing to hypotension and hypoperfusion. When

TABLE 27-15

Inflammatory Cells and Multisystem Organ Failure (MSOF)

Cell	Activators	Contribution to MSOF
Neutrophils	Complement kinins, endotoxin, clotting factors	Release of phagocytic products: toxic oxygen free radicals, superoxide ion, hydrogen peroxide, hydroxyl radicals, proteases, platelet-activating factor (PAF), arachidonic acid metabolites (prostaglandins, thromboxane, leukotrienes)
		Endothelial damage, vasodilation, vasopermeability, microvascular coagulation, selective vasoconstriction, hypotension, shock
Macrophages	Complement, endotoxin, chemotactic factors	Release of same phagocytic products as neutrophils
		Release of monokines: tumor necrosis factor (TNF), interleukin-1 (IL-1)
		TNF produces fever, anorexia, hyperglycemia, weight loss
Mast cells	Direct injury, endotoxin, complement	Release of histamine, PAF, arachidonic acid metabolites
		Vasodilation, vasopermeability, hypotension, shock

damaged, the endothelium loses much of its ability to prevent blood clotting and releases tissue thromboplastin, resulting in microvascular coagulation. (Function of the endothelium is discussed in Chapter 26.)

Because of the initial insult and release of mediators, three major plasma enzyme cascades are activated: complement, coagulation, and kallikrein/kinin. Complement components, particularly the anaphylatoxins, C3a and C5a, activate phagocytes and induce further inflammation, particularly damage to the endothelium. Because tissue injury and endothelial cell damage are extensive, coagulation is uncontrolled, resulting in microvascular thrombus formation and tissue ischemia. Fibrinolytic mechanisms are activated concurrently, and the combination of precoagulant and anticoagulant processes can lead to disseminated intravascular coagulation (DIC) (see Chapter 24). The kallikrein/kinin system also is activated, resulting in the release of bradykinin, a potent vasodilator that contributes to low systemic vascular resistance. The overall effect of the activation of these three systems is a hyperinflammatory and hypercoagulant state that maintains the edema formation, cardiovascular instability, endothelial damage, and clotting abnormalities. Once inflammatory mediators have been released and the plasma enzyme cascades have been activated, a massive systemic immune/inflammatory response develops. The major cells participating in the response are neutrophils, macrophages, and mast cells (Table 27-15). The pathway by which neutrophils and macrophages are activated is variable and involves multiple events rather than individual insults. It is the multiple stimulation that sets the stage for MODS (Anderson & Harken, 1990).

The numerous inflammatory processes operating in MODS cause maldistribution of blood flow, which is a major component in the pathophysiology of MODS, and hypermetabolism. Alterations in blood flow can occur in the microvascular, organ, or regional circulations, resulting in a hyperdynamic circulation with increased venous return. There is a decrease in oxygen delivery to the tissues, however, despite the supranormal systemic blood flow, for several reasons. First is the shunting of blood past selected regional capillary beds. Shunting is caused by autoregulation in some organs that occurs because inflammatory mediators override the normal vascular tone to cause selective vasoconstriction, and because injured endothelial cells are unable to respond to normal vasodilator mediators. Second, interstitial edema resulting from microvascular changes in permeability contributes to decreased oxygen delivery by creating a relative hypovolemia and by increasing the distance oxygen must travel to reach the cells. Third, capillary obstruction occurs because of formation of microvascular thrombi and the aggregation of inflammatory cells.

Hypermetabolism in MODS with accompanying alterations in carbohydrate, fat, and lipid metabolism is initially a compensatory measure to meet the body's increased demands for energy. Over time, hypermetabolism becomes detrimental, placing enormous demands on the heart. Energy expenditure increases to 1.5 to 2 times the base level, and cardiac output increases to 10 to 12 L/min (normal resting output is 5 L/min) (Cerra, 1990). Hypermetabolism is the result of the neuroendocrine response to stress with the release of catecholamines and cortisol and the action of TNF and IL-1. The alterations in metabolism affect all aspects of substrate utilization. Most important is the catabolism of protein, primarily of skeletal muscle and visceral organs. Lean body mass can be significantly depleted in 7 to 10 days (Lekander & Cerra, 1990). Hyperglycemia develops as gluconeogenesis by the liver increases and glucose use by the cells decreases. Fatty acids are mobilized from adipose tissue. The net result of the hypermetabolism is depletion of oxygen and fuel supplies.

Myocardial depression also accompanies MODS. The cause remains unclear, but possible explanations are the effect of myocardial depressant factor (MDF) on myocardial contractility and a decrease in the number of beta-adrenergic receptors.

The decrease in oxygen delivery to the cells caused by maldistribution of blood flow, myocardial depression, and the hypermetabolic state combine to create an imbalance in oxygen supply and demand. This imbalance is critical in the pathogenesis of MODS because it results in a pathologic condition known as **supply-dependent oxygen consumption**. Ordinarily, the amount of oxygen consumed by the cells depends only on the needs of the cells because there is an adequate reserve of oxygen that can be delivered if needed. The reserve, however, has been exhausted in MODS, and the amount of oxygen consumed becomes dependent on the amount the circulation is able to delivery; this amount is inadequate in MODS. Therefore, tissue hypoxia with cellular acidosis and impaired cellular function ensue and result in the multiple organ failure characteristic of MODS.

Clinical Manifestations

There is a well-established clinical pattern in the development of MODS. After the inciting event and aggressive resuscitation of the individual for approximately 24 hours, the individual develops a low-grade fever, tachycardia, dyspnea, altered mental status, and hyperdynamic and hypermetabolic states. The lung is the first organ to fail, resulting in adult respiratory distress syndrome (ARDS) (see Chapter 30). Between 7 and 10 days, the hypermetabolic and hyperdynamic states intensify, bacteremia with enteric organisms is common, and signs of liver and kidney failure appear. During days 14 to 21, renal and liver failures become more severe and the gastrointestinal and immune systems fail. Ultimately, there is cardiovascular collapse. If the individual's condition has not improved by the end of the third week, survival is unlikely. Death usually occurs between days 21 and 28 (Bone, 1991b; Lekander & Cerra, 1990).

The clinical manifestations of individual organ failure in MODS are inflammation, tissue hypoxia, and hypermetabolism. Respiratory failure progresses early to ARDS and is characterized by tachypnea, pulmonary edema with crackles and diminished breath sounds, use of accessory muscles, and hypoxemia. Ventilatory demand is increased to 15 to 20 L/min ventilation (Lekander & Cerra, 1990). Liver failure, although developing early, is not clinically detectable until later stages of MODS when jaundice, abdominal distention, liver tenderness, muscle wasting, and hepatic encephalopathy appear. All facets of metabolism, substance detoxification, and immune response are impaired; albumin and clotting factor synthesis decreases, protein wastes accumulate, and liver tissue macrophages (Kupffer cells) no longer function effectively.

Progressive oliguria, azotemia, and edema mark the development of renal failure. Anuria, hyperkalemia, and metabolic acidosis may occur if renal shutdown is severe. The gastrointestinal system is very sensitive to ischemic and inflammatory injury. Clinical manifestations of bowel involvement are hemorrhage, ileus, malabsorption, diarrhea or constipation, vomiting, anorexia, abdominal pain, and pancreatitis. Compounding the damage caused by injury to the bowel is the phenomenon of bacterial translocation. When mediators and severe ischemia injure the mucosal epithelium, bacteria and endotoxin pass from the gut into the portal circulation. The overwhelmed liver is unable to clear these products and they move into the systemic circulation. Thus, whether infection or some other injury was the precipitating cause of MODS, once the systemic response is initiated, infection occurs (Cerra, 1990).

The signs and symptoms of cardiac failure in the hypermetabolic, hyperdynamic phase of MODS are similar to those of septic shock: tachycardia, bounding pulse, increased cardiac output, decrease in systemic vascular resistance, hypotension, warm skin, and supraventricular arrhythmias (see p. 1066 for a discussion of septic shock). In the terminal stages, hypodynamic circulation with bradycardia, profound hypotension, and ventricular arrhythmias may develop. Ischemia and inflammation are responsible for the central nervous system manifestations, which include apprehension, confusion, disorientation, restlessness, agitation, headache, decreased cognitive ability and memory, and decreased level of consciousness. Seizures and coma can occur when ischemia is severe.

Evaluation and Treatment

Because there is no specific therapy for MODS, early detection is extremely important so that supportive measures can be initiated immediately. Frequent assessment of the clinical status of individuals at known risk is essential. Once organ failure develops, monitoring of laboratory values and hemodynamic parameters also can be used to assess the degree of impairment. Criteria for the determination of organ failure were proposed by Knaus and Wagner (1989).

Therapeutic management of MODS consists of prevention and support. First, if the initial insult is known,

CLINICAL CRITERIA FOR MODS

Cardiovascular failure	Heart rate ≤ 54/min
	Mean arterial pressure ≤ 49 mm Hg
	Ventricular tachycardia; fibrillation
Respiratory failure	Respiratory rate ≤ 5/min or ≥ 49/min
	Paco₂ ≤ 50 mm Hg
	Ventilatory- or CPAP-dependent on 2nd day of organ failure
Renal failure	Urine output ≤ 480 ml/24 hours
	BUN ≥ 100 mg/dl
	Creatinine ≥ 3.5 mg/dl
Neurologic failure	Glasgow Coma Score ≤ 6 in absence of sedation

it is aggressively treated and sources of infection are removed. Antibiotics are often used. Although corticosteroids have beneficial antiinflammatory effects, they are not used in MODS because of their immunosuppressive properties. The second priority is restoration and maintenance of tissue oxygenation. Because of the low systemic vascular resistance, large volumes of fluid (crystalloid or colloid) are given to maintain adequate preload. Inotropic agents, such as dopamine and dobutamine, are used to counteract myocardial depression. To optimize oxygen transport, the hemoglobin level is maintained at 10 to 12 g/dl. In addition, supplemental oxygen and mechanical ventilation are used to keep the SaO₂ ≥ 90%. Third, nutritional support must be provided. Because enteral feedings help preserve the gut microbial barrier function, the feeding formula is carefully calculated to meet the each individual's nutritional requirements. Lastly, individual organs must be supported.

Fortunately, recent scientific knowledge about inflammatory mediators has led to several promising investigational therapies for MODS. An important area of research is the development of monoclonal antibodies to modulate or inhibit the immune and inflammatory responses. Monoclonal antibodies against endotoxin, endotoxin receptors, TNF, and TNF receptors have been developed. Another area of research is drug therapy. Ibuprofen, which inhibits the production of prostaglandins and thromboxanes, and pentoxifylline, which suppresses the inflammatory effects of neutrophils, are among the most effective of these drugs. Numerous an-

tioxidants and free radical scavengers also are being tested. Because it is improbable that a single agent will be able to control or block the effects of systemic inflammation, it is likely that any therapies found to be safe and effective will be used in combination.

Impairment of Cellular Metabolism

The final common pathway in all types of shock is impairment of cellular metabolism, which is a complex concept in itself. Fig. 27-43 illustrates the pathophysiology of shock at the cellular level.

Impairment of Oxygen Use

In all types of shock, the cell either is not receiving an adequate amount of oxygen or is unable to use oxygen (Fig. 27-43). In cardiogenic shock, cardiac output is too low to deliver adequate oxygen to the cell. In hypovolemic shock, oxygen delivery is impaired by inadequate numbers of red cells or inadequate volume of intravascular fluid. In neurogenic, anaphylactic, and septic shock, SVR is too low and perfusion pressure in the capillaries is inadequate to drive oxygen across cell membranes. In septic shock, hypoxia is made worse by fever, which increases the cell's oxygen consumption rate, and by endotoxic and inflammatory chemical disruption of cells' metabolism, which impairs the cells' ability to use oxygen.

Without oxygen, the cell shifts from aerobic to anaerobic metabolism. Anaerobic metabolism is a less efficient method of extracting energy from carbon bonds, and the cell begins to use its stores of adenosine triphosphate (ATP) faster than stores can be replaced. Without ATP, the cell loses its ability to maintain an electrochemical gradient across its selectively permeable membrane. Specifically, the cell cannot operate the sodium-potassium pump. Sodium and chloride accumulate inside the cell, and potassium exits. Cells of the nervous system and myocardium are profoundly and immediately affected. The resting potentials of these cells are reduced, and action potentials decrease in amplitude. Myocardial depressant factor also decreases the contractility of the heart. A variety of clinical manifestations of impaired central nervous system and myocardial function result.

As sodium moves into the cell, water follows. Throughout the body, the water drawn from the interstitium into the cells is "replaced" by water that is, in turn, drawn out of the vascular space. This decreases circulatory volume. Within the cells, water causes cellular edema that disrupts cellular membranes, releasing lysosomal enzymes that injure the cells internally and leak into the interstitium.

Three positive-feedback loops now begin that further impair oxygen use: (1) activation of the clotting cascade, (2) decreased circulatory volume, and (3) lysosomal en-

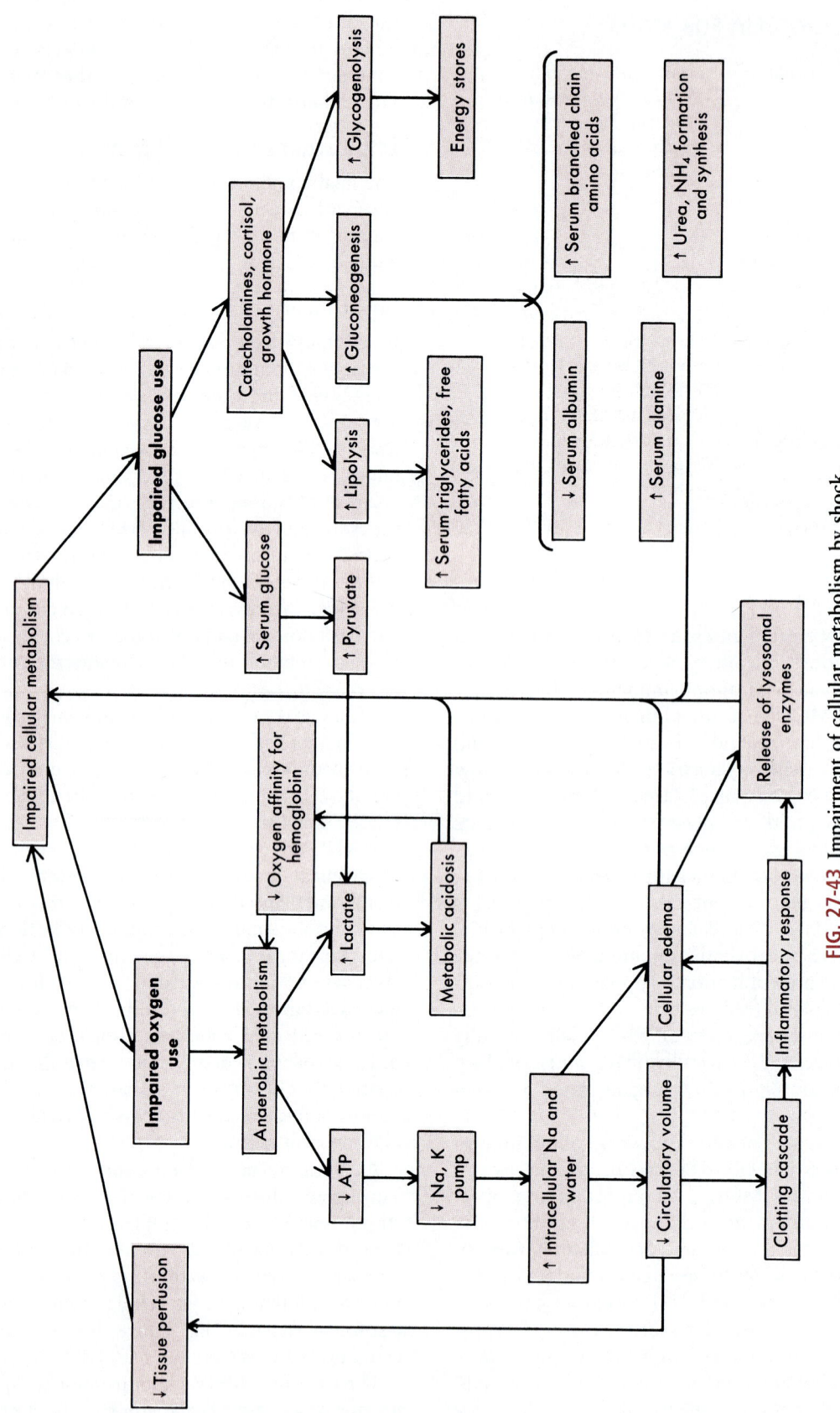

FIG. 27-43 Impairment of cellular metabolism by shock.

zyme release. First, enzymatic processes are disrupted by the change in the normal ionic and osmotic levels in the cell, as are those processes governed by the physical laws of diffusion. Diffusion of nutrients and wastes into and out of the cell takes longer, and cellular metabolism is further altered. At the same time, diffusion across capillary membranes occurs more slowly as blood flow in the capillary beds becomes sluggish. Sluggish capillary flow decreases tissue perfusion further and activates the clotting cascade (see Chapter 22). The clotting cascade activates the inflammatory response and also accounts for common complications of shock, such as acute tubular necrosis, adult respiratory distress syndrome, and disseminated intravascular coagulation.

Decreased circulatory volume causes the second positive-feedback loop and magnifies decreased tissue perfusion in all types of shock. Decreased intravascular volume causes decreased cardiac output in septic shock and further decreases cardiac output in cardiogenic shock. In individuals with anaphylactic, neurogenic, or septic shock and an already dilated vasculature, hypotension worsens as a result of decreased circulatory volume.

The third positive-feedback loop involves the release of lysosomal enzymes. Lysosomal enzymes not only injure the cell that released them, but also injure adjacent cells. By damaging the mechanisms of surrounding cells, lysosomal enzymes extend areas of impaired metabolism and cellular injury.

In addition to decreasing ATP stores, anaerobic metabolism affects the pH of the cell and metabolic acidosis develops (Siegel, 1983). A compensatory mechanism is initiated that enables cardiac and skeletal muscles to use lactic acid as a fuel source, but only for a limited time.

The decreasing pH of the cell that is functioning anaerobically has serious consequences. Enzymes necessary for cellular function dissociate under acid conditions. Enzyme dissociation stops cell function, repair, and division. As lactic acid is released systemically, blood pH drops, reducing the oxygen-carrying capacity of the blood (see Chapter 2). Therefore, less oxygen is delivered to the cells. Further acidosis triggers the release of more lysosomal enzymes because the low pH disrupts lysosomal membrane integrity.

Impairment of Glucose Use

Impaired glucose use can be caused by either impaired glucose delivery or impaired glucose uptake by the cells (Fig. 27-43). The reasons for inadequate glucose delivery are the same as those enumerated for inadequate oxygen delivery. Additionally, in septic and anaphylactic shock, glucose metabolism may be increased or disrupted because of fever or bacteria, and glucose uptake

can be prevented by the presence of vasoactive toxins, endotoxins, histamine, and kinins.

Some of the compensatory mechanisms activated by shock contribute to decreased glucose uptake by the cells. High serum levels of cortisol, growth hormone, and catecholamines account for hyperglycemia and insulin resistance, tachycardia, increased SVR, and increased cardiac contractility. Cells shift to glycogenolysis, gluconeogenesis, and lipolysis to generate fuel for survival (see Chapter 1). Except in the liver, kidneys, and muscles, the body's cells have extremely limited stores of glycogen. In fact, total body stores can only fuel the metabolism for about 10 hours. The depletion of fat and glycogen stores is not itself a cause of organ failure, but the energy costs of glycogenolysis and lipolysis are considerable and contribute to the cells' failure.

The depletion of protein is, however, a cause of organ failure. When gluconeogenesis causes proteins to be used for fuel, these proteins are no longer available to maintain cellular structure, function, repair, and replication. The breakdown of protein occurs in starvation states, hyperdynamic metabolic states, and septic shock. The breakdown of protein into amino acids that occurs with septicemia is called septic autocannibalism (Siegel, 1983). Under anaerobic metabolism, protein breakdown liberates alanine, which is converted to pyruvate. In sepsis, pyruvic acid is changed into lactic acid, and a positive feedback loop is formed.

As proteins are broken down anaerobically, ammonia and urea are produced. Ammonia is toxic to living cells. Uremia develops and uric acid further disrupts cellular metabolism.

Proteins are broken down preferentially. Serum albumin and other plasma proteins are consumed for fuel first. Serum protein consumption decreases capillary osmotic pressure and contributes to the development of interstitial edema, creating another positive-feedback loop that decreases circulatory volume. In septic shock, plasma protein breakdown includes breakdown of immunoglobulins (Siegel, 1983), thereby impairing immune system function when it is most needed.

Muscle wasting caused by protein breakdown weakens skeletal and cardiac muscle. Skeletal muscle wasting impairs the muscles that facilitate breathing. Muscle wasting therefore alters the actions of both heart and lungs. The delivery of oxygen and glucose to the cells is directly reduced, as is the removal of waste products, forming another positive-feedback loop.

A final outcome of impaired cellular metabolism is the buildup of metabolic end-products in the cell and interstitial spaces. Waste products are toxic to the cells and further disrupt cellular function and membrane integrity. In septic shock, for example, a deficiency in cellular metabolism and the buildup of toxins may precede and cause decreased tissue perfusion.

Treatment for Shock

The first treatment for shock is to discover and correct or remove the underlying cause. Although this seems a simple tenet, it is one that is not always remembered. Thus, treatment for cardiogenic shock begins with treatment of heart failure or at least enhancement of cardiac output. If hypovolemia is the cause of shock, hemorrhage and other causes of fluid loss must be stopped. In neurogenic shock, as a result of spinal cord trauma, stabilization of the spine and surrounding tissue is a beginning, and pain usually can be decreased to a level at which neurally mediated decreases of SVR cease. The initial treatment for anaphylactic shock is to remove or neutralize the antigen. Treatment for septic shock begins with eradication of the infective agent, usually with antibiotics.

After the underlying cause or condition is corrected as far as possible, treatment is supportive. Intravenous fluid is administered to expand intravascular volume, except in cardiogenic shock, which requires diuresis to reduce preload. Supplemental oxygen is always given. Cardiotonic drugs are given early in cardiogenic shock, and later in other forms of shock. Steroid use in septic shock remains unproven, although there is evidence that a single, high dose early in the illness improves mortality rates (Sjolin, 1991).

Once positive-feedback loops are established, intervention in shock is difficult. Prevention and very early treatment offer the best prognosis.

SUMMARY REVIEW

Diseases of the Arteries and Veins

1 Arteriosclerosis is a thickening and hardening of the arteries, involving the intimal layer and leading to hypertension. It seems to be a part of the normal aging process, but is a disease state when occurring to the point of symptom development.

2 Arteriosclerosis raises the systolic pressure by decreasing arterial distensibility and lumen diameter. With arteriosclerotic changes in the artery causing narrowing and decreased elasticity, diastolic blood pressure is elevated.

3 Hypertension is the elevation of systemic arterial blood pressure resulting from increases in cardiac output or total peripheral resistance or both.

4 Hypertension can be primary, without a known cause, or secondary, caused by a primary disease.

5 The risk factors for hypertension include a positive family history, male gender, advancing age, black race, obesity, high sodium intake, diabetes mellitus, labile blood pressure, cigarette smoking, and heavy alcohol consumption.

6 The pathophysiology of hypertension includes damage and inflammation of the vessel walls that stimulates the vessels to thicken, harden, and become narrow. Narrowing causes vasoconstriction and increases the permeability of the vessel walls, leading to the influx of sodium, calcium, water, plasma proteins, and other substances. Calcium further increases smooth muscle contraction.

7 The exact cause of primary hypertension is unknown, although several hypotheses are proposed, including increases in blood volume, inappropriate autoregulation, an increase in sympathetic stimula-

tion, water and sodium retention by the kidneys, and inhibition of the sodium-potassium active pump.

8 Clinical manifestations of hypertension result from damage of organs and tissues outside the vascular system. These include heart disease, renal disease, central nervous system problems, and musculoskeletal dysfunction.

9 Hypertension is managed with both pharmacologic and nonpharmacologic methods, for example, dietary alterations.

10 Orthostatic hypotension is a drop in blood pressure that occurs on standing. The compensatory vasoconstriction response to standing is altered by a marked vasodilation and blood pooling in the muscle vasculature.

11 Orthostatic hypotension may be acute or chronic. The acute form is caused by a delay in the normal regulatory mechanisms. The chronic forms are secondary to a specific disease or are idiopathic in nature.

12 The clinical manifestations of orthostatic hypotension include fainting and may involve cardiovascular symptoms, as well as impotence and bowel and bladder dysfunction.

13 An aneurysm is a localized dilatation of a vessel wall, to which the aorta is particularly susceptible.

14 A thrombus is a clot that remains attached to a vascular wall. Arteriosclerosis can generate thrombus formation through roughening of the intima that activates the clotting cascade. Thrombus formation may be discrete or diffuse.

15 An embolus is a mobile aggregate of a variety of substances that occludes the vasculature. Sources of emboli include clots, air, amniotic fluid, bacteria, fat, and foreign matter.

16 The most common cause of arterial thrombotic emboli is the heart, as a result of mitral and aortic valvular disease and atrial fibrillation, followed by myxomas. Tissues affected include the lower extremities, the brain, and the heart.

17 Emboli to the central organs cause tissue death in lungs, kidneys, and mesentery.

18 The generation of air emboli requires a connection between the vascular compartment and a source of air. These emboli cause ischemia and necrosis when a vessel is totally blocked.

19 Amniotic fluid may be forced into the bloodstream and generate an embolus during the labor and delivery of pregnancy.

20 Aggregates of bacteria in the vasculature may be large enough to form an embolus.

21 Fat emboli are caused mainly by trauma to the long bones, either through defective fat metabolism after trauma or through the release of fat globules from bone marrow exposed by fracture.

22 The introduction of foreign matter into the vasculature can occur with trauma and also can occur in a hospital setting in which intravenous and intraarterial lines are being used.

23 Vasospastic disorders include Raynaud disease, involving arterioles of the extremities; Prinzmetal angina, involving coronary arteries; and Buerger disease, involving arteries of the hands and feet.

24 Diabetic lesions of the arteries may be caused by a defect in glycoprotein metabolism that involves the capillary basement membranes in kidneys, retinas, and extremities.

25 Varicosities are areas of veins in which blood has pooled, usually in the saphenous veins. Varicosities may be caused by damaged valves as a result of trauma to the valve, or by chronic venous distention involving gravity and venous constriction.

26 Chronic venous insufficiency is inadequate venous return over a long period of time that causes pathologic ischemic changes in the vasculature, skin, and supporting tissues.

27 Venous stasis ulcers follow the development of chronic venous insufficiency and probably develop as a result of the borderline metabolic state of the cells in the affected extremities.

28 The pathophysiology of thrombus formation in the veins is the same as for thrombus formation in the arteries. Because of the triggering of the inflammatory response at the site of formation, deep vein thrombi are characterized by tenderness, swelling, and redness.

29 Superior vena cava syndrome is a progressive occlusion of the superior vena cava that leads to venous distention in the upper extremities and head. Because this syndrome is usually caused by bronchogenic cancer, it is generally not a vascular emergency, but is an oncologic emergency.

30 Coronary artery disease (CAD) is any disorder that narrows or occludes the coronary arteries. Many risk factors contribute to the onset and escalation of CAD, including: hyperlipidemia (primarily hypercholesterolemia), smoking, hypertension, male gender, diabetes mellitus, advancing age, obesity, sedentary lifestyle, psychosocial factors, hormone therapy, and heavy consumption of alcohol.

31 The three risk factors most predictive of CAD are hypercholesterolemia, cigarette smoking, and hypertension.

32 Ischemic heart disease is most commonly the result of coronary artery disease and the resultant decrease in myocardial blood supply.

33 Angina pectoris is chest pain caused by myocardial ischemia.

34 Therapeutic interventions for CAD include use of vasodilators and medications to reduce cardiac workload (e.g., beta-blockers), as well as surgical procedures.

35 Myocardial infarction is caused by prolonged, unrelieved ischemia that interrupts blood supply to the myocardium. After about 20 minutes of myocardial ischemia, irreversible hypoxic injury causes cellular death and tissue necrosis.

36 A transient increase in plasma enzyme levels may diagnose the occurrence of myocardial infarction and indicate its severity. Elevations of the isoenzymes creatine kinase (CK-MB) and lactic dehydrogenase (LDH-1) are those most predictive of a myocardial infarction.

37 Treatment of a myocardial infarction includes bed rest, pain relief, and drug interventions to limit infarct size, prevent thrombus formation, and augment repair. Dysrhythmias and cardiac failure are the most common complication of acute myocardial infarction.

Disorders of the Heart Wall

1 Inflammation of the pericardium, pericarditis, may result from innumerable sources (infection, drug therapy, tumors). Pericarditis presents with symptoms that are physically troublesome, but in and of themselves are not life-threatening.

2 Fluid may collect within the pericardial sac (pericardial effusion). Cardiac function may be severely impaired if the accumulation of fluid occurs rapidly and involves a large volume.

3 Cardiomyopathies are a diverse group of primary myocardial disorders that are poorly understood. The cardiomyopathies are categorized as dilated (congestive), restrictive (rigid and noncompliant), and hypertrophic (asymmetric). Size of the cardiac

muscle walls and chambers may increase or decrease, depending on the type of cardiomyopathy, thereby altering contractile activity.

4 Hemodynamic integrity of the cardiovascular system depends to a great extent on properly functioning cardiac valves. Congenital or acquired disorders that result in stenosis or incompetence or both can structurally alter the valves.

5 Characteristic heart sounds, cardiac murmurs, and systemic complaints assist in determination of which valve is abnormal. If severely compromised function exists, a prosthetic heart valve may be surgically implanted to replace the faulty one.

6 Mitral valve prolapse (MVP) is a common finding, especially in young women. Although not grossly abnormal, the mitral valve leaflets do not position themselves properly during systole. Mitral valve prolapse may be a completely asymptomatic condition or could result in severe subjective symptoms. Afflicted valves may be at greater risk for developing infective endocarditis.

7 Rheumatic fever is an inflammatory disease that results from a delayed immune response to a streptococcal infection. The disorder usually resolves without sequelae if treated early.

8 Severe or untreated cases of rheumatic fever may progress to rheumatic heart disease, a potentially disabling cardiovascular disorder.

9 Infective endocarditis is a general term for inflammation of the endocardium, especially the cardiac valves. A wide range of conditions predispose to the development of this disorder. In the mildest cases, valvular function may be slightly impaired by vegetations that collect on the valve leaflets. If left unchecked, severe valve abnormalities, chronic bacteremia, and systemic emboli may occur as vegetations break off the valve surface and travel through the bloodstream. Antibiotic therapy can limit the extension of this disease.

10 Human immunodeficiency virus is associated with cardiac abnormalities including myocarditis, endocarditis, pericarditis, and cardiomyopathy. Congestive heart failure is the most frequent clinical manifestation.

Manifestations of Heart Disease

1 A dysrhythmia (arrhythmia) is a disturbance of heart rhythm. Dysrhythmias range in severity from occasional missed beats or rapid beats to disturbances that impair myocardial contractility and are life-threatening.

2 Dysrhythmias can occur because of an abnormal rate of impulse generation or the abnormal conduction of impulses.

3 Heart failure is an inability of the heart to supply the metabolism with adequate circulatory volume and pressure.

4 The supply/demand oxygen ratio is one of the major components of heart failure. A decrease in the ratio can precipitate, exacerbate, or follow heart failure.

5 The most common cause of right heart failure is left heart failure, followed by pulmonary disease with an elevated pulmonary vascular resistance.

6 Because the right ventricle normally has a high oxygen supply/demand ratio, and the pulmonary vasculature is normally low, right ventricular infarction is rare, and left ventricular failure or pulmonary disease may be present for quite some time before the right ventricle begins to fail.

7 As oxygen supply/demand ratio falls and pulmonary vascular resistance increases, right ventricular preload increases, and the right heart begins to fail.

8 Symptoms of right heart failure arise in the systemic venous system because of elevated venous pressures and volumes.

9 The most common causes of left ventricular failure are myocardial infarction, systemic hypertension, and valvular incompetence or stenosis.

10 The pathophysiology of left heart failure resembles that of right heart failure.

11 Biventricular failure is failure of the right and left ventricles.

12 A decrease in left ventricular output triggers sodium and water retention through renal, adrenal, and posterior pituitary hormone actions. This increases vascular volume and preload, and contributes to additional failure.

13 Epinephrine and norepinephrine release is triggered by a lowered ventricular output. These neurotransmitters increased oxygen demand through cardiotonic and vascular resistance increases.

14 Left ventricular failure in the aged does not necessarily include a reduction in left ventricular ejection force.

15 The earliest clinical indicator of left heart failure is a rise in the left ventricular end-diastolic pressure or pulmonary capillary wedge pressure.

16 Low-output failure is (1) biventricular, (2) commonly caused by cardiomyopathies and myocarditis, and (3) usually refractory to treatment.

17 High-output failure is the inability of the heart to adequately supply the metabolism with blood, despite adequate blood volume and a normal myocardial contractility. Common causes are anemia, sepsis, hyperthyroidism, and beriberi.

Shock

1 Shock is a widespread impairment of cellular metabolism involving positive-feedback loops that places the individual on a downward physiologic spiral leading to multiple organ dysfunction syndrome.

2 Types of shock are cardiogenic, hypovolemic, neurogenic, anaphylactic, and septic. Multiple organ

dysfunction syndrome can develop from all types of shock.

3 Cardiogenic shock is attributable to heart failure and is characterized by a decrease in cardiac output and impaired cellular metabolism.

4 Hypovolemic shock is caused by loss of blood or fluid in large amounts. The use of compensatory mechanisms may be vigorous, but tissue perfusion ultimately decreases and results in impaired cellular metabolism.

5 Neurogenic shock results from massive vasodilation, causing a relative hypovolemia, even though cardiac output may be high, and results in impaired cellular metabolism.

6 Anaphylactic shock is caused by physiologic recognition of a foreign substance. The inflammatory response is triggered, and a massive vasodilation with fluid shift into the interstitium follows. The relative hypovolemia leads to impaired cellular metabolism.

7 Septic shock begins with impaired cellular metabolism caused by uncontrolled septicemia. The infecting agent triggers the inflammatory and immune responses. Four major chemicals have been implicated in the cause of shock: (1) interleukins, (2) platelet-activating factor, (3) tumor necrosis factor, and (4) myocardial depressant substance.

8 Toxic shock syndrome is a form of septic shock caused by *S. aureus*.

9 Multiple organ dysfunction syndrome (MODS) is the progressive failure of two or more organ systems after a severe illness or injury. It can be triggered by chronic inflammation, necrotic tissue, severe trauma, burns, adult respiratory distress syndrome, acute pancreatitis, and other severe injuries.

10 The mortality rate of MODS is very high, ranging from 60% to 100%.

11 Multiple organ dysfunction syndrome involves the stress response; changes in the vascular endothelium resulting in microvascular coagulation; release of complement, coagulation, and kinin proteins; and numerous inflammatory processes. Consequences of all these mediators are a maldistribution of blood flow, hypermetabolism, hypoxic injury, and myocardial depression.

12 Clinical manifestations of MODS include inflammation, tissue hypoxia, and hypermetabolism. The lung is usually the first organ to fail.

13 The final common pathway in all types of shock is impaired cellular metabolism—cells switch from aerobic to anaerobic metabolism. Energy stores drop and cellular mechanisms relative to membrane permeability, action potentials, and lysozyme release fail.

14 Anaerobic metabolism results in activation of the inflammatory response, decreased circulatory volume, and decreasing pH.

15 Impaired cellular metabolism results in cellular inability to use glucose because of impaired glucose delivery or impaired glucose intake, resulting in a shift of glycogenolysis, gluconeogenesis, and lipolysis for fuel generation.

16 Glycogenolysis is affected for up to 10 hours. Gluconeogenesis results in the use of proteins necessary for structure, function, repair, and replication that leads to more impaired cellular metabolism. Lipolysis is ineffective because of a lack of transport serum proteins and malfunction of the Krebs cycle.

17 Gluconeogenesis contributes to lactic acid, uric acid, and ammonia buildup, interstitial edema, and impairment of the immune system, as well as general muscle weakness leading to decreased respiratory function and cardiac output.

KEY TERMS

REFERENCES

Acierno, L. J. (1989). Cardiac complications in acquired immunodeficiency syndrome (AIDS): A review. *Journal of the American College of Cardiology, 13,* 1144-1154.

Adams, J. E. III, Bodor, G. S., Dávila-Román, V. G., Delmez, J. A., Apple, F. S., Landenson, J. H., Jaffe, A. S. (1993). Cardiac troponin I: A marker with high specificity for cardiac injury. *Circulation, 88* (July), 101-106.

Ahumada, G. G. (Ed.). (1987). *Cardiovascular pathophysiology.* New York: Oxford University Press.

American Heart Association. (1982). *Jones criteria (revised) for guidance in the diagnosis of rheumatic fever.* Dallas, TX: Author.

American Heart Association. (1991). *1992 heart and stroke facts.* Dallas, TX: Author.

Anderson, B. O., Bernsard, D. D., & Harken. A. H. (1991). The role of platelet activating factor and its antagonists in shock, sepsis, and multiple organ failure. *Surgery, Gynecology, & Obstetrics, 172*(5), 415-424.

Anderson, B. O., & Harken, A. H. (1990). Multiple organ failure: Inflammatory priming and activation sequences promote autologous tissue injury. *Journal of Trauma, 30*(12), S44-S49.

Archer, G. L. (1977). Experimental endocarditis. In R. J. Duma (Ed.), *Infections of prosthetic heart valves and vascular grafts. Prevention, diagnosis, and treatment.* Baltimore: University Park Press, pp. 43-57.

Assmann, G. (1987). Lipoproteins and apolipoproteins in the prediction of coronary artery disease. *Acta Medica Scandinavica* [Supplement], 715, 67-77.

Baim, D. S. (1992). Interventional catheterization techniques: Percutaneous transluminal balloon angioplasty, valvuloplasty, and related procedures. In E. Braunwald (Ed.), *Heart disease: A textbook of cardiovascular medicine* (4th ed., pp. 1365-1381). Philadelphia: Saunders.

Baue, A. E. (1975). Multiple, progressive, or sequential systems failure: A syndrome of the 1970s. *Archives of Surgery, 11*(7), 779-781.

Blackburn, G. L., & Kanders, B S. (1987). Medical evaluation and treatment of the obese patient with cardiovascular disease. *American Journal of Cardiology, 60,* 55G-58G.

Blair, S. N., Kohl, H. W. III, Paffenbarger, R. S., Jr., Clark, D. G., Cooper, K. H., & Gibbons, L. W. (1989). Physical fitness and all-cause mortality: A perspective study of healthy men and women. *Journal of the American Medical Association, 252*(17), 2395-2401.

Blumenthal, J. A., Williams, R. G. J., Kong, Y., Schanberg, S. M., & Thompson, L. W. (1978). Type A behavior pattern and coronary atherosclerosis. *Circulation, 58,* 634-639.

Bone, R. C. (1991a). Let's agree on terminology: Definition of sepsis. *Critical Care Medicine, 19*(7), 973-976.

Bone, R. C. (1991b). The pathogenesis of sepsis. *Annals of Internal Medicine, 115*(6), 457-469.

Bone, R. C., Fisher, C. J., Clemmer, T. P. (1987). A controlled clinical trial of high-dose methylprednisone in the treatment of severe sepsis and septic shock. *New England Journal of Medicine, 317,* 653-658.

Boudoulas, H., & Wooley, C. F. (1988). Mitral valve prolapse syndrome: Neuroendocrinological aspects. *Hertz, 13*(4), 249-258.

Braunwald, E. (Ed.). (1988). *Heart disease: A textbook of cardiovascular medicine* (3rd ed.). Philadelphia: Saunders.

Braunwald, E. (Ed.). (1992). *Heart disease: A textbook of cardiovascular medicine* (4th ed.). Philadelphia: Saunders.

Braunwald, E., & Sobel, B. E. (1992). Coronary blood flow and myocardial ischemia. In E. Braunwald (Ed.), *Heart disease: A textbook of cardiovascular medicine* (4th ed., pp. 1161-1199). Philadelphia: Saunders.

Brischetto, C. S., Connor, W. E., Connor, S. L., & Matarazzo, J. D. (1983). Plasma lipid and lipoprotein profiles of cigarette smokers from randomly selected families: Enhancement of hyperlipidemia and depression of high density lipoprotein. *American Journal of Cardiology, 52,* 675.

Castaner, A., Betriu, A., Sanz, G., Paré, J. C., Coll, S., Soler, J., Roig, E., & Navarro-López, F. (1984). Natural history of severe left ventricular hypertrophy after myocardial infarction. *Chest, 85*(6), 744-750.

Cerami, A. (1991). Inflammatory cytokines. *Clinical Immunology and Immunopathology, 62*(1), S3-S10.

Cerra, F. B. (1990). The multiple organ failure syndrome. *Hospital Practice, 25*(8), 169-176.

Cheng, T. O. (1986). *The international textbook of cardiology.* New York: Pergamon Press.

Cheng, T. O. (1989). Mitral valve prolapse. *Annual Review of Medicine, 40,* 201-211.

Cheng, T. O. (1990). Cardiac failure in coronary heart disease. *American Heart Journal, 120*(2), 396-412.

Cody, R. J., Covit, A. B., Schaer, G. L., & Laragh, J. H. (1984). Estimation of angiotensin II receptor activity in chronic congestive heart failure. *American Heart Journal, 108*(1), 81-89.

Cotran, R. S., Kumar, V., & Robbins, S. L. (1989). *Robbins' pathological basis of disease* (4th ed.). Philadelphia: Saunders.

Crimi, G., Conti, G., Bufi, M., Antonelli, M., deBlasi, R. A., Mattia, C., Romano, R., & Gasparetto, A. (1988). A high frequency jet ventilation (HFJV) has no better haemodynamic tolerance than controlled mechanical ventilation (CMV) in cardiogenic shock. *Intensive Care Medicine, 14*(4), 359-363.

Criqui, M. H. (1986). Epidemiology of atherosclerosis: an updated overview. *American Journal of Cardiology, 57*(5), 18C-23C.

Crouse, J. R. III. (1989, February). Gender, lipoproteins, diet, and cardiovascular risk. *Lancet, 1,* 318-320.

Cunnion, R. E., & Parrillo, J. E. (1989). Myocardial dysfunction in sepsis: Recent insights. *Chest, 95,* 941-945.

Dajani, A. S., Bisno, A. L., Chung, K. J., Durack, D. T., Freed, M., Gerber, M. A., Karchmer, A. W., Millard, H. D., Rahimtoola, S., Shulman, S. T., Watanakunakorn, C., & Taubert, D. A. (1990). Prevention of bacterial endocarditis. Recommendations by the American Heart Association. *Journal of the American Medical Association, 264*(22), 2919-2922.

Dal Nogare, A. R. (1991). Southwestern internal medicine conference: Septic shock. *American Journal of Medical Science, 302*(1), 50-65.

Danielson, M., & Dammstrom, B. G. (1981). The prevalence of secondary and curable hypertension. *Acta Medica Scandinavica, 209,* 451-455.

Das, B. N., & Banka, V. S. (1992). Coronary artery disease in women. *Postgraduate Medicine, 91*(4), 197-200, 203-204, 206.

Demeules, J. E. (1984). A physiological explanation for cardiac deterioration in septic shock. *Journal of Surgical Research, 36*(6), 533-562.

DeSanctis, R. W. (1990). Cardiomyopathies. *Scientific American Medicine, 1*(1-XIV), 1-23.

Detre, K. M. (1984). Hypertension in women—a review. In E. G. Gold (Ed.), *The changing risk of disease in women: An epidemiologic approach.* Lexington, MA: D. C. Heath Co.

Devereaux, R. B., Kramer-Fox, R., & Kligfield, P. (1989). Mitral valve prolapse: Causes, clinical manifestations, and management. *Annals of Internal Medicine, 111*(4), 305-317.

Dimsdale, J. E. (1988). A perspective on type A behavior and coronary disease. *New England Journal of Medicine, 318*(2), 110-112.

Dujovne, V. F. (1991). Hostility-related variables and plasma lipid levels. *Journal of Behavioral Medicine, 14*(6), 555-565.

Esposito, T. J., Gens, D. R., Smith, L. G., Scorpio, R., & Buchanan, T. (1991). Trauma during pregnancy: A review of 79 cases. *Archives of Surgery, 126*(9), 1073-1078.

Estok, P. J., & Rudy, E. B. (1986). Jogging: cardiovascular benefits and risks. *Nurse Practitioner, 11*(5), 21-28.

Fackelmann, K. A. (1991). The African gene? *Science News, 140*(16), 254-255.

Farmer, J. A., & Gotto, A. M. (1992). Risk factors for coronary artery disease. In E. Braunwald (Ed.), *Heart disease: A textbook of cardiovascular medicine* (4th ed., pp. 1125-1161). Philadelphia: Saunders.

Feinleib, M., & Garrison, R. J. (1979). The contribution of family studies to the partitioning of population variation of blood pressure. In C. F. Sing, M. Skolnick, & A. R. Liss (Eds.), *Genetic analysis of common diseases: Application to predictive factors in coronary disease.* New York: Alan R. Liss, p. 653.

Fitzmaurice, J. B. (1980). *Rheumatic heart disease and mitral valve disease.* New York: Appleton-Century-Crofts.

Frank, K. A., Heller, S. S., Kornfield, D. S., Sporn, A. A., & Weiss, M. B. (1978). Type A behavior pattern and coronary angiographic findings. *Journal of the American Medical Association, 240,* 761-763.

Friedman, L. R. (1987). The pathogenesis of infective endocarditis. *Journal of Antimicrobial Chemotherapy, 20*(Suppl. A), 1-6.

Friedman, M., & Rosenman, R. H. (1974). *Type A behavior and your heart.* New York: Knopf.

Fuster, V., Badimon, L., Badimon, J. J., & Chesebro, J. H. (1992a). The pathogenesis of coronary artery disease and the acute coronary syndromes. First of 2 parts. *New England Journal of Medicine, 326*(4), 242-250.

Fuster, V., Badimon, L., Badimon, J. J., & Chesebro, J. H. (1992b). The pathogenesis of coronary artery disease and the acute coronary syndromes. Second of 2 parts. *New England Journal of Medicine, 326*(4), 310-318.

Ganz, P., & Alexander, R. W. (1985). New insights into the cellular mechanisms of vasospasm. *American Journal of Cardiology, 56*(9), 11E-15E.

Goldstein, J. L. & Brown, M. S. (1989). Familial hypercholesterolemia. In C. R. Scriver, A. L. Beaudet, W. S. Sly, & D. Valle (Eds.), *The metabolic basis of inherited disease* (6th ed., pp. 1215-1250). New York: McGraw-Hill.

Gould, K., Ramirez-Ronda, C. J., Holmes, R. K., & Stanford, J. P. (1975). Adherence of bacteria to heart valves in vitro. *Journal of Clinical Investigation, 56,* 1364-1370.

Hamby, J. I., Weissman, R. H., Prakash, M. N., & Hoffman, I. (1983). Left bundle branch block: a predictor of poor left ventricular function in CAD. *American Heart Journal, 106*(3), 471-477.

Hancock, E. W. (1989). Diseases of the pericardium. *Scientific American Medicine, 1*(1-XIII), 1-9.

Hancock, E. W. (1991). Coronary artery disease—epidemiology and prevention. *Scientific American Medicine, 1*(1-VIII), 1-10.

Hancock, E. W. (1992). Valvular heart disease. *Scientific American Medicine, 1*(1-XI), 1-4.

Harris, E. D. (1991). Acute rheumatic fever. *Scientific American Medicine, 3*(15-VII), 1-4.

Haynes, S., Eaker, E. D., & Feinleib, M. (1984). The effects of employment, family, and job stress on coronary heart disease patterns in women. In E. B. Gold (Ed.), *The changing risk of disease in women: An epidemiological approach.* Lexington, MA: D. C. Heath Co.

Hazzard, W. R. (1989). Why do women live longer than men? Biologic influences that influence longevity. *Post Graduate Medicine 85* (5), 271-278, 281-283.

Hershman, W. Y., Moskowitz, M. A., Marton, K. I., & Balady, G. J. (1989). Utility of endocardiography in patients with suspected mitral valve prolapse. *American Journal of Medicine, 87*(4), 371-376.

Hibbard, M. D., Holmes, D. R., Bailey, K. R., Reeder, G. S., Bresnahan, J. F., & Gersh, B. J. (1992). Percutaneous transluminal coronary angioplasty in patients with cardiogenic shock. *Journal of the American College of Cardiology, 19*(3), 639-646.

Hilbert, P., Lindpaintner, K., Beckmann, J. S., Serikawa, R., Soubrier, F., Dubayu, C., Cartwright, P., DeGouyon, B., Julier, C., & Takahasi, S. (1992). Chromosomal mapping of two genetic loci associated with blood-pressure regulation in hereditary hypertensive rats. *Nature, 353*(6344), 521-529.

Hjermann, I., Velve Byrek, K., Holm, I., & Leren, P. (1981). Effect of diet and smoking intervention on the incidence of cardiac heart disease: Report from the Oslo study group of a randomized trial of healthy men. *Lancet, 2*(8259)m, 1303-1310.

Howard, M., Puri, V. K., & Paidipaty, B. B. (1984). The effects of fluid resuscitation in the critically ill patient. *Heart & Lung, 13*(6), 649-654.

Huddleston, V. B. (1992). Multisystem organ failure: Background and etiology. In V. B. Huddleston (Ed.), *Multisystem organ failure* (pp. 3-15). St. Louis: Mosby–Year Book.

Hunt, A. H. (1985). Mitral valve prolapse: Physical assessment, complications, and management. *Nurse Practitioner,* April, 15-21.

Hurst, J. W., Logue, R. B., Rackley, C. E., Schlant, R. B., Sonnenblick, E. H., Wallace, A. G., & Wenger, N. K. (Eds.). (1986). *The heart, arteries, and veins* (6th ed.). New York: McGraw-Hill.

Hurst, J. W., Schlant, R. C., Rackley, C. E., Sonnenblick, E. H., & Wenger, N. K. (Eds.). (1990). *The heart, arteries, and veins* (7th ed.). New York: McGraw-Hill.

Jacobs, R. F., Shelhamer, J. H., Kaliner, M., & Parrillo, J. E. (1989). Blood histamine concentrations are not elevated in humans with septic shock. *Critical Care Medicine, 17,* 30-36.

Jaffe, A. S., Spandaro, J. J., Schechtman, K., Roberts, R., Gettman, E. M., & Sobel, B. E. (1984). Incidence of congestive heart failure after MI of modest extent in patients with DM. *American Heart Journal, 108*(1), 31-37.

Jenkins, C. D., Zyzanski, S. J., & Rosenman, R. H. (1976). Risk of new myocardial infarction in middle-aged men with manifest coronary heart disease. *Circulation, 53,* 342-347.

Joint National Committee. (1988). The 1988 report of the Joint National Committee on detection, evaluation, and treatment of high blood pressure. *Archives of Internal Medicine, 148*(5), 1023-1038.

Kafka, K. R., Meltzer, A. H., & Frishman, W. H. (1985). Antianginal agents part I: Ischemic heart disease and the role of nitrates. *Hospital Formulary 20*(1), 1144-1153.

Kannel, W. B., Feinleib, M., McNamara, P. M., Garrison, J. R., & Castelli, W. P. (1979). An investigation of coronary heart disease in families. The Framingham offspring study. *American Journal of Epidemiology, 110,* 281.

Kaplan, N. M. (1990). *Clinical hypertension* (5th ed.). Baltimore: Williams & Wilkins.

Kaplan, N. M. (1992). Systemic hypertension: Mechanisms and diagnosis. In E. Braunwald (Ed.), *Heart disease: A textbook of cardiovascular medicine* (4th ed., pp. 817-851). Philadelphia: Saunders.

Khan, A. H. (1992). The postcardiac injury syndromes. *Clinical Cardiology, 15*(2), 67-72.

Kinney, M. (1991). *Comprehensive cardiac care* (7th ed.). St. Louis: Mosby–Year Book.

Kissane, J. M. (Ed.). (1985). *Anderson's pathology* (8th ed.). St. Louis: Mosby–Year Book.

Kissane, J. M. (Ed.). (1990). *Anderson's pathology* (9th ed.). St. Louis: Mosby–Year Book.

Knaus, W. A., & Wagner, D. P. (1989). Multiple systems organ failure: Epidemiology and prognosis. *Critical Care Clinics, 5*(2), 221-232.

Korzeniowski, O. M., & Kaye, D. (1992). Infective endocarditis. In E. Braunwald (Ed.), *Heart disease: A textbook of cardiovascular medicine* (4th ed., pp. 1078-1105). Philadelphia: Saunders.

LaRosa, J. C. (1990). At what levels of total low or high density lipoprotein cholesterol should diet therapy be initiated? United States guidelines. *American Journal of Cardiology, 65*(12), 7F-10F.

Lekander, B. J., & Cerra, F. B. (1990). The syndrome of multiple organ failure. *Critical Care Nursing Clinics of North America, 2*(2), 331-342.

Liebermann, E. (1990). Hypertension in childhood and adolescence. In N. M. Kaplan (Ed.), *Clinical hypertension* (5th ed.). Baltimore: Williams & Wilkins.

Lifton, R. P., Dluhy, R. G., Powers, M., Rich, G. M., Cook, S., Ulick, S., & Lalouel, J. M. (1992). A chimeric 11 beta-hydroxylase/aldosterone synthase gene causes glucocorticoid-remediable aldosteronism and human hypertension. *Nature, 355*(6357), 262-265.

Luchi, R. J., Snow, E., Luchi, J. M., Nelson, C. S., & Pircher, F. J. (1982). Left ventricular function in hospitalized geriatric patients. *Journal of the American Geriatric Society, 30*(11), 700-705.

MacDougall, J. M., Dembroski, T. M., Dimsdale, J. B., & Hackett, T. P. (1985). Components of type A, hostility, and anger in further relationships to angiographic findings. *Health Psychology, 4,* 137-150.

Markowitz, M. (1988). Evolution and critique of changes in the Jones criteria for the diagnosis of rheumatic fever. *New Zealand Medical Journal, 101,* 392-394.

Mattox, K. L., Bickell, W., Pepe, P. E., Burch, J., & Feliciano, D. (1989). Prospective MAST study in 911 patients. *Journal of Trauma, 29*(8), 1104-1112.

McCance, K. L. (1983). Genetics: Implications for preventative nursing practice. *Journal of Advanced Nursing, 8,* 359-364.

McFadden, E. P., Clarke, J. G., Davies, G. J., Kaski, J. C., Halder, A. W., & Maseri, A. (1991). Effect of intracoronary serotonin on coronary vessels in patients with stable angina and patients with variant angina. *New England Journal of Medicine, 324*(10), 648-654.

Mizock, B. A., & Falk, J. F. (1992). Lactic acidosis in critical illness. *Critical Care Medicine, 20*(1), 80-93.

Ognibene, F. P., Parker, M. M., Natanson, C., Shelhamer, J. H., & Parrillo, J. E. (1988). Depressed left ventricular performance. Response to volume infusion in patients with sepsis and septic shock. *Chest, 93*(5), 903-910.

Page, I. H. (1987). *Hypotension mechanisms.* New York: Grune & Stratton.

Parker, M. M., & Parrillo, J. E. (1983). Septic shock: Hemodynamics and pathogenesis. *Journal of the American Medical Association, 250,* 3324-3327.

Parker, M. M., McCarthy, K. E., Ognibene, F. P., & Parrillo, J. E. (1990). Right ventricular dysfunction and dilatation, similar to left ventricular changes, characterize the cardiac depression of septic shock in humans. *Chest, 97*(1), 126-131.

Parsonnet, J. (1989). Mediators in the pathogenesis of toxic shock syndrome: Overview. *Review of Infectious Diseases, 11,* S263-S269.

Pasternak, R. C., Braunwald, E., & Sobel, B. E. (1992). Acute myocardial infarction. In E. Braunwald (Ed.), *Heart disease: A textbook of cardiovascular medicine* (4th ed., pp. 1200-1291). Philadelphia: Saunders.

Pilz, G., Kaab, S., Neeser, G., Class, I., Schweigart, U., Brahler, A., Bujdoso, O., Neumann, R., & Werdan, K. (1991). Supplemental immunoglobulin (IV IgG) treatment in 163 patients with sepsis and septic shock—An observational study as a prerequisite for placebo-controlled clinical trials. *Infection, 19,* 216-227.

Powell, K. E., Thompson, P. D., Caspersen, C. J., & Kendrick, J. S. (1987). Physical activity and the incidence of coronary heart disease. *Annual Review of Public Health, 8,* 253-287.

Ragland, D. R., & Brand, R. J. (1988). Type A behavior and mortality from coronary heart disease. *New England Journal of Medicine, 318,* 5-9.

Rahe, R. H., Romo, M., Bennett, L., & Sietonen, P. (1974). Recent life changes, myocardial infarction, and abrupt coronary death. *Archives of Internal Medicine, 133,* 221.

Ranjadayalan, K., Umachandran, V., & Timmis, A. D. (1992). Clinical impact of introducing thrombolytic and aspirin therapy into the management policy of a coronary care unit. *American Journal of Medicine, 93*(3), 233-238.

Rimm, E. B., Giovannucci, E. L., Willett, W. C., Golditz, G. A., Ascherio, A., Rosner, B., & Stampfer, M. J. (1991). Prospective study of alcohol consumption and risk of coronary disease in men. *Lancet, 338*(8765), 464-468.

Reingold, A. L. (1991). Toxic shock syndrome: An update. *American Journal of Obstetrics & Gynecology, 165*(4), 1236-1239.

Robson, W. L. M., & Leung, A. K. C. (1991). Hypertension in young patients. *Postgraduate Medicine, 90*(30), 191-200.

Rose, M. I. (1987). Type A behavior pattern: A concept revisited. *Canadian Medical Association Journal, 136*(4), 345-350.

Ross, R. (1992). The pathogenesis of atherosclerosis. In E. Braunwald (Ed.), *Heart disease: A textbook of cardiovascular medicine* (4th ed., pp. 1106-1124). Philadelphia: Saunders.

Rudnick, K. V., Sackett, D. L., Hirst, S., & Holmes, C. (1977). Hypertension in a family practice. *Canadian Medical Association Journal, 117*(5), 492-497.

Ruokonen, E., Takala, J., Kari, A., & Alhava, E. (1991). Septic shock and multiple organ failure. *Critical Care Medicine, 19*(9), 1146-1151.

Salonen, J. T., Nyyssonen, K., Korpela, H., Tuomilehto, J., Seppanen, R., & Salonen. R. (1992). High stored iron levels are associated with excess risk of myocardial infarction in eastern Finnish men. *Circulation, 86*(3), 803-811.

Schlievert, P. M. (1989). TSST-1: Structure, function, purification, and detection. Role of toxic shock syndrome toxin 1 in toxic shock syndrome: Overview. *Review of Infectious Diseases, 11,* S107-S109.

Schrott, H. G., Bucker, K. A., Clarke, W. R., & Lauer, R. M. (1979). The Muscatine hyperlipidemia family study program. In C. F. Sing & M. Skolnick (Eds.), *Genetic analysis of common diseases: Application to preventive factors in coronary disease.* New York: Alan R. Liss, p. 629.

Schuchat, A., & Broome, C. V. (1991). Toxic shock syndrome and tampons. *Epidemiologic Reviews, 13,* 99-112.

Sclarovsky, S., Strasberg, B., Hirshberg, A., Arditi, A., Lewin, R. J., & Agman, J. (1984). Advanced early and late atrioventricular block in acute inferior wall MI. *American Heart Journal, 108*(1), 19-24.

Scragg, R., Stewart, A., Jackson, R., & Beaglehole, R. (1987). Alcohol and exercise in myocardial infarction and sudden coronary death in men and women. *American Journal of Epidemiology, 126*(1), 77-85.

Scrogin, K. E., Hatton, D. C., & McCarron, D. A. (1992). The interactive effects of dietary sodium chloride and calcium on cardiovascular stress responses. *American Journal of Physiology, 261*(4), R945-R949.

Seeman, T. E. (1991). Personal control and coronary artery disease: How generalized expectancies about control may influence disease risk. *Journal of Psychosomatic Research, 35*(6), 661-669.

Shabetai, R. (1990). Acute pericarditis. *Cardiology Clinics, 8*(4), 639-644.

Shah, P. K., & Forrester, J. S. (1991). Pathophysiology of acute coronary syndromes. *American Journal of Cardiology, 68*(12), 16C-23C.

Shaper, A. G., Phillips, A. N., Pocock, S. J., & Walker, M. (1987). Alcohol and ischaemic heart disease in middle aged British men. *British Medical Journal, 294,* 733-737.

Sheehy, T. W. (1992). Alcohol and the heart. How it helps, how it harms. *Postgraduate Medicine, 91*(5), 271-277.

Siegel, J. H. (1983). Cardiorespiratory manifestations of metabolic failure in sepsis and multiple organ failure syndrome. *Surgical Clinics of North America, 63*(2), 379-399.

Silber, E. N. (1987). *Heart disease* (2nd ed.). New York: Macmillan.

Sjolin, J. (1991). High-dose corticosteroid therapy in human septic shock: Has the jury reached a correct verdict? *Circulatory Shock, 35,* 139-151.

Sleight, P. (1984). Hemodynamics in hypertension and heart failure. *American Journal of Medicine, 76*(58), 3-13.

Smith, C., Arregui, L. M., Promnitz, D. A., & Feldman, C. (1991). Septic shock in the intensive care unit, Hillbrow Hospital, Johannesburg. *South African Medical Journal, 80*(4), 181-184.

Snell, R. J., & Parrillo, J. E. (1991). Cardiovascular dysfunction in septic shock. *Chest, 99*(4), 100-109.

Stollerman, G. H. (1975). *Rheumatic fever and streptococcal infection.* New York: Grune & Stratton.

Stollerman, G. H. (1992). Rheumatic fever and other rheumatic diseases of the heart. In E. Braunwald (Ed.), *Heart disease: A textbook of cardiovascular medicine* (4th ed., pp. 1721-1741). Philadelphia: Saunders.

Sullam, P. M., Drake, T. A., & Sande, M. A. (1985, June). Pathogenesis of endocarditis. *The American Journal of Medicine* [Supplement], *78*(6B), 110-115.

The Expert Panel. (1988). Report of the National Cholesterol Education Program Expert Panel in detection, evaluation, and treatment of high blood cholesterol in adults. *Archives of Internal Medicine, 148*(1), 36-69.

The Expert Panel. (1991). National Cholesterol Education Program. Report of the Expert Panel on population strategies for blood cholesterol reduction: Executive summary. *Achives of Internal Medicine, 151*(6), 1071-1084.

The Review Panel on Coronary Prone Behavior and Coronary Heart Disease. (1981). Coronary prone behavior and coronary heart disease: a critical review. *Circulation, 63,* 1199-1215.

Tiefenbrunn, A. J. (1992). Clinical benefits of thrombolytic therapy in acute myocardial infarction. *American Journal of Cardiology, 69*(2), 3A-11A.

Titus, J. L., & Kim, H. (1990). Blood vessels and lymphatics. In J. M. Kissane (Ed.), *Anderson's pathology* (9th ed., pp. 752-801). St. Louis: Mosby—Year Book.

Tracey, K. J. (1991). Trends in shock research: Tumor necrosis factor (cachectin) in the biology of septic shock syndrome. *Circulatory Shock, 35*(2), 123-128.

Varricchio, C. (1985). Clinical management of superior vena cava syndrome. *Heart & Lung, 14*(4), 411-416.

Virchow, R. (1862). Phlogose und thrombose in geyfassystem. *Gesammelte abhandlungen zur wissen chaftlichen medizin.* Berlin: Max Hirsch.

von Rokitansky, C. (1852). *A manual of physiological anatomy* (vol 4, p. 204). London: Sydenham Society.

Wenger, N. K., Ablemann, W. H., & Roberts, W. C. (1990). Cardiomyopathy and specific heart muscle disease. In J. W. Hurst, R. C. Schlant, C. E. Rackley, E. H. Sonnenblick, & N. K. Wenger, (Eds.), *The heart, arteries, and veins* (7th ed., pp. 1278-1347). New York: McGraw-Hill.

Williams, R. R. (1984). Understanding genetic and environmental risk factors in susceptible persons. *Western Journal of Medicine, 141*(6), 799-806.

Williams, R. R., Hunt, S. C., Hasstedt, S. J., Hopkins, P. N., Wu, L. L., Berry, T. D., Stults, B. M., Barlow, G. K., & Kuida, H. (1990). Genetics of hypertension: What we know and don't know. *Clinical and Experimental Hypertension: Theory and Practice, A12*(5), 865-876.

Williams, R. R., Hunt, S. C., Hasstedt, S. J., Hopkins, P. N., Wu, L. L., Berry, T. D., Stults, B. M., Barlow, G. K., Schumacher, M. C., Lifton, R. P., et al. (1991). Are there interactions and relations between genetic and environmental factors predisposing to high blood pressure? *Hypertension, 18*(3 Suppl. I), I29-I37.

Woo, M. A. (1992). Clinical management of the patient with acute myocardial infarction. *Nursing Clinics of North America, 27*(10), 189-203.

Wynne, J., & Braunwald, E. (1992). The cardiomyopathies and myocarditides. In E. Braunwald (Ed.), *Heart disease: A textbook of cardiovascular medicine* (4th ed., pp. 1394-1450). Philadelphia: Saunders.

Zabriskie, J. B., & Friedman, J. E. (1983). The role of heart binding antibodies in rheumatic fever. *Advances in Experimental Medicine and Biology, 161,* 457-470.

Zentella, A., Kanogue, K., & Cerami, A. (1991). The role of cachectin/TNF and other cytokines in sepsis. *Progress in Clinical and Biological Research, 367,* 9-24.

SUGGESTED READINGS

Anversa, P., Olivett, G., & Capasso, J. M. (1991). Cellular basis of ventricular remodeling after myocardial infarction. *American Journal of Cardiology, 68,* 7D-16D.

Baddour, L. M., Meyer, J., & Henry, B. (1991). Polymicrobial infective endocarditis in the 1980s. *Review of Infectious Diseases, 13*(5), 963-970.

Barco, C. T. (1991). Prevention of infective endocarditis: A review of the medical and dental literature. *Journal of Periodontology, 62*(8), 510-523.

Baue, A. E. (1990). *Multiple organ failure: Patient care and prevention.* St. Louis: Mosby—Year Book.

Baxendale, L. M. (1992). Pathophysiology of coronary artery disease. *Nursing Clinics of North America, 27*(1), 143-152.

Blaustein, M. P., & Grim, C. E. (1991). The pathogenesis of hypertension: Black-white differences. *Cardiovascular Clinics, 21*(3), 97-114.

Cercek, B., Sharifi, B., Barath, P., Bailey, L., & Forrester, J. S. (1991). Growth factors in pathogenesis of coronary arterial restenosis. *American Journal of Cardiology, 68,* 24C-33C.

Chung, E. K. (1987). *Cardiovascular diseases, quick reference to.* Baltimore: Williams & Wilkins.

Cunningham, S. (1992). The epidemiological basis of coronary disease prevention. *Nursing Clinics of North America, 27*(1), 153-170.

Doll, R., & Peto, R. (1976). Mortality in relation to smoking: 20 years observations on male British doctors. *British Medical Journal, 2,* 1525-1536.

Esler, M., Ferrier, C., Lambert, G., Eisenhofer, G., Cox, H., & Jennings, G. (1991). Biochemical evidence of sympathetic hyperactivity in human hypertension. *Hypertension, 17*(4 Suppl. III), III29-III35.

Forrester, J. (1991). Intimal disruption and coronary thrombosis: Its role in the pathogenesis of human coronary disease. *American Journal of Cardiology, 68,* 69B-77B.

Goldstein, J. L., & Brown, M. S. (1985). Familial hypercholesterolemia. A genetic receptor disease. *Hospital Practice, 20*(11), 35-46.

Haber, E., & Slater, E. E. (1988). High blood pressure. *Scientific American Medicine, 1*(I-VII), 1-30.

Hazzard, W. R. (1989). Why do women live longer than men? Biologic differences that influence longevity. *Postgraduate Medicine, 85,* 271-278, 281-283.

Huddleston, V. B. (1992). Conclusion: Collaborative management and overview of multisystem organ failure. In V. B. Huddleston (Ed.), *Multisystem organ failure* (pp. 293-313). St. Louis: Mosby–Year Book.

Huddleston, V. B. (1992). Inflammatory mediators and multisystem organ failure. In V. B. Huddleston (Ed.), *Multisystem organ failure* (pp. 37-56). St. Louis: Mosby–Year Book.

Jacobs, R. F., & Tabor, D. R. (1989). Immune cellular interactions during sepsis and septic injury. *Critical Care Clinics, 5*(1), 9-26.

Kramer, H. J., Meyer-Lehnert, H., Michel, H., & Predel, H. (1991). Endogenous natriuretic and ouabain-like factors. Their roles in body fluid volume and blood pressure regulation. *American Journal of Hypertension, 4*(1), 81-89.

Lerman, A., Edwards, B. S., Hallett, J. W., Heublein, D. M., Sandberg, S. M., & Burnett, J. C., Jr. (1991). Circulating and tissue endothelin immunoreactivity in advanced atherosclerosis. *New England Journal of Medicine, 325*(14), 997-1001.

Mehta, J. L., Nicolini, F. A., Donnelly, W. H., & Nichols, W. W. (1992). Platelet-leukocyte-endothelial interactions in coronary artery disease. *American Journal of Cardiology, 69*(7), 8B-13B.

Schultheis, A. H. (1990). Hypercholesterolemia: Prevention, detection, and management. *Nurse Practitioner, 15*(2), 50-56.

Sugiishi, M., & Takatsu, F. (1993). Cigarette smoking is a major risk factor for coronary spasm. *Circulation, 87,* 76-79.

Alterations of Cardiovascular Function in Children

Sharon L. Sims

Chapter Outline

C*ardiovascular disorders in children can be classified as congenital or acquired. Although this is an oversimplification in some ways, it does facilitate discussion. Certainly the most dramatic and most highly documented cardiovascular disorders in* children *are the congenital defects. The acquired cardiovascular disorders of childhood are less studied and less well documented. They include heart failure (left heart failure), rheumatic heart disease, Kawasaki disease, and hypertension.*

DEVELOPMENT OF THE CARDIOVASCULAR SYSTEM

To understand the pathophysiology of congenital heart defects, it is first necessary to have a clear idea of how the heart develops, the fetal circulation, and changes occurring in the circulation after birth. Heart defects often can be traced to disturbances in these events.

Development of the Heart

The heart arises from the mesenchyme and begins its development as an enlarged blood vessel with a large lumen and a muscular wall (Fig. 28-1, *A*). During the fifth week of gestation, the midsection of this tube begins to grow faster than its ends. This causes the tube to bulge and twist (Fig. 28-1, *B* and *C*) until both ends of the tube come together and fuse (Fig. 28-1, *B* to *D*). The part of the tube at the cranial end of the embryo is the **truncus arteriosus,** which divides longitudinally into the pulmonary artery and aorta. The part of the tube at the caudal end of the embryo becomes the superior and inferior venae cavae.

Inside the developing heart, other changes occur that result in the eventual formation of the four chambers. These changes are illustrated in Fig. 28-2. The development of the cardiac septa, which eventually divide the four chambers, is an intricate process. If the parts of the septa do not develop or fuse properly, several types of

FIG. 28-1 Embryologic development of the heart. The earliest heart structure, **A,** consists of a muscular tube with a large lumen. About the fifth week of gestation, **B,** the tube bulges and, **C,** twists until, **D,** the ends come together and fuse.

defects may occur, among them abnormal openings between chambers, formation of a single atrium or ventricle, or a lack of septa between atria and ventricles. If development of the septa proceeds normally, the four-chambered heart is present by the sixth or seventh week of gestation. Examples of crucial times in fetal heart development with regard to specific defects described in this chapter are listed in Table 28-1.

Development of the Circulation

The anatomic features and direction of fetal blood flow are illustrated in Fig. 28-3. Blood for the fetus is oxygenated in the placenta and returns to the fetus through the umbilical vein. Part of this blood passes through the liver, but approximately half the flow is diverted from the liver through the **ductus venosus** (a connection between the hepatic vessels and the inferior vena cava) into the inferior vena cava, where it is mixed with the blood from the lower extremities. This blood flows into the heart through the **foramen ovale** (the opening between the right and left atria), through the left ventricle, and into the aorta. From there it flows to the head and upper extremities. Because this blood is mainly from the placenta, it has the highest oxygen concentration, or saturation. The brain and coronary arteries therefore receive the blood with the highest oxygen saturation.

Blood returning from the upper body (head, neck, and arms) collects in the superior vena cava. A small portion of this blood passes into the left atrium through the foramen ovale, but most of the blood flows into the right ventricle and out through the pulmonary artery. A small amount of this blood enters the lungs. The largest amount, however, flows through the **ductus arteriosus** (a connection between the pulmonary artery and the aorta) into the descending aorta, to the body, and then back to the placenta through the two umbilical arteries.

It is important to note that the right and left sides of the fetal heart are connected in parallel, rather than in series. That is, they work side by side as almost separate systems, connected only by the foramen ovale and ductus arteriosus. Therefore, the distribution of blood through the body depends on vascular resistance. Fetal pulmonary vascular resistance is high because of vasoconstriction in the lungs caused by low oxygen saturation. (This phenomenon is sometimes called hypoxic va-

TABLE 28-1

Critical Times in Fetal Heart Development Related to Specific Defects

Defect	Critical time in gestation
Transposition of the great vessels	Third to fourth week
Patent ductus arteriosus	Third to eighth week
Anomalous pulmonary venous connection	Third to eighth week
Tricuspid or mitral atresia	Third to sixth week
Ventricular septal defect (muscular)	Fourth to sixth week
Coarctation of the aorta	Fourth week on
Truncus arteriosus	Sixth to seventh week
Ventricular septal defect (membranous)	Sixth to seventh week
Persistent foramen ovale	Eighth week on

From Keith, Roe, & Vlad, 1978.

FIG. 28-2 Development of the cardiac septa. (From Thompson, McFarland, Hirsch, & Tucker, 1993.)

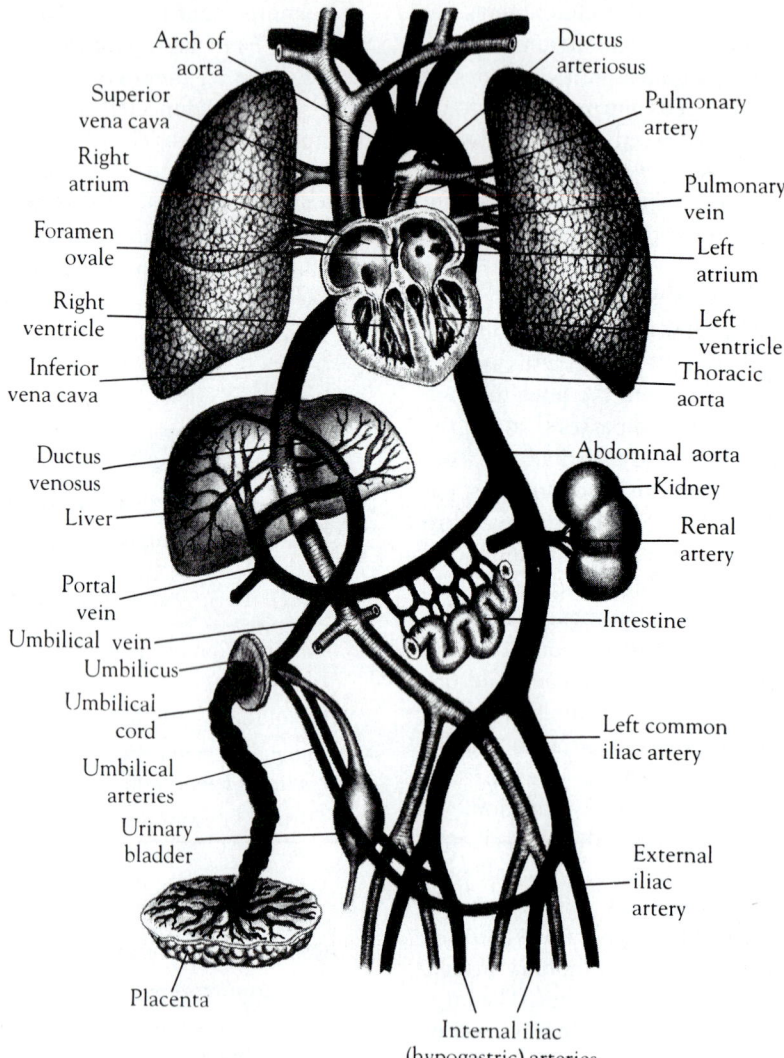

FIG. 28-3 **Fetal circulation.** Circulation of the fetus reflects the fact that oxygenation of fetal blood does not take place in the lungs, but rather in the placenta. Therefore, the pulmonary circulatory system is essentially "bypassed." Instead of traveling from the right heart to the lungs, as occurs after birth, most blood entering the right heart passes through the ductus arteriosus and into the systemic circulation. (From Thompson et al., 1993.)

soconstriction.) Oxygen saturation is low because no gas exchange is taking place in the fetus's uninflated lungs. Conversely, fetal systemic resistance is low because the large-volume placenta is a low-resistance organ. High resistance impedes blood flow and low resistance encourages it. Because of this, very little blood flows into the high-resistance lungs, and most of the blood flows into the low-resistance systemic circulation. High pulmonary resistance diverts most of the blood flow into the pulmonary artery, through the ductus arteriosus, and into the aorta, thereby equalizing the pressure in those two vessels. Because resistance determines the flow when pressure is equal, the blood returns to the low-resistance placenta.

Changes in Circulation at Birth

At birth, a series of circulatory changes occurs, some sudden and some gradual, that affect blood flow dramatically. The most important change taking place in the circulation at birth is the shift of gas exchange from the placenta to the lungs. In addition, changes in pressure and volume of blood flowing through the heart's chambers functionally close the ductus arteriosus, ductus venosus, and foramen ovale. A decrease of pulmonary vascular resistance and an increase of systemic vascular resistance lead to changes in the size and shape of the heart's chambers. The most immediate changes are caused by the severing of the umbilical cord. This removes the low-resistance placenta from the neonate's circulation and causes an immediate increase in systemic vascular resistance, to about twice that before birth. The absence of the placenta also causes a decrease in blood flow through the inferior vena cava because the ductus venosus no longer receives blood from the placenta. Only blood returning to the heart from the lower body now enters the inferior vena cava. Pulmonary vascular resistance decreases suddenly after birth, partly because the lungs expand with breathing, but mostly because exposure to blood with a higher oxygen saturation dilates the pulmonary vessels.

Increased pulmonary venous return and decreased inferior vena caval return cause immediate functional closure of the foramen ovale. In the fetus, the foramen ovale is held open because blood is pushed through it by the relatively greater pressure of inferior vena caval (systemic) return to the right atrium. After birth, this pressure difference is reversed, and the valve flaps of the foramen ovale are closed by the now relatively greater pressure of pulmonary return to the left atrium. Over the course of several months, or even years, the valve flaps of the foramen ovale adhere to the atrial septum and the foramen ovale closes permanently.

The ductus arteriosus closes a little more gradually than the foramen ovale. Increased oxygen saturation in the systemic arterial blood is thought to cause the muscular wall of the ductus arteriosus to constrict, which occludes the opening within 15 to 18 hours after birth. Permanent closure of the ductus arteriosus is complete within about 10 to 21 days after birth (Rudolph, 1974). Low arterial oxygen saturation at birth stimulates the ductus arteriosus to remain open.

Another change that occurs in the first week of life is the closure of the ductus venosus. The mechanism by which this happens is unclear, but closure is usually complete within 7 days of birth. Blood flow through the ductus venosus falls instantly when the umbilical cord is cut, because the umbilical veins no longer bring placental blood to it.

Other more gradual changes combine to decrease pulmonary vascular resistance during the 6 to 8 weeks after birth. The inner medial linings of the small pulmonary arterioles thin out in response to decreased pulmonary arterial pressure. The resulting larger diameters of these vessels cause a decrease in pulmonary resistance. As the lungs grow, so does the pulmonary arterial bed, which further decreases resistance to flow. Finally, increased oxygen saturation causes vasodilation in the pulmonary bed.

The high pulmonary vascular resistance during fetal life affects the anatomy of the ventricles in a significant way. Before birth, high pressure in the pulmonary circulation causes high pressure in the right ventricle. The right ventricle is subject to high afterload, which causes the right ventricular myocardium to become as thick

FIG. 28-4 Oxygen saturation. Schematic representation of normal oxygen saturation (%) and hemodynamics in the neonatal heart and great vessels. This and similar schematics throughout the chapter are extremely simplified; see Chapter 26, Figure 26-5, for correct placement of the great vessels. *RA,* Right atrium; *LA,* left atrium; *RV,* right ventricle. Percentages equal the percentage of hemoglobin (per unit of blood) that is bound with oxygen molecules, or saturated.

and strong as the left. In addition, the fetal right ventricle is heavier than the left ventricle. After birth, when the pulmonary vascular resistance decreases, the right ventricular myocardium begins to thin out. By 1 month of age, the neonate's ventricles are approximately equal in weight. As systemic resistance increases, the left ventricular myocardium becomes thicker than the right, and the ventricles begin to assume the relative size and shape of maturity (Whaley & Wong, 1991). Fig. 28-4 represents normal hemodynamics and oxygen saturation in the neonatal heart.

CONGENITAL HEART DEFECTS

Statistics on the incidence of congenital heart defects have been kept with some consistency since the late 1930s. These figures have been shown to vary widely from medical center to medical center, however, and they depend on criteria used for diagnosis, thoroughness of follow-up, the child's age, and autopsy findings. Reviews of such data for the past 20 years indicate that the overall incidence of congenital heart defects is 1%

TABLE 28-2

Environmental Factors and Associated Congenital Heart Defects

Cause	Type of congenital heart defect
Infection	
Intrauterine	Patent ductus arteriosus (PDA), pulmonary stenosis, coarctation of aorta
Systemic viral	PDA, pulmonary stenosis, coarctation of aorta
Rubella	PDA, pulmonary stenosis, coarctation of aorta
Coxsackie B	Endocardial fibroelastosis
Radiation	Specific cardiovascular effect not known
Metabolic disorders	
Diabetes	Ventricular septal defect (VSD), cardiomegaly, transposition of the great vessels
Phenylketonuria (PKU)	Coarctation of aorta, PDA
Hypercalcemia	Supravalvular aortic stenosis, pulmonic stenosis; aortic hyperplasia
Drugs	
Thalidomide	No specific lesion
Dextroamphetamine	One case of reported transposition
Alcohol	Tetralogy of Fallot, atrial septal defect, ventricular septal defect
Peripheral conditions	
Increased maternal age	VSD, tetralogy of Fallot (relationship unclear)
Antepartal bleeding	Various defects (relationship unclear)
Prematurity	PDA, VSD
High altitude	PDA, atrial septal defect (increased incidence)

Modified from Doyle & Rutkowski, 1970; Whaley & Wong, 1991.

to 2% of all live births (Keith, Rowe, & Vlad, 1978). Other sources estimate the overall incidence of congenital heart defects at 8 in 1000 live births (Behrman, Kliegman, Nelson, & Vaughn, 1992). Stillbirths and spontaneous abortions are generally excluded from these estimates because the incidence of heart defects is much higher in this group.

Although their incidence is significant, the morbidity and mortality rates for congenital heart defects are more significant. It is currently estimated that most deaths caused by congenital heart defects occur in the first year of life (35%) and that more than one third of all children with such defects eventually die of congenital heart disease (Moller & Neal, 1990).

Several environmental and genetic risk factors are associated with the incidence of various types of congenital heart defects. Among the environmental factors are maternal conditions, such as intrauterine viral infection (especially rubella), diabetes mellitus, phenylketonuria, maternal alcoholism, maternal hypercalcemia, drugs (e.g., thalidomide, lithium, dilantin, and dextroamphet-

amine), and complications of increased maternal age, antepartal bleeding, and prematurity. These risk factors and associated heart defects are summarized in Table 28-2.

Genetic factors also have been implicated in the incidence of congenital heart defects, although the mechanism of causation is often unknown. Family studies have shown that the incidence of congenital heart defects in siblings of affected children is three to four times higher than in the general population (Doyle & Rutkowski, 1970). Chromosomal aberrations account for about 6% of all congenital heart defects (Doyle & Rutkowski, 1970). Down syndrome, trisomy 13-15 syndrome, Turner syndrome, and cri du chat syndrome all have been associated with a relatively high incidence of heart defects. (Genetic inheritance is discussed in Chapter 4.) These syndromes and their associated defects are summarized in Table 28-3. Other disorders associated with congenital heart defects are presented in Table 28-4. Only a small percentage of congenital heart defects are clearly linked solely to genetic or to environmental fac-

TABLE 28-3

Genetic Factors and Congenital Heart Defects

Chromosomal aberrations or syndrome	Incidence of defects	Type of defect
Trisomy 13-15	80%	Ventricular septal defect (VSD), atrial septal defect (ASD), patent ductus arteriosus (PDA), anomalous pulmonary venous connection, bicuspid aorta, overriding aorta
Trisomy 18	90%	VSD, PDA, patent foramen ovale, bicuspid aorta, dextrocardia
Down syndrome	12%-44%	Endocardial cushion defects, VSD, PDA, ASD, transposition of great vessels, tetralogy of Fallot, persistent truncus arteriosus, coarctation of aorta, endocardial fibroelastosis
Cri du chat syndrome	20%	PDA, mixed defects
Turner syndrome	20%-40%	Coarctation of aorta, pulmonary stenosis, subaortic and aortic stenosis, PDA, septal defects

From Doyle & Rutkowski, 1970.

TABLE 28-4

Disorders Coexistent with Congenital Heart Defects

Disorder	Associated cardiovascular defect
Connective tissue disorders	
Marfan syndrome	Aortic or mitral regurgitation, aortic aneurysm
Hurler syndrome	Pseudoatherosclerosis
Hunter syndrome	Pseudoatherosclerosis, hypertension
Osteogenesis imperfecta	Incompetent aortic valve
Complex syndromes	
Kartagener syndrome	Dextrocardia
Holt-Oram syndrome	Atrial septal defect (ASD), ventricular septal defect (VSD)
Ellis-van Creveld syndrome	Defect or absence of atrial septum
Laurence-Moon-Biedl syndrome	Tetralogy of Fallot, single ventricle, transposition of aorta
Inborn errors of metabolism	
Pompe disease	Cardiomegaly, left heart failure
Homocuptinuria	Thromboembolic episodes, pulmonic and aortic regurgitation
Phakomatosis	
Neurofibromatosis (von Recklinghausen disease)	Hypertension, pheochromocytoma
von Hippel-Lindau disease	Hypertension, pheochromocytoma
Sturge-Weber-Dimitri disease	Anomalies of carotid and meningeal arteries
Vascular malformations	
Osler-Weber-Rendu disease (hereditary hemorrhagic telangiectasia)	Atrioventricular fistula, telangiectasia
Milroy disease (lymphedema)	Hypoplasia of lymphatic vessels

From Doyle & Rutkowski, 1970.

tors. The cause of most defects is probably multifactorial.

Congenital heart defects can be described with respect to anatomic abnormality, hemodynamic abnormality, or the status of tissue oxgenation. Possible anatomic defects include valvular abnormalities; abnormal openings in the septa, including persistence of the foramen ovale; continued patency of the ductus arteriosus; and malformation or abnormal placement of the great vessels. The hemodynamic alterations caused by these anatomic defects consist of (1) increases or decreases of blood flow through the pulmonary or systemic circulatory systems and (2) the mixing of pulmonary and systemic blood through an abnormal communication that permits flow between the two circulatory systems. The movement of blood between the normally separate pulmonary and systemic circulations is termed a **shunt.** Movement from the pulmonary to the systemic circulation (i.e., from the right heart to the left heart) is called a **right-to-left shunt.** Movement from the systemic to the pulmonary circulation (from the left heart to the right heart) is a **left-to-**

right shunt. Shunt direction depends on relative pressures and resistances (see Chapter 26), and can be obligatory or dependent. In an obligatory shunt, pressure gradients determine the direction of blood flow through an opening, whereas in a dependent shunt, vascular resistance or ventricular compliance determines the direction of flow.

The status of tissue oxygenation is gauged by the presence or absence of cyanosis. **Cyanosis** is a bluish discoloration of the skin. It is a sign that the tissues are not receiving enough oxygen, a condition known as hypoxia. (See Chapter 29 for more discussion about cyanosis and hypoxia. Hypoxic injury to cells is described in Chapter 2.) Hypoxia may be the result of any disorder that prevents oxygen from reaching the body's cells. Ischemia, for example, is hypoxia from lack of blood flow. Congenital heart defects that cause hypoxia, and therefore cyanosis, usually involve a right-to-left shunt, which directs blood flow away from the lungs, or **stenosis** (restrictive narrowing) of structures in the right heart, which restricts outflow to the lungs. Such defects

TABLE 28-5

Classification of Congenital Heart Defects

Pulmonary blood flow	Shunt direction	Specific defects
Acyanotic		
Normal pulmonary flow	None	Pulmonary stenosis; pulmonary valvular dysplasia; peripheral pulmonary arterial stenosis; obstruction to left ventricular outflow (coarctation of aorta, interruption of aortic arch, vascular aortic stenosis, systemic hypertension); endocardial fibroelastosis; myocarditis
Increased pulmonary flow	Left to right	Ventricular septal defect (VSD); patent ductus arteriosus; corrected transposition of the great vessels with VSD; aorticopulmonary septal defect; aortic origin of pulmonary artery; atrial shunts (endocardial cushion defect, atrial septal defect)
Decreased pulmonary flow*	Usually none	Cor triatriatum; parachute mitral valve; supravalvular stenosing ring; pulmonary vein stenosis
Cyanotic		
Increased pulmonary flow	Either direction	Admixture lesions; persistent truncus arteriosus; transposition of great vessels; single ventricle; tricuspid atresia; total anomalous pulmonary venous connection (TAPVC) without obstruction
Decreased pulmonary flow	Right to left	Ventricular septal communications (tetralogy of Fallot and variants); mixed lesions (e.g., single ventricle with pulmonary stenosis); atrial septal communications (pulmonary valve atresia, tricuspid valve atresia, Ebstein anomaly, tricuspid insufficiency)
Increased pulmonary venous markings	Left to right	TAPVC with obstruction

Modified from Moller & Neal, 1990.

*Decreased pulmonary flow causes a characteristic x-ray finding called pulmonary venous markings. The pulmonary veins become distended, which makes them more visible on x-ray films.

are commonly called **cyanotic defects.** Congenital defects that do not cause cyanosis, or **acyanotic defects,** usually involve a left-to-right shunt, which directs blood toward the lungs, or no shunt at all. For the sake of convenience, congenital heart defects can be categorized according to (1) whether they cause cyanosis, (2) whether they increase or decrease blood flow into the pulmonary circulation, and (3) shunt direction. Table 28-5 categorizes the congenital heart defects based on these three characteristics (Moller & Neal, 1990). Many, but not all, of these defects are described in this chapter.

Restriction of Ventricular Outflow

Acyanotic defects with normal pulmonary blood flow are those that cause **right ventricular outflow obstruction,** such as pulmonary stenosis, and those that cause left ventricular outflow obstruction, such as coarctation of the aorta.

Pulmonary Stenosis

Right ventricular outflow can be obstructed by any anatomic abnormality that affects the pulmonic semilunar valve, also called the pulmonary valve. The pulmonic valve is located between the right ventricle and the pulmonary artery. **Pulmonary stenosis** is the narrowing of the valvular opening, by either partial fusing or abnormal thickening of the valve leaflets. Sometimes the annulus, or muscular ring around the valve, is severely narrowed, a variation of pulmonic stenosis termed **pulmonary atresia.** Narrowing also can occur on the arterial side of the valve (**supravalvular stenosis**) or on the ventricular side (**infundibular stenosis**). Pulmonic stenosis accounts for 5% to 8% of all congenital heart defects (Park, 1988).

Pathophysiology

Whatever the anatomic features in a given child, their effect is to create an opening too small for normal outflow during systole (Fig. 28-5, A). Less blood can pass through the pulmonary valve under normal systolic pressure, and some of it remains in the right ventricle, causing increased afterload (see Chapter 26). Essentially, valvular stenosis causes the whole system to "back up," which further increases pressures in the right ventricle. The smaller the valve opening, the harder it will be for the right ventricle to maintain output. To do so, the right ventricular myocardium undergoes hypertrophy. If the outflow obstruction is very severe, blood backs up in the right atrium, causing dilation and hypertrophy, and leads to the reopening of the foramen ovale. Higher pressures in the right atrium can create a right-to-left shunt across the foramen ovale. Children with this condition also develop cyanosis, because the blood shunting from right to left is deoxygenated (Fig.

FIG. 28-5 Pulmonary stenosis. A, Obstruction of right ventricular outflow due to pulmonary stenosis. Pressure on the ventricular side of the pulmonic semilunar valve (pulmonary valve) is much greater than that on the pulmonary arterial side. This difference disrupts the normal pressure gradient across the valve. Pulmonary stenosis increases ventricular afterload by decreasing blood flow through the valve *(dashed arrows),* which causes ventricular hypertrophy. **B,** The backup of ventricular afterload into the right atrium reopens the foramen ovale. Venous blood then flows from the area of higher pressure (the right atrium) to the area of lower pressure (the left atrium) causing a right-to-left shunt. Cyanosis occurs if enough venous blood shunts from right to left to reduce oxygen saturation in the systemic circulation by 3% to 5%. (From Whaley & Wong, 1991.)

28-5, *B*). Related conditions with similar cardiac effects are stenosis of the peripheral pulmonary arteries and dysplasia of the pulmonary valve.

Clinical Manifestations

In mild to moderate cases of right ventricular outflow obstruction, the right ventricle and atrium remain almost normal in size, and the foramen ovale does not reopen, so that shunting and cyanosis do not occur. The child looks healthy and may be asymptomatic. Growth and development usually are normal. A systolic murmur is heard because blood flow through the narrowed valve is turbulent. The electrocardiogram (ECG) is likely to be normal or indicates some right ventricular hypertrophy. X-ray films show a normal-sized heart and normal pulmonary vessels.

In severe cases of right ventricular outflow obstruction, decreased growth and development, cyanosis, dyspnea, and breathlessness caused by congestive heart failure may be evident. The systolic murmur is louder than in a mild case, and the ECG indicates hypertrophy of the right ventricle and, perhaps, of the right atrium.

Evaluation and Treatment

Besides electrocardiography and chest x-ray films, diagnostic procedures include cardiac catheterization, angiocardiography, and echocardiogram. The treatment of pulmonary stenosis consists of pulmonary valvotomy, in which fused pulmonary valve leaflets are freed from one another or the narrow opening is widened.

Coarctation of the Aorta
Pathophysiology

Obstruction of outflow from the left ventricle often is the result of a localized malformation of the aorta that narrows its lumen sufficiently to impede blood flow. This congenital defect, termed **coarctation of the aorta,** may occur anywhere between the origin of the aortic arch and bifurcation of the aorta in the lower abdomen. Coarctation is most common (98% of cases) in the aortic arch, just below the origin of the left subclavian artery (Behrman et al., 1992). Narrowing may occur before, at, or after the opening of the ductus arteriosus.

The location of the coarctation determines its hemodynamic consequences. When the narrowing is distal to the opening of the ductus arteriosus, and the ductus is closed, it is called **postductal coarctation** (Fig. 28-6). When the narrowing is proximal to the ductus arteriosus, it is called a **preductal coarctation.**

Postductal coarctation. Closure of the ductus arteriosus, which occurs 10 to 21 days after birth, proceeds from its pulmonary to its aortic end. While the aortic end of the ductus arteriosus is open, blood can flow around the coarctation through the orifice of the ductus arteriosus. As the opening of the ductus arteriosus

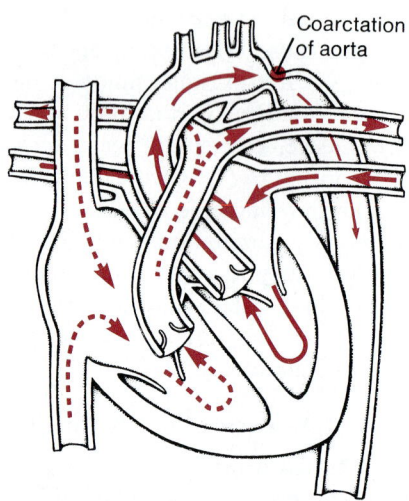

FIG. 28-6 **Postductal and preductal coarctation of the aorta.** Postductal coarctation occurs distal to ("after") the insertion of the closed ductus arteriosus into the aortic arch. Preductal coarctation occurs proximal to ("before") insertion of the patent ductus arteriosus. The coarctation consists of a flap of tissue that protrudes from the tunica media of the aortic wall. (From Whaley & Wong, 1991.)

closes, the degree of obstruction increases. Systolic pressure increases in the ascending aorta and the left ventricle and decreases in the descending aorta beyond the coarctation (Fig. 28-7). Because the vessels branching off the ascending aorta (the subclavian arteries) supply the head and upper extremities, systolic blood pressure in these parts of the body *may* be elevated, and because the descending aorta ultimately supplies the lower extremities, systolic blood pressure in the legs *may* be depressed. The classic clinical manifestations of postductal coarctation are decreased or absent pulses in the femoral arteries and lower extremities, sometimes accompanied by mottled skin or cyanosis of the lower extremities and epistaxis (nosebleeds).

The likelihood of congestive left heart failure depends on the severity and location of the coarctation and the age of the child. In the first month of life, the ventricles have a limited ability to compensate for the higher afterload that occurs with coarctation. As a consequence of the increased afterload, the left ventricle and atrium enlarge. To bypass the coarctation, collateral circulation develops around the obstruction. Small arteries bypass the coarctation by branching from the subclavian arteries and joining the intercostal arteries that branch from the descending aorta. This bypass around the coarctation supplies more oxygenated blood to the lower extremities. The collateral vessels become enlarged and kinked, and leave telltale "notches" that are visible on x-ray films where they pass over the ribs.

Preductal coarctation. Preductal coarctation of the

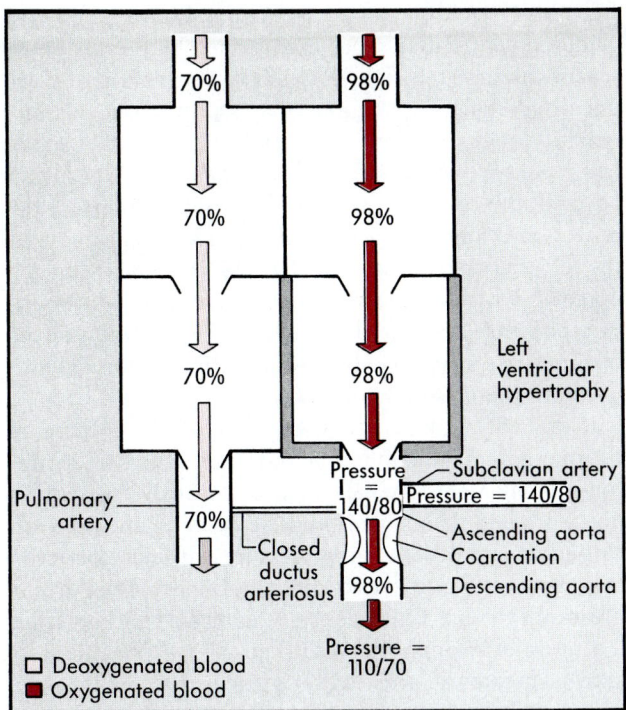

FIG. 28-7 Hemodynamics of postductal coarctation of the aorta. Blood pressure increases in the ascending aorta and subclavian artery and decreases in the descending aorta. These pressure changes eventually occur in the parts of the systemic circulation served by arteries that branch from the aorta before and after the coarctation.

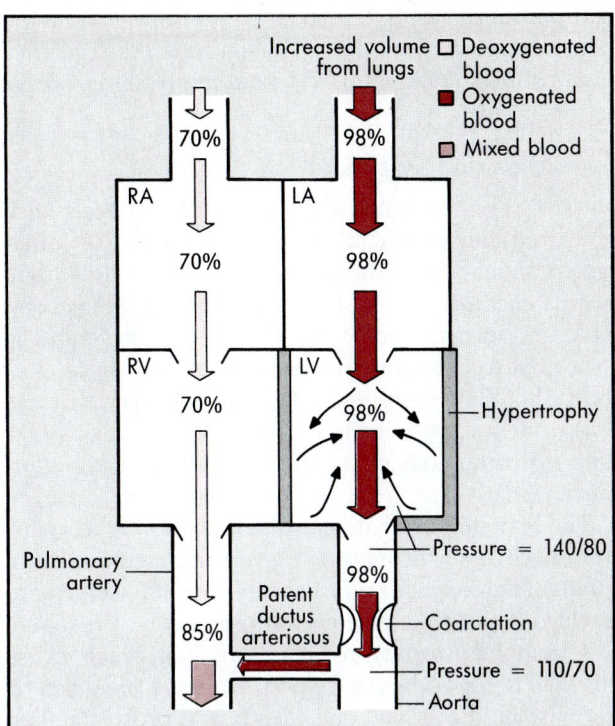

FIG. 28-8 Hemodynamics of preductal coarctation of the aorta with a patent ductus arteriosus. The left-to-right shunt through the ductus arteriosus increases the volume of blood in the pulmonary circulation. Afterload (indicated by dashed arrows) is increased in the left heart by (1) increased return from the lungs and (2) decreased ventricular outflow caused by the coarctation. The outcome is left heart failure (congestive heart failure).

aorta (infantile coarctation) occurs proximal to the opening of the ductus arteriosus (see Fig. 28-6). Preductal coarctation is often associated with other congenital defects, particularly continued patency of the ductus arteriosus and openings in the interventricular septum.

A shunt is created if the ductus remains patent. The direction of the shunt depends first on the difference in blood pressure between the aorta and pulmonary artery. If there is no difference in pressure between these vessels, the direction of the shunt is determined by differences in total pulmonary and systemic resistance. For example, if pulmonary vascular resistance is higher than systemic resistance (as it is in the neonate before pulmonary vascular resistance decreases), blood flow through the patent ductus arteriosus will be from right to left. The right ventricle acts as a systemic pump, sending unoxygenated blood through the ductus into the descending aorta below the coarctation. When this occurs, the classic difference between pulses in the upper and lower extremities disappears.

If the blood pressure is greater in the aorta than in the pulmonary artery, blood flow through the ductus will be left to right, toward the lungs (Fig. 28-8). This can cause more than the normal amount of blood to be

sent to the lungs. As the increased pulmonary blood volume reaches the left heart, it puts a strain on the left atrium and ventricle, often leading to congestive heart failure. The left heart has two sources of afterload: increased volume from the pulmonary circulation and obstruction to outflow caused by coarctation of the aorta. Both cause left ventricular hypertrophy.

Clinical Manifestations

The most important clinical manifestation of coarctation of the aorta is left heart failure (see p. 1108). Its onset and associated problems depend on how soon after birth the neonate's pulmonary vascular resistance decreases and the ductus arteriosus closes, the location and degree of coarctation, and whether the neonate has associated cardiac defects.

Usually the first manifestations of coarctation of the aorta are manifestations of congestive heart failure (see p. 1108 and Chapter 27). Once heart failure has developed, cyanosis occurs in the whole body, not just in the lower extremities. Fine crackles can be heard in the lungs. If the heart failure is advanced, insufficient cardiac output causes decreased blood pressures in both the upper and lower extremities, obliterating the difference in pressures that might otherwise result from the coarctation.

Evaluation and Treatment

Chest x-ray examinations show an enlarged heart with left atrial and ventricular hypertrophy. Cardiac catheterization may be performed to measure pressures in the heart's chambers, the pulmonary artery, and the aorta. Oxygen saturation of blood within these structures is measured to determine the direction of the shunt. Angiocardiography also may be performed to visualize the aorta, the location of the coarctation, and any associated malformations of the interventricular septum and aortic valve.

The first step in treatment of coarctation is to stabilize the child's vital signs and treat the congestive heart failure. High concentrations of supplemental oxygen are avoided because the ductus arteriosus (unlike other vessels) responds to oxygen by constricting, which worsens the effects of the coarctation. Diuretics are given to decrease fluid overload and edema, and prostaglandins may be given to dilate the ductus arteriosus.

Resection of the coarctation is the classic surgical treatment for localized postductal coarctation. Surgery is performed when the congestive heart failure is under control or when the child's aorta has grown to near-maximum size, between the ages of 3 and 5 years (Moller & Neal, 1990). Preductal coarctation requires resection of a larger portion of the aorta, closure of the ductus arteriosus, and closure of interventricular septal openings, which are commonly associated with preductal coarctations. Bypass grafts and subclavian flap aortoplasty are examples of other surgical techniques used to correct coarctations.

Acyanotic Heart Defects with Increased Pulmonary Blood Flow

Acyanotic heart defects with increased pulmonary blood flow result in a left-to-right shunt. Some of the most common conditions in this category are ventricular septal defects, patent ductus arteriosus, and atrial septal defects. Other such defects, which are not discussed here, are endocardial cushion defect and systemic arteriovenous fistulous connection.

Ventricular Septal Defect

A **ventricular septal defect** (VSD) is a hole in the interventricular septum. As an isolated (single) defect, VSD occurs at a rate of 1.5 to 2.6 per 1000 live births and as 25% to 30% of all congenital heart defects (Behrman et al., 1992). Ventricular septal defects occur in conjunction with other heart defects in about 50% of children who have congenital heart disease.

Pathophysiology

The interventricular septum is formed by the fusion of several tissues: the right and left bulbar ridges, the endocardial cushions, the muscular septum, and the aorticopulmonary system (Fig. 28-2). Fusion is usually complete by the seventh week of gestation. A VSD can occur if any of these tissues fail to fuse with any of the others, creating an opening almost anywhere between the left and right ventricles (Fig. 28-9). The size of the opening, which can vary widely, determines the amount of blood that is shunted through it. The position of the opening also can vary, but its size affects hemodynamics more than its location does.

If the VSD is very small, the flow of blood through the opening may be minimal and often causes no symptoms. Small VSDs often close spontaneously and require no treatment. The controlling factor in shunt direction through a small VSD is the pressure difference between the right and left ventricles. Normally, pressure is greater in the left ventricle, causing blood to shunt from left to right through the VSD (Fig. 28-9, B). If the pressure is greater in the right ventricle than in the left, blood shunts from right to left through the VSD.

Hemodynamics are quite different if the VSD is large (Fig. 28-9, C). With a large VSD, the blood flows through the opening unimpeded, leading to equal pressure in both ventricles. Because there is no pressure gradient to produce a shunt, the difference between pulmonary and systemic vascular resistance becomes the determinant of shunt direction through a large VSD. Because systemic resistance is usually higher than pulmonary resistance, blood flows from the left (the area of greatest resistance) to the right (the area of lowest resistance).

When a large amount of blood shunts from left to right through a VSD, it has nowhere to go except into the lungs through the pulmonary artery and then back to the left side of the heart, where it creates serious strain. To compensate for volume overload, the left ventricle enlarges. Enlargement (hypertrophy) reduces compliance and increases contractility. For a time, the larger ventricle pumps more effectively. Eventually, however, the heart can no longer handle the increased volume, and heart failure ensues.

The pulmonary vascular bed also undergoes changes due to the increased volume it receives. In an attempt to maintain normal blood volume, the vessels undergo changes that increase their resistance to flow. The smooth muscle layer in the arteriolar walls increases and extends farther than normal into the metarterioles. Proliferation of the intimal layer also occurs. The effect of these changes is to decrease the diameter of the vessels, which increases their resistance to blood flow. This protective mechanism of pulmonary hypertension succeeds at first, because it helps to decrease the volume of blood flowing into the lungs. Eventually, however, the changes become permanent, and pulmonary vascular resistance

Ventricular septal defect

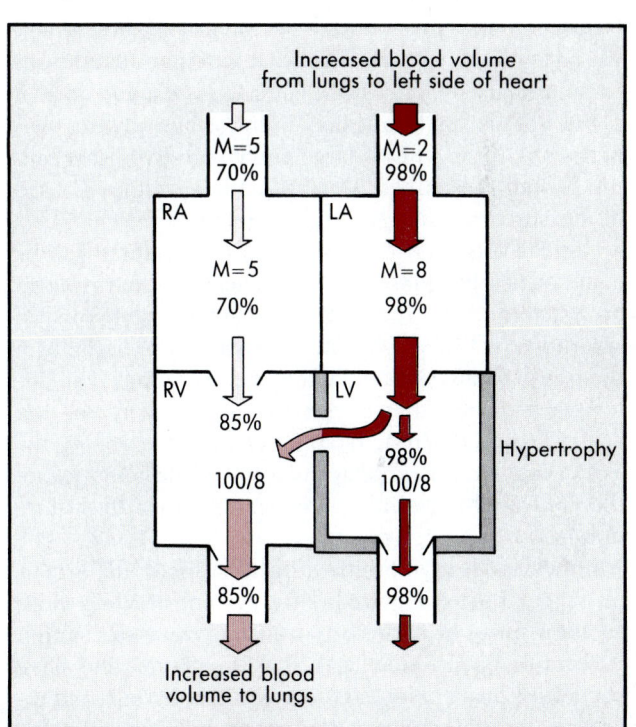

FIG. 28-9 **Ventricular septal defects. A,** Ventricular septal defect (VSD) with left-to-right shunt. **B,** Hemodynamics of a small VSD with left-to-right shunt. Mean (M) indicates mean of pressure; systolic/diastolic pressures are in mm Hg; and percentages indicate oxygen saturation. **C,** Hemodynamics of a large VSD with left-to-right shunt. Like the shunting that occurs in preductal coarctation of the aorta, the shunting pictured here causes left ventricular overload and hypertrophy. (From Whaley & Wong, 1991.)

continues to rise. In some cases, it eventually exceeds systemic vascular resistance, causing the shunt through the VSD to reverse directions. At this point, deoxygenated blood is forced into the systemic circulation, and cyanosis occurs. This phenomenon, known as **Eisenmenger syndrome,** is a late and usually fatal complication of a VSD.

Clinical Manifestations

Neonates with small VSDs are usually acyanotic and have no symptoms. Those with large VSDs have obvious manifestations. The murmur is usually heard shortly after birth, and is a harsh, loud, holosystolic murmur heard at the left lower sternal border. The loudness of the murmur is not directly correlated with the size of the VSD; rather, the smaller the opening, the louder the murmur. This is because there is a greater pressure gradient across a small VSD, which creates greater turbulence of blood flow through the opening. The more turbulent the flow, the louder the murmur. Congestive heart failure develops when the infant is 4 to 12 weeks of age (Keith et al., 1978). Cyanosis is caused by low cardiac output caused by heart failure and not by the VSD itself. Cyanosis does not result directly from a left-to-right shunt. Only in the case of Eisenmenger syndrome, in which the shunt is reversed, does the VSD itself cause cyanosis.

Evaluation and Treatment

Diagnosis of a VSD is made on the basis of chest x-ray films, ECGs, cardiac catheterization, angiography, or echocardiogram. Chest x-ray films will show cardiac enlargement and pronounced or intensified pulmonary vascular markings, which indicate vascular adaptations to pulmonary hypertension. The ECG is usually normal if the VSD is small, but may indicate biventricular hypertrophy if the VSD is large and congestive heart failure is well established. Cardiac catheterization is used to measure pressures and oxygen levels in the chambers and great vessels. If the VSD is large, pressures will be equal or nearly equal in both ventricles and in the aorta at systemic levels. If the shunt is left to right, oxygen saturation will be higher in the right ventricle than in the right atrium. (Normally they are the same.) The difference indicates that oxygenated blood from the left ventricle has entered the right ventricle through the VSD. Angiography is performed to visualize and locate the VSD and to determine whether any other defects are present.

If the child is asymptomatic or has a small VSD, treatment may not be required. Fifty percent of VSDs close spontaneously or shrink to an insignificant size within 5 years of birth (Arciniegas, 1985). Infants who have congestive heart failure are treated with digoxin and diuretics until surgery can be performed. Although the surgical closure is sometimes performed on an infant, many surgeons prefer to wait until the child is 1 to 3 years old, provided that the VSD is asymptomatic. Waiting until the heart is larger lowers the risks of surgery. The surgery must, however, be done before increases in pulmonary vascular resistance become permanent. In some cases, the pulmonary artery is banded, or artificially constricted, before the VSD is closed. This decreases the left-to-right shunt and protects the pulmonary vasculature from overload. Permanent repair is made with a synthetic patch over the VSD. Because the conduction system of the heart runs through the ventricular septum, surgical manipulation carries some risk of heart block.

Patent Ductus Arteriosus

The aortic arch system develops between the fifth and sixth weeks of gestation. Six pairs of arches branch off the truncus arteriosus and connect with the dorsal aorta. Eventually, most of these arches develop into arteries, such as the right and left pulmonary arteries, and lose their connection to the aorta. The sixth arch on the left side, however, retains an attachment to the aorta and becomes the ductus arteriosus. Its function is to shunt blood away from the fetal lungs and into the systemic circulation. Normally, the ductus arteriosus becomes functionally closed shortly after birth and anatomically by constriction and fibrosis within 10 to 21 days after birth. Sometimes closure does not occur and the ductus arteriosus remains open, or patent. This condition is termed **patent ductus arteriosus** (PDA).

Estimates of incidence vary. Patent ductus arteriosus occurs in isolation or with other defects in approximately 10% of children with congenital heart defects (Moller & Neal, 1990). The incidence of PDA is greater in females than in males, and it is greater in premature infants than in full-term infants.

Pathophysiology

The pathogenesis of PDA is not known. Because it is not known precisely what causes the ductus arteriosus to close, it is difficult to pinpoint what might cause it to remain open.

The PDA may be long and narrow or short and wide. At the short extreme, it consists of only a "window" between the aorta and pulmonary artery. Its hemodynamic effects depend on the size of its lumen and, as always, the relative resistance in the pulmonary and systemic circulations (Behrman et al., 1992) (Fig. 28-10, A). In general, as pulmonary resistance decreases and systemic resistance increases at birth, blood flow through the PDA reverses, becoming left to right. This shunts oxygenated blood into the pulmonary circulation. The hemodynamic effect of a left-to-right shunt is to increase pulmonary blood flow (Fig. 28-10, B). The hemodynamic effects of a PDA are similar to those of a VSD, and so are the possible complications: pulmonary hypertension and congestive heart failure. Subacute bacterial endocarditis is also seen as a complication of PDA. These complications are most common in premature infants who also have respiratory distress syndrome (see Chapter 31).

Clinical Manifestations

Full-term infants do not exhibit clinical manifestations of PDA at birth. No murmur is heard at birth because the systemic and pulmonary vascular resistances are still approximately equal, which prevents shunting of blood through the PDA. As the pulmonary and systemic resis-

FIG. 28-10 Patent ductus arteriosus. **A,** Patent ductus arteriosus with left-to-right shunt. **B,** Changes in oxygen saturation, left ventricular volume, and the myocardium due to left-to-right shunt through a patent ductus arteriosus. (From Whaley & Wong, 1991.)

tances approach mature values—between 2 and 6 weeks after birth—left-to-right shunting begins. With its onset, a murmur is heard. The murmur begins as a systolic murmur, but both systolic and diastolic components of the typical "machinery" murmur are evident by the end of the first year. This occurs because the shunting begins to take place during both phases of the cardiac cycle (Fink, 1991). If the left ventricle does not

accommodate the increased load of blood returning from the lungs, the infant may develop left heart failure (see p. 1108).

Evaluation and Treatment

Chest x-rays usually show cardiomegaly and intensified pulmonary vascular markings. Cardiac catheterization and angiography may be performed to determine the size and location of the PDA. These procedures are used if the child has congestive heart failure or pulmonary hypertension, or if the diagnosis cannot be made on the basis of the characteristic murmur.

Digoxin and diuretics are given if the infant has congestive heart failure. Drug therapy is followed by ligation of the PDA. Ligation has a mortality rate of less than 1% (Behrman et al., 1992). The procedure does not require cardiopulmonary bypass or incisions into the heart itself. The ductus arteriosus is simply ligated with a suture and allowed to fibrose. In older children, the ductus may be ligated and oversewn (Arciniegas, 1985). Catheter-delivered occlusion devices have also been shown to be safe and effective in the closure of PDAs. In critically ill infants, medical closure is attempted through the use of prostaglandin inhibitors, such as indomethacin (Whaley & Wong, 1991).

Atrial Septal Defect

An **atrial septal defect** (ASD) is an abnormal opening in the interatrial septum (Fig. 28-11, *A*). Atrial septal defects account for approximately 8% of congenital heart defects. The interatrial septum develops during the fourth to sixth weeks of gestation, from a series of tissue walls (septum primum and septum secundum) that are laid down and resorbed (Fig. 28-2). The fetal atrial septum contains one opening, the foramen ovale, which is covered by a flap of tissue on the left side, creating a one-way valve from right to left. During fetal life, blood flows through the foramen ovale from right to left, shunting blood away from the pulmonary circulation into the systemic circulation (Fig. 28-3). Normal development of the atrial septum involves a delicate balance between the laying down of tissue and its reabsorption.

Pathophysiology

The hemodynamics of ASDs are similar to those of VSDs. The size of the ASD determines the direction of blood flow through the opening. If the opening is small, the normal pressure difference between the right and left atria is maintained; that is, pressure is greater on the left side. This gradient causes blood to shunt from left to right through the ASD. If the opening is large, however, pressures in the atria are equalized and shunt direction is determined by relative resistance in the ventricles. In this respect, the hemodynamics of ASDs dif-

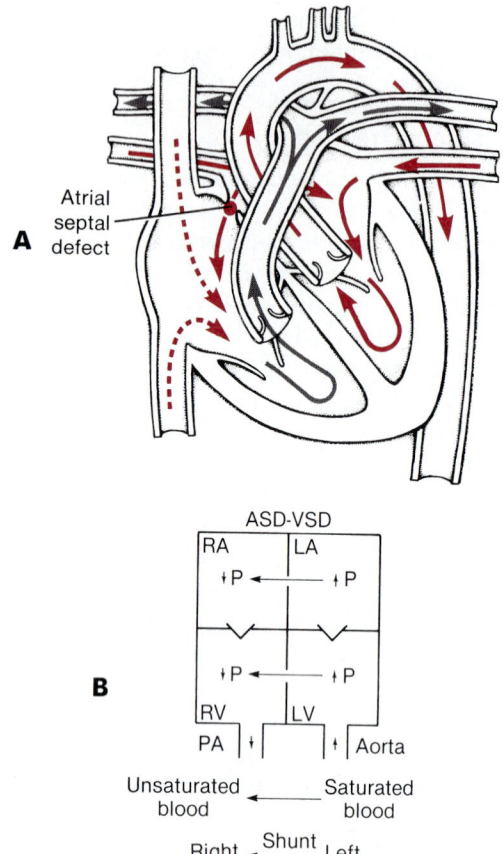

FIG. 28-11 **Atrial septal defect. A,** Atrial septal defect. **B,** Hemodynamics of atrial septal defect with left-to-right shunt. (From Whaley & Wong, 1991.)

Clinical Manifestations

Because the shunt through a simple ASD is from left to right, cyanosis does not occur. Most neonates and infants with isolated ASDs are asymptomatic until changes in myocardial thickness affect compliance. Therefore the defect may go undetected until the child is of preschool age. Only approximately 2% of children with ASDs develop congestive heart failure (Moller & Neal, 1990). (Manifestations of left heart failure are described on p. 1108.) Children with congestive heart failure attributable to ASDs are prone to develop respiratory infections, such as pneumonia. The soft murmur associated with ASD is usually heard at the second intercostal space and is caused by the increased flow of blood across the pulmonic semilunar valve. The second heart sound may have a fixed, wide split because the right ventricle is always overloaded, which causes continuous delayed closure of the pulmonic valve. (In the normal heart, delayed closure is only detected on inspiration.)

Evaluation and Treatment

Chest x-ray films of symptomatic children show an enlarged heart and increased pulmonary vascular markings. Electrocardiograms often indicate right axis deviation and diastolic overload of the right ventricle (Behrman et al., 1992). Cardiac catheterization may not be performed unless the cause of the congestive heart failure is undetermined. Because oxygenated blood enters the right atrium, oxygen saturation in the right heart is greater than normal. Pressures will be equal in both atria if the ASD is large. Two-dimensional echocardiography is often used to determine the features of a given ASD (Moller & Neal, 1990).

Congestive heart failure must be stabilized before surgery can be performed. Stabilization includes administration of digoxin and diuretics, sometimes for several months. If the pharmacologic treatment is effective, respiratory infections will decrease, and the child will be able to eat and grow more normally while awaiting surgery. If the child is too stressed to eat, gastrostomy feedings become part of the medical management. Surgery consists of patching the ASD with a synthetic graft or simply stitching it shut. Although surgery has been performed on very young infants, the preferred approach is to wait until the child is older and risk decreases. There is also the possibility that the defect will close spontaneously.

Cyanotic Heart Defects with Increased Pulmonary Blood Flow
Persistent Truncus Arteriosus

Persistent truncus arteriosus (PTA) is the failure of the large embryonic artery, the truncus arteriosus, to divide into the pulmonary artery and the aorta. Instead, the

fer somewhat from the hemodynamics of VSDs. Shunt direction through a large VSD is determined by relative resistance in the pulmonary and systemic circulation, because these circuits receive ventricular outflow. Because atrial outflow is received by the ventricles, relative ventricular resistance is the crucial factor determining shunt direction through a large ASD.

Resistance to blood flow from the atria to the ventricles is determined by ventricular compliance. Ventricular compliance, or elasticity, depends on the thickness of the ventricular walls: the thicker the myocardium, the less compliant it is (see Chapter 26). At birth, the walls of both ventricles are about equal in thickness, so they are equally compliant, and no blood flows through the ASD. As the infant grows, the left ventricular wall thickens and the right ventricular wall thins. Compliance decreases on the left and increases on the right, causing blood to flow through the ASD from left to right (Fig. 28-11, *B*).

truncus arteriosus persists and, through a single valve, empties both ventricles, which communicate through a large VSD at the top of the interventricular septum (Fig. 28-12, *A*). This single valve takes the place of the aortic and pulmonic valves. Persistent truncus arteriosus causes the combined output of the ventricles to flow into both the systemic and pulmonary circulations. Persistent truncus arteriosus is fairly rare, accounting for approximately 2% of congenital heart defects.

Pathophysiology

The truncus arteriosus normally divides into the aorta and pulmonary trunk through the development of a spiral septum, which also closes the upper part of the interventricular septum. Any interruption of this process of division results in a large, single artery (the truncus arteriosus), which overrides a VSD.

The truncus arteriosus usually lies over both ventricles and all blood flowing from both chambers enters through the truncal valve. A mixture of oxygenated and deoxygenated blood is thus pumped to the lungs and to the body (Fig. 28-12, *B*). Because the VSD is usually high on the septal wall, just below the truncal valve, the mitral valve adjoins the truncal valve. Occasionally, the tricuspid valve is part of this complex as well. (Normally, all of the valves are part of the heart's fibrous skeleton; see Chapter 26.) The truncal valve is often stenosed and thickened or has defective leaflets. The pulmonary arteries originate in various abnormal sites. For example, they may originate on the left side of the truncus arteriosus, just above the truncal valve; on the posterior side of the truncus; or on the sides of the truncus (Fig. 28-12, *B*). Sometimes the pulmonary arteries are absent or stenotic.

All of the blood from both ventricles flows into the truncus, after which the volume of flow that enters the aorta and pulmonary arteries depends on the difference between pulmonary and systemic resistance. In most cases, blood pressures in the pulmonary arteries and aorta are equal, so that relative total systemic and pulmonary resistances determine which system receives the greatest amount of blood. The hemodynamic pattern is basically that of a VSD. If, however, the ductus arteriosus is stenosed, a natural pulmonary artery banding occurs that limits blood flow to the lungs. If pulmonary vascular resistance is high and blood flow to the lungs is low, less oxygenated blood returns to the left heart, and cyanosis is increased. If pulmonary vascular resistance decreases, cyanosis decreases because more blood flows to the lungs.

Clinical Manifestations

Congestive heart failure is a common manifestation of persistent truncus arteriosus, and the child may fail to thrive from an early age. Fine crackles in the lungs are

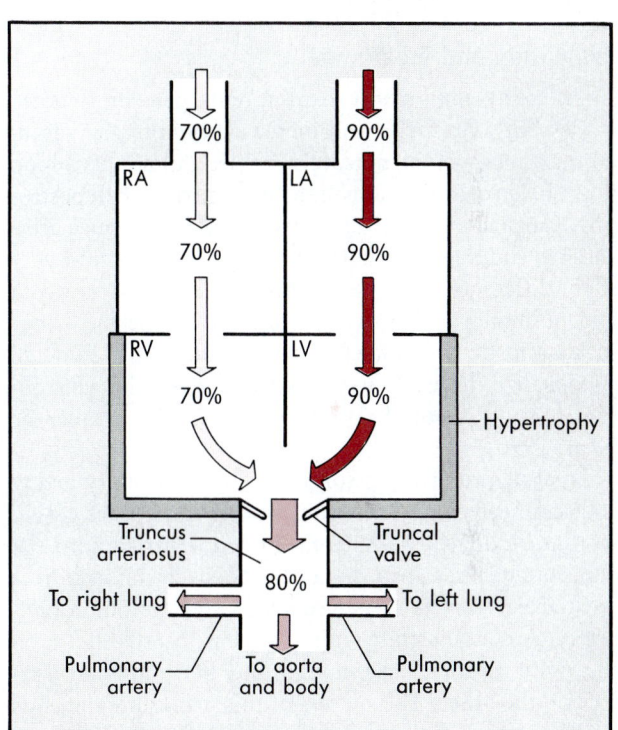

FIG. 28-12 Truncus arteriosus. A, Persistent truncus arteriosus. The truncus arteriosus fails to divide into the pulmonary artery and aorta, and the interventricular septum fails to close at the top. Blood from both ventricles mixes in the truncus arteriosus and then enters the pulmonary and systemic circuits. **B,** Alterations of hemodynamics and oxygen saturation by persistent truncus arteriosus. (From Whaley & Wong, 1991.)

common. Cyanosis is present in varying degrees. It usually is mild in the neonate, but increases with age. The degree of cyanosis depends on the amount of blood flowing to the lungs. Usually, PTA causes an increase in pulmonary blood flow, so cyanosis is mild or absent. If, however, blood flow to the lungs is significantly restricted over time, the child develops polycythemia (overproliferation of red blood cells), plethora (reddened skin caused by excessive blood volume), and clubbing of the fingers, as well as bluish lips and mucous membranes. Like a large VSD, PTA can increase pulmonary vascular resistance to the point of causing Eisenmenger syndrome (see p. 1097). Cyanosis then becomes chronic.

Persistent truncus arteriosus causes a wide pulse pressure (a greater-than-average difference between systolic and diastolic blood pressures). Systolic pressure is increased because the output of *both* ventricles enters the truncus arteriosus with each systolic contraction. Diastolic pressure is lower than usual because blood is diverted from the aorta (systemic circulation) into the pulmonary arteries (pulmonary circulation) during the diastolic phase of the cardiac cycle.

Evaluation and Treatment

Chest x-ray films show cardiac enlargement that includes both ventricles and increased pulmonary vascular markings, which indicate increased pulmonary blood flow. Electrocardiograms indicate ventricular hypertrophy. Cardiac catheterization usually detects equal pressures in the right and left ventricles and aorta and very slight differences in oxygen saturation between the aorta and pulmonary arteries. Angiography is the most useful diagnostic technique because it enables the clinician to visualize the PTA, hypertrophied ventricles, and location and size of the pulmonary arteries (Moller & Neal, 1990).

Treatment of PTA is surgical. The pulmonary artery is disconnected from the truncus, and the VSD is closed so that blood will flow from the left ventricle into the truncus and then into the aorta. Next, a connection is created between the right ventricle and the pulmonary artery. A conduit graft with a valve is inserted between the right ventricle on one end and the pulmonary artery on the other. The success of this procedure depends on the status of the child's pulmonary vascular resistance. Mortality rate is 39% if pulmonary vascular resistance is high and 14% if it is low (Arciniegas, 1985). Untreated PTA is fatal, usually within the first few months of life.

Complete Transposition of the Great Vessels

Complete transposition of the great vessels (TGA) is a defect in which the aorta and pulmonary arteries are completely switched; that is, the aorta arises from the right ventricle, and the pulmonary artery arises from the left ventricle. Complete transposition of the great vessels accounts for 8% to 9% of congenital heart disorders. Various studies have shown that the incidence of this condition is 1 in 4000 to 4500 live births (Moller & Neal, 1990). Males are affected twice as often as females, and maternal diabetes is a risk factor. Until an

effective treatment was developed in the 1960s, transposition of the great vessels was fatal in 95% of cases. By the early 1980s, the mortality rate had dropped to less than 10% (Guzzetta & Dossey, 1984).

Pathophysiology

It is not known precisely which embryologic events lead to transposition, but researchers have proposed that the fault lies in the development of conal tissue in the fibrous skeleton of the heart (Moller & Neal, 1990). The conus is a segment of muscle that separates the atrioventricular (tricuspid and mitral) valves from the semilunar (aortic and pulmonic) valves. (The fibrous skeleton and heart valves are described and illustrated in Chapter 26; see Figure 26-4.) Normally, this conus grows more on the left side, under the pulmonic valve. This pushes the pulmonic valve anteriorly and to the left of the aortic valve. Some researchers believe that in transposition of the great vessels, nearly the opposite occurs; that is, the conus beneath the aortic valve grows more, pushing the aortic valve until it is anterior (forward) and superior to the pulmonic valve. This causes the aorta to rise anteriorly and to the right of the pulmonary artery (Fink, 1991; Keith et al., 1978). The interventricular septum is intact in about 60% of cases of transposition; a VSD is present in the remaining 40%. Pulmonary stenosis is associated with the transposition in about 4% to 6% of children with intact septums and in 28% to 31% of children with VSDs (Keith et al., 1978). The discussion that follows is limited to the pathophysiology of complete transposition with an intact interventricular septum.

The outstanding feature of complete transposition is that it creates two closed systems: blood from the pulmonary circulation does not enter the systemic circulation, and vice versa (Fig. 28-13). This, of course, is not conducive to life, because unoxygenated blood circulates continuously through the systemic circulation, and oxygenated blood circulates repeatedly through the pulmonary circulation.

Two factors allow neonates with complete transposition to survive long enough to be treated. First, blood from the two closed systems can mix through the ductus arteriosus for a short time after birth if pulmonary vascular resistance remains high. Some mixing also may occur through the foramen ovale. If the child has a VSD, mixing occurs through that opening as well.

Clinical Manifestations

The degree of mixing permitted by fetal structures determines the type and severity of clinical manifestations. The neonate with complete transposition and an intact ventricular septum develops cyanosis within 24 hours of birth. Cyanosis may be mild shortly after and worsen during the first day because of functional closure of the ductus arteriosus. Breathing is not effective because the oxygen taken in by the lungs never reaches the systemic circulation. Low oxygen levels in the blood (hypoxemia) cause metabolic acidosis, tachycardia, and tachypnea.

The first heart sound is normal and the second sound may be heard as a single sound, even though both the aortic and pulmonic valves are functioning. The single sound (S_2) may occur because transposition places the aortic valve closer to the chest wall than the pulmonic valve. A systolic murmur is heard in about 50% of cases, even if no other lesion, such as a VSD, is present. The murmur is fairly nonspecific, and varies in loudness.

Evaluation and Treatment

On chest x-ray films, the heart is seen to have a characteristic shape—like an egg on its side—and pulmonary vascular markings are increased. The heart may be enlarged if the infant is a few weeks old and has a VSD. Electrocardiogram findings in the neonate are usually normal; that is, they indicate a right-axis deviation and some right ventricular hypertrophy. These findings reflect the initially larger and heavier right ventricle of the neonate. In the normal infant, however, the ECG pattern changes, reverting to an axis more to the left. In the infant with transposition, the axis remains to the right (Moller & Neal, 1990).

The neonate's response to supplemental oxygen indicates whether cyanosis is the result of pulmonary disease or transposition of the great vessels. If the infant has pulmonary problems, inhalation of supplemental oxygen increases arterial oxygen saturation. Arterial oxygen saturation remains unchanged in an infant with transposition.

Cardiac catheterization and angiography are usually performed on an emergency basis if transposition is indicated, to (1) confirm the diagnosis, (2) check for other lesions, such as VSD or pulmonary stenosis, and (3) enlarge the foramen ovale to increase mixing of the circulations, a procedure termed balloon septostomy. Before the septostomy, catheterization is used to measure the percentage of desaturated blood in the peripheral system, to measure pressure in the right ventricle, and to confirm that the aorta and pulmonary artery are transposed (Fink, 1991).

The age at which surgical repair of TGA is done has steadily decreased over the years, and significant changes in repair procedures also have occurred. Twenty years ago the age for repair was 2 years; 10 years ago it was 3 to 6 months. Some procedures are now done at 2 weeks or less (Moller & Neal, 1990).

In the early 1960s, atrial switching techniques were developed by Senning and Mustard. Through the use of intraatrial baffles, blood flow is rerouted so oxygenated blood flows out through the aorta and deoxygenated blood exits through the pulmonary artery. The arteries

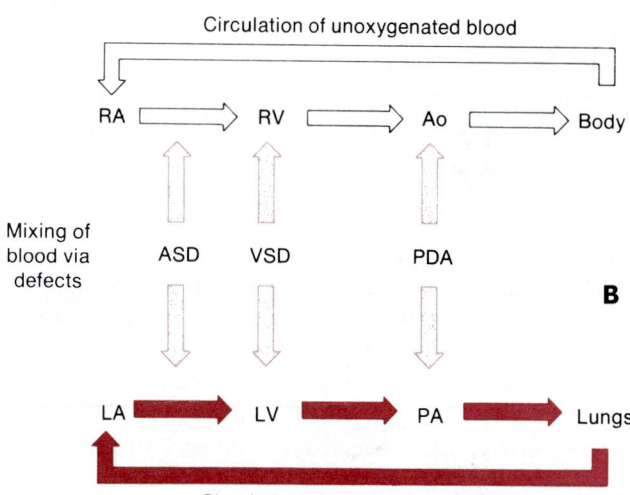

Hemodynamics in transposition of great vessels.

FIG. 28-13   Transposition of the great vessels (TGV). A, Complete transposition of the great vessels with an intact interventricular septum. The aorta arises from the right ventricle and the pulmonary artery from the left. **B,** Oxygen saturation in the two parallel circuits. (From Whaley & Wong, 1991.)

remain transposed but a physiologic repair is effected (Behrman et al., 1992). Currently, the procedure of choice is the Jatene arterial switch, wherein the arteries are physically reversed. It is done at less than 2 weeks of age, before the left ventricular muscle begins to decrease in mass because of decreasing pulmonary resistance. The procedure has a survival rate of 80% to 90% and has fewer long-term complications than the atrial switch (Moller & Neal, 1992).

Total Anomalous Pulmonary Venous Connection

Total anomalous pulmonary venous connection (TAPVC), also called total anomalous pulmonary venous return, is a condition in which blood from the pulmonary circulation enters the right atrium instead of the left. Several developmental defects can cause TAPVC, which is thought to account for approximately 2% of all congenital cardiac defects.

Pathophysiology

During about the third week of fetal life, the lung buds begin to develop a venous drainage system. This system consists of indirect connections to embryonic vessels— the umbilical vitelline veins (veins that return blood from the yolk sac to the heart of the embryo) and the cardinal veins—through the splanchnic plexus. At the same time, another embryonic vessel, the common pulmonary vein, grows out of the common atrium of the embryo. There is no direct connection between the lungs and the common pulmonary vein at this time. As the common pulmonary vein grows from the atrium toward the lung buds, the cardinal and umbilical vitelline veins lose their connection with the splanchnic plexus, which develops into the four pulmonary veins that eventually enter the left atrium. The common pulmonary vein continues to grow into these veins, establishing a direct connection between the lungs and the pulmonary vein. Ultimately, the common pulmonary vein is reabsorbed, leaving the four pulmonary veins that enter the heart at the left atrium. If the common pulmonary vein fails to develop fully from the left atrium, the earlier connections between the cardinal and umbilical vitelline veins may persist and cause a TAPVC.

Total anomalous pulmonary venous connections can take various forms, depending on the vascular abnormality that causes pulmonary venous return to the right atrium. The four common forms are (1) drainage of the pulmonary veins into the superior vena cava and right atrium through the right anterior cardinal vein; (2) drainage into the right atrium through the coronary sinus through a remnant of the left anterior cardinal vein; (3) attachment of the four pulmonary veins directly to the right (instead of the left) atrium; or (4) drainage into the right atrium from the common pulmonary vein through the portal system into the inferior vena cava and right atrium. This particular connection is caused by persistence of a remnant of the umbilical vitelline veins (Fink, 1991). Atrial septal defects accompany all forms of TAPVC, and pulmonary venous obstruction accompanies most forms. Obstruction is most common with the fourth form, however.

Pulmonary venous obstruction limits the return of oxygenated blood to the heart. The obstruction may be caused by external compression of the venous channel where it passes through the diaphragm, stenosis at the junction of the pulmonary venous channel and portal vein, or narrowing of the channel at any point along the route to the inferior vena cava. The blood that cannot pass the obstruction exerts pressure backward into the pulmonary capillary bed, causing pulmonary hypertension. As hydrostatic pressure increases in the pulmonary capillaries, plasma extravasates into the lung tissues, causing pulmonary edema. Obstruction also increases pulmonary vascular resistance, which in turn inhibits blood flow to the lungs from the right ventricle.

Oxygenated blood that enters the right atrium from the lungs mixes with unoxygenated blood returning from the body through the venae cavae. After that, the blood can flow (1) into the right ventricle and back to the lungs to be oxygenated or (2) through the ASD into the left atrium, the left ventricle, and out to the body. Ventricular compliance is a major determinant of the path the blood takes. Because pulmonary vascular resistance does not decrease to normal levels in infants with TAPVC, the right ventricular wall does not thin out and become more compliant as it should. Lack of right ventricular compliance limits the amount of blood that will flow from the right atrium into the right ventricle and out to the lungs. Therefore, much of the mixed blood in the right atrium shunts through the ASD into the left ventricle. This hemodynamic pattern causes mixed blood to be pumped throughout the systemic circulation (Fig. 28-14).

Clinical Manifestations

Because TAPVC causes a mixture of oxygenated and deoxygenated blood to enter the systemic circulation, cyanosis is the predominant clinical manifestation. The degree of cyanosis ultimately depends on pulmonary blood flow, that is, pulmonary vascular resistance. The higher the resistance, the lower the flow; and the lower the flow, the greater the cyanosis. The cyanosis may worsen with feeding, elimination, or any strain that increases intrathoracic pressure by causing exhalation against a closed glottis (Valsalva maneuver). Pressure on the pulmonary venous channel further decreases the amount of oxygenated blood that flows to the right atrium.

Tachypnea and dyspnea are other early signs of TAPVC. These respiratory manifestations, which are attributable to pulmonary edema, cause poor feeding. The respiratory signs of TAPVC are identical to those of left heart failure (see p. 1108), although their underlying cause is different. If the infant survives long enough, the increased workload of the right heart may cause congestive heart failure.

Heart sounds may be normal and there may be no murmur because the amount of blood returning to the right atrium is often limited by obstruction. (Murmurs are caused by turbulence, which is created by high volumes.) The volume of blood flowing out of the right

FIG. 28-14 Hemodynamics of total anomalous venous connection (TAPVC). In the form of TAPVC represented here, the pulmonary veins enter the left anomalous vertical vein instead of the left atrium. From the left anomalous vertical vein, the mixed blood from the lungs flows into the superior vena cava through an innominate vein (literally, a "vein without a name"). Oxygen saturation within the four heart chambers, the pulmonary artery, and the aorta is the same. Blood pressure in the right heart exceeds that in the left heart because the right heart is receiving blood from both the pulmonary and systemic circulatory systems. (Abnormal vessels are shaded.) (From Whaley & Wong, 1991.)

ventricle is not increased; therefore, right ventricular ejection time is not increased, and the second heart sound is normal.

Evaluation and Treatment

Electrocardiograms indicate right ventricular hypertrophy. Chest x-ray films show a normal-sized heart with increased pulmonary venous markings and a prominent pulmonary trunk. Pulmonary edema is apparent in the lung fields. Cardiac catheterization and angiography are the most useful diagnostic procedures. Catheterization shows that oxygen saturation is equally low in all chambers of the heart, the aorta, and the pulmonary artery. Normally, the oxygen saturation of blood in the aorta is approximately 97%. In an infant with TAPVC, aortic oxygen may range from 20% to 70% (Fink, 1991). Catheterization also indicates pulmonary hypertension. Total anomalous pulmonary venous connection often causes pulmonary arterial pressure to exceed systemic arterial pressure. Pressures in the right atrium and ventricle also may be higher than normal. Angiography shows the route of the anomalous pulmonary venous blood flow and right-to-left atrial shunting through the ASD.

If not treated surgically, most infants with TAPVC and pulmonary venous obstruction die within months of birth. Surgical treatment consists of attaching the common pulmonary vein to the left atrium and tying off the anomalous connecting vein. The atrial septal defect is usually closed at this time. The likelihood of postoperative death depends on the infant's condition before surgery, for example, degree of pulmonary hypertension, nutritional status, condition of the lungs, presence or absence of obstruction, and the size of the left atrium.

Cyanotic Heart Defects with Decreased Pulmonary Blood Flow

Malformations of the chambers or valves of the right heart can cause cyanosis by reducing the volume of blood that flows to the lungs to be oxygenated. Several congenital heart defects restrict pulmonary blood flow. They include endocardial fibroelastosis of the right ventricle, in which ventricular hypertrophy and endocardial fibrosis reduce flow by reducing ventricular compliance; Ebstein anomaly, in which the tricuspid valve is malformed; tricuspid atresia, in which the tricuspid opening is abnormally narrow; and **tetralogy of Fallot,** which consists of four defects involving the valves, the aorta, the interventricular septum, and the right ventricular myocardium. Tetralogy of Fallot and tricuspid atresia are useful examples of right heart defects that cause cyanosis by restricting pulmonary blood flow.

Tetralogy of Fallot

Tetralogy of Fallot, a syndrome of four defects, is the most common of the cyanotic heart defects and accounts for approximately 10% of all congenital heart defects. Tetralogy of Fallot has been associated with Down syndrome, first-trimester rubella, and Noonan syndrome (male Turner syndrome, in which stature and overall appearance are altered because the gonads fail to develop). The risk for recurrence of tetralogy of Fallot in a family with an affected child is approximately 3%.

Pathophysiology

The anatomic features of tetralogy of Fallot are (1) a ventricular septal defect, which is high on the septum and usually large, (2) an overriding aorta, which straddles the VSD, (3) pulmonary stenosis, usually caused by hypertrophy of the arterial infundibulum (funnel-shaped opening at the entrance of the pulmonary artery), and (4) right ventricular hypertrophy (Fig. 28-15, A). Right ventricular hypertrophy develops because afterload is increased by the obstruction of flow from the right ventricle.

Tetralogy of Fallot develops during two phases of embryologic growth: (1) during the division of the truncus

FIG. 28-15 Tetralogy of Fallot. A, Anatomic defects in tetralogy of Fallot. **B,** Hemodynamics of tetralogy of Fallot with right-to-left shunt. (**A** from Whaley & Wong, 1991.)

arteriosus by the spiral septum in the third or fourth week of gestation and (2) during the division of the ventricles between the fourth and eighth weeks of gestation (Fig. 28-2). Normally, as these events progress, the truncal septum fuses with the bulbar ridges and, in turn, with the endocardial cushions. The membranous portion of the interventricular septum grows upward to meet the endocardial cushions and, ultimately, all of these tissues come together to complete the interventricular septum.

The embryologic error that causes tetralogy of Fallot is not known for certain, but two theories have been proposed (Fink, 1991). The first is that the truncus arteriosus divides unevenly, resulting in great vessels of unequal size. Because of this asymmetry, the part of the spiral septum that normally fuses with the atrioventricular septa is not where it should be, causing a VSD. Concomitantly, pulmonary stenosis develops because there is a larger than normal amount of tissue in the infundibulum of the right ventricle. (This infundibulum is on the ventricular side of the pulmonic valve.) The second theory proposes that infundibular overgrowth in the right ventricle is the major developmental anomaly. The extra tissue restricts the blood flow through the pulmonary artery, causing the artery to be smaller than normal at birth. Concomitantly, the aorta is subjected to greater-than-normal blood flow during fetal life, causing it to be larger than normal at birth. In addition, infundibular overgrowth in the right ventricle prevents normal closure of the ventricular septum, causing the VSD.

The pathophysiology associated with tetralogy of Fallot varies widely, depending primarily on the degree of pulmonary stenosis, but also on the size of the VSD and the pulmonary and systemic resistance to flow. Because the VSD is usually large, pressures may be equal in the right and left ventricles. Therefore the major determinant of shunt direction through the VSD is the difference between pulmonary and systemic vascular resistance. If pulmonary vascular resistance is higher than systemic resistance, the shunt is from right to left. If systemic resistance is higher than pulmonary resistance, the shunt is from left to right. Because many factors can alter the balance between pulmonary and systemic resistance, shunt direction is not necessarily constant (Fig. 28-15, *B*).

Stenosis decreases blood flow to the lungs and, consequently, the amount of oxygenated blood that returns to the left heart. If blood also shunts from right to left through the VSD, deoxygenated blood mixes with the small amount of relatively oxygenated blood returning from the lungs. The result is low O_2 saturation (hypoxemia) in the systemic circulation. The body attempts to compensate for hypoxemia by producing more red cells (thereby causing polycythemia) and by increasing blood flow to the lungs through collateral bronchial vessels.

Clinical Manifestations

As long as the ductus arteriosus remains open, the neonate's pulmonary blood flow may be adequate. As the ductus closes, however, cyanosis becomes apparent. Many factors can affect the degree of cyanosis, especially those that change the balance between systemic and pulmonary resistance. For example, a hot environment causes peripheral vessels to dilate, thereby lowering systemic vascular resistance and shifting more un-oxygenated blood through the VSD into the aorta. (This increases cyanosis.) Physical exertion (e.g., playing or eating) also lowers systemic resistance as blood travels to the muscles. Chronic cyanosis causes clubbing of the fingers and toes (see Chapter 30).

A common manifestation of tetralogy of Fallot is the sudden onset of dyspnea, cyanosis, and restlessness, sometimes called a hypoxic spell or a "tet spell." These spells generally occur in the morning or early evening and in the summer, often with crying and exertion. No one knows for sure what causes these episodes, but it is theorized that the right ventricular outflow tract goes into spasm or the systemic resistance drops suddenly (Moller & Neal, 1990; Perloff, Friedman, Laks, & Child, 1983). In either case, the relative or actual increase in pulmonary vascular resistance increases the right-to-left shunt and the cyanosis. Other signs associated with these episodes, such as loss of consciousness and seizures, are the result of hypoxia (lack of tissue oxygenation).

Squatting is a spontaneous compensatory mechanism used by older children to alleviate hypoxic spells. Squatting and its variants increase systemic resistance while decreasing venous return to the heart from the inferior vena cava. The decrease of systemic return makes relatively more oxygenated blood available to the body. The increase of systemic resistance also reverses the shunt through the VSD to a left-to-right shunt, which has the effect of increasing pulmonary blood flow. Through both of these mechanisms, squatting decreases cyanosis temporarily. Infants do not squat, but may assume a knee-chest position, which accomplishes the same thing. Infants and children also experience slow growth and failure to thrive. Infants often have difficulty with feeding because the exertion required increases hypoxia.

Left heart failure is not usually a manifestation of tetralogy, because blood can exit from the right heart through the overriding aorta. This prevents afterload from building in the right heart, despite pulmonary stenosis.

Polycythemia can lead to iron-deficiency anemia if the child's iron intake does not keep pace with the increased production of red blood cells (see Chapter 23). Polycythemia also may cause thromboembolism by making the blood more viscous, which slows flow and promotes clotting. The brain is particularly vulnerable to thromboembolism in children with tetralogy of Fallot.

The typical heart murmur of tetralogy is a pulmonary systolic ejection murmur caused by the obstruction in the outflow tract, which creates turbulence during systole. The smaller the obstruction, the louder the murmur. This explains why the murmur often disappears during a hypoxic spell, when obstruction increases. The second heart sound seems to be single, but in fact it is

not. The pulmonary component is very soft and delayed and is usually not heard, although it is present. The enlarged right ventricle may cause the left side of the chest to be more prominent, and a "heave" also may be felt.

Evaluation and Treatment

The ECG indicates right ventricular hypertrophy. Chest x-ray examination shows that the heart is shaped like a boot and that pulmonary vascular markings are decreased. Measurements made during cardiac catheterization demonstrate normal systemic pressure in the right ventricle, decreased pressure in the right ventricular outflow tract, and low oxygen saturation in the aorta. Angiograms enable the clinician to see the size and position of the VSD, the stenotic pulmonary infundibulum or valve, the smaller-than-normal pulmonary artery, and the overriding aorta.

Children who are not treated surgically have a life expectancy of about 12 years (Keith et al., 1978). Pulmonary stenosis tends to progress with age. Surgical treatment has been available since the mid-1940s, and the age at which surgery is performed has decreased steadily. Surgical correction may be performed in two stages. In the first stage, palliation is achieved by creating one of three types of anastomoses (Blalock-Taussig shunt) between the aorta and the pulmonary artery. Anastomosis increases pulmonary blood flow and decreases hypoxia. In the second step, correction is achieved by patching the VSD and enlarging the right ventricular outflow tract.

Tricuspid Atresia

Tricuspid atresia consists of an imperforate tricuspid valve, resulting in no communication between the right atrium and right ventricle. There may be a small "dimple" on the floor of the right atrium, but there is no opening (Roberts, 1987). This defect accounts for 2% to 3% of congenital heart defects and is the third most common cyanotic heart defect (Adams, Emmanouilides, & Reimenschneider, 1989; Arciniegas, 1985). Tricuspid atresia is really a complex of defects, including the imperforate tricuspid valve, as well as an atrial septal defect, hypoplastic or absent right ventricle, enlarged mitral valve and left ventricle, and varying degrees of pulmonic stenosis (Arciniegas, 1985; Roberts, 1987). Tricuspid atresia also may be associated with transposition of the great vessels. The most common type of tricuspid atresia involves a hypoplastic right atrium with decreased pulmonary blood flow and a VSD, and is not associated with transposition (Adams et al., 1989). The pathophysiology of this type is presented here.

Pathophysiology

Systemic blood returns through the superior and inferior venae cavae to the right atrium. Because there is no opening between the right atrium and right ventricle, blood flows through the atrial septal defect into the left atrium, mixing with blood returning from the pulmonary circulation. The blood then enters the left ventricle. Most of this blood goes out into the systemic circulation through the aorta, but varying amounts pass through the VSD into the hypoplastic right atrium and then out through the pulmonary valve to the lungs. Pulmonary circulation depends on the presence of a VSD, which in turn assumes a right ventricle of some size is present. If the right ventricle is absent, the pulmonary valve is usually imperforate as well. If this is the case, a PDA is necessary to ensure that some blood flows into the pulmonary circulation (Adams et al., 1989).

As is the case with tetralogy of Fallot, pulmonary circulation also depends on the relationship between pulmonary and systemic vascular resistance. As long as pulmonary resistance is lower than systemic resistance, blood flows through the VSD from left to right, feeding the pulmonary circulation. If pulmonary resistance rises above systemic resistance, blood will not reach the pulmonary circulation through the VSD.

Clinical Manifestations

Central cyanosis in some degree is a common manifestation in tricuspid atresia. Growth failure is also common. As with tetralogy of Fallot, these children also experience exertional dyspnea and squatting. Long-term effects of hypoxia are polycythemia and clubbing. These children also may display hypoxic "spells," like the tet spells. It is not coincidental that the clinical manifestations of tricuspid atresia (type 1-b) described here are so similar to the clinical manifestations of tetralogy. Although the anatomic features are somewhat different, the hemodynamic effects are the same.

The ECG in tricuspid atresia shows right atrial and left ventricular hypertrophy, and left axis deviation. There is a single first heart sound because there is no tricuspid valve to make a sound on closing. The second sound also may be single because of the presence of pulmonic stenosis. The murmur heard with tricuspid atresia may have several components, depending on the anatomic features of each case. Pulmonic stenosis produces a systolic murmur, the loudness of which depends on the degree of stenosis. A severely stenotic valve produces a soft murmur because very little blood flows through the valve. A less stenotic valve produces a louder murmur from more blood flow. The VSD also causes a murmur that is systolic; the larger the VSD, the softer and shorter the murmur is likely to be.

Evaluation and Treatment

Although cardiac catheterization and angiocardiography still are done frequently to ascertain the anatomic and hemodynamic features of tricuspid atresia, echocardiography and magnetic resonance imaging are gaining popularity in the evaluation of this and most other congenital heart defects (Roberts, 1987). These techniques are noninvasive and can provide information about anatomy and some information about hemodynamic characteristics.

Surgical treatment of tricuspid atresia consists of maximizing systemic and pulmonary blood flow and increasing pulmonary blood flow (Arciniegas, 1985). The Fontan procedure, developed in the early 1970s, establishes a more normal circulation by creating a four-chambered, four-valve heart and eliminates systemic-pulmonary mixing (Behrman et al., 1992; Roberts, 1987).

ACQUIRED CARDIOVASCULAR DISORDERS

Acquired heart diseases in children include left heart failure, rheumatic heart disease, Kawasaki disease, and essential or primary hypertension. (Rheumatic heart disease is discussed in Chapter 27, as are adult forms of heart failure and primary hypertension.)

Left Heart Failure

Left heart failure (LHF) is a common complication of many congenital heart defects. The effect of left heart failure is the same in all age groups: the heart is unable to maintain sufficient output to meet the body's metabolic needs. The most common causes of LHF in infancy are pressure and volume overloads secondary to congenital disease. (Table 28-6 lists the congenital heart defects that cause LHF, by age.) Ninety percent of children who develop LHF do so within 12 months of birth (Guzzetta & Dossey, 1984), often by the age of 6 months (Park, 1988).

In general, the pathophysiologic mechanisms of LHF in infants and children are very similar to those in adults. The same compensatory mechanisms are activated in the face of inadequate cardiac output. A decrease in blood pressure stimulates stretch receptors and baroreceptors in the aorta and carotid arteries, which in turn stimulate the sympathetic nervous system. With the release of catecholamines and the stimulation of β receptors, heart rate and the force of myocardial contraction increase. Venous smooth muscle tone also increases, which increases return of venous blood to the heart. Sympathetic stimulation also decreases blood flow to the kidneys, skin, spleen, and extremities, so that maximum flow to the brain, heart, and lungs can be maintained. Decreased blood flow to the kidneys causes the release of renin, angiotensin, and aldosterone. This cycle results in retention of sodium and fluid by the kid-

TABLE 28-6

Congenital Heart Defects Causing Left Heart Failure

Age	Congenital heart defect
Time of birth	Hypoplastic left heart syndrome Volume overload caused by tricuspid regurgitation Arterial venous fistula
Birth to 1 week	Hypoplastic left heart syndrome Aortic atresia Transposition of the great vessels Coarctation of the aorta Total anomalous pulmonary venous connection (TAPVC) with obstruction Patent ductus arteriosus (PDA) in premature infants
First 4 weeks	Coarctation of the aorta TAPVC Large left-to-right shunt caused by ventricular septal defect (VSD), PDA in premature infants Tricuspid atresia All previously mentioned defects
4-6 weeks	Transposition of the great vessels Large left-to-right shunt caused by endocardial cushion defect
6 weeks to 6 months	VSD
6 months	Endocardial fibroelastosis Persistent truncus arteriosus with large left-to-right shunt

Data from Keith, Rowe, & Vlad, 1978; Park, 1988.

neys, which in turn increases volume in the circulatory system.

The myocardium hypertrophies in LHF, which increases ventricular pressure. The myocardium fibers also stretch to accommodate the increased volume. This increases contractility and hence the force of ventricular contraction. Both hypertrophy and increased stretch eventually fail to maintain cardiac output as LHF progresses. A review of the Frank-Starling law of the heart is useful for an understanding of the cycle of compensation and decompensation that occurs in LHF. (The Frank-Starling law is described in Chapter 26.)

Despite its different causes, LHF in infants is not generally differentiated as right or left ventricular failure. Usually, both ventricles are involved by the time signs and symptoms are apparent (Mott, James, & Sperhac, 1990; Smith, 1983).

Left heart failure in infants is manifested as poor feeding and sucking (leading to failure to thrive), diaphoresis (increased perspiration), breathlessness (dyspnea), and irritability. Most of the symptoms of congestive heart failure are attributable to low cardiac output and venous congestion (see Chapter 27). The body tries to compensate for low output by increasing the pulse rate until the infant has tachycardia even at rest. Any increase in exertion, such as eating, has the same effect. Blood flow to all peripheral organs, including the skin, diminishes to conserve flow to the brain and heart. This causes peripheral hypotension, cool extremities, and muscular flaccidity. Decreased flow to the skin decreases elimination of body heat through radiation, and the body compensates by increasing perspiration. (Mechanisms of temperature regulation are described in Chapter 13.)

The failing heart eventually causes venous congestion throughout the body, resulting in hepatomegaly, edema, and dyspnea. Edema may appear in the periorbital area early in left heart failure and progress to peripheral edema later in the course of the condition. Dyspnea occurs when the hydrostatic pressure in the pulmonary veins exceeds that in the surrounding tissue, enabling fluid to leak out into the lung tissue. Edema decreases lung compliance, in effect creating a stiff lung and increasing the work of breathing. (Dyspnea and pulmonary edema are defined in Chapter 30.) Cyanosis is sometimes a sign of congestive heart failure in children, but other skin changes, such as pallor or mottling, are more common.

Dyspnea on exertion is manifested in infants as difficulty with feeding. When the infant tries to suck and swallow, breathing is interrupted, and the child becomes exhausted. Poor feeding, coupled with failure to thrive, is one of the primary indicators of LHF in infants. The child's growth is slowed, and parents report that it can take 45 to 60 minutes for the infant to finish 1 to 2 ounces of formula.

The infant's respiratory rate may be greater than 40 breaths per minute. In severe LHF, tachypnea may be accompanied by retractions, grunting, nasal flaring, wheezing, coughing, and rales (Smith, 1983).

Hepatomegaly (enlargement of the liver) is typically attributable to systemic venous congestion caused by right ventricular failure. In infants, the normal liver is sharp-edged and palpable 1 to 2 cm below the costal margin. In the infant with CHF, the liver has a dull, rounded edge that is felt more than 3 cm below the costal margin, and may be tender (Guzzetta & Dossey, 1984; Keith et al., 1978).

Although peripheral edema is a common finding in adults with LHF, it is unusual in infants and young children. Periorbital tissue may be the only site of obvious edema in infants. Another manifestation in adults, distention of the jugular veins, is seldom apparent in infants because of their relatively short necks. Fluid retention in infants is usually manifested by a weight gain without any increase in calorie intake. The clinical manifestations of LHF are illustrated in the box at right.

A chest x-ray examination is performed to ascertain the presence of cardiomegaly (a reflection of hypertrophy). An ECG is also performed to determine the presence of arrhythmias and as an indirect indicator of heart size. Plotting the child's growth (height, weight, and head circumference) is an important method of assessing failure to thrive. A thorough physical examination indicates the extent of tachycardia, tachypnea, dyspnea, diaphoresis, edema, and hepatomegaly.

Treatment is aimed at decreasing cardiac workload and increasing the efficiency of the heart (Moller & Neal, 1990). Digitalis and diuretics are prescribed for these same reasons. Other treatments may include the administration of oxygen, sedation, gastrostomy feedings, and keeping the child in a semi-upright position. The semi-upright position causes fluid to pool in the lung bases, limiting areas of fluid reabsorption by lymphatic vessels in the lungs. This decreases the volume of blood that returns to the heart (Smith, 1983). Diuretics usually make salt and fluid restrictions unnecessary for infants (Guzzetta & Dossey, 1984; Park, 1988).

Rheumatic Heart Disease

The incidence of rheumatic fever and rheumatic heart disease has a wide geographic variation. In many Third World countries, it remains a common, virulent disease with early cardiac sequelae and a much-shortened lifespan. In the United States, this disease has decreased

---

CLINICAL MANIFESTATIONS OF LEFT HEART FAILURE

Impaired myocardial function

Tachycardia	Anorexia
Sweating (inappropriate)	Pale, cool extremities
Decreased urine output	Weak peripheral pulses
Fatigue	Decreased blood pressure
Weakness	
Restlessness	Gallop rhythm
	Cardiomegaly

Pulmonary congestion

Tachypnea	Orthopnea
Dyspnea	Cough, hoarseness
Retractions (infants)	Cyanosis
Flaring nares	Wheezing
Exercise intolerance	Grunting

Systemic venous congestion

Weight gain	Ascites
Hepatomegaly	Neck vein distention
Peripheral edema, especially periorbital	(children)

(From Whaley & Wong, 1991, p. 1548.)

---

markedly in the last 50 to 60 years. In the late 1920s, it was estimated that rheumatic heart disease accounted for 40% of all heart disease, but by the 1950s, this estimate was only 23% (Keith et al., 1978). One estimate of incidence of rheumatic heart disease in the 1970s was two cases per 1000 children, with an equal number contracting rheumatic fever without cardiac complications (Keith et al., 1978). In recent years, there has been a dramatic increase in the incidence of rheumatic fever in some regions of the United States, such as the Intermountain West, Ohio, Texas, and Hawaii (Kaplan, 1988; Ruttenberg, 1986; Whaley & Wong, 1991). The incidence figures for the nation as a whole remain very low. Nonetheless, rheumatic fever remains one of the leading *causes* of acquired heart disease in children.

The usual age of onset is between 5 and 10 years, although some cases occur before the age of 5. Demographic characteristics, such as race and sex, are not strongly related to the incidence of rheumatic fever (Keith et al., 1978). The possibility of a genetic predisposition has been discussed but not proven (Behrman et al., 1992).

The initiating cause of rheumatic fever is infection by group A β-hemolytic streptococcus. The streptococcal infection usually precedes the onset of rheumatic fever by several days. It has been suggested that rheumatic fever may be the result of a hypersensitivity reaction to some antigen in the streptococcus or its toxins. If this is so, rheumatic fever could be categorized as an autoimmune disease. Other theories of pathogenesis include actual infection of the cardiac valves with living bacteria in altered forms. (See Chapter 27 for a detailed discussion of rheumatic fever and its sequelae.)

Kawasaki Disease

Kawasaki disease is an acute, self-limiting systemic vasculitis that may result in cardiac sequelae. It was identified in 1967 by Kawasaki and described as mucocutaneous lymph node syndrome. Although it certainly occurs throughout the world, the greatest number of cases are seen in Japan (Moller & Neal, 1990).

There appears to be no particular pattern in the incidence of Kawasaki disease. Although it seems more prevalent in Asian populations, it occurs in other ethnic groups as well. It seems to be a condition of young children, with 80% of cases seen in children younger than 5 years of age, peaking in the toddler age group. Currently, it is the leading cause of pediatric acquired heart disease in the United States (Whaley & Wong, 1991). Males are affected slightly more often than females.

Because Kawasaki disease occurs in "mini epidemics," an infectious cause has been suggested but has not been substantiated. Current etiologic theories center on an immunologic response to an infectious, toxic, or antigenic substance (Moller & Neal, 1990).

Pathophysiology

Kawasaki disease progresses pathologically and clinically in stages. In stage I (day 0-12), small capillaries, arterioles, and venules become inflamed, as does the heart itself (pancarditis). In stage II (day 12-25), the inflammation spreads to larger vessels, and aneurysms of the coronary arteries develop. In stage III (day 26-40), the medium-sized arteries begin the granulation process and inflammation resolves in the microcirculation. In stage IV (day 40 and beyond), the vessels develop scarring, intimal thickening, calcification, and formation of thrombi. Although arteritis occurs most commonly in the coronary arteries, it also can develop in renal mesenteric, subclavian, and other arteries. The development of aneurysms is the major pathologic feature of this illness and is seen in 10% to 20% of children with Kawasaki disease.

Clinical Manifestations

There are six major clinical features of Kawasaki disease, and the diagnosis is made if five of the six are evident. The diagnostic criteria for Kawasaki disease are outlined in the following box. They include fever with temperature spikes of greater than 104° F, bilateral conjunctivitis, erythema and other changes of the oral mu-

cosa, erythema of palms and soles with desquamation, polymorphous erythematous rash, and cervical lymphadenopathy (Whaley & Wong, 1991). Some children also develop arthralgias in large joints and gastrointestinal symptoms.

The clinical course of the disease progresses in three stages: acute, subacute, and convalescent. In the acute phase, the child has fever, conjunctivitis, oral changes, rash, and lymphadenopathy. During this phase, myocarditis may develop. The subacute phase begins when the fever ends and continues until the clinical signs have resolved. It is at this time that the child is most at risk for coronary artery aneurysm development. Desquamation of the palms and soles occurs at this time. The convalescent phase is marked by the continued elevation of laboratory values, although all clinical signs have resolved. Arthritis still may be present. This phase continues until all laboratory values return to normal—usually about 6 to 8 weeks after onset (Whaley & Wong, 1991).

Evaluation and Treatment

There are no specific laboratory tests for Kawasaki disease, so the diagnosis is made clinically and on the basis of nonspecific laboratory values. These children usually have leukocytosis, increased erythrocyte sedimentation rates, and elevated liver enzymes. Echocardiograms are done to monitor the condition of the coronary arteries.

As with diagnosis, there is no specific treatment of this disease. The goals of treatment include symptomatic management of the acute phase and prevention of cor-

---

DIAGNOSTIC CRITERIA FOR KAWASAKI DISEASE

The child must exhibit five of the following six criteria, including fever:
1. Fever for 5 or more days (often diagnosed with shorter duration of fever if other symptoms are present)
2. Bilateral conjunctival infection without exudation
3. Changes in the oral mucous membranes, such as erythema, dryness, and fissuring of the lips; oropharyngeal reddening; or "strawberry tongue"
4. Changes in the extremities, such as peripheral edema, peripheral erythema, and desquamation of palms and soles, particularly periungual peeling
5. Polymorphous rash, often accentuated in the perineal area
6. Cervical lymphadenopathy

(From Whaley & Wong, 1991, p. 1585.)

onary artery thrombosis. Gamma globulin and aspirin are used to reduce the coronary artery abnormalities and to decrease inflammation (Whaley & Wong, 1991). Hospitalization and bed rest are the usual course for the acute phase, along with fluid replacement and nutritional support. Although most children recover completely from Kawasaki disease, those with cardiovascular sequelae may experience serious problems later—most notably, coronary thrombosis. Because the disease has only been recognized since 1967, the long-term effects are unknown.

Primary Hypertension

In the past, most hypertension in children was thought to be secondary to other diseases, such as chronic glomerulonephritis or renal tumors, to name but two (see the box below). In the 1950s, this opinion began to

change because autopsies done on young Korean War casualties disclosed significant arterial disease, which is known to cause hypertension. It was discovered that many of these young men (and later, young casualties of the Vietnam War) had significant atherosclerosis in major blood vessels. The autopsies showed that even the late lesions of atherosclerosis, fibrous plaques, can be present by late adolescence (Berenson, 1980). Since then, autopsies on infants have shown fatty streaks—the earliest lesions of atherosclerosis—in the intimal lining of blood vessels (Engle, 1981). Evidently, hypertension-causing arterial disease can begin extremely early in life.

The incidence of primary (or essential) hypertension in childhood is a controversial topic, partly because normal blood pressure values, a consistent definition, and diagnostic criteria are still being established.

Pathophysiology

It is unclear whether the pathophysiologic mechanisms of primary hypertension in adults and children are the same, or even exactly what those mechanisms are. Primary hypertension is thought to result from a complex interaction of disturbances in sympathetic vascular smooth muscle tone, humoral agents (angiotensin, catecholamines), renal sodium excretion, and cardiac output. (See Chapter 26 for a full discussion of these mechanisms.) Ultimately, these factors impair the ability of the peripheral vascular bed to adjust its own resistance to meet tissue perfusion needs (Kotchen & Kotchen, 1983).

Clinical Manifestations

An increase in peripheral vascular resistance decreases the body's ability to perfuse its tissues at normal arterial pressures. Over time, the increased pressures resulting from those changes cause permanent thickening of vessel walls, which in turn leads to further increases in resistance, setting up a vicious cycle. This cycle serves as another illustration of Poiseuille's equation in action, where thickening of vessel walls causes a decreased radius, which in turn results in increased resistance to flow (see Chapter 26).

Changes in cardiac output provide the other hemodynamic element in hypertension. The aorta is a distensible tube that is subjected to intermittent pressure increases with each systole. These pressure increases drive the blood through the arterial system to the capillaries and then back to the heart through the veins. The distensibility of the aorta determines how easily it can adjust to systemic pressure changes. If the walls of the aorta become less distensible (i.e., more rigid), greater systolic pressure will be generated within it, even if the volume remains the same.

CONDITIONS ASSOCIATED WITH SECONDARY HYPERTENSION IN CHILDREN

Cardiovascular

Coarctation of the aorta
Hypoplastic aorta
Abnormalities of renal artery
Renal vein thrombosis

Renal

Hydronephrosis
Chronic glomerulonephritis
Chronic pyelonephritis
Dysplastic kidney
Hydronephrosis
Polycystic kidneys
Renal trauma
Renal tumors
Medullary cystic disease
Posttransplantation

Adrenal

Neuroblastoma
Cushing disease
Pheochromocytoma
Adrenogenital syndrome
Primary aldosteronism
Adrenal carcinoma

Other

Intracranial tumors
Chronic use of steroids
Excessive intake of licorice
Renal disease secondary to irradiation
Lead neuropathy

(From Adams, Emmanuoilides, & Riemenschneider, 1989.)

Peripheral vascular resistance helps to determine diastolic pressure. Because increased resistance causes decreased flow, any increase in peripheral vascular resistance results in decreased flow to the microcirculation from the arteries. This in essence creates a pressure backup and results in a smaller than usual decrease in blood pressure during diastole.

Risk factors (such as smoking, obesity, hypercholesteremia, diabetes mellitus, positive family history, poor fitness, and increased sodium intake) have been correlated with the development of hypertension in adults. In recent years, much research has been done to assess the importance and interrelatedness of these factors in the development of hypertension (and coronary artery disease) in children (Fig. 28-16).

Obesity has been identified as one of these factors (Berenson, 1986). Approximately 50% to 60% of hypertensive children are obese. Obesity in the high school population as a whole is approximately 10% to 15%. For many hypertensive children, a weight loss of 15 pounds can cause a decrease in diastolic pressure of 15 mm Hg. Conversely, another study showed that weight gain was associated with the development of hypertension in a group of adolescents (Kotchen & Kotchen,

1983). Sodium intake is also a known correlate of hypertension. In industrialized nations with a high salt intake, the incidence of hypertension is greater than in those countries with low salt intake (Berenson, 1980). This correlation gains strength in those individuals with a family history of hypertension—there may be a genetic interaction as well.

Some differences in the development of hypertension in children are race related (Berenson et al., 1984). Black children generally develop a greater body mass than white children and also have a decreased ability to achieve sodium and water balance. (Imbalances of sodium and water are described in Chapter 3.) Increased body mass could increase blood volume and cardiac output, both of which can increase blood pressure (Berenson et al., 1984). In addition, if sodium intake is high, the decreased sodium-handling ability in blacks may contribute to the earlier onset of hypertension. The race-related risk factors differ slightly for white children. White children have a greater percentage of body fat for their weight (as opposed to greater body mass), more of a tendency toward obesity, faster heart rates, higher levels of blood sugar, and higher renin and dopamine-β-hydroxylase levels than black children.

FIG. 28-16 Mechanisms believed to influence blood pressure in childhood. According to this model, a critical factor in the development of hypertension is obesity during childhood. Increased body mass, coupled with excessive sodium intake, can cause primary hypertension in children or set the stage for its development later in life. (Adapted from Voors & Berenson, 1981.)

These findings suggest that hypertension in black children is associated with body mass and renal mechanisms, whereas hypertension in white children is associated with obesity and neurohumoral factors (Berenson et al., 1984).

High cholesterol levels also may be a significant risk factor for hypertension in children because high cholesterol levels are associated with atherosclerosis. Several studies in different areas of the United States show that 5% to 9% of school-age children tested have serum cholesterol levels of 220 mg/dl or more (Engle, 1981). Although it is hard to say with certainty that all of those children are at risk for atherosclerosis, it is known that the incidence of hypercholesteremia is much greater in children with a family history of heart disease and hypercholesteremia than in children with no such history (Croft et al., 1988).

Smoking doubles the risk of hypertension and other cardiovascular diseases at any age. The number of children who smoke seems to be increasing. It is estimated that approximately 40% of both black and white adolescents are smoking by high school age (Berensen et al., 1984).

The interrelationships among these risk factors are currently being studied in children. The precise relevance of each is not yet known. It seems logical to assume that the more factors present, the greater the risk of hypertension. What remains to be seen is how assessment of these factors can be used to identify and treat children at risk for hypertension and the later development of cardiovascular disease.

Evaluation and Treatment

Diagnosis of primary hypertension in children is difficult because (1) the early stages of primary hypertension (which children are likely to have) are asymptomatic, and (2) normal blood pressures vary from child to child and change continuously as the child grows. It is not surprising that "normal" blood pressure in children is still being debated. Longitudinal studies in which blood pressure was measured under controlled conditions in children of various races and economic backgrounds indicated that normal systolic and diastolic values are considerably lower than was previously thought (Berenson, 1980; Kotchen & Kotchen, 1983). Currently, normal values are usually computed by age, but research indicates that height and weight (body mass) are more important than age in determining normal blood pressure in children (Berenson, 1986).

Blood pressure tends to remain at about the same percentile as the child grows older. A child who is consistently at the 95th percentile may well be at risk for adult hypertension and cardiovascular disease. Some clinicians base their treatment of childhood hypertension on this belief, and prescribe antihypertensive medications for children whose blood pressures are above the 90th or 95th percentile. The preventive efficacy of antihypertensive therapy during childhood is debated among researchers and clinicians, some of whom prefer to emphasize the control or elimination of risk factors.

SUMMARY REVIEW

Development of the Cardiovascular System

1 The heart arises from the mesenchyme and begins as an enlarged blood vessel with a large lumen and a muscular wall. By approximately the eighth week of gestation, all of the structures of the fetal heart and vascular system are present.

2 Fetal blood is oxygenated in the placenta and returned to the fetus through the umbilical vein.

3 In the fetus, the pulmonary and systemic circulatory systems are connected by the foramen ovale, an opening between the atria; by the ductus arteriosus, a fetal vessel that joins the pulmonary artery to the aorta; and by the ductus venosus, a fetal vessel that connects the inferior vena cava to the umbilical vein.

4 Fetal blood flow depends on resistance for its distribution through the body. Resistance in the pulmonary circulation is higher than resistance in the systemic circulation, so myocardial thickness is about the same in the right heart and the left heart.

5 After birth, systemic resistance increases and pulmonary resistance decreases.

6 Pulmonary vascular resistance drops suddenly at birth because the lungs expand and the pulmonary vessels dilate. It continues to decrease gradually over the first 6 to 8 weeks after birth. Decreased resistance causes the right myocardium to thin out.

7 Systemic vascular resistance increases markedly at birth because severance of the umbilical cord removes the low-resistance placenta from the systemic circulation. Increased systemic resistance causes the right myocardium to thicken.

8 Changes in resistance cause the fetal connections between the pulmonary and systemic circulatory systems to disappear. The foramen ovale closes functionally at birth and anatomically several months later; the ductus arteriosus closes functionally 15 to 18 hours after birth and anatomically within 10 to 21 days; and the ductus venosus closes within 1 week after birth.

Congenital Heart Defects

1 Most congenital cardiovascular defects have begun to develop by the eighth week of gestation, and most have many causes, both environmental and genetic.

2 Environmental risk factors associated with the incidence of congenital heart defects typically are maternal conditions. Among these are viral infections, diabetes, drug intake, and advanced maternal age.

3 Genetic factors associated with congenital heart defects include but are not limited to Down syndrome, trisomy 13-16, trisomy 18, cri du chat syndrome, and Turner syndrome.

4 Classification of congenital heart defects is based on (a) whether they cause blood flow to the lungs to increase, decrease, or remain normal and (b) whether they cause cyanosis.

5 Cyanosis, a bluish discoloration of the skin, indicates that the tissues are not receiving adequate oxygenated blood. Cyanosis can be caused by defects that (a) restrict blood flow into the pulmonary circulation, (b) overload the pulmonary circulation, causing pulmonary hypertension, pulmonary edema, and respiratory difficulty, or (c) cause large amounts of unoxygenated blood to shunt from the pulmonary to the systemic circulation.

6 Congenital defects that maintain or create direct communication between the pulmonary and systemic circulatory systems cause blood to shunt from one system to another, mixing oxygenated and unoxygenated blood and increasing blood volume and pressure on the receiving side of the shunt.

7 The direction of shunting through an abnormal communication depends on differences in pressure and resistance between the two systems. Flow is always from an area of high pressure to an area of low pressure.

8 Obstruction of ventricular outflow is commonly caused by pulmonary stenosis (right ventricle) or coarctation of the aorta (left ventricle).

9 Despite obstruction, ventricular outflow remains normal because of compensatory ventricular hypertrophy stimulated by increased afterload and, in postductal coarctation of the aorta, development of collateral circulation around the coarctation.

10 Congestive heart failure can develop as a result of right ventricular obstruction if afterload backs up into the pulmonary circulation. Congestive heart failure can result from left ventricular obstruction in preductal coarctation of the aorta in which left-to-right shunting through the patent ductus arteriosus greatly increases blood flow into the pulmonary circulation.

11 Acyanotic congenital defects that increase pulmonary blood flow consist of abnormal openings (ventricular septal defect, patent ductus arteriosus, or atrial septal defect) that permit blood to shunt from left (systemic circulation) to right (pulmonary circulation). Cyanosis does not occur because the left-to-right shunt does not interfere with the flow of oxygenated blood through the systemic circulation.

12 If the abnormal communication between the left and right circuits is large, volume and pressure overload in the pulmonary circulation leads to congestive heart failure.

13 Cyanotic congenital defects that increase pulmonary blood flow are caused by abnormal development of the great vessels. These defects include persistent truncus arteriosus, complete transposition of the great vessels, and total anomalous pulmonary venous connection.

14 In persistent truncus arteriosus, the truncus arteriosus fails to divide longitudinally into the aorta and pulmonary artery. All of the blood from both ventricles enters the truncus, so that mixed blood is delivered to both circulatory systems, causing cyanosis and failure to thrive.

15 In complete transposition of the great vessels, the circulatory systems are not connected serially or through a shunt, so that oxygenated blood remains permanently in the pulmonary circulation and unoxygenated blood remains permanently in the systemic circulation. Life is possible while the ductus arteriosus remains patent; after that, surgical intervention is mandatory.

16 Total anomalous pulmonary venous connection is caused by the persistence of the fetal common pulmonary artery and the lack of pulmonary venous return to the left atrium. All blood from the pulmonary and systemic circulations enters the right atrium. Mixed blood enters the left atrium through an atrial septal defect, then flows into the systemic circulation and causes cyanosis. Obstruction in the common pulmonary vein causes pressure to back up into the lungs, leading to congestive heart failure.

17 In cyanotic heart defects that decrease pulmonary blood flow (tetralogy of Fallot, tricuspid atresia), myocardial hypertrophy cannot compensate for restricted right ventricular outflow. Flow to the lungs decreases, and cyanosis is caused by an insufficient volume of oxygenated blood.

18 Treatment for all congenital defects is surgical correction of the anomaly and management of cyanosis and congestive heart failure.

Acquired Cardiovascular Disorders

1 The most common acquired cardiovascular disorders of childhood are congestive heart failure, rheumatic heart disease, and hypertension.

2 Congestive heart failure is usually the result of congenital heart defects that increase blood volume and pressure in the pulmonary circulation. Clinical manifestations are almost the same as the manifestations of congestive heart failure in adults. Unique manifestations in children include failure to thrive and periorbital edema.

3 Rheumatic heart disease, like rheumatic heart disease in adults, begins with acute pharyngeal infection by a group A β-hemolytic streptococcus that leads to valvular dysfunction.

4 Kawasaki disease is an acute systemic vasculitis that also may result in the development of coronary artery aneurysms and thrombosis.

5 Primary hypertension in children is the same as that in adults, except that it is more likely to be in its early, asymptomatic stage.

KEY TERMS

Acyanotic defect, 1093
Atrial septal defect (ASD), 1099
Coarctation of the aorta , 1094
Complete transposition of the great vessels (TGA), 1102
Cyanosis, 1092
Cyanotic defect, 1093
Ductus arteriosus, 1087
Ductus venosus, 1087
Eisenmenger syndrome, 1097
Foramen ovale, 1087
Infundibular stenosis, 1093

Kawasaki disease, 1111
Left-to-right shunt, 1092
Patent ductus arteriosus (PDA), 1098
Persistent truncus arteriosus (PTA), 1100
Postductal coarctation, 1094
Preductal coarctation (infantile coarctation), 1094
Pulmonary atresia, 1093
Pulmonary stenosis, 1093
Right-to-left shunt, 1092
Right ventricular outflow obstruction, 1093

Shunt, 1092
Stenosis, 1092
Supravalvular stenosis, 1093
Tetralogy of Fallot, 1105
Total anomalous pulmonary venous connection (TAPVC), 1104
Tricuspid atresia, 1107
Truncus arteriosus, 1086
Ventricular septal defect (VSD), 1096

REFERENCES

Adams, F. H., Emmanouilides, G. C., & Riemenschneider, T. A. (Eds.). (1989). *Moss' heart disease in infants, children, and adolescents.* (4th ed.). Baltimore: Williams & Wilkins.

Arciniegas, E. (Ed.). (1985). *Pediatric cardiovascular surgery.* Chicago: Year Book Medical Publishers.

Behrman, R. E., Kleigman, R. M., Nelson, W. E., & Vaughn, V. C. (Eds.). (1992). *Nelson textbook of pediatrics* (14th ed.). Philadelphia: Saunders.

Berenson, G. S. (1980). *Cardiovascular risk factors in children.* New York: Oxford University Press.

Berenson, G. S. (Ed.). (1986). *Causation of cardiovascular risk factors in children.* New York: Raven.

Berenson, G. S., Webber, L. S., Srinivasan, S. R., Cresanta, J. L., Frank, G. C., & Farris, R. P. (1984). Black-white contrasts as determinants of cardiovascular risk in childhood: Precursors of coronary artery and primary hypertensive diseases. *American Heart Journal, 108,* 3.

Croft, J. B., Cresanta, J. L., Webber, L. S., Srinivasan, S. R., Freedman, D. S., Burke, G. L., & Berenson, G. S. (1988). Cardiovascular risk in parents of children with extreme lipoprotein cholesterol levels: The Bogalusa Heart Study. *Southern Medical Journal, 81*(3), 341-349, 353.

Doyle, E. F., & Rutkowski, M. (1970). Etiology of congenital heart disease. *Cardiovascular Clinics, 2,* 2.

Engle, M. E. (Ed.). (1981). *Pediatric cardiovascular disease.* Philadelphia: Davis.

Fink, B. W. (1991). *Congenital heart disease* (3rd ed.). St. Louis: Mosby–Year Book.

Guzzetta, C., & Dossey, B. M. (Eds.). (1984). *Cardiovascular nursing: Bodymind tapestry.* St. Louis: Mosby–Year Book.

Kaplan, E. L. (1988). A comeback for rheumatic fever? *Patient Care, 22*(5), 80-84.

Keith, J. D., Rowe, R. D., & Vlad, P. (Eds.). (1978). *Heart disease in infancy and childhood* (3rd ed.). New York: Macmillan.

Kotchen, T. A., & Kotchen, J. M. (Eds.). (1983). *Clinical approaches to high blood pressure in the young.* Boston: John Wright PSG Inc.

Moller, J. H., & Neal, W. A. (Eds.). (1990). *Fetal, neonatal, and infant cardiac disease.* Norwalk, CT: Appleton & Lange.

Mott, W. R., James, S. R., & Sperhac, A. M. (Eds.). (1990). *Nursing care of children and families* (2nd ed.). Redwood City, CA: Addison-Wesley.

Park, M. K. (1988). *Pediatric cardiology for practitioners* (2nd ed.). Chicago: Year Book Medical Publishers.

Perloff, J. K., Friedman, W. F., Laks, H., & Child, J. S. (1983). From cyanotic infant to a cyanotic adult—The odyssey of blue babies. *The Western Journal of Medicine, 139*(5), 673-687.

Roberts, W. C. (1987). *Adult congenital heart disease.* Philadelphia: F. A. Davis.

Rudolph, A. M. (1974). *Congenital diseases of the heart: Clinical-physiologic considerations in diagnosis and management.* Chicago: Year Book Medical Publishers.

Ruttenberg, A. D. (1986). Acute rheumatic fever in the 1980s. *Pediatrician, 13*(4), 180-188.

Smith, J. B. (Ed.). (1983). *Pediatric critical care.* New York: John Wiley & Sons.

Thompson, J. M., McFarland, G. K., Hirsch, J. E., & Tucker, S. M. (1993). *Mosby's clinical nursing* (3rd ed.). St. Louis: Mosby–Year Book.

Whaley, L. F., & Wong, D. L. (1991). *Nursing care of infants and children* (4th ed.). St. Louis: Mosby–Year Book.

SUGGESTED READINGS

Lieberman, E. (1990). Hypertension in childhood and adolescence. In N. C. Kaplan (Ed.), *Clinical hypertension* (5th ed.). Baltimore: Williams & Wilkins.

Park, M. K. (1991). *The pediatric cardiology handbook.* St. Louis: Mosby–Year Book.

UNIT X

The Pulmonary System

ALTHOUGH PULMONARY DISEASE has been documented as a significant problem since the time of Hippocrates, human understanding and knowledge of respiratory physiology, pathology, and therapy were extremely limited until the end of the nineteenth and beginning of the twentieth century. At the time of Hippocrates it was believed that the purpose of the lungs was to cool the heart. Early physicians thought air entered the heart directly through the lungs and pulmonary vein, bringing to the body "vital forces" responsible for life. An imbalance of these forces, or "humors," was believed to cause disease. In the second century AD, asthma, the term then used to describe most respiratory diseases, was thought to be the result of excessive and thick secretions that dripped into the lung from the brain.

Leonardo DaVinci was the first to document that the airways of the lungs had no direct connection to the heart, and in the 1600s William Harvey accurately described the pulmonary circulation. Oxygen and carbon dioxide were not identified until the 1700s. In the 1800s the hemoglobin molecule was discovered, and Adolph Fick described the relationship of blood oxygen content, metabolism, and

THE PULMONARY SYSTEM

Inside your lungs. (Courtesy National Library of Medicine.)

for tuberculosis in the first century AD, rest and a good diet, remained essentially the same for centuries. It was not until the Middle Ages that tuberculosis was even considered to be contagious. By the 1800s contagion was feared to the extent that individuals with tuberculosis were sent to sanitoriums, where they were isolated from the general population. The tubercle bacillus was not identified by Robert Koch until 1890, and there was little change in treatment until 1944, when streptomycin was developed.

Within the last 100 years, mortality and morbidity rates from pulmonary diseases have decreased dramatically, yet these diseases are a major cause of death and disability today. Such diseases as asthma, bronchitis, and emphysema are now better understood, but a definitive treatment for them has not yet been discovered. Others, particularly lung cancer and occupational diseases, are on the increase. Some respiratory diseases, such as respiratory distress syndrome, are "new" in that they occur in individuals whose treatments have enabled them to survive other disorders that proved fatal in the past. Today progress is being made toward (1) further understanding of the mechanisms of pulmonary disease, (2) early detection and treatment of disease, (3) development of new therapies, and (4) prevention of disease through public education, improvements in environmental and occupational safety standards, and air quality.

cardiac output. It was not until 1910 that the mechanism for the exchange of oxygen and carbon dioxide in the lung was established. Pulmonary mechanics and the principles of acid-base physiology were first understood in the early 1900s.

Misconceptions about the structure and function of the pulmonary system severely limited early attempts to treat respiratory disease. For example, during the time of the Romans, tuberculosis was treated with a special root that was dug up before dawn and wrapped in the wool of a sheep who had just given birth to a ewe lamb. The treatment recommended

Structure and Function of the Pulmonary System

Sheryl S. Davey
Sue E. Huether
Marjorie Budd*

Chapter Outline

The pulmonary system consists of the lungs, airways, chest wall, and pulmonary circulation. Its primary function is the exchange of gases between the environmental air and the blood. There are three steps in this process: (1) ventilation, the movement of air into and out of the lungs; (2) diffusion, the movement of gases between air spaces in the lungs and the bloodstream; and (3) perfusion, the movement of blood into and out of the capillary beds of the lungs to body organs and tissues. The first two functions are carried out by the pulmonary system and the third by the cardiovascular system (see Chapter 26). Normally the pulmonary system functions efficiently under a variety of conditions and with little energy expenditure.

STRUCTURES OF THE PULMONARY SYSTEM

The pulmonary system is made up of two lungs, their airways, and the blood vessels that serve them (Fig. 29-1) and the chest wall, or thoracic cage. The lungs are divided into lobes, three in the right lung (upper, middle, and lower) and two in the left lung (upper and lower). Each lobe is further divided into segments and lobules. The space between the lungs, which contains the heart, great vessels, and esophagus, is called the mediastinum. A set of tubes, or conducting airways, delivers air to each section of the lung. The lung tissue that surrounds the airways supports them, preventing their

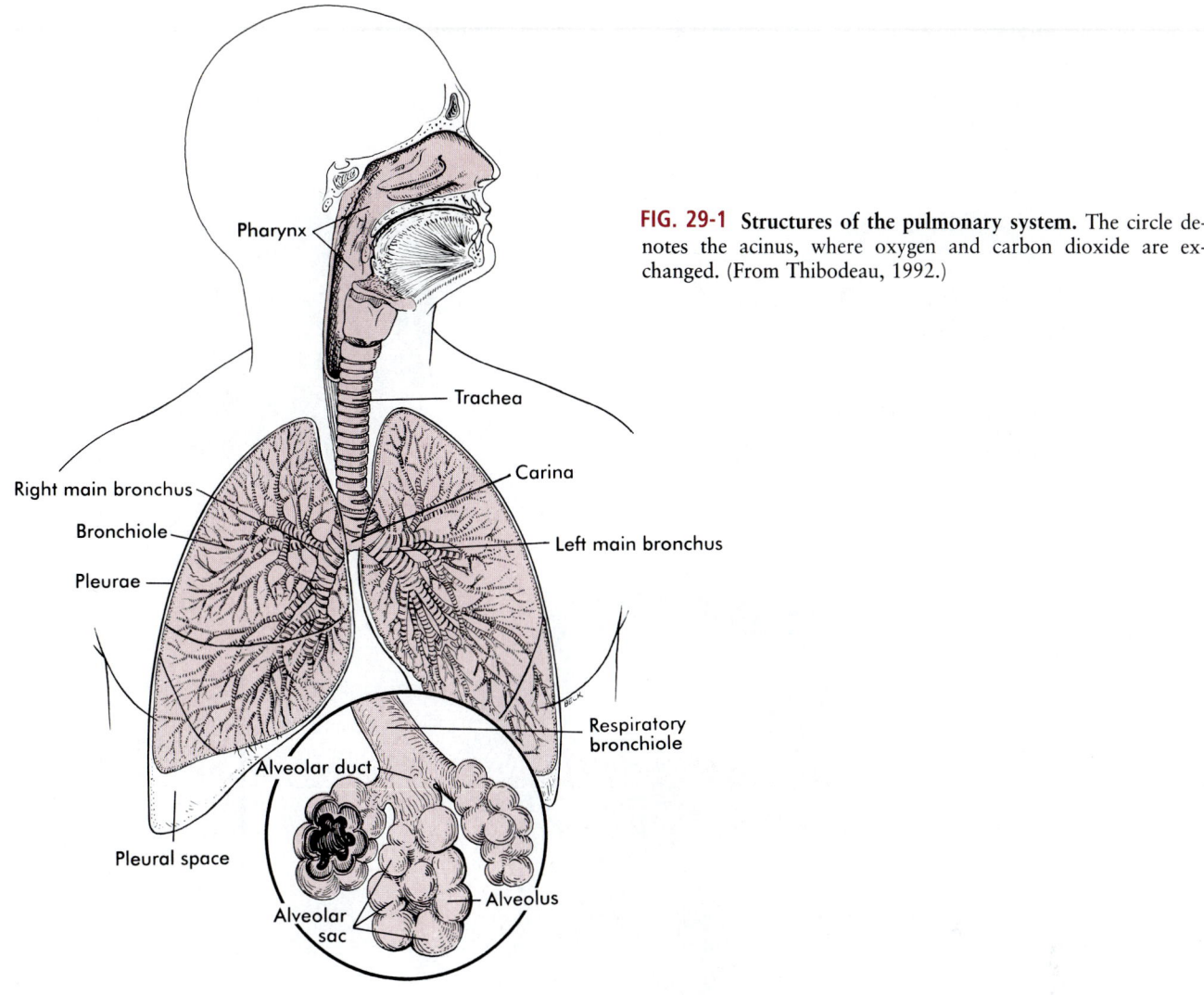

FIG. 29-1 **Structures of the pulmonary system.** The circle denotes the acinus, where oxygen and carbon dioxide are exchanged. (From Thibodeau, 1992.)

TABLE 29-1

Pulmonary Defense Mechanisms

Structure or substance	Mechanism of defense
Upper respiratory tract mucosa	Maintains constant temperature and humidification of gas entering the lungs; traps and removes foreign particles, some bacteria, and noxious gases from inspired air
Nasal hairs and turbinates	Trap and remove foreign particles, some bacteria, and noxious gases from inspired air
Mucous blanket	Protects trachea and bronchi from injury; traps most foreign particles and bacteria that reach the lower airways
Cilia	Propel mucous blanket and entrapped particles toward the oropharynx, where they can be swallowed or expectorated
Alveolar macrophages	Ingest and remove bacteria and other foreign material from alveoli by phagocytosis (see Chapters 6 and 7)
Irritant receptors in nares (nostrils)	Stimulation by chemical or mechanical irritants triggers sneeze reflex, which results in rapid removal of irritants from nasal passages
Irritant receptors in trachea and large airways	Stimulation by chemical or mechanical irritants triggers cough reflex, which results in removal of the irritant from the lower airways

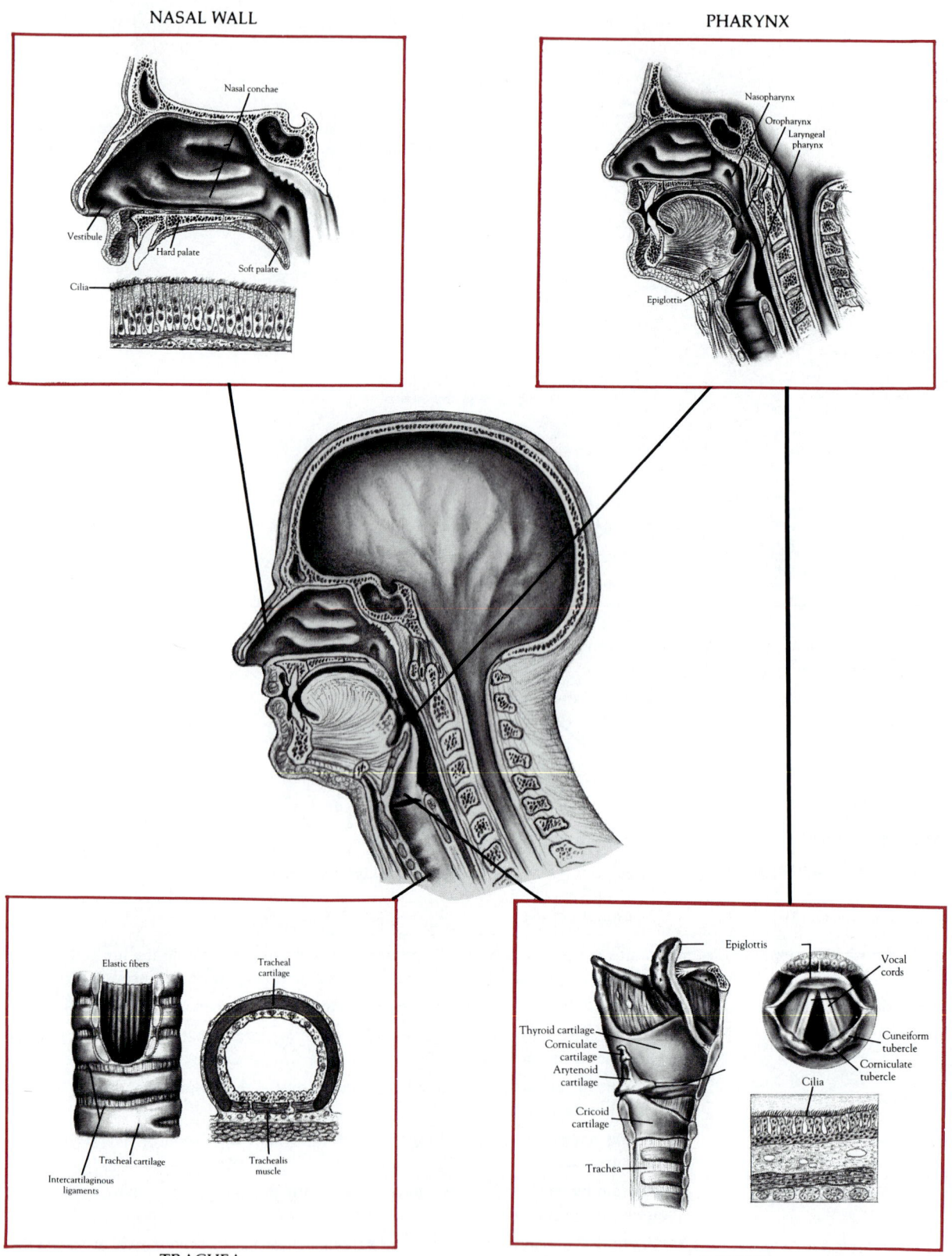

FIG. 29-2 **Structures of the upper airway.** (From Thompson, McFarland, Hirsch, & Tucker, 1993.)

distortion or collapse as gas moves in and out during ventilation.

The lungs are protected from a variety of exogenous contaminants by a series of mechanical barriers (Table 29-1). These defense mechanisms are so effective that contamination of the lung tissue itself, particularly by infectious agents, is rare. (Other mechanisms of self-defense are discussed in Chapters 6 and 7.)

Conducting Airways

The conducting airways are the portion of the pulmonary system that provides a passage for the movement of air into and out of the gas-exchange portions of the lung. They consist of upper and lower airways. The **nasopharynx** and **oropharynx** and related structures are often called the upper airway (Fig. 29-2). These structures are lined with a ciliated mucosa with a very rich vascular supply. The mucosal lining warms and humidifies inspired air and removes foreign particles from it as it passes into the lungs. During quiet breathing, gas usually flows through the nose, nasopharynx, and oropharynx to the lower airways. The mouth and oropharynx are also used for ventilation when the nose is obstructed or when increased flow is required, for example, during exercise. Filtering and humidifying are not, however, as efficient with mouth breathing.

The **larynx** connects the upper and lower airways. The structure of the larynx consists of the endolarynx and its surrounding triangular-shaped bony and cartilaginous structures. The endolarynx is formed by two pairs of folds that form the false vocal cords (supraglottis) and the true vocal cords. The slit-shaped space between the true cords forms the glottis (Fig. 29-3). The vestibule is the space above the false vocal cords. The laryngeal box is formed of three large cartilages—the epiglottis, thyroid, and cricoid—and three smaller cartilages— the arytenoid, corniculate, and cuneiform— that are connected by ligaments. The supporting cartilages prevent collapse of the larynx during inspiration and swallowing. The internal laryngeal muscles control vocal cord length and tension, and the external laryngeal muscles move the larynx as a whole. Both sets of muscles are important to swallowing, respiration, and vocalization. The internal muscles contract during swallowing to prevent aspiration into the trachea and also contribute to voice pitch.

The **trachea,** which is supported by U-shaped cartilage, connects the larynx to the **bronchi,** the conducting airways of the lungs. The trachea divides into the two main airways, or bronchi, at the **carina** (Fig. 29-1). This area is very sensitive and when stimulated can cause coughing and airway narrowing. The right main bronchus extends from the trachea more vertically than the left main bronchus, so that aspirated fluids or foreign particles tend to enter the right lung rather than

FIG. 29-3 Larynx in quiet respiration. (From Thompson, McFarland, Hirsch, & Tucker, 1993.)

the left. The right and left main bronchi enter the lungs at the **hili,** or "roots" of the lungs, along with the pulmonary blood and lymphatic vessels. From the hili the main bronchi branch into lobar bronchi, then to segmental and subsegmental bronchi, and finally end at the sixteenth division in the smallest of the conducting airways, the terminal **bronchioles** (Fig. 29-5).

The bronchial walls have three layers: an epithelial lining, a smooth muscle layer, and a connective tissue layer. In the large bronchi (to approximately the tenth division), the connective tissue layer contains cartilage. The epithelial lining of the bronchi contains single-celled exocrine glands—the mucus-secreting **goblet cells**—and ciliated cells. High columnar pseudostratified epithelium lines the larger airways, changing to columnar cuboidal epithelium in the bronchioles (types of epithelium are illustrated in Chapter 1). The submucosal glands of the bronchial lining also produce mucus, contributing to the mucus blanket that covers the bronchial epithelium. The ciliated epithelial cells rhythmically beat this mucus blanket toward the trachea and pharynx, where it can be swallowed or expectorated by coughing. Foreign particles and microorganisms that are not expelled by mucociliary clearance and coughing are attacked by cellular components of the inflammatory response and antibodies of the secretory immune system (see Unit III). The biochemical mediators released early in inflammation also play a part in antibody-mediated hypersensitivity reactions, such as asthma, because they stimulate bronchial smooth muscles and blood vessels to constrict.

With branching, the layers of epithelium that line the bronchi become thinner (Fig. 29-4). Mucus-producing glands are found only in the bronchi, and goblet cells are not found past the terminal bronchioles (seventeenth division). Ciliated cells become more sparse, and

(Longitudinal section)

Bronchus

Ciliated cell   Goblet cells   Serous cell

Pseudo-stratified epithelium
Basement membrane
Lamina propria
Smooth muscle layer
Submucosal glands
Cartilage

Bronchiole

Cuboidal epithelium
Ciliated cells   Clara cell

Alveoli

Alveolar macrophage
Surfactant
Capillary
C
A
C
Type II alveolar cell
Alveolus
Surfactant
C

Cartilage
Alveoli
Smooth muscle
Submucosal glands
Capillary
Ciliated columnal epithelium with goblet cells

Alveoli
Smooth muscle

(Cross section)   **Bronchus**   **Bronchiole**   **Alveoli**

FIG. 29-4 Changes in the bronchial wall with progressive branching.

CONDUCTING AIRWAYS				RESPIRATORY UNIT
TRACHEA	SEGMENTAL BRONCHI	SUBSEGMENTAL BRONCHI (BRONCHIOLES)		ALVEOLAR DUCTS
		Nonrespiratory	Respiratory	
GENERATIONS	8	16	24	26

FIG. 29-5 Structures of the lower airway. (From Thompson, McFarland, Hirsch, & Tucker, 1993.)

smooth muscle and connective tissue layers thin toward the terminal bronchioles (Bergofsky, 1991).

Gas-Exchange Airways

The conducting airways terminate in gas-exchange airways, where oxygen (O_2) enters the blood and carbon dioxide (CO_2) is removed from it. The gas-exchange airways are made up of **respiratory bronchioles, alveolar ducts,** and **alveoli.** These structures together are sometimes called the **acinus** (Fig. 29-5), and all of them participate in gas exchange.

Because the walls of bronchioles from the sixteenth through the twenty-third divisions contain increasing numbers of alveoli, the bronchioles at this level are called respiratory bronchioles. The walls of the respiratory bronchioles are very thin, consisting of an epithelial layer devoid of cilia and goblet cells, very little smooth muscle fiber, and a very thin and elastic connective tissue layer. The respiratory bronchioles end in alveolar ducts, which lead to alveolar sacs made up of numerous alveoli.

The alveoli are the primary gas-exchange units of the lung, where oxygen enters the blood and carbon dioxide is removed. They are thin-walled, spherical structures about 3 mm in diameter and have shared walls, or septa (Fig. 29-6). Tiny passages called pores of Kohn permit some air to pass through the septa from alveolus to alveolus, promoting collateral ventilation and even distribution of air among the alveoli. In cross sections, alveoli appear similar to common sponges. The lungs contain approximately 25 million alveoli at birth and 300 million by adulthood.

The alveolar septa consist of an epithelial layer and a thin, elastic basement membrane, but no muscle layer (Fig. 29-7). Two major types of epithelial cells appear in the alveolus. Type I alveolar cells provide structure, and type II alveolar cells secrete **surfactant,** a lipopro-

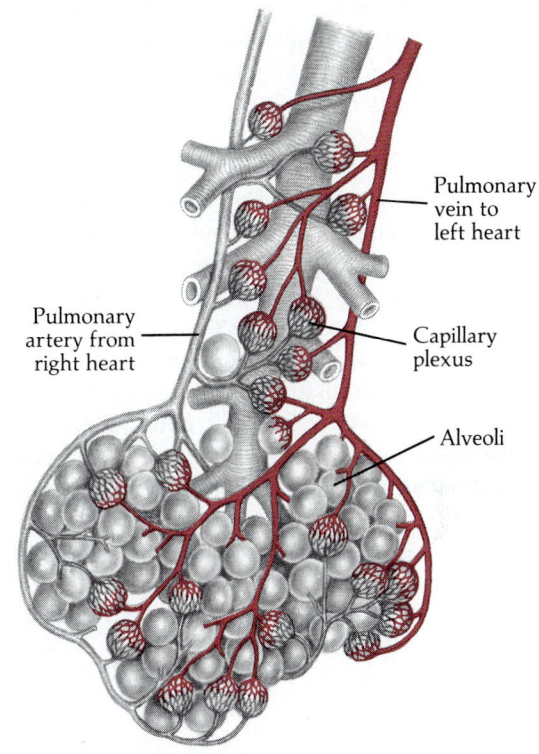

FIG. 29-6 **Terminal respiratory units.** (From Thompson, McFarland, Hirsch, & Tucker, 1993.)

FIG. 29-7 **Photomicrograph of lung, showing several alveoli.** Note the proximity of the capillary to the alveolar wall ($\times 140$). (From Thibodeau, G. A. [1987]. *Anatomy and physiology.* St. Louis: Mosby–Year Book.)

tein that coats the inner surface of the alveolus and facilitates its expansion during inspiration.

Like the bronchi, alveoli contain cellular components of inflammation and immunity, particularly the mononuclear phagocytes. The mononuclear phagocytes of the lungs are called alveolar macrophages. These cells ingest foreign material that reaches the alveolus and prepare it for removal through the lymphatics. (Phagocytosis and the mononuclear phagocyte system are described in Chapters 6 and 7.)

Pulmonary and Bronchial Circulation

The main function of the pulmonary circulation is to facilitate gas exchange. Its other functions are to deliver nutrients to lung tissues, act as a reservoir for the left ventricle, and serve as a filtering system that removes clots, air, and other debris from the circulation. The pulmonary circulation is illustrated in Fig. 29-8.

The pulmonary circulation has a lower pressure and resistance than the systemic circulation. Pulmonary arteries are exposed to about one fifth the pressure of the systemic circulation. (Mean pulmonary artery pressure is 18 mm Hg; mean aortic pressure is 90 mm Hg.) The smooth muscle layer in normal pulmonary artery walls is much thinner than that in systemic vessel walls, and pulmonary arteries are more distensible than their systemic counterparts. (Systemic vessels are described in Chapter 26.)

Usually approximately one third of the pulmonary vessels are filled with blood (perfused) at any given time. Additional vessels become perfused when right ventricular cardiac output increases. Therefore, increased delivery of blood to the lungs does not normally increase mean pulmonary artery pressure.

The pulmonary artery divides and enters the lung at the hilus with each main bronchus and branches with the bronchus at every division, so that every bronchus and bronchiole has an accompanying artery or arteriole. The arterioles, less than 1 mm in diameter, regulate blood flow through their respective capillary beds.

The arterioles divide at the terminal bronchiole to form a network of pulmonary capillaries around the acinus. The capillaries are an integral part of the alveolar septa. Capillary walls consist of an endothelial layer and a thin basement membrane, which often fuses with the basement membrane of the alveolar septum. This results in very little separation between blood in the capillary and gas in the alveolus.

The shared alveolar and capillary walls compose the **alveolocapillary membrane,** a very thin membrane made up of the alveolar epithelium, the alveolar basement membrane, an interstitial space, the capillary basement

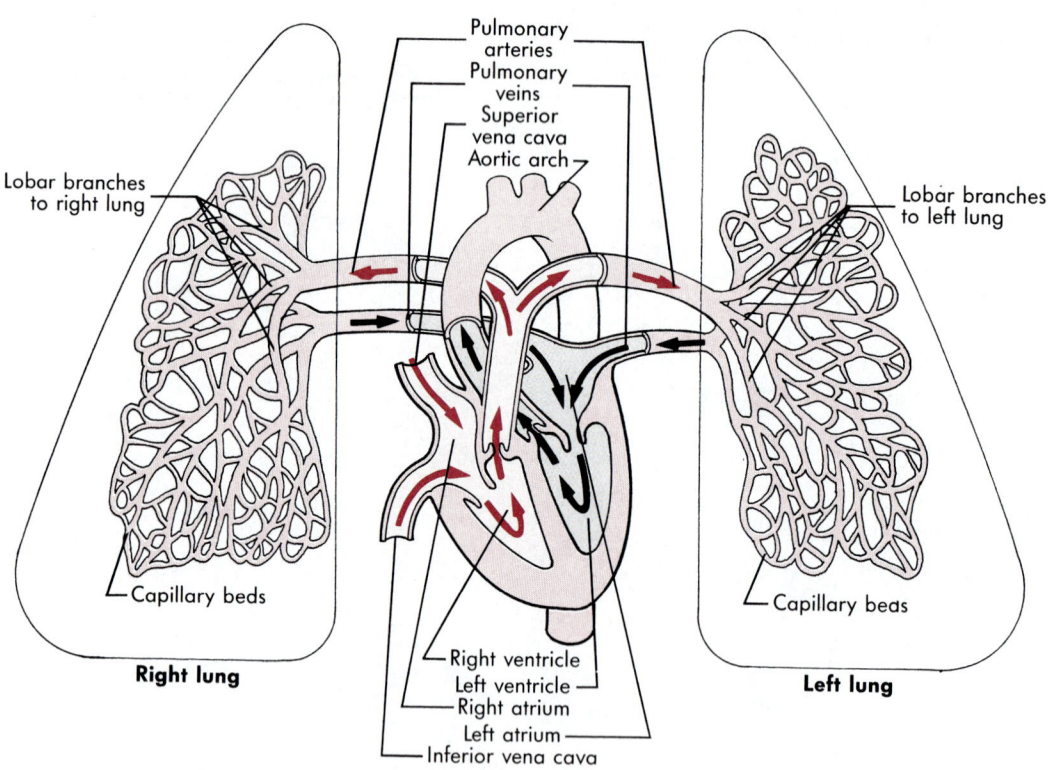

FIG. 29-8 The pulmonary circulation. The right and left pulmonary veins and arteries and the branching capillaries are illustrated.

membrane, and the capillary endothelium (Fig. 29-9). Gas exchange occurs across the alveolocapillary membrane. With normal perfusion, approximately 100 ml of blood in the pulmonary capillary bed is spread very thinly over 70 to 100 m^2 of alveolar surface area. This could be compared with spreading 100 ml of blood over a tennis court and covering it with a sheet of cellophane to separate it from the air. The alveolocapillary membrane efficiently exposes large quantities of blood to gas in the alveoli. Any disorder that thickens the membrane impairs gas exchange.

Each pulmonary vein drains several pulmonary capillaries. Unlike the pulmonary arteries, which follow the branching bronchi, pulmonary veins are dispersed randomly throughout the lung, then leave the lung at the hili and enter the left atrium. They are similar to veins in the systemic circulation but have no valves.

The bronchial circulation is part of the systemic circulation. It supplies nutrients to the conducting airways, large pulmonary vessels, and membranes (pleurae) that surround the lungs. The bronchial circulation is unique in that not all of its capillaries drain into its own venous system. Some of the bronchial capillaries empty into the pulmonary vein and contribute to the normal venous admixture (mixing of oxygenated and deoxygenated blood) or right-to-left shunt (right-to-left shunts are described in Chapter 30). The bronchial circulation does not participate in gas exchange but warms and moistens inspired air and provides airway nourishment (Charan & Carvalho, 1992).

Lung vasculature also includes deep and superficial lymphatic capillaries. The deep lymphatic capillaries begin at the level of the terminal bronchioles; there are no lymphatic structures in the acinus. Fluid and alveolar macrophages migrate from the alveoli to the terminal bronchioles, where they enter the lymphatic system. The superficial lymphatic capillaries drain the membrane that surrounds the lungs. Both deep and superficial lymphatic vessels leave the lung at the hilus. The lymphatic system plays an important role in keeping the lung free of fluid. (The lymphatic system is described in Chapter 26.)

Chest Wall and Pleura

The chest wall (thoracic cage) protects the lungs from injury, and its muscles, in conjunction with the diaphragm, perform the muscular work of breathing. The **thoracic cavity** is contained by the chest wall and en-

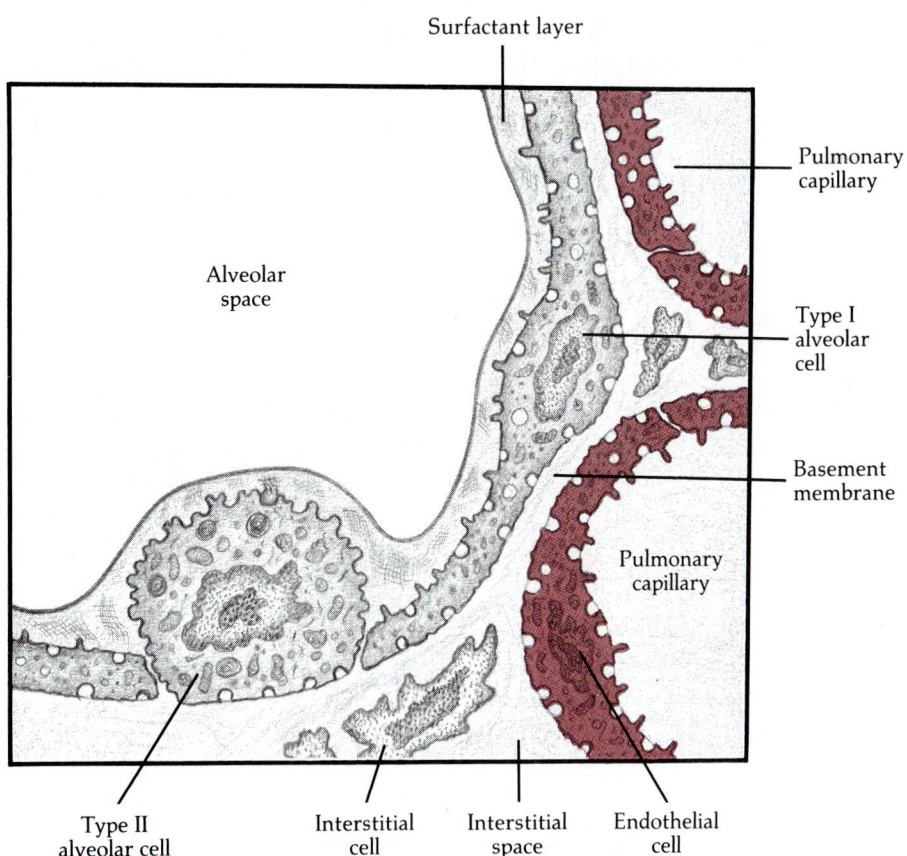

FIG. 29-9 Alveolar wall and space. (From Thompson, McFarland, Hirsch, & Tucker, 1993.)

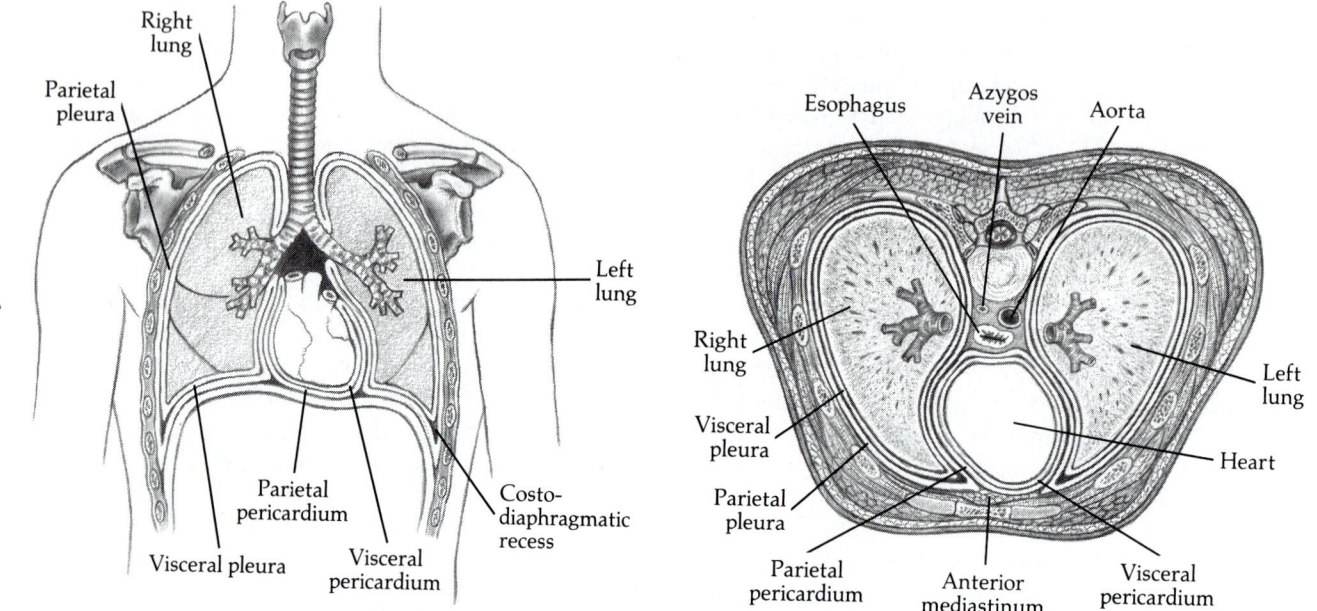

FIG. 29-10 Chest cavity and related structures. **A,** Anterior view; **B,** cross section. (From Thompson, McFarland, Hirsch, & Tucker, 1993.)

cases the lungs (Fig. 29-10). A serous membrane called the **pleura** adheres firmly to the lungs. It then folds over itself and attaches firmly to the chest wall. The pleural membrane covering the lungs is the visceral pleura; that lining the thoracic cavity is the parietal pleura. The area between the two pleurae is called the **pleural space**, or pleural cavity. Normally only a thin layer of fluid secreted by the pleura (pleural fluid) fills the pleural space. This lubricates the pleural surfaces, allowing the two layers to slide over each other without separating. Pressure in the pleural space is usually negative or subatmospheric (−4 to −10 mm Hg).

FUNCTION OF THE PULMONARY SYSTEM

Ventilation

Ventilation is the mechanical movement of gas or air into and out of the lungs. Ventilation is often misnamed respiration, which is actually the exchange of oxygen and carbon dioxide during cellular metabolism. "Respiratory rate" is actually the ventilatory rate, or the number of times gas is inspired and expired per minute.

Measurement of Gas Pressure

A few physical characteristics of gas are important for an understanding of ventilation. A gas is made up of millions of molecules moving randomly. As they move,

they collide with each other and the wall of the space in which they are contained. These collisions exert pressure. If more molecules are present in the space, the pressure, or number of collisions, increases (Fig. 29-11). If the same number of gas molecules is contained in a small and a large container, the pressure is greater in the small container because more collisions occur in the smaller space. Increases in temperature increase the speed of the molecules, which increases the number of collisions. Therefore, pressure also increases at higher temperatures.

Barometric pressure (P_B) (atmospheric pressure) is the pressure exerted by gas molecules in air at specific altitudes. At sea level, barometric pressure is 760 mm Hg. This number is the sum of the pressure exerted by each gas in the air at sea level. The portion of the total pressure exerted by any individual gas is its **partial pressure** (see Fig. 29-11). At sea level the air is made up of oxygen (20.9%), nitrogen (78.1%), and a few other trace gases. The partial pressure of oxygen is equal to the percentage of oxygen in the air (20.9) times the total pressure (760 mm Hg), or 159 mm Hg (760 × 0.209 = 158.84). (Symbols used in the measurement of gas pressures and pulmonary ventilation are defined in Table 29-2.)

The amount of water vapor contained in a gas mixture is determined by the temperature of the gas and is unrelated to barometric pressure. Gas that enters the lungs becomes saturated with water vapor (humidified) as it passes through the upper airway. At body temper-

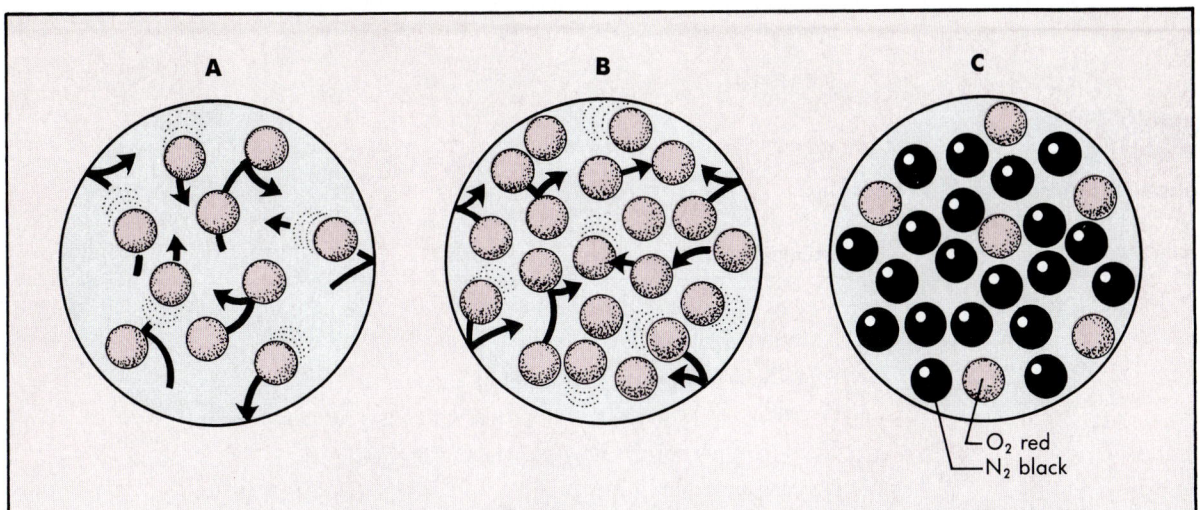

FIG. 29-11 Relationship between number of gas molecules and pressure exerted by the gas in an enclosed space. **A,** Theoretically 10 molecules of the same gas exert a total pressure of 10 within the space. **B,** If the number of molecules is increased to 20, total pressure is 20. **C,** If there are different gases in the space, each gas exerts a partial pressure: Here the partial pressure of nitrogen (N_2) is 18, that of oxygen (O_2) is 6, and total pressure is 24.

Measure	TLC	V_t	FRC	IC	IRV	ERV	RV	VC
Value (ml)	5800	500	2300	3500	3000	1100	1200	4600
	6000		2400	3600	3100	1200	1300	4800

FIG. 29-12 **Lung volume measurements.** All values are approximately 25% lower in women. *TLC,* Total lung capacity; *V_T,* tidal volume; *FRC,* functional residual capacity; *IC,* inspiratory capacity; *IRV,* inspiratory reserve volume; *ERV,* expiratory reserve volume; *RV,* residual volume; *VC,* vital capacity. (From Thompson, McFarland, Hirsch, & Tucker, 1993.)

TABLE 29-2

Common Pulmonary Abbreviations

Symbol	Definition
V	Volume or amount of gas
Q	Perfusion or blood flow
P	Pressure (usually partial pressure) of a gas
S	Percentage of hemoglobin saturation with a gas (usually oxygen)
F	Fraction of gas, or gas flow (in a laboratory test)
C	Content or amount of gas
C_T	Thoracic compliance
E	Expired gas
i	Inspired gas
A	Alveolar gas
a	Arterial blood
$\bar{v}$	Mixed venous or pulmonary artery blood
D	Dead space
Pa_{O_2}	Partial pressure of oxygen in arterial blood
PA_{O_2}	Partial pressure of oxygen in alveolar gas
Pa_{CO_2}	Partial pressure of carbon dioxide in arterial blood
$P\bar{v}_{O_2}$	Partial pressure of oxygen in mixed venous or pulmonary artery blood
$P(A - a)_{O_2}$	Difference between alveolar and arterial partial pressure of oxygen (A − a gradient)
P_B	Barometric or atmospheric pressure
Sa_{O_2}	Saturation of hemoglobin (in arterial blood) with oxygen
$S\bar{v}_{O_2}$	Saturation of hemoglobin (in mixed venous blood) with oxygen
Ca_{O_2}	Content or amount (volume) of oxygen in arterial blood
$C\bar{v}_{O_2}$	Content of oxygen in mixed venous blood
$C(a - \bar{v})_{O_2}$	Oxygen content difference between arterial and mixed venous blood
$\dot{V}_A$	Alveolar ventilation
$\dot{V}_D$	Dead-space ventilation
$\dot{V}_E$	Minute volume
VC	Vital capacity
V_T	Tidal volume or average breath
$\dot{Q}T$	Total perfusion or blood flow (cardiac output)
$\dot{V}/\dot{Q}$	Ratio of ventilation to perfusion
Fi_{O_2}	Fraction of inspired oxygen
FRC	Functional residual capacity
IC	Inspiratory capacity

NOTE: Subscripts identify the particular gas, volume, or pressure being discussed. A dot (˙) means measurement over time, usually 1 minute.

ature (37° C), water vapor exerts a pressure of 47 mm Hg. Because this is true regardless of total (barometric) pressure, the partial pressure of water vapor (always 47 mm Hg) must be subtracted from the barometric pressure before the partial pressure of other gases in the mixture can be determined. In saturated air at sea level, the partial pressure of oxygen is, therefore, $(760 - 47) \times 0.209 = 149$. All pressure and volume measurements made in pulmonary function laboratories specify the temperature and humidity of a gas at the time of measurement.

Many pressure measurements are stated as variations from barometric pressure, rather than percentages of it. On such scales, barometric pressure is considered zero, and pressure varies up or down from zero. Physiologic pressure measurements that involve fluids, rather than gases, are measured as variations from barometric pressure. For example, a systolic blood pressure of 120 mm Hg indicates that systolic pressure is 120 mm Hg above barometric pressure.

Measurement of Lung Volumes and Capacities

Tidal volume (V_T) is the amount of gas inspired and expired during normal breathing (Fig. 29-12). **Inspiratory reserve volume (IRV)** is the amount of gas that can be inspired in addition to tidal volume. **Expiratory reserve volume (ERV)** is the amount of gas that can be expired after a passive (relaxed) expiration. **Residual volume (RV)** is the volume of gas that cannot be expired and is always present in the lungs.

Total lung capacity (TLC) is the total gas volume in the lung when it is maximally inflated. It is made up of RV, ERV, V_T, and IRV. **Vital capacity (VC)** is the maximum amount of gas that can be displaced (expired) from the lung. It includes IRV, V_T, and ERV. **Functional residual capacity (FRC)** is the amount of gas remaining in the lung at the end of a passive expiration (RV and ERV). At this point the lungs are at rest, or in a state of mechanical equilibrium. **Inspiratory capacity (IC)** is the amount of gas that can be inspired after a passive expiration (from FRC). It includes V_T and IRV. The lung capacities are always the sum of two or more volumes. Norms for volumes and capacities are based on age, sex, and height and are referred to as predicted values. Changes from predicted or baseline values are taken into account in diagnosing and assessing respiratory disorders.

Not all of the air entering the airways and lungs participates in gas exchange. This volume of wasted ventilation is called **dead-space ventilation ($\dot{V}_D$)**. There are two types of dead space, anatomic and alveolar. With each breath, a portion of the tidal volume remains in the conducting airways. This is the **anatomic dead space**. Anatomic dead space averages about 1 ml per pound of lean body weight or approximately one third of each breath. In certain disease conditions, some of the respiratory bronchioles and alveoli receive adequate ventilation but do not participate in gas exchange because they are not perfused by the pulmonary circulation. The volume of gas in unperfused alveoli is known as **alveolar dead space**. Physiologic dead space is the sum of the normal anatomic dead space and the abnormal alveolar dead space (Scanlan, 1990b).

Alveolar ventilation ($\dot{V}_A$) is that portion of the tidal volume that reaches the alveoli. Adequate alveolar ventilation is required for sufficient gas exchange. During expiration, a portion of this alveolar gas remains in the conducting airways and moves back into the alveoli with the next inspiration.

Carbon dioxide (CO_2), the gaseous form of carbonic acid (H_2CO_3), is a product of cellular metabolism. The lung eliminates about 10,000 milliequivalents (mEq) of carbonic acid per day in the form of CO_2, which is produced at the rate of approximately 200 ml/min. Carbon dioxide elimination is necessary to maintain a normal arterial CO_2 (Pa_{CO_2}) of 40 mm Hg and normal acid-base balance (see Chapter 3 for a discussion of acid-base regulation).

The adequacy of alveolar ventilation *cannot* be determined by observation of ventilatory rate, pattern, or effort. If a health professional has a question about the adequacy of ventilation, an arterial blood gas analysis must be performed to measure Pa_{CO_2}.

Mechanics of Breathing

The mechanical aspects of inspiration and expiration are known collectively as the mechanics of breathing. The mechanics of breathing involve (1) major and accessory muscles of inspiration and expiration, (2) elastic properties of the lungs and chest wall, and (3) resistance to air flow through the conducting airways. Alterations in any of these properties increase the work of breathing, or the metabolic energy that must be expended to achieve adequate ventilation and oxygenation of the blood (see p. 1140).

Major and accessory muscles

The major muscles of inspiration are the diaphragm and the external intercostal muscles (muscles between the ribs) (Fig. 29-13). The diaphragm is a dome-shaped muscle that separates the abdominal and thoracic cavities. When the diaphragm contracts, it flattens downward, increasing the volume of the thoracic cavity, and creates a negative pressure that draws gas into the lungs. Contraction of external intercostal muscles elevates the anterior portion of the ribs. This increases the volume of the thoracic cavity by increasing its front-to-back (anterior-posterior [AP]) diameter. Although the exter-

FIG. 29-13 **Muscles of ventilation.** **A,** Anterior view; **B,** posterior view. (From Thompson, McFarland, Hirsch, & Tucker, 1993.)

nal intercostals may contract during quiet breathing, inspiration at rest is usually assisted by the diaphragm alone.

The accessory muscles of inspiration are the sternocleidomastoid and scalene muscles. Like the external intercostals, these muscles enlarge the thorax by increasing its AP diameter. The accessory muscles of inspiration assist inspiration when minute volume (volume of air inspired and expired per minute) is very high, as during strenuous exercise, or when the work of breathing is increased because of disease. The accessory muscles do not increase the volume of the thorax as efficiently as the diaphragm does.

There are no major muscles of expiration because normal, relaxed expiration is passive and requires no muscular effort. The accessory muscles of expiration, the abdominal and internal intercostal muscles, assist expiration when minute volume is high, when expiration exceeds FRC, or when airway obstruction is present. When the abdominal muscles contract, intraabdominal pressure increases, pushing up the diaphragm and decreasing the volume of the thorax. The internal intercostal muscles pull down the anterior ribs, decreasing the AP diameter of the thorax.

Alveolar surface tension

Surface tension occurs at any gas-liquid interface. **Surface tension** is the tendency for liquid molecules that are exposed to air to adhere to one another. This phenomenon can be seen, for example, in a glass of liquid that is about to overflow or in the way liquids "bead" when splashed on a waterproof surface. In both examples, this phenomenon decreases the surface area exposed to the air.

Within a sphere, such as an alveolus, surface tension tends to make expansion difficult. According to the law of Laplace, the pressure (P) required to inflate a sphere is equal to two times the surface tension (2T) divided by the radius (r) of the sphere, or $P = (2T/r)$. As the radius of the sphere (or alveolus) becomes smaller, more and more pressure is required to inflate it. If the alveoli were lined with a waterlike fluid, taking breaths would be extremely difficult.

Alveolar ventilation, or distention, is made possible by surfactant, which lowers surface tension by coating the air-liquid interface in the alveoli. Surfactant, a lipoprotein produced by type II alveolar cells, has a detergentlike effect that separates the liquid molecules, thereby decreasing alveolar surface tension.

Surfactant lines the alveolar side of the alveolocapillary membrane and, in effect, reverses the law of Laplace. In the lung, the relationship between surface tension and radius is opposite to that of the law of Laplace. As the radius of a surfactant-lined sphere (alveolus) grows smaller, the surface tension *decreases*, and as the radius grows larger, the surface tension *increases*. This occurs because the smaller radius causes surfactant molecules to crowd together, then repel one another strongly. A larger radius spreads them apart, decreasing their mutual repellence. Therefore, the alveoli are much easier to inflate at low lung volumes (i.e., after expiration) than at high volumes (i.e., after inspiration). If surfactant production is disrupted or surfactant is not produced in adequate quantities, alveolar surface tension increases and results in alveolar collapse, decreased lung expansion, increased work of breathing, and severe gas-exchange abnormalities.

The decrease in surface tension caused by surfactant is also responsible for keeping the alveoli free of fluid. In the absence of surfactant, the surface tension tends to attract fluid into the alveoli.

Elastic properties of the lung and chest wall

The lung and chest wall have elastic properties that permit expansion during inspiration and return to resting volume (FRC) during expiration. The elasticity of the lungs is caused both by elastin fibers in the alveolar walls and surrounding the small airways and pulmonary capillaries, and by surface tension at the alveolar air-liquid interface. The elasticity of the chest wall is the result of the configuration of its bones and musculature.

Elasticity, or elastance, is the tendency of a structure to resist stretching and, when stretched, to return to its original shape. In the lung, elasticity is a measure of the pressure required to inflate the lungs and the volume of inflation achieved. Elasticity can be calculated using the formula

$$E = \frac{\Delta P}{\Delta V}$$

where E = elasticity, ΔP = change in pressure applied to the lungs, and ΔV = change in volume (Scanlan, 1990b).

Elastic recoil is the tendency of the lungs to return to the resting state after inspiration. Normal elastic recoil permits passive expiration, eliminating the need for major muscles of expiration. Passive elastic recoil may be insufficient during labored breathing (high minute volume), in which case the accessory muscles of expiration are used. The accessory muscles are also used if disease compromises elastic recoil (e.g., in emphysema) or blocks the conducting airways.

Normal elastic recoil depends on an equilibrium between opposing forces of recoil in the lungs and chest wall. Under normal conditions the chest wall tends to recoil by expanding outward. This can be observed readily during open heart surgery. When the sternum is split to open the thoracic cavity, the chest wall moves outward laterally. The tendency of the chest wall to recoil by expanding is balanced by the tendency of the lungs to recoil or collapse around the hili. The tendency of the lungs to collapse can be demonstrated if the chest is opened without mechanically ventilating the lungs (for example, at postmortem examination). As the thorax is opened, the lungs immediately collapse like in-

flated balloons that have been released. This reaction is caused by elastic recoil and surface tension in the alveoli. The opposing forces of the chest wall and lungs create, in part, the negative intrapleural pressure.

Balance between the outward recoil of the chest wall and inward recoil of the lungs occurs at the resting level, the end of expiration, where the functional residual capacity is reached. During inspiration, the diaphragm and intercostal muscles contract, air flows into the lungs, and the chest wall expands. Muscular effort is needed to overcome the resistance of the lungs to expansion. During expiration, the muscles relax and the elastic recoil of the lungs causes the thorax to decrease in volume until, once again, balance between the chest wall and lung recoil forces is reached (Scanlan, 1990b) (Fig. 29-14).

Compliance is the measure of lung and chest wall distensibility. It represents the relative ease with which these structures can be stretched. Compliance is, therefore, the reciprocal of elasticity. Compliance is determined by alveolar surface tension and the elastic recoil of the lung and chest wall and can be measured by using the formula

$$C = \frac{\Delta V}{\Delta P}$$

where C = compliance in liters/centimeter of water, ΔV = volume change (usually tidal volume), and ΔP = pressure change (airway or pleural pressure) in centimeters of water (Altose, 1988).

Compliance of the lung and chest wall can be measured separately. The value used in the clinical setting is *lung* compliance, which is measured under conditions of airflow (static compliance) because airflow resistance contributes to the pressure gradient. Normal static lung compliance is 100 ml/cm H_2O or 0.1 liter/cm H_2O. The volume-pressure curve shown in Fig. 29-15 depicts the mechanical forces of ventilation or thoracic compliance at varying lung volumes. An increase in compliance indicates that the lungs or chest wall is abnormally easy to inflate and has lost some elastic recoil. A decrease indicates that the lungs or chest wall is abnormally stiff or difficult to inflate. Compliance is increased in emphysema and decreased in adult respiratory distress syndrome, pneumonia, pulmonary edema, or fibrosis. (These disorders are described in Chapter 30.)

Airway resistance

Airway resistance, which is similar to resistance to blood flow (described in Chapter 26), is determined by the length, radius, and cross-sectional area of the airways and density, viscosity, and velocity of the gas (Poiseuille's law). Resistance is computed by dividing change in pressure *(P)* by rate of flow *(F)*, or R = P/F (Ohm's law). Airway resistance is normally very low.

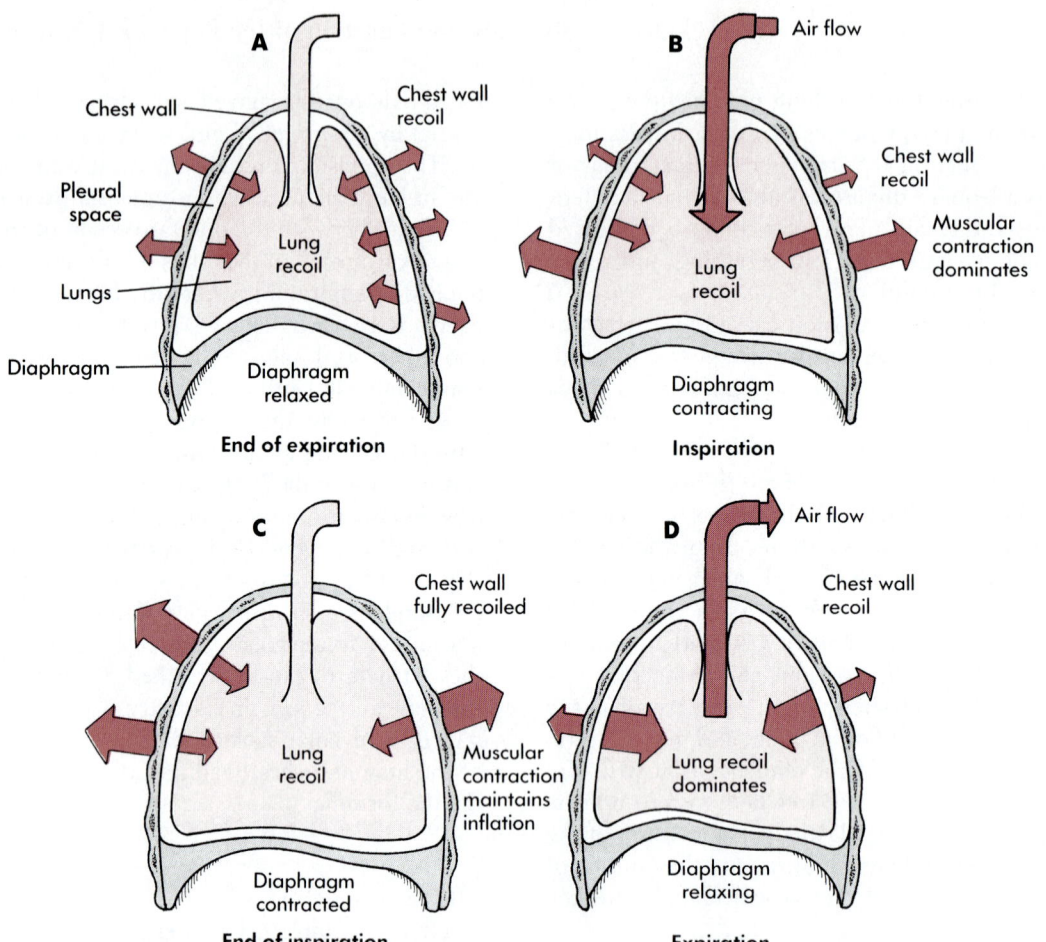

FIG. 29-14 Interaction of forces during inspiration and expiration. Outward recoil of the chest wall equals inward recoil of the lungs at the end of expiration (**A**). During inspiration, contraction of respiratory muscles, assisted by chest wall recoil, overcomes tendency of lungs to recoil (**B**). At the end of inspiration, respiratory muscle contraction maintains lung expansion (**C**). During expiration, respiratory muscles relax, allowing elastic recoil of the lungs to deflate the lungs (**D**).

FIG. 29-15 Volume-pressure curves of the chest wall and lung. The elastic recoil pressure of the respiratory system (chest wall and lungs together) is the sum of the recoil pressure of the chest wall and the recoil pressure of the lung. At FRC, the recoil pressure of the lung equals the recoil pressure of the chest wall.

One half to two thirds of total airway resistance occurs in the nose. The next highest resistance is in the oropharynx and larynx. There is very little resistance in the conducting airways of the lungs because of their large cross-sectional area. The most common causes of increased airway resistance are swelling (edema), obstruction (i.e., mucus plugging), and spasm of bronchial smooth muscle (bronchospasm), all of which decrease the radius of the airways. Resistance is inversely proportional to the fourth power of the radius.

Work of breathing

The work of breathing is determined by the muscular effort (and therefore oxygen and energy) required for ventilation. The work of breathing is normally very low but may increase considerably in diseases that disrupt the equilibrium between forces exerted by the lung and chest wall. More muscular effort is required when lung compliance is decreased (e.g., in pulmonary edema), chest wall compliance is decreased (e.g., in spinal deformity or obesity), or airways are obstructed by bronchospasm or mucus plugging (e.g., in asthma or bronchitis). An increase in the work of breathing can be life-threatening when oxygen delivery also is impaired (e.g., in anemia).

Neurochemical Control of Ventilation

Although breathing is usually involuntary, voluntary breathing is necessary for talking, singing, laughing, and deliberately holding one's breath, because homeostatic changes in ventilatory rate and volume are adjusted automatically by the nervous system to maintain normal gas exchange. The mechanisms that control respiration are very complex.

The **respiratory center** in the brainstem controls respiration by transmitting impulses to the respiratory muscles, causing them to contract and relax (Fig. 29-16). The respiratory center is composed of several groups of neurons located bilaterally in the brainstem: the dorsal respiratory group (DRG), the ventral respiratory group (VRG), the pneumotaxic center, and the apneustic center (Fraser, Paré, Paré, Fraser, & Genereux, 1988). The basic automatic rhythm of respiration is set by the DRG, a cluster of inspiratory nerve cells located in the medulla that sends efferent impulses to the diaphragm and inspiratory intercostal muscles (Guyton, 1992). The DRG also receives afferent input from **peripheral chemoreceptors** in the carotid and aortic bodies and from several different types of receptors in the lungs. The VRG, also located in the medulla, contains both inspiratory and expiratory neurons. It is almost inactive during normal, quiet respiration, becoming active when increased ventilatory effort is required. The pneumotaxic center and apneustic centers, situated in the pons, do not generate primary rhythm but rather act as modifiers of the rhythm established by the medullary centers.

Lung Receptors

Three types of lung receptors send impulses from the lungs to the dorsal respiratory group: (1) irritant receptors, (2) stretch receptors, and (3) J-receptors. **Irritant receptors** are found in the epithelium of all conducting airways. They are sensitive to noxious aerosols (vapors), gases, and particulate matter (inhaled dusts, etc.), which cause them to initiate the cough reflex. When stimulated, irritant receptors cause bronchoconstriction and increased ventilatory rate. **Stretch receptors** are located in the smooth muscles of airways and are sensitive to increases in the size or volume of the lungs. Stretch receptors decrease ventilatory rate and volume when stimulated, an occurrence sometimes referred to as the Hering-Breuer expiratory reflex. This reflex is not thought to play a major role in the regulation of ventilation in adults, although it may be important in infants (Scanlan, 1990a). J-receptors (juxtapulmonary capillary receptors) are located near the capillaries in the alveolar septa. They are sensitive to increased pulmonary capillary pressure, which stimulates them to initiate rapid, shallow breathing.

The lung is innervated by the autonomic nervous system (ANS). Fibers of the sympathetic division of the ANS in the lung branch from the upper thoracic and cervical ganglia of the spinal cord. Fibers of the parasympathetic division of the ANS travel in the vagus nerve to the lung. (Structures and function of the autonomic nervous system are covered in detail in Chapter 12.) The parasympathetic and sympathetic divisions of the ANS control airway caliber (interior diameter of the airway lumen) by stimulating bronchial smooth muscle to contract or relax. The parasympathetic receptors cause smooth muscle to contract, whereas sympathetic receptors cause it to relax. Bronchial smooth muscle tone depends on equilibrium, that is, equal stimulation of contraction and relaxation. The parasympathetic division of the ANS is the main controller of airway caliber under normal conditions. Constriction occurs if the irritant receptors in the airway epithelium are stimulated by irritants in inspired air, by endogenous substances (e.g., histamine, serotonin, prostaglandins), by many drugs, and by humoral substances. The balance between parasympathetic and sympathetic stimulation of the airway is important in many pathologic conditions, the most important of which is asthma.

Chemoreceptors

Chemoreceptors monitor the pH, $Paco_2$, and Pao_2 of arterial blood. **Central chemoreceptors** monitor arterial blood indirectly by sensing changes in the pH of cerebrospinal fluid (CSF). They are located in the myelen-

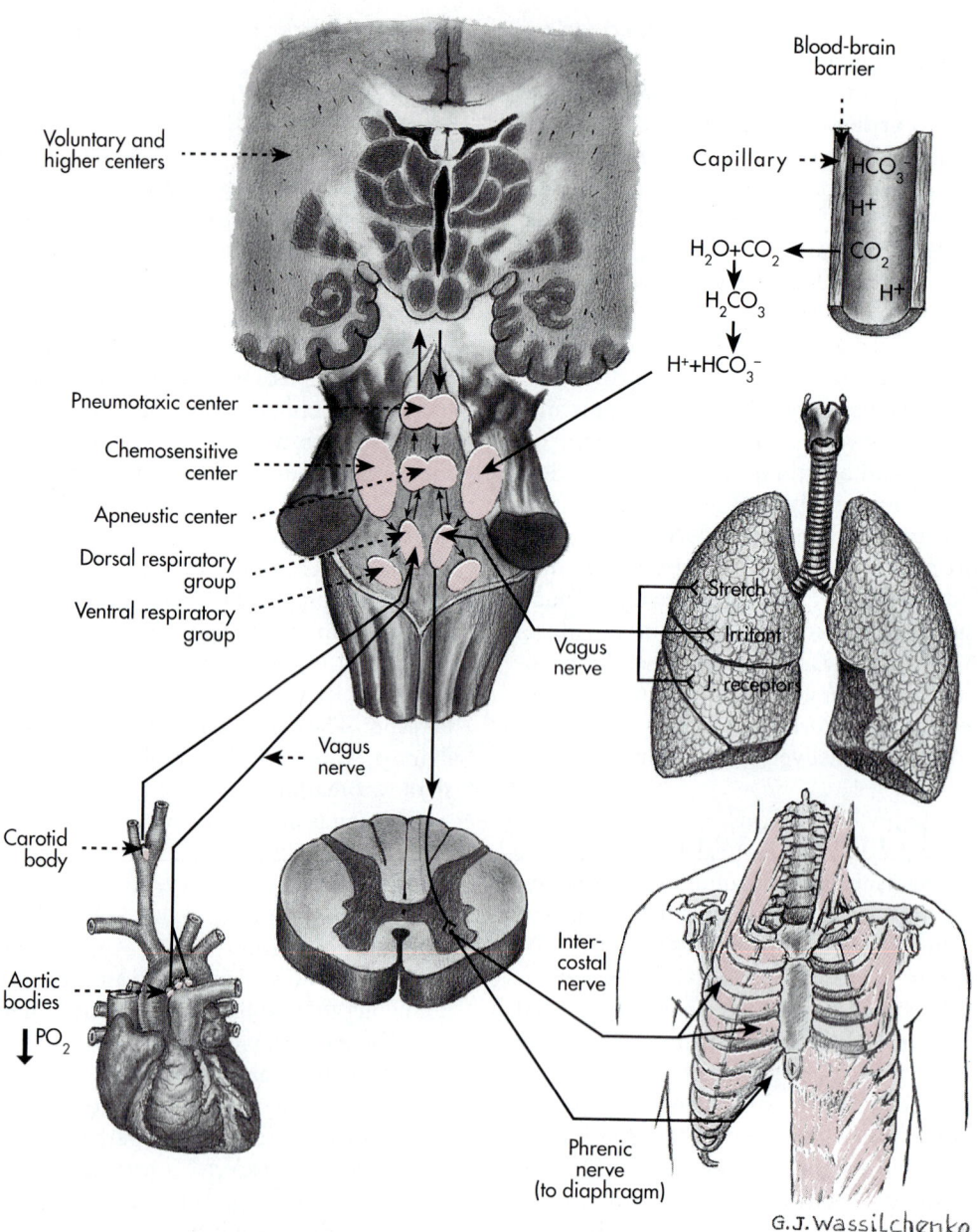

FIG. 29-16 Neurochemical respiratory control system. (Adapted from Thompson, McFarland, Hirsch, & Tucker, 1993.)

cephalon, near the respiratory center, and are sensitive to hydrogen ion concentration in the CSF. (Chapter 3 describes the relationship between ions and the pH, or acid-base status, of body fluids.) The pH, or concentration of hydrogen ions in the CSF, reflects $Paco_2$ because, unlike H^+ ions, carbon dioxide in arterial blood diffuses across the blood-brain barrier (the barrier separating blood from cells of the central nervous system) into the CSF until the partial pressure of carbon dioxide (Pco_2) is equal on both sides. Carbon dioxide that has entered

the CSF combines with H_2O to form carbonic acid, which subsequently dissociates into hydrogen ions that are capable of stimulating the central chemoreceptors. In this way $Paco_2$ regulates ventilation through its impact on the pH (hydrogen ion content) of the CSF (Guyton, 1992).

If alveolar ventilation is inadequate, $Paco_2$ increases. Carbon dioxide diffuses across the blood-brain barrier until Pco_2 in blood and CSF reaches equilibrium. As the central chemoreceptors sense the resulting decrease in pH (increase in hydrogen ion concentration), they stimulate the respiratory center to increase the depth and rate of ventilation. Increased ventilation causes the P_{CO_2} of arterial blood to decrease below that of the CSF, and carbon dioxide diffuses back out of the CSF, returning its pH to normal.

The central chemoreceptors are sensitive to very small changes in the pH of CSF (equivalent to a 1 to 2 mm Hg change in P_{CO_2}) and are able to maintain a normal Pa_{CO_2} under many different conditions, including strenuous exercise. If inadequate ventilation, or hypoventilation, is long-term, for example, in chronic obstructive pulmonary disease, these receptors become insensitive to small changes in Pa_{CO_2} and become poor regulators of ventilation.

The **peripheral chemoreceptors** are located in aortic bodies, the aortic arch, and carotid bodies at the bifurcation of the carotids, near the baroreceptors (see Chapter 26). Although the peripheral chemoreceptors are sensitive to changes in Pa_{CO_2} and pH, they are primarily sensitive to oxygen levels in arterial blood (Pa_{O_2}). As Pa_{O_2} and pH decrease, peripheral chemoreceptors, particularly in the carotid bodies, send signals to the respiratory center to increase ventilation. The peripheral chemoreceptors are not as sensitive as the central chemoreceptors. The Pa_{O_2} must drop well below normal (to approximately 60 mm Hg) before the peripheral chemoreceptors have much influence on ventilation. If Pa_{CO_2} is elevated as well, however, ventilation increases much more than it would in response to either abnormality alone. The peripheral chemoreceptors become the major stimulus to ventilation when the central chemoreceptors are "reset" by chronic hypoventilation.

Control of the Pulmonary Circulation

The caliber of pulmonary artery lumina decreases as smooth muscle in arterial walls contracts. Contraction increases pulmonary artery pressure. Caliber increases as these muscles relax, decreasing blood pressure. Contraction (vasoconstriction) and relaxation (vasodilation) apparently occur in response to local humoral conditions, even though the pulmonary circulation is innervated by the ANS in the same manner as the systemic circulation.

The most important cause of pulmonary artery constriction is a low alveolar P_{O_2} (PA_{O_2}). Vasoconstriction caused by alveolar hypoxia, often termed **hypoxic vasoconstriction,** can affect only one portion of the lung (i.e., one lobe that is obstructed, decreasing its PA_{O_2}) or the entire lung. If only one segment of the lung is involved, the arterioles to that segment constrict, shunting blood to other, well-ventilated portions of the lung. This reflex improves the lung's efficiency by better matching ventilation and perfusion. If hypoventilation

affects all segments of the lung, however, pulmonary hypertension (elevated pulmonary artery pressure) can result. The pulmonary vasoconstriction caused by low alveolar P_{O_2} is reversible if the alveolar P_{O_2} is corrected. Chronic alveolar hypoxia can result in permanent pulmonary artery hypertension, which eventually leads to cor pulmonale and heart failure.

Acidemia also causes pulmonary artery constriction. If the acidemia is corrected, the vasoconstriction is reversed. (Respiratory acidosis and metabolic acidosis are described in Chapter 3.) It is important to note that an elevated Pa_{CO_2} without a drop in pH does not cause pulmonary artery constriction. Other biochemical factors that affect the caliber of vessels in pulmonary circulation are histamine, prostaglandins, serotonin, and bradykinin.

Gas Transport

Gas transport, the delivery of oxygen to the cells of the body and the removal of carbon dioxide, has four steps: (1) ventilation of the lungs, (2) diffusion of oxygen from the alveoli into the capillary blood, (3) perfusion of systemic capillaries with oxygenated blood, and (4) diffusion of oxygen from systemic capillaries into the cells. Steps in the transport of carbon dioxide occur in reverse order: (1) diffusion of carbon dioxide from the cells into the systemic capillaries, (2) perfusion of the pulmonary capillary bed by venous blood, (3) diffusion of carbon dioxide into the alveoli, and (4) removal of carbon dioxide from the lung by ventilation. If any step in gas transport is impaired by a respiratory or cardiovascular disorder, gas exchange at the cellular level is compromised.

Distribution of Ventilation and Perfusion

Effective gas exchange depends on an approximately even distribution of gas (ventilation) and blood (perfusion) in all portions of the lungs. Gas exchange would not be very efficient if most of each inspired breath went to the right lung and most of the pulmonary blood flow went to the left lung.

The lungs are suspended from the hili in the thoracic cavity. When the individual is in an upright position (sitting or standing), gravity pulls the lungs down toward the diaphragm and compresses their lower portions or bases. As a result the alveoli in the upper portions, or apices, of the lungs contain a greater residual volume of gas and are larger and less numerous than those in the lower portions. Because surface tension increases as the alveoli become larger, the larger alveoli in the upper portions of the lung are more difficult to inflate (less compliant) than the smaller alveoli in the lower portions of the lung. Therefore, during ventilation most of the tidal volume is distributed to the bases of the lungs, where compliance is greater.

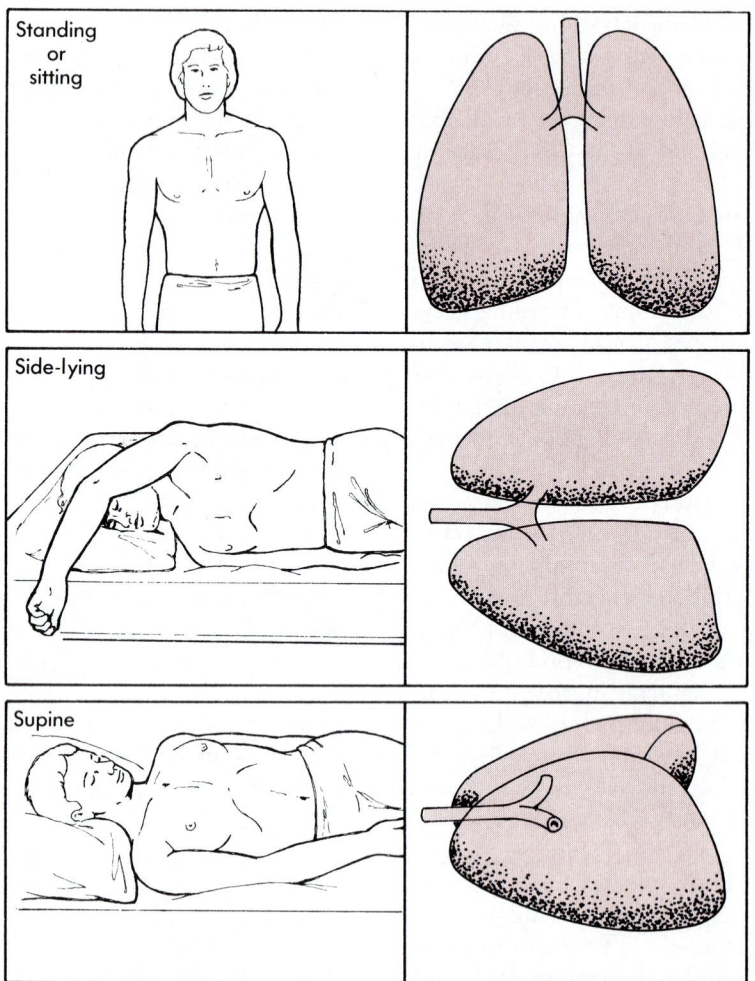

FIG. 29-17 Pulmonary blood flow and gravity. The greatest volume of pulmonary blood flow will normally occur in the gravity-dependent areas of the lung. Body position has a significant effect on the distribution of pulmonary blood flow.

The heart pumps against gravity to perfuse the pulmonary circulation. As blood is pumped into the lung apices of a sitting or standing individual, some blood pressure is dissipated in overcoming gravity. As a result, blood pressure at the apices is lower than that at the bases. Because greater pressure causes greater perfusion, the bases of the lungs are better perfused than the apices (Fig. 29-17). Thus, ventilation and perfusion are greatest in the same lung portions: the lower lobes. Ventilation and perfusion are dependent on body position. If a standing individual assumes a supine or side-lying position, the areas of the lungs that are then most dependent become the best ventilated and perfused.

Distribution of perfusion in the pulmonary circulation also is affected by alveolar pressure (gas pressure in the alveoli). The pulmonary capillary bed differs from the systemic capillary bed in that it is surrounded by gas-containing alveoli. If the gas pressure in the alveoli ex-

ceeds the blood pressure in the capillary, the capillary collapses and flow ceases. This is most likely to occur in portions of the lung where blood pressure is lowest and alveolar gas volume, and therefore pressure, is greatest: that is, the apex of the lung.

The lungs have been divided into three zones on the basis of the relationships among all the factors affecting pulmonary blood flow. Alveolar pressure plus the forces of gravity, arterial blood pressure, and venous blood pressure affect the distribution of perfusion, as shown in Fig. 29-18.

Zone I is that portion of the lung in which alveolar pressure exceeds pulmonary arterial and venous pressures. The capillary bed collapses, and normal blood flow ceases. Normally zone I is a very small part of the lung at the apex. Zone II is the portion where alveolar pressure is greater than venous pressure but not arterial pressure. Blood flows through zone II, but it is impeded

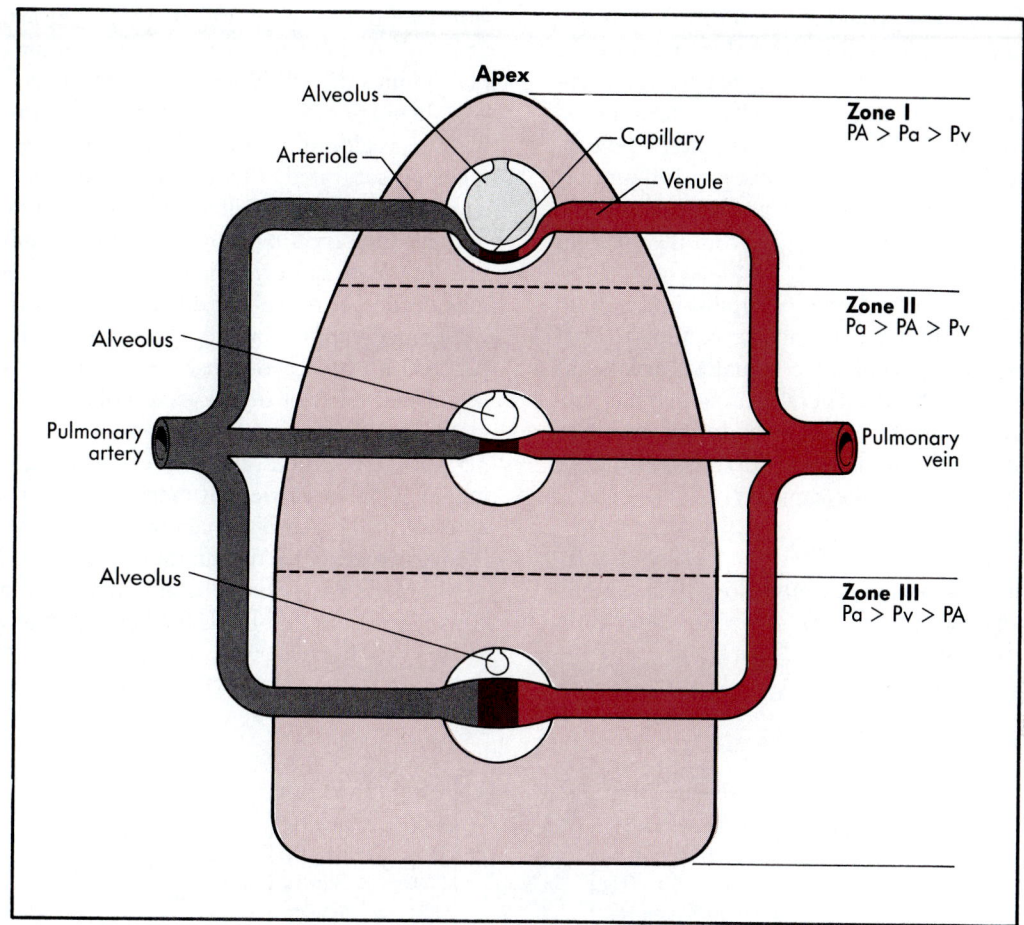

FIG. 29-18 Gravity and alveolar pressure. Effects of gravity and alveolar pressure on pulmonary blood flow in the three lung zones. In zone I, alveolar pressure (P_A) is greater than arterial and venous pressure, and no blood flow occurs. In zone II, arterial pressure (P_a) exceeds alveolar pressure, but alveolar pressure exceeds venous pressure (P_V). Blood flow occurs in this zone, but alveolar pressure compresses the venules (venous ends of the capillaries). In zone III, both arterial and venous pressures are greater than alveolar pressure, and blood flow fluctuates, depending on the difference between arterial and venous pressure.

to a certain extent by alveolar pressure. Zone II is normally above the level of the left atrium. In zone III both arterial and venous pressures are greater than alveolar pressure and blood flow is not affected by alveolar pressure. Zone III is in the base of the lung. Blood flow through the pulmonary capillary bed increases in regular increments from the apex to the base.

Although both blood flow and ventilation are greater at the base of the lungs than at the apices, they are not perfectly matched in any of the zones. Perfusion exceeds ventilation in the bases and ventilation exceeds perfusion in the apices of the lung. The relationship between ventilation and perfusion is expressed as a ratio called the **ventilation-perfusion ratio,** or $\dot{V}/\dot{Q}$. The normal $\dot{V}/\dot{Q}$ ratio is 0.8. This is the amount by which perfusion exceeds ventilation under normal conditions.

Oxygen Transport

Approximately 1000 ml (1 liter) of oxygen is transported to the cells each minute. Oxygen is transported in the blood in two forms. A small amount dissolves in plasma, and the remainder binds to hemoglobin molecules. Without hemoglobin, oxygen would not reach the cells in amounts sufficient to maintain normal metabolic function. (Hemoglobin is discussed in detail in Chapter 22; cellular metabolism in Chapter 1.)

Diffusion across the alveolocapillary membrane

The alveolocapillary membrane is the ideal medium for oxygen diffusion because it has a large total surface area (70 to 100 m²) and is very thin (0.5 micrometer [μm]). In addition, the partial pressure of oxygen molecules (P_{O_2}) is much greater in alveolar gas than in capillary blood, a condition that promotes rapid diffusion down the concentration gradient from the alveolus into the capillary. The partial pressure of oxygen (oxygen tension) in mixed venous or pulmonary artery blood ($P\bar{v}O_2$) is approximately 40 mm Hg as it enters the capillary, and alveolar oxygen tension (PAO_2) is 100 mm Hg at sea level. Therefore, a pressure gradient of 60 mm Hg facilitates the diffusion of oxygen from the alveolus into the capillary.

Blood remains in the pulmonary capillary for about 0.75 seconds, but only 0.25 seconds is required for oxygen concentration to equilibrate (equalize) across the alveolocapillary membrane. Therefore, oxygen has ample time to diffuse into the blood, even during increased cardiac output, which speeds blood flow, shortening the time the blood remains in the capillary.

Determinants of arterial oxygenation

As oxygen diffuses across the alveolocapillary membrane, it dissolves in the plasma, where it exerts pressure (the partial pressure of oxygen in arterial blood, or PaO_2). As the PaO_2 increases, oxygen moves from the plasma into the red blood cells (erythrocytes) and binds with hemoglobin molecules. Oxygen continues to bind with hemoglobin until the hemoglobin binding sites are filled or saturated. Oxygen then continues to diffuse across the alveolocapillary membrane until the PaO_2 (oxygen dissolved in plasma) and PAO_2 equilibrate, eliminating the pressure gradient across the alveolocapillary membrane. At this point diffusion ceases (Fig. 29-19).

Normally approximately 20 ml oxygen is transported per 100 ml blood. Because oxygen is not very soluble in plasma, most of the oxygen molecules bind with hemoglobin. Plasma carries only about 0.3 ml of oxygen per 100 ml of blood (at sea level). Although the remaining 19.7 ml is carried by hemoglobin, it is the small amount of oxygen dissolved in plasma that is responsible for oxygen's partial pressure (PaO_2) in the blood.

Although PaO_2 is important in that it provides the driving pressure that loads the hemoglobin with oxygen,

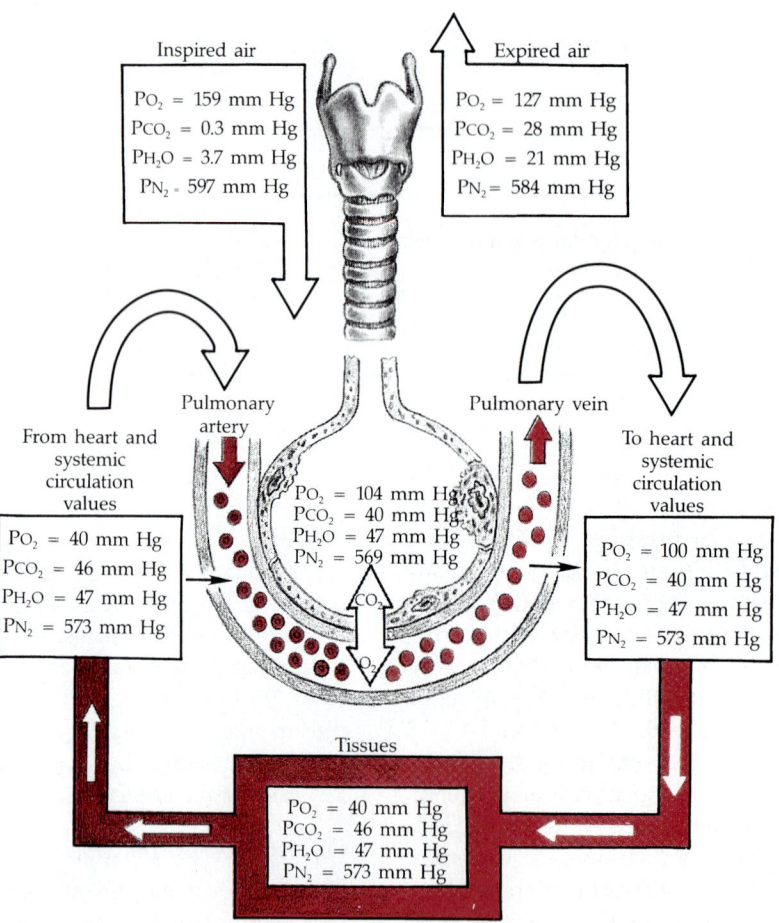

FIG. 29-19 Partial pressure of respiratory gases in normal respiration. The above are average values. The values of PO_2, PCO_2, and PN_2 fluctuate from breath to breath. (Adapted from Thompson, McFarland, Hirsch, & Tucker, 1993.)

it gives little information about the *amount* of oxygen carried in the blood. This amount, which is measured in milliliters per deciliter (100 ml) of blood, is the **oxygen content** of the blood. The total oxygen content of the blood depends on the amount of oxygen chemically combined with hemoglobin, as well as that dissolved in the blood. To calculate the total arterial oxygen content, we must know (1) hemoglobin concentration, or the amount of hemoglobin that is available to bind with oxygen (Hb in g/dl); (2) the oxygen saturation or percentage of available hemoglobin that is bound to oxygen (SaO_2); and (3) the partial pressure of oxygen (PaO_2). The maximum amount of oxygen that can be transported by hemoglobin is 1.34 ml/g. The amount of oxygen that can be physically dissolved in blood is 0.003 ml/dl per mm Hg PO_2. If these specific values are known, the oxygen content of arterial blood can be calculated (Gross & Scanlan, 1990). The basic formula is

O_2 content
$= O_2$ bound to Hb + dissolved O_2
$= (Hb \times 1.34 \times SaO_2) + (PaO_2 \times 0.003)$
$\quad (g/dl \times ml/g \times \%) + (mm\ Hg \times ml/dl/mm\ Hg)$

If hemoglobin concentration (Hb) = 15 g/dl, arterial oxygen saturation = 97%, and PaO_2 = 100 mm Hg, then arterial oxygen content is calculated as follows:

O_2 content
$= (15\ g/dl \times 1.34\ ml/g \times 0.97) +$
$\quad (100\ mm\ Hg \times 0.003\ ml/dl/mm\ Hg)$
$= 19.5\ ml/dl + 0.3\ ml/dl$
$= 19.8\ ml/dl$

Normal arterial oxygen content is 19 to 20 ml/dl blood. Note that the amount of dissolved oxygen (0.3 ml/dl) is a very small fraction of the total oxygen content of 19.8 ml/dl.

The basic formula also can be used to calculate the oxygen content of venous blood by substituting the partial pressure of mixed venous blood ($P\bar{v}O_2$) and venous oxygen saturation ($S\bar{v}O_2$) for the arterial values in the basic formula. Normal venous oxygen content is 15 to 16 ml/dl.

Because hemoglobin transports all but a small fraction of the oxygen carried in arterial blood, increases in hemoglobin concentration affect the oxygen content of the blood. Decreases in hemoglobin concentration below the normal value of 15 ml/dl blood reduce oxygen content, and increases in hemoglobin concentration may minimize the impact of impaired gas exchange. In fact, an increase in hemoglobin concentration is a major compensatory mechanism in pulmonary diseases that impair gas exchange. For this reason, measurement of hemoglobin concentration is important in the assessment of individuals with pulmonary disease. If cardiovascular function is normal, the body's initial response

to low oxygen content is to speed up cardiac output. In individuals who also have cardiovascular disease, this compensatory mechanism does not work, making increased hemoglobin concentration an even more important compensatory mechanism. (Hemoglobin structure and function are described in Chapter 22.)

Oxyhemoglobin association and dissociation

The binding of hemoglobin molecules with oxygen forms a compound known as **oxyhemoglobin (HbO_2)**. The process of binding occurs in the lungs and is called oxyhemoglobin association or hemoglobin saturation with oxygen (SaO_2). The reverse process, where oxygen is released from hemoglobin, occurs in the body tissues at the cellular level and is called hemoglobin desaturation. When hemoglobin saturation and desaturation are plotted on a graph the result is a distinctive **S**-shaped curve known as the **oxyhemoglobin dissociation curve** (Fig. 29-20).

The horizontal or flat segment of the curve at the top of the graph is sometimes called the arterial portion, or that part of the curve where oxygen is bound to hemoglobin. This portion of the curve is flat because partial pressure changes of oxygen between 60 and 100 mm Hg do not significantly alter the percent saturation of hemoglobin with oxygen. The wide range of partial pressures of oxygen (PaO_2)—60 to 100 mm Hg, represented by the flat part of the curve—allows adequate hemoglobin saturation at a variety of altitudes. For example, a PaO_2 of 100 mm Hg at sea level results in a hemoglobin saturation with oxygen of 98%. At an altitude of 5000 feet the PaO_2 is about 70 mm Hg and hemoglobin saturation is 94%, only 4% less than at sea level. If the relationship between SaO_2 and PaO_2 were linear (in a downward sloping straight line) instead of flat shaped between 60 and 100 mm Hg, there would be inadequate saturation of hemoglobin with oxygen. For example, with a PaO_2 of 70 mm Hg the saturation would be only 70%, which is equivalent to normal *venous* oxygen saturation, and life could not be sustained at altitudes much above sea level.

The steep part of the oxyhemoglobin dissociation curve occurs after the PaO_2 drops below 60 mm Hg and represents the rapid dissociation of oxygen from hemoglobin. During this phase there is rapid diffusion of oxygen from the blood into tissue cells.

Several factors can change the relationship between PO_2 and SO_2, causing the oxyhemoglobin dissociation curve to shift to the right or left (Fig. 29-20). A shift to the right depicts hemoglobin's decreased affinity for oxygen or an increase in the ease with which oxyhemoglobin dissociates and oxygen moves into the cells. A shift to the left depicts hemoglobin's increased affinity for oxygen, which promotes association in the lungs and inhibits dissociation in the tissues.

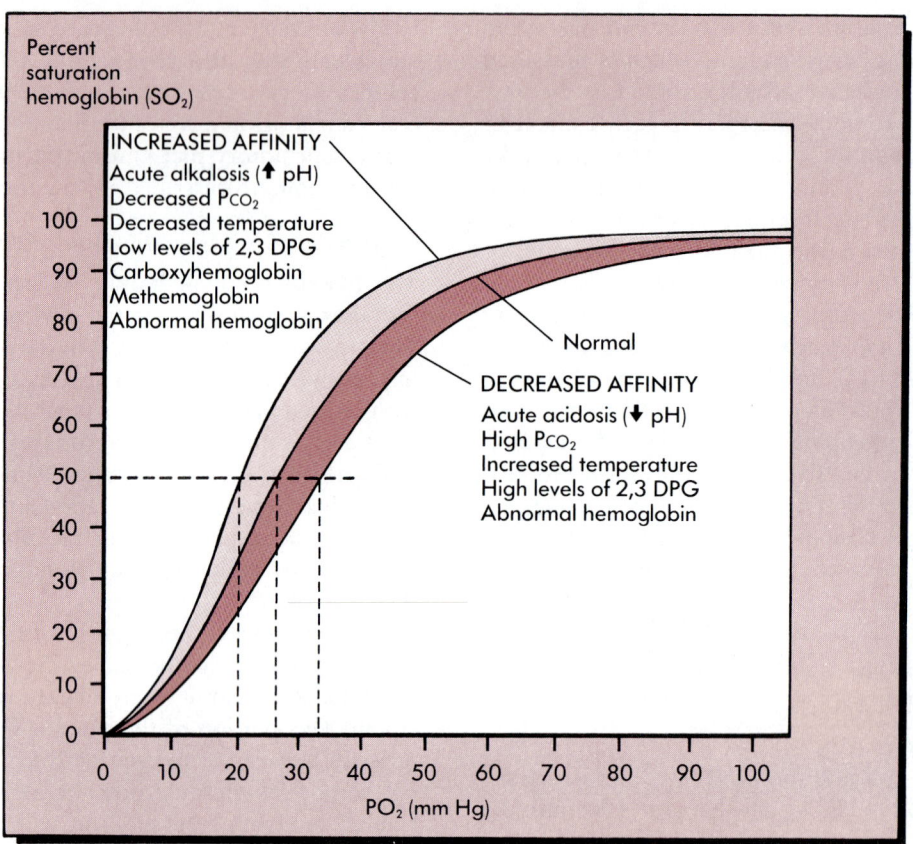

FIG. 29-20 Oxyhemoglobin dissociation curve. Conditions associated with altered affinity of hemoglobin for O_2. P_{50} is the Pa_{O_2} at which hemoglobin is 50% saturated, normally 26.6 mm Hg. A lower than normal P_{50} represents increased affinity of hemoglobin for O_2; a high P_{50} is seen with decreased affinity. Note that variation from the normal is associated with decreased (low P_{50}) or increased (high P_{50}) availability of O_2 to tissues *(dotted lines)*. The shaded area shows the entire oxyhemoglobin dissociation curve under the same circumstances. (From Lane & Walker, 1987.)

The oxyhemoglobin dissociation curve is shifted to the right by acidosis (low pH) and hypercapnia (increased Pa_{CO_2}). In the tissues, the increased levels of carbon dioxide and hydrogen ions produced by metabolic activity decrease the affinity of hemoglobin for oxygen. The curve is shifted to the left by alkalosis (high pH) and hypocapnia (decreased Pa_{CO_2}). In the lungs, as carbon dioxide diffuses from the blood into the alveoli, the blood carbon dioxide level is reduced and the affinity of hemoglobin for oxygen is increased. The shift in the oxyhemoglobin dissociation curve by changes in carbon dioxide and hydrogen ion concentrations in the blood is called the **Bohr effect** (Guyton, 1991).

The oxyhemoglobin curve is also shifted by changes in body temperature and increased or decreased levels of 2,3-diphosphoglycerate (2,3-DPG), a substance normally present in erythrocytes. Hyperthermia and increased 2,3-DPG levels shift the curve to the right. Hypothermia and decreased 2,3-DPG levels shift the curve to the left.

Carbon Dioxide Transport

Approximately 200 ml of CO_2 is produced by the tissues per minute as a by-product of cellular metabolism. This CO_2 equilibrates with carbonic acid ($H_2O + CO_2 \rightleftharpoons H_2CO_3 \rightleftharpoons H^+ HCO_3^-$) and must be eliminated continuously to prevent acidosis. The elimination of carbon dioxide by the lungs plays an important role in the regulation of acid-base balance (see Chapter 3).

Carbon dioxide is carried in the blood in three ways: (1) dissolved in plasma (P_{CO_2}), (2) as bicarbonate, and (3) as carbamino compounds. As CO_2 diffuses out of the cells into the blood, it dissolves in the plasma. Approximately 10% of the total CO_2 in venous and 5% of the CO_2 in arterial blood is carried dissolved in the plasma (P_{CO_2}). As CO_2 moves into the blood, it diffuses into the red blood cells. Within the red blood cells, carbon dioxide, with the help of the enzyme carbonic anhydrase, combines with water to form carbonic acid and then quickly dissociates into H^+ and HCO_3^-. As carbonic acid dissociates, the H^+ binds to hemoglobin, where it is buffered, and the HCO_3^- moves out of the red blood cell into the plasma. Approximately 60% of the CO_2 in venous blood and 90% of the CO_2 in arterial blood are carried in the form of bicarbonate. The remainder combines with blood proteins, hemoglobin in particular, to form carbamino compounds. Approximately 30% of the CO_2 in venous blood and 5% of the CO_2 in arterial blood is carried as carbamino compounds (see Fig. 3-9, Chapter 3).

Carbon dioxide is 20 times more soluble than O_2 and diffuses very quickly from the tissue cells into the blood. The amount of CO_2 that is able to enter the blood is enhanced by diffusion of oxygen out of the blood and into the cells. Reduced hemoglobin (hemoglobin that is dissociated from oxygen) is able to carry more CO_2 than hemoglobin that is saturated with O_2. Therefore, the drop in So_2 at the tissue level increases the ability of hemoglobin to carry CO_2 back to the lung.

The diffusion gradient for CO_2 in the lung is only approximately 6 mm Hg (venous Pco_2 = 46 mm Hg; alveolar Pco_2 = 40 mm Hg). Yet CO_2 is so soluble in the alveolocapillary membrane that the CO_2 in the blood quickly diffuses into the alveoli, where it is removed from the lung with each expiration. Diffusion of CO_2 in the lung is so efficient that diffusion defects that cause hypoxemia (low oxygen content of the blood) do not cause hypercapnia (excessive carbon dioxide in the blood).

The diffusion of CO_2 out of the blood is also enhanced by oxygen binding with hemoglobin in the lung. As hemoglobin binds with O_2, the amount of CO_2 carried by the blood is decreased. Thus, in the tissue capillaries, O_2 dissociation from hemoglobin facilitates the pickup of CO_2, and the binding of O_2 to hemoglobin in the lungs facilitates the release of CO_2 from the blood. This effect of oxygen on carbon dioxide transport is called the **Haldane effect** (Guyton, 1991).

TESTS OF PULMONARY FUNCTION

Several laboratory tests aid in the diagnosis and evaluation of pulmonary system abnormalities. Most of them are easy to perform and are performed in most hospitals and many clinics. They provide valuable information as to the possible cause of a respiratory abnormality and are also helpful in evaluating the progression or resolution of disease.

Spirometry is an important test of pulmonary function. It is used to measure forced expiration, which is frequently affected by diffuse pulmonary disease. Because the pulmonary system has remarkable reserves, disease may become well established before clinical manifestations appear. Spirometry enables clinicians to detect restrictive or obstructive deficits early in the course of disease. Restrictive lung diseases restrict the lung's volume: the lungs are unable to expand normally, diminishing the amount of gas that can be inspired. Obstructive diseases affect gas flow: air flow into and out of the lungs is obstructed.

Spirometry measures both volume and flow. The test is performed with a spirometer, which is a water-filled cylinder into which an inverted cylinder or bell has been inserted. A length of tubing runs from the inverted bell to a mouthpiece through which a person breathes during testing. The bell is attached to a pen that writes on calibrated paper rotating at a constant speed. As the person performs various breathing maneuvers, the inverted bell moves up and down, causing the pen to move on the calibrated paper. This produces a spirogram, which records the individual's ventilation in relation to time. (Values measured by spirometry are listed in Table 29-3.)

Diffusing capacity is a measure of the rate of gas diffusion across the alveolocapillary membrane. Oxygen, or more commonly carbon monoxide, is used to mea-

TABLE 29-3

Values Measured by Spirometry

Symbol	Ventilatory property measured
FVC	Forced vital capacity: maximum amount of gas that can be displaced from the lung during a forced expiration
FEV_1	Forced expiratory volume in 1 second: maximum amount of air that can be expired from the lung in 1 second
FEV_1/FVC	Percentage of maximum inspiration that is expired in 1 second, usually 80% of FVC
FEV_3	Forced expiratory volume in 3 seconds; maximum amount of gas that can be expired in 3 seconds
FEV_3/FVC	Percentage of FVC that is expired in 3 seconds; usually 95% of FVC
$FEF_{25\%-75\%}$	Forced expiratory flow rate during the middle 50% of expiration; is sometimes reported as maximum midexpiratory flow rate (MMFR)

TABLE 29-4

Normal Ranges for Arterial and Mixed Venous Blood Gases

Measurement	Arterial blood	Mixed venous blood*	Clinical notes
Acid-base status (pH)	7.35-7.45	7.33-7.43	Most important acid-base value; detects acidosis or alkalosis
Partial pressure of carbon dioxide (P_{CO_2})	35-45 mm Hg	41-57 mm Hg	Measures adequacy of ventilation and respiratory contribution to acid-base abnormality (respiratory acidosis)
Bicarbonate (HCO_3^-)	22-26 mEq/L	24-28 mEq/L	Measures metabolic contribution to acid-base abnormality (metabolic acidosis); calculated from pH and P_{CO_2}
Base excess (BE)	−2-+2	0-+4	Reflects deviation of bicarbonate concentration from normal
Partial pressure of oxygen (P_{O_2}) (sea level)	80-100 mm Hg	35-40 mm Hg	Indicates driving pressure that causes oxygen-hemoglobin binding; varies with age and barometric pressure
Saturation of hemoglobin with oxygen (S_{O_2})	96%-98%	70%-75%	Indicates abnormalities of oxyhemoglobin association and dissociation; may be measured directly or calculated from P_{O_2}, pH, and body temperature
Concentration of hemoglobin in the blood	15 g/100 ml	15 g/100 ml	Detects alterations of gas transport caused by anemia
Oxygen content of the blood	19-20 ml/100 ml	14-15 ml/100 ml	Detects hypoxemia

*Mixed venous (pulmonary artery) blood is analyzed for critically ill individuals and those undergoing cardiac catheterization (it is not practical to withdraw samples except from a pulmonary artery catheter). Mixed venous blood gas analysis, in conjunction with arterial analysis, provides important information about the adequacy of cardiac output and tissue oxygenation.

sure diffusing capacity. The measurement is made by determining how much carbon monoxide is taken up by the blood and dividing this amount by the pressure gradient across the alveolocapillary membrane. Helium is often added to the gas mixture to obtain a simultaneous measurement of RV, FRC, and TLC. Individuals are asked to perform ventilatory maneuvers similar to those of spirometry. A decreased diffusing capacity can be the result of an abnormal ventilation/perfusion ratio or an actual diffusion defect. Diffusing capacity is decreased in individuals with emphysema.

Arterial blood gas analysis is commonly performed for individuals with suggested or diagnosed pulmonary disease. Direct analysis of the pH and gas concentrations in arterial blood provides valuable information about an individual's gas exchange and acid-base status. Acidosis (low pH), alkalosis (high pH), ventilatory alterations, and decreased Pa_{O_2} can be only diagnosed by arterial blood gas analysis. A blood gas report may be divided into an acid-base/ventilation portion and an oxygenation portion. (Normal values for arterial blood

gases can be seen in Table 29-4.) (Acid-base alterations are described in Chapter 3.)

Signs and symptoms of most respiratory abnormalities first appear when the system is stressed during exercise. Therefore, if pulmonary disease is suspected, the individual is evaluated at rest and during exercise. During exercise the usual procedures are spirometry and withdrawal of arterial blood for gas analysis. The exercise usually consists of riding a stationary bicycle or walking on a treadmill. Exercise testing enables clinicians to detect early changes in respiratory function and begin treatment. Exercise tests are also used in planning and evaluating exercise and rehabilitation programs.

Chest radiograms are among the most common examinations of the pulmonary system. A few of the abnormalities detected in chest radiographs are air trapping in the alveoli and airways (e.g., in asthma or emphysema), consolidation of lung tissue (in pneumonia or pulmonary edema), cavities (abscesses or tuberculosis), and nodules (lung cancer). Often pulmonary abnormalities are detected in routine chest radiographs of asymptomatic individuals. A variety of radiographic techniques are available for the diagnosis and evaluation of respiratory disorders.

AGING and the Pulmonary System

Most knowledge about pulmonary structure and function is based on norms for the middle years. Less is known about structure and function in the very young (see Chapter 31) and the elderly, but a few normal physiologic (developmental and degenerative) changes are known to occur from birth to old age. An understanding of these changes is needed to provide appropriate care and to differentiate between normal alterations and disease. Normal alterations include (1) loss of elastic recoil, (2) stiffening of the chest wall, and (3) alterations in gas exchange. These changes are influenced by environmental factors, respiratory disease, body size, and race (Crapo, 1993).

During adulthood and as age advances, the alveoli tend to lose alveolar wall tissue and capillaries. This process diminishes alveolar surface area available for gas diffusion and decreases airway support provided by normal lung tissues. Mechanical changes involve elastic properties of the lungs and chest wall. Chest wall compliance decreases with age because the ribs become ossified (less flexible) and joints become stiffer. As a result the chest wall loses some of its ability to expand. Elastic recoil diminishes with advancing age, possibly because of loss of elastic fibers in the lung tissue. This leads to an increase in lung compliance. These mechan-

ical changes in the lung and chest wall, along with structural changes in the alveoli, reduce ventilatory capacity in old age. Vital capacity decreases and residual volume increases; however, total lung capacity remains unchanged. These changes decrease ventilatory reserves and lead to decreased ventilation/perfusion ratios (Knudson, 1991).

Alterations in gas exchange are reflected by blood gas analysis. With advancing age, pH and P_{CO_2} do not change much, even though it has been documented that the chemoreceptors become less sensitive to gas partial pressures with age. P_{O_2}, however, does decline with age as a result of structural and mechanical changes, such as loss of alveolar surface area and increased ventilation/perfusion mismatch. The maximum Pa_{O_2} in an elderly individual at sea level can be estimated by multiplying the person's age by 0.3 and subtracting the product from 100. For example, an 80-year-old individual would have an estimated maximum P_{O_2} of 76 mm Hg ($0.3 \times 80 = 24$; $100 - 24 = 76$).

The decrease in Pa_{O_2} and diminished ventilatory reserve in the elderly lead to a decrease in exercise tolerance. Changes in respiratory function can vary considerably from person to person, however. Changes are also affected by activity and fitness earlier in life. A very active, physically fit individual will, all else being equal, have fewer changes in function at any age than one who has been sedentary. Respiratory muscle strength and endurance decrease with age but can be enhanced with exercise (Chen & Kuo, 1989).

SUMMARY REVIEW

Structures of the Pulmonary System

1 The pulmonary system consists of the lungs, airways, chest wall, and pulmonary and bronchial circulation.

2 Air is inspired and expired through the conducting airways, which include the nasopharynx, oropharynx, trachea, bronchi, and bronchioles to the sixteenth division.

3 Gas exchange occurs in structures beyond the sixteenth division: the respiratory bronchioles, alveolar ducts, and the alveoli. Together these structures compose the acinus.

4 The chief gas-exchange units of the lungs are the alveoli. The membrane that surrounds each alveolus and contains the pulmonary capillaries is called the alveolocapillary membrane.

5 The gas-exchange airways are served by the pulmonary circulation, a separate division of the circulatory system. The bronchi and other lung structures are served by a branch of the systemic circulation called the bronchial circulation.

6 The chest wall, which contains and protects the contents of the thoracic cavity, consists of the skin, ribs, and intercostal muscles, which lie between the ribs.

7 The chest wall is lined by a serous membrane called the parietal pleura; the lungs are encased in a separate membrane called the visceral pleura. The area where these two pleurae come into contact and slide over one another is called the pleural space.

Function of the Pulmonary System

1 The pulmonary system enables oxygen to diffuse into the blood and carbon dioxide to diffuse out of the blood.

2 Ventilation is the process by which air flows into and out of the gas-exchange airways.

3 Successful ventilation involves the mechanics of breathing: the interaction of forces and counterforces involving the muscles of inspiration and expiration, alveolar surface tension, elastic properties of the lungs and chest wall, and resistance to airflow.

4   The major muscle of inspiration is the diaphragm. When the diaphragm contracts, it moves downward in the thoracic cavity, creating a vacuum that causes air to flow into the lungs.

5   The alveoli produce surfactant, a lipoprotein that lines the alveoli. Surfactant reduces alveolar surface tension and permits the alveoli to expand as air flows in.

6   Compliance is the ability of the lungs and chest wall to expand during inspiration. Lung compliance is ensured by adequate production of surfactant, whereas chest wall expansion depends on flexibility.

7   Elastic recoil is the tendency of the lungs and chest wall to return to their resting state after inspiration. The elastic recoil forces of the lungs and chest wall are in opposition and pull on each other, creating the normally negative pressure of the pleural space.

8   Most of the time ventilation is involuntary. It is controlled by the sympathetic and parasympathetic divisions of the autonomic nervous system, which adjust airway caliber (by causing bronchial smooth muscle to contract or relax) and control the rate and depth of ventilation.

9   Neuroreceptors in the lungs (lung receptors) monitor the mechanical aspects of ventilation. Irritant receptors sense the need to expel unwanted substances, stretch receptors sense lung volume (lung expansion), and J-receptors sense alveolar size.

10 Chemoreceptors in the circulatory system and brain stem sense the effectiveness of ventilation by monitoring the pH status of cerebrospinal fluid and the oxygen content (Po_2) of arterial blood.

11 The pulmonary circulation is innervated by the ANS, but vasodilation and vasoconstriction are controlled mainly by local and humoral factors, particularly arterial oxygenation and acid-base status.

12 Gas transport depends on ventilation of the alveoli, diffusion across the alveolocapillary membrane, perfusion of the pulmonary and systemic capillaries, and diffusion between systemic capillaries and tissue cells.

13 Efficient gas exchange depends on an even distribution of ventilation and perfusion within the lungs. Both ventilation and perfusion are greatest in the bases of the lungs because the alveoli in the bases are more compliant (their resting volume is low) and perfusion is greater in the bases as a result of gravity.

14 Almost all of the oxygen that diffuses into pulmonary capillary blood is transported by hemoglobin, a protein contained within red blood cells. The remainder of the oxygen is transported dissolved in plasma.

15 Oxygen enters the body by diffusing down the concentration gradient, from high concentrations in the alveoli to lower concentrations in the capillaries. Diffusion ceases when alveolar and capillary oxygen pressures equilibrate.

16 Oxygen is loaded onto hemoglobin by the driving pressure exerted by Pao_2 in the plasma. As pressure decreases at the tissue level, oxygen dissociates from hemoglobin and enters tissue cells by diffusion, again down the concentration gradient.

17 Carbon dioxide is more soluble in plasma than oxygen is. Therefore, carbon dioxide diffuses readily from tissue cells into plasma. Carbon dioxide returns to the lungs dissolved in plasma, as bicarbonate, or in carbamino compounds (e.g., bound to hemoglobin).

Tests of Pulmonary Function

1   Spirometry measures both volume and flow rate during forced expiration.

2   The alveolar-arterial oxygen gradient is used to evaluate the cause of hypoxia.

3   Diffusing capacity is a measure of the gas diffusion rate at the alveolocapillary membrane.

4   Arterial blood gas (ABG) analysis can be used to determine pH and oxygen and carbon dioxide concentrations.

5   Radiographic examination of the chest evaluates air trapping, consolidation, cavity formation, or presence of tumors.

Aging and the Pulmonary System

1   Aging affects the mechanical aspects of ventilation by decreasing chest wall compliance and elastic recoil of the lungs. Changes in these elastic properties reduce ventilatory reserve.

2   Aging causes the Pao_2 to decrease but does not affect the $Paco_2$.

KEY TERMS

Acinus, 1125

Alveolar dead space, 1131

Alveolar duct, 1125

Alveolar ventilation ($\dot{V}_A$), 1131

Alveolocapillary membrane, 1126

Alveolus (pl., alveoli), 1125

Anatomic dead space, 1131

Arterial blood gas analysis, 1144

Bohr effect, 1142

Bronchiole, 1123

Bronchus (pl., bronchi), 1123

Carina, 1123

Central chemoreceptor, 1135

Chest radiogram, 1144

Compliance, 1133

Dead-space ventilation ($\dot{V}_D$), 1131

Diffusing capacity, 1143

Elasticity (elastance), 1133

REFERENCES

Altose, M. D. (1988). Pulmonary mechanisms. In A. P. Fishman (Ed.), *Pulmonary diseases and disorders* (2nd ed.). New York: McGraw-Hill.

Bergofsky, E. H. (1991). The lung mucosa. A critical environmental battleground. *American Journal of Medicine, 91*(Suppl. 4A), 4S-10S.

Charan, N. B., & Carvalho, P. G. (1992). Anatomy of the normal bronchial circulatory system in humans and animals. In J. Butler (Ed.), *The bronchial circulation* (pp. 45-77). New York: Marcel Dekker, Inc.

Chen, H. I., & Kuo, C. S. (1989). Relationship between respiratory muscle function and age, sex, and other factors. *Journal of Applied Physiology, 66,* 943-948.

Crapo, R. O. (1993). The aging lung. In D. A Mahler (Ed.), *Pulmonary disease in the elderly patient* (pp. 1-25). New York: Marcel Dekker, Inc.

Fraser, R. G., Paré, J. A. P., Paré, P. D., Fraser, R. S., & Genereux, G. P. (1988). *Diagnosis of diseases of the chest* (3rd ed.). Philadelphia: Saunders.

Gross, G. W., & Scanlan, C. L. (1990). Gas exchange and transport. In C. L. Scanlan, C. B. Spearman, & R. L. Sheldon (Eds.), *Egan's fundamentals of respiratory care* (5th ed.). St. Louis: Mosby—Year Book.

Guyton, A. (1991). *Textbook of medical physiology* (8th ed.). Philadelphia: Saunders.

Guyton, A. (1992). *Human physiology and mechanisms of disease* (5th ed.). Philadelphia: Saunders.

Knudson, R. S. (1991). Physiology of the aging lung. In R. J. Crystal & J. B. West (Eds.), *The lung* (pp. 1749-1759). New York: Raven Press.

Lane, E. E., & Walker, J. F. (1987). *Clinical arterial blood gas analysis.* St. Louis: Mosby—Year Book.

Scanlan, C. L. (1990a). Acid-base balance and the regulation of respiration. In C. L. Scanlan, Spearman, C. G., Sheldon, R. L. (Eds.), *Egan's fundamentals of respiratory care* (5th ed.). St. Louis: Mosby—Year Book.

Scanlan, C. L. (1990b). Ventilation. In C. L. Scanlan, Spearman, C. G., Sheldon, R. L. (Eds.), *Egan's fundamentals of respiratory care* (5th ed.). St. Louis: Mosby—Year Book.

Thibodeau, G. A. (1992). *Structure and function of the body.* St. Louis: Mosby—Year Book.

Thompson, J. M., McFarland, G., Hirsch, J., Tucker, S., & Bowers, A. (1989). *Mosby's manual of clinical nursing* (2nd ed.). St. Louis: Mosby—Year Book.

Bates, D. V. (1989). *Respiratory function in disease* (3rd ed.). Philadelphia: Saunders.

Bogartz, L. J. (1983). Control of respiration: A review and update. *Current Revue of Respiratory Theory, 8*(21), 167-172.

Brian, I. (1965). *A history of medicine.* Cleveland: World Publishing Company.

Carrieri, V. K., Murdaugh, C., & Janson-Bjerklie, S. (1984, April). A framework for assessing pulmonary disease categories. *Focus on Critical Care, 11*(2), 10-24.

Clemmer, T. P. (1982). Oxygen transport. *International Anesthetic Clinics, 19*(3), 21-38.

Collett, P. W., Rousos, C., & Macklem, P. T. (1988). Respiratory mechanics. In J. F. Murray & J. A. Nadel (Eds.), *Textbook of respiratory medicine* (vol. 1). Philadelphia: Saunders.

Des Jardins, T. R. (1993). *Cardiopulmonary anatomy and physiology: essentials for respiratory care.* Albany, Delmar Publishers.

Drain, C. B., & Cristoph, S. S. (Eds.). (1987). *The recovery room: A critical care approach to post anesthesia nursing* (2nd ed.). Philadelphia: Saunders.

Hlastala, M. P. (1991). Ventilation. In R. G. Crystal, & J. B. West (Editors-in-chief); Barres, P. J., Cherniak, N. S., & Weibel, E. R. (Assoc. Eds.), *The lung: Scientific foundations* (vol. 2). New York: Raven Press.

Kacmarek, R. M., Hess, D., & Stoller, J. K. (Eds.). (1993). *Monitoring in respiratory care.* St. Louis: Mosby—Year Book.

Murray, J. F. (1986). *The normal lung.* Philadelphia: Saunders.

Roussos, C. (1985, August). Function and fatigue of respiratory muscles. *Chest, 88*(2), 1245.

Ruppel, G. L. (1991). *Manual of pulmonary function testing.* St. Louis: Mosby—Year Book.

Shapiro, B. A., Harrison, R. A., & Cane, R. D. (1989). *Clinical application of blood gases* (4th ed.). Chicago: Year Book Medical.

Staub, N. C., & Albertine, K. H. (1988). The structure of the lungs relative to their principal function. In J. F. Murray & J. A. Nadel (Eds.), *Textbook of respiratory medicine* (vol. 1). Philadelphia: Saunders.

Tesoriero, J. V., & Dail, D. H. (1990). Functional anatomy of the respiratory system. In C. L. Scanlan, C. G. Spearman, & R. L. Sheldon. (Eds.), *Egan's fundamentals of respiratory care* (5th ed.). St. Louis: Mosby—Year Book.

Thurlbeck, W. M. (1988). Growth, aging, and adaption. In J. F. Murray & J. A. Nadel (Eds.), *Textbook of respiratory medicine* (vol. 1). Philadelphia: Saunders.

West, J. B. (1988). Ventilation, blood flow, and gas exchange. In J. F. Murray & J. A. Nadel (Eds.), *Textbook of respiratory medicine* (vol. 1). Philadelphia: Saunders.

SUGGESTED READINGS

Altose, M. D. (1988). Pulmonary mechanics. In A. P. Fishman (Ed.), *Pulmonary diseases and disorders* (2nd ed.). New York: McGraw-Hill.

Alterations of Pulmonary Function

Sheryl S. Davey

Kathryn L. McCance

Marjorie Cengiz Budd*

Chapter Outline

*Contributing author to first edition.

1148

Pulmonary disease is often classified as acute or chronic, obstructive or restrictive, infectious or noninfectious, and is caused by lung or heart failure. Because skillful and knowledgeable clinical care plays a major role in decreasing respiratory mortality and morbidity, the clinician who has a clear understanding of the pathophysiology of common respiratory problems can greatly affect the outcome for each individual.

CLINICAL MANIFESTATIONS OF PULMONARY ALTERATIONS

Signs and Symptoms of Pulmonary Disease

Pulmonary disease is associated with many common signs and symptoms. The most common of these are cough and dyspnea. Other manifestations include chest pain, abnormal sputum, hemoptysis, altered breathing patterns, cyanosis, and fever. The signs and symptoms present and their specific characteristics often help in identifying the underlying disorder.

Dyspnea

Dyspnea is the subjective sensation of uncomfortable breathing, the feeling of inability to get enough air. It is often described as breathlessness, air hunger, shortness of breath, labored breathing, and preoccupation with breathing. Dyspnea is a very common symptom of respiratory disease.

Dyspnea is usually caused by diffuse and extensive rather than focal pulmonary disease. Disturbances of ventilation, gas exchange, or ventilation-perfusion relationships can cause dyspnea, as can increased work of breathing or diseases that severely damage lung tissue (lung parenchyma).

Many mechanisms have been proposed to explain the complex sensation of dyspnea, but no single mechanism has been found to be responsible in all situations. The most commonly accepted explanation is the length-tension inappropriateness theory, which involves stimulation of receptors in respiratory muscles. According to this theory, the perception of dyspnea develops when muscle spindles in intercostal muscles are stimulated by a disparity between the tension generated by the muscles and the tidal volume (change in muscle fiber length) that results. This can occur if increased airway resistance or decreased compliance results in respiratory effort that is greater than appropriate for the ventilation achieved. A second explanation involves the stimulation of central and peripheral chemoreceptors. It has long

been known that decreased pH, hypercapnia, and hypoxemia can cause dyspnea. Stimulation of chemoreceptors is a cause of dyspnea in many lung diseases in which oxygenation and gas exchange are impaired. A third explanation is stimulation of the afferent receptors in the lung, the stretch, irritant, and J-receptors, which send impulses to the central nervous system through the vagus nerve. J-receptors, for example, trigger dyspnea in individuals with pulmonary edema and pulmonary microemboli. (The neurochemical control of ventilation is described in Chapter 29.) Other factors contributing to the sensation of dyspnea include increased work of breathing, respiratory muscle fatigue, decreased breathing reserve, and strong emotions, particularly anxiety and anger. There is general agreement that the neurologic control and function of respiratory muscles are the common element in most clinical experiences of dyspnea and that the sensation perceived is that of increased respiratory effort.

The signs of dyspnea include flaring of the nostrils, use of accessory muscles of respiration, and retraction (pulling back) of the intercostal spaces. In dyspnea caused by parenchymal disease (e.g., pneumonia), retractions of tissue between the ribs (subcostal and intercostal retractions) are observed more frequently than supercostal retractions (retractions of tissues above the ribs), which predominate in upper-airway obstruction.

Dyspnea can occur transiently or in specific circumstances. Frequently the first episode occurs with exercise and is called dyspnea on exertion. Pulmonary congestion tends to cause dyspnea when the individual is lying down. This type is called **orthopnea**. Orthopnea is caused by the horizontal position, which redistributes body water, causes the abdominal contents to exert pressure on the diaphragm, or decreases the efficiency of the respiratory muscles. Orthopnea is generally relieved by sitting up in a forward-leaning posture or supporting the upper body on several pillows. Some individuals with left ventricular failure wake up at night gasping for air and have to sit up or stand to relieve the dyspnea. This type of positional dyspnea is termed **paroxysmal nocturnal dyspnea (PND)**. Paroxysmal nocturnal dyspnea results from fluid in the lungs caused by the redistribution of body water while the individual is recumbent.

Abnormal Breathing Patterns

Normal breathing (eupnea) is rhythmic and effortless. Ventilatory rate is 8 to 16 breaths per minute, and tidal volume ranges from 400 to 800 ml. A short expiratory pause occurs with each breath, and the individual takes an occasional deeper breath or sighs. Sigh breaths, which help to maintain normal lung function, are usually one and one-half to two times the normal tidal volume and occur approximately 10 to 12 times per hour.

The rate, depth, regularity, and effort of breathing undergo characteristic alterations in response to physiologic and pathophysiologic conditions. Patterns of breathing automatically adjust to minimize the work of respiratory muscles. Strenuous exercise or metabolic acidosis induces **Kussmaul respiration** (hyperpnea). Kussmaul respiration is characterized by a slightly increased ventilatory rate, very large tidal volumes, and no expiratory pause.

Labored, or obstructed, breathing occurs if the airways are obstructed, as in chronic obstructive pulmonary disease. Obstructed breathing consists of slow ventilatory rate, large tidal volume, increased effort, and prolonged inspiration or expiration, depending on the site of obstruction. Audible wheezing (whistling sounds) or stridor (high-pitched sounds made during inspiration) is often present.

Restricted breathing is commonly caused by disorders, such as pulmonary fibrosis, that stiffen the lungs or chest wall and decrease compliance. Restricted breathing is characterized by small tidal volumes and rapid ventilatory rate (tachypnea).

Panting occurs with exercise. Shock and severe cerebral hypoxia (insufficient oxygen in the brain) contribute to gasping respirations that consist of irregular, quick inspirations with an expiratory pause. Sighing respirations consist of irregular breathing characterized by frequent, deep sighing inspirations. Sighing respirations are caused by anxiety.

Cheyne-Stokes respirations are characterized by alternating periods of deep and shallow breathing. Apnea lasting from 15 to 60 seconds is followed by ventilations that increase in volume until a peak is reached, after which ventilation (tidal volume) decreases again to apnea. Cheyne-Stokes respirations result from any condition that slows the blood flow to the brainstem, which, in turn, slows impulses sending information to the respiratory centers of the brainstem. Neurologic impairment above the brainstem is also a contributing factor.

Hypoventilation/Hyperventilation

Hypoventilation is inadequate alveolar ventilation in relation to metabolic demands. It is caused by alterations in pulmonary mechanics or in the neurologic control of breathing. When alveolar ventilation is normal, carbon dioxide is removed from the lungs at the same rate as it is produced by cellular metabolism. This maintains arterial and alveolar P_{CO_2} at normal levels (40 mm Hg). With hypoventilation, CO_2 removal does not keep up with CO_2 production and Pa_{CO_2} increases, causing **hypercapnia** (Pa_{CO_2} greater than 44 mm Hg). (See Chapter 29, Table 29-2, for a definition of gas partial pressures and other pulmonary abbreviations.)

Hypoventilation is often overlooked until it is severe because breathing pattern and ventilatory rate may appear to be normal. Hypoventilation can only be determined by blood gas analysis (i.e., by measurement of the Pa_{CO_2} of arterial blood). Pronounced hypoventilation can cause somnolence or disorientation. Pa_{O_2} may be reduced in those breathing room air.

Hyperventilation is alveolar ventilation that exceeds metabolic demands. The lungs remove CO_2 at a faster rate than it is produced by cellular metabolism, resulting in decreased Pa_{CO_2}, or **hypocapnia** (Pa_{CO_2} less than 36 mm Hg). Like hypoventilation, hyperventilation can be determined only by arterial blood gas analysis. Hyperventilation commonly occurs with severe anxiety, acute head injury, and conditions that cause insufficient oxygenation of the blood.

Cough

A **cough** is a protective reflex that cleanses the lower airways by an explosive expiration. Inhaled particles, accumulated mucus, inflammation, or presence of a foreign body initiates the cough reflex by stimulating the irritant receptors in the airway. The cough consists of inspiration, closure of the glottis and vocal cords, contraction of the expiratory muscles, and reopening of the glottis, causing a sudden, forceful expiration that removes the offending matter. The effectiveness of the cough depends on the depth of the inspiration and the degree to which the airways narrow, increasing the velocity of expiratory gas flow. Cough occurs frequently in healthy individuals.

A persistent cough indicates the presence of a disorder or disease. An acute nonproductive cough often indicates bronchitis or viral pneumonia. Aspiration of a foreign body or irritating fumes can cause a dry cough. A persistent dry cough is commonly caused by a tumor, congestion, or hypersensitive airways. A cough that produces purulent sputum usually indicates infection, whereas a cough that produces nonpurulent sputum is nonspecific and merely indicates irritation. It is important to remember that many individuals swallow their sputum, and a lack of expectorated sputum does not mean that a cough is nonproductive.

Hemoptysis

Hemoptysis is the coughing up of blood or bloody secretions. Hemoptysis is sometimes confused with hematemesis, which is the vomiting of blood. Blood that is coughed up is usually bright red, has an alkaline pH, and is mixed with frothy sputum, whereas blood that is vomited is dark, has an acidic pH, and is mixed with food particles.

Hemoptysis indicates a localized abnormality, usually infection or inflammation that damages the bronchi (bronchitis, bronchiectasis) or the lung parenchyma (tuberculosis, lung abscess). Other causes include cancer and pulmonary infarction. The amount and duration of bleeding (i.e., a sudden large amount versus a persistent slight amount) provide important clues about the source of the bleeding. Bronchoscopy is used to confirm the site of bleeding.

Cyanosis

Cyanosis is a bluish discoloration of the skin and mucous membranes caused by increasing amounts of desaturated or reduced hemoglobin (which is bluish) in the blood. Cyanosis generally develops when 5 g of hemoglobin is desaturated, regardless of hemoglobin concentration. For example, if total hemoglobin concentration is 15 g/100 ml blood, then 5 g/100 ml must be desaturated to cause cyanosis. If total Hb is 11 g/100 ml, 5 g/100 ml must still be desaturated for cyanosis to occur.

Cyanosis can result from decreased arterial oxygenation (low PaO_2), pulmonary or cardiac right-to-left shunts, or decreased cardiac output. A cold environment or anxiety can cause cyanosis because of peripheral vasoconstriction. Lack of cyanosis does not necessarily indicate that oxygenation is normal. Sometimes impaired cellular oxygenation is not accompanied by cyanosis. For example, severe anemia (inadequate hemoglobin concentration) and carbon monoxide poisoning (in which hemoglobin binds to carbon monoxide instead of to oxygen) can cause inadequate oxygenation of tissues without causing cyanosis. Individuals with polycythemia (an abnormal increase in numbers of red blood cells), however, may have cyanosis when oxygenation is adequate. Because polycythemia causes hemoglobin concentration to be greater than normal, 5 g/100 ml can be desaturated, causing cyanosis, without having much effect on oxygenation. Therefore, the significance of cyanosis as a clinical finding must be interpreted in relation to the underlying pathophysiology. If cyanosis is suggested, the PaO_2 should be measured. Central cyanosis, decreased oxygen saturation of hemoglobin in arterial blood, is best seen in buccal mucous membranes and lips. Peripheral cyanosis, slow blood circulation in fingers and toes, is best seen in nail beds.

Pain

Pain caused by pulmonary disorders originates in the pleurae, airways, or the chest wall. Pleural pain is the most common pain caused by pulmonary disease. Infection and inflammation of the parietal pleura cause pain when the pleura stretches during inspiration. The pain is usually localized to a portion of the chest wall, where a unique breath sound called a pleural friction rub can be heard over the painful area. Laughing or coughing makes pleural pain worse. Pleural pain is also common with pulmonary infarction (tissue death) caused by pulmonary embolism. In the case of infarction, the pain emanates from the area around the infarction.

Pulmonary pain is central chest pain that is pronounced after coughing and occurs in individuals with infection and inflammation of the trachea or bronchi (tracheitis or tracheobronchitis). Central chest pain has to be differentiated from cardiac pain (see Chapter 27). High blood pressure in the pulmonary circulation (pulmonary hypertension) can cause pain during exercise that is often mistaken for cardiac pain (angina pectoris).

Pain in the chest wall is muscle pain or rib pain (costochondritis). The common causes of chest wall pain are excessive coughing, which makes the muscles sore, and rib fractures. Chest wall pain often mimics pleural pain.

Clubbing

Clubbing is the selective bulbous enlargement of the end (distal segment) of a digit (finger or toe) (Fig. 30-1). Usually it is painless. Clubbing is commonly associated with diseases that interfere with oxygenation, such as lung cancer, bronchiectasis, cystic fibrosis, pulmonary fibrosis, lung abscess, and congenital heart disease. Its pathogenesis is unknown.

Abnormal Sputum

The color, consistency, odor, and amount of sputum vary with different pulmonary disorders. A distinctive color or odor may indicate infection by a specific microorganism. Changes in the amount and consistency of sputum provide information about progression of dis-

Clubbing—early

Clubbing—middle

Clubbing—severe

FIG. 30-1 **Clubbing of fingers caused by chronic hypoxemia.** (From Seidel, Ball, Dains, & Benedict, 1991.)

ease and effectiveness of therapy. The gross and microscopic appearances of sputum enable the clinician to identify cellular debris or microorganisms that aid in diagnosis and choice of therapy.

Conditions Caused by Pulmonary Disease or Injury
Hypoxemia

Hypoxemia, or reduced oxygenation of arterial blood (reduced Pao_2), is caused by respiratory alterations, whereas **hypoxia,** or reduced oxygenation of cells in tissues, may be caused by alterations of other systems as well. (Hypoxia can occur anywhere in the body; if it occurs in arterial blood, it is correctly called hypoxemia.) Although hypoxemia can lead to tissue hypoxia, tissue hypoxia can result from other abnormalities, such as low cardiac output or cyanide poisoning, that have no relation to alterations of pulmonary function.

There are five causes of hypoxemia: (1) decreased oxygen content (Po_2) of inspired gas, (2) hypoventilation, (3) diffusion abnormalities, (4) abnormal ventilation/perfusion ratios, and (5) pulmonary right-to-left shunt (Table 30-1). The physiologic mechanisms for each cause of hypoxemia are different, and each requires different clinical management.

The Po_2 of arterial blood depends on the Po_2 of inspired gas (Pio_2). If the Po_2 of inspired gas is below normal, then less oxygen is available to diffuse into the blood. The most common cause of a decrease in inspired oxygen is the drop in atmospheric pressure that occurs at high altitudes. Pio_2 drops proportionately with atmospheric pressure, resulting in a decrease in Pao_2. Hypoxemia caused by high altitude is prevented by the use of supplemental oxygen.

Hypoventilation of the alveoli causes elevated $Paco_2$ (hypercapnia). If oxygen-rich gas is not delivered to the alveoli, the oxygen content of alveolar gas (PAo_2) decreases as $Paco_2$ increases. As PAo_2 decreases, less oxygen diffuses into the blood, causing hypoxemia. This type of hypoxemia can be completely corrected if alveolar ventilation is improved by increases in the rate and depth of breathing. Hypoventilation is a common cause of hypoxemia in unconscious persons and in individuals who have chronic obstructive pulmonary disease.

Diffusion of oxygen through the alveolocapillary membrane is impaired if the alveolocapillary membrane is thickened or the surface area available for diffusion is decreased. Abnormal thickness, such as that which occurs with edema (tissue swelling) and fibrosis (formation of fibrous lesions), increases the time required for diffusion across the alveolocapillary membrane. If diffusion is slowed enough, the Po_2 of alveolar gas and capillary blood does not have time to equilibrate during the fraction of a second that blood remains in the capillary. Destruction of alveoli, such as that which occurs in emphysema, decreases the surface area available for diffusion. Hypoxemia caused by impaired diffusion alone is rare, however, and hypercapnia is rarely produced by impaired diffusion because carbon dioxide diffuses so easily from capillary to alveolus that the indi-

TABLE 30-1

Causes of Hypoxemia

Mechanism	Common clinical cause
Decrease in inspired oxygen	High altitude Low oxygen content of gas mixture Enclosed breathing space (suffocation)
Hypoventilation	Lack of neurologic stimulation of the respiratory center (oversedation, drug overdose, neurologic damage) Chronic obstructive pulmonary disease
Alveolocapillary diffusion abnormality	Emphysema Fibrosis Edema
Ventilation-perfusion mismatch	Asthma Chronic bronchitis Pneumonia
Shunting	Adult respiratory distress syndrome Respiratory distress syndrome of the newborn (hyaline membrane disease) Atelectasis

vidual with impaired diffusion would succumb from hypoxemia before hypercapnia could occur.

An abnormal ventilation/perfusion ratio ($\dot{V}/\dot{Q}$) is the most common cause of hypoxemia (Fig. 30-2). Normally, alveolocapillary lung units receive almost equal amounts of ventilation and perfusion. The normal $\dot{V}/\dot{Q}$ is 0.8 to 0.9 because perfusion is somewhat greater than ventilation in the lung bases. $\dot{V}/\dot{Q}$ mismatch refers to an abnormal distribution of ventilation and perfusion. Hypoxemia can be caused by inadequate ventilation of well-perfused areas of the lung (low $\dot{V}/\dot{Q}$). Blood passing through pulmonary capillaries is exposed to less oxygen than normal. Mismatching of this type occurs in asthma as a result of bronchoconstriction, and in pulmonary edema and pneumonia when alveoli are filled with fluid. A pulmonary right-to-left shunt exists when blood passes through portions of the pulmonary capillary bed that receive no ventilation, either because the airway leading to the alveoli is completely obstructed or because the alveoli are collapsed or filled with fluid and cellular debris. Blood flows through the pulmonary circulation without being oxygenated. This results in decreased systemic Pao_2 and hypoxemia. $Paco_2$ is usually not affected except by severe shunting. Hypoxemia resulting from shunting does not respond to increases in supplemental inspired oxygen concentration because a portion of the pulmonary capillary blood is never exposed to the oxygen-rich gas. This makes hypoxemia produced by shunting very difficult to treat. Shunting is the cause of hypoxemia in adult respiratory distress syndrome and respiratory distress syndrome of the newborn.

Hypoxemia also can be caused by poor perfusion of well-ventilated portions of the lung (high $\dot{V}/\dot{Q}$), resulting in wasted ventilation. In this case, oxygen in the alveoli is not exposed to circulating blood. The result is a decrease in Pao_2. The most common cause of high $\dot{V}/\dot{Q}$ is a pulmonary embolus that impairs blood flow to a segment of the lung. An area where alveoli are ventilated but not perfused is termed alveolar dead space. (Alveolar dead space is described in Chapter 29.)

Pulmonary Edema

Pulmonary edema is excess water in the lung. The normal lung contains very little water or fluid. It is kept dry by lymphatic drainage and a balance among capillary hydrostatic pressure, capillary oncotic pressure, and capillary permeability. In addition, surfactant lining the alveoli repels water, keeping fluid from entering the alveoli. (The mechanisms that determine this balance and water movement across the capillary membrane are described in Chapters 1 and 3.) Predisposing factors for pulmonary edema include heart disease, adult respiratory distress syndrome, and inhalation of toxic gases. The pathogenesis of pulmonary edema is shown in Fig. 30-3.

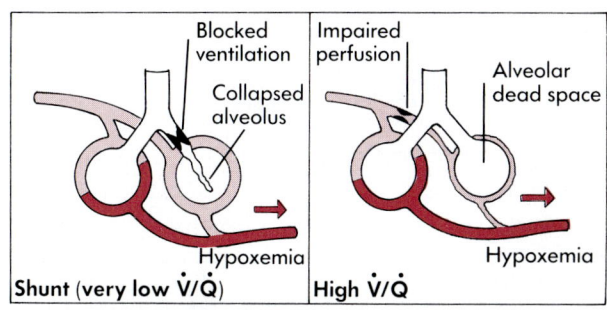

FIG. 30-2 Ventilation-perfusion abnormalities.

The most common cause of pulmonary edema is heart disease. When the left ventricle fails, filling pressures on the left side of the heart increase and cause a concomitant increase in pulmonary capillary hydrostatic pressure. When the hydrostatic pressure push exceeds oncotic pressure, which holds fluid in the capillary, fluid moves out into the interstitium, or interstitial space (the space within the alveolar septum between alveolus and capillary). Initially fluid is picked up by lymphatic vessels and removed from the lung. When the flow of fluid out of the capillaries exceeds the lymphatic system's ability to remove it, pulmonary edema develops.

Pulmonary edema usually begins to develop at a pulmonary capillary wedge pressure or left atrial pressure of 20 mm Hg. If the capillary oncotic pressure is decreased for any reason (such as anemia or decreased plasma proteins), pulmonary edema develops at a lower hydrostatic pressure. Individuals with chronically elevated hydrostatic pressure tend to develop pulmonary edema at higher left atrial pressures.

Another cause of pulmonary edema is capillary injury that increases capillary permeability. Capillary injury causes edema in cases of adult respiratory distress syndrome or inhalation of toxic gases, such as ammonia. Capillary injury causes water and plasma proteins to leak out of the capillary and move into the interstitium. When plasma proteins move into the lung interstitium, they increase the interstitial oncotic pressure, which is usually very low. As the interstitial oncotic pressure begins to equal capillary oncotic pressure, water moves

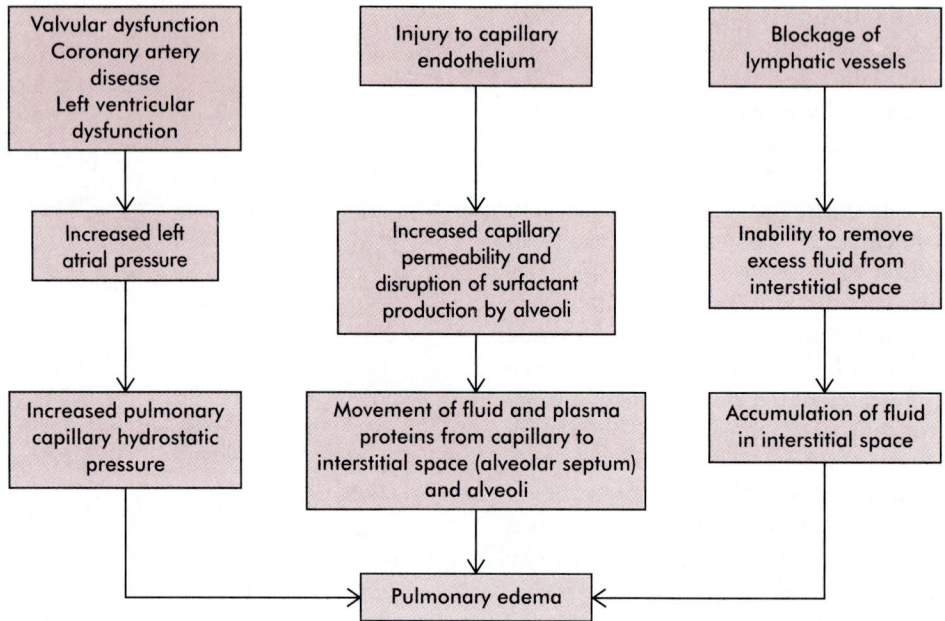

FIG. 30-3 Pathogenesis of pulmonary edema.

out of the capillary and into the lung. (This phenomenon is discussed in Chapter 3, Fig. 3-1.)

Pulmonary edema also can result from obstruction of the lymphatic system. When lymph drainage is blocked, fluid accumulates in the lungs. Drainage can be blocked by an increase in systemic venous pressure, which elevates the hydrostatic pressure of the large pulmonary veins into which the pulmonary lymphatic system drains. This can happen in left heart failure. Drainage also can be obstructed by compression of lymphatic vessels by edema, tumors, and fibrotic tissue.

Clinical manifestations of pulmonary edema include dyspnea, hypoxemia, and increased work of breathing. In severe edema, pink frothy sputum is expectorated and PCO_2 increases.

The treatment of pulmonary edema depends on its cause. If the edema is caused by increased hydrostatic pressure, therapy is geared toward reducing blood pressure with diuretics, vasodilators, and drugs that improve the contraction of the heart muscle. If edema is the result of increased capillary permeability resulting from injury, the treatment is focused on removing the offending agent and supportive therapy to maintain adequate ventilation and circulation. Individuals with either type of pulmonary edema require supplemental oxygen. Positive-pressure mechanical ventilation is also used if edema significantly impairs ventilation and oxygenation.

Aspiration

Aspiration is the passage of fluid and solid particles into the lung. It tends to occur in individuals whose normal swallowing mechanism and cough reflex are impaired by a decreased level of consciousness or central nervous system abnormalities. Predisposing factors include altered level of consciousness caused by substance abuse, sedation, or anesthesia; seizure disorders; cerebrovascular accident; myasthenia gravis (a neuromuscular disorder); and Guillain-Barré syndrome (inflammation of the nerves). Aspiration is also common in children with tracheoesophageal fistula (a congenital abnormality in which the trachea and esophagus communicate; see Chapter 37). The right lung, particularly the right lower lobe, is more susceptible to aspiration than the left lung because the branching angle of the right main stem bronchus is straighter than the branching angle of the left main stem bronchus.

The effects of aspiration depend on the material aspirated. The aspiration of large food particles or gastric fluid with pH of less than 2.5 has serious consequences. Solid food particles can obstruct a bronchus, resulting in bronchial inflammation and collapse of airways distal to the obstruction. If the aspirated solid is not identified and removed by bronchoscopy, a chronic, local inflammation develops that may lead to recurrent infection and bronchiectasis (permanent dilatation of the bronchus). Once the pathologic process has progressed to bronchiectasis, surgical resection of the affected area is usually required.

Aspiration of acidic gastric fluid may cause severe pneumonitis (localized lung inflammation). Bronchial damage includes inflammation, loss of ciliary function, and bronchospasm. In the alveoli, acidic fluid damages the alveolocapillary membrane. This allows plasma and blood cells to move from capillaries into the alveoli, resulting in hemorrhagic pneumonitis. Movement of serous transudate into the lung causes systemic hypovolemia and hypotension. The lung becomes stiff and noncompliant as surfactant production is disrupted, leading to further edema and collapse.

Preventive measures for individuals at risk are more effective than treatment of known aspiration. Surgical patients do not receive food or fluid for several hours before surgery. Antacids are sometimes given to persons at risk to keep gastric pH above 2.5. Individuals who have difficulty swallowing are fed with extreme caution and positioned so as to minimize the likelihood of aspiration. Nasogastric tubes, which are often used to remove stomach contents, can also cause aspiration if fluid and particulate matter are regurgitated.

The rate of deaths caused by aspiration-caused pneumonitis is greater than 50%. Treatment includes supplemental oxygen and mechanical ventilation with positive end-expiratory pressure (PEEP). Fluids are restricted to decrease blood volume and minimize pulmonary edema. Steroids are often administered during the first 72 hours after aspiration, although their effectiveness is not well documented. Bacterial pneumonia may develop as a complication of aspiration pneumonitis. If bacterial pneumonia occurs, it is treated with organism-specific antibiotics.

Atelectasis

Atelectasis is the collapse of lung tissue. There are two types of atelectasis: compression atelectasis and absorption atelectasis. **Compression atelectasis** is caused by the external pressure exerted by a tumor, fluid, or air in the pleural space or by an abdominal distension that presses on a portion of the lung, causing collapse of alveoli. **Absorption atelectasis** is collapse resulting from removal of air from obstructed or hypoventilated alveoli. If a bronchus is obstructed, atelectasis occurs as air in the alveoli is slowly absorbed into the bloodstream. Absorption atelectasis also can be caused by inhalation of concentrated oxygen or anesthetic agents, which are quickly absorbed into the bloodstream and can lead to collapse of alveoli in dependent portions of the lung, particularly when tidal volumes are small. Clinical manifestations of atelectasis are similar to those of pulmonary infection: dyspnea, cough, fever, and leukocytosis.

Atelectasis tends to occur after surgery. Postoperative patients may have received supplemental oxygen or inhaled anesthetics, and they are usually in pain, breathe shallowly, are reluctant to change position, and produce viscous secretions that tend to pool in dependent portions of the lung. Prevention and treatment of postoperative atelectasis usually include deep breathing, frequent position changes, and early ambulation. Deep breathing is beneficial because it (1) promotes the cili-

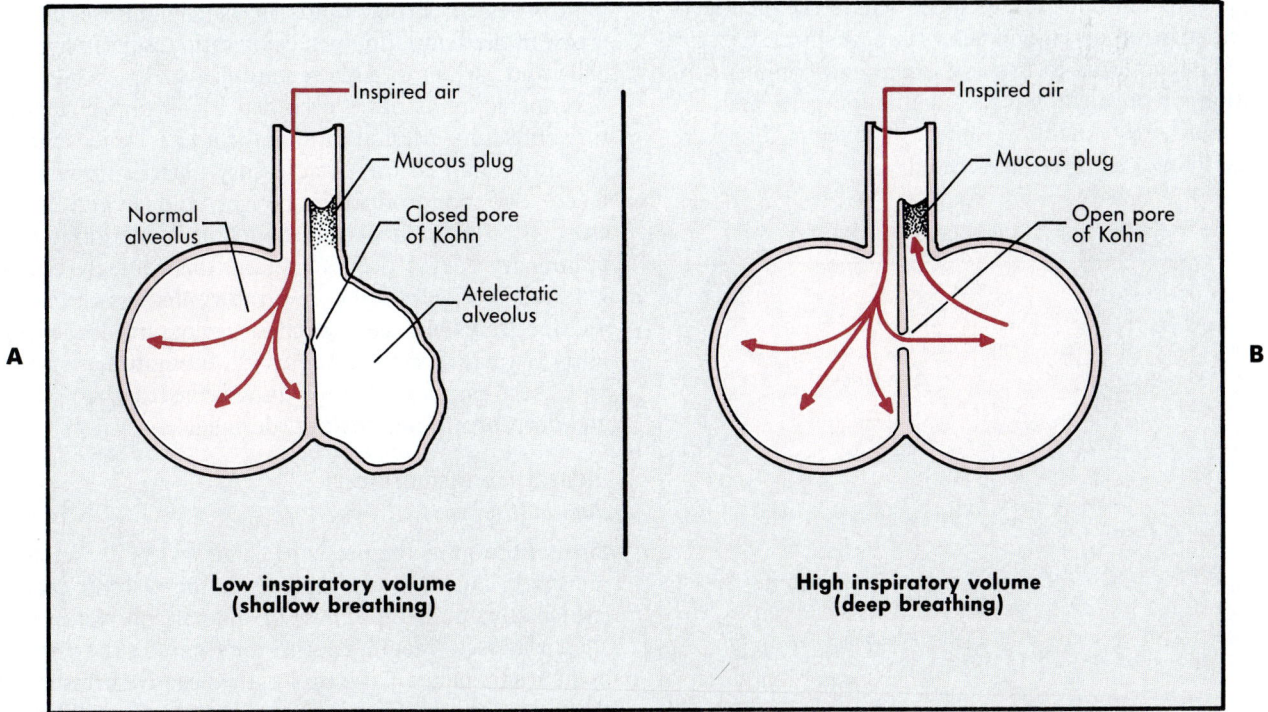

FIG. 30-4 Pore of Kohn. A, Absorption atelectasis caused by lack of collateral ventilation through pores of Kohn; **B,** restoration of collateral ventilation during deep breathing.

ary clearance of secretions, (2) stabilizes the alveoli by redistributing surfactant, and (3) permits collateral ventilation of the alveoli, through pores of Kohn in the alveolar septa. The pores of Kohn, which open only during deep breathing, allow air to pass from well-ventilated alveoli to obstructed alveoli, minimizing their tendency to collapse and facilitating obstruction removal (Fig. 30-4).

Bronchiectasis

Bronchiectasis is persistent abnormal dilatation of the bronchi. It usually occurs in conjunction with other respiratory conditions and can be caused by obstruction of an airway with mucous plugs, atelectasis, aspiration of a foreign body, infection, cystic fibrosis, tuberculosis, congenital weakness of the bronchial wall, or impaired defense mechanisms. Bronchiectasis is frequently associated with inflammation of the bronchi (bronchitis) and has similar symptoms (see p. 1175).

Bronchial dilatation may be cylindrical, saccular, or varicose (Fig. 30-5). In **cylindrical bronchiectasis,** the airways are symmetrically dilated. Cylindrical bronchiectasis is commonly seen after pneumonia and is reversible. In **saccular bronchiectasis** the bronchi become large and balloon like. In **varicose bronchiectasis,** constrictions and dilatations deform the bronchi. In both varicose and saccular bronchiectasis, the smaller bronchial divisions are plugged with secretions or obliterated by fibrosis. Large anastomoses (connections) develop between the bronchial and pulmonary blood vessels, increasing blood flow through the bronchial circulation. These anastomoses are thought to cause the hemoptysis experienced by individuals with bronchiectasis. Airway damage leads to bronchospasm and copious production of purulent mucus. Ventilation-perfusion abnormalities develop and result in hypoxemia. In severe cases, $Paco_2$ also may be elevated.

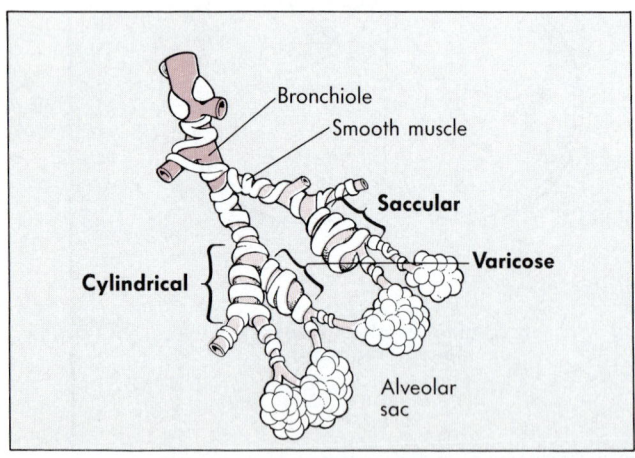

FIG. 30-5 Types of bronchiectasis.

The symptoms of bronchiectasis may date back to a childhood illness or infection. The disease is commonly associated with recurrent lower respiratory tract infections and expectoration of voluminous amounts of purulent sputum (measured in cupfuls). If the individual is not receiving antibiotics, the sputum has a foul odor. Hemoptysis and clubbing of the fingers are common. Pulmonary function studies show a decrease in vital capacity (VC) and in expiratory flow rates. Bronchiectasis is often associated with bronchitis and atelectasis. Hypoxemia eventually leads to cor pulmonale (see p. 1178).

The goals of treatment for bronchiectasis are removal of secretions and prevention of infection. Adequate hydration, percussion, and postural drainage are essential parts of therapy. Bronchodilators are administered to relieve spasms of bronchial smooth muscle, and appropriate antibiotics are given. Hemoptysis is monitored closely, and lung resection may be required to stop severe bleeding. If symptoms are severe and disease is confined to one lobe or area of the lung, surgical resection is sometimes the treatment of choice.

Bronchiolitis

Bronchiolitis is an inflammatory obstruction of the small airways or bronchioles. It is most common in children (see Chapter 31). In adults, it usually occurs with chronic bronchitis but can occur in otherwise healthy individuals in association with an infection or inhalation of toxic gases. Atelectasis or emphysematous destruction of the alveoli may develop distal to the inflammatory lesion. Bronchiolitis is usually diffuse. A decrease in the ventilation/perfusion ratio results in hypoxemia and carbon dioxide retention.

Bronchiolitis is often preceded by an upper respiratory infection. Manifestations include a rapid ventilatory rate, marked use of accessory muscles, low-grade fever, dry nonproductive cough, and hyperinflated chest. If bronchiolitis is caused by an inhalation injury, pulmonary edema occurs rapidly, then quickly clears. One to two weeks later, respiratory distress develops, and infiltrates are seen on chest radiographs. Bronchiolitis is treated with appropriate antibiotics, steroids, and chest physical therapy (humidified air, coughing and deep breathing, postural drainage).

Pleural Abnormalities
Pneumothorax

Pneumothorax is the presence of air or gas in the pleural space caused by a rupture in the visceral pleura (which surrounds the lungs) or the parietal pleura and chest wall (see Chapter 29). As air separates the visceral and parietal pleurae, it destroys the negative pressure of the pleural space. This disrupts the state of equilibrium that normally exists between elastic recoil forces of the lung and chest wall. No longer held in check by the recoil forces of the chest wall, the lung fulfills its tendency to recoil by collapsing toward the hilus (Fig. 30-6).

In **open pneumothorax** (communicating pneumothorax), air pressure in the pleural space equals barometric pressure because air that is drawn into the pleural space during inspiration (through the damaged chest wall and parietal pleura or through the lungs and damaged visceral pleura) is forced back out during expiration. In **tension pneumothorax,** however, the site of pleural rupture acts as a one-way valve, permitting air to enter on inspiration but preventing its escape by closing up during expiration. As more and more air enters the pleural space, air pressure in the pneumothorax begins to exceed barometric pressure. The pathophysiologic effects of tension pneumothorax are life-threatening. Air pressure in the pleural space pushes against the already recoiled lung, causing compression atelectasis, and against the mediastinum, compressing and displacing the heart and great vessels.

Spontaneous pneumothorax, which occurs unexpectedly in healthy individuals (usually men) between the ages of 20 and 40, is caused by the spontaneous rupture of blebs (blisterlike formations) on the visceral pleura. Bleb rupture can occur during sleep, rest, or exercise. The ruptured bleb or blebs are usually located in the apices of the lungs. The cause of bleb formation is

not known. Tension pneumothorax can develop with bleb rupture.

Clinical manifestations of spontaneous pneumothorax begin with sudden pleural pain, tachypnea, and possibly mild dyspnea. The manifestations depend on the size of the pneumothorax. If the pneumothorax is large or if there is a tension pneumothorax, it may push the mediastinum toward the unaffected lung, causing the chest to appear asymmetrical. Hypoxemia may develop. Lung collapse causes diminished breath sounds over the affected lung. Diagnosis is made with chest radiographs.

A secondary pneumothorax can be caused by chest trauma, such as a rib fracture or stab and bullet wounds that tear the pleura; rupture of a bleb or bulla (larger vesicle), as occurs in chronic obstructive pulmonary disease; or mechanical ventilation, particularly if it includes PEEP.

The pathophysiology and clinical manifestations of secondary pneumothorax are similar to those of spontaneous pneumothorax. Occasionally air enters the mediastinum. Secondary pneumothorax (and other open pneumothoraces if large enough) is treated with a chest tube that is attached to a water-seal drainage system with suction. After the pneumothorax is evacuated and the pleural rupture is healed, the chest tube is removed.

Tension pneumothorax, in which air in the pleural space cannot escape through the rupture, is a life-

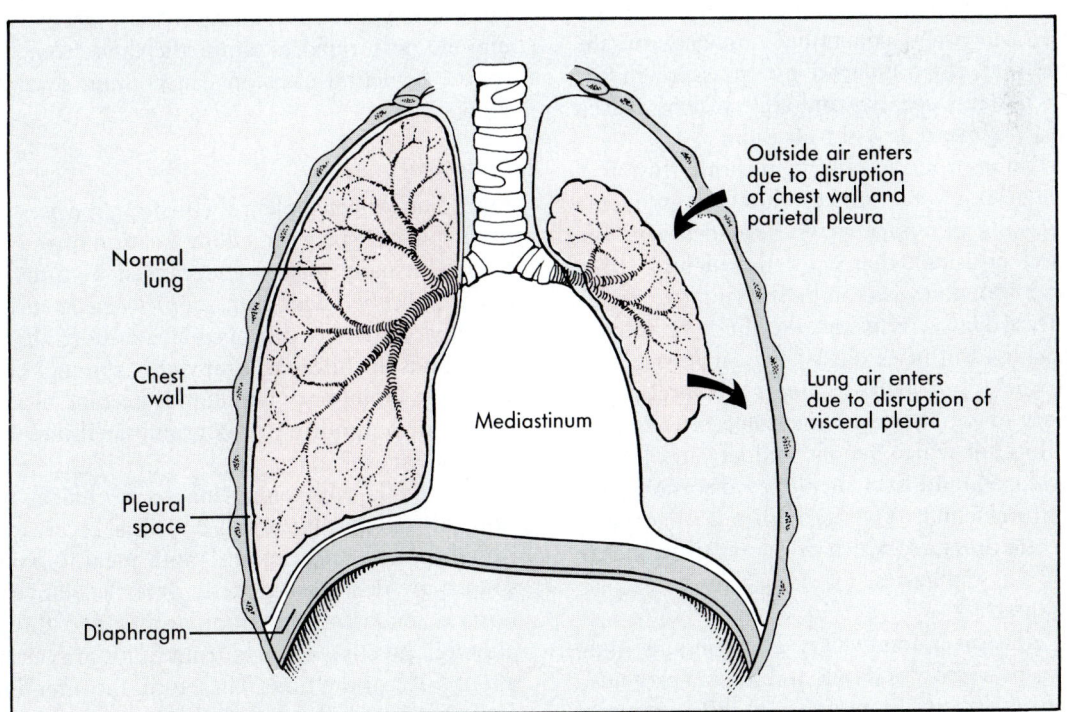

FIG. 30-6 **Pneumothorax.** Air in the pleural space causes the lung to collapse around the hilus and may push mediastinal contents (heart and great vessels) toward the other lung.

threatening emergency. As increasing positive pressure in the pleural space compresses lung tissue and thoracic blood vessels, venous return and cardiac output decrease. Clinical manifestations of tension pneumothorax include severe hypoxemia, dyspnea, and hypotension (low blood pressure), as well as the other signs and symptoms of pneumothorax. Deterioration occurs rapidly, and shock and bradycardia (reduced heart rate) may develop.

Tension pneumothorax requires immediate treatment. A chest tube is placed quickly, usually after physical examination alone. If a chest tube is not readily available, a large-bore needle is inserted into the pleural space to decompress it until a chest tube can be placed. An outward gush of air as the needle or chest tube is inserted confirms the presence of tension pneumothorax. The chest tube is connected to a water-seal drainage and suction until the damaged pleura is healed.

Pleural effusion

Pleural effusion is the presence of fluid in the pleural space. The source of the fluid is usually blood vessels or lymphatic vessels lying beneath either pleura, but occasionally the source is an abscess or other lesion that drains into the pleural space. Because the pleura is a relatively permeable membrane, fluids that accumulate in the lung can cross into the pleural space.

Like pneumothorax, pleural effusion can cause compression atelectasis and displace mediastinal contents. Unlike pneumothorax, however, pleural effusion does not cause the lung to collapse as a result of elastic recoil. Because there is no communication between the pleural space and environmental air, pressure in the pleural space remains negative and atelectasis is caused solely by pressure exerted by the effusion.

The most common mechanism of pleural effusion is migration of fluids and other blood components through the walls of intact capillaries bordering the pleura. Pleural effusions that enter the pleural space from the intact blood vessels can be transudative or exudative. In **transudative effusion,** the fluid, or transudate, is watery and diffuses out of the capillaries as a result of disorders that increase blood pressure or decrease capillary oncotic pressure. Examples are congestive heart failure, in which venous and left atrial pressures are increased, and liver or kidney disorders that cause hypoproteinemia. Hypoproteinemia decreases capillary oncotic pressure, which promotes diffusion of water out of the capillaries. (This mechanism is discussed in Chapter 3.)

Exudative effusion is less watery and contains high concentrations of white blood cells and plasma proteins. Exudative effusion occurs in response to inflammation, infection, or malignancy and involves inflammatory processes that increase capillary permeability (see Chap-

ter 7). When stimulated by biochemical mediators of inflammation, junctions in the capillary endothelium separate slightly, enabling leukocytes and plasma proteins to migrate out into affected tissues.

Other fluids occasionally accumulate in the pleural space. Overproduction of the serous fluid that enables the pleurae to slide over one another can cause pleural effusion. Rupture of a blood vessel or leakage of blood from an injured vessel causes a form of pleural effusion termed **hemothorax.**

Lymphatic blockage from any cause can result in drainage of the contents of lymphatic vessels into the pleural space. Lymphatic contents, which can include pus being drained from infectious lesions in the lungs or substances being transported from other areas of the body to the thoracic duct (which lies near the pleural space), sometimes drain to the pleural space. (Mechanisms of pleural effusion are summarized in Table 30-2.)

Small collections of fluid can normally be drained away by the lymphatics. Large effusions cause clinical manifestations related to their volume and the rate at which they accumulate in the pleural space. Dyspnea, compression atelectasis with impaired ventilation, and mediastinal shift occur with large effusions. Pleural pain is present if the pleura is inflamed, and cardiovascular manifestations occur in large, rapidly developing hemothorax. A pleural friction rub can be heard over areas of extensive effusion.

If the effusion is causing considerable impairment of pulmonary function, thoracentesis (needle aspiration) may be performed to drain the fluid from the pleural space. A pleural effusion can contain several liters of fluid.

Empyema

Empyema (infected pleural effusion), the presence of pus in the pleural space, is a complication of respiratory infection, usually pneumonia caused by *Staphylococcus aureus, Escherichia coli,* or *Klebsiella pneumoniae.* (*Staphylococcus* is responsible for more than 90% of empyemas in children.) Empyema is thought to develop when the pulmonary lymphatics become blocked, leading to an outpouring of contaminated lymphatic fluid into the pleural space.

Individuals with empyema have clinical manifestations of toxicity, including cyanosis, fever, tachycardia (rapid heart rate), cough, and pleural pain. Breath sounds are decreased directly over the empyema. Diagnosis is made by chest radiographs and thoracentesis, although positive cultures from fluids are obtained only about 50% of the time. Therefore, the offending microorganism is usually identified by its preponderance in a sputum culture.

The treatment for empyema is similar to that for

TABLE 30-2

Mechanism of Pleural Effusion

Type of fluid/effusion	Source of accumulation	Primary or associated disorder
Transudate (hydrothorax)	Watery fluid that diffuses out of capillaries beneath the pleurae (i.e., capillaries in lung or chest wall)	Cardiovascular disease that causes high blood pressure; liver or kidney disease that disrupts plasma protein production, causing hypoproteinemia (decreased oncotic pressure in the blood vessels)
Exudate	Fluid rich in proteins (leukocytes, plasma proteins of all kinds; see Chapter 34) that migrates out of the capillaries	Infection, inflammation, or malignancy of the pleurae that stimulates mast cells to release biochemical mediators that increase capillary permeability
Pus (empyema)	Detritus of infection (microorganisms, leukocytes, and cellular debris) dumped into the pleural space by blocked lymphatic vessels	Pulmonary infections, such as pneumonia; lung abscesses; infected wounds
Blood (hemothorax)	Hemorrhage into the pleural space	Traumatic injury, surgery, rupture, or malignancy that damages blood vessels
Chyle (chylothorax)	Chyle (milky fluid containing lymph and fat droplets) that is dumped by lymphatic vessels into the pleural space instead of passing from the gastrointestinal tract to the thoracic duct	Traumatic injury, infection, or disorder that disrupts lymphatic transport

NOTE: The principles of diffusion are described in Chapter 1; mechanisms that increase capillary permeability and cause exudation of cells and proteins are discussed in Chapter 7.

---

pneumonia (see p. 1172). Antibiotics are given, and thoracentesis is performed to drain the pleural space. Chest tube placement and continuous drainage also may be required. In severe cases, surgical debridement of the pleural space is performed to prevent reaccumulation.

Pleurisy

Pleurisy (pleuritis) is inflammation of the pleura. Pleurisy causes pleura to become reddened and covered with an exudate of lymph, fibrin, and cellular elements and may lead to pleural effusion. The most common signs and symptoms of pleurisy are chills, fever, and pain on inspiration. Often a pleural friction rub can be heard over the affected area. Pleurisy is frequently preceded by upper respiratory infection.

Abscess Formation and Cavitation

An **abscess** is a circumscribed area of suppuration and destruction of lung parenchyma. Abscess formation follows **consolidation** of lung tissue, in which inflammation causes alveoli to fill with fluid, pus, and microorganisms. Necrosis (death and decay) of consolidated tissue may progress proximally until it communicates with a bronchus. If this occurs, the abscess empties into the bronchus, leaving a cavity that has a radiographic appearance similar to that of a lesion of tuberculosis. **Cavitation** is the process of abscess emptying and cavity formation. The diagnosis is made by radiography.

Pneumonia caused by aspiration, *Klebsiella,* or *Staphylococcus* is the most common cause of abscess formation. Aspiration abscess is usually associated with alcohol abuse, seizure disorders, general anesthesia, and swallowing disorders. The clinical manifestations of abscess formation are similar to those of pneumonitis: fever, cough, chills, sputum production, and pleural pain. Abscess communication with a bronchus causes a severe cough, copious amounts of often foul-smelling sputum, and occasionally hemoptysis.

Treatment includes the administration of appropriate antibiotics and chest physical therapy, including chest percussion and postural drainage. Sometimes bronchoscopy is performed to drain the abscess. Mortality is influenced by the severity of the primary disease that initially caused consolidation.

Pulmonary Fibrosis

Pulmonary fibrosis is an excessive amount of fibrous or connective tissue in the lung. It can be caused by healing (formation of scar tissue) after active disease (e.g., adult respiratory distress syndrome or tuberculosis) or by inhalation of harmful substances (such as coal dust or asbestos). When no cause for the development of fibrosis is known, it is called idiopathic pulmonary fibrosis.

Fibrosis causes a marked loss of lung compliance. The lung becomes stiff and difficult to ventilate, and the diffusing capacity of the alveolocapillary membrane may decrease, causing hypoxemia. Diffuse pulmonary fibrosis has a very poor prognosis.

Chest Wall Restriction

If the chest wall is deformed, immobilized, or made heavy by fat, the work of breathing is increased and ventilation may be compromised. The degree of ventilatory impairment depends on the severity of the chest wall abnormality. Grossly obese individuals are often dyspneic on exertion or when recumbent. Individuals with severe kyphoscoliosis (lateral bending and rotation of the spinal column, with distortion of the thoracic cage) often present with dyspnea on exertion that can progress to respiratory failure. Such individuals are also susceptible to lower respiratory tract infections. Both obesity and kyphoscoliosis are risk factors for respiratory disease in hospital patients admitted for other problems, particularly those who require surgery. Other musculoskeletal abnormalities that can impair ventilation are ankylosing spondylitis (rheumatoid arthritis of the spine; see Chapters 39 and 40) and pectus excavatum, or funnel chest (a deformity characterized by depression of the sternum).

Impairment of respiratory muscle function caused by neuromuscular disease can also restrict the chest wall and impair pulmonary function. Muscle weakness can result in hypoventilation, inability to remove secretions, and hypoxemia. The most common cause of hospital admission for individuals with such neuromuscular diseases as poliomyelitis, muscular dystrophy, myasthenia gravis, and Guillain-Barré syndrome is respiratory difficulty. (See Unit V for a more complete discussion of these disorders.)

Flail Chest

Flail chest results from the fracture of several consecutive ribs in more than one place, or the fracture of the sternum plus several consecutive ribs. These multiple fractures result in instability of a portion of the chest wall, causing paradoxical movement of the chest with breathing. During inspiration the unstable portion of the chest wall moves inward, and during expiration it moves outward, impairing movement of gas in and out of the lungs (Fig. 30-7).

The clinical manifestations of flail chest are pain, dyspnea, unequal chest expansion, hypoventilation, and hypoxemia. Treatment is internal fixation by controlled mechanical ventilation until the chest wall has stabilized.

Inhalation Disorders
Exposure to toxic gases

Inhalation of gaseous irritants can cause significant respiratory dysfunction. Commonly encountered toxic gases include smoke, ammonia, hydrogen chloride, sulfur dioxide, chlorine, phosgene, and nitrogen dioxide. Inhalation of a toxic gas results in severe inflammation of the airways, alveolar and capillary damage, and pulmonary edema. (The cellular effects of toxic gases are described in Chapter 2.) Initial symptoms include burning of the eyes, nose, and throat; coughing; chest tightness; and dyspnea. Hypoxemia is common. Treatment includes supplemental oxygen, mechanical ventilation with PEEP, and support of the cardiovascular system. Steroids are sometimes used, although their effectiveness has not been well documented. Most individuals respond very quickly to therapy. Some, however, may improve initially and then deteriorate as a result of bronchiectasis or bronchiolitis (inflammation of the bronchioles).

Prolonged exposure to high concentrations of supplemental oxygen can result in a relatively rare iatrogenic condition known as **oxygen toxicity**. Although there is great individual variation in susceptibility to oxygen toxicity, generally the higher the concentration and longer the exposure, the more likely the occurrence of toxicity. Oxygen concentrations of 50% to 75% for greater than 24 to 48 hours have been associated with injury to cells of the lungs. The basic underlying mechanism of injury is a severe inflammatory response mediated primarily by oxygen radicals (Hankins, 1990). The result is damage to alveolocapillary membranes, disruption of surfactant production, interstitial and alveolar edema, and decrease in compliance. Toxicity is often undetected because it occurs in individuals who are already in acute respiratory failure. Clinical manifestations are indistinguishable from those of adult respiratory distress syndrome (see p. 1162). Treatment involves ventilatory support and reduction of inspired oxygen concentration to less than 60% as soon as tolerated by the individual.

Pneumoconiosis

Pneumoconiosis represents any change in the lung caused by inhalation of inorganic dust particles, usually in the workplace (Scanlan & Gupta, 1990). As in all cases of environmentally acquired lung disease, the individual's history of exposure is important in determining the diagnosis. Pneumoconiosis often occurs after years of exposure to the offending dust, and manifestations are often difficult to differentiate from those resulting from smoking.

The dusts of silica, asbestos, and coal are the most common causes of pneumoconiosis. Others include talc, fiberglass, clays, mica, slate, cement, cadmium, beryllium, tungsten, cobalt, aluminum, and iron. No matter

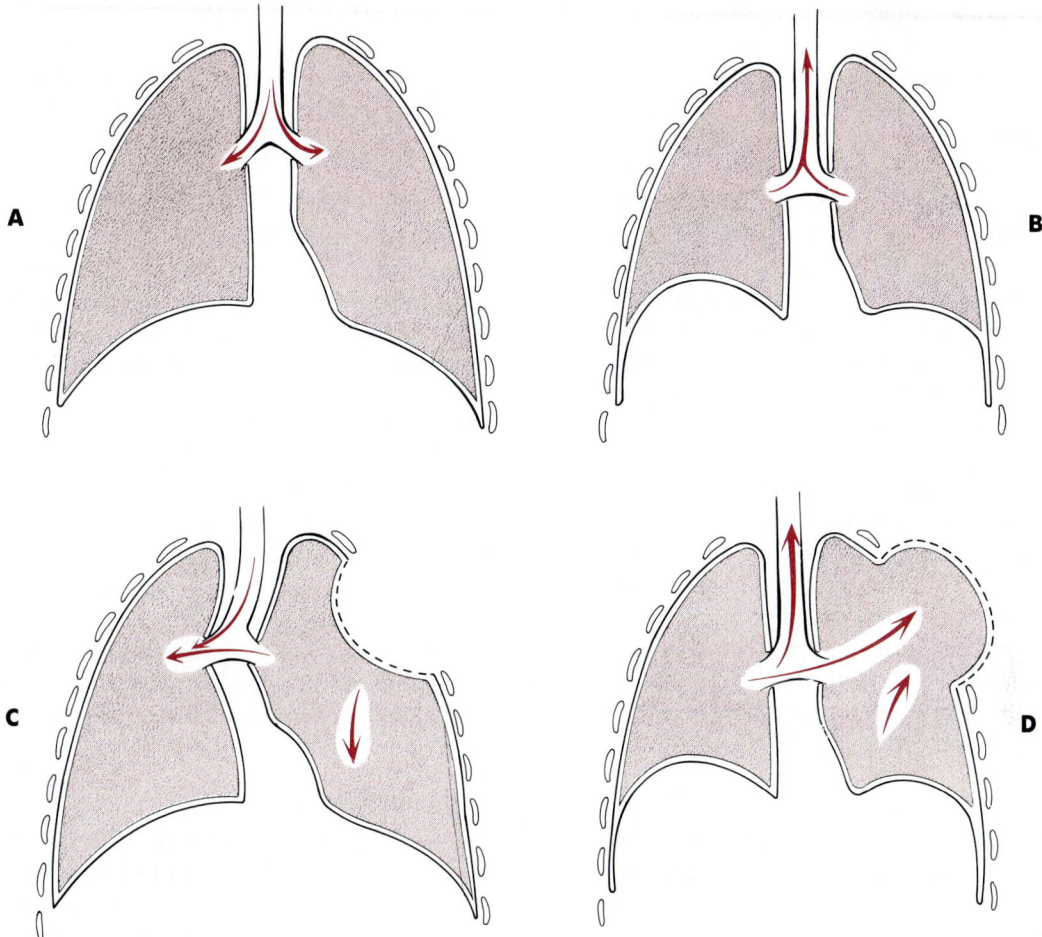

FIG. 30-7 **Flail chest.** Normal respiration: **A,** inspiration; **B,** expiration. Paradoxical motion: **C,** inspiration, area of lung underlying unstable chest wall sucks in on inspiration; **D,** expiration, unstable area balloons out. Note movement of mediastinum toward opposite lung during inspiration.

what the substance, the dust deposits are permanent. Treatment, therefore, is palliative and focuses on preventing further exposure and improving working conditions.

Silicosis is a type of pneumoconiosis resulting from the inhalation of free silica (silicon dioxide) and silica-containing compounds (Scanlan & Gupta, 1990). The silica produce fibrous nodules within the lung. Exposed individuals usually remain asymptomatic long after the nodules are visible on chest radiography. When they do appear, clinical manifestations include cough and dyspnea. Silicosis is also a predisposing factor for lower respiratory tract infection. There is no specific treatment for the disease, although corticosteroids may produce some improvement. Silica exposure occurs in mining and other industries involved with the extraction and processing of ores; preparation and use of sand; and manufacture of pipe, building, and roofing material.

Coal worker pneumoconiosis, sometimes called coal miner lung or black lung, is caused by coal dust deposits in the lung. Its mild form is asymptomatic, except

for possible chronic bronchitis. Its advanced form consists of severe pulmonary fibrosis. Individuals usually are seen with a productive cough and wheezing. Symptoms are more severe with advanced disease and mimic those of chronic bronchitis (see p. 1167). Diagnosis is made by history of exposure and characteristic chest radiographs. There is no specific treatment for coal worker pneumoconiosis. Individuals with the mild form of the disease usually do well. Those with more complicated forms often develop marked cardiopulmonary dysfunction.

Asbestos exposure affects not only factory workers but also individuals who live in areas of asbestos emission. Asbestos exposure can result in a type of pulmonary fibrosis called **asbestosis** or in tumor formation, depending on the amount of exposure. It is caused by inhalation of hydrous silicates of various metals in fibrous form (Scanlan & Gupta, 1990). The most prominent clinical manifestations of fibrosis are dyspnea on exertion, a nonproductive cough, hypoxemia, and decreased lung volume. Progressive disease may lead to respiratory failure and cardiac complications. Asbestos workers who smoke have a marked increase in risk for developing bronchogenic cancer (see p. 1181).

Allergic alveolitis

Inhalation of organic dusts can result in an allergic inflammatory response called **extrinsic allergic alveolitis,** or hypersensitivity pneumonitis. Many allergens can cause this disorder, including grains, silage, bird droppings or feathers, wood dust (particularly redwood and maple), cork dust, animal pelts, coffee beans, fish meal, mushroom compost, and molds that grow on sugarcane, barley, and straw. The lung inflammation, or pneumonitis, occurs after repeated, prolonged exposure to the allergen.

Allergic alveolitis can be acute, subacute, or chronic. The acute form causes a fever, cough, and chills a few hours after exposure. In the subacute form, coughing and dyspnea are common and sometimes necessitate hospital care. Recovery is complete if the offending agent can be avoided in the future. With continued exposure, the disease becomes chronic and pulmonary fibrosis develops. (The mechanisms of hypersensitivity reactions are discussed in Chapter 8.)

Systemic Disorders

Several systemic diseases affect the airways, pleurae, or lung parenchyma, causing fibrosis, vasculitis, pulmonary hemorrhage, or granuloma formation. Clinical manifestations of lung involvement are usually nonspecific, and the diagnosis is based on involvement of other organs. There is usually no specific treatment, although corticosteroids are frequently used. Some of the systemic diseases affecting the lung are granulomatous disorders such as sarcoidosis, Wegener granulomatosis, lymphomatoid granulomatosis, and eosinophilic granuloma; connective tissue diseases such as rheumatoid disease, systemic lupus erythematosus, scleroderma, polymyositis or dermatomyositis, Sjögren syndrome, and polyarteritis nodosa; angioimmunoblastic or immunoblastic lymphadenopathy, a disease of the lymph nodes; cystic fibrosis (see Chapter 31); and Goodpasture syndrome, a renal disorder.

PULMONARY DISORDERS

Acute Respiratory Failure

Respiratory failure is defined as inadequate gas exchange, that is, hypoxemia, where $Pao_2 \leq 50$ mm Hg or where $Paco_2 \geq 50$ mm Hg with pH ≤ 7.25. Respiratory failure can result from direct injury to the lungs, airways, or chest wall or to another body system. It can occur in individuals who have an otherwise normal re-

spiratory system or in those with underlying chronic pulmonary disease. Most pulmonary diseases can cause episodes of acute respiratory failure. Whatever the cause of acute respiratory failure, its pathophysiologic results and treatment are quite similar.

Adult Respiratory Distress Syndrome

Adult respiratory distress syndrome (ARDS) is a fulminant form of respiratory failure characterized by acute lung inflammation and diffuse alveolocapillary injury. Identified within the last 25 years, the syndrome affects an estimated 200,000 to 250,000 people per year in the United States and has a mortality rate close to 65%, despite therapy (Raffin, 1987). Most survivors, however, have almost normal lung function 1 year after the acute illness. Adult respiratory distress syndrome is the result of injury to the lung by numerous unrelated causes. Predisposing factors commonly associated with ARDS are shock, pneumonia, sepsis, trauma, burns, aspiration, cardiopulmonary bypass surgery, pancreatitis, massive blood transfusions, drug overdose, inhalation of smoke or noxious gases, fat emboli, high concentrations of supplemental oxygen, radiation therapy, and intravascular coagulation.

Pathophysiology

All disorders that result in ARDS acutely injure the alveolocapillary membrane and cause severe pulmonary edema (Fig. 30-8). The alveolocapillary damage can occur directly, as with the aspiration of highly acidic gastric contents or inhalation of toxic gases, or indirectly from chemical mediators released in response to systemic disorders. Whether the damage is direct or indirect, the common pathway for alveolocapillary membrane is a massive inflammatory response by the lungs. Several cell types and inflammatory mediators play key roles in the lung injury. The most important of these are neutrophils, complement, endotoxin, and tumor necrosis factor (TNF) (Dal Nogare, 1989; Neuhof, 1991; Rinaldo & Christman, 1990).

The initial injury to the lungs damages the pulmonary capillary endothelium, stimulating platelet aggregation and intravascular thrombus formation. Platelets release substances that attract and activate neutrophils. One of the identified neutrophil chemotactic factors is endotoxin, present in sepsis, a common cause of ARDS. Others are TNF and interleukin-1 (IL-1), cytokines released by macrophages mobilized by endotoxin, bacteria, activated neutrophils, or foreign substances in the alveoli. Endothelial damage also initiates the complement cascade. One component of the cascade, C5a, is a strong stimulator of neutrophil activity.

The role of neutrophils is central to the development of ARDS (Rinaldo & Christman, 1990). Activated neutrophils release a battery of inflammatory mediators,

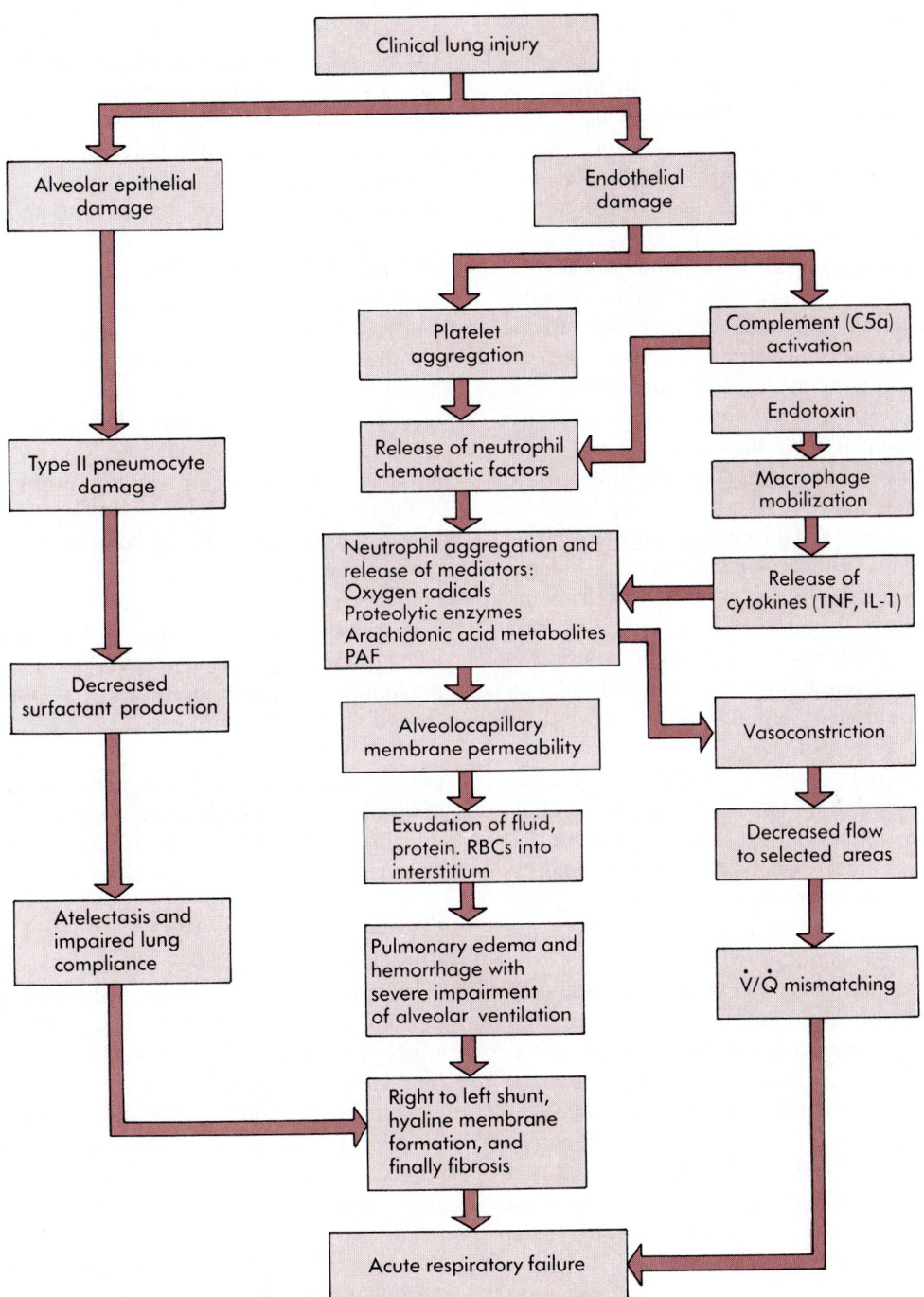

FIG. 30-8 **Pathogenesis of adult respiratory distress syndrome (ARDS).** *TNF,* tumor necrosis factor; *IL-1,* interleukin-1; *PAF,* platelet-activating factor; *RBCs,* red blood cells.

among them proteolytic enzymes, oxygen free radicals (superoxide radicals, hydrogen peroxide, hydroxyl radicals), arachidonic acid metabolites (prostaglandins, thromboxanes, leukotrienes), and platelet-activating factor. These mediators cause extensive damage of the alveolocapillary membrane and greatly increase capillary membrane permeability.

Increased capillary permeability, a hallmark of ARDS, allows fluids, proteins, and blood cells to leak from the capillary bed into the pulmonary interstitium and alveoli. The resulting pulmonary edema and hemorrhage severely reduce lung compliance and impair alveolar ventilation.

Mediators released by neutrophils, and to a certain extent by macrophages, also cause pulmonary vasoconstriction. Pulmonary hypertension occurs early in the course of the disease secondary to vasoconstriction and to vascular occlusion by aggregated neutrophils, macrophages, and platelets. Because vasoconstriction occurs more in some vascular beds than others, there is decreased blood flow to selected areas of the lungs resulting in $\dot{V}/\dot{Q}$ mismatching.

The initial lung injury damages the alveolar epithelium and the vascular endothelium. Surfactant is inactivated and its production by type II alveolar cells is impaired as alveoli and respiratory bronchioles fill with fluid or collapse. The lungs become less compliant, resulting in decreased ventilation of alveoli and right-to-left shunting of pulmonary blood flow.

Twenty-four to forty-eight hours after the acute, hemorrhagic phase of ARDS, hyaline membranes form, and after approximately 7 days fibrosis progressively obliterates the alveoli, respiratory bronchioles, and interstitium. This leads to a decrease in functional residual capacity and even more severe right-to-left shunting. The end result of this overwhelming inflammatory response by the lungs is acute respiratory failure.

It has been recognized in recent years that besides the respiratory effects of ARDS, there are significant systemic components (Rinaldo & Christman, 1990). Neutrophils and inflammatory mediators cause generalized endothelial damage and capillary permeability throughout the body, resulting in multiple organ dysfunction syndrome (MODS). In fact, death may not be caused by respiratory failure alone but by MODS associated with ARDS. (Multiple organ dysfunction syndrome is discussed in Chapter 27.)

Clinical Manifestations

The classic signs and symptoms of ARDS are rapid, shallow breathing; respiratory alkalosis; marked dyspnea; decreased lung compliance; hypoxemia unresponsive to oxygen therapy (refractory hypoxemia); and diffuse alveolar infiltrates seen on chest radiographs, without evidence of cardiac disease. Symptoms develop as the disease progresses. Initially individuals hyperventilate, causing respiratory alkalosis. As the work of breathing increases because of the decrease in compliance caused by alveolar filling and collapse, the individual experiences dyspnea and hypoxemia. Hypoxemia worsens despite oxygen therapy, and diffuse crackles can be heard on auscultation. Eventually metabolic acidosis develops because of the increased work of breathing and cellular hypoxia, and fluffy infiltrates appear on chest radiographs. If ARDS is not reversed, respiratory acidosis develops and further hypoxemia results in hypotension, decreased cardiac output, and death.

Evaluation and Treatment

Diagnosis is made on the basis of physical examination, analysis of blood gases, and radiologic examination. Initial physical examination may show fine crackles, and the chest film may be clear or show a few scattered infiltrates. With progressive respiratory involvement, crackles are heard throughout the lungs and radiographs show extensive bilateral infiltrates.

Treatment is based on early detection, supportive therapy, and prevention of complications. Traditional therapy involves mechanical ventilation with PEEP and high oxygen concentrations. Sedation may be employed to decrease oxygen consumption. If necessary, drugs are given to increase cardiac output. Steroid administration remains controversial because it has not been demonstrated to alter the outcome of ARDS.

Many studies are under way investigating new ways to prevent or treat ARDS. Prophylactic immunotherapy, antibodies against endotoxin, and inhibition of various inflammatory mediators are among the possibilities being tested (Lankin, 1990; Morris, 1992).

Postoperative Respiratory Failure

Although usually not as severe as ARDS, postoperative respiratory failure can result in the same pathophysiology and clinical manifestations as ARDS. Smokers are at risk, particularly if they have preexisting lung disease. Limited cardiac reserve, chronic renal failure, chronic hepatic disease, and infection also increase the tendency to develop postoperative respiratory failure. Surgical procedures involving the thorax or abdomen carry the greatest risk.

The most common postoperative pulmonary problems are atelectasis, pneumonia, pulmonary edema, and pulmonary emboli. These problems usually result in reduced functional residual capacity, decreased compliance, and decreased ventilation/perfusion ratio. Individuals in whom respiratory failure develops have usually had a period of hypotension during surgery, and many have sepsis.

Prevention of postoperative respiratory failure includes frequent turning, deep breathing, and early ambulation to prevent atelectasis and accumulation of secretions. Humidification of inspired air can help loosen secretions. Incentive spirometry gives individuals immediate feedback about tidal volumes, which encourages them to breathe deeply. Supplemental oxygen is given for hypoxemia, and antibiotics are given as appropriate to treat infection. If respiratory failure develops, the individual may require mechanical ventilation for a time. Treatment is then very similar to that for ARDS.

Obstructive Pulmonary Disease

Obstructive pulmonary disease is characterized by difficult expiration. Either more force (i.e., use of accessory muscles of expiration) is required to expire a given volume of air, or emptying of the lungs is slowed, or both. The most common obstructive diseases are asthma, chronic bronchitis, and emphysema. Because many individuals have both chronic bronchitis and emphysema, these diseases together are often called **chronic obstructive pulmonary disease (COPD)**. Asthma is more acute and intermittent than COPD, even though it can be chronic (Fig. 30-9).

Chronic obstructive pulmonary disease is second only to heart disease as a cause of disability in adults younger than 65 years of age. More than one third of all patients admitted to VA hospitals have evidence of COPD. The primary cause of COPD is cigarette smoking. Air pollution and occupational exposure to noxious dusts and gases also may contribute to the development of obstructive pulmonary disease.

Asthma

Asthma is an inflammatory disease characterized by hyperresponsiveness of the airways and episodic periods of **bronchospasm** (spasm, or prolonged contractions, of the bronchial smooth muscle). It is a complex disorder involving biochemical, autonomic, immunologic, infectious, endocrine, and psychologic factors in varying degrees in different individuals. Most attacks of asthmatic bronchospasm are short-lived, with freedom from symptoms between episodes, although airway inflammation is present even in asymptomatic individuals.

Asthma occurs in families and affects 4% to 5% of the population. There are at least two genetic influences,

A

Emphysema

Walls of individual air sacs
torn; repair not possible
Bronchioles collapse,
trapping air;
exhalation difficult
Lung tissue becomes inelastic;
lungs enlarged, resulting
in barrel-chest appearance

B

Chronic bronchitis

Bronchial tubes narrowed as a result of
thickened mucous membrane;
surrounding tissue inflamed
Mucus and pus impede action
of respiratory cilia
Characterized by cough

C

Bronchial asthma

Swollen mucous membranes
of bronchial tubes and surrounding
tissue
Muscles of bronchial tubes become
spastic, causing narrowing
Thick mucus fills bronchial
tubes and sacs; breathing
becomes labored; expiration
difficult

FIG. 30-9 Airway obstruction caused by emphysema, chronic bronchitis, and asthma. A, Emphysema: enlargement and destruction of alveolar walls with loss of elasticity and trapping of air; **B,** chronic bronchitis: inflammation and thickening of mucous membrane with accumulation of mucus and pus leading to obstruction; **C,** bronchial asthma: thick mucus, mucosal edema, and smooth muscle spasm causing obstruction of small airways.

one associated with the capacity to develop allergies (atopy) and the other with the tendency to develop hyperresponsiveness of the airways independent of atopy. Apparently environmental factors interact with inherited factors to cause attacks of bronchospasm. For example, asthma can develop when "predisposed" individuals are infected by viruses or exposed to allergens or pollutants. The severity of asthma attacks varies among individuals, over time, and with the degree of exposure to inciting factors.

Bronchial asthma occurs at all ages. Approximately half of all cases develop during childhood, another third before age 40. It has been estimated that 5% of adults and 7% to 10% of children in the United States have asthma (McFadden, 1991). Complete remission is relatively common among children. Remissions are less common among adults and symptomatic episodes tend to occur more frequently. Despite the recent increased numbers and availability of antiasthma drugs, especially bronchodilators, asthma morbidity and mortality rates have risen in the past 20 years.

Types of asthma

Asthma is described as extrinsic if it is triggered by allergens and intrinsic if it is not. **Extrinsic asthma** (atopic or allergic asthma) is more common than intrinsic. It is distinguished from other inflammatory responses of the airways by mast cell activation, eosinophil infiltration, and epithelial sloughing. Extrinsic asthma is triggered by environmental antigens, such as dust, pollen, molds, animal dander, and foods. The initial encounter with the inciting allergen stimulates plasma cells to produce antigen-specific IgE antibodies that bind to mast cells in the airways (see Fig. 31-6). With subsequent exposure to the allergen, IgE-antigen binding causes mast cell degranulation and release of inflammatory mediators. Most important of the mediators released are histamine; bradykinin; leukotrienes C, D, and E; platelet-activating factor; prostaglandins; thromboxane A_2; and chemotactic factors for eosinophils, platelets, neutrophils, and T lymphocytes. These mediators initiate an intense inflammatory response of the airways. Eosinophils play a key role in extrinsic asthma. In addition to releasing inflammatory mediators, eosinophils produce a protein, major basic protein, that stops ciliary beating, disrupts mucosal integrity, and causes damage and sloughing of epithelial cells. Epithelial cell damage is correlated with airway hyperresponsiveness (Berman & Weller, 1992).

In extrinsic asthma, bronchoconstriction occurs within minutes, then usually resolves within a short time. In some individuals, however, a second episode, called the late reaction, develops 4 to 8 hours after the first. Late reaction symptoms are less responsive to bronchodilator drugs and are of longer duration. Eosinophils predominate and are responsible for increased bronchial inflammation.

Intrinsic asthma (nonatopic asthma) has no known allergic cause. Attacks usually occur in adults older than age 35 and are often severe. Factors known to precipitate intrinsic asthma attacks are respiratory tract infections; drugs (aspirin, beta-adrenergic antagonists); environmental irritants (occupational chemicals, air pollution); cold, dry air; exercise; and emotional stress. Although the causes have been identified, the mechanisms by which they initiate an asthma attack are not completely understood. An hypothesis for the pathogenesis of intrinsic asthma implicates abnormalities in the autonomic neural regulation of airway function (Leatherman & Ingram, 1992). Proponents of this hypothesis believe that bronchospasm is caused by an imbalance between the sympathetic and parasympathetic divisions of the autonomic nervous system. Because airway caliber is controlled by a balance between the sympathetic division, which causes dilation, and the parasympathetic division, which causes constriction, parasympathetic domination would cause bronchospasm. Increased stimulation of the parasympathetic system might develop as the result of exposure of sensory nerve endings within inflamed or damaged epithelium. Explanations for decreased sympathetic stimulation might be a deficiency in the number or function of beta-adrenergic receptors or an increase in alpha-adrenergic responsiveness. Chemical mediators are thought to interact with the autonomic nervous system to produce inflammation and bronchoconstriction.

Pathophysiology

Inflammation resulting in hyperresponsiveness of the airways is the common factor and major pathologic feature of all types of asthma (see Fig. 31-6). The release of inflammatory mediators produces bronchial smooth muscle spasm; vascular congestion; increased vascular permeability; edema formation; production of thick, tenacious mucus; and impaired mucociliary function (Fig. 30-9). Several mediators also cause thickening of airway walls and increased contractile response of bronchial smooth muscle. These changes in the bronchial musculature, combined with the epithelial cell damage caused by eosinophil infiltration, result in the airway hyperresponsiveness characteristics of asthma (McFadden & Gilbert, 1992).

Airway obstruction increases resistance to airflow and decreases flow rates, including expiratory flow. Impaired expiration causes hyperinflation distal to obstructions, altered pulmonary mechanics, and increased work of breathing. Changes in resistance to airflow are not uniform throughout the lungs. Because of regional differences in airway resistance, the distribution of inspired air is uneven, with more air flowing to the less resistant portions.

Hyperventilation is eventually triggered by lung receptors responding to increased lung volume and obstruction. Continued air trapping increases intrapleural and alveolar gas pressures and causes decreased perfusion of the alveoli. Increased alveolar gas pressure, decreased ventilation, and decreased perfusion lead to variable and uneven ventilation-perfusion relationships within different lung segments. The result is early hypoxemia without CO_2 retention (hypercapnia). Hypoxemia further increases hyperventilation through stimulation of the respiratory center, causing $Paco_2$ to decrease and pH to increase (respiratory alkalosis). As the obstruction becomes more severe, however, the number of alveoli being inadequately ventilated and perfused increases, a point at which CO_2 retention and respiratory acidosis develop. Respiratory acidosis signals respiratory failure.

Clinical Manifestations

During full remission, individuals are asymptomatic and pulmonary function tests are normal. During partial remission, there are no clinical symptoms but pulmonary function tests are abnormal. During attacks, individuals are dyspneic and respiratory effort is marked. Breath sounds are decreased except for considerable wheezing. Because the severity of alterations in blood gases is difficult to evaluate by clinical signs alone, arterial blood gas tensions should be measured.

At the beginning of an attack there are a sensation of chest constriction, inspiratory and expiratory wheezing, dyspnea, nonproductive coughing, prolonged expiration, tachycardia, and tachypnea. With severe attacks the accessory muscles of respiration are prominent. As the episode resolves, coughing produces a thick, stringy mucus with casts of the small airways that can be seen microscopically.

Evaluation and Treatment

Spirometry shows decreases in expiratory flow rate, forced expiratory volume (FEV), and forced vital capacity (FVC) (see Chapter 29). Functional residual capacity (FRC) and total lung capacity (TLC) are increased. Blood gas analysis shows hypoxemia with early respiratory alkalosis or late respiratory acidosis.

The most successful treatment of asthma is elimination of the causative agents. Acute episodes are treated with drugs that are geared toward reversing bronchospasm and airway inflammation. Over the years, powerful beta-adrenergic agonists have been relied on to control asthma. Recently, concern has been expressed that overuse of beta-agonists may mask the underlying inflammatory process and lead to worsening of the individual's condition. New recommended management is anti-inflammatory therapy followed by treatment of breakthrough symptoms with bronchodilators as needed (Lee, 1992; Rachelefsky, 1992). Recommended anti-inflammatory drugs include cromolyn sodium, which stabilizes mast cells and suppresses activation of

other inflammatory cells; and low-dose, inhaled corticosteroids, which decrease the inflammatory response and bronchial reactivity in the airways.

If bronchospasm is not reversed by usual measures, the individual is considered to have severe bronchospasm or **status asthmaticus.** With severe bronchospasm, the work of breathing can be 5 to 10 times that of normal. When air trapping is severe, paradoxic pulse (a systolic blood pressure decrease of more than 10 mm Hg during inspiration) and pneumothorax are common. If status asthmaticus continues, hypoxemia worsens, expiratory flows and volumes decrease further, and the individual begins to tire. Acidosis develops as arterial Pco_2 begins to rise. Asthma becomes life-threatening at this point if treatment does not reverse this process quickly. A silent chest (no audible air movement) and a Pco_2 over 70 mm Hg are ominous signs.

Chronic bronchitis

Bronchitis is inflammation of the bronchi caused by irritants (cigarette smoke, air pollutants) or infection. Bronchitis can be acute or chronic and is characterized by mucous gland hyperplasia, muscle hypertrophy, bronchial wall thickening, and inflammation. The consequences are narrowing of the bronchial lumen caused by excess mucus and thickening of the airway walls, which lead to obstruction of airflow (Mahler, 1993).

Pathophysiology

Chronic bronchitis is defined as hypersecretion of mucus and chronic productive cough that continues for at least 3 months of the year (usually the winter months) for at least 2 consecutive years. Incidence is increased in smokers (up to 20-fold) and even more so in workers exposed to air pollution. It is a major health problem for the elderly (Mahler, 1993). Repeated infections are common.

Inspired irritants not only increase mucus production but also increase the size and number of mucous glands and goblet cells in airway epithelium. The mucus produced is thicker and more tenacious than normal. Ciliary function is impaired, reducing mucus clearance further. The lung's defense mechanisms are therefore compromised, increasing susceptibility to pulmonary infection and injury. As infection and injury increase mucus production further, the bronchial walls become inflamed and thickened from edema and accumulation of inflammatory cells. (The pathogenesis of chronic bronchitis is shown in Fig. 30-10.)

Initially chronic bronchitis affects only the larger bronchi, but eventually all airways are involved. The thick mucus and hypertrophied bronchial smooth muscle obstruct the airways and lead to closure, particularly during expiration, when the airways are narrowed (Fig. 30-11). The airways collapse early in expiration, trapping gas in the distal portions of the lung. Obstruction

FIG. 30-10 Pathogenesis of chronic bronchitis and emphysema (chronic obstructive pulmonary disease [COPD]). (Dashed arrows indicate role of α_1-antitrypsin deficiency, if present.)

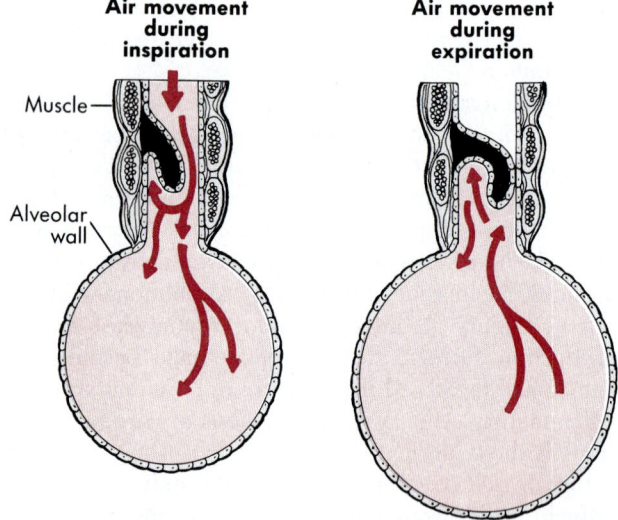

FIG. 30-11 Mechanisms of air trapping in COPD. Mucus plugs and narrowed airways cause air trapping and hyperinflation on expiration. During inspiration the airways enlarge, allowing gas to flow past the obstruction. During expiration the airways narrow and prevent gas flow. This mechanism of air trapping, known as "ball valving," occurs in asthma and chronic bronchitis.

TABLE 30-3

Clinical Manifestations of Chronic Obstructive Lung Disease

Clinical manifestations	Bronchitis	Emphysema
Productive cough	Classic sign	Late in course with infection
Dyspnea	Late in course	Common
Wheezing	Intermittent	Minimal
History of smoking	Common	Common
Barrel chest	Occasionally	Classic
Prolonged expiration	Always present	Always present
Cyanosis	Common	Uncommon
Chronic hypoventilation	Common	Late in course
Polycythemia	Common	Late in course
Cor pulmonale	Common	Late in course

eventually leads to ventilation-perfusion mismatch, hypoventilation (increased $Paco_2$), and hypoxemia.

Clinical Manifestations

The symptoms that lead individuals with chronic bronchitis to seek medical care include decreased exercise tolerance, wheezing, and shortness of breath. Individuals usually have a productive cough ("smoker's cough"), and evidence of airway obstruction (decreased FEV_1) is shown by spirometry. Hypoxemia may occur with exercise. As the disease progresses, copious amounts of sputum are produced, accompanied by frequent pulmonary infections. Forced vital capacity and FEV_1 become markedly reduced, and FRC and residual volume (RV) are increased as airway obstruction and air trapping become more pronounced.

Airway obstruction results in decreased alveolar ventilation and increased $Paco_2$. Marked hypoxemia leads to polycythemia (overproduction of erythrocytes) and cyanosis. If not reversed, hypoxemia leads to pulmonary hypertension and eventually results in cor pulmonale and congestive heart failure (see Chapter 27) and can lead to severe disability or death. (Table 30-3 lists the common clinical manifestations of chronic bronchitis.)

Evaluation and Treatment

Diagnosis is made on the basis of physical examination, chest radiograph, pulmonary function tests, and blood gas analyses; these tests reflect the progressive nature of the disease. The best "treatment" for chronic bronchitis is prevention, because pathologic changes are not reversible. By the time an individual seeks medical care for symptoms, considerable airway damage is present. If the individual stops smoking, disease progression can be halted. If smoking is stopped before symptoms occur, the risk of chronic bronchitis decreases considerably and eventually reaches that of nonsmokers.

Bronchodilators and expectorants are prescribed to increase airway caliber, improve secretion removal, and maximize gas exchange. Chest physical therapy, including deep breathing, postural drainage when 30 ml or more of sputum is produced per day, and percussion, is also used to remove secretions and open airways. Teaching of individuals includes nutritional counseling, respiratory hygiene, recognition of the early signs of infection, and techniques that relieve dyspnea, such as pursed-lip breathing. Some individuals receive prophylactic antibiotic therapy, particularly during the winter months. Steroids are often used late in the course of the disease.

Low-flow oxygen is administered with care to individuals with severe hypoxemia and CO_2 retention. Because of the chronic elevation of $Paco_2$, the central chemoreceptors no longer act as the primary stimulus for breathing. (Chemoreceptors are described in Chapter 29.) This role is taken over by the peripheral chemoreceptors, which are sensitive to changes in Pao_2. Peripheral chemoreceptors do not stimulate breathing if the Pao_2 is much over 60 mm Hg. Therefore, if oxygen therapy causes Pao_2 to exceed 60 mm Hg, the stimulus to breathe is lost, $Paco_2$ increases, and apnea results. Oxygen is used only to keep Pao_2 above 50 mm Hg.

Emphysema

Emphysema is abnormal permanent enlargement of gas-exchange airways (acini) accompanied by destruction of alveolar walls (Snider, Kleinerman, Thurlbeck, & Bengali, 1985). In emphysema, obstruction results from changes in lung tissues, rather than mucus production and inflammation, as in chronic bronchitis. The major mechanism of airflow limitation in emphysema is loss of elastic recoil (Mahler, 1993). Some degree of emphysema is considered normal in elderly individuals. When it occurs earlier in life, however, it is usually secondary to chronic bronchitis and cigarette smoking, but may be primary emphysema.

Primary emphysema is commonly linked to an inherited deficiency of the enzyme α_1-antitrypsin. α_1-Antitrypsin is a major component of α_1 globulin, a plasma protein. Normally α_1-antitrypsin inhibits the action of many proteolytic enzymes (enzymes that break down proteins). Individuals who have α_1-antitrypsin deficiency (an autosomal recessive trait) have an increased likelihood of developing emphysema because proteolysis in lung tissues is not inhibited. Homozygous individuals have a 70% to 80% likelihood of developing lung

Normal expiration   Impaired expiration

Reduced airway patency

Easy expiration due to normal elastic recoil of alveolus and open bronchiole

Difficult expiration due to decreased elastic recoil of alveolus and narrowed bronchiole

FIG. 30-12 **Mechanisms of air trapping in emphysema.** Damaged or destroyed alveolar walls no longer support and hold open the airways, and alveoli lose their property of passive elastic recoil. Both of these factors contribute to collapse during expiration.

Normal lungs

Centriacinar emphysema

Panacinar emphysema

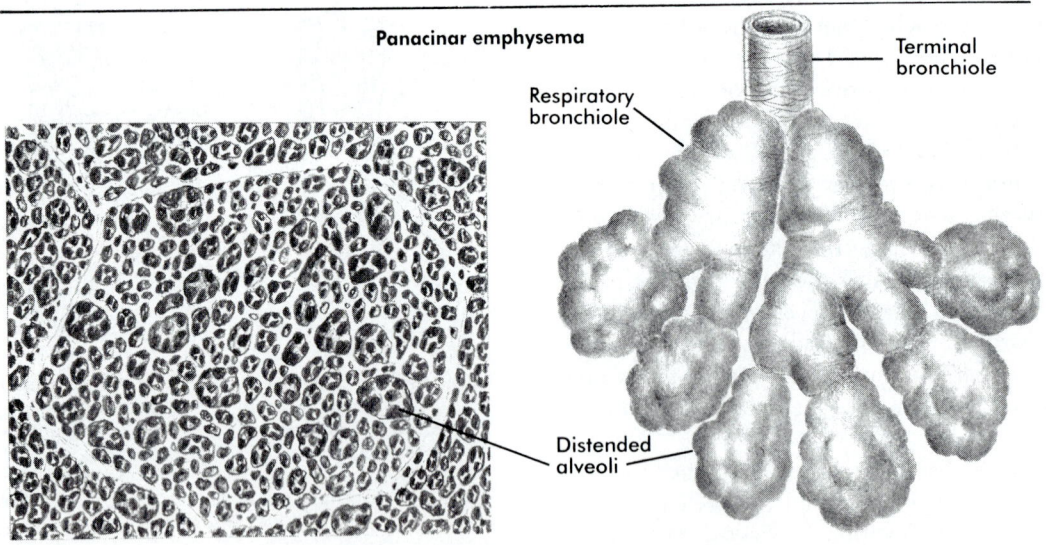

FIG. 30-13 Types of emphysema.

disease. (Mechanisms of genetic inheritance are described in Chapter 4.) Persons with α_1-antitrypsin deficiency who smoke are even more susceptible to emphysema than those with the deficiency alone (Janus, Philipps, & Carrell, 1985). α_1-Antitrypsin deficiency is suggested in individuals who develop emphysema before age 40 or in their early 40s and in nonsmokers who develop the disease. (The principles of risk-factor analysis are discussed in Chapter 5.)

Pathophysiology

Emphysema begins with destruction of alveolar septa, probably because of elastin breakdown within the septa. Septal destruction eliminates portions of the pulmonary capillary bed and increases the volume of air in the acinus. Expiration becomes difficult because loss of elastic recoil reduces the volume of air that can be expired passively. Hyperinflation of alveoli causes large air spaces (bullae) and air spaces adjacent to pleura (blebs) to develop. Septal destruction also affects airway caliber because the force that normal alveoli exert on bronchiolar walls is diminished. The combination of increased residual volume in the alveoli and diminished caliber of the bronchioles causes part of each inspiration to be trapped in the acinus (Fig. 30-12).

Emphysema can be centriacinar (centrilobular) or panacinar (panlobular), depending on site of involvement (Fig. 30-13). In **centriacinar emphysema,** septal destruction occurs in the respiratory bronchioles and alveolar ducts, usually in the upper lobes of the lung. Inflammation develops in the bronchioles, but the alveolar sac (alveoli distal to respiratory bronchiole) remains intact. Smokers tend to develop centriacinar emphysema, and it tends to occur with chronic bronchitis. In **panacinar emphysema,** the whole acinus is involved (Fig. 30-14). The damage is more randomly distributed and tends to involve the lower lobes of the lung. Panacinar emphysema occurs in the elderly and in patients with α_1-antitrypsin deficiency (Mahler, 1993).

Clinical Manifestations

Individuals with emphysema usually present with dyspnea on exertion that later progresses to marked dyspnea, even at rest (Table 30-3). There is no cough and very little sputum production. The individual is often thin, has tachypnea with prolonged expiration, and must use accessory muscles for ventilation. The anterior-posterior diameter of the chest is increased and has a hyperresonant sound with percussion. To increase lung capacity, the individual often leans forward with arms extended and braced on knees when sitting.

Evaluation and Treatment

The most definitive evidence for the presence of emphysema is obtained from the chest radiograph. Pulmonary

FIG. 30-14 Paracinar emphysema. Uniformly enlarged air spaces. (From Kissane, 1990.)

function measurements are helpful in determining a prognosis. On radiographs the diaphragm appears flattened and the lung fields translucent. Marked and persistent overdistention of the lungs is suggestive of emphysema. Pulmonary function tests indicate obstruction to gas flow during expiration. Airway collapse and air trapping in distal portions of the lung lead to a decrease in FVC and FEV_1 and an increase in FRC, RV, and TLC. Total lung capacity can increase to twice normal. Diffusing capacity is decreased because of destruction of the alveolocapillary membrane. Arterial blood gases are usually normal until late in the disease. The disease course is usually prolonged, with increasing dyspnea and intermittent bouts of infection that culminate in failure of the right side of the heart (cor pulmonale) and death.

Treatment for emphysema is similar to that for chronic bronchitis. Like chronic bronchitis, emphysema is not reversible, although its progression can be slowed if the individual stops smoking. Treatment focuses on minimizing air trapping and relieving dyspnea. Dyspnea is relieved by relaxation exercises, reconditioning exercises, and breathing retraining. The individual is taught to maximize ventilation, avoid respiratory irritants, and stay away from people with upper respiratory infections. Because infection can prove life-threatening, prophylactic antibiotics may be prescribed, particularly during the winter months.

Respiratory Tract Infections

Respiratory tract infections are the most common cause of short-term disability in the United States. Most of these infections—the common cold, pharyngitis (sore throat), and laryngitis—involve only the upper airways. Although the lungs have direct contact with the atmosphere, they remain sterile under most circumstances. Infections of the lower respiratory tract occur most frequently in the young, the very old, or individuals with impaired immunity or underlying disease. In all cases, the body's normal defense mechanisms are impaired.

Pneumonia

Pneumonia is an acute infection of the lung caused by bacteria or viruses. More than 1 million cases of pneumonia are diagnosed each year. Pneumonia primarily occurs during the winter months and is frequently associated with recent upper respiratory tract infection.

Many microorganisms can cause pneumonia. Most of them are carried in the oropharynx of normal individuals. The most common causal microorganisms are the following:

Gram-positive bacteria	Gram-negative bacteria	Nonbacterial organisms
Streptococcus pneumoniae	Escherichia coli	Pneumocystis carinii
Mycoplasma pneumoniae	Pseudomonas aeruginosa	Fungi
Klebsiella pneumoniae	Proteus species	Viruses
Staphylococcus aureus	Bacteroides species	
Streptococcus pyogenes	Haemophilus species	Legionella species

Fungi are an uncommon cause of pneumonia, but fungal pneumonia can be caused in immunosuppressed individuals by *Candida*, *Mucor*, and *Aspergillus*. Fungi associated with histoplasmosis and coccidioidomycosis can infect both normal and immunosuppressed individuals.

The microorganisms that cause "community-acquired" pneumonia usually differ in identity, virulence, and mortality from those that cause hospital-acquired, or nosocomial, pneumonia. The most common cause of community-acquired pneumonia is *Streptococcus pneumoniae*. This microorganism causes more than 70% of all diagnosed cases of pneumonia (community-acquired and nosocomial). *Mycoplasma*

pneumoniae is the next most common cause of community-acquired pneumonia. Mortality rate from these two organisms is very low (less than 5%). *Staphylococcus aureus* and *Klebsiella pneumoniae* cause some community-acquired disease, usually in individuals with other health problems, such as COPD or alcoholism. *Staphylococcus aureus* and *Klebsiella pneumoniae* also can cause secondary infection in individuals with a primary viral illness. Viral pneumonia is usually caused by influenza viruses.

Most nosocomial pneumonias are caused by gram-negative bacteria, commonly *Escherichia coli*, *Klebsiella pneumoniae*, and *Pseudomonas aeruginosa*, although *Staphylococcus aureus*, which is gram-positive, also causes pneumonia in some hospitalized individuals. The gram-positive organisms result in more serious infection, with an average mortality rate of 50%. They are also more likely to result in lung necrosis, abscess, or empyema.

The *Legionella* species are widely distributed in water environments and are present in cooling systems, condensers, shower heads, and water reservoirs. Infections may occur in outbreaks, as with the 1976 incident at the American Legion Convention in Philadelphia, or more sporadically.

Pathophysiology

Pathogenic microorganisms can reach the lung by several routes. A common mode of transmission is inspiration. When an infected individual coughs, sneezes, or talks, microorganisms are released into the air in tiny droplets that can be inhaled by other people. Microorganisms also can be inspired with aerosols (nebulized gas) from contaminated respiratory therapy equipment. One of the few microorganisms transmitted by inhalation outside the hospital is influenza.

Another common pathway is aspiration of oropharyngeal secretions. Aspiration of small amounts is normal, particularly during sleep. The oropharynx is normally colonized by a variety of potential pathogens, mostly gram-positive bacteria. In illness or cases of poor dental hygiene, the oropharynx is often colonized by gram-negative bacteria. Whether pneumonia develops depends on the virulence of microorganisms aspirated and the effectiveness of the individual's immune system.

Infection also can be spread by the circulation. *Staphylococcus* and gram-negative bacteria are the most common organisms transmitted by this route. The source is usually systemic infection, sepsis, or contaminated needles of intravenous drug abusers.

In healthy individuals pathogens that reach the lung are expelled or held in check by mechanisms of self-defense (see Chapters 6 and 7). The lungs' defense mechanisms—the cough reflex, mucociliary clearance, and phagocytosis by alveolar macrophages—are backed up by the body's immune system and various components of the inflammatory response, including the release of biochemical mediators by alveolar mast cells. In susceptible individuals the invading pathogen is not held in check but multiplies, releasing damaging toxins and stimulating full-scale inflammatory and immune responses, both of which have damaging side effects. The immune response (antigen-antibody reaction) and the endotoxins released by some microorganisms damage bronchial mucous membranes and alveolocapillary membranes. Inflammation and edema cause the acini and terminal bronchioles to fill with infectious debris and exudate, leading to ventilation-perfusion abnormalities. If the pneumonia is caused by *Staphylococcus* or gram-negative bacteria, necrosis of lung parenchyma may also occur.

Pneumococcal pneumonia. The pathogenesis of pneumococcal pneumonia *(Streptococcus pneumoniae)* is best understood (Fig. 30-15). *Streptococcus pneumoniae* organisms initiate the inflammatory response (see Chapter 7), and inflammatory exudate causes alveolar edema. Edema creates a medium for the multiplication of bacteria and aids in the spread of infection into adjacent portions of the lung. The involved lobe undergoes consolidation (solidification of the tissue caused by filling with exudate). There follows a stage of red hepatiza-

tion in which alveoli fill with blood cells, fibrin, edematous fluid, and pneumococci, giving lung tissue a red appearance. This passes into the stage of gray hepatization, in which affected tissues become gray because of fibrin deposition over the pleural surfaces and the presence of fibrin and leukocytes (neutrophils) in the consolidated alveoli, where phagocytosis is rapidly taking place. With resolution, increasing numbers of macrophages appear in the alveolar spaces, the neutrophils degenerate, and the fibrin threads and remaining bacteria are digested by macrophages and removed by lymphatic vessels. Usually infection is limited to one or two lobes.

Viral pneumonia. Viral pneumonia is usually mild and self-limiting but can set the stage for a secondary bacterial infection by providing an ideal environment for bacterial growth and by damaging ciliated epithelial cells, which normally prevent pathogens from reaching the lower airways. Viral pneumonia can be a primary infection or a complication of another viral illness (such as chickenpox or measles). The virus not only destroys the ciliated epithelial cells but also invades the goblet cells and bronchial mucous glands. Sloughing of destroyed bronchial epithelium occurs throughout the respiratory tract, preventing mucociliary clearance. Bronchial walls become edematous and infiltrated with leukocytes.

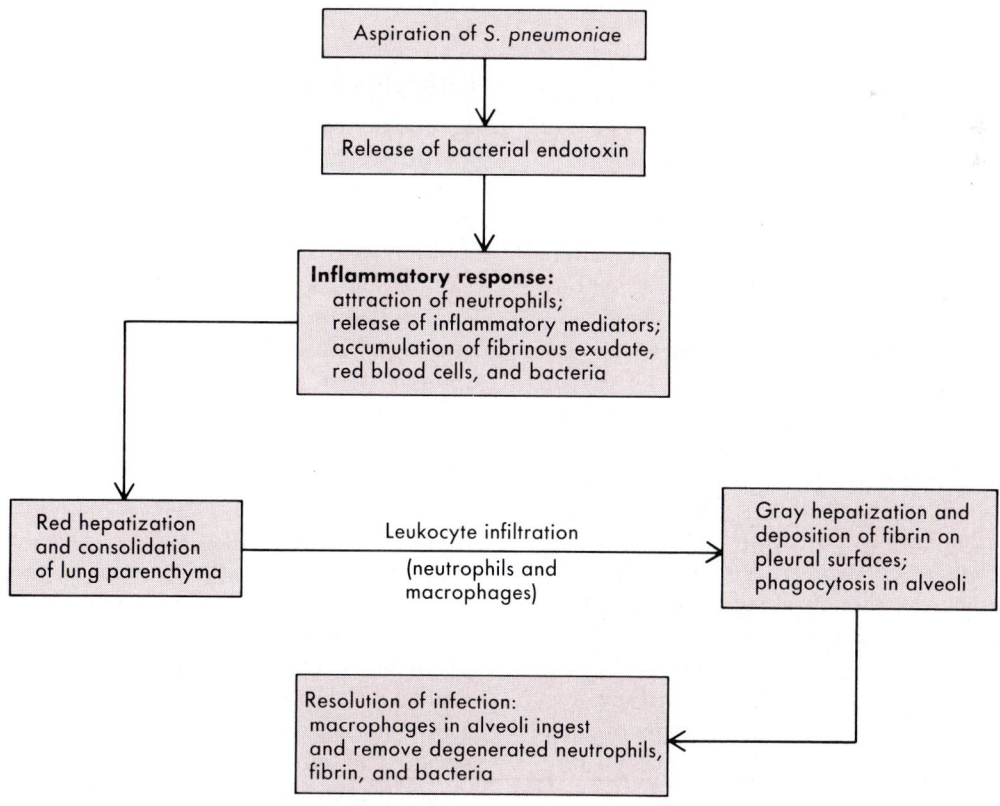

FIG. 30-15 Pathophysiologic course of bacterial pneumonia.

Clinical Manifestations

Most cases of pneumonia are preceded by an upper respiratory infection, which is frequently viral. Individuals then develop fever, chills, productive or dry cough, malaise, pleural pain, and sometimes dyspnea and hemoptysis.

The white blood count is usually elevated (greater than 10,000/mm³), although it may be low (less than 6000/mm³) if the individual is debilitated. Chest radiographs show infiltrates that may involve a single lobe of the lung (**lobar pneumonia**) or may be more diffuse (**bronchopneumonia**).

Once the diagnosis of pneumonia has been made, the pathogen is identified by means of sputum characteristics (Gram stain, color, odor) and cultures or, if sputum is absent, blood cultures. Purulent sputum is expectorated by individuals with bacterial pneumonia, and the appearance and odor of the sputum aid in pathogen identification. For example, infection by *Streptococcus pneumoniae* results in rusty-colored sputum, infection by *Staphylococcus aureus* results in salmon-pink sputum, and infection by *Pseudomonas aeruginosa* causes greenish sputum with a distinctive odor. Viral pneumonia and pneumonia caused by *Mycoplasma pneumoniae* characteristically result in scanty sputum production. Because many pathogens are part of the normal flora in the oropharynx, the specimen may be contaminated with pathogens from oral secretions. Transtracheal aspiration is used to obtain an uncontaminated sputum specimen.

If sputum studies fail to identify the pathogen, pneumonia is assumed to be viral. Positive identification of the virus is often difficult. Blood cultures often help to identify the virus if systemic disease is present.

Evaluation and Treatment

Diagnosis is made on the basis of physical examination, cultures of blood, and cultures of respiratory secretions. Antibiotics are used to treat bacterial pneumonia. Selection of the appropriate antibiotic is based on the sputum culture and specific bacterial sensitivity. The individual's condition usually begins to improve 24 hours after antibiotic therapy is instituted. The duration of antibiotic therapy depends on the identity of the microorganism and the severity of the illness. The development of a complication, such as abscess or empyema, necessitates longer antibiotic therapy. Viral pneumonia is treated with supportive therapy alone, unless secondary bacterial infection is present.

Adequate hydration and good pulmonary hygiene (deep breathing, coughing, chest physical therapy, etc.) are important aspects of treatment for all types of pneumonia. Mechanical ventilation and supplemental oxygen are provided as needed to maintain adequate gas exchange. Severe pneumonia may develop into ARDS, in which case PEEP is added to ventilatory support measures.

Tuberculosis

Tuberculosis is an infection caused by *Mycobacterium tuberculosis*, an acid-fast bacillus that usually affects the lungs but may invade other body systems. Before the advent of specific antimicrobial therapy, tuberculosis was an important cause of death and disability in North America. During the decades from 1950 to 1980 there was a decrease in the incidence of tuberculosis. In the last decade the number of reported cases has alarmingly increased to nearly 16%. The largest increases have occurred in men 25 to 44 years old and, to a lesser extent, in children younger than 15 years of age and in Hispanic, black, and Asian populations (Jereb, Kelly, Dooley, Cauther, & Snider, 1990). The major reason for this trend is the epidemic of acquired immune deficiency syndrome (AIDS). Individuals with AIDS are highly susceptible to respiratory infections, including tuberculosis. A second important reason is the growing number of drug-resistant strains of tuberculosis bacillus that have developed because a large number of individuals do not consistently take their medications, allowing resistant strains to be selected and spread. Emigration of infected individuals from high-prevalence counties, transmission in crowded institutional settings, homelessness, substance abuse, and lack of access to medical care have also contributed to the problem. There has been a reduction in the number of cases in recent years among the elderly. The case rate in this age group is still higher than in any other, however (Dutt & Stead, 1993).

Pathophysiology

Like some types of pneumonia, tuberculosis is transmitted from person to person in airborne droplets. Microorganisms lodge in the lung periphery, usually in the upper lobe. Once the bacilli are inspired into the lung, they multiply and cause nonspecific pneumonitis (lung inflammation). Some bacilli migrate through the lymphatics and become lodged in the lymph nodes, where they encounter lymphocytes and initiate the immune response.

Inflammation in the lung causes neutrophils to migrate to the area, then alveolar macrophages. These cells are phagocytes that engulf the bacilli and begin the process by which the body's defense mechanisms isolate the bacilli, preventing their spread. The neutrophils and macrophages seal off the colonies of bacilli, forming a granulomatous lesion called a tubercle (see Chapter 7). Infected tissues within the tubercle die, forming cheese-like material called caseation necrosis. (Necrosis is described in Chapter 2.) Collagenous scar tissue then grows around the tubercle, completing isolation of the bacilli. The immune response is complete after 10 days or so, preventing further multiplication of the bacilli (Bloom & Murray, 1992).

Once the bacilli are isolated in tubercles and immunity develops, tuberculosis may remain dormant for life. If the immune system is impaired, however, or if live bacilli escape into the bronchi, active disease occurs and may spread through the blood and lymphatics to other organs. Endogenous reactivation of dormant bacilli in the elderly may be caused by poor nutritional status, insulin-dependent diabetes, long-term corticosteroid therapy, and other debilitating diseases (Dutt & Stead, 1993).

Clinical Manifestations

In many infected individuals, tuberculosis is asymptomatic. In others, symptoms develop so gradually that they are not noticed until the disease is advanced. However, symptoms can appear in immunosuppressed individuals within weeks of exposure to the bacillus. Common clinical manifestations include fatigue, weight loss, lethargy, anorexia (loss of appetite), and a low-grade fever that usually occurs in the afternoon. (These are common signs and symptoms of all chronic infections.) A cough that produces purulent sputum develops slowly and becomes more frequent over several weeks or months. "Night sweats" and general anxiety are often present. Dyspnea, chest pain, and hemoptysis are uncommon findings.

Evaluation and Treatment

Tuberculosis is diagnosed by a positive tuberculin skin test, sputum culture, and chest radiographs. A positive tuberculin skin test indicates that an individual has been infected and has produced antibodies against the bacillus. By itself the positive skin test does not indicate the presence of active disease. It is important that the material used for skin testing be standardized to minimize the number of false-positive and false-negative results.

When active disease is present, the tubercle bacillus can be cultured from the sputum and may be seen with an acid-fast stain. Chest radiographs of individuals with current or previous active disease demonstrate characteristic changes. Nodules, calcifications, cavities, and hilar enlargement (enlarged mediastinal lymph nodes) are commonly seen in the upper lobes. A positive skin test indicates the need for yearly chest radiographs to detect active disease.

Tuberculosis is graded as follows to aid in evaluation and determination of appropriate therapy (American Thoracic Society, 1990):

0 No tuberculosis, no exposure, no infection
1 Exposure to tuberculosis, no infection
2 Tuberculosis infection, no disease
3 Tuberculosis, active disease
4 Tuberculosis, no active disease
5 Tuberculosis suspected

Treatment consists of antibiotic therapy to control active or dormant tuberculosis and prevent transmission.

The choice of drugs and the duration of treatment depend on the individual's health history, the likelihood of bacterial resistance to certain drugs, and the presence of active disease. The waxy coat of *M. tuberculosis* renders it impermeable to many common drugs. Before the increase in tuberculosis incidence during the past decade, treatment with two effective drugs was generally sufficient. Isoniazid with either rifampin or ethambutol was usually used for 6 to 9 months. Today, with the increased numbers of immunosuppressed and susceptible individuals and drug-resistant bacilli, the recommended treatment for those at high risk is a combination of four drugs: isoniazid, rifampin, pyrazinamide, and ethambutol ("Drugs for tuberculosis," 1992).

In the past, individuals with active tuberculosis were isolated from the community and their families in sanitariums. Today individuals remain at home or, rarely, in the hospital, until sputum cultures show that the active bacilli have been eliminated. This usually takes a few weeks to 2 months if the antibiotics are taken conscientiously. If the individual's cooperation is in question, it is advisable for the administration of the drugs to be supervised by health care workers.

Acute Bronchitis

Acute bronchitis is acute infection or inflammation of the airways or bronchi. Acute bronchitis commonly follows a viral illness and is usually self-limiting. Many of the clinical manifestations are similar to those of pneumonia (i.e., fever, cough, chills, and malaise), but chest radiographs show no infiltrates. Individuals with viral bronchitis present with a nonproductive cough that frequently occurs in paroxysms and is aggravated by cold, dry, or dusty air. Purulent sputum may be produced. Chest pain often develops from the effort of coughing. Treatment consists of rest, aspirin, humidity, and a cough suppressant, such as codeine.

Individuals with bacterial bronchitis present with a productive cough, fever, and pain behind the sternum (breastbone) that is aggravated by coughing. It is rare in previously healthy adults except after viral infection but is common in patients with COPD. Bacterial bronchitis is treated with rest, aspirin, humidity, and antibiotics (usually a penicillinase-resistant penicillin). If the cough is nonproductive, a cough suppressant is given, because a dry cough can cause bronchial irritation and damage. Acute bronchitis may progress to pneumonia.

Pulmonary Vascular Disease

Blood flow through the lungs can be disrupted by a number of disorders that result in occlusion of the vessels, an increase in pulmonary vascular resistance, or destruction of the vascular bed. The consequences of altered pulmonary blood flow may be of no functional significance or can result in severe and life-threatening changes in ventilation/perfusion ratios. Major disorders include pulmonary embolism, pulmonary hypertension, and cor pulmonale.

Pulmonary Embolism

Pulmonary embolism is occlusion of a portion of the pulmonary vascular bed by an embolus: a thrombus (blood clot), tissue fragment, lipids (fats), or air bubble. The most common emboli are thrombi dislodged from deep veins in the calf. They can also originate in the pelvis, particularly in pregnant women.

Risk factors for **pulmonary thromboembolism,** the obstruction of a pulmonary vessel by a thrombus, include many conditions and disorders that promote blood clotting (see Chapter 22). Clotting within the vessels is promoted by venous stasis (slowing or stagnation of blood flow through the veins), hypercoagulability (increased tendency of the blood to form clots), and injuries that cause bleeding. Venous stasis is usually caused by immobility associated with prolonged bed rest or sitting, obesity, and old age, but it can also be caused by pregnancy, congestive heart failure, sickle cell disease, and systemic lupus erythematosus. Hypercoagulability can result from coagulation disorders of the blood or oral contraceptive use. Clot formation also proceeds if vessel damage occurs, as in traumatic injury, surgery, or spontaneous rupture (e.g., cerebrovascular accident).

No matter what its source, a blood clot becomes an embolus when all or part of it breaks away from the site of formation and begins to travel in the bloodstream. (Thromboembolism is described further in Chapter 24.)

Pulmonary emboli are the most common cause of acute pulmonary disease in hospital patients. They are the third leading cause of death in the United States, accounting for 100,000 deaths per year and are a major contributor to another 100,000 deaths per year (Kinasewitz, 1993). One half of the deaths occur within 2 hours of embolization, which often is undetected and therefore untreated.

Pathophysiology

The impact or effect of the embolus depends on the extent of pulmonary blood flow obstruction, the size of the affected vessels, the nature of the embolus, and the secondary effects. Pulmonary emboli can occur as any of the following:

1. Massive occlusion, an embolus that occludes a major portion of the pulmonary circulation (i.e., main pulmonary artery embolus)
2. Embolus with infarction, an embolus that is large enough to cause infarction (death) of a portion of lung tissue
3. Embolus without infarction, an embolus that is not severe enough to cause permanent lung injury
4. Multiple pulmonary emboli, which may be chronic or recurrent

Depending on its pattern of occurrence and severity, pulmonary embolism causes varying degrees of hypoxic vasoconstriction, pulmonary edema, decrease in surfactant, atelectasis, and release of neurohumoral substances such as histamine, serotonin, and thromboxane. The embolus also may cause systemic hypotension, decreased cardiac output, and pulmonary hypertension, which, when severe, results in acute right ventricular failure and death. The pathogenesis of pulmonary embolism due to a thrombus is summarized in Fig. 30-16.

If the embolus does not cause infarction, the clot is dissolved by the fibrinolytic system (see Chapter 24), and pulmonary function returns to normal. If pulmonary infarction occurs, shrinking and scarring develop in the affected area of the lung. (Infarction, or cellular death caused by lack of blood supply, is described in detail in Chapter 27.)

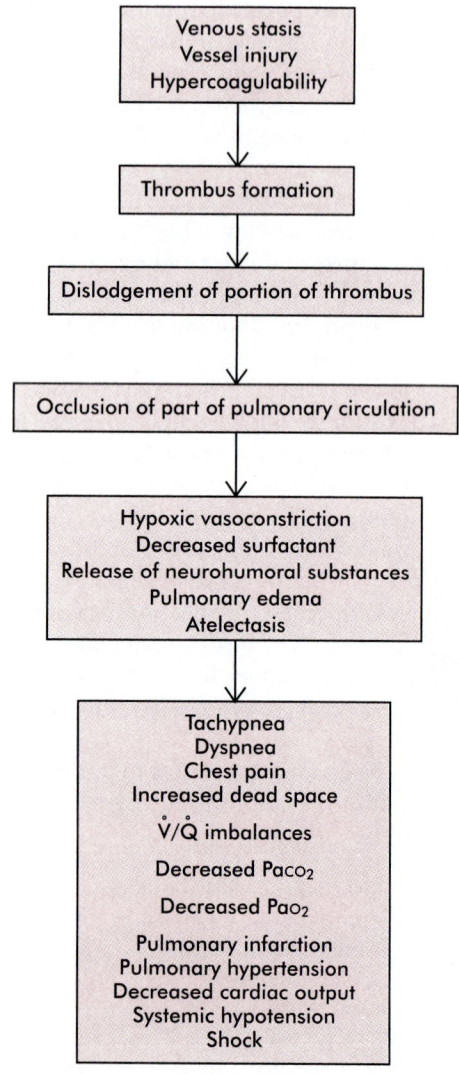

FIG. 30-16 Pathogenesis of massive pulmonary embolism caused by a thrombus (pulmonary thromboembolism).

Clinical Manifestations

In most cases the clinical manifestations of pulmonary embolism are nonspecific, so that evaluation of risk factors and predisposing factors is an important aspect of diagnosis. More than 90% of pulmonary emboli are the consequence of clots that were initially formed in the veins of the legs and pelvis (Kenasewitz, 1993). The characteristic signs of deep vein thrombosis are leg swelling, duskiness, and a positive Homans sign (calf pain on palpation and dorsiflexion of the foot). Sometimes the thrombus is palpable, but quite often the legs appear normal or signs are masked by superficial thrombophlebitis.

The clinical manifestations of pulmonary embolism vary, depending on its type. Massive occlusion causes profound shock, hypotension, tachypnea, tachycardia, severe pulmonary hypertension, and chest pain. Diagnosis can be difficult because the signs mimic those of other cardiopulmonary problems (Kinasewitz, 1993). Once these manifestations occur, death is imminent.

Manifestations of emboli that cause infarction are pleural pain, dyspnea, pleural friction rub, pleural effusion, hemoptysis, fever, and leukocytosis. On chest radiographs, the infarcted portion of the lung shows up as a nonspecific infiltrate in a classic wedge shape bordering the pleura. Pulmonary infarction is most likely in individuals with underlying pulmonary disease.

Pulmonary embolism without infarction is the most common type and is the most difficult to evaluate. The individual usually presents with tachypnea, tachycardia, dyspnea, and unexplained anxiety. Occasionally syncope (fainting) or pleural pain occurs. Recurrent pulmonary emboli occur in individuals who have had a history of previous emboli. Recurrent emboli may not be detected until progressive incapacitation, precordial pain, anxiety, dyspnea, and right ventricular enlargement are exhibited.

Evaluation and Treatment

Routine chest radiographs and pulmonary function tests are not definitive tests for pulmonary embolism. Pulmonary embolism is suggested if arterial blood gas analyses demonstrate unexplained hypoxemia and hyperventilation. A perfusion scan, in which lungs are scanned after injection of a radioactive substance into the venous circulation, may indicate embolism.

The ideal treatment for pulmonary embolism is prevention through risk factor analysis and elimination of predisposing factors for individuals at risk. (Risk factor analysis is described in Chapter 5.) Venous stasis in hospital patients is minimized by leg elevation, bed exercises, position changes, early postoperative ambulation, and pneumatic calf compression. Clot formation is also prevented by prophylactic low-dose anticoagulant therapy; less anticoagulant is required to prevent a clot than to treat one.

Anticoagulant therapy is the primary treatment for pulmonary embolism. Intravenous administration of heparin is begun immediately and is followed by oral doses of coumarin. If massive life-threatening embolism occurs, a fibrinolytic agent, such as streptokinase, is sometimes used. (Streptokinase is contraindicated for 10 days after surgery.)

Pulmonary Hypertension

Pulmonary hypertension is high blood pressure in the pulmonary arteries. Normally pulmonary artery pressure is lower than systemic artery pressure. Pulmonary hypertension is defined as a rise in pulmonary artery pressure (normally 15 to 18 mm Hg) of 5 to 10 mm Hg above normal.

Primary pulmonary hypertension is very rare. It has no known cause, usually occurs in women between the ages of 20 and 40, and may be hereditary in some cases. Primary pulmonary hypertension has a very poor prognosis: most individuals die within 5 years of diagnosis.

Secondary pulmonary hypertension is more common. It can be secondary to any respiratory or cardiovascular disorder that (1) increases the volume or pressure of blood entering the pulmonary arteries or (2) narrows or obstructs the pulmonary arteries. The first cause overloads the pulmonary circulation from without; the second elevates blood pressure by increasing resistance to flow within the lungs.

Pathophysiology

In primary hypertension, the small pulmonary arteries (arterioles) become narrow or obliterated as a result of hypertrophy (enlargement) of smooth muscle in the vessel walls and formation of fibrous lesions around the vessels. The mechanisms that cause these changes are not known. Vessel narrowing or obliteration increases resistance and causes the pulmonary hypertension. Pressures in the left ventricle, which receives blood from the lungs, remain normal, but high pressures generated in the lungs are transmitted to the right ventricle, which supplies the pulmonary arteries. Eventually the right ventricle fails. Right ventricular disease resulting from pulmonary hypertension is termed **cor pulmonale**. Oxygenation is not severely affected, although mild hypoxia and cyanosis do occur. Death eventually results from cor pulmonale. (Mechanisms of heart failure are described in Chapter 27.)

There are four causes of secondary pulmonary hypertension. The first is elevated left ventricular filling pressures, such as occur with coronary artery disease and mitral valve disease. When pressures on the left side of the heart are elevated, the pulmonary artery pressure rises proportionally to maintain normal blood flow. The second cause of secondary pulmonary hypertension is increased blood flow through the pulmonary circulation (left-to-right shunts), as occurs with a ventricular septal

FIG. 30-17 Pathogenesis of pulmonary hypertension and cor pulmonale.

defect or patent ductus arteriosus. (These congenital heart defects are discussed in Chapter 28.) The third cause is obliteration or obstruction of the pulmonary vascular bed by a pulmonary embolus, and the fourth is vasoconstriction of the vascular bed. Vasoconstriction is usually caused by hypoxemia, acidosis, or both.

Secondary pulmonary hypertension can be reversed if the primary disorder is resolved. If hypertension persists, hypertrophy occurs in the medial smooth muscle layer of the arterioles. The larger arteries stiffen, and hypertension progresses until pulmonary artery pressure equals systemic blood pressure. The result is right ventricular hypertrophy and eventual cor pulmonale. The pathogenesis of heart failure caused by secondary pulmonary hypertension is shown in Fig. 30-17.

Clinical Manifestations

Pulmonary hypertension may not be detected until pulmonary artery pressure is equal to systemic blood pressure. The symptoms are often masked by primary pulmonary or cardiovascular disease. The first indication of pulmonary hypertension is often an abnormality seen on a chest radiograph (enlarged right heart border) or an electrocardiogram that shows right ventricular hypertrophy. Manifestations of fatigue, chest discomfort, tachypnea, and dyspnea, particularly with exercise, are common.

Evaluation and Treatment

Diagnosis of pulmonary hypertension can be made only with right heart catheterization. The diagnosis of primary pulmonary hypertension is made when all other causes of hypertension, such as mitral stenosis (see Chapter 27), COPD, and pulmonary embolus, have been ruled out.

There is no effective treatment for primary pulmonary hypertension except lung transplantation, but supplemental oxygen, digitalis, and diuretics are used as palliatives. α-Blockers, vasodilators, β-receptor stimulants,

and prostaglandins are currently being evaluated, but none of these agents has been proved to affect mortality.

The most effective treatment for secondary pulmonary hypertension is treatment of the primary disorder. If the underlying cause is removed, pulmonary hypertension disappears. Once pulmonary hypertension has persisted long enough for hypertrophy of the medial smooth muscle layer to develop, however, as it does with chronic hypoxemia, it is no longer reversible. Treatment often includes supplemental oxygen to reverse hypoxic vasoconstriction. Diuretics and digitalis are used judiciously to treat right ventricular failure.

Cor Pulmonale

Cor pulmonale, also called pulmonary heart disease, consists of right ventricular enlargement (hypertrophy, dilatation, or both). It is secondary to pulmonary hypertension caused by disorders of the lungs or chest wall.

Pathophysiology

Cor pulmonale develops as pulmonary hypertension creates chronic pressure overload in the right ventricle similar to that created in the left ventricle by systemic hypertension. (Systemic hypertension is discussed in Chapter 27.) Pressure overload increases the work of the right ventricle and causes hypertrophy of the normally

FIG. 30-18 **Lip cancer.** Carcinoma of lower lip with central ulceration and raised, rolled borders. (From del Regato, Spjut, & Cox, 1985.)

STAGING OF LIP CANCER

Stage I

Primary tumor less than 2 cm; no palpable nodes

Stage II

Primary tumor 2 to 4 cm; no palpable nodes

Stage III

Primary tumor over 4 cm; metastatic lymph nodes

Stage IV

Large primary tumors; nodes fixed to mandible or
 distant metastases

thin-walled heart muscle. Acute hypoxemia, such as might occur with pneumonia, can exaggerate pulmonary hypertension and dilate the ventricle as well. Right ventricular filling pressures are normal until failure occurs. The right ventricle usually fails when pulmonary artery pressure equals systemic blood pressure.

Clinical Manifestations

The clinical manifestations of cor pulmonale may be obscured by primary respiratory disease and appear only during exercise testing. The heart appears normal at rest, but with exercise cardiac output falls and the electrocardiogram shows right ventricular hypertrophy. Chest pain is common. The pulmonary component of the second heart sound, which represents closure of the pulmonic valve, may be accentuated, and a pulmonic valve murmur also may be present. Tricuspid valve murmur may accompany the development of right ventricular failure.

Evaluation and Treatment

Diagnosis is made on the basis of physical examination, radiologic examination, and electrocardiogram or echocardiography, or both. Physical examination findings are often similar to those of chronic lung disease with dyspnea and distended neck veins. The goal of treatment for cor pulmonale is to decrease the workload of the right ventricle by lowering pulmonary artery pressure. Treatment is the same as that for pulmonary hypertension, and its success depends on reversal of the underlying lung disease.

Lip Cancer

Cancer of the lip is more prevalent in men, with 3000 new cases per year accounting for about 1% of all cancers in men (American Cancer Society [ACS], 1993). Chronic exposure to sun, wind, and cold over a period of years results in dryness, chapping, hyperkeratosis, and predisposition to malignancy. The lower lip is the most common site.

Pathophysiology

The most common form of lower lip cancer is termed exophytic. The lesion usually develops in the outer part of the lip along the vermilion border. The lip becomes thickened and evolves to an ulcerated center with a raised border (Fig. 30-18). Verrucous-type lesions are less common. They have an irregular surface, follow cracks in the lip, and tend to extend toward the inner surface. Squamous cell carcinoma is the most common cell type. Basal cell carcinoma does not develop unless there is extension beyond the mucous membrane or vermilion border of the lip.

Clinical Manifestations

Malignant lesions are often preceded by the development of a blister that evolves into a superficial ulceration. In some cases there is a history of recurrent scales that precede development of a bleeding ulceration. Metastases to the cervical lymph nodes have a low rate of occurrence (2% to 8%) and are more likely when the primary lesion is larger and exists for a longer period.

Evaluation and Treatment

Diagnosis is commonly made by clinical history and presentation of the lesion. Biopsy confirms the presence of malignant cells. The staging for lip cancer is summarized in the box above. Surgical excision is effective for smaller lesions. Larger lesions that require extensive resection may be followed by subsequent cosmetic surgeries. Interstitial irradiation and radioactive implants have been proved effective for control of primary lesions (Pigneaux, Richard, & LaGarde, 1979). The prognosis for recovery is excellent, and deaths are usually the result of inadequate treatment.

Laryngeal Cancer

Cancer of the larynx represents approximately 2% to 3% of all cancers in the United States. There are approximately 12,600 new cases per year, 10,000 of them in men (ACS, 1993). The risk of laryngeal cancer is increased by the amount of tobacco smoked; risk is further heightened with the combination of smoking and alcohol consumption. The highest incidence is in men between 50 and 75 years of age (Newell & Hong, 1991).

Pathophysiology

Carcinoma of the true vocal cords (glottis) is more common than that of the supraglottic structures (epiglottis, aryepiglottic folds, arytenoids, and false cords). Tumors of the subglottic area are rare. Squamous cell carcinoma is the most frequent cell type, although small cell carcinomas also occur (Fig. 30-19). Metastasis develops by spread to the draining lymph nodes, and distant metastasis, usually to the lung, is rare.

Clinical Manifestations

The presenting symptoms of laryngeal cancer include hoarseness, dyspnea, and cough. Progressive hoarseness is the most significant symptom and can result in voice loss. Dyspnea is rare in the case of supraglottic tumors, but can be severe in subglottic tumors. Cough occurs less commonly and may follow swallowing. Laryngeal pain or a sore throat is likely to be present with supraglottic lesions (Wang, 1990).

Evaluation and Treatment

Evaluation of the larynx includes external inspection and palpation of the larynx and the lymph nodes of the neck. Indirect laryngoscopy provides a stereoscopic view of the structure and movement of the larynx. A biopsy can also be obtained during this procedure. Direct laryngoscopy provides specific visualization of the tumor. Plain films of the larynx and computed tomography facilitate the identification of tumor boundaries and the degree of extension to surrounding tissue.

Radiation therapy has shown good results for early carcinoma of the vocal cords. Partial laryngectomies are the preferred treatment for small supraglottic and subglottic malignancies. Total laryngectomy is required when lesions are extensive and involve the cartilage.

Lung Cancer

Lung cancers (bronchogenic carcinomas) arise from the epithelium of the respiratory tract. As such, the term *lung cancer* excludes other pulmonary tumors, including sarcomas, lymphomas, blastomas, hematomas, and mesotheliomas. Lung cancer is an epidemic in the United States, with an estimated 170,000 new cases in 1993 (ACS, 1993) (see box on p. 1181). It is the most frequent cause of cancer death and is responsible for 6% of all deaths in the United States and, along with malignant melanoma, is the only major cancer type whose incidence is rapidly increasing (ACS, 1993; Fontana et al., 1991). Although there has been some slowing of deaths caused by lung cancer in men, the increase among women has been extraordinarily high. The lung cancer death rate for women is now higher than that of any other cancer because of increased cigarette smoking by women (ACS, 1993). Deaths of lung cancer appear at ages 35 to 44 years; a sharp increase occurs between the ages of 45 and 55, and the incidence rate continues to increase through ages 65 to 74, after which it levels off and decreases among the very old.

The most common cause of lung cancer is cigarette

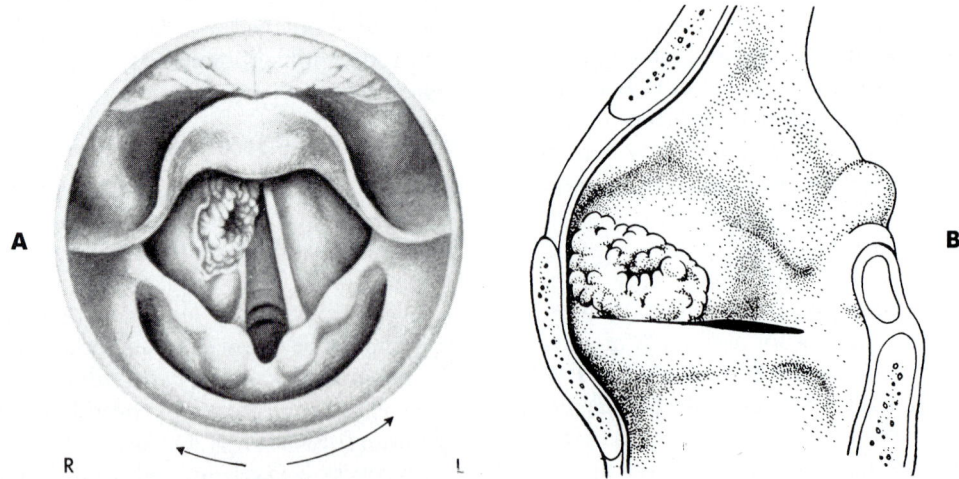

FIG. 30-19 Laryngeal cancer. **A,** Mirror view of carcinoma of right false cord partially hiding true cord; **B,** lateral view. (From del Regato, Spjut, & Cox, 1985.)

smoking. Heavy smokers have about 25 times greater chance of developing lung cancer than nonsmokers. Cigarette smoke contains several organ-specific carcinogens, and smoking has been causally related to carcinogenesis at several sites, including the larynx, oral cavity, esophagus, and urinary bladder. Genetic predisposition to developing lung cancer, which is evident in analysis of pedigrees, also plays a role in its pathophysiology (see Chapter 5).

The cancer death rates for pipe and cigar users are about equal to those of cigarette smokers for cancer of the larynx, oral cavity, and esophagus. The incidence of lung cancer decreases among people who stop smoking, and it reaches a level almost as low as that of nonsmokers 15 years after smoking has stopped. Theories of carcinogenesis are discussed in Chapter 11.

Environmental or occupational risk factors associated with lung cancer include benzopyrene and radon particles associated with uranium mining, radiation, and nuclear bombs. Others are polycyclic aromatic hydrocarbons and arsenicals, asbestos fibers, diesel exhaust, nitrogen mustard gases, nickel, silica, vinyl chloride, and chloromethyl methyl ether. Air pollution, coal, and iron mining are also considered risk factors (Matthews & Linniola, 1988).

Types of Lung Cancer

At least a dozen different cell types of tumors are included under the broad heading of lung cancer. The four major histologic types are squamous cell carcinoma, small cell carcinoma, large cell carcinoma, and adenocarcinoma (including bronchioloalveolar cell carcinoma). For clinical and therapeutic reasons, however, lung cancers are frequently classified in small cell lung cancer (SCLC, 25% of all lung cancers) and non-SCLC (NSCLC, 75% of all lung cancers). Characteristics of these tumors, including evaluation and treatment, are listed in Table 30-4. Some controversy exists as to the most frequently encountered cell type of bronchogenic carcinoma. In the past, squamous cell carcinoma was considered the most common type, but the incidence of adenocarcinoma is currently greater. Common sites of involvement for all four types of bronchogenic carcinoma are shown in Fig. 30-20. (Tumor biology is the subject of Chapter 10.)

Primary carcinomas of the lung and large metastatic tumors receive their blood supply from the bronchial arteries. The advancing tumor edge and small metastatic lesions receive their blood supply from the pulmonary circulation. Regional chemotherapeutic perfusion has not been very successful palliation for lung cancer (Hyde, 1992).

Squamous cell carcinoma

Squamous cell carcinoma accounts for about 30% of bronchogenic carcinomas, representing a sharp decline

IMPORTANT TRENDS FOR LUNG CANCER

Incidence

An estimated 170,000 new cases in 1993: 100,000 in males and 70,000 in females.

Mortality

An estimated 149,000 deaths in 1993: 93,000 in males and 56,000 in females. The death rate for women is now higher than that of any other cancer.

Risk Factors

Heavy cigarette smoking (more than 20 cigarettes/day) is the number one risk factor. Passive smoking (exposure to someone else's cigarette smoke) increases the risk of lung cancer. Occupational risk factors include exposure to asbestos dust, arsenic, chromium, nickel, ionizing radiation, chloromethyl ethers, coal products, mustard gas, and vinyl chloride. Cigarette smoking and exposure to asbestos may have a synergistic effect on the production of lung cancer.

Warning Signs

A persistent cough, sputum streaked with blood, chest pain, recurring attacks of pneumonia or bronchitis.

Early Detection and Prevention

Lung cancer is very difficult to detect early. If a smoker quits at the time of early cellular changes, altered bronchial lining often returns to normal. Periodic chest x-ray films and sputum cytologic analysis can detect presymptomatic, early-stage lung cancers, particularly of the squamous cell type; however, no conclusive evidence of reduction in lung cancer mortality as a consequence of screening has been found.

Treatment

Surgery, radiation therapy, and chemotherapy are all used. Surgery is usually the treatment of choice, and with improved ventilation machinery and antibiotics, surgical complications are infrequent. Tumor spread requiring chemotherapy or radiation therapy is evident in about one third of all surgical lung cancer patients.

Survival

Only 13% of white and black patients live 5 or more years after diagnosis. Non–small cell carcinomas are considered separately from small cell carcinomas (see text). Rates have improved only sightly over a recent 10-year period.

(From American Cancer Society. [1993]. Cancer statistics 1993. *Ca—A Cancer Journal for Clinicians*, 43[1].)

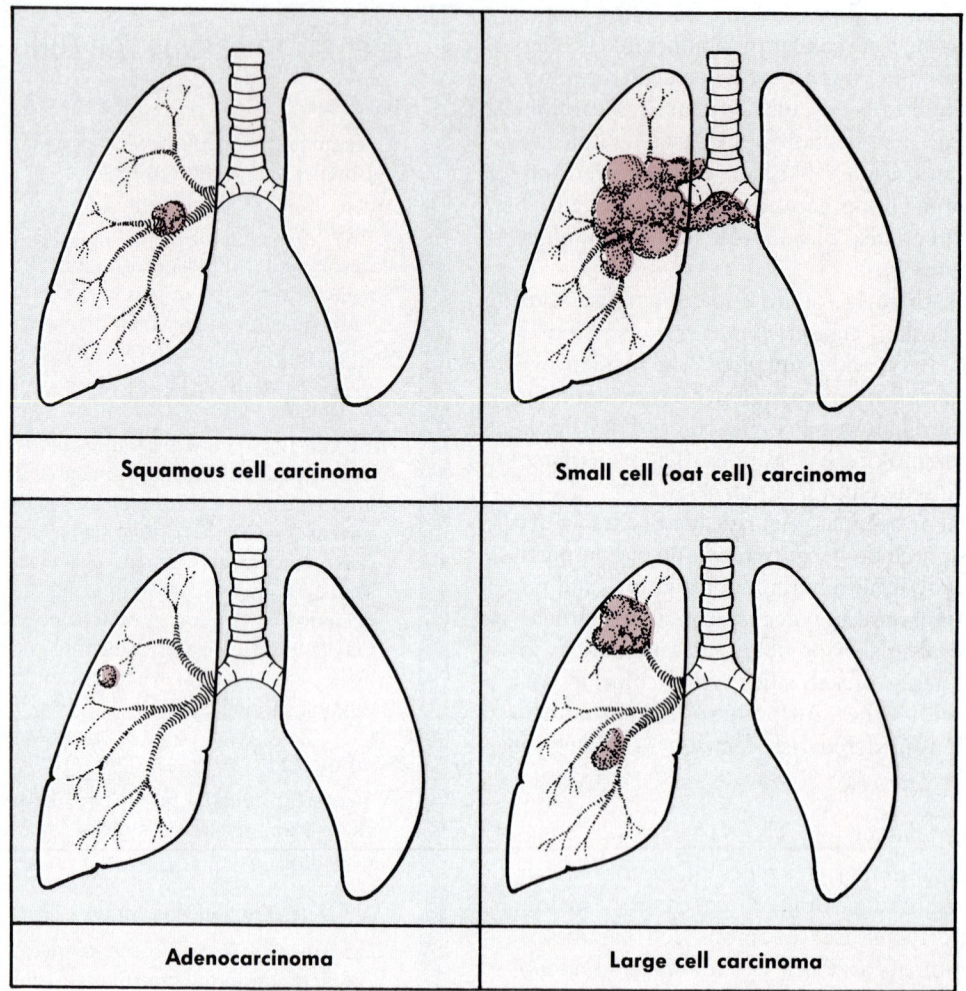

FIG. 30-20 Predominant sites of types of lung cancer. (Tumor characteristics are summarized in Table 30-4.)

in incidence in the past two decades. These tumors are typically located near the hilus and project into bronchi (Fig. 30-21).

Because of the location in the central bronchi, obstructive manifestations are nonspecific and include nonproductive cough. Pneumonia and atelectasis are often associated with squamous cell carcinoma (Fig. 30-21). Chest pain is a late symptom associated with large tumors. These tumors can remain fairly well localized and tend not to metastasize until late in the course of the disease. The preferred treatment is surgical resection, although once metastasis has taken place, total surgical resection is most difficult and survival rates dramatically decrease.

Small cell carcinoma

Small cell carcinomas constitute between 20% and 25% of bronchogenic carcinomas. It is estimated that most of these tumors are central in origin (Fig. 30-20). Cell

sizes range from 6 to 8 μm. When almost no cytoplasm is present (because of density of cells) and the cells are compressed into an ovoid mass, the tumor is called **oat cell carcinoma**. This cell type has the strongest correlation with cigarette smoking. Because these tumors show a rapid rate of growth and tend to metastasize early and widely, small cell carcinomas have the worst prognosis. The most frequent survival time for small cell carcinoma is between 9 and 10 months. Fewer than 5% of individuals are alive 2 years after diagnosis.

Small cell carcinoma is most often associated with ectopic hormone production, production of hormones by tumors of nonendocrine origin, or production of an inappropriate hormone by an endocrine gland. Neuroendocrine cells (NE cells) containing neurosecretory granules exist throughout the tracheobronchial tree (MacKay, Lukeman, & Ordonez, 1991). Ectopic hormone production is important to the clinician because resulting signs and symptoms may be the first manifes-

FIG. 30-21 **Lung cancer.** Bronchogenic carcinoma extending into a major bronchial airway. Bronchogenic squamous cell carcinoma arising in major bronchus. Tumor disrupts bronchial wall and extends into surrounding tissue. Pneumonia can be seen at periphery. (From Rosai, 1989.)

tation of the underlying cancer. Small cell carcinomas commonly produce gastrin-releasing peptide, calcitonin, arginine vasopressin, and adrenocorticotropic hormone (ACTH) (Matthews & Linnoila, 1988). As a result of ACTH secretion, lung cancer patients secrete large quantities of 17-hydroxysteroids and 17-ketosteroids, leading to the development of an atypical Cushing syndrome. Signs and symptoms related to this condition include muscular weakness, facial edema, hypokalemia, alkalosis, hyperglycemia, hypertension, and increased pigmentation. They are primarily treated with chemotherapy and radiation therapy with temporary remission.

Adenocarcinoma

Adenocarcinoma (tumor arising from glands) of the lung constitutes 30% to 35% of all bronchogenic carcinomas. The recent increase in incidence of adenocarcinoma has been ascribed to the increasing frequency of lung cancer in women, environmental and occupational carcinogens, and changes in the histologic criteria for diagnosis. These tumors, which are usually smaller than 4 cm, more commonly arise in the peripheral regions of the pulmonary parenchyma. They are asymptomatic

and discovered by routine chest roentgenogram in the early stages.

Included in the category of adenocarcinoma is bronchioloalveolar cell carcinoma. These tumors tend to arise from the terminal bronchioles and alveoli. They are slow-growing tumors with an unpredictable pattern of metastasis. Metastasis occurs through the pulmonary arterial system and mediastinal lymph nodes (MacKay et al., 1991). This cell type has the weakest association with smoking.

Surgical resection is possible in a high proportion of cases, but because metastasis occurs early, the 5-year survival rate is less than 10%. Neither chemotherapy nor radiation therapy has, as yet, increased the survival rate.

Large cell carcinoma (undifferentiated)

Undifferentiated large cell carcinomas constitute between 10% and 15% of bronchogenic carcinomas. This cell type has lost all evidence of differentiation and is therefore commonly referred to as **undifferentiated large cell anaplastic cancer.** Because large cell carcinomas show none of the histologic findings of squamous cell carcinoma or adenocarcinoma, this type is diagnosed by a process of exclusion. The cells are generally larger than leukocytes and contain large, darkly stained nuclei. These tumors commonly arise peripherally but are found centrally and can grow to distort the trachea and cause widening of the carina.

Once metastasis has occurred, surgical therapy is limited to palliative procedures (comfort measures) designed to relieve obstructive pneumonitis or prevent recurrence of pleural effusion. Neither radiation therapy nor chemotherapy has been successful in increasing survival.

Pathogenesis

A number of investigators have stressed that at sites of segmental bronchial bifurcations airflow and mucus production are altered and bronchial epithelium becomes very susceptible to injury (Matthews & Linnoila, 1988). It is proposed that carcinogenic agents are likely to be deposited and absorbed in these areas. Saccomanno and others (1971), who studied uranium miners, reported that metaplastic squamous cells were replaced in a progressive manner over time by dysplastic, in situ, and invasive neoplastic cells.

The single most important risk factor in lung cancer is tobacco smoke. The effects of smoking include structural, functional, malignant, and toxic changes. DNA-mutating agents in cigarettes produce alterations in both oncogenes and tumor-suppressor genes (Carbone, 1992). For example, there are specific central nervous system receptor sites for nicotine that produce an opiatelike state (Smoking & Health, 1979). Individuals with lung cancer demonstrate bronchial epithelial changes progressing from squamous cell alteration or metaplasia to carcinoma in situ. Histologic changes are evident with bronchitis and emphysema. Thickening of the bronchial epithelium, mucous gland hypertrophy, and alveolar cell rupture occur more frequently in smokers that nonsmokers. Cigarette smokers also have altered alveolar macrophage functions or phagocytosis, which may increase the risk of pulmonary infections.

Clinical Manifestations

Symptoms of early-stage, localized disease are nonspecific and are likely to be attributed by the individual to the effects of smoking. The clinical manifestations are ambiguous and insidious; they include coughing, sputum production, hemoptysis, pneumonia, airway obstruction, and pleural effusions. Table 30-4 summarizes the clinical manifestations according to tumor type. By the time there are manifestations severe enough to mo-

TABLE 30-4

Characteristics of Lung Cancers

Tumor type	Growth rate	Metastasis	Means of diagnosis	Clinical manifestations and treatment
Squamous cell carcinoma	Slow	Late; mostly to hilar lymph nodes	Biopsy, sputum analysis, bronchoscopy, electron microscopy, immunohistochemistry	Cough, sputum production, airway obstruction; treated surgically
Small cell (oat cell) carcinoma	Very rapid	Very early; to mediastinum or distally in lung	Radiography, sputum analysis, bronchoscopy, electron microscopy, immunohistochemistry, and clinical manifestations (cough, chest pain, dyspnea, hemoptysis, localized wheezing)	Airway obstruction caused by pneumonitis, signs and symptoms of excessive hormone secretion; treated by chemotherapy and ionizing radiation to thorax and central nervous system
Adenocarcinoma	Moderate	Early	Radiography, fiber-optic bronchoscopy, electron microscopy	Pleural effusion; treated surgically
Large cell carcinoma	Rapid	Early and widespread	Sputum analysis, bronchoscopy, electron microscopy (by exclusion of other cell types)	Chest wall pain, pleural effusion, cough, sputum production, hemoptysis, airway obstruction caused by pneumonia (if airways involved); treated surgically

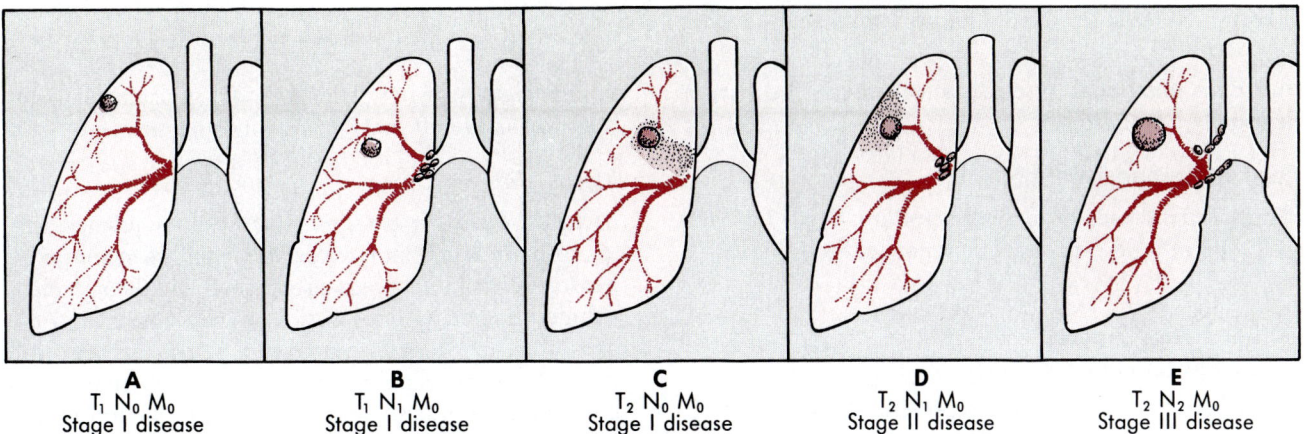

A	**B**	**C**	**D**	**E**
$T_1 N_0 M_0$	$T_1 N_1 M_0$	$T_2 N_0 M_0$	$T_2 N_1 M_0$	$T_2 N_2 M_0$
Stage I disease	Stage I disease	Stage I disease	Stage II disease	Stage III disease

FIG. 30-22 **Staging of lung cancer by the TNM classification system. A** and **B,** Stage I disease includes tumors classified at T_1, with or without metastasis to the lymph nodes in the ipsilateral hilar region. **C,** Also included in stage I are tumors classified as T_2, but having no nodal or distant metastases. **D,** Stage II disease includes those tumors classified as T_2, with metastasis only to the ipsilateral hilar lymph nodes. **E,** Stage III includes all tumors more extensive than T_2, or any tumor with metastasis to the lymph nodes in the mediastinum or with distant metastasis.

TABLE 30-5

TNM Classification of Lung Cancer

Symbol	Definition
Primary tumors (T)	
T_0	No evidence of primary tumor
T_x	Presence of tumor proved by malignant cells in bronchopulmonary secretions but not visualized by x-ray films or bronchoscopy
T_{is}	Carcinoma in situ
T_1	Tumor 3.0 cm or less in diameter, surrounded by lung or visceral pleura, no evidence of invasion proximal to a lobar bronchus at bronchoscopy
T_2	Tumor more than 3.0 cm in diameter, or a tumor of any size that invades the visceral pleura or has associated atelectasis or obstructive pneumonitis to the hilar regions
T_3	Tumor of any size with direct extension into an adjacent structure, such as chest wall, diaphragm, or mediastinum; or tumor demonstrated bronchoscopically to involve a main bronchus less than 2.0 cm to the carina; any tumor associated with atelectasis or obstructive pneumonitis of an entire lung or pleural effusion
T_4	Tumor of any size with invasion of the mediastinum or involvement of heart, great vessels, trachea, esophagus, vertebral body, carina, or presence of malignant pleural effusion
Lymph node involvement (N)	
N_0	No demonstrable metastasis to regional lymph nodes
N_1	Metastasis to nodes in the peribronchial and/or ipsilateral hilar region
N_2	Metastasis to ipsilateral lymph nodes within the mediastinum
N_3	Metastasis to contralateral mediastinal or hilar lymph nodes, or contralateral ipsilateral scalene or supraclavicular nodes
Metastasis (M)	
M_0	No distant metastasis
M_1	Distant metastasis, such as to scalene or contralateral hilar lymph nodes, brain, bones, lung, liver

tivate the individual to seek medical advice, the disease is usually advanced.

Evaluation and Treatment

The specific means of diagnosis and treatment for each cell type of lung cancer are summarized in Table 30-4.

Other Lung Cancers

Bronchial Carcinoid Tumors

Bronchial carcinoid tumors represent about 1% of all lung tumors. The tumor cells have dense granules containing neuroendocrinelike hormones, but they rarely produce endocrine symptoms (carcinoid syndrome) (MacKay et al., 1991).

Carcinoid tumors tend to occur earlier in life than bronchogenic carcinoma. The average age at diagnosis is about 45 years and they are not related to smoking. The tumors arise more commonly in the main or segmental bronchi, are easily visualized bronchoscopically, and are found on routine chest radiographs. Cells are not recovered from bronchial washings because the tumor is covered with normal mucosa. These tumors are slow-growing cancers, so that 50% of individuals with bronchial carcinoid tumors are asymptomatic. Local surgical resection is curative if metastasis has not occurred (Marchevsky, 1990).

Adenocystic tumors (cylindromas) and **mucoepidermoid carcinomas** are rare bronchial gland tumors. They predominately arise in the trachea or large airways and cause obstruction. They can be malignant and metastasize early, although distal pulmonary metastases are usually slow-growing. Thus it is not unusual for a patient to survive 10 to 15 years after diagnosis.

Mesotheliomas

Mesotheliomas are benign or malignant sarcomas arising from the epithelium covering the serous membranes. Most arise from the pleural surface (80%). Benign pleural mesotheliomas have a slow clinical onset and are usually asymptomatic, but over a period of years can cause dyspnea and mild pleuritic pain. These tumors can grow to be very large and fill the entire pleural cavity. Mesotheliomas are more likely to be malignant than benign. Survival for diffuse untreated mesothelioma is approximately 1 year.

Recently of more concern is the reported excess incidence of malignant mesotheliomas in asbestos workers (Antman & Corson, 1985). Some individuals develop mesothelioma after minimal asbestos exposure. A long latent interval between exposure to asbestos and appearance of mesothelioma usually occurs, and onset of symptoms may take 20 to 30 years (MacKay et al., 1991).

Staging of Lung Cancer

The histologic cell type and the stage of the disease are the major factors that influence choice of therapy for patients. The current accepted system for the staging of lung cancer is the **TNM classification** (Table 30-5). This system is a code in which *T* denotes the extent of the primary tumor, *N* indicates the nodal involvement, and *M* describes the extent of metastasis. Staging of lung cancer is illustrated in Fig. 30-22.

SUMMARY REVIEW

Clinical Manifestations of Pulmonary Alterations

1 Dyspnea is the feeling of breathlessness and increased respiratory effort.
2 Abnormal breathing patterns are adjustments made by the body to minimize the work of respiratory muscles. They include Kussmaul, obstructed, restricted, gasping, and Cheyne-Stokes respirations, and sighing.
3 Hypoventilation is decreased alveolar ventilation caused by airway obstruction, chest wall restriction, or altered neurologic control of breathing. Hypoventilation causes increased $Paco_2$.
4 Hyperventilation is increased alveolar ventilation produced by anxiety, head injury, or severe hypoxemia. Hyperventilation causes decreased $Paco_2$.
5 Coughing is a protective reflex that expels secretions and irritants from the lower airways.
6 Hemoptysis is expectoration of bloody mucus, which can be caused by bronchitis, tuberculosis, abscess, neoplasms, and other conditions that cause hemorrhage from damaged vessels.
7 Cyanosis is a bluish discoloration of the skin caused by desaturation of hemoglobin, polycythemia, or peripheral vasoconstriction.
8 Chest pain can result from inflamed pleurae, trachea, bronchi, or respiratory muscles.
9 Clubbing of the fingertips is associated with diseases that interfere with oxygenation of the tissues.
10 Hypoxemia is a reduced Pao_2 caused by (a) decreased oxygen content of inspired gas, (b) hypoventilation, (c) diffusion abnormality, (d) ventilation-perfusion mismatch, or (e) shunting.

11 Pulmonary edema is excess water in the lung caused by disturbances of capillary hydrostatic pressure, capillary oncotic pressure, or capillary permeability. A common cause is left heart failure that increases the hydrostatic pressure in the pulmonary circulation.

12 Atelectasis is the collapse of alveoli resulting from compression of lung tissue or absorption of gas from obstructed alveoli.

13 Bronchiectasis is abnormal dilatation of the bronchi secondary to another pulmonary disorder, usually infection or inflammation.

14 Pneumothorax is the accumulation of air in the pleural space. It can be caused by spontaneous rupture of weakened areas of a pleura or secondary to pleural damage caused by disease, trauma, or mechanical ventilation.

15 Pleural effusion is the accumulation of fluid in the pleural space, usually resulting from disorders that promote transudation or exudation from capillaries underlying the pleura, but occasionally from blockage or injury that causes lymphatic vessels to drain into the pleural space.

16 Empyema is the presence of pus in the pleural space (infected pleural effusion). The source of the pus is usually lymphatic drainage from sites of bacterial pneumonia.

17 Pleurisy is inflammation of the pleura.

18 Pulmonary fibrosis is an excessive amount of connective tissue in the lung. It diminishes lung compliance and may be idiopathic or caused by disease.

19 Chest wall compliance is diminished by obesity and kyphoscoliosis, which compress the lungs, and by neuromuscular diseases that impair chest wall muscle function.

20 Flail chest results from rib or sternal fractures that disrupt the mechanics of breathing.

21 Inhalation of noxious gases or prolonged exposure to high concentrations of oxygen can damage the bronchial mucosa or alveolocapillary membrane and cause inflammation or acute respiratory failure.

22 Pneumoconiosis, which is caused by inhalation of dust particles in the workplace, can cause pulmonary fibrosis, susceptibility to lower airway infection, and tumor formation.

23 Allergic alveolitis is an allergic or hypersensitivity reaction to many allergens.

24 Bronchiolitis is the inflammatory obstruction of small airways. It is most common in children.

Pulmonary Disorders

1 Acute respiratory failure is caused by inadequate gas exchange or ventilation (Pao_2 equal to or less than 50 mm Hg or $Paco_2$ equal to or greater than 50 mm Hg and pH equal to or less than 7.25).

2 Adult respiratory distress syndrome (ARDS) results from an acute, diffuse injury to the alveolocapillary membrane and decreased surfactant production, which increases membrane permeability and causes edema and atelectasis.

3 Postoperative respiratory failure is most common in surgical patients who smoke or have chronic disease.

4 Obstructive pulmonary disease is characterized by airway obstruction that causes difficult expiration. Obstructive disease can be acute or chronic in nature and includes asthma, chronic bronchitis, and emphysema.

5 In asthma obstruction is caused by episodic attacks of bronchospasm, bronchial inflammation, mucosal edema, and increased mucus production.

6 Extrinsic asthma is caused by an immune response to allergens or other irritants.

7 Intrinsic asthma is not caused by allergens and occurs in adults older than age 35.

8 A local imbalance between the parasympathetic and sympathetic divisions of the autonomic nervous system is thought to facilitate bronchospasm in individuals with intrinsic asthma.

9 Chronic bronchitis causes airway obstruction resulting from bronchial smooth muscle hypertrophy and production of thick, tenacious mucus.

10 In emphysema destruction of the alveolar septa and loss of passive elastic recoil lead to airway collapse and obstruct gas flow during expiration.

11 Emphysema in which septal deterioration is caused by α_1-antitrypsin deficiency or old age tends to be panacinar.

12 Emphysema in which septal deterioration results from smoking tends to be centriacinar.

13 Chronic obstructive pulmonary disease (COPD) is the coexistence of chronic bronchitis and emphysema.

14 Upper respiratory tract infections, which are the most common cause of short-term disability in the United States, include rhinitis (the common cold), pharyngitis, and laryngitis.

15 Serious lower respiratory tract infections, which occur most frequently in the very old and individuals with impaired immunity or underlying disease, include pneumonia and tuberculosis.

16 Pneumococcal pneumonia is an acute lung infection resulting in an inflammatory response with four phases: (a) consolidation, (b) red hepatization, (c) gray hepatization, and (d) resolution.

17 Viral pneumonia is an acute, self-limiting lung infection usually caused by the influenza virus.

18 Tuberculosis is a lung infection caused by *Mycobacterium tuberculosis* (tubercle bacillus).

19 In tuberculosis the inflammatory response proceeds to isolate colonies of bacilli by enclosing them in tubercles and surrounding the tubercles with scar tissue.

20 Bacilli may remain dormant within the tubercles for life or, if the immune system breaks down, cause recurrence of active disease.

21 Pulmonary vascular diseases are caused by embolism or hypertension in the pulmonary circulation.

22 Pulmonary embolism is occlusion of a portion of the pulmonary vascular bed by a thrombus (most common), tissue fragment, or air bubble. Depending on its size and location, the embolus can cause hypoxic vasoconstriction, pulmonary edema, atelectasis, pulmonary hypertension, shock, and even death.

23 Pulmonary hypertension (pulmonary artery pressure 5 to 10 mm Hg above normal) is caused by (a) elevated left ventricular pressure, (b) increased blood flow through the pulmonary circulation, (c) obliteration or obstruction of the vascular bed, or (d) active constriction of the vascular bed produced by hypoxemia or acidosis.

24 Cor pulmonale is right ventricular enlargement caused by chronic pulmonary hypertension. Cor pulmonale progresses to right ventricular failure if the pulmonary hypertension is not reversed.

25 Lip cancer is most common in men and represents about 1% of all cancers. In the most common cell type, squamous cell, metastasis is rare when lesions are diagnosed and treated early.

26 Laryngeal cancer occurs primarily in men and represents 2% to 3% of all cancers. Squamous cell carcinoma of the true vocal cords is most common and presents with a clinical symptom of progressive hoarseness.

27 Lung cancer, the most frequent cause of cancer death in the United States, is commonly caused by cigarette smoking.

28 Cancer cell types include squamous cell carcinoma, small cell (oat cell) carcinoma, adenocarcinoma, large cell carcinoma, bronchial adenoma, and mesothelioma. Each type arises in a characteristic site or type of tissue, causes distinctive clinical manifestations, and differs in likelihood of metastasis and prognosis.

29 Bronchial carcinoid and adenocystic tumors are rare tumors of the bronchial airways.

KEY TERMS

Abscess, 1159

Absorption atelectasis, 1155

Adenocarcinoma, 1183

Adenocystic tumor (cylindroma), 1186

Adult respiratory distress syndrome (ARDS), 1162

Asbestosis, 1161

Aspiration, 1154

Asthma, 1165

Atelectasis, 1155

Bronchial carcinoid tumor, 1186

Bronchiectasis, 1156

Bronchiolitis, 1156

Bronchitis, 1167

Bronchopneumonia, 1174

Bronchospasm, 1165

Cavitation, 1159

Centriacinar (centrilobular) emphysema, 1171

Cheyne-Stokes respirations, 1150

Chronic obstructive pulmonary disease (COPD), 1165

Clubbing, 1151

Coal worker pneumoconiosis (coal miner lung, black lung), 1161

Compression atelectasis, 1155

Consolidation, 1159

Cor pulmonale, 1177

Cough, 1150

Cyanosis, 1151

Cylindrical bronchiectasis, 1156

Dyspnea, 1149

Emphysema, 1169

Empyema (infected pleural effusion), 1158

Extrinsic allergic alveolitis (hypersensitivity pneumonitis), 1162

Extrinsic asthma (atopic or allergic asthma), 1166

Exudative effusion, 1158

Flail chest, 1160

Hemoptysis, 1150

Hemothorax, 1158

Hypercapnia, 1150

Hyperventilation, 1150

Hypocapnia, 1150

Hypoventilation, 1150

Hypoxemia, 1152

Hypoxia, 1152

Intrinsic asthma (nonatopic asthma), 1166

Kussmaul respiration (hyperpnea), 1150

Lobar pneumonia, 1174

Mesothelioma, 1186

Mucoepidermoid carcinoma, 1186

Oat cell carcinoma, 1182

Open pneumothorax (communicating pneumothorax), 1157

Orthopnea (positional dyspnea), 1149

Oxygen toxicity, 1160

Panacinar (panlobular) emphysema, 1171

Paroxysmal nocturnal dyspnea (PND), 1149

Pleural effusion, 1158

Pleurisy (pleuritis), 1159

Pneumoconiosis, 1160

Pneumonia, 1172

Pneumothorax, 1156

Pulmonary edema, 1153

Pulmonary embolism, 1176

Pulmonary fibrosis, 1159

Pulmonary thromboembolism, 1176

Saccular bronchiectasis, 1156

Silicosis, 1161

Small cell carcinoma, 1182

Squamous cell carcinoma, 1181

Status asthmaticus, 1167

Tension pneumothorax, 1157

TNM classification, 1186

Transudative effusion, 1158

Tuberculosis, 1174

Undifferentiated large cell carcinoma (undifferentiated large cell anaplastic cancer), 1183

Varicose bronchiectasis, 1156

REFERENCES

American Cancer Society (ACS). (1993). Cancer statistics 1993. *Ca—A Cancer Journal for Clinicians, 43*(1).

American Thoracic Society (ATS). (1990). Diagnostic standards and classification of tuberculosis. *American Review of Respiratory Diseases, 142*(3), 725-735.

Antman, K. H., & Corson. J. M. (1985). Benign and malignant pleural mesotheliomas. *Clinics in Chest Medicine, 6,* 127.

Berman, J. S., & Weller, P. F. (1992). Airway eosinophils and lymphocytes in asthma: Birds of a feather? *American Review of Respiratory Disease, 145*(6), 1246-1248.

Bloom, B. R., & Murray, C. J. L. (1992). Tuberculosis: Commentary on a recurrent killer. *Science, 257,* 1055-1078.

Carbone, D. (1992). Smoking and cancer. *American Journal of Medicine, 93*(Suppl. 1A), 135-175.

Dal Nogare, A. R. (1989). Southwestern internal medicine conference: Adult respiratory distress syndrome. *The American Journal of the Medical Sciences, 298*(6), 413-430.

del Regato, J. A., Spjut, H. J., & Cox, J. D. (1985). *Ackerman and del Regato's cancer* (2nd ed.). St. Louis: Mosby—Year Book.

Drugs for tuberculosis. (1992). *The Medical Letter on Drugs and Therapeutics, 34*(863), 10-12.

Dutt, A. K., & Stead, W. W. (1993). Tuberculosis in the elderly. In D. A. Mahler (Ed.), *Pulmonary disease in the elderly.* New York: Marcel Dekker.

Fontana, R. S., Saunderson, D. R., Woolner, L. B., Taylor, W. F., Miller, E. W., Muhm, J. R., Bernatz, P. E., Payne, S. W., Pairdero, P. C., & Bergstralh, E. J. (1991). Screening for lung cancer. *Cancer, 67,* 1155-1164.

Hankins, G. D. V. (1990). Acute respiratory failure. *Clinical Obstetrics and Gynecology, 33*(3), 493-501.

Hyde, R. W. (1992). Circulation of lung neoplasms. In J Butler (Ed.), *The bronchial circulation* (pp. 551-578). New York: Marcel Dekker, Inc.

Janus, E. D., Philipps, N. T., & Carrell, R. N. (1985). Smoking, lung function, and alpha-1-antitrypsin deficiency. *Lancet, 1*(8421), 152.

Jereb, J. A., Kelly, G. D., Dooley, S. W., Cauther, G. M., & Snider, D. E., Jr. (1991). Tuberculosis morbidity in the United States: Final data, 1990. In CDC surveillance summaries, Dec 1991, *MMWR* 1991:40(No. SS-3), 23-27.

Kinasewitz, G. T. (1993). Thromboembolism in the elderly. In D. A. Mahler (Ed.), *Pulmonary disease in the elderly.* New York: Marcel Dekker.

Kissane, J. M. (Ed.). (1990). *Anderson's pathology* (9th ed.). St. Louis: Mosby—Year Book.

Lankin, P. N. (1990). New therapeutic approaches for ARDS. *Hospital Practice,* October 30, 42-45.

Leatherman, J. W., & Ingram, R. J. (1992). 14 respiratory medicine: II asthma. In E. Rubenstein & D. D. Federman (Eds.), *Scientific American medicine.* New York: Scientific American, Inc.

Lee, T. H. (1992). Airway inflammation in asthma: Conclusions and summary. *American Review of Respiratory Disease, 145*(2, Part 2), S58.

MacKay, B., Lukeman, J. M., & Ordonez, N. G. (1991). *Tumors of the lungs.* Philadelphia: Saunders.

Mahler, D. A. (1993). Chronic obstructive pulmonary disease. In D. A. Mahler (Ed.), *Pulmonary disease in the elderly.* New York: Marcel Dekker.

Marchevsky, A. M. (1990). Neuroendocrine tumors of the lung. In A. M. Marchevsky (Ed.), *Surgical pathology of lung neoplasms* (pp. 247-288). New York: Marcel Dekker.

Matthews, M. J., & Linnoila, R. I. (1988). Pathology of lung cancer. An update. In J. D. Britan, H. M. Golomb, A. G. Little (Eds.), *Lung cancer: A comprehensive treatise.* New York: Grune & Stratton.

McFadden, E. R., Jr. (1991). Asthma. In J. D. Wilson, E. Braunwald, K. J. Isselbacher, R. G. Petersdorf, J. B. Martin, A. S. Fauci, & R. K. Root (Eds.), *Harrison's principles of internal medicine* (12th ed., vol. 2). New York: McGraw-Hill.

McFadden, E. R., Jr., & Gilbert, I. A. (1992). Asthma. *New England Journal of Medicine, 327,* 1928-1937.

Morris, M. T. (1992). Adult respiratory distress syndrome. In V. Huddleston (Ed.), *Multisystem organ failure: Pathophysiology and clinical implications.* St. Louis: Mosby—Year Book.

Neuhof, H. (1991). Actions and interactions of mediator systems and mediators in the pathogenesis of ARDS and multiorgan failure. *Acta Anaesthesiologica Scandinavica, 35*(95S), 7-14.

Newell, G. R., & Hong, W. K. (1991). *The biology and prevention of aerodigestive tract cancers.* New York: Plenum Press.

Pigneaux, J., Richard, P. M., & LaGarde, C. (1979). The place of interstitial therapy using 192 iridium in the management of carcinoma of the lip. *Cancer, 43,* 1073-1077.

Rachelefsky, G. S. (1992). The inflammatory response in asthma. *American Family Physician, 45*(1), 153-160.

Raffin, T. A. (1987, Nov. 15). ARDS: Mechanisms and management. *Hospital Practice,* 65-80.

Rinaldo, J. E., & Christman, J. W. (1990). Mechanisms and mediators of the adult respiratory distress syndrome. *Clinics in Chest Medicine, 11*(4), 621-632.

Rosai, J. (1989). *Ackerman's surgical pathology* (7th ed.). St. Louis: Mosby—Year Book.

Saccomanno, G., Archer, V. E., Auerbach, O., Kuschner, M., Saunders, R. P., & Klein, M. P. (1971). Histologic types of lung cancer among uranium miners. *Cancer, 27,* 515-523.

Scanlan, C. L., & Gupta, T. L. (1990). Synopsis of cardiopulmonary diseases. In C. L. Scanlan, C. B. Spearman, & R. L. Sheldon (Eds.), *Egan's fundamentals of respiratory care* (5th ed.). St. Louis: Mosby—Year Book.

Seidel, H. M., Ball, J. W., Dains, J. E., & Benedict, G. W. (1991). *Mosby's guide to physical examination* (2nd ed.). St. Louis: Mosby—Year Book.

Smoking and Health. (1979). A report of the surgeon general. Rockville, Md.: U.S. Department of Health, Education, and Welfare (DHEW).

Snider, G. L., Kleinerman, J., Thurlbeck, W. M., & Bengali, Z. H. (1985). The definition of emphysema. Report of a national heart, lung, blood institute, division of lung diseases workshop. *American Review of Respiratory Diseases, 132*(1), 182.

Wang, C. C. (1990). *Radiation therapy for head and neck neoplasms.* Chicago: Year Book Medical Publishers.

SUGGESTED READINGS

Bardana, E. J. (1992). What characterizes allergic asthma? *Annals of Allergy, 68*(5), 371-373.

Burrows, B., Martinez, F. D., Halonen, M., Barbee, R. A., & Cline, M. G. (1989, February). Association of asthma with serum IgE levels and skin-test reactivity to allergens. *New England Journal of Medicine, 310*(5), 271-277.

Busse, W. W., & Sedgwick, J. B. (1992). Eosinophils in asthma. *Annals of Allergy, 68*(3), 286-290.

Campbell, E. J. M., & Guz, A. (1981). Breathlessness. In T. F. Hornbein (Ed.), *Regulation of breathing, part 2.* New York: Marcel Dekker.

Carrieri, V. K., & Janson-Bjerklie, S. (1986). Dyspnea. In V. K. Carrieri, A. M. Lindsey, & C. M. West (Eds.), *Pathophysiological phenomena in nursing: Human responses to illness.* Philadelphia: Saunders.

Cherniack, N. S. (1988). Chest pain. In J. F. Murray & J. A. Nadel (Eds.), *Textbook of respiratory medicine* (vol. 1). Philadelphia: Saunders.

Cherniack, N. S. (1988). Dyspnea. In J. F. Murray & J. A. Nadel (Eds.), *Textbook of respiratory medicine* (vol. 1). Philadelphia: Saunders.

Colice, G. L. (1986). Pulmonary edema. *Clinical Geriatric Medicine, 2*(2), 411-432.

Elliot, C. G. (1990). Pulmonary sequelae in survivors of the adult respiratory distress syndrome. *Clinics in Chest Medicine, 11*(4), 789-800.

Flick, M. R. (1988). Pulmonary edema and acute lung injury. In J. F. Murray & J. A. Nadel (Eds.), *Textbook of respiratory medicine* (vol. 2). Philadelphia: Saunders.

Fox, C. W., & George, R. B. (1992). Current concepts in the management and prevention of tuberculosis. *Journal Louisiana State Medical Society 144*(8):363-368.

Fracica, P. J., Piantadosi, C. A., & Crapo, J. D. (1991). Oxygen toxicity. In R. G. Crystal & J. B. West (Eds.), *The lung: Scientific foundations* (vol. 2). New York: Raven Press.

Goldsmith, M. F. (1992). Medical exorcism required as revitalized remnant of tuberculosis haunts and harries the land. *Journal of the American Medical Association, 268*(2), 174-175.

Goldstein, G., & Luce, J. M. (1990). Pharmacologic treatment of the adult respiratory distress syndrome. *Clinics in Chest Medicine, 11*(4), 773-787.

Heim, C. R., & Des Prez, R. M. (1986). Pulmonary embolism: A review. *Advances in Internal Medicine, 31,* 187-212.

Killian, K. J., & Campbell, E. J. M. (1991). Dyspnea. In R. G. Crystal & J. B. West (Eds.), *The lung: Scientific foundations* (vol. 2). New York: Raven Press.

McCord, M., & Cronin-Stubbe, D. (1992). Operationalizing dyspnea: Focus on measurement. *Heart & Lung, 21*(2), 167-179.

McFadden, E. P., Jr., & Gilbert, I. A. (1992). Asthma. *New England Journal of Medicine 327*(27),1928-1937.

Murray, J. F., Matthay, M. A., Luce, J. M., & Flick, M. R. (1988). An expanded definition of the adult respiratory distress syndrome. *American Review of Respiratory Disease, 138*(Sept), 720-723.

Piper, P. J., & Krell, R. D. (1991). Advances in the understanding and treatment of asthma. *Annals of the New York Academy of Sciences* (vol. 629). New York: New York Academy of Sciences.

Platts-Mills, T. A. E. (1992). Mechanisms of bronchial reactivity: The role of immunoglobulin E. *American Review of Respiratory Disease, 145*(2, Part 2), S44-S47.

Realy, A. M. (1990). Hyperinflation therapy. In C. L. Scanlan, C. B. Spearman, & R. L. Sheldon (Eds.), *Egan's fundamentals of respiratory care* (5th ed.). St. Louis: Mosby–Year Book.

Scanlan, C. L. (1990). Patterns of cardiopulmonary dysfunction. In C. L. Scanlan, C. B. Spearman, & R. L. Sheldon (Eds.), *Egan's fundamentals of respiratory care* (5th ed.). St. Louis: Mosby–Year Book.

Seale, D. D., & Beaver, B. M. (1992). Pathophysiology of lung cancer. *Nursing Clinics of North America, 27*(3), 603-613.

Snider, D. E., Jr., & Roper, W. L. (1992). The new tuberculosis. *New England Journal of Medicine, 326*(10), 703-705.

Strunk, R. (1992). Understanding asthma mortality. *Annals of Allergy, 68*(4), 291-292.

Tomashefski, J. F. (1990). Pulmonary pathology of the adult respiratory distress syndrome. *Clinics in Chest Medicine, 11*(4), 593-619.

West, J. B. (1992). *Pulmonary pathophysiology* (4th ed.). Philadelphia: Williams & Wilkins.

CHAPTER 31

Alterations of Pulmonary Function in Children

Sue E. Huether
Margaret M. Andrews*

Alterations of respiratory function in children are influenced by age, sex, race, genetic alterations, geographic location, season of the year, environmental conditions, and the presence of structural anomalies. Premature infants have immature lungs placing them at risk for respiratory failure. Both premature infants and newborns have limited abilities to form antibodies, increasing their vulnerability to respiratory infection, particularly viral pneumonia (Graham, 1990). The shorter and straighter eustachian tube and the smaller lumen of both the upper and lower airways of young children increase the incidence of otitis media and bronchiolitis. Asthma occurs during times of high pollen currents, and respiratory infections are more common in the winter when there is confinement and more crowded living conditions. Nutritional state, occurrence of other systemic diseases, environmental air pollution, and access to medical care are other variables important to the development of respiratory diseases in children.

STRUCTURE AND FUNCTION OF THE PULMONARY SYSTEM IN CHILDREN

There are a number of structural differences between mature and immature upper airways and lungs that influence the way in which children respond to respiratory disturbances. Children are less well equipped than adults to overcome pulmonary infections. Their airways are shorter and narrower from the trachea through the terminal bronchioles, so that a relatively small amount of mucus or mucosal edema can cause obstruction. The trachea bifurcates higher in infants than in adults (Fig. 31-1), the accessory muscles of respiration are not fully developed in infants, and respiratory and coughing efforts are not as effective or sustained. The upper airway is narrow, and its caliber may be reduced further by hypertrophied tonsils and adenoids, or by posterior displacement of the tongue, which diminishes airflow. Infants breathe primarily through the nose until they are about 4 weeks old.

All the conducting airways are present at birth and change only in size through adulthood. During the first 5 years of life, the respiratory tract grows longer, but the lumen remains narrow. Therefore, any obstruction of the airway greatly increases resistance to airflow and increases the work of breathing and oxygen requirements. Only after age 5 does lumen caliber increase. Infants do not have as many alveoli as older children and adults. There are only about 25 million alveoli at birth, and they are less complex than alveoli in an adult. The lack of development and the reduced number of pores of Kohn make collateral ventilation of alveoli less efficient than in adults. Until age 8, alveoli and their vascular supply multiply until there are several hundred million (approximately 300,000,000). The alveoli then increase in size and complexity through puberty.

Surfactant production is thought to begin during the twenty-fourth week of gestation. Production continues to increase through term (fortieth week of gestation). At term, surfactant production is comparable to that of an adult and remains so throughout life. If an infant is born prematurely, however, surfactant production is frequently inadequate to maintain normal alveolar surface tension. Without surfactant, the alveoli do not inflate sufficiently. This leads to alveolar edema and collapse, resulting in respiratory distress syndrome of the newborn, or hyaline membrane disease (see p. 1203).

At birth, because the chest wall is soft and compliant, the intercostal muscles stabilize the chest wall. Chest wall compliance decreases with bone and muscle development throughout childhood until adult compliance is approached at puberty. Compliance increases to adult values by approximately age 20.

The thoracic cage (chest wall) is less rigid in childhood as well, and its contents are more easily displaced by the abdominal organs. This reduces its efficiency in assisting or preserving ventilation. Fig. 31-2 shows developmental differences in chest wall shape and rigidity.

Lung mechanics, or the interaction and equilibrium between compliance and elastic recoil, differ in adults and infants, as can be seen in Fig. 31-2, B. (Lung mechanics are described in Chapter 29.) The adult's wider and more rigid chest wall expands during inspiration because the vacuum (negative pressure) created by downward movement of the diaphragm draws air inward. In the preterm infant, or the infant with respiratory disease, the chest wall is so flexible that the vacuum created by downward movement of the diaphragm not only draws in air, but also causes the chest wall to be drawn inward with retraction of the intercostal and supraclavicular spaces. Expiration relieves the force that drew the infant's chest wall inward, and it expands. The diaphragm relaxes and is pushed upward by pressure from abdominal contents. In adults, an equilibrium is reached between elastic recoil of the lungs and compliance of the chest wall, which keeps the lungs from collapsing further and prevents the relaxed diaphragm from pushing against the lungs. At the end of expiration, the adult's residual volume is 50% greater than the residual volume of the infant. (Lung volumes and capacities are defined in Chapter 29.)

The infant's tracheobronchial cartilaginous rings are also more flexible than those of an older child or adult. The rings collapse easily, and the lumina of the upper airways are not sufficiently wide to permit airflow around obstructions. Overall, airway resistance in infancy is 15 times greater than in adulthood.

Physiologic differences involve metabolic rate and immunologic competence. Children rely on respiratory function to a greater extent than do adults because metabolic rate and oxygen consumption in children are

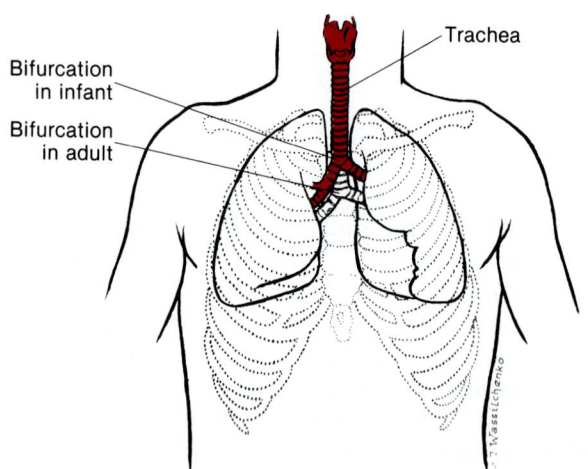

FIG. 31-1 Level of bifurcation of the trachea in infants and adults. (From Whaley & Wong, 1991.)

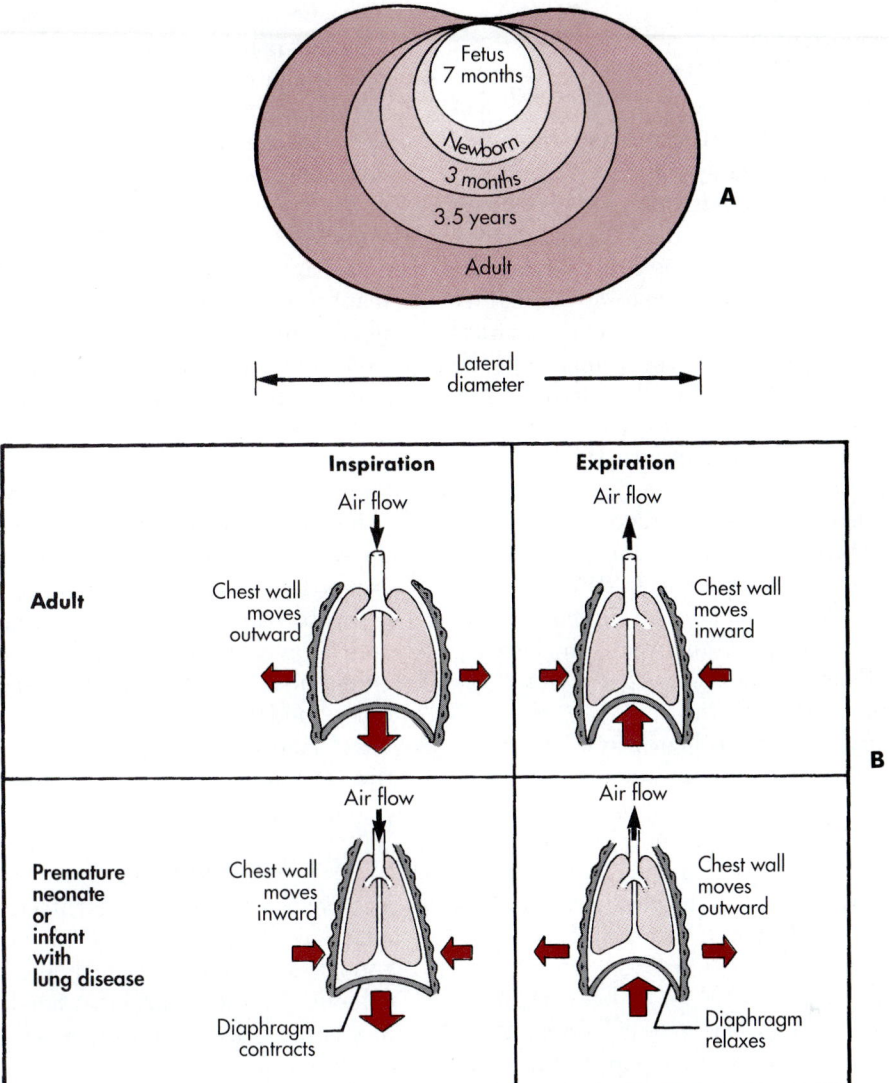

Lateral diameter

FIG. 31-2 **Developmental difference in the chest wall and lung mechanics. A,** Changes in chest wall shape and lung mechanics with age. **B,** Differences in lung mechanics caused by differences in chest wall compliance (degree of rigidity) in premature neonates and adults. (Arrows indicate direction of airflow, chest wall movement, and diaphragm movement.)

much higher. Children have less muscle glycogen in reserve. Consequently, the accessory muscles of inspiration tire relatively quickly, as lactic acidosis develops. The proportionately greater body surface area and respiratory rate of children lead to rapid heat and water loss during infection and fever. Dehydration and acidosis occur rapidly during times of decreased oral intake as a result of respiratory distress and vomiting, which frequently accompany acute infections in children.

Children are more susceptible than adults to infections of the respiratory tract because their immune systems are immature, they have not had time to develop immunity to most microorganisms, and they are frequently exposed to respiratory tract infections through contact with other children with similar immunologic incompetence. (The development of immunity is discussed in Chapter 6.) The physiology of children and adults is otherwise the same. Within a few hours of birth, the infant achieves normal arterial pH, P_{CO_2}, and P_{O_2}. However, the neonate and young child do not increase ventilation in response to increased carbon dioxide or hypoxemia the way adults do (Behrman, Kliegman, Nelson, & Vaughan, 1992). The reason for the differences in function is unknown.

PULMONARY DISORDERS

Disorders of the Upper Airways
Croup Syndrome

Croup is a syndrome of clinical manifestations caused by infection of the upper airways. Croup is characterized by inspiratory stridor, hoarseness, and a resonant cough described as "barking," "brassy," or "croupy." The clinical manifestations are caused by varying degrees of laryngeal obstruction due to inflammatory edema and spasm (Fig. 31-3). Because the upper airways of young children are easily occluded, croup can be life threatening. The conditions frequently referred to as croup include **viral croup, epiglottitis, laryngitis, acute laryngitis,** and **laryngotracheobronchitis (LTB)** (Table 31-1).

The actual incidence of these disorders is difficult to determine, but they comprise a significant number of respiratory illnesses in young children. In 85% of cases, croup is caused by a virus and affects children between 3 months and 5 years of age. Croup caused by bacteria (*Haemophilus influenzae* and *Corynebacterium diphtheriae*) occurs more rarely and in children aged 3 to 7 years. The incidence of croup is higher in males and is most common during the winter months. Approximately 15% of affected children have a strong family history of croup, with laryngitis tending to recur in the same child. Acute epiglottitis is usually caused by *H. influenzae* type b, with the peak incidence at 3.5 years of age (Behrman et al., 1992).

Pathophysiology

The anatomic differences between the larynx of the child and of the adult explain why croup is principally a disease of children. Not only are the diameter and surface area of the immature airway relatively smaller, but the mucous membrane is more loosely attached and more vascular. The glottis is small and is rapidly compromised by inflammatory edema and spasm. The negative pressure of inspiration is transmitted to the inflamed and edematous upper airway, causing it to collapse and resulting in obstruction of airflow (Fig. 31-4). Turbulent airflow across inflamed vocal cords causes inspiratory stridor. The obstruction is in contrast to inflammation of the lower airways, which tend to obstruct during inspiration when positive pressure inside the thorax narrows the airways causing expiratory wheezes. (Lymphoid tissues are described in Chapters 24 and 26.)

Children with viral croup may have a preceding infection of the upper respiratory passages (e.g., rhinitis or the common cold), which primarily involves the nasal mucosa. After 3 or 4 days, the infection spreads to the larynx, where the true vocal cords and subglottic structures become inflamed and edematous. In addition, spasms of smooth muscle in laryngeal walls contribute to the laryngeal obstruction.

In infections caused by *H. influenzae,* the primary site of inflammation is the **epiglottis. Epiglottitis** is a serious, life-threatening condition, because the inflammatory edema can obstruct the airway. Inflammation may spread above and below the epiglottis to involve the trachea and bronchi. If this occurs, respiratory distress is more severe and the outcome of the disease is less favorable.

In bacterial croup caused by *C. diphtheriae,* inflammation and infection of the upper airways, including pharyngitis and rhinitis, proceed to laryngeal inflammation. Diphtheria causes the mucosa of the larynx to become coated with a fibrous exudate, occluding the airway. Fortunately, immunization against diphtheria has made this serious disease a rare occurrence in the United States.

Regardless of the causal microorganism, certain endogenous factors are believed to predispose a child to croup. Evidence for this includes (1) the tendency for croup to recur in children who have had one episode and (2) the likelihood that the same virus will cause croup in susceptible children while causing a variety of other, milder illnesses in children who are not susceptible (Baugh & Gilmore, 1986). An anatomically defective or abnormally immature larynx may be a predisposing factor for croup.

Clinical Manifestations

The clinical manifestations of croup are mainly produced by inflammation and obstruction of the larynx. Soon after the onset of cough and hoarseness, the child exhibits inspiratory stridor, a harsh, high crowing noise that is most distinct during inspiration. Unlike wheezing, inspiratory stridor originates high in the respiratory tract, usually in the trachea or larynx. It indicates obstruction and may be combined with cough, dyspnea, hoarseness, retractions of the chest wall with respiration, and tachypnea. The degree of nasal flaring, tracheal tugging, and retraction of the chest muscles depends on the degree of airway resistance (Fig. 31-5). The child becomes apprehensive and agitated as dyspnea and airway obstruction worsen. Agitation, cyanosis, pallor, weakness, rapid pulse, low tidal volumes, and stridor are all signs of hypoxemia. Death may occur from hypoventilation.

Most cases of croup progress only as far as stridor and slight dyspnea, and the child recovers from the acute crisis in a few hours. Complete recovery from croup often requires 24 to 48 hours.

Evaluation and Treatment

Diagnosis is made on the basis of physical examination and radiologic examination. Treatment for croup consists of (1) restricting the child's activity to avoid aggravating respiratory distress, (2) administering humidifier and oxygen (25% to 30%) to alleviate anxiety and

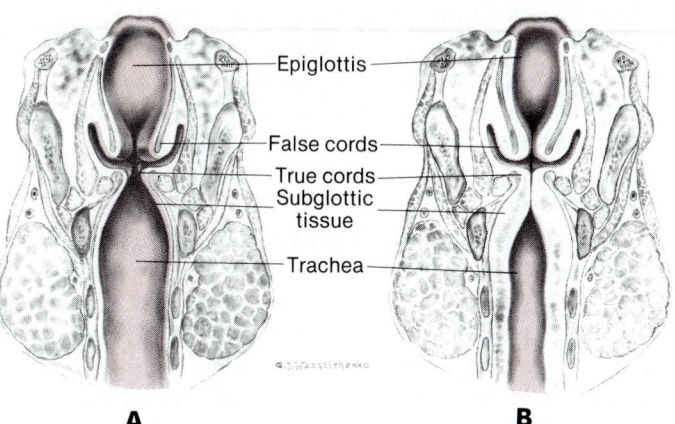

FIG. 31-3 The larynx. A, Normal larynx. B, Narrowing and obstruction from edema of croup. (From Whaley & Wong, 1991.)

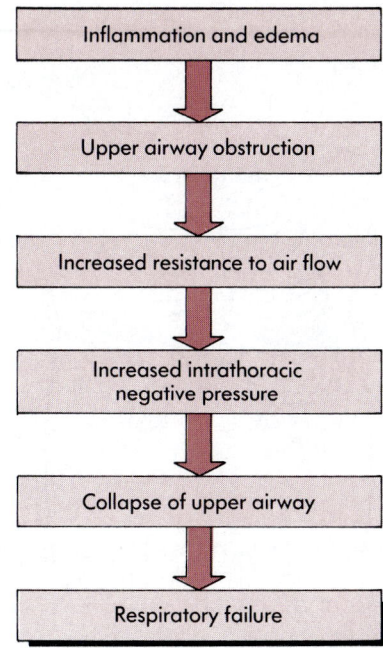

FIG. 31-4 Upper airway obstruction with croup.

TABLE 31-1

Croup Syndromes

Syndrome	Etiology	Age	Onset	Pathophysiology	Signs/symptoms
Acute tracheitis	*Staphylococcus aureus* (bacterial)	1 mo-6 yr	Gradual, previous upper respiratory infection	Inflammation of upper trachea	Stridor; high fever; croupy cough; thick, purulent secretions
Epiglottitis	*Haemophilus influenzae* (bacterial)	2-7 yr	Rapidly progressive	Inflammation of supraglottic structures with increasing airway obstruction	Respiratory distress, drooling, stridor, agitation, muffled voice, retractions, red inflamed throat
Acute infectious laryngitis	Virus	2 yr	Sudden	Brassy cough, low-grade fever, restless, agitated, occurs at night	Inflammation below vocal cords
Acute laryngotracheobronchitis	Virus	6 mo-3 yr	Gradual, previous rhinitis, conjunctivitis	Croupy cough, stridor, low-grade fever, restless, lower rib retractions, pale, worse at night	Inflammation of vocal cords, bronchi, bronchioles; airway obstruction with prolonged expiration

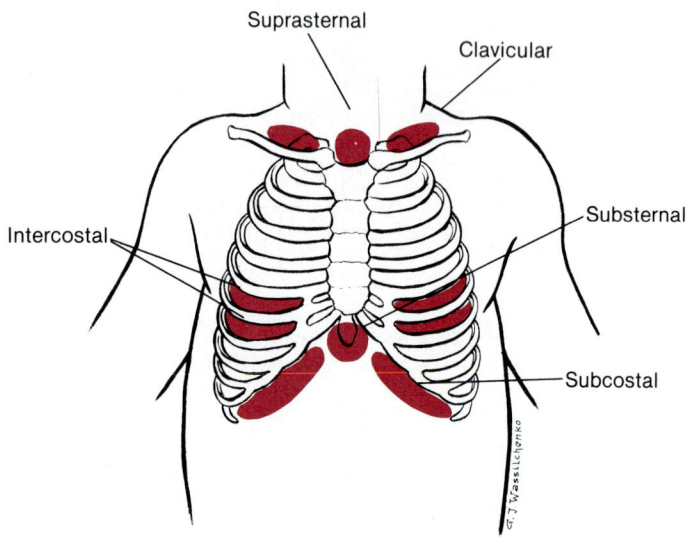

FIG. 31-5 Areas of chest muscle retraction. (From Whaley & Wong, 1991.)

reverse hypoxemia, (3) administering intravenous fluids to ensure adequate hydration, (4) aerosolized epinephrine to relieve destruction, (5) instituting mechanical ventilation (intermittent positive-pressure breathing) with aerosol epinephrine to relieve obstruction, (6) administering antibiotics (if croup is bacterial in origin), and (7) tracheotomy or nasal intubation for laryngeal obstruction.

With the exception of epiglottitis, which is a localized and frequently fatal infection, the likelihood of death increases as the infection extends to involve a greater portion of the respiratory tract. Most deaths from croup are the result of laryngeal obstruction or the complications of tracheotomy, most commonly mediastinal emphysema (air in the mediastinum) and pneumothorax. Untreated epiglottitis has a mortality rate of up to 25%. The prognosis of acute laryngitis and LTB is excellent.

Types of Croup
Acute epiglottitis

Acute epiglottitis is a severe, life-threatening, rapidly progressive infection of the epiglottis and surrounding area. Mortality is between 8% and 12% of children admitted to hospitals. In the classic form of the disease, a child between 2 and 7 years of age suddenly develops fever, inspiratory stridor, and severe respiratory distress. The child appears anxious and has a voice that sounds muffled. Drooling and dysphagia (inability to swallow) are common. Death can occur in a few hours. Nasotracheal intubation or tracheotomy is mandatory in in-

stances of rapidly increasing obstruction. Examination of the throat may trigger laryngospasm and cause respiratory collapse. Pneumonia, cervical lymph node inflammation, otitis, and, rarely, meningitis or septic arthritis may occur during the course of epiglottitis.

Viral croup and acute laryngotracheobronchitis

Viral croup and acute laryngotracheobronchitis are frequently caused by the same virus. Viral croup usually occurs in children between the ages of 6 months and 3 years. It follows an upper respiratory infection consisting of rhinorrhea, coryza (severe infection, with discharge, of the nasal mucosa), and fever. After 2 to 3 days, the child suddenly develops symptoms of croup, with inspiratory stridor and a harsh, barking cough. Difficulty in breathing makes the child apprehensive and restless. In viral croup, the obstruction is caused by inflammatory swelling of the subglottic tissues with impingement on the airway below the level of the glottis. Spasm of the vocal cords occurs with tracheobronchitis as the inflammatory process extends.

Acute laryngotracheobronchitis (LTB) (sometimes called acute laryngotracheitis) is the most common form of croup. Affected children have frequent recurrences between ages 3 and 6 years, after which airway growth decreases susceptibility. Symptoms characteristically appear worse at night. A considerable number of children with LTB require tracheotomy for the establishment of an adequate airway.

Complications occur in approximately 15% of children with viral croup or LTB. The most common complication is extension of the infection to other regions of the respiratory tract, such as the middle ear, terminal bronchioles, or pulmonary parenchyma.

Aspiration Syndromes
Aspiration of foreign bodies

Aspiration of foreign bodies into the airways is a common occurrence among children. Most objects are expelled by the cough reflex, but some objects may lodge in the larynx, trachea, or bronchus. Large objects (a bite of hot dog, toy balloons, coins, bottle caps, and nuts) may occlude the airway and are life-threatening. Lodging of smaller objects may be asymptomatic initially. Symptoms of cough, hoarseness, and dyspnea are consistent with a foreign body in the larynx. Similar symptoms with blood-streaked sputum are associated with a foreign body in the bronchus. The obstruction can progress to atelectasis, or there can be a ball-valve effect with air accumulation distal to the obstruction. Chronic infection, bronchiectasis, asthma, or lung abscess occurs with late diagnosis (Mu, He, & Sun, 1991). Lodged objects require endoscopic removal and treatment of the consequent problem.

Aspiration of foreign substances

Infants may aspirate amniotic fluid contaminated with meconium, bacteria, or cells from the birth canal that can cause pneumonia or respiratory distress. Aspiration of baby powder can also produce dyspnea and respiratory distress. Infants with tracheoesophageal fistulas (see Chapter 37) or gastroesophageal reflux may aspirate gastric fluids and develop chemical pneumonia. Treatment is related to the severity of the aspiration. Most important for preventing aspiration is suctioning airways when the baby's head is delivered, controlling the use of baby powder, proper positioning during feeding, and avoiding overfeeding.

Sudden Infant Death Syndrome (SIDS)

The greatest single cause of death among infants between 1 week and 1 year of age is **sudden infant death syndrome (SIDS),** also called crib death or cot death. The syndrome refers to the sudden, unexpected death of any infant or young child in whom a postmortem examination fails to demonstrate a cause for death. The incidence is 2 to 3 per 1000 live births (Gilbert-Barness & Barness, 1992).

The highest incidence of SIDS is between 2 and 4 months of age; it almost always occurs during sleep, with higher frequencies during the winter months. Sudden infant death syndrome is the leading cause of postneonatal death and claims 700 to 10,000 lives each year (Little & Peterson, 1990). The occurrence rate varies between 1 and 3 per 1000 live births. Risk factors associated with SIDS include (1) poor mothers younger than 20 years of age; (2) low birth weight; (3) preterm delivery; (4) multiple pregnancies; (5) siblings who died of SIDS; (6) smoking during pregnancy; (7) anemia during pregnancy; and (8) lack of prenatal care (Kraus, Greenland, & Bultery, 1989).

The cause of SIDS is unknown, and no single factor is predictive of the sudden death. There is no treatment because the death is sudden and unexplained. Apnea is a common finding in infants with apparent life-threatening events, and these infants have survived with successful resuscitation. The apnea leads to manifestations of asphyxia, including pallor or cyanosis, bradycardia, gasping respiratory efforts, limpness, and unresponsiveness. Home monitoring of respiratory and cardiovascular functions has been successful for infant apnea. Research is continuing to find the cause and prevention of this mysterious syndrome.

Sudden infant death syndrome occurs most often between 2 and 6 months of age, with fewer than 1% of deaths occurring during the first 2 months of life, and more than 90% of the deaths occurring within the first 6 months. Sudden infant death syndrome is known to occur more frequently in males (60%), in siblings of

SIDS victims (2 of 100 live births), in twins of SIDS victims (5 to 10 of 100 live births) (Spitzer & Fox, 1984), and in low birth weight or small for gestational age infants (Shannon & Kelly, 1982). Sudden infant death syndrome is reportedly more frequent in families of low socioeconomic status and occurs often during the winter months when upper respiratory infections are most prevalent. It occurs most often during sleep, with 50% to 80% of deaths occurring between midnight and 6:00 AM (Aranda, Trippenbach, Turmen, & Lopes, 1983; Meadow, 1990; Nuttall, 1986).

Despite much medical controversy, it is likely that SIDS has many causes. In studies of infants who have almost succumbed, several abnormalities have been identified: hypoventilation, depressed ventilatory response to carbon dioxide, prolonged sleep apnea, frequent short apneic episodes, excessive periodic breathing, and heart rate variability during sleep (Nuttall, 1986; Schechtman et al., 1988; Schechtman, Harper, Wilson, & Southall, 1991; Ward et al., 1986).

Although the procedure can be burdensome to parents, infants considered at risk are often placed on home apnea monitors during sleep until they are past the age of vulnerability and demonstrate normal lung functioning as evidenced by normal pneumatograms (Nuttall, 1986). The American Academy of Pediatrics recommends that healthy infants be positioned on their side or back to sleep, not in a prone position (American Academy of Pediatrics Task Force on Infant Positioning and SIDS, 1992).

Disorders of the Lower Airways

Lung disease is the single major cause of death in the first year of life, accounting for 46% of deaths. Death is usually caused by lower airway obstruction by foreign bodies, inflammation, mucus, and edema. In addition, the child's poorly supported large airways may collapse during forced expiration, such as in crying, or as a result of disturbance of lung pressures caused by acceleration of expired gas past a partially occluded segment of the large bronchi.

Asthma

Asthma is characterized by hyperresponsive airways and mild to severe obstruction of air movement into and out of the lungs (Larsen, 1992) (see Chapter 30). It is a leading chronic illness in childhood, affecting 5% to 10% of children to some degree, and is the most frequent cause of hospital admission. Inner city black and Hispanic children have higher morbidity and mortality rates (Weiss, Gergen, & Crain, 1992). Before puberty, approximately twice as many boys as girls are affected. After puberty, the incidence of asthma is evenly divided between the sexes. Approximately 80% to 90% of asthmatic children have their first symptoms before 4 or 5 years of age. Children with asthma have increased wheezing during viral respiratory infections. Mortality rates among children and young adults with asthma were higher in 1987 than in 1969 (Hurd & Lenfant, 1992).

Pathophysiology

Allergy plays a major role in the pathogenesis and inflammatory processes of childhood asthma, particularly in children older than 5 years of age (Morgan & Fernando, 1992). Edema of the bronchial mucosa, bronchospasm, cellular infiltration, and mucus plugging vary in severity depending on the age of the child, the size and anatomy of the airways, the type of irritant that precipitates obstruction, and the duration and severity of the asthma attack (see Chapter 30). The increased work of breathing caused by use of accessory muscles during an asthma attack increases oxygen consumption and cardiac output. This level of exertion is difficult for young children to maintain because of their small glycogen reserves and the likelihood that caloric intake is inadequate because of illness. Hyperventilation can be severe and prolonged and cause permanent anatomic changes (e.g., barrel chest, prominent sternum, and malformation of the ribs), particularly in young children with soft, developing rib cages.

The site and degree of obstruction may differ in a given child from one asthma attack to another. In most children, both larger and smaller airways are obstructed. Even when the bronchi at all levels are involved, the large and small airways can respond differently to inciting agents. Acute, relatively short-lived asthma attacks may chiefly involve the large bronchi. Obstruction of the small airways occurs more slowly. It follows that relief of obstruction occurs more rapidly in larger than in smaller airways. Chronic, partially irreversible small airway obstruction may occur in asymptomatic children with asthma.

There can be both an early and late phase to an asthma attack. The early phase is the result of IgE-mediated mast cell degranulation. The late phase results from inflammatory mediators released from cells attracted to the small airways during the acute phase, such as leukotrienes, prostaglandins, and platelet-activating factor from mast cells; neutrophils; macrophages; and T lymphocytes. There may be an initial relief of the acute phase of obstruction which is followed 6 to 8 hours later by an increase in obstruction to airflow (Hill, Szefler, & Larsen, 1992; Kalinger, Barnes, & Persson, 1991; Walker, Virchow, & Bruijnzeel, 1991) (Fig. 31-6).

The severity, location, and sites of obstruction by asthma are related to age. In general, the younger the child, the greater the risk of morbidity and mortality.

Infants in particular are at an anatomic and physiologic disadvantage because of (1) their relatively small alveolocapillary surface area; (2) the increased resistance to airflow in their narrow airways; (3) the horizontal insertion angle of their diaphragm, which is mechanically disadvantageous and increases the work of breathing; (4) the relatively large number of mucous glands per square centimeter of bronchial mucosa; and (5) a deficiency in the numbers of pores of Kohn and Lambert canals that promote atelectasis distal to obstructed airways (Behrman et al., 1992). The one anatomic advantage of infants is the relatively small amount of smooth muscle in their smaller airways, making bronchospasm less severe. In infants, mechanical obstruction from edema, mucus, and inflammatory cell infiltrates, which is slow to resolve, is a more important component of airway obstruction than bronchospasm, which can be reversed with drugs. This difference is reflected in the higher number of infants and very young children requiring hospitalization for control of asthma.

The effects of asthma also depend on the duration of attacks. In short attacks of acute asthma, bronchospasm or mucosal edema usually predominates, and obstruction from secretions is of secondary importance. Mucous secretions become a more important cause of obstruction if inflammation is intense and prolonged, such as in viral infections of the lung.

Clinical Manifestations

The course and severity of asthma are difficult to predict. In typical cases, previously well infants or young children develop what seems to be a cold with rhinorrhea, which is rapidly followed by signs and symptoms of asthma. These include the high-pitched, wheezing sound heard mostly on expiration; cough, sometimes so severe as to induce gagging and vomiting; an anxious facial expression; irritability or restlessness; dyspnea; labored breathing; tachypnea; use of accessory muscles of respiration; nasal flaring; assumption of an upright posture, with raised shoulder, expanded upper chest, and arms extended behind to prop the upper torso; and, in severe attacks, cyanosis, pallor, and diaphoresis (sweating). Obstruction is more severe during expiration because airways become smaller from the elastic forces of expiration. Respiratory symptoms may be preceded by exposure to irritants, animals, molds or dusty areas, pollens, tobacco smoke, or cold air. Sometimes exercise precipitates an asthma attack (see Chapter 30) or the attack follows bronchitis or recurrent chest colds. Most children have only occasional attacks of mild to moderate severity and are easily treated. Chronic asthma causes chest abnormalities, such as pectus excavatum (funnel chest), or barrel chest, an abnormal prominence of the ribs. Growth may be retarded, resulting in abnormally small stature or low weight, and puberty may

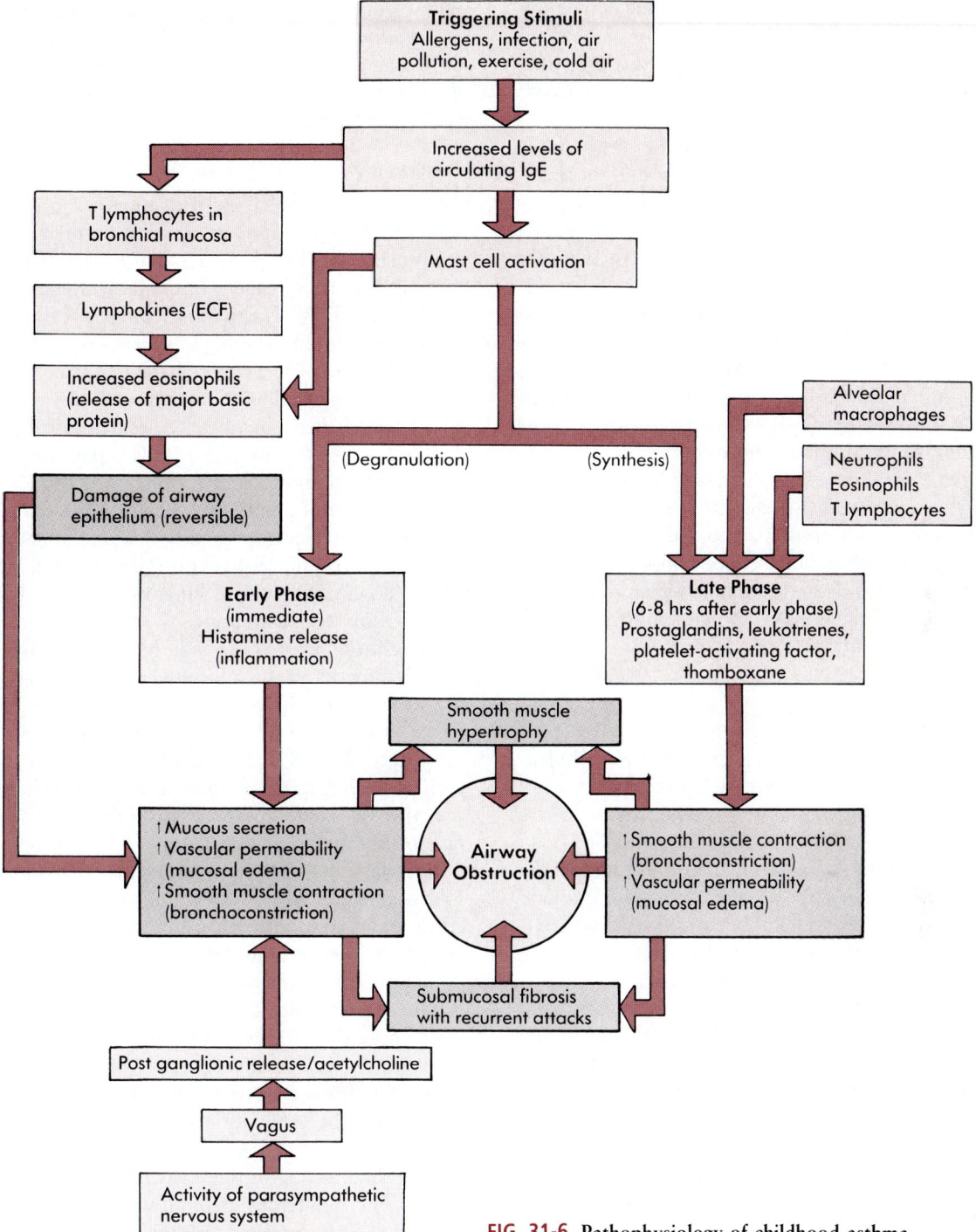

FIG. 31-6 Pathophysiology of childhood asthma.

be delayed. Although there are an increasing number of medications to treat asthma, asthma-related deaths are increasing (Evans, Mullally, & Wilson, 1987).

Evaluation and Treatment

Diagnosis is determined on the basis of history, clinical manifestations, physical examination, and to a lesser ex-

tent, laboratory tests. Treatment for mild and moderate asthma consists of avoidance of contact with suggested allergens or irritants; hyposensitization therapy; promotion of liquefication and expectoration of mucus through adequate hydration, administration of adrenergic aerosols, postural drainage; administration of oral or aerosol bronchodilators; correction of metabolic acidosis; and administration of corticosteroids (prednisone) in severe acute and chronic asthma unresponsive to other measures. Between attacks, the child is encouraged to exercise, and prophylactic medication (theophylline or cromolyn sodium or adrenergic aerosol) may be prescribed.

Severe asthma or status asthmaticus (intractable asthma in which the child continues to have incapacitating dyspnea, cough, and obstruction of airways despite treatment) is a life-threatening emergency requiring admission to an intensive care unit. Emergency care includes administration of epinephrine, oxygen, corticosteroids, methylxanthines, sedatives (contraindicated in status asthmaticus), intravenous hydration, correction of acidosis, and administration of antibiotics.

Although there is a widespread notion that children usually "outgrow" their asthma in adolescence, half of them do not. Many children whose overt symptoms disappear continue to have persistent airway obstruction. The recurrence of overt asthma after years of freedom from symptoms is not unusual. Thus, asthma is often a lifelong disorder with periodic exacerbations and remissions. The likelihood of becoming asymptomatic is greater if the asthma is mild and the child is free of symptoms between attacks.

Respiratory Infection

Children have approximately six to eight upper respiratory infections a year. The incidence of lower respiratory infections is approximately 50 infections per 1000 individuals each year for children younger than 6 years of age. Most of these illnesses are pneumonia.

The cause of lower airway infection depends on the infectious microorganism, the age of the child, immune function, seasonal and geographic variables, and environment. Microorganisms transmitted from the maternal genital tract during childbirth, particularly gram-negative bacteria, group B streptococci, and *Chlamydia trachomatis*, can cause pulmonary infections in infants up to 3 months of age. Later in infancy and during early childhood, viral rather than bacterial infections predominate. Respiratory syncytial virus and parainfluenza 3 virus infections are most common. Ninety percent of bacterial pneumonias in children are caused by *S. pneumoniae*, with the remainder caused by *Staphylococcus* and *H. influenzae*. The incidence of *Mycoplasma pneumoniae* infection peaks between the ages of 5 and 10 years, and as the incidence of all pneumonia decreases during adolescence, *M. pneumoniae* becomes the most common cause of bacterial pneumonia.

In infants and young children, viral infections tend to be more common during the winter and early spring, with other minor peaks in the fall. During influenza epidemics, pneumonia and croup may develop in infants and children of all ages.

Familial and environmental factors are associated with certain types of respiratory infection. For example, *M. pneumoniae* infections tend to occur with overcrowding and affect multiple members of a family. (Predisposing environmental and familial risk factors are described in Unit X.)

Pneumonia

The more common types of pneumonia in children are viral and bacterial (pneumococcal, staphylococcal, and streptococcal) (Table 31-2). *Viral pneumonia* causes varying degrees of illness in children. Respiratory syncytial virus (RSV) is the most common cause of pneumonia in children. The highest rates are between 2 and 3 years of age. In severe cases, the child may rapidly become dangerously ill with fever, respiratory distress, and circulatory failure. Death may occur in 1 to 3 days because of marked tissue necrosis. This pattern occurs primarily with adenovirus infection and is rare. The mildest cases of viral pneumonia occur in infants or young children, who develop a cough, fever, and tachypnea with mild systemic disturbance after a cold. There are few or no clinical signs of lung involvement, but radiographs show consolidation.

Bacterial pneumonia (pneumococcal, staphylococcal, and streptococcal) in children is usually lobar pneumonia caused by *Streptococcus pneumoniae* (90% of cases). It occurs at all ages but is most common in children aged 3 to 8 years during late winter and early spring, when respiratory infections are at their peak. Often, there is a preceding or an underlying chronic illness or immunologic deficiency.

The classic clinical manifestations of a shaking chill followed by a high fever, cough, and chest pain may occur in older children with streptococcal pneumonia but are rarely observed in infants and young children, in whom the clinical picture is considerably more variable. A mild upper respiratory tract infection characterized by stuffy nose, irritability, and poor feeding usually precedes the onset of streptococcal pneumonia in infants. This mild illness of several days' duration ends with an abrupt onset of fever, restlessness, apprehension, and respiratory distress. The respiratory distress is manifested by grunting; flaring of the nostrils; retraction of the supraclavicular, intercostal, and subcostal areas; tachypnea; and tachycardia. Cyanosis is often apparent.

Clinical manifestations in children and adolescents are similar to those in adults. A brief, mild upper respiratory infection is followed by the onset of a shaking chill, then fever. These manifestations are accompanied by drowsiness, intermittent periods of restlessness, tachypnea, a dry, hacking, unproductive cough, anxiety, and cyanosis around the mouth. Many children splint the affected side to minimize pleural pain and improve ventilation and may lie on their side with knees drawn up to the chest. Children with pneumonia may have

TABLE 31-2

More Common Types of Pneumonia in Children

Type	Causal agent	Age	Onset	Signs/symptoms	Pathophysiology
Viral pneumonia	Respiratory syncytial virus (most common)	All ages	Acute or gradual, winter and early spring	Mild to high fever, cough, rhinorrhea, malaise, fine rales, diffuse rhonchi, wheezing, diffuse areas of consolidation	Bronchiolitis with edema, increased mucus, and interstitial pneumonia
Pneumococcal pneumonia	Pneumococci (*Streptococcus pneumoniae*)	1-4 yr	Acute, follows an upper respiratory infection, winter and early spring	High fever, productive cough, pleuritic pain, increased respiration rate, decreased breath sounds in area of consolidation	Inflammation of bronchial mucosa with alveolar exudate; consolidation of all or part of a lobe. Early: red hepatization with WBCs, RBCs, and fibrin consolidation. Late: gray hepatization with fibrin and neutrophils in alveoli. Resolution: many phagocytic macrophages
Staphylococcal pneumonia	*Staphylococcus aureus* *S. epidermidis*	1 wk-2 yr	Acute, winter months	High fever, cough, respiratory distress (retractions, nasal flaring, cyanosis, anxiety, increased respirations, grunting, shocklike state may be present)	Unilateral edema and hemorrhagic necrosis of one or more lobes, exudate on pleural surface may develop multiple abscesses
Streptococcal pneumonia	Group A β-hemolytic streptococci	All ages, acute, any season	Acute, any season	High fever, chills, respiratory distress	Tracheitis, bronchitis, and interstitial pneumonia with ulcers, exudate, edema, and localized hemorrhage

pain referred to the abdomen. Abdominal distention may occur because of swallowed air or air ileus (intestinal blockage by gas) associated with the pneumonia.

S. pneumoniae is treated with penicillin alone or combined with ampicillin and gentamicin. Supplemental oxygen is given for significant respiratory distress, and acetaminophen for high fever. With appropriate antibiotic therapy instituted early in the course of illness, the mortality rate from bacterial pneumonia is now less than 1% (Arguedas, Stutman, & Marks, 1990).

Bronchitis

Bronchitis in children tends to occur in association with a number of other conditions of the upper and lower airways, including asthma and cystic fibrosis. Bronchitis occurs most commonly after a respiratory illness, such as croup, pneumonia, or even a mild upper respiratory tract infection, and it is aggravated by dry environmental air (e.g., in homes with forced-air heating). Viruses produce most attacks of chronic bronchitis. When the dry, hacking cough is severe enough to interfere with eating or resting, demulcents such as lollipops or cough drops are quite effective. Recurring bronchitis in childhood may be a predisposing factor for later bronchial lesions that cause chronic obstruction. Treatment of viral bronchitis is palliative and treatment of bacterial pneumonia is related to the causing microorganism (Loughlin, 1990).

Bronchiolitis

Bronchiolitis is a common disease of the lower respiratory tract in infants. Caused by inflammatory obstruction of the bronchioles, it tends to occur during the first 2 years of life, with a peak incidence at approximately 6 months of age, particularly during the winter and spring. Bronchiolitis is a major reason for hospital admission of infants less than 1 year of age.

Respiratory syncytial virus causes more than 50% of cases of bronchiolitis, but parainfluenza 3 virus, mycoplasma, some adenoviruses, and occasionally other viruses or bacteria cause acute bronchiolitis. Infection is usually transmitted to the infant from a family member with a minor respiratory illness.

Pathophysiology

Viral infection causes necrosis of the bronchial epithelium and destruction of ciliated epithelial cells. There is infiltration with lymphocytes around the bronchioles, a cell-mediated hypersensitivity to viral antigens with release of lymphokines causing inflammation, and necrosis of bronchiolar epithelium, as well as activation of monocytes. As the submucosa becomes edematous, cellular debris and fibrin form plugs within the bronchioles.

Edema of the bronchiolar wall, accumulation of mucus and cellular debris, and bronchospasm narrow many peripheral airways. Other airways become partially or completely occluded. Obstruction varies in degree and location. Atelectasis occurs in some areas of the lung and hyperinflation in others.

The mechanics of breathing are disrupted by bronchiolitis. Tidal volume is high and functional residual capacity is approximately twice normal. Compliance is decreased because the lungs are already highly inflated and because airway resistance within the lung is uneven and increased. The decrease in compliance and the increase in airway resistance result in a substantial increase in the work of breathing.

Serious alterations in gas exchange occur because of airway obstruction and patchy atelectasis. Hypoxemia and hypercapnia develop due to ventilation-perfusion abnormalities (see Chapter 30), and hypercapnia is increased further because the increased work of breathing causes hypoventilation. Although pH varies, metabolic acidosis occurs more frequently than respiratory alkalosis. The cause of metabolic acidosis is complex. Hypoxemia can produce lactic acidosis. Poor caloric and fluid intake may contribute to ketoacidosis, and carbon dioxide retention can produce respiratory acidosis. (Acid-base disturbances are discussed in Chapter 3.)

Clinical Manifestations

Older children and adults can tolerate bronchiolar edema better than infants and thus seldom develop the clinical manifestations of bronchiolitis. In infants and young children, bronchiolitis is characterized by difficulty in expiration, wheezing, tachypnea, chest wall retractions, and cyanosis around the mouth. Severely affected infants appear anxious and distressed because of dyspnea. The thoracic cage is overexpanded, particularly in its anteroposterior diameter. The infant takes rapid, short breaths, and wheezing and rales are often heard on auscultation. With overexpansion of the lungs, the diaphragm is flattened, causing downward displacement of the liver and spleen. Abdominal distention results from air swallowing. The tidal volume decreases. Some individuals have persistent airway resistance and airway hyperresponsiveness (Castleman, Sovkness, Lemanske, & McAllister, 1990).

Evaluation and Treatment

Diagnosis of bronchiolitis is made on the basis of physical examination (e.g., rhinitis, cough, wheezing, chest retractions, and tachypnea) and radiologic examination. Humidification of inspired air is the traditional treatment for bronchiolitis in children. Cold and humidified oxygen relieves hypoxemia and possibly reduces the insensible water loss caused by tachypnea. Placing the child in a croup tent with the head elevated at a 30- to 34-degree angle relieves dyspnea, cyanosis, anxiety, and restlessness.

Some children recover from bronchiolitis within 3 to 4 days, whereas others require a week or more. Long-term follow-up of infants who have had bronchiolitis shows an increased incidence of asthma during childhood (Wohl, 1990).

Bronchiolitis obliterans

In **bronchiolitis obliterans,** injured bronchioles and some small bronchi are partially or completely obliterated by nodular masses containing granulomatous and fibrotic tissue (Epler, 1992). In adults, some cases can be related to chemical injury by nitrogen oxide or other toxic gases, although it is not related to smoking. Most cases in children are associated with pulmonary infections, such as influenza, adenoviral infection, or pertussis (whooping cough), or to measles. Cough, respiratory distress, and cyanosis occur initially, followed by a brief period of improvement. The progression of disease is then reflected by increasing dyspnea, cough, sputum production, and wheezing.

There is no specific treatment for bronchiolitis obliterans. Some children deteriorate rapidly and die within weeks, whereas others follow a more chronic course.

Respiratory Distress Syndrome of the Newborn

The names **respiratory distress syndrome of the newborn (RDS)**, idiopathic respiratory distress syndrome (IRDS), and hyaline membrane disease (HMD) all refer to the severe lung disorder that is responsible for more neonatal deaths than any other condition. Respiratory distress syndrome of the newborn affects 5% to 10% of premature infants, or 0.05% to 0.1% of all neonates. Respiratory distress syndrome of the newborn or its complications are responsible for 30% to 50% of all neonatal deaths and up to 70% of deaths in premature infants (Washington Office of Technology Assessment, 1987).

The chief predisposing factor is premature birth, but several other factors are important. The condition is twice as common in males as in females. It frequently follows delivery by cesarean section, particularly if the procedure is done before labor has begun. Infants of diabetic mothers are five times more likely to develop RDS than infants of nondiabetic mothers, regardless of gestational age, sex, and mode of delivery. Asphyxia increases the possibility that a premature infant will develop RDS because acidosis (caused by hypoxemia) interferes with production of alveolar surfactant, increasing the likelihood of atelectasis. Other predisposing factors are hypovolemia or hypervolemia, maternal antepartum hemorrhage, and shock.

Pathophysiology

During the third trimester of gestation, the final unfolding of the alveolar septum takes place, an event that significantly increases the alveolocapillary surface area of the lungs. Because alveolar septal unfolding is incomplete in premature infants, they are born with many underdeveloped and uninflatable alveoli. In addition, pulmonary blood flow is limited by fetal atelectasis and incomplete vascular development, particularly of the alveolocapillary network. Because of increased pulmonary vascular resistance, most fetal blood is shunted from the lungs through the fetal cardiac structures, the ductus arteriosus and foramen ovale. (These structures are described in Chapter 28.)

At birth, the infant must initiate breathing and keep the previously fluid-filled lungs inflated with air. With the onset of ventilation, a marked increase in pulmonary blood flow occurs because oxygen dilates the constricted pulmonary blood vessels. Pulmonary venous return is thus increased and, consequently, so is left ventricular output. In the normal neonate, ductal closure and the decrease of pulmonary vascular resistance result in a decrease of pulmonary arterial and right ventricular pressures. The major decline from the high fetal pressures to low adult pressures usually occurs within the first 2 to 3 days after birth but may be prolonged for 7 or more days (Behrman et al., 1992). At the same time, the volume of pulmonary capillary blood flow must increase approximately 10 times to provide adequate pulmonary perfusion and alter intracardiac pressure enough to close the ductus arteriosus and foramen ovale. Most full-term infants are successful in making these changes, but the premature infant with RDS is not.

The primary problem in RDS is atelectasis, which develops in premature infants as a result of three interrelated developmental factors: (1) small alveoli that are difficult to inflate; (2) a weak, compliant chest wall (see Fig. 31-2, *B*); and (3) insufficient production of pulmonary surfactant, which is needed to reduce surface tension and permit alveolar inflation. (The principles that govern alveolar inflation are described in Chapter 29.) These factors combined contribute to the greater respiratory effort required to expand the alveoli of premature infants and the greater end-expiratory pressure (functional residual capacity) required to prevent chest wall collapse. Incomplete initial inflation and small lung volume at end-inspiration both promote atelectasis.

Premature infants who do not have RDS have developed sufficient alveolar surface area to meet their metabolic needs and have produced and accumulated sufficient surfactant to permit alveolar inflation. Infants with RDS have not developed the ability to synthesize, store, and secrete surfactant onto the alveolocapillary membrane. Surfactant reaches the alveolar surface of the membrane at approximately 28 to 38 weeks of gestation, as demonstrated by its detection in amniotic fluid. This variation in ages at detection is evidence that the lung matures at different rates in different individuals. It also explains why some infants with a gestational age of <30 weeks do not acquire RDS, whereas other infants with greater gestational age may do so.

Without surfactant, each breath requires as much negative pressure as the initial lung expansion at birth. The infant uses more oxygen to sustain the work of breathing than is gained from ventilation. This leads to exhaustion and a decreased ability to maintain lung expansion. The result is widespread atelectasis, one of the characteristics of RDS.

In the absence of alveolar stability (normal functional

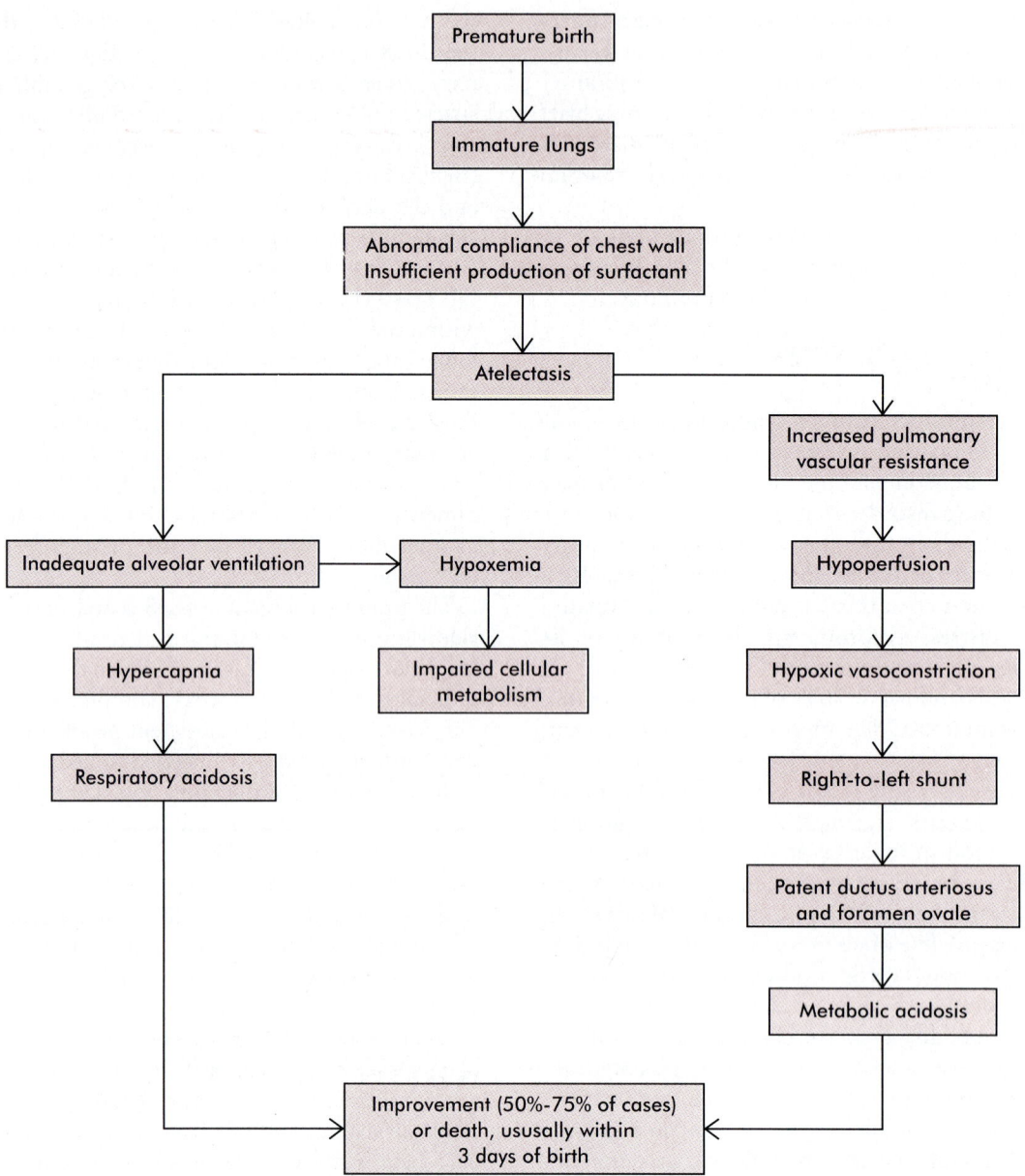

FIG. 31-7 Pathogenesis of respiratory distress syndrome of the newborn (RDS), also known as hyaline membrane disease.

residual capacity) and with progressive atelectasis, pulmonary vascular resistance is increased instead of decreased, as in normal lungs. This results in hypoperfusion of the lung and a decrease in effective pulmonary blood flow. Increased pulmonary vascular resistance causes a partial return to fetal circulation, with right-to-left shunting of blood through the ductus arteriosus and foramen ovale. Inadequate pulmonary perfusion and ventilation produce hypoxemia and hypercapnia. Because the thick muscular layer of the pulmonary arterioles is sensitive to diminished oxygen concentration and decreased blood pH, hypoxic vasoconstriction oc-

curs. Hypoxic vasoconstriction contributes to further increases in pulmonary vascular resistance.

Capillary permeability increases, resulting in the leakage of plasma proteins into the interstitium, where clotting causes fibrin formation. Fibrin deposited in the alveolocapillary interstitium creates the hyaline appearance seen on histologic examination; hence the name hyaline membrane disease.

To make the situation more complex, prolonged hypoxemia activates anaerobic glycolysis, which produces increased amounts of lactic acid and promotes metabolic acidosis. Because the collapsed alveoli are unable

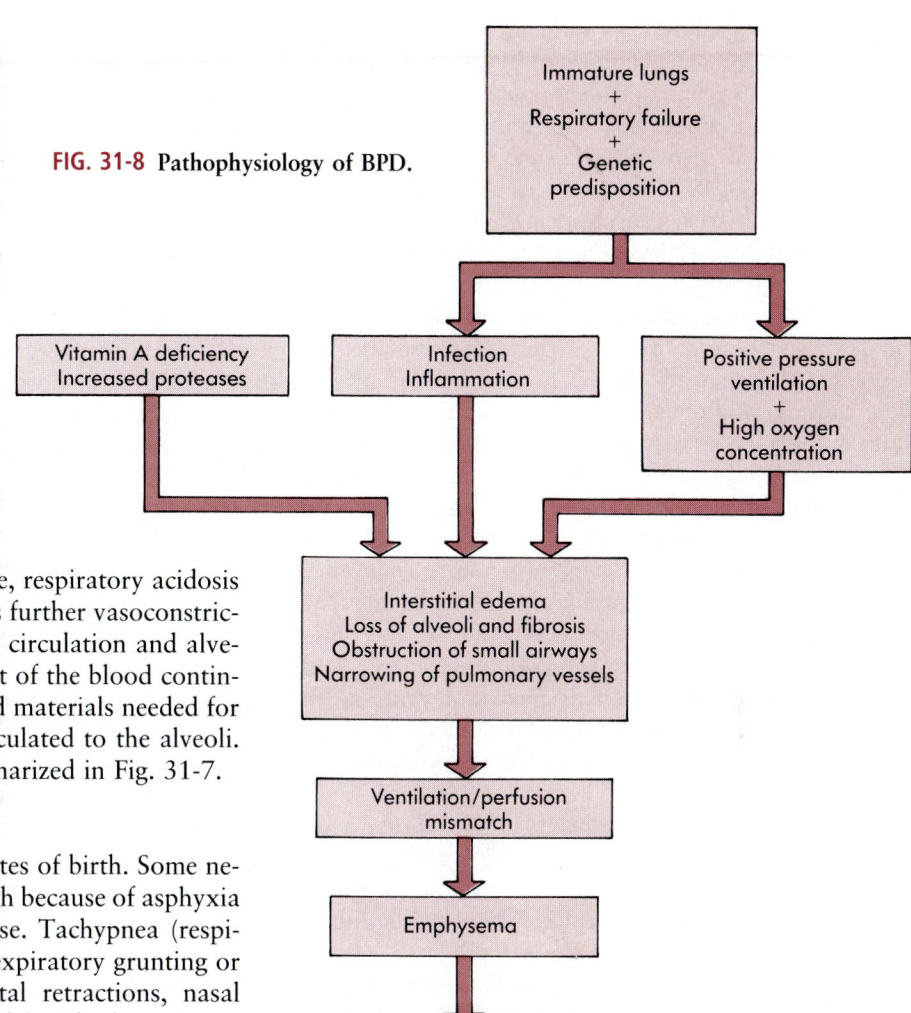

FIG. 31-8 Pathophysiology of BPD.

to get rid of excess carbon dioxide, respiratory acidosis also develops. Lowered pH causes further vasoconstriction. With inadequate pulmonary circulation and alveolar perfusion, the oxygen content of the blood continues to decrease, pH decreases, and materials needed for surfactant production are not circulated to the alveoli. The pathogenesis of RDS is summarized in Fig. 31-7.

Clinical Manifestations

Signs of RDS appear within minutes of birth. Some neonates require resuscitation at birth because of asphyxia or initial severe respiratory disease. Tachypnea (respiratory rate over 20 per minute), expiratory grunting or whining, intercostal and subcostal retractions, nasal flaring, duskiness of the skin, and low body temperature are the most striking clinical manifestations of RDS. The natural course is characterized by progressive hypoxemia and dyspnea. Blood pressure and body temperature decrease. Fatigue, cyanosis, and pallor increase, and grunting decreases or disappears as the condition worsens. Apnea and irregular respirations occur as the infant tires. Edema of the extremities, ileus, and oliguria may also occur during the first 2 to 3 days of life. Signs of asphyxia as a result of apnea or partial respiratory failure indicate rapid progression of the disease. Respiratory distress syndrome can progress to death in severe cases, but in milder cases the clinical manifestations reach a peak within 3 days, after which time gradual improvement is seen. Death is rare after 3 days.

Evaluation and Treatment

Diagnosis is made on the basis of clinical manifestations, blood gas analysis, shunting, and chest radiographs. The course of RDS can be altered dramatically by supportive treatment that maintains adequate oxygenation, circulation, acid-base balance, nutrition, and administration of exogenous surfactant (Fujiwara, Kon-

ishi, & Chida, 1991). Mechanical ventilation, often used successfully in managing RDS, can create such secondary problems as bronchopulmonary dysplasia, however. Approximately 50% to 70% of infants survive with treatment. Even in severe cases, recovery may be complete within 10 to 14 days. The long-term prognosis for normal pulmonary function in most infants is excellent. Neurologic deficits, however, occur in about 20% of neonates weighing less than 1500 g.

Bronchopulmonary Dysplasia

Bronchopulmonary dysplasia (BPD) is a more severe form of lung damage associated with neonatal chronic lung disease (Northway, Rosan, & Porter, 1967). Risk factors for BPD include premature birth and immature lungs, oxygen toxicity (see Chapter 29), positive pressure ventilation, respiratory infection, vitamin A deficiency, α_1-antiprotease deficiency, genetic predisposition, and persistent patent ductus arteriosus.

The incidence of BPD is difficult to ascertain. The most common clinical definition of BPD includes infants who remain oxygen-dependent and have respiratory symptoms and radiographic abnormalities after 28 days of life (Northway, Rosan, & Porter, 1967).

The process of BPD is one of continuous injury and repair of lung tissue, causing delays in both lung and body growth (Fig. 31-8). Pulmonary alterations include scarring and emphysema. Alveoli fail to multiply, and alveolar walls or capillaries become inflamed and may be destroyed. The pulmonary arteries have smaller lumina and thicker walls than is normal for the infant's age, causing pulmonary hypertension. Ciliated epithelium is lost, and mucus plugs and debris clog the airways. Ventilation-perfusion mismatch is severe, and the infant may develop an infection, cor pulmonale, and right heart failure (Behrman et al., 1992).

Episodes of atelectasis, hyperinflation, pneumothorax, and air in the interstitium are characteristic. The infant may seem to be improving but suddenly becomes apneic, or develops more severe respiratory distress and cyanosis. Bronchopulmonary dysplasia can cause death within a few weeks or can continue for months or years. Either death or recovery is possible regardless of the length of disease.

The goals of treatment are to maintain normal oxygenation, prevent further lung damage, and promote lung repair. Regulation of the environmental temperature, monitoring of oxygen requirements, prevention of infection, and maintenance of nutritional status are essential aspects of care. Steroids may be used to control an acute inflammatory response. Other drug therapy is evolving (Fanaroff & Martin, 1992).

Cystic Fibrosis

Cystic fibrosis (CF) (mucoviscidosis) is an inherited disease of the exocrine glands resulting in the production of excessive, thick mucus that obstructs the gastrointestinal system and lungs. (The gastrointestinal component of CF is discussed in Chapter 37.) Although CF is a multiorgan disease, pulmonary failure is the most common cause of death. Cystic fibrosis is the most common fatal genetic disease and it affects about 1 of every 2500 white children; it is much less prevalent in black populations and other populations of color. The disease is characterized by pancreatic enzyme deficiency, progressive obstructive infectious pulmonary disease, and elevated sodium chloride concentrations in the sweat. The incidence is highest in white children, although occurrence in any race is possible. Genetic transmission follows an autosomal recessive mode of inheritance (a child must inherit a defective gene from each parent). The cystic fibrosis gene is located in the middle of the long arm of chromosome 7 (Rommens et al., 1989) and

codes for the protein CF transmembrane regulator (CFTR). Mutation of the gene results in the abnormal expression of the CFTR protein in airway epithelial cells and respiratory manifestations of CF (Crystal, 1992). Clinical manifestations are only present in homozygotes. Approximately 2% to 5% of the white population are carriers. The biochemical defect of CF remains unknown.

Pathophysiology

CF is a generalized disease with complications that affect nearly every organ system. Four alterations contribute to the presentation of the disease: thick, tenacious mucous secretions; stasis of mucous secretions; excess sodium chloride in serous secretions and sweat; and chronic respiratory tract infection. Alteration in CFTR protein results in abnormal regulation of the sodium and chloride ion channels across apical membranes resulting in dehydrated secretions, primarily in the lungs, pancreas, intestine, and sweat glands.

The exocrine, or mucus-producing, glands secrete an abnormally thick mucus that coagulates in the ducts of organs or the airways of the lung with obstruction and dilation that alter or destroy structure and function. Bronchiolar obstruction with thick mucus is the first stage of pulmonary involvement. The obstruction predisposes the lung to infection, primarily with *Staphylococcus aureus* and *Pseudomonas aeruginosa*. With chronic inflammation there is hyperplasia of goblet cells with enlargement and destruction of airway walls causing bronchiectasis. The disease progresses from bronchiolitis (mucus plugging and inflammation of small airways) to bronchitis, followed by bronchiectasis, pneumonia, peribronchial fibrosis, and the formation of large cystic dilations that involve all bronchi. Alveolar involvement ensues with infection, atelectasis, and hemorrhagic pneumonia. Recurrent pneumothorax, hemoptysis, pulmonary hypertension, and cor pulmonale are serious and life-threatening complications of severe and diffuse pulmonary disease.

Clinical Manifestations

Children with CF may have few or numerous clinical manifestations. Chronic cough and sputum production are symptomatic of lung involvement. Mucus is usually purulent. There is labored ventilation resulting in hypoxia, clubbing of the fingers, and cyanosis. The chronic pulmonary infection and malabsorption can lead to secondary manifestations of barrel chest, pectus carinatum, and kyphosis. Chronic rhinitis is common among children with CF. Although diffuse organ involvement can be characteristic of the complications of CF, the pulmonary disorders are the most common cause of morbidity and mortality.

Evaluation and Treatment

Recently, new genetic markers make it possible to diagnose CF prenatally and to detect carriers in more than 70% of families with a history of CF (O'Connell et al., 1987). Cystic fibrosis is traditionally diagnosed when a sweat test discloses a sodium chloride concentration greater than 60 mEq/L. The sweat test is performed when there is a family history of CF or when there are pulmonary or gastrointestinal symptoms consistent with the disease.

Management of CF requires a multidisciplinary effort to relieve symptoms from generalized organ involvement and the social and financial burdens of the disease. The management plan includes judicious use of antibiotics to control pulmonary infection; aggressive pulmonary therapy with drugs to thin mucous secretions, humidified air, postural drainage, respiratory treatments, and oxygen.

Cystic fibrosis was first described in 1936, and the natural history of the disease has changed from death in early childhood to a mean life expectancy approaching 30 years, primarily as a function of improved clinical management (Behrman et al., 1992). There is a need to provide genetic counseling, in addition to educating the entire family about the nature of the disease with instruction in pulmonary and nutritional therapy. Once a couple has a child with CF, the risk for a subsequent child with CF is 1:4 (25%) and 2:4 (50%) will be carriers. The chance of a healthy sibling being a carrier is 2:3 (66%).

SUMMARY REVIEW

Structure and Function of the Pulmonary System in Children

1 The airways of infants and children are shorter and narrower from the trachea through the terminal bronchioles, thus making them more prone to obstruction than the airways of adults.
2 The accessory muscles of respiration are not fully developed in infants and children, making respiratory efforts and coughing less effective than those of adults.
3 Infants have fewer alveoli than older children and adults.
4 The immature chest wall is soft and compliant, contributing to inefficient mechanisms of breathing.

Pulmonary Disorders

1 Croup is a syndrome of clinical manifestations due to acute obstruction of the larynx caused by infection, aspiration of a foreign body, or allergy.
2 Acute epiglottitis is the most life-threatening type of croup. Acute laryngotracheobronchitis, which is less dangerous, is the most common type.
3 Aspiration of foreign bodies that lodge in the airways may cause cough, hoarseness, dyspnea, and can cause chronic infection, asthma, or lung abscess. Pneumonia and respiratory distress also can result from aspiration of contaminated fluids or gastric reflux.
4 The severity of asthma in children depends on the child's age (because age determines the caliber of airway lumina), the child's hypersensitivity to the variant, and the duration of the asthma attack.
5 Children are less well equipped than adults to sustain the work of breathing during asthma attacks.

6 Viral and bacterial pneumonia cause varying degrees of illness in children; symptoms range from mild respiratory distress to rapid death.
7 Bronchiolitis, the inflammatory obstruction of the bronchioles, is most common in infants and is usually caused by infection by a virus that would cause only mild illness in older children or adults.
8 In bronchiolitis obliterans, the bronchioles and some small bronchi are partially or completely obliterated by nodular masses containing granulomatous or fibrous tissue.
9 Respiratory distress syndrome (RDS) of the newborn usually occurs in premature infants who are born before surfactant production and alveolocapillary development are complete. Atelectasis and hypoventilation cause shunting, hypoxemia, and hypercapnia.
10 Bronchopulmonary dysplasia (BPD) is an iatrogenic abnormality of pulmonary and bronchial development in premature neonates. It is caused by administration of oxygen via positive pressure, which injures tissues and delays both lung and body growth. Alterations include scarring of the alveoli and emphysema.
11 Cystic fibrosis is an autosomal recessive genetic disease characterized by excessive secretion of thick, tenacious mucus resulting in bronchiolar obstruction and infection with progression to bronchiectasis, pneumonia, pneumothorax, pulmonary hypertension, and cor pulmonale.

KEY TERMS

Acute laryngitis, 1194
Asthma, 1197
Bronchiolitis obliterans, 1202
Bronchopulmonary dysplasia (BPD) (chronic or respiratory lung disease), 1205
Croup, 1194

Cystic fibrosis (CF), 1206
Epiglottis, 1194
Epiglottitis, 1194
Laryngitis, 1194
Laryngotracheobronchitis (LTB), 1194

Respiratory distress syndrome of the newborn (RDS, idiopathic RDS, hyaline membrane disease), 1203
Sudden infant death syndrome (SIDS), 1197
Viral croup, 1194

REFERENCES

American Academy of Pediatrics Task Force on Positioning and SIDS. (1992). Positioning and SIDS. *Pediatrics, 89*(6), 1120-1126.

Aranda, J. B., Trippenbach, T., Turmen, T., Lopes J. M. (1983). Apnea and control of breathing in newborn infants. In L. Stern (Ed.), *Diagnosis and management of respiratory disorders in the newborn* (pp. 134-157). Reading, MA: Addison-Wesley.

Arguedas, A. G., Stutman, H. R., & Marks, M. I. (1990). Bacterial pneumonias. In V. Chermick & E. L. Kendig (Eds.), *Disorders of the respiratory tract in children* (pp. 371-380). Philadelphia: Saunders.

Baugh, R., & Gilmore, B. B. (1986). Infectious croup: A critical review. *Otolaryngology: Head & Neck Surgery, 95*, 40.

Behrman, R. E., Kliegman, R. M., Nelson, W. E., & Vaughan, V. C. (1992). *Nelson textbook of pediatrics* (14th ed.). Philadelphia: Saunders.

Boule, M., Gaultier, C., Tournier, G., Allaire, Y., & Girard, F. (1979). Lung function in children with recurrent bronchitis. *Respirations, 38*, 127-129.

Castleman, W. L., Sovkness, R. L., Lemanske, R. F., & McAllister, P K. (1990). Viral bronchiolitis during early life induces increased number of bronchiolar mast cells and airway hyperresponsiveness. *American Journal of Pathology, 137*(4), 821-831.

Crystal, R. G. (1992). In vivo gene transfer strategies for the respiratory manifestations of cystic fibrosis. *Pediatric Pulmonology, Suppl. 8*, 67.

Eisen, A. H., & Bacal, H. L. (1963). The relationship of acute bronchiolitis to bronchial asthma: A 4 to 14-year follow-up. *Pediatrics, 31*, 859.

Epler, G. R. (1992). Bronchiolitis obliterans organizing pneumonia: Definition and clinical features. *Chest, 102*(1 Suppl.), 2S-6S.

Evans, R., III, Mullally, P. I., & Wilson, R. W. (1987). National trends in the morbidity and mortality of asthma in the US: Prevalence, hospitalization, and death from asthma over two decades 1965-1984. *Chest, 91*(Suppl.), 65S-74S.

Fanaroff, A. A., & Martin, R. (1992). *Neonatal and perinatal medicine* (pp. 860-876). St. Louis: Mosby–Year Book.

Fujiwara, T., Konishi, M., & Chida, S. (1991). Surfactant therapy in neonatal respiratory distress syndrome. In T. F. Yeh (Ed.), *Neonatal therapeutics* (2nd ed., pp. 70-86). St. Louis: Mosby–Year Book.

Gilbert-Barness, E., & Barness, L. A. (1992). Cause of death: SIDS or something else. *Contemporary Pediatrics, 9*, 13.

Graham, N. M. H. (1990). The epidemiology of acute respiratory infections in children and adults: A global perspective. *Epidemiologic Reviews, 12*, 149-178.

Hill, M., Szefler, S. J., & Larsen, G. L. (1992). Asthma pathogenesis and the implications for therapy in children. *Pediatric Clinics of North America, 39*(6), 1205-1224.

Hurd, S. S., & Lenfant, C. (1992). The national heart, lung, and blood institute asthma program. *Chest, 101*(6, Suppl.), 359S-361S.

Kalinger, M. A., Barnes, P. J., & Persson, C. G. A. (1991). *Asthma: Its pathology and treatment.* New York: Marcel Dekker, Inc.

Kraus, J. F., Greenland, S., & Bultery, S. M. (1989). Risk factors for sudden infant death syndrome in the US collaborative perinatal project. *International Journal of Epidemiology, 18*(1), 113-120.

Larsen, G. L. (1992). Asthma in children. *New England Journal of Medicine, 326*(23), 1540-1545.

Little, R E., & Peterson, D. R. (1990). Sudden infant death syndrome epidemiology: A review and update. *Epidemiologic Reviews, 12*, 241-246.

Loughlin, G. M. (1990). Bronchitis. In V. Chermick & E. L. Kendig (Eds.), *Disorders of the respiratory tract in children*. Philadelphia: Saunders.

Meadow, R. (1990). Suffocation, recurrent apnea, and sudden infant death. *Journal of Pediatrics, 117*, 351.

Morgan, W. J., & Fernando, M. D. (1992). Risk factors for developing wheezing and asthma in childhood. *Pediatric Clinics of North America, 39*(6), 1185-1203.

Mu, L., He, P., & Sun, D. (1991). The causes and complications of late diagnosis of foreign body aspiration in children. *Archives of Otolaryngology: Head & Neck Surgery, 117*, 876-879.

Northway, W. H., Rosan, R. C., & Porter, D. Y. (1967). Pulmonary disease following respiratory therapy of hyaline membrane disease: Bronchopulmonary dysplasia. *New England Journal of Medicine, 276*, 357.

Nuttall, P. (1986). Maternal and infant responses to home apnea monitoring (Doctoral dissertation). Salt Lake City: University of Utah.

O'Connell, D. M., Leppert, M., Park, A., Amos, J. A., Phillips, D. G., White, R., & Vande Woude, G. F. (1987). Three additional polymorphisms in the *met* gene and D758 locus: Use in prenatal diagnosis of cystic fibrosis. *The Journal of Pediatrics, III*(4), 490-495.

Rommens, J. M., Iannuzzi, M. C., Kerem, B., Drumm, M. L., Melmer, G., Dean, M., Rozmahel, R., Cole, J. L., Kennedy, D., Hidaka, N., Zsiga, M., Buchwald, M., Riordan, J. R., Tsui, L. C., & Collins, F. S. (1989). Identification of the cystic fibrosis gene: Chromosome walking and jumping. *Science, 245*, 1059.

Rudolph, A. M. (1987). *Pediatrics* (18th ed.). Norwalk, CT: Appleton & Lange.

Schechtman, V. L., Harper, R. M., Kluge, K. A., Wilson, A. F., Hoffman, H. J., & Southhall, D. P. (1988). Cardiac and respiratory patterns in normal infants and victims of sudden infant death syndrome. *Sleep, 11*, 413-424.

Schechtman, V. L., Harper, R. M., Wilson, A. J., & Southhall, D. P. (1991). Sleep apnea in infants who succumb to the sudden infant death syndrome. *Pediatrics, 87*, 841-846.

Shannon, D. C., & Kelly, D. H. (1982). SIDS and near SIDS (Part I). *New England Journal of Medicine, 306*(16), 959-965.

Spitzer, A. R., & Fox, W. W. (1984). Sudden infant death syndrome: Guidelines for averting tragedy. *Post Graduate Medicine, 23*(7), 374-380.

Walker, C., Virchow, J. C., & Bruijnzeel, P. L. B. (1991). T-cell subsets and their soluble products regulate eosinophilia in allergic and non-allergic asthma. *Journal of Immunology, 146,* 1829-1835.

Ward, L., Keens, T., Chan, L. S., Chipps, B., Carson, S., Deming, D., Krishna, V., MacDonald, H. M., Martin, G., Meredith, K. S., Merritt, T. A., Nickerson, B. G., Stoddard, R. A., & van der Hall, A. L. (1986). Sudden infant death syndrome in infant evaluated by apnea programs in California. *Pediatrics, 77*(840), 451-458.

Washington Office of Technology Assessment. (1987). Neonatal intensive care for low birthweight infants: Costs and effectiveness. Washington, DC: U. S. Congress [Pub. No. OTA-HCS-38].

Weiss, K. B., Gergen, P. J., & Crain, E. E. (1992). Inner city asthma: The epidemiology of an emerging US public health concern. *Chest, 101*(6, Suppl.), 362S-267S.

Whaley, L. F. & Wong, D. L. (1991). *Nursing care of infants and children* (4th ed.). St. Louis: Mosby—Year Book.

Wohl, M. G. (1990). Bronchiolitis. In V. Chermick & E. L. Kendig (Eds.), *Disorders of the respiratory tract in children.* Philadelphia: Saunders.

SUGGESTED READINGS

Avery, G. B. (Ed.). (1987). *Neonatology: Pathophysiology and management of the newborn* (3rd ed.). Philadelphia: Lippincott.

Custer, J. R. (1993). Croup and related disorders. *Pediatric Reviews, 14*(1):19-29.

DiMaio, A. M., & Singh, J. (1992). The infant with cyanosis in the emergency room. *Pediatric Clinics of North America, 39*(5), 987-1006.

Furhman, B. P., & Zimmerman, J. J. (1992). *Pediatric critical care.* St. Louis: Mosby—Year Book.

Godfrey, S. (1993). Airway inflammation, bronchial reactivity and asthma. *Agents and Actions: Supplement 40:*109-143.

Hegyi, T. (1992). Sudden infant death syndrome in 1992: the known and the unknown. Unpublished.

Hoekelman, R. A., Friedman, S. B., Nelson, N. M., & Seidel, H. M. (1992). *Primary pediatric care.* St. Louis: Mosby—Year Book.

Hoffman, H. J., & Hillman, L. S. (1992). Epidemiology of the sudden infant death syndrome. *Clinics in Perinatology, 19*(4):717-737.

Kaliner, M. A., Barnes, P. J., Persson, C. G. A. (1991). *Asthma, its pathology and treatment.* New York: Dekker.

Landau, L. I. (1993). Evolution of asthma. *Journal of Paediatric Child Health 29*(1):4-5.

North American Cystic Fibrosis Conference. (1991). *Pediatric pulmonology* (Suppl. 6, pp. 1-326).

Sferra, T. J., & Collins, F. S. (1993). The molecular biology of cystic fibrosis. *Annual Review of Medicine, 44:*133-144.

Taeush, W. H., Ballard, R. H., & Avery, M. E. (1991). *Schaffer and Avery's diseases of the newborn.* Philadelphia: Saunders.

Wainwright, B. J., Scrambler, R. J., Schmidtke, J., Watson, E. A., Law, H., Farrall, M., Cooke, H. J., Eiberg, H., & Williamson, R. (1985). Localization of cystic fibrosis locus to human chromosome 7 cen-q 22. *Nature, 318,* 384.

West, J. B. (1992). *Pulmonary pathophysiology* (4th ed.). Philadelphia: Williams & Wilkins.

Wiswell, T. E., & Mendiola, J., Jr. (1993). Respiratory distress syndrome in the newborn: Innovative therapies. *American Family Physician, 47*(2):407-414.

UNIT XI

The Renal and Urologic Systems

HIPPOCRATES (400 BC) first wrote descriptions of the characteristics of urine as a basis for the appearance or progression of disease. Galen (AD 130-200) dissected the kidney, ureters, and bladder in humans and animals and evolved a theory of how the kidneys "attract" waste products from the blood. After the pre-scientific era, Malpighi (1628-1694) made the greatest contribution to defining the anatomy of the kidney by using the microscope to describe the glomeruli (malpighian corpuscles). He described the glomeruli as glands but was unable to identify them as capillary tufts.

Bladder stones were removed during ancient and medieval times, but it was not until the invention of instruments that could be passed

Detail of the urogenital system. (From Jakob & Rueff, De conceptu et generatione hominis, 1580; courtesy National Library of Medicine.)

gen introduced x-rays, a technique was devised to adequately visualize the urologic tract.

Physicians before Richard Bright (1789-1858) had observed albuminuria (albumin in the urine), but Bright was the first to associate a coagulable urine with kidney disease and granular-appearing kidneys. Lorenzo Bellini had previously described the tubules of the kidney, and William Bowman (1816-1892) described the microscopic anatomy of the kidney, including the spheric capsule still known as Bowman's capsule. From his understanding of the proximity of the glomerular blood flow to the fluid in Bowman's capsule, he proposed a theory of the movement of water and salts to form urine. But this description, which was based on anatomy, was incomplete without physiologic experimentation.

Filtration as a function of hydrostatic pressure in the glomerular capillaries was described by Carl Ludwig in 1842, and tubular secretion was demonstrated by Rudolf Heidenhain (1834-1897). The processes of filtration, reabsorption, and secretion then were synthesized by Robert Cushny (1866-1926), thus completing a foundation for the advancement of modern renal physiology and a continued understanding of disease.

into the bladder for observation that modern urology was born. Cheselden (1688-1752), an expert anatomist from England, was especially adept in the removal of bladder stones (lithotomy), and it was reputed that he performed a lithotomy in less than 1 minute. In Germany, Nitze and Leiter invented the first practical cystoscope in 1879. In the 1920s, after Roent-

Structure and Function of the Renal and Urologic Systems

Sue E. Huether

Chapter Outline

*T*he primary function of the kidney is to maintain a stable internal environment for optimal cell and tissue metabolism. The kidneys accomplish these life-sustaining tasks by balancing solute and water transport, excreting metabolic waste products, conserving nutrients, and regulating acids and bases. The kidney also has an endocrine function and secretes the hormones renin, erythropoietin, and 1,25-dihydroxyvitamin D for regulation of blood pressure, erythrocyte production, and calcium metabolism, re-

spectively. In times of severe fasting the kidney also can synthesize glucose from amino acids, performing the process of gluconeogenesis. The formation of urine is achieved through the process of filtration, reabsorption, and secretion by the glomeruli and tubules within the kidney. The bladder stores the urine that it receives from the kidney by way of the ureters. Urine is then removed from the body through the urethra.

STRUCTURES OF THE RENAL SYSTEM

Structures of the Kidney

The **kidneys** are paired organs located on the posterior abdominal wall outside the peritoneal cavity. They lie on either side of the vertebral column with their upper and lower poles extending from the twelfth thoracic to the third lumbar vertebrae (Fig. 32-1). Each kidney is approximately 11 cm long, 5 to 6 cm wide, and 3 to 4 cm thick. A tightly adhering capsule (the **renal capsule**) surrounds each kidney, and the kidney then is embedded in a mass of fat. The capsule and fatty layer are covered with a double layer of **renal fascia,** fibrous tissue that attaches the kidney to the posterior abdominal wall.

The cushion of fat and the position of the kidney between the abdominal organs and muscles of the back protect it from trauma. The right kidney is slightly lower than the left; it is displaced downward by the overlying liver. A medial indentation (the **hilum**) contains the entry and exit for the renal blood vessels, nerves, lymphatic vessels, and ureter.

The gross structure of the kidney can be identified when it is divided from top to bottom in a coronal plane (Fig. 32-2). The major components are the outer **renal cortex** and the inner **renal medulla.** The cortex contains all the glomeruli and portions of the tubules. The medulla consists of a series of wedges, called **renal pyramids,** with an outer zone close to the cortex and an inner zone. **Renal columns** extend from the cortex down between the renal pyramids. The apices of the pyramids project into a **minor calyx** (a cup-shaped cavity), which joins together to form a **major calyx.** The major calyces join to form the **renal pelvis,** an extension of the upper end of the ureter.

Nephron

The **nephron** is the functional unit of the kidney. Approximately 1.2 million nephrons are contained in each kidney. The nephron is a tubular structure with subunits that include the renal corpuscle, proximal convoluted tubule, loop of Henle, distal convoluted tubule, and collecting duct, all of which contribute to the formation of final urine (Fig. 32-3). The different structures of the epithelial cells lining various segments of the tubule facilitate the special functions of secretion and reabsorption (Fig. 32-4).

The kidney has two kinds of nephrons: (1) **cortical nephrons** (85% of all nephrons), which extend only partially into the medulla, and (2) **juxtamedullary nephrons,** which lie close to and extend deep into the medulla and are important for the concentration of urine (Fig. 32-5). The **glomerulus** is a tuft of capillaries, the glomerular capillaries, that loop into a circular capsule, called **Bowman's capsule,** like fingers pushed into bread

FIG. 32-1 Organs of the urinary system. (From Thompson et al., 1993.)

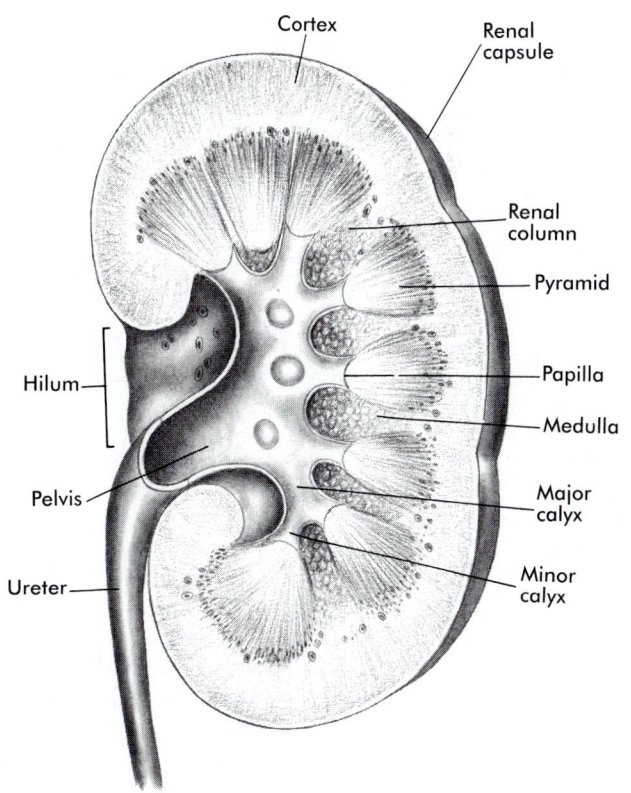

FIG. 32-2 Kidney structure. (From Thompson et al., 1993.)

FIG. 32-3 Components of nephron.
(From Thompson et al., 1993.)

FIG. 32-4 Epithelial cells of the various segments of nephron tubules. (From Berne & Levy, 1993.)

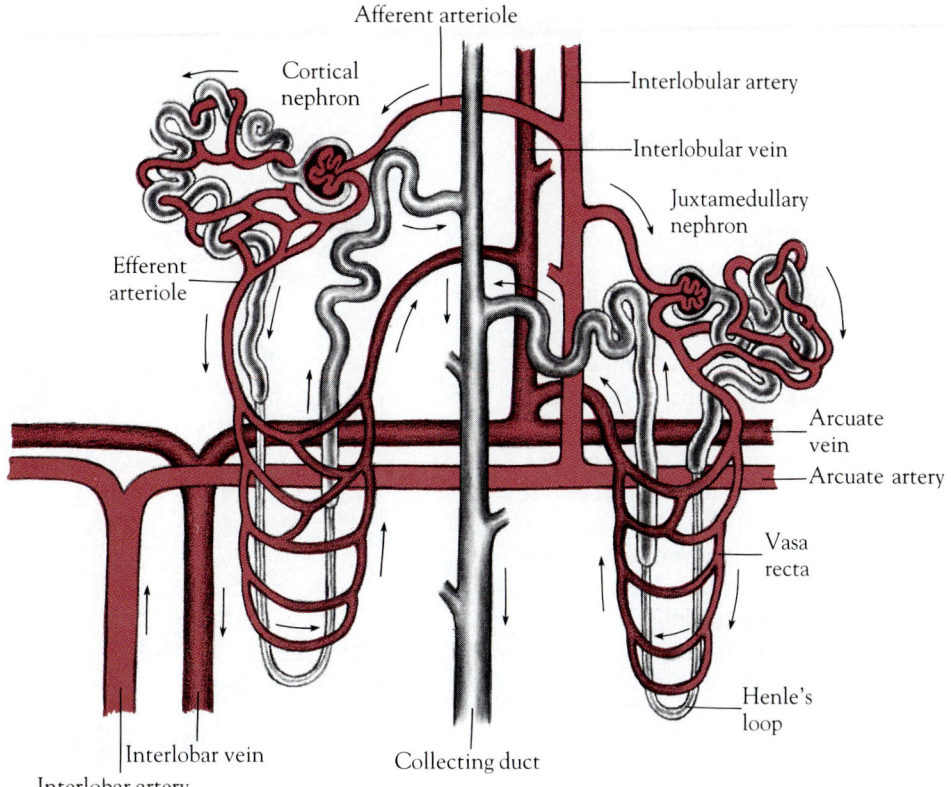

FIG. 32-5   The nephron unit with its blood vessels. Blood flows through nephron vessels as follows: interlobular artery, afferent arteriole, glomerulus, efferent arteriole, peritubular capillaries (around the tubules), venules, interlobular vein. (From Thompson et al., 1993.)

dough. Together, the glomerulus and Bowman's capsule are called the renal corpuscle. **Mesangial cells** (shaped like smooth muscle cells) and some macrophages lie between and support the capillaries. The space inside of Bowman's capsule is called **Bowman's space.**

The wall of the glomerular capillary serves as a filtration membrane (the **glomerular filtration membrane**) and has three layers: (1) an inner capillary endothelium, (2) a middle basement membrane, and (3) an outer layer of capillary epithelium. Each layer has unique structural properties that allow all components of the blood to filter through, with the exception of blood cells and plasma proteins with a molecular weight greater than 70,000 (Figs. 32-6 and 32-7). The capillary endothelium is composed of cells in continuous contact with the basement membrane. It is perforated by many small openings or windows, called fenestrae. The middle basement membrane is a selectively permeable network of glycoproteins and mucopolysaccharides. The epithelium has specialized cells called **podocytes.** Footlike processes, or pedicles, radiate from the podocytes and adhere to the basement membrane. The pedicles of one podocyte interlock with the pedicles of adjacent podocytes, form-

ing an elaborate network of intercellular clefts. These clefts are called **filtration slits** or slit membranes. The glomerular filtration membrane separates the blood of the glomerular capillaries from the fluid in Bowman's space. The glomerular filtrate passes through the three layers of the glomerular membrane and forms the primary urine.

The glomerulus is supplied by the afferent arteriole and drained by the efferent arteriole. A group of specialized cells known as **juxtaglomerular cells** are located around the afferent arteriole where it enters the renal corpuscle (Fig. 32-3). Between the afferent and efferent arteriole is a portion of the distal convoluted tubule with specialized cells known as **macula densa** (Fig. 32-6). Together the juxtaglomerular cells and macula densa cells form the **juxtaglomerular apparatus** (see Fig. 32-3). Control of renal blood flow, glomerular filtration, and renin secretion occurs at this site.

The **proximal tubule** continues from Bowman's space and has an initial convoluted segment (pars convoluta) and then a straight segment (pars recta) that descends toward the medulla (Fig. 32-3). The proximal tubular lumen consists of one layer of cuboidal cells. This is the only surface inside the nephron where the cells are covered with microvilli (a brush border). The microvilli create a brushlike surface that greatly expands the surface area of the tubule and enhances its reabsorptive function (Fig. 32-4). The proximal tubule joins the **loop of Henle,** a hairpin loop composed of thick and thin portions of a descending segment that goes into the medulla. The tube then loops and becomes the thickening ascending segment that extends toward the cortex. The thin segment is composed of thin squamous cells with no active transport function. The cells of the thick segment are cuboidal and actively transport several solutes.

The more numerous cortical nephrons have glomeruli originating close to the surface of the cortex or in the midcortex unlike the juxtamedullary nephrons, whose glomeruli are located deep in the cortex close to the medulla. The major structural difference between the glomeruli in the two types of nephrons is the length of the loop of Henle. In cortical nephrons, the loop is short and may not extend into the medulla. The loops of Henle for the juxtamedullary nephrons, however, may extend the whole length of the medulla (40 mm). Juxtamedullary nephrons represent about 12% of the total number of nephrons.

The **distal tubule** has straight and convoluted segments. It extends from the macula densa to the **collecting duct.** The collecting duct is a large tubule that descends down the cortex, through the renal pyramids of the inner and outer medulla, and into the minor calyx.

Blood Vessels of the Kidney

The blood vessels of the kidney closely parallel nephron structure. The **renal arteries** arise as the fifth branches of the abdominal aorta. At the renal hilum they divide into anterior and posterior branches and then subdivide into lobar arteries that supply blood to the lower, middle, and upper thirds of the kidney. The **interlobar arteries** are further subdivisions that travel down the renal columns and between the pyramids. At the cortical medullary junction, interlobar arteries branch into the **arcuate arteries,** which arch over the base of the pyramids and run parallel to the surface of the kidney.

The interlobular arteries arise from the arcuate arteries and extend through the cortex toward the periphery and form the afferent glomerular arterioles (Fig. 32-5). The afferent arteriole subdivides into a fistlike structure of four to eight **glomerular capillaries** (Fig. 32-6). The glomerular capillaries empty into the efferent arteriole, which conveys blood to a second capillary bed, the peritubular capillaries. This is the only place in the body where an arteriole is positioned between two capillary beds. Increases or decreases in the resistance of the afferent and efferent arterioles increase or decrease glomerular filtration.

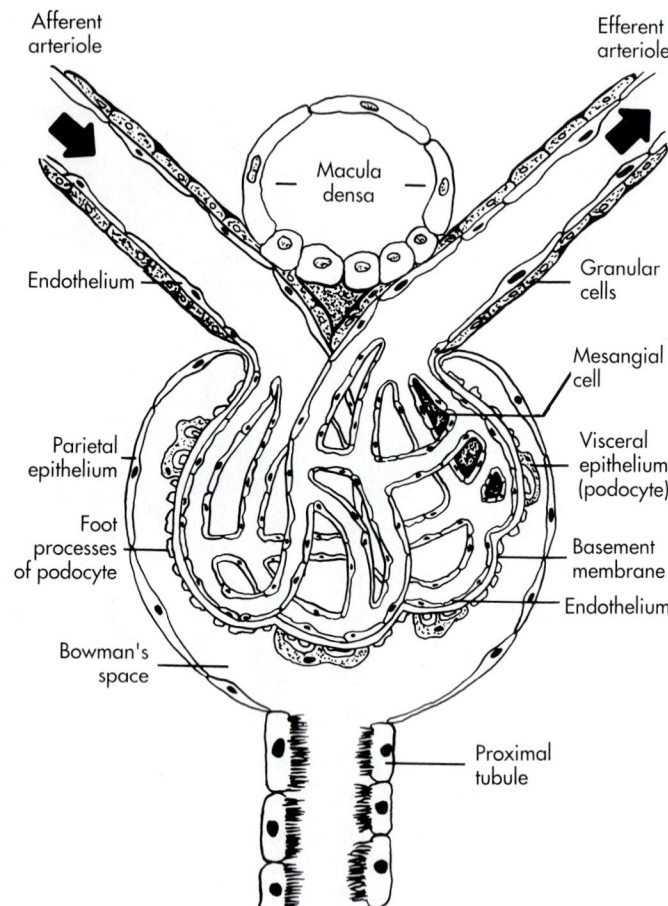

FIG. 32-6 Anatomy of the glomerulus and juxtaglomerular apparatus. (From Berne & Levy, 1993.)

The peritubular capillaries surround the convoluted portions of the proximal and distal tubules and the loop of Henle (Fig. 32-5). The peritubular capillaries are adapted differently for the cortical and juxtamedullary nephrons. The peritubular capillaries surrounding the tubules of the cortical nephrons are similar to capillaries in other tissues. For the juxtamedullary nephrons, a network of capillaries called the **vasa recta** forms loops and closely follows the loops of Henle. The capillaries of the vasa recta are the only blood supply to the medulla. They influence the osmolar concentration of the medullary extracellular fluid, which is important to the formation of a concentrated urine. All capillaries then drain into the venous system. The renal veins follow the arterial path in a reverse direction and have the same names as the arteries. The renal vein empties into the inferior vena cava. The lymphatic vessels tend also to follow the distribution of the blood vessels.

FIG. 32-7 Glomerular capillary. A, Scanning electron micrograph of normal glomerular capillary *(C)* enclosed by podocytes *(P)* with primary processes and interdigitating foot processes. (×5200.) **B,** Glomerular capillary wall showing foot processes of endothelial podocytes *(F),* filtration slit membrane *(arrow),* basement membrane *(M),* and fenestrated endothelium *(E).* (×40,000.) **C,** Portion of human glomerulus showing endothelial cell *(E),* mesangial cell *(M),* and capillaries *(C).* Basement membrane *(B)* is somewhat thickened by hypertension. (×3600.) (From Kissane, 1990.)

Urinary Structures
Ureters

The urine formed by the nephrons flows from the distal tubules and collecting ducts through the duct of Bellini, the **renal papillae** (projections of the ducts), and into the calyces, and is collected in the renal pelvis (Fig. 32-2). From the renal pelvis, urine is funneled into the **ureters.** Each adult ureter is approximately 30 cm long and is composed of long, intertwining muscle bundles. The lower ends of the ureters pass obliquely through the posterior aspect of the bladder wall. The close approximation of muscle cells permits the direct transmission of electrical stimulation, and the resulting peristaltic activity propels urine into the bladder. Peristaltic activity is affected by urine volume. When urine flow is slow, the contraction is segmented, with downward propulsion of urine. Increasing flow rates increase peristalsis. Peristalsis is maintained even when the ureter is denervated, so that ureters can be transplanted.

Sensory innervation for the upper part of the ureter arises from the tenth thoracic nerve roots, with referred pain to the umbilicus. The innervation of lower segments arises from the sacral nerves with referred pain to the vulva or penis. The ureters have a rich blood supply. The primary arteries come from the kidney with contributions from the lumbar and superior vesical artery. Contraction of the bladder during **micturition** (urination) compresses the lower end of the ureter, preventing reflux.

Bladder and Urethra

The **bladder** is a bag composed of a basket weave of smooth muscle fibers that forms the **detrusor muscle** and its smooth lining of transitional epithelium. As the bladder fills with urine, it distends and the layers of transitional epithelium slide past each other and become thinner as the volume of the bladder increases. The **trigone** is a smooth triangular area lying between the openings of the two ureters and the urethra (Fig. 32-8). The position of the bladder varies with age and sex. In infants and young children, the bladder rises above the symphysis pubis, providing easy access for percutaneous aspiration. In adults it lies in the true pelvis, in front of the rectum and in front of the uterus in women. Inferiorly, the bladder sits on the prostate in men and on the anterior vagina in women. The bladder has a profuse blood supply, accounting for the bleeding that readily occurs with trauma, surgery, or inflammation.

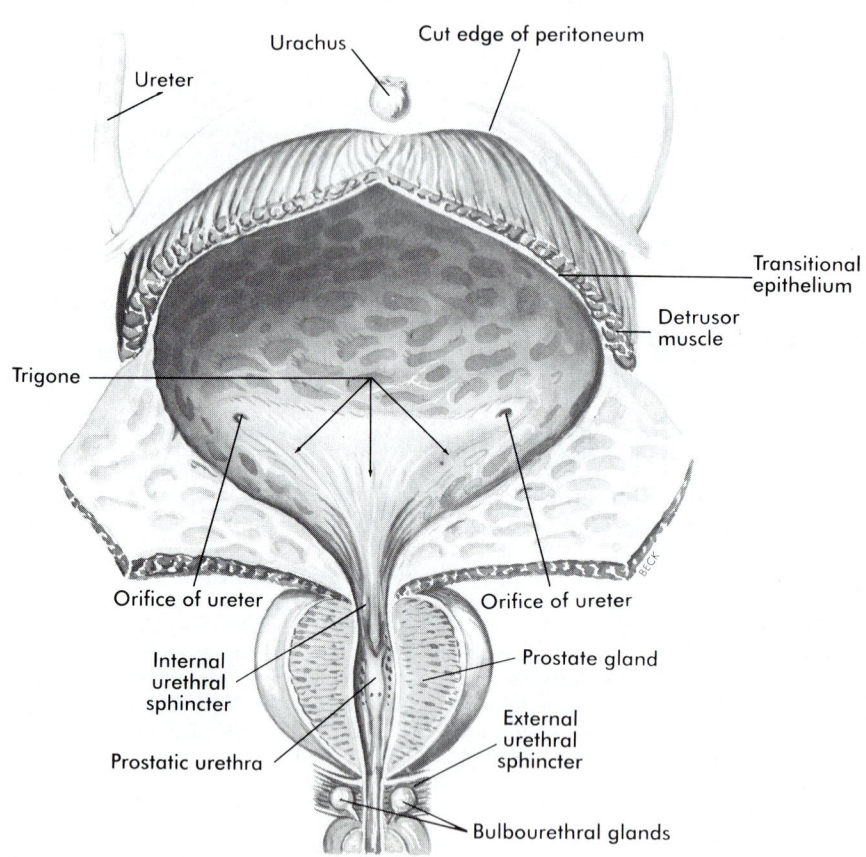

FIG. 32-8 **The male urinary bladder cut to show the interior.** (From Thibodeau & Patton, 1993.)

The **urethra** extends from the inferior side of the bladder to the outside of the body. Two muscles called sphincters control excretion of urine from the bladder through the urethra. A ring of smooth muscle forms the **internal urethral sphincter** at the junction of the urethra and bladder. The **external urethral sphincter** is composed of striated muscles and is under voluntary control. The entire urethra is lined with mucus-secreting glands. The female urethra is short (3 to 4 cm). The male urethra is long (18 to 20 cm) and has three segments: prostatic, membranous, and cavernous. The prostatic urethra is closest to the bladder. It passes through the prostate gland and contains the openings of the ejaculatory ducts. The membranous urethra is the segment that passes through the floor of the pelvis. The cavernous segment forms the remainder of the tube. The cavernous segment is surrounded by erectile tissue and contains the openings of the bulbourethral mucous glands.

The innervation of the bladder and internal urethral sphincter is supplied by parasympathetic fibers of the autonomic nervous system. They primarily pass with the arteries to and from the sacral levels of the spinal cord. Sensory fibers may extend as high as the T6 portion of the spinal cord. Motor fibers from the pudendal nerve supply the external urethral sphincter. The reflex arc required for micturition is stimulated by mechanoreceptors, which respond to stretching of tissue. The mechanoreceptors sense bladder fullness and send impulses to the sacral level of the cord with bladder filling. When the bladder accumulates 250 to 300 ml of urine, the bladder contracts, and the internal urethral sphincter relaxes through activation of the spinal reflex arc (known as the micturition reflex). At this time a person feels the urge to void. In older children and adults, the reflex can be inhibited or facilitated by impulses coming from the brain, resulting in voluntary control of micturition.

RENAL BLOOD FLOW

The kidneys are highly vascular organs and usually receive 1000 to 1200 ml of blood/min, or about 20% to 25% of the cardiac output. With a normal hematocrit of 45%, about 600 to 700 ml of blood flowing through the kidney per minute is plasma. From the renal plasma flow (RPF), 20% (approximately 120 to 140 ml/min) is filtered at the glomerulus and passes into Bowman's capsule. The filtration of the plasma per unit of time is known as the **glomerular filtration rate** (GFR), and the GFR is directly related to the perfusion pressure in the glomerular capillaries.

The remaining 80% (about 480 ml) of plasma flows through the efferent arterioles to the peritubular capillaries. The ratio of glomerular filtrate to renal plasma flow per minute (125/600 = 0.20) is called the filtration fraction. All but 1 to 2 ml of the glomerular filtrate is normally reabsorbed and returned to the circulation by the peritubular capillaries.

The GFR is directly related to renal blood flow (RBF), which is regulated by intrinsic autoregulatory mechanisms, by neural regulation, and by hormonal regulation. In general, blood flow to any organ is determined by the arteriovenous pressure differences across the vascular bed. If there is a decrease in mean arterial pressure or an increase in vascular resistance, there is a decrease in RBF.

Autoregulation

In the kidney, a local mechanism tends to keep the rate of blood flow and therefore the GFR fairly constant over a range of arterial pressures between 80 and 180 mm Hg (Fig. 32-9). This means that changes in afferent arteriolar resistance and arteriolar pressure occur in the same direction. For example, as systemic blood pressure increases, the afferent arterioles constrict, preventing an increase in glomerular blood flow and filtration pressure. Opposite processes occur with a decrease in systemic blood pressure. Therefore RBF and GFR are relatively constant. This "constant" state is maintained by some intrinsic autoregulatory mechanism mediating the arteriolar resistance changes. The purpose of renal autoregulation is to prevent wide fluctuations in systemic arterial pressure from being transmitted to the glomerular capillaries. In this way, large fluctuations in GFR are prevented, and solute and water excretion is constantly maintained when arterial pressure changes.

One mechanism responsible for the autoregulatory response in the kidney is probably a myogenic mechanism. As arterial pressure declines, the stretch on the afferent

FIG. 32-9 Renal autoregulation. Blood flow and glomerular filtration rate are stabilized in the face of changes in perfusion pressure. (From Berne & Levy, 1993.)

arteriolar wall decreases and the arteriole relaxes, with an increase in renal blood flow; an increase in arteriolar pressure causes the arteriole to contract and decreases renal blood flow. Other mechanisms may operate to influence autoregulation, including changes in flow through the macula densa and the presence of metabolites (i.e., kinins and prostaglandins) (Brenner, Katz, & Ishikawa, 1991).

Neural Regulation

The blood vessels of the kidney are innervated by the autonomic nervous system through sympathetic fibers that cause vasoconstriction. The innervation of the kidney comes primarily from the celiac ganglion and greater splanchnic nerve (see Fig. 12-23). Adrenergic fibers are mainly present and are generally distributed with the arteries and arterioles. The afferent and efferent arterioles are richly innervated, but nerves have not been observed in the glomerular capillaries.

The RBF is reflexly related to the systemic arterial pressure. When systemic arterial pressure decreases, increased renal sympathetic nerve activity is mediated reflexively through the carotid sinus and the baroreceptors of the aortic arch. This stimulates renal arteriolar vasoconstriction and decreases both RBF and GFR. Thus, RBF still changes when systemic arterial pressure is significantly reduced, although autoregulatory processes dampen the response. The decreased renal blood flow decreases the GFR and diminishes excretion of sodium and water, promoting an increase in blood volume and thus an increase in systemic pressure.

Exercise, body position, and hypoxia also influence RBF. Exercise and change of body position activate renal sympathetic neurons and cause mild vasoconstriction. Severe hypoxia stimulates the chemoreceptors of the carotid and aortic bodies and decreases RBF by means of sympathetic stimulation. Hemorrhage induces intense sympathetic stimulation and vasoconstriction and both glomerular filtration rate and blood flow are reduced.

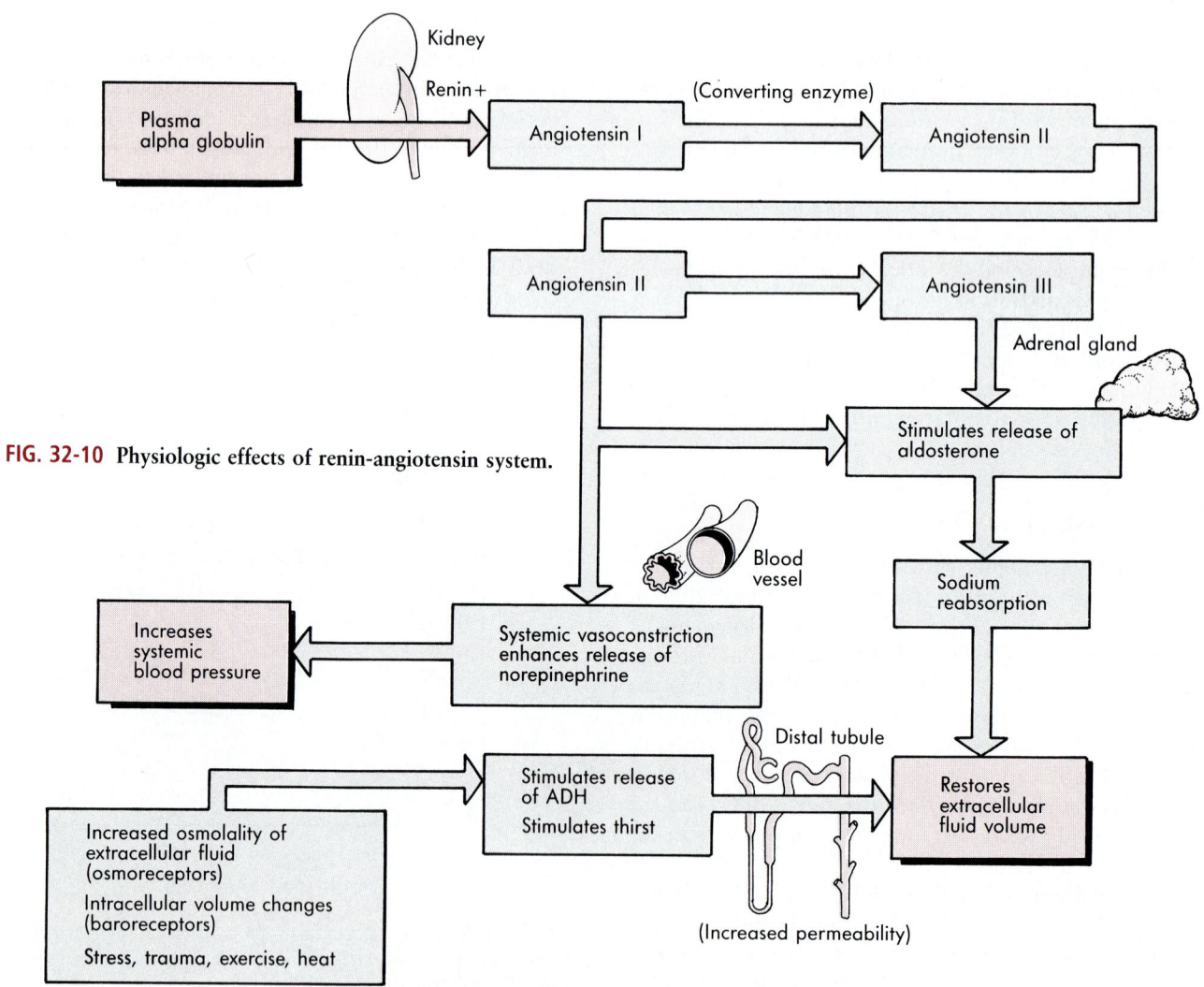

FIG. 32-10 Physiologic effects of renin-angiotensin system.

Hormonal Regulation

Hormonal factors can alter the resistance of the renal vasculature by stimulating vasodilation or vasoconstriction. A major hormonal regulator of renal blood flow is the **renin-angiotensin system,** which can increase systemic arterial pressure and change renal blood flow. Renin is an enzyme formed and stored in the cells of the arterioles of the juxtaglomerular apparatus (Fig. 32-3). Several complex physiologic mechanisms stimulate the release of renin. These mechanisms are principally decreased blood pressure in the afferent arterioles, which reduces stretch of the juxtaglomerular cells; decreased sodium chloride concentration in the distal convoluted tubule; and sympathetic nerve stimulation of β-adrenergic receptors on the juxtaglomerular cells (Re, 1987).

When renin is released, it cleaves an α-globulin (angiotensinogen) in the plasma to form angiotensin I, which is physiologically inactive. In the presence of a converting enzyme, angiotensin I is converted to angiotensin II and angiotensin III. Angiotensin II stimulates secretion of aldosterone by the adrenal cortex (see Chapter 17), is also a potent vasopressor, and inhibits renin release. Angiotensin III has less of an effect than angiotensin II. Numerous physiologic effects of the renin-angiotensin system serve the purpose of stabilizing systemic blood pressure and preserving the extracellular fluid volume during hypotension or hypovolemia, including sodium reabsorption, systemic vasoconstriction, sympathetic nerve stimulation, thirst stimulation, and drinking. (The effects are summarized in Fig. 32-10.)

Atrial natriuretic factor (ANF) is a hormone secreted from cells in the right atrium when right atrial blood pressure increases. Atrial natriuretic factor inhibits adrenocorticotropic hormone (ADH) secretion and leads to the formation of a large volume of dilute urine that decreases blood volume and blood pressure (Sagnalla & MacGregor, 1990).

Prostaglandins and kinins are other hormones that are formed in and act on the kidneys. The precise effect of locally produced prostaglandins is not clear, but different types of prostaglandins appear to have different actions. For example, prostaglandin E_2 in the kidney is a vasodilator. Other renal hormones are discussed on p. 1228.

KIDNEY FUNCTION

Nephron Function

The nephron is able to perform many functions simultaneously. It filters the plasma at the glomerulus and reabsorbs and secretes different substances at various parts of its tubular structure (Fig. 32-11). The function of the nephron is to form a filtrate of protein-free plasma. This process, known as **ultrafiltration,** occurs across the glomerular capillaries. The nephron then regulates the filtrate to maintain body fluid volume, electrolyte composition, and pH within narrow limits.

Regulation of the filtrate occurs through two processes: tubular reabsorption and tubular secretion. **Tubular reabsorption** is the movement of fluids and solutes from the tubular lumen to the peritubular capillary plasma. Transfer of substances from the plasma of the peritubular capillary to the tubular lumen is **tubular secretion.** The transport mechanisms are both active and passive (processes defined in Chapter 3). The elimination of a substance in the final urine is known as **excretion** (Fig. 32-12).

Glomerular Filtration

The fluid filtered by the glomerular capillary filtration membrane is protein free but contains electrolytes such as sodium, chloride, and potassium and organic molecules such as creatinine, urea, and glucose in the same concentrations as in plasma. Like other capillary membranes, the glomerulus is freely permeable to water and relatively impermeable to large colloids such as plasma proteins. The size of the molecules and their electrical charge are important factors affecting the permeability of substances crossing the glomerulus. The small size of the filtration slits or pores in the membrane restricts the passage of proteins and other macromolecules. The negative charge along the filtration membrane further impedes the passage of negatively charged macromolecules (because like forces repel each other). Positively charged macromolecules therefore permeate the membrane more readily than neutrally charged particles.

Capillary pressure, as well as electrical charge, has an effect on glomerular filtration. The hydrostatic pressure within the capillary is the major force for inducing water and solutes across the filtration membrane and into Bowman's capsule. This pressure is determined indirectly by the efficiency of cardiac contraction and directly by the systemic arterial pressure and the resistances to blood flow in the afferent and efferent arterioles. Two forces oppose the filtration effects of the glomerular capillary hydrostatic pressure (P_{GC}): (1) the hydrostatic pressure in Bowman's space (P_{BC}) and (2) the effective oncotic pressure of the glomerular capillary blood (π_{GC}). (As explained in Chapter 3, hydrostatic pressure is a pushing force in relation to water, and oncotic pressure is a pulling force.) Because the fluid in Bowman's space normally contains only minute amounts of protein, it does not normally have an oncotic influence on the plasma of the glomerular capillary (Fig. 32-13).

The combined effect of forces favoring and forces opposing filtration determines the filtration pressure. The

FIG. 32-11 Major functions of nephron segments. (From Whaley & Wong, 1991.)

net filtration pressure (NFP) is the sum of forces favoring and opposing filtration and is expressed by the following equation:

$$NFP = [P_{GC} + \pi_{BC}] - [B_{BC} + \pi_{GC}]$$
Forces favoring − Forces opposing
filtration   filtration

(The estimated values contributing to the forces of net filtration are presented in Table 32-1.)

As the protein-free fluid is filtered into Bowman's capsule, the plasma oncotic pressure increases, and the hydrostatic pressure decreases. The increase in glomerular capillary oncotic pressure is great enough to reduce the net filtration pressure to zero at the efferent end of the capillary and to stop the filtration process effectively. The low hydrostatic pressure and increased oncotic pressure in the efferent arteriole then are transferred to the peritubular capillaries and facilitate reabsorption of fluid from the proximal tubules.

Filtration rate

The total volume of fluid filtered by the glomeruli averages 180 L/day, or approximately 120 ml/min, a phe-

nomenal amount considering the size of the kidneys. Because only 1 to 2 L of urine is excreted per day, 99% of the filtrate is reabsorbed into the peritubular capillaries and returned to the blood. The factors determining the GFR are directly related to the pressures that favor or oppose filtration. Any changes in afferent or efferent arteriolar resistance will alter glomerular capillary hydrostatic pressure and GFR. Vasoconstriction of one or the other of these two arterioles produces opposite effects on glomerular pressure. For example, if the afferent arteriole constricts, blood flow decreases with a corresponding drop in glomerular pressure. The GFR then decreases, and body fluids are conserved. Conversely, constriction of the efferent arteriole increases the net filtration pressure, and the GFR increases. When both afferent and efferent arterioles constrict, little change occurs in filtration pressure, but renal blood flow is reduced and so is the GFR.

Obstruction to the outflow of urine (caused by strictures, stones, or tumors along the urinary tract) can cause a retrograde increase in pressure at Bowman's capsule and a decrease in GFR. Excessive loss of protein-free fluid from vomiting, diarrhea, use of diuretics, or excessive sweating can increase glomerular cap-

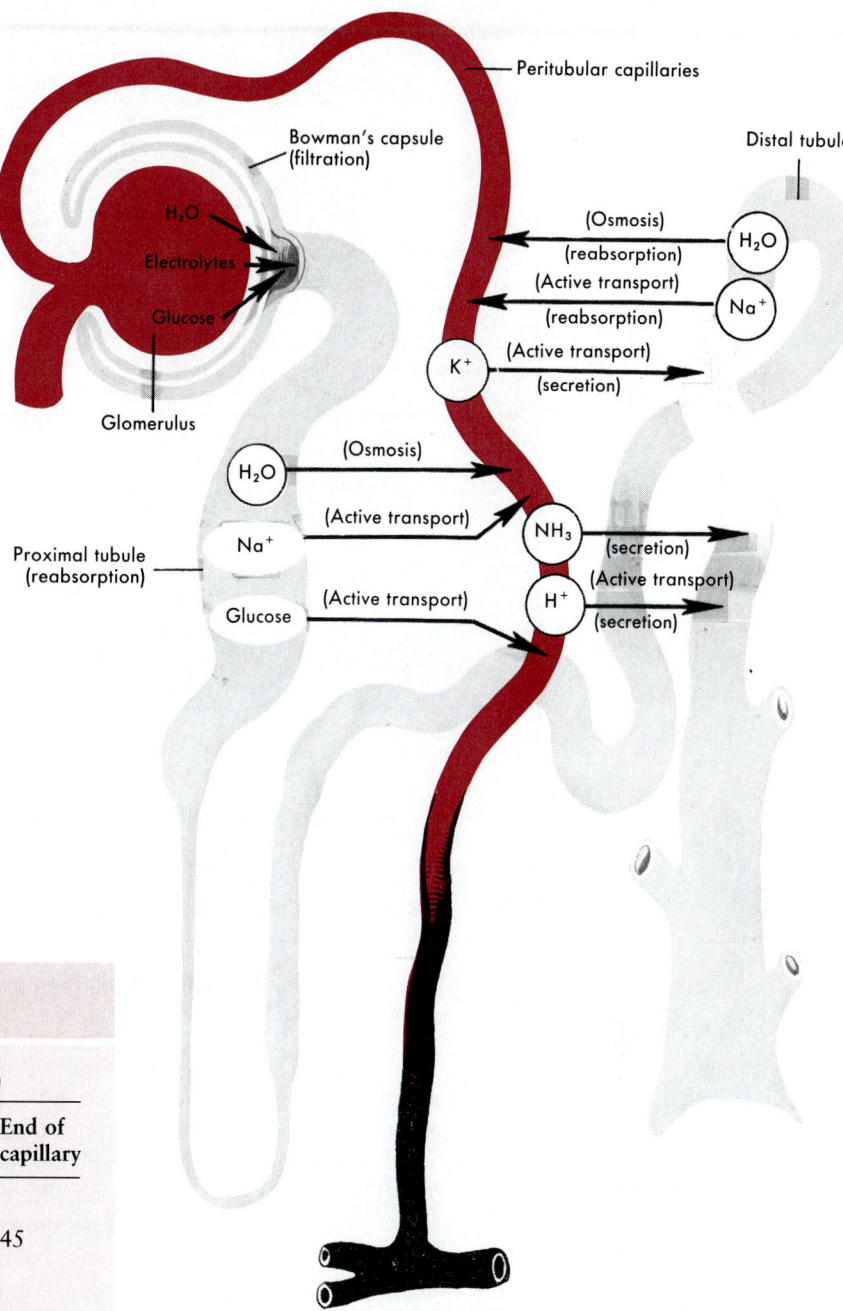

FIG. 32-12 Glomerular filtration, tubular reabsorption, and tubular secretion. The three processes by which the kidneys excrete urine. From proximal convoluted tubules, sodium and glucose are reabsorbed into peritubular capillaries by active transport. Water reabsorption by osmosis follows. From distal convoluted tubules, sodium is reabsorbed by active transport. Osmotic reabsorption of water from them occurs when ADH is present. Secretion of ammonia and hydrogen occurs from peritubular capillaries into distal tubules by active transport. (From Thibodeau, G. A. [1987]. *Anatomy and physiology.* St. Louis: Mosby–Year Book.)

TABLE 32-1

Glomerular Filtration Pressures

Forces	Pressures	Pressures (mm Hg)	
		Beginning of capillary	End of capillary
Promoting filtration			
Glomerular capillary hydrostatic pressure	P_{GC}	47	45
Bowman's capsule oncotic pressure	π_{BC}	Negligible effect	
Opposing filtration			
Bowman's capsule hydrostatic pressure	P_{BC}	10	10
Glomerular capillary oncotic pressure	π_{GC}	<u>25</u>	<u>35</u>
Net filtration pressure		12	0

FIG. 32-13 Glomerular filtration pressures.

illary oncotic pressure and decrease the GFR. Renal disease can also cause changes in pressure relationships by altering capillary permeability and the surface area available for filtration (see Chapter 33).

Tubular transport

By the end of the proximal tubule, approximately 60% to 70% of filtered sodium and water and about 50% of urea have been reabsorbed, along with 90% or more of potassium, glucose, bicarbonate, calcium, phosphate, amino acids, and uric acid. All this occurs by active transport. Chloride, water, and urea are reabsorbed passively but are linked to the active transport of sodium (cotransport). Active transport in the renal tubules can be limited as the carrier molecules become saturated, a phenomenon known as **transport maximum** (Tm). Transport maximums exist for most substances actively transported by the tubular epithelium. The reabsorption of glucose is a significant example. Glucose is coupled to sodium transport and is almost completely reabsorbed in the proximal tubule. Like other actively transported substances, glucose has a maximal transport capacity, or renal threshold. This means that when the carrier molecules for glucose become saturated, the excess will be excreted in the urine. Normally, the plasma level and filtered glucose load are not high enough to saturate the carrier mechanism. When the plasma glucose reaches 180 mg/dl, however, as occurs in the individual with uncontrolled diabetes mellitus, the threshold for glucose is achieved. Any further increase in the plasma level causes loss of glucose in the urine.

Proximal tubule. Active reabsorption of sodium is the primary function of the proximal tubule. Water, most electrolytes, and organic substances are cotransported with sodium. The osmotic force generated by active sodium transport promotes the passive diffusion of water out of the tubular lumen and into the peritubular capillaries. Passive transport of water is further enhanced by the elevated oncotic pressure of the blood in the peritubular capillaries. The reabsorption of water leaves an increased concentration of urea within the tubular lumen, creating a gradient for its passive diffusion to the peritubular plasma.

As the positively charged sodium ions leave the tubu-

FIG. 32-14 Bicarbonate conservation. Cellular mechanism of bicarbonate (HCO_3^-) conservation (reabsorption) by the proximal tubule. *CA,* Carbonic anhydrase. (From Berne & Levy, 1993.)

lar lumen, negatively charged chloride ions passively follow to maintain electroneutrality. Because the luminal membrane (the inside of the tubule) of the proximal tubular cell has a limited permeability to chloride, however, chloride reabsorption lags behind sodium.

Hydrogen ions are actively exchanged for sodium ions. The hydrogen ions (H^+) then combine with bicarbonate (HCO_3^-). Bicarbonate is completely filtered at the glomerulus, and approximately 90% is reabsorbed in the proximal tubule. This process also occurs to a lesser extent in the ascending loop of Henle and the distal tubule.

In the tubular lumen, hydrogen and bicarbonate ions form carbonic acid (H_2CO_3). The carbonic acid rapidly breaks down, or dissociates, to carbon dioxide (CO_2) and water (H_2O) in the presence of the enzyme carbonic anhydrase, which is in the luminal membrane. The CO_2 and H_2O then diffuse into the tubular cell, where carbonic anhydrase again catalyzes the CO_2 and H_2O to form HCO_3^- and H^+. The H_2CO_3 thus produces H^+ and HCO_3^-. The H^+ is secreted again, and HCO_3^- combines with sodium and is transported to the peritubular capillary blood.

Thus, because bicarbonate is not highly permeable at

the peritubular capillary membrane, it is reabsorbed as $CO_2 + H_2O$, which are readily diffusible. One of the unusual aspects of this process is that the bicarbonate molecule filtered at the glomerulus is not the same molecule that is reabsorbed (because it dissociates) and the hydrogen ion secreted by the proximal tubule is not excreted in the urine. Bicarbonate is thus conserved, and the hydrogen is reabsorbed as water. Therefore these ions normally do not contribute to the urinary excretion of acid or the addition of acid to the blood (Fig. 32-14).

In addition to the proximal tubular secretion of hydrogen ions, secretory transport mechanisms exist for creatinine, other organic bases, and endogenous and exogenous organic acids including para-aminohippurate (PAH) and penicillin (Table 32-2). These secretory mechanisms are important for eliminating drugs and other exogenous chemical products from the body. Frequently, exogenous substances are conjugated with sulfate and glucuronic acid by the liver and then actively secreted by the renal tubules. This has important clinical implications because many drugs and their metabolites are eliminated from the body in this way. When the renal tubules are damaged, metabolic byproducts

TABLE 32-2

Substances Transported by Renal Tubules

Reabsorption	Secretion
Albumin	Choline
Ascorbate	Creatinine
Fructose	Histamine
Galactose	Methyl guanidine
Glutamate	Para-aminohippurate
Glucose	Penicillin
Phosphate	Steroid glucuronides
Sulfate	Thiamine
Xylose	

and drugs may accumulate, causing toxic levels in the body.

Loop of Henle and distal tubule. The filtrate entering and leaving the proximal tubule is essentially isoosmotic with the plasma and has a concentration of about 285 mOsm. Although approximately 65% of salt and water is reabsorbed along the proximal tubule, they are reabsorbed in equal amounts, causing only minor changes in the osmotic and electrolyte concentrations of the fluid flowing into the loop of Henle. Therefore any concentration or dilution of urine occurs at more distal sites of the nephron, principally in the loop of Henle and collecting ducts. Near the top of the renal pyramids, the interstitial osmolality reaches 1200 mOsm/L.

These quantitative changes taking place in the loop of Henle are related to the length of the loop and its depth of penetration into the medulla. The structural features of the medullary hairpin loops provide the kidney with the ability to concentrate urine and conserve water for the body. The transition of the filtrate into urine is a function of the concentrating ability of the loops and final adjustments in urine composition made by the distal tubule and collecting duct.

The primary function of the loop of Henle is to establish a hyperosmotic state within the medullary interstitial fluid. This is achieved by reabsorbing more solute than water into the interstitium. The fluid leaving the ascending limb of the loop is therefore hypoosmotic, or more dilute than the fluid that entered. This dilution allows the distal tubule and collecting duct to make final adjustments in the concentration or dilution of the excreted urine according to body needs. The vasa recta act to maintain the high osmotic gradient established by the loop of Henle.

Different transport or permeability functions of the

loop of Henle are important for dilution and concentration of urine. The thin, descending segment of the loop of Henle is highly permeable to water and moderately permeable to sodium, urea, and other solutes. The thin, ascending segment is more permeable to solutes and almost impermeable to water. The thick portion of the ascending segment is highly permeable to sodium, potassium, and chloride and significantly less permeable to water and urea.

The convoluted portion of the distal tubule is poorly permeable to water but readily absorbs ions and contributes to the dilution of the tubular fluid. The later, straight segment of the distal tubule and the collecting duct are permeable to water as controlled by ADH. Sodium is readily absorbed by the later segment of the distal tubule and collecting duct under the regulation of the hormone aldosterone (see Chapter 17). Potassium is actively secreted in these segments and is also controlled by aldosterone and other factors related to the concentration of potassium in body fluids.

Hydrogen is also secreted by the distal tubule and combines with nonbicarbonate buffers for the elimination of acids in the urine. (See Chapter 3 for further discussion of renal regulation of acid-base balance.) The distal tubule thus contributes to the regulation of acid-base balance by excreting hydrogen ions into the urine and by adding new bicarbonate to the plasma. The mechanism is similar to the conservation of bicarbonate by the proximal tubule, except that the hydrogen ion is excreted in the urine. (The specific mechanisms of acid-base balance and acid excretion are described in Chapter 3.)

Glomerulotubular balance

To regulate body fluid balance, the kidney must not reabsorb or excrete too much sodium or water. Normally, 99% of the glomerular filtrate is reabsorbed. When the GFR decreases or increases, the renal tubules, primarily the proximal tubules, automatically adjust their rate of reabsorption of sodium and water to balance the change in GFR and regulate the quality and quantity of water delivered to the distal tubules.

Concentration and Dilution of Urine

The production of a concentrated urine involves a **countercurrent exchange system,** in which fluid flows in opposite directions through parallel tubes. A concentration gradient causes fluid to be exchanged across the parallel pathways. In the nephron, the fluid moves up and down the parallel sides of the hairpin loop of Henle in the medulla. The longer the loop, the greater the concentration gradient because the concentration gradient increases from the cortex to the tip of the medulla. The loops of Henle serve as multipliers of the concentration gradient, and the vasa recta act as a countercurrent exchanger for maintaining the gradient (Knepper, Chou, & Layton, 1993).

Water, Sodium, and Chloride

The process is initiated in the thick ascending limb of the loop of Henle with the active transport of chloride and sodium out of the tubular lumen and into the medullary interstitium (Fig. 32-15). Because the lumen of the ascending limb is impermeable to water, water cannot follow the sodium-chloride transport. This lack of luminal permeability causes the ascending tubular fluid to become hypoosmotic and the medullary interstitium to become hyperosmotic. The descending limb of the loop, which receives fluid from the proximal tubule, is highly permeable to water, but it is the only place in the nephron that does not actively transport either sodium or chloride. Sodium and chloride may, however, diffuse into the descending tubule from the interstitium. The hyperosmotic interstitium causes water to move out of the descending limb, and the remaining fluid in the descending tubule becomes increasingly concentrated as it flows toward the tip of the medulla. As the tubular fluid rounds the loop and enters the ascending limb, sodium and chloride are removed, and water is retained. The fluid then becomes more and more dilute as it encounters the distal tubule.

The slow rate of blood flow and the hairpin structure of the vasa recta allow blood to flow through the medullary tissue without disturbing the osmotic gradient. As blood flows into the descending limb of the vasa recta, it encounters the increasing osmotic concentration gradient of the medullary interstitium. Water moves out, and sodium and chloride diffuse into the descending vasa recta. The plasma becomes increasingly concentrated as it flows toward the tip of the medulla.

As the blood flow passes into the ascending limb and back toward the cortex, the surrounding interstitial fluid becomes comparatively more dilute. Water then moves back into the vasa recta, and sodium and chloride diffuse out. The net result is a preservation of the medullary osmotic gradient. If blood were to flow rapidly through the vasa recta, as occurs in some renal diseases, the medullary concentration gradient would be washed away, and the ability to concentrate urine and conserve water would be lost. The efficiency of water conservation is related to the length of the loops: the longer the loops, the greater the ability to concentrate the urine. Many desert animals have very long loops and can reabsorb water so efficiently that they rarely need to drink.

Urea

Urea is an end-product of protein metabolism and is the major constituent of urine along with water. The glo-

FIG. 32-15 Countercurrent mechanism for concentrating and diluting urine.

merulus freely filters urea, and tubular reabsorption of urea depends on urine flow rate with less reabsorption at higher flow rates. Approximately 50% of urea is excreted in the urine and 50% is recycled within the kidney. The recycling of urea from the tubules and collecting ducts contributes to the osmotic gradient within the medulla and is necessary for the concentration and dilution of urine. Because urea is an end-product of protein metabolism, individuals with protein deprivation are not able to maximally concentrate their urine.

Antidiuretic Hormone (ADH)

The distal tubule in the cortex receives the hypoosmotic urine from the ascending limb of the loop of Henle. The concentration of the final urine is controlled by antidiuretic hormone (ADH), which is secreted from the posterior pituitary or neurohypophysis. Antidiuretic hormone increases water permeability in the last segment of the distal tubule and along the entire length of the collecting ducts, which pass through the inner and outer zones of the medulla.

In the presence of ADH, water reabsorption is high. Most of the water is reabsorbed in the medullary collecting ducts because of the high osmotic gradient in the medullary interstitium. The water diffuses into the ascending limb of the vasa recta and returns to the systemic circulation. The excreted urine can have a high osmotic concentration, up to 1400 mOsm. The volume is normally reduced to about 1% of what was filtered at the glomerulus.

Antidiuretic hormone secretion is therefore one cause of **oliguria,** or diminished excretion of urine that is less than 400 ml/day or 30 ml/hr. Fluid imbalance may be related to the syndrome of inappropriate secretion of ADH, which is a cause of water excess (see Chapter 3). Inadequate secretion of ADH results in diabetes insipidus, the excretion of a large volume of dilute urine.

In the absence of ADH, **water diuresis,** an increase in excretion of a highly dilute urine, takes place. The distal tubules and collecting ducts become impermeable to water. Water remains in the tubular lumen and is excreted as a dilute and large volume of urine. Because ADH has no effect on sodium reabsorption, it continues to be actively transported from the distal tubule. (The mechanism for the regulation of ADH and plasma osmolality is described in Chapter 3.)

Diuretics as a Factor in Urine Flow

A **diuretic** is any agent that enhances the flow of urine. Clinically, diuretics interfere with renal sodium reabsorption and reduce extracellular fluid volume. Diuretics are commonly used to treat hypertension and edema caused by heart failure, cirrhosis, and nephrotic syndrome.

Different diuretics affect different sites of tubular

function and may produce side effects that alter acid-base and electrolyte balance. Therefore health professionals need to understand their indications for use, mechanisms of action, and toxic side effects. Diuretics are divided into four general categories: (1) osmotic diuretics, (2) carbonic anhydrase inhibitors (inhibitors of urinary acidification), (3) inhibitors of loop sodium or chloride transport, and (4) aldosterone antagonists. (The physiologic mechanism related to each category is summarized in Table 32-3.)

Renal Hormones

Certain hormones are either activated or synthesized by the kidney. These hormones have significant systemic effects and include the active form of vitamin D, erythropoietin, and natriuretic hormone.

Vitamin D

Vitamin D is a hormone that can be obtained in the diet or synthesized by the action of ultraviolet radiation on cholesterol in the skin. These forms of vitamin D_3 (cholecalciferol) are inactive and require two hydroxylations to establish a metabolically active form. The first step occurs in the liver with hydroxylation at the twenty-fifth carbon, and the second hydroxylation occurs at the first carbon position in the kidneys. The end product is l,25-dihydroxycholecalciferol, or more simply l,25-dihydroxyvitamin D_3 (1,25-OH_2D_3).

Vitamin D is necessary for the absorption of calcium and phosphate by the small intestine. The renal hydroxylation step is stimulated by parathyroid hormone. A decreased plasma calcium level (less than 10 mg/dl) stimulates the secretion of parathyroid hormone. Parathyroid hormone then stimulates a sequence of events that help restore plasma calcium back toward normal:

Calcium mobilization from bone

Synthesis of l,25-dihydroxyvitamin D
↓
Absorption of calcium from the intestine
↓
Increased renal calcium reabsorption
↓
Decreased renal phosphate reabsorption

Serum phosphate fluctuations also influence the renal hydroxylation of vitamin D. Decreased levels stimulate active 1,25-OH_2D_3 formation and increased levels inhibit formation. This results in compensatory changes in phosphate absorption from bone and the intestine. The clinical significance of the role of the kidney in calcium and phosphate metabolism is evident in renal disease. Patients with renal disease have a deficiency of

TABLE 32-3

Action of Diuretics

Diuretic	Site of action	Action	Side effects
Osmotic diuretic			
Mannitol Glycerol Urea	Proximal tubule	Freely filtered but not reabsorbed; osmotically attracts water and diminishes sodium reabsorption	Hypokalemia, dehydration
Carbonic anhydrase inhibitors			
Acetazolamide	Proximal tubule	Inhibits carbonic anhydrase; blocks hydrogen ion secretion and reabsorption of sodium and bicarbonate	Hypokalemia, systemic acidosis, alkaline urine
Inhibitors of sodium/chloride reabsorption			
Thiazides	Between end of ascending loop and beginning of distal tubule	Blocks sodium and chloride reabsorption; mildly suppresses carbonic anhydrase	Hypokalemia, metabolic alkalosis
Furosemide Ethacrynic acid Bumetanide	Thick ascending limb of Henle's loop	Blocks active transport of chloride, sodium, and potassium	Hypokalemia, uric acid retention
	Cortical vasodilation	Increased rate of urine formation	Hypokalemia, uric acid retention
Aldosterone antagonists			
Spironolactone	Distal tubule	Inhibits aldosterone, blocks sodium reabsorption, and results in potassium retention	Hyperkalemia, nausea, confusion, gynecomastia
Triamterene and amiloride	Distal tubule	Blocks sodium reabsorption and inhibits potassium excretion	Nausea, vomiting, headache, granulocytopenia, skin rash

1,25-OH$_2$D$_3$ and manifest symptoms of disturbed calcium and phosphate balance (see Chapter 3).

Erythropoietin

Erythropoietin stimulates the bone marrow to produce red blood cells in response to tissue hypoxia. (Erythrocyte production is discussed in Chapter 22.) The stimulus for erythropoietin release is decreased oxygen delivery in the kidneys. The anemia of chronic renal failure, in which kidney cells have become nonfunctional, may be related to the lack of this hormone.

Natriuretic Hormone

Atrial natriuretic hormone (ANF) probably also contributes to the loss of sodium and water and the regulation of fluid balance by inhibiting ADH secretions and the effect of ADH on the collecting ducts. When ECF volume is expanded, ANF secretion is increased, and a large volume of dilute urine is excreted. Natriuretic hormone is released from cardiocyte granules located in the right atria of the heart in response to increased atrial stretch (Genest & Cantin, 1986).

TESTS OF RENAL FUNCTION

The Concept of Clearance

A number of specific renal functions can be measured by renal clearance. Renal clearance techniques determine how much of a substance can be cleared from the blood by the kidneys per given unit of time. The application of this principle permits an indirect measure of GFR, tubular secretion, tubular reabsorption, and renal blood flow.

Clearance and Glomerular Filtration Rate

The GFR provides the best estimate of functioning renal tissue. Loss or damage to nephrons leads to a corresponding decrease in GFR. The measurement of GFR requires use of a substance that has a stable plasma concentration, is freely filtered at the glomerulus, and is not secreted, reabsorbed, or metabolized by the tubules. Inulin (a fructose polysaccharide) is one substance that meets the criteria for measurement of GFR.

The kidney "clears" inulin from the plasma by filtering it at the glomerulus, reabsorbing nearly all of the fluid, and excreting the inulin left behind in the urine. The amount of inulin filtered is equal to the volume of plasma filtered (GFR) multiplied by the plasma concentration of inulin (P_{in}). The amount of inulin in the urine is equal to a volume of urine per unit of time ($\dot{V}$) (usually 24 hours) multiplied by the inulin concentration of urine (U_{in}). Because all the inulin filtered is excreted in the urine:

$$GFR \times P_{in} = U_{in} \times \dot{V}$$

GFR can be calculated by rearranging the formula:

$$GFR(ml/min) = \frac{U_{in} \times \dot{V}}{P_{in}}$$

The accurate determination of inulin clearance requires constant infusion to maintain a stable plasma level. This is time-consuming and inconvenient. Therefore the clearance of creatinine, a natural substance produced by muscle and released into the blood at a relatively constant rate, is commonly used clinically. It is freely filtered at the glomerulus, but a small amount is secreted by the renal tubules. Therefore creatinine clearance overestimates the GFR but within tolerable limits. Creatinine clearance provides a good measure of GFR because only one blood sample is required in addition to a 24-hour volume of urine. The GFR estimated by creatinine clearance is

$$GFR \times \frac{U_{cr}\dot{V}}{P_{cr}}$$

Similar calculations can be made for all solutes excreted in the urine per unit of time. Substances freely filtered at the glomerulus but with a clearance less than inulin or creatinine have been reabsorbed along the tubules. For example, glucose is completely reabsorbed and has a clearance rate of nearly zero. Conversely, substances secreted by the tubules have a clearance rate greater than inulin or creatinine (i.e., greater than 1.0).

Clearance and Renal Blood Flow

The standard clearance formula can also be used to estimate renal plasma flow (RPF) and renal blood flow (RBF). The substance used for this evaluation is paraaminohippurate (PAH). Some PAH is filtered at the glomerulus, and most of the remainder is secreted into the tubules in one circulation through the kidney. If all of the PAH were removed from the plasma during a single pass through the kidney, then total renal plasma flow could be determined. Because the supporting and nonsecreting structures of the kidney receive 10% to 15% of renal blood flow, clearance of PAH (CPAH) only measures what is known as the **effective renal plasma flow** (ERPF), which is 85% to 90% of the true renal plasma flow:

$$ERBF = ERPF$$
$$1 - Hematocrit$$
$$(1.0 - 0.45)$$

The estimation of effective renal blood flow (ERBF) can then be calculated by considering the hematocrit in the formula:

$$ERPF = C_{PAH} = \frac{U_{PAH}\,\dot{V}}{B_{PAH}}$$

Blood Tests
Plasma Creatinine Concentration

A chronic decline in the GFR over weeks or months is reflected in the **plasma creatinine (P_{cr}) concentration** (normal value = 0.7 to 1.2 mg/dl). The P_{cr} concentration has a stable value when the GFR is stable because creatinine has a constant rate of production as a product of muscle metabolism. The amount filtered is approximately equal to the amount excreted. When the GFR declines, the P_{cr} increases proportionately. Thus, the GFR and P_{cr} are inversely related. If the GFR were to decrease by 50%, the filtration and excretion of creatinine would be reduced by 50%, and creatinine would accumulate in plasma to twice the normal value. Therefore elevated P_{cr} values represent decreasing GFR. In the new steady state, however, the total amount of creatinine excreted in the urine would remain the same because of the proportionate decrease in GFR and increase in P_{cr}.

The application of this principle is simple and useful for monitoring progressive changes in renal function. The test is most valuable for monitoring the progress of chronic rather than acute renal disease because it takes 7 to 10 days for the plasma creatinine level to stabilize when GFR declines. Serial measures can be obtained over a long time and plotted as a curve of glomerular function. The P_{cr} also becomes elevated during trauma or breakdown of muscle tissue. In such instances the value is then not useful for estimating GFR.

Blood Urea Nitrogen

The concentration of urea nitrogen in the blood reflects glomerular filtration and urine-concentrating capacity. Because urea is filtered at the glomerulus, blood urea nitrogen (BUN) levels increase as glomerular filtration drops. Because urea is reabsorbed by the blood through the permeable tubules, the BUN rises in states of dehydration and acute and chronic renal failure when passage of fluid through the tubules is slowed. Blood urea nitrogen also changes as a result of altered protein intake and protein catabolism. The normal range for BUN in the adult is 10 to 20 mg/dl of blood.

Urinalysis

Urinalysis is a noninvasive and relatively inexpensive diagnostic procedure. The best results are obtained from a fresh, clearly voided specimen, because decay permits changes in the composition of urine. Urinalysis includes evaluation of color, turbidity, protein, pH, specific gravity, sediment, and supernatant.

Urine normally has a clear light yellow color because of urochrome and other pigments. When formed substances (crystals, blood cells, or casts) are in the urine, it appears turbid. Protein in the urine creates marked foaming when shaken, and the foam is yellow when the urine contains bile pigments.

Urine pH normally ranges between 5.0 and 6.5, but may vary from 4.5 to 8.0. Urine is more alkaline after eating and then declines before the next meal. Because sleep is accompanied by intermittent hypoventilation, a person produces more acidic urine after awakening.

Specific Gravity

Specific gravity is an estimated measure of the solute concentration of the urine. Specific gravity of any solution is measured by comparing the weight of the solution compared with an equal volume of distilled water. Hence, specific gravity is not a true measure of the number or concentration of particles but it correlates well with osmolality and is a useful clinical tool. Specific gravity is usually measured with a hydrometer in a cylinder of urine; the normal value is 1.016 to 1.022.

The final urine osmolality is primarily a function of ADH, which controls water reabsorption in the collecting ducts. If the kidney is unable to concentrate or dilute urine, given a stimulus, the cause is usually a malfunction of the renal tubules or inappropriate ADH secretion by the posterior pituitary gland. The state of hydration also affects the urine specific gravity, so that hydration status should be evaluated before making a diagnosis. This determination is helpful for differentiating oliguria caused by intrinsic renal disease from hypovolemia as a result of dehydration.

Urine Sediment

The urine sediment is examined microscopically and may contain cells, casts, crystals, and bacteria. Epithelial cells may be seen in the microscopic field as they are shed naturally throughout the urinary tract.

Red blood cells

Normal urine contains few or no red blood cells. If large numbers of red cells are present, this is known as **hematuria** and the sediment may be red. An alkaline or hypotonic urine causes lysis of red cells, however, so that the cells will not be seen. Urine then will be positive for hemoglobin, and the specific gravity will be elevated. Hematuria can occur with the administration of anticoagulants and with several renal diseases.

Casts

Casts (accumulations of cellular precipitates) originate in the renal tubules, from which they take their shape. They are cylindric with distinct borders. All casts have a precipitated microprotein matrix and arise primarily from the ascending limb of the distal tubule. Red cell casts indicate bleeding into the tubules; white cell casts are associated with an inflammatory process. Epithelial cell casts indicate degeneration of the tubular lumen or necrosis of the renal tubules. The type of cast identified suggests the disease process occurring in the kidney.

Crystals

Numerous kinds of crystals can be observed in the urine. They may be composed of cystine, uric acid, calcium oxalate, or phosphate. They may not be initially observable, but as the urine cools, crystals will form. Crystals tend to form in a concentrated acidic or alkaline urine. Generally, they are not clinically significant. Crystal formation is diagnostically significant, usually indicating inflammation, infection, or a metabolic disorder.

White blood cells

White blood cells (WBC) in the urine (a condition termed **pyuria**) are primarily indicative of urinary tract infection, particularly when bacteria are present. Glomerulonephritis and nephrotic syndrome also may demonstrate pyuria, but usually in combination with proteinuria, red cells, and casts. The finding of white blood cell casts reflects a kidney infection, because these casts are not formed in the bladder or prostate. The presence of white cells in the urine should be followed by a culture for specific identification of bacteria and sensitivity of bacteria to antibiotics.

☐ AGING and Renal Function

Throughout life, the kidney responds to an increased work load by compensatory hypertrophy. This hypertrophy is marked in individuals who have donated a kidney for transplant or have lost functioning nephrons from trauma or disease. The glomeruli increase in diameter, and the tubules enlarge effectively to maintain the regulatory functions of the kidney. Hypertrophy occurs more rapidly and with a larger size increase in younger individuals and in those with high protein intake.

Changes in the kidneys occur throughout life, with a linear decrease in renal blood flow and GFR. With aging, the number of nephrons decreases. The primary mechanism appears to be a change in the renal vasculature and perfusion pattern, which leads to a reduction in numbers of nephrons. The rate of nephron loss accelerates between 40 and 80 years. By 75 years of age the nephron population is reduced by 30% to 50%. Degenerative changes within nephrons also occur with aging. The glomerular capillaries atrophy with a reduction in the branching vessels. The glomeruli then may disappear completely. The arcuate and interlobular arteries become tortuous, contributing to ischemia. The loss of the glomerular tuft may cause a shunt between the afferent and efferent arterioles. Although loss of juxtaglomerular nephrons still allows the vasa recta to be perfused, the combination of events contributes to a decreasing ability to excrete a concentrated urine. Thus the specific gravity of the urine in older individuals tends to be on the low side of normal.

Tubular transport changes with aging. Glucose and bicarbonate are not as efficiently reabsorbed. Response to acid or base loads is delayed and prolonged. Sudden or large changes in pH or fluid load may lead to serious imbalances. Thus acute losses or chronic fluid deficits can lead to renal insufficiency in the elderly person. Administration of drugs eliminated by renal processes may require dose modifications and more astute observations for toxic side effects. The T_m for glucose reabsorption decreases with age, contributing to a greater amount of glucose in the urine. This is an important consideration when glycosuria is used for screening or monitoring the process of diabetes mellitus in the elderly. These changes occur independently of disease, however, indicating a normal process of aging. Previous or concurrent renal disease or urinary tract obstruction may amplify age-related changes in function.

SUMMARY REVIEW

Structures of the Renal System

1 The kidneys are paired structures lying bilaterally between the twelfth thoracic and third lumbar vertebrae.
2 The kidney is composed of an outer cortex and an inner medulla.
3 The calyces join to form the renal pelvis, which is continuous with the upper end of the ureter.
4 The nephron is the urine-forming unit of the kidney and is composed of the glomerulus, proximal tubule, hairpin loops of Henle, distal tubule, and collecting duct.
5 The glomerulus contains loops of capillaries. The capillary walls serve as a filtration membrane for the formation of the primary urine.
6 The proximal tubule is lined with microvilli to increase surface area and enhance reabsorption.
7 The hairpin loops of Henle transport solutes and water, contributing to the hypertonic state of the medulla.
8 The distal tubule adjusts acid-base balance by excreting acid into the urine and forming new bicarbonate ions.

9 The ureters extend from the renal pelvis to the posterior wall of the bladder. Urine flows through the ureters by means of peristaltic contraction of the ureteral muscles.
10 The bladder is a bag composed of the detrusor and trigone muscles and innervated by parasympathetic fibers. When accumulation of urine reaches 250 to 300 ml, mechanoreceptors, which respond to stretching of tissue, stimulate the micturition reflex.

Renal Blood Flow

1 Renal blood flows at about 1000 to 1200 ml/min, or 20% to 25% of the cardiac output.
2 Blood flow through the glomerular capillaries is maintained at a constant rate in spite of a wide range of arterial pressures.
3 The glomerular filtration rate (GFR) is the filtration of plasma per unit of time and is directly related to the perfusion pressure of renal blood flow.
4 Autoregulation of renal blood flow and neural regulation of vasoconstriction maintain a constant GFR.

5 Renin is an enzyme secreted from the juxtaglomerular apparatus and causes the generation of angiotensin, a potent vasoconstrictor. The renin-angiotensin system is thus a regulator of renal blood flow.

Kidney Function

1 The major function of the nephron is urine formation, which involves the processes of glomerular filtration, tubular reabsorption, and tubular secretion and excretion.

2 Glomerular filtration is favored by capillary hydrostatic pressure and opposed by oncotic pressure in the capillary and hydrostatic pressure in Bowman's capsule. The balance of favoring and opposing filtration forces is known as net filtration pressure (NFP).

3 The GFR is approximately 120 ml/min, and 99% of the filtrate is reabsorbed.

4 The proximal tubule reabsorbs about 60% to 70% of the filtered sodium and water and 90% of other electrolytes.

5 Because most molecules are reabsorbed by active transport, the carrier mechanism can become saturated at a point known as the transport maximum (Tm). Molecules not reabsorbed are excreted with the urine.

6 The distal tubules actively reabsorb sodium and secrete potassium and hydrogen for the regulation of electrolyte and acid-base balance.

7 The concentration of the final urine is a function of the level of antidiuretic hormone (ADH) that stimulates the distal tubules and collecting ducts to reabsorb water. The countercurrent exchange system of the long loops of Henle and their accompanying capillaries establishes a concentration gradient within the renal medulla to facilitate the reabsorption of water from the collecting duct.

8 The distal nephron regulates acid-base balance by excreting hydrogen ions and forming new bicarbonate.

9 The kidney secretes or activates a number of hormones that have systemic effects, including $1,25\text{-}OH_2D_3$, erythropoietin, and natriuretic hormone.

Tests of Renal Function

1 Tests that measure renal clearance indicate how much of a substance can be cleared from the blood by the kidneys per given amount of time.

2 Creatinine, a substance produced by muscle, is measured in both plasma and urine to calculate a commonly used clinical measurement of GFR.

3 Both the plasma creatinine concentration and the blood urea nitrogen (BUN) levels indicate glomerular function. Plasma creatinine is measured to monitor progressive renal dysfunction; BUN is an indicator of hydration status.

4 Urinalysis involves evaluation of color, turbidity, protein, pH, specific gravity, sediment, and supernatant.

5 Presence of bacteria, red blood cells, white blood cells, casts, or crystals in the urine sediment may indicate a renal disorder.

Aging and Renal Function

1 As a person grows older, a decrease occurs in the number of nephrons. Both renal blood flow and GFR decline.

2 Tubular transport and reabsorption decrease with age. Response to acid-base changes and reabsorption of glucose are delayed. Drugs eliminated by the kidney can accumulate in the plasma, causing toxic reactions.

KEY TERMS

REFERENCES

Berne, R. M. & Levy, M. N. (Eds.). (1993). *Principles of physiology* (3rd ed.). St. Louis: Mosby–Year Book.

Brenner, B. M., Katz, R., & Ishikawa, I. (1986). The renal circulation. In B. M. Brenner & F. C. Rector (Eds.), *The kidney* (pp. 115-117). Philadelphia: Saunders.

Genest, J. & Cantin, M. (1986). Regulation of body fluid volume: The atrial natriuretic factor. *News in Physiological Sciences, 1,* 3-5.

Kissane, J. M. (Ed.). (1990). *Anderson's pathology* (9th ed.). St. Louis: Mosby–Year Book.

Knepper, M. A., Chou, C-L., & Layton, H. B. (1993). How is urine concentrated by the renal inner medulla? In E. Bourke, N. P. Mallick, & V. E. Pollak (Eds.), *Moving points in nephrology* (vol. 102, pp. 144-160). Basel: Karger.

Re, R. N. (1987). The renin-angiotensin system. *Medical Clinics of North America, 71*(5), 877-895.

Sagnalla, G. A., & MacGregor, G. A. (1990). Atrial natriuretic peptides. *Quarterly Journal of Medicine, 77,* 1001.

Thibodeau, G. A., & Patton, K. T. (1992). *The human body in health and disease.* St. Louis: Mosby–Year Book.

Thompson, J., et al. (1989). *Clinical nursing* (2nd ed.). St. Louis: Mosby–Year Book.

Whaley, L. F. & Wong, D. L. (1991). *Nursing care of infants and children* (4th ed.). St. Louis: Mosby–Year Book.

SUGGESTED READINGS

Berlyne, G. M. (1992). *The kidney today: Selected topics in renal science.* Basel: Karger.

Brenner, B. M., & Rector, F. C., Jr. (Eds.). (1991). *The kidney* (4th ed.). Philadelphia: Saunders.

Kass, E. H. (1978). Horatio at the orifice: The significance of bacteriuria. *Journal of Infectious Disease, 138,* 546-557.

Koeppen, B. M., & Stanton, B. A. (1992). *Renal physiology.* St. Louis: Mosby–Year Book.

Schmidt, R. A. (1985). The urethral syndrome. *Urologic Clinics of North America, 12*(2), 349-354.

Schrier, R. W. (Ed.). (1992). *Renal and electrolyte disorders* (4th ed.). Boston: Little, Brown & Co.

Seldin, D. W., & Giebish, G. (Eds.). (1985). *The kidney: Physiology and pathophysiology* (2nd ed.). New York: Raven Press.

Windhager, E. E. (Ed.). (1992). *Handbook of physiology: Renal physiology* (vols. 1 & 2, 2nd ed.). New York: Oxford University Press.

CHAPTER 33

Alterations of Renal and Urinary Tract Function

Sue E. Huether

Chapter Outline

R*enal and urinary function can be affected by a variety of disorders. The most common type of urinary dysfunction is infection of the bladder. The urinary tract also can be obstructed by stones or tumors. Renal function can be impaired by disorders of the kidney itself or by many other systemic diseases. Because the kidney filters the blood, it is directly linked to every other organ system. Renal failure, whether acute or chronic, is therefore a life-threatening condition.*

URINARY TRACT OBSTRUCTION

Urinary tract obstruction, or obstructive uropathy, is an interference with the flow of urine at any site along the urinary tract (Fig. 33-1). The obstruction causes stasis and accumulation of urine behind the obstruction that can lead to infection or damage to involved organs. Obstruction can be either congenital or acquired. (Congenital obstruction is discussed in Chapter 34.) Among the numerous causes of acquired obstruction are tumors,

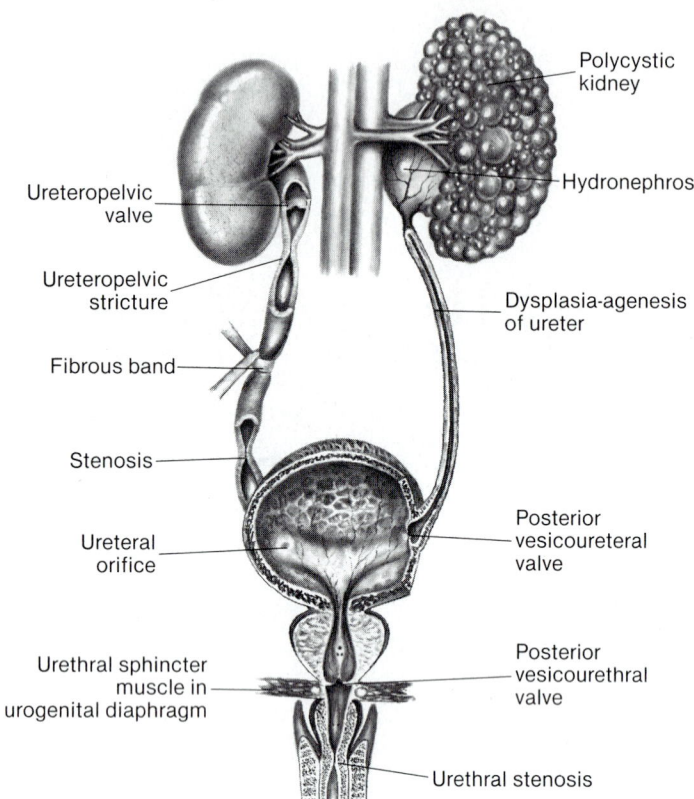

Polycystic kidney

Hydronephrosis

Ureteropelvic valve

Ureteropelvic stricture

Dysplasia-agenesis of ureter

Fibrous band

Stenosis

Ureteral orifice

Posterior vesicoureteral valve

Urethral sphincter muscle in urogenital diaphragm

Posterior vesicourethral valve

Urethral stenosis

FIG. 33-1 **Major sites of urinary tract obstruction.** (From Whaley & Wong, 1991.)

stones (calculi), and trauma. The obstruction can be within the urinary tract (as with renal calculi) or within the ureteral strictures. It can be caused by edema associated with infection or by tumors of the bladder or urethra. Obstructions arising from outside the urinary tract can be related to pregnancy, benign prostatic hyperplasia or carcinoma, and inflammation of the gastrointestinal tract. Functional causes of obstruction are caused by loss of ureteral peristaltic activity or bladder muscle function, which occur with vesicoureteral reflux (reflux of urine from the bladder into the ureter) or with neurogenic bladder. (Vesicoureteral reflux is discussed in Chapter 34.)

Urinary tract obstructions can develop acutely or evolve insidiously over weeks or months. Early recognition of obstruction is important to the prevention of infection and permanent loss of renal function. The pathophysiology of obstructive disorders frequently can be reversed by alleviating the obstruction.

Consequences of Obstruction

The pathophysiologic consequences of urinary tract obstruction are related to (1) location within the urinary tract, (2) unilateral or bilateral involvement, (3) partial or complete obstruction, (4) acute or chronic duration, and (5) the underlying cause. Whenever the flow of urine is obstructed, hydrostatic pressure increases, and structures behind the site of occlusion dilate. Obstructions lower in the urinary tract cause less severe pressure increases because more surface area is available for dilation.

Obstruction of the ureter causes **hydroureter** (accumulation of urine in the ureter). Retrograde increases in hydrostatic pressure involving the renal pelvis and calyces produce **hydronephrosis** (accumulation of urine in the renal collecting system). Acute, complete obstructions cause an increase in pressure that is transmitted to the proximal tubule and decreases glomerular filtration. If the obstruction is complete, the glomerular filtration rate (GFR) will decline to zero, with resulting renal failure. Partial obstructions generally do not cause a cessation of glomerular filtration (Wilson & Schrier, 1986). Complete unilateral obstruction may reduce the GFR to 30% of normal and is reflected by an increased plasma creatinine level (see Chapter 35).

Chronic partial obstruction causes compression of the kidney structures from accumulation of urine, with ischemic atrophy of the papilla and medulla. Although the kidneys initially increase in size, progressive atrophy follows, with eventual loss of renal mass and smaller kidneys. The accompanying tubular damage decreases renal ability to conserve sodium and water and to excrete hydrogen ion and potassium. The resulting failure to concentrate the urine may produce excessive urine volumes even though the GFR has declined. Sodium and bicarbonate are wasted with an increased risk of dehydration and metabolic acidosis.

The relief of urinary tract obstruction—in one or both kidneys—is usually followed by a variable period of diuresis (commonly called postobstructive diuresis) with losses of large amounts of urine. The diuresis is related to salt and water retention during the period of obstruction and a return to a normal GFR. The diuresis lasts for a few days, usually without symptoms of volume depletion such as postural hypotension or elevated blood urea nitrogen (BUN) and plasma creatinine levels.

An uncommon result of obstruction relief is an excessive loss of sodium and water (greater than 10 L/day). These losses are particularly unusual when intake is matched with output. In such cases reducing fluid intake until output decreases to normal is appropriate while monitoring for volume deficit. In some cases of chronic obstruction, diuresis may not be significant after relief of obstruction because the GFR returns to normal slowly or not at all.

Complications of urinary tract obstruction include infection and renal failure. The type of complication depends on the site of obstruction. Obstructions below the bladder cause infection because the accumulated urine is an excellent medium for bacterial growth. Acute or chronic renal failure occurs with prolonged bilateral obstruction (see p. 1254). Acute renal failure can be prevented if the obstruction is relieved within 1 week. Chronic renal failure may be insidious.

Obstructive Disorders
Kidney Stones

Calculi, or **renal stones** (nephrolithiasis), are masses of crystals and protein and are a common cause of urinary tract obstruction in adults. Renal stones account for 1 of 1000 hospitalizations, with an incidence at autopsy of approximately 5%. A significant number of patients are treated in outpatient settings. Approximately 1% of the U.S. population will have a renal stone at some time.

Three major kinds of renal stones are (1) calcium oxalate (75% to 80%); (2) struvite (magnesium, ammonium, phosphate) (15%); and (3) uric acid (7%). Cystine stones are relatively rare and account for less than 1% of all renal stones.

Pathophysiology

The formation of stones is complicated and not entirely understood. The factors that contribute to stone formation include high urinary concentration of stone-forming substances, urine pH that affects solubility, and facilitators and inhibitors of crystal growth. Various diseases, drugs, and diet can contribute to stone development, so each person has to be reviewed carefully to establish the specific causes. Inhibitors of crystal aggregation (nephrocalcin) are normally present in the urine. One theory of stone formation is a reduced excretion of these inhibitors in the urine (Coe & Parks, 1988; Wickham & Buck, 1990).

The formation of a stone begins with a nucleus, or nidus. A **nidus** is a crystal that evolves in the presence of stone-forming substances such as calcium oxalate, calcium phosphate, or struvite. After the nidus is formed, it may become trapped within the urinary tract. There it attracts other crystals and eventually grows into a stone. A high urinary saturation of stone-forming substances enhances crystal formation and stone growth (Fig. 33-2).

Some types of stones are aggregates of different substances. For example, people with high concentrations of uric acid attract calcium oxalate crystals onto a uric acid nidus even though urinary calcium and oxalate levels are normal. An aggregate stone composed of these different substances then forms. The pH of the urine affects the solubility of many stone-forming substances. For instance, an alkaline urine decreases the solubility and enhances the crystallization of calcium carbonate and calcium phosphate. Keeping the urine more acidic increases the solubility of these substances and therefore

FIG. 33-2 Hydronephrosis. Hydronephrosis with renal stones in renal pelvis and calyces. (From Kissane, 1990.)

helps to prevent supersaturation and stone formation. Uric acid tends to crystallize in an acidic urine, particularly when the pH remains below 5.5 and urine volume is low. Calcium oxalate and cystine stones form independently of the urine pH.

Stones usually grow on the papillae or in the renal tubules, calyces, or renal pelvis. Stones also may form in the ureter or bladder. Many stones are less than 5 mm in diameter and are readily passed with the urine. Large stones are sometimes called **staghorn calculi**, as they grow in the pelvis and extend into the calyces to form branching stones. Renal failure may be a consequence, unless they are surgically removed.

Calcium stones are the smallest and most common stones. They occur most commonly in middle-aged men with a familial history of stone formation. Most of these stones are formed of calcium oxalate or an aggregate of calcium oxalate and calcium phosphate. Approximately 80% of them are idiopathic, although they frequently are associated with hypercalciuria and hyperuricosuria (a high level of uric acid in urine). Prolonged immobilization resulting in bone demineralization can precipitate hypercalciuria and stone formation. Struvite stones (magnesium, ammonium, and phosphate) are precipitated by infection with urea-splitting organisms (e.g., *Pseudomonas* and *Proteus*) and are more common in women. With such infections, an alkaline urine is produced and the stones tend to form large stones in the kidney or bladder and, although rarely, in the ureter.

Uric acid stones are caused by gout, an increase in uric acid production and hyperuricosuria. High-purine diets (consisting of meat, fish, and poultry) also can contribute to elevated levels of uric acid. Formation of uric acid stones is enhanced by a concentrated and acidic urine. Thus regional enteritis and ulcerative colitis can precipitate the formation of uric acid stones. Both of these diseases may cause fluid loss and a metabolic acidosis that develops from loss of bicarbonate (see Chapter 3). Patients with the rare hereditary disorder cystinuria develop cystine stones. In cystinuria, an error in cystine metabolism causes decreased tubular reabsorption of cystine with an increased amount of this relatively insoluble substance in the urine.

Clinical Manifestations

Pain is the hallmark symptom of a renal stone. The location and severity vary with the site of occurrence. The presence of stones above the ureters is usually asymptomatic unless an infection or obstruction occurs. When a stone migrates into the ureter and obstructs the lumen, however, a colicky pain occurs as the rhythmic contractions of the ureter attempt to advance the stone. Distention and spasm of the ureter follow from the accumulation of urine behind the stone. The pain may be in the flank, or at the costovertebral angle (between the last rib and the lumbar vertebrae), or it may radiate into the groin if the stone is lower in the ureter. The pain can be exquisitely severe, requiring narcotic analgesia for relief, and is frequently accompanied by nausea and vomiting. Gross or microscopic hematuria (blood in the urine) may be present.

Evaluation and Treatment

The diagnosis of renal stones requires a thorough medical and family history, diet history, previous history of urinary tract disease, and use of medications. Each of these factors may singularly or in combination contribute to stone formation. Both blood and urine tests should be performed to evaluate the presence of stone-forming substances. Urine pH and the presence of red or white blood cells should be evaluated. The GFR can be estimated by assessing the BUN and plasma creatinine (see Chapter 32). A plain (flat plate) film of the abdomen and an intravenous pyelogram will identify the presence of radiopaque stones and confirm the anatomic location.

The purpose of treatment is to prevent new stone formation and to reduce the size of stones that have already formed (Preminger, 1992). Calcium stones reduce with difficulty, but struvite, uric acid, and cystine stones may dissolve with appropriate therapy. The principal components of treatment include (1) reducing the concentration of stone-forming substances by increasing the flow of urine with a high fluid intake or (2) decreasing

the amount of the substance in the urine by decreasing dietary intake or endogenous production. The solubility of stone-forming substances often can be enhanced by altering the pH of the urine. Surgical removal may be required for large stones, obstruction, recurrent infections, or intractable pain. Smaller stones may pass spontaneously, or they can be extracted by instrumentation. Extracorporeal ultrasonic lithotripsy is a relatively noninvasive procedure that uses high-frequency sound waves to fragment stones for excretion in the urine (Bierkens et al., 1992). Lasers also are being used for the treatment of renal stones (Dretler, 1988).

Neurogenic Bladder

Neurogenic bladder is a functional urinary tract obstruction caused by an interruption of the nerve supply to the bladder. The neurologic disruption can occur in the central nervous system or at the level of the spinal cord.

Pathophysiology

The resulting bladder paralysis interferes with the normal flow of urine. This type of urinary dysfunction is related to the level of the neural lesion. Upper motor neuron lesions occur in the cortex or below the cortex but above the sacral level of the spinal cord. An upper motor neuron lesion causes loss of voluntary control of voiding. Lower motor neuron lesions affecting the bladder occur at the sacral level of the spinal cord and disrupt the sacral reflex arc. These lesions cause loss of both voluntary and involuntary control of urination. Some disease states or trauma may affect only the sensory or motor innervation of the bladder. (The types of neurogenic bladder are reviewed in Table 33-1.)

Clinical Manifestations

Infection with a neurogenic bladder may be associated with bladder distention and urine retention, placement of catheters, or the development of stones caused by bone resorption from physical immobility. Symptoms of infection in neurogenic bladder are often difficult to interpret because of disordered sensation and the presence of other neurologic disturbances. The condition may cause symptoms. Pain may not be experienced, but the individual may experience a burning sensation. The development of fever is frequently accompanied by chills and shivering, which aid in differentiating fever caused by other neurologic lesions. Neurogenic bladder must be properly diagnosed and treated or it can lead to deterioration of renal function (Amis & Blaives, 1991).

Evaluation and Treatment

Sterile sampling of urine for bacterial analysis confirms the presence of bacteriuria. Antibiotic treatment for specific organisms is required.

TABLE 33-1				
Classification of Neurogenic Bladder				
Type of neurogenic bladder	**Cause**	**Neural lesion**	**Clinical manifestations**	**Treatment**
Uninhibited (loss of cortical inhibition)	Lack of voluntary control in infancy, multiple sclerosis	Upper motor neuron	Smaller urine volume, frequency, urgency, incontinence, enuresis	
Reflex or automatic (reflex arc maintained below lesion with spontaneous voiding)	Spinal cord transection, cord tumors, multiple sclerosis above level T_{12} of cord	Upper motor neuron	Involuntary voiding that may include incomplete emptying with retention and infection	Catheter or condom drainage; stimulation of reflex arc by stroking perineum, abdomen, or rectum
Autonomous (loss of cortical inhibition and interruption of spinal reflex arc)	Sacral cord trauma, tumors, herniated disk, abdominal surgery with transection of pelvic parasympathetic nerves	Lower motor neuron	Overflow incontinence in which bladder does not empty spontaneously with stretch-fullness	Catheter, urinary diversion surgery
Motor paralysis (sensory functions intact)	Lesions at levels S_2, S_3, S_4; poliomyelitis; trauma; tumors	Lower motor neuron	Overflow incontinence caused by loss of bladder contraction	Manual compression (Credé maneuver)
Sensory paralysis (motor functions intact)	Posterior lumbar nerve roots, diabetes mellitus, tabes dorsalis	Lower motor neuron	Dribbling, overflow incontinence; loss of sensation of bladder fullness	Bladder training to empty at regular intervals (i.e., every 3 hr)

Tumors

Renal Tumors

Renal adenomas (benign tumors) are uncommon. The tumors are encapsulated and are usually located near the cortex of the kidney. Because they can become malignant, they are usually surgically removed. **Renal cell carcinoma** is the most common renal neoplasm (85% of all renal neoplasms) and represents about 2% of cancer deaths. Renal cell carcinoma usually occurs in men (two times greater than women) between 50 and 60 years of age (Boring, Squires, & Tony, 1991).

Pathogenesis

A moderate association has been identified between tobacco use and the incidence of renal cell carcinoma (LaVecchia, Negri, & D'Avanzo, 1990). Diethylstilbestrol and estrogen administration is linked to renal cell carcinoma in animals.

Renal cell carcinomas are adenocarcinomas and are classified according to cell type and extent of metastasis. Clear cell tumors present a better prognosis than granular cell or spindle tumors. Confinement within the renal capsule, together with treatment, is associated with a better survival rate. The tumors usually occur unilaterally and spread through the lymph nodes and blood vessels to the lungs, liver, lymph nodes, and bone (Fig. 33-3) (Fidler, 1992).

Clinical Manifestations

The classic clinical manifestations of renal cell carcinoma are hematuria, flank pain, palpable flank mass, and weight loss, but these symptoms occur in fewer than 10% of cases. Such signs and symptoms represent an advanced stage of disease, whereas earlier stages are often silent. Hematuria is the most common presenting symptom. The flank pain is usually dull and aching, and frequently associated with bleeding within the tumor. Tumor palpation is generally difficult but easier in thin people. Systemic manifestations include weight loss and fatigue; intermittent fever from tumor toxins; anemia from hematuria and lack of erythropoietin or polycythemia from secretion of erythropoietic factor; altered liver function with elevated serum alkaline phosphatase, prothrombin, and bilirubin; and hypertension from el-

FIG. 33-3 Papillary carcinoma of renal pelvis. (From Kissane, 1990.)

evated renin levels. The most common sites of distant metastasis are the lung, lymph nodes, liver, bone, thyroid, and central nervous system (Vetter, 1990).

Evaluation and Treatment

Diagnosis is based on the clinical symptoms, plain x-ray films of the abdomen, intravenous pyelography, renal angiography, and computed tomography. (Staging of renal cell carcinoma is presented in Table 33-2.) Treatment is usually surgical removal of the affected kidney (radical nephrectomy) with combined use of chemotherapeutic agents and, less effectively, hormonal agents (antiestrogen drugs). Radiation therapy may also be used. Immediate relief of obstruction caused by invading tumors can be obtained by placing ureteral catheters past the obstruction or by inserting a nephrostomy tube percutaneously into the renal pelvis. If the obstruction is not treatable, urinary diversion procedures may be required to prevent chronic infection. Survival is related to tumor grade, tumor cell type, and extent of metastasis.

Bladder Tumors

Bladder tumors represent about 2% of all malignant tumors and are the fifth most common malignancy (American Cancer Society [ACS], 1993). Approximately 49,000 people develop bladder cancer each year and

TABLE 33-2

Staging of Renal Cell Carcinoma

Stage	Metastasis
I	Tumor confined within kidney capsule
II	Invasion through renal capsule but within surrounding fascia
III	Involvement of regional lymph nodes, renal vein, or vena cava
IV	Distant metastases

9700 die of it (Silverman, Hartge, Morrison, & Devesa, 1992). The development of bladder cancer is highest in men older than 60 years of age.

Pathogenesis

The risk of bladder cancer is greater for people who smoke or work in the chemical, rubber, and textile industry and among women who take large amounts of phenacetin. Bladder cancer results from a genetic alteration in normal bladder epithelium (Borland, Brendler, & Issacs, 1992; Kantoff, 1990). The tumor is usually composed of transitional cells (the cells lining the bladder) and may or may not have a papillary growth pattern (a tuftlike lesion attached to a stalk) (Fig. 33-4). Nonpapillary tumors (representing 10% of bladder tumors) are not as common as papillary tumors, but they tend to be more invasive and have a poorer prognosis. Metastasis is usually to lymph nodes, liver, bones, and lungs. Staging for bladder carcinoma is presented in Table 33-3. Secondary bladder cancer develops by invasion of cancer from bordering organs, such as cervical carcinoma in women or prostatic carcinoma in men.

Clinical Manifestations

Bladder tumors may be asymptomatic or accompanied by hematuria. Advanced cancers are associated with pelvic pain and frequent urination.

Evaluation and Treatment

Diagnosis is made by cystoscopy (visual examination of the urinary tract through a cystoscope), cell studies, urograms (x-ray examinations), and transurethral biopsy. Treatment is related to the type and size of the lesion. Transurethral resection is the treatment of choice for superficial tumor because of the high propensity for bladder tumors to recur. Endoscopic treatment with Nd:YAG laser has also proven very effective (Hofstetter, 1992). Intravesicular (inside the bladder) chemotherapeutic agents also have been used with some suc-

FIG. 33-4 Cystectomy specimen. Multiple papillary tumors cover greater part of bladder wall. (From Kissane, 1990.)

TABLE 33-3

Staging of Bladder Carcinoma

Stages	Metastasis
O	Limited to mucosal involvement
A	Submucosal involvement
B	Involvement of the muscularis layer
C	Invasion of the perivesical fat
D_1	Spread to regional lymph nodes
D_2	Spread to distant sites, bone, and visceral organs

cess to prevent recurrence. Radiation therapy is not as effective, and candidates for radiation must be carefully selected based on tumor type. Chemotherapy may be combined with radiation and surgical resection. Cystectomy is a standard for invasive bladder cancer (Whitmore, 1990). Because of the risk of recurrence, cystoscopic evaluations are performed every 3 to 6 months after initial treatment. Clinical trials are currently in progress for treatment with photodynamic therapy (Nseyo, 1992).

URINARY TRACT INFECTION

Causes of Urinary Tract Infection

Urinary tract infections (UTIs) are usually caused by bacteria. At risk are premature newborns, prepubertal children, sexually active young women, diaphragm spermatocide use, and elderly males and females (Nev, 1992). Infections are diagnosed by culture of specific organisms with counts of 100,000 bacteria/ml of freshly voided urine. Bacterial contamination of the normally sterile urine usually occurs by retrograde movement of gram-negative bacilli (*Escherichia coli, Pseudomonas,* or *Proteus*) into the urethra and bladder and then to the ureter and kidney. Gram-positive organisms (*Staphylococcus*), fungi, or tubercular bacillus are less common causes of infection. A UTI can occur anywhere along the urinary tract, including the urethra, prostate, bladder, ureter, and kidney. Infections of the lower urinary tract affect 10% to 20% of all women (Fihn, 1992).

Several factors normally combine to protect against UTIs. Most bacteria are washed out of the urethra during micturition. The low pH and presence of urea in the urine provide a bactericidal effect. The ureterovesical junction closes during bladder contraction, preventing reflux of urine to the ureters and kidneys. Both the longer urethra and prostatic secretion decrease the risk of infection in men.

Types of Urinary Tract Infection
Cystitis

Cystitis is an inflammation of the bladder, the most common site of UTI. The morphologic appearance of the bladder through cystoscopy describes different types of cystitis. With mild inflammation the mucosa is hyperemic (red). More advanced cases may show diffuse hemorrhage (called hemorrhagic cystitis) or pus formation, suppurative exudate (called suppurative cystitis) on the epithelial surface of the bladder. Prolonged infection may lead to sloughing of the bladder mucosa with ulcer formation (termed ulcerative cystitis). The most severe infections may cause necrosis of the bladder wall (termed gangrenous cystitis). Generally, the infections are uncomplicated and resolve spontaneously.

Pathophysiology

The most common infecting organisms are *Escherichia coli, Klebsiella, Proteus, Pseudomonas,* and *Staphylococcus.* The disease may occur alone or in association with pyelonephritis or prostatitis. Cystitis is more common in women because of the shorter urethra, the closeness of the urethra to the anus, and the possibility of bacterial contamination from vaginal secretions. Introduction of bacteria and an environment that promotes bacterial growth are the common factors in cystitis. Sexually active and pregnant women, individuals with indwelling catheters, and persons with diabetes mellitus, neurogenic bladder, poor hygiene, and urinary tract obstruction are at greater risk for developing cystitis. Prostatitis and urethral obstruction from prostatic hypertrophy are predisposing factors to bacteriuria, particularly in men older than 50 years of age.

Clinical Manifestations

Many individuals with bacteriuria are asymptomatic. The clinical manifestations of cystitis, however, usually include frequency, urgency, dysuria (painful urination), and suprapubic and low back pain. Hematuria, cloudy urine, and flank pain are more serious symptoms. Approximately 10% of individuals with bacteriuria have no symptoms, and 30% of individuals with symptoms are abacteriuric (Stanford, 1975). Cystitis in the elderly may be asymptomatic (Kaye, 1980).

Evaluation and Treatment

Evaluation of the urine for bacteria is the most important diagnostic procedure. Risk factors, such as urinary tract obstruction, should be identified and treated. Evidence of bacteria from urine culture and sensitivity warrants treatment with an organism-specific antibiotic. A single large dose of antibiotic may be effective when there are a short duration of symptoms and no complications. Three to five days of treatment is most common. Elderly people with obstructive disorders may require 7 to 14 days of treatment. Twenty percent to 25% of women have relapsing infection within 7 to 10 days, requiring prolonged antibiotic therapy (Fero, 1992). Follow-up urine cultures should be obtained 1 week after initiation of treatment and again at monthly intervals for 3 months. Clinical symptoms frequently are relieved but bacteriuria may still be present. Repeated cultures should be obtained every 3 to 4 months until 1 year after treatment for evaluation of recurrent infection.

"Nonbacterial" Cystitis

A significant number of women have symptoms of cystitis but a negative urine culture. This is more common in women 20 to 30 years of age and is called acute **urethral syndrome** (O'Dowd et al., 1984). Its cause is obscure, but dysfunction of the external sphincter, vaginitis, urethritis, and inflammation of glands near the vagina and urethra are associated findings. Bacteria may develop in 60% of individuals up to 9 months after the initial symptoms. Symptoms are frequently relieved by a course of treatment with antibiotics, use of drugs that relax the external sphincter, or retraining of voiding habits.

A persistent and chronic form of "nonbacterial" cystitis occurring primarily in women is **interstitial cystitis.** The cause is not clearly known, but an autoimmune reaction may cause the inflammatory response. The inflammation is associated with a derangement of the bladder mucosa that makes it more susceptible to penetration by bacteria. Inflammation and fibrosis of the bladder wall are accompanied by the presence of hemorrhagic ulcers (Hunner's ulcers). Characteristic symptoms include bladder fullness, frequency, small urine volume, and lower abdominal pain. Response to treatment is generally good with fluid distention of the bladder followed by weekly instillations of dimethyl sulfoxide for up to 12 weeks.

Acute Pyelonephritis

Pyelonephritis is an infection of the renal pelvis and interstitium. The causative organism is usually bacterial but can be fungi or viruses. (Common causes of pyelonephritis are summarized in Table 33-4.) Urinary obstruction and reflux of urine from the bladder (vesicoureteral reflux) are the most common underlying risk factors. (See Chapter 34 for vesicoureteral reflux in children.) One or both kidneys may be involved. Most cases occur in women. The responsible organism is usually *E. coli, Proteus,* or *Pseudomonas.* The latter two organisms are more commonly associated with infections after urethral instrumentation or urinary tract surgery. These organisms also split urea to ammonia, making an alkaline urine that increases the risk of stone formation.

Pathophysiology

The infection is probably spread by ascending organisms along the ureters, but spread also may occur by way of the bloodstream. The inflammatory process is usually focal and irregular, primarily affecting the pelvis, calyces, and medulla. The infection causes medullary infiltration of white blood cells with renal inflammation, renal edema, and purulent urine. In severe infections, localized abscesses may form in the medulla

FIG. 33-5 Acute pyelonephritis. Papillary necrosis resulting from acute pyelonephritis and obstruction. Note necrotic papillae *(arrows),* mottled patchy cortical infiltrate of acute pyelonephritis, and congested, dilated renal pelvis. (From Kissane, 1990.)

TABLE 33-4	
Common Causes of Pyelonephritis	
Predisposing factors	**Pathologic mechanisms**
Kidney stones	Obstruction and stasis of urine contributing to bacteriuria and hydronephrosis; irritation of epithelial lining with entrapment of bacteria
Vesicoureteral reflux	Chronic reflux of urine up the ureter and into kidney during micturition contributing to bacterial infection
Pregnancy	Dilation and relaxation of ureter with hydroureter and hydronephrosis; partly caused by obstruction from enlarged uterus and partly from ureteral relaxation caused by higher progesterone levels
Neurogenic bladder	Neurologic impairment interfering with normal bladder contraction with residual urine and ascending infection
Instrumentation	Introduction of organisms into urethra and bladder by catheters and endoscopes introduced into the urinary tract for diagnostic purposes
Female sexual trauma	Movement of organisms from the urethra into the bladder with infection and retrograde spread to kidney

and extend to the cortex. The tubules are primarily affected, but the glomeruli are usually spared. Necrosis of renal papillae can develop (Fig. 33-5). After the acute phase, healing occurs with deposition of scar tissue and atrophy of affected tubules. The number of bacteria decreases until the urine again becomes sterile. Acute pyelonephritis rarely causes renal failure (Jones, 1992).

Clinical Manifestations

The onset of symptoms is usually acute, with fever, chills, flank or groin pain, frequency, dysuria, and costovertebral tenderness. Children and older adults may have nonspecific symptoms such as fever and malaise.

Evaluation and Treatment

Differentiating symptoms of cystitis from pyelonephritis by clinical symptoms alone is very difficult. The specific diagnosis is established by urine culture. The presence of antibody-coated bacteria is associated more closely with pyelonephritis (Ratner, Thomas, Sanford, & Forland, 1981). White blood cell casts indicate pyelonephritis, but they are not always present in the urine.

Uncomplicated acute pyelonephritis responds well to 2 weeks of organism-specific antibiotic therapy. Follow-up urine cultures are obtained at 1 and 4 weeks after treatment if symptoms recur. Antibiotic-resistant organisms or reinfection may occur in cases of urinary tract obstruction or reflux. Intravenous pyelography and voiding cystourethrography identify surgically correctable lesions.

Chronic Pyelonephritis

Chronic pyelonephritis is a persistent or recurrent autoimmune infection of the kidney with inflammation and scarring of the kidney. One or both kidneys may be involved. The specific cause of chronic pyelonephritis is more difficult to determine, and controversy surrounds the criteria for constituting the diagnosis (Ronald & Simonsen, 1988). Recurrent infections from acute pyelonephritis may be associated with chronic pyelonephritis. The urine in chronic pyelonephritis may, however, contain only a few white cells and bacteria (Rubin, Tolkoff-Rubin, & Cotran, 1986). Generally, chronic pyelonephritis is more likely to occur in patients who have renal infections associated with some type of obstructive pathologic condition. This includes renal stones and vesicoureteral reflux.

Pathophysiology

Chronic urinary tract obstruction prevents elimination of bacteria in the normal flow of urine, resulting in progressive inflammation that causes fibrosis and scarring. The renal pelvis and calyces become dilated and blunted. Gradual destruction of the tubules occurs, with areas of atrophy or dilation and diffuse scarring. Impair-

ment of function may affect urine-concentrating ability, with the excretion of a dilute urine, and can lead to chronic renal failure.

The lesions of chronic pyelonephritis are sometimes termed "chronic interstitial nephritis" because the inflammation and fibrosis are located in the interstitial spaces between the tubules. Chronic interstitial nephritis occurs from causes other than chronic pyelonephritis, including drug toxicity from analgesics such as phenacetin, aspirin, and acetaminophen; ischemia; irradiation; and immune complex diseases.

Clinical Manifestations

The early symptoms of chronic pyelonephritis are often minimal and may include hypertension. They may be similar to acute pyelonephritis with frequency, dysuria, and flank pain, although milder and more vague. Progression of the disease leads to renal failure.

Evaluation and Treatment

The urinalysis usually shows white blood cells and less commonly white blood cell casts. Bacteriuria may or may not be associated with the presenting symptoms. The diagnosis is commonly established by intravenous pyelogram and ultrasound, which reveals a small kidney with a characteristic "clubbing" of the affected calyces.

The choice of treatment is related to the underlying cause. When obstruction occurs, it must be relieved. Appropriate antibiotic treatment is important and requires regular surveillance of the urine for bacterial growth. Antibiotics may be given in short courses when urine cultures are positive. Recurrent infection may require prolonged antibiotic therapy.

GLOMERULAR DISORDERS

Immunologic mechanisms are primarily responsible for glomerular disease with the exception of hereditary disorders, nephritis associated with systemic diseases, and vascular pathologic conditions. Most information has been derived from animal studies and microscopic examination of renal biopsies.

The onset of glomerular disease may be sudden or insidious with hypertension, edema, and an elevated BUN. Some individuals are asymptomatic, and the disease is detected through the presence of microscopic hematuria from a routine urinalysis. The most definitive indication of glomerular disease is microscopic evaluation of tissue obtained by renal biopsy. The presence of clinical symptoms such as edema, hypertension, urinary changes, or systemic diseases associated with glomerular injury provides supporting evidence for the diagnosis.

Different types of glomerular disease may be associated with patterns of urinary sediment. Urine in diseases associated with a **nephrotic sediment** has massive proteinuria, lipiduria, and microscopic or no hematuria. Urine in diseases associated with **nephritic sediment** is characterized by hematuria with red cell casts, white cell casts, and varying degrees of proteinuria, which is usually not severe. The sediment of chronic glomerular disease has waxy casts, granular casts, and less proteinuria and hematuria than nephrotic or nephritic sediment. Severe glomerular disease is usually associated with diffuse lesions and may demonstrate oliguria, hypertension, and renal failure. Focal lesions tend to produce less severe clinical symptoms. In some instances a combination of hematuria may occur with excessive amounts of urine protein (as in renal symptoms of lupus erythematosus and membranous proliferative glomerulonephritis).

Reduced GFR during glomerular disease is evidenced by the plasma creatinine concentration or creatinine clearance (see Chapter 32). Glomerular damage causes a decrease in glomerular membrane surface area, glomerular capillary blood flow, and driving hydrostatic pressure. In the presence of hypoalbuminemia plasma fluid tends to move to the interstitial spaces, contributing to decreased blood volume, decreased renal blood flow, and decreased glomerular capillary hydrostatic pressure with a decline in GFR.

Edema is commonly associated with nephrotic syndrome (see p. 1251) or may be caused by salt and water retention from reduced GFR. Excessive fluid retention may cause systemic and pulmonary edema, requiring the use of diuretics or dialysis. The volume expansion that accompanies salt and water retention leads to hypertension. Generally excessive renin production is not a cause of hypertension in glomerular diseases unless it is associated with ischemia, as in uremia (see p. 1253), or with profound hypovolemia.

Death occurs in 2% to 5% of all persons during acute glomerular disease. During the first few weeks, the major life-threatening problems are acute renal insufficiency with fluid, electrolyte, and acid-base imbalances; acute hypertension that may cause hypertensive encephalopathy; circulatory failure; and pulmonary edema.

Glomerulonephritis

Glomerulonephritis is an inflammation of the glomerulus that can be caused by a variety of factors including immunologic abnormalities, effects of drugs or toxins, vascular disorders, and systemic diseases. In some cases, the exact cause of glomerular injury may be unknown. Immunologic alterations are most frequently responsible for glomerular injury (Fig. 33-6) (Couser, 1991; Sax-

ena, Johansson, Bygren, & Wieslander, 1992). Glomerular disease is the most common cause of chronic and end-stage renal failure.

Types of Glomerulonephritis

The classification of glomerulonephritis is arbitrary and can be described according to cause, pathologic lesions, disease progression, or clinical presentation. (Types of glomerular lesions are reviewed in Table 33-5 and features of types of glomerulonephritis are summarized in Table 33-6.)

Acute glomerulonephritis

Acute glomerulonephritis is frequently associated with a poststreptococcal infection (acute poststreptococcal glomerulonephritis). The disease has an abrupt onset and usually occurs 7 to 10 days after a streptococcal infection of the throat (5% to 10% incidence) or skin (25% incidence), commonly in children (see Chapter 34). Sporadic occurrences have been observed after bacterial endocarditis, which may be associated with streptococcal or staphylococcal organisms, or after viral diseases such as varicella and hepatitis B.

TABLE 33-5

Types of Glomerular Lesions

Lesion	Characteristics
Diffuse	Relatively uniform involvement of most (>50%) or all glomeruli; most common form of glomerulonephritis
Focal	Changes in only some glomeruli (<50%), whereas others are normal
Segmental-local	Changes in one part of the glomerulus with other parts unaffected
Mesangial	Deposits of immunoglobulins in the mesangial matrix
Membranous	Thickening of the glomerular capillary wall
Proliferative	An increase in the number of glomerular cells
Sclerotic	Glomerular scarring from previous glomerular injury
Crescentic	The accumulation of proliferating cells within Bowman's space making the appearance of a crescent

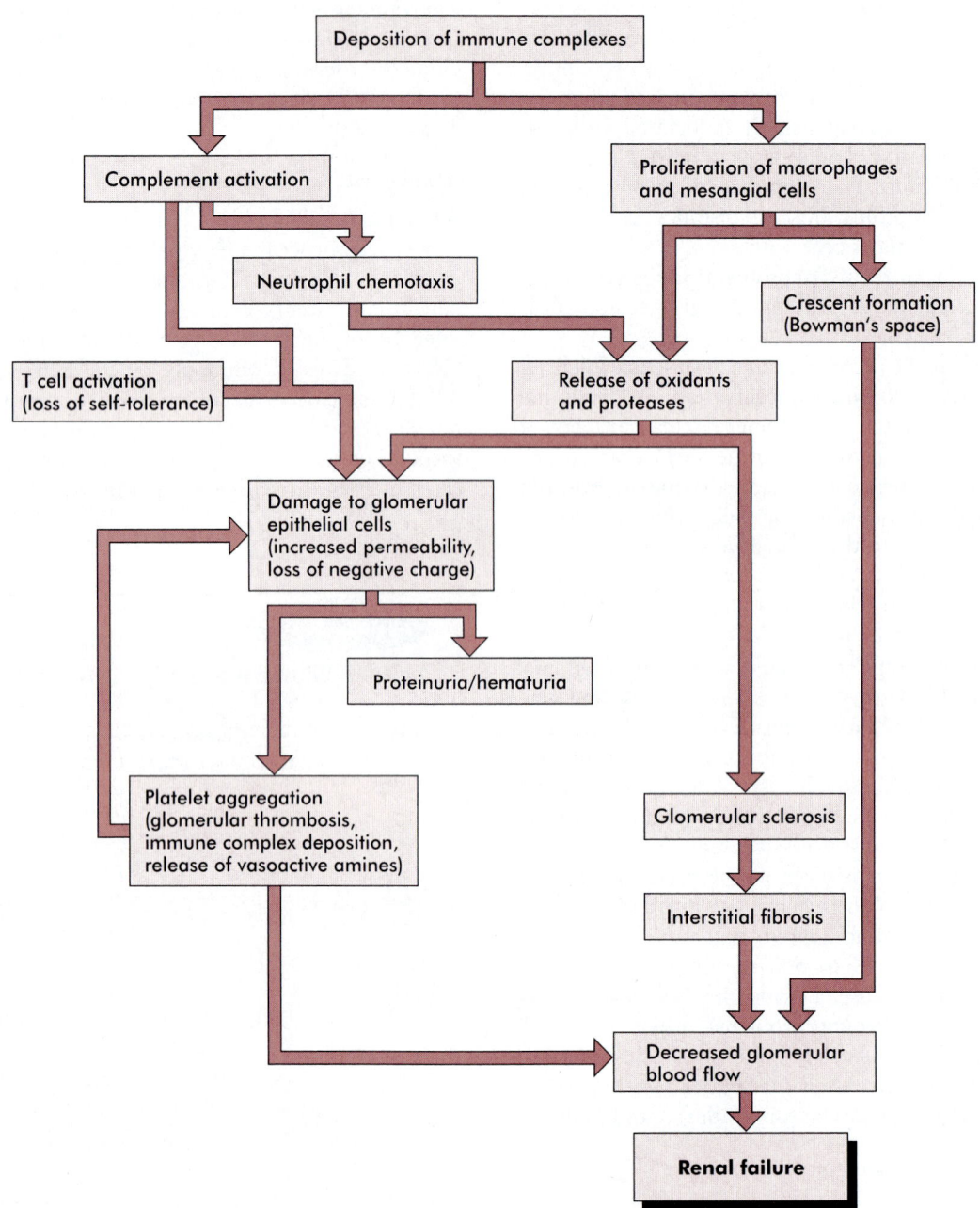

FIG. 33-6 **Mechanisms of glomerular injury.** (Modified from Couser, 1991.)

TABLE 33-6

Features of the Common Types of Glomerulonephritis

Type and cause	Pathophysiology
Poststreptococcal Group A-beta hemolytic streptococcus	Usually diffuse lesions; subepithelial deposits of IgG and complement complexes; infiltration of neutrophils and monocytes; proliferation of mesangial and epithelial cells; with occlusion of glomerular capillary blood flow and decreased glomerular filtration
Rapidly progressive or crescentic Nonspecific response to glomerular injury; can occur in any severe glomerular disease	Diffuse lesions; accumulation of fibrin, macrophages, and epithelial cell proliferation into Bowman's space forms crescents and occludes glomerular capillary blood flow decreasing glomerular filtration; anti–glomerular basement membrane antibodies lead to necrotizing, proliferative GN and renal failure

Membranoproliferative
  Usually idiopathic; associated with hypocomplementemia
  Type I: activation of classical complement pathway
  Type II: activation of alternate complement pathway
	Diffuse lesions; mesangial cell proliferation; thickening of basement membrane; subendothelial deposits of immune complex occlude glomerular capillary blood flow and decrease glomerular filtration

IgA nephropathy (Berger disease) Usually idiopathic; elevated IgA plasma levels	Usually focal, some diffuse lesions; mesangial cell proliferation with IgA deposits; release of inflammatory mediators with crescent formation, sclerosis, interstitial fibrosis, and decreased GFR
Minimal change disease (lipoid nephrosis) Usually idiopathic	Diffuse fusion of epithelial foot processes; loss of negative charge in basement membrane and increased permeability lead to severe proteinuria and nephrotic syndrome
Focal glomerulosclerosis Usually idiopathic	Similar pathology to minimal change disease with focal glomerulosclerosis from hyaline deposits in the glomerular membrane resulting in proteinuria and nephrotic syndrome
Membranous nephropathy Usually idiopathic; can be associated with systemic diseases, i.e., hepatitis B virus, systemic lupus erythematosus, solid malignant tumors	Diffuse thickening of glomerular basement membrane and capillary wall from deposits of antibody and complement; increased permeability with proteinuria and nephrotic syndrome

The presenting symptoms are related to the preceding illness, and the manifestations of renal disease are variable. Symptoms usually occur 10 to 21 days after infection. Acute onset of hematuria, red blood cell casts, proteinuria, decreased GFR, oliguria, edema, and hypertension is common. The edema of acute glomerulonephritis tends to be around the eyes but may involve dependent areas such as the feet and ankles. Occasionally, ascites or pleural effusions develop. Serum complement levels are usually low because they are consumed by the initial infection. Immunofluorescent findings from renal biopsy indicate the presence of immune complex deposits in the glomerulus, with diffuse mesangial cell and capillary endothelial cell proliferation (Fig. 33-7). The thickening of the glomerular membrane contributes to the decreased GFR. More severe renal disease is observed after a prolonged infection before antibiotic therapy. Antibiotic therapy prevents the spread of infection, but there is no specific treatment for the glomerulonephritis. Most individuals, especially children, recover without significant loss of renal function or recurrence of the disease.

Proximal
convoluted
tubule

Renal
corpuscle

Distal
convoluted
tubule

FIG. 33-7 **Acute poststreptococcal glomerulonephritis. A,** Photomicrograph of kidney showing normal glomerulus surrounded by profiles of sectioned renal tubules. (×140.) **B,** Acute poststreptococcal glomerulonephritis. Swollen, hypercellular glomerular lobules with few open capillaries. (×250.) **C,** Acute poststreptococcal glomerulonephritis. "Humps" of immune complex stained with fluorescent antihuman complement (C3). (×1000; courtesy Dr. Claude Cornwall, Syracuse, NY.) (**A** from Thibodeau, G. A. [1987]. *Anatomy and physiology.* St. Louis: Mosby–Year Book. **B** and **C** from Kissane, 1990.)

Rapidly progressive glomerulonephritis

Rapidly progressive glomerulonephritis (RPGN) is also known as subacute, crescentic, or extracapillary glomerulonephritis. The disease primarily affects adults in their 50s and 60s. Rapidly progressive glomerulonephritis may be idiopathic or associated with a number of proliferative glomerular diseases (with diffuse proliferation of extracapillary cells), such as poststreptococcal glomerulonephritis and Goodpasture syndrome.

Goodpasture syndrome is an example of RPGN. The disease is associated with antibody formation against both pulmonary capillary and glomerular basement membranes. The relationship between these two antibodies is unknown. Goodpasture syndrome is rare but occurs in men 20 to 30 years of age.

By the time RPGN is diagnosed, renal insufficiency is apparent. The disease is characterized by extensive proliferation of cells into Bowman's space with crescent formation. The cells become mixed with fibrin and form crescent-shaped deposits (Fig. 33-8). Typically, the glomerular injury is accompanied by a rapid decline in glomerular function progressing to renal failure in a few weeks or months (Couser, 1988). Hematuria is common and may or may not be accompanied by proteinuria, edema, or hypertension.

Rapidly progressive glomerulonephritis has a relatively poor prognosis. Prednisone alone or combined with immunosuppressant drugs such as cyclophosphamide or azathioprine has not been very effective. Pulsed methylprednisolone administration, which is given once a day for 3 to 5 days before prednisone therapy, is helpful in some cases. Anticoagulants, such as heparin or warfarin, may be of some benefit in reducing the fibrin component of crescent formation. Plasmapheresis (separation of the cells from the plasma) has been useful for removal of antibodies in Goodpasture syndrome and other causes of RPGN. Plasmapheresis is usually combined with prednisone and cyclophosphamide to suppress a rebound antibody production. Dialysis or transplantation is required when failure is irreversible.

Chronic glomerulonephritis

Chronic glomerulonephritis includes a variety of glomerular diseases, each with a progressive course leading to chronic renal failure. Chronic glomerulonephritis may occur with no history of renal disease before the diagnosis, although several years of proteinuria and hematuria may have preceded the diagnosis. Various pathologic changes are evident in the glomerulus. Proliferation of mesangial cells (cells in connective tissue supporting the glomerular capillaries; see Fig. 32-8, *B*) may be focal or diffuse with segmental fibrosis and glomerular deterioration. Secondary tubular dilation and atrophy may develop. Hypercholesterolemia has also been associated with progressive glomerular injury. The

FIG. 33-8 Rapidly progressive glomerulonephritis, anti-glomerular basement membrane type. Note crescent of epithelial cells encircling compressed glomerular tuft. (From Kissane, 1990.)

FIG. 33-9   End-stage chronic glomerulonephritis. Pebbly surface corresponds to surviving hypertrophied nephrons amid atrophy. (From Kissane, 1990.)

proposed mechanism is related to glomerulosclerosis (Diamond & Karnovsky, 1992). The primary cause may be difficult to establish because advanced pathologic changes may obscure specific disease characteristics (Fig. 33-9).

Pathophysiology

Patterns of antigen-antibody complex deposition within the glomerular capillary filtration membrane have been established using light, electron, and immunofluorescent microscopy for different disease processes. The findings on light microscopy provide information about the distribution and extent of immune response injury (Table 33-7). Electron microscopy differentiates morphologic changes within the glomerular capillary wall. Staining with fluorescein identifies different antibodies (i.e., IgG or IgA) and their configurations when viewed under ultraviolet (black) light with a microscope (see Fig. 33-7, C).

Two types of immune mechanisms commonly contribute to glomerular injury: (1) deposition of circulating soluble antigen-antibody complexes and (2) formation of antibodies specific for the anti–glomerular basement membrane (anti-GBM antibodies). The former is the more prevalent. Other immune mechanisms may also operate, but they have not been as clearly substantiated in humans. The severity of glomerular damage and renal insufficiency is related to the size, number, location (focal or diffuse), duration of exposure, and type of antigen-antibody complexes.

Glomerular damage generally occurs from activation of biochemical mediators of inflammation (complement, leukocytes, fibrin), which begins after the antibody or antigen-antibody complexes have localized in the glomerular capillary wall. Complement is deposited with the antibodies, followed by a sequence of metabolic events that initiate an attack on the glomerular membrane. Complement activation can serve as a chemotactic stimulus for attraction of neutrophils and monocytes. The neutrophils and monocytes further the inflammatory reaction by releasing lysosomal enzymes, which damage glomerular cell walls.

These processes alter membrane permeability and may cause loss of the negative electrical charge across the glomerular filtration membrane. Membrane damage can lead to platelet aggregation and degranulation, whereby platelets release vasoactive amines such as serotonin or histamine. These substances then increase glomerular permeability. Changes in membrane permeability and electrical charge permit the passage of protein molecules or red blood cells into the urine, causing proteinuria or hematuria. The coagulation system also may be activated and lead to fibrin deposition in Bowman's space, contributing to crescent formation (deposition of substance in Bowman's space). (Coagulation is discussed in Chapter 22.) Membrane proliferation, de-

TABLE 33-7	
Immunologic Pathogenesis of Glomerulonephritis	
Glomerular injury	**Mechanism**
Soluble immune-complex glomerulonephritis (90%)	Formation of antibodies stimulated by the presence of endogenous or exogenous antigens results in circulating soluble antigen-antibody complexes, which are deposited in glomerular capillaries; glomerular injury occurring with complement activation and release of immunologic substances that lyse cells and increase membrane permeability; immune deposits with a microscopic appearance that fluoresce in a *granular pattern* when stained with fluorescein and viewed under ultraviolet light; severity of glomerular injury related to the number of complexes formed; a type III hypersensitivity
Anti–glomerular basement membrane glomerulonephritis (5%)	Antibodies are formed and act directly against the glomerular basement membrane; immune response that causes crescent formation and a *linear pattern* of immunofluorescence; generally associated with rapidly progressive renal failure such as Goodpasture syndrome
Alternative complement pathway	A relatively obscure mechanism associated with low levels of complement and membranoproliferative glomerulonephritis
Cell-mediated immunity	A delayed hypersensitivity response that damages the glomerulus; actual cellular mechanism not clearly understood

posits in the membrane, mesangial proliferation, and swelling reduce renal blood flow and depress glomerular filtration.

Clinical Manifestations

Two major changes in the urine are distinctive of glomerulonephritis: (1) hematuria with red blood cell casts and (2) proteinuria exceeding 3 to 5 g/day, with albumin as the major protein. Several disorders may produce hematuria because bleeding can occur anywhere along the urinary tract. The characteristics of hematuria from red blood cells escaping through the glomerular membrane include a smoky brown-tinged urine, red blood cell casts, and an accompanying proteinuria. Bleeding from sites lower in the urinary tract may produce a pink- or red-colored urine. Glomerular bleeding provides prolonged contact with the acidic urine and transforms hemoglobin to methemoglobin, which has a brownish color and no blood clots. The immune-mediated inflammatory response with cellular infiltration decreases GFR, which leads to fluid retention. Salt and water are also reabsorbed, contributing to fluid volume expansion and hypertension. Additionally, the history and physical examination may disclose findings that differentiate glomerular disease from another source of urinary tract bleeding. Gross proteinuria is associated with nephrotic syndrome; a decrease in urine output accompanies a decreased GFR.

Mild proteinuria and hematuria may occur during the early years of the disease. Blood pressure may be normal. After 10 or 20 years, renal insufficiency begins to develop, followed by nephrotic syndrome and an accelerated progression to end-stage renal failure. Symptom patterns vary depending on the underlying cause. Steroids usually do not change the course of the disease, and dialysis or kidney transplantation ultimately may be necessary.

Evaluation and Treatment

The diagnosis of glomerular disease is confirmed by the progressive development of clinical manifestations and laboratory findings of abnormal urinalysis with proteinuria, red blood cells, white blood cells, and casts. In acute poststreptococcal glomerulonephritis, the streptococcal exoenzymes are elevated, such as antistreptolysin-O (ASO) and antistreptokinase (ASK). Serum complement is decreased. Creatinine clearance evaluates the extent of glomerular damage. Microscopic evaluation from renal biopsy provides a specific determination of renal injury and type of pathology.

The basic principles for treating glomerulonephritis are related to treating the primary disease, preventing or minimizing immune responses, and correcting accompanying problems such as edema, hypertension, and hyperlipidemia. Specific treatment regimens are necessary for particular types of glomerulonephritis.

Antibiotic therapy is essential for management of underlying infections, which may be contributing to ongoing antigen-antibody responses. Several approaches have been instituted to control immune-mediated glomerular injury. Corticosteroids decrease antibody synthesis and suppress inflammatory responses. Different administrative protocols are implemented, including pulsed therapy (high doses once per day for 3 to 5 days) or more prolonged administration until clinical improvement is sustained.

Cytotoxic agents may be used cautiously because of their severe side effects. These drugs destroy lymphocytes or prevent their proliferation, and they are used more commonly when lupus erythematosus involves renal function. Immune complexes may be removed by removing the plasma and replacing it with fresh frozen plasma. Anticoagulants may be useful for controlling fibrin crescent formation in rapidly progressive glomerulonephritis.

Nephrotic Syndrome
Types of Nephrotic Syndrome

Nephrotic syndrome is simply defined as the excretion of 3.5 g or more of protein in the urine per day. This large amount of urine protein is characteristic of glomerular injury. A constellation of other clinical findings is usually associated with the proteinuria. These include hypoalbuminemia, edema, hyperlipidemia, and lipiduria (Table 33-8). Lipoid nephrosis (minimal change disease), membranous glomerulonephritis, and focal glomerulosclerosis are directly related to nephrotic syndrome, although these conditions can occur with other types of glomerular disease (Carome & Moore, 1992).

Secondary forms of nephrotic syndrome occur as a result of other organic pathologic processes. Systemic diseases often implicated in secondary nephrotic syndrome include diabetes mellitus, amyloidosis, systemic lupus erythematosus, and Henoch-Schönlein purpura. Nephrotic syndrome also is seen in association with certain drugs, infections, malignancies, and vascular disorders. When present as a secondary complication with renal diseases, nephrotic syndrome often signifies a more serious prognosis.

Pathophysiology

The pathophysiology of nephrotic syndrome is primarily related to loss of plasma proteins, particularly albumin and some immunoglobulins, across the injured glomerular filtration membrane. Disturbances in the glomerular basement membrane, which may be metabolic, biochemical, or physiochemical, lead to increased permeability to protein. Hypoalbuminemia is a conse-

TABLE 33-8

Clinical Manifestations of Nephrotic Syndrome

Manifestation	Contributing factors	Result
Proteinuria	Increased glomerular permeability, decreased proximal tubule reabsorption	Edema, increased susceptibility to infection from loss of immunoglobulins
Hypoalbuminemia	Increased urinary losses of protein	Edema
Edema	Hypoalbuminemia (decreased oncotic pressure, sodium and water retention, increased aldosterone and ADH secretion), unresponsiveness to atrial natriuretic peptides	Soft, pitting, generalized edema
Hyperlipidemia	Decreased serum albumin; increased hepatic synthesis of very low-density lipoproteins; increased cholesterol, phospholipids, triglycerides	Increases atherogenesis
Lipiduria	Sloughing of tubular cells containing fat (oval fat bodies); free fat from hyperlipidemia	Fat droplets that may float in urine
Decreased vitamin D	The globulin to which 1,25-vitamin D is attached for transport passes through the glomerulus and is lost in the urine	Decreased absorption of calcium from gut

quence of the urinary loss of albumin combined with a diminished synthesis of replacement albumin by the liver. Albumin is lost in the greatest quantity because of its high plasma concentration and low molecular weight.

Although synthesis of plasma proteins may be increased, the synthesis is insufficient to compensate for losses. Factors such as decreased dietary intake of protein from anorexia or malnutrition, or accompanying liver disease, may contribute to lower levels of plasma albumin. Loss of immunoglobulins may increase susceptibility to infections.

Clinical Manifestations

Proteinuria is an excessive amount of protein in the urine (up to 10 g/24 hours). Many of the clinical manifestations of nephrotic syndrome are related to loss of serum proteins (Table 33-8).

Edema may be the first symptom noticed by the patient (see Chapter 3). Renal edema is usually associated with hypoalbuminemia and is soft, pitting, and in areas of low tissue pressure, such as the periorbital regions. According to Starling's law, hydrostatic pressure acts to force fluid into the interstitial space at the arterial end of the capillaries. The hydrostatic pressure is balanced by the oncotic pressure of the plasma proteins, which tends to draw the fluid back into the capillaries at the venous end (see Chapter 3). Plasma albumin concentra-

tion in nephrotic syndrome is often reduced to 20% of normal, with a considerable decrease in the plasma oncotic pressure. The threat of decreased plasma volume from the accumulation of fluid in the tissues stimulates compensatory mechanisms. Among these mechanisms are activation of the renin-angiotensin-aldosterone system and antidiuretic hormone, which together lead to excessive sodium and water retention. The nephrotic kidney is also unresponsive to atrial natriuretic peptide with increased sodium and water retention (Coe et al., 1992). Increased lymph flow may allow some compensation. Edema in the interstitial space may facilitate lymph flow by elevating tissue pressure, facilitating the return of interstitial fluid into the plasma compartment.

Levels of all the plasma lipids (triglycerides, phospholipids, and cholesterol) are elevated, producing a hyperlipidemia. The inverse relationship between plasma albumin and plasma lipids indicates that hypoalbuminemia and the associated decrease in plasma oncotic pressure may play a causative role in hyperlipidemia. Hyperlipidemia is primarily related to increased synthesis by the liver and decreased lipoprotein catabolism (Coe et al., 1992). **Lipiduria** is manifested by lipid casts or free fat droplets that leak across the glomerular capillary walls and into the urine. Tubular epithelial cells that reabsorb lipoprotein also may be shed and appear in the urine as "oval fat bodies."

Vitamin D deficiency also may be related to the proteinuria of nephrotic syndrome. The hormone 25-hydroxycholecalciferol is normally bound to a circulating globulin. If this is lost in the urine, there will be decreased absorption of intestinal calcium and hypocalcemia (see Chapter 3). Symptoms of vitamin D deficiency will develop, including low plasma levels of ionized calcium, secondary hyperparathyroidism, and osteomalacia.

Evaluation and Treatment

Nephrotic syndrome is diagnosed when the protein level in a 24-hour urine collection is greater than 3.5 g. Serum albumin decreases (to less than 3 g/dl), and serum cholesterol, phospholipids, and triglycerides increase. Fat bodies may be present in the urine. The specific pathology is identified by renal biopsy.

Nephrotic syndrome is commonly treated with a normal-protein, low-fat diet; salt restriction; diuretics; steroids; and occasionally albumin replacement. Because the nephrotic state is primarily caused by protein depletion, dietary protein supplements (up to 100 g) are essential, unless renal failure has occurred. Diuretics may be used, particularly loop diuretics such as furosemide or ethacrynic acid, to control edema or hypertension. Care must be taken to observe for hypovolemia and hypokalemia or potassium toxicity in the presence of renal insufficiency. Aldactone may be combined with loop diuretics to suppress aldosterone activity and conserve potassium.

Because hyperlipidemia is associated with hypoalbuminemia, correction occurs when normal plasma albumin levels are reestablished. A low–saturated-fat diet may be helpful in chronic nephrosis as a way of slowing down atherogenic processes. Drugs such as clofibrate are not safe to use when renal insufficiency exists. The underlying cause of nephrotic syndrome should be treated specifically if it is known.

RENAL FAILURE

Classification of Renal Dysfunction

The terms *renal insufficiency, renal failure, azotemia,* and *uremia* are all associated with decreasing renal function. Often, they are used synonymously, although with some distinctions. Generally, **renal insufficiency** refers to a decline in renal function to about 25% of normal or a GFR of 25 to 30 ml/min. Levels of serum creatinine and urea are mildly elevated. **Renal failure** often refers to significant loss of renal function. When less than 10% of renal function remains, this is termed **end-stage renal failure** (ESRF).

Renal failure may be acute and rapidly progressive, although the process may be reversible. Renal failure also can be chronic, progressing to ESRF over a period of months or years. **Uremia** is a syndrome of renal failure and includes elevated blood urea and creatinine levels accompanied by fatigue, anorexia, nausea, vomiting, pruritus, and neurologic changes. Azotemia and uremia are sometimes incorrectly used interchangeably. **Azotemia** means increased serum urea levels and frequently increased creatinine levels as well. Renal insufficiency or renal failure causes azotemia. Uremia represents the numerous consequences related to renal failure, including retention of toxic wastes, deficiency states, and electrolyte disorders. Both azotemia and uremia indicate an accumulation of nitrogenous waste products in the blood, a common characteristic that explains the overlap in definitions of terms.

Types of Renal Failure
Acute Renal Failure

Acute renal failure (ARF) is an abrupt reduction in renal function with elevation of BUN and plasma creatinine levels. Acute renal failure is usually associated with oliguria (urine output of less than 30 ml/hr or less than 400 ml of urine per day), although urine output may be normal or increased. Most types of acute renal failure are reversible if diagnosed and treated early. Acute renal failure can be caused by different clinical conditions, severe hypotension including vascular obstruction, or severe glomerular disease, and commonly is classified as prerenal, intrarenal, or postrenal (Table 33-9). A combination of ischemic or hepatotoxic factors may combine to produce ARF (Agmon & Brezis, 1993).

Pathophysiology

Prerenal acute renal failure is caused by impaired renal blood flow. The GFR declines because of the decrease in filtration pressure. Poor perfusion can result from renal vasoconstriction, hypotension, hypovolemia, hemorrhage, or inadequate cardiac output. Acute prerenal failure may occur when chronic renal failure exists if a sudden stress is imposed on already marginally functioning kidneys. Failure to restore blood volume or blood pressure may cause acute tubular necrosis or acute cortical necrosis.

Intrarenal acute renal failure may result from prerenal acute renal failure (e.g., acute tubular necrosis or cortical necrosis) or many other diseases, including acute glomerulonephritis, malignant hypertension, disseminated intravascular coagulation, and renal vasculitis. **Acute tubular necrosis** (ATN) is the most common cause of acute renal failure (Douglas, 1992). Acute tubular necrosis and acute renal failure are sometimes used interchangeably but they are not the same as acute renal failure that can occur without ATN. Acute tubular necrosis is generally described as postischemic or nephrotoxic.

Acute tubular necrosis caused by ischemia occurs

TABLE 33·9

Classifications of Acute Renal Failure

Area of dysfunction	Possible causes

Prerenal	Hypovolemia
	  Hemorrhagic blood loss (trauma, gastrointestinal bleeding, complications of childbirth)
	  Loss of plasma volume (burns, peritonitis)
	  Water and electrolyte losses (severe vomiting or diarrhea, intestinal obstruction, uncontrolled diabetes mellitus, inappropriate use of diuretics)
	Hypotension or hypoperfusion
	  Septic shock
	  Cardiac failure or shock
	  Massive pulmonary embolism
	  Stenosis or clamping of renal artery

Intrarenal	Acute tubular necrosis (postischemic or nephrotoxic) Glomerulopathies Malignant hypertension Coagulation defects

Postrenal	Obstructive uropathies (usually bilateral)
	  Ureteral destruction (edema, tumors, stones, clots)
	  Bladder neck obstruction (enlarged prostate)

most frequently after surgery (40% to 50% of cases), but ATN is also associated with sepsis, obstetric complications, or severe burns. A severe episode of hypotension often associated with hypovolemia is a significant contributing event. The ischemia generates toxic oxygen free radicals that cause cell swelling, injury, and necrosis, a form of reperfusion injury (Canavese, Stratta, & Varcellone, 1988; Yoshioka, Bills, & Moore-Jarrett, 1990). Nephrotoxic ATN can be produced by numerous antibiotics, but the aminoglycosides (neomycin, gentamicin, tobramycin) are the major culprits. The drugs tend to accumulate in the renal cortex and may not cause renal failure until after treatment is complete. Radiocontrast media (x-ray media) also may be neph-

rotoxic. Dehydration, advanced age, concurrent renal insufficiency, and diabetes mellitus tend to enhance nephrotoxicity from either agent. Other substances such as excessive myoglobin (oxygen-transporting substance in muscles), carbon tetrachloride, heavy metals (mercury, arsenic), or methoxyflurane anesthesia may promote renal failure. Necrosis caused by nephrotoxins is usually uniform and limited to the proximal tubules. Ischemic necrosis tends to be patchy and may be distributed along any part of the nephron.

Three pathophysiologic explanations have been proposed to account for the oliguria of ATN. All three mechanisms probably contribute to oliguria in varying degrees throughout the course of the disease (Fig. 33-10). The most classic explanation is the *tubular obstruction theory*. This theory suggests that necrosis of the tubules causes sloughing of cells, cast formation (composed of granular and epithelial cells), or ischemic edema, resulting in tubular obstruction. Obstruction then causes a retrograde increase in pressure and reduces the GFR. Renal failure can occur within 24 hours. The theory does not always hold, however, because in some cases no cellular debris or casts can be observed in the urine.

The *back leak theory* suggests that glomerular filtration remains normal but that tubular reabsorption of filtrate is accelerated because of changes in permeability caused by ischemia. Most studies of renal function in ATN, however, indicate a decrease in glomerular filtration, and back leak may be only a minor aspect of acute failure.

Alterations in renal blood flow are considered by some authorities to be a major cause of decreased glomerular filtration. The exact mechanism is unknown, although afferent arteriolar constriction may be produced by an intrarenal release of angiotensin II or by a redistribution of blood flow from the cortex (where the glomeruli are located) to the medulla. Ischemia also may contribute to changes in glomerular permeability and decreased GFR.

Postrenal acute renal failure usually occurs with urinary tract obstruction that affects the kidneys bilaterally (e.g., bladder outlet obstruction, prostatic hypertrophy, or bilateral ureteral obstruction). A pattern of several hours of anuria with flank pain followed by polyuria is a characteristic finding. This type of renal failure can occur after diagnostic catheterization of the ureters, a procedure that may cause edema of the tubular lumen.

Clinical Manifestations

The clinical progression of acute renal failure with recovery of renal function occurs in three phases: oliguria, diuresis, and recovery. The initial phase of oliguria may begin within a day after a hypotensive event, although it may be delayed with exposure to nephrotoxic

FIG. 33-10 Mechanisms of oliguria in acute renal failure.

substances. Generally, the oliguria lasts for 1 to 3 weeks, but it may regress in several hours or extend for several weeks, depending on the duration of ischemia or severity of toxic injury. Anuria (urine output less than 50 ml/ day) is uncommon in ATN, but 10% to 20% of cases have nonoliguric failure. Anuria suggests bilateral renal artery occlusion, obstructive uropathy, or acute cortical necrosis. Nonoliguric failure usually represents less severe injury. The urine output may vary in volume, but the BUN and plasma creatinine concentrations increase (plasma creatinine is inversely proportional to the GFR).

Other early manifestations depend on the underlying cause of renal failure. Individuals who have experienced trauma or surgery, or those in a catabolic state, may have more rapid elevations in BUN. They are prone to hyperkalemia and hyperphosphatemia from cellular breakdown. Fluid retention may cause edema. Symptoms of congestive heart failure develop in persons with cardiac disease. Nausea, vomiting, and fatigue accompany uremia and electrolyte imbalances. Wound healing is delayed, and the risk of infection, particularly pneumonia, is greater. Nonoliguric renal failure generally has a better prognosis because of fewer complica-

tions. Oliguric patients may require maintenance dialysis to attenuate symptoms of renal failure.

As renal function improves, increase in urine volume (diuresis) is progressive. During the early diuretic phase, the tubules are still damaged. Sodium and potassium are lost in the urine and there is a greater risk for hypokalemia. Volume depletion may ensue, with fluid losses of 3 to 4 L/day. Fluid and electrolyte balance must be carefully monitored and excessive urinary losses replaced.

Serial measurements of plasma creatinine provide an index of renal function during the recovery phase. Return to normal status may take from 3 to 12 months, and approximately 30% of individuals do not have full recovery of a normal GFR or tubular function.

Evaluation and Treatment

The diagnosis of ATN is related to the cause of the disease. A history of surgery, trauma, or cardiovascular disorders is common. Exposure to nephrotoxins also must be considered. The diagnostic challenge is to differentiate prerenal acute renal failure from intrarenal acute renal failure. Urine composition provides helpful diagnostic clues to changes in tubular function. Urine

TABLE 33-10

Differentiation of Acute Oliguric Renal Failure

	Urine volume	Urine specific gravity	Urine osmolality	Urine sodium	BUN/plasma creatinine	FE$_{Na}$*
Prerenal failure	<400 ml	1.16-1.020	>500 mOsm	<10 mEq/L	>15:1	<1% (also seen in acute glomerulonephritis)
Acute tubular necrosis	<400 ml	1.010-1.012	<400 mOsm	>30 mEq/L	<15:1	>1% (also seen in urinary tract obstruction and renal parenchymal disease)

$$*FE_{Na} = \frac{Urine\ Na/plasma\ Na}{Urine\ creatinine/plasma\ creatine} \times 100$$

osmolarity and specific gravity tend to be high in prerenal acute renal failure and are accompanied by low urinary sodium concentrations (Table 33-10). The ratios of the BUN to plasma creatinine concentration and fractional excretion of sodium (the ratio of filtered sodium to excreted sodium) are also helpful diagnostic indicators. The tests reflect renal tubular reabsorption ability. In prerenal failure, tubular function is maintained and salt, water, and urea are reabsorbed. With ATN, reabsorption and urinary concentration abilities are compromised. Other causes of renal failure also may exhibit similar clinical findings.

Prevention of acute renal failure is a major treatment factor. Maintenance of fluid volume before and after surgery or diagnostic procedures may significantly reduce acute renal failure precipitated by hypovolemia. Good hydration reduces the nephrotoxic risk of drugs, such as gentamicin or radiocontrast media, and sustains an adequate GFR. Mannitol has been used before surgery in patients at high risk for developing acute renal failure (heart or aortic surgery) or during the oliguric phase of failure. Mannitol causes renal vasodilation with increased renal blood flow and glomerular filtration rate. The osmotic diuretic effect decreases sodium and water reabsorption and increases urine output. The net effect is a maintenance of renal blood flow and urine output with the prevention of accumulated tubular debris and obstruction. This drug is relatively safe but should be discontinued if the response is not immediate because it disrupts the distribution of body fluids if not excreted.

The use of loop diuretics, furosemide and ethacrynic acid, to treat acute renal failure is more controversial (Kjellstrand, Berkseth, & Klinkmann, 1988). These drugs increase renal blood flow and urine output but do not change the GFR. The therapeutic intent is to wash out cellular casts and relieve tubular obstruction. Whether these drugs alter the course of acute renal failure, however, has not been clearly established (Kjellstrand et al., 1988). In some instances a combination of diuretics may be successful.

The primary goal of therapy is to maintain the individual's life until renal function has been recovered. Management principles directly related to physiologic alterations generally include (1) correcting fluid and electrolyte disturbances, (2) treating infections, (3) maintaining nutrition, and (4) remembering that drugs or their metabolites are not excreted. Fluid replacement must be carefully calculated with consideration of urine losses, insensible losses (up to 1000 ml/day), and production of endogenous water by oxidation (450 ml/day). Overhydration of patients dilutes their plasma sodium concentration. **Dialysis** (mechanical removal of water, electrolytes, and toxins from the blood) is indicated for uncontrollable hyperkalemia or acidosis, or severe fluid overload.

Hyperkalemia can be managed by restricting dietary sources of potassium or using cation-ion exchange resins, which may be administered orally or rectally. These resins exchange potassium for another cation, such as sodium in the bowel, and the potassium then is excreted attached to the resin. With tissue trauma or catabolic states, large amounts of potassium may be liberated from cells. Dialysis may be required or potassium can temporarily be driven back into the cells by administering glucose and insulin or by infusing sodium bicarbonate. Glucose metabolism causes potassium to move to the intracellular fluid, and insulin infusions therefore can be effective in shifting potassium from the extracellular to intracellular space, along with the transport of glucose, within 30 minutes. (Glucose metabolism is discussed in Chapter 19.) Causing alkalemia with sodium bicarbonate also shifts potassium into cells in exchange for hydrogen ions.

Careful monitoring of the electrocardiogram for peaking T waves is essential for patients with hyperkalemia. Intravenous infusion of calcium is the most rapid method of treating cardiac effects of hyperkalemia. Calcium decreases the threshold potential and reduces the membrane excitability caused by hyperkalemia (see Chapter 3). Calcium should be used only in emergencies, however, because hypercalcemia also may cause cardiac arrest.

Azotemia is generally controlled and nutrition maintained with a low-protein, high-carbohydrate diet. Essential amino acid replacement can be given orally or parenterally. Adequate carbohydrate intake slows protein catabolism and helps to prevent hyperkalemia. Because sepsis is a common serious or fatal complication of renal failure, observation for signs of infection and early treatment with antibiotics are necessary. Drug dosage levels may require adjustment if they are metabolized or excreted by the kidneys. Recovery may take up to 1 year.

Chronic Renal Failure

The kidney has many important regulatory functions, including body fluid volume, solute concentration and dilution, acid-base balance, excretion of waste products, and secretion of hormones that regulate red blood cell production, blood pressure, and calcium metabolism. Progressive and irreversible loss of renal function (**chronic renal failure**), regardless of the cause, affects these vital processes with changes manifest throughout all organ systems. The kidneys, however, exhibit remarkable adaptive abilities, and symptomatic changes resulting from increased creatinine, urea, potassium, and alterations in salt and water balance usually do not become apparent until the renal function declines to less than 25% of normal.

Pathophysiology

Two theories have been proposed to account for the adaptation to loss of renal function. One view suggests that the adaptive response depends on the particular location of kidney damage. For example, tubular interstitial diseases primarily damage the tubular or medullary parts of the nephron, producing problems such as renal tubular acidosis, salt wasting, and difficulty diluting or concentrating the urine. Conversely, when there is primarily vascular or glomerular damage, proteinuria, hematuria, and nephrotic syndrome are more prominent. This theory is useful for planning treatment in early stages of renal failure when symptomatic differences in renal disease may be distinct.

A second theory (the intact nephron hypothesis) proposes that loss of nephron mass with progressive kidney damage causes the remaining nephrons to sustain normal kidney function. These nephrons are capable of

a compensatory expansion in their rates of reabsorption and secretion. They also can maintain a constant rate of excretion in the presence of a declining GFR. The increased work load is achieved primarily by hypertrophy and hyperfunction of the remaining nephrons.

The intact nephron hypothesis explains adaptive changes in solute and water regulation that occur with advancing renal failure. Although the urine of an individual with chronic renal failure may contain abnormal amounts of protein and red and white blood cells or casts, the major end products of excretion will be similar to normally functioning kidneys until advanced stages of renal failure when there is a significant reduction of functioning nephrons.

Creatinine and urea clearance. Creatinine is constantly released from muscle and excreted primarily by glomerular filtration with relatively no reabsorption and some secretion. In a steady state, the amount produced equals the amount filtered and excreted. If either the rate of production or the GFR changes, the plasma concentration of creatinine changes until the amount excreted again equals the amount produced. Therefore, if the GFR falls, as in chronic renal failure, the plasma creatinine level increases by a reciprocal amount to maintain a constant rate of excretion. Because no significant tubular adjustment occurs for creatinine (i.e., tubular secretion), the plasma levels continue to increase as the GFR decreases. This relationship allows the plasma creatinine concentration to serve as an index of changing glomerular function (Perrone, Madias, & Levy, 1992). (This relationship is represented in Fig. 33-11.)

The clearance of urea is similar, although urea is both filtered and reabsorbed and varies with the state of hy-

FIG. 33-11 Plasma creatinine and glomerular filtration rate.

dration and diet. Urea clearance, therefore, is less than the GFR. If protein intake and metabolism are constant, however, plasma levels increase as the GFR declines. Thus, no tubular adaptation modifies urea levels because urea is excreted primarily by glomerular filtration.

Sodium and water balance. Levels of sodium must be regulated within narrow limits, because sodium is the major extracellular solute. In chronic renal failure, the sodium load delivered to each remaining nephron is greater than normal, so that the fractional excretion of sodium (the ratio of excreted to filtered sodium) must increase to maintain normal sodium balance. Increased excretion of sodium is accomplished by a decrease in the fractional reabsorption of sodium (ratio of reabsorbed to filtered sodium). Although the tubules exhibit a compensatory increased reabsorption, a large obligatory loss remains. The exact regulatory mechanism, however, remains obscure.

Although the nephron is quite efficient at excreting sodium, it has difficulty conserving sodium when GFR decreases to 25% (approximately 25 ml/min) of normal. At this GFR an obligatory loss of 20 to 40 mEq of sodium per day occurs. If dietary intake is less than this amount, sodium deficits and volume depletion occur. These may be caused by osmotic diuresis from loss of urea or by an inability to inhibit natriuretic hormone after a sudden decrease in sodium intake.

The regulation of water balance and osmolality is normally achieved by urinary concentration mediated by ADH. As GFR is reduced, ability to concentrate and dilute the urine diminishes. In earlier stages of renal failure, this may be caused by osmotic diuresis produced by increased fractional excretion of solutes by the remaining nephrons or by a decreased tubular response to ADH. Individual nephrons can maintain water balance until severe renal failure occurs and GFR declines to 15% to 20% of normal with extensive loss of nephron and tubular function. At this stage the urinary concentration becomes fixed and approaches that of the plasma at 285 mOsm/L with a specific gravity of about 1.010.

Potassium balance. Urinary excretion of potassium is primarily related to distal tubular secretion mediated by aldosterone and sodium-potassium adenosine triphosphatase (see Chapter 3). In renal failure there is increased tubular secretion that provides effective regulation until the onset of oliguria. Larger amounts of potassium are also lost through the bowel (Kupin & Narins, 1993). Although nonoliguric patients can maintain potassium excretion with normal dietary intake, they are more prone to develop hyperkalemia with increased loading (i.e., use of salt substitutes). Use of potassium-sparing diuretics, such as spironolactone (Aldactone), volume depletion, acute infection, severe acidosis, or marked hyperglycemia, also may precipitate elevated levels of serum potassium. With progression of disease to end-stage renal failure, total-body potassium can increase to life-threatening levels and has to be controlled by dialysis (Giovannetti, Cupisti, & Barsotti, 1992).

Acid-base balance. The intake of a normal diet produces 50 to 100 mEq hydrogen per day. These ions are secreted from the renal tubules and excreted in the urine combined with phosphate and ammonia buffers (buffering is described in Chapter 3). During early stages of renal insufficiency, normal pH is maintained by an increased rate of acid excretion and bicarbonate reabsorption by individual nephrons. Metabolic acidosis begins to develop when the GFR decreases by 30% to 40%, primarily because of decreased ammonia synthesis and decreased bicarbonate reabsorption. Phosphate buffers remain effective until late stages of chronic renal failure. When end-stage renal failure develops, serum bicarbonate levels stabilize at 15 to 20 mEq/L, partly because the excess hydrogen is buffered by anions in bone. Individuals with end-stage renal failure develop metabolic acidosis, which may be severe enough to require dialysis.

Phosphate and calcium balance. The metabolism of calcium and phosphate is mediated by parathyroid hormone (PTH) and vitamin D. Changes in acid-base balance also influence the status of calcium and phosphate (see Chapter 3). The major calcium and phosphate disorders associated with chronic renal failure are reduced renal phosphate excretion, decreased renal synthesis of 1,25-$(OH)_2$ vitamin D_3 (the active form of vitamin D), and hypocalcemia (Table 33-11).

In early chronic renal failure, excreted phosphate levels decrease and the plasma phosphate concentration increases because of the decrease in GFR. The elevated plasma phosphate binds calcium ($CaHPO_4$), causing hypocalcemia. The decreased calcium stimulates the secretion of PTH. The PTH causes release of calcium from bone and enhanced urinary excretion of phosphate. The adaptive effect is a secondary hyperparathyroidism with return of phosphate and calcium levels toward normal (see Chapter 18). With each incremental loss of GFR, however, the effectiveness of PTH in maintaining phosphate balance diminishes. Reducing the dietary intake of phosphate and providing calcium supplementation is helpful at this early stage of failure. When the GFR declines to 25% of normal, however, PTH is no longer effective in maintaining serum phosphate levels. The persistent decreased GFR and hyperparathyroidism causes progressive hyperphosphatemia, hypocalcemia, and dissolution of bone (e.g., osteitis fibrosa and osteomalacia).

Hypocalcemia and bone disease are accelerated by impaired synthesis of 1,25-vitamin D_3 when loss of functioning nephrons is significant and GFR is less than 25% of normal. Lack of the active form of vitamin D

TABLE 33-11

Calcium and Phosphate Metabolism in Chronic Renal Failure

Kidney	Plasma	Bone
Decreased renal production of vitamin D_3	Decreased source of calcium from gut Increased PTH secretion	Decreased calcium deposition
Decreased phosphate excretion	Elevated phosphate Formation of $CaPO_4$ Decreased ionized calcium	
Increased phosphate excretion (phosphaturia)	Increased PTH secretion (secondary hyperparathyroidism)	Release of calcium and phosphate
Increased calcium reabsorption and increased vitamin D formation (increased intestinal absorption of calcium)	Increased calcium	Osteitis fibrosa, osteomalacia, calcium deposits in soft tissue (occurs when kidney fails to respond to PTH secretion because of loss of renal mass and calcium and phosphate continues to be absorbed from bone)

reduces intestinal absorption of calcium and impairs the effectiveness of calcium and phosphate resorption from bone by PTH. The toxicity of uremia also may suppress vitamin D action in the gut. This depletion can be treated with vitamin D supplements, but larger than normal doses are required. A negative calcium balance also occurs when acidosis is present, which is common in chronic renal failure. Generally, patients with advanced chronic renal failure have high phosphate and low serum calcium concentrations. The secondary hyperparathyroidism, however, may cause calcium levels to approach normal, and in a small percentage of cases they may be elevated.

Hematocrit. Anemia accompanies chronic renal failure because of inadequate production of erythropoietin by diseased kidneys and the uremic state. Lethargy, dizziness, and low hematocrit are common findings (Levin, 1992).

Clinical Manifestations

The clinical manifestations of chronic renal failure are often described using the term *uremia*. Uremia refers to a number of symptoms caused by decline in renal function with the accumulation of toxins in the plasma. The specific mechanisms contributing to toxic symptoms are unknown, although studies have shown that urea and creatinine are only minimally responsible. A combination of other end products of metabolism is associated with toxic symptoms and accompanies accumulations of urea and creatinine. Generally, the symptoms include anorexia, nausea, vomiting, diarrhea, weight loss, pruritus, edema, and neurologic changes (Table 33-12).

Evaluation and Treatment

Evaluation of chronic renal failure is based on the history and presenting signs and symptoms. Elevated serum creatinine concentrations and urea nitrogen are consistent with chronic renal failure. Ultrasound, intravenous pyelogram, or plain x-ray films will show small kidney size. Renal biopsy confirms the diagnosis.

Dietary management. The management of nutrition is essential for the person with chronic renal failure. Generally, nutritional management requires limiting the intake of some nutrients. Loss of renal function causes retention of end products of protein metabolism, and alterations in the ability to maintain fluid and electrolyte balance. Regulation of food and fluid intake may delay the need for dialysis. Diet therapy is planned according to individual needs by considering the type and severity of renal disease. The major objective is to maintain adequate nutrition while preventing the accumulation of metabolic waste products.

Sodium and fluids. Sodium requirements for individuals with renal failure may vary widely depending on the type of renal disease and use of diuretics. Glomerular disease tends to cause sodium retention, whereas tubulointerstitial diseases lead to sodium wasting. Sodium requirements can be evaluated by determining 24-hour urinary sodium levels. Usually sodium and fluids are restricted in patients with renal failure.

Fluid intake is usually limited to the amount of urine output, plus an additional amount for insensible water losses (500 to 1000 ml). Higher insensible losses occur with fever, excessive sweating, and elevations greater than 5000 feet.

Potassium.   Potassium is usually retained in chronic renal failure and requires dietary restriction. In the presence of anuria or oliguria, potassium is restricted to 0.5 mEq/kg of body weight/day (i.e., 50 mEq or about 2 g/day). Many individuals with renal failure are able to maintain normal serum potassium levels if foods high in potassium are avoided.

Caloric intake.   Adequate caloric intake is necessary to maintain ideal body weight. Calories are usually supplied in the form of fats and carbohydrates when protein intake is restricted. Individuals with chronic renal failure often have anorexia as a result of nausea, altered taste sensation, or psychologic depression, making it difficult to maintain an adequate caloric intake. A caloric intake of 35 kcal/kg of body weight/day usually spares tissue protein as a source of calories. Activity levels and metabolic rate also should be considered when calculating caloric intake.

TABLE 33-12

Systemic Effects of Uremia

System	Manifestations	Mechanisms	Treatment
Skeletal	Osteitis fibrosa (bone inflammation with fibrous degeneration); bone demineralization (principally subperiosteal loss of cortical bone in the fibers, lateral ends of the clavicles, and lamina dura of the teeth); spontaneous fractures, bone pain; osteomalacia (rickets) with end-stage renal failure	Bone resorption associated with hyperparathyroidism, vitamin D deficiency, and demineralization; lowered calcium and raised phosphate levels	Control of hyperphosphatemia to reduce hyperparathyroidism; administration of calcium and aluminum hydroxide antacids, which bind phosphate in the gut, together with a phosphate-restricted diet; vitamin D replacement; avoidance of magnesium antacids because of impaired magnesium excretion
Cardiopulmonary	Hypertension, pericarditis with fever, chest pain, and pericardial friction rub, pulmonary edema, Kussmaul's respirations	Extracellular volume expansion as cause of hypertension; hypersecretion of renin also associated with hypertension; fluid overload associated with pulmonary edema and acidosis leading to Kussmaul respirations	Volume reduction with diuretics that are not potassium sparing (to avoid hyperkalemia); ACE inhibitors; combination of propranolol, hydralazine, and minoxidil for those with high levels of renin; bilateral nephrectomy with dialysis or transplantation
Neurologic	Encephalopathy (fatigue, loss of attention, difficulty problem solving); peripheral neuropathy (pain and burning in the legs and feet, loss of vibration sense and deep tendon reflexes); loss of motor coordination, twitching, fasciculations, stupor, and coma with advanced uremia	Uremic toxins associated with end-stage renal disease	Dialysis

During dialysis, most water-soluble vitamins are lost into the dialysis bath, requiring replacement to maintain normal body requirements. Minerals, such as zinc and magnesium, also may be lost. Zinc replacement improves taste sensation and appetite.

When conservative management of chronic renal failure with diet, diuretics, and fluid restriction is no longer effective, dialysis or transplantation becomes a necessary form of treatment. Indications for initiating dialysis include uncontrollable hypertension, hyperkalemia, and signs of uremia, particularly neuropathies. When signs of neuropathy develop, dialysis should be initiated as soon as possible to prevent permanent damage.

Erythropoietin. Anemia of renal failure can be successfully treated with recombinant human erythropoietin. Symptoms of lethargy are significantly improved with increased sense of well-being, appetite, and sleep. Supplemental iron and vitamin B_{12} may be required (Humphries, 1992).

TABLE 33-12

Systemic Effects of Uremia—cont'd

System	Manifestations	Mechanisms	Treatment
Hematologic	Anemia, usually normochromic normocytic; platelet disorders with prolonged bleeding times	Reduced erythropoietin secretion associated with loss of renal mass, leading to reduced red cell production in the bone marrow; uremic toxins associated with shortened red cell survival	Dialysis; recombinant human erythropoietin and iron supplementation; conjugated estrogens; DDAVP (1-desamino-8-D-arginine vasopressin); transfusion
Gastrointestinal	Anorexia, nausea, vomiting; mouth ulcers, stomatitis, urinous breath (uremic fetor), hiccups, peptic ulcers, gastrointestinal bleeding, and pancreatitis associated with end-stage renal failure	Retention of metabolic acids and other metabolic waste products	Protein-restricted diet for relief of nausea and vomiting
Integumentary	Abnormal pigmentation and pruritus	Retention of urochromes, contributing to sallow, yellow color; high plasma calcium levels associated with pruritus	Dialysis with control of serum calcium levels
Immunologic	Increased risk of infection that can cause death	Suppression of cell-mediated immunity; reduction in number and function of lymphocytes, diminished phagocytosis	Routine dialysis
Reproductive	Sexual dysfunction: menorrhagia, amenorrhea, infertility, and decreased libido in women; decreased testosterone levels, infertility, and decreased libido in men	Probably related to dysfunction of ovaries and testes	No specific treatment

SUMMARY REVIEW

Urinary Tract Obstruction

1 Obstruction can occur anywhere in the urinary tract and is usually caused by renal stones or tumors. The most serious complications are hydronephrosis, hydroureter, and infection caused by accumulation of urine behind the obstruction.

2 The most common kidney stone is formed from calcium and most often causes obstruction by lodging in the urethra.

3 Obstruction can be caused by a neural lesion that interrupts innervation of the bladder. The dysfunction is called a neurogenic bladder.

4 Renal cell carcinoma is the most common renal neoplasm. The larger neoplasms tend to metastasize to the lung, liver, and bone.

5 Bladder tumors are commonly composed of transitional cells with a papillary appearance and a high rate of recurrence.

Urinary Tract Infection

1 Urinary tract infections (UTIs) are usually caused by bacteria, commonly from the retrograde movement of bacteria into the urethra and bladder.

2 Cystitis is an inflammation of the bladder commonly caused by bacteria, although types of "nonbacterial" cystitis may be caused by other conditions or by an autoimmune reaction.

3 Pyelonephritis is an acute or chronic inflammation of the renal pelvis that may cause abscess formation and scarring with an alteration in renal function. Pyelonephritis may be acute or chronic.

Glomerular Disorders

1 Glomerulonephritis is a group of related diseases of the glomerulus that can be caused by immune responses, toxins or drugs, vascular disorders, and other systemic diseases.

2 Acute glomerulonephritis commonly results from inflammatory damage to the glomerulus as a consequence of immune reactions after a streptococcal infection.

3 Rapidly progressive glomerulonephritis (RPGN) is associated with injury that results in proliferation of glomerular capillary endothelial cells and rapid loss of renal function.

4 Chronic glomerulonephritis is related to a variety of diseases that cause deterioration of the glomerulus and progressive loss of renal function.

5 Immune mechanisms in glomerulonephritis are the deposition of antigen-antibody complexes and the formation of antibodies specific for the glomerular basement membrane.

6 Nephrotic syndrome is the excretion of at least 3.5 g protein in the urine per day. Its principal symptoms are hypoproteinuria, hyperlipidemia, and edema.

7 Nephrotic syndrome is caused by a loss of plasma proteins, principally albumin and some immunoglobulins, across the injured glomerular filtration membrane.

Renal Failure

1 Acute renal failure is classified as prerenal, intrarenal, or postrenal and is usually accompanied by oliguria with an elevated plasma BUN and plasma creatinine levels.

2 Prerenal acute renal failure is caused by decreased renal perfusion with a decreased GFR, ischemia, and tubular necrosis.

3 Intrarenal acute renal failure is associated with several systemic diseases but is commonly related to acute tubular necrosis (ATN).

4 Postrenal failure is associated with diseases that obstruct the flow of urine from the kidneys.

5 Chronic renal failure represents a progressive loss of renal function. Plasma creatinine levels gradually become elevated as GFR declines; sodium is lost in the urine; potassium is retained; acidosis develops; and calcium and phosphate metabolism is altered.

KEY TERMS

REFERENCES

Agmon, Y., & Brezis, M. (1993). Acute renal failure: A multifactorial syndrome. In E. Bourke, N. P. Mallick, & B. E. Pollak (Eds.), *Moving points in nephrology*. Basel: Karger.

American Cancer Society (ACS). (1990). Cancer statistics 1990. *CA—A Cancer Journal for Clinicians, 40*, 9-26.

Amis, E. S., Jr., & Blaives, J. G. (1991). Neurogenic bladder simplified. *Radiologic Clinics of North America, 29*(3), 571-580.

Bierkens, A. F., Hendriks, A. J. M., deKort, V. J. W., deReyke, T., Bruynen, C. A. H., Bouve, E. R., Beek, T. V. D., Vos, P., & Berkel, H. V. (1992). Efficacy of second generation lithotriptors: A multicenter comparative study of 2206 extracorporeal shock wave lithotripsy treatments with the Siemens Lithostar, Dornier HM4, Wolf piezolith 2300, Divex Tripter X-1, and Breakstone Lithotriptors. *Journal of Urology, 148*, 1052-1057.

Boring, C. C., Squires, T. S., & Tony, T. (1991). Cancer statistics 1991. *CA—A Cancer Journal for Clinicians, 41*, 19.

Borland, R. N., Brendler, C. B., & Isaacs, W. B. (1992). Molecular biology of bladder cancer. *Hematology and Oncology Clinics of North America, 6*(1), 31-39.

Canavese, C., Stratta, P., & Varcellone, A. (1988). The case for oxygen free radicals in the pathogenesis of ischemic acute renal failure. *Nephron, 49*, 9.

Carome, M. A., & Moore, J. (1992). Nephrotic syndrome in adults. *Postgraduate Medicine, 92*(22), 209-215, 218, 220.

Coe, F. L., Favus, M. J., Henderson, L., Kashgarian, M., Luke, R. G., Myers, B., & Strom, T. (Eds.). (1992). *The yearbook of nephrology*. St. Louis: Mosby–Year Book.

Coe, F. L., & Parks, J. H. (1988, March 15). Pathophysiology of kidney stones and strategies for treatment. *Hospital Practice, 185*, 207.

Couser, W. G. (1988). Rapidly progressive glomerulonephritis: Classification, pathogenic mechanisms, and therapy. *American Journal of Kidney Disease, 11*, 449.

Couser, W. G. (1991). Mechanisms of glomerular injury: An overview. *Seminars in Nephrology, 11*(3), 254-258.

Diamond, J. R., & Karnovsky, M. J. (1992). A putative role of hypercholesterolemia in progressive glomerular injury. *Annual Review of Medicine, 43*, 83-92.

Douglas, S. (1992). Acute tubular necrosis: Diagnosis, treatment, and nursing implications. *Critical Care Nursing, 3*(3), 688-697.

Dretler, S. (1988). Laser lithotripsy: A review of 20 years of research and clinical applications. *Lasers in Surgery and Medicine, 8*, 341-356.

Fero, S. (1992). New considerations in treatment of urinary tract infections in adults. *Urology, 39*(1), 1-11.

Fidler, I. J. (1992). The biology of renal carcinoma metastasis. *Seminars in Urology, 10*(1), 3-11.

Fihn, S. D. (1992). Lower urinary tract infection in women. *Current Opinions in Obstetrics and Gynecology, 4*(4), 571-578.

Giovannetti, S., Cupisti, A., & Barsotti, G. (1992). The metabolic acidosis of chronic renal failure: Pathophysiology and treatment. In G. M. Berlyn (Ed.), *The kidney today*. Basel: Karger.

Hofstetter, A. G. (1992). Application of lasers in bladder cancer. *Seminars in Surgical Oncology, 8*(4), 214-216.

Humphries, J. E. (1992). Anemia of renal failure: Use of erythropoietin. *Medical Clinics of North America, 76*(3), 711-725.

Jones, S. R. (1992). Acute renal failure in adults with uncomplicated acute pyelonephritis: Case reports and review. *Clinics in Infectious Disease, 14*(1), 243-246.

Kantoff, P. W. (1990). Bladder cancer. *Current Problems in Cancer, 14*(5), 233-291.

Kaye, D. (1980). Urinary tract infection in the elderly. *Bulletin of the New York Academy of Medicine, 56*, 209.

Kissane, J. M. (Ed.). (1990). *Anderson's pathology* (9th ed.). St. Louis: Mosby–Year Book.

Kjellstrand, C. M., Berkseth, R. O., & Klinkmann, H. (1988). Treatment of acute renal failure. In R. W. Schrier & C. W. Gottschalk (Eds.), *Diseases of the kidney* (4th ed.) (pp. 1510-1511). Boston: Little, Brown, & Co.

Kupin, W. L., & Narins, R. G. (1993). The hyperkalemia of renal failure: Pathophysiology, diagnosis, and therapy. In E. Bourke, N. P. Mallick, & B. E. Pollak (Eds.), *Moving points in nephrology*. Basel: Karger.

LaVecchia, C., Negri, E., & D'Avanzo, B. F. (1990). Smoking and renal cell carcinoma. *Cancer Research, 50*, 5231-5233.

Levin, N. W. (1992). Quality of life and hematocrit level. *American Journal of Kidney Disease, 20*(1 Suppl. 1), 16-20.

Nev, H. C. (1992). Urinary tract infections. *American Journal of Medicine, 92*(4A), 635-705.

Nseyo, U. O. (1992). Photodynamic therapy. *Urologic Clinics of North America, 19*(3), 591-599.

O'Dowd, T. C., Ribiero, C. D., Munro, J., West, R. R., Howells, C. H. L., & Davis, R. H. (1984). Urethral syndrome: A self-limiting illness. *British Medical Journal, 288*, 1349.

Perrone, R. D., Madias, N. E., & Levy, A. S. (1990). Serum creatinine as an index of renal function: New insights into old concepts. *Clinical Chemistry, 38*(10), 1933-1953.

Preminger, G. M. (1992). Renal calculi: Pathogenesis, diagnosis, and medical therapy. *Seminars in Nephrology, 12*(2), 200-216.

Ratner, J. J., Thomas, V. L., Sanford, B. A., & Forland, M. (1981). Bacteria-specific antibody in the urine of patients with acute pyelonephritis and cystitis. *Journal of Infectious Diseases, 143,* 404.

Ronald, A. R., & Simonsen, N. (1988). Infections of the upper urinary tract. In R. W. Schrier & C. W. Gottschalk (Eds.), *Diseases of the kidney* (4th ed.) (p. 1084). Boston: Little, Brown, & Co.

Rubin, R. H., Tolkoff-Rubin, N. E., & Cotran, R. S. (1986). Urinary tract infection, pyelonephritis, and reflux nephropathy. In B. M. Brenner & R. C. Rector (Eds.), *The kidney* (3rd ed.) (p. 1115). Philadelphia: Saunders.

Sanford, J. P. (1975). Urinary tract symptoms and infection. *Annual Review of Medicine, 26,* 485.

Saxena, R., Johansson, C., Bygren, P., & Weislander, J. (1992). Autoimmunity and glomerulonephritis. *Postgraduate Medical Journal, 68*(798), 242-250.

Silverman, D. T., Hartge, P., Morrison, A. S., & Devesa, S. S. (1992). Epidemiology of bladder cancer. *Hematology and Oncology Clinics of North America, 6*(1), 1-30.

Thibodeau, G. A., & Patton, K. T. (1992). *The human body in health and disease.* St. Louis: Mosby–Year Book.

Vetter, J. M. (1990). Metastasis of renal-cell carcinoma: A pathologist's theoretical view. In C. G. Bollack & D. Jacqmin (Eds.), *Basic research and treatment of renal cell carcinoma metastasis.* New York: Wiley-Liss.

Whaley, L. F. & Wong, D. L. (1991). *Nursing care of infants and children* (4th ed.). St. Louis: Mosby–Year Book.

Whitmore, W. F. (1990). Current therapy of bladder cancer. *Journal of Occupational Medicine, 32*(9), 921-925.

Wickham, J. E. A., & Buck, C. A. (1990). *Renal tract stone: Metabolic basis and clinical practice.* London: Churchill Livingstone.

Wilson, D. R., & Schrier, R. S. (1986). Obstructive nephropathy: Pathophysiology and management. In R. Seiver (Ed.), *Renal electrolyte disorders.* Boston: Little, Brown, & Co.

Yoshioka, T., Bills, T., & Moore-Jarrett, T. (1990). Role of intrinsic antioxidant enzymes in renal oxidant injury. *Kidney International, 38,* 282.

SUGGESTED READINGS

Andriole, V. T. (1992). Urinary tract infection in the 90's: Pathogenesis and management. *Infection 20*(suppl 4), 5251-5256.

Dretler, S., Watson, G., & Parrish, J. (1986). Laser fragmentation of ureteral calculi: Clinical experience. *Lasers in Surgery and Medicine 62*(2), 191.

Druml, W. (1992). Metabolic alterations in acute renal failure. *Contributions in Nephrology 98,* 59-66.

Fugelso, P., & Neal, P. M. (1991). Endoscopic laser lithotripsy: Safe effective therapy for ureteral calculi. *Journal of Urology, 145,* 950.

Gitte, S. (1991). Carcinoma of the prostate. *New England Journal of Medicine, 324,* 236.

Leaf, A. L., & Cotran, R. S. (1985). *Renal pathophysiology* (3rd ed.) (p. 304). New York: Oxford University Press.

Nicholls, K. M., Fairley, K. P., & Dowling, J. P. (1984). The clinical course of meningeal IgA nephropathy in adults. *Quarterly Journal of Medicine, 53,* 227.

Piper, J. M., Tonascia, J., & Matanoski, G. M. (1985). Heavy phenacetin use and bladder cancer in women aged 20 to 40 years. *New England Journal of Medicine, 313,* 292.

Rambausek, M. H., Waldherr, R., & Ritz, E. (1993). Immunogenetic findings in glomerulonephritis. *Kidney International 39* (suppl), 33-38.

Reiselbach, R. E., & Garnick, M. B. (Eds.). (1982). *Cancer and the kidney.* Philadelphia: Lea & Febiger.

Rosenberg, S. J., & Williams, R. D. (1986). Photodynamic therapy of bladder carcinoma. *Urologic Clinics of North America 13*(3), 435-444.

Vandeursen, H., Pittomvils, G., Boving, R., & Baert, L. (1991, June). High energy pulsed dye laser lithotripsy: Management of ureteral calcium oxalate monohydrate calculi. *Journal of Urology, 145,* 1148.

Webster, D. C. (1993). Sex and interstitial cystitis: Explaining the pain and planning self-care. *Urology Nursing 13*(1), 4-11.

Alterations of Renal and Urinary Tract Function in Children

Cyrena M. Gilman
Kathleen Hardin Mooney
Margaret M. Andrews*

Chapter Outline

Some renal and urinary disorders occur in children as well as adults. In childhood, however, the kidney and genitourinary structures continue to develop, so that renal dysfunction may be associated with mechanisms and manifestations that are different from those in adults. In addition, some renal and urinary disorders are congenital. Many of these involve structural anomalies of the renal system.

STRUCTURE AND FUNCTION OF THE RENAL SYSTEM IN CHILDREN

Development of the Renal System

The embryonic kidneys develop as three sets of sequentially replaced organs (Fig. 34-1). First, the pronephros arise at the level of the cervical and upper thoracic regions during the third fetal week. The mesonephros begin development more caudally about the fourth fetal week and begin excretory function in the sixth week.

FIG. 34-1 Topography of the pronephros, mesonephros, and metanephric primordium. (From Netter et al., 1973.)

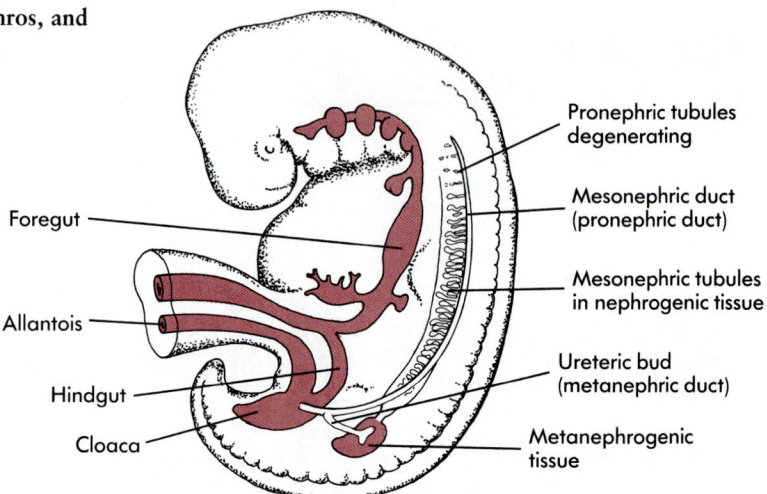

Metanephros, the permanent kidneys, arise distal to the bifurcation of the aorta. The metanephros have two parts, the metanephric duct that buds off the mesonephric duct and metanephrogenic tissue. The ureteric bud (metanephric duct) grows dorsocranially and starts subdividing to become the collecting system for the kidneys. By the fifth fetal month, it will have progressively branched into the collecting ducts. The metanephrogenic tissue atop the terminal branches of the collecting ducts develops into primitive glomeruli and uriniferous tubules. Establishing the connection between the uriniferous tubules and the collecting ducts is a vital part of kidney development; errors in this stage can result in polycystic kidneys.

After glomeruli and tubules form, the tissues organize and progressively differentiate over approximately 30 days. Initial glomerular development is staggered, so there are glomeruli in various stages. In fact, a few of the first glomeruli formed degenerate and disappear during the later stages of pregnancy. Progressive development continues into the tenth fetal month when all metanephrogenic tissue disappears.

As the embryo develops and the vertebral column straightens, the kidneys appear to ascend to the sacral area at about 6 weeks, to the third lumbar area by the third month, and to the first lumbar area at term. The kidneys rotate 90° as they ascend so that renal tissue is lateral and the collecting system is medial.

While the kidneys mature, the cloaca becomes the urogenital sinus. It then differentiates into the vesicourethral canal, which forms the bladder and the upper urethra, and the urogenital sinus, which forms the main part of the urethra.

At birth, the kidneys occupy a large portion of the posterior abdominal wall, and the ureters are proportionately shorter than those of an adult. All the nephrons are present at birth, and their number does not increase as the kidney grows and matures. The kidney reaches adult size by adolescence and, because of maturation of the tubular system, increases in weight 10-fold from birth.

Urine formation and excretion begin by the third month of gestation, contributing to the amniotic fluid. In infancy, the bladder lies close to the abdominal wall, making urinary bladder aspiration for diagnostic purposes a relatively simple procedure. The bladder descends into the pelvis with growth, changing from a cylindric organ to the adult pyramidal shape. Although small amounts of urine are found in the bladder at birth, the newborn may not void for 12 to 24 hours. (The average daily urine output is shown in Table 34-1.)

Immediately at birth the renal blood flow and glomerular filtration rate (GFR) increase because of a decrease in vascular resistance and the need to perform excretory functions no longer performed by the placenta. Renal vascular resistance remains higher in newborns and infants, however, which may be attributed to increased levels of circulating renin. The resistance progressively declines during the first year of development, with an increasing fraction of the cardiac output going to the kidney. The GFR continues to increase, becoming stable at 1 or 2 years but retaining 30% to 50% of adult levels until the end of the first year. Although glomerular filtration is important in removing nitrogenous and other wastes, the amount of urea to be removed is small.

Fluid and Electrolyte Balance in Children

Because the kidney develops from the center toward the periphery, renal distribution of blood flow during the newborn period is primarily to the renal medulla. The result is a preferential flow to the medullary nephrons, which have comparatively short loops at this stage of development. The combination of higher blood flow and shorter loops produces a more dilute urine, approximately 600 to 700 mOsm. The dilute urine is accentuated by a low rate of urea excretion because urea is nec-

TABLE 34-1

Average Daily Urine Output in Children

Age	Output (ml/day)
1 and 2 days	15-50
3-10 days	50-300
10 days to 2 mo	250-400
2 mo to 1 yr	400-500
1-3 yr	500-600
5-8 yr	700-1000
8-14 yr	700-1500

From Kempe, Silver, & O'Brien, 1982.

essary to establish the concentration gradient in the medulla. Urea excretion is low primarily because infants are in a high anabolic state and use their protein for growth.

Because of a high hydrogen ion concentration, limited ability to regulate the internal environment, and lowered osmotic pressure, the infant's renal system has a narrow chemical safety margin. The immaturity and smaller surface area of the tubules also may diminish the water reabsorption response to antidiuretic hormone. An immature tubular transport capacity means that the ability to excrete a potassium load, reabsorb bicarbonate, or buffer hydrogen with ammonia does not become efficient until approximately 2 years of age. Consequently, any disturbance, such as diarrhea, infection, fasting for diagnostic tests, or improper feeding, can rapidly lead to severe acidosis and fluid imbalance because the infant can rapidly develop overhydration, or edema.

After birth, the proportion of total body water to body weight does not change markedly. Considerable change occurs, however, in the location of that body water as the child matures (see Chapter 3). The percentage of extracellular fluid volume of the newborn infant is nearly double that of the adult. Decrease in extracellular fluid volume occurs in two different periods of rapid growth, infancy and adolescence.

Not only does the infant have a greater content of extracellular fluid, but the fluid exchange rate also is greater. The adult takes in and excretes approximately 2000 ml water daily, representing 5% of the total body fluid and 14% of the extracellular fluid. In contrast, the infant's daily exchange of 600 to 700 ml represents 290% of the total or nearly 50% of the extracellular volume, making control of dehydration and overhydration more difficult.

The composition of body fluids differs slightly with age. The total electrolyte concentration in extracellular fluids is greater in the newborn than in the adult. The

concentration of sodium, chloride, phosphates, and organic acids is also greater. The concentration of bicarbonate ions is lower in the infant than in the older child, with a mild acidosis evidenced by a lowered pH. These variations, combined with a lowered plasma protein level, cause a reduced oncotic pressure of the vascular compartment and favor accumulation of fluid in the tissue spaces and an increased GFR. In the healthy child, these differences remain for a few weeks or months. The premature infant and the normal newborn infant are usually in a state of well-compensated acidosis and potential edema.

ALTERATIONS IN RENAL FUNCTION IN CHILDREN

Structural Abnormalities

Variations from the normal anatomic structure of the urinary tract occur in 10% to 15% of the total population. The structural abnormalities range from minor, nonpathologic, or easily correctable anomalies to those that are incompatible with life. For example, the kidneys may fail to ascend from the pelvis to the abdomen, causing ectopic kidneys—which usually function normally. The kidneys also may fuse as they ascend, causing a single, U-shaped **horseshoe kidney**. Approximately one third of individuals with horseshoe kidneys are asymptomatic, and the most common problems are hydronephrosis, infection, and stone formation (Permutter, Retik, & Bauer, 1986). Collectively, structural anomalies of the renal system account for approximately 45% of cases of renal failure in children.

Some anomalies are obvious at birth, whereas others remain latent. Certain structural anomalies are commonly associated with urinary tract malformations (James, 1972). These include:

Low-set malformed ears
Chromosomal disorders, especially trisomy 13 (Patau syndrome) and trisomy 18
Absent abdominal muscles (prune belly syndrome)
Anomalies of the spinal cord and lower extremities
Imperforate anus or genital deviation
Wilms tumor
Congenital ascites
Cystic disease of the liver
Positive family history of renal disease (hereditary nephritis or cystic disease)

Hypospadias

Hypospadias is a congenital condition in which the urethral meatus is located on the ventral side or undersurface of the penis. The meatus can be located anywhere on the glans, the penile shaft, at the base of the penis,

FIG. 34-2 Hypospadias. (Courtesy M. C. Gleason, M.D., San Diego, California; from Ingalls & Salerno, 1979.)

FIG. 34-3 Hypospadias with significant chordee. (From Shirkey, 1980.)

the penoscrotal junction, or the perineum (Fig. 34-2). This is the most common anomaly of the penis and occurs in about 1 in 300 infant boys. **Chordee** or penile torsion may accompany most cases of hypospadias. In chordee, a tough band of fibrous tissue replaces the normal tissue, causing the penis to bend or to "bow" ventrally (Fig. 34-3). Penile torsion is a counterclockwise twist of the penile shaft. Partial absence of the foreskin and cryptorchidism (undescended testicles, see Chapter 20) are associated with the anomaly (Speakman & Azmy, 1992).

The goals for corrective surgery on the child with hypospadias are (1) a straight penis when erect to facilitate intercourse as an adult, (2) a uniform urethra of adequate caliber, (3) a cosmetic appearance, and (4) repair completed in as few procedures as possible. Surgery is most effective between 18 and 30 months of age when the penis has reached sufficient size. Psychologically, the preferred time to perform the correction is before the child enters school and before he develops castration and mutilation anxiety.

Epispadias

Epispadias and exstrophy of the bladder are the same congenital defect but expressed to a different degree. In male epispadias, the urethral opening is on the dorsal surface of the penis. In females, a cleft along the ventral urethra usually extends to the bladder neck. The incidence of epispadias is about 1 in 200,000 infant boys and 1 in 400,000 infant girls.

In boys, the urethral opening may be small and situated behind the glans (anterior epispadias) or a fissure may extend the entire length of the penis and into the bladder neck (posterior epispadias). Children with anterior epispadias can be continent with perhaps only stress incontinence, but those with posterior epispadias will experience constant dribbling of urine.

Exstrophy of the Bladder

Exstrophy of the bladder is an extensive congenital anomaly in which the lower urinary tract is exposed directly to the surface of the body (Fig. 34-4). The posterior portion of the bladder mucosa is exposed and appears bright red through a fissure in the abdominal wall. The incidence of exstrophy of the bladder is 1 in 40,000 live births. Boys are predominant by 3:1.

Exstrophy of the bladder is caused by intrauterine failure of the abdominal wall and the mesoderm of the anterior bladder to fuse. The rectus muscles below the umbilicus are separated and the pubic rami (bony projections of the pubic bone) are not joined. The lack of bone fusion causes a waddling gait when the child first learns to walk, but most quickly learn to compensate. Urine seeps onto the abdominal wall from the ureters, causing a constant odor of urine and excoriation of the surrounding skin. Because the exposed bladder mucosa becomes hyperemic and edematous, it bleeds easily and is painful. It should be covered with Silastic or a plastic dressing (Glad Wrap or Saran Wrap) for protection from diaper irritation while permitting urine drainage.

The unrepaired exstrophic bladder is cosmetically unacceptable and prone to cancerous changes as soon as

FIG. 34-4 **Exstrophy of bladder.** (Courtesy E. S. Tank, M.D., Division of Urology, University of Oregon Health Sciences Center, Portland, Oregon; from Whaley & Wong, 1991.)

1 year after birth. Ideally, the bladder and pubic defect should be closed before the infant is 48 hours old. The secondary bladder neck reconstruction, ureteral reimplantation, and bladder augmentation can be done when the child reaches 2 or 3 years. Any associated genital, inguinal, and rectal defects can be repaired at that time or somewhat later. Objectives of management include preservation of renal function, attainment of urinary control, prevention of infection, reconstructive repair of the defect, and improvement of sexual function.

Hypoplastic/Dysplastic Kidneys

During embryologic development, the ureteric duct grows into the metanephric tissue, triggering the formation of the kidneys. If this growth does not occur, the kidney is absent, a condition called **renal aplasia**. Occasionally, a **hypoplastic kidney**, a very small normal kidney, may develop. These aberrations may be unilateral or bilateral; the occurrence may be incidental or familial. Bilateral hypoplastic kidneys are a common cause of chronic renal failure in children. Segmental hypoplasia, the Ask-Upmark kidney, is not the result of developmental abnormalities but a deformity acquired secondary to intrarenal reflux (Gauthier, Edelmann, & Barnett, 1982).

Renal dysplasia usually results from abnormal differentiation of the renal tissues; for example, primitive glomeruli and tubules, cysts, and nonrenal tissue, such as cartilage, are found in the dysplastic kidney. Dysplasia is usually also associated with a functional or organic obstruction of the collecting system. The obstruction may begin before birth, as in prune-belly syndrome, posterior urethral valves, or ureteroceles.

Renal Agenesis

Renal agenesis (failure of a kidney to grow or develop) may be unilateral or bilateral, randomly occurring or clearly hereditary. The kidney is usually polycystic and dysplastic. The condition may occur as an isolated entity or as a problem associated with other unrelated disorders.

Unilateral renal agenesis occurs in approximately 1 of 1000 live births. Males are more often affected and it is usually the left kidney that is absent. The single kidney is often completely normal so that the child can expect a normal, healthy life. The normal solitary kidney grows because of compensatory hypertrophy after birth, and by the time the child is several years older, the volume of this kidney may approach twice the normal size.

In some instances, however, the single kidney is abnormally formed and associated with abnormalities of its collecting system. Extrarenal congenital abnormalities are relatively more common with unilateral renal agenesis.

Bilateral renal agenesis (also called **Potter syndrome**) occurs in about 1 in 3000 live births, 75% being male. Bilateral renal agenesis results either from an abnormal development of the normal progression from pronephros to mesonephros to metanephros or from an isolated bilateral failure of development of the ureteral buds. The term *Potter syndrome* refers to the association with a specific group of facial anomalies (wide-set eyes, parrot-beak nose, low-set ears, and receding chin). Affected infants rarely live more than a few hours. Most die of respiratory distress caused by associated pulmonary hypoplasia rather than from renal failure. Approximately 40% of affected infants are stillborn.

Glomerular Disorders
Nephrotic Syndrome

Nephrotic syndrome is a term used to describe a symptom complex characterized by proteinuria, hypoproteinemia, hyperlipidemia, and edema. Transient hematuria or hypertension may occur. Nephrotic syndrome is a clinical and biochemical state that may develop during the course of several different renal or systemic diseases. (The pathophysiology and common clinical manifestations of nephrotic syndrome in adults are described in Chapter 33.)

Pathophysiology

In children with nephrotic syndrome, the kidney is usually the only or principal organ involved. This condi-

FIG. 34-5 Child with nephrotic syndrome. (From Shirkey, 1980.)

TABLE 34-2

Corticosteroid Treatment in Children with Nephrotic Syndrome

Response to corticosteroid	Incidence (%)	Outcomes
Steroid responders	93	Single course of therapy, low recurrence rate
Steroid nonresponders	7	Intermittent exacerbations with remissions over several years
Steroid-resistant	Rare	Resistance to steroids, eventual development of chronic renal failure

tion is termed **primary nephrotic syndrome.** If it is caused by a systemic disease or other causes (drugs, toxins, etc.), it is called **secondary nephrotic syndrome** (see Chapter 33).

Approximately 95% of nephrotic syndrome in children occurs in the absence of systemic or preexisting renal disease. Primary nephrotic syndrome is found predominantly in the preschool child, with a peak incidence of onset between 2 and 3 years of age. It is rare after 8 years of age. Boys are affected more frequently than girls. No prevalent racial or geographic distributions are evident. The incidence is approximately 3 per 100,000 children per year.

Clinical Manifestations

Onset of nephrotic syndrome is insidious, with periorbital edema as the first sign. The edema is most noticeable in the morning but subsides during the day as fluid shifts to the abdomen and lower extremities (Fig. 34-5). Because toddlers have picky eating habits, parents are often pleased with the weight gain associated with edema. Parents become alerted to an abnormality when they notice diminished, "frothy," or "foamy" urine output and when edema becomes pronounced with ascites, respiratory difficulty from pleural effusion, and labial or scrotal swelling.

Edema of the intestinal mucosa may cause diarrhea, anorexia, and poor absorption. Edema often masks the malnutrition caused by malabsorption and protein loss. Because of protein deficiency, changes in the quality of hair indicates a malnourished state. Pallor, with shiny skin and prominent veins, is also common. Blood pressure is usually normal or slightly decreased. The child has an increased susceptibility to infection, especially pneumonia, peritonitis, cellulitis, and septicemia. Irritability, fatigue, and lethargy are common.

Evaluation and Treatment

The diagnosis of nephrotic syndrome is evident from the finding of proteinuria, hyperlipidemia, and lipiduria. Several different diagnostic tests, including kidney biopsy, may be required to determine whether the cause is an intrinsic renal disease or a consequence of systemic disease.

The goals of treatment are to reduce the excretion of protein and to maintain a protein-free urine. Prevention or treatment of infection, control of edema, establishment of a balanced nutritional state, and restoration of normal metabolic processes are also important in managing the disorder. Corticosteroids are the primary therapeutic agents, and children are often described according to their response to steroid therapy (Table 34-2). Basic management of nephrotic syndrome includes activity as tolerated; a low-sodium, well-balanced diet; glucocorticosteroids (prednisone), diuretics (Lasix), and immunosuppressive agents (Cytoxan, Imuran); paracentesis (for ascites); and skin care.

Adults and children respond differently to management. Most children, as opposed to few adults, have complete remission. Most children have minimal or no pathologic renal changes. The prognosis for ultimate recovery is quite good. Although relapses are common, usually after respiratory infections or immunizations, most children can look forward to a healthy future. Even those with frequent relapses usually have a spontaneous resolution before age 30.

Glomerulonephritis

Glomerulonephritis includes a number of renal disorders in which proliferation and inflammation of the glomeruli are secondary to an immune mechanism (Table 34-3). (The major glomerulopathies are described in

Chapter 33.) Chronic glomerulonephritis accounts for 53% of renal failure in children and is responsible for most school-aged and teen-aged children requiring dialysis and kidney transplantation.

Poststreptococcal glomerulonephritis

Acute poststreptococcal glomerulonephritis is one of the most common noninfectious renal diseases in children. It is characterized by a sudden onset of gross hematuria, edema, hypertension, and renal insufficiency that occurs after a throat or skin infection with certain strains of group A beta-hemolytic streptococci.

Pharyngeal infections are most common during cold weather; skin infections from impetigo, infected insect bites, or varicella sores usually occur during warm weather. Symptoms of varying severity develop about 1 to 3 weeks after the streptococcal infection. As many as half the children affected are asymptomatic and show only microscopic hematuria with otherwise normal renal function. The most severely affected develop acute renal failure with oliguria.

Typically, a child is in good health until the onset of an upper respiratory or skin infection. One to 2 weeks later, mild proteinuria (< 2g/24 hr), hematuria, and periorbital edema appear. The urine is usually smoky brown or "cola" colored because of the presence of red blood cells, and the volume is reduced. The onset of symptoms in the child is abrupt and consists of flank or midabdominal pain, irritability, general malaise, and fever. Acute hypertension may cause headache, vomiting, somnolence, and other central nervous system manifestations, including seizures. Cardiovascular symptoms are related to circulatory overload and are compounded by hypertension. These include dyspnea, tachypnea, and an enlarged, tender liver.

The disease usually runs its course in a month, but urine abnormalities may be found for up to a year after the onset. Some children become oliguric and develop rapidly progressive glomerulonephritis, whereas others slowly progress to chronic glomerulonephritis. Prolonged proteinuria and abnormal GFR indicate an unfavorable prognosis. More than 95% recover completely.

Treatment is symptom-specific. Because oliguria and hypertension are common, fluid, sodium, and potassium intake are restricted. Bed rest, antihypertensive medication, and diuretic agents are indicated during the acute phase.

Acute glomerulonephritis (AGN) may be accompanied by a positive throat or skin culture for *Streptococcus*. The urine usually contains red blood cells and proteins. As a precautionary measure, penicillin is given in therapeutic doses for 10 to 14 days to eradicate residual streptococci. Early treatment of streptococcal infec-

TABLE 34-3

Primary Glomerulonephritis in Children

Classification	Findings
Cause	Poststreptococcal infection
	Related to other bacterial or viral infection
	Unknown
Immunologic mechanism	Antigen-antibody complex
	Anti-GMB disease
	No immunologic cause established
Histopathology	No lesion
	Diffuse, focal, or segmented
	Membranous, proliferative, or combination of types
	Lobular, exudative, necrotizing, and other types
	Chronic with glomerular proliferation
Clinical manifestations of disease	Acute glomerulonephritis
	Persistent (chronic) glomerulonephritis
	Idiopathic nephrotic syndrome

Adapted from James, 1972.

tions with antibiotics does not preclude the development of the disease. Family members of the child should be cultured and treated if positive, however (Behrman, Kliegman, Nelson, & Vaughan, 1992).

IgA nephropathy

Immunoglobulin A nephropathy is one of the many types of glomerulonephritis. It is characterized by deposition mainly of the immunoglobulin IgA, but also some IgM, in the mesangium of the glomerular capillaries, even though there is no evidence of systemic immunologic disease such as systemic lupus erythematosus or anaphylactoid purpura. Immunoglobulin A neuropathy occurs almost twice as frequently in males as in females.

Children with the disease have recurrent gross hematuria, often after a respiratory infection. Most continue to have microscopic hematuria between the attacks of gross hematuria. Many have a mild proteinuria as well in spite of otherwise normal renal function. Treatment is supportive because kidney damage is generally insignificant. Approximately 20% of affected children develop the progressive form of the disease, however, with hypertension and decreasing renal function. These children eventually require dialysis and transplantation.

Hemolytic Uremic Syndrome

Hemolytic uremic syndrome is an acute disorder characterized by hemolytic anemia originating in the microcirculation, thrombocytopenia, and acute renal failure. The cause remains unknown although an association between hemolytic uremic syndrome and both bacterial and viral agents has been established. Hemolytic uremic syndrome is the most frequent cause of acute renal failure in children. The disease occurs in infants and children younger than 4 years of age. When it occurs in adults, it is often associated with pregnancy and with use of oral contraceptives. The prognosis has improved dramatically in recent years, with more than 90% of children surviving and most regaining normal renal function.

Pathophysiology

In hemolytic uremic syndrome, the endothelial lining of the glomerular arterioles becomes swollen and occluded with platelets and fibrin clots. Narrowed vessels damage erythrocytes as they pass through. These damaged burr cells, helmet cells, and fragmented red blood cells are removed by the spleen, causing acute hemolytic anemia. Fibrinolysis, the process of dissolution of a clot, acts on precipitated fibrin, causing the fibrin-split products to appear in serum and urine. The platelet clustering within damaged vessels, combined with the damage and removal of platelets, produces thrombocytopenia.

Clinical Manifestations

A prodromal gastrointestinal illness (fever, vomiting, diarrhea) or, less frequently, an upper respiratory infection often precedes the onset of hemolytic uremic syndrome by 1 to 2 weeks. After a symptom-free 1- to 5-day period, the sudden onset of pallor, bruising or purpura, irritability, and oliguria heralds the onset of the disease. Slight fever, anorexia, vomiting, and diarrhea, with the stool characteristically watery and blood stained, abdominal pain, mild jaundice, and circulatory overload are accompanying symptoms. Seizures and lethargy indicate central nervous system (CNS) involvement. Renal failure is apparent within the first days of onset. The renal failure causes metabolic acidosis, azotemia, hyperkalemia, and often hypertension.

Evaluation and Treatment

Clinical evaluation includes history of preexisting illness, presenting symptoms, and urine and blood analysis. Management is supportive. When renal failure occurs, early and frequent peritoneal dialysis is indicated. Blood transfusions with packed red cells are needed to maintain reasonable hemoglobin levels.

Obstructive Disorders
Urinary Tract Infections

Urinary tract infections (UTIs) are rare in newborns and are usually caused by bacteria from the bloodstream settling in the urinary tract. Urinary tract infections are most common in 7- to 11-year-old girls as a result of bacteria ascending the urethra. Individual susceptibility, bacterial virulence, and the host's anatomy (presence of reflux, obstruction, stasis, or stones) affect the severity of the disease.

Cystitis, infection of the bladder, results in mucosal inflammation and congestion. This causes detrusor muscle hyperactivity and a resulting decrease in the bladder capacity. It also can lead to reflux or urine up the ureters. This transient reflux caused by the cystitis or chronic reflux can send bacteria all the way to the kidney, causing acute or chronic pyelonephritis. Either of these can cause renal abscesses or scarring.

Differentiating whether an infection is in the bladder or the kidneys is difficult based on symptoms alone. Infants usually develop nausea, vomiting, diarrhea, or jaundice. Children may present with fever of undetermined origin, frequency, urgency, enuresis or incontinence in a previously dry child, abdominal pain, foul-smelling urine, and, sometimes, hematuria. Acute pye-

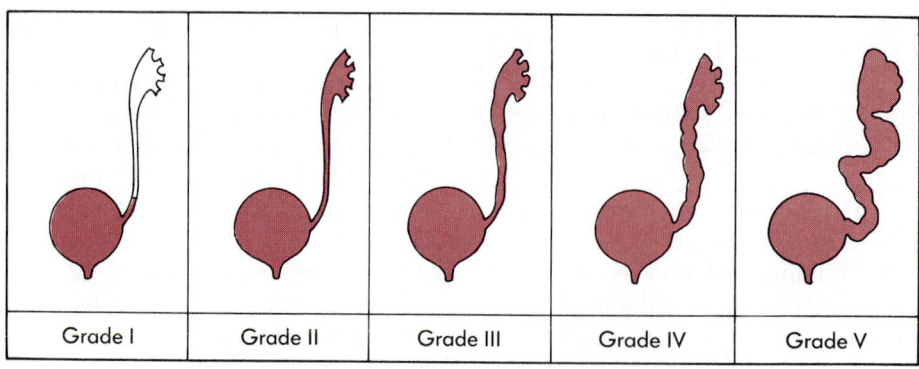

FIG. 34-6 **Grades of reflux.** (From Retik & Cukier, 1987.)

lonephritis usually causes chills, fever, and flank or abdominal pain along with enlarged kidney caused by edema. Chronic pyelonephritis may be asymptomatic.

Diagnosis of UTIs is by urine culture. An accompanying urinalysis can show pyuria and microscopic hematuria. The presence of casts in the urine can indicate pyelonephritis. Ultrasound may be necessary to rule out obstructions or abscesses.

With treatment, UTI symptoms are usually relieved in 1 to 2 days and the urine becomes sterile. Sulfonamides are the drug of choice, with the usual treatment lasting 7 to 10 days. More potent medications may be required if the child has been previously treated for UTI or has congenital abnormalities of the urinary tract. About 3 to 6 weeks after treatment is completed, all children with a first UTI should have a voiding cystourethrogram done to rule out reflux. It is important not to rush this test because the UTI can cause mild to severe reflux. If reflux is found, an intravenous pyelogram may be done to check for renal damage or scarring. Follow-up cultures should be done 2 to 3 weeks after the medication is completed and every 3 months for the next 1 to 2 years to monitor for recurrence, even if the child is asymptomatic.

Surgical correction of reflux or obstruction is necessary before the urinary tract can be sterilized. Children who develop frequent recurrences and who do not have surgically correctable anomalies may need prophylactic antibiotic therapy. A low dose (one-half to one-third usual dose) of the antibiotic is given at bedtime for 1 year to keep high levels of antibiotic in bladder urine. These children also require regular cultures to rule out asymptomatic infections with resistant microorganisms.

Vesicoureteral Reflux

Vesicoureteral reflux is the retrograde flow of bladder urine into the ureters. Reflux allows infected urine from the bladder to be repeatedly swept up into the kidneys. The reflux perpetuates infection by preventing complete emptying of the bladder, because infected, refluxed urine drains back into the bladder at the end of each voiding. In addition, the reflux allows the maximal intravesical pressure to be transmitted to the renal calyces and pyramids (Fig. 34-6). The combination of reflux and infection is an important cause of pyelonephritis, especially in children younger than 5 years of age.

Vesicoureteral reflux occurs more frequently in girls by a ratio of 10:1 and is uncommon in blacks. Its incidence is approximately 1 in 1000 children, and siblings of those affected have a 25% chance of developing reflux. Although reflux is considered abnormal at any age, the shortness of the submucosal segment of the ureter during infancy and childhood renders the antireflux mechanism relatively inefficient and delicate. Thus, reflux is seen commonly in association with infections during early childhood but rarely in older children and adults. (Among adults with urinary tract infections, the incidence of reflux is approximately 5%.)

Reflux may be unilateral or bilateral, and it can be classified or graded for comparative purposes:
Grade I—Reflux into a nondilated distal ureter
Grade II—Reflux into the upper collecting system without dilation
Grade III—Reflux into dilated ureter or blunting of calyceal fornices
Grade IV—Reflux into a grossly dilated ureter
Grade V—Massive reflux with urethral dilation and tortuosity and effacement of the calyceal details

Pathophysiology

Primary reflux results from a congenitally abnormal or ectopic insertion of the ureter into the bladder. Occasionally, the condition is hereditary. Secondary reflux is of more serious importance and may be transient or persistent. It develops in association with infection, malformations of the ureterovesical (UV) junction, increased intravesical pressures, and surgery on the UV junction (Fig. 34-7).

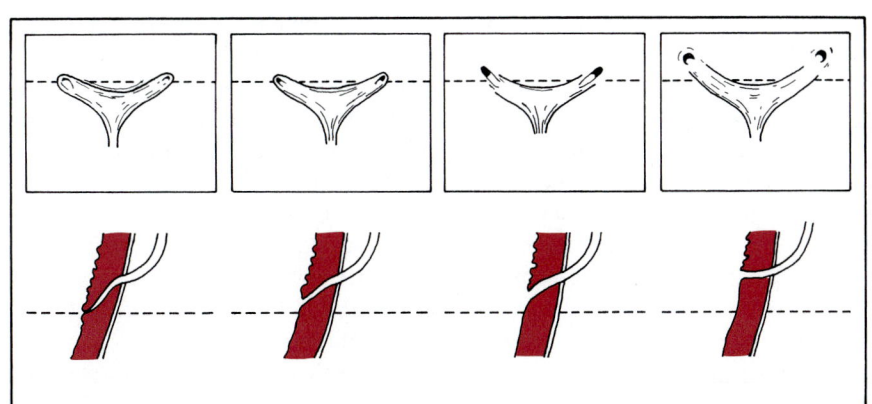

FIG. 34-7 Normal and abnormal configuration of the ureteral orifices. Shown from left to right, progressive lateral displacement of the ureteral orifices and shortening of the intramural tunnels. *Top,* Endoscopic appearance. *Bottom,* Sagittal view through the intramural ureter. (From Behrman et al., 1992.)

Clinical Manifestations

Children with reflux have recurrent urinary tract infection or unexplained fever, poor growth and development, irritability, and feeding problems. Both children and adults may have a family history of reflux or urinary tract infection, pain with voiding, and signs of urinary obstruction or neuropathy.

Evaluation and Treatment

In addition to the history of recurrent urinary tract infection and other symptoms, a voiding cystourethrogram and an intravenous pyelogram may be required for diagnosis. Most children with vesicoureteral reflux respond to nonoperative management aimed at prevention and treatment of infection. Spontaneous remission of grade I and II reflux may occur in 30% to 60% of children younger than 5 years of age. Children with grades III and IV reflux need careful monitoring. Recurrent infection requires surgical intervention. In cases of grade V reflux, early surgical intervention is indicated to prevent renal scarring.

Wilms Tumor

Wilms tumor is an embryonal tumor of the kidney. Although the tumor was first described in 1814, it was named after Max Wilms, a German surgeon who wrote a detailed explanation of the tumor in 1899. At that time, Wilms proposed that the tumor was of embryonic origin and arose from undifferentiated mesoderm. Because it is an embryonal tumor of the kidney, Wilms tumor is also known by the histologic name of nephroblastoma.

The incidence of Wilms tumor remains constant in the United States, with 7.8 cases per million population aged 1 to 14 years. This means that approximately 400 children are diagnosed each year in the United States. Most children are between 1 and 5 years of age when they are diagnosed. The peak incidence occurs between 2 and 3 years of age. Wilms tumor is the most common childhood cancer of the urinary tract. There are no associations between frequency and gender; however, Wilms tumor is slightly more common in black children than in white children.

Microscopically, Wilms tumor is composed of three cellular components: (1) stromal, (2) epithelial, and (3) blastemic. This occurs because blastemic cells, which are primitive and undifferentiated, may have partially developed into epithelial or stromal tissue. With each of these three cellular components, varying stages of differentiation may be evident.

Pathogenesis

Wilms tumor has both sporadic and inherited origins. The sporadic form occurs in children with no known genetic predisposition. Inherited cases, which are rela-

tively rare, are transmitted in an autosomal dominant fashion. In both cases, Wilms tumor has been linked to the deletion or inactivation of genes on the short arm of chromosome 11 (Huff et al., 1991). The deletion or inactivation of these genes demonstrates that the mechanism for development of Wilms tumor involves a tumor-suppressor gene (D'Angio, 1991). The pathogenesis of both the sporadic and inherited forms of Wilms tumor is similar to retinoblastoma. In the inherited form of the disease, the child inherits the loss of one copy of the Wilms tumor—suppressor gene in all of the primitive metanephric blastemic (fetal renal) cells that normally differentiate into the renal tubules and glomeruli. All that is needed is the loss of the other copy of the gene for a Wilms tumor to develop. Because many cells are vulnerable to the loss of this second copy of the gene, bilateral presentation of Wilms tumor (tumor in both kidneys) occurs occasionally in the inherited form of the disease. In the sporadic form of Wilms tumor, both copies of the gene are lost during fetal development. Because normal renal development occurs during the eighth to the thirty-fourth week of gestation, gene loss likely occurs during this time (Belasco, Chatten, & D'Angio, 1984).

Eighteen percent of children who have Wilms tumor also have a number of congenital anomalies. Children with these abnormalities are usually found to have large deletions of the short arm of chromosome 11. Besides loss of the Wilms tumor—suppressor genes, several other important genes are lost, resulting in the anomalies. The anomalies associated with Wilms tumor are aniridia (lack of an iris in the eye), hemihypertrophy (an asymmetry of the body), and genitourinary malformations (i.e., horseshoe kidneys, hypospadias, ureteral duplication, and polycystic kidneys) (Breslow & Beckwith, 1982). Children with both congenital anomalies and Wilms tumor are more likely to have the inherited bilateral form of the disease.

Clinical Manifestations

Most Wilms tumors are enlarging asymptomatic abdominal masses at the time of diagnosis. Many tumors are actually discovered by the child's parent, who feels or notices an abdominal swelling, usually while dressing or bathing the child. The child appears healthy and thriving. Other presenting complaints include vague abdominal pain (37%), hematuria (21%), and fever (23%) (Green, 1985). Hypertension also may be present. The reported frequency is quite variable, from 25% to as high as 63% in one report (Sukarochana, Tolentino, & Kiesewetter, 1972). Hypertension is probably caused by either encroachment by the tumor on the blood supply or secretion of renin by the tumor.

Wilms tumor may occur in any part of the kidney and varies greatly in size at the time of diagnosis. The tumor generally appears as a solitary tumor surrounded by a smooth, fibrous external capsule and also may contain cystic or hemorrhagic areas. A pseudocapsule generally separates the tumor from the renal parenchyma.

Evaluation and Treatment

On physical examination, the tumor feels firm, nontender, and smooth. The mass is generally confined to one side of the abdomen. Should the tumor be palpable past the midline of the abdomen, it may be very large or may be arising from a horseshoe or ectopic kidney. Once an abdominal mass is detected, an abdominal ultrasound may be the initial study and demonstrate a solid intrarenal mass. Abdominal computed tomography scan or magnetic resonance imaging also may be obtained before biopsy and surgical removal of the tumor.

Diagnosis is based on surgical biopsy. Additional laboratory and radiologic studies are used to evaluate the presence or absence of metastasis. The most common sites of metastasis are regional lymph nodes and the lungs. Metastases also occur in the liver, brain, and bone.

Several staging systems for Wilms tumor have been developed. The most widely accepted system was developed by the National Wilms Tumor Study Group (Table 34-4). The system is based on surgical findings and the extent of disease at diagnosis (Farewell, D'Angio, Breslow, & Norkool, 1981).

Surgical exploration and resection begin the treatment of Wilms tumor. The abdomen is explored to determine the extent of disease. In the case of bilateral disease, surgical intervention may include heminephrectomy of the less involved kidney and nephrectomy of the other. Wilms tumor is considered radiosensitive, and radiation therapy has been found to be most effective if begun within 1 to 3 days after surgery. Radiation is not needed for stages I or II disease; it is used in stages III and IV disease. Radiation therapy also is used for lung, nonresectable liver, brain, bone, and lymph node metastases should they be present.

The optimal protocol for chemotherapy is still under study for each stage of Wilms tumor. A combination of vincristine and actinomycin D currently appears to be more effective than either drug alone. Vincristine, actinomycin D, and doxorubicin hydrochloride (Adriamycin) together improve survival rates in children with stage III. Cyclophosphamide also has shown some benefit in very aggressive tumors.

Tremendous advances have been made in the treatment and cure of Wilms tumor. Before the 1930s, 90% of children died of Wilms tumor. Today, with modern treatment, the overall cure rate is as high as 90% for children with stage I through stage III disease. Prognosis is generally poor for children with metastases, al-

though this is one of the few tumors for which lung metastases have been cured.

A variety of factors affect the child's prognosis. These include tumor weight at diagnosis, the age of the child, lymph node invasion, and histologic category. The most important prognostic factors, however, appear to be the histologic category and regional lymph node involvement (Table 34-5). Children with favorable history and no metastatic sites have a 90% survival rate. Even those children with less favorable results do very well, with up to an 80% survival rate (D'Angio, Breslow, & Beckwith, 1989).

TABLE 34-4

Staging of Wilms Tumor

Stage	Tumor characteristics
Stage I	Tumor limited to the kidney, completely resected
Stage II	Tumor ascending beyond the kidney but appearing to be totally resected
Stage III	Residual nonhematogenous tumor confined to the abdomen
Stage IV	Hematogenous metastases
Stage V	Bilateral disease either at diagnosis or later

NOTE: Staging system of the National Wilms Tumor Study Group.

TABLE 34-5

National Wilms Tumor Study Survival Rates

	Relapse-free survival, 4 years (percent)	Four-year survival (percent)
Stage I/FH	90	96
Stage II/FH	88	92
Stage III/FH	79	87
Stage IV/FH	75	82
Stage I, II, III/UH	65	68
Stage IV/UH	55	55

The treatment results of the Third National Wilms Tumor Study (NWTS-3) are now being analyzed and prepared for publication. Between May 1979 and May 1985, 2496 patients were registered. The above data were available as of June 1988.
Abbreviations: *FH*, favorable histology; *UH*, unfavorable histology.
From Ashcraft, 1990.

Enuresis

Enuresis refers to the involuntary passage of urine by a child who is beyond the age when voluntary bladder control should have been acquired. Bladder control is accomplished by most children before the age of 4 years. Five years of age is more accurate and widely accepted, however, being largely determined by cultural beliefs and practices of parents regarding toilet training. In 80% of children, enuresis occurs at night only and is then called **nocturnal enuresis.**

Types of Enuresis

Primary enuresis refers to a condition in which the child has never been continent. **Secondary enuresis,** or acquired enuresis, occurs when a child who has experienced a period of dryness of at least 3 to 6 months after toilet training becomes incontinent again. Secondary enuresis may be diurnal (daytime), nocturnal, or a combination of both. (Types of incontinence are defined in Table 34-6.)

The incidence of enuresis is difficult to determine because it is not a problem that parents readily share with others and because definitions vary according to cultural norms and family practices. Some families start toilet training before 1 year of age and expect continence by the age of 1 or 1½, whereas other families do not expect dryness earlier than 5 years. According to research data, the incidence of enuresis in children older than 5 years ranges from 15% to 26%. Boys are more enuretic than girls by a ratio of 3:2. Teenage enuresis is usually a continuation of childhood bed-wetting. Sours (1978) reports that approximately 2% of men in the armed forces are enuretic.

Theories of Enuresis

Theories about the cause of enuresis abound. A combination of factors is likely to be responsible for enuresis. All or part of each one might be operating in a given child. Reasonable evaluation is to eliminate organic or physiologic causes for enuresis before exploring the psychologic ones.

Organic causes of enuresis account for 2% to 10% of cases. The causes include urinary tract infections; neurologic disturbances; congenital defects of the meatus, urethra, and bladder neck; and allergies. Disorders that increase the normal output of urine, such as diabetes mellitus and diabetes insipidus, or disorders that impair the concentrating ability of the kidney, such as chronic renal failure or sickle cell disease, must be considered in the evaluation of enuresis.

Enuresis in children is possibly caused by a maturational lag. Studies have demonstrated that the child with enuresis has a smaller functional bladder capacity than a nonenuretic child (Troup & Hodgson, 1971). A number of children show a general developmental delay along with elevated intravesical pressure and spikelike detrusor contractions during bladder filling. Enuresis may spontaneously disappear in these children as they get older.

Genetic factors as a cause of enuresis are speculative, but the condition does show a familial tendency (Koff, 1986). Bed-wetting does occur with high frequency among parents, siblings, and other near relatives of symptomatic children. These observations are further supported by a high concordance rate in enuretic monozygotic twins. Family studies indicate that the closer the relationship, the higher the incidence of enuresis.

TABLE 34-6

Classification of Incontinence

Types of incontinence	Definition
Total incontinence	Inability to store any urine; indicates an anatomic or functional absence of urinary sphincters (e.g., epispadias or myelomeningocele) or a bypassing of urinary sphincters (e.g., vesicovaginal fistula)
Overflow incontinence	Frequent dribbling that relieves a constantly full bladder; occurs when urinary outlet is obstructed
Urge incontinence	Sudden and uncontrollable need to void that cannot be suppressed; suggests bladder irritation
Precipitate voiding	Voiding without a preceding urge to void; suggests neurologic origin
Stress incontinence	Uncontrollable voiding that occurs when intravesical pressure momentarily exceeds intravesical resistance, as in "giggle incontinence"
Paradoxic incontinence	Incontinence in spite of normal voiding; suggests an ectopic ureteral orifice outside the urinary sphincter mechanism (e.g., a girl who is constantly wet, yet voids normally)

A significant number of nocturnal enuretic episodes have been related to deep sleep. These children sleep more soundly than others. Many demonstrate increased frequency and magnitude of spontaneous bladder contractions during the non-rapid-eye-movement (non-REM) stage of sleep preceding bed-wetting. Nocturnal enuresis occurs as the child moves from the deeper stages of non-REM sleep into the REM stage. Bed-wetting incidents are incorrectly associated with dreaming. Laboratory studies of sleep have demonstrated that very few incidents of bed-wetting occur when the child is dreaming (Kales & Kales, 1970). If the bed is not changed, however, the child may incorporate the feeling of wetness with the next REM dream cycle and may, therefore, incorrectly associate the enuresis with the dream. As the child develops, the deep sleep period, which is associated with a physiologic dysfunction of the reticular activating system, resolves, and the child "outgrows" the problem.

A variety of psychosocial theories have also been postulated as explanation of enuresis. Enuresis has been associated with temper tantrums, fear reactions, excitability, low birth weight, and minimal brain dysfunction (Knopf, 1984; Retik & Cukier, 1987).

Therapeutic management of enuresis includes conditioning devices, drug therapy (Tofranil), bladder training, withholding fluids, sleep interruption, and diet therapy. Psychotherapy and behavior modification are recommended when enuresis is associated with psychologic stress.

SUMMARY REVIEW

Structure and Function of the Renal System in Children

1 Because of high hydrogen ion concentration, limited ability to regulate the internal environment, and lowered osmotic pressure, children have a narrow chemical safety margin.

2 Any disturbance, such as diarrhea, infection, fasting, or feeding alterations, can lead rapidly to severe acidosis and fluid imbalance.

3 The composition of body fluids differs with age, thus making children more vulnerable to pathophysiologic changes.

4 Because the kidney develops from the medulla to the cortex, blood flow to the medullary nephrons is limited in infancy, and infants thus have limited urine-concentrating capacity.

Alterations in Renal Function in Children

1 Congenital renal disorders affect 10% to 15% of the population. These disorders range in severity from minor, easily correctable anomalies to those incompatible with life.

2 Hypospadias is a congenital condition in which the urethral meatus is located on the undersurface of the penis; epispadias is a congenital condition in which the urethral opening is located on the dorsal surface of the penis.

3 Epispadias is a mild form of exstrophy, a congenital condition that affects the urethra and bladder neck. The urethral opening in boys is on the dorsal surface of the penis.

4 Exstrophy of the bladder is a congenital malformation in which the pubic bones are separated, the lower portion of the abdominal wall and anterior wall of the bladder are missing, and the back wall of the bladder is everted through the opening.

5 A dysplastic kidney is the result of abnormal differentiation of renal tissues. The hypoplastic kidney is a very small but otherwise normal kidney.

6 Renal agenesis is the failure of a kidney to grow or develop. (The condition may be unilateral or bilateral and may occur as an isolated entity or in association with other disorders.)

7 Nephrotic syndrome is a term used to describe a symptom complex characterized by proteinuria, hypoproteinemia, hyperlipidemia, and edema. Metabolic, biochemical, or physiochemical disturbance in the glomerular basement membrane may lead to increased permeability to protein.

8 Glomerulonephritis is an inflammation of the glomeruli characterized by hematuria, edema, and hypertension. (The cause is unknown, but glomerulonephritis may follow other infections, especially those of the upper respiratory tract). Deposition of immunoglobulins in the mesangium of the glomerular capillaries leads to another type of glomerulonephritis.

9 Hemolytic uremic syndrome is an acute disorder characterized by hemolytic anemia, acute renal failure, and thrombocytopenia.

10 Urinary tract infections can result from general sepsis in the newborn but are caused by bacteria ascending the urethra in older children. The bladder, alone, is infected in cystitis. The infection ascends to the kidney(s) in pyelonephritis. Urinary tract anomalies must be surgically corrected to prevent frequent recurrent infections.

11 Vesicoureteral reflux, which refers to the retrograde flow of bladder urine into the ureters, provides mechanisms for bladder infection in children, whose ureters are shorter than those of adults.

12 Wilms tumor is an embryonal tumor of the kidney that usually presents between birth and 5 years of age. The tumor can be successfully treated by surgery, with a combination of drugs, and, sometimes, radiation therapy.

13 Enuresis refers to the involuntary passage of urine.

14 Enuresis may occur during the daytime (diurnally) or during the night (nocturnally). The disorder tends to occur during non-REM sleep and can have a variety of organic and psychologic causes.

KEY TERMS

Chordee, 1268
Enuresis, 1276
Epispadias, 1268
Exstrophy of the bladder, 1268
Glomerulonephritis, 1270
Hemolytic uremic syndrome, 1272
Horseshoe kidney, 1267
Hypoplastic kidney, 1269

Hypospadias, 1267
Nocturnal enuresis, 1276
Potter syndrome, 1269
Primary enuresis, 1276
Primary nephrotic syndrome, 1270
Renal agenesis, 1269
Renal aplasia, 1269

Renal dysplasia, 1269
Secondary enuresis, 1276
Secondary nephrotic syndrome, 1270
Urinary tract infection (UTI), 1272
Vesicoureteral reflux, 1273
Wilms tumor (nephroblastoma), 1274

REFERENCES

Ashcraft, K. (1990). *Pediatric urology*. Philadelphia: Saunders.

Behrman, R., Kliegman, R., Nelson, W., & Vaughan, V., III (Eds.). (1992). *Nelson textbook of pediatrics*. Philadelphia: Saunders.

Belasco, J., Chatten, J., & D'Angio, G. (1984). Wilms' tumor. In W. Sutow, D. Fernbach, & T. Vietti (Eds.), *Clinical pediatric oncology* (3rd ed.). St. Louis: Mosby—Year Book.

Breslow, N. E., & Beckwith, J. B. (1982). Epidemiological features of Wilms' tumor: Results of the national Wilms' tumor study. *Journal of the National Cancer Institute, 68*, 429-436.

D'Angio, G. J. (1991). Wilms tumor: Status report. *Journal of Clinical Oncology, 9*, 877-887.

D'Angio, G. J., Breslow, N. E., & Beckwith, J. B. (1989). Treatment of Wilms tumor: Results of the third national Wilms tumor study. *Cancer, 64*, 349-360.

Farewell, V. T., D'Angio, G. J., Breslow, N. E., & Norkool, P. (1981). Retrospective validation of a new staging system for Wilms' tumor. *Cancer Clinic Trials, 4*, 167-171.

Gauthier, B., Edelmann, C., & Barnett, H. (1982). *Nephrology and urology for the pediatrician*. Boston: Little, Brown, & Co.

Green, D. M. (1985). The diagnosis and management of Wilms' tumor. *Pediatric Clinics of North America, 32*, 735-754.

Huff, V., Miwa, H., Haber, D. A., Call, K. M., Housman, D., Strong, L. C., & Saunders, G. F. (1991). Evidence for WTI as a Wilms tumor (WT) gene: Iatrogenic germinal deletion in bilateral WT. *American Journal of Human Genetics, 48*, 997-1003.

Ingalls, A. J., & Salerno, M. C. (1979.) *Maternal and child health nursing* (4th ed.). St. Louis: Mosby—Year Book.

James, J. A. (1972). *Renal disease in childhood* (2nd ed. p. 84.) St. Louis: Mosby—Year Book.

Kales, A., & Kales, J. D. (1970, September). Evaluation, diagnosis, and treatment of clinical conditions related to sleep. *Journal of the American Medical Association, 11*, 2229-2235.

Kempe, C. H., Silver, K. H., & O'Brien, D. (1982). *Current pediatric diagnosis and treatment*. Los Altos, CA: Lange Medical Publishers.

Knopf, I. J. (1984). *Childhood psychopathology: A developmental approach* (2nd ed.). Englewood Cliffs, NJ: Prentice-Hall.

Koff, S. A. (1986). Enuresis [Chapter 54]. In P. C. Walsh, G. F. Ruben, A. D. Permutter, & T. A. Stanley (Eds.), *Campbell's urology* (vol. 2, 5th ed.). Philadelphia: Saunders.

Netter, F., Shapter, R., & Yonkman, F. (Eds.). (1973). *The Ciba collection of medical illustrations, volume 6: Kidneys, ureters, and urinary bladder*. Summit: Ciba Pharmaceutical Corporation.

Permutter, A. D., Retik, A. B., & Bauer, S. B. (1986). Anomalies of the upper urinary tract [Chapter 38, p. 1165]. In P. C. Walsh, G. F. Ruben, A. D. Permutter, & T. A. Stanley (Eds.), *Campbell's urology* (vol. 2, 5th ed.). Philadelphia: Saunders.

Retik, A., & Cukier, J. (Eds.). (1987). *Pediatric urology*. Baltimore: Williams & Wilkins.

Shirkey, H. C. (Ed.). (1980). *Pediatric therapy* (6th ed.). St. Louis: Mosby—Year Book.

Sours, J. (1978). Enuresis. In B. Wolman (Ed.), *Handbook of treatment of mental disorders in childhood and adolescence* (pp. 153-160). New Jersey: Prentice-Hall.

Speakman, M. J., & Azmy, A. F. (1992). Skin chordee without hypospadias—An under recognized entity. *British Journal of Urology, 69*(4), 428-429.

Sukarochana, K., Tolentino, W., & Kiesewetter, W. B. (1972). Wilms' tumor and hypertension. *Journal of Pediatric Surgery, 7*, 573-578.

Troup, C. W., & Hodgson, N. B. (1971, January). Nocturnal functional bladder capacity in enuretic children. *Journal of Urology, 105*, 129-136.

Whaley, L. F. & Wong, D. L. (1991). *Nursing care of infants and children* (4th ed.). St. Louis: Mosby—Year Book.

SUGGESTED READINGS

Robson, W. L., Leung, A. K., & Kaplan, B. S. (1993). Hemolytic-uremic syndrome. *Current Problems in Pediatrics, 23*(1), 16-33.

Zelikovic, I., Adelman, R. D., Nancarrow, P. A. (1992). Urinary tract infections in children: An update. *Western Journal of Medicine, 157*(5), 554-561.

UNIT XII

The Digestive System

GASTROINTESTINAL DISORDERS have been a source of human misery since ancient times. Hippocrates (460-370 BC) described clinical symptoms of dysentery, intestinal obstruction, and liver disease. Detailed descriptions of tumors and ulcers of the esophagus and stomach and hardening of the liver and ascites were made by Galen (131-201 AD). As one of the earliest physiologists, he offered ideas about processes of digestion and functions of the liver that provided the basis for his discussion of gastrointestinal diseases. Although his descriptions contained fundamental misconceptions, 1400 years passed before a Florentine physician, Antonius Benivenius (1507), accurately wrote about gastric ulcers, intestinal carcinoma, and gallstones on the basis of postmortem examinations.

By 1761, Morgagni had described the pathologic anatomy of gastritis, gastric and intestinal ulcers, and tumors and cirrhosis of the liver. The pathologic anatomy of gastrointestinal disease was advanced by Karl Rokitansky (1804-1878) from descriptions based on more than 30,000 autopsies. Microscopic classifications of intestinal disease were first published by Rudolf Virchow in 1856.

THE DIGESTIVE SYSTEM

Anatomy of the gastrointestinal system. (From Bidlow & Govard, Anatomia system humani corporis, 1685; courtesy National Library of Medicine.)

Chemical processes of digestion were first introduced in the 1600s. Regner de Graaf (1641-1673) isolated pancreatic and salivary juices by creating parotid and pancreatic fistulas in a dog. Two hundred years later, Claude Bernard (1813-1878) described the storage of sugar in the liver as glycogen and its release as glucose, as well as the digestive function of the pancreas. Pepsin was isolated in 1861, and the pancreatic enzyme trypsin was isolated in 1867. The first intestinal hormone, secretin, was identified in 1902, and the field of endocrinology began. Since that time more than two dozen intestinal hormones have been described. During World War II, a Dutch physician observed that children with celiac sprue (gluten intolerance) who were deprived of bread had a great improvement in their symptoms. From this observation, gluten was identified as the cause of celiac sprue. The virus causing serum hepatitis was discovered by B. S. Blumberg in 1965; for this work he was awarded the Nobel Prize in 1976.

The functions of gastric juice were studied by the swallowing and retrieval of sponges from which the juice was squeezed. Swallowing linen bags or perforated metal tubes filled with food allowed analysis of gastric digestion. The presence of hydrochloric acid in gastric juice was established by an English physiologic chemist, William Prout, in 1824. An American frontier physician, William Beaumont (1785-1853), studied gastric function over many years by observing the gastric mucosa of a patient he treated who survived a gunshot wound in the abdomen. The wound healed, leaving a permanent gastric fistula, allowing Beaumont the opportunity to collect gastric secretions and study gastric activity under a variety of circumstances. He is credited as the father of American physiology and gastroenterology.

Structure and Function of the Digestive System

Sue E. Huether

Chapter Outline

T he digestive system breaks down ingested food, prepares it for uptake by the body's cells, provides body water, and eliminates wastes. This system consists of the gastrointestinal tract, a long tube that extends from the mouth to the anus, and accessory organs of digestion: the liver, gallbladder, and exocrine pancreas.

Food breakdown begins in the mouth with chewing and continues in the stomach, where food is churned and mixed with acid, mucus, enzymes, and other secretions. From the stomach the fluid and partially digested food passes into the small intestine, where biochemicals and enzymes secreted by the liver

and exocrine pancreas break it down into absorbable components of proteins, carbohydrates, and fats. These nutrients pass through the walls of the small intestine into blood vessels and lymphatics that carry them to the liver for storage or further processing.

Ingested substances and secretions that are not absorbed in the small intestine pass into the large intestine, where fluid continues to be absorbed. Fluid wastes travel to the kidneys and are eliminated in the urine. Solid wastes pass into the rectum and are eliminated from the body through the anus.

Except for chewing, swallowing, and defecation of solid wastes, the movements of the digestive system *(gastrointestinal motility) are all controlled by hormones and the autonomic nervous system. As ingested substances move through the gastrointestinal tract, they trigger the release of hormones that stimulate or inhibit (1) the muscular contractions that mix and propel food from the esophagus to the anus and (2) the timely secretion of substances that aid in digestion. The autonomic innervation, both sympathetic and parasympathetic, is controlled by centers in the brain and by local stimuli that are mediated at plexuses (networks of nerve fibers) within the gastrointestinal walls.*

THE GASTROINTESTINAL TRACT

The alimentary canal, or **gastrointestinal tract,** consists of the mouth, esophagus, stomach, small intestine, large intestine, rectum, and anus (Fig. 35-1). It carries out the following digestive processes:

1. Ingestion of food
2. Propulsion of food and wastes from the mouth to the anus
3. Secretion of mucus, water, and enzymes
4. Mechanical digestion of food particles
5. Chemical digestion of food particles
6. Absorption of digested food
7. Elimination of waste products by defecation

The histologic organization of the gastrointestinal tract consists of four layers. From the inside out they are the mucosa, submucosa, muscularis, and serosa or adventitia. They are organized into concentric layers that vary in thickness. Each layer has sublayers (Fig. 35-2). Intrinsic nerves are located solely within the gastrointestinal tract and are controlled by local and autonomic nervous system stimuli through the **enteric plexus,** three nerve plexuses located in different layers of the gastrointestinal walls. The **submucosal plexus** (Meissner plexus) is located in the muscularis mucosae, the **myenteric plexus** (Auerbach plexus) in the muscle layers (tunica muscularis), and the **subserosal plexus** just beneath the serosa.

Mouth and Esophagus

The **mouth** is a reservoir for the chewing and mixing of food with saliva. As food particles become smaller and move around in the mouth, the taste buds and olfactory nerves are continuously stimulated, adding to the satisfaction of eating. The tongue's surface contains thousands of chemoreceptors, or taste buds, which can distinguish salty, sour, bitter, and sweet tastes. Tastes and food odors help to initiate salivation and the secretion of gastric juice in the stomach. There are 32 per-

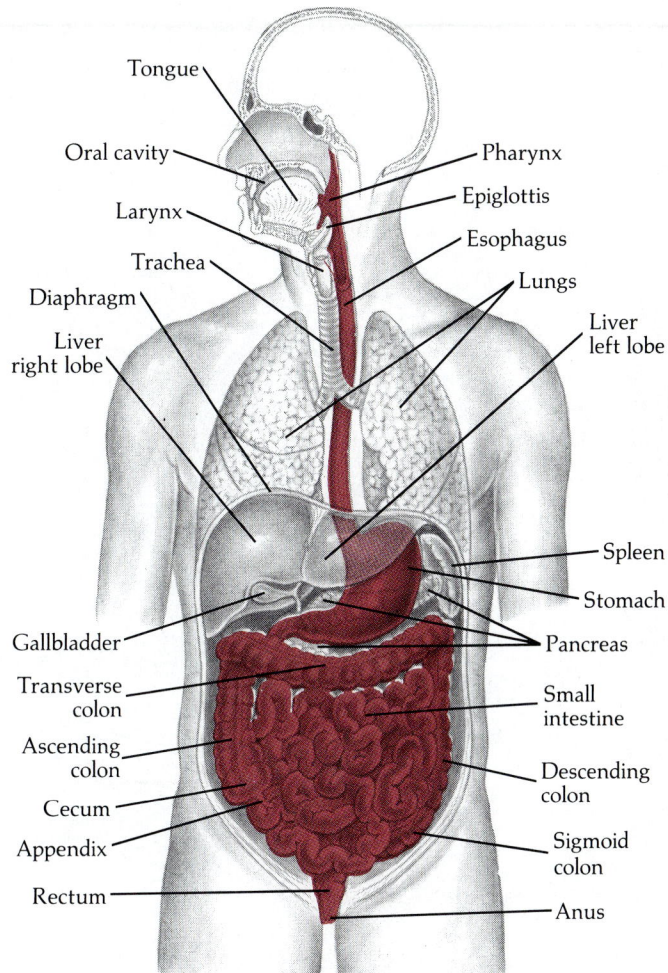

FIG. 35-1 Structure and function of the digestive system. Digestion begins in the mouth with chewing, which breaks down food mechanically and mixes it with saliva. Swallowing propels chewed food through the esophagus to the stomach, where acids and stomach motility liquefy it further. Next the liquefied food enters the small intestine, where secretions of the intestinal walls, liver, gallbladder, and pancreas digest it into absorbable nutrients. Nutrients are absorbed through intestinal walls, and unabsorbed wastes enter the large intestine (colon), where fluids are removed. Solid wastes then enter the rectum and leave the body through the anus. (From Thompson et al., 1993.)

manent teeth in the adult mouth, and they are important for speech and mastication.

Salivation

There are three pairs of **salivary glands,** the submandibular, sublingual, and parotid glands (Fig. 35-3). Together they secrete about 1 L of saliva per day. **Saliva** consists mostly of water that contains varying amounts of mucus, sodium, bicarbonate, chloride, potassium,

FIG. 35-2 A cross section of the small intestine. There are four concentric tissue layers: the serosa, muscularis, submucosa, and mucosa. The muscularis is subdivided into longitudinal and circular layers of smooth muscle fibers. A network of nerve fibers called the myenteric plexus is located between the muscle layers. The submucosa contains a variety of exocrine glands. Between the submucosa and the circular muscle is the submucosal neural plexus. The mucosa is subdivided into the epithelium, lamina propria, and muscularis mucosae. (From Schauff, Moffett, & Moffett, 1990.)

and **salivary α-amylase** (ptyalin), an enzyme that initiates carbohydrate digestion in the mouth and stomach.

Both sympathetic and parasympathetic divisions of the autonomic nervous system control salivation. Because cholinergic parasympathetic fibers stimulate the salivary glands, atropine (an anticholinergic agent) inhibits salivation and makes the mouth dry. β-Adrenergic stimulation from sympathetic fibers also increases salivary secretion. The salivary glands, unlike other secretory glands of the gastrointestinal tract, are not regulated by hormones.

The composition of saliva depends on the rate of secretion. At low rates of flow, such as those between meals, sodium, chloride, and bicarbonate are reabsorbed in the collecting ducts of the salivary glands, and the saliva contains fewer of these electrolytes (i.e., is more hypotonic). At higher flow rates, which are stimulated by food, reabsorption is decreased and there is more sodium, chloride, and bicarbonate in the saliva, making it hypertonic (Fig. 35-4). By this mechanism, sodium, chloride, and bicarbonate are recycled until they are released to help with digestion and absorption. Potassium secretion is fairly constant, independent of flow rate. Aldosterone, however, can increase an exchange of sodium for potassium, increasing sodium conservation and potassium excretion. The bicarbonate concentration of saliva sustains a pH of about 7.4, which neutralizes bacterial acids and prevents tooth decay. Saliva also contains IgA, which helps prevent infection. Exog-

---

STRUCTURAL LAYERS OF THE GASTROINTESTINAL TRACT

Mucosa: a mucous membrane composed of three layers
- Epithelium
- Lamina propria: connective tissue containing blood vessels, lymph nodes, and glands
- Muscularis mucosa: thin layer of smooth muscle between mucosa and submucosa

Submucosa: connective tissue containing blood vessels, lymph channels, nerves, and glands (in some regions)

Tunica muscularis: layers of smooth muscle with a myenteric nerve plexus (Auerbach plexus) lying between them
- Oblique muscle layer (stomach only)
- Circular muscle layer
- Longitudinal muscle layer

Serosa or adventitia: a serous membrane covered with an outer layer of squamous epithelial cells enous fluoride (e.g., fluoride in drinking water) is also secreted in the saliva, providing additional protection against tooth decay.

Swallowing

The **esophagus** is a hollow muscular tube approximately 25 cm long that conducts substances from the oropharynx to the stomach (Fig. 35-1). Swallowed food is moved to the stomach by **peristalsis,** the sequential contraction and relaxation of outer longitudinal and inner circular layers of muscles. The upper third of the esophagus contains striated muscle that is directly innervated by motor neurons. The lower two thirds contains smooth muscle that is innervated by preganglionic cholinergic fibers from the vagus nerve. The fibers are activated in a downward sequence. Peristalsis is stimulated when afferent fibers distributed along the length of the esophagus sense changes in wall tension caused by stretching as food passes. The greater the tension, the greater the intensity of esophageal contraction. Occasionally, intense contractions cause pain similar to "heartburn" or angina.

Each end of the esophagus is opened and closed by a sphincter. The **upper esophageal sphincter** prevents entry of air into the esophagus during respiration. The **lower esophageal sphincter** (cardiac sphincter) prevents regurgitation from the stomach. This is a necessary function because intraabdominal pressure is greater than intrathoracic or atmospheric pressure. The lower esophageal sphincter is located near the esophageal hiatus, the opening in the diaphragm where the esophagus ends at the stomach.

Swallowing is a complex event mediated by the swallowing center, which is located in the reticular formation of the brainstem. Swallowing occurs in two phases, the oropharyngeal (voluntary) phase and the esophageal (involuntary) phase. During the **oropharyngeal phase** of swallowing, food is segmented into a bolus by the tongue and forced posteriorly toward the pharynx as the tongue pushes upward against the hard palate. The superior constrictor muscle of the pharynx contracts, preventing movement of food into the nasopharynx. At the same time, respiration is inhibited and the epiglottis slides downward to prevent the bolus from entering the larynx and trachea. The movements of the tongue and pharyngeal constrictors propel the food into the esophagus in a series of coordinated events taking less than 1 second (Christensen, 1987).

The **esophageal phase** of swallowing begins as the bolus of food enters the esophagus. The bolus is transported by peristalsis, the sequential waves of muscular contractions that travel down the esophagus and are preceded by receptive waves of relaxation. The wave of relaxation reduces resistance and allows food to pass, after which the wave of contraction pushes food farther

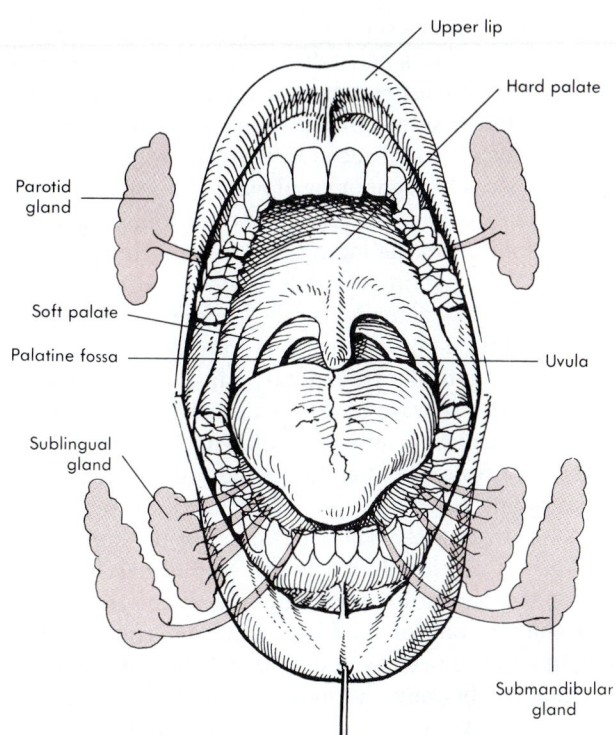

FIG. 35-3 Structures of the mouth. (From Phipps, Long, Woods, & Cassmeyer, 1991.)

FIG. 35-4 Salivary electrolyte concentrations and flow rate. Changes in concentration of sodium (Na^+), potassium (K^+), chloride (Cl^-), and bicarbonate (HCO_3^-) with increases in flow rate of saliva. Black dotted line = sodium; solid black line = bicarbonate; solid red line = chloride; dotted red line = potassium.

along. The lower esophageal sphincter relaxes just before the arrival of a peristaltic wave. The sphincter muscles return to their resting tone after the bolus of food passes into the stomach. The esophageal phase of swallowing takes 5 to 10 seconds, with the bolus moving 2 to 6 cm/sec. Throughout swallowing the sphincters and esophagus work in concert with the peristaltic wave that moves food from the mouth to the stomach.

Peristalsis that immediately follows the oropharyngeal phase of swallowing is called **primary peristalsis.** If a bolus of food becomes stuck in the esophageal lumen, the distention of the esophageal wall stimulates **secondary peristalsis,** a wave of contraction and relaxation that is independent of voluntary swallowing. Secondary peristalsis is a response to stretch receptors that are stimulated by increased wall tension, causing an increase in impulses from the swallowing center of the brain.

When it is closed, the lower esophageal sphincter serves as a barrier between the stomach and esophagus. The muscle tone of the lower sphincter changes with neural and hormonal stimulation. Cholinergic vagal input and the digestive hormone gastrin increase sphincter tone. Nonadrenergic, noncholinergic vagal impulses relax the lower esophageal sphincter, as do the hormones progesterone, secretin, and glucagon. Relaxation during swallowing is mediated by the vagus.

Stomach

The **stomach** is a hollow, muscular organ that stores food during eating, secretes digestive juices, mixes food with these juices, and propels partially digested food, called **chyme,** into the duodenum of the small intestine. The anatomy of the stomach is presented in Fig. 34-5.

The stomach's major anatomic boundaries are the lower esophageal sphincter, where food passes through the **cardiac orifice** into the stomach; the greater and lesser curvatures; and the **pyloric sphincter,** which relaxes as food is propelled through the **pylorus** into the duodenum. Functional areas of the stomach are the **fundus** (upper portion), **body** (middle portion), and **antrum** (lower portion).

The tunica muscularis consists of a circular muscle layer and a longitudinal layer (Fig. 35-5). The stomach wall is unique in that it also contains a layer of oblique muscle between the submucosa and the circular muscle layer. The oblique muscle is prominent in the anterior and posterior walls of the stomach. The circular and longitudinal layers of muscle are thinnest in the fundus, where the stomach relaxes and expands to store food received from the esophagus. These layers become progressively thicker in the body and antrum, where food is mixed, churned, and pushed out into the duodenum. The mucosa of the stomach consists of glandular epithelium. This layer is discussed in the section about secretory functions of the stomach (p. 1288).

Blood is supplied to the stomach by a branch of the celiac artery. Major arteries lie along the greater and lesser curvatures. They branch and penetrate the serosa and muscle layers to form a rich collateral circulation throughout the mucosa, submucosa, and tunica muscularis. The blood supply is so abundant that nearly all arterial vessels must be occluded before ischemic changes occur in the stomach wall. The splenic vein drains the right side of the stomach, and the gastric vein drains the left side.

The stomach is innervated by sympathetic and para-

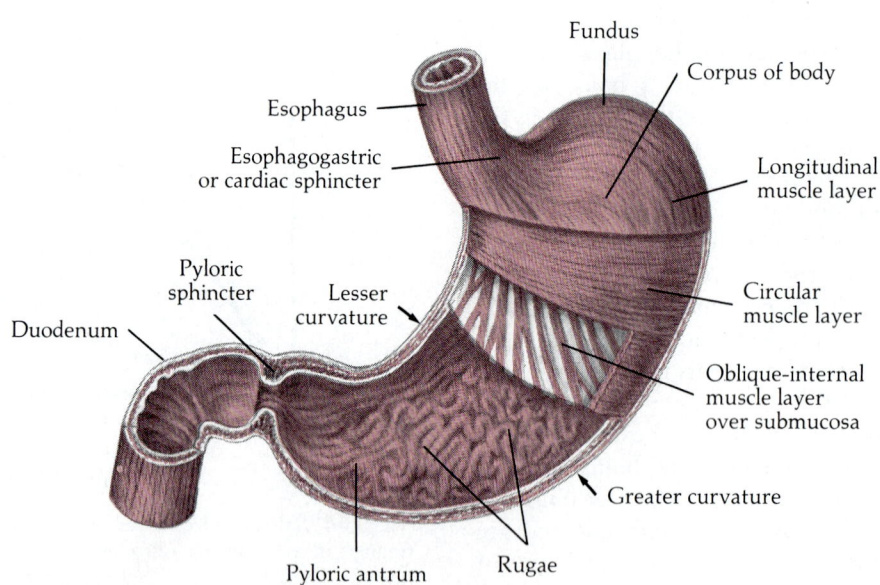

FIG. 35-5 Muscle layers and interior of the stomach. (From Thompson et al., 1993.)

sympathetic divisions of the autonomic nervous system. Some of the autonomic fibers are extrinsic: that is, they originate outside the stomach and are controlled by nerve centers in the brain. Others are intrinsic: they originate within the stomach and also respond to local stimuli. Extrinsic sympathetic fibers reach the stomach through the celiac plexus (solar plexus), whereas extrinsic parasympathetic fibers enter through the gastric branch of the vagus nerve.

Gastric Motility

In its resting state, the stomach is small and contains about 50 ml fluid. There is no wall tension, and the muscle layers in the fundus contract very little. Swallowing causes the fundus to relax (receptive relaxation) to receive a bolus of food from the esophagus. Relaxation is coordinated by efferent, nonadrenergic, noncholinergic vagal fibers and is facilitated by **gastrin** and **cholecystokinin,** two polypeptide hormones secreted by the gastrointestinal mucosa. (The actions of digestive hormones are summarized in Table 35-1.) Food is stored in vertical or oblique layers as it arrives in the fundus, whereas fluids flow relatively quickly down to the antrum.

Gastric (stomach) motility increases with the initiation of peristaltic waves, which sweep over the body of the stomach toward the antrum. The rate of peristaltic contractions is approximately three per minute and is influenced by neural and hormonal activity. Gastrin,

motilin (an intestinal hormone), and the vagus nerve increase contraction by lowering the threshold potential of muscle fibers. (The neural and biochemical mechanisms of muscle contraction are described in Chapter 12.) Sympathetic activity and **secretin** (another intestinal hormone) are inhibitory and raise the threshold potential. The rate of peristalsis is mediated by pacemaker cells that initiate a wave of depolarization (basic electrical rhythm), which moves from the upper part of the stomach to the pylorus.

The mixing and emptying of food (chyme) from the stomach take several hours. Mixing occurs as food is propelled toward the antrum. As food approaches the pylorus, the velocity of the peristaltic wave increases. The passage of the contractile wave over the gastric contents forces the contents back toward the body of the stomach. This action, which is known as **retropulsion,** effectively mixes food with digestive juices, and the oscillating motion breaks down large food particles. With each peristaltic wave, a small portion of the gastric contents (chyme) passes through the pylorus and into the duodenum. The pylorus is about 1.5 cm long and is always open about 2.0 mm. It opens wider during antral contraction. Normally there is no regurgitation from the duodenum into the antrum.

The rate of **gastric emptying** (movement of gastric contents into the duodenum) depends on the volume, osmotic pressure, and chemical composition of the gastric contents. Larger volumes of food increase gastric

TABLE 35-1

Hormones of the Digestive System

Source	Hormone	Stimulus for secretion	Action
Mucosa of the stomach	Gastrin	Presence of partially digested proteins in the stomach	Stimulates gastric glands to secrete hydrochloric acid and pepsinogen
Mucosa of the small intestine	Motilin	Presence of acid and fat in the duodenum	Increases gastrointestinal motility
	Secretin	Presence of chyme (acid, partially digested proteins, and fats) in the duodenum	Stimulates pancreas to secrete alkaline pancreatic juice and liver to secrete bile; decreases gastrointestinal motility
	Cholecystokinin	Same as for secretin	Stimulates gallbladder to eject bile and pancreas to secrete alkaline fluid; decreases gastric motility
	Enterogastrone	Presence of fat in the duodenum	Inhibits gastric secretion and motility
	Entero-oxyntin	Presence of chyme in small intestine	Stimulates gastric glands to secrete hydrochloric acid
	Gastric-inhibitory peptide	Stretching of the duodenum and fatty acids	Decreases gastric motility and secretion of pepsin and HCl

Adapted from Thibodeau.
NOTE: The digestive hormones are not secreted into the gastrointestinal lumen, but rather into the bloodstream, in which they travel to target tissues.

pressure, peristalsis, and rate of emptying. Solids, fats, and nonisotonic solutions delay gastric emptying. (Osmotic pressure and tonicity are described in Chapters 1 and 3.) Products of fat digestion, which are formed in the duodenum by the action of bile from the liver and enzymes from the pancreas, stimulate the secretion of cholecystokinin. This hormone inhibits gastric motility and decreases gastric emptying so that fats are not emptied into the duodenum at a rate that exceeds the rate of bile and enzyme secretion. Osmoreceptors in the wall of the duodenum are sensitive to the osmotic pressure of duodenal contents. The arrival of hypertonic or hypotonic gastric contents activates the osmoreceptors, which delay gastric emptying to facilitate formation of an isoosmotic duodenal environment. The rate at which acid enters the duodenum also influences gastric emptying. Secretions from the pancreas, liver, and duodenal mucosa neutralize gastric acid in the duodenum. The rate of emptying is adjusted to the duodenum's ability to neutralize the incoming acidity (Berne & Levy, 1993).

Gastric Secretion

Stimulated by eating, the stomach secretes large volumes of gastric juices or gastric secretions. Specialized cells located throughout the gastric mucosa produce mucus, acid, enzymes, hormones, and intrinsic factor. (Intrinsic factor is necessary for the intestinal absorption of vitamin B_{12}.) The hormones are secreted into the blood and travel to target tissues in the bloodstream. The other gastric secretions are released directly into the stomach lumen. Different areas of the stomach mucosa secrete different substances, with the exception of mucus, which is secreted by epithelial and mucous cells in all parts of the stomach. Mucus covers the entire mucosa, forming a protective barrier against acid and proteolytic enzymes, which otherwise would damage the gastric lining.

In the fundus and body of the stomach the **gastric glands** of the mucosa are the primary secretory units (Fig. 35-6). Several of these glands (three to seven) empty into a common duct known as the **gastric pit**. The **parietal cells** (oxyntic cells) within the glands secrete hydrochloric acid and intrinsic factor. The **chief cells** within the glands secrete **pepsinogen**, an enzyme precursor that is readily converted to **pepsin** (a proteolytic enzyme) in the gastric juice.

Like that of the secretions of salivary glands, the composition of gastric juice depends on volume and flow rate (Fig. 35-7). At low rates of secretion, hydrogen and chloride concentrations are low and sodium concentra-

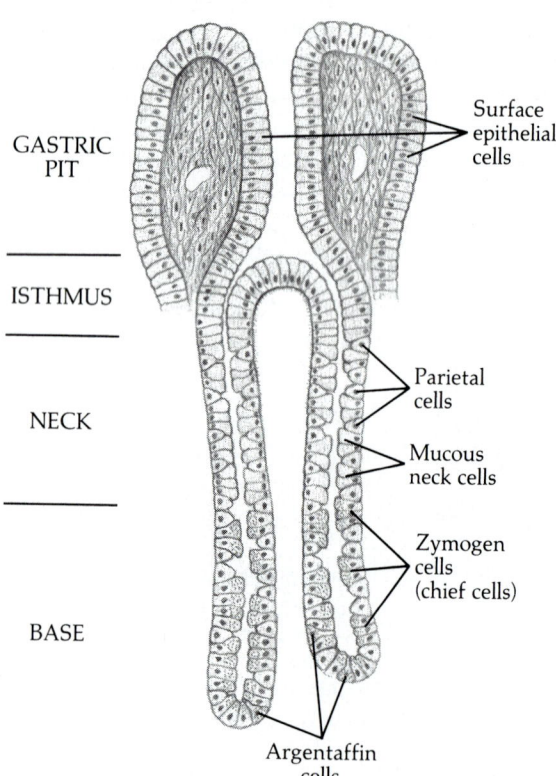

FIG. 35-6 Gastric gland. The gastric gland empties cellular secretions into a gastric pit. Secretions flow from the gastric pit into the lumen of the stomach. Surface epithelial cells have tight junctions and mucous coating. Parietal cells (oxyntic cells) secrete hydrochloric acid and intrinsic factor. Mucous neck cells secrete mucus. Chief cells (zymogen cells) secrete pepsinogen. Argentaffin cells secrete serotonin. (From Thompson et al., 1993.)

FIG. 35-7 Relationship between secretory rate and electrolyte composition of the gastric juice. Sodium (Na^+) concentration is lower in the gastric juice than in the plasma, whereas hydrogen (H^+), potassium (K^+), and chloride (Cl^-) concentrations are higher. Solid red line = chloride; solid black line = hydrogen; dotted black line = sodium; dotted red line = potassium.

tion is high. The reverse is true at high flow rates. Potassium remains relatively constant, but its concentration is greater in gastric juice than in plasma. The rate of secretion varies with the time of day. Generally the rate and volume of secretion are lowest in the morning and highest in the afternoon and evening. Loss of gastric juices through vomiting, drainage, or suction may decrease body stores of sodium and potassium.

Gastric secretion is inhibited by unpleasant odors and tastes and by rage, fear, or pain. These sensations and emotions cause a discharge of sympathetic impulses and inhibit parasympathetic impulses. Increased secretions may be associated with feelings of aggression or hostility and may contribute to some forms of gastric pathology.

Acid

The major functions of gastric acid are to dissolve food fibers, act as a bactericide against swallowed organisms, and convert pepsinogen to pepsin. The production of acid by the parietal cells requires the transport of hydrogen and chloride from the parietal cells to the stomach lumen. Acid is formed in the parietal cells, primarily through the hydrolysis of water (Fig. 35-8). At a high rate of gastric secretion, bicarbonate moves into the plasma, producing an "alkaline tide" in the venous blood, which also may result in a more alkaline urine (Helander & Keeling, 1993).

Acid secretion is stimulated by acetylcholine (a neurotransmitter), gastrin (a hormone), and histamine (a biochemical mediator), and is inhibited by somatostatin (a hormone). The vagus nerve releases acetylcholine and stimulates the secretion of gastrin, probably in response to histamine. Histamine is stored in enterochromaffin cells (mast cells; see Chapter 7) in the gastric mu-

cosa. Histamine receptors in the gastric mucosa are H2 receptors (unlike those in the bronchial mucosa, which are H1 receptors). The drug cimetidine is an H2 antagonist and is therefore effective in suppressing acid secretion in persons with ulcers. Prostaglandins inhibit the secretion of acid (Wolfe & Soll, 1988).

Pepsin secretion

Acetylcholine, gastrin, and secretin stimulate the chief cells to release pepsinogen during eating. Gastrin indirectly stimulates pepsinogen secretion through a cholinergic reflex that it causes while stimulating acid secretion. Pepsinogen is quickly converted to pepsin in the acid gastric environment. Conversion to pepsin occurs at any pH below 5.0, but the optimum pH for pepsin activation is 2.0. Pepsin is a proteolytic enzyme: that is, it breaks down protein. Pepsin hydrolyzes peptide bonds at the anterior of protein molecules, thereby forming polypeptides. This action occurs in the stomach. Once chyme has entered the duodenum, the alkaline environment of the duodenum inactivates pepsin.

Mucus

The gastric mucosa is protected from the digestive actions of acid and pepsin by a coating of mucus called the **mucosal barrier.** The quality and quantity of mucus and the tight junctions between epithelial cells make gastric mucosa relatively impermeable to acid. Prostaglandins protect the mucosal barrier by stimulating the secretion of mucus and bicarbonate and by inhibiting secretion of acid. A break in the protective barrier may occur because of exposure to aspirin, ethanol, regurgitated bile, or ischemia. Breaks cause inflammation and ulceration.

FIG. 35-8 One mechanism for secretion of hydrochloric acid. (From Berne & Levy, 1993.)

Phases of Gastric Secretion

The secretion of gastric juice is influenced by numerous stimuli that together facilitate the process of digestion. The phases of gastric secretion are the cephalic phase, the gastric phase, and the intestinal phase (Fig. 35-9).

Cephalic phase

The anticipatory and sensory experiences of smelling, seeing, tasting, chewing, and swallowing food contribute to the **cephalic phase** of secretion. Sensory experiences stimulate the secretion of acid, pepsinogens, and mucus in the body of the stomach and the release of gastrin from **G cells** (gastrin-secreting cells) in the antral region. The cephalic phase of gastric secretion is mediated by the vagus nerve through the myenteric plexus. Acetylcholine (ACh) is liberated and stimulates the parietal and chief cells to secrete acid and pepsinogen, respectively. The G cells in the antrum release gastrin into the bloodstream, through which it travels to the gastric glands and stimulates acid secretion. The secretion of gastric juice before the arrival of food in the stomach contributes to the desire for and enjoyment of food.

Insulin secretion by the endocrine pancreas, which is stimulated by hyperglycemia, is also a strong stimulus for gastric secretion. Acid secretion in response to insulin is mediated by the vagus through sensors located in the hypothalamus. These sensors respond to the decreased levels of serum glucose caused by insulin release. Maintenance of steady serum glucose levels suppresses the gastric response to insulin.

Gastric phase

The **gastric phase** of secretion begins with the arrival of food in the stomach. The presence of food in the stomach is the most powerful stimulus of gastric secretion. Two major stimuli have a secretory effect: (1) distention of the stomach and (2) the presence of digested protein. Mechanoreceptors are activated as the stomach becomes distended with food, thereby stimulating secretions mediated by the vagus nerve. The enteric nerve plexus is also stimulated by distention and contributes to gastric secretion through a local reflex. Because both neural reflexes are mediated by acetylcholine, they can be blocked by atropine. As digestion proceeds, products of protein breakdown come in contact with the pyloric mucosa and stimulate the release of gastrin from G cells in the antrum. Proteins activate the release of gastrin indirectly as well. Proteins in the stomach buffer the acid gastric juice and increase the gastric pH. The rise in pH promotes the secretion of gastrin because it cancels out the inhibitory effect of low pH on gastrin release in the antrum. Caffeine stimulates acid secretion, as does calcium.

Intestinal phase

The movement of chyme from the stomach into the duodenum initiates the **intestinal phase** of gastric secretion. This phase represents a slowdown of the gastric secretory response and appears to be hormonally mediated. Apparently the presence of chyme in the small intestine causes a hormone called entero-oxyntin to be released

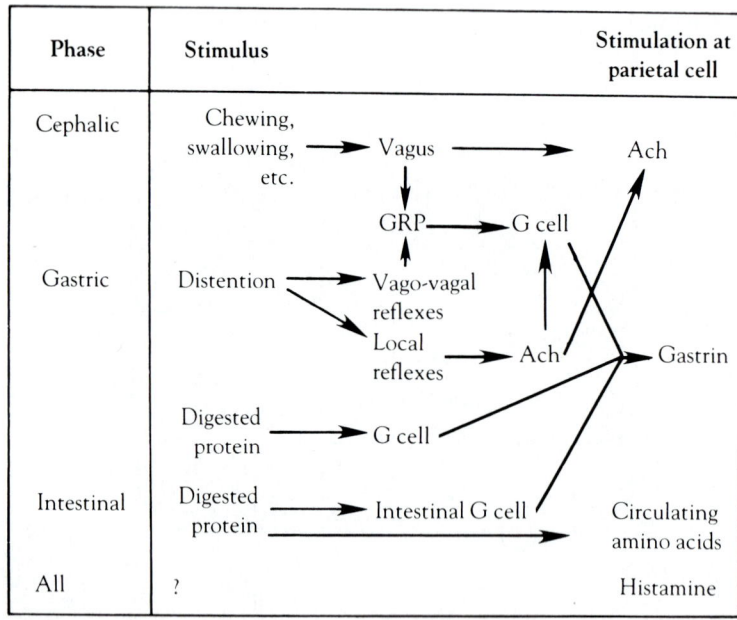

FIG. 35-9 The phases of gastric acid secretion. *GRP*, Gastrin-releasing peptide. (From Johnson, 1991.)

into the bloodstream and travel to the gastric mucosa, where it causes the parietal cells to secrete acid. Gastric inhibitory peptide decreases gastric motility and the secretion of acid and pepsin when chyme enters the duodenum. The intestinal absorption of some amino acids (products of protein breakdown) also stimulates gastric secretion. The intestinal phase of gastric secretion is limited by the fact that acidic chyme in the duodenum tends to inhibit both gastric acid secretion and gastric motility. Acid in the duodenum stimulates the release of hormones that inhibit acid secretion while stimulating pepsinogen secretion. One of these hormones, cholecystokinin-pancreozymin, inhibits gastrin-stimulated acid production. There are probably other intestinal hormones that act synergistically to regulate gastric secretion.

Small Intestine

The **small intestine** is about 5 meters long and is functionally divided into three segments: the **duodenum, jejunum,** and **ileum** (see Fig. 35-10). The duodenum begins at the pylorus and ends where it joins the jejunum at a suspensory ligament called the Treitz ligament. The end of the jejunum and beginning of the ileum are not distinguished by an anatomic marker. These structures are not grossly different, but the jejunum has a slightly larger lumen. The **ileocecal valve,** or sphincter, controls the flow of digested material from the ileum into the large intestine and prevents reflux into the small intestine.

The **peritoneum** is the serous membrane surrounding the organs of the abdomen and pelvic cavity. It is analogous to the pericardium and pleura that surround the heart and lungs, respectively. The peritoneum has two layers: the visceral peritoneum lies over the organs, and the parietal peritoneum lines the wall of the abdominal cavity. The space between these two layers is called the **peritoneal cavity.** This cavity normally contains just enough fluid to lubricate the two layers and prevent friction during organ movement. Inflammation of the peritoneum, called peritonitis, may occur with perforation of the large intestine or after abdominal surgery. As the inflammatory process resolves, adhesions may form and cause colonic obstruction.

The duodenum lies behind the peritoneum, or retroperitoneally, and is attached to the posterior abdominal wall. The ileum and jejunum are suspended in loose folds from the posterior abdominal wall by a peritoneal membrane called the **mesentery.** The mesentery facilitates intestinal motility and supports blood vessels, nerves, and lymphatics.

The arterial supply to the duodenum arises primarily from the gastroduodenal artery. The jejunum and ileum are supplied by branches of the superior mesenteric ar-

tery. The superior mesenteric vein joins the splenic vein and empties into the portal circulation to the liver. The regional lymph nodes and lymphatics drain into the thoracic duct. Both divisions of the autonomic nervous system innervate the small intestine. Secretion, motility, pain sensation, and intestinal reflexes (e.g., relaxation of the lower esophageal sphincter) are mediated by parasympathetic nerves. Sympathetic activity inhibits motility and produces vasoconstriction. Intrinsic motor innervation is mediated by the myenteric plexus (Auerbach plexus) and the submucosal plexus (Meissner plexus).

The smooth muscles of the small intestine are arranged in two layers: a longitudinal outer layer and a thicker inner circular layer (Fig. 35-10, *A*). Mucosal folds (plica) within the small intestine slow the passage of food, thereby providing more time for digestion and absorption. The folds are most numerous and prominent in the jejunum and upper ileum (Fig. 35-10).

Absorption occurs through **villi,** which cover the mucosal folds and are the functional units of the intestine. (A single villus is shown in Fig. 35-10.) Each villus secretes some of the enzymes necessary for digestion and absorbs nutrients. A villus is composed of absorptive columnar cells and mucus-secreting goblet cells of the mucosal epithelium. Near the surface columnar cells closely adhere to each other at sites called tight junctions. Water and electrolytes are absorbed through these intercellular spaces. The surface of each columnar epithelial cell contains tiny projections called **microvilli** (Fig. 35-10). Together the microvilli create a mucosal surface known as the **brush border.** The villi and microvilli greatly increase the surface area available for absorption. Coating the brush border is an "unstirred" layer of fluid that is important for the absorption of substances other than water and electrolytes. The **lamina propria** (a connective tissue layer of the mucous membrane) lies beneath the epithelial cells of the villi and contains lymphocytes; plasma cells, which produce immunoglobulins; and macrophages.

Central arterioles ascend within each villus and branch into a capillary array that extends around the base of the columnar cells and cascades down to the venules that lead to the portal circulation. The opposing ascending and descending blood flow provides a countercurrent exchange system for absorbed substances and blood gases. A central **lacteal,** or lymphatic channel, is also contained within each villus and is important for the absorption and transport of fat molecules. Contents of the lacteals flow to regional nodes and channels that eventually drain into the thoracic duct (Kvietys, Barrowman, & Granger, 1987).

Between the bases of the villi are the crypts of Lieberkühn, which extend to the submucosal layer. Undif-

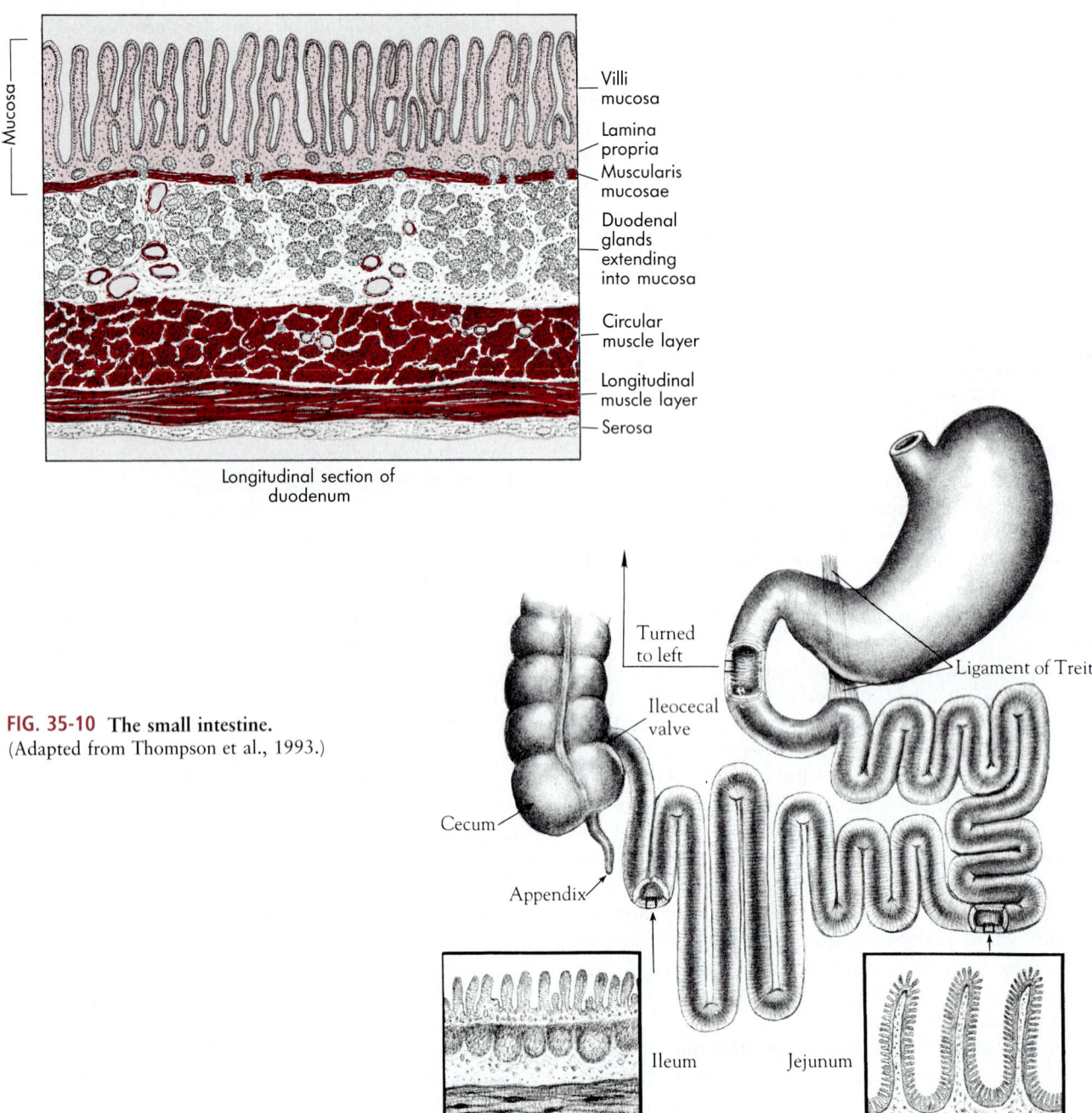

Longitudinal section of
duodenum

Mucosa

Villi
mucosa

Lamina
propria

Muscularis
mucosae

Duodenal
glands
extending
into mucosa

Circular
muscle layer

Longitudinal
muscle layer

Serosa

FIG. 35-10 **The small intestine.**
(Adapted from Thompson et al., 1993.)

Turned
to left

Ligament of Treitz

Ileocecal
valve

Cecum

Appendix

Ileum

Jejunum

ferentiated and secretory cells are located here. The undifferentiated cells are precursors of columnar epithelial cells. These cells arise from the base of the crypt and move toward the tip of the villus, maturing in shape and function as they progress. After becoming columnar cells and completing their migration to the tip of the villus, they function for a few days and then are sloughed into the intestinal lumen and digested. Sloughed epithelial cells are an important source of endogenous protein. The entire epithelial population is replaced about every 4 to 7 days. Many factors can influence this process of cellular proliferation. Starvation, vitamin B_{12} deficiency, and cytotoxic drugs or irradiation suppress cell division and shorten the villi. The decreased absorption that results can cause diarrhea and malnutrition. Nutrient intake and intestinal resection stimulate cell production.

Intestinal Digestion and Absorption

The process of digestion is initiated in the stomach by the actions of hydrochloric acid and pepsin, which break down food fibers and proteins. The chyme that passes into the duodenum is a liquid that contains small particles of undigested food. Digestion is continued in the proximal portion of the small intestine by the action of pancreatic enzymes, intestinal enzymes, and bile salts. Here carbohydrates are broken down to monosaccharides and disaccharides; proteins are degraded further to amino acids and peptides; and fats are emulsified and reduced to fatty acids and monoglycerides (Fig. 35-11). These nutrients, along with water, vitamins, and electrolytes, are absorbed across the intestinal mucosa by active transport, diffusion, or facilitated diffusion. Products of carbohydrate and protein breakdown move into villus capillaries and then to the liver through the portal vein. Digested fats move into the lacteals and eventually reach the liver through the systemic circulation. Intestinal motility exposes nutrients to a large mucosal surface area by mixing chyme and moving it through the lumen. Different segments of the gastrointestinal tract absorb different nutrients. Sites of absorption are shown in Fig. 35-12.

Water and electrolytes

The epithelial cell membranes of the small intestine are formed of lipids and therefore are hydrophobic, or tend to repel water. (The properties of cell membranes are described in Chapter 1.) Therefore, water and electrolytes are transported in both directions (toward the capillary blood or toward the intestinal lumen) through the tight junctions and intercellular spaces rather than across cell membranes. Water diffuses passively according to hydrostatic pressure and in relation to osmotic gradients established by the active transport of sodium and other substances. Approximately 85% to 90% of the water that enters the gastrointestinal tract each day

is absorbed in the small intestine. Sodium passes through the tight junctions and is actively transported across cell membranes. The proximal part of the small intestine is more permeable to sodium than the distal part. Sodium is transported into the intestinal cells in exchange for hydrogen at the brush border, and chloride actively enters the cell in exchange for bicarbonate to maintain electroneutrality in the ileum. There is also a sodium pump at the basolateral membrane. Sodium and glucose share a common carrier mechanism, so that sodium absorption is enhanced by glucose transport (Fig. 35-13). Potassium moves passively across the tight junctions with changes in the electrochemical gradient.

Carbohydrates

Carbohydrate (starch, table sugar, milk, sugar, and maltose) accounts for at least 50% of the American diet. Because only monosaccharides (galactose, glucose, and fructose) are absorbed by the intestinal mucosa, the complex carbohydrates (polysaccharides and oligosaccharides) must be hydrolyzed to their simplest form (Fig. 35-10). Ribose, a 5-carbon sugar that forms part of RNA, ATP, and DNA, is an important part of the diet. Salivary and pancreatic amylases break down starches to oligosaccharides by splitting α-1,4-glucosidic linkages of long-chain molecules. The major oligosaccharides are sucrose (glucose-fructose), maltose (glucose-glucose), and lactose (glucose-galactose). Approximately half of starch hydrolysis occurs in the stomach and about half in the duodenum. In the small intestine the oligosaccharides are hydrolyzed by brush-border enzymes, mainly sucrase, maltase, and lactase, to their respective monosaccharides (fructose, glucose, and galactose). The sugars then pass through the unstirred layer by diffusion. At the cell membrane glucose and galactose are actively transported with a sodium carrier and fructose is absorbed passively. Consequently glucose and galactose are absorbed more rapidly than fructose. Insulin is not required for the intestinal absorption of carbohydrates. Fructose passes by diffusion into the bloodstream, and glucose and galactose enter by diffusion or active transport. The sugars are primarily absorbed in the duodenum and upper jejunum. Cellulose is a glucose polysaccharide found in plants. Humans do not have enzymes to digest cellulose but the undigested material contributes to volume and stimulates large intestine motility.

Proteins

Protein intake varies among different populations. Adults require 44 to 56 g protein per day. Approximately 20 to 30 g of protein is derived endogenously from shed epithelial cells and small amounts of plasma proteins. Most protein is absorbed; only 5% to 10% is eliminated in the stool.

Gastric digestion of protein by pepsin and acid is not

Action	Foodstuff	Enzymes/source	Site of action

FIG. 35-11 Digestion and absorption of foodstuffs.

FIG. 35-12 Sites of absorption of major nutrients.

FIG. 35-13 **Glucose and sodium transport.** Schematic showing glucose and sodium (Na^+) transport through the intestinal epithelium. Glucose and sodium are transported into the epithelial cell by a joint carrier.

essential. Major protein hydrolysis is accomplished in the small intestine by the pancreatic enzymes: trypsin, chymotrypsin, and carboxypeptidase (Fig. 35-10). **Trypsin** and **chymotrypsin** (endopeptidase) hydrolyze the interior bonds of the large molecules, and **carboxypeptidases** break away the end amino acids (exopeptidase). Hydrolysis of proteins is also carried out by the brush-border enzymes and enzymes in the epithelial cytosol (intracellular fluid). The brush border enzymes hydrolyze the large oligopeptides (proteins composed of three to six amino acids) into smaller peptides, which can cross cell membranes. The cytosol then breaks them down to amino acids. Amino acids are actively transported by a carrier at the basal membrane. Protein absorption is directly linked to the active transport of sodium. There are three groups of free amino acids:

1. Neutral amino acids (methionine, glycine, phenylalanine, and tryptophan)
2. Basic amino acids (arginine, ornithine, lysine, and cystine)
3. Proline and hydroxyproline

Each group enters the circulation through a specific mechanism of transport. A small amount of protein may be taken into the cells by pinocytosis (see Chapter 1).

Like the sugars, proteins are absorbed primarily in the proximal area of the small intestine. Protein absorption is impaired if inadequate amounts of proteolytic enzymes are secreted from the pancreas, as occurs with cystic fibrosis.

Fats

Approximately 90 to 100 g of fat is consumed daily by the average American. Fat is an important source of calories and is a primary structural component of cell membranes and organelles. Sources of dietary fat are reviewed in the following box. Although triglycerides are the major dietary lipids, cholesterol, phospholipids, and fat-soluble vitamins also have nutritional importance. The digestion and absorption of fat occur in four phases: (1) emulsification and lipolysis, (2) micelle formation, (3) fat absorption, and (4) resynthesis of triglycerides and phospholipids.

The mechanical action of the stomach and small intestine disperses the triglyceride droplets into small particles. **Emulsification** is the process by which emulsifying agents (fatty acids, monoglycerides, lecithin, cholesterol, protein, and bile salts) in the intestinal lumen cover the small fat particles and prevent them from reforming into fat droplets. Emulsified fat is then ready for **lipolysis** (lipid hydrolysis) by pancreatic lipase, phospholipase, and hydrolase. **Lipase** breaks down triglycerides to diglycerides, monoglycerides, free fatty acids, and glycerol (Fig. 35-11). The action of lipase requires the presence of colipase, a pancreatic enzyme that al-

lows lipase to penetrate the triglyceride molecule. **Phospholipase** cleaves fatty acids from phospholipids, and **hydrolase** breaks cholesterol esters into fatty acids and cholesterol.

The products of lipid hydrolysis must be made water soluble if they are to be absorbed efficiently from the intestinal lumen. This is accomplished by the formation of water-soluble molecules known as **micelles** (Fig. 35-14). Micelles are formed of bile salts, the products of fat hydrolysis, fat-soluble vitamins, and cholesterol. The

DIETARY FAT

Saturated fatty acid (palmitic acid [$C_{16}H_{32}O_2$])
Each carbon atom in the chain is linked by single bonds to adjacent carbon and hydrogen atoms; atoms are solid at room temperature and found in animal fat and tropical oils (coconut and palm oil); they increase low-density lipoprotein (LDL) cholesterol ("bad" cholesterol) blood levels and increase the risk of coronary artery disease

Unsaturated fatty acid
Unsaturated fatty acids are soft or liquid at room temperature; omega 6 fatty acids are found in plants and vegetables (olive, canola, and peanut oils), and omega 3 fatty acids are found in fish and shellfish
1. Monounsaturated fatty acids (oleic acid [$C_{18}H_{34}O_2$])
   Contain one double bond in the carbon chain and are found in both plants and animals; may be beneficial in reducing blood cholesterol, glucose levels, and systolic blood pressure (Trevisan et al., 1990); do not lower high-density lipoprotein (HDL) cholesterol ("good" cholesterol) level. Low HDL levels have been associated with coronary heart disease (National Institutes of Health Consensus, 1992)
2. Polyunsaturated fatty acids (linoleic acid [$C_{18}H_{32}O_2$])
   Contain two or more double bonds in the carbon chain and are found in plants and fishoils; omega 6 fatty acids lower total and LDL cholesterol blood levels; high levels of polyunsaturated fatty acids may lower LDL; omega 3 fatty acids lower blood triglyceride levels and reduce platelet aggregation and reduce blood clotting tendency; are necessary for growth and development and may prevent coronary artery disease, hypertension, cancer, inflammatory and immune disorders (Simopoulos, 1991)

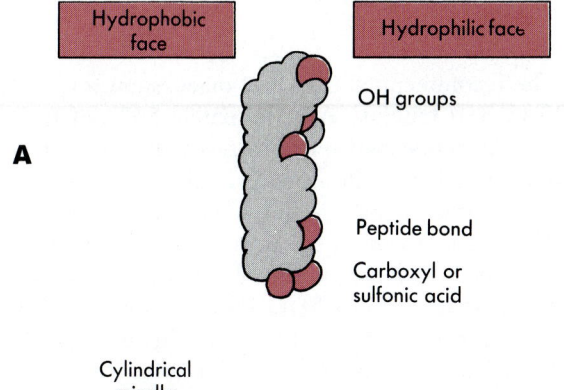

Hydrophobic face   Hydrophilic face

OH groups

A

Peptide bond

Carboxyl or sulfonic acid

Cylindrical micelle

Cross section

B

Bile acids

Cholesterol

Phospholipids

Free fatty acids

2-Monoglycerides

FIG. 35-14 Structure of bile acid and micelle. A, A bile acid molecule in solution. The molecule is amphipathic in that it has a hydrophilic face and a hydrophobic face. The amphipathic structure is key in the ability of the bile acids to emulsify lipids and form micelles. **B,** A model of the structure of a bile acid–lipid mixed micelle, an emulsified fat. (From Berne & Levy, 1993.)

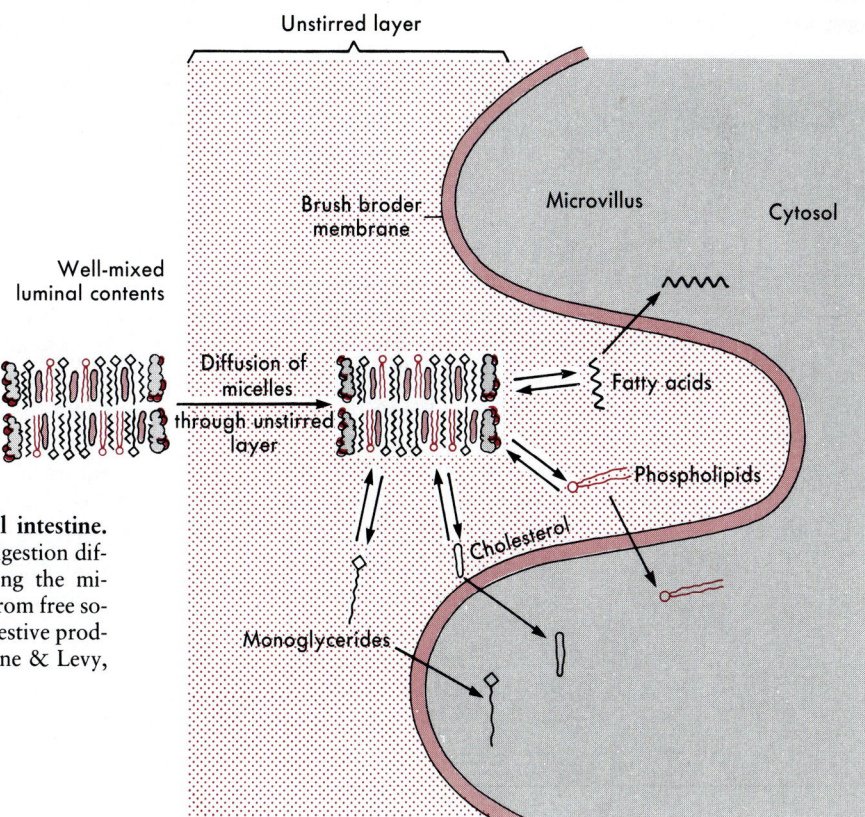

Unstirred layer

Brush broder membrane

Microvillus

Cytosol

Well-mixed luminal contents

Diffusion of micelles through unstirred layer

Fatty acids

Phospholipids

Cholesterol

Monoglycerides

FIG. 35-15 Lipid absorption in the small intestine. Micelles of bile salts and products of lipid digestion diffuse through the unstirred layer and among the microvilli. As digestive products are absorbed from free solution by epithelial cells of the villi, more digestive products dissociate from the micelles. (From Berne & Levy, 1993.)

fats form the core of the micelle and the polar bile salts form an outer shell, with the hydrophobic ("water-hating") side facing the interior and the hydrophilic ("water-loving") side facing the aqueous (waterlike) content of the intestinal lumen. Because the unstirred layer of the brush border is aqueous, the micelles readily diffuse through it. The micelles maintain the fat molecules in the dissolved or solubilized form, which allows them to move more rapidly from the micelle toward the absorbing surface of the intestinal epithelium. The fat products of the micelle then readily diffuse through the epithelial cell membrane, while the bile salts remain in the lumen and proceed to the ileum, where they are absorbed into the circulation and returned to the liver (Fig. 35-15). Almost all of the bile salts are recycled in this way.

When the fat products reach the inside of the epithelial cell, they are resynthesized into triglycerides and phospholipids. The triglycerides are covered with phospholipids, lipoproteins, and cholesterol to become particles called **chylomicrons**. The chylomicrons travel to the basolateral membrane of the columnar epithelial cells, where they are extruded into the intercellular spaces of the villus. From here they enter the lacteals and lymphatic channels and, eventually, the systemic circulation.

Minerals and vitamins

The recommended intake of calcium ranges from 1000 to 1500 mg/day. Between 500 and 600 mg is secreted or shed into the lumen with desquamated epithelial cells. Not all this calcium is absorbed. Daily absorption of calcium is approximately 600 mg. This amount increases with increased intake. When its concentration in the lumen is greater than 5 mmol/L, calcium is absorbed by passive diffusion. At concentrations less than 5.0 mmol/L, calcium is transported actively across cell membranes, bound to a carrier protein. The carrier formation requires the presence of the active form of vitamin D (1,25-dihydroxy vitamin D). The calcium-protein complex moves into the epithelial cell, where the calcium binds to proteins or other substances. Then these complexes move through the basolateral membrane to the interstitial fluid by diffusion or active transport. Calcium is absorbed throughout the small intestine, but primarily in the ileum.

That calcium is absorbed more rapidly in children and pregnant or lactating women is evidence that increased demand results in increased uptake. Bile salts enhance calcium absorption indirectly by facilitating the absorption of vitamin D. Additionally bile salts promote the absorption of free fatty acids, which, at high concentrations, bind calcium and form soaps in the intestinal lumen. In older individuals, calcium is absorbed less readily because of inadequate amounts of the active form of vitamin D.

The recommended intake of **magnesium** for adults is 300 to 350 mg/day. Approximately 50% of it is absorbed by active transport or passive diffusion in the jejunum and ileum. Phosphate is also absorbed in the small intestine by passive diffusion and active transport.

The levels of **iron** in the body are regulated primarily by intestinal absorption and secretion. The average intake ranges from 15 to 30 mg/day. Of this amount, menstruating women absorb 1.0 to 1.5 mg and men absorb 0.15 to 1.0 mg. Generally the amount of iron absorbed is equal to the amount required. Iron is absorbed more rapidly if a deficiency exists. The primary sources of iron are heme from hemoglobin and myoglobin from animal protein. This iron is rapidly absorbed by the epithelial cells of the duodenum and jejunum. Inorganic iron (e.g., iron in fruits, cereals, eggs, vegetables) is also readily absorbed. The presence of vitamin C reduces ferric iron to ferrous iron, which is the form more easily absorbed. Calcium phosphate and phosphoproteins (milk and antacids) in the intestinal lumen bind iron and reduce absorption. Tea also binds iron by forming iron tannate complexes.

Iron is primarily bound to the protein ferritin and to amino acid chelates in the cytosol of epithelial cells. Transport of iron across the basolateral membrane is determined by the amount of iron in the circulation. During hemorrhage, pregnancy, or growth, iron is actively transported from the epithelial cell to the plasma, where it is carried by the globulin protein transferrin (see Chapter 22). When there is less need for iron, it remains in the cell and is carried into the lumen when the cell is sloughed from the end of the villus. The intestinal cells require 3 days to increase their rate of iron absorption after hemorrhage. This is because the need for iron is perceived by the precursor cells in the crypts of Lieberkühn and they take 3 days to mature and migrate to the tips of the villi, where they absorb more iron.

The absorption of **vitamins** is summarized in Table 35-2. Most of the water-soluble vitamins are absorbed by sodium-dependent active transport. Most vitamin B_{12} (cobalamin) is bound to intrinsic factor and absorbed in the terminal ileum, although a small amount of the vitamin is absorbed in its free (unbound) form. Because intrinsic factor is secreted by gastric cells of the stomach, gastric resection and gastric atrophy with achlorhydria diminish the secretion of intrinsic factor and hence the absorption of vitamin B_{12}. Lack of vitamin B_{12} prevents normal erythrocyte maturation and causes pernicious (macrocytic) anemia. (Anemias are discussed in Chapter 23.)

Vitamin B_{12} is present in animal protein and is particularly abundant in liver and kidney. Gastric and pancreatic enzymes release vitamin B_{12} from food, after which the vitamin binds to intrinsic factor through an intermediary transport protein. The intrinsic factor–vi-

TABLE 35-2

Intestinal Absorption of Vitamins

Vitamin	Mechanisms of absorption	State of absorption
Fat-soluble vitamins		
A (retinol)	Micelle formation with bile salts	Upper small intestine
D (1,25 dihydroxycalciferol)		
E (tocopherol)		
K		
Water-soluble vitamins		
B_1 (thiamine)	Active transport (sodium-dependent)	Duodenum and jejunum
B_2 (riboflavin)	Unknown	Duodenum and jejunum
Niacin (nicotinic acid)	Passive diffusion	Jejunum
C (ascorbic acid)	Active transport (sodium-dependent)	Ileum
Folic acid	Active transport (sodium-dependent)	Jejunum
B_{12} (cobalamin)	Active transport (intrinsic-factor–dependent)	Terminal ileum
B_6 (pyridoxine, pyridoxamine, pyridoxal)	Passive diffusion	Jejunum
Pantothenic acid	Passive diffusion	Duodenum and jejunum
Biotin	Unknown	Unknown

tamin B_{12} complex then attaches to specific receptor sites on epithelial cells of the terminal ileum, where it is absorbed. After several hours the vitamin enters the plasma, attaches to the carrier protein transcobalamin, and is transported to tissues.

Intestinal Motility

The movements of the small intestine facilitate both digestion and absorption. Chyme coming from the stomach stimulates intestinal movements that mix in secretions from the liver, pancreas, and intestinal glands. A churning motion brings the luminal content into contact with the absorbing cells of the villi. Propulsive movements then advance the chyme toward the large intestine.

Intestinal motility is affected by two movements: haustral segmentation and peristalsis. **Haustral segmentation,** which occurs more frequently than peristalsis, consists of localized rhythmic contractions of the circular smooth muscles. The contractions occur at different rates in different parts of the small intestine. Frequency is greatest (12 per minute) in the upper small intestine and least (8 per minute) in the distal part of the ileum. Haustral segmentation divides and mixes the chyme, bringing it into contact with the absorbent mucosal surface. It also helps to propel the chyme toward the large intestine. The frequency of the haustral segmentation is regulated intrinsically by the frequency of the basic electrical rhythm (BER), which arises in the myenteric plexus of longitudinal smooth muscle. Although the basic rate of contraction is controlled intrin-

sically, the force of contraction can be enhanced by vagal stimulation (i.e., extrinsically).

Peristaltic movements involve short segments (about 10 cm) of longitudinal smooth muscle. The wave of contraction moves slowly (1 to 2 cm/sec) to allow time for digestion and absorption.

The intestinal villi move with contractions of the muscularis mucosae, a very thin layer of muscle that separates the mucosa and submucosa. Absorption is promoted by the swaying of villi in the luminal contents. Contractile activity also helps to empty the central lacteals, which contain products of fat digestion.

Neural reflexes along the length of the small intestine facilitate motility, digestion, and absorption. Through reflex action, receptors in one part of the intestine transmit signals that influence the function of another part. The **ileogastric reflex** inhibits gastric motility when the ileum becomes distended. This prevents the continued movement of chyme into an already distended intestine. The **intestinointestinal reflex** inhibits intestinal motility when one part of the intestine is overdistended. Both of these reflexes require extrinsic innervation. The **gastroileal reflex,** which is activated by an increase in gastric motility and secretion, stimulates an increase in ileal motility. This empties the ileum and prepares it to receive more chyme. The gastroileal reflex is probably regulated by the hormone gastrin.

During prolonged fasting or between meals, particularly overnight, slow waves sweep along the entire length of the intestinal tract from the stomach to terminal ileum. This is known as the interdigestive myoelectric complex, and it appears to propel residual gastric and intestinal contents into the colon.

The ileocecal valve (sphincter) marks the junction between the terminal ileum and the large intestine. This valve is intrinsically regulated and is normally closed. The arrival of peristaltic waves from the last few centimeters of the ileum causes the ileocecal valve to open, allowing a small amount of chyme to pass through. Distention of the upper large intestine causes the sphincter to constrict, preventing further distention or retrograde flow of intestinal contents.

Large Intestine

The **large intestine** is approximately 1.5 m long and consists of the cecum, appendix, colon (ascending, transverse, descending, and sigmoid), rectum, and anal canal (Fig. 35-16). The **cecum** is a pouch that receives chyme from the ileum. Attached to the cecum is the **vermiform appendix,** an appendage having little or no physiologic function. From the cecum, chyme enters the **colon,** a four-part length of intestine that loops upward, traverses the abdominal cavity, and descends to the anal canal. The four parts of the colon are the **ascending colon, transverse colon, descending colon,** and **sigmoid colon.** Two sphincters control the flow of intestinal contents through the cecum and colon: the ileocecal valve, which admits chyme from the ileum to the cecum, and the **O'Beirne sphincter,** which controls the movement of wastes from the sigmoid colon into the rectum. A thick (2.5 to 3 cm) portion of smooth muscle surrounds the anal canal, forming the **internal anal sphincter.** Overlapping it distally is the striated muscle of the **external anal sphincter.**

In the cecum and colon, the longitudinal muscle layer consists of three longitudinal bands called **teniae coli** (Fig. 35-16). The teniae coli are shorter than the colon, giving the colon its "gathered" appearance. The circular muscles of the colon separate the gathers into outpouchings called **haustra.** The haustra become more or less prominent with the contractions and relaxations of the circular muscles. The mucosal surface of the colon has rugae (folds), particularly between the haustra, and **Lieberkühn crypts** but no villi. Columnar epithelial cells and mucus-secreting goblet cells form the mucosa throughout the large intestine. The columnar epithelium absorbs fluid and electrolytes, and the mucus-secreting cells lubricate the mucosa.

Intrinsic innervation in the colon is mediated by the myenteric plexus, which can regulate motor and secretory activity independently of the extrinsic system. Extrinsic parasympathetic innervation occurs through the vagus and extends from the cecum up to the first part of the transverse colon. Vagal stimulation increases rhythmic contraction of the proximal colon. Extrinsic parasympathetic fibers reach the distal colon through the pelvic nerves and can increase motility throughout the colon. The internal anal sphincter is usually in a state of contraction, and its reflex response is to relax when the rectum is distended. The intrinsic nerve plexuses provide the major innervation of the internal anal sphincter, which also receives sympathetic innervation to maintain contraction and parasympathetic innervation that facilitates relaxation when the rectum is full. The external anal sphincter is innervated by branches of the sacral division of the spinal cord. Sympathetic innervation of this sphincter arises from the celiac and superior mesenteric ganglia and the sphincter nerve. The external anal sphincter is paralyzed after destruction of the lower spinal cord, but the internal sphincter is not. Sympathetic activity in the entire large intestine modulates intestinal reflexes, conveys somatic sensation of fullness and pain, participates in the defecation reflex, and constricts blood vessels.

The primary type of colonic movement is segmental and is termed haustral shuttling, segmental propulsion, or multihaustral propulsion. The circular muscles contract and relax at different sites, shuttling the intestinal contents back and forth between the contracting and relaxing haustra, most commonly during fasting. The movements massage the intestinal contents, now called **fecal mass,** and facilitate the absorption of water. Propulsive movement occurs with the proximal-to-distal contraction of several haustral units. Peristaltic movements also occur and promote the emptying of the colon. The **gastrocolic reflex** initiates propulsion in the entire colon, usually during or immediately after eating, when chyme enters from the ileum. The gastrocolic reflex causes the fecal mass to pass rapidly into the sigmoid colon and rectum, stimulating defecation. Gastrin may participate in stimulating this reflex.

Approximately 500 to 700 ml chyme flows from the ileum to the cecum per day. Most of the water is absorbed in the colon by diffusion and active transport. The electrochemical gradient established by sodium movement enhances the diffusion of serum potassium from the capillaries in the lumen. Aldosterone increases membrane permeability to sodium, thereby increasing both the diffusion of sodium into the cell and its active transport across the basolateral membrane to the interstitial fluid. (See Chapter 17 for a discussion of aldosterone secretion.) This increases the cell-to-lumen diffusion gradient for potassium. Potassium moves outward, and chloride is absorbed with sodium as the complementary anion. Chloride also enters the cell in exchange for bicarbonate. Sugars and amino acids are not absorbed by the colon, but some short-chain free fatty acids, which are produced by fermentation, are absorbed.

Absorption and epithelial transport occur in the cecum, ascending colon, transverse colon, and descending colon. By the time the fecal mass enters the sigmoid co-

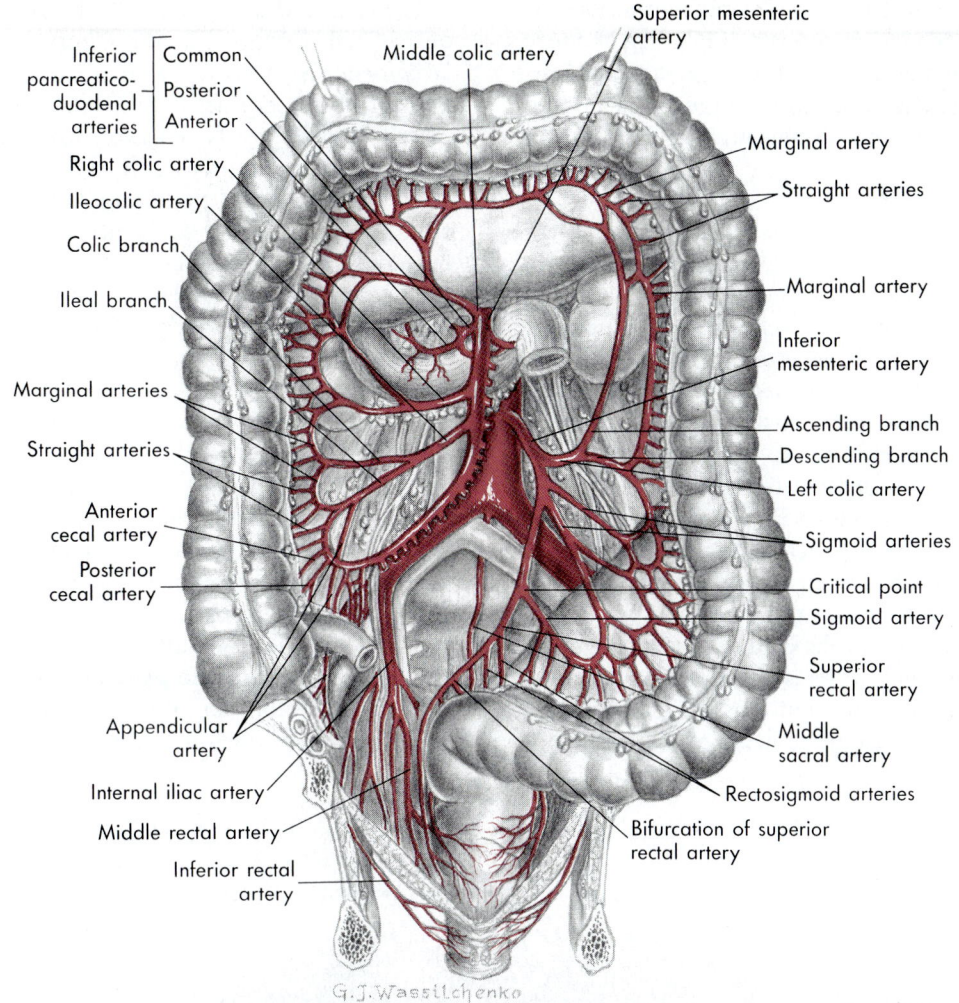

Inferior pancreatico-duodenal arteries { Common / Posterior / Anterior

Right colic artery

Ileocolic artery

Colic branch

Ileal branch

Marginal arteries

Straight arteries

Anterior cecal artery

Posterior cecal artery

Appendicular artery

Internal iliac artery

Middle rectal artery

Inferior rectal artery

Middle colic artery

Superior mesenteric artery

Marginal artery

Straight arteries

Marginal artery

Inferior mesenteric artery

Ascending branch

Descending branch

Left colic artery

Sigmoid arteries

Critical point

Sigmoid artery

Superior rectal artery

Middle sacral artery

Rectosigmoid arteries

Bifurcation of superior rectal artery

G.J.Wassilchenko

FIG. 35-16 Arterial and venous blood supply to primary and accessory organs of the alimentary canal. (From Thompson et al., 1993.)

lon, the mass consists entirely of wastes and is called the feces. **Feces,** or excrement, consists of food residue, unabsorbed gastrointestinal secretions, shed epithelial cells, and bacteria.

The **rectum** receives feces from the sigmoid colon. The movement of feces into the sigmoid colon and rectum stimulates the **defecation reflex** (rectal reflex). Increased volume and pressure cause peristalsis in the sigmoid colon, forcing the feces into the normally empty rectum. This stretches the rectal wall and relaxes the tonically constricted internal anal sphincter (smooth muscle with autonomic nervous system control), creating the urge to defecate. If the external anal sphincter (striated muscle with voluntary and autonomic control) is relaxed or paralyzed, defecation occurs. The defecation reflex can be overridden voluntarily by contraction of the exter-

nal anal sphincter and muscles of the pelvic floor. The rectal wall gradually relaxes, reducing tension, and the urge to defecate passes. Retrograde contraction of the rectum may displace the feces out of the rectal vault until a more convenient time for evacuation. Pain or fear of pain associated with defecation, e.g., rectal fissures or hemorrhoids, can inhibit the defecation reflex. The defecation reflex is regulated by parasympathetic and cholinergic fibers. Voluntary inhibition or facilitation of defecation is mediated from cortical projections onto the medulla and down to sacral segments of the cord. Habit and diet affect the pattern of frequency.

Defecation is facilitated by squatting or sitting because these positions straighten the angle between the rectum and anal canal and increase the efficiency of straining (increasing intraabdominal pressure). Intraabdominal pressure is increased by initiating the Valsalva maneuver. This maneuver consists of inhaling and forcing the diaphragm and chest muscles against the closed glottis. This increases both intrathoracic and intraabdominal pressure, which is transmitted to the rectum.

Intestinal Bacteria

The type and number of bacteria vary greatly throughout the normal gastrointestinal tract. There is an increasing number of bacteria from the stomach to the distal colon. The stomach is relatively sterile because of the secretion of acid that kills ingested pathogens or inhibits bacterial growth. Bile acid secretion, intestinal motility, and antibody production suppress bacterial growth in the duodenum, and in the duodenum and jejunum there is a low concentration of aerobes (10^{-1} to 10^{-4}/ml), primarily streptococci, lactobacilli, staphylococci, and enterobacteria. There are no anaerobes proximal to the ileum. The largest number of anaerobes are found distal to the ileocecal valve. They constitute about 95% of the fecal flora in the colon and contribute one third of the solid bulk of feces. *Bacteroides*, clostridia, anaerobic lactobacilli, and coliforms are the most common microorganisms from the ileum to the cecum.

The intestinal tract is sterile at birth but becomes colonized with *Escherichia coli, Clostridium welchii,* and *Streptococcus* within a few hours. Within 3 to 4 weeks after birth, the normal flora is established. The intestinal bacteria do not have major digestive or absorptive functions. They do play a role in the metabolism of bile salts, contributing to the intestinal reabsorption of bile and the elimination of toxic bile metabolites. Intestinal bacteria are also involved in the metabolism of estrogens and androgens, lipid metabolism, conversion of unabsorbed carbohydrates to absorbable organic acids, and metabolism of various nitrogenous substances and drugs.

Endogenous infections of the gastrointestinal tract occur by three major mechanisms: proliferation or overgrowth of bacteria, perforation of the intestine, and contamination of neighboring structures. Proliferation of bacteria occurs whenever there is obstruction to normal peristaltic flow of intestinal contents. The overpopulation of bacteria results in malabsorption of nutrients; bacterial utilization of folic acid and vitamin B_{12} may cause anemia. Ruptured appendix or external trauma can lead to perforation of the intestine, releasing bacteria into the peritoneum, and can lead to peritonitis or

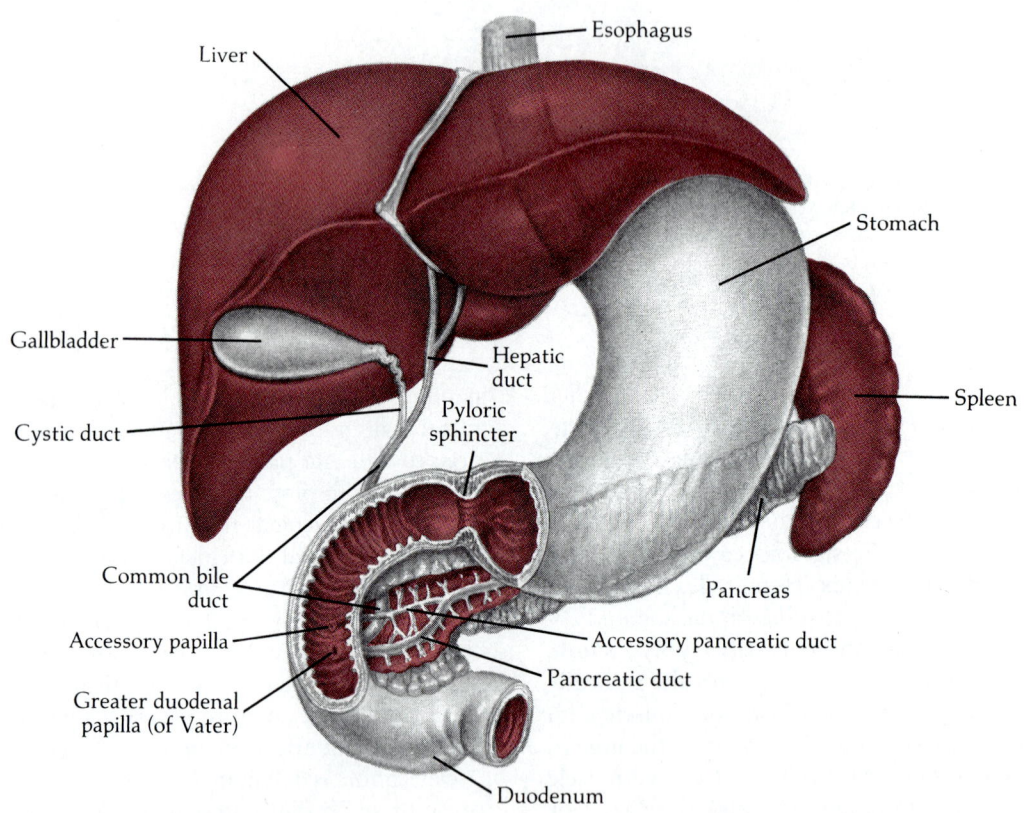

FIG. 35-17 Location of the liver, gallbladder, and exocrine pancreas, which are the accessory organs of digestion. (From Thompson et al., 1993.)

bacteremia. Movement of bacteria from the intestinal tract into the biliary tree can lead to cholangitis (inflammation of the bile ducts). Colonization of the female urethra and bladder can result from fecal contamination caused by the close proximity of structures.

ACCESSORY ORGANS OF DIGESTION

The liver, gallbladder, and exocrine pancreas all secrete substances necessary for the digestion of chyme. These secretions are delivered to the duodenum through ducts (Fig. 35-17). The liver produces bile, which contains salts necessary for fat digestion and absorption. Between meals, bile is stored in the gallbladder. The exocrine pancreas produces enzymes needed for the complete digestion of carbohydrates, proteins, and fats. The exo-

crine pancreas also produces an alkaline fluid that neutralizes chyme, creating a duodenal pH that supports enzymatic action.

The liver has many important functions besides bile secretion. It receives nutrients absorbed by the small intestine and metabolizes or synthesizes these nutrients into forms that can be absorbed by the body's cells. Having completed these processes, the liver releases the nutrients into the bloodstream or stores them for later use.

Liver

The **liver,** which weighs 1200 to 1600 g, is the largest organ in the body. It is located under the right diaphragm and is divided into right and left lobes. The larger, right lobe is divided further into the caudate and quadrate lobes (Fig. 35-18). The falciform ligament sep-

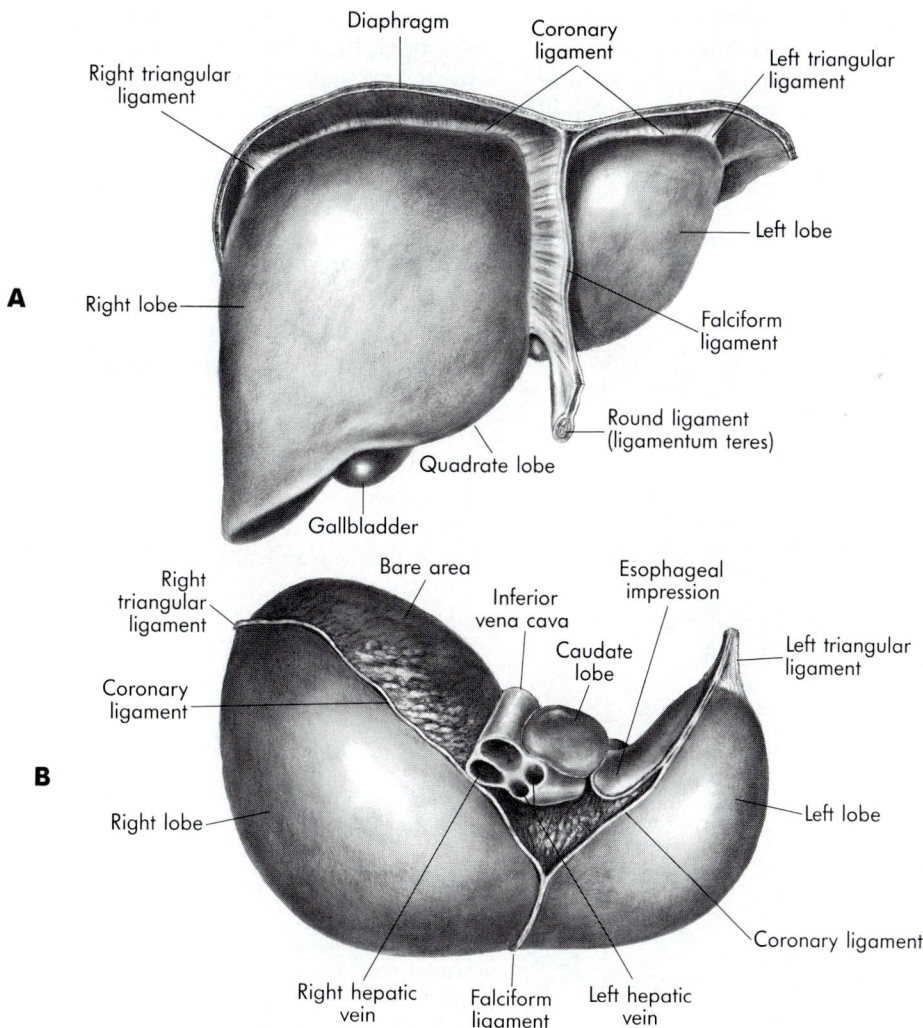

FIG. 35-18 Gross structure of the liver. A, Anterior view, showing supporting ligaments. **B,** Superior (diaphragmatic) surface of the liver.

arates the right and left lobes and attaches the liver to the anterior abdominal wall. A fibrous cord called the round ligament (ligamentum teres) extends along the free edge of the falciform ligament. The round ligament is the remnant of the umbilical vein and extends from the umbilicus to the inferior surface of the liver. The coronary ligament branches from the falciform ligament and extends over the superior surface of the right and left lobes, adhering the liver to the inferior surface of the diaphragm. The liver is covered by a fibroelastic capsule called the **Glisson capsule.** The Glisson capsule contains blood vessels, lymphatics, and nerves. When the liver is diseased or swollen, distention of the capsule causes pain and the lymphatics may ooze fluid into the peritoneal space.

The metabolic functions of the liver require a large amount of blood. The liver receives blood from both arterial and venous sources. The hepatic artery branches from the abdominal aorta and provides oxygenated blood at the rate of 400 to 500 ml/min (about 25% of the cardiac output). The hepatic portal vein, which receives deoxygenated blood from the inferior and superior mesenteric veins and the splenic vein, delivers about 1000 to 1200 ml/min to the liver. Portal venous blood constitutes 70% of the blood supply to the liver. This blood carries some oxygen and is rich in nutrients that have been absorbed from the digestive tract.

Within the liver lobes are multiple, smaller anatomic units called **liver lobules** (Fig. 35-19). The lobules are formed of cords or plates of **hepatocytes,** which are the functional cells of the liver. These cells are capable of regeneration; therefore, damaged or resected liver tissue can regrow. Small capillaries, or **sinusoids,** are located between the plates of hepatocytes. The sinusoids receive a mixture of venous and arterial blood from branches of the hepatic artery and portal vein. Blood from the sinusoids drains to a central vein in the middle of each liver lobule. Venous blood from all the lobules then flows into the hepatic vein, which empties into the inferior vena cava. Small channels known as **bile canaliculi** conduct bile, which is produced by the hepatocytes, outward to bile ducts and eventually drain into the **common bile duct** (Fig. 35-19). The common bile duct empties bile into the duodenum through an opening called the **major duodenal papilla** (sphincter of Oddi).

The sinusoids of the liver lobules are lined with highly permeable endothelium. This permeability enhances the transport of nutrients from the sinusoids into the hepatocytes, where they are metabolized. The sinusoids are also lined with phagocytic cells known as **Kupffer cells.** Kupffer cells are part of the mononuclear phagocyte system (see Chapter 22). They remove foreign substances from the blood and trap bacteria. Between the endothelial lining of the sinusoid and the hepatocyte is the **Disse space,** which drains interstitial fluid into the hepatic lymph system.

Secretion of Bile

The liver assists intestinal digestion by secreting 700 to 1200 ml bile per day. **Bile** is an alkaline, bitter-tasting, yellowish green fluid that contains bile salts (conjugated bile acids), cholesterol, bilirubin (a pigment), electrolytes, and water. It is formed by hepatocytes and secreted into the canaliculi. **Bile salts,** which are conjugated bile acids, are required for the intestinal emulsification and absorption of fats. Having facilitated fat emulsification and absorption, most bile salts are ac-

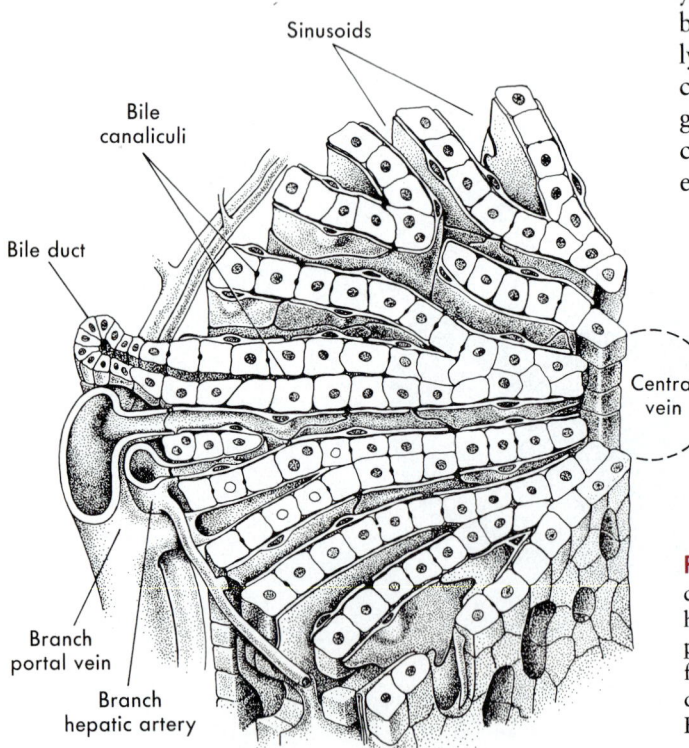

Sinusoids

Bile canaliculi

Bile duct

Central vein

Branch portal vein

Branch hepatic artery

FIG. 35-19 Diagrammatic representation of a liver lobule. A central vein is located in the center of the lobule with plates of hepatic cells disposed radially. Branches of the portal vein and hepatic artery are located on the periphery of the lobule, and blood from both perfuses the sinusoids. Peripherally located bile ducts drain the bile canaliculi that run between the hepatocytes. (From Berne & Levy, 1993.)

tively absorbed in the terminal ileum and returned to the liver through the portal circulation for resecretion. The recycling of bile salts is termed the **enterohepatic circulation** (Fig. 35-20).

Bile has two fractional components: the acid-dependent fraction and the acid-independent fraction. Hepatocytes secrete the **bile acid–dependent fraction** of the bile. This fraction consists of bile acids, cholesterol, lecithin (a phospholipid), and bilirubin (a bile pigment). The **bile acid–independent fraction** of the bile, which is secreted by the hepatocytes and epithelial cells of the bile canaliculi, is a bicarbonate-rich aqueous fluid that gives bile its alkaline pH.

Bile salts are conjugated in the liver from primary and secondary bile acids. The **primary bile acids** are cholic acid and chenodeoxycholic (chenic) acid. These acids are synthesized from cholesterol by the hepatocytes. The **secondary bile acids** are deoxycholic and lithocholic acid. These acids are formed in the small intestine by the action of intestinal bacteria, after which they are ab-

sorbed and flow to the liver (Fig. 35-20). Both forms of bile acids are conjugated with amino acids (glycine or taurine) in the liver to form bile salts. Conjugation makes the bile acids more water-soluble, thus restricting their diffusion from the duodenum and ileum. The primary and secondary bile acids together form the **bile acid pool.**

Bile salts are planar molecules: that is, they are hydrophobic on one end and hydrophilic on the other. When the concentration of bile salts is adequate or has reached the **critical micelle concentration,** the molecules form micelles with their hydrophilic side toward the watery chyme of the intestine and their hydrophobic side surrounding fat molecules such as cholesterol, free fatty acids, and phospholipids (Fig. 35-14). Micelle formation facilitates the absorption of fat by the intestinal mucosa.

When they reach the terminal ileum, bile salts are actively transported into the portal blood and returned to the liver for resecretion. Some bile salts are deconju-

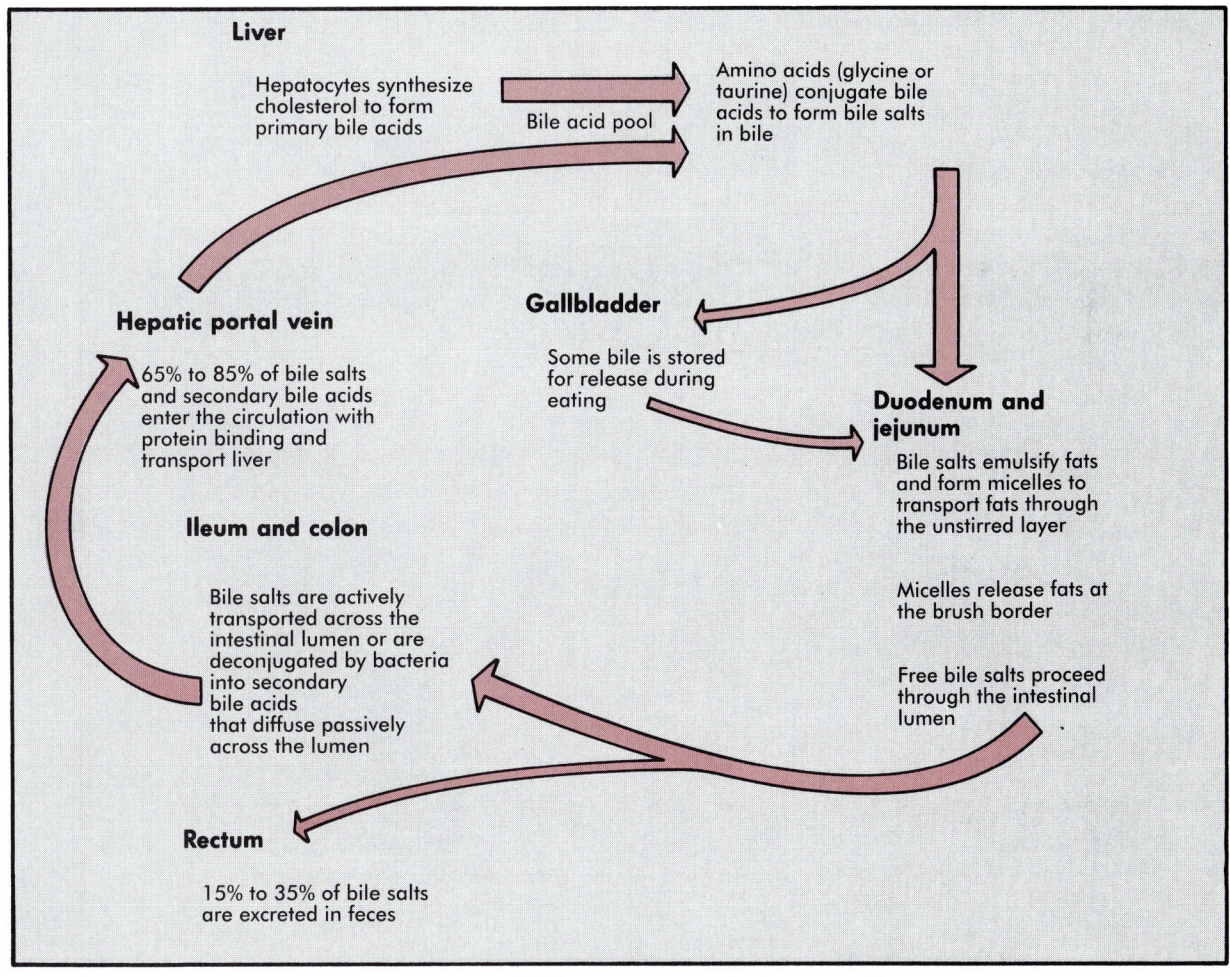

FIG. 35-20 The enterohepatic circulation of bile salts.

gated by intestinal bacteria to secondary bile acids. These acids diffuse passively into the portal blood from both small and large intestines. An increase in the plasma concentration of bile acids accelerates the uptake and resecretion of bile acids and salts by the hepatocytes. The cycle of hepatic secretion, intestinal absorption, and hepatic resecretion of bile acids completes the enterohepatic circulation.

Bile secretion is called **choleresis**. A **choleretic agent** is a substance that stimulates the liver to secrete bile. One strong stimulus is a high concentration of bile salts.

Other choleretics include secretin, which increases the rate of bile flow by promoting the secretion of bicarbonate from canaliculi and other intrahepatic bile ducts; cholecystokinin; and vagal stimulation.

Metabolism of Bilirubin

Bilirubin is a byproduct of destruction of aged red blood cells. It gives bile a greenish black color and produces the yellow tinge of jaundice. Aged red blood cells are taken up and destroyed by macrophages of the mononuclear phagocyte system (also called the reticuloendo-

FIG. 35-21 Bilirubin metabolism.

thelial system), primarily in the spleen and liver. (In the liver these macrophages are Kupffer cells.) Within these cells hemoglobin is separated into its component parts, heme and globin (Fig. 35-21). The globin component is further degraded into its constituent amino acids, which are recycled to form new protein. The heme moiety is converted to biliverdin by the enzymatic cleavage of iron. The iron attaches to transferrin in the plasma and can be stored in the liver or used by the bone marrow to make new red blood cells. The biliverdin is enzymatically converted to bilirubin in the macrophage of the mononuclear phagocytic system and then is released into the plasma. In the plasma, bilirubin binds to albumin and is known as **unconjugated bilirubin,** or free bilirubin, which is lipid soluble.

In the liver, unconjugated bilirubin moves from plasma in the sinusoids into the hepatocyte. Within hepatocytes it joins with glucuronic acid to form **conjugated bilirubin,** which is water-soluble. Conjugation transforms bilirubin from a lipid-soluble substance that can cross biologic membranes to a water-soluble substance that can be excreted in the bile. When conjugated bilirubin reaches the distal ileum and colon, it is deconjugated by bacteria and converted to **urobilinogen.** Most of the urobilinogen is then excreted in the urine, and a small amount is eliminated in feces.

Vascular and Hematologic Functions

Because of its extensive vascular network the liver can store a large volume of blood. The amount stored at any one time depends on pressure relationships in the arteries and veins. Increased central venous pressure, such as that caused by congestive heart failure, expands the venous capacity of the liver by several hundred milliliters. The liver can also release blood to maintain systemic circulatory volume in the event of hemorrhage.

Plasma proteins synthesized by the liver, particularly albumin, maintain blood volume and pressure by maintaining plasma oncotic pressure. Reduced concentrations of plasma proteins resulting from altered liver function or leakage of plasma proteins into interstitial spaces cause fluid to shift from the vascular compartment to the extravascular compartment (interstitial space). The consequence is reduced blood volume.

Kupffer cells in the sinusoids of the liver remove bacteria and foreign particles from the portal blood. Because the liver receives all of the venous blood from the gut and pancreas, the Kupffer cells play an important role in destroying intestinal bacteria and preventing infections.

The liver also has hemostatic functions. It synthesizes prothrombin, fibrinogen, and factors I, II, VII, IX, and X, all of which are necessary for effective clotting (see Chapter 22). Vitamin K, a fat-soluble vitamin, is essential for the synthesis of other clotting factors. Because bile salts are needed for reabsorption of fats, vitamin K

absorption depends on adequate bile production in the liver. Impairment of vitamin K absorption diminishes production of clotting factors and increases risk of bleeding.

Metabolism of Nutrients
Fats

Fat is synthesized from carbohydrate and protein, primarily in the liver. Fat absorbed by lacteals in the intestinal villi enters the liver through the lymphatics, primarily as triglycerides. In the liver, the triglycerides can be hydrolyzed to glycerol and free fatty acids and used to produce metabolic energy (adenosine triphosphate [ATP]), or they can be released into the bloodstream as lipoproteins (lipids bound to proteins). The lipoproteins are carried by the blood to adipose cells for storage. The liver also synthesizes phospholipids and cholesterol, which are needed for the hepatic production of bile salts, steroid hormones, components of plasma membranes, and other special molecules.

Proteins

Protein synthesis requires the presence of all of the essential amino acids (obtained only from food), as well as nonessential amino acids. Proteins perform many important roles in the body and are summarized in Table 35-3.

TABLE 35-3

Proteins in the Body

Role	Example
Contraction	Actin and myosin enable muscle contraction
Energy	Proteins can be metabolized for energy
Fluid balance	Albumin, a major source of plasma oncotic pressure
Protection	Antibodies and complement protect against infection and foreign substances
Regulation	Enzymes control chemical reactions; hormones regulate many physiologic processes
Structure	Collagen fibers provide structural support to many part of the body; keratin strengthens skin, hair, and nails
Transport	Hemoglobin transports oxygen and carbon dioxide in the blood; plasma proteins serve as transport molecules; proteins in cell membranes control movement of materials into and out of cells

Adapted from Seeley, Stephens, & Tate, 1992, p. 53.

Within hepatocytes, amino acids are converted to carbohydrates (ketoacids) by the removal of ammonia (NH_3), a process known as **deamination.** The ammonia is converted to urea by the liver and passes into the blood to be excreted by the kidneys. Depending on need, the ketoacids are converted to fatty acids for fat synthesis and storage or are oxidized by the Krebs tricarboxylic acid cycle (see Chapter 1) to provide energy for the liver cells.

The plasma proteins, including albumins and globulins (with the exception of γ-globulin, which is formed in lymph nodes and lymphoid tissue), are synthesized by the liver. The liver also synthesizes several nonessential amino acids and serum enzymes, including aspartate aminotransferase (AST; previously SGOT), alanine aminotransferase (ALT; previously SGPT), lactate dehydrogenase (LDH), and alkaline phosphatase.

Carbohydrates

The liver contributes to the stability of blood glucose levels by releasing glucose during states of hypoglycemia (low blood sugar) and taking up glucose during states of hyperglycemia (high blood sugar) and storing it as glycogen (glyconeogenesis) or converting it to fat. When all glycogen stores have been used, the liver can convert amino acids and glycerol to glucose.

Metabolic Detoxification

The liver alters exogenous and endogenous chemicals (e.g., drugs), foreign molecules, and hormones to make them less toxic or less biologically active. This process, called **metabolic detoxification,** or biotransformation, diminishes intestinal or renal tubular reabsorption of potentially toxic substances and facilitates their intestinal and renal excretion. In this way alcohol, barbiturates, amphetamines, steroids, and hormones (including estrogens, aldosterone, antidiuretic hormone, and testosterone) are metabolized or detoxified, preventing excessive accumulation and adverse effects.

Although metabolic detoxification is usually protective, sometimes the end products of metabolic detoxification become toxins. Those of alcohol metabolism, for example, are acetaldehyde and hydrogen. Excessive intake of alcohol over a prolonged period causes these end products to damage hepatocytes. Acetaldehyde damages cellular mitochondria, and the excess hydrogen promotes fat accumulation. This is how alcohol impairs the liver's ability to function.

Storage of Minerals and Vitamins

The liver stores certain vitamins and minerals, including iron and copper, in times of excessive intake and releases them in times of need. The liver can store vitamins B_{12} and D for several months and vitamin A for several years. The liver also stores vitamins E and K.

Iron is stored in the liver as ferritin, an iron-protein complex, and is released as needed for red blood cell production.

Gallbladder

The **gallbladder** is a saclike organ that lies on the inferior surface of the liver (Fig. 35-22). The primary function of the gallbladder is to store and concentrate bile between meals. During the interdigestive period, bile flows from the liver through the right or left hepatic duct into the common hepatic duct and meets resistance at the closed **sphincter of Oddi,** which controls flow into the duodenum. Bile then flows to the **cystic duct** into the gallbladder, where it is concentrated and stored. The mucosa of the gallbladder wall readily absorbs water and electrolytes, leaving a high concentration of bile salts, bile pigments, and cholesterol. The gallbladder holds about 90 ml of bile.

Within 30 minutes after eating, the gallbladder begins to contract and the sphincter of Oddi relaxes, forcing bile into the duodenum through the major duodenal papilla. During the cephalic and gastric phases of digestion, gallbladder contraction is mediated by cholinergic branches of the vagus nerve. Hormonal regulation of gallbladder contraction is derived from the release of cholecystokinin and motilin secreted by the duodenal mucosa in the presence of fat.

Exocrine Pancreas

The **pancreas** is approximately 20 cm long, with its head tucked into the curve of the duodenum and its tail touching the spleen. The body of the pancreas lies deep in the abdomen, behind the stomach (Fig. 35-22). The pancreas is unique in that it has both endocrine and exocrine functions. The endocrine pancreas secretes hormones, primarily insulin and glucagon.

The **exocrine pancreas** is composed of acini and networks of ducts that secrete enzymes and alkaline fluids with important digestive functions. The acinar cells are organized into spherical lobules around small secretory ducts (Fig. 35-22). Secretions drain into a system of ducts that leads to the **pancreatic duct** (Wirsung duct), which empties into the common bile duct at the **ampulla of Vater.** In some individuals an accessory duct (the duct of Santorini) branches off the pancreatic duct and drains directly into the duodenum at an opening called the minor duodenal papilla.

Arterial blood is supplied to the pancreas by branches of the celiac and superior mesenteric arteries. Venous blood leaves the head of the pancreas through the portal vein, with the body and tail being drained through the splenic vein. All hormonal pancreatic secretions also pass through the portal vein into the liver.

Pancreatic innervation arises from preganglionic parasympathetic fibers of the vagus nerve. The pregan-

Neck of gallbladder

Right and left hepatic ducts

Corpus (body) of gallbladder

Common hepatic duct

Cystic duct

Common bile duct

Accessory duct of pancreas

Pancreas

Fundus of gallbladder

Minor duodenal papilla

Sphincter muscles

Pancreatic duct

Superior mesenteric artery and vein

Major duodenal papilla

Duodenum

Beck

Duct cells secrete bicarbonate

Acinar cells secrete enzymes

Centroacinar cells secrete electrolytes and water

FIG. 35-22 Associated structures of the gallbladder and pancreas.

glionic fibers activate postganglionic fibers, which stimulate enzymatic and hormonal secretion. Sympathetic postganglionic fibers from the celiac and superior mesenteric plexuses innervate the blood vessels and cause vasoconstriction. Generally the sympathetic nerves inhibit pancreatic secretion and the parasympathetic nerves stimulate it.

The aqueous secretions of the exocrine pancreas are isotonic and contain potassium, sodium, bicarbonate, and chloride. Sodium and potassium concentrations are about equal to those in the plasma. The concentration of bicarbonate in pancreatic juice varies from 50 mEq/L at low secretory flow rates to 120 mEq/L at high flow rates. As bicarbonate secretion increases, chloride secretion decreases to maintain a constant anionic concentration. The highly alkaline pancreatic juice neutralizes

the acidic chyme that enters the duodenum from the stomach and provides the alkaline medium needed for the actions of digestive enzymes.

In the pancreas, transport of water and electrolytes through the ductal epithelium involves both active and passive mechanisms. The secretory cells of the acini actively transport hydrogen into the blood and bicarbonate into the duct lumen. Hydrogen (H^+) and bicarbonate (HCO_3^-) are produced in the cell from the dissociation of carbonic acid (H_2CO_3), which is formed from the combination of CO_2 and H_2O through the action of carbonic anhydrase. Hydrogen is secreted into the blood in exchange for sodium. Bicarbonate enters the duct lumen by an active transport process. Potassium and chloride are secreted by diffusion according to changes in electrochemical potential gradients. As the secretion flows down the duct, water is osmotically transported into the juice until it becomes isoosmotic. At low flow rates, bicarbonate is exchanged passively for chloride, but at higher flow rates there is less time for this exchange and bicarbonate concentration increases. Because eating stimulates the flow of pancreatic juice, the juice is most alkaline when it needs to be: during digestion.

The enzymes of the pancreas are capable of hydrolyzing proteins, carbohydrates, and fats. The proteolytic (protein-digesting) enzymes include trypsin, chymotrypsin, and carboxypeptidase. These enzymes are secreted in their inactive forms, that is, as trypsinogen, chymotrypsinogen, and procarboxypeptidase. This is necessary to protect the pancreas from the digestive effects of its own enzymes. For further protection the pancreas produces **trypsin inhibitor,** which prevents the activation of proteolytic enzymes while they are in the pancreas. Once in the duodenum, the inactive forms (proenzymes) are activated by **enterokinase,** an enzyme secreted by the duodenal mucosa. Trypsinogen is the first proenzyme to be activated. Its conversion to trypsin stimulates the conversion of chymotrypsinogen to chymotrypsin and procarboxypeptidase to carboxypeptidase. Each of these enzymes cleaves specific peptide bonds to reduce polypeptides to smaller peptides.

Pancreatic α-amylase is secreted in active form. Like salivary amylase, it participates in carbohydrate digestion by cleaving interior α-1,4-glucosidic bonds. The optimum pH for α-amylase action is approximately 6.9, although enzymatic activity is supported at a pH of 4 to 11.

Several pancreatic enzymes digest fats. **Pancreatic lipase** (glycerol ester hydrolase) hydrolyzes triglycerides to one free fatty acid and two monoglycerides. Cholesterol ester hydrolase and phospholipase A and B produce free fatty acids and cholesterol or phosphate products. These enzymes require an alkaline pH ranging from 7 to 9.

Secretion of the aqueous and enzymatic components of pancreatic juice is controlled by hormonal and vagal stimuli. The hormone secretin stimulates the acinar and duct cells to secrete the bicarbonate-rich fluid that neutralizes chyme and prepares it for enzymatic digestion. As chyme enters the duodenum, its acidity (pH of 4.5 or less) stimulates the **S cells** (secretin-producing cells) of the duodenum to release secretin, which is absorbed by the intestine and delivered to the pancreas in the bloodstream. In the pancreas, secretin causes ductal and acinar cells to release alkaline fluid. Secretin also inhibits the actions of gastrin, thereby decreasing gastric acid secretion and motility. The overall effect is to neutralize contents of the duodenum.

Enzymatic secretion follows, stimulated by cholecys-tokinin and acetylcholine. Cholecystokinin is released in the duodenum in response to the essential amino acids and fatty acids already present in chyme. Cholecystokinin and acetylcholine both act on the acinar cells, causing enzyme release. Once in the small intestine, activated pancreatic enzymes inhibit the release of more cholecystokinin and acetylcholine. This feedback mechanism inhibits the secretion of more pancreatic enzymes. Acetylcholine is liberated from pancreatic branches of the vagus nerve during the cephalic phase of digestion. (See Table 35-1 for a summary of hormonal stimulation of pancreatic secretions.)

TESTS OF DIGESTIVE FUNCTION
Gastrointestinal Tract

Although important diagnostic information can be obtained from the history and presenting symptoms, numerous disease-specific tests must be performed to evaluate the structure and function of the gastrointestinal tract. A description of selected studies is presented in Tables 35-4 and 35-5. X-ray films and imaging techniques, including ultrasound and radionuclide and computed tomography (CT scanning), are common procedures for evaluating structure and function. Plain x-ray films using contrast media such as barium- or iodine-containing compounds can be used to outline the gastrointestinal lumen, biliary tree and pancreatic ducts, fistulas, and arteriovenous systems. Computed tomography scanning is particularly useful for diagnosis of pancreatic or hepatic tumors or cysts. Ultrasonic scanning is a safe, simple, and relatively inexpensive technique used to detect liver-related jaundice and intraabdominal masses, particularly abscesses.

Fiberoptic endoscopy, using flexible endoscopes, allows direct visualization of the gastrointestinal tract. A biopsy channel allows tissue sampling, and suction can be applied to remove gastrointestinal secretions or blood. Analysis of stool, gastric secretions, and plasma provides important clues to infection, malabsorption syndromes, ulcerative lesions, and tumor growth.

Liver

A variety of diagnostic tests can be performed to evaluate liver function (Table 35-6). Imaging techniques similar to those described for the gastrointestinal tract are also useful to evaluate liver structure and function. Plasma chemistry findings are also altered with many liver diseases because of release of cytoplasmic enzymes into the circulation when there is damage to the hepatocyte. Of particular importance are elevations of aminotransferases and LDH. Obstruction of bile canaliculi

TABLE 35-4

Selected Studies of Gastrointestinal Structure

Test	Description	Application
Plain x-ray films	Use of high-energy electromagnetic radiation to evaluate tissue structure by radiopacity or radiolucency	Visualization of the position, size, and structure of abdominal contents
Air or barium contrast x-ray films	Introduction of radiopaque substances into the upper or lower gastrointestinal tract	Enhanced visualization of the contours, position, and size of the gastrointestinal tract to detect umbilical hernia, ulcers, diverticula, congenital anomalies, polyps, tumors, strictures, obstructions
Endoscopy Esophagoscopy (esophagus) Gastroscopy (stomach) Duodenoscopy (duodenum) Colonoscopy (large intestine) Sigmoidoscopy (sigmoid colon)	Passage of rigid or flexible (fiberoptic) endoscope into the gastrointestinal tract for visualization of biopsy	Visualization or biopsy of inflamed hernias, polyps, ulcers, strictures, varices, tumors, sites of bleeding, mucosal or neoplastic lesions and for culture of *Helicobacter pylori* from stomach
Ultrasound	Use of piezoelectric crystal to generate sound waves that are reflected from tissue interfaces to provide an image	Imaging of abdominal organs (gallbladder, liver, pancreas, spleen), masses, stones, abscesses, structural abnormalities
Computed tomography (CT)	Use of a computer to integrate differences in absorption of a large number of x-rays to produce a cross-sectional image; may be done with contrast agents	Imaging of gallbladder, liver, pancreas, spleen, cysts, hematomas, abscesses, stones, extrahepatic bile ducts, and portal vein
Magnetic resonance imaging (MRI)	Projection of differences in magnetic properties of molecules within different cells and tissues, using the field of a large magnet	Same applications as CT scan; can also detect blood flow and vessel patency

or ducts results in regurgitation of bile back into the hepatic sinusoids and into the circulation with elevation of bilirubin levels. Prothrombin times are often prolonged with both hepatitis and chronic liver disease. In severe disease, other plasma proteins, such as albumin and globulins, may be diminished as a result of hepatocyte damage. Liver biopsies are often performed to evaluate the extent of liver involvement or degeneration with cirrhosis or hepatitis.

Gallbladder

Evaluation of structural alterations in the gallbladder may be achieved by the use of different imaging techniques. Table 35-7 summarizes these techniques. Obstruction of the common ducts from stones, tumors, or inflammation prevents the flow of bile from the liver and gallbladder from reaching the gastrointestinal tract.

Both the conjugated and total serum bilirubin values are elevated, urine urobilinogen is increased, stools are clay-colored, and jaundice develops. Fat absorption can be impaired and the prothrombin time prolonged if vitamin K is not absorbed. With inflammation of the gallbladder, the white cell count is elevated.

Exocrine Pancreas

Tests of pancreatic function are summarized in Table 35-8. Evaluation of plasma and urinary amylase provides particularly significant measures of pancreatic function. Inflammation or obstruction of the pancreas results in an increase in serum amylase levels. Decreased renal absorption of amylase results in increased urine amylase levels. Increased stool fat can reflect pancreatic insufficiency caused by decreased lipase secretion when biliary function is normal.

TABLE 35-5

Selected Tests of Gastrointestinal Function

Test	Normal findings	Clinical significance of abnormal findings
Stool studies	Resident microorganisms: clostridia, enterococci, *Pseudomonas,* a few yeasts	Detection of *Salmonella typhi* (typhoid fever), *Shigella* (dysentery), *Vibrio cholerae* (cholera), *Yersinia* (enterocolitis), *Escherichia coli* (gastroenteritis), *Staphylococcus aureus (food poisoning), Clostridium botulinum* (food poisoning), *Clostridium perfringens* (food poisoning), *Aeromonas* (gastroenteritis)
	Fat: 2-6 g/24 hr	Steatorrhea (increased values) can result from intestinal malabsorption or pancreatic insufficiency
	Pus: none	Large amounts of pus are associated with chronic ulcerative colitis, abscesses, and anal-rectal fistula
	Occult blood: none (Ortho-Tolidin or guaiac test)	Positive tests associated with bleeding
	Ova and parasites: none	Detection of *Entamoeba histolytica* (amebiasis), *Giardia lamblia* (giardiasis), and worms
D-Xylose absorption	5-Hr urinary excretion: r4.5 g/L Peak blood level: >30 mg/dl	Differentiation of pancreatic steatorrhea (normal D-xylose absorption) from intestinal steatorrhea (impaired D-xylose absorption)
Gastric acid stimulation	11-20 mEq/hr after stimulation	Detection of duodenal ulcers, Zollinger-Ellison syndrome (increased values), gastric atrophy, gastric carcinoma (decreased values)
Manometry (use of water-filled catheters connected to pressure transducers passed into the esophagus, stomach, colon, or rectum to evaluate contractility)	Values vary at different levels of the intestine	Inadequate swallowing, motility, sphincter function
Culture and sensitivity of duodenal contents	No pathogens	Detection of *Salmonella typhi* (typhoid fever)

TABLE 35-6

Common Liver Function Tests

Test	Normal value	Interpretation
Serum enzymes		
Alkaline phosphatase	13-39 U/ml	Increases with biliary obstruction and cholestatic hepatitis
Aspartate amino transferase (AST; previously SGOT)	5-40 U/ml	Increases with hepatocellular injury
Alanine amino transferase (ALT; previously SGPT)	5-35 U/ml	Increases with hepatocellular injury
LDH (lactate dehydrogenase)	200-500 U/ml	Isoenzyme LD$_5$ is elevated with hypoxic and primary liver injury
5'-Nucleotidase	2-11 U/ml	Increases with increase in alkaline phosphatase and cholestatic disorders
Bilirubin metabolism		
Serum bilirubin		
Indirect (unconjugated)	<0.8 mg/dl	Increases with hemolysis (lysis of red blood cells)
Direct (conjugated)	0.2-0.4 mg/dl	Increases with hepatocellular injury or obstruction
Total	<1.0 mg/dl	Increase with biliary obstruction
Urine bilirubin	0	Decreases with biliary obstruction
Urine urobilinogen	0-4 mg/24 hr	Increases with hemolysis or shunting of portal blood flow
Serum proteins		
Albumin	3.5-5.5 g/dl	Reduced with hepatocellular injury
Globulin	2.5-3.5 g/dl	Increases with hepatitis
Total	6-7 g/dl	
A/G ratio	1.5:1-2.5:1	Ratio reverses with chronic hepatitis or other chronic liver disease
Transferrin	250-300 μg/dl	Liver damage with decreased values, iron deficiency with increased values
α-Fetoprotein	6-20 ng/ml	Elevated values in primary hepatocellular carcinoma
Blood clotting functions		
Prothrombin time	11.5-14 sec or 90%-100% of control	Increases with chronic liver disease (cirrhosis) or vitamin K deficiency
Partial thromboplastin time	25-40 sec	Increases with severe liver disease or heparin therapy
BSP (bromsulphalein) excretion	<6% retention in 45 min	Increased retention with hepatocellular injury

TABLE 35-7

Diagnostic Evaluation of the Gallbladder

Test	Application
Plain film of the abdomen	Visualization of calcified gallstones
Oral cholecystogram (use of an oral contrast medium such as iodopanoic acid, which is excreted with bile and concentrated in the gallbladder for visualization by radiography; may be administered as a double dose)	Visualization of gallstones; evaluation of filling and emptying of gallbladder
Intravenous cholangiography (use of intravenous contrast agents for visualization of gallbladder and bile ducts)	Diagnosis of acute gallbladder inflammation (cholecystitis) or disease of bile ducts
Cholecystosonography (ultrasound imaging of gallbladder and bile ducts)	Preferred method for detecting gallstones; differentiation of hepatic disease from biliary obstruction; diagnosis of chronic cholecystitis
Cholescintigraphy (radioisotope imaging of gallbladder)	Diagnosis of cholecystitis in individuals allergic to iodine-containing contrast agents; diagnosis of cystic duct obstruction
Endoscopic retrograde cholangiography (instillation of contrast medium through cannulation of ampulla of Vater with a duodenoscope)	Differentiation of intrahepatic or extrahepatic obstructive jaundice
Computed tomography (CT)	Diagnosis of biliary obstruction or malignancy when ultrasound is not successful

TABLE 35-8

Selected Tests of Pancreatic Function

Test	Normal value	Clinical significance
Serum amylase	60-180 Somogyi units/ml	Elevated levels with pancreatic inflammation
Serum lipase	1.5 Somogyi units/ml	Elevated levels with pancreatic inflammation (may be elevated with other conditions; differentiates with amylase isoenzyme study)
Urine amylase	35-260 Somogyi units/hr	Elevated levels with pancreatic inflammation
Secretin test	Volume r1.8 ml/kg/hr; Bicarbonate concentration: >80 mEq/L; Bicarbonate output: >10 mEq/L/30 sec	Decreased volume with pancreatic disease as secretin stimulates pancreatic secretion
Stool fat	2-5 g/25 hr	Measures fatty acids; decreased pancreatic lipase increases stool fat

❑ AGING and the Gastrointestinal System

Age-related changes in gastrointestinal function begin to occur before the age of 50. Tooth enamel and dentin wear down, making the teeth vulnerable to cavities. Teeth are lost, frequently as a result of periodontal (gum) disease. Taste buds decline in number, and the sense of smell diminishes. Together these losses decrease the sense of taste. Salivary secretion decreases and contributes to dry mouth. In the very old, these oral and sensory changes make eating less pleasurable and reduce appetite. Food may not be chewed or lubricated sufficiently, making swallowing difficult.

Age also diminishes gastric motility and volume and acid content of gastric juice. These alterations cause hypochlorhydria (insufficient hydrochloric acid) and delayed gastric emptying, which are best managed with frequent and small meals. The villi of the small intestine become broader and shorter, perhaps because of a decrease in cell turnover. Intestinal absorption, motility, and blood flow decrease, impairing nutrient absorption. Proteins, fats, minerals (including iron and calcium), and vitamins are absorbed more slowly and in lesser amounts, and there is decreased absorption of carbohydrates. Although constipation is often described as a condition of old age, it is probably caused by life-style factors rather than physiologic decline. Lifelong bowel habits, current diet, lack of fluid intake, and immobility are likely causes of constipation in the elderly (Shamburek & Farrar, 1990).

The liver decreases in size and weight with advancing age, but liver function test results remain within normal ranges. Any alterations in liver function in older individuals are therefore signs of pathology. Liver blood flow decreases with age and can influence efficiency of drug metabolism. There may be decreased oxidative metabolism of drugs (Brocklehurst, Tallis & Fillit, 1992). The pancreas undergoes structural changes, such as fibrosis, fatty acid deposits, and atrophy. Pancreatic secretion decreases, but there is usually no observable dysfunction. Aging does not cause apparent changes in the structure and function of the gallbladder and bile ducts.

SUMMARY REVIEW

The Gastrointestinal Tract

1. The major functions of the gastrointestinal tract are the mechanical and chemical breakdown of food and the absorption of digested nutrients.
2. The gastrointestinal tract is a hollow tube that extends from the mouth to the anus.
3. The walls of the gastrointestinal tract have several layers: mucosa, muscularis mucosae, submucosa, tunica muscularis (circular muscle and longitudinal muscle), and serosa.
4. The peritoneum is a double layer of membranous tissue. The visceral layer covers the abdominal organs, and the parietal layer extends along the abdominal wall.
5. Except for swallowing and defecation, which are controlled voluntarily, the functions of the gastrointestinal tract are controlled by extrinsic and intrinsic autonomic nerves and intestinal hormones.
6. Digestion begins in the mouth, with chewing and salivation. The digestive component of saliva is α-amylase, which initiates carbohydrate digestion.
7. The esophagus is a muscular tube that transports food from the mouth to the stomach. The tunica muscularis in the upper part of the esophagus is striated muscle and that in the lower part is smooth muscle.
8. Swallowing is controlled by the swallowing center in the reticular formation of the brain. The two phases of swallowing are the oropharyngeal phase (voluntary swallowing) and the esophageal phase (involuntary swallowing).
9. Food is propelled through the gastrointestinal tract by peristalsis: waves of sequential relaxations and contractions of the tunica muscularis.
10. The lower esophageal sphincter opens to admit swallowed food into the stomach, then closes to prevent regurgitation of food back into the esophagus.
11. The stomach is a baglike structure that secretes digestive juices, mixes and stores food, and propels partially digested food (chyme) into the duodenum.
12. The vagus nerve stimulates gastric (stomach) secretion and motility.
13. The hormones gastrin and motilin stimulate gastric emptying; the hormones secretin and cholecystokinin delay gastric emptying.
14. Mucus is secreted throughout the stomach and protects the stomach wall from acid and digestive enzymes.
15. Gastric glands in the fundus and body of the stomach secrete intrinsic factor, which is needed for vitamin B_{12} absorption, and hydrochloric acid, which

dissolves food fibers, kills microorganisms, and activates the enzyme pepsin.

16 Chief cells in the stomach secrete pepsinogen, which is converted to pepsin in the acid environment created by hydrochloric acid.

17 Acid secretion is stimulated by the vagus nerve, gastrin, and histamine and inhibited by sympathetic stimulation and cholecystokinin.

18 The three phases of acid secretion by the stomach are the cephalic phase (anticipation and swallowing), the gastric phase (food in the stomach), and the intestinal phase (chyme in the intestine).

19 The small intestine is 5 m long and has three segments: the duodenum, jejunum, and ileum.

20 The duodenum receives chyme from the stomach through the pyloric valve. The presence of chyme stimulates the liver and gallbladder to deliver bile and the pancreas to deliver digestive enzymes. Bile and enzymes flow through an opening guarded by the sphincter of Oddi.

21 Bile is produced by the liver and is necessary for fat digestion and absorption. Bile's alkalinity helps to neutralize chyme, thereby creating a pH that enables the pancreatic enzymes to digest proteins, carbohydrates, and sugars.

22 Enzymes secreted by the small intestine (maltase, sucrose, and lactase), pancreatic enzymes, and bile salts act in the small intestine to digest proteins, carbohydrates, and fats.

23 Digested substances are absorbed across the intestinal wall and then transported to the liver, where they are metabolized further.

24 The ileocecal valve connects the small and large intestines and prevents reflux into the small intestine.

25 Villi are small fingerlike projections that extend from the small intestinal mucosa and increase its absorptive surface area.

26 Sugars, amino acids, and fats are primarily absorbed by the duodenum and jejunum; bile salts and vitamin B_{12} are absorbed by the ileum. Vitamin B_{12} absorption requires the presence of intrinsic factor.

27 Bile salts emulsify and hydrolyze fats and incorporate them into water-soluble micelles, which transport them through the unstirred layer to the brush border of the intestinal mucosa. The fat content of the micelles readily diffuses through the epithelium into lacteals (lymphatic ducts) in the villi. From there fats flow into lymphatics and into the systemic circulation, which delivers them to the liver.

28 Minerals and water-soluble vitamins are absorbed by both active and passive transport throughout the small intestine.

29 Peristaltic movements created by longitudinal muscles propel the chyme along the intestinal tract, while contractions of the circular muscles (haustral segmentation) mix the chyme.

30 The ileogastric reflex inhibits gastric motility when the ileum is distended.

31 The intestinointestinal reflex inhibits intestinal motility when one intestinal segment is overdistended.

32 The gastroileal reflex increases intestinal motility when gastric motility increases.

33 The large intestine consists of the cecum, appendix, colon (ascending, transverse, descending, and sigmoid), rectum, and anal canal.

34 The teniae coli are three bands of longitudinal muscle that extend the length of the colon.

35 Haustra are pouches of colon that are formed with alternating contraction and relaxation of the circular muscles.

36 The mucosa of the large intestine contains mucus-secreting cells and mucosal folds, but no villi.

37 The large intestine massages the fecal mass and absorbs water and electrolytes.

38 Distention of the ileum with chyme causes the gastrocolic reflex, or the mass propulsion of feces to the rectum.

39 Defecation is stimulated when the rectum is distended with feces. The conically contracted internal anal sphincter relaxes and, if the voluntarily regulated external sphincter relaxes, defecation occurs.

40 The largest number of intestinal bacteria are in the colon. They are anaerobes consisting of *Bacteroides*, clostridia, coliforms, and lactobacilli.

41 The intestinal tract is sterile at birth and becomes totally colonized within 3 to 4 weeks.

42 Endogenous infections of the gastrointestinal tract occur by excessive proliferation of bacteria, perforation of the intestine, or contamination from neighboring structures.

Accessory Organs of Digestion

1 The liver is the largest organ in the body. It has digestive, metabolic, hematologic, vascular, and immunologic functions.

2 The liver is divided into the right and left lobes and is supported by the falciform, round, and coronary ligaments.

3 Liver lobules consist of plates of hepatocytes, which are the functional cells of the liver.

4 The hepatocytes synthesize 700 to 1200 ml of bile per day and secrete it into the bile canaliculi, which are small channels between the hepatocytes. The bile canaliculi drain bile into the common bile duct and then into the duodenum through an opening called the major duodenal papilla (sphincter of Oddi).

5 Sinusoids are capillaries located between the plates of hepatocytes. Blood from the portal vein and hepatic artery flows through the sinusoids to a central vein in each lobule and then to the hepatic vein and inferior vena cava.

6 Kupffer cells, which are part of the mononuclear phagocyte system, line the sinusoids and destroy microorganisms in sinusoidal blood.

7 The primary bile acids are synthesized from cholesterol by the hepatocytes. The primary acids are then conjugated to form bile salts. The secondary bile acids are the product of bile salt deconjugation by bacteria in the intestinal lumen.

8 Most bile salts and acids are recycled. The absorption of bile salts and acids from the terminal ileum and their return to the liver are known as the enterohepatic circulation of bile.

9 Bilirubin is a pigment liberated by the lysis of aged red blood cells in the liver and spleen. Unconjugated bilirubin is fat-soluble and can cross cell membranes. Unconjugated bilirubin is converted to water-soluble, conjugated bilirubin by hepatocytes and is secreted with bile.

10 The gallbladder is a saclike organ located in the inferior surface of the liver. The gallbladder stores bile between meals and ejects it when chyme enters the duodenum.

11 Stimulated by cholecystokinin, the gallbladder contracts and forces bile through the cystic duct and into the common bile duct. The sphincter of Oddi relaxes, enabling bile to flow through the major duodenal papilla into the duodenum.

12 The pancreas is a gland located behind the stomach. The exocrine pancreas produces hormones (glucagon and insulin) that facilitate the formation and cellular update of glucose. The endocrine pancreas secretes an alkaline solution and the enzymes (trypsin, chymotrypsin, carboxypeptidase, α-amylase, and lipase) that digest proteins, carbohydrates, and fats.

13 Secretin stimulates pancreatic secretion of alkaline fluid, and cholecystokinin and acetylcholine stimulate secretion of enzymes. Pancreatic secretions originate in acini and ducts of the pancreas and empty into the duodenum through the common bile duct or an accessory duct that opens directly into the duodenum.

Tests of Digestive Function

1 Numerous diagnostic tests are performed to evaluate structure and function (digestion, secretion, and absorption) of the gastrointestinal tract. X-rays and scans are most commonly used to evaluate structure, in addition to direct observation by endoscopy. Gastric and stool analysis and blood studies provide important information about digestion, absorption, and secretion.

2 Plasma chemistries and imaging procedures are commonly used to diagnose alterations in liver function. Of particular importance are the enzymes LDH, AST, and GPT. Plasma bilirubin levels reflect alterations in bilirubin and bile metabolism, and prothrombin times are prolonged in hepatitis and chronic liver disease.

3 Obstructive diseases of the gallbladder are evident by elevated serum bilirubin, elevated urine urobilinogen, and increased stool fat. The serum leukocytes become elevated with inflammation of the gallbladder.

4 The most significant indicators of pancreatic dysfunction are serum amylase and stool fat. Both values are increased with diseases of the pancreas.

Aging and the Gastrointestinal System

1 Advancing age is often associated with the loss or wearing down of teeth, diminished senses of taste and smell, and diminished salivary secretions, all of which may make eating difficult and reduce appetite.

2 Aging reduces gastric motility and secretions, particularly of hydrochloric acid. These changes slow gastric digestion and emptying.

3 Intestinal motility and absorption of carbohydrates, proteins, fats, and minerals decrease with age.

KEY TERMS

Ampulla of Vater, 1308
Antrum of stomach, 1286
Ascending colon, 1300
Bile, 1304
Bile acid–dependent fraction, 1305
Bile acid–independent fraction, 1305
Bile acid pool, 1305
Bile canaliculi, 1304
Bile salts, 1304
Bilirubin, 1306
Body of stomach, 1286
Brush border, 1291
Carboxypeptidase, 1296
Cardiac orifice, 1286
Cecum, 1300
Cephalic phase of secretion, 1290
Chief cell, 1288
Cholecystokinin, 1287
Choleresis, 1306
Choleretic agent, 1306
Chylomicron, 1298
Chyme, 1286
Chymotrypsin, 1296
Colon, 1300
Common bile duct, 1304
Conjugated bilirubin, 1307
Critical micelle concentration, 1305
Cystic duct, 1308
Deamination, 1308
Defecation reflex (rectal reflex), 1301
Descending colon, 1300
Disse space, 1304
Duodenum, 1291
Emulsification, 1296
Enteric plexus, 1283
Enterohepatic circulation, 1305
Enterokinase, 1310
Esophageal phase of swallowing, 1285
Esophagus, 1285
Exocrine pancreas, 1308
External anal sphincter, 1300
Fecal mass, 1300
Feces, 1301
Fundus of stomach, 1286
Gallbladder, 1308
Gastric emptying, 1287
Gastric gland, 1288
Gastric phase of secretion, 1290

Gastric pit, 1288
Gastrin, 1287
Gastrocolic reflex, 1300
Gastroileal reflex, 1299
Gastrointestinal tract (alimentary canal), 1283
G cell, 1290
Glisson capsule, 1304
Haustral segmentation, 1299
Haustrum (pl., haustra), 1300
Hepatocyte, 1304
Hydrolase, 1296
Ileocecal valve (sphincter), 1291
Ileogastric reflex, 1299
Ileum, 1291
Internal anal sphincter, 1300
Intestinal phase of secretion, 1290
Intestinointestinal reflex, 1299
Iron, 1298
Jejunum, 1291
Kupffer cell, 1304
Lacteal, 1291
Lamina propria, 1291
Large intestine, 1300
Lieberkühn crypts, 1300
Lipase, 1296
Lipolysis, 1296
Liver, 1303
Liver lobule, 1304
Lower esophageal sphincter (cardiac sphincter), 1285
Magnesium, 1298
Major duodenal papilla, 1304
Mesentery, 1291
Metabolic detoxification (biotransformation), 1308
Micelle, 1296
Microvillus, 1291
Motilin, 1287
Mouth, 1283
Mucosal barrier, 1289
Myenteric plexus (Auerbach plexus), 1283
O'Beirne sphincter, 1300

Oropharyngeal phase of swallowing, 1285
Pancreas, 1308
Pancreatic α-amylase, 1310
Pancreatic duct (Wirsung duct), 1308
Pancreatic lipase, 1310
Parietal cell (oxyntic cell), 1288
Pepsin, 1288
Pepsinogen, 1288
Peristalsis, 1285
Peritoneal cavity, 1291
Peritoneum, 1291
Phospholipase, 1296
Primary bile acid, 1305
Primary peristalsis, 1286
Pyloric sphincter, 1286
Pylorus, 1286
Rectum, 1301
Retropulsion, 1287
Saliva, 1283
Salivary α-amylase (ptyalin), 1284
Salivary gland, 1283
S cell, 1310
Secondary bile acid, 1305
Secondary peristalsis, 1286
Secretin, 1287
Sigmoid colon, 1300
Sinusoid, 1304
Small intestine, 1291
Sphincter of Oddi, 1308
Stomach, 1286
Submucosal plexus (Meissner plexus), 1283
Subserosal plexus, 1283
Swallowing, 1285
Teniae coli, 1300
Transverse colon, 1300
Trypsin, 1296
Trypsin inhibitor, 1310
Unconjugated bilirubin, 1307
Upper esophageal sphincter, 1285
Urobilinogen, 1307
Vermiform appendix, 1300
Villus, (pl., villi), 1291
Vitamin, 1298

REFERENCES

Berne, R. M. & Levy, M. N. (Eds.). (1993). *Principles of physiology* (3rd ed.). St. Louis: Mosby–Year Book.

Brocklehurst, J. C., Tallis, R. C., & Fillit, H. M. (1992). *Textbook of geriatric medicine and gerontology* (4th ed.). New York: Churchill-Livington.

Christensen, J. (1987). Motor functions of the pharynx and esophagus. In L. R. Johnson (Ed.), *Physiology of the gastrointestinal tract* (vol. 7) (pp. 600-601). New York: Raven Press.

Davenport, H. W. (1982). *Physiology of the digestive tract* (8th ed., p. 119). Chicago: Year Book Medical.

Helander, H. F., & Keeling, D. J. (1993). Cell biology of gastric acid secretion. *Baillieres Clinical Gastroenterology* 7(1):1-21.

Johnson, L. R. (1991). *Gastrointestinal physiology* (4th ed.). St. Louis: Mosby–Year Book.

Kvietys, P. R., Barrowman, J. A., & Granger, N. D. (1987). *Pathophysiology of the splanchnic circulation* (p. 5). Boca Raton, FL: CRC Press.

National Institutes of Health. (1991). Consensus development conference statement: Triglyceride, high-density lipoprotein, and coronary heart disease. Washington, DC: Author.

Phipps, W. J., Long, B. C., & Woods, W. F. (1987). *Medical surgical nursing: Concepts and clinical practice.* St. Louis: Mosby–Year Book.

Schauf, C. L., Moffett, D. F., & Moffett, S. B. (1990). *Human physiology: Foundations and frontiers.* St. Louis: Mosby–Year Book.

Seeley, R. S. Stephens, T. D., & Tate, P. (1992). *Anatomy and physiology* (2nd ed., p. 53). St. Louis: Mosby–Year Book.

Shamburek, R. D., & Farrar, J. T. (1990). Disorders of the digestive system in the elderly. *New England Journal of Medicine, 322*(7), 438-443.

Simopoulos, A. P. (1991). Omega-3 fatty acids in health and disease and in growth and development. *American Journal of Clinical Nutrition, 54,* 438-463.

Thibodeau, G. A., & Patton, G. A. (1992). *Structure and function of the body.* St. Louis: Mosby–Year Book.

Thompson, J. M., McFarland, G. K., Hirsch, J. E., & Tucker, S. M. (1993). *Mosby's clinical nursing* (ed. 3). St. Louis: Mosby–Year Book.

Trevisan, M., Krough, V., Freudenheim, J., Blake, A., Muti, P., Panico, S., Farinaro, E., Mancini, M., Menotti, A., & Ricci, G. (1990). Consumption of olive oil, butter, and vegetable oils and coronary heart disease risk factors. *Journal of the American Medical Association, 263,* 688.

Wolf, M. M., & Soll, A. H. (1988). The physiology of gastric acid secretion. *New England Journal of Medicine, 319*(26), 1707-1715.

SUGGESTED READINGS

Derek, P. M., & Sandstead, H. H. (1989). Nutrition and aging. In *Proceedings of the 1988 international conference on nutrition and aging.* New York: Liss.

Gordon, D. J., & Rifkind, B. M. (1989). High-density lipoprotein— The clinical implications of recent studies. *New England Journal of Medicine, 321*(19), 1311-1316.

Henry, J. B. (1991). *Clinical diagnosis and management of laboratory methods.* Philadelphia: Saunders.

Alterations of Digestive Function

Sue E. Huether
Kathryn L. McCance
Mary Suzanne Tarmina*

Chapter Outline

*Contributing author to first edition.

The gastrointestinal tract is a continuous, hollow organ that extends from the mouth to the anus. It includes the esophagus, stomach, small intestine (duodenum, jejunum, and ileum), large intestine (ascending, transverse, descending, and sigmoid colon), and rectum.

Disorders of the gastrointestinal tract disrupt one or more of its functions. Structural and neural abnormalities can slow, obstruct, or accelerate the movement of chyme at any level of the gastrointestinal tract. Inflammatory and ulcerative conditions of the gastrointestinal wall disrupt secretion, motility, and absorption. Many clinical manifestations of gastrointestinal tract disorders are nonspecific: that is, they can be caused by a variety of impairments. These manifestations are described in the next section.

DISORDERS OF THE GASTROINTESTINAL TRACT

Clinical Manifestations of Gastrointestinal Dysfunction

Anorexia

Anorexia is lack of a desire to eat despite physiologic stimuli that would normally produce hunger. Anorexia is a nonspecific symptom that is often associated with nausea, abdominal pain, and diarrhea. Disorders of other organ systems, including cancer, heart disease, and renal disease, are often accompanied by anorexia.

Vomiting

Vomiting is the forceful emptying of stomach and intestinal contents (chyme) through the mouth. Several types of stimuli initiate the vomiting reflex, including the presence of ipecac or copper salts in the duodenum; severe pain; distention of the stomach or duodenum; torsion or trauma affecting the ovaries, testes, uterus, bladder, or kidney; and activation of the chemoreceptor trigger zone in the medulla.

Nausea and retching usually precede vomiting. **Nausea** is a subjective experience that is associated with many different conditions. Specific neural pathways have not been identified with nausea. Hypersalivation and tachycardia are common associated symptoms. **Retching** begins with deep inspiration. The glottis closes, intrathoracic pressure falls, and the esophagus becomes distended. Simultaneously the abdominal muscles contract, creating a pressure gradient from abdomen to thorax. The lower esophageal sphincter and body of the stomach relax, but the duodenum and an-

trum of the stomach go into spasm. The reverse peristalsis and pressure gradient force chyme from the stomach and duodenum up into the esophagus. Because the upper esophageal sphincter is closed, chyme does not enter the mouth. As the abdominal muscles relax, the contents of the esophagus drop back into the stomach. This process may be repeated several times before vomiting occurs. A diffuse sympathetic discharge causes the tachycardia, tachypnea, and sweating that accompany retching and vomiting. The parasympathetic system mediates copious salivation, increased gastric motility, and relaxation of the upper and lower esophageal sphincters.

Vomiting usually follows retching. The duodenum and antrum of the stomach produce retrograde peristalsis, while the body of the stomach and esophagus relax. When the stomach is full of gastric contents, the diaphragm is forced high into the thoracic cavity by strong contractions of the abdominal muscles. The higher intrathoracic pressure forces the upper esophageal sphincter to open, and chyme is expelled from the mouth. Then the stomach relaxes and the upper part of the esophagus contracts, forcing the remaining chyme back into the stomach. The lower esophageal sphincter then closes. The cycle is repeated if there is a volume of chyme remaining in the stomach.

Spontaneous vomiting that is not preceded by nausea or retching is called **projectile vomiting**. Projectile vomiting is caused by direct stimulation of the vomiting center by neurologic lesions (e.g., tumors or aneurysms) involving the brainstem. The metabolic consequences of vomiting are fluid, electrolyte, and acid-base disturbances (see Chapter 3).

Constipation

Constipation is difficult or infrequent defecation. It is a common complaint caused by personal habits and a variety of disorders and drugs. Because patterns of bowel evacuation differ greatly among individuals, constipation must be individually defined. It usually means a decrease in the number of bowel movements per week, hard stools, and difficult evacuation. Normal bowel habits range from two or three evacuations per day to one per week.

Pathophysiology

Constipation can be caused by neurogenic disorders of the large intestine in which neural pathways are absent or degenerated. An example is Hirschsprung disease (congenital megacolon), the absence of ganglion cells in the myenteric plexus of the large intestine. Constipation is usually evident from birth, because the colon is incapable of the propulsive movements that move feces into the rectum (see Chapter 37). Other disorders associated with constipation include acquired megacolon (enlarged or dilated colon), multiple sclerosis, spinal cord trauma, and cerebrovascular disease.

Many functional or mechanical conditions can cause constipation. Muscle weakness or pain caused by abdominal surgery can impair or inhibit defecation. Normally the abdominal muscles are used to create the intraabdominal pressure required to evacuate the rectum. Weakness or pain can interfere with the generation of adequate intraabdominal pressure. Lesions of the anus, such as inflamed hemorrhoids, fissures, or fistulas, make defecation painful because of stretching. With the urge to defecate, the sphincter becomes hypertonic, and the stool is not eliminated.

A low-residue diet (the habitual consumption of highly refined foods) decreases the volume and number of stools and causes constipation. Increased consumption of cereals, fruits, and vegetables adds nonabsorbable fiber to the feces and is conducive to regular and easy evacuations.

A sedentary lifestyle and lack of regular exercise are frequent causes of constipation. Lack of access to toilet facilities and consistent suppression of the urge to empty the bowel are other causes. Depression often impairs bowel evacuation, partly because depressed individuals tend to be sedentary and lack the motivation to eat healthfully. The problem is made worse if antidepressant drugs (e.g., anticholinergics) are used to treat the depression. Anticholinergics block parasympathetic impulses in the gastrointestinal tract, thereby impairing motility.

Excessive use of antacids containing calcium carbonate or aluminum hydroxide often results in constipation. Opiates, particularly codeine, tend to inhibit bowel motility.

CAUSES OF CONSTIPATION

Megacolon (enlarged or dilated colon)
Abdominal muscle weakness
Painful anal lesions
Low-residue diet
Sedentary lifestyle
Delayed spontaneous defecation
Emotional depression
Selected drugs
  Opiates
  Anticholinergics
  Antacids (calcium carbonate, aluminum hydroxide)
Systemic diseases
  Hypothyroidism
  Diabetic neuropathy

Clinical Manifestations

Any change in bowel evacuation patterns may be significant. Changes such as less frequent defecation, smaller stool volume, difficulty in evacuating the rectum, or a feeling of bowel fullness and discomfort require investigation.

Evaluation and Treatment

The history and physical examination provide precise clues regarding the nature of constipation. Functional constipation, that is, constipation resulting from lifestyle or bowel habits, usually has a long history. Dysfunctional constipation is more likely to be sudden. Sudden-onset constipation can accompany the development of organic lesions and requires careful evaluation.

The individual's description of frequency, stool consistency, associated pain, and presence of blood is significant. Blood may be present as a result of bleeding hemorrhoids or a neoplastic lesion of the colon. Cramping abdominal pain may be symptomatic of partial bowel obstruction. In assessing frequency, it is important to discover whether evacuation was stimulated by enemas or cathartics (laxatives). Palpation discloses colonic distention, masses, and tenderness. Digital examination of the rectum is performed to assess sphincter tone and detect anal lesions. Proctosigmoidoscopy is used to visualize the lumen directly. A barium enema may be required if no lesions are directly visualized and symptoms continue after simple treatment.

The treatment for dysfunctional constipation is to manage the underlying lesion or disease. Management of functional constipation likewise depends on its cause. Treatment usually consists of bowel retraining, in which the individual establishes a satisfactory bowel evacuation routine without becoming preoccupied with bowel movements. The best time for defecation is during the period after a meal. The individual also may need to engage in moderate exercise, drink more fluids, and increase fiber intake. Bulk supplements (i.e., Metamucil or Konsyl), stool softeners, and laxative agents are useful for some individuals. Enemas can be used to establish bowel routine, but they should not be used habitually. Fluid instilled into the rectum causes distention, which stimulates propulsive movements and defecation. High colonic irrigations with large volumes of fluid should be avoided.

Diarrhea

Diarrhea is an increase in the frequency of defecation and the fluidity and volume of feces. Many factors determine stool volume and consistency, including water content of the colon and the presence of unabsorbed food, unabsorbable material, and intestinal secretions. Stool volume in the normal adult averages less than 200 g/day. Stool volume in children depends on age and size.

An infant may pass up to 100 g/day. The adult intestine processes approximately 9 L of luminal content per day: 2 L is ingested, and the remaining 7 L consists of intestinal secretions. Of this volume, 99% of the fluid is absorbed: 90% (7 to 8 L) in the small intestine and 9% (1 to 2 L) in the colon. Normally, approximately 150 ml water is excreted daily in the stool.

Pathophysiology

Diarrhea in which the volume of feces is increased is called large-volume diarrhea. Large-volume diarrhea generally is caused by excessive amounts of water or secretions or both in the intestines. Small-volume diarrhea, in which the volume of feces is not increased, usually results from excessive intestinal motility.

The three major mechanisms of diarrhea are osmotic, secretory, and motile. (Specific mechanisms of diarrhea in children are described in Chapter 37.)

In **osmotic diarrhea,** the presence of a nonabsorbable substance in the intestine causes it to be drawn into the lumen by osmosis. The excess water is retained in the intestine and, along with the nonabsorbable substance, increases stool weight and volume. This causes large-volume diarrhea. Lactase deficiency is the most common cause of osmotic diarrhea. In this condition, the nonabsorbable substance is milk sugar, or lactose. The intestine does not produce enough lactase, the lactose-digesting enzyme. Lactose remains in the intestinal lumen because it is not digested and absorbed (see p. 1339). Excessive ingestion of synthetic, nonabsorbable sugars (e.g., sorbitol) has a similar effect.

Secretory diarrhea is a form of large-volume diarrhea caused by excessive mucosal secretion of fluid and electrolytes. Primary stimuli of intestinal secretion are bacterial enterotoxins, particularly those released by cholera or strains of *Escherichia coli*. Secretory diarrhea can also be caused by neoplasms, such as gastrinoma or thyroid carcinoma. These tumors produce hormones that stimulate intestinal secretion.

Large-volume diarrhea also can result from excessive motility of the intestine. The cause is usually a lesion that impairs autonomic control of motility, such as diabetic neuropathy. Excessive motility decreases transit time, mucosal surface contact, and opportunities for fluid absorption. Therefore, a larger volume of stool reaches the rectum, producing urgency and frequency of elimination.

Small-volume diarrhea is usually caused by an inflammatory disorder of the intestine, such as ulcerative colitis or Crohn disease. Inflammation of the colon causes cramping pain, urgency, and frequency. Small-volume diarrhea can also be caused by fecal impaction, a severe form of constipation. In this case, the diarrhea consists of secretions (mucus and fluid) produced by the colon to lubricate the impacted feces and move it toward the

anal canal. These secretions flow around the impaction and cause low-volume, secretory diarrhea.

Motility diarrhea is caused by resection of the small intestine, surgical bypass of an area of the intestine, or fistula formation between loops of intestine. Food is not mixed properly and there is impaired digestion and increased motility.

Clinical Manifestations

Diarrhea can be acute or chronic, depending on its cause. Systemic effects of prolonged diarrhea are dehydration, electrolyte imbalance, and weight loss. Manifestations of acute bacterial or viral infection include fever, with or without cramping pain. Fever, cramping pain, and bloody stools accompany diarrhea caused by inflammatory bowel disease. Steatorrhea (fat in the stools) and diarrhea are common signs of malabsorption syndromes.

Evaluation and Treatment

A thorough history is taken to document the onset and frequency of diarrhea. Exposure to contaminated food or water is indicated if the individual has traveled in foreign countries or areas where drinking water might be contaminated. Iatrogenic diarrhea is suggested if the individual has undergone abdominal radiation therapy, intestinal resection, or treatment with selected drugs (e.g., antibiotics, diuretics, antihypertensives, or laxatives). Physical examination helps the clinician to identify underlying systemic disease. Stool culture, examination of stool specimens for blood, abdominal x-ray films, and intestinal biopsies provide more specific data.

Treatment for diarrhea includes restoration of fluid and electrolyte balance, management of distressing symptoms, and treatment of causal factors. In older adults and children, dehydration and electrolyte imbalance may be severe and require intravenous fluid therapy. Nutritional deficiencies need to be corrected in cases of chronic diarrhea or malabsorption. Substances that solidify stools decrease frequency and water content. Natural bran and commercial preparations of psyllium, such as Konsyl and Metamucil, are inexpensive and effective treatments for mild diarrhea. Opium alkaloids such as Lomotil suppress motility, relieve cramping, and reduce stool volume and frequency.

Abdominal Pain

Abdominal pain is the presenting symptom of a number of gastrointestinal diseases. (The physiology of pain is described in Chapter 13.) The causal mechanisms of abdominal pain are mechanical, inflammatory, or ischemic. Generally the abdominal organs are not sensitive to mechanical stimuli, such as cutting, tearing, or crushing. These organs are, however, sensitive to stretching and distention, which activate nerve endings in both hollow and solid structures. The onset of pain is associated with rapid distention; gradual distention causes little pain. Traction on the peritoneum caused by adhesions, distention of the common bile duct, or forceful peristalsis resulting from intestinal obstruction causes pain because of increased tension. Capsules that surround solid organs, such as the liver and gallbladder, contain pain fibers that are stimulated by stretching if these organs swell.

Biochemical mediators of the inflammatory response, such as histamine, bradykinin, and serotonin, stimulate organic nerve endings and produce abdominal pain. The edema and vascular congestion that accompany chemical, bacterial, or viral inflammation also cause painful stretching. Obstruction of blood flow from the distention of bowel obstruction or mesenteric vessel thrombosis produces the pain of ischemia, and increased concentrations of tissue metabolites stimulate pain receptors.

Abdominal pain can be parietal (somatic), visceral, or referred. **Parietal pain** arises from the parietal peritoneum. This pain is more localized and intense than visceral pain, which arises from the organs themselves. Nerve fibers from the parietal peritoneum travel with peripheral nerves to the spinal cord, and the sensation of pain corresponds to skin dermatomes T_6 and L_1. Parietal pain lateralizes because, at any particular point, the parietal peritoneum is innervated from only one side of the nervous system.

Visceral pain arises from a stimulus acting on an abdominal organ. It is usually felt near the midline in the epigastrium (upper midabdomen), midabdomen, or lower abdomen. The pain is poorly localized and is dull rather than sharp. Its location is generally related to the corresponding skin dermatomes of the affected organ. Visceral pain is diffuse and vague because nerve endings in abdominal organs are sparse and multisegmented. Pain arising from the stomach, for example, is experienced as a sensation of fullness, cramping, or gnawing in the midepigastric area.

Referred pain is visceral pain felt at some distance from a diseased or affected organ. Referred pain is usually well localized and is felt in skin or deeper tissues that share a central afferent pathway with the affected organ. Generally referred pain develops as the intensity of a visceral pain stimulus increases. Intense gallbladder pain is, for example, referred to the back between the scapulae (shoulder blades). The pain may begin as a vague discomfort in the right epigastric region and then, as inflammation worsens, progress to a sharp, localized, referred pain between the shoulder blades.

Gastrointestinal Bleeding

Numerous disorders cause bleeding in the gastrointestinal tract. Upper **gastrointestinal bleeding,** which is de-

fined as bleeding in the esophagus, stomach, or duodenum, is commonly caused by bleeding varices (varicose veins) in the esophagus, peptic ulcers, or a Mallory-Weiss tear at the esophageal gastric junction from severe retching. Lower gastrointestinal bleeding, or bleeding from the jejunum, ileum, colon, or rectum, can be caused by polyps, inflammatory disease, cancer, or hemorrhoids. Acute, severe gastrointestinal bleeding is life-threatening. Mortality depends on the volume and rate of blood loss, associated disease, age, and effectiveness of treatment.

The signs of gastrointestinal bleeding are defined in Table 36-1. Acute blood loss is usually characterized by **hematemesis** (the presence of blood in the vomitus), **hematochezia** (frank bleeding from the rectum), or **melena** (dark, tarry stools). **Occult bleeding** is usually caused by slow, chronic blood loss that results in iron-deficiency anemia as iron stores in the bone marrow are slowly depleted. Physiologic response to gastrointestinal bleeding depends on the amount and rate of the loss (Fig. 36-1). Changes in blood pressure and heart rate are the best indicators of massive blood loss in the gastrointestinal tract. Blood losses of 1000 ml or more over a short time cause a decrease in cardiac output, a decrease in systolic and diastolic blood pressure, and an increase in pulse rate. With losses of 1000 ml or more, the heart rate is greater than 100 beats/min and systolic blood pressure is less than 100 mm Hg. During the early stages of blood volume depletion, the peripheral vascular compartment constricts to shunt blood to vital organs, including the brain (see Chapter 26). A sign that this is

TABLE 36-1

Presentations of Gastrointestinal Bleeding

Presentations	Definition
Acute bleeding	
Hematemesis	Bloody vomitus; either fresh, bright red blood or dark, grainy digested blood with "coffee grounds" appearance
Melena	Black, sticky, tarry, foul-smelling stools caused by digestion of blood in the gastrointestinal tract
Hematochezia	Fresh, bright red blood passed from the rectum
Occult bleeding	Trace amounts of blood in normal-appearing stools or gastric secretions; detectable only with a guaiac test

FIG. 36-1 Pathophysiology of gastrointestinal (GI) bleeding.

happening is postural hypotension, a drop in blood pressure that occurs with a change from the recumbent position to a sitting or upright position, lightheadedness, and loss of vision. If blood loss continues, hypovolemic shock progresses. Diminished blood flow to the kidneys causes decreased urine output and may lead to oliguria (low urine output), tubular necrosis, and renal failure. Ultimately, insufficient cerebral and coronary blood flow causes irreversible anoxia and death.

The accumulation of blood in the gastrointestinal tract is irritating and increases peristalsis, causing diarrhea. If bleeding is from the lower gastrointestinal tract, the diarrhea is frankly bloody. Bleeding from the upper gastrointestinal tract also can be rapid enough to produce bright red stools, but generally some digestion of the blood components will have occurred, producing melena. The digestion of blood proteins originating from massive upper gastrointestinal bleeding is reflected by an increase in blood urea nitrogen (BUN) levels (Fig. 36-1).

The hematocrit and hemoglobin values are not the best indicators of acute gastrointestinal bleeding because plasma and red cell volume are lost proportionately. As the plasma volume is replaced, the hematocrit and hemoglobin values begin to reflect the extent of blood loss. The interpretation of these values is modified to account for exogenous replacement of fluids and the hydration status of the tissues.

Disorders of Motility
Dysphagia
Pathophysiology

Dysphagia is difficulty swallowing. It can result from mechanical obstruction of the esophagus or a disorder that impairs esophageal motility. Mechanical obstructions can be intrinsic or extrinsic. Intrinsic obstructions originate in the wall of the esophageal lumen. Tumors, strictures, and diverticular herniations (outpouchings) are all causes of intrinsic mechanical obstruction. Extrinsic mechanical obstructions originate outside the esophageal lumen and narrow the esophagus by pressing inward on the esophageal wall. The most common cause of extrinsic mechanical obstruction is tumor.

Functional dysphagia is caused by neural or muscular disorders that interfere with voluntary swallowing or peristalsis (Merlo & Cohen, 1988). Disorders that affect the striated muscles of the upper esophagus interfere with the oropharyngeal (voluntary) phase of swallowing. Typical causes of functional dysphagia in the upper esophagus are dermatomyositis (a muscle disease) and neurologic impairments caused by cerebrovascular accidents, Parkinson disease, or achalasia.

Achalasia is a form of dysphagia that impairs (1) peristalsis of smooth muscle in the middle and lower portions of the esophagus and (2) lower esophageal sphinc-

ter (LES) functioning. Achalasia results from neural dysfunction, probably a decrease in the number of ganglion cells in the myenteric plexus and atrophy of smooth muscle cells or lesions along the vagus nerve. Disrupted innervation results in loss of neuromuscular coordination and muscle tone at the lower end of the esophagus. The three mechanisms that impair swallowing are decreased peristalsis of the middle esophagus, loss of tone in the lower esophageal sphincter, and decreased relaxation of the lower esophageal sphincter after swallowing. Food accumulates above the obstruction and distends the esophagus (Fig. 36-2). As hydrostatic pressure increases, food is slowly forced past the obstruction into the stomach.

Clinical Manifestations

Clinical manifestations of dysphagia vary according to the cause and location of the obstruction. Distention and spasm of the esophageal muscles during eating or drinking may cause a mild or severe stabbing pain at the level of obstruction. Discomfort occurring 2 to 4 seconds after swallowing is associated with upper esophageal obstruction. Discomfort occurring 10 to 15 seconds after swallowing is more common in obstructions of the lower esophagus. If the cause of obstruction is a growing tumor, dysphagia begins with difficulty swallowing solids and advances to difficulty swallowing semisolids and liquids (McCallum, 1987). If the cause is loss of motor function, dysphagia is experienced with both solids and liquids. Regurgitation of undigested food, unpleasant taste, vomiting, and weight loss are common man-

FIG. 36-2 Achalasia. Decreased muscle tone and peristaltic function prevent food from entering the stomach, causing esophageal distention. (From Phipps, Long, Woods, & Cassmeyer, 1991.)

ifestations of all types of dysphagia. Aspiration of esophageal contents can lead to pneumonia.

Evaluation and Treatment

Knowledge of the patient's history and clinical manifestations contributes significantly to a diagnosis of dysphagia. A barium swallow is used to visualize the contours of the esophagus and identify structural defects. Manometry documents the duration and amplitude of abnormal pressure changes associated with obstruction or loss of neural regulation. Esophageal endoscopy is performed to examine the esophageal mucosa and obtain biopsy specimens.

The individual is taught to manage symptoms by eating slowly, eating small meals, taking fluid with meals, and sleeping with the head elevated to prevent regurgitation and aspiration. Anticholinergic drugs, such as dicyclomine (Bentyl), may alleviate achalasia. Definitive treatments include mechanical dilation of the esophageal sphincter and surgical separation of the lower esophageal muscles with a longitudinal incision (myotomy). Myotomy widens the passage into the stomach.

Gastroesophageal Reflux

Gastroesophageal reflux is the reflux of chyme from the stomach to the esophagus. The lower esophageal sphincter may relax spontaneously and transiently 1 to 2 hours after eating, permitting gastric contents to regurgitate into the esophagus. The acid is usually neutralized and cleared from the esophagus by peristaltic action within 1 to 3 minutes and sphincter tone is restored. Gastroesophageal reflux that does not cause symptoms is known as physiologic reflux. In some individuals, however, a combination of factors causes an inflammatory response to reflux called **reflux esophagitis.**

Pathophysiology

Normally the resting tone of the lower esophageal sphincter maintains a zone of high pressure that prevents gastroesophageal reflux. In individuals who develop reflux esophagitis, this pressure tends to be lower than normal (Gelfand, 1991). Vomiting, coughing, lifting, or bending that increases abdominal pressure can contribute to the development of reflux esophagitis. The severity of the esophagitis depends on the composition of the gastric contents and the length of time they are in contact with the esophageal mucosa. If the chyme is highly acidic or contains bile salts and pancreatic enzymes, reflux esophagitis can be severe. In individuals with weak esophageal peristalsis, refluxed chyme remains in the esophagus longer than usual. This increases the amount of time the esophageal mucosa is exposed to acids, bile, and enzymes. Finally, delayed gastric emptying contributes to reflux esophagitis by (1) lengthening the period during which reflux is possible and (2)

increasing the acid content of chyme. Disorders that delay emptying include gastric or duodenal ulcers, which can cause pyloric edema; strictures that narrow the pylorus; and hiatal hernia, which can weaken the lower esophageal sphincter.

Reflux esophagitis causes inflammatory responses in the esophageal wall, such as hyperemia, increased capillary permeability, edema, tissue fragility, and erosion. Fibrosis and thickening may develop.

Clinical Manifestations

The clinical manifestations of reflux esophagitis are heartburn and regurgitation of acidic chyme within an hour of eating. The symptoms worsen if the individual lies down or if intraabdominal pressure increases (e.g., as a result of coughing, vomiting, or straining at stool). Edema, fibrosis, esophageal spasm, or decreased esophageal motility may result in dysphagia. Alcohol or acid-containing foods, such as citrus fruits, can cause discomfort during swallowing.

Evaluation and Treatment

Diagnosis of reflux esophagitis is based on clinical manifestations, esophageal endoscopy that shows edema and erosion, and a 24-hour monitor of acidity near the LES. A barium swallow is used to identify associated conditions, such as hiatal hernia, gastric ulcers, and abnormal contours of the esophageal lumen.

Antacids relieve symptoms by neutralizing gastric contents. Weight reduction and cessation of smoking also help to alleviate symptoms. Cimetidine (or another H_2 blocker) may be used to decrease nocturnal acid secretion; sucralfate will coat ulcerated tissue; smooth muscle stimulants, such as bethanechol chloride (Urecholine) or metoclopramide (Reglan), can increase lower esophageal sphincter gastric motility and rate of gastric emptying. If other treatments fail, or if erosive esophagitis fails to heal, the lower esophageal sphincter may be narrowed surgically.

Hiatal Hernia
Pathophysiology

Hiatal hernia is the protrusion (herniation) of the upper part of the stomach through the diaphragm and into the thorax. There are two types of hiatal hernia: (1) sliding (direct) hiatal hernia and (2) paraesophageal (rolling) hiatal hernia (Fig. 36-3). **In sliding hiatal hernia** the stomach slides or moves into the thoracic cavity through the esophageal hiatus, an opening in the diaphragm for the esophagus and vagus nerves. A congenitally short esophagus, trauma, or weakening of the diaphragmatic muscles at the gastroesophageal junction contributes to the hernia. While the individual is in the supine position, the lower esophagus and stomach are pulled into the thorax. Standing causes the stomach to "slide" back

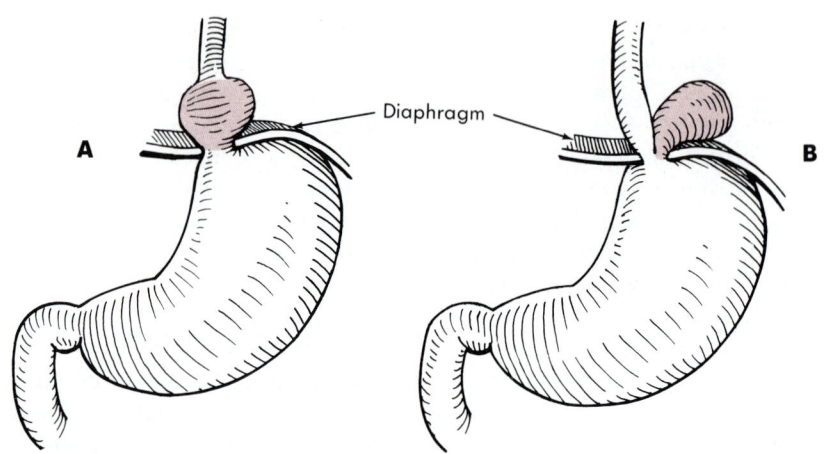

FIG. 36-3 **Types of hiatal hernia. A,** In sliding hiatal hernia the visceral peritoneum remains intact and restrains the size of the hernia. **B,** In paraesophageal hernia, the membrane becomes thinned out or defective, allowing a true peritoneal sac to protrude into the posterior mediastinum, where negative intrathoracic pressure causes it to enlarge. (From Phipps, Long, Woods, & Cassmeyer, 1991.)

into the abdomen. Sliding hiatal hernia is exacerbated by factors that increase intraabdominal pressure. Therefore, coughing, bending, tight clothing, ascites, or pregnancy accentuates the hernia. This type of hernia is associated with gastroesophageal reflux and esophagitis because the hernia diminishes the resting pressure of the lower esophageal sphincter. In pregnant women with sliding hiatal hernia, progesterone and estrogen may lower the resting pressure of the lower esophageal sphincter further.

Paraesophageal hiatal hernia (rolling hiatal hernia) is herniation of the greater curvature of the stomach through a secondary opening in the diaphragm (Fig. 36-3). As the stomach protrudes through the opening into the thorax, it lies alongside the esophagus. The gastroesophageal junction remains below the diaphragm. With paraesophageal hernia, reflux is uncommon. The position of a portion of the stomach above the diaphragm, however, causes congestion of mucosal blood flow and can lead to gastritis and ulcer formation. A mechanical strangulation of the hernia is a major complication. Strangulation occludes blood vessels and causes vascular engorgement, edema, ischemia, and hemorrhage. Hiatal hernias of both types tend to occur in conjunction with several other diseases, including peptic ulcer, cholecystitis (gallbladder inflammation), cholelithiasis (gallstones), chronic pancreatitis, and diverticulosis.

Clinical Manifestations

Hiatal hernias are often asymptomatic. Generally a wide variety of symptoms develop later in life and are associated with other gastrointestinal disorders as well.

Manifestations of the different types of hiatal hernia are difficult to distinguish and include gastroesophageal reflux, dysphagia, heartburn, and epigastric pain. Regurgitation and substernal discomfort after eating are common.

Evaluation and Treatment

Diagnostic procedures include barium x-rays and endoscopy. A chest x-ray film often will show the protrusion of the stomach into the thorax, indicating paraesophageal hiatal hernia.

Treatment for sliding hiatal hernia is usually conservative. The individual can diminish reflux by eating small, frequent meals and avoiding the recumbent position after eating. Abdominal supports and tight clothing are avoided, and weight control is recommended for obese individuals. Antacids alleviate reflux esophagitis. Anticholinergic drugs are contraindicated because they relax the lower esophageal sphincter and delay gastric emptying. Individuals who are uncomfortable at night benefit from sleeping in a semi-Fowler position. Surgery (fundoplication) may be performed if medical management fails to control symptoms.

Pyloric Obstruction
Pathophysiology

Pyloric obstruction is the narrowing or blocking of the opening between the stomach and the duodenum. This condition can be congenital (see Chapter 37) or acquired. Acquired obstruction is caused by peptic ulcer disease or carcinoma near the pylorus. Duodenal ulcers are more likely than gastric ulcers to obstruct the pylorus. Ulceration causes obstruction resulting from inflammation, edema, spasm, fibrosis, or scarring. Tumors cause obstruction by growing into the pylorus.

Clinical Manifestations

Early in the course of pyloric obstruction, the individual experiences vague epigastric fullness, which becomes more distressing after eating and later in the day. Nausea and epigastric pain may occur as the muscles of the stomach contract in attempts to force chyme past the obstruction. These symptoms disappear when the chyme finally moves into the duodenum. As obstruction progresses, anorexia develops, sometimes accompanied by weight loss. Severe obstruction causes gastric distention and atony (lack of muscle tone and gastric motility). Gastric distention stimulates gastric secretion, which increases the feeling of fullness. Rolling or jarring of the abdomen produces a sloshing sound called the succussion splash. At this stage vomiting is a cardinal sign of obstruction. It is usually copious and occurs several hours after eating. The vomitus contains undigested food but no bile. Prolonged vomiting leads to dehydration, which is accompanied by a hypokalemic and hypochloremic metabolic alkalosis caused by loss of potassium and gastric acid. Because food does not enter the intestine, stools are infrequent and small. Prolonged pyloric obstruction causes malnutrition, dehydration, and extreme debilitation.

Evaluation and Treatment

Diagnosis is based on clinical manifestations, a history of ulcer disease, and examination of residual gastric contents. Endoscopy is performed if gastric carcinoma is the suggested cause of pyloric obstruction. Barium studies are contraindicated because the barium may harden and be retained in the stomach.

Obstructions resulting from ulceration often resolve with conservative management. A large-bore tube is used to aspirate stomach contents and relieve distention. Then nasogastric suction is maintained for 2 to 3 days to decompress the stomach and restore normal motility. Gastric secretions that contribute to inflammation and edema can be suppressed with intravenous cimetidine. Fluids and electrolytes (saline and potassium) are given intravenously to effect rehydration and correct hypokalemia and alkalosis (see Chapter 3). Severely malnourished individuals may require parenteral hyperalimentation (intravenous nutrition). Surgery may be required to treat gastric carcinoma or persistent obstruction caused by fibrosis and scarring.

Intestinal Obstruction

Intestinal obstruction can be caused by any condition that prevents the normal flow of chyme through the intestinal lumen (Table 36-2). Criteria for classifying intestinal obstruction are summarized in Table 36-3. Intestinal obstruction is classified by cause as simple or

TABLE 36-2

Common Causes of Intestinal Obstruction

Cause	Pathophysiology
Hernia	Protrusion of the intestine through a weakness in the abdominal muscles or through the inguinal ring
Intussusception	Telescoping of one part of the intestine into another; this usually causes strangulation of the blood supply; more common in infants 10-15 months of age than in adults
Torsion (volvulus)	Twisting of the intestine on its mesenteric pedicle, with occlusion of the blood supply; often associated with fibrous adhesions; occurs most frequently in middle-aged and elderly men
Diverticulosis	Inflamed saccular herniations (diverticuli) of the mucosa and submucosa through the tunica muscularis of the colon; diverticuli are interspersed between thick, circular, fibrous bands; most common in obese individuals older than 60 years of age
Tumor	Tumor growth into the intestinal lumen; adenocarcinoma of the colon and rectum is the most common tumoral obstruction; most common in individuals older than 60 years of age
Paralytic (adynamic) ileus	Loss of peristaltic motor activity in the intestine; associated with abdominal surgery, peritonitis, hypokalemia, ischemic bowel, spinal trauma, or pneumonia

TABLE 36-3

Classification of Intestinal Obstruction

Criteria for classification	Definition
Onset	
Acute	Sudden onset; often caused by torsion, intussusception, or herniation
Chronic	Protracted onset; more commonly from tumor growth or progressive formation of strictures
Extent of obstruction	
Partial	Incomplete obstruction of intestinal lumen
Complete	Complete obstruction of intestinal lumen
Location of obstructing lesion	
Intrinsic	Obstruction develops within intestinal lumen; examples: luminal edema or hemorrhage, foreign bodies (gallstones), tumors, or intraluminal fibrosis
Extrinsic	Obstruction originates outside the intestine; examples: tumors, torsion, fibrosis, hernia, intussusception
Effects on intestinal wall	
Simple	Luminal obstruction without impairment of blood supply
Strangulated	Luminal obstruction with occlusion of blood supply
Closed loop	Obstruction at each end of a segment of the intestine
Causal factors	
Mechanical	Blockage of the intestinal lumen by intrinsic or extrinsic lesions; usually treated surgically
Functional (paralytic ileus)	Paralysis of the intestinal musculature due to trauma, peritonitis, electrolyte imbalances, or spasmolytic agents; usually treated surgically

functional. Simple obstruction is mechanical blockage of the lumen by a lesion; functional obstruction is a failure of motility. Simple obstruction of the small intestine is the most common type of intestinal obstruction. Acute obstructions usually have mechanical causes, such as adhesions or hernias. Chronic or partial obstructions are more often associated with tumors or inflammatory disorders, particularly of the large intestine. Common causes of intestinal obstruction in children are presented in Chapter 37.

Pathophysiology

The consequences of intestinal obstruction are related to its onset and location and the length of intestinal tract proximal to the obstruction. The major pathophysiologic alterations are presented in Fig. 36-4. Usually the first symptoms of obstruction result from distention and the loss of fluids and electrolytes. Distention begins almost immediately, as gases and fluids accumulate proximal to the obstruction. The major source of gas is swallowed air, but some is contributed by bacterial fermentation. Distention decreases the intestine's ability to absorb water and electrolytes and increases the net secretion of these substances into the lumen. Within 24 hours, up to 8 L of fluid and electrolytes enters the lumen in the form of saliva, gastric juice, bile, pancreatic juice, and intestinal secretions. Copious vomiting or sequestration of fluids in the intestinal lumen prevents their reabsorption and produces severe fluid and electrolyte disturbances. Extracellular fluid volume and plasma volume decrease, causing dehydration. Hemoconcentration (decreased plasma volume) elevates hematocrit, decreases central venous pressure, and causes tachycardia. Severe dehydration leads to hypovolemic shock.

If the obstruction is at the pylorus or high in the small intestine, metabolic alkalosis develops initially as a result of excessive loss of hydrogen ions that normally would be reabsorbed from the gastric juice. With prolonged obstruction or obstruction lower in the intestine, metabolic acidosis is more likely to occur because bicarbonate from pancreatic secretions and bile cannot be reabsorbed. Hypokalemia can be extreme, promoting acidosis and atony of the intestinal wall. Metabolic acidosis also may be accentuated by ketosis, the result of declining carbohydrate stores caused by starvation. If

FIG. 36-4 Pathophysiology of intestinal obstruction.

pressure from the distention is severe enough, it occludes the arterial circulation and causes strangulation. Lack of circulation permits the buildup of significant amounts of lactic acid, which worsen the metabolic acidosis.

Clinical Manifestations

Signs and symptoms of intestinal obstruction are consistent with the pathophysiology. Colicky pains followed by vomiting are the cardinal symptoms. Typically the pain occurs intermittently. Pain intensifies for seconds or minutes as a peristaltic wave of muscle contraction meets the obstruction. The passing of the wave is followed by a pain-free interval. With severe distention, the pain may diminish in intensity. If strangulation occurs, the pain loses its colicky character, becoming more constant and severe as ischemia progresses to necrosis or perforation.

Vomiting and distention vary, depending on the level of the obstruction. Obstruction at the pylorus causes early, profuse vomiting of clear gastric fluid. Obstruction in the proximal small intestine causes mild distention and vomiting of bile-stained fluid. Obstruction lower in the intestine causes more pronounced distention because a greater length of intestine is proximal to the obstruction. In this case vomiting may not occur or may occur later and contain fecal material. Partial obstruction can cause diarrhea or constipation, but complete obstruction usually causes constipation only. Complete obstruction increases the number of bowel sounds, which may be tinkly and accompanied by peristaltic rushes and crampy, abdominal pain. Signs of dehydration, hypovolemia, and metabolic acidosis may be observed as early as 24 hours after the occurrence of complete obstruction. Distention may be severe enough to push against the diaphragm and decrease lung volume. This can lead to atelectasis and pneumonia, particularly in debilitated individuals.

Evaluation and Treatment

Evaluation is based on clinical manifestations. Successful management requires early identification of the site and type of obstruction. Replacement of fluid and electrolytes and decompression of the lumen with gastric or intestinal suction are essential forms of therapy. Immediate surgical intervention is required for strangulation and complete obstruction.

Gastritis

Gastritis is an inflammatory disorder of the gastric mucosa. It can be acute or chronic and affect the fundus or antrum or both. **Acute gastritis** erodes the surface epithelium in a diffuse or localized pattern. The erosions are usually superficial.

The cause of acute gastritis is usually injury of the protective mucosal barrier by drugs or chemicals. Anti-inflammatory drugs, such as aspirin and indomethacin, are known to cause gastritis, perhaps because they inhibit prostaglandins, which normally stimulate the secretion of mucus. Alcohol, histamine, digitalis, and metabolic disorders such as uremia are contributing factors. The clinical manifestations of acute gastritis can include vague abdominal discomfort, epigastric tenderness, and bleeding. Healing usually occurs spontaneously within a few days. Discontinuing injurious drugs, using antacids, or decreasing acid secretion with cimetidine facilitates healing.

Chronic gastritis is a progressive disease that tends to occur in elderly individuals. Chronic gastritis causes thinning and degeneration of the stomach wall. The gastric mucosa becomes thin, and the muscle layers atrophy. Chronic gastritis is classified as type A (fundal) or type B (antral), depending on the pathogenesis and location of the lesions.

Chronic fundal gastritis, also called atrophic gastritis, is the most severe type. The gastric mucosa degenerates extensively in the body and fundus of the stomach, leading to gastric atrophy. Loss of chief cells and parietal cells diminishes secretion of pepsinogen, hydrochloric acid, and intrinsic factor. Because acid secretion is insufficient, the feedback mechanism that normally inhibits gastrin secretion is impaired, causing elevated plasma levels of gastrin. Pernicious anemia develops because intrinsic factor is unavailable to facilitate vitamin B_{12} absorption.

A significant number of individuals with chronic fundal gastritis have antibodies to parietal cells, intrinsic factor, and gastric cells in their sera, suggesting that an

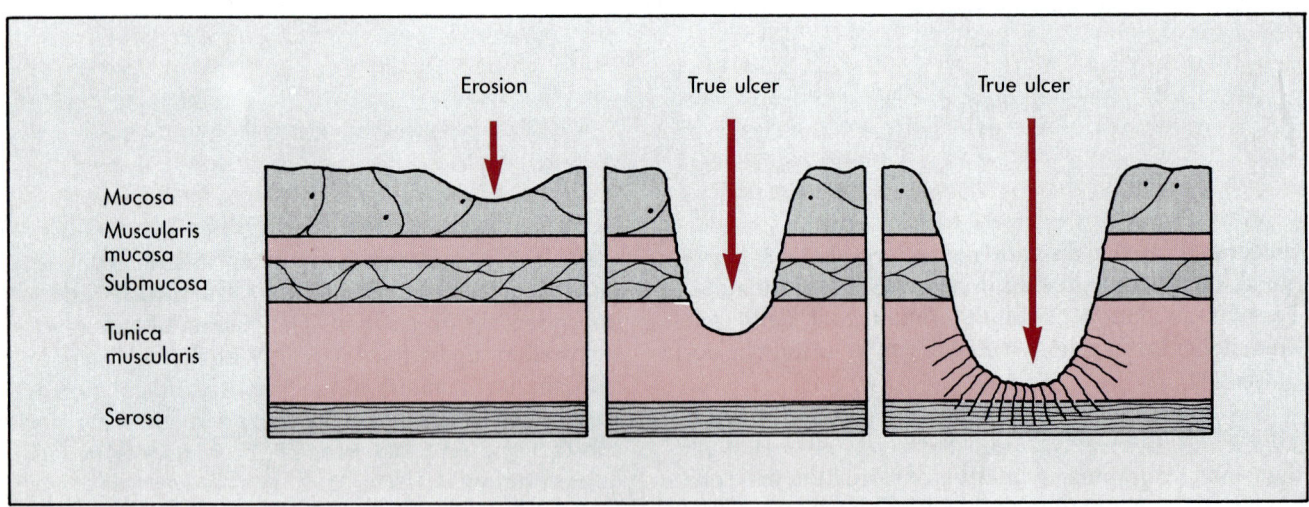

FIG. 36-5 Lesions caused by peptic ulcer disease.

autoimmune mechanism is involved in pathogenesis of the disease. The fact that chronic fundal gastritis occurs in association with other autoimmune diseases, such as diabetes, Addison disease, and thyroid disease, strengthens this association. Chronic fundal gastritis is a risk factor for gastric carcinoma, particularly in individuals who develop pernicious anemia.

Chronic antral gastritis generally involves the antrum only and is approximately four times more frequent than fundal gastritis. It is not associated with decreased hydrochloric acid secretion, pernicious anemia, or presence of parietal cell antibodies. *Helicobacter pylori* is a major causative factor associated with the inflammation of chronic gastritis (Collins, 1992). Mucosal atrophy is a rare finding. In approximately 10% of cases, antibodies to gastrin-secreting cells are found in the serum. Chronic reflux of bile may contribute to the gastritis by persistently disrupting the mucosal barrier (Fig. 36-5).

Signs and symptoms of chronic gastritis often do not correlate with the severity of the disease. Gastroscopic examination and biopsy may show a long-standing inflammatory process and gastric atrophy in an individual with no history of abdominal distress. Failure to stimulate acid secretion confirms achlorhydria (diminished secretion of hydrochloric acid). The gastric secretions also can be evaluated for the presence of intrinsic factor. Individuals may report vague symptoms, including anorexia, fullness, nausea, vomiting, and epigastric pain. Gastric bleeding may be the only clinical manifestation of gastritis.

Symptoms can usually be managed with smaller meals; a soft, bland diet; and avoidance of alcohol and aspirin. Vitamin B_{12} is administered to correct pernicious anemia.

Peptic Ulcer Disease

Normally, the gastric and duodenal mucosa is protected from acid and pepsin by mucus and bicarbonate that are secreted by surface epithelial cells, and by cellular tight junctions that prevent back-diffusion of acid. A **peptic ulcer** is a break, or ulceration, in the protective mucosal lining of the lower esophagus, stomach, or duodenum. Such breaks expose submucosal areas to gastric secretions and autodigestion. Peptic ulcers can be acute or chronic, superficial or deep. Superficial ulcerations are called erosions because they erode the mucosa but do not penetrate the muscularis mucosae (Fig. 36-5). True ulcers extend through the muscularis mucosae and damage blood vessels, causing hemorrhage, or perforate the gastrointestinal wall.

Risk factors for peptic ulcer disease are smoking and habitual use of nonsteroidal antiinflammatory drugs (NSAIDs), or alcohol. Some chronic diseases, such as emphysema, rheumatoid arthritis, and cirrhosis, are associated with the development of peptic ulcers. Infec-

tion of the gastric and duodenal mucosa with *H. pylori* also is proposed as a cause of peptic ulcers (Ateshkadi, Lam, & Johnson, 1993). Psychologic stress may be a risk factor for peptic ulcer disease, although studies of life stress and ulcer disease are inconclusive. Individuals with multiple stressors, poor coping skills, and persistent anxiety and depression in the presence of recurrent peptic ulcers may require psychiatric management (Schineller & Ramchandani, 1991). The exact mechanism of causation is not known.

Duodenal Ulcers

Duodenal ulcers occur with greater frequency than other types of peptic ulcers. The incidence of duodenal ulcers is approximately the same among men and women (Schineller & Ramchandani, 1991). Duodenal ulcers tend to develop in younger persons and in individuals with type O blood.

Pathophysiology

Hypersecretion of acid and pepsin is the primary cause of duodenal ulcers, but inadequate secretion of bicarbonate by the duodenal mucosa also may be a factor. Other factors that contribute to ulcer formation are:

1. A greater than usual number of parietal cells (acid-secreting cells) in the gastric mucosa
2. High serum gastrin levels that remain high longer than normal after eating and continue to stimulate secretion of acid (may be caused by *H. pylori*)
3. Failure of the feedback mechanism whereby acid in the gastric antrum inhibits gastrin release
4. Rapid gastric emptying, which overwhelms the buffering capacity of the bicarbonate-rich pancreatic secretions
5. Alteration in the protective mucosal layer (may be caused by *H. pylori*)
6. *H. pylori* may release a toxin that promotes inflammation and ulceration (McQuaid & Isenberg, 1992; Tytgat et al., 1993)
7. Use of NSAIDs
8. Cigarette smoking
9. Decreased mucosal bicarbonate secretion

All of these factors, singly or in combination, cause acid and pepsin concentrations in the duodenum to penetrate the mucosal barrier and cause ulceration (Fig. 36-6).

Clinical Manifestations

The characteristic manifestation of a duodenal ulcer is chronic intermittent pain in the epigastric area. The pain begins 2 or 3 hours after eating, when the stomach is empty. It is not unusual for pain to occur in the middle of the night and disappear by morning. The pain results from sensorineural stimulation by acid, muscle spasm, or both. Pain is relieved rapidly by ingestion of food or antacids, creating a typical "pain-food-relief" pattern.

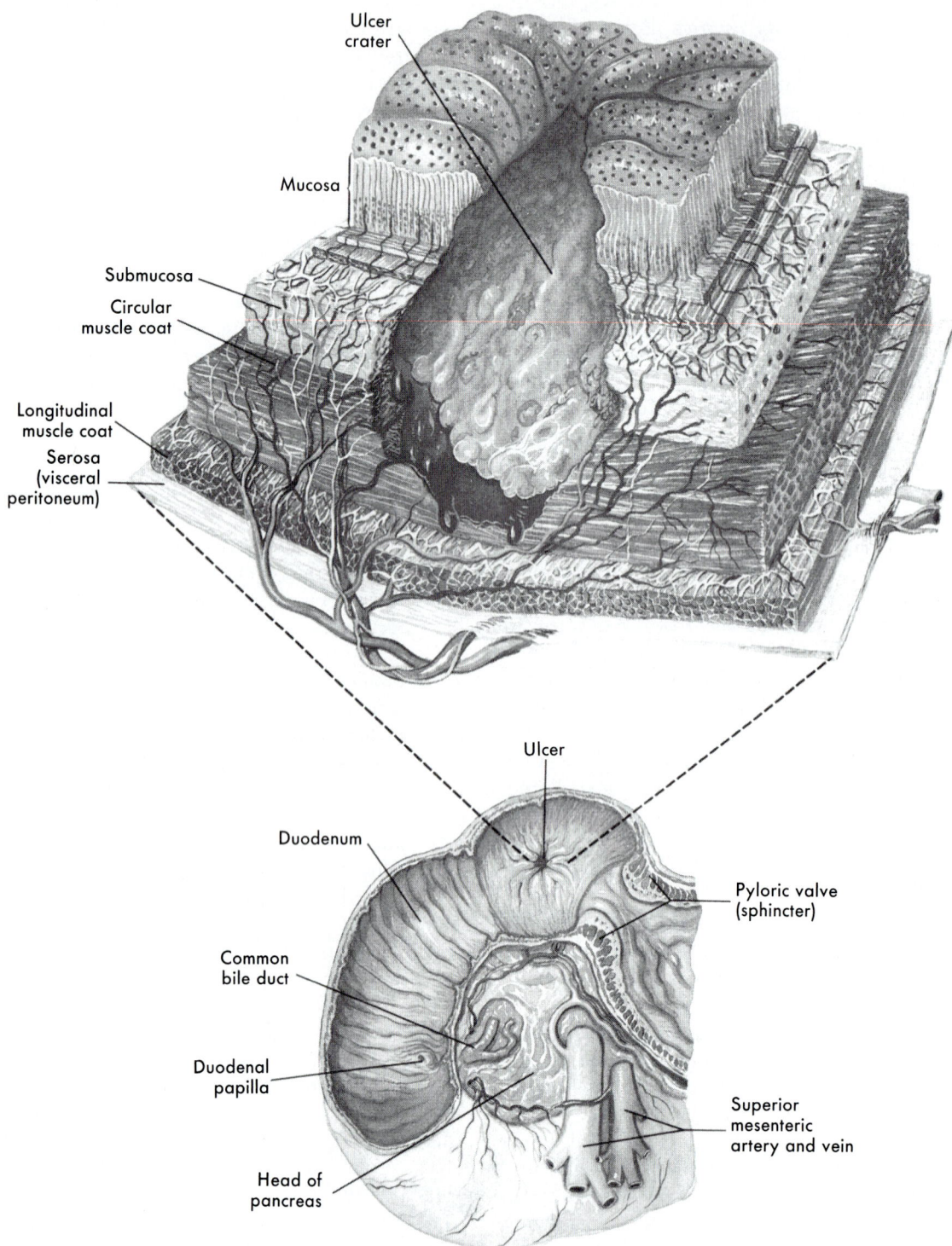

FIG. 36-6 Duodenal ulcer. The illustration depicts a deep ulceration in the duodenal wall extending as a crater through the entire mucosa and into the muscle layers. (From Thibodeau. [1993]. *Anatomy and physiology*. St. Louis: Mosby–Year Book.)

Some individuals with duodenal ulcer may have no symptoms; the first manifestation may be hemorrhage or perforation.

Duodenal ulcers often heal spontaneously but recur within months. Exacerbations tend to develop in the spring and fall. Healing is accompanied by relief of pain. Constant, unremitting pain may be caused by complications, such as intestinal obstruction or perforation. Bleeding from duodenal ulcers causes hematemesis or melena.

Evaluation and Treatment

Several diagnostic approaches are used to differentiate duodenal ulcers from gastric ulcers or gastric carcinoma. Barium x-ray films may show an anatomic deformity created by the ulcer crater. If the x-ray examination is inconclusive, flexible endoscopic evaluations may be performed. Radioimmune assays of gastrin levels are evaluated to identify ulcers associated with gastric carcinomas.

Management of duodenal ulcers is aimed at relieving the causes and effects of hyperacidity. Antacids neutralize gastric contents, elevate pH, inactivate pepsin, and relieve pain. Acid secretion can be suppressed with drugs (e.g., cimetidine) that block histamine (H_2) receptors and inhibit the secretion of acid. Omeprazole inhibits acid production and may have bacteriologic action on *H. pylori*. Triple therapy with bismuth, metronidazole, and either amoxicillin or tetracycline for *H. pylori* produces better clinical outcomes (Ateshkadi et al., 1993). Ulcer-coating agents, such as sucralfate and colloidal bismuth, promote healing. Anticholinergic drugs may be used to inhibit gastric secretion, suppress gastric motility, and delay gastric emptying. Surgical resection may be required for bleeding or perforating ulcers.

Gastric Ulcers

Gastric ulcers are ulcers of the stomach. They occur about equally in males and females, usually between the ages of 55 and 65 years, and are about one fourth as common as duodenal ulcers (Table 36-4).

Pathophysiology

Generally gastric ulcers develop in the antral region, adjacent to the acid-secreting mucosa of the body. The primary defect is an abnormality that increases the muco-

---

TABLE 36-4

Characteristics of Gastric and Duodenal Ulcers

Characteristics	Gastric ulcer	Duodenal ulcer
Incidence		
Age at onset	50-70 years	20-50 years
Family history	Usually negative	Positive
Sex (prevalence)	Equal in women and men	Greater in men
Stress factors	Increased	Average
Ulcerogenic drugs	Normal use	Increased use
Cancer risk	Increased	Not increased
Pathophysiology		
Abnormal mucus	May be present	May be present
Parietal cell mass	Normal or decreased	Increased
Acid production	Normal or decreased	Increased
Serum gastrin	Increased	Normal
Serum pepsinogen	Normal	Increased
Associated gastritis	More common	Usually not present
Helicobacter pylori	May be present (60%-80%)	Often present (95%-100%)
Clinical manifestations		
Pain	Located in upper abdomen	Located in upper abdomen
	Intermittent	Intermittent
	Pain-antacid-relief pattern	Pain-antacid or food-relief pattern
	Food-pain pattern	Nocturnal pain common
Clinical course	Chronic ulcer without pattern of remission and exacerbation	Pattern of remissions and exacerbations for years

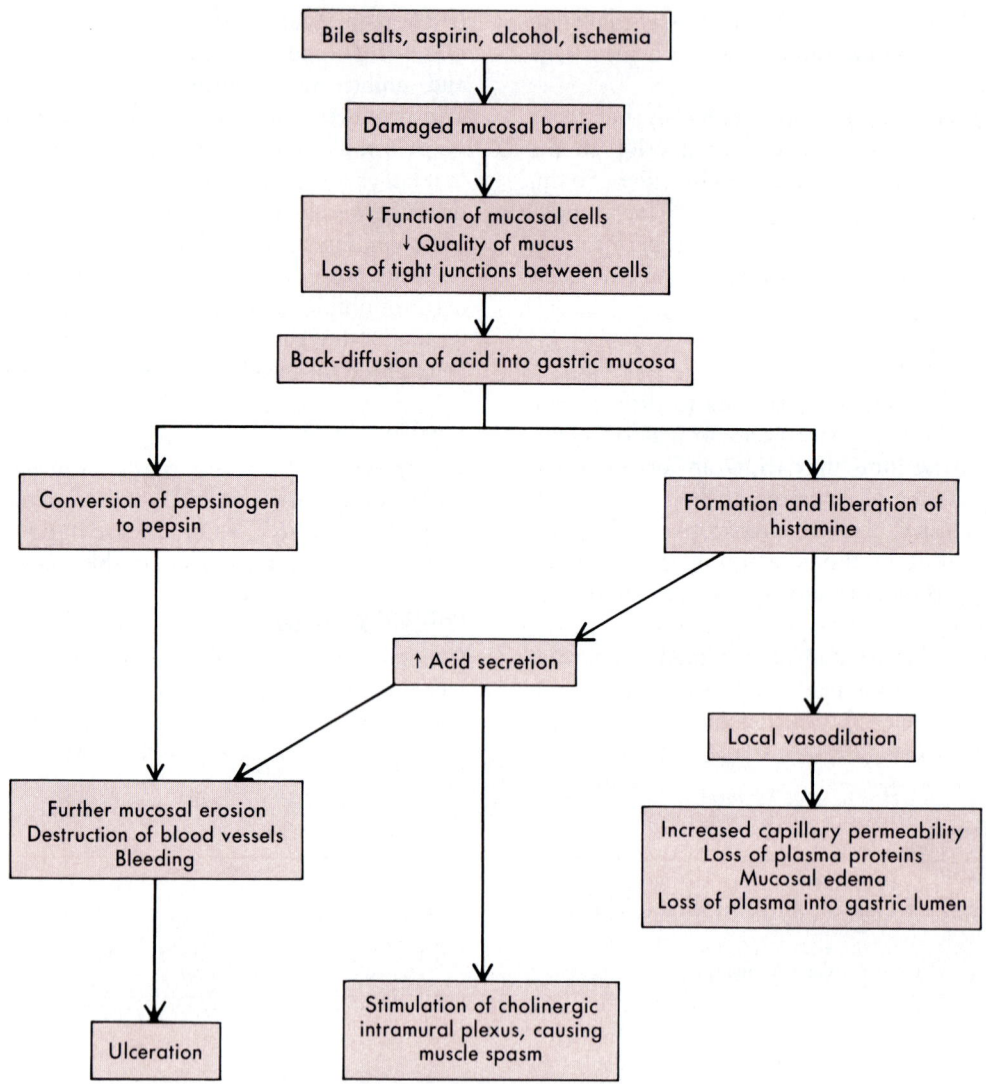

FIG. 36-7 Pathophysiology of gastric ulcer formation.

sal barrier's permeability to hydrogen ions. Gastric secretion may be normal or less than normal.

Chronic gastritis is often associated with development of gastric ulcers and may precipitate ulcer formation by limiting the mucosa's ability to secrete a protective layer of mucus (Fig. 36-7). Decreased mucosal synthesis of prostaglandin may be one factor causing decreased mucus secretion (Miller & Victor, 1990).

Other factors associated with gastric ulcer development include duodenal reflux of bile and use of ulcerogenic drugs (aspirin and indomethacin). Reflux of bile is caused by loss of tone at the pyloric sphincter. The pyloric sphincter may fail to respond to stimuli that normally increase resting tone, such as entry of acid, protein, and fat into the duodenum.

An increased concentration of bile salts disrupts the gastric mucosa; this disruption may decrease the electrical potential across the gastric mucosal membrane. The break damages the mucosal barrier by permitting hydrogen ions to diffuse into the mucosa, where they disrupt permeability and cellular structure. A vicious cycle can be established as the damaged mucosa liberates histamine, which stimulates the increase of acid and pepsinogen production, blood flow, and capillary permeability. The disrupted mucosa becomes edematous and loses plasma proteins. Destruction of small vessels causes bleeding.

Clinical Manifestations

The clinical manifestations of gastric ulcers are similar to those of duodenal ulcers (Table 36-4). The pattern of "pain-food-relief" is common, but the pain of gastric ulcers also may occur immediately after eating. Another difference is that gastric ulcers tend to be chronic rather than alternate between periods of remission and exacerbation. Gastric ulcers also cause more anorexia, vomiting, and weight loss than duodenal ulcers. The evaluation and treatment of gastric ulcers are similar to the evaluation and treatment of duodenal ulcers.

Stress Ulcers

A **stress ulcer** is an acute form of peptic ulcer that tends to accompany severe illness, systemic trauma, or neural injury. Usually multiple sites of ulceration are distributed within the stomach or duodenum. Decreased mucosal blood flow is an important contributing event in stress ulcer formation (Durham & Shapiro, 1991). Stress ulcers may be classified as ischemic ulcers and Cushing ulcers.

Ischemic ulcers develop within hours of an event, such as hemorrhage, multisystem trauma, severe burns, heart failure, or sepsis, that causes ischemia of the stomach and duodenal mucosa. Stress ulcers that develop as a result of burn injury are frequently called **Curling ulcer.**

The shock, anoxia, and sympathetic responses produced by the precipitating event decrease mucosal blood flow, leading to ischemia. Because the metabolism of the mucosal cells declines as a result of lack of arterial blood, the mucosal lining degenerates. Acid diffuses back into the mucosa, causing inflammation, ulceration, hemorrhage, and necrosis. The ulcerative process is accelerated if bile or pancreatic enzymes are regurgitated from the duodenum.

Cushing ulcer is a stress ulcer associated with severe head trauma or brain surgery. This ulcer results from decreased mucosal blood flow and hypersecretion of acid caused by overstimulation of the vagal nuclei. Excessive acid damages the mucosal barrier, initiating the processes summarized in Fig. 36-7.

The primary clinical manifestation of stress ulcers is bleeding. Other symptoms may not be present. The bleeding may be slight or, if a small vessel is perforated, amount to hundreds of milliliters. Use of prophylactic antacids, H_2 receptor blockers, and suppression of vagal stimulation with anticholinergic drugs are effective forms of therapy. Stress ulcers seldom become chronic.

Ulcer Disease

Advances in the medical treatment of peptic ulcer disease have reduced the number of cases requiring surgery to 10% to 15%. Despite this small percentage, clinicians care for a significant number of individuals who undergo upper gastrointestinal surgery and experience long-term complications. The most common indications for ulcer surgery are recurrent or uncontrolled bleeding and perforation of the stomach or duodenum. The primary objectives of surgical treatment are to reduce stimuli for acid secretion, decrease the number of acid-secreting cells in the stomach, and correct complications of ulcer disease (Table 36-5).

Acute complications of gastrectomy or anastomosis, such as poor wound healing, abscess formation, or suture failure, are relatively uncommon except in the debilitated person. Chronic complications, however, occur more often and are likely to develop if a large portion

TABLE 36-5

Surgical Management of Peptic Ulcer Disease

Procedure	Definition	Purpose
Neural surgery		
Vagotomy	Severance of the vagus nerve	Eliminate neural stimulus of acid secretion
Selective vagotomy	Severance of vagal branches supplying acid-secreting (parietal) cells	Eliminate neural stimulus of acid secretion
Gastric surgery		
Pyloroplasty	Surgical widening or removal of obstruction of the pylorus	Facilitate gastric emptying
Antrectomy (partial gastrectomy)	Removal of the antrum	Eliminate hormonal stimulus of acid secretion; that is, the gastrin-secreting cells of the antral mucosa
Subtotal gastrectomy	Removal of most of the body and all of the antrum of the stomach	Remove acid-secreting and gastrin-secreting mucosa
Anastomosis (Billroth operation)	Reattachment of stomach to duodenum (Billroth I) or jejunum (Billroth II)	Restore continuity of the gastrointestinal tract after resection

of the stomach has been removed. These complications and their pathophysiologic mechanisms are described in the next section.

Postgastrectomy Syndromes

Postgastrectomy syndromes are a group of signs and symptoms that occur after gastric resection. They are caused by changes in motor and control functions of the stomach and upper small intestine (Eagon, Miedema, & Kelly, 1992).

Dumping syndrome

Dumping syndrome is the rapid emptying of hypertonic chyme from the surgically residual stomach into the small intestine 10 to 20 minutes after eating. It occurs with varying severity in 5% to 10% of individuals who have undergone partial gastrectomy or pyloroplasty. It is not common in individuals who have undergone a Billroth II anastomosis accompanied by vagotomy. Factors that promote dumping syndrome include (1) loss of gastric capacity, (2) loss of emptying control when the pylorus is removed, and (3) loss of feedback control by the duodenum when it is removed. Rapid gastric emptying and creation of a high osmotic gradient within the small intestine cause a sudden shift of fluid from the vascular compartment to the intestinal lumen. Plasma volume decreases, causing vasomotor responses, such as increased pulse rate, hypotension, weakness, pallor, sweating, and dizziness. Rapid distention of the intestine produces a feeling of epigastric fullness, cramping, nausea, vomiting, and diarrhea.

A less common form of dumping syndrome, termed late dumping syndrome, occurs 1 to 2 hours after eating. The symptoms include weakness, diaphoresis, and confusion, but they cannot be explained by rapid gastric emptying. After a high-carbohydrate meal, individuals who have undergone gastrectomy may develop hypoglycemia, which causes the symptoms. The hypoglycemia is caused by an increase in insulin secretion stimulated by the hyperglycemia that follows eating. Other hormonal responses may also participate in the development of hypoglycemia.

Most cases of dumping syndrome respond well to dietary management. Frequent small meals that are high in protein and low in carbohydrates relieve symptoms. Other measures include drinking fluids between meals instead of at mealtime and reclining on the left side after eating. Some cases require surgical intervention including reconstruction of the pylorus or a gastrojejunostomy (Eagon et al., 1992).

Alkaline reflux gastritis

Alkaline reflux gastritis is a stomach inflammation caused by reflux of bile and alkaline pancreatic secretions that contain proteolytic enzymes and disrupt the mucosal barrier. This form of gastritis occurs in 5% to 20% of individuals who have undergone gastrectomy or pyloroplasty. Clinical manifestations include nausea, bilious vomiting (vomiting in which the vomitus contains bile), and sustained epigastric pain that worsens after eating and is not relieved by antacids. Endoscopy shows a hemorrhagic and friable gastric mucosa. Conservative management is often difficult because antacids do not consistently improve symptoms. Avoidance of use of aspirin and alcohol may decrease gastric irritation, and a low-fat diet may limit bile secretion. Surgical correction may ultimately be required.

Afferent loop obstruction

Afferent loop obstruction is an unusual problem that may occur after gastrojejunostomy (Billroth II; Table 36-5). The problem is caused by volvulus, hernia, adhesion, or stenosis in the duodenal stump on the proximal side of the gastrojejunostomy. Partial obstruction causes bile and pancreatic secretions to accumulate and distend the loop. Obstruction also causes delayed emptying. The symptoms of afferent loop obstruction include intermittent severe pain and epigastric fullness after eating. Vomiting usually relieves symptoms. Conservative management consists of a low-fat diet. Surgical correction is required for complete obstruction.

Diarrhea

Diarrhea is one of the most common long-term alterations caused by gastric surgery. Diarrhea can accompany dumping syndrome or occur as a solitary symptom. Two forms of diarrhea can occur after gastrectomy. The first is the frequent, persistent elimination of liquid stool. The second is the intermittent, precipitous, and unpredictable elimination of a large volume of stool. Both types can be either mild or severe. Postgastrectomy diarrhea appears to be related to rapid gastric emptying, particularly after intake of large amounts of high-carbohydrate liquids, which increase the osmotic gradient and attract water into the intestinal lumen. Small, dry meals and anticholinergic drugs are effective control measures.

Weight loss

Weight loss frequently follows gastric resection. Inadequate food intake is a common cause, because many individuals cannot tolerate carbohydrates or a normal-sized meal. Foods may be poorly absorbed because the stomach is less able to mix, churn, and break down food particles. Vomiting, diarrhea, and malabsorption of fats also contribute to weight loss.

Anemia

Anemia after gastrectomy results from iron, vitamin B_{12}, or folate deficiency. Iron malabsorption may be caused by decreased acid secretion. Acid changes iron from a trivalent to a divalent molecule, making it easier to absorb. Iron absorption is also compromised in individuals who have undergone a Billroth II procedure because the duodenum is no longer available to absorb iron.

Vitamin B_{12} deficiency may occur several years after gastrectomy. Contributing factors include loss of parietal cells, which secrete intrinsic factor. (Intrinsic factor facilitates absorption of vitamin B_{12}; see Chapter 35.) Vitamin B_{12} absorption is also compromised if gastric contents are not mixed adequately with pancreatic enzymes, as may occur after Billroth II anastomosis.

Folate deficiency is related to poor intake or malabsorption. Management of deficiencies consists of replacement of iron and folate with supplements. Vitamin B_{12} can be administered monthly by injection.

Malabsorption Syndromes

Malabsorption syndromes interfere with nutrient absorption in the small intestine. Historically malabsorption disorders have been classified as maldigestion or malabsorption. **Maldigestion** is failure of the chemical processes of digestion that take place in the intestinal lumen or at the brush border of the intestinal mucosa. **Malabsorption** is the failure of the intestinal mucosa to absorb (transport) the digested nutrients. Frequently maldigestion and malabsorption are interrelated or occur together, making classification difficult. Generally, however, maldigestion is caused by deficiencies of enzymes, such as pancreatic lipase or intestinal lactase, that are necessary for digestion. Inadequate secretion of bile salts and inadequate reabsorption of bile in the ileum also contribute to maldigestion. Malabsorption is the result of mucosal disruption caused by gastric or intestinal resection, vascular disorders, or intestinal disease.

Pancreatic Insufficiency

The pancreatic enzymes (lipase, amylase, trypsin, and chymotrypsin) are required for the digestion of proteins, carbohydrates, and fats. **Pancreatic insufficiency** is the deficient production of these enzymes by the pancreas. Causes of pancreatic insufficiency include chronic pancreatitis, pancreatic carcinoma, pancreatic resection, and cystic fibrosis. Significant damage to or loss of pancreatic tissue must occur before enzyme levels decrease sufficiently to cause maldigestion. Although pancreatic insufficiency causes poor digestion of all nutrients, fat maldigestion is the chief problem. Salivary amylase and enzymes secreted by the intestinal brush border assist in carbohydrate and protein digestion, but these enzymes do not digest fats. Absence of pancreatic bicarbonate in the duodenum and jejunum causes an acidic pH that worsens maldigestion by preventing activation of pancreatic enzymes that are present. A large amount of fat in the stool (steatorrhea) is the most common sign of pancreatic insufficiency.

Lactase Deficiency

Deficiency of disaccharidase at the brush border of the small intestine is caused by a congenital defect in which a single enzyme, usually lactase, is lacking. **Lactase deficiency** inhibits the breakdown of lactose (milk sugar) into monosaccharides and therefore prevents lactose digestion and absorption across the intestinal wall. Lactase deficiency is most common in blacks. The deficiency usually does not develop until adulthood. Secondary (acquired) lactase deficiency can be caused by several diseases of the intestine, including gluten-sensitive enteropathy (see Chapter 37), enteritis, and bacterial overgrowth.

The undigested lactose remains in the intestine, where bacterial fermentation causes gases to form. Undigested lactose also increases the osmotic gradient in the intestine, causing irritation and osmotic diarrhea. Clinical manifestations of lactase deficiency are bloating, crampy pain, diarrhea, and flatulence. The disorder is diagnosed by a lactose-tolerance test. Avoiding milk and adhering to a lactose-free diet relieve symptoms.

Bile Salt Deficiency

Conjugated bile acids (bile salts) are necessary for the digestion and absorption of fats. Bile salts are conjugated in the bile that is secreted from the liver. When bile enters the duodenum, the bile salts aggregate with fatty acids and monoglycerides to form micelles. Micelle formation solubilizes fat molecules and allows them to pass through the unstirred layer at the brush border (see Chapter 35). A minimum concentration of bile salts, termed the critical micelle concentration, is required to allow micelles to form. Therefore, conditions that decrease the production or secretion of bile result in decreased micelle formation and fat malabsorption. These conditions include advanced liver disease, which decreases production of bile salts; obstruction of the common bile duct, which decreases flow of bile into the duodenum; intestinal stasis (lack of motility), which permits overgrowth of intestinal bacteria that deconjugate bile salts; and diseases of the ileum, which prevent the reabsorption and recycling of bile salts (enterohepatic circulation).

Clinical manifestations of bile salt deficiency are related to poor intestinal absorption of fat and fat-soluble vitamins (A, D, E, K). Increased fat in the stools (steatorrhea) leads to diarrhea and decreased plasma proteins. The losses of fat-soluble vitamins and their effects include the following:

1. Vitamin A deficiency results in night blindness.
2. Vitamin D deficiency results in decreased calcium

absorption with bone demineralization (osteoporosis), bone pain, and fractures.

3. Vitamin K deficiency prolongs prothrombin time, leading to spontaneous development of purpura (bruising) and petechiae.
4. Vitamin E deficiency has uncertain effects but may cause testicular atrophy and neurologic defects in children.

The most effective treatment for fat-soluble vitamin deficiency is to increase medium-chain triglycerides in the diet, for example, by using coconut oil for cooking. Vitamins A, D, and K are given parenterally.

Ulcerative Colitis

Ulcerative colitis is a chronic inflammatory disease that causes ulceration of the colonic mucosa, usually in the rectum and sigmoid colon. The lesions appear in susceptible individuals between 20 and 40 years of age. Risk factors include family history of disease and Jewish descent, and the disease is more prevalent among white populations.

Although the cause of ulcerative colitis is unknown, infectious, genetic, and immunologic factors are all suggested causes (Selby, 1993). The hypothesis that inflammation is caused by infectious agents is not supported by consistent identification of specific viruses or bacteria in affected individuals. The familial tendency to develop ulcerative colitis and the occurrence of disease in identical twins support a genetic theory of causation. Perhaps most significant are immunologic factors associated with the disease. Anticolon antibodies have been identified in the sera of individuals with ulcerative colitis. Lymphocytes (T cells) in individuals with ulcerative

FIG. 36-8 **Chronic ulcerative colitis.** (From Kissane, 1990.)

colitis may have cytotoxic effects on the epithelial cells of the colon. Furthermore, autoimmune disorders, such as systemic lupus erythematosus and erythema nodosum, often accompany ulcerative colitis.

Pathophysiology

The primary lesion of ulcerative colitis begins with inflammation at the base of the crypt of Lieberkühn in the large intestine. The disease is most severe in the rectum and sigmoid colon. The mucosa is hyperemic and may appear dark red and velvety (Fig. 36-8). Small erosions form and coalesce into ulcers. Abscess formation, necrosis, and ragged ulceration of the mucosa ensue. Edema and thickening of the muscularis mucosae may narrow the lumen of the involved colon. Mucosal destruction causes bleeding, cramping pain, and urge to defecate. Frequent diarrhea, with passage of small amounts of blood and purulent mucus, is common. Loss of the absorptive mucosal surface and decreased colonic transit time cause large volumes of watery diarrhea.

Clinical Manifestations

The course of ulcerative colitis consists of intermittent periods of remission and exacerbation. Clinical manifestations vary with the severity and extent of disease. Mild ulcerative colitis involves less mucosa, so that frequency of bowel movements, bleeding, and pain are minimal. Severe forms may involve the entire colon and are characterized by fever, elevated pulse rate, frequent diarrhea (10 to 20/day), urgency, obviously bloody stools, and continuous, crampy pain. Dehydration, weight loss, anemia, and fever result from fluid loss, bleeding, and inflammation. Complications include anal fissures, hemorrhoids, and perirectal abscess. Severe hemorrhage is rare, but chronic blood loss can precipitate hypotension and shock. Edema, strictures, or fibrosis can obstruct the colon. Perforation is an unusual but possible complication. The risk of colon cancer increases significantly after 10 years of ulcerative colitis.

Evaluation and Treatment

Diagnosis of ulcerative colitis is based on the medical history and clinical manifestations. Sigmoidoscopy shows an inflamed and hemorrhagic mucosa. A barium enema and x-ray films may show loss of haustra, ulceration, and irregular mucosa. The laboratory data include low hemoglobin values, hypoalbuminemia, and low serum potassium levels. Infectious causes are ruled out by stool culture. The symptoms of ulcerative colitis are very similar to those of Crohn disease, making differential diagnosis difficult.

Treatment depends on the severity of symptoms and the extent of mucosal involvement. The disease is often treated with sulfasalazine (a combination of a sulfa drug and aspirin). Steroids and salicylates suppress the inflammatory response and help to alleviate the cramping pain. Broad-spectrum antibiotics may be prescribed if bacterial infection is suggested. Severe, unremitting disease can require hospital admission and administration of intravenous fluids. Extreme malnutrition may require intravenous hyperalimentation. Surgical resection of the colon or a colostomy may be performed if other forms of therapy are unsuccessful (Hastings & Weber, 1993).

Crohn Disease

Crohn disease (granulomatous colitis or regional enteritis) is an inflammatory disorder that affects both the large and small intestines. In a small percentage of cases, Crohn disease is difficult to differentiate from ulcerative colitis (Table 36-6). The rectum is seldom involved, and the development of colon cancer is rare. Risk factors and theories of causation are the same as those for ulcerative colitis. Like ulcerative colitis, Crohn disease tends to run in families. Ten percent to 20% of affected individuals have a positive family history. Increased suppressor T cell activity and alterations in IgA production are the immunologic factors associated with Crohn dis-

ease. Psychologic stresses have been suggested as a cause of both inflammatory bowel diseases. Although stressful events may exacerbate illness, stress is probably not a cause of disease.

Pathophysiology

The inflammation process of Crohn disease begins in the intestinal submucosa and spreads inward and outward to involve the mucosa and serosa. The ascending and transverse colon is the most common site of the disease, but both the large and small intestine may be involved. The inflammation can affect some haustral segments but not others, creating a pattern called "skip lesions." One side of the intestinal wall may be affected and not the other.

The ulcerations of Crohn disease produce fissures that extend inflammation into lymphoid tissue. The typical lesion is a granuloma having projections of inflamed tissue surrounded by fibrous scarring. (Granulomas are described in Chapter 7.) Fistulas may form in the perianal area between loops of intestine or extend into the bladder.

TABLE 36-6

Features of Ulcerative Colitis and Crohn Disease

Feature	Ulcerative colitis	Crohn disease
Incidence		
Age at onset	Any age; 10-40 years most common	Any age; 10-30 years most common
Family history	Less common	More common
Gender (prevalence)	Equal in women and men	About equal in women and men
Cancer risk	Increased	Not increased
Pathophysiology		
Location of lesions	Large intestine, no "skip" lesions	Large or small intestine, "skip" lesions common
Inflammation and ulceration	Mucosal layer involved	Entire intestinal wall involved
Granulomas	Rare	Common
Friable mucosa	Common	Less common
Anal and perianal fistulas and abscesses	Rare	Common
Narrowed lumen and possible obstruction	Rare	Common
Clinical manifestations		
Abdominal pain	Mild to severe	Mild to severe
Diarrhea	Common	Common
Bloody stools	Common	Less common
Abdominal mass	Rare	Common
Small intestinal malabsorption	Rare	Common
Steatorrhea	Rare	Common
Clinical course	Remissions and exacerbations	Remissions and exacerbations

Clinical Manifestations

Individuals with Crohn disease may have no specific symptoms other than an "irritable bowel" for several years. Nonbloody diarrhea is the most common sign. Other manifestations are related to the location and extent of intestinal involvement. Inflammation of the ileum, for example, causes tenderness in the lower right side of the abdomen. Weight loss and lower abdominal pain accompany Crohn disease. If the ileum is involved, the individual may be anemic as a result of malabsorption of vitamin B_{12}. There also may be deficiencies in folic acid and vitamin D absorption. Proteins also may be lost, leading to hypoalbuminemia.

Evaluation and Treatment

The diagnosis and treatment of Crohn disease are similar to the diagnosis and treatment of ulcerative colitis. Surgery is generally performed to manage complications such as fistula, abscess, or relief of obstruction (Fazio, 1990).

Diverticular Disease

Diverticula are herniations or saclike outpouchings of mucosa through the muscle layers of the colon wall (Fig. 36-9). **Diverticulosis** is asymptomatic diverticular disease. **Diverticulitis** represents inflammation. Diverticular disease is most common in the elderly, particularly in those who live in developed countries where much of the diet consists of refined foods.

Pathophysiology

Although diverticula can occur anywhere in the gastrointestinal tract, the most frequent site is the sigmoid colon. The diverticula form at weak points in the colon wall, usually where arteries penetrate the tunica muscularis to nourish the mucosal layer. A common associated finding is thickening of the circular and longitudinal (teniae coli) muscles surrounding the diverticula. Hypertrophy and contraction of these muscles increase intraluminal pressure and degree of herniation. Habitual consumption of a low-residue diet reduces fecal bulk, thus reducing the diameter of the colon. According to the Law of Laplace (see Chapter 26), wall pressure increases as the diameter of a cylindrical structure decreases. Therefore, pressure within the narrow lumen can increase enough to rupture the diverticula. Diverticulitis can cause abscess formation or peritonitis (Jones, 1992b).

Clinical Manifestations

Symptoms of diverticular disease may be vague or absent. Cramping pain of the lower abdomen can accompany constriction of the hypertrophied colonic muscles. Diarrhea, constipation, distention, or flatulence may occur. If the diverticula become inflamed or abscesses form, the individual develops fever, leukocytosis (increased white blood cell count), and tenderness of the lower left quadrant. Severe complications, such as hemorrhage, peritonitis, bowel obstruction, and fistula formation, are rare.

FIG. 36-9 Multiple diverticula in resected section of the colon. Weak spots in the muscle layers of the intestinal wall permitted the mucosa to bulge outward (herniate) into the pelvic cavity. (From Rosai, 1989.)

Evaluation and Treatment

Diverticula are often discovered during diagnostic procedures performed for other problems. Sigmoidoscopy permits direct observation of the lesions. Barium enema reveals the muscle hypertrophy, but there is some risk that the barium will become trapped in the diverticula and form hard masses.

An increase of dietary fiber intake frequently relieves symptoms. Surgical resection may be required if there are severe complications.

Appendicitis

Appendicitis is an inflammation of the vermiform appendix, which is a projection from the apex of the cecum. It is the most common surgical emergency of the abdomen and affects 7% to 12% of the population. The most common occurrence is between 20 and 30 years of age, although it may develop at any age.

Pathophysiology

The exact mechanism of the cause of appendicitis is controversial. Obstruction of the lumen with stool, tumors, or foreign bodies with consequent bacterial infection is the most common theory. The obstructed lumen does not allow drainage of the appendix, and, as mucosal secretion continues, intraluminal pressure increases. The resultant increased pressure decreases mucosal blood flow and the appendix becomes hypoxic. The mucosa ulcerates, promoting bacterial or other microbial invasion with further inflammation and edema. Inflammation may involve the distal or entire appendix. Gangrene develops from thrombosis of the luminal blood vessels, followed by perforation (Jones, 1992a).

Clinical Manifestations

Epigastric or periumbilical pain is the typical symptom of an inflamed appendix. The pain may be vague at first, increasing in intensity over a period of 3 to 4 hours. It may subside and then recur with a shift of location to the right lower quadrant. Right lower quadrant pain is associated with extension of the inflammation to the surrounding tissues. Nausea, vomiting, and anorexia follow the onset of pain, and a low-grade fever is common. Diarrhea occurs in some individuals, particularly children; others have a sensation of constipation. Perforation, peritonitis, and abscess formation are the most serious complications of appendicitis.

Evaluation and Treatment

In addition to clinical manifestations, the clinician can usually locate the painful site with one finger. Rebound tenderness is usually referred to the right lower quadrant. The white blood cell count ranges from 10,000 to 16,000 cells/mm^3 with increased neutrophils. Plain films of the abdomen and computed tomography (CT) scans can assist in differentiating appendicitis from perforated ulcer or cholecystitis.

Appendectomy is the treatment for simple or perforated appendicitis. Surgery provides quick recovery for simple appendicitis. Recovery is more complicated in cases of perforation or abscess formation.

Vascular Insufficiency

The stomach and intestines are supplied by three branches of the abdominal aorta: the celiac axis and the superior and inferior mesenteric arteries. Because of the rich collateral circulation, at least two of the supplying vessels must be compromised to cause ischemia (Patel, Kaleya, & Sammartano, 1992). Atherosclerotic lesions, thrombi, and emboli can develop in these vessels, occluding blood flow and causing ischemia or necrosis in the gastrointestinal tract.

Chronic mesenteric insufficiency can develop secondary to congestive heart failure, acute myocardial infarction, hemorrhage, stenosis, thrombus formation, or any condition that decreases arterial blood flow. Elderly individuals with arteriosclerosis are particularly susceptible. Chronic occlusion is often accompanied by formation of collateral circulation. The collateral vessels may be able to nourish the resting intestine. After eating, however, when the intestine requires more blood, the arterial supply may be insufficient. Ischemia develops, causing a cramping abdominal pain, called abdominal angina, after meals. Progressive vascular obstruction eventually causes continuous abdominal pain and necrosis of the intestinal tissue.

Acute occlusion of mesenteric blood flow results from dissecting aortic aneurysms or emboli. Embolic obstruction is associated with atrial fibrillation, mitral valve disease, and heart valve prostheses. The superior mesenteric artery has a more direct line of flow from the aorta; therefore, emboli enter it more readily than the inferior branch, causing ischemia and necrosis of the small intestine. Ischemia and necrosis alter membrane permeability. Initially, there is increased motility followed by absence of motility from the ischemia. The damaged intestinal mucosa cannot produce enough mucus to protect itself from digestive enzymes (Kvietys, Barrowmand, & Granger, 1987). Mucosal dysfunction causes fluid to move from the blood vessels into the bowel wall and peritoneum. Fluid loss causes hypovolemia and further decreases in intestinal blood flow. As intestinal infarction progresses, shock, fever, bloody diarrhea, leukocytosis, and abdominal distention develop. Abdominal pain may be severe.

Colicky abdominal pain after eating is a cardinal symptom of chronic mesenteric insufficiency. Some individuals suffer significant weight loss because they stop eating to control the pain. Acute mesenteric insufficiency causes severe continuous pain, rigid abdomen, and bloody diarrhea. Manifestations of unrelieved acute obstruction are distended abdomen, loss of bowel sounds, shock, peritonitis, fever, and tachycardia.

Diagnosis of mesenteric artery occlusion is based on clinical manifestations, mesenteric artery angiography, and abdominal radiography. Frequently bruit can be heard over the occluded artery. After angiography, a vasodilating agent may be injected into the vessels to improve the circulation. Surgery is required to remove necrotic tissue or repair sclerosed vessels. The mortality rate is high for individuals with acute occlusion and compromised cardiac output.

Disorders of Nutrition
Overnutrition

Overnutrition, or excessive caloric intake, is a major nutritional problem in the United States. It leads to **obesity** (excessive body fat), which is associated with the three leading causes of death: cardiovascular disease, cancer, and diabetes mellitus.

Obesity is classified by cause as either exogenous (resulting from an excess of ingested calories) or endogenous (resulting from inherent metabolic problems) (Ravussin & Swinburg, 1992). Physiologically obesity can be classified according to the structure and distribution of the adipose tissue itself. Child-onset obesity is both hyperplastic (caused by a greater-than-normal number of fat cells) and hypertrophic (caused by a greater-than-normal size of fat cells). In children, the adipose tissue is dispersed over the entire body, and few metabolic abnormalities exist. Adult-onset obesity is hypertrophic, the adipose tissue is centrally located, and metabolic abnormalities are more common. Genotype is an important predisposing factor (Stunkard, Harris, Pederson, & McClearn, 1990).

A number of theories have been postulated to explain the physiology of obesity. The fat-cell theory proposes that individuals with hyperplastic fat (adipose) cells are overweight or obese because they have an excessive number of fat cells. The number of fat cells increases whenever a positive energy balance occurs (Faust, Johnson, Stern, & Hirsch, 1978).

The lipoprotein-lipase (LPL) theory involves biochemical mechanisms within the fat cells. Lipoprotein lipase is an enzyme synthesized by fat cells. It hydrolyzes triglycerides into glycerol and free fatty acids, which then enter the fat cells and are reesterified into triglycerides. In other words, LPL promotes fat storage. According to theorists, obese individuals have elevated levels of LPL in their fat cells, and these levels rise even higher after weight reduction. The LPL works against the maintenance of reduced body weight and stimulates the fat cells to return to their hypertrophic size (Schwartz & Brunzell, 1981).

The lipostatic theory states that every individual has a biologic "set point" that maintains body weight. The set point is controlled by the ventromedial hypothalamus, which regulates an individual's appetite. Obese individuals are proposed to have a higher set point, which makes it difficult for them to maintain weight loss (Keesey, 1986).

Another theory of obesity is based on the thermogenesis of brown adipose tissue, the mitochondria-rich fat cells responsible for heat production. Individuals with a large number of subcutaneous brown fat cells release excess energy through heat production instead of converting the energy to fat stores. Obese people are believed to have very few brown fat cells compared with the average individual (Himms-Hagen, 1985; Miller, 1979).

The sodium–potassium–adenosine triphosphatase (ATPase) pump is believed to play a major role in the development of obesity. This enzyme pump transports sodium out of the cell and potassium into the cell and splits adenosine triphosphate, releasing energy. De Luise and colleagues (1980) discovered that obese people have an average of 22% fewer ATPase pumps than nonobese individuals. This lack could lead to less energy release and obesity.

The type II or non–insulin-dependent type of diabetes mellitus is often associated with obesity. Excessive food intake stimulates hyperinsulinemia. Through a negative-feedback mechanism, excessive insulin levels decrease the number of insulin receptor sites on adipose cells. The decrease of insulin receptor sites decreases the amount of glucose that can enter the cells. This promotes high blood levels of glucose. The excess glucose is stored as glycogen in the liver or as triglycerides in adipose cells, thereby enhancing hypertrophy and hyperplasia of fat cells in the already obese person. Weight reduction reverses this process.

Obesity probably has psychologic as well as physiologic causes (Wadden & Stunkard, 1985). One theory of psychologic causation proposes that obese people are directed more by external cues, such as the sight, smell, and taste of food, than by internal cues, such as hunger and satiety (Stunkard, 1980). Another psychologic theory is that eating creates the desire to eat more. Several studies have shown that some obese individuals eat more food after a snack or preload meal than nonobese individuals, who compensate for the preload meal by reducing food intake afterward.

Pathophysiology

Obese individuals are at risk for coronary artery disease resulting from hypercholesterolemia and hypertension. Abnormal obesity increases risks for diabetes, hypertension, and cardiovascular disease (Despres et al., 1992). Obesity is also a risk factor for breast, cervical, endometrial, and liver cancer in women. Obese men are at greater risk for prostatic, colon, and rectal cancer (American Cancer Society [ACS], 1986). Pulmonary function can be compromised by a large amount of adipose tissue overlying the chest cage. Gas exchange, vital capacity, and expiratory volume all decrease, causing low arterial oxygen tension and high carbon dioxide tension. Sleep apnea can occur. Exercise intolerance and pain in the fingers and weight-bearing joints, particularly the knees, are common. Joint pain may be caused by premature erosion of cartilage (Bray, 1985).

Evaluation and Treatment

Obesity is evaluated by a number of methods, including use of height and weight tables, body mass index (ratio of weight to height), skinfold thickness, hydrostatic weighing, measurement of oxygen intake, and bioelectric impedance analysis. If excess fat interferes with physiologic or psychologic functioning, treatment may be initiated.

The treatment for obesity caused by excessive nutrient intake is a regimen of reduced nutrient intake and increased energy expenditure. Age at onset, laboratory data about metabolic function (e.g., glucose tolerance tests, serum triglyceride, and cholesterol analyses), and distribution of adipose tissue determine the weight-reduction goal. Individuals with adult-onset obesity can reduce the size of their adipose cells and achieve a standard weight. Those with child-onset obesity may never achieve a standard weight.

The goal of weight reduction is to return the adipose cells to normal size and correct any associated metabolic abnormalities. The diet-exercise regimen is tailored to the unique problems of each obese individual. Self-motivation and a support system are critical aspects of treatment. Additional treatments, such as psychotherapy, behavioral modification, medications, and surgery, are prescribed as needed (Garrow, 1992).

Anorexia Nervosa and Bulimia

Many young adults and adolescents, as many as 1% of women and adolescent girls (Szmuckler, 1985), in the United States are affected by two complex and related eating disorders, anorexia nervosa and bulimia (American Psychiatric Association [APA], 1988). **Anorexia nervosa** is a psychologic and physiologic syndrome characterized by the following:

1. A fear of becoming obese despite progressive weight loss
2. A distorted body image; the perception that the body is fat when it is actually underweight
3. Body weight 15% less than normal for age and height because of refusal to eat
4. In women and girls, absence of three consecutive menstrual periods

Persons with anorexia nervosa frequently deny they have any eating problem. As the disease progresses, muscle and fat depletion give the individual a skeleton-like appearance. Postural hypotension, edema, brady-

cardia, hypothermia, constipation, and sleep disturbances may ensue. The loss of 25% to 30% of ideal body weight can eventually lead to death caused by starvation-induced cardiac failure. Diagnosis of anorexia nervosa involves a thorough medical history, physical and psychologic examination, and ruling out other causes of anorexia and malnutrition.

There are no universally accepted treatments. Treatment objectives for anorexia nervosa include reversing the compromised physical state, promoting insights and knowledge about the disorder, mutual goals, interaction with family members, restoring developmental growth, and modifying food habits. Correction of nutritional status can require hospitalization. When the individual demonstrates the willingness to eat food for nourishment, dietary protein, carbohydrate, and fat are introduced in tolerable amounts. Psychotherapy begins as soon as the physical symptoms are stabilized and may continue for several years.

Bulimia is characterized by binging—the consumption of normal to large amounts of food, often several thousand calories at a time—followed by self-induced vomiting or purging of the intestines with laxatives. The group at risk is the same as that for anorexia nervosa, except that bulimia tends to occur in slightly older, less affluent women. Approximately 50% of individuals with anorexia nervosa are bulimic as well (Halmi, 1987). Many young women stimulate vomiting inappropriately to control weight but are not classified as bulimic unless the pattern is obsessional or normal health or activity is interrupted. Diagnosis of bulimia is based on these findings:

1. Recurrent episodes of binge eating during which the individual fears not being able to stop
2. Self-induced vomiting, use of laxatives, or fasting to oppose the effect of binge eating
3. Two binge-eating episodes per week for at least 3 months

Although individuals with bulimia are afraid of gaining weight, their weight usually remains within normal range. Because of negative connotations associated with self-stimulated vomiting and purging, individuals who have bulimia binge and purge secretly. Bulimics may binge and purge as often as 20 times a day. Continual vomiting of acidic chyme can cause pitted teeth, pharyngeal and esophageal inflammation, and tracheo-esophageal fistulas. Overuse of laxatives can cause rectal bleeding. Secret binging isolates the bulimic individual and leads to depression and anger that is turned inward. A vicious cycle of depression, overeating to try to feel better, vomiting and purging to maintain a normal weight, and returning depression perpetuates this eating disorder.

Because bulimics are usually older than individuals with anorexia nervosa and have usually separated from a family core, individual or group counseling is the treatment focus. Individuals with bulimia rarely have physical problems requiring hospital care.

Bulimarexia combines the major components of anorexia nervosa and bulimia. Individuals with bulimarexia binge and gorge with food, vomit and purge with laxatives, and starve themselves intermittently. Risk factors and treatment objectives for bulimarexia are the same as for anorexia nervosa.

Starvation

Short-term starvation and long-term starvation have different effects. Therapeutic short-term starvation is part of many weight-reduction programs because it causes an initial rapid weight loss that reinforces the individual's motivation to diet. Therapeutic long-term starvation is used in medically controlled environments to facilitate rapid weight loss in morbidly obese individuals. Pathologic long-term starvation can be caused by poverty; chronic diseases of the cardiovascular, pulmonary, hepatic, and digestive systems; malabsorption syndromes; and cancer.

Short-term starvation, or extended fasting, consists of several days of total dietary abstinence or deprivation. For 4 to 6 hours after the last meal, the body is in a well-fed state, and its energy requirements are supplied by glucose from recently ingested carbohydrates. Once all available energy has been absorbed from the intestine, glycogen in the liver is converted to glucose through **glycogenolysis,** the splitting of glycogen into glucose. This process peaks within 4 to 8 hours, and gluconeogenesis begins. **Gluconeogenesis** is the formation of glucose from noncarbohydrate molecules: lactate, pyruvate, amino acids, and the glycerol portion of fats. Like glycogenolysis, gluconeogenesis takes place within the liver. Both of these processes deplete stored nutrients and thus cannot meet the body's energy needs indefinitely. Proteins continue to be catabolized to a minimal degree, providing carbon for the synthesis of glucose.

Long-term starvation begins after several days of dietary abstinence and eventually causes death. The major characteristic of long-term starvation is a decreased dependence on gluconeogenesis and an increased use of ketone bodies (products of lipid and pyruvate metabolism) as a cellular energy source. During long-term starvation, depressed insulin and glucagon levels promote lipolysis in adipose tissue. Lipolysis liberates fatty acids, which supply energy to cardiac and skeletal muscle cells, and ketone bodies, which sustain brain tissue. Fatty acid or ketone body oxidation meets most of the energy needs of the cells. (Some glucose is still needed as fuel for brain tissue.) Once the supply of adipose tissue is depleted, proteolysis begins. The breakdown of muscle protein is the last process to supply energy for life. Death results from severe alterations in electrolyte balance and loss of renal, pulmonary, and cardiac function.

Adequate ingestion of appropriate nutrients is the obvious treatment for starvation. In medically induced starvation, the body is maintained in a ketotic state until the desired amount of adipose tissue has been lysed. Starvation imposed by chronic disease, long-term illness, or malabsorption is treated with enteral or parenteral nutrition.

DISORDERS OF THE ACCESSORY ORGANS OF DIGESTION

The accessory organs of digestion, the liver, gallbladder, and pancreas, secrete substances necessary for digestion and, in the case of the liver, carry out metabolic functions needed to maintain life. Inflammatory disease is a common cause of accessory organ dysfunction. Inflammation disrupts secretory function and prevents secretions from flowing into the duodenum. Lack of accessory organ secretions is a major cause of maldigestion and malabsorption in the small intestine. Other causes of accessory organ dysfunction are obstruction of ducts by aggregates in the secretions themselves (e.g., obstruction of bile flow by gallstones) or by tumors. (Cancers of the digestive tract are described at the end of the chapter.)

Clinical Manifestations of Liver Disorders

Of all the accessory organ disorders, acute or chronic liver disease leads to the most systemic, life-threatening complications. These complications include portal hypertension, ascites, hepatic encephalopathy, jaundice, and hepatorenal syndrome.

Portal Hypertension

Portal hypertension is abnormally high blood pressure in the portal venous system. Pressure in this system is normally 3 mm Hg; portal hypertension is an increase to at least 10 mm Hg. The portal veins carry blood from the gastrointestinal tract, pancreas, and spleen to the liver. In the liver the blood flows through the sinusoids and empties into the hepatic veins, which carry it into the inferior vena cava. The inferior vena cava delivers blood to the right atrium. The portal veins, sinusoids, and hepatic veins compose the portal venous system.

Pathophysiology

Portal hypertension is caused by disorders that obstruct or impede blood flow through any component of the portal venous system or vena cava. The obstruction can occur in the liver as a result of thrombosis, inflammation, or fibrosis of the sinusoids, as occurs in cirrhosis of the liver, viral hepatitis, or schistosomiasis (a parasitic infection). Portal outflow to the vena cava can be impeded by hepatic vein thrombosis or cardiac disorders, such as failure of the right side of the heart or constrictive pericarditis, that impair the pumping ability of the right heart. This causes blood to "back up" and increase pressure in the portal system. The most common cause of portal hypertension is obstruction caused by cirrhosis of the liver (see p. 1356).

High pressure in the portal veins causes collateral vessels to open between the portal veins and the systemic veins, in which blood pressure is considerably lower (Fig. 36-10). This enables blood to bypass the ob-structed portal vessels. The collateral veins develop in the esophagus, anterior abdominal wall, and rectum. High pressure and increased flow volume are transmitted through these veins from the portal to the systemic venous circulation.

Long-term portal hypertension causes several problems that are difficult to treat and can be fatal:

1. **Varices** (distended, tortuous, collateral veins). Prolonged elevation of pressure in collateral veins causes their transformation into varices, particularly in the lower esophagus and stomach, but also in the rectum.

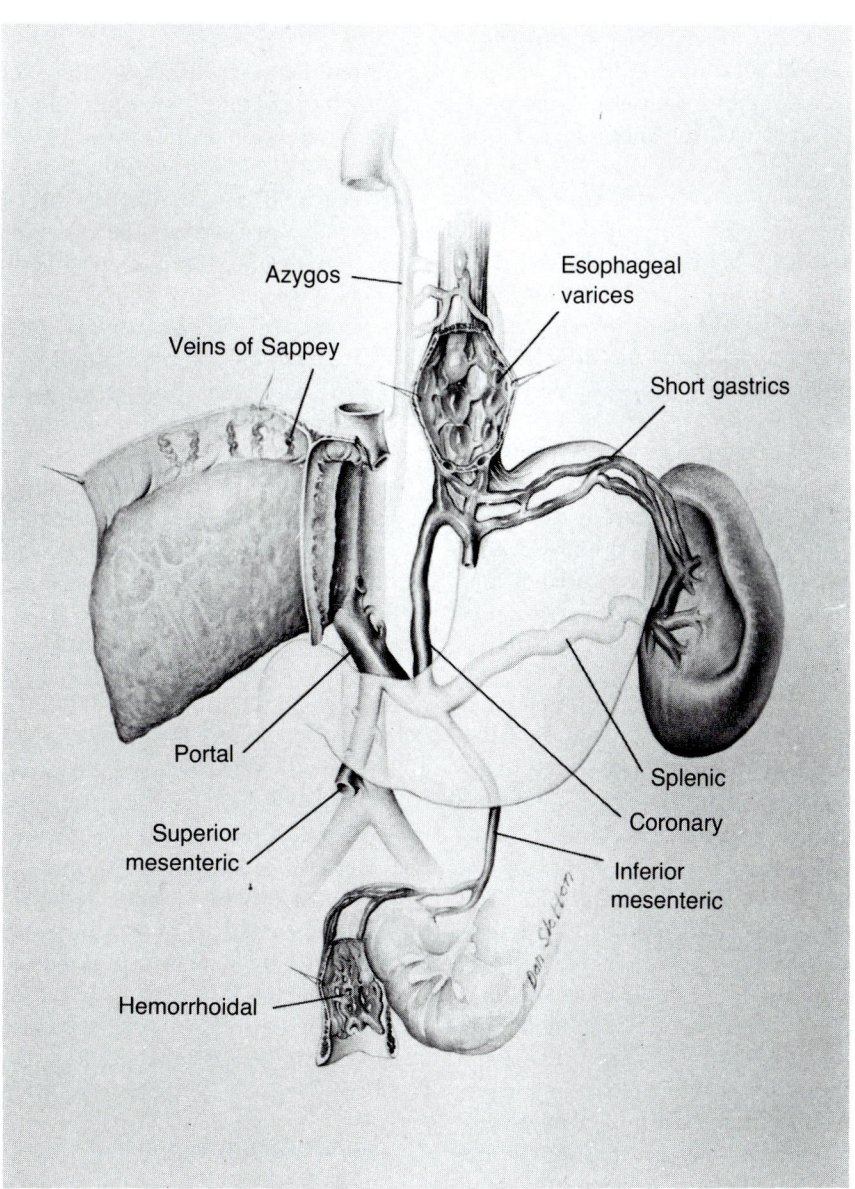

FIG. 36-10 Varices related to portal hypertension. Portal vein, its major tributaries, and the most important shunts (collateral veins) between the portal and caval systems. (From Kissane, 1990.)

2. **Splenomegaly** (enlargement of the spleen) caused by increased pressure in the splenic vein, which branches from the portal vein.
3. **Ascites** (the accumulation of fluid in the peritoneal cavity, which is the space between the visceral peritoneum and the parietal peritoneum). Ascites is caused by increased pressure in the mesenteric tributaries of the portal vein. Hydrostatic pressure forces water out of these vessels and into the peritoneal cavity. (This process, termed transudative effusion, is described in Chapter 30.)
4. **Hepatic encephalopathy,** also called portal-systemic encephalopathy. This condition is characterized by central nervous system disturbances, particularly reversible alterations of consciousness.

Blood that is shunted through collateral vessels to the systemic veins bypasses the liver, where toxins, hormones, and other harmful substances normally are removed. Hepatic encephalopathy results from the presence of these substances, particularly ammonia, in blood that reaches the brain.

Clinical Manifestations

The vomiting of blood from bleeding esophageal varices is the most common clinical manifestation of portal hypertension. Slow, chronic bleeding from varices causes anemia or melena. Usually the bleeding is from varices that have developed slowly over a period of years.

Rupture of esophageal varices causes hemorrhage and voluminous vomiting of dark-colored blood. The ruptured varices are usually painless. Rupture is caused by a combination of erosion by gastric acid and elevated venous pressure. The mortality rate of ruptured esophageal varices ranges from 30% to 60%. Recurrent bleeding of esophageal varices indicates a poor prognosis. Most individuals die within 1 year.

Evaluation and Treatment

Diagnosis of portal hypertension is often made at the time of variceal bleeding and confirmed by endoscopy and evaluation of portal venous pressure. Distended collateral veins may radiate over the abdomen, giving rise to the description caput medusae (Medusa's head). The individual usually has a history of jaundice, hepatitis, or alcoholism.

Emergency management of bleeding varices includes compression of the varices with an inflatable Sengstaken-Blakemore tube, which is shaped like a cylindrical balloon with a bulb at the end. In some cases the varices are obliterated by injection of a sclerosing agent. Surgical construction of a portacaval shunt (anastomosis of the portal vein to the inferior vena cava) may decompress the varices, but this treatment can precipitate encephalopathy or liver failure resulting from re-

duced hepatic blood flow. There is no effective, definitive treatment for portal hypertension.

Ascites

Ascites is the accumulation of fluid in the peritoneal cavity. Ascites traps body fluid in a "third space" from which it cannot escape. The effect is to reduce the amount of fluid available for normal physiologic functions. Cirrhosis is the most common cause of ascites. Other diseases associated with ascites include heart failure, constrictive pericarditis, abdominal malignancies, nephrotic syndrome, and malnutrition. Twenty-five percent of individuals who develop ascites caused by cirrhosis die within 1 year. Continued heavy drinking is associated with this mortality rate.

Pathophysiology

Several factors contribute to the development of ascites. Impaired excretion of sodium by the kidneys promotes water retention. Portal hypertension and reduced serum albumin levels cause capillary hydrostatic pressure to exceed capillary osmotic pressure. This imbalance tends to push water into the peritoneal cavity. Portal hypertension also increases the production of hepatic lymph, which "weeps" into the peritoneal cavity.

In cases of cirrhosis, both portal hypertension and decreased production of albumin by hepatocytes contribute to the ascites. Besides reducing albumin synthesis, deranged liver metabolism permits the accumulation of hormones that regulate sodium and water balance. Excessive amounts of aldosterone and antidiuretic hormone remain in the blood, stimulating the kidneys to retain sodium and water. High aldosterone levels can be attributed also to increased secretion mediated by excessive plasma renin activity. The increased plasma renin activity may develop because of decreased metabolic function of the liver, increased renal secretion stimulated by low blood flow, or both.

As ascites sequesters more and more bodily fluid, the kidneys respond by retaining sodium and water in amounts exceeding intake. Retention of sodium and water expands plasma volume, thereby accelerating portal hypertension and ascites formation.

Ascites can be complicated by bacterial peritonitis. Peritonitis involves an inflammatory response that worsens ascites by increasing mesenteric capillary permeability. As plasma seeps out of the permeable mesenteric capillaries, it adds to the volume of ascitic fluid. Fig. 36-11 summarizes the mechanisms by which cirrhosis of the liver causes ascites.

Clinical Manifestations

The accumulation of ascitic fluid causes weight gain, abdominal distention, and increased abdominal girth (Fig. 36-12). Large volumes of fluid (10 to 20 L) displace the

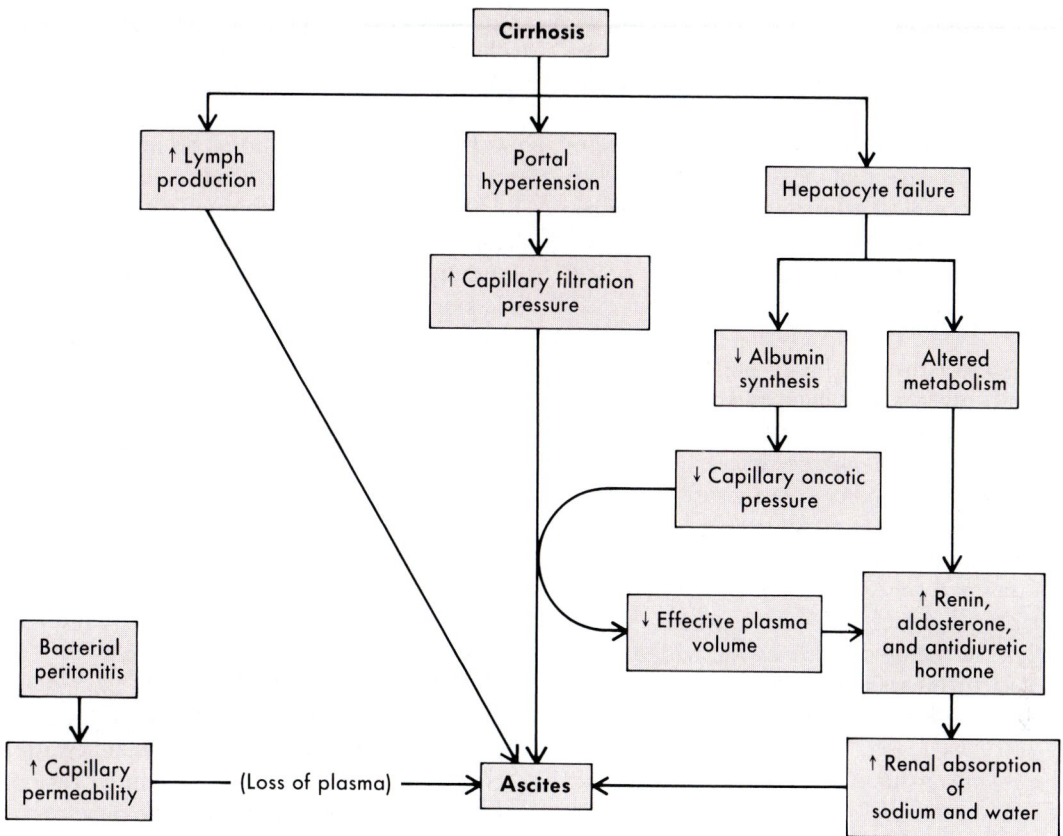

FIG. 36-11 Mechanisms of ascites caused by cirrhosis.

FIG. 36-12 Massive ascites in an individual with cirrhosis. Distended abdomen, dilated upper abdominal veins, and inverted umbilicus are classic manifestations. (From Prior, Silberstein, & Stang, 1981.)

diaphragm and cause dyspnea by decreasing lung capacity. Respiratory rate increases, and the individual assumes a semi-Fowler position to relieve the dyspnea. Some peripheral edema is usually present. Approximately 10% of individuals with ascites develop bacterial peritonitis, either spontaneously or as a result of paracentesis (needle aspiration of ascitic fluid). Peritonitis causes fever, chills, abdominal pain, decreased bowel sounds, and cloudy ascitic fluid.

Evaluation and Treatment

Diagnosis of ascites is usually based on clinical manifestations and identification of liver disease. Paracentesis is used to aspirate ascitic fluid for bacterial culture, biochemical analysis, and microscopic examination. The goal of treatment is to relieve discomfort. If the restoration of liver function is possible (e.g., in ascites caused by viral hepatitis), the ascites diminishes spontaneously. In the meantime, dietary salt restriction and potassium-sparing diuretics can reduce ascites. Strong diuretics, such as furosemide or ethacrynic acid, may be used. Serum electrolytes are monitored carefully because the individual is at risk for hyponatremia and hypokalemia.

Palliative measures include paracentesis to remove 1 or 2 L ascitic fluid and relieve respiratory distress. This procedure can have serious complications, however. The removal of too much fluid relieves pressure on blood vessels and carries the risk of hypotension, shock, or death. Despite repeated paracentesis, ascitic fluid reaccumulates in individuals with irreversible disease, drawing more albumin and electrolytes out of the vascular compartment. Paracentesis is also likely to cause peritonitis. Individuals with ascites and portal hypertension have a poor prognosis.

Hepatic Encephalopathy

Hepatic encephalopathy (portal-systemic encephalopathy) is a complex neurologic syndrome characterized by impaired cerebral function, flapping tremor (asterixis), and electroencephalogram (EEG) changes. The syndrome may develop rapidly during acute fulminant hepatitis or slowly during the course of chronic liver disease.

Pathophysiology

Hepatic encephalopathy probably results from a combination of biochemical alterations that affect neurotransmission. Liver dysfunction and collateral vessels that shunt blood around the liver to the systemic circulation both permit toxins absorbed from the gastrointestinal tract to circulate freely to the brain. The most hazardous substances are end products of intestinal protein digestion, particularly ammonia. The digestion of blood from leaking or ruptured varices adds to the amount of ammonia present in systemic blood, as does the action of ammonia-forming bacteria in the colon. Ammonia that reaches the brain may alter cerebral energy metabolism or interfere with neurotransmitters.

Blood levels of ammonia do not account for all symptoms associated with hepatic encephalopathy. The accumulation of short-chain fatty acids, serotonin, tryptophan, and false neurotransmitters probably contributes to neural derangement (Schafer & Jones, 1990). Infection, hemorrhage, electrolyte imbalance, sedatives, and analgesics can also precipitate stupor and coma in the presence of liver disease.

Clinical Manifestations

Subtle changes in personality, memory loss, irritability, lethargy, and sleep disturbances are common initial manifestations of hepatic encephalopathy. Symptoms then can progress to confusion, flapping tremor of the hands, stupor, convulsions, and coma. Coma is usually a sign of liver failure and ultimately results in death.

Evaluation and Treatment

Diagnosis of hepatic encephalopathy is based on a history of liver disease and clinical manifestations. Electroencephalography and blood chemistry tests provide supportive data. There is no specific diagnostic test.

Correction of fluid and electrolyte imbalances and withdrawal of depressant drugs metabolized by the liver are first steps in the treatment of hepatic encephalopathy. Reduction of blood ammonia levels is a major objective. This is accomplished by restricting dietary protein intake and eliminating intestinal bacteria. Neomycin is effective in sterilizing the bowel, but it can be nephrotoxic. Lactulose may be administered to prevent ammonia absorption in the colon. Lactulose passes unabsorbed into the large intestine, where bacteria hydrolyze it to a watery acid. The acid (1) converts ammonia to nonabsorbable ammonium and (2) produces diarrhea, which limits the amount of time feces are available for ammonia production by intestinal bacteria.

Jaundice

Jaundice, or icterus, is a yellow or greenish pigmentation of the skin caused by hyperbilirubinemia (plasma bilirubin concentrations above 1.2 mg/dl). Hyperbilirubinemia and jaundice can result from excessive hemolysis of red blood cells or disorders of the bile ducts or liver cells (Fig. 36-13). Jaundice in newborns is caused by impaired bilirubin uptake and conjugation (see Chapter 37).

Pathophysiology

Obstructive jaundice can result from extrahepatic or intrahepatic obstruction. Extrahepatic obstructive jaundice develops if the common bile duct is occluded by a

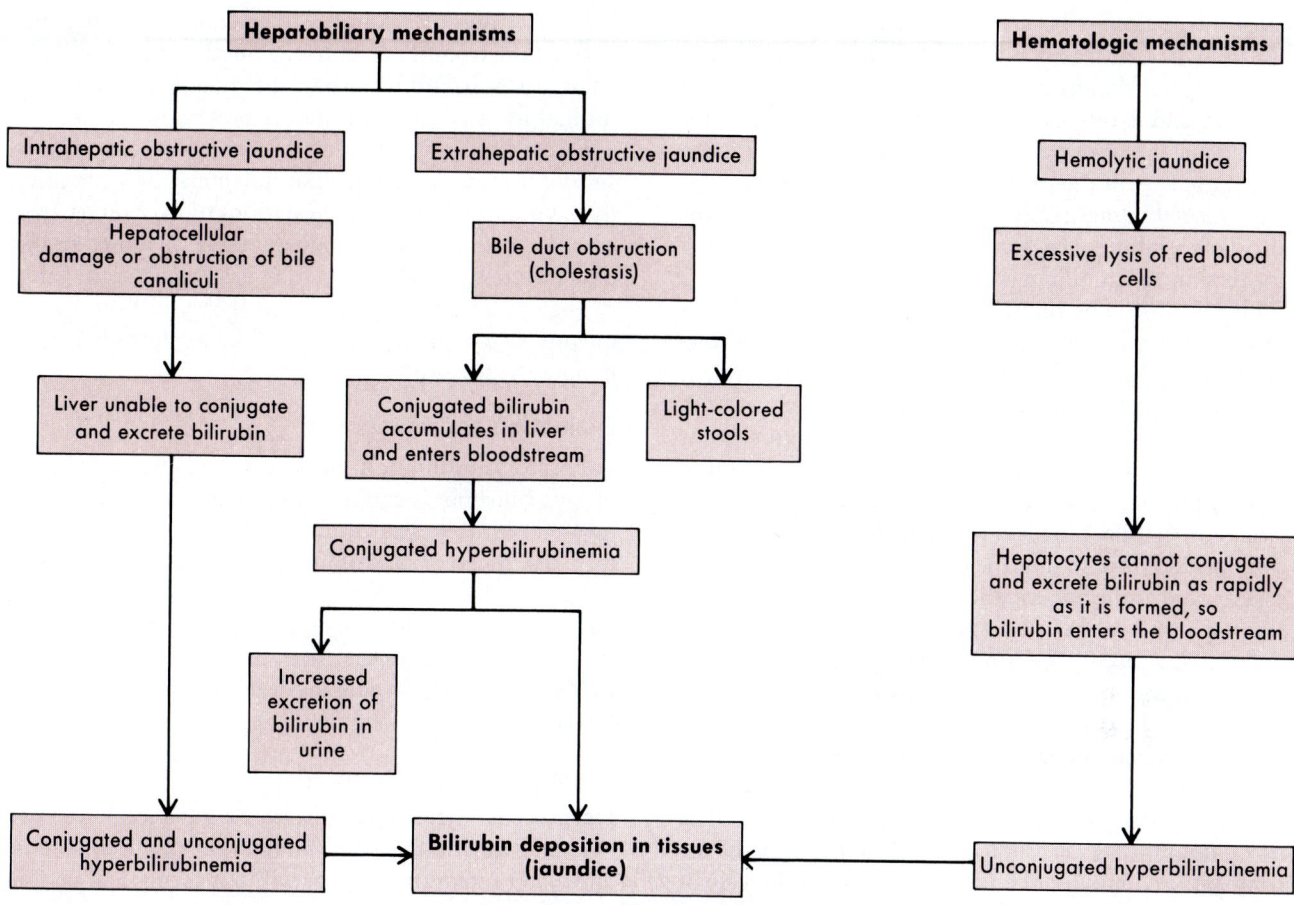

FIG. 36-13 Mechanisms of jaundice.

TABLE 36-7

Three Common Types of Jaundice

Type	Mechanism	Causes
Hemolytic jaundice (predominately un-conjugated bilirubin)	Destruction of erythrocytes	Membrane defect of erythrocytes Immune reaction Severe infection Toxic substances in the circulation (e.g., snake venom) Transfusion of incompatible blood
Obstructive jaundice (predominately conjugated bilirubin)	Obstruction of passage of conjugated bilirubin from liver to intestine	Obstruction of bile duct by gallstones or tumor (extrahepatic obstructive jaundice) Obstruction of bile flow through the liver (intrahepatic obstructive jaundice) Drugs
Hepatocellular jaundice	Failure of liver cells (hepatocytes) to conjugate bilirubin and of bilirubin to pass from liver to intestine	Genetic defect of hepatocyte (decreased enzymes), such as occurs in premature infants (see Chapter 37) Severe infections

gallstone or tumor. Because the bile duct is obstructed, bilirubin is conjugated by the hepatocytes but cannot flow into the duodenum. Therefore, it accumulates in the liver and enters the bloodstream, causing hyperbilirubinemia. Because conjugated bilirubin is water soluble, it appears in the urine. The stools may be light- or clay-colored because they lack bile pigments. The stools also lack urobilinogen because bile is not available for conversion to urobilinogen.

Intrahepatic obstructive jaundice involves disturbances in hepatocyte function and obstruction of bile canaliculi. The uptake, conjugation, and excretion of bilirubin are affected, because of elevated levels of both conjugated and unconjugated bilirubin. Hepatocellular damage increases plasma concentrations of unconjugated bilirubin. The major disorder, however, is obstruction of bile canaliculi, which diminishes flow of conjugated bilirubin into the common bile duct. In mild cases, some of the bile canaliculi open. Consequently the amount of bilirubin in the intestinal tract may be only slightly decreased. The stools may appear normal or light-colored.

Excessive hemolysis (breakdown) of red blood cells can cause **hemolytic jaundice.** An increased amount of unconjugated bilirubin is formed through metabolism of the heme component of destroyed red blood cells. The extra amount of unconjugated bilirubin exceeds the conjugation ability of the liver, causing blood levels of unconjugated bilirubin to rise. Unconjugated bilirubinemia is the major cause of hemolytic jaundice. Because unconjugated bilirubin is not water-soluble, it is not excreted in the urine. The reserve conjugation ability of the liver usually prevents long-term unconjugated hyperbilirubinemia greater than 4 to 5 mg/dl. Severe hemolytic crisis, such as that which occurs with sickle cell disease (see Chapter 25), is a cause of hemolytic jaundice. Hemolytic drugs can also cause jaundice. If unconjugated hyperbilirubinemia exceeds 5 mg/dl, both hemolytic and liver disorders are indicated.

Hyperbilirubinemia and jaundice can be caused also by metabolic defects that impair the uptake or conjugation of unconjugated bilirubin in the liver. Gilbert disease, for example, causes an elevation of unconjugated bilirubin in the plasma but no other symptoms of liver disease. Gilbert disease is probably caused by an inherited deficiency of glucuronyltransferase enzyme, which is required for the hepatic uptake of unconjugated bilirubin. The causes of jaundice are summarized in Table 36-7.

Clinical Manifestations

The clinical manifestations of jaundice vary and are related to the underlying pathology. Conjugated hyperbilirubinemia may cause the urine to darken several days before the onset of jaundice. The complete obstruction of bile flow from the liver to the duodenum causes light-colored stools. With partial obstruction the stools are normal in color and bilirubin is present in the urine.

Fever, chills, and pain often accompany jaundice resulting from viral or bacterial inflammation of the liver (e.g., viral hepatitis). Manifestations of liver injury from any cause commonly include anorexia, malaise, and fatigue. Yellow discoloration may first occur in the sclera of the eye and then progress to the skin. Pruritus frequently accompanies jaundice because bilirubin accumulates in the skin.

Evaluation and Treatment

Laboratory evaluation of serum establishes whether plasma bilirubin is conjugated or unconjugated. Unconjugated bilirubinemia results from hemolysis or hereditary disorders of bilirubin metabolism. Elevations of conjugated bilirubin indicate liver injury or extrahepatic obstruction. The history and physical examination identify underlying disorders, such as alcoholism, exposure to hepatitis virus, or gallbladder disease. The treatment for jaundice consists of correcting the cause.

Hepatorenal Syndrome

Hepatorenal syndrome consists of advanced liver disease and functional renal failure with oliguria, sodium and water retention (with or without ascites and peripheral edema), hypotension, and peripheral vasodilation. Renal disorders associated with liver disease can have numerous causes, but hepatorenal syndrome is usually associated with alcoholic cirrhosis and fulminant hepatitis. The renal failure is not caused by primary renal disease or other extrinsic factors, but rather by circulatory alterations.

Pathophysiology

Oliguric hepatic failure generally accompanies a sudden decrease in blood volume secondary to massive gastrointestinal bleeding or hypotension caused by failing liver function. Hypotension also can be caused by the excessive use of diuretics to treat ascites. The diuretics may decrease renal blood flow and glomerular filtration rate and cause oliguria. A significant number of individuals with advanced liver disease develop oliguria unrelated to any precipitating event. Liver failure is the apparent cause of functional renal failure in hepatorenal syndrome. Inappropriate constriction of renal arterioles is proposed as the causative mechanism. Intrarenal vasoconstriction may result from the selective effects of vasoactive substances that accumulate in the blood because of liver failure. The diseased liver fails to remove excessive angiotensin, vasopressin, prostaglandins, and catecholamines from the blood. These substances travel to the kidneys and cause vasoconstriction. Vasoconstriction also may be a compensatory response to portal hypotension and the pooling of blood in the splanchnic circulation. The exact reason for the vasoconstriction is unknown (Mudge & Carlson, 1992; Punukollu & Gopalswamy, 1990).

Clinical Manifestations

The onset of hepatorenal manifestations may be gradual or acute. Oliguria and complications of advanced liver disease, including jaundice, ascites, and gastrointestinal bleeding, are usually present. Systolic blood pressure is usually below 100 mm Hg. Nonspecific symptoms of hepatorenal syndrome include anorexia, weakness, and fatigue.

Evaluation and Treatment

Despite oliguria, serum potassium levels do not become dangerously elevated until the terminal stages of the hepatorenal syndrome. Blood urea increases, followed by an increase in creatinine concentration. Urine osmolality is increased, but urine sodium concentrations are below normal. Urine specific gravity is above 1.015.

The prognosis is usually poor and is related to liver function. Secondary problems, including fluid and electrolyte disorders, bleeding, infections, and encephalopathy, are vigorously treated.

Disorders of the Liver
Viral Hepatitis

Viral hepatitis is a relatively common systemic disease that primarily affects the liver. Five strains of viruses cause different types of hepatitis: hepatitis A virus (HAV), hepatitis B virus (HBV), hepatitis D virus (HDV), hepatitis C virus (HCV), and hepatitis E virus (HEV). Hepatitis A used to be known as infectious hepatitis, and hepatitis B as serum hepatitis. Characteristics of the different types are presented in Table 36-8.

Types of hepatitis

Hepatitis A. The hepatitis A virus can be recovered from the feces, bile, and sera of infected individuals. The usual mode of transmission is the fecal-oral route (contaminated food or water), but the virus can also be spread by the transfusion of infected blood. Approximately 45% of adults in urban areas have HAV antibodies in their blood. The disease spreads readily in crowded, unsanitary conditions, usually through contaminated food or water. Person-to-person spread is more likely to occur in settings such as day care centers or institutions for the mentally retarded, where there is close contact between clients and caregivers (Shulman, 1992).

The incubation period (the time between exposure and onset of symptoms) for hepatitis A is 4 to 6 weeks

TABLE 36-8
Characteristics of Viral Hepatitis

Characteristic	Hepatitis A	Hepatitis B	Hepatitis D	Hepatitis C	Hepatitis E
Size of virus	27 mm RNA virus	42 mm DNA virus	36 mm RNA virus, defective virus with HB$_s$Ag coat	Unknown RNA virus	32 mm RNA virus
Incubation period	30 days	60-180 days	30-180 days	35-60 days	15-60 days
Route of transmission	Fecal-oral parenteral, sexual	Parenteral, sexual	Parenteral, ? fecal-oral, sexual	Parenteral	Fecal-oral
Onset	Acute with fever	Insidious	Insidious	Insidious	Acute
Carrier state	Negative	Positive	Positive	Positive	Negative
Severity	Mild	Severe; may be prolonged or chronic	Severe	Unknown	Severe in pregnant women
Chronic hepatitis	No	Yes	Yes	Yes	No
Age group affected	Children and young adults	Any	Any	Any	Children and young adults
Prophylaxis	Hygiene, immune serum globulin	Hygiene, HBV vaccine	Hygiene, HBV vaccine	Hygiene, screening blood, interferon alpha	Hygiene, safe water

Course of infection with the hepatitis A virus (HAV).

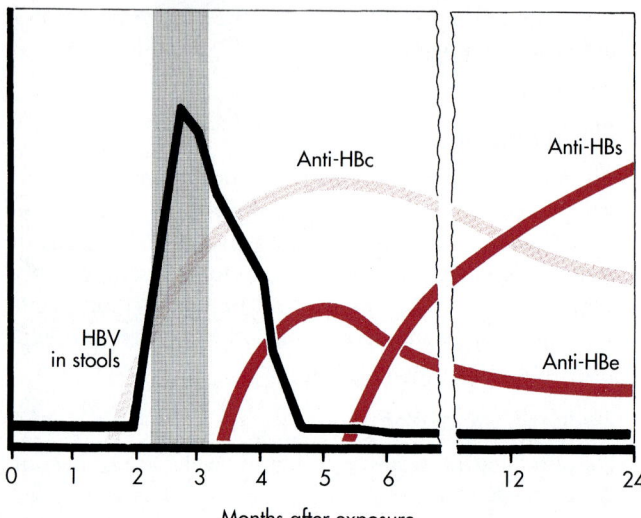

FIG. 36-15 Course of infection with the hepatitis B virus (HBV). *HB$_s$Ag*, Hepatitis B surface antigen; *anti-HBs*, antibody to HB$_s$Ag; *HB$_e$Ag*, hepatitis Be antigen; *anti-HBe*, antibody to HB$_e$Ag; *anti-HB$_c$*, antibody to hepatitis B core antigen. The antibody to HB$_s$ (anti-HB$_s$) is IgG, the immunoglobulin that creates immunity.

(Fig. 36-14). Fecal shedding of the virus is greatest for 10 to 14 days before the onset of symptoms and during the first week of symptoms. The disease is most contagious during this time. Antibodies to HAV (anti-HAV) develop about 4 weeks after infection. The serum IgM concentration increases initially and is followed by an increase of serum IgG. IgG levels remain elevated for several years after infection, creating immunity to the disease. (See Chapter 6 for a description of immune functions.)

Hepatitis B. Hepatitis B is transmitted through contact with infected blood, body fluids, or contaminated needles. Hepatitis B is also considered to be a sexually transmitted disease (see Chapter 21). Transmission among homosexual men may be by oral or genital contact with bleeding lesions in the rectal mucosa. People receiving hemodialysis, multiple blood transfusions, or immunosuppressive drugs have a greater risk of exposure or less resistance to HBV. Mother-infant transmission occurs if the mother becomes infected during the third trimester of pregnancy. Approximately 0.3% of adults in the United States carry the HB$_s$Ag marker for active HBV (Gerety, 1985).

Three types of viral particles are involved in HBV infection. The larger (47 nm) Dane particle probably represents the intact HBV. The Dane particle has a double-layered outer coat and carries the hepatitis B surface antigen (HB$_s$Ag), which was originally called the Australia antigen. HB$_s$Ag can be identified in the serum by radioimmune assay. Hepatitis B core antigen (HB$_c$Ag)

is usually not detected in the serum. The HB$_e$Ag is a derivative of HB$_c$Ag and is a marker of HBV replication. The HBV has an incubation period of 6 to 8 weeks. The initial serologic change is a transient increase in IgM. Levels of IgG antibodies to HB$_s$Ag elevate more slowly and remain elevated for years (Fig. 36-15).

Hepatitis C. Hepatitis C virus (non-A, non-B hepatitis) causes most cases of posttransfusion hepatitis. Hepatitis C antibody is present in 44% of blood donors with increased aminotransferase levels (Kuo et al., 1989). The risk for developing hepatitis C is greater with large volumes of blood replacement and among intravenous drug users. HCV is an RNA virus and the federal Food and Drug Administration (FDA) has approved an assay for screening hepatitis C antibodies in blood products.

Hepatitis D. The hepatitis D virus (HDV) occurs in individuals with hepatitis B. The delta virus depends on the hepatitis B virus for its replication because the coat of the delta virus consists of HB$_s$Ag molecules that are on the surface of the HBV virus. Parenteral drug users have a high incidence of HDV infection. Hepatitis D has been shown to suppress replication of hepatitis B virus (DeCock, Govindarajan, & Redeker, 1985). The clinical course of HDV is similar to that of hepatitis A and B, although it is sometimes more severe.

Hepatitis E. Hepatitis E is most common in developing countries and is transmitted by the fecal-oral route, usually by contaminated water. It is more prevalent among adults and has the highest mortality in pregnant women. Clinically, it resembles HAV.

Pathophysiology

The pathologic lesions of hepatitis are similar to those caused by other viral infection. Hepatic cell necrosis, scarring, Kupffer cell hyperplasia, and infiltration by mononuclear phagocytes occur with varying severity. Cellular injury is promoted by cell-mediated immune mechanisms (i.e., cytotoxic T cells and natural killer cells). Regeneration of hepatic cells begins within 48 hours of injury. The inflammatory process can damage and obstruct bile canaliculi, leading to cholestasis and obstructive jaundice. In milder cases the liver parenchyma is not damaged. Damage tends to be most severe in cases of hepatitis B and C. Hepatitis B is also associated with acute fulminating hepatitis, a rare form of the disease that is characterized by massive hepatic necrosis. Acute fulminating hepatitis causes severe encephalopathy, which is manifested as confusion, stupor, and coma. Liver failure can occur, leading to intestinal bleeding, cardiorespiratory insufficiency, and renal failure. The mortality rate is high, but recovery can be complete.

Clinical Manifestations

The clinical manifestations of the different types of hepatitis are very similar. The spectrum of manifestations ranges from absence of symptoms to fulminating hepatitis, with rapid onset of liver failure and coma. Acute viral hepatitis causes abnormal liver function test results. The serum aminotransferase values, AST and ALT, are elevated, but their elevation may not be consistent with the extent of cellular damage. The clinical course of hepatitis usually consists of three phases: the prodromal, icteric, and recovery phases.

Prodromal phase.   The **prodromal phase** of hepatitis begins about 2 weeks after exposure and ends with the appearance of jaundice. Fatigue, anorexia, malaise, nausea, vomiting, headache, hyperalgia, cough, and low-grade fever are prodromal symptoms that precede the onset of jaundice. Food odors often cause nausea, and changes in taste suppress the desire to smoke and drink alcohol. Right upper abdominal pain is common, and a weight loss of 2 to 4 kg is not unusual. The infection is highly transmissible during this phase.

Icteric phase (jaundice).   The **icteric phase** begins about 1 to 2 weeks after the prodromal phase and lasts 2 to 6 weeks. Hepatocellular destruction and intrahepatic bile stasis cause jaundice (icterus). The urine may be dark and the stools clay-colored before the onset of jaundice. The icteric phase is the actual phase of illness. The liver is enlarged, smooth, and tender, and percussion over the liver causes pain. During the icteric phase

gastrointestinal and respiratory symptoms subside, but fatigue and abdominal pain may persist or become more severe. Serum bilirubin levels range from 5 to 10 mg/dl, with both conjugated and unconjugated fractions increasing. The jaundice may last 2 to 6 weeks or longer. Mild and transient itching often accompanies jaundice. The prothrombin time may be prolonged in individuals with more serious forms of the disease.

Recovery phase.   The posticteric or **recovery phase** begins with resolution of jaundice, about 6 to 8 weeks after exposure. Although the liver may still be enlarged and tender, symptoms diminish. In most cases liver function test results return to normal within 2 to 12 weeks after the onset of jaundice.

Chronic hepatitis may begin at this point and is associated with HBV infection. **Chronic active hepatitis** is the persistence of clinical manifestations and liver inflammation after acute hepatitis B, hepatitis C, and hepatitis D. Liver function tests remain abnormal for longer than 6 months, and HB_sAg persists. Chronic, active hepatitis B is a predisposition to cirrhosis and primary hepatocellular carcinoma.

Evaluation and Treatment

The most specific diagnostic test for viral hepatitis is serologic analysis for HB_sAg, which is the marker for HBV. Diagnosis of type A hepatitis is based on the presence of anti-HAV, as is the diagnosis of HCV. The assay HDV is the total antibody to hepatitis D and antigen (anti-HDV). A test for HEV has not been developed. Liver function tests also can indicate other viral liver diseases, drug toxicity, or alcoholic hepatitis.

There is no specific treatment for acute viral hepatitis. Physical activity may be restricted. A low-fat, high-carbohydrate diet is beneficial if bile flow is obstructed. Interferon can be useful in the treatment of chronic hepatitis B and C (Lamboise & Davis, 1992).

To prevent transmission of hepatitis A, hand washing and use of gloves for disposing of bed pans and fecal matter are imperative. There should be no direct contact with blood or body fluids of patients with hepatitis B or non-A, non-B hepatitis. The administration of immune globulin before exposure or early in the incubation period can prevent hepatitis A. A vaccine for hepatitis A is being investigated. Prophylactic immune globulin administered before exposure can also prevent hepatitis B. A vaccine is available to protect against HBV infection. Alpha interferon is used for the treatment of chronic hepatitis B. Prophylaxis is recommended for health care workers and others who are at risk for contact with infected body fluids.

Fulminant Hepatitis

Fulminant hepatitis is a clinical syndrome resulting in severe impairment or necrosis of liver cells and potential liver failure. The disorder may occur as a complication of hepatitis C or hepatitis B, particularly HBV infection compounded by infection with the delta virus. Toxic reactions to drugs and congenital metabolic disorders also can cause fulminant hepatitis.

Causative mechanisms of fulminant hepatic failure are poorly understood. Hepatocytes become edematous, and patchy areas of necrosis and inflammatory cell infiltrates disrupt the parenchyma. The death of hepatocytes may be caused by viral or immunologic damage.

Fulminant hepatitis usually develops 6 to 8 weeks after the initial symptoms of viral hepatitis or a metabolic liver disorder. Anorexia, vomiting, abdominal pain, and progressive jaundice are initial signs, followed by ascites and gastrointestinal bleeding. Hepatic encephalopathy is manifested as lethargy, altered motor functions, and coma. Liver function tests show elevations of both direct and indirect serum bilirubin, serum transaminases, and blood ammonia. Prothrombin time is prolonged.

Treatment of fulminant hepatitis is supportive. The hepatic necrosis is irreversible, and 60% to 90% of affected children die. Liver transplantation may be lifesaving. Survivors usually do not develop cirrhosis or chronic liver disease.

Cirrhosis

Cirrhosis is an irreversible inflammatory disease that disrupts liver structure and function. It is a leading cause of death in the United States. Cirrhosis is the disorganization of hepatic tissues caused by diffuse fibrosis and nodular regeneration. Nodules of regenerated tissue form between fibrous bands, giving the liver a cobbly appearance. The liver may be larger or smaller than normal, and usually it is firm or hard when palpated. A variety of disorders can cause cirrhosis. Therefore, it is often classified by cause (Table 36-9). In many cases the cause of cirrhosis is unknown.

The precise cause of cellular injury depends on the type of cirrhosis, and the causes are not all clearly understood. Structural changes result from fibrosis, which is a consequence of inflammation. The parenchyma of the liver becomes distorted, and biliary channels may be altered or obstructed, producing jaundice. Obstruction caused by cirrhosis can cause portal hypertension. New vascular channels can form shunts, and blood from the portal vein bypasses the liver. These vascular changes compromise liver function further, and the process of regeneration is replaced by hypoxia, necrosis, atrophy, and, ultimately, liver failure.

Cirrhosis develops slowly over a period of years. Its severity and rate of progression depend on the cause. If toxins, such as alcohol, are involved, the rate of cell death and the severity of inflammation depend on the amount of toxin present. Removal of the toxin slows the progression of liver damage and enhances the process of regeneration (Carithers, 1992).

TABLE 36-9

Cirrhosis of the Liver

Type and disease name	Causal mechanisms	Pathophysiology
Alcoholic cirrhosis, Laennec cirrhosis, portal cirrhosis, fatty cirrhosis	Toxic effects of chronic, excessive alcohol intake; acetylaldehyde formed by alcohol metabolism damages hepatocytes	Fatty liver, inflammation (alcoholic hepatitis), and derangement of the lobular architecture by necrosis and fibrosis (cirrhosis)
Biliary cirrhosis (intrahepatic or extrahepatic obstruction of bile flow)		
Primary biliary cirrhosis	Unknown; possibly an autoimmune mechanism	Inflammation and scarring of lobular bile ducts
Secondary biliary cirrhosis	Obstruction by neoplasms, strictures, or gallstones	Inflammation and scarring of bile ducts proximal to the obstruction
Postnecrotic cirrhosis	Viral hepatitis due to HAV or hepatitis C; drugs or other toxins; autoimmune destruction	Replacement of necrotic tissue with cirrhotic tissue, particularly fibrous, nodular scar tissue
Metabolic cirrhosis	Metabolic defects and storage disease, such as α_1-antitrypsin deficiency, glycogen storage disease, hemochromatosis, Wilson disease, galactosemia	Inflammation and scarring with specific morphologic changes related to cause

Alcoholic cirrhosis

Alcoholic hepatitis is a precursor of cirrhosis characterized by inflammation, degeneration, and necrosis of hepatocytes and infiltration of polymorphonuclear leukocytes and lymphocytes. The injured hepatocytes contain Mallory bodies (hyaline endoplasmic reticulum). The presence of Mallory bodies indicates the onset of fibrosis. The mechanism of hepatocyte injury is not clearly understood, but immunologic factors are suggested. Serum IgA is often elevated in individuals with alcoholic hepatitis, and liver antigens and antibodies have been identified in those with progressive alcoholic liver disease. The inflammation and necrosis caused by alcoholic hepatitis stimulate the fibrosis characteristic of the cirrhotic stage of disease.

Deaths from alcohol-related liver disease have increased over the past decade. The incidence of alcoholic cirrhosis is greatest in middle-aged men. In the United States mortality resulting from cirrhosis is highest among nonwhites. Although alcoholic cirrhosis is the most prevalent of the different types of cirrhosis, the occurrence of cirrhosis among alcoholics is relatively low

FIG. 36-16 Liver injury. A, Submassive hepatic necrosis from viral hepatitis, with bulging areas of residual liver and much shrinkage and collapse of left lobe. Individual lived 24 days after onset of clinical manifestations. **B,** Hypertrophic, firm, smooth alcoholic fatty liver. **C,** Eutrophic, hard, finely pseudolobular alcoholic cirrhosis in a 65-year-old man. **D,** Cut surface of alcoholic cirrhosis showing pseudolobular pattern. **E,** Atrophic, firm, megalonodular lupoid cirrhosis, quiescent in 20-year-old woman. **F,** Suppurative cholangitis with multiple abscesses resulting from carcinomatous obstruction of common duct. (From Kissane, 1990.)

(approximately 25%). The amount and duration of alcohol consumption are positively related to the extent of liver damage. Abuse of any type of alcoholic beverage can cause cirrhosis. Malnutrition may add to the risk of cirrhosis in alcohol abusers.

Pathophysiology

Alcoholic cirrhosis is caused by the toxic effects of alcohol on the liver. The oxidative metabolism of alcohol occurs primarily in the liver (see Chapter 2, p. 62). Alcohol is transformed to acetaldehyde. Excessive amounts of acetaldehyde significantly alter hepatocyte function. Mitochondrial function is impaired, decreasing oxidation of fatty acid. Enzyme and protein synthesis may be depressed or altered, and hormone and ammonia degradation is diminished. Acetaldehyde inhibits export of proteins from the liver, alters metabolism of vitamins and minerals, and induces malnutrition (Zakim, Boyer, & Montgomery, 1990). Cellular damage initiates an inflammatory response. Inflammation and necrosis result in excessive collagen formation. (Collagen is the protein component of fibrous tissues.) Fibrosis and scarring alter the structure of the liver and obstruct biliary and vascular channels (Domurat & Elias, 1992). Examples of liver damage are shown in Fig. 36-16.

Alcoholic cirrhosis begins with fatty infiltration and cirrhosis. The relationship among these stages of alcoholic liver disease is not clear. Fatty infiltration can occur without subsequent hepatitis or cirrhosis. Fat deposition (deposition of triglycerides) within the liver is primarily caused by increased lipogenesis and decreased fatty acid oxidation by hepatocytes. Lipids mobilized from adipose tissue or dietary fat intake may contribute to fat accumulation. Cessation of alcohol intake reverses the fatty accumulation.

Clinical Manifestations

Fatty infiltration causes no specific symptoms or abnormal liver function test results. The liver is usually enlarged, however, and the individual has a history of continuous alcohol intake during the previous weeks or months. Anorexia, nausea, jaundice, and edema develop with advanced fatty infiltration or the onset of alcoholic hepatitis (Fig. 36-17).

The clinical manifestations of alcoholic hepatitis can be mild or severe. Nonspecific symptoms include fatigue, weight loss, and anorexia (Woods et al., 1993). Toxic effects of alcohol also can cause testicular atrophy, reduced libido, azoospermia, and decreased testosterone in men (Gavaler & van Thiel, 1983). Manifestations of acute illness include nausea, anorexia, fever, abdominal pain, and jaundice. Cirrhosis is a multiple-system disease and causes hepatomegaly, splenomegaly, ascites, gastrointestinal hemorrhage, portal hyperten-

sion, hepatic encephalopathy, and esophageal varices. Anemia results from blood loss, poor nutrition, and hypersplenism. The presence of numerous and severe manifestations increases the risk of death. The clinical features of alcoholic cirrhosis depend on the duration of the disease and the severity of liver damage.

Evaluation and Treatment

The diagnosis of alcoholic hepatitis is based on the individual's history and clinical manifestations. The results of liver function tests are abnormal, and serologic studies show elevated serum enzymes and bilirubin, decreased serum albumin, and prolonged prothrombin time.

Liver biopsy can confirm the diagnosis of cirrhosis, but biopsy is not necessary if clinical manifestations of cirrhosis are evident. Liver function test results are usually abnormal and reflect the severity of liver damage. In severe disease with a poor prognosis, the serum albumin concentration is very low, prolonged prothrombin times cannot easily be corrected with vitamin K therapy, and serum bilirubin levels are high.

There is no specific treatment for alcoholic cirrhosis. Rest, a nutritious diet, and management of complications, such as ascites, gastrointestinal bleeding, and encephalopathy, are essential. Cessation of drinking slows the progression of liver damage, improves clinical symptoms, and prolongs life. Although the liver damage is irreversible, measures that halt the inflammation and destruction of liver cells prolong life.

Biliary cirrhosis

Biliary cirrhosis differs from alcoholic cirrhosis in that the damage and inflammation leading to cirrhosis begin in bile canaliculi and bile ducts, rather than in the hepatocytes. There are two types of biliary cirrhosis: primary and secondary. Although both involve bile duct pathology, they differ with respect to cause, risk factors, and mechanisms of obstruction and inflammation.

Primary biliary cirrhosis. Primary biliary cirrhosis causes inflammation and destruction of the intrahepatic bile ducts. Women are affected more commonly than men. Symptoms rarely develop before the age of 30 years. Primary biliary cirrhosis frequently accompanies collagen diseases, leading to speculation that autoimmune mechanisms initiate inflammation. The cause of the disease is unknown.

Primary biliary cirrhosis develops insidiously. It begins with inflammation, destruction, and fibrosis of the intrahepatic bile ducts. Nodular regeneration and cirrhosis follow. Portal hypertension develops during the later stages of the disease (Manns, 1992).

A significant number of individuals with primary biliary cirrhosis are asymptomatic. The earliest manifestations are pruritus, hyperbilirubinemia, jaundice, and

FIG. 36-17 Clinical manifestations of cirrhosis.

light-colored stools. These symptoms are caused by intrahepatic obstruction of bile flow. Steatorrhea and fat-soluble vitamin deficiencies are present in some cases. Cirrhosis and symptoms of portal hypertension and encephalopathy ultimately develop. Life expectancy is approximately 5 to 10 years after onset of symptoms.

Serologic tests show elevated alkaline phosphatase levels and hyperlipidemia, with or without other clinical manifestations. Most individuals have a circulating IgG antimitochondrial antibody that is not found in other types of liver disease. Evaluation involves ruling out biliary obstruction caused by gallstones, tumor, or inflammation of the common bile duct (i.e., secondary biliary cirrhosis). Liver biopsy usually confirms the diagnosis of primary biliary cirrhosis.

No specific treatment is available. The distressing pruritus may be relieved by cholestyramine, which binds bile salts in the intestine. Intramuscular injections of vitamins D and K alleviate the vitamin deficiency. The

other symptoms of cirrhosis are managed as they develop.

Secondary biliary cirrhosis. Secondary biliary cirrhosis develops when there is prolonged partial or complete obstruction of the common bile duct or its branches. The obstruction may be caused by gallstones, tumors, fibrotic strictures, or chronic pancreatitis. Biliary atresia and cystic fibrosis cause secondary biliary cirrhosis in children.

Chronic obstruction to bile flow increases pressure in the hepatic bile duct and results in the accumulation of bile in the centrilobular spaces. Necrotic areas develop and are followed by proliferation and inflammation of the portal ducts that result in edema and fibrosis. Pools of bile form when the portal ducts rupture into surrounding necrotic areas. Injury is accompanied by regeneration of hepatic cells with the development of finely nodular cirrhosis.

Clinical manifestations are similar to those of primary

biliary cirrhosis, with jaundice and pruritus the most distressing. Right upper quadrant pain is common, and there may be a low-grade fever from bile duct inflammation (cholangitis).

Cholangiography provides the most definitive diagnosis. Laboratory tests usually show elevated conjugated bilirubin and alkaline phosphatase levels. Aminotransferase increases if there is an accompanying cholangitis. Surgery or endoscopy relieves obstruction, prolongs survival, and diminishes or resolves symptoms. Continued obstruction leads to advanced cirrhosis and liver failure.

Postnecrotic cirrhosis

Postnecrotic cirrhosis is a consequence of many types of chronic, severe liver disease. Twenty-five percent of individuals with hepatitis C progress to postnecrotic cirrhosis. Liver injury results from drugs or toxins; inherited metabolic disorders, such as Wilson disease; α_1-antitrypsin deficiency; advanced alcoholic cirrhosis; or primary biliary cirrhosis that progresses to postnecrotic cirrhosis.

Clinical manifestations represent a progression of symptoms associated with an earlier stage of liver disease. Portal hypertension with ascites, bleeding varices, hypersplenism, and encephalopathy are the most prominent symptoms. As a consequence of progressive liver injury, broad and dense bands of fibrosis separate islands of liver cells, giving the liver a nodular appearance. The liver is small in size and distorted in shape.

Diagnosis is confirmed by needle biopsy, and treatment is directed toward relief of symptoms. Death usually occurs as a result of bleeding or encephalopathy.

Disorders of the Gallbladder

Obstruction and inflammation are the most common disorders of the gallbladder. Obstruction is caused by **gallstones,** which are aggregates of substances in the bile. The gallstones may remain in the gallbladder or be ejected, with bile, into the cystic duct. Gallstones that become lodged in the cystic duct obstruct the flow of bile into and out of the gallbladder and cause inflammation. Gallstone formation is termed **cholelithiasis.** Inflammation of the gallbladder or cystic duct is known as **cholecystitis.**

Cholelithiasis

Cholelithiasis is a prevalent disorder in developed countries, where incidence is 10% to 20%. The actual incidence is unknown because many individuals who have gallstones are asymptomatic. Gallstones are of two types: cholesterol and pigmented. Cholesterol stones are the most common. Risk factors include obesity, middle age, female gender, American Indian ancestry, and gallbladder, pancreatic, or ileal disease. Pigmented stones, which are common, occur later in life and are associated with cirrhosis.

Pathophysiology

Cholesterol gallstones form in bile that is supersaturated with cholesterol produced by the liver. Supersaturation sets the stage for cholesterol crystal formation, or the formation of "microstones." More crystals then aggregate on the microstones, which grow to form "macrostones." This process usually occurs in the gallbladder, which may have decreased motility. The stones may lie "silent" or become lodged in the cystic or common duct, causing pain and cholecystitis. Gallstone formation may be such that the stones accumulate and fill the entire gallbladder (Fig. 36-18).

It is not known why the hepatocytes secrete bile that is supersaturated with cholesterol. Proposed mechanisms include (1) an enzymatic defect that affects the hepatocytes' synthesis of cholesterol; (2) diminished secretion of bile acids, which normally promote cholesterol solubility; (3) decreased resorption of bile salts from the ileum, which decrease the bile acid pool; and (4) some combination of these mechanisms. In obese individuals the mechanism appears to involve cholesterol synthesis, whereas in nonobese individuals, it appears to involve decreased secretion of bile acids.

Pigmented stones are created by cholesterol, calcium bilirubinate, or pigmented polymers. The formation of pigmented stones is associated with biliary infection and increased amounts of unconjugated bilirubin in bile. The unconjugated bilirubin precipitates in the gallbladder or bile ducts to form the stones (Carey, 1993).

Clinical Manifestations

Abdominal pain and jaundice are the cardinal manifestations of cholelithiasis. Vague symptoms include heartburn, flatulence, epigastric discomfort, and food intolerances, particularly to fats and cabbage. The pain, frequently called biliary colic, is caused by the lodging of one or more gallstones in the cystic or common duct. The pain can be intermittent or steady. It usually is located in the right upper quadrant and radiates to the mid-upper back. Jaundice indicates that the stone is located in the common bile duct. Abdominal tenderness and fever indicate cholecystitis.

Evaluation and Treatment

Diagnosis is based on the history, physical examination, and radiographic evaluation. An oral cholecystogram usually outlines the stones. Intravenous cholangiography is used to differentiate cholelithiasis from other causes of extrahepatic biliary obstruction if the cholecystogram is negative. Endoscopic or percutaneous cholangiography is also a diagnostic option.

Laparoscopic cholecystectomy is the preferred treatment for gallstones that cause obstruction or inflammation. An alternative treatment is the administration of drugs that dissolve the stones. For example, the bile acid chenodeoxycholic acid (CDCA) can completely or par-

FIG. 36-18 Resected gallbladder containing mixed gallstones. (From Kissane, 1990.)

tially dissolve cholesterol gallstones. Ursodeoxycholic acid (UDCA), which is structurally similar to CDCA, is also effective, is less toxic to hepatocytes, and does not cause fatty diarrhea, as does CDCA.

Cholecystitis

Cholecystitis can be acute or chronic. Both forms are almost always caused by the lodging of a gallstone in the cystic duct. Obstruction causes the gallbladder to become distended and inflamed. The pain is similar to that caused by gallstones. Pressure against the distended wall of the gallbladder decreases blood flow. Ischemia, necrosis, and perforation of the gallbladder are possible. Fever, leukocytosis, rebound tenderness, and abdominal muscle guarding are common findings. Serum bilirubin and alkaline phosphatase levels may be elevated. Nevertheless, the acute abdominal pain of cholecystitis must be differentiated from the pain caused by other disorders, such as pancreatitis, myocardial infarction, and acute pyelonephritis of the right kidney. Cholangiography or radioactive scan can confirm a diagnosis of cholecystitis.

Narcotics may be required to control pain, and antibiotics (e.g., gentamicin and clindamycin) are often prescribed to manage bacterial infection in severe cases. Persistent symptoms or development of chronic cholecystitis punctuated by recurrent, acute attacks usually requires gallbladder resection (cholecystectomy). If pancreatic abscesses develop, they are usually resected (Domschke, 1987).

Disorders of the Pancreas

Pancreatitis, or inflammation of the pancreas, is a relatively rare and potentially serious disorder. Incidence is about equal in men and women. The disease is most common during the fifth decade of life (Trapnell & Duncan, 1975). Pancreatitis can be acute or chronic. It is associated with several other clinical conditions, in-

cluding alcoholism, obstructive biliary tract disease (particularly cholelithiasis), peptic ulcers, trauma, hyperlipidemia, and certain drugs (Steer, 1992).

Acute Pancreatitis
Pathophysiology

Acute pancreatitis, also called acute hemorrhagic pancreatitis, is a severe pancreatic inflammation requiring hospital care. In many cases the precise pathogenic mechanism or sequence of events that triggers acute pancreatitis is unknown (Steinberg, 1992). Many causal factors are probably involved. The most common theory is that pancreatitis develops because of an injury or disruption of the pancreatic ducts or acini, which permits leakage of pancreatic enzymes into pancreatic tissue. The leaked enzymes become activated in the tissue, initiating autodigestion and acute pancreatitis. The exact mechanism of enzyme activation remains to be described (Steer, 1992), but activation is known to occur in the presence of bile. Bile reflux into the pancreas occurs if gallstones obstruct the common bile duct and hidden gallstones can contribute to attacks of acute pancreatitis (Lee, Nicholls, & Park, 1992). The activated proteolases (trypsin, elastase, and lipases) break down tissue and cell membranes causing edema, vascular damage, hemorrhage, and necrosis (Nevalainen & Aho, 1987). (Fatty necrosis is described in Chapter 2.) Toxic enzymes also are released into the bloodstream and cause injury to vessels and other organs, such as the lungs and kidneys. These systemic effects are major causes of morbidity and mortality.

Clinical Manifestations

Epigastric or midabdominal pain is the cardinal symptom of acute pancreatitis. It can range from mild abdominal discomfort to severe, incapacitating pain. The pain may radiate to the back because of the retroperitoneal location of the pancreas. The pain is caused by edema, which distends the pancreatic ducts and capsule; chemical irritation and inflammation of the peritoneum; and irritation or obstruction of the biliary tract. Fever and leukocytosis accompany the inflammatory response.

Nausea and vomiting are common. These gastrointestinal symptoms are caused by hypermotility or paralytic ileus secondary to the pancreatitis or peritonitis.

Abdominal distention accompanies bowel hypermotility and the accumulation of fluids in the peritoneal cavity. Hypotension and shock occur frequently because plasma volume is lost as enzymes and kinins released into the circulation increase vascular permeability and dilate vessels. The results are hypovolemia, hypotension, and myocardial insufficiency. A small percentage of individuals develop tachypnea and hypoxemia secondary to pulmonary edema, atelectasis, or pleural effusions caused by circulating pancreatic enzymes. In severe cases hypovolemia decreases renal blood flow sufficiently to impair renal function. Tetany may develop as a result of deposition of calcium in areas of fat necrosis or as a decreased response to parathormone. Transient hyperglycemia also can occur if glucagon is released from damaged alpha cells in the pancreatic islets.

Evaluation and Treatment

Diagnosis of pancreatitis is based on clinical findings, identification of associated disorders, and laboratory studies. Elevated serum amylase is a characteristic diagnostic feature. The amylase level usually rises within 12 hours after the onset of symptoms and returns to normal within 3 to 5 days in most cases. Urine amylase and serum lipase are also elevated. The ratio of amylase clearance to creatinine clearance by the kidney can be diagnostic because, in cases of pancreatitis, amylase clearance increases significantly compared with creatinine clearance. Acute pancreatitis is difficult to diagnose because several other disorders can cause similar clinical and laboratory findings. These disorders include perforating duodenal ulcer, acute cholecystitis, small bowel obstruction, and kidney stones.

The goal of treatment for acute pancreatitis is to stop the process of autodigestion and prevent systemic complications. Narcotic medications may be needed to relieve pain. Demerol is used instead of morphine because it causes less spasm of the sphincter of Oddi than morphine. To decrease pancreatic secretions and "rest the gland," oral food and fluids are withheld and continuous gastric suction is instituted. Nasogastric suction may not be necessary with mild pancreatitis, but it helps to relieve pain and prevent paralytic ileus in individuals who are nauseated and vomiting. Parenteral fluids are given to restore blood volume and prevent hypotension and shock. Parenteral hyperalimentation should be initiated to reverse the catabolic state associated with se-

vere pancreatitis (Pisters & Ranson, 1992). Drugs that decrease gastric acid production (e.g., cimetidine) can decrease stimulation of the pancreas by secretin. Severe, unremitting pancreatitis may require peritoneal lavage to remove toxic exudates or surgical drainage of the pancreas. The risk of mortality increases significantly with the development of pulmonary, cardiac, and renal complications.

Chronic Pancreatitis

Structural or functional impairment of the pancreas leads to **chronic pancreatitis.** Chronic alcohol abuse is the most common cause (Holt, 1993). Chronic pancreatitis causes continuous or intermittent abdominal pain, which usually intensifies after a meal. Individuals who require narcotic medications to relieve pain are at high risk for narcotic addiction. Occasionally manifestations of pancreatic enzyme deficiency, such as steatorrhea or a malabsorption syndrome, are present. To correct enzyme deficiencies and prevent malabsorption, oral enzyme replacements are taken before and during meals. Loss of islet cell function can cause insulin-dependent diabetes. Cessation of alcohol intake is essential for the management of chronic pancreatitis.

Pancreatic cysts are common lesions of chronic pancreatitis. The cysts are walled-off areas or pockets of pancreatic juice, necrotic debris, or blood within or adjacent to the pancreas. Surgical drainage or partial resection of the pancreas may be required to relieve pain and prevent cystic rupture.

CANCER OF THE DIGESTIVE SYSTEM
Cancer of the Gastrointestinal Tract
Cancer of the Esophagus

Carcinoma of the esophagus is a rare disease. The incidence in the United States and Europe is less than 1% of new cancers per year (ACS, 1993). The incidence in the United States is higher in blacks than in whites and peaks at about 60 years of age.

Dietary factors, particularly deficiencies of trace elements and vitamins, possibly influence carcinogenesis. Esophageal cancer is strongly associated with malnutrition caused by poor economic conditions, special dietary habits, or alcoholism (Dowlatshahi et al., 1984). Alcohol and tobacco use have long been established as risk factors for esophageal cancer. The risk of esophageal cancer increases with the amount of alcohol consumed. Alcohol abuse, in combination with dietary zinc deficiency, renders the esophageal mucosa susceptible to carcinogens. Although heavy cigarette smoking is known to increase the risk of esophageal cancer, esophageal cancer is found more frequently in pipe and cigar smokers than cigarette smokers.

Reflux esophagitis is associated with carcinomas of the esophagus, as is sliding hiatal hernia. Both of these conditions can cause erosive esophagitis and ulceration that can eventually lead to metaplasia and neoplastic changes.

Pathogenesis

Carcinoma of the esophagus is usually squamous cell carcinoma or, less commonly, adenocarcinoma. Adenocarcinomas of the esophagus are frequently secondary to infiltration by a gastric carcinoma or to the presence of Barrett's epithelium (columnar rather than squamous epithelium in the lower esophagus), which is associated with chronic gastroesophageal reflux. Carcinomas can occur at any level of the esophageal tract but are most common where the esophagus joins the stomach (the gastroesophageal junction) (Mufti, Zirvi, & Garewal, 1991).

The pathogenesis of esophageal carcinoma is facilitated by (1) alterations of esophageal structure and function that permit food and drink to remain in the esophagus for prolonged periods of time, (2) ulceration and metaplasia caused by esophageal reflux, and (3) chronic exposure to irritants, such as alcohol and tobacco, that cause neoplastic transformation (see Chapter 11). Chronic inadequate nutrition can impair both structure and function of the esophagus. Nutritional deprivation, particularly deficiencies of vitamin A and zinc, results in mucosal changes that make the esophageal mucosa vulnerable to neoplastic changes.

Clinical Manifestations

The two main manifestations of esophageal carcinoma are chest pain and dysphagia. The most common type of pain is heartburn (pyrosis). It is initiated by eating spicy or highly seasoned foods and by lying down. Dysphagia (pain on swallowing), another common symptom, is usually pressurelike and may radiate posteriorly between the scapulae. Odynophagia may be initiated by the swallowing of cold liquids. Spontaneous chest pain is more difficult to diagnose positively. Some individuals with esophageal cancer complain of a constant retrosternal pain that radiates to the back. Dysphagia usually progresses rapidly. It is mostly painless during the early stages of esophageal carcinoma.

Evaluation and Treatment

Individuals who present with dysphagia undergo endoscopy so that specimens can be obtained and examined for neoplastic change. Computed tomography (CT) studies of the thorax are also used for diagnosis. Esophageal cancer metastasizes rapidly and therefore has a poor prognosis. The lymphatic vessels of the esophagus are continuous with vital mediastinal structures and drain to the lymph nodes from the neck of the celiac axis, making it impossible to remove all the lymph nodes with the tumor. Removal of the primary lesion and the local lymph nodes, however, can benefit the individual with esophageal cancer. If the malignancy has not spread beyond these sites, cure is likely. If spread has occurred, however, an incomplete resection is of little benefit.

Cancer of the Stomach

Although the incidence of gastric cancer has declined in the United States, it still represents about 2% of all new cancer cases annually (ACS, 1993). In countries such as Japan, the British Isles, and Iceland, the incidence of stomach cancer has remained high consistently. The incidence rate in Japan is one of the highest in the world. Studies of Japanese immigrants to the United States show that offspring who are born and raised in the United States have an incidence rate comparable to that of other Americans. These data illustrate the importance of environmental factors, such as diet, to carcinogenesis.

The most important environmental factors in the cause of gastric cancer are (1) salt added to food; (2) food additives (e.g., nitrates) in pickled or salted foods (e.g., bacon); and (3) food factors found in water and vegetables, such as vitamin C (vitamin C is possibly a protective factor). Dietary salt enhances the conversion of nitrates to carcinogenic nitrosamines in the stomach. Salt is also caustic to the stomach and can cause chronic atrophic gastritis. Finally, hypertonic salt solutions delay gastric emptying. Delayed emptying increases the time during which carcinogenic nitrosamines can exert their effects on the stomach mucosa.

The metabolism of nitrates and nitrites is very complex. Nitrates interact with amino acids in the stomach to form nitrosamines. The conversion of these carcinogenic nitrosamines is enhanced at a low pH by iodides and thiocyanates. Nitrates are thought to be active only when converted to nitrites and to cause stomach cancer once atrophic gastritis has occurred.

The incidence of gastric cancer is greater in males than in females. Other nonenvironmental risk factors are a family history of gastric adenocarcinoma, blood type (blood group A), and pernicious anemia, which causes atrophy of the gastric mucosa in the same locations where gastric tumors arise.

Pathogenesis

Gastric cancer usually begins in the glands of the stomach mucosa. Approximately 50% of all gastric cancers develop in the prepyloric antrum (Fig. 36-19). Atrophic gastritis and intestinal metaplasia are strongly linked to the development of gastric cancer. Insufficient acid secretion by the atrophic mucosa creates a relatively alkaline environment that permits bacteria to multiply

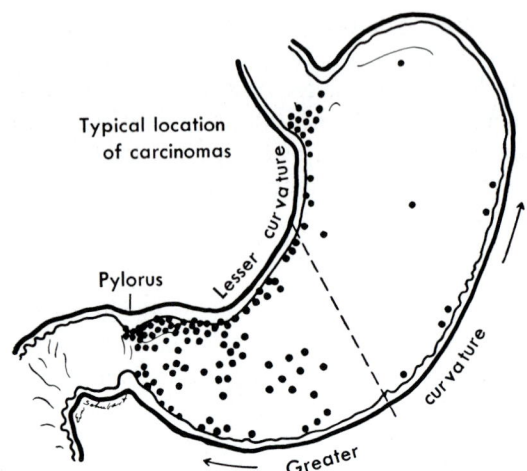

FIG. 36-19   Typical sites of stomach cancer. (From del Regato, Spjut, & Cox, 1985.)

and act on nitrates. The resulting increase in nitrosoamines damages the DNA of mucosal cells further, promoting metaplasia and neoplasia. Duodenal reflux may also contribute to intestinal metaplasia. The reflux contains caustic bile salts that destroy the mucosal barrier that normally protects the stomach.

Clinical Manifestations

The early stages of gastric cancer are generally asymptomatic or produce vague symptoms such as loss of appetite (especially for meat), malaise, and "indigestion." Later manifestations of gastric cancer include unexplained weight loss, upper abdominal pain, vomiting, change in bowel habits, and anemia caused by persistent occult bleeding. The prognosis is poor because symptoms do not occur until the tumor has penetrated the muscle layers of the stomach, spread to surrounding tissues, and entered the draining lymph nodes and veins, causing distant metastases. Generally the first manifestations of carcinoma are caused by distant metastases.

Evaluation and Treatment

The choice of diagnostic tests depends on the clinical manifestations at the time of presentation. Most symptoms suggest a problem in the upper gastrointestinal tract, and the lesion is shown by a barium x-ray film. Direct endoscopic visualization and biopsy usually establish the diagnosis. Another definitive technique is microscopic examination of exfoliated cells obtained by lavage during endoscopy.

Surgery is the usual treatment for gastric cancer. Staging is determined by pathologic findings after resection. Radiation therapy is generally unsuccessful, and immunotherapy is still experimental. Chemotherapy some-

times reduces the tumor. Individuals who respond well to chemotherapy generally live longer than those who do not.

Cancer of the Colon and Rectum

Cancer of the lower intestinal tract (colorectal cancer) is the second most frequent cause of cancer death in the United States, for both men and women. Colorectal cancer accounts for 10% to 15% of all cancer deaths (ACS, 1993). Cancer of the colon tends to occur in individuals older than 50 years of age. It is rare in children. Worldwide, the prevalence of colorectal cancer is highest in populations with high socioeconomic standards, possibly because of dietary habits.

Pathogenesis

Genetic events are associated with the development of colonic cancer. Allelic deletion on chromosomes 5, 17, and 18 appears to promote transition from normal to malignant colon mucosa. The chromosome 17 deletion is a mutation of the gene for transformation of associated protein, P53. Dietary factors, including high fat, low fiber, and low calcium, may promote somatic mutations. Promoting mechanisms are related to prolonged contact of the fecal mass with colon mucosa (Ahnen, 1991).

Colorectal polyps are closely associated with development of cancer. A polyp, or papilloma, is a fingerlike projection arising from the mucosal epithelium. Most polyps are benign. The two major types of neoplastic polyps are pedunculated (stalk), adenomatous polyps, and sessile (papillary or villous) adenomas (Fig. 36-20). Once the adenoma traverses the muscularis mucosae, it becomes invasive and highly malignant. Adenomas can be detected early, however, and the submucosa may not be penetrated for several years. The larger the polyp, the greater the risk of colorectal cancer. Although lesions larger than 1.5 cm occur less frequently, they are more likely to be malignant than those smaller than 1.0 cm. For other conditions commonly confused with colorectal cancer see Table 36-10.

Most colorectal cancers are moderately differentiated adenocarcinomas. These tumors have a long preinvasive phase, and when they invade they tend to grow slowly. Colorectal carcinoma starts in the glands of the mucosal lining. Because the lymphatic channels are located underneath the muscularis mucosae, the lesions must traverse this layer before metastasis can occur.

Clinical Manifestations

Tumors of the right (ascending) and left (descending) colon evolve into two distinct tumor types. On the right side the lesions are polypoid and extend along one wall of the cecum and ascending colon. Clinical manifestations include pain, palpable mass in the lower right

Adenomatous polyp

Focal atypia
(cancer in situ)

Focal cancer
(malignant adenoma)

FIG. 36-20 Development of cancer of the colon from adenomatous polyps. The tumor becomes invasive if it penetrates the muscularis mucosae and enters the submucosal layer. (From del Regato, Spjut, & Cox, 1985.)

Focal cancer invading stalk with some "benign" polyp still in body

Invasive cancer containing piece of polyp

Polypoid invasive cancer without polyp remnant

Ulcerated invasive cancer without polyp remnant

TABLE 36-10

Conditions Commonly Confused with Colorectal Cancer

Condition	Significant characteristics
Diverticulitis	Left-sided pain similar to that of appendicitis; tender lower left quadrant. Associated findings: nausea, vomiting, fever, obstruction, anorexia, and leukocytosis; mucosa is intact, and perforation, peritonitis, and abscesses occur more frequently than in cancer; protosigmoidoscopy or barium enema used to distinguish from cancer
Chronic ulcerative colitis	Younger people with chronic attacks of bloody diarrhea, crampy abdominal pain, fever, malnutrition, and dehydration; usually involves the left colon and rectum; endoscopy, barium enema, and biopsy performed for definitive diagnosis
Crohn disease (granulomatous colitis)	Generally involves the right colon; chronic diarrhea with abdominal cramps, fever, weight loss, and often a palpable abdominal mass; difficult at times to distinguish Crohn disease from ulcerative colitis; endoscopic examination and barium enema used to distinguish from cancer
Appendicitis	Vague abdominal symptoms, often with a tender or nontender mass in the lower right quadrant; associated symptoms: mild fever and leukycytosis; barium enema used to distinguish cancer of the cecum from appendiceal abscess
Thrombosed hemorrhoids	Examination shows a tender, swollen, bluish painful mass in the anus; patient will have a history of hemorrhoids

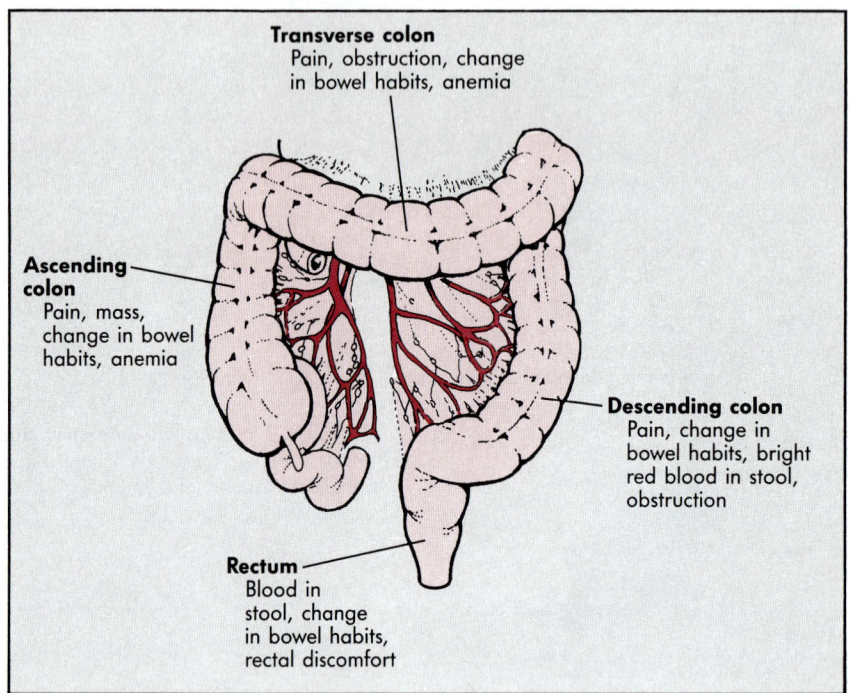

FIG. 36-21 Signs and symptoms of colorectal cancer by location of primary lesion. Clinical manifestations are listed in order of frequency for each region (lymphatics of colon also shown).

quadrant, anemia, and dark red or mahogany-colored blood mixed with the stool (Fig. 36-21). These large, bulky tumors become necrotic and ulcerated, contributing to persistent blood loss and anemia. Obstruction is unusual because the growth does not readily encircle the colon.

Tumors of the left or descending colon start as small, elevated buttonlike masses. This type grows circumferentially and spreads along the entire bowel wall, eventually ulcerating in the middle as the tumor penetrates the blood supply. Obstruction is frequent but occurs slowly. Manifestations include progressive abdominal distention, pain, vomiting, constipation, need for laxatives, cramps, and bright red blood on the surface of the stool.

Systematic lymphatic spread occurs along the aorta to the mesenteric and pancreatic lymph nodes. Liver metastasis follows invasion of the mesenteric veins (left colon) or superior veins (right colon), which drain into the portal circulation.

Rectal carcinomas are defined as tumors occurring up to 15 cm from the anal opening. Tumors of the rectum can spread through the rectal wall to nearby structures: the prostate in men and the vagina in women. Penetration occurs more readily in the lower third of the rectum because it has no serosal covering. Systemic and pulmonary metastases occur through the hemorrhoidal plexus, which drains into the vena cava.

Evaluation and Treatment

Individuals with family history of polyps should be screened using colonoscopy with removal of the polyp when they are found. A diet rich in vegetables, grains, fruit, and calcium and low in fat can modify cancer risk (Trock, Lanza, & Greenwald, 1990; Vargas & Alberts, 1992). Genetic markers are being developed to identify at-risk populations (Shike et al., 1990).

The staging of colorectal cancer involves preoperative testing and operative exploration. Preoperative testing begins with physical examination of the abdomen to detect liver enlargement and ascites and palpate appropriate lymph nodes. Elevations of carcinoembryonic antigen (CEA) are often detected in the sera of individuals with colorectal carcinoma. The amount of CEA in the serum is a function of the stage of the disease and the type of tumor. Operative staging consists of careful exploration during surgery and biopsy of possible metastases. The Dukes classification for staging of colorectal cancer is as follows:

Stage A: cancer limited to the bowel wall
Stage B: cancer extending through the bowel wall
Stage C: nodal metastases regardless of extension into bowel wall
Stage D: distant metastases regardless of primary size

Treatment for cancer of the colon is always surgical. The location and amount of colon resected depend on the site of the cancer. Resection and anastomosis can be performed for cancer of the ascending, transverse, descending, or sigmoid colon and upper rectum. These surgeries are performed through abdominal incisions, and natural defecation is preserved.

Growths in the lower portion of the rectum require removal of the entire rectum. The proximal end of the descending colon is brought out through a small incision in the abdominal wall and becomes a permanent colostomy. Prognosis after surgery depends on the stage and location of the tumor.

Radiation therapy is often given before surgery in the hope that it will shrink the tumor, alter the malignant cells, or do both, so that these cells will not survive after surgery. Chemotherapy is used to treat metastatic disease and cases with a high risk of recurrence. Immunotherapy can boost the immune response.

Cancer of the Accessory Organs of Digestion

Cancer of the Liver

Cancer of the liver is usually caused by metastatic spread from a primary site elsewhere in the body. Primary liver cancer is relatively rare in the United States but is common in densely populated parts of the Far East, Southern Africa, China, and Greece. In the United States, the incidence of primary liver cancer is higher in blacks than in whites (2 to 10 per 100,000 per annum). For reasons not understood, incidence is higher in males than in females. Primary liver cancer is rare before the age of 40 and most common during the sixth decade. Together, primary and secondary liver cancer accounts for 2% of all cancer deaths in the United States (ACS, 1993).

Risk factors for primary liver cancer include the following:

1. Exposure to mycotoxins. The most significant mycotoxins are the aflatoxins, particularly those produced by *Aspergillus flavus,* a mold found on spoiled corn, peanuts, and grain.
2. Chronic liver disease, especially cirrhosis.
3. Infection with hepatitis B virus (HBV), hepatitis C virus (HCV), and hepatitis D virus (HDV), particularly in conjunction with cirrhosis, acts either as a carcinogen or as a cocarcinogen in chronically infected hepatocytes.

Pathogenesis

Primary carcinomas of the liver are hepatocellular or cholangiocellular. **Hepatocellular carcinoma** (hepatocarcinoma) develops in the hepatocytes, whereas **cholangiocellular carcinoma** (cholangiocarcinoma) develops in the bile ducts. Hepatocellular carcinoma can be nodular (consisting of multiple, discrete nodules), massive (consisting of a large tumor mass having satellite nodules), or diffuse (consisting of very small nodules distributed throughout most of the liver). Hepatocellu-

lar carcinoma is the type of primary liver cancer that is closely associated with cirrhosis. Because carcinoma of the liver invades the hepatic and portal veins, it often spreads to the heart and lungs. Other sites of metastases are the brain, kidney, and spleen.

Cholangiocellular carcinomas occur less frequently than hepatocellular carcinomas. This type of primary liver cancer is most common in areas where liver fluke infestation is prevalent, such as Southeast China. The mechanism by which fluke infestation causes cholangiocellular carcinoma is unknown. Cholangiocellular carcinoma can occur anywhere along the bile duct and extend directly into the liver, usually as a solitary lesion. It is difficult to distinguish an invasion of cholangiocellular carcinoma from a metastatic adenocarcinoma except by neoplastic changes found in nearby ducts.

Clinical Manifestations

The clinical presentation of liver cancer in adults is characterized by vague abdominal symptoms, such as nausea and vomiting, fullness, pressure, and dull ache in the right hypochondrium. Manifestations of hepatocellular carcinoma can occur slowly or abruptly. In individuals with cirrhosis, deepening jaundice or abrupt lack of appetite is a sign of hepatocellular carcinoma. Obstruction by the tumor can cause sudden worsening of portal hypertension and development of ascites. As the tumor enlarges, it causes pain. Cholangiocellular carcinoma more commonly presents insidiously as pain, loss of appetite, weight loss, and gradual onset of jaundice. Some carcinomas of the liver rupture spontaneously, causing hemorrhage. Others are discovered accidentally during evaluation of a bone fracture or surgical exploration.

Evaluation and Treatment

There is no specific test for the diagnosis of liver cancer. The diagnosis is based on clinical manifestations, laboratory findings, radiologic examination, and exploratory laparotomy.

Levels of alkaline phosphatase, serum glutamic oxaloacetic transaminase (AST), and serum glutamic pyruvic transaminase (ALT) are commonly elevated in individuals with hepatocellular carcinoma. α-Fetoprotein is elevated (in excess of 400 ng/ml) in individuals with advanced hepatocellular carcinoma. Excessive levels of α-fetoprotein have been correlated with hepatitis B antigen, rapid tumor growth, and poor tumor differentiation. Erythrocytosis is secondary to erythropoietin production.

In individuals without cirrhosis, liver scans can document filling defects. Computed tomography or ultrasonography is used to detect solid tumors, but neither can distinguish benign from malignant tumors. A liver biopsy can be diagnostic unless scattered nodules are missed by the examiner.

Surgical resection is possible only if the tumor is localized to a removable lobe of the liver. Tumors of the posterior segment of the right lobe are not resectable because this segment contains the right hepatic vein. Chemotherapeutic agents are administered systemically or locally. Radiation is not part of the treatment regimen because the dosages needed for effectiveness exceed the tolerance of liver tissue.

The overall median survival rate for those with symptomatic liver cancer is only 3 to 4 months. Surgery is hazardous and usually not undertaken if the individual has cirrhosis. Most individuals develop metastases after surgical resection, but long-term survival is possible.

Cancer of the Gallbladder

Cancer of the gallbladder is more common in women than in men by a ratio of about 3 to 1. It occurs rarely before the age of 40 and is most common between the ages of 50 and 60. Most gallbladder cancer is caused by metastasis. Primary carcinoma of the gallbladder is rare and is usually associated with cholelithiasis.

Pathogenesis

Most primary carcinomas of the gallbladder are adenocarcinomas. A few are squamous cell carcinomas. Invasion of the liver occurs early. Spreading occurs to the cystic and periportal lymph nodes with invasion of the pancreas and retroperitoneal lymph nodes. Direct invasion of the stomach and the duodenum can cause pyloric obstruction. Infection often accompanies cancer of the gallbladder. Generalized peritonitis, gangrene, perforation, and liver abscesses are potential complications of infection.

Clinical Manifestations

A typical presentation of carcinoma of the gallbladder is steady, upper-right-quadrant pain for a couple of months. Other manifestations include diarrhea, belching, weakness, loss of appetite, weight loss, and vomiting. Obstructive jaundice can occur if an enlarging tumor presses on the extrahepatic ducts.

Evaluation and Treatment

Early diagnosis of cancer of the gallbladder is not possible. Therefore, individuals with gallstones, especially older women, are evaluated carefully. Inflammatory disorders, such as cholangitis (bile duct inflammation) and peritonitis, often obscure an underlying malignancy. Diagnostic procedures include upper gastrointestinal barium study, ultrasonography, cholangiography, and CT.

Complete surgical resection of the gallbladder is the only effective treatment. Because advanced malignancies cannot be resected, gallbladders containing stones are removed as a preventive measure. The prognosis of gallbladder cancer is extremely poor; most individuals die 1 year after surgery (Nadhler & McSheny, 1992).

Cancer of the Pancreas

Pancreatic cancer now ranks fifth as a cause of cancer deaths in the United States. The incidence of pancreatic cancer rises steadily with age. Males are affected slightly more often than females, and blacks more often than whites. Pancreatic cancer accounts for about 25,000 deaths annually in the United States (ACS, 1993). The mortality rate is nearly 100%. The cause of pancreatic cancer is not known, and with the exception of an association of risk with cigarette smoking, no external risk factors have been identified (ACS, 1988).

Pathogenesis

Cancer of the pancreas can arise from exocrine or endocrine cells. Most pancreatic tumors arise from exocrine cells in the ducts and are called ductal adenocarcinomas. Tumors arising in small ducts invade nearby glandular tissue, penetrate the covering of the pancreas, and extend into surrounding tissues (Poston, Gillespie, & Guillou, 1991).

Ductal adenocarcinomas can occur in the head, body, or tail of the pancreas. Tumors of the head quickly spread to obstruct the common bile duct and portal vein. These tumors can then infiltrate the superior mesenteric artery, the vena cava, and the aorta. Cancer cells that enter the blood vessels can form emboli. Tumors of the body and tail infiltrate the posterior abdominal wall. Lymphatic invasion occurs early and rapidly and involves local and regional lymph nodes. Venous invasion causes metastases to the liver. Tumor implants on the peritoneal surface can obstruct veins and promote development of ascites.

Ductal adenocarcinomas arising in the head of the pancreas cause biliary obstruction somewhat early in the disease. Individuals with such tumors survive slightly longer than those with cancer of the body and tail, presumably because they seek medical attention earlier.

Tumors of the endocrine pancreas are rare neoplasms of the islets of Langerhans known as "apudomas." The *apud* in *apudoma* is an acronym for *amine precursor uptake* and *decarboxylation*. The apudomas are so named because they contain neurosecretory granules. Endocrine neoplasms are fatal because they secrete abnormal amounts of hormones, such as insulin.

Clinical Manifestations

Cancer of the body and tail of the pancreas is generally asymptomatic until the tumor invades adjacent tissue. Frequently vague back pain is an initial symptom. Jaundice develops in most cases, usually caused by obstruction of the bile duct (Krech & Walsh, 1991). Because it impairs enzyme secretion and flow to the duodenum, pancreatic cancer causes fat and protein malabsorption, resulting in weight loss. Distant metastases are found in

TABLE 36-11

Cancer of the Gut, Liver, and Pancreas

Organ	Deaths of all cancers	Risks	Cell type	Common manifestations
Esophagus	2%	Malnutrition Alcohol Tobacco Chronic reflux	Squamous cell Adenocarcinoma	Chest pain Dysphagia
Stomach	2%	Salty food Nitrates-nitrosamines Gastric atrophy	Adenocarcinoma Squamous cell	Anorexia Malaise Weight Upper abdominal pain Vomiting Occult blood
Colorectal	12%	Polyps Ulcerative colitis Diverticulitis High refined CHO, low-fiber/high-fat diet	Adenocarcinoma (left colon grows in ring; right colon grows as mass)	Pain Mass Anemia Bloody stool Obstruction Distention
Liver	2%	HBV, HCV, HDV Cirrhosis Intestinal parasite Aflatoxin from moldy peanuts	Hepatomas Cholangiomas	Pain Anorexia Bloating Weight loss Portal hypertension Ascites ± jaundice
Pancreas	5%	Chronic pancreatitis Cigarette smoking Alcohol (?) Diabetic women	Adenocarcinoma (exocrine part of gland, ductal epithelium)	Weight loss Weakness Nausea Vomiting Abdominal pain Depression ± jaundice May have insulin-secreting tumors with symptoms of hypoglycemia

All the above cancers are within the top 10 causes of death from cancer.
From: American Cancer Society (ACS). (1993). Cancer statistics 1993. *CA—A Cancer Journal for Clinicians,* 43(1).

the neck nodes, the lungs, and the brain. Most individuals die of hepatic failure, malnutrition, or systemic diseases.

Evaluation and Treatment

A laparotomy is often performed, particularly if jaundice is present. Ultrasonography and computed tomography may be needed to confirm the need for a laparotomy, especially in individuals without jaundice. Laparotomy is used to establish a definitive diagnosis, evaluate the extent of disease, and determine whether palliative bypass surgery (i.e., cholecystojejunostomy

and gastrojejunostomy) is needed. Most individuals require palliative double bypass of the blocked bile ducts, as well as gastrojejunostomy to prevent duodenal obstruction.

Many surgeons recommend a total pancreatectomy because cancer of the pancreas seldom consists of a single lesion. Chemotherapy and radiation therapy are seldom beneficial, except as palliative measures. Because almost all pancreatic cancers are advanced at the time of diagnosis, staging has little relevance in determining treatment. Cancers of the gastrointestinal tract are summarized in Table 36-11.

Disorders of the Gastrointestinal Tract

1. Anorexia (loss of appetite), vomiting, constipation, diarrhea, abdominal pain, and evidence of gastrointestinal bleeding are clinical manifestations of many disorders of the gastrointestinal tract.

2. Vomiting is the forceful emptying of the stomach effected by gastrointestinal contraction and reverse peristalsis of the esophagus. It is usually preceded by nausea and retching, with the exception of projectile vomiting, which is associated with direct stimulation of the vomiting center in the brain.

3. Constipation is frequently caused by unhealthy dietary and bowel habits combined with lack of exercise. Constipation also can result from a disorder that impairs intestinal motility or obstructs the intestinal lumen.

4. Diarrhea can be caused by excessive fluid drawn into the intestinal lumen by osmosis (osmotic diarrhea), excessive secretion of fluids by the intestinal mucosa (secretory diarrhea), or excessive gastrointestinal motility.

5. Abdominal pain is caused by stretching, inflammation, or ischemia (insufficient blood supply). Abdominal pain originates in the organs themselves (visceral pain) or in the peritoneum (parietal pain). Visceral pain is frequently referred to the back.

6. Obvious manifestations of gastrointestinal bleeding are hematemesis (vomiting of blood), melena (dark, tarry stools), and hematochezia (frank bleeding from the rectum). Occult bleeding can only be detected by testing stools or vomitus for presence of blood.

7. Dysphagia is difficulty in swallowing. It can be caused by a mechanical or functional obstruction of the esophagus. Functional obstruction is an impairment of esophageal motility.

8. Achalasia is a form of functional dysphagia caused by loss of esophageal innervation.

9. Gastroesophageal reflux is the regurgitation of chyme from the stomach into the esophagus. An inflammatory response (reflux esophagitis) ensues if the esophageal mucosa is repeatedly exposed to acids and enzymes in the regurgitated chyme.

10. Hiatal hernia is the protrusion of the upper part of the stomach through the hiatus (esophageal opening in the diaphragm) at the gastroesophageal junction. Hiatal hernia can be sliding or paraesophageal.

11. Pyloric obstruction is the narrowing or blockage of the pylorus, which is the opening between the stomach and the duodenum. It can be caused by a congenital defect, inflammation and scarring secondary to a gastric ulcer, or tumor growth.

12. Intestinal obstruction prevents the normal movement of chyme through the intestinal tract. It is usually mechanical, that is, caused by torsion, herniation, or tumor.

13. The most severe consequences of intestinal obstruction are fluid and electrolyte losses, hypovolemia, shock, intestinal necrosis, and perforation of the intestinal wall.

14. Gastritis is an acute or chronic inflammation of the gastric mucosa.

15. Regurgitation of bile, use of antiinflammatory drugs or alcohol, and some systemic diseases are associated with gastritis.

16. Chronic gastritis of the fundus and body is the most severe form of gastritis. It can result in gastric atrophy and decreased secretion of hydrochloric acid, pepsinogen, and intrinsic factor.

17. Chronic gastritis of the antrum, the most common type, is not usually associated with impaired secretion or gastric atrophy.

18. Appendicitis is the most common surgical emergency of the abdomen. Obstruction of the lumen leads to increased pressure, ischemia, and inflammation of the appendix. Inflammation may progress to gangrene, perforation, and peritonitis without surgical resection.

19. A peptic ulcer is a circumscribed area of mucosal inflammation and ulceration caused by excessive secretion of gastric acid, disruption of the protective mucosal barrier, or both.

20. There are three types of peptic ulcers: duodenal, gastric, and stress ulcers.

21. Duodenal ulcers, the most common peptic ulcers, are associated with increased numbers of parietal (acid-secreting) cells in the stomach, elevated gastrin levels, and rapid gastric emptying. Pain occurs when the stomach is empty, and it is relieved with food or antacids. Duodenal ulcers tend to heal spontaneously and recur frequently.

22. Gastric ulcers develop near parietal cells, generally in the antrum, and tend to become chronic. Gastric secretions may be normal or decreased, and pain may occur after eating.

23. Ischemic stress ulcers develop suddenly after severe illness, systemic trauma, or neural injury. Ulceration follows mucosal damage caused by ischemia (decreased blood flow to the gastric mucosa).

24. Cushing ulcer is a stress ulcer caused by head trauma. Ulceration follows hypersecretion of hydrochloric acid caused by overstimulation of the vagal nuclei.

25 Postgastrectomy syndromes are long-term complications that follow gastrectomy, the resection of all or part of the stomach. The postgastrectomy syndromes include dumping syndrome, alkaline reflux gastritis, afferent loop obstruction, diarrhea, weight loss, and anemia.

26 Dumping syndrome is the rapid emptying of chyme into the small intestine. It causes an osmotic shift of fluid from the vascular compartment to the intestinal lumen, which decreases plasma volume.

27 Alkaline reflux gastritis is stomach inflammation caused by the reflux of bile and pancreatic secretions from the duodenum into the stomach. These substances disrupt the mucosal barrier and cause inflammation.

28 Afferent loop obstruction is an obstruction of the duodenal stump on the proximal side of a gastrojejunostomy. Biliary and pancreatic secretions accumulate in the stump, causing distention, intermittent pain, and vomiting.

29 Malabsorption syndromes result in impaired digestion or absorption of nutrients.

30 Pancreatic insufficiency causes malabsorption associated with impaired digestion. The pancreas does not produce sufficient amounts of the enzymes that digest protein, carbohydrates, and fats into components that can be absorbed by the intestine.

31 Deficient lactase production in the brush border of the small intestine inhibits the breakdown of lactose. This prevents lactose absorption and causes osmotic diarrhea.

32 Bile salt deficiency causes fat malabsorption and steatorrhea (fatty stools). Bile salt deficiency can result from inadequate secretion of bile, excessive bacterial deconjugation of bile, or impaired reabsorption of bile salts caused by ileal disease.

33 Ulcerative colitis is an inflammatory disease that causes ulceration, abscess formation, and necrosis of the colonic and rectal mucosa. Cramping pain, bleeding, frequent diarrhea, dehydration, and weight loss accompany severe forms of the disease. A course of frequent remissions and exacerbations is common.

34 Crohn disease is similar to ulcerative colitis, but it affects both the large and small intestines, and ulceration tends to involve all the layers of the lumen. "Skip lesion" fissures and granulomas are characteristic of Crohn disease. Abdominal tenderness, nonbloody diarrhea, and weight loss are the usual symptoms.

35 Diverticula are outpouchings of colonic mucosa through the muscle layers of the colon wall. Diverticulosis is the presence of these outpouchings; diverticulitis is inflammation of the diverticula.

36 Vascular insufficiency in the intestine is most often associated with occlusion or obstruction of the mesenteric vessels or insufficient arterial blood flow. The resulting ischemia and necrosis produce abdominal pain, fever, bloody diarrhea, hypovolemia, and shock.

37 Obesity can be classified as exogenous or endogenous, and adipose (fat) cells as hyperplastic or hypertrophic.

38 Susceptibility to obesity may involve an excessive number of fat cells, increased amounts of lipoprotein in fat cells, high biologic set point controlled by the hypothalamus, presence of relatively few brown (thermoregulating) fat cells, high blood glucose levels associated with type II diabetes, or decreased action of the ATPase pump.

39 Obesity increases the risk of developing coronary artery disease, cancer, and pulmonary disorders.

40 Anorexia nervosa, or self-imposed starvation, is a psychogenic disorder of adolescent and young women. It causes significant weight loss and developmental delays and can be fatal.

41 Bulimia, or binging and purging, involves eating normal or large amounts of food and then purging by inducing vomiting or abusing laxatives. Severe weight loss is rare, but frequent vomiting causes tooth decay, pharyngitis, and esophagitis.

42 Short-term starvation, or lack of dietary intake for 3 or 4 days, stimulates mobilization of stored glucose by two metabolic processes: glycogenolysis (splitting of glycogen into glucose) and gluconeogenesis (formation of glucose from noncarbohydrate molecules).

43 Long-term starvation triggers the breakdown of ketone bodies and fatty acids. Eventually proteolysis (protein breakdown) begins, and death ensues if nutrition is not restored.

Disorders of the Accessory Organs of Digestion

1 Portal hypertension, ascites, hepatic encephalopathy, jaundice, and hepatorenal syndrome are complications of many liver disorders.

2 Portal hypertension is an elevation of portal venous pressure to at least 10 mm Hg. It is caused by increased resistance to venous flow in the portal vein and its tributaries, including the sinusoids and hepatic vein.

3 Portal hypertension is the most serious complication of liver disease because it can cause potentially fatal complications, such as bleeding varices, ascites, and hepatic encephalopathy.

4 Ascites is the accumulation and sequestration of fluid in the peritoneal cavity, often as a result of portal hypertension and decreased concentrations of plasma proteins.

5 Hepatic encephalopathy (portal systemic encephalopathy) is impaired cerebral function caused by blood-borne toxins (particularly ammonia) not metabolized by the liver. Toxin-bearing blood may bypass the liver in collateral vessels opened as a result of portal hypertension, or diseased hepatocytes may be unable to carry out their metabolic functions.

6 Manifestations of hepatic encephalopathy range from confusion and asterixis (flapping tremor of the hands) to loss of consciousness, coma, and death.

7 Jaundice (icterus) is a yellow or greenish pigmentation of the skin or sclera of the eyes caused by increases in plasma bilirubin concentration (hyperbilirubinemia).

8 Obstructive jaundice is caused by obstructed bile canaliculi (intrahepatic obstructive jaundice) or obstructed bile ducts outside the liver (extrahepatic obstructive jaundice). Bilirubin accumulates proximal to sites of obstruction, enters the bloodstream, and is carried to the skin and deposited.

9 Hemolytic jaundice is caused by destruction of red blood cells at a rate that exceeds the liver's ability to metabolize unconjugated bilirubin.

10 Hepatorenal syndrome is functional kidney failure caused by advanced liver disease, particularly cirrhosis with portal hypertension. Renal failure is caused by a sudden decrease in blood flow to the kidneys, usually caused by massive gastrointestinal hemorrhage or liver failure. Its chief clinical manifestation is oliguria.

11 Viral hepatitis is an infection of the liver caused by a strain of the hepatitis virus: hepatitis A virus (HAV), hepatitis B virus (HBV), or non-A, non-B hepatitis. Although they differ with respect to modes of transmission and severity of acute illness, all cause hepatic cell necrosis, Kupffer cell hyperplasia, and infiltration of liver tissue by mononuclear phagocytes. These changes obstruct bile flow and impair hepatocyte function.

12 The clinical manifestations of viral hepatitis depend on the stage of infection. Fever, malaise, anorexia, and liver enlargement and tenderness characterize the prodromal phase (stage 1). Jaundice and hyperbilirubinemia mark the icteric phase (stage 2). During the recovery phase (stage 3), symptoms resolve. Recovery takes several weeks.

13 Fulminant hepatitis is a complication of hepatitis B (with or without hepatitis D infection) or non-A, non-B hepatitis. It causes widespread hepatic necrosis and is often fatal.

14 Cirrhosis is an inflammatory disease of the liver that causes disorganization of lobular structure, fibrosis, and nodular regeneration. Cirrhosis can result from hepatitis or exposure to toxins, such as acetylaldehyde (a product of alcohol metabolism). The disease causes progressive irreversible liver damage, usually over a period of years.

15 Alcoholic cirrhosis impairs the hepatocytes' ability to oxidize fatty acids, synthesize enzymes and proteins, degrade hormones, and clear portal blood of ammonia and toxins. The inflammatory response includes excessive collagen formation, fibrosis, and scarring, which obstruct bile canaliculi and sinusoids. Bile obstruction causes jaundice. Vascular obstruction causes portal hypertension, shunting, and varices.

16 Primary biliary cirrhosis is the inflammatory destruction of intrahepatic bile ducts. Its cause is unknown.

17 Secondary biliary cirrhosis develops from prolonged obstruction of bile flow with increased pressure in the hepatic bile ducts that causes pooling of bile and necrosis of tissue. Relief of obstruction relieves symptoms of jaundice and pruritus. Continued obstruction causes cirrhosis and liver failure.

18 Postnecrotic cirrhosis is the consequence of many severe, chronic liver diseases. Fibrosis, atrophy, and nodular regeneration are characteristic of liver structure with severely altered liver function and manifestations, including portal hypertension, ascites, bleeding varices, and encephalopathy.

19 Cholelithiasis (the formation of gallstones) is a common disorder of the gallbladder. Gallstones form in the bile as a result of the aggregation of cholesterol crystals (cholesterol stones) or precipitates of unconjugated bilirubin (pigmented stones). Gallstones that fill the gallbladder or obstruct the cystic or common bile duct cause abdominal pain and jaundice.

20 Cholecystitis is an inflammation of the gallbladder. It is usually associated with obstruction of the cystic duct by gallstones.

21 Acute pancreatitis (pancreatic inflammation) is a serious but relatively rare disorder. Some unknown factor injures the pancreatic ducts or acini. Injury permits leakage of digestive enzymes into pancreatic tissue, where they become activated and begin the process of autodigestion, inflammation, and destruction of tissues. Release of pancreatic enzymes into the bloodstream or abdominal cavity causes damage to other organs.

22 Chronic pancreatitis results from structural or functional impairment of the pancreas. It causes recurrent abdominal pain and digestive disorders.

Cancer of the Digestive System

1 Cancer of the esophagus is rare and tends to occur in people older than 60 years of age. Alcohol and tobacco use, reflux esophagitis, and nutritional deficiencies are associated with esophageal carcinoma.

2 Dysphagia and chest pain are the primary manifestations of esophageal cancer. Early treatment of tumors that have not spread into the mediastinum or lymph nodes results in a good prognosis.

3 Gastric carcinoma is associated with high salt intake, food preservatives (nitrates and nitrites), and atrophic gastritis.

4 Approximately 50% of all gastric cancers are located in the prepyloric antrum. Clinical manifestations (weight loss, upper abdominal pain, vomiting, hepatemesis, and anemia) develop only after the tumor has penetrated the wall of the stomach.

5 Cancer of the colon and rectum (colorectal cancer) is the second most common cause of cancer death in the United States. Preexisting polyps are highly associated with adenocarcinoma of the colon.

6 Tumors of the right (ascending) colon are usually large and bulky; tumors of the left (descending, sigmoid) colon develop as small, buttonlike masses. Manifestations of colon tumors include pain, bloody stools, and change in bowel habits.

7 Rectal carcinoma is located up to 15 cm from the opening of the anus. The tumor spreads transmurally to the vagina in women or prostate in men.

8 Metastatic invasion of the liver is more common than primary cancer of the liver.

9 Primary liver cancers are associated with chronic liver disease (cirrhosis and hepatitis B). Hepatocellular carcinomas arise from the hepatocytes, whereas cholangiocellular carcinomas arise from the bile ducts. Primary liver cancer spreads to the heart, lungs, brain, kidney, and spleen through the circulation.

10 Cancer of the gallbladder is relatively rare and tends to occur in women over 50. Adenocarcinoma is most common. Because clinical manifestations occur late in the disease, metastases to lymph channels have usually occurred by the time of diagnosis, and the prognosis is poor.

11 Cancer of the pancreas now ranks fifth as a cause of cancer deaths. The one known risk factor is heavy cigarette smoking. Most tumors are adenocarcinomas that arise in the exocrine cells of ducts in the head, body, or tail of the pancreas. Symptoms may not be evident until the tumor has spread to surrounding tissues. Treatment is palliative, and mortality is nearly 100%.

KEY TERMS

Achalasia, 1326
Acute gastritis, 1332
Acute pancreatitis (acute hemorrhagic pancreatitis), 1361
Afferent loop obstruction, 1338
Alcoholic cirrhosis, 1358
Alcoholic hepatitis, 1357
Alkaline reflux gastritis, 1338
Anorexia, 1321
Anorexia nervosa, 1345
Appendicitis, 1343
Ascites, 1348
Biliary cirrhosis, 1358
Bulimarexia, 1346
Bulimia, 1345
Cholangiocellular carcinoma (cholangiocarcinoma), 1367
Cholecystitis, 1360
Cholelithiasis (gallstone), 1360
Chronic active hepatitis, 1355
Chronic gastritis, 1332
Chronic pancreatitis, 1362
Cirrhosis, 1356
Constipation, 1321

Crohn disease, 1341
Curling ulcer, 1337
Cushing ulcer, 1337
Diarrhea, 1322
Diverticula, 1342
Diverticulitis, 1342
Diverticulosis, 1342
Dumping syndrome, 1338
Duodenal ulcer, 1333
Dysphagia, 1326
Fulminant hepatitis, 1355
Gallstone, 1360
Gastric ulcer, 1355
Gastritis, 1332
Gastroesophageal reflux, 1327
Gastrointestinal bleeding, 1324
Gluconeogenesis, 1346
Glycogenolysis, 1346
Hematemesis, 1324
Hematochezia, 1324
Hemolytic jaundice, 1352
Hepatic encephalopathy, 1348
Hepatocellular carcinoma (hepatocarcinoma), 1367

Hepatorenal syndrome, 1352
Hiatal hernia, 1327
Hyperbilirubinemia, 1350
Icteric phase of hepatitis, 1355
Intestinal obstruction, 1329
Ischemic ulcer, 1337
Jaundice (icterus), 1350
Lactase deficiency, 1339
Long-term starvation, 1346
Malabsorption, 1339
Maldigestion, 1339
Melena, 1324
Motility diarrhea, 1323
Nausea, 1321
Obesity, 1344
Obstructive jaundice, 1350
Occult bleeding, 1324
Osmotic diarrhea, 1323
Overnutrition, 1344
Pancreatic insufficiency, 1339
Pancreatitis, 1361
Paraesophageal hiatal hernia, 1328
Parietal pain, 1324
Peptic ulcer, 1333

REFERENCES

Ahnen, D. J. (1991). Genetics of cancer. *Western Journal of Medicine, 154*(6), 700-705.

American Cancer Society (ACS). (1986). *Cancer facts and figures, 1986.* New York: American Cancer Society.

American Cancer Society (ACS). (1988). *Cancer facts and figures, 1988.* New York: American Cancer Society.

American Cancer Society (ACS). (1993). Cancer statistics 1993. *CA—A Cancer Journal for Clinicians, 43*(1).

American Psychiatric Association (APA). (1988). *Diagnostic and statistical manual of mental disorders* (3rd ed.). Washington, DC: American Psychiatric Press.

Ateshkadi, A., Lam, N. P., & Johnson, C. A. (1993). Helicobacter pylori and peptic ulcer disease. *Clinical Pharmacology 12*(1):34-38.

Bray, G. A. (1985). The obese patient. In L. H. Smith (Ed.), *Major problems in internal medicine,* (Vol. 9). Philadelphia: Saunders.

Carey, M. C. (1993). Pathogenesis of gallstones. *American Journal of Surgery 165*(4):410-419.

Carithers, R. L. (1992). Alcoholic hepatitis and cirrhosis. In N. Kaplowitz (Ed.), *Liver and biliary diseases* (pp. 334-346). Baltimore: Williams & Wilkins.

Collins, J. S. (1992). Role of *Helicobacter pylori* in gastritis and duodenitis in man. *Agents-Actions* (Spec. No. C47-9).

DeCock, K. M., Govindarajan, S., & Redeker, A. G. (1985). Acute delta hepatitis without circulating HB$_s$Ag. *Gut, 25,* 212-214.

del Regato, J. A., Spjut, H. J., & Cox, J. D. (1985). *Cancer: Diagnosis, treatment, and prognosis* (2nd ed.). St. Louis: Mosby—Year Book.

De Luise, M., Blackburn, G. L., & Flier, J. S. (1980). Reduced activity of the red cell sodium-potassium pump in human obesity. *New England Journal of Medicine, 303,* 1017.

Despres, J. P., Moorjani, S., Lupien, P. J., Tramblay, A., Nadeau, A., & Bouchard, C. (1992). Genetic aspects of susceptibility to obesity and related dyslipidemias. *Molecular & Cellular Biochemistry, 113*(2), 151-169.

Domschke, W. (1987). Medical and/or surgical treatment of severe pancreatitis. In H. G. Berger & M. Buchler (Eds.), *Acute pancreatitis* (pp. 295-302). New York: Springer-Verlag.

Domurat, E. S., & Elias, A. N. (1992). The endocrinology and pathophysiology of alcoholic cirrhosis and renal failure. *Journal of the National Medical Association, 84*(2), 153-162.

Dowlatshahi, K., Mehta, R. G., Levin, B., Gerny, W. L., Skinner, D. B., & Moon, R. C. (1984). Retinoic-acid-binding protein in normal and neoplastic human esophagus. *Cancer, 54*(2), 308-311.

Durham, R. M., & Shapiro, M. C. (1991). Stress gastritis revisited. *Surgical Clinics of North America, 71*(40), 791-810.

Eagon, J. C., Miedema, B. W., & Kelly, K. A. (1992). Postgastrectomy syndromes. *Surgical Clinics of North America, 72*(2), 445-465.

Faust, I. M., Johnson, P. R., Stern, J. S., & Hirsch, J. (1978). Diet-induced adipocyte number increases in adult rats: A new model for obesity. *American Journal of Physiology, 235,* E279-E286.

Fazio, V. W. (1990). Crohn's disease. In F. G. Moody, L. C. Carey, S. R. Jones, K. A. Kelly, D. L. Nahrwold, & D. R. Skinner (Eds.), *Surgical treatment of digestive diseases* (2nd ed., pp. 655-683). Chicago: Year Book Medical.

Garrow, J. S. (1992). Treatment of obesity. *Lancet, 340,* 409-413.

Gavaler, J. S., & van Thiel, D. H. (1983). Ethanol: Its adverse effects upon the hypothalamic pituitary-gonadal axis. *Journal of Laboratory and Clinical Medicine, 101,* 21-33.

Gelfand, M. D. (1991). Gastroesophageal reflux disease. *Medical Clinics of North America, 75*(4), 923-941.

Gerety, R. J. (1985). *Hepatitis B* (pp. 94, 121). Orlando, FL: Academic Press.

Halmi, K. A. (1987). Anorexia nervosa and bulimia. *Annual Review of Medicine, 38,* 373-380.

Hastings, G. E., & Weber, R. J. (1993). Inflammatory bowel disease: Part II. Medical and surgical management. *American Family Physician 47*(4), 811-818.

Himms-Hagen, J. (1985). Brown adipose tissue metabolism and thermogenesis. *Annual Review of Nutrition, 5,* 69-84.

Holt, S. (1993). Chronic pancreatitis. *Southern Medical Journal 86*(2):201-207.

Jones, D. S. (1992a). Appendicitis. *British Journal of Medicine, 305,* 44-47.

Jones, D. S. (1992b). Diverticular disease. *British Journal of Medicine, 304,* 1435-1437.

Keesey, R. E. (1986). A set-point theory of obesity. In K. D. Brownell & J. P. Foreyt (Eds.), *Handbook of eating disorders* (pp. 63-87). New York: Basic Books.

Kissane, J. M. (Ed.). (1990). *Anderson's pathology* (9th ed.). St. Louis: Mosby—Year Book.

Krech, R. L., & Walsh, D. (1991). Symptoms of pancreatic cancer. *Journal of Pain Symptom Management, 6*(6), 360-367.

Kuo, G., Choo, Q. L., Alter, H. J., Gitnick, G. L., Redeker, A. G., Purcell, R. H., Miyamura, T., Dienstag, J. L., Alter, M. J., & Stevens, C. E. (1989). An assay for circulating antibodies to a major etiologic virus of human non-A, non-B hepatitis. *Science, 21;244*(4901), 362-364.

Kvietys, P. R., Barrowmand A., & Granger, N. D. (1987). *Pathophysiology of the splanchnic circulation* (Vol. 1, p. 129). Boca Raton, FL: CRC Press.

Lamboise, L., & Davis, G. L. (1992). Treatment of chronic hepatitis. *Gastroenterology Clinics of North America, 21*(3), 659-677.

Lee, S. P., Nicholls, S. F., & Park H. Z. (1992). Biliary sludge as a cause of acute pancreatitis. *New England Journal of Medicine, 326,* 589-593.

Manns, M. P. (1992). Autoimmune diseases of the liver. *Clinical and Laboratory Medicine, 12*(1), 25-40.

McCallum, R. W. (1987). The spectrum of esophageal motility disorders. *Hospital Practice,* (December 15), 22(12), 71-83.

McQuaid, K. R., & Isenberg, J. I. (1992). Medical therapy of peptic ulcer disease. *Surgical Clinics of North America, 72*(2), 285-316.

Merlo, A., & Cohen, S. (1988). Swallowing disorders. *Annual Review of Medicine, 39*, 17-28.

Miller, D. S. (1979). Thermogenesis and obesity. *Bibliotheca Nutritio et Dieta, 27*, 25-32.

Miller, T. A., & Victor, B. E. (1990). Gastritis and gastric ulcer. In F. G. Moody, L. C. Carey, S. R. Jones, K. A. Kelly, D. L. Nahrwold, & D. R. Skinner (Eds.), *Surgical treatment of digestive diseases* (2nd ed.). Chicago: Year Book Medical.

Mudge, C., & Carlson, L. (1992). Hepatorenal syndrome. *Critical Care Nurse, 3*(3), 614-632.

Mufti, S. I., Zirvi, K. A., & Garewal, H. S. (1991). Precancerous lesions and biologic markers in esophageal cancer. *Cancer Detection and Prevention, 15*(4), 291-301.

Nadhler, L. J., & McSheny, C. K. (1992). Carcinoma of the gallbladder: Review of the literature and report on 56 cases at Beth Israel Medical Center. *Mt. Sinai Journal of Medicine, 59*(1), 47-52.

Patel, A., Kaleya, R. N., & Sammartano, J. R. (1992). Pathophysiology of mesenteric ischemia. *Surgical Clinics of North America, 72*(1), 31-41.

Phipps, W. J., Long, B. C., & Woods, W. F. (1991). *Medical surgical nursing: Concepts and clinical practice* (4th ed.). St. Louis: Mosby–Year Book.

Pisters, P. W., & Ranson, J. H. (1992). Nutritional support for acute pancreatitis. *Surgical Gynecology and Obstetrics, 175*(3), 275-284.

Poston, G. J., Gillespie, J., & Guillou, P. J. (1991). Biology of pancreatic cancer. *Gut, 32*(7), 800-812.

Prior, J. A., Silberstein, J. S., & Stang, J. M. (1981). *Physical diagnosis: The history and examination of the patient* (6th ed.). St. Louis: Mosby–Year Book.

Punukolla, R. C., & Gopalswamy, N. (1990). The hepatorenal syndrome. *Medical Clinics of North America, 74*(4), 933-943.

Ravussin, E., & Swinburg, G. A. (1992). Pathophysiology of obesity. *Lancet, 340*, 404-408.

Rosai, J. (1989). *Ackerman's surgical pathology* (7th ed.). St. Louis: Mosby–Year Book.

Schafer, D. F., & Jones, E. A. (1990). Hepatic encephalopathy. In D. Zakim & T. D. Boyer (Eds.), *Hepatology: A textbook of liver disease* (Vol. 1, p. 455). Philadelphia: Saunders.

Schineller, B. A., & Ramchandani, D. (1991). Psychologic factors associated with peptic ulcer disease. *Medical Clinics of North America, 75*(4), 865-875.

Schwartz, R. B., & Brunzell, J. D. (1981). Increase of adipose tissue lipoprotein lipase activity with weight loss. *Journal of Clinical Investigation, 67*, 1425.

Selby, W. (1993). Current management of inflammatory bowel disease. *Journal of Gastroenterology and Hepatology 8*(1), 70-83.

Shike, M., Winewar, S. J., Greenwald, P. H., Bloch, A., Hill, M. S., & Swaroop, S. V. (1990) Primary prevention of colorectal cancer. *Bulletin of the World Health Organization, 68*(3), 377-385.

Shulman, S. T. (1992). Viral hepatitis. In S. T. Shulman, J. P. Phair, & H. M. Sommers (Eds.), *The biological and clinical basis for infectious diseases* (p. 316). Philadelphia: Saunders.

Steer, M. L. (1992). How and where does acute pancreatitis begin? *Archives of Surgery 127*(11):1350-1353.

Steinberg, W. M. (1992). Acute pancreatitis: Never leave a stone unturned. *New England Journal of Medicine, 326*(9), 635-637.

Stunkard, A. J. (Ed.). (1980). *Obesity*. Philadelphia: Saunders.

Stunkard, A. J., Harris, J. R., Pederson, N. L., & McClearn, G. E. (1990). The body-mass index of twins who have been reared apart. *New England Journal of Medicine, 322*, 1483-1487.

Szmuckler, G. I. (1985). The epidemiology of anorexia nervosa and bulimia. *Journal of Psychiatric Research, 19*, 143-154.

Thibodeau, G. A., & Patton, K. T. (1992). *The human body in health and disease*. St. Louis: Mosby–Year Book.

Trapnell, J. E., & Duncan, E. J. L. (1975). Patterns of incidence in acute pancreatitis. *British Journal of Medicine*, (January), 2, 179-183.

Trock, B., Lanza, E., & Greenwald, P. (1990). Dietary fiber, vegetables, and colon cancer: Critical review and meta-analysis of the epidemiologic evidence. *Journal of the National Cancer Institutes, 82*(8), 650-661.

Tutgat, G. N., Noach, L. A., & Rauws, E. A. (1993). *Helicobacter pylori* infection and duodenal ulcer disease. *Gastroenterology Clinics of North America 22*(1), 127-139.

Vargas, P. A., & Alberts, D. S. (1992). Primary prevention of colorectal cancer through dietary modification. *Cancer, 70*(5 Suppl.), 1229-1235.

Wadden, T. A., & Stunkard, A. J. (1985). Social and psychological consequences of obesity. *Annuals of Internal Medicine 103*, 1062-1067.

Woods, S. E., Hitchcock, M., & Meyer, A. (1993). Alcoholic hepatitis. *American Family Physician 47*(5):1171-1178.

Zakim, D., Boyer, T. D., & Montgomery, C. (1990). Alcoholic liver disease. In D. Zakim & T. D. Boyer (Eds.), *Hepatology: A textbook of liver disease* (2nd ed., p. 822). Philadelphia: Saunders.

SUGGESTED READINGS

Bray, G. A. (1991). Obesity: A disorder of nutrient partitioning the MONA LISA hypothesis. *Journal of Nutrition, 121*, 1146-1162.

Cello, J. P., & Schneiderman, D. L. (1989). Ulcerative colitis. In M. H. Sleisenger & J. S. Fortran (Eds.), *Gastrointestinal disease: Pathophysiology, diagnosis, and management* (4th ed., pp. 1436-1438). Philadelphia: Saunders.

Contie, V. L. (1991). Scrutinizing the life cycle of hepatitis delta virus. *Research Resources Reporter: National Center for Research Resources, 15*(12), 6-8.

Feldman, M., Walker, P., Green, J. L., & Weingarden, K. (1986). Life events stress and psychosocial factors in men with peptic ulcer disease: A multidimensional case-controlled study. *Gastroenterology, 91*, 1370.

Hirsch, J., & Liebel, R. L. (1988). New light on obesity. *New England Journal of Medicine, 318*(8), 509-510.

Mertz, H. R., & Walsh, J. H. (1991). Peptic ulcer pathology. *Medical Clinics of North America 75*(4):799-814.

CHAPTER 37

Alterations of Digestive Function in Children

Gale D. Danek
Sue E. Huether
Margaret M. Andrews*

D isorders of the gastrointestinal tract in children include anomalies with structural and
functional alterations as well as enzyme deficiencies.
Structural alterations can occur throughout the gastrointestinal tract and include cleft lip and palate,
esophageal atresia, tracheoesophageal fistulae, pylo-

ric stenosis, aganglionic megacolon, and imperforate
anus. Gastroesophageal reflux, hepatic and pancreatic enzyme deficiencies, and bacterial or viral inva-
sions of the gastrointestinal tract also contribute to
the diseases and gastrointestinal clinical manifestations in children.

DISORDERS OF THE GASTROINTESTINAL TRACT

Congenital Impairment of Motility
Cleft Lip and Cleft Palate

Cleft lip (**harelip**) and **cleft palate** are developmental anomalies of the first branchial arch (Fig. 37-1). These defects, which occur during embryonic development, vary in severity. Some are barely perceptible, and others are exceedingly handicapping functionally, cosmetically, and psychologically.

In whites, the incidence of cleft lip or cleft palate ranges from 1 in 600 to 1 in 1250 births. The incidence of cleft lip, with or without cleft palate, is 1 in 1000 births, whereas the incidence of cleft palate alone is about 1 in 2500 births. Incidence is lower in black and higher in Japanese populations. Cleft lip, with or without cleft palate, is more frequent in females. Both anomalies can be unilateral or bilateral, partial or complete.

In most cases, cleft lip and cleft palate are caused by multiple factors, both genetic and nongenetic, each of which contributes only a minor developmental defect. (This phenomenon, called multifactorial inheritance, is discussed in Chapter 4.) Together, these factors reduce the amount of neural crest mesenchyme that migrates into the area that will develop into the face of the em-

FIG. 37-1 Variations in clefts of the lip and palate. **A,** Notch in vermilion border. **B,** Unilateral cleft lip and palate. **C,** Bilateral cleft lip and cleft palate. **D,** Cleft palate. (From Whaley & Wong, 1991.)

bryo. If the amount is sufficiently reduced, clefting occurs (Mitchell & Risch, 1992). The cleft can be part of a syndrome determined by single mutant genes or part of a chromosomal defect, usually trisomy 13. Rarely, the cleft is caused by a teratogenic agent, such as an anticonvulsant drug (Mosher, 1986).

Pathophysiology

Cleft lip. Cleft lip is caused by the incomplete fusion of the nasomedial or intermaxillary process during the second month of embryonic development. The deformity develops during a period of very rapid fetal growth. The cleft causes structures of the face and mouth to develop without the normal restraints of encircling lip muscles. A characteristic depression or flattening of the infant's midfacial contour may occur because normal antagonistic forces across the midline are absent, and growth of the involved facial segments is disturbed. The facial cleft may affect not only the lip but also the external nose, the nasal cartilages, the nasal septum, and the alveolar processes.

The cleft is usually just beneath the center of one nostril. The defect may occur bilaterally and may be symmetric or asymmetric. The cleft can range in severity from a slight indentation of the lip to a fissure that extends to the nostril, causing a sagging and flattening of the nose. The failure of lip fusion by 35 days of gestation may impair closure of the palatal shelves. The more complete the cleft lip, the greater the chance that teeth in the line of the cleft will be missing or malformed.

Cleft palate. Cleft palate is often associated with cleft lip but may occur without it. The fissure may affect only the uvula and soft palate or may extend forward to the nostril and involve the hard palate and the maxillary alveolar ridge. It may be unilateral or bilateral, with the cleft occupying the midline posteriorly and as far forward as the alveolar process, where it deviates to the involved side. Clefts involving the palate only are usually but not necessarily in the midline. In some cases, the vomer and nasal septum are partly or completely undeveloped. When these facial bones are involved, the nasal cavity may freely communicate with the oral cavity.

Clinical Manifestations

Feeding the infant with cleft lip usually presents no difficulty if the cleft lip is simple and the palate intact. Nursing at breast or bottle depends on suction developed by pressing the nipple against the hard palate with the tongue. Closure of the lips is not necessary, but the tongue must work harder if the infant cannot purse its lips. A baby with cleft palate usually requires large, soft nipples with cross-cut openings. Breast feeding may be impossible for some infants. An orthodontic prosthesis for the roof of the mouth may facilitate sucking for some infants.

Evaluation and Treatment

Facial x-ray films confirm the extent of bone deformity. Soft tissue alterations are evaluated by history and physical examination.

The nature and extent of the cleft, the infant's condition, and the method of surgical correction proposed determine the course of treatment. Surgical correction is often planned in stages. The lip is united first. Although this can be done within a few weeks of birth, most surgeons prefer to wait until the infant is 2 to 3 months old to allow for sufficient growth to occur. The initial repair may be revised when the child is 4 to 5 years old.

Repair of a cleft lip that is accompanied by bilateral cleft palate is technically more difficult, and so the procedure is often performed in two steps. The lip is repaired when the infant is a few weeks old. The palate is closed after the child is weaned from the nipple but before he or she has begun to talk, usually at about 12 to 18 months of age. The aim of surgery is to obtain an airtight closure of the palatal cleft and to preserve the mobility and length of the soft palate. Even with early closure, the child may experience difficulty sealing off the nasopharynx from the buccal cavity during swallowing and while pronouncing certain consonants. Speech training and special attention by a prosthodontist and orthodontist are almost always required.

Both before and after surgery, children with cleft palate tend to suffer from repeated infections of the paranasal sinuses. Excessive dental decay is not unusual. Hypertrophy of tonsils and adenoids and otitis media are frequent accompaniments, and the child should be evaluated for hearing loss (Suslak & Desposito, 1988).

Esophageal Malformations

Congenital malformations of the esophagus occur in 1 of 3000 to 4500 live births. **Esophageal atresia** is a condition in which the esophagus ends in a blind pouch. Esophageal atresia is usually accompanied by a fistula between the esophagus and the trachea. This connection is called a **tracheoesophageal fistula** (**TEF**). Either defect can occur alone, however (Fig. 37-2).

Pathophysiology

The esophageal abnormalities are thought to arise from defective differentiation as the trachea separates from the esophagus during the fourth to sixth weeks of embryonic development. Defective growth of endodermal cells leads to atresia. Incomplete fusion of the lateral walls of the foregut leads to incomplete closure of the laryngotracheal tube and fistula formation.

Clinical Manifestations

Polyhydramnios is reported to occur in 14% to 90% of mothers of affected infants (Faranoff & Martin, 1987). The blind end of the proximal esophagus has a capac-

FIG. 37-2 **Five types of esophageal atresia and tracheoesophageal fistula. A,** Simple esophageal atresia. Proximal and distal esophagus end in blind pouches, and there is tracheal communication. Nothing enters the stomach; regurgitated food and fluid may enter the lungs. **B,** Proximal and distal esophageal segments end in blind pouches, and a fistula connects the proximal esophagus to the trachea. Nothing enters the stomach; food and fluid enter the lungs. **C,** Proximal esophagus ends in a blind pouch, and a fistula connects the trachea to the distal esophagus. Air enters the stomach; regurgitated gastric secretions enter the lungs through the fistula. **D,** Fistula connects both proximal and distal esophageal segments to the trachea. Air, food, and fluid enter the stomach and the lungs. **E,** Simple tracheoesophageal fistula between otherwise normal esophagus and trachea. Air, food, and fluid enter the stomach and the lungs. Between 90% and 95% of esophageal anomalies are type **C;** 6% to 8% are type **A;** 3% to 5% are type **E;** and fewer than 1% are type **B** or **D.** (From Whaley & Wong, 1991.)

ity of only a few milliliters. As the infant with esophageal atresia swallows oral secretions, the pouch fills and overflows into the pharynx, resulting in drooling and occasionally in aspiration (Fig. 37-2, *A* and *B*).

If a fistula connects the trachea with the distal esophagus, the abdomen fills with air and becomes distended. The distention may be great enough to interfere with breathing (Fig. 37-2, *C* to *E*). If the fistula connects the proximal esophagus to the trachea, the first feeding after birth will be problematic (Fig. 37-2, *B* to *E*). As the infant drinks, the blind end of the esophagus and the mouth fill with fluid. When the infant tries to take a breath, the fluid is aspirated into the lungs, which triggers protective cough and choke reflexes. Intermittent cyanosis may result. Plain water or glucose is recommended for the initial feeding to minimize the dangers associated with aspiration. If an abnormality of the esophagus is indicated, oral feedings are withheld until a diagnosis is confirmed.

Pulmonary complications are compounded by reflux of air and gastric secretions into the tracheobronchial tree through the fistula, causing severe chemical irritation. The upper lobe of the right lung is most commonly involved because of its proximity to the tracheoesophageal fistula. Infants with esophageal atresia but no fistula have scaphoid (boat-shaped), gasless abdomens. In fistula with atresia (Fig. 37-2, *B*), the usual symptoms are recurrent aspiration, pneumonia, and atelectasis that remains "silent" for days or even months.

In at least 30% of infants with esophageal defects, other congenital anomalies are present as well. Cardio-

vascular anomalies are the most common, but other digestive tract, urinary, vertebral, and central nervous system defects can accompany esophageal atresia and tracheoesophageal fistula.

Evaluation and Treatment

Esophageal atresia is usually diagnosed at birth, when attempts to pass a catheter into the stomach fail. X-ray films will show the catheter coiled in the upper esophageal pouch. Barium x-ray examinations are used by some investigators (Beasley & Meyers, 1988).

Treatment is surgical. Esophageal continuity is restored and the fistula is eliminated. Surgery is usually undertaken after birth, sometimes in stages. First, the tracheoesophageal fistula is ligated and a gastrostomy is created for feeding. Second, the two ends of the esophagus are joined. The child may continue to have problems with aspiration, gastroesophageal reflux, and esophagitis after surgical repair (Nakazato, Landing, & Wells, 1986). The overall survival rate for infants with esophageal defects is approximately 75%.

Pyloric Stenosis

Pyloric stenosis is an obstruction of the pyloric sphincter caused by hypertrophy of the sphincter muscle. Pyloric stenosis is one of the most common disorders of early infancy. It affects infants between the ages of 1 and 2 weeks or 3 and 4 months (Welch, 1986). The incidence of pyloric stenosis among males is approximately 5 in 1000, whereas that among females is only 1 in 1000. Whites are affected more frequently than blacks or Orientals, and full-term infants are affected more frequently than premature infants. Increased gastrin secretion by the mother in the last trimester of pregnancy increases the likelihood of pyloric stenosis in the infant. The overproduction of gastric secretions in the infant may be due to stress-related factors in the mother.

Pathophysiology

The cause of the increased pyloric hypertrophy is unknown, but hereditary factors may be involved (Carter, 1961). There is an increased incidence in children with Down syndrome; 6.9% of children have a parent who had pyloric stenosis, and 4.9% have a close relative affected (Levy, 1991; Welch, 1986). Individual muscle fibers thicken, so that the whole pyloric sphincter becomes enlarged and inelastic. The mucosal lining of the pyloric opening is folded and narrowed by the encroaching muscle. Because of the extra peristaltic effort necessary to force the gastric contents through the narrow pylorus, the muscle layers of the stomach may become hypertrophied as well.

Clinical Manifestations

The clinical manifestations of pyloric stenosis usually evolve as follows: Between 2 and 3 weeks after birth, an infant who has fed well and gained weight begins to vomit without apparent reason. The vomiting gradually becomes more forceful. In some cases, stomach contents may shoot out 3 or 4 feet. Food is often regurgitated through the nose. The forceful, or projectile vomiting, usually occurs immediately after eating, and the vomitus consists of the bulk of the feeding plus some food retained from previous feedings but is almost always free of bile.

Prolonged retention of food in the stomach is a characteristic feature of pyloric stenosis. In healthy infants, the stomach empties within 2 to 3 hours after eating. In infants with pyloric stenosis, food is present after 4 hours unless vomiting has occurred. Constipation is the rule because not much food reaches the intestine.

In severe untreated cases, increased gastric peristalsis and vomiting lead to severe fluid and electrolyte imbalances, malnutrition, and weight loss that can be fatal within 4 to 6 weeks. Infants with pyloric stenosis are irritable because of hunger, and they may have esophageal discomfort caused by repeated vomiting and esophagitis. The vomitus may be blood streaked because of rupture of gastric and esophageal vessels.

Evaluation and Treatment

Diagnosis is based on the history of clinical manifestations. Occasionally, gastric peristalsis is observable over the abdomen. A firm, small, movable mass, approximately the size of an olive, is felt in the right upper quadrant in 70% to 90% of infants with pyloric stenosis. Sonography is routinely done because this clearly shows

the hypertrophied pyloric muscles and narrowed pyloric channel. This technique is replacing contrast x-ray examinations (O'Keeffe, Stansberry, Swischuk, & Hayden, 1991).

The standard treatment for hypertrophic pyloric stenosis is a pyloromyotomy, in which the muscles of the pylorus are split and separated. Preoperative medical management to correct fluid and electrolyte imbalance has been the key to the high success rate and low complication rates with this surgery (Bissonnette & Sullivan, 1991).

Some infants respond to medical and nutritional management, which is based on the theory that the pylorus will open spontaneously by 6 to 8 months of age if nutrition can be maintained. To maintain nutrition, antispasmodic drugs are given to relax the pylorospasm, and the infant is refed after vomiting.

Malrotation

During the tenth week of embryonic development, the emerging ileum and cecum normally rotate, so that the cecum moves into the lower right quadrant of the abdomen and is fixed there by the mesentery. **Malrotation** is a condition in which rotation does not occur, and the colon remains in the upper right quadrant, where an abnormal membrane may press on and obstruct the duodenum. The obstructing band over the duodenum, called a **periduodenal band,** is one of the most significant findings in malrotation. Associated abnormalities are seen in 30% to 62% of children in a reported series; 50% of children with duodenal atresia and 33% of those with jejunal atresia have associated malrotation (Filston & Kirks, 1981).

Pathophysiology

The small intestine lacks a normal posterior fixation in malrotation because it has only a rudimentary attachment near the origin of the superior mesenteric artery. Therefore the entire mass can twist when the mobile loops of intestine from the duodenojejunal junction to the middle of the transverse colon twist on themselves. The twisting is known as volvulus. Intestinal twisting around the rudimentary mesentery angulates and obstructs the intestinal lumen and partly or completely occludes the superior mesenteric artery, causing infarction and necrosis of the entire midgut.

Clinical Manifestations

Although most cases of malrotation-associated volvulus and infarction develop during the neonatal period (50%) or infancy (85% are younger than 1 year of age), some develop during childhood or even adulthood. In infants the obstruction causes intermittent or persistent bile-stained vomiting after feedings. Abdominal distention is limited initially to the epigastrium because only the stomach and duodenum are dilated. The degree of distention depends on the pressure of swallowed air and the degree of obstruction caused by the volvulus. Dehydration and electrolyte imbalance may occur rapidly because large amounts of pancreatic juice, bile, and gastric secretions are lost through vomiting. Fever usually ensues. Scanty stools, diarrhea, and bloody stools are associated with progressive volvulus, vascular compression, and infarction of the intestine in infants. Intermittent or partial volvulus may be seen in older children and adults. This may be asymptomatic and discovered during unrelated abdominal surgery or cause minor abdominal complaints, such as nausea after meals, vomiting, or abdominal pain (Welch, 1986).

Evaluation and Treatment

Diagnosis of malrotation with volvulus and infarction is based on a review of the clinical manifestations. X-ray films of the abdomen show gas bubbles and distention proximal to the site of obstruction.

Treatment consists of opening the abdomen and reducing the volvulus manually. The surgeon takes the entire intestinal mass in hand and rotates it in a counterclockwise direction. Necrotic bowel may be resected and a primary anastomosis performed. When there is gangrene and question of viability of the bowel ends, an enterostomy may be performed. Second-look operations may be done to avoid resection of viable bowel. In cases of malrotation without duodenal obstruction, operative survival is 80%. Operative survival is 40% to 50% in cases of malrotation complicated by obstruction caused by periduodenal bands or other intraabdominal anomalies. Resection of large segments of the small intestine results in short bowel syndrome and its long-term sequelae.

Meconium Ileus

Meconium is a substance that fills the entire intestine before birth. It consists of intestinal gland secretions and some amniotic fluid. Normally, meconium is passed from the rectum during the first 12 to 72 hours after birth.

Meconium ileus is intestinal obstruction caused by meconium formed in utero that is abnormally sticky and adheres firmly to the mucosa of the small intestine, resisting passage beyond the terminal ileum. The cause is usually a lack of digestive enzymes during fetal life. This meconium is also found to contain albumin, which is not normally found in meconium. The detection of albumin in meconium has been used as a screening test for cystic fibrosis. Most cases of meconium ileus are due to cystic fibrosis, but a few are not. In the cases *not* associated with cystic fibrosis, the cause usually is unknown. Partial aplasia of the pancreas is an associated factor, however, and one fifth of infants with meconium ileus are premature or have a history of maternal hydramnios (excessive amniotic fluid). After intestinal

atresia and malrotation with volvulus, meconium ileus is the most common cause of small intestinal obstruction in newborns.

Pathophysiology

In infants with meconium ileus, the terminal ileum is plugged with thick, viscous meconium. The viscosity of the meconium is caused by the formation of an insoluble, calcium-glycoprotein compound in abnormal mucus. The segment of the ileum proximal to the obstruction is distended with liquid contents, and its walls may be hypertrophied. The segment distal to the obstruction is collapsed and filled with small pellets of pale-colored stool. Meconium in the obstructed segment has the consistency of thick syrup or glue. Peristalsis fails to propel this viscous material through the ileum, and so it becomes impacted. Volvulus, atresia, or perforation of the bowel sometimes accompanies meconium ileus.

Clinical Manifestations

Abdominal distention usually develops during the first few days after birth. The infant does not pass meconium and begins to vomit within hours or days of birth. Infants with cystic fibrosis may have signs of pulmonary involvement, such as tachypnea, intercostal retractions, and grunting respirations. The distended abdomen shows patterns of dilated intestinal loops that feel doughlike when palpated. Some of the loops contain scattered, firm, movable masses. Despite hyperactive peristalsis, the rectal ampulla is empty.

Evaluation and Treatment

Radiologic examination is used to confirm the presence of meconium ileus. The sweat test, which is accurate in 90% of infants, is performed to detect or rule out cystic fibrosis. In approximately 50% of cases not complicated with volvulus or perforation, a hyperosmolar enema, such as Gastrografin or Hypaque, done under fluoroscopy, evacuates the meconium. If this is not possible, the meconium is removed surgically.

Survival of infants with meconium ileus is improving, with 85% to 100% survival at 1 year (DelPina, Czyrko, Ziegler, Scanlin, & Bishop, 1992; Rescorla, Grosfeld, West, & Vane, 1989). The mortality rate increases to 70% if obstruction is complicated by peritonitis. After recovery from neonatal meconium ileus, the long-term outlook depends on the severity and progression of pulmonary disease. Meconium ileus does not adversely affect the long-term nutritional outcome of cystic fibrosis.

Meconium Ileus Equivalent

Meconium ileus equivalent affects approximately 10% of older children with cystic fibrosis. Intestinal contents may become abnormally thick and impact the intestinal lumen, particularly after episodes of dehydration or lack of pancreatic enzymes. The child displays signs and symptoms of intestinal obstruction. In most cases, the obstruction is relieved by hypertonic enemas. Meconium ileus and meconium ileus equivalent have been shown to be risk factors for the development of cirrhosis in individuals with cystic fibrosis (Maurage et al., 1989).

Obstructions of the Duodenum, Jejunum, and Ileum

Congenital obstruction of the duodenum can be caused by intrinsic malformations or external pressure. Intrinsic duodenal obstruction is caused by failure of canalization, which may be partial or complete. During embryonic development, the duodenal lumen does not become patent. The obstruction usually is located at or near the major duodenal papilla. Extrinsic obstructions can be caused by peritoneal bands that constrict the duodenum. This type of obstruction is associated with a partial failure of intestinal rotation and fixation during embryonic development. The duodenum can be obstructed by an annular pancreas, a defect in which the head of the pancreas surrounds part of the duodenum. Congenital obstructions of the jejunum and ileum can be attributable to atresia, stenosis, meconium ileus, megacolon (Hirschsprung disease), intussusception, Meckel diverticulum, intestinal duplication, or strangulated hernia.

In **ileal** or **jejunal atresia**, the intestine ends blindly proximal and distal to an interruption in its continuity, with or without a gap in the mesentery. Stenosis (narrowing of the lumen) causes dilation proximal to the obstruction and luminal collapse distal to it.

Congenital Aganglionic Megacolon

Congenital aganglionic megacolon (Hirschsprung disease) is a functional obstruction of the colon caused by inadequate motility. Congenital megacolon is the most common cause of colon obstruction; it accounts for about one third of all gastrointestinal obstructions in infants. The incidence is 1 in 5000, with a preponderance in males. There is an increase in children with Down syndrome (Levy, 1991).

Pathophysiology

Congenital aganglionic megacolon is caused by a malformation of the parasympathetic nervous system. It is characterized by absence of the intramural ganglion cells in the enteric nerve plexuses (Meissner and Auerbach plexuses). Lacking neural stimulation, the muscle layers of the colon wall fail to propel feces through the colon. In 80% of cases the aganglionic segment is limited to the rectal end of the sigmoid colon. In 3% of cases the entire colon lacks ganglion cells. The abnormally innervated colon obstructs fecal movements, caus-

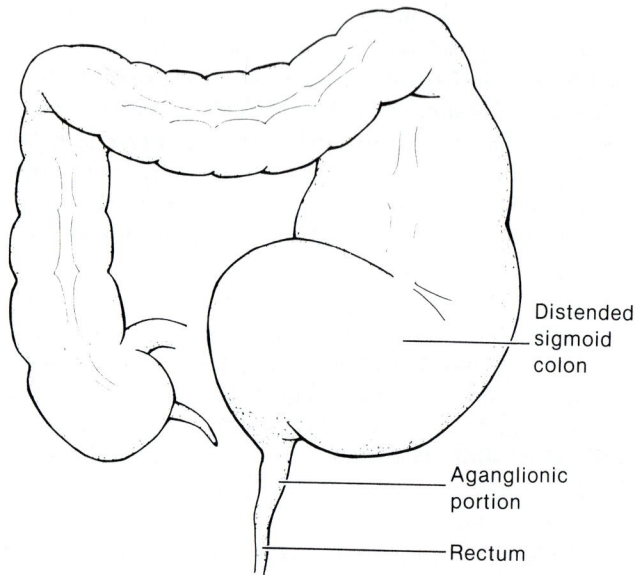

Distended sigmoid colon

Aganglionic portion

Rectum

FIG. 37-3 Congenital aganglionic megacolon (Hirschsprung disease). (From Whaley & Wong, 1991.)

ing the proximal colon to become distended; hence the term megacolon (Fig. 37-3).

The ganglia normally develop between the muscle layers (tunica muscularis) in the submucosal area (muscularis mucosae) of the intestinal wall. In cases of congenital megacolon, large, nonmyelinated fibers develop in place of these ganglion cells. The segment of colon that lacks ganglion cells has a relatively normal lumen caliber and wall thickness. In the segment of the colon proximal to it, the lumen is dilated and the muscle hypertrophied. Therefore, the abnormal portion of the colon appears to be normal and the normal portion appears to be diseased.

The mechanism of propulsive failure is not entirely clear. Some investigators believe that the aganglionic segment simply fails to participate in normal peristalsis. Others suggest that tonic contraction of smooth muscle in the wall of the aganglionic colon narrows the lumen (Milla, 1988).

Clinical Manifestations

Mild to severe constipation is the usual manifestation of congenital aganglionic megacolon. Diarrhea may be the first sign, however, because only water can travel around the impacted feces.

The most serious complication in the neonatal period is enterocolitis related to fecal impaction. Bowel dilation stretches and partly occludes the encircling blood and lymphatic vessels, causing edema, ischemia, infarction of the mucosa, and significant outflow of fluid into the bowel lumen. Copious, liquid stools result. Infarction and destruction of the mucosa enable enteric microorganisms to penetrate the bowel wall. Frequently, gram-negative sepsis occurs, accompanied by fever and vomiting. Severe and rapid electrolyte changes may take place, causing collapse and rapid death.

Evaluation and Treatment

Anorectal manometry is a reliable screening tool for the diagnosis of Hirschsprung disease. Serial manometries may be required in neonates. This test has uncovered ultrashort-segment Hirschsprung disease in older children with a history of constipation (Iwai et al., 1988). The definitive diagnosis is made by rectal biopsy showing an absence of ganglion cells in the submucosa of the colon. X-ray films show dilated loops of colon and contrast films show aganglionic areas. The infant usually cannot expel the barium.

The involved segment is resected within the first few months of life. Alternatively, enemas are given until the lumen is clear, and then stool softeners are prescribed for life. The child is not treated for diarrhea.

After surgery, enterocolitis sometimes recurs. If the postoperative enterocolitis is allowed to persist,

pseudopolyps may appear. Because these are essentially identical to the lesions of ulcerative colitis, they have malignant potential. Therefore, a colectomy is indicated if pseudopolyps develop.

In general, the prognosis of congenital megacolon is satisfactory for children who undergo surgical treatment. Bowel training may be prolonged, but most children achieve bowel continence before puberty.

Anorectal Malformations

Several congenital malformations of anorectal structures can obstruct the passage of feces. The incidence of minor abnormalities is approximately 1 in 500, and that of major anomalies is approximately 1 in 5000.

Congenital anorectal malformations range from mild anal stenosis, which is corrected by simple dilation, to complex deformities, such as anal or rectal agenesis, atresia, and fistula (Fig. 37-4). Deformities that cause complete obstruction are known collectively as **imperforate anus**.

Approximately 40% of infants with anorectal malformations have other developmental anomalies as well.

FIG. 37-4 Anorectal stenosis and imperforate anus. **A,** Congenital anal stenosis. **B,** Anal membrane atresia. **C,** Anal agenesis. **D,** Rectal atresia. **E,** Rectoperineal fistula. **F,** Rectovaginal fistula. (From Whaley & Wong, 1991.)

The most commonly associated major anomalies are Down syndrome, congenital heart disease, renal abnormalities, esophageal atresia, and malformations of the spine.

Imperforate anus may not be obvious. It can be detected by gentle insertion of a rectal tube. X-ray films show dilations throughout the intestinal tract. Anal stenosis can be treated by dilations, but all other anorectal malformations require surgical correction. The overall mortality rate is approximately 10%. Children with a low (anal) anomaly usually achieve bowel continence, but those with a high (rectal) anomaly rarely do.

Acquired Impairment of Motility
Intussusception

The most frequent cause of acquired intestinal obstruction in infants is intussusception. **Intussusception** is the telescoping or invagination of one portion of the intestine into another. Usually, the ileum invaginates the cecum and part of the ascending colon by collapsing through the ileocecal valve. Intussusception involving the ileum and colon (ileocolic intussusception) accounts for 80% to 90% of intestinal obstructions in infants and is two to three times more frequent in males than in females. Nearly 75% of intussusceptions occur before the age of 2 years; 70% occur before the age of 1 year. Intussusception is rare in infants younger than 3 months

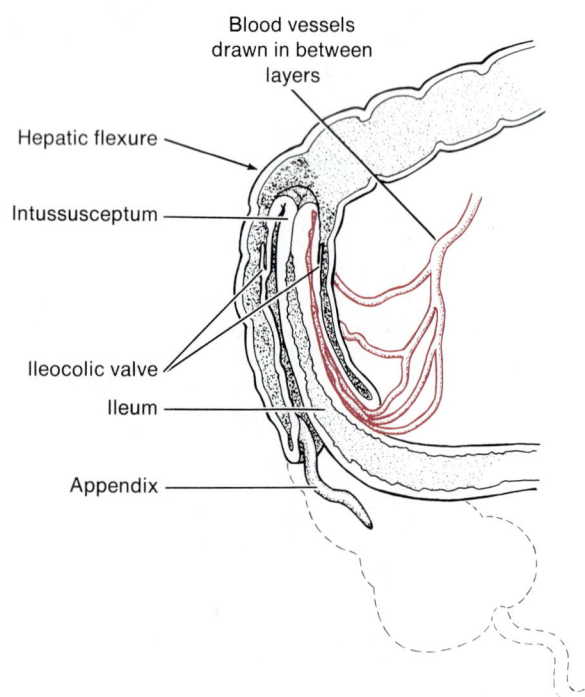

FIG. 37-5 Ileocolic intussusception. (From Whaley & Wong, 1991.)

Blood vessels drawn in between layers

Hepatic flexure

Intussusceptum

Ileocolic valve

Ileum

Appendix

of age and is infrequent after 36 months. Intussusception has occurred in children of all ages recovering from abdominal surgery; intussusception has been found in children with cystic fibrosis and symptoms of bowel obstruction that were initially misdiagnosed as meconium ileus equivalent (Holcomb, Ross, & O'Neill, 1991; Holmes, Murphy, Taylor, & Denham, 1991).

Pathophysiology

The proximal portion of the intestine, the intussusceptum, collapses into the distal portion, the intussuscipiens, in the direction of peristaltic flow (Fig. 37-5). As it does so, the intussusceptum drags its mesentery into the enveloping lumen. Initially, the mesentery is constricted, obstructing venous return. Compression of the mesenteric vessels between the two layers of intestinal wall and at the U-shaped angle at either end of the intussusceptum leads within hours to venous stasis, engorgement, edema, exudation, and further vascular compression. Unless the intussusception is treated, gangrene ensues. The tension of the mesentery on the intussusceptum tends to arch the bowel in a curve having its center at the mesenteric root. Edema and compression obstruct the flow of chyme through the intestine.

Clinical Manifestations

Typically, intussusception occurs in thriving, previously healthy infants. The affected infant suddenly develops abdominal pain, becomes irritable (colicky), and draws up the knees. Vomiting occurs soon afterward. A single normal stool may be passed, evacuating the colon distal to the apex of the intussusception. After that, 60% of infants pass "currant jelly" stools, which appear dark and gelatinous because of their blood and mucus content. Most infants have a tender, sausage-shaped abdominal mass. Abdominal tenderness and distention develop as intestinal obstruction becomes more acute.

Evaluation and Treatment

Diagnosis of intussusception is based on clinical manifestations, onset of symptoms, and contrast x-rays. Reduction of the intussusception is an emergency procedure. Reduction is accomplished by hydrostatic pressure exerted by an enema given under fluoroscopic guidance, which is successful 60% to 70% of the time. Free intraperitoneal air, peritonitis, and evidence of infarcted bowel are contraindications to nonsurgical reduction (Barr, Stansberry, & Swischuk, 1990; Skipper, Boeckman, & Klein, 1990). Surgical reduction is done on children who fail or are not candidates for hydrostatic reduction. Untreated intussusception in infants is nearly always fatal. Most infants recover if the intussusception is reduced within 24 hours. The mortality rate increases rapidly after that time.

Gastroesophageal Reflux

Gastroesophageal reflux (GER) is the return of stomach contents into the esophagus because of relaxation or incompetence of the lower esophageal sphincter (see Chapter 36). In newborns, reflux is normal because neuromuscular control of the gastroesophageal sphincter is not fully developed. The frequency of reflux is highest in premature infants and decreases during the first 6 to 12 months of life. Normal infants and children have been shown to have some reflux but may be asymptomatic (Sterling, Jolley, Besser, & Matteson-Kane, 1991).

In a small percentage of infants and children, reflux causes clinical manifestations. There is an increased incidence of symptomatic reflux in children with neurologic impairment. It is thought to be a factor in the stimulation of apnea and reactive airway disease in some children. Reflux is thought to be a contributing cause in infant deaths and sudden infant death syndrome (Jolly, Halpern, Tunell, Johnson, & Sterling, 1991).

Pathophysiology

The cause of gastroesophageal reflux in infants is unknown. Delayed maturation of the lower esophageal sphincter or impaired hormonal response mechanisms are possible causes. In addition, several factors besides pressure maintain lower esophageal sphincter integrity in children. These factors include location of the gastroesophageal junction in a high-pressure zone within the abdomen, mucosal gathering within the sphincter, and the angle at which the esophagus is inserted into the stomach. Reflux persists if any of these pressure-maintaining factors is altered. Irritation of the mucosa by acidic gastric contents results in deterioration of the esophageal epithelium and stimulation of the vomiting reflex.

Clinical Manifestations

The signs and symptoms of gastroesophageal reflux are caused by exposure of the esophageal epithelium to refluxed gastric contents. Eighty-five percent of affected infants vomit excessively during the first week of life, and usually have other symptoms by 6 weeks.

Vomiting may be forceful. Aspiration pneumonia develops in one third of infants with gastroesophageal reflux. In cases that persist into childhood, chronic cough, wheezing, and recurrent pneumonia are common. Repeated vomiting leads to inadequate retention of nutrients, adversely impacting on growth and weight gain. Esophagitis results from exposure of the esophageal mucosa to acidic gastric contents. This is manifested by pain, bleeding, and eventually stricture formation and abnormal motility. Approximately 25% suffer from iron deficiency anemia caused by frank or occult blood loss.

Evaluation and Treatment

The clinical manifestations are often adequate to confirm a diagnosis of gastroesophageal reflux. A barium swallow and esophageal pH monitoring with a probe are useful diagnostic procedures in complex cases.

Mild gastroesophageal reflux resolves without treatment. Prone elevated positioning or upright sitting of an older child, particularly for the hour after a feeding, decreases episodes of reflux (Orenstein & Whittington, 1983). Thickened feedings have not been shown to consistently help infants with reflux and may make it worse (Bailey, Andres, Danek, & Pineiro-Carrero, 1987). Medications to increase motility, to increase lower esophageal sphincter pressure, or to decrease gastric acid production have been used to treat GER. If no improvement is seen with medical management or the child has life-threatening events with reflux, an antireflux surgical procedure, including gastropexy and fundoplication, is performed. A fundoplication recreates a valve by wrapping the fundus of the stomach around the lower esophagus (Sterling et al., 1991).

Impairment of Digestion, Absorption, and Nutrition

Cystic Fibrosis

Cystic fibrosis (CF) of the pancreas, also called mucoviscidosis or fibrocystic disease of the pancreas, is a genetically transmitted disease that involves many organs and systems and usually causes death in childhood or young adulthood. It is the most frequent cause of chronic suppurative lung disease in children and is the most common life-threatening inherited disease in the white population. This section focuses on the deficiency of pancreatic enzymes. (Chapter 31 discusses the pulmonary consequences of cystic fibrosis.)

Pathophysiology

Dysfunction of the exocrine glands, which secrete such substances as digestive enzymes, mucus, sweat, and tears onto internal and external body surfaces, is the predominant pathogenic mechanism in CF. The pathophysiologic triad that is the hallmark of CF includes (1) pancreatic enzyme deficiency, which causes maldigestion; (2) overproduction of mucus in the respiratory tract, and inability to clear secretions that cause progressive chronic obstructive pulmonary disease; and (3) abnormally elevated sodium and chloride concentrations in sweat. Exocrine secretions tend to be abnormally thick and to precipitate in the glandular ducts, obstructing flow. Almost all clinical manifestations of CF are a result of overproduction of extremely viscous mucus and pancreatic enzyme deficiency. The full spectrum of involvement is evident from Table 37-1.

TABLE 37-1

Pathophysiology, Clinical Manifestations, and Complications of Cystic Fibrosis

Organ involved	Secretory dysfunction	Clinical manifestations	Complications
Sweat glands	Elevated concentration of sodium and chloride in sweat	Hyponatremia; hypochloremia	Heat prostration; shock
Intestine 　Newborn	Viscid meconium	Meconium ileus with intestinal obstruction	Meconium peritonitis
Older child and adult	Inspissated (dried out) mucofecal masses (intestinal sludging)	Partial intestinal obstruction with severe cramping pains	Volvulus (obstruction), intussusception (prolapse)
Pancreas (enzyme deficiency)	Inspissation and precipitation of pancreatic secretions, causing obstruction of pancreatic ducts	Absence of pancreatic enzymes, causing malabsorption of food and fatty, bulky stools	Hypoproteinemia; iron deficiency anemia; malnutrition
		Decreased vitamin A, D, E, K absorption	Vitamin A, D, E, and K deficiency and rectal prolapse
	Insulin deficiency	Glucose intolerance	Diabetes mellitus
Liver	Inspissation and precipitation of bile in biliary system	Focal biliary cirrhosis; shrunken, "hob-nail" liver	Portal hypertension with esophageal varices and hematemesis
Salivary glands	Inspissation and precipitation of secretions in small ducts of submaxillary and sublingual salivary glands	Mild patchy fibrosis of salivary glands	None
Paranasal structures	Viscid mucus	Retention of mucus; clouding seen on sinus roentgenograms	Mucopyoceles (pus accumulations) with nasal deformity or orbital cavity extension
Nose	Nasal polyps	Obstruction of nasal airflow	None
Lungs	Viscid mucus in bronchioles and bronchi	Obstruction of bronchioles causing bronchiolectasis, bronchiectasis, and chronic lung infection	Hemoptysis; pneumothorax; cor pulmonale; respiratory failure
Reproductive tract 　Male	Viscid genital tract secretions during embryologic development, causing failure of formation of normal vas deferens	Sterility	None
Female	Distention of endocervical epithelial cells with cytoplasmic mucin	Decreased fertility	Polypoid cervicitis (cervical inflammation) while taking oral contraceptives

From Rudolph & Hoffman, 1982.

Pancreatic function may range from normal to completely ablated. Approximately 85% have pancreatic insufficiency (Forstner & Durie, 1991). Individuals with near-normal pancreatic function have normal fat absorption, lower chloride values in sweat, and better pulmonary function. When pancreatic function is compromised, severe problems with maldigestion of proteins, carbohydrates, and fats occur because of insufficient secretion of pancreatic enzymes. Obstruction of the pancreatic ducts with thick mucus blocks the flow of pancreatic enzymes and causes degenerative and fibrotic changes in the pancreas. This pancreatic damage eventually can affect the beta cells, resulting in diabetes mellitus in some children.

Clinical Manifestations

Inadequate pancreatic secretions result in steatorrhea (fatty stools) and azotorrhea (excess nitrogen in stools). Maldigestion results in malnutrition and **failure to thrive.** Children may have short stature, pitting edema, and anemia from untreated hypoproteinemia. Purpura and telangiectasia may develop from vitamin K deficiency related to fat malabsorption. Secondary biliary cirrhosis (see Chapter 36) may develop because of obstruction of the bile channels. Stomatitis (inflammation of the mucosa of the mouth) occurs with vitamin B_2 (riboflavin) deficiency. Renal prolapse, thought to be related to the passage of large bulky stools, occurs in 20% of children, usually between 1 and 2½ years of age.

Evaluation and Treatment

Seventy-two-hour stool fat measurements are used to determine the extent of pancreatic function. Stools also may be examined for absence of pancreatic enzymes, particularly trypsin and chymotrypsin. Pancreatic replacement enzymes are administered before or with meals. High-caloric, high-protein diets with frequent snacks are used to treat the malnutrition.

Gluten-Sensitive Enteropathy

Gluten-sensitive enteropathy, formerly called **celiac sprue** or celiac disease, is the loss of mature villous epithelium caused by ingestion of gluten, the protein component of cereal grains. The gluten in wheat, rye, barley, and oats is toxic to the intestinal epithelial cells of genetically susceptible individuals (Auricchio, Greco, & Troncone, 1988). The disease occurs largely in whites and has been documented in Asians from India and Pakistan, but is almost nonexistent in native Africans, Japanese, and Chinese. Prevalence rates in Europe range from 1:1000 to 1:3000 (Trier, 1991).

Although it is known that the α-gliadin fraction of gluten induces the mucosal damage, the exact mechanism of injury is unknown. Pathogenesis appears to be complex, involving dietary, genetic, and immunologic factors, as well as requiring exposure of susceptible individuals to environmental agents in addition to gluten.

Pathophysiology

The mucosa of the upper small intestine appears shiny, cobble-stoned, and thin in children with gluten-sensitive enteropathy. The major pathophysiologic characteristics of the disease are atrophy of villi in the upper small intestine and malabsorption of most nutrients in the presence of cereal gluten (Fig. 37-6). The atrophy is caused by accelerated shedding of epithelial cells from the villi. To compensate for this loss, epithelial cell production increases, causing hypertrophy of the crypts of Leiberkühn. Increased cell production is not sufficient to keep pace with cell loss, however. Inflammation and edema develop around the enlarged cysts. The villi shorten and atrophy, and their surface cells are not mature enough to sustain absorptive functions. The microvilli and brush border disappear, leaving patches of bald mucosa. The loss of mucosal surface area and brush border enzymes leads to severe malabsorption. The pathologic process is most pronounced in the duodenum and jejunum. The ileum may be spared.

Damage to the mucosa of the duodenum and jejunum has secondary effects that exacerbate malabsorption. The secretion of intestinal hormones, such as secretin and cholecystokinin-pancreozymin, may be diminished. Because these chemical messengers are scarce, secretion of pancreatic enzymes and expulsion of bile from the gallbladder decrease.

Destruction of mucosal cells causes inflammation. The inflamed mucosa secretes rather than absorbs water and electrolytes, leading to watery diarrhea. In addition, absorption that normally occurs by sodium-dependent active transport or facilitated diffusion is impaired. Carbohydrates, amino acids, dipeptides, water-soluble vitamins, bile salts, and cations are not absorbed from the intestinal lumen. Potassium loss, which is more severe than sodium loss, leads to muscle weakness. Magnesium and calcium malabsorption can cause seizures or tetany. Unabsorbed fatty acids combine with calcium, and secondary hyperparathyroidism increases phosphorus excretion, resulting in bone reabsorption. Calcium is no longer available to bind oxalate in the intestine and is absorbed, which causes hyperoxaluria. Gallbladder function may be abnormal, and bile salt conjugation may be decreased.

Fat malabsorption in the jejunum is the major cause of steatorrhea (fatty stools). Malabsorption may be mild early in the disease. Fecal nitrogen is elevated because peptidase deficiencies impair protein absorption. Pancreatic function is decreased, not only because of decreased hormonal levels but also because of malnutrition.

Deficiencies of fat-soluble vitamins are common in

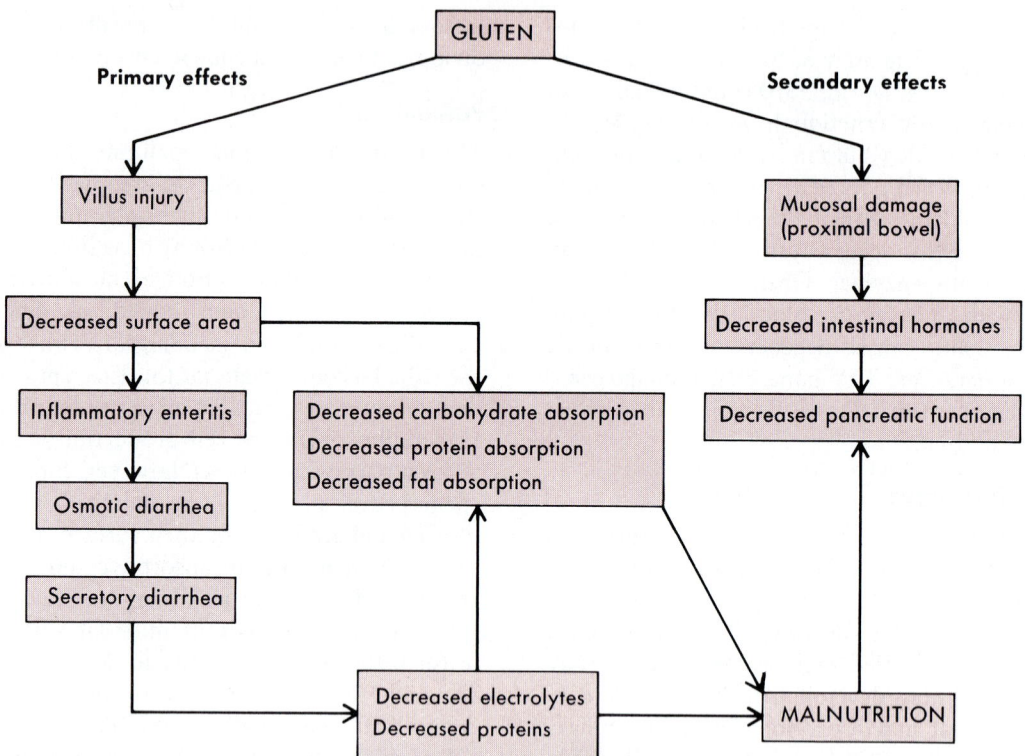

FIG. 37-6 Pathophysiology of gluten-sensitive enteropathy.

children with gluten-sensitive enteropathy. Vitamin K malabsorption leads to hypoprothrombinemia. In one third of cases, iron and folic acid malabsorption are manifested as cheilosis, anemia, and a smooth red tongue. Vitamin B_{12} absorption is impaired in those with extensive ileal disease. Because the absorption of folate and iron is greatest in the proximal small intestine, deficiencies of these substances are common.

Clinical Manifestations

The onset of clinical manifestations of gluten-sensitive enteropathy depends on the age of the infant when gluten-containing substances are added to the diet. In 50% of affected children, onset occurs by 18 months of age, with latent intervals varying from months to years. Severity of symptoms can vary tremendously.

Diarrhea is an early sign in most infants. The stools are pale, bulky, greasy, and foul-smelling, and they may contain oil droplets. Three to five such movements occur daily. As early as 3 or 4 months of age, growth failure, anorexia, and constipation can begin. In older children, constipation is occasionally seen despite steatorrhea. Vomiting and abdominal pain are prominent in infants, but unusual in older children. Anorexia is prevalent. The classic physical manifestations of organic failure to thrive, such as abdominal protuberance, wasted buttocks and limbs, and hypotonia, occur in fewer than

50% of infants with gluten-sensitive enteropathy. Growth is usually diminished (Greco, Tozzi, & Mayer, 1987).

Manifestations of malabsorption, such as rickets, anemia, tetany, frank bleeding, or anemia, may be obvious. Some children urinate more at night. The tongue is smooth and red, and the child may bruise and bleed easily. Hypomagnesemia and hypocalcemia cause irritability, tremor, convulsions, tetany, bone pain, osteomalacia, and dental abnormalities. If vitamin D deficiency is prolonged, rickets and clubbing of the terminal phalanges are likely. Eighty-six percent of older children have fingerprint changes (ridge atrophy). Fingerprint changes are unusual before 5 years of age, and, if present, they resolve with treatment. In older children, delayed puberty and infertility may be a manifestation of otherwise subtle gluten-sensitive enteropathy.

An unusual complication of gluten-sensitive enteropathy in infancy is celiac crisis. Celiac crisis is characterized by severe diarrhea, dehydration, and hypoproteinemia as a result of malabsorption and protein loss.

Evaluation and Treatment

An intestinal biopsy is mandatory to detect the classic mucosal changes caused by gluten-sensitive enteropathy. The initial biopsy is generally followed by a second intestinal biopsy to demonstrate regeneration of intestinal villi after treatment with a gluten-free diet. Occasionally, the child will be rechallenged with gluten at a later point and a biopsy performed a third time to demonstrate return of intestinal mucosal damage. A wide variety of screening tests for malabsorption also may be useful. The best-known tests are the serum D-xylose assay, which is used to assess upper intestinal surface area, and the quantitative, 72-hour stool fat determination, which is used to detect steatorrhea. Steatorrhea is present in 80% of infants with gluten-sensitive enteropathy. Serum IgA and IgG antigliaden (from gluten) antibodies also are measured.

Treatment consists of the immediate and permanent institution of a diet free of cereal grains (wheat, rye, barley, oats, and malt). Lactose intolerance is presumed; therefore, lactose (milk sugar) is also excluded from the diet. Tolerance to lactose improves with removal of gluten and healing of the mucosa and may be reintroduced at a later point. Infants are routinely given vitamin D, iron, and folic acid supplements to treat deficiencies.

Approximately 25% of children suffer from recurrent relapses that interfere with growth. For most children, however, the long-term prognosis is excellent. There is an increased incidence in malignant disease, particularly lymphoma, in individuals who fail to respond to gluten-free diets.

Protein Energy Malnutrition

Kwashiorkor and marasmus are the two most common types of malnutrition in children. These disorders are known collectively as **protein energy malnutrition (PEM)**. Both are states of long-term starvation (see Chapter 36). **Kwashiorkor** is a severe protein deficiency, and **marasmus** is a severe deficiency of all nutrients. Kwashiorkor is a widespread nutritional problem among children in developing countries and economically destitute populations. The disease usually occurs in infants or children from 1 to 4 years of age who have been weaned from breast milk to a high-starch, protein-deficient diet.

Marasmus, which means "to waste," can occur at any age, but it is common in children younger than 1 year of age. In marasmus, starvation is attributable to lack of protein and carbohydrates. In developing countries and impoverished populations, early weaning of breast-fed infants to overdiluted commercial formulas is a risk factor for marasmus (Hegsted, 1976).

Protein energy malnutrition is also a complication of diseases, such as chronic fever, tuberculosis, malignancy, digestive and malabsorptive disorders, and psychogenic illness. Radiation therapy and chemotherapy can also contribute to protein energy malnutrition.

Pathophysiology

In cases of kwashiorkor, the deficit of dietary amino acids reduces protein synthesis in all tissues. Physical and mental growth are stunted, and maintenance of minimal life processes is in jeopardy. The lack of sufficient plasma proteins, particularly albumin, causes systemic pressure changes that result in generalized edema. The volume of total body water and extracellular fluid increases, causing a substantial loss of potassium. The liver swells with stored fat because no hepatic proteins are synthesized to form and release lipoproteins. Pancreatic atrophy and fibrosis may be present. Kwashiorkor also causes malabsorption, reduced bone density, and impaired renal function. If the condition is not reversed, the prognosis is very poor.

Because the intake of all dietary nutrients is reduced to a minimum in marasmus, metabolic processes, including liver function, are preserved, and growth is severely retarded. Caloric intake is too low to support protein synthesis for growth or the storage of fat. If more protein is needed than is ingested, muscle wasting occurs. Fat wasting and anemia are common and can be severe. The volume of total body water is high, extracellular fluid is somewhat increased, and potassium is depleted slightly. The serum lipoprotein level is high, but other serum values are normal or slightly reduced. Severe vitamin A deficiency commonly results in blindness (Widdowson, 1991).

Clinical Manifestations

Retarded physical, mental, and psychologic development; muscle wasting; diarrhea; dermatosis; and infection characterize marasmus. The presence of subcutaneous fat, hepatomegaly, and fatty liver distinguishes kwashiorkor from marasmus. These manifestations are missing in marasmus because caloric intake is not sufficient to support fat synthesis and storage (Latham, 1991).

Evaluation and Treatment

Evaluation of PEM is based on nutritional history and clinical manifestations. The provision of deficient nutrients will resolve clinical symptoms in 4 to 6 weeks. Physical and mental retardation may not be reversible, however. Reversibility depends on the duration of PEM and the child's developmental status when the deficiency occurred. Nutritional rehabilitation with appropriate environmental stimulation for infants and young children has been shown to resolve or improve cerebral shrinkage, physical growth, and psychomotor development (Gunston, Burkimsher, Malan, & Sive, 1992; Proos, Hofvander, Wennqvist, & Tuvemo, 1992).

Failure to Thrive

Failure to thrive (FTT) is the inadequate physical development of an infant or child. It is manifested as a deceleration in weight gain, a low weight/height ratio, or a low weight/height/head circumference ratio. In the United States, FTT usually affects infants and young children. Failure to thrive is a nutritional disorder having organic or nonorganic causes. Nonorganic FTT is most common among psychosocially and economically deprived populations, whereas organic FTT occurs equally in all populations. The incidence of nonorganic FTT is greater than that of organic FTT (Cupoli, 1980).

Pathophysiology

Organic FTT has a pathophysiologic cause. Gastroesophageal reflux and pyloric stenosis, for example, cause nutrients to be lost through persistent vomiting. Gastroenteritis and infection by intestinal parasites cause nutrients to be lost through vomiting, diarrhea, and interference with mucosal absorption. Congenital anomalies or chronic diseases of major body systems can inhibit enzyme and hormone secretion, digestion, absorption, and the transport of nutrients to tissues. All of these factors reduce the availability of nutrients for maintenance and growth. Psychosocial problems can develop as a result of organic FTT. A chronic disease or congenital anomaly that causes weakness or reduced stature can create developmental, psychosocial, and emotional problems for the child.

Nonorganic FTT is a syndrome with many psychosocial causes and may be complicated by inadequate economic resources and lack of knowledge. The problem in nonorganic FTT is ineffective nurturing by primary caregivers. Infants and children are at risk for nonorganic FTT if their parents or primary caregivers are unable to provide nurturance. A variety of parental stressors may be involved, for example:

Lack of nurturance in the parents' own childhood
Unwanted pregnancy
Inability to bond with the infant because of health or other problems
Postpartum depression
Family crisis, such as a death or marital problems
Stress caused by single parenthood or social isolation
Mental, emotional, or physical illness

Clinical Manifestations

Clinical manifestations of organic FTT are retarded growth accompanied by manifestations of the underlying disease. Manifestations of nonorganic FTT are retarded growth plus reduced energy level, reduced responsiveness and interaction with the environment, social isolation, spasticity and rigidity when held or touched, inability to make eye contact or smile, refusal to eat, and rejection of foods. Weight loss and decelerated growth are accompanied by developmental retardation in many areas. Nonorganic FTT is a complex syndrome involving psychosocial, emotional, and parent-child problems that compound the pathophysiologic abnormalities (Chow, Durand, Feldman, & Mills, 1984).

Evaluation and Treatment

Failure to thrive is often complex and difficult to assess. The condition is suggested if a child falls below the third percentile on the growth curve or is falling off a previously established growth curve. Organic FTT is manifested in infancy by weight, height, and head circumference growth that may be parallel to but below the normal ranges. If no genetic, endocrine, or other systemic disorder is identified, and if the physical and laboratory examinations show no abnormalities other than delayed growth, an environmental cause is indicated.

Hospital admission is recommended if the diagnosis is unclear or the child is in nutritional or emotional jeopardy. Eating patterns, food preferences, caloric intake, and family interactions can be assessed during the hospital stay. If the cause is environmental, the hospitalized child with FTT usually begins to gain weight.

If an organic problem has been identified, management of FTT consists of treating the cause. Management of nonorganic FTT involves the immediate total care of the child and measures to address (1) the psychosocial and emotional problems of the caretakers, and (2) parent-child interactions. Counseling, parental modeling, and long-term family support are sometimes required.

Necrotizing Enterocolitis

Necrotizing enterocolitis is a potentially fatal condition that, if untreated, causes bowel necrosis or perforation. Its cause is unknown. The incidence reported in one study was 3 per 1000 live births and 30 per 1000 low-weight births (Pokorny, Garcia-Pratts, & Yvonne, 1986). It occurs primarily in premature infants; affected infants have a mean gestational age of 31 weeks and weigh less than 1500 g (Welch, 1986). The risk of necrotizing enterocolitis decreases as the gastrointestinal tract matures.

Pathophysiology

A number of factors can contribute to the development of necrotizing enterocolitis, including infections, immunologic injury, perinatal stress, and the effects of medications and feeding practices. This is not clear, however, because these factors describe the population of very sick, very small, vulnerable infants (Yu, Joseph, Bajuk, Orgill, & Astbury, 1984). Reduced mucosal blood flow leading to hypoxic injury to intestinal mucosa is thought to be the cause. This injury allows bacterial invasion of the bowel wall (Welch, 1986). Accumulation of gas in the mucosa and submucosa leads to ischemia and necrosis of intestinal segments.

Clinical Manifestations

Manifestations of necrotizing enterocolitis usually appear within 2 weeks of birth. They range from mild abdominal distention to bowel perforation, sepsis, and death. Abdominal pain, unstable temperature, brady-cardia, and apnea are nonspecific signs. Affected infants have occult or grossly bloody stools (80%), gastric retention (70%), and abdominal distention (70% to 90%). Premature infants often have more severe disease and other disorders, such as hyaline membrane disease (Barnard, Cotton, & Lutin, 1985).

Evaluation and Treatment

Diagnosis of necrotizing enterocolitis is based on clinical manifestations and plain films of the abdomen that show gas accumulation in the intestine. Treatments include cessation of feeding, gastric suction to decompress the intestines, fluid and electrolyte maintenance, and administration of antibiotics to control sepsis. Surgical resection is the treatment of choice for perforation (Cooper, Ross, O'Neill, & Schnaufer, 1988). Overall mortality rate is 20% to 40% (Walsh, Kleigman, & Fanaroff, 1988). Low-birth-weight infants are at greatest risk of death.

Diarrhea

Diarrhea is a frequent gastrointestinal problem during infancy and early childhood. Severe diarrhea occurs between one and three times during the first 3 years of life. Most episodes are self-limiting and resolve within 72 hours.

The pathophysiologic mechanisms of diarrhea in children are similar to those described in Chapter 36 for adults. Prolonged diarrhea is more dangerous in children, however, because they have much smaller fluid reserves than adults. Therefore, dehydration can develop rapidly if any disturbance increases fluid secretion into the gastrointestinal lumen (secretory diarrhea), draws fluid into the lumen by osmosis (osmotic diarrhea), or prevents fluid absorption in the intestine.

Infant diarrhea is of special concern because its cause may be a congenital or metabolic anomaly. Infants have low fluid reserves and relatively rapid peristalsis and metabolism. Therefore, the danger of dehydration is great.

Common causes of acute diarrhea in infants include congenital aganglionic megacolon, infections, milk protein allergies, and necrotizing enterocolitis. Less common causes are adrenogenital syndrome, impaired chloride-bicarbonate exchange, congenital lactase deficiency, glucose-galactose malabsorption, and sucrase-isomaltase deficiency.

Infectious diarrhea in newborns is usually associated with nursery epidemics involving such pathogens as *Escherichia coli*, *Klebsiella*, staphylococci, *Salmonella*, and *Shigella*. Diarrhea caused by these agents has a rapid onset, and acidosis and shock can occur quickly. *Clostridium difficile*, often associated with previous antibiotic therapy, can cause acute profuse watery diarrhea and symptoms of colitis (Niyogi, Dutta, Dutta, Mitra, &

Sikdar, 1991.) True milk protein allergy, which is uncommon, causes bloody, explosive stools after the introduction of milk into the diet.

Acute Diarrhea in Children

Acute diarrhea in children is almost synonymous with acute viral or bacterial gastroenteritis. Viral gastroenteritis tends to be self-limiting. Bacterial gastroenteritis is treated with antibiotics if the causal pathogen can be identified. Other causes of acute diarrhea in the older child include antibiotic therapy, appendicitis, chemotherapy, inflammatory bowel disease, parasitic infestation, parenteral infections, and ingestion of toxic substances.

Chronic Diarrhea in Children

In adults, diarrhea is considered to be chronic if it lasts longer than 2 weeks. This definition does not apply to children, because children with acute gastroenteritis frequently remain mildly symptomatic for up to 4 weeks. In children, diarrhea that persists longer than 4 weeks is considered to be chronic.

Children with chronic diarrhea can be divided into two groups: (1) otherwise well children whose growth is normal and (2) ill children whose growth is retarded. Causes of chronic diarrhea in the first group include abnormal colonic motility, lactose intolerance, encopresis, parasitic infestation, and antibiotic use. Chronic diarrhea in the second group is usually caused by a disease that impairs absorption.

Chronic nonspecific diarrhea

Chronic nonspecific diarrhea is a condition in which uncoordinated colonic motility causes forceful expulsion of feces. Apparently, the lower sigmoid colon remains in a tonically contracted state. Defecation occurs when pressure in the upper sigmoid colon and distal descending colon becomes great enough to force feces through the nonmotile, contracted segment.

In some instances, there is a family history of bowel complaints. As an infant, the child is likely to have experienced colic and diarrhea associated with teething and immunizations. In more than 90% of cases, chronic nonspecific diarrhea resolves by 40 to 50 months of age. The cure frequently accompanies toilet training. Many children with chronic nonspecific diarrhea develop irritable bowel syndrome (also called mucous colitis) as adults (Levine, 1987). Children with chronic nonspecific diarrhea usually do well with normal food and fluid intake. Special diets and medications are used with caution (Behrman, Kleigman, Nelson, & Vaughan, 1992).

Primary lactose intolerance

Lactose intolerance, the inability to digest milk sugar, is caused by inadequate production of lactase (see Chapter 36). Lactose intolerance is a common cause of diarrhea in children, particularly black children. The malabsorption of lactose results in osmotic diarrhea, in which fluids move by osmosis from the vascular compartment into the intestinal lumen. As the undigested sugar is acted on by the colonic bacteria, intestinal gas is produced. The diarrhea is accompanied by abdominal pain, bloating, and flatulence. These symptoms begin before the age of 7 in half of affected blacks. Treatment consists of reducing milk consumption. Some children can tolerate lactose in fermented forms, such as cheese and yogurt.

DISORDERS OF THE LIVER
Disorders of Biliary Metabolism and Transport
Physiologic Jaundice of the Newborn

Physiologic jaundice of the newborn is usually a transient, benign icterus that occurs during the first week of life in otherwise healthy, full-term infants. It is caused by mild unconjugated (indirect-reacting) hyperbilirubinemia. A high level of indirect hyperbilirubinemia (15 mg/dl) is considered pathologic. There is a risk of brain damage (kernicterus) with persistent high indirect hyperbilirubinemia. (Hyperbilirubinemia is described in Chapter 36.)

Pathophysiology

Physiologic jaundice results from the complex interaction of factors that cause (1) increased bilirubin production, (2) impaired hepatic uptake and excretion of bilirubin, and (3) reabsorption of bilirubin in the small intestine. Serum bilirubin values increase to 5 to 6 mg/dl by the second to fourth day after birth in full-term infants, and 10 to 15 mg/dl by the fifth to seventh day in premature infants.

Clinical Manifestations

Physiologic jaundice develops during the second or third day after birth. It usually subsides in 1 to 2 weeks in full-term infants and 2 to 4 weeks in premature infants. After this, increasing bilirubin values and persistent jaundice indicate pathologic hyperbilirubinemia. Bilirubin encephalopathy (kernicterus), which is caused by the deposition of toxic, unconjugated bilirubin in brain cells, usually does not occur in healthy, full-term infants. Premature infants with respiratory distress, acidosis, or sepsis are at greater risk for encephalopathy. The mechanism by which bilirubin crosses the blood-brain barrier and precipitates into brain cells is not known (Stern & Brodersen, 1987).

Evaluation and Treatment

Laboratory tests are conducted to determine bilirubin levels. Both total and direct (conjugated) bilirubin levels are measured; the direct bilirubin should not exceed 1 mg/dl (Behrman et al., 1992). Other causes of jaundice must be eliminated to confirm physiologic jaundice. Treatment depends on the degree of hyperbilirubinemia. Physiologic jaundice is usually treated by phototherapy (ultraviolet light). Pathologic jaundice requires an exchange transfusion.

Biliary Atresia

Biliary atresia is a congenital malformation characterized by the absence or obstruction of intrahepatic or extrahepatic bile ducts. Extrahepatic ducts may end in a blind pouch. The cause of the intrauterine injury to the ducts is not clear but is thought to be related to chromosomal abnormality or active agents, such as infection or drugs (Glaser & Morecki, 1987; Silveira, Salzano, Howard, & Mowat, 1991). The disease expression is a continuum in which the principal process is one of bile duct destruction. The points of destruction are influenced by the stage of intrauterine development in which injury occurs (Raweily, Gibson, & Burt, 1990).

The atresia or obstruction of the bile ducts leads to plugging, inflammation, and fibrosis of the bile canaliculi. Progressive obstruction may lead to biliary cirrhosis (see Chapter 36), portal hypertension, or liver failure (Treem, 1991).

Jaundice is the primary clinical manifestation of biliary atresia. Other signs are hepatomegaly and acholic (clay-colored) stools. Fat absorption is impaired for lack of bile salts, and the infant may fail to gain weight. Cirrhosis and liver failure can lead to death.

Diagnosis of biliary atresia is based on clinical manifestations and liver biopsy. Liver function test results are abnormal. Serum transaminase and alkaline phosphatase values are elevated, and conjugated (direct) serum bilirubin levels rise progressively.

Extrahepatic atresia can be relieved by surgical drainage and correction in approximately 10% of cases. Some infants benefit from the Kasai procedure, in which a hepatic duct remnant is anastomosed to the jejunum or a jejunal segment is anastomosed to the porta hepatis if the patent hepatic duct remnant is not available (Fig. 37-7). This procedure has a 71% success rate in establishing bile flow if the infant is younger than 2 months of age; establishment of bile flow is achieved in 25% of infants older than 2 months of age. Even with initial restoration of bile flow, however, obliteration of intrahepatic bile ducts continues and cirrhosis results. Liver transplantation is the long-term therapy for biliary atresia. Half to two thirds of children receiving liver transplantation have biliary atresia. Approximately

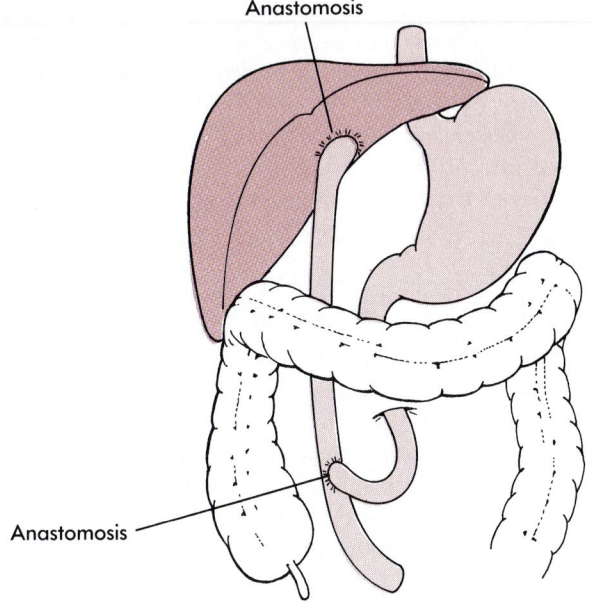

FIG. 37-7 **Kasai procedure.** Surgical correction for extrahepatic biliary atresia. The jejunal segment between the liver and bowel may be externalized, creating a double-barrel portoenterostomy.

40% of children with biliary atresia are immediate candidates for transplantation. Eighty percent of children with biliary atresia die before the age of 3 years if transplantation is not done (Treem, 1991).

Inflammatory Disorders
Hepatitis

Hepatitis A, B, C, and D (delta) and fulminant hepatitis affect children and adults. Hepatitis also can result from infection with other viruses, for example, herpesvirus, varicella, cytomegalovirus, rubella, Coxsackie B, and Epstein-Barr virus. The pathophysiology of viral and fulminant hepatitis is described in Chapter 36.

Hepatitis A

Approximately one third of the reported cases of hepatitis A occur in children (Francis et al., 1984). Incidence is highest among young children of nursery school age. Outbreaks tend to occur in day care centers with large numbers of children who are not toilet trained and staff members who practice poor hand washing techniques (Hadler & McFarland, 1986). Hepatitis A in children is usually mild and asymptomatic. Clinical manifestations, however, may include nausea, vomiting, and diarrhea. Because jaundice is absent, infected children appear to have the "flu." Almost all children recover from hepatitis A without residual liver damage (Lesnicar, 1988).

Hepatitis B

Infection with the hepatitis B virus (HBV) usually occurs among children in high-risk situations. Infants of mothers who are chronic HB$_s$Ag carriers, hemophiliacs who receive frequent blood transfusions, children who abuse parenteral drugs, and children who live in institutions for the mentally retarded are all at risk for HBV infection. Ninety percent of newborns infected by their mothers develop chronic hepatitis and become carriers. Chronic hepatitis may develop because the infant's immune system is immature. Infected infants are at risk for cirrhosis and hepatocellular carcinoma (Balistreri, 1988). The most serious consequence of HBV infection is fulminant hepatitis, which occurs in 1% of cases. Hepatitis D infection depends on active infection with HBV. There is evidence that the risk of fulminant hepatitis is higher in individuals with combined infection of HBV and HDV than in those with HBV infection alone (Treem, 1991).

Hepatitis C

Hepatitis C in children is primarily associated with blood transfusions. Children who receive frequent transfusions are at highest risk. Because there are no serologic markers for hepatitis C, other causes of acute hepatitis must be ruled out (Hay et al., 1987). Between 10% and 50% of affected children develop chronic liver disease.

Chronic hepatitis

Chronic hepatitis in adults is usually defined as liver disease lasting longer than 6 months. Chronic hepatitis in children is more difficult to define because the clinical manifestations of illness are milder than they are in adults. Hepatitis A, which is prevalent in childhood, neither persists nor progresses to chronic liver disease (Bortollotti et al., 1987). The cause of chronic hepatitis is unknown in most cases, but an autoimmune mechanism is suggested because inflammatory findings are commonly seen in biopsy specimens of the liver.

Manifestations of chronic hepatitis include malaise, anorexia, fever, gastrointestinal bleeding, hepatomegaly, edema, and transient joint pain. Serum transaminase and bilirubin levels are elevated. There may be evidence of impairment of synthetic functions of the liver: prolonged prothrombin time and hypoalbuminemia. The diagnosis of chronic hepatitis is based on the clinical manifestations and liver biopsy. There is no effective therapy for chronic hepatitis B or chronic hepatitis C. Some success has been achieved with human alpha interferon; improvement in liver function is seen in approximately 50% of children with HBV infection treated. Young children may respond to alternate-day treatment with steroids (Behrman et al., 1992).

Cirrhosis

Most forms of chronic liver diseases in children can progress to cirrhosis, but they seldom do so. Cirrhosis is the excessive formation of fibrous tissue in response to inflammation and tissue damage (see Chapter 36). The complications of cirrhosis in children are the same as those in adults: portal hypertension, the opening of collateral vessels between the portal and systemic veins, and varices. In addition, children with cirrhosis experience growth failure caused by nutritional deficits and developmental delay, particularly in gross motor function because of ascites and weakness. The cause of cirrhosis may influence its severity and course. Some types of cirrhosis can be stabilized if the cause is identified and treated early.

Portal Hypertension

Portal hypertension is a persistent increase in portal venous pressure (see Chapter 36). Because the portal system is relatively inaccessible, pressures in children are not often measured or are measured in unique ways. There are no standard values for portal pressure in children. In adults, however, portal hypertension is often defined as the presence of a pressure gradient of 10 to 15 cm H_2O between the portal and the systemic venous system.

There are two basic causes of portal hypertension in children: (1) increased resistance to blood flow within

the portal system or (2) increased volume of portal blood flow. The second cause is quite rare in children and is not discussed here. Increased resistance to flow can occur anywhere in the portal circulatory system. Portal hypertension can accompany cirrhosis, intraabdominal infections, portal vein thrombosis, congenital anomalies of the portal vein, and congenital hepatic fibrosis.

Types of Portal Hypertension
Extrahepatic portal hypertension

Extrahepatic (prehepatic) portal venous obstruction causes 50% to 70% of extrahepatic portal hypertension in children. In approximately two thirds of these children, no specific cause can be found (Behrman et al., 1992). Obstruction is almost always in the portal vein and is usually caused by thrombosis. Portal vein thrombosis can occur as a complication of abdominal trauma, pancreatitis, abdominal infections, and some systemic disorders; however, these causes are rare. The liver is usually normal in cases of extrahepatic portal hypertension.

Intrahepatic portal hypertension

Cirrhosis is the primary cause of intrahepatic portal hypertension. In some cases of severe cirrhosis, the portal flow is thought to be reversed; whether this actually happens is controversial (Whitington, 1985). The most common finding is fibrosis, which increases resistance to portal blood flow by constricting and reducing the compliance of the hepatic sinusoids.

Course of the Disease

The important consequences of portal hypertension in children are the development of collateral circulation, with portal-systemic shunting; hypersplenism; and ascites. The pathophysiology of portal hypertension is described in Chapter 36.

Clinical Manifestations

The clinical manifestations of portal hypertension are (1) splenomegaly, (2) upper gastrointestinal bleeding, (3) ascites, and (4) hepatic encephalopathy. Splenomegaly is the most frequent sign of portal hypertension in children. The spleen may be firm or hard, depending on the duration of portal hypertension. Hematemesis, which may or may not be associated with abdominal pain, is often associated with sudden pallor. Melena is observed, either at the time of hematemesis or soon afterward. In children, most episodes of gastrointestinal bleeding are caused by rupture of esophageal varices. Clotting abnormalities caused by altered liver function promote the bleeding. If plasma volume is increased, esophageal varices readily rupture during activities, such as coughing, that increase blood pressure. Acetyl-salicylic acid (aspirin), which should not be administered to children, can trigger bleeding, but its exact mechanisms of action are not known. Severe bleeding episodes can cause hypovolemic shock and death. Symptoms of ascites include weight gain, protruding abdomen, and reduced tidal volumes if the ascites is severe.

Hepatic encephalopathy in children can be acute or chronic. Acute encephalopathy is characterized by major disorders of consciousness, which may progress to coma. This may follow an acute episode of variceal bleeding as the impaired liver attempts to metabolize the large protein (nitrogenous) load from the blood. Chronic, or minimal, encephalopathy is characterized by emotional or psychiatric disorders, decreased intellectual functioning, personality disorders caused by minimal brain dysfunction, and spatial disorientation.

Evaluation and Treatment

Assessment of portal hypertension in children must be thorough because the cause dictates the management. The objectives of the clinical investigation are to (1) locate the site of the venous block and (2) identify the disease responsible for the portal hypertension. Thorough physical examination, laboratory tests of liver function, imaging procedures, and biopsy may be included in the diagnostic evaluation (see Chapter 35). Severe liver disease is characterized by hypoalbuminemia, prolonged prothrombin times, hyperbilirubinemia, electrolyte imbalance, and hypoglycemia. Sclerotherapy is the initial treatment of choice for severe esophageal varices in children. Surgical venous shunts are rarely performed on small children because of the high failure rate secondary to vessel occlusion, but may be an alternative in older children (Behrman et al., 1992).

The outcome of portal hypertension depends almost entirely on its cause. Children with extrahepatic disease are expected to recover with little morbidity. For children with intrahepatic disease, the prognosis varies. For example, stable postnecrotic cirrhosis, complicated by variceal bleeding, has a much better prognosis than does cirrhosis with chronic acute liver disease and variceal bleeding. Postsinusoidal hypertension (high pressure generated in the hepatic veins or vena cava) generally results in extreme morbidity and mortality. Encephalopathy has been reported in 22% to 29% of children (Voorhes & Price, 1974).

Metabolic Disorders

More than 5000 genetically determined metabolic pathways have been identified in liver tissue. The earliest possible identification of metabolic disorders is essential because (1) early treatment may prevent permanent damage to vital organs, such as the liver or brain; (2)

precise genetic counseling may be possible with prenatal diagnosis; and (3) complications can be minimized, even if cure is not possible. Galactosemia, fructosemia, and Wilson disease are treatable metabolic disorders that have hepatic clinical manifestations.

Galactosemia

Galactosemia is a rare disorder caused by a deficiency of the enzyme galactose-1-phosphate uridyltransferase (a hepatic enzyme needed to convert galactose to glucose). This deficiency is inherited as an autosomal recessive trait. Because galactose cannot be incorporated into carbohydrate metabolism, it accumulates in all body tissues together with metabolites, which may be toxic. Galactosuria may occur after the ingestion of lactose.

Pathophysiology

A deficiency of galactose-1-phosphate uridyltransferase results in the accumulation of galactose-1-phosphate in body cells. These accumulations are most injurious in the liver, where they cause cirrhosis, and in the brain, where they cause mental retardation. Increasing accumulations cause severe and irreversible damage. Cataracts form because of increasing concentrations of galactitol resulting from uridyltransferase deficiency (Silverman & Roy, 1983).

Clinical Manifestations

Signs of galactosemia appear in early infancy because milk (particularly breast milk) contains lactose. Some infants have mild failure to thrive, recurrent hypoglycemia, and manifestations of cirrhosis that become evident at 2 to 6 months of age. Rarely are the early signs mental retardation, cataracts, or both.

Evaluation and Treatment

Diagnosis is based on a test for the presence of a reducing substance in the urine while the infant is receiving a formula containing lactose. Treatment consists of a galactose-free diet. Removal of dietary lactose causes rapid improvement in the infant's condition, including regression of jaundice, gastrointestinal symptoms, bleeding, and other symptoms of cirrhosis. Most infants have no subsequent liver problems. Cataracts are stabilized and may regress slightly with treatment. Brain damage is irreversible. Long-term follow-up of adequately treated children shows that their mental development is often impaired. Children with galactose-1-phosphate uridyltransferase deficiency must continue a lactose-free diet for life.

Fructosemia

Fructosemia (hereditary fructose intolerance) is an inherited, autosomal recessive deficiency of the enzyme fructose-1-phosphate aldolase. If fructose is ingested, it has profound secondary effects on carbohydrate and nucleotide metabolism, particularly within the liver cells. Affected individuals develop an extreme aversion to fructose-containing foods.

Pathophysiology

Because of the fructose-1-phosphate aldolase deficiency, fructose-1-phosphate accumulates in hepatocytes. This accumulation is toxic in some children and results in severe, progressive liver disease. The accumulation of fructose-1-phosphate transiently inhibits the conversion of glycogen to glucose, causing severe hypoglycemia.

Clinical Manifestations

Signs of fructosemia include jaundice, vomiting, irritability, hepatomegaly, coagulation disorders, and convulsions that begin as soon as fructose is ingested. Onset occurs when breast milk is replaced by cow's milk, formula, or foods containing fructose, sucrose, or honey. In an older child, fructosemia may be seen as a feeding difficulty because ingestion of a fructose-containing food will cause anorexia and malaise. Older children and adults may develop manifestations when given intravenous fructose during an illness. Some children can tolerate a small amount of sucrose, but in most, sucrose ingestion provokes progressive liver damage, abdominal distention, and, ultimately, cirrhosis.

Evaluation and Treatment

A detailed dietary history is essential. The diagnosis is confirmed if low enzymatic activity is demonstrated in a liver or intestinal mucosal biopsy specimen.

Withdrawal of fructose from the diet causes vomiting to regress almost immediately, and other signs of liver disease improve within a few days. A fructose-free and sucrose-free diet must be maintained for life, and vitamin C supplements must be taken. If fructosemia causes acute liver failure, exchange transfusions, plasma and blood transfusions, and intravenous glucose may be required. With the institution of a fructose-free diet, the liver gradually decreases in size, and liver function tests return to normal. Fatty changes in liver tissue diminish but never disappear completely.

Wilson Disease

Wilson disease (hepatolenticular degeneration) is an autosomal recessive defect of copper metabolism that causes toxic amounts of copper to accumulate in the liver, brain, kidneys, and corneas. This defect in the uptake and excretion of copper by hepatocytes is an important cause of progressive liver disease in children and young adults. Wilson disease is very rare, with an incidence between 1 in 100,000 and 1 in 500,000 persons.

Between 1 in 200 and 1 in 500 persons are carriers (Behrman et al., 1992).

Pathophysiology

Two major abnormalities in copper metabolism have been identified: (1) diminished biliary excretion of copper and (2) impaired production of ceruloplasmin (a glycoprotein that transports copper in the blood). A positive copper balance is present from birth in children with Wilson disease, despite increased excretion of copper in the urine.

Early in the disease, intestinal absorption of copper is normal, as is hepatic clearance of albumin-bound, absorbed copper. As copper-binding proteins in the liver become saturated, hepatic uptake of copper diminishes. Decreased hepatic metabolism of copper causes elevated serum copper levels and biochemical and clinical evidence of liver damage caused by copper accumulation. In later stages of the disease, copper accumulates in extrahepatic tissues, including the eyes, brain, and kidneys.

Controversy exists over the pathogenesis of Wilson disease. One theory holds that the synthesis of the copper-binding protein, ceruloplasmin, may be deficient or abnormal; another suggests that biliary excretion of copper is impaired (Scheinberg & Sternlieb, 1984). When copper accumulating in liver cells (hepatocytes) reaches toxic levels, the liver cells die. Copper is released and accumulates in and damages other tissues.

When cerebral copper-binding proteins become saturated, a characteristic pattern of brain damage develops, particularly in the basal ganglia. Neural effects include intention tremor, unsteady gait, dystonia, and behavioral changes. Manifestations of renal tubular injury usually appear simultaneously. The uptake of copper by red blood cells is thought to cause hemolytic anemia, a condition sometimes seen early in the clinical course of Wilson disease.

Clinical Manifestations

The clinical manifestations of Wilson disease begin at about 4 years of age, the age by which control mechanisms responsible for copper homeostasis and biliary excretion should have matured. Some individuals, however, do not develop signs and symptoms until later in life.

The classic clinical presentation of Wilson disease is a triad of neuromuscular abnormalities, intention tremors, dysarthria (indistinct speech), and dystonia (disordered muscular tonicity): (1) Kayser-Fleischer rings (accumulation of copper in the limbus of the cornea, causing a greenish yellow ring), (2) cirrhosis associated with elevated serum copper, and (3) low ceruloplasmin levels. Initial symptoms vary from malaise and abdominal pain to jaundice and changes in mental performance. The earliest signs of liver involvement include enlargement of the liver and spleen, jaundice, and anorexia. Edema and ascites may develop suddenly, or gastrointestinal hemorrhage may be the initial sign of the disease. Occasionally, Wilson disease begins with a hemolytic crisis caused by the toxic effects of copper on the red blood cells. Cirrhosis develops in all untreated cases. Copper deposition in the kidneys causes a proximal renal tubular defect that results in losses of glucose, amino acids, phosphate, and uric acid in the urine and renal tubular acidosis.

Evaluation and Treatment

Because Wilson disease is rare, it may not be diagnosed until clinical manifestations develop. Laboratory tests detect a serum ceruloplasmin concentration less than 30 mg/dl. Serum copper values may be normal or high, and urine copper values are elevated. Liver biopsy is used to assess structural changes and measure copper concentrations.

Definitive treatment of Wilson disease is chelation therapy, the removal of excess copper from the tissues. Chelation is accomplished with *d*-penicillamine, an agent that incorporates copper into a complex that is readily eliminated in the urine. Children receiving penicillamine are given vitamin supplements, especially vitamin B_6. Copper intake is reduced by eliminating organ meats, nuts, legumes, shellfish, and chocolate from the diet. Physiotherapy may accelerate the recovery of gait and muscular coordination.

Children with untreated Wilson disease die of neural, hepatic, renal, or hematologic complications. The success of *d*-penicillamine therapy depends on early treatment and individual responsiveness. Therapy is seldom successful in children with chronic active liver disease, acute liver failure, or severe neuromuscular alterations. Failure of a 2- to 3-month course of chelation therapy in individuals with Wilson disease and decompensated cirrhosis is considered an indication for liver transplantation (Treem, 1991).

SUMMARY REVIEW

Disorders of the Gastrointestinal Tract

1 Most alterations of digestive function in children are caused by congenital obstructions of the intestinal tract; disorders of digestion, absorption, or nutrition; or liver disease.

2 Cleft lip (harelip) and cleft palate (failure of the bony palate to fuse in the midline) may occur separately or together. The fissure may affect the uvula, soft palate, hard palate, nostril, and maxillary alveolar ridge.

3 Esophageal atresia, a condition in which the esophagus ends in a blind pouch, may occur with or without tracheoesophageal fistula, or connection between the esophagus and the trachea. As the infant swallows oral secretions or ingests milk, the pouch fills, causing either drooling or aspiration into the lungs.

4 Pyloric stenosis, one of the most common disorders requiring surgery in early infancy, is an obstruction of the pyloric outlet caused by hypertrophy of circular muscles in the pyloric sphincter.

5 Malrotation of the intestine, with an obstructing band and volvulus (twisting of the bowel on itself), may partly or completely occlude the gastrointestinal tract and its blood vessels.

6 Meconium ileus is a condition in the newborn in which intestinal secretions and amniotic waste products produce a thick, tarry plug that obstructs the intestine. Ten percent to 20% of children with cystic fibrosis present with meconium ileus as a neonate.

7 Duodenal, jejunal, and ileal obstructions can be due to meconium ileus, atresia, congenital aganglionic megacolon, and acquired obstructive disorders.

8 Congenital aganglionic megacolon (Hirschsprung disease) is caused by a malformation of the parasympathetic nervous system in a segment of the colon. It is characterized by the absence of nerves needed for peristalsis.

9 Malformations of the anus and rectum range from mild congenital stenosis of the anus to complex deformities, all of which are classified as imperforate anus.

10 The most frequent cause of acquired intestinal obstruction in infants is intussusception, a condition in which one portion of the bowel telescopes, or invaginates, into another, most commonly in the area of the ileocecal junction.

11 Gastroesophageal reflux is caused by the relaxation or incompetence of the lower esophageal sphincter. Infants are susceptible to reflux because the sphincter is not fully mature, their diet consists of liquids, and they are seldom in an upright position.

12 Cystic fibrosis is an inherited exocrine gland abnormality that causes chronic suppurative lung disease and abnormalities in other organs that contain exocrine glands.

13 The pathophysiologic triad that is the hallmark of cystic fibrosis includes pancreatic enzyme deficiency (which causes maldigestion), overproduction of mucus in the respiratory tract, and abnormally elevated sodium and chloride concentrations in sweat. Older children with cystic fibrosis also may have diabetes mellitus caused by damage to endocrine function of the pancreas and chronic liver disease. Affected individuals seldom survive beyond their 20s.

14 Gluten-sensitive enteropathy is a lifelong disease characterized by the loss of mature villous epithelium in the presence of a gluten-containing diet. It results in malabsorption and growth failure.

15 Protein energy malnutrition is a group of disorders resulting from a severe dietary deficiency of proteins, carbohydrates, or both. Starvation causes stunted mental and physical development.

16 Kwashiorkor is a severe protein deficiency that occurs in children who have stopped breast feeding and subsist on a high-carbohydrate diet. Marasmus is a deficiency of all dietary nutrients, including carbohydrates.

17 Failure to thrive is inadequate physical growth of a child. Organic failure to thrive is caused by genetic, anatomic, or pathophysiologic factors that retard normal growth and development. Nonorganic failure to thrive is caused by nutritional deficits associated with inadequate nurturing.

18 Necrotizing enterocolitis is a disorder in neonates, particularly premature infants, thought to result from stress and anoxia of the bowel wall. Bacteria invade the mucosa and submucosa resulting in colitis, necrosis, and even perforation of the intestinal wall.

19 Diarrhea in infants and children can rapidly cause dehydration and electrolyte imbalances because fluid reserves are relatively small.

20 The most common cause of acute diarrhea in children is bacterial or viral enterocolitis (infection of the gastrointestinal tract).

21 Chronic diarrhea (diarrhea persisting longer than 4 weeks) can be caused by a wide variety of underlying conditions and frequently leads to growth failure and slow development.

Disorders of the Liver

1 Physiologic jaundice of the newborn is caused by mild hyperbilirubinemia that subsides in a week or two. Pathologic jaundice is caused by severe hyperbilirubinemia and can cause brain damage.

2 Biliary atresia is a congenital malformation of the bile ducts that obstructs bile flow. Atresia causes jaundice, cirrhosis, and liver failure. Biliary atresia is the most common reason for liver transplantation in children.

3 Acute hepatitis has the same clinical course in children and adults, but children have milder cases of the disease. Hepatitis A is the most common form of childhood hepatitis.

4 Cirrhosis is rare in children, but it can develop from most forms of chronic liver disease.

5 Portal hypertension in children usually is caused by extrahepatic obstruction. Thrombosis of the portal vein is the most common cause of portal hypertension in children, and splenomegaly is the most frequent sign.

6 The three most common metabolic disorders that cause liver damage in children are galactosemia, fructosemia, and Wilson disease. All three are inherited as genetic traits and permit the accumulation of toxins in the liver.

7 Galactosemia is caused by a deficiency of the enzyme galactose-1-phosphate uridyltransferase. Galactose cannot be metabolized and accumulates in the liver, kidney, and brain, causing damage. When the diagnosis is not made at birth and lactose is not removed from the diet, damage to the liver (cirrhosis) and brain (mental retardation) becomes increasingly severe and irreversible.

8 Fructosemia is caused by a deficiency of the enzyme fructose-1-phosphate aldolase. Lack of this enzyme causes ingested fructose to disrupt carbohydrate and nucleotide metabolism. The infant is asymptomatic until fructose and sucrose are introduced into the diet.

9 Wilson disease causes defective copper uptake and metabolism. Unexcreted copper accumulates in the liver, brain, kidney, and corneal cells. Damage from accumulated copper is gradual; the disease is not diagnosed before the age of 4 or 5 years.

KEY TERMS

Biliary atresia, 1392
Chronic nonspecific diarrhea, 1391
Cleft lip (harelip), 1377
Cleft palate, 1377
Congenital aganglionic megacolon (Hirschsprung disease), 1382
Cystic fibrosis (CF), 1385
Esophageal atresia, 1378
Failure to thrive (FTT), 1387, 1389
Fructosemia (hereditary fructose intolerance), 1395
Galactosemia, 1395
Gluten-sensitive enteropathy (celiac sprue), 1387

Ileal atresia, 1382
Imperforate anus, 1383
Infant diarrhea, 1391
Intussusception, 1384
Jejunal atresia, 1382
Kwashiorkor, 1389
Lactose intolerance, 1391
Malrotation, 1380
Marasmus, 1389
Meconium, 1381
Meconium ileus, 1381
Meconium ileus equivalent, 1381
Necrotizing enterocolitis, 1390
Nonorganic FTT, 1390

Organic FTT, 1390
Periduodenal band, 1380
Physiologic jaundice of the newborn, 1392
Protein energy malnutrition (PEM), 1389
Pyloric stenosis, 1379
Tracheoesophageal fistula (TEF), 1378
Wilson disease, 1396

REFERENCES

Auricchio, S., Greco, L., & Troncone, R. (1988). Gluten-sensitive enteropathy in childhood. *Pediatric Clinics of North America, 35*(1), 157-187.

Bailey, D. J., Andres, J. M., Danek, G. D., & Pineiro-Carrero, V. M. (1987). Lack of efficacy of thickened feeding as treatment for gastroesophageal reflux. *Journal of Pediatrics, 110,* 187-189.

Balistreri, W. F. (1988). Viral hepatitis. *Pediatric Clinics of North America, 35,* 375-407.

Barnard, J. A., Cotton, B. C., & Lutin, W. (1985). Necrotizing enterocolitis: Variables associated with severity of disease. *American Journal of Diseases of the Child, 139,* 375-377.

Barr, L. L., Stansberry, S. D., & Swischuk, L. E. (1990). Significance of age, duration, obstruction, and the dissection sign in intussusception. *Pediatric Radiology, 20,* 454-456.

Beasley, S. W., & Meyers, W. A. (1988). The diagnosis of congenital tracheoesophageal fistula. *Journal of Pediatric Surgery, 23*(5), 415-417.

Behrman, R. E., Kleigman, R. M., Nelson, W. E., & Vaughan, V. C. (1992). *Nelson textbook of pediatrics* (14th ed.). Philadelphia: Saunders.

Bissonnette, B., & Sullivan P. J. (1991). Pyloric stenosis. *Canadian Journal of Anaesthesiology, 38,* 668-676.

Bortollotti, P., Cadrobbi, P., Armigliato, M., Rude, L., Rugge, M., & Realdi, G. (1987). Prognosis of chronic hepatitis B transmitted from HB$_s$Ag positive mother. *Archives of Disease in Childhood, 62,* 201-203.

Carter, C. O. (1961). The inheritance of congenital pyloric stenosis. *British Medical Bulletin, 17,* 251-254.

Chow, M. P., Durand, B. A., Feldman, M. N., & Mills, M. A. (1984). Failure to thrive. In M. P. Chow, B. Durand, M. N. Feldman, & M. A. Mills (Eds.), *Handbook of pediatric primary care* (pp. 1185-1205). New York: Wiley & Sons.

Cooper, A., Ross, A. J., O'Neill, J. A., & Schnaufer, L. (1988). Resection with primary anastomosis for necrotizing enterocolitis: A contrasting view. *Journal of Pediatric Surgery, 23,* 64-68.

Cupoli, J. (1980). Failure to thrive. *Current Problems in Pediatrics, 10,* 2-43.

DelPina, C. A., Czyrko, C., Ziegler, M. M., Scanlin, T. F., & Bishop, H. C. (1992). Management and survival of meconium ileus: A 30 year review. *Annals of Surgery, 215,* 179-185.

Fanaroff, A. F., & Martin, R. J. (1987). *Neonatal-perinatal medicine: Diseases of the fetus and newborn* (4th ed.). St. Louis: Mosby–Year Book.

Filston, H. C., & Kirks, D. R. (1981). Malrotation: The ubiquitous anomaly. *Journal of Pediatric Surgery, 16*(4 Suppl. 1), 614-620.

Forstner, G., & Durie, P. R. (1991). Cystic fibrosis. In W. A. Walker, P. R. Durie, J. R. Hamilton, J. A. Walker-Smith, & J. B. Watkins I (Eds.), *Pediatric gastrointestinal disease.* Burlington, Ontario: B. C. Decker.

Francis, D. P., Hadler, S. C., Prendergast, T. J., Peterson, E., Ginsberg, M. M., Loockbaugh, C., Holmes, J. R., & Maynard, J. E. (1984). Occurrence of hepatitis A, B, and non-A/non-B in the United States: CDC sentinel county hepatitis study I. *American Journal of Medicine, 76,* 69-74.

Glaser, J. H., & Morecki, R. (1987). Retrovirus type 3 and neonatal cholestasis. *Seminars in Liver Disease, 7,* 100.

Greco, L., Tozzi, A. E., & Mayer, M. (1987). Growth status of coeliac patients in the florid phase. *Italian Journal of Pediatrics, 13,* 161.

Gunston, G. D., Burkimsher, D., Malan, H., & Sive, A. A. (1992). Reversible cerebral shrinkage in kwashiorkor: An MRI study. *Archives of Disease in Childhood, 67,* 1030-1032.

Hadler, S. C., & McFarland, L. (1986). Hepatitis in day care centers. *Review of Infectious Diseases, 8,* 548-557.

Hay, C. R. M., Preston, F. E., Triger, D. R., Greaves, M., Underwood, J. C. E., & Westlake, L. (1987). Predictive markers of chronic liver disease in hemophilia. *Blood, 69,* 1595-1599.

Hegsted, D. M. (1976). Protein needs and possible modification of the American diet. *Journal of the American Dietetic Association, 68,* 317.

Holcomb, G. W., Ross, A. J., & O'Neill, J. A. (1991). Postoperative intussusception: Increasing frequency or increasing awareness? *Southern Medical Journal, 84,* 1334-1339.

Holmes, M., Murphy, V., Taylor, M., & Denham, B. (1991). Intussusception in cystic fibrosis. *Archives of Disease in Childhood, 66,* 726-727.

Iwai, N., Yanagihara, J., Tokiwa, K., Deguchi, E., Perdzynski, W., & Takahashi, T. (1988). Reliability of anorectal manometry in the diagnosis of Hirschsprung disease. *Zeitschrift fur Kinderchirurgie, 43,* 405-407.

Jolley, S. G., Halpern, L. M., Tunell, W. P., Johnson, D. G., & Sterling, C. E. (1991). The risk of sudden infant death from gastroesophageal reflux. *Journal of Pediatric Surgery, 26,* 691-696.

Latham, M. C. (1991). The dermatosis of kwashiorkor in young children. *Seminars in Dermatology, 10,* 270-272.

Lesnicar, C. (1988). A prospective study of viral hepatitis A and the question of chronicity. *Hepatogastroenterology, 35*(2), 69-72.

Levine, J. J. (1987). Chronic nonspecific diarrhea. *Pediatric Annals, 10,* 822-829.

Levy, J. (1991). The gastrointestinal tract in Down's syndrome. *Progress in Clinical Biology, 373,* 245-256.

Maurage, C., Lenaerts, C., Weber, A., Brochu, P., Yousef, I., & Roy, C. C. (1989). Meconium ileus and its equivalent as a risk factor for the development of cirrhosis: An autopsy study in cystic fibrosis. *Journal of Pediatric Gastroenterology and Nutrition, 9,* 17-20.

Milla, P. J. (1988). Gastrointestinal motility disorders in children. *Pediatric Clinics of North America, 35*(5), 311-330.

Mitchell, L. E., & Risch, N. (1992). Mode of inheritance of nonsyndromic cleft lip with or without cleft palate: A reanalysis. *American Journal of Human Genetics, 51,* 323-332.

Mosher, M. S. (1986). Genetic counseling in cleft lip and palate. *Ear, Nose, and Throat Journal, 65,* 330-336.

Nakazato, Y., Landing, B. H., & Wells, T. R. (1986). Abnormal Auerbach plexus in the esophagus and stomach of patients with esophageal atresia and tracheoesophageal fistula. *Journal of Pediatric Surgery, 21,* 831-837.

Niyogi, S. K., Dutta, P., Dutta, D., Mitra, U., & Sikdar, S. (1991). *Clostridium difficile* and its cytotoxin in hospitalized children with acute diarrhea. *Indian Pediatrician, 28,* 1129-1132.

O'Keeffe, F. N., Stansberry, S. D., Swischuk, L. E., & Hayden, C. K. (1991). Antropyloric muscle thickness in U. S. in infants: What is normal. *Radiology, 178,* 827-830.

Orenstein, S. R., & Whittington, P. F. (1983). Positioning for prevention of infant gastroesophageal reflux. *Journal of Pediatrics, 103,* 534-537.

Pokorny, W. J., Garcia-Pratts, J. A., & Yvonne, B. N. (1986). Necrotizing enterocolitis: Incidence, operative care, and outcome. *Journal of Pediatric Surgery, 21,* 1149-1154.

Proos, L. A., Hofvander, Y., Wennqvist, K., & Tuvemo, T. (1992). A longitudinal study on anthropometric and clinical development of Indian children adopted in Sweden: Growth, morbidity, and development during two years after arrival in Sweden. *Uppsala Journal of Medical Sciences, 97,* 93-106.

Raweily, E. A., Gibson, A. A., & Burt, A. D. (1990). Abnormalities of intrahepatic bile ducts in extrahepatic biliary atresia. *Histopathology, 17,* 521-527.

Rescorla, F. J., Grosfeld, J. L., West, K. J., & Vane, D. W. (1989). Changing patterns of treatment and survival in neonates with meconium ileus. *Archives of Surgery, 124,* 837-840.

Rudolph, A. M., & Hoffman, J. I. E. (1982). *Pediatrics*. Norwalk, CT: Appleton-Century-Crofts.

Scheinberg, H. I., & Sternlieb, I. (1984). *Wilson's disease* (pp. 29-30). Philadelphia: Saunders.

Silveira, T. R., Salzano, F. M., Howard, E. R., & Mowat, A. P. (1991). Congenital structural abnormalities in biliary atresia: Evidence for etiopathogenic heterogeneity and therapeutic implications. *Acta Paediatrica Scandinavica, 80,* 1192-1199.

Silverman, A., & Roy, C. C. (1983). *Pediatric clinical gastroenterology* (3rd ed.). St. Louis: Mosby–Year Book.

Skipper, R. P., Boeckman, C. R., & Klein, R. L. (1990). Childhood intussusception. *Surgery, Gynecology, and Obstetrics, 171,* 151-153.

Sterling, C. E., Jolley, G. G., Besser, A. S., & Matteson-Kane, M. (1991). Nursing responsibility in the diagnosis, care, and treatment of the child with gastroesophageal reflux. *Journal of Pediatric Nursing, 6,* 435-441.

Stern, L., & Brodersen, R. (1987). Kernicterus research and the basic sciences: A project for future development. *Pediatrics, 79,* 154-155.

Suslak, L., & Desposito, F. (1988). Infants with cleft lip/palate. *Pediatric Review, 9,* 331-334.

Treem, W. R. (1991). Hepatic failure. In W. A. Walker, P. R. Durie, J. R. Hamilton, J. A. Walker-Smith, & J. B. Watkins (Eds.), *Pediatric gastrointestinal disease*. Philadelphia: B. C. Decker, Inc.

Trier, J. S. (1991). Celiac sprue. *New England Journal of Medicine, 325,* 1709-1719.

Voorhes, A. B., & Price, J. B. (1974). Extra-hepatic portal hypertension: Retrospective analysis of 127 cases and associated clinical implications. *Archives of Surgery, 108,* 138-144.

Walsh, M. C., Kleigman, R. M., & Fanaroff, A. A. (1988). Necrotizing enterocolitis: A practitioner's perspective. *Pediatric Review, 9,* 219-226.

Welch, K. J. (1986). *Pediatric surgery* (4th ed.). Chicago: Year Book Medical Publishers.

Whaley, L. F. & Wong, D. L. (1991). *Nursing care of infants and children* (4th ed.). St. Louis: Mosby–Year Book.

Whitington, P. F. (1985). Portal hypertension in children. *Pediatric Annals, 14,* 494-499.

Widdowson, E. M. (1991). Contemporary human diets and their relation to health and growth: Overview and conclusions. *Philosophical Transactions of the Royal Society of London, 334,* 289-295.

Yu, V. Y., Joseph, R., Bajuk, B., Orgill, A., Astbury, J. (1984). Perinatal risk factors for necrotizing enterocolitis. *Archives of Diseases in Children, 59,* 430-434.

SUGGESTED READING

Bithoney, W. G., Dubowitz, H., & Egan, H. (1992). Failure to thrive—growth deficiency. *Pediatric Review,* 13(12), 453-460.

Goepp, J. G., & Katz, S. A. (1993). Oral rehydration therapy. *American Family Physician,* 47(4), 843-851.

UNIT XIII

The Musculoskeletal System

MUSCULOSKELETAL SYSTEM alterations are among the oldest known conditions. Evidence of bone disease can be found in the earliest skeletal specimens of humans. The femur of Java man evidences a large, benign osteochondroma, a common bone tumor today. Evidence of a healed fracture is present in the ulna of a Neanderthal skeleton. Egyptian mummies from the Fifth Dynasty have been unearthed with fractured limbs bound in splints. Apparently fractures of the forearm and femur were fairly common during that time, probably as a result of constant warfare. Some fractures were healed, others not united, but usually some attempt had been made to immobilize the fracture. By the time Hippocrates (460-370 BC) wrote his books, *On Fractures* and *On Articulations*, the diagnosis and treatment of fractures had reached quite a level of sophistication. Closed fractures were differentially

An orthopedic specialist stands with his hand on the head of a young boy; he gestures to the boy's parents with his other hand; a young girl stands with her parents; a skeleton and general orthopedic devices are hanging on the wall. (Courtesy National Library of Medicine.)

the Ape man, who lived 2 million years ago. Joint disease can be traced further from the Ape man through the Java and Lansing men of 500,000 years ago to Egyptian mummies dating to 8000 BC. The prevalence of chronic joint disease can be traced also through the Roman civilization and is believed to be one of the reasons that Romans built extensive baths throughout their empire.

By far the most important description of muscle fibers was first made by Louis-Antoine Ranvier (1835-1922) more than 100 years ago. In his study of animal muscle fibers, he noted that "when electrically stimulated," red or dark muscle fibers fired less frequently and for longer duration than the rapid firing in white muscle. The fact that muscle fibers are not homogenous and differ on the basis of color has been further refined by modern histochemical techniques.

diagnosed from open fractures, and many types of fracture-dislocations of the clavicle, elbow, and hip were described. Along with bandages and splints, the books contained a carefully prescribed method of traction for reducing fractures. Maintaining a limb in its "natural" (anatomic) position during healing and early mobility after inflammation subsided were well-recognized fundamental principles of treatment. Both of these principles still underlie much of orthopedic treatment today.

The earliest evidence of joint disease (arthritides) is found in a fossil vertebrate (platycarpus) that lived about 100 million years ago. In the primitive species of humans, the earliest evidence of joint disease is found in the spine of

An understanding of the structure and function of normal skeletal muscle has been enhanced by the study of pathologic changes in muscle tissue. In 1861, the French neurologist Guillaume Benjamin Armand Duchenne introduced the skeletal muscle biopsy technique, similar to the technique still in use today. The report of this procedure sparked a lively debate in the nineteenth century press over the morality of studying living *human* tissue! Advances in the muscle and nerve biopsy technique, as well as biochemical electrical study, have immeasurably changed the understanding of skeletal muscle function.

Structure and Function of the Musculoskeletal System

Leona A. Mourad
Katherine Hoare*
Katharine M. Donohoe*

Chapter Outline

*Contributing authors to first edition.

The way an individual functions in daily life, moves about, or manipulates objects physically depends on the integrity of the musculoskeletal system. The musculoskeletal system is actually composed of two systems: (1) the skeleton proper, which is composed of bones and joints, and (2) skeletal mus-cles. Each of the systems contributes to mobility. The skeleton supports the body and provides leverage to the skeletal muscles so that movement of various parts of the body is possible. Movement of the various body parts is accomplished by contraction of the skeletal muscles and bending or rotation at the joints.

STRUCTURE AND FUNCTION OF BONES

Bones give form to the body, support tissues, and permit movement by providing points of attachment for muscles. Many bones meet in movable joints that determine the type and extent of movement possible. Bones also protect many of the body's vital organs. For example, the bones of the skull, thorax, and pelvis are hard exterior shields that protect the brain, heart, lungs, and reproductive and urinary organs.

The marrow cavities within certain bones serve as sites of blood cell formation. In adults, blood cells originate exclusively in the marrow cavities of the skull, vertebrae, ribs, sternum, shoulders, and pelvis. Bones also have a crucial role in mineral homeostasis. They store minerals (i.e., calcium, phosphate, carbonate, magnesium) that are essential for the proper working of many delicate cellular mechanisms throughout the body. Through the action of certain cells within bone, the stored minerals can be mobilized and distributed as needed by the body.

Elements of Bone Tissue

Mature bone is a rigid connective tissue. Like other connective tissues, bone consists of cells, fibers, and a gelatinous material termed **ground substance.** Unlike other connective tissue, however, bone contains large amounts of crystallized minerals, mostly calcium, that give bone its rigidity. The structural elements of bone are summarized in Table 38-1.

Bone cells enable bone to grow, repair itself, and change shape. Even in mature bone, these cells continuously synthesize new bone tissue and resorb (dissolve or digest) old tissue. The fibers in bone are made of collagen, a protein that is synthesized and secreted by certain bone cells. The fibers give bone its tensile strength (the ability to hold itself together). Ground substance acts as a medium for the diffusion of nutrients, oxygen, metabolic wastes, biochemicals, and minerals between bone tissue and blood vessels.

Bone also contains blood vessels and nerves. Bone tissue is nourished by a network of capillaries, and major vessels serve the marrow cavities. The nerves in bone

TABLE 38-1

Structural Elements of Bone

Structural element	Function
Bone cells	
Osteoblasts	Synthesize collagen and proteoglycans; stimulate osteoclast resorptive activity
Osteocytes	Maintain bone matrix
Osteoclasts	Resorb bone; assist with mineral homeostasis
Bone matrix	
Collagen fibers	Lend support and tensile strength
Proteoglycans	Control transport of ionized materials through matrix

Bone morphogenic proteins
  BMP-1
  BMP-2A
  BMP-3
	Induce cartilage formation

Glycoproteins	
Sialoprotein	Promotes calcification
Osteocalcin	Inhibits calcium-phosphate precipitation; promotes bone resorption
Laminin	Stabilizes basement membranes in bones
Osteonectin	Binds calcium in bones
Albumin	Transports essential elements to matrix; maintains osmotic pressure of bone fluid
Alpha-glycoprotein	Promotes calcification
Minerals (elements)	
Calcium	Crystallizes to lend rigidity and compressive strength
Phosphate	Regulates vitamin D and thereby promotes mineralization

send messages to the central nervous system about stresses and pain stimuli that affect bone.

Bone formation begins during fetal life with the growth of cartilage—the precursor of bone tissue. In mature bone the formation of new tissue begins with the production of organic matrix by the bone cells. The organic components of bones' intercellular matrix, or **bone matrix,** consist of ground substances; collagen, which forms the fibers; and other proteins, which have several functions in bone formation and maintenance.

The next step in bone formation is **calcification,** the process of mineral deposition and crystallization. Minerals present in the matrix precipitate within and around the collagen fibers. A tight bond between the crystals and collagen fibers gives tensile and compressional strength (the ability to withstand pressure and weight bearing) to bone.

Bone Cells

Bone contains three types of cells: osteoblasts, osteocytes, and osteoclasts. **Osteoblasts** are the bone-forming cells. Their primary function is to lay down new bone. Once this function is complete, osteoblasts become osteocytes. **Osteocytes** are osteoblasts that have become "imprisoned" within the mineralized bone matrix. They have an ill-defined role in maintaining the inorganic (mineral) and organic elements of bone matrix. **Osteoclasts** function primarily to resorb (remove) bone during processes of growth and repair.

Osteoblast

Osteoblasts are active on the outer surfaces of bones, where they form a single layer of cells. They bring about the formation of new bone by their synthesis of **osteoid** (nonmineralized bone matrix). Stimulation of bone formation has been demonstrated by a direct effect of fluoride ions on osteoblasts to attract osteoblast precursors to the resorption defect in the bone (Mundy, 1991). The mechanism of osteoblast stimulation is reported to be the production of so-called coupling factors generated during the resorption process. Osteoblasts bring about the formation of new bone and the orderly mineralization of bone matrix by concentrating some of the plasma proteins found in the bone matrix and by facilitating the deposit and exchange of calcium and other ions at the site. As new bone is formed, it is shaped and remodeled through the effects of transforming growth factor-β (TGF-β), as well as other plasma proteins found in the bone marrow (Table 38-2).

The concept of coupling bone formation with bone resorption has been extensively studied, yet is still not entirely clear. Recent studies have shown that osteoblasts are responsive to and have receptors for parathyroid hormone (PTH), which stimulates osteoblasts to release a factor that induces osteoclastic activity by stimulating osteoblasts to remove nonmineralized organic material from native bone surfaces, exposing resorption-inducing bone mineral to osteoclastic contact. In contact with bone mineral, osteoclasts can be

TABLE 38-2

Effects of Selected Cytokines (Growth Factors) on Skeletal Tissues

Cytokine (growth factor)	Target tissue	Formation	Resorption
Transforming growth factor-β	Bone	+, −	+, −
	Cartilage	+, −	−
Transforming growth factor-α or epidermal growth factor	Bone	+, −	+
	Cartilage	+	
Insulin-like growth factor	Bone	−	0
	Cartilage	−	?
Fibroblast growth factor	Bone	+, −	0
	Cartilage		?
Colony-stimulating factors	Bone	0	+
	Cartilage	?	?
Interferon-γ	Bone	−	−
	Cartilage	−	?
Tumor necrosis factor	Bone	−	+
	Cartilage	−	+
Interleukin-1	Bone	+, −	+
	Cartilage	−	+

Modified from Goldring, M. B., & Goldring, S. R. (1990). Skeletal tissue response to cytokines. *Clinical Orthopaedics, 258*(9), 245-263.

further stimulated by colony-stimulating factor and interleukins 1, 3, and 6 produced by macrophage cells in the presence of PTH (Russell, 1992). Thus, the cells of the osteoblastic lineage (osteoblasts and osteocytes) form a network of cells in bone that seems to sense the shape and structure of bone and to determine where it is appropriate that bone be formed or resorbed, according to Wolfe's law (bone is shaped according to its function).

Osteoblasts have two states, an active state and a resting state. When active, osteoblasts synthesize and secrete osteoid. When in the resting state, they appear dormant. If appropriately stimulated, however, the resting osteoblasts are capable of resuming activity.

Osteocyte

An osteocyte is an osteoblast that is trapped or surrounded in osteoid as it hardens from minerals that enter during calcification. The osteocyte is within a space in the hardened bone matrix called a **lacuna.** Each osteocyte has a thin layer of nonmineralized osteoid around it, like the egg white surrounding an egg yolk.

The function of osteocytes is still somewhat unclear, but they are thought to participate in the maintenance of bone matrix by helping to concentrate nutrients in the matrix. Osteocytes obtained from nutrients from capillaries in the canaliculi contain nutrient-rich fluids. Osteocytes also may help synthesize and replace needed elements of the matrix, thus helping maintain mineral homeostasis with the help of the parathyroid hormone and osteoblast cells. Through exchanges between these cells, hormone catalyst, and minerals, optimal levels of calcium, phosphorus, and other minerals are maintained in blood plasma. The osteocyte also aids in modifying bone matrix through release of enzymes to dissolve the mineralized walls of the lacunae to prepare the bone for remodeling. Remodeling is described on p. 1410.

Osteoclast

The osteoclast is a large, multinucleated cell with a short life span. Osteoclasts develop from the hematopoietic stem cell in the bone marrow stroma (Beresford, 1989) and adjacent vessels and from mononuclear phagocytic cells. Osteoclasts contain lysosomes (digestive vacuoles) filled with hydrolytic enzymes. Fine projections, or microvilli, fan out from the osteoclast cell's surface, terminating in the area of bone being resorbed, referred to as the "ruffled border" (Mundy, 1991). Osteoclasts are found in shallow, self-made excavations known as Howship's lacunae on the undersurfaces of bones, where their electropositive action contrasts with the electronegative action of the osteoblasts (Einhorn, 1991). Electropositivity occurs on the convex surface and electronegativity on the concave surface (Bucholz, 1991).

The function of osteoclasts is to resorb bone. Presumably, osteoclasts secrete citric and lactic acids, which help dissolve bone minerals, and collagenase, which aids in digesting collagen, along with the action of cytokines, to bring about bone resorption (Table 38-2). Osteoblasts also aid in bone resorption. Once resorption is completed, the osteoclast disappears from degeneration either by reversing to its parent cell or through cell mobility from the site.

Bone Matrix

Bone matrix is made of the extracellular elements of bone tissue, composed of about 35% organic and 65% inorganic materials (Seeley, Stephens, & Tate, 1990). The major organic components are collagen fibers, and the major inorganic components are the calcium and phosphate minerals. Other parts of the bone matrix are the proteins, carbohydrate-protein complexes, and ground substances.

Collagen fibers

Collagen fibers make up the major organic component of bone matrix. The fibers are made of type I collagen synthesized and secreted by osteoblasts. Once secreted, the collagen molecules assemble into thin chains called alpha chains, which combine in threes to form **fibrils.** The fibrils form a staggered pattern, overlapping nearby fibrils by approximately one fourth their length. This staggered, overlapping pattern creates regular gaps into which mineral crystals are deposited. After mineral deposition, the fibrils link together and twist to form rope-like fibers. Collagen fibers then join to form a framework that gives bone its tensile strength and enables it to bear weight.

Proteoglycans

Proteoglycans are large complexes of numerous polysaccharides attached to a common protein core. They strengthen bone by forming compression-resistant networks between the collagen fibrils. Proteoglycans also control the transport and distribution of electrically charged particles (ions), particularly calcium, through the bone matrix, thereby playing a role in bone calcium deposition and calcification.

Glycoproteins

Glycoproteins are also carbohydrate-protein complexes of bone. Glycoproteins control the collagen interactions that lead to fibril formation. They also may play a role in calcification.

Some of the glycoproteins in bone matrix include bone sialoprotein, osteocalcin, osteonectin, laminin, albumin, and alpha-glycoprotein. Other proteins recently found in bone matrix are the compounds currently called **bone morphogenic proteins (BMPs)** (Table 38-1).

| TABLE 38-3 |

Sequence of Calcium and Phosphate Compound Formation and Crystallization

Formula	Name	Abbreviation
$Ca(HPO_4) \cdot 2 H_2O$	Dicalcium phosphate dihydrate	DCPD
$Ca_4H(PO_4)_3$	Octacalcium phosphate	OCP
$Ca_9(PO_4)_6$ (var.)	Amorphous calcium phosphate	ACP
$Ca_3(PO_4)_2$	Tricalcium phosphate	TCP
$Ca_5(PO_4)_3OH$	Hydroxyapatite	HAP

NOTE: Compounds are listed in the order in which precipitation and crystal formation occur.

Sialoprotein, also known as osteopontin, makes up about 8% of the noncollagenous matrix of bone, and its function is to enhance cell attachment (Bonewald & Mundy, 1990).

Osteocalcin is also a calcium-binding protein that binds preferentially to calcium that has already crystallized. The roles of osteocalcin may be to inhibit calcium phosphate precipitation and play a part in bone resorption by recruiting osteoclasts.

Osteonectin is also thought to bind calcium in bones, and **laminin** stabilizes basement membranes in bones. It is the most abundant bone matrix protein in humans (Boskey, 1990).

Bone albumin is identical to serum albumin (see Chapter 22). In calcified matrix, bone albumin is permanently fixed to bone mineral crystals and remains so until the bone is resorbed. Researchers believe bone albumin transports essential elements such as hormones, ions, and other metabolites to and from the bone cells and maintains the osmotic pressure of **bone fluid** (fluid surrounding mineral crystals and osteoblasts).

Alpha-glycoprotein is thought to be synthesized in the liver, to be released into blood plasma, and to circulate to bone matrix, where it accumulates. Alpha-glycoprotein's affinity for calcium is 40 times greater than that of albumin. Therefore, it probably plays an important role in the calcification of growing bone. Alpha-glycoprotein also may facilitate bone resorption by activating osteoclasts.

Bone Minerals

Mineralization is the final step in bone formation, after collagen synthesis and fiber formation. During mineral-ization, some unknown mechanism triggers calcium and phosphate precipitation and subsequent crystallization.

Table 38-3 lists the sequence in which calcium and phosphate form amorphous (fluid) calcium phosphate compounds that are converted, in stages, to solid hexagonal crystals of **hydroxyapatite** (**HAP**). As the calcium and phosphorus concentrations increase in the bone matrix, the first precipitate to form is dicalcium phosphate dihydrate (DCPD). Once DCPD precipitation begins, the remaining phases of bone crystal formation proceed until insoluble HAP is produced with approximately 80% to 90% of the HAP incorporated into the collagen fibers. Amorphous calcium phosphate is distributed throughout the bone matrix.

Types of Bone Tissue

Bone is made up of two types of bony (osseous) tissue: **compact bone** (cortical bone) and **spongy bone** (cancellous bone) (Fig. 38-1). Both types of bone tissue contain the same structural elements and, with a few exceptions, both compact and spongy tissue are present in every bone. The major difference between the two types of tissue is the organization of the elements.

Compact bone is highly organized, solid, and extremely strong. The basic structural unit in compact bone is the **haversian system** (Fig. 38-2). Each haversian system is made up of the following:

1. A central canal called the **haversian canal**
2. Concentric layers of bone matrix called **lamellae**
3. Tiny spaces (lacunae) between the lamellae
4. Bone cells (osteocytes) within the lacunae
5. Small channels or canals called **canaliculi**

Each haversian system is a separate cylindrical entity that looks like a set of concentric rings. In the center of the haversian system is the haversian canal. The haversian canal runs through the long axis of bone and contains one or two blood vessels and nerve fibers. The blood vessels in the canal communicate with blood vessels in the periosteum (surface cover) and marrow cavity to transport nutrients and wastes to and from the osteocytes contained within the lacunae. Surrounding each haversian canal are the concentric lamellae. Between the lamellae are the lacunae, each of which contains one osteocyte. The lacunae are connected to each other and to the haversian canal by the canaliculi, which run parallel to the horizontal axis of the bone. Each canaliculus encloses a small extension (cytoplasmic process) from the osteocyte contained in the lacuna.

Spongy bone is less complex and lacks haversian systems. In spongy bone the lamellae are not arranged in concentric layers but in plates or bars termed **trabeculae** that branch and unite with one another to form an irregular meshwork. The pattern of the meshwork is determined by the direction of stress on the particular bone. The spaces between the trabeculae are filled with red bone marrow. The osteocyte-containing lacunae are distributed between the trabeculae and interconnected by canaliculi. Capillaries pass through the marrow to nourish the osteocytes.

All bones are covered with a double-layered connective tissue called the **periosteum.** The outer layer of the periosteum contains blood vessels and nerves, some of which penetrate to the inner structures of the bone through channels called Volkmann's canals (Fig. 38-2). The inner layer of the periosteum is anchored to the bone by collagenous fibers (Sharpey's fibers) that penetrate the bone. Sharpey's fibers also help hold or attach tendons and ligaments to the periosteum of bones (Seeley et al., 1990).

Characteristics of Bone

The human skeleton consists of 206 bones, which constitute the axial skeleton and the appendicular skeleton (Fig. 38-3). The **axial skeleton** consists of 80 bones that make up the skull, vertebral column, and thorax. The **appendicular skeleton** consists of 126 bones that make up the upper and lower extremities, the shoulder girdle (pectoral girdle), and the pelvic girdle. The skeleton contributes about 14% of the weight of the adult body.

Bones can be classified by shape as long, flat, short (cuboidal), or irregular. **Long bones** are longer than they are wide and consist of a narrow tubular midportion

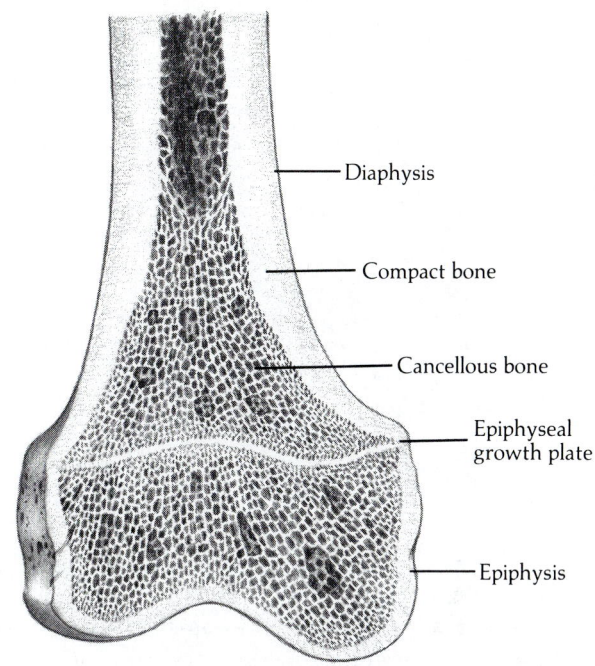

FIG. 38-1 Cross section of bone. Bone showing relationships of compact and cancellous bone, epiphysis, epiphyseal plate, and diaphysis. (From Thompson, McFarland, Hirsch, & Tucker, 1993.)

FIG. 38-2 Structure of bone. (**1**) Three-dimensional view of compact bone; (**2**) transverse section of compact bone depicting lamellae, lacunae, and canaliculi; (**3**) longitudinal section of bone with lacunae and canaliculi; (**4**) lacunae occupied by osteocyte. (From Thompson, McFarland, Hirsch, & Tucker, 1993.)

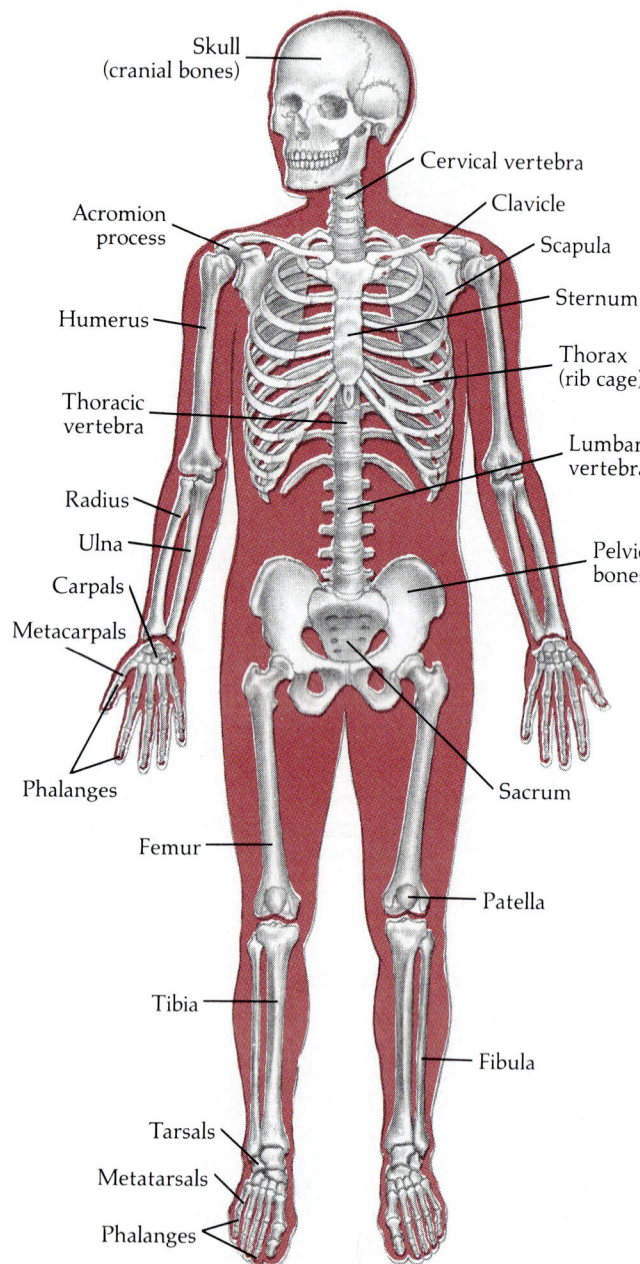

Skull
(cranial bones)

Cervical vertebra

Acromion
process

Clavicle

Scapula

Sternum

Humerus

Thorax
(rib cage)

Thoracic
vertebra

Lumbar
vertebra

Radius

Ulna

Carpals

Pelvic
bones

Metacarpals

Phalanges

Sacrum

Femur

Patella

Tibia

Fibula

Tarsals

Metatarsals

Phalanges

FIG. 38-3 **Axial and appendicular skeleton.** (From Thompson, McFarland, Hirsch, & Tucker, 1993.) See text for explanation.

(**diaphysis**) that merges into a broader neck (**metaphysis**) and a broad end (**epiphysis**) (Fig. 38-1).

The diaphysis consists of a shaft of thick, rigid compact bone that is able to tolerate bending forces. Contained within the diaphysis is the elongated marrow (medullary) cavity. The marrow cavity of the diaphysis contains primarily fatty tissue, which is referred to as yellow marrow. The yellow marrow assists red bone marrow in hematopoiesis only during times of stress.

The yellow marrow cavity of the diaphysis is continuous with marrow cavities in the spongy bone of the metaphysis and diaphysis. The marrow contained within the epiphysis is red because it contains primarily blood-forming tissue (see Chapter 22). A layer of connective tissue, **endosteum,** lines the outer surfaces of both types of marrow cavity.

The broadness of the epiphysis allows weight bearing to be distributed over a wide area. The epiphysis is made up of spongy bone covered by a very thin layer of compact bone. In a child, the epiphysis is separated from the metaphysis by a cartilaginous **growth plate,** the **epiphyseal plate.** After puberty, the epiphyseal plate calcifies and the epiphysis and metaphysis merge. By adulthood, the line of demarcation between the epiphysis and metaphysis is undetectable.

In **flat bones,** such as the ribs or scapulae, two plates of compact bone are roughly parallel to each other. Between the compact bone plates is a layer of spongy bone. **Short bones (cuboidal bones),** such as the bones of the wrist or ankle, are often cuboidal in shape. They consist of spongy bone covered by a thin layer of compact bone.

Irregular bones, such as the vertebrae, mandibles, or other facial bones, have various shapes that include thin and thick segments. The thin part of an irregular bone consists of two plates of compact bone with spongy bone in between. The thick part consists of spongy bone surrounded by a layer of compact bone.

Maintenance of Bone Integrity
Remodeling

The internal structure of bone is maintained by **remodeling,** a three-phase process in which existing bone is resorbed and new bone is laid down to replace it. Remodeling is carried out by clusters of bone cells termed **basic multicellular units.** The basic multicellular units are made up of bone precursor cells that differentiate into osteoclasts and osteoblasts. Precursor cells are located on the free surfaces of bones and along the vascular channels (especially the marrow cavities).

In phase 1 of the remodeling cycle, a stimulus (e.g., hormone, drug, vitamin, physical stressor) activates the bone cell precursors in a localized area of bone to osteoclasts. In phase 2, the osteoclasts form a "cutting cone," which gradually resorbs bone, leaving behind an elongated cavity termed a resorption cavity. The resorption cavity in compact bone follows the longitudinal axis of the haversian system, whereas the resorption cavity in spongy bone parallels the surface of the trabeculae.

Phase 3 is the laying down of new bone, termed secondary bone, by osteoblasts lining the walls of the resorption cavity. The osteoblasts lay down new bone. Successive layers (lamellae) in compact bone are laid

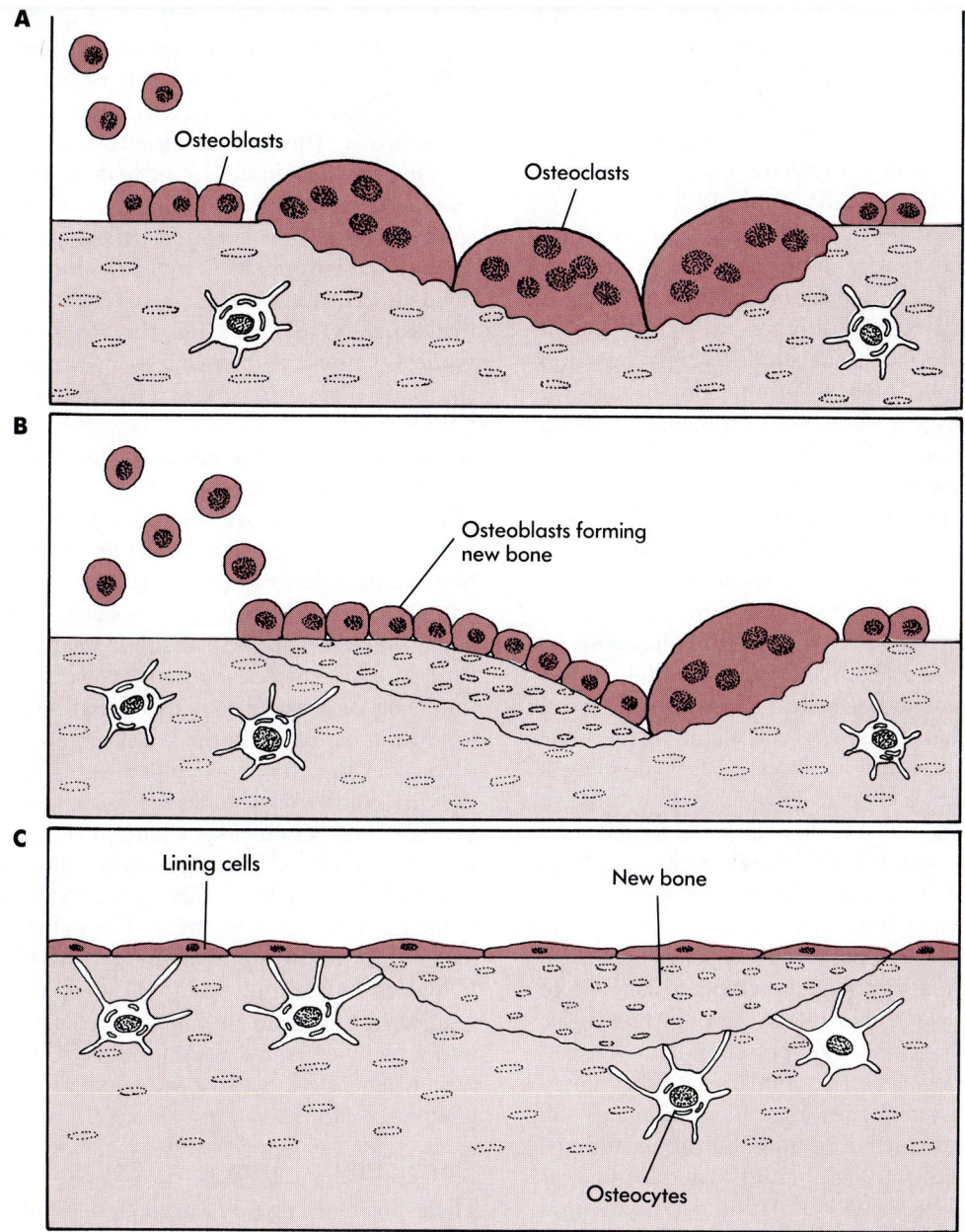

FIG. 38-4 Bone remodeling. In the remodeling sequence, bone sections are removed by the bone-resorbing cells, osteoclasts, and replaced with a new one laid down by bone-forming cells, osteoblasts. The cells work in response to signals generated in that environment. The first phase of remodeling is mediated only by the multinucleated osteoclastic cells. They are activated, scoop out bone, **A**, and resorb it; then the work of the osteoblasts begins, **B**. They form new bone that replaces bone removed by the resorption process, **C**. The sequence takes 4 to 5 months. (From Mundy, 1991; used with permission.)

down, until the resorption cavity is reduced to a narrow haversian canal around a blood vessel. In this way, old haversian systems are destroyed and new haversian systems are formed. New trabeculae are formed in spongy bone. The entire process of remodeling takes about 4 months.

Repair

The remodeling process can repair microscopic bone injuries, but gross injuries, such as fractures and surgical wounds (osteotomies), heal by the same stages as soft tissue injuries, except that new bone, instead of scar tissue, is the final result (see Chapter 7). In bone the stages of wound healing are as follows.

1. Hematoma formation. This occurs if vessels have been damaged, causing hemorrhage. Fibrin and platelets within the hematoma form a meshwork, which is the initial framework for healing, with the help of hematopoietic growth factors such as platelet-derived growth factor and transforming growth factor-β (TGF-β) (Table 38-2).
2. Procallus formation. Fibroblasts, capillary buds, and osteoblasts move into the wound to produce granulation tissue called **procallus**. Cartilage is formed as a precursor of bone. Types I, II, and III collagen are formed (Einhorn, 1991). Enzymes and growth factors, such as insulin and insulin-like growth factors, plus bone morphogenic protein and osteogenin, aid in this stage of healing.
3. Callus formation. Osteoblasts in the procallus form membranous or **woven bone** (callus). Enzymes increase the phosphate content and permit the phosphate to join with calcium to be deposited as mineral to harden the callus.
4. Osteoblasts continue to replace the callus with lamellar bone or trabecular bone (Fig. 38-4).
5. The periosteal and endosteal surfaces of the bone are remodeled to the size and shape of the bone before injury. Synthesis of other types of collagen recedes in favor of type I, which is the collagen found in bone. This final stage of healing, or remodeling, is vital because bone that has not been remodeled does not have good mechanical properties for weight bearing and mobility.

The speed with which bone heals depends on the severity of the bone disruption; the type and amount of bone tissue that needs to be replaced (spongy bone heals faster); blood supply to the site; presence of growth and thyroid hormones, insulin, vitamins, and other nutrients; presence of systemic disease; effects of aging; and effective treatment, including immobilization and the prevention of complications such as infection. In general, however, hematoma formation occurs within hours of fracture or surgery; formation of procallus by osteoblasts within days; callus formation within weeks; and replacement and contour modeling within years—up to 4 years in some cases.

STRUCTURE AND FUNCTION OF JOINTS

The site where two or more bones are attached is called a **joint,** or **articulation.** The primary function of joints is to provide stability and mobility to the skeleton. Whether a joint provides stability or mobility depends on its location and its structure. Generally, joints that stabilize the skeleton have a simpler structure than those that enable the skeleton to move. Most joints provide both stability and mobility to some degree (Fig. 38-5).

Joints are classified based on the degree of movement they permit or on the connecting tissues that hold them together. Based on movement, a joint is classified as a **synarthrosis (immovable joint),** an **amphiarthrosis (slightly movable joint),** or a **diarthrosis (freely movable joint).** On the basis of connective structures, joints are classified broadly as fibrous, cartilaginous, and synovial. Each of these three structural classifications can be subdivided according to the shape and contour of the articulating surfaces (ends) of the bones and the type of motion the joint permits.

Fibrous Joints

A joint in which bone is united directly to bone by fibrous connective tissue is called a **fibrous joint.** Generally, fibrous joints are synarthroses (immovable), but many fibrous joints allow some movement. The degree of movement depends on the distance between the bones and the flexibility of the fibrous connective tissue.

Fibrous joints are further subdivided into three types: sutures, syndesmoses, and gomphoses. A **suture** has a thin layer of dense fibrous tissue that binds together interlocking flat bones in the skulls of young children. Sutures form an extremely tight union that permits no motion. By adulthood, the fibrous tissue has been replaced by bone. A **syndesmosis** is a joint in which the two bony surfaces are united by a ligament or membrane. The fibers of ligaments are flexible and stretch, permitting a limited amount of movement. The paired bones of the lower arm (radius and ulna) and the lower leg (tibia and fibula) are syndesmotic joints. A **gomphosis** is a special type of fibrous joint in which a conical projection fits into a complementary socket and is held there by a ligament. The teeth held in the maxilla or mandible are gomphosis joints.

Cartilaginous Joints

There are two types of cartilaginous joints—symphyses and synchondroses. A **symphysis** is a cartilaginous joint in which bones are united by a pad or disk of fibrocartilage. The articulating surfaces of the two bones are usually covered by a thin layer of hyaline cartilage, and the thick pad of fibrocartilage acts as a shock absorber and stabilizer. Examples of symphyses are the symphysis pubis, which joins the two pubic bones, and the intervertebral disks, which join the bodies of the vertebrae. A **synchondrosis** is a joint in which hyaline cartilage, rather than fibrocartilage, connects the two bones. The joints between the ribs and the sternum are synchondroses. The hyaline cartilage of these joints is called costal cartilage (Fig. 38-5). Slight movement at the synchondroses between the ribs and the sternum allows the chest to move outward and upward during breathing.

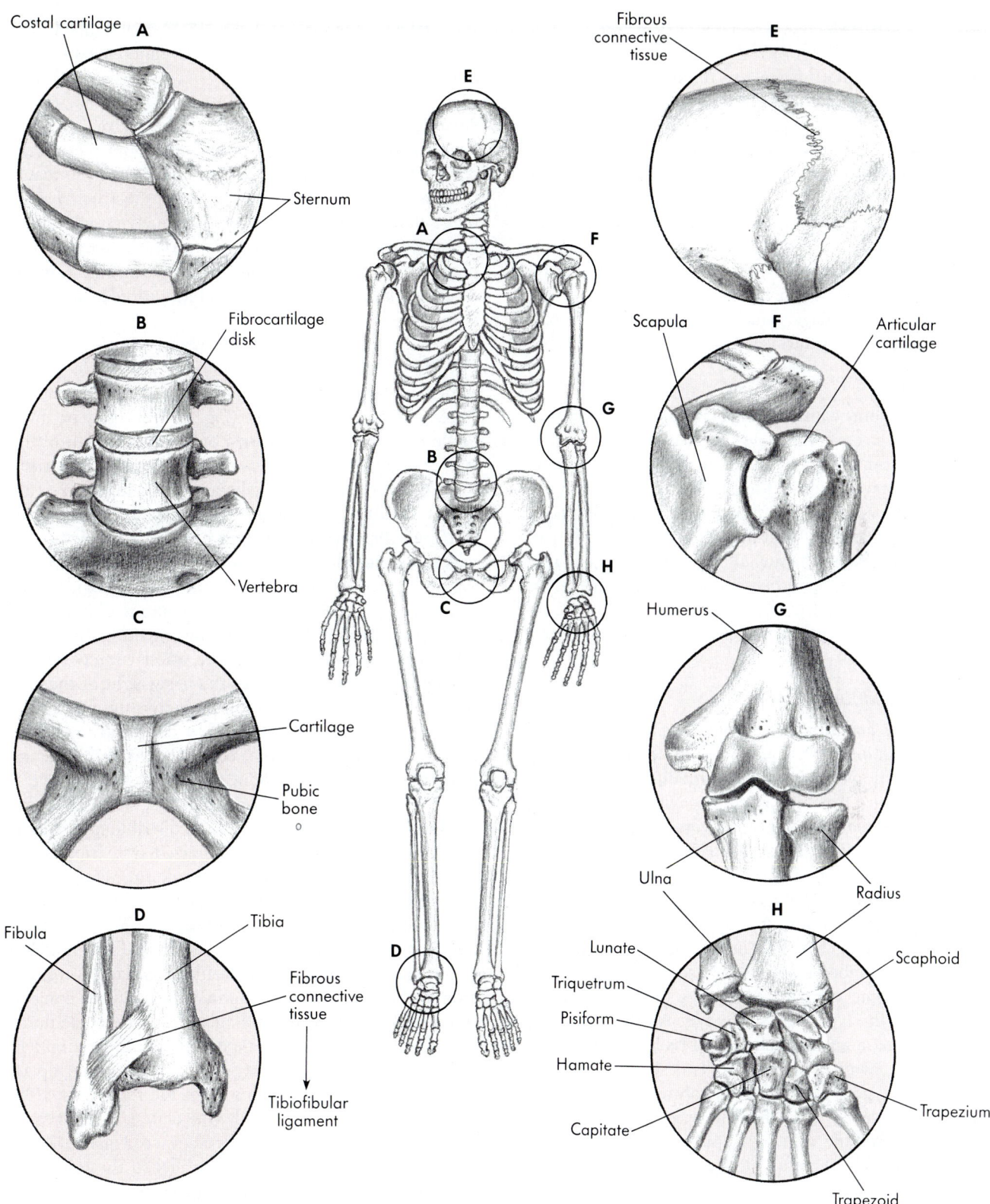

FIG. 38-5 Types of joints. Cartilaginous (amphiarthrodial) joints, which are slightly movable, include (**A**) a synchondrosis that attaches ribs to costal cartilage, (**B**) a symphysis that connects vertebrae, and (**C**) the symphysis that connects the two pubic bones. Fibrous (synarthrodial) joints, which are immovable, include (**D**) the syndesmosis between the tibia and fibula, (**E**) sutures that connect the skull bones, and the gomphosis (not shown), which holds teeth in their sockets. The synovial joints include (**F**) the spheroid type at the shoulder, (**G**) the hinge type at the elbow, and (**H**) the gliding joints of the hand.

Synovial Joints
Structure of Synovial Joints

Synovial joints (diarthroses) are the most movable and the most complex joints in the body (Fig. 38-6). A synovial joint consists of:

1. A fibrous joint capsule (articular capsule)
2. A synovial membrane that lines the inner surface of the joint capsule
3. A joint cavity (synovial cavity), a space formed by the capsule
4. Synovial fluid, which fills the joint cavity and lubricates the joint surface
5. Articular cartilage, which covers and pads the articulating bony surfaces

Joint capsule

The fibrous **joint capsule (articular capsule)** is connective tissue that covers the ends of the bones where they meet in the joint. Sharpey's fibers firmly attach the proximal and distal capsule to the periosteum and ligaments and tendons, which also reinforce the capsule. The joint capsule is made up of parallel, interlacing bundles of dense, white fibrous tissue. It is richly supplied with nerves, blood vessels, and lymphatic vessels. The nerves in and around the joint capsule are sensitive to the rate and direction of motion, compression, tension, vibration, and pain.

Synovial membrane

The **synovial membrane (synovium)** is the smooth, delicate inner lining of the joint capsule. It lines the nonarticular portion of the synovial joint and any ligaments or tendons that traverse the joint cavity. The synovial membrane is made up of two layers, a vascular layer called the **subintima** and a thin cellular layer called the **intima**. The vascular subintima merges with the fibrous joint capsule and is composed of loose fibrous connective tissue, elastin fibers, fat cells, fibroblasts, macrophages, and mast cells. The intima consists of rows of synovial cells embedded in a fiber-free intercellular matrix. The intima contains two types of synovial cells, type A cells and type B cells. The **type A cells** ingest and remove bacteria and particles of debris by phagocytosis in the joint cavity. (Phagocytosis is described in Chapter 7.) The **type B cells** secrete **hyaluronate,** a binding agent that gives synovial fluid its viscous quality. The synovial membrane is richly supplied with blood and lymphatic vessels; therefore, it is capable of rapid repair and regeneration.

Joint cavity

The **joint cavity (synovial cavity)** is an enclosed, fluid-filled space between the articulating surfaces of the two bones. This small cavity, often called the **joint space,** enables the two bones to move "against" one another. The synovial cavity is surrounded by the synovial membrane and filled with a clear, viscous, slick fluid called the synovial fluid.

Synovial fluid

Synovial fluid is superfiltrated plasma from blood vessels in the synovial membrane. Synovial fluid lubricates the joint surfaces, nourishes the pad of the articular cartilage that covers the ends of the bones, and contains free-floating synovial cells and various leukocytes that phagocytose joint debris and microorganisms. Loss of synovial fluid leads to rapid deterioration of articular cartilage.

Articular cartilage

Articular cartilage is a layer of hyaline cartilage that covers the end of each bone (Fig. 38-7). It may be thick or thin, depending on the size of the joint, the fit of the two bone ends, and the amount of weight and shearing force the joint normally withstands. The function of articular cartilage is to reduce friction in the joint and to distribute the forces of weight bearing. Articular cartilage is composed of **chondrocytes** (cartilage cells) (making up about 2% of the tissue) and an intercellular matrix made up of collagen (making up about 10% to 30% of weight), protein polysaccharides (making up 5% to 10% of weight), and water. The water content ranges from 60% to almost 80% of the net weight of the cartilage, and individual molecules rapidly enter or exit the articular cartilage to contribute to the resiliency of the tissue (Kuettner, Aydelotte, & Thonar, 1991). The intercellular matrix is produced by the chondrocytes, which synthesize and extrude collagen, which, like the collagen produced by bone cells, is distributed throughout the cartilage in a highly organized system of fibers. Collagen fibers in cartilage are made up of many fine fibrils that, like bone fibrils, are assembled in an orderly fashion that makes them resistant to physical, metabolic, or chemical breakdown. The main differences between bone collagen and cartilage collagen are the amino acid content of the alpha chains and the composition of the fibrils. Bone collagen fibrils are made up of two type I chains and one type II chain. Approximately 90% of the cartilage collagen fibrils are made up of three identical type II chains, with the remaining 10% made up of types VI, IX, and XI (Kuettner et al., 1991).

At the surface of articular cartilage (see Figs. 38-7 and 38-8), the collagen fibers run parallel to the joint surface and are closely compacted into a dense, protective mat called the reserve zone (Iannotti, 1990). (Loss of this dense, compacted configuration at the surface subjects the underlying fibers to splitting and thinning, in which case the cartilage is unable to tolerate weight bearing.) In the middle layer (the proliferative zone) of the cartilage, the fibers are arranged tangential to the

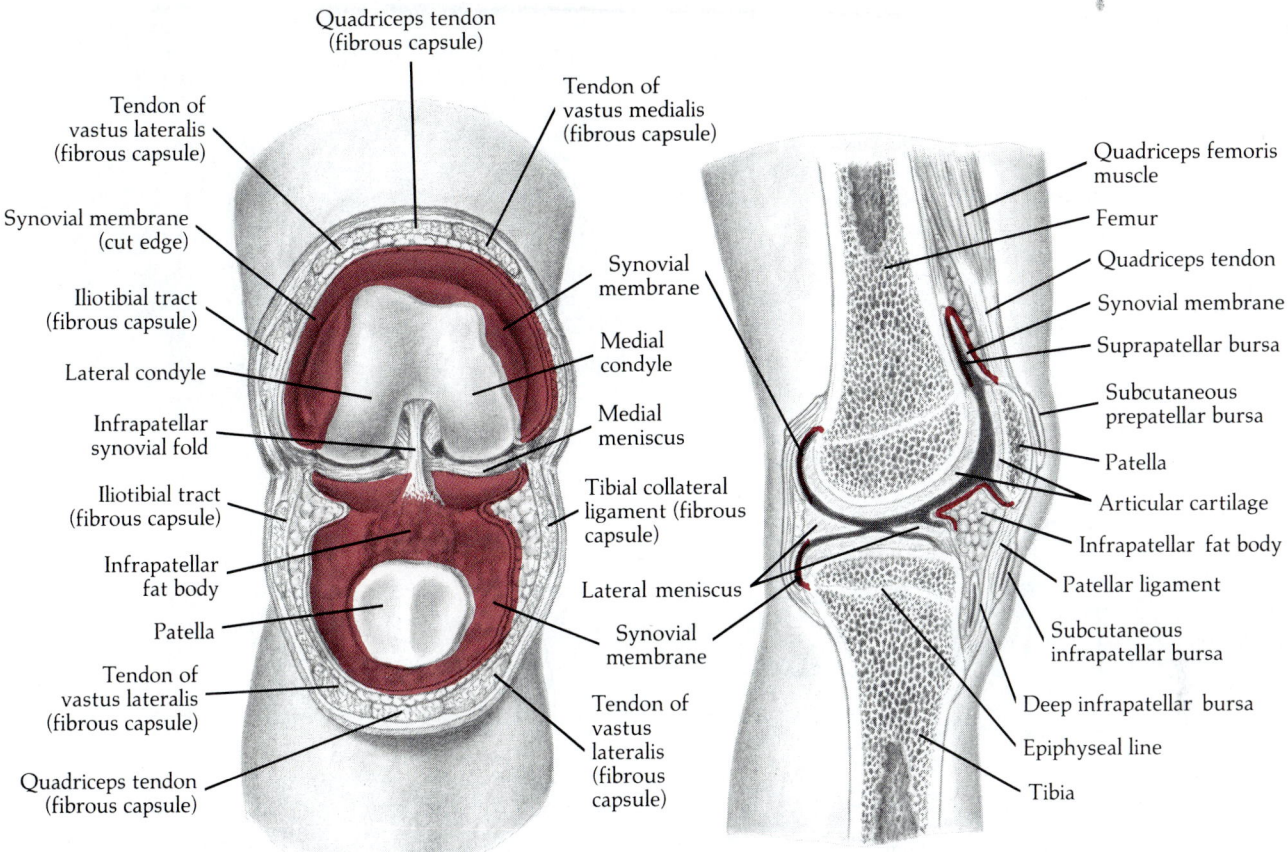

FIG. 38-6 Knee joint (synovial joint). (From Thompson, McFarland, Hirsch, & Tucker, 1993.)

FIG. 38-7 Organization of collagen fibers in articular cartilage.

FIG. 38-8 **Collagen fibers.** Each fiber is composed of many collagen strands. (From Mourad, 1991.)

Uniaxial (elbow)

Biaxial (finger)

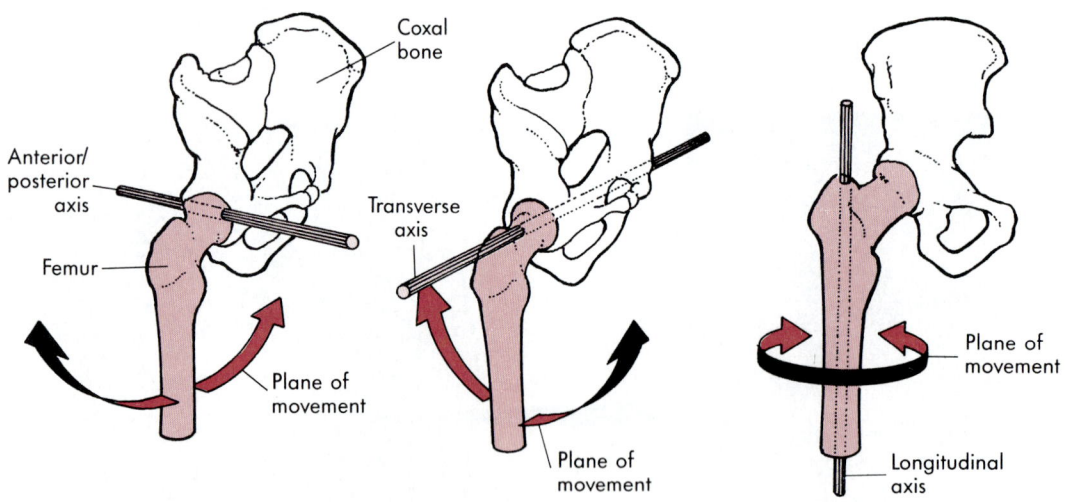

Multiaxial (hip)

FIG. 38-9 Movements of synovial (diarthrodial) joints.

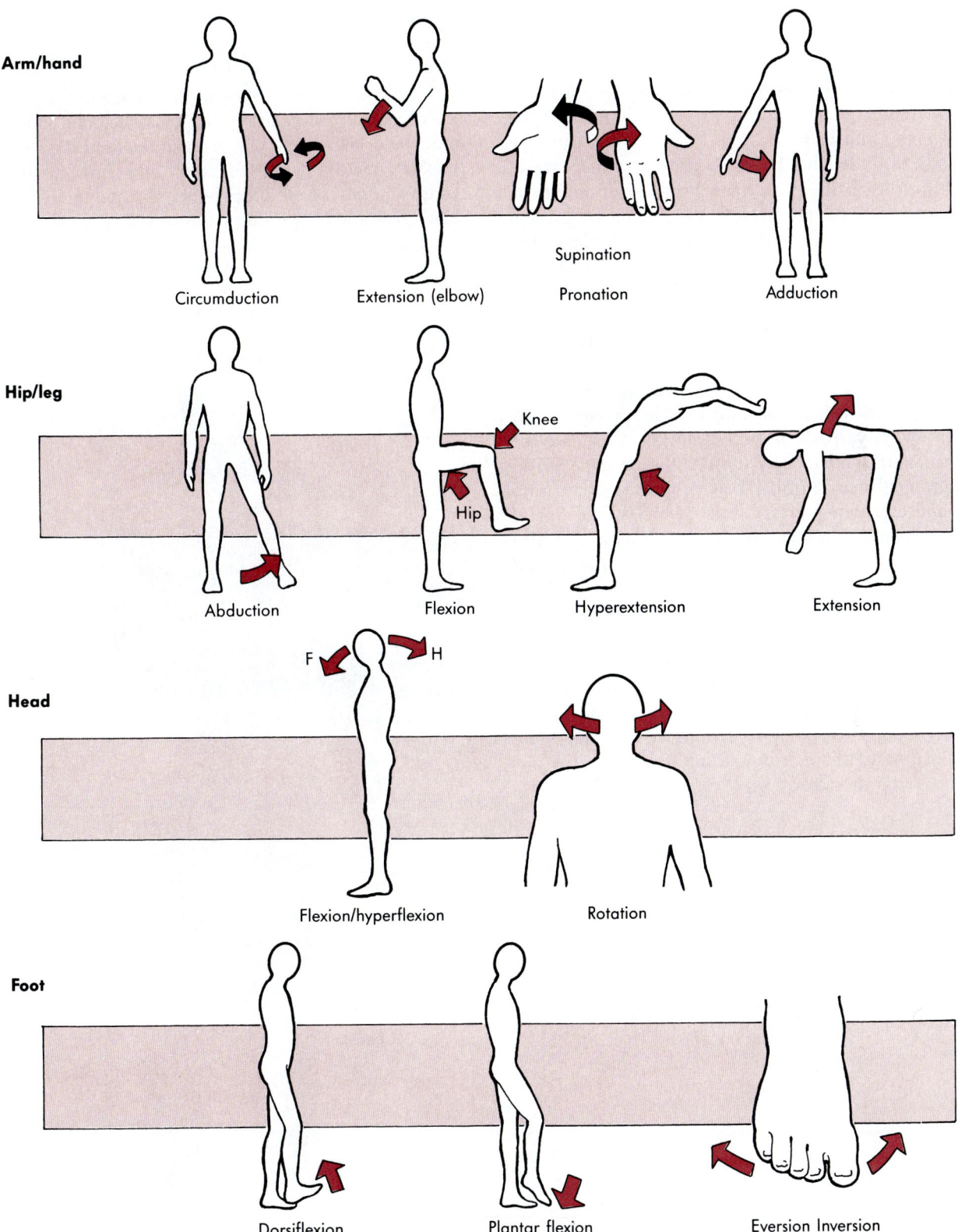

FIG. 38-10 Body movements provided by synovial (diarthrodial) joints.

surface, which allows them to deform and absorb some of the force of weight bearing. In the bottom layer (the hypertrophic zone) of the cartilage, the fibers are perpendicular to the joint surface, allowing them to resist shear forces, and are embedded in a calcified layer of cartilage called the **tidemark**. The tidemark anchors the collagen fibers to the underlying (subchondral) bone. Collagen fibers are important components of the cartilage matrix, accounting for approximately 60% of the dry weight, and because they (1) anchor the cartilage securely to underlying bone, (2) provide a taut framework for the cartilage, (3) control the loss of fluid from the cartilage, and (4) prevent the escape of protein polysaccharides (proteoglycans) from the cartilage. The proteoglycans are macromolecules consisting of proteins, carbohydrates (**glycosaminoglycans**), and hyaluronic acid. The glycosaminoglycans (keratan sulfate and chondroitin sulfate) are attached to the **protein core**, and several protein cores (with their attached glycosaminoglycans) are bound to a hyaluronic acid chain by a special protein called **link protein**. The proteoglycans give articular cartilage its stiff quality and regulate the movement of synovial fluid through the cartilage. Without proteoglycans, normal weight bearing would rapidly and completely press all the synovial fluid out of the cartilage. The proteoglycans act as a pump, permitting enough fluid to be pressed out to ensure that a fluid film is always present on the surface of the cartilage, even after hours of weight bearing. The pumping action of proteoglycans also draws synovial fluid back into the cartilage after a weight-bearing load is released. Mobility and weight bearing are necessary for the pumping action of proteoglycans to occur. Nonuse of a joint quickly reduces the pumping action, which changes the composition of the matrix and interferes with the nutrition of the chondrocytes.

FIG. 38-11 **Skeletal muscles of body. A,** Anterior view. **B,** Posterior view. (From Thompson, McFarland, Hirsch, & Tucker, 1993.)

Articular cartilage has no blood vessels, lymph vessels, or nerves. Therefore it is insensitive to pain and regenerates slowly and minimally after injury. Regeneration occurs primarily at sites where the articular cartilage meets the synovial membrane.

Movement of Synovial Joints

Synovial joints are described as uniaxial, biaxial, or multiaxial according to the shapes of the bone ends and the type of movement occurring at the joint (Fig. 38-9). Usually, one of the bones is stable and serves as an axis for the motion of the other bone. The body movements made possible by various synovial joints are either circular or angular (Fig. 38-10).

A

Trapezius
Deltoid
Serratus anterior
Internal oblique
External oblique
Transversus abdominis
Tensor of fascia lata
Sartorius
Adductor magnus
Iliotibial tract
Vastus lateralis
Tendon of rectus femoris
Patella
Peroneus longus
Tibialis anterior
Extensor digitorum longus

Sternocleidomastoid
Pectoralis major
Biceps brachii
Rectus abdominis
Brachioradialis
Flexor carpi radialis
Iliopsoas
Pectineus
Adductor longus
Gracilis
Rectus femoris
Vastus lateralis
Patellar ligament
Gastrocnemius
Soleus

STRUCTURE AND FUNCTION OF SKELETAL MUSCLES

The skeletal muscles are made up of millions of individual fibers that, by the process of contraction and relaxation, do the work necessary to complete movements as varied as a ballerina's pirouette or an artist's deft stroke (Fig. 38-11). Muscle constitutes 40% of adults' body weight and 50% of children's. Muscle is 75% water, 20% protein, and 5% organic and inorganic compounds. Thirty-two percent of all protein stores for energy and metabolism are contained in muscle.

Whole Muscle

There are more than 350 named muscles; almost all are paired. The body's muscles vary dramatically in size and shape. They range from 2 to 60 cm in length and are shaped according to function. **Fusiform muscles** are elongated muscles shaped like straps and can run from one joint to another. **Pennate muscles** are broad, flat, and slightly fan shaped, with fibers running obliquely to the muscle's long axis. The multipennate deltoid muscle, which flexes and extends the arm, is a good example of a muscle shaped according to its function.

FIG. 38-11, cont'd For legend see opposite page.

B

Sternocleidomastoid
Trapezius
Rhomboideus minor
Deltoid
Latissimus dorsi
Triceps (long and short head)
Brachioradialis
Extensor carpi radialis longus
Extensor digitorum communis
Gluteus medius
Gluteus maximus
Gracilis
Semitendinosus
Biceps femoris (short head)
Peroneus longus
Peroneus brevis

Splenius capitis
Levator scapulae
Supraspinatus
Rhomboideus major
Infraspinatus
Teres minor
Teres major
Serratus anterior
External oblique
Anconeus
Flexor carpi ulnaris
Extensor carpi ulnaris
Abductor pollicis longus
Extensor pollicis brevis
Adductor magnus
Iliotibial tract
Semimembranosus
Biceps femoris (long head)
Semimembranosus
Gastrocnemius
Soleus

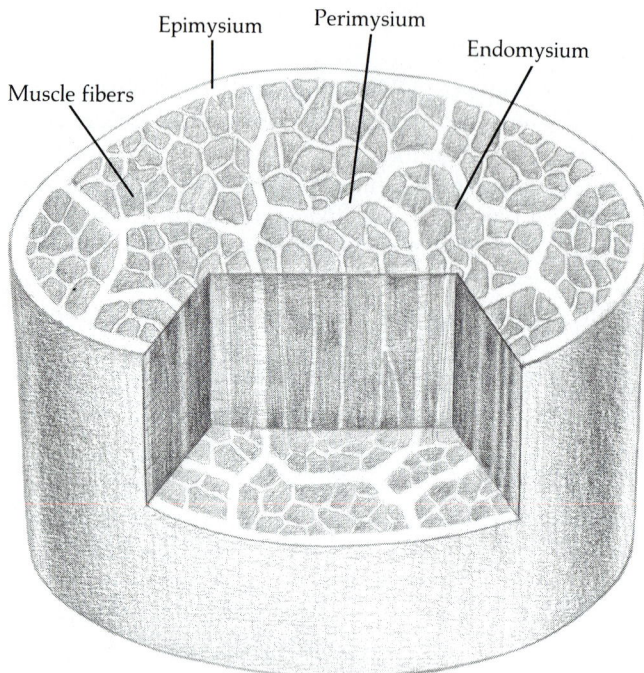

Epimysium   Perimysium

Muscle fibers   Endomysium

FIG. 38-12 Cross section of skeletal muscle showing muscle fibers and their coverings. (From Thompson, McFarland, Hirsch, & Tucker, 1993.)

Each skeletal muscle is a separate organ, encased in a three-part connective tissue framework called **fascia.** The layers of connective tissue protect the muscle fibers, attach the muscle to bony prominences, and provide a structure for a network of nerve fibers, blood vessels, and lymphatic channels.

The outermost layer, the **epimysium,** is located on the surface of the muscle and tapers at each end to form the **tendon** (Fig. 38-12). Tendons allow a short muscle to exert power on a distant joint where a thick muscle would interfere with joint mobility. The next layer, the **perimysium,** further subdivides the muscle fibers into bundles of connective tissue, or **fascicles.** The **endomysium** surrounds the muscle fascicles, the smallest unit of muscle fibers visible without a microscope. The ligaments, tendons, and fascia are made up of connective tissue that also serves to buffer the limbs from the effects of sudden strains or changes in speed. The rapid recovery necessary for strenuous exercise is supported by the elastic property of muscle and its connective tissue.

Skeletal muscle is described, almost interchangeably, as **voluntary, striated,** or **extrafusal.** "Voluntary" indicates that the muscle is controlled directly by the central nervous system. "Striated" describes the striated, or striped, pattern of skeletal muscle viewed under a light microscope. The striations result from the organization of the muscle fibers into the contractile units called sar-

comeres. "Extrafusal" distinguishes the skeletal muscle fibers from other contractile fibers located within the sensory organs of the muscle.

Other components that are visible on gross inspection of the whole muscle include the motor and sensory nerve fibers. These function together with the muscle, innervating portions of it and providing the electrical impulses needed for motor function.

Motor Unit

From the anterior horn cell of the spinal cord, the axons of motor nerves branch out to innervate a specific group of muscle fibers. Each anterior horn cell, its axon (part of lower motor neuron, see Chapter 12), and the muscle fibers innervated by it are called a **motor unit** (Fig. 38-13). The motor units are composed of lower motor neurons, which extend to skeletal muscles. Often termed the functional unit of the neuromuscular system, the motor unit behaves as a single entity and contracts as a whole when it receives an electrical impulse.

The whole muscle may be controlled by several motor nerve axons. These branch to innervate many motor units within the muscle. The whole muscle then may be made up of many motor units. The number of motor units per individual muscle varies greatly. In the calf, for example, one motor axon will innervate approximately 2000 muscle fibers, out of a total of 1,200,000 muscle fibers. This is a high innervation ratio of muscle fibers to axons, and it contrasts markedly with the low innervation ratio in the laryngeal muscles. There, two to three muscle fibers constitute each motor unit, and the innervation ratio can be of great functional significance. The greater the innervation ratio of a particular organ, the greater its endurance. Higher innervation ratios prevent fatigue, whereas lower innervation ratios allow for precision of movement.

Sensory receptors

Although muscles function as effector organs, they also contain sensory receptors and are involved in sending different signals to the central nervous system. Among these are the muscle spindles and Golgi tendon organs. **Spindles** are mechanoreceptors that lie parallel to muscle fibers and respond to muscle stretching. **Golgi tendon organs** are dendrites that terminate and branch to tendons near the neuromuscular junction. The muscle spindles, Golgi tendon organs, and free nerve endings provide a means of reporting changes in length, tension, velocity, and tone in the muscle. This system of afferent signals is responsible for the muscle stretch response and maintenance of normal muscle tone.

Muscle fibers

Each **muscle fiber** is a single **muscle cell.** This long cell is cylindrical in structure surrounded by a membrane ca-

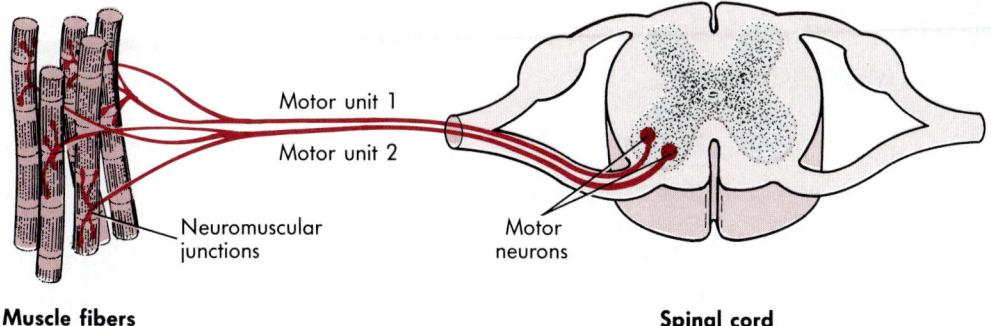

FIG. 38-13 **Motor units of a muscle.** Each motor unit consists of a motor neuron and all the muscle fibers (cells) supplied by the neuron.

FIG. 38-14 Myofibrils of a skeletal muscle fiber (cell) and overall organization of skeletal muscle. (From Seeley, Stephens, & Tate, 1990.)

pable of excitation and impulse propagation. The muscle fiber contains bundles of **myofibrils,** the fiber's functional subunits, in a parallel arrangement along the longitudinal axis of the muscle (Fig. 38-14). At birth, the muscle fibers have completed development from precursor cells called **myoblasts.** All voluntary muscles are derived from the mesodermal layer of the embryo.

The type of peripheral nerve influences the muscle fiber and motor unit considerably. Whether motor nerves are fast or slow determines the type of muscle fibers in the motor unit. Type II fibers, also called white fast-motor fibers, are innervated by relatively large type II alpha motor neurons with fast conduction velocities. These fibers rely on a short-term anaerobic glycolytic system for rapid energy transfer, whereas type I fibers depend on aerobic oxidative metabolism. Histochemical stains are now routinely used to describe the structure of muscle fibers and contractile elements of muscle

TABLE 38-4

Characteristics of Muscle Fibers

Characteristic	Type I (red)	Type II (white)
Anatomic location	Deep axial portion of surface muscle	Surface portion of surface muscle
Contraction speed	Slow	Fast
Motor neuron type	Type I, small alpha	Type II, large alpha
Firing frequency	Low, long duration	Rapid, short duration
Resistance to fatigue	High	Low
Myoglobin	High	Low
Capillary supply	Profuse	Intermediate to sparse
Metabolism	Oxidative	Glycolysis
Mitochondria	Many	Few
Enzymes	Lactate dehydrogenase, types 1-3	Lactate dehydrogenase types, 4-5
Creatine kinase	Cardiac type	Fast, skeletal
Example (most muscles are mixed)	Greater proportion of slow-contracting fibers in soleus	Greater proportion of fast-contracting fibers in laryngeal and ocular muscles
Mitochondria	Many	Few
Glycogen content	Low	High
Intensity of contraction	Low	High
Aerobic metabolic capacity	High	Low
Fiber diameter	Small	Large
Myosin-ATPase activity	Low	High

From Spence, A. P., & Mason, E. E. (1992). *Human anatomy and physiology* (4th ed.). St. Paul, MN: West Publishing Company.

biopsy specimens. White muscle, or **type II fibers,** stains dark in the enzyme stain adenosine triphosphatase (ATPase) at a pH of 9.4. Red muscle, or **type I fibers,** appears lightly stained.

The overlap of muscle fibers that appears with staining gives the checkerboard appearance of muscle biopsy specimens and provides an equal distribution of fiber types throughout the muscle. This overlap also helps to compensate for muscle fiber loss and fatigue of individual motor units during activity. In spite of this, some muscles contain proportionally more of one fiber type than another. The postural muscles have more type I fibers, allowing them the high resistance to fatigue that is necessary to maintain the same position for extended periods. The ocular muscles have more type II muscle fibers, allowing them to respond rapidly to visual changes. (Table 38-4 describes the specific characteristics of type I and type II fibers.)

The number of muscle fibers varies according to location. Large muscles, such as the gastrocnemius, have more fibers (1,200,000) than the smaller muscles, such as the lumbrical muscles in the hand (10,000). The diameter of muscle fibers also varies. The closely packed polygons are small (10 to 20 μm) until puberty, when they attain the normal adult diameter of 40 to 80 μm. Women usually have smaller diameter fibers than men. Small muscles, such as the ocular muscles, are 15 μm in diameter; larger more proximal muscles are 40 μm. Fiber size can have functional significance. Studies have shown that larger fiber diameter is associated with generation of greater forces. Fiber diameter can be increased by exercise, or occupational overuse, activities that cause hypertrophied muscle.

The major components of the muscle fiber include the muscle membrane, myofibrils, sarcotubular system, sarcoplasm, and mitochondria (Fig. 38-14). The **muscle membrane** is a two-part membrane. It includes the **sarcolemma,** which contains the plasma membrane of the muscle cell, and the cell's **basement membrane.** The sarcolemma is 7.5 nm thick and is capable of propagating electrical impulses to initiate contraction. At the motor nerve end plate, where the nerve impulse is transmitted, the sarcolemma forms the highly convoluted synaptic cleft. The sarcolemma is made up of lipid molecules and protein systems. The protein systems perform special functions, such as transport of nutrients and protein synthesis. They also provide the sodium-potassium pump and include the cell's cholinergic receptor. The basement membrane is 50 nm thick and is composed primarily of proteins and polysaccharides. It also serves as the cell's microskeleton and maintains the shape of the muscle cell. The basement membrane also may function in some way to restrict further diffusion of electrolytes once they have crossed the sarcolemma.

The **sarcoplasm** is the cytoplasm of the muscle cell and contains the intracellular components that are common to all cells (see Chapter 1). The sarcoplasm is an aqueous substance that provides a matrix that surrounds the myofibrils. It contains numerous enzymes and proteins that are responsible for the cell's energy production, protein synthesis, and oxygen storage. The mitochondria house enzyme systems for energy production, particularly those that regulate such processes as the citric acid cycle and adenosine triphosphate (ATP) formation. Many other structures are present in the sarcoplasm. The ribosomes are primarily composed of RNA and participate in the process of protein synthesis. The cell nucleus, satellite cells, glycogen granules, and lipid droplets are suspended in the sarcoplasmic matrix. Blood vessels, nerve endings, muscle spindles, and Golgi tendon organs are also directly located within this structure.

Unique to the muscle is the **sarcotubular system,** a network that includes the transverse tubules and the sarcoplasmic reticulum, which crosses the interior of the cell. The **sarcoplasmic reticulum** is made like the endoplasmic reticulum in other cells. In the muscle cells, the sarcoplasmic reticulum is involved in calcium transport, which initiates muscle contraction at the **sarcomere,** a portion of the myofibril (Fig. 38-14). The sarcoplasmic reticulum is composed of tubules that run parallel to the myofibrils. The longitudinal tubules are termed **sarcotubules.** The **transverse tubules,** which are closely associated with the sarcotubules, run across the sarcoplasm and communicate with the extracellular space. Together, the tubules of this membrane system allow for intracellular calcium uptake, regulation, release during muscle contraction, and storage of calcium during muscle relaxation.

Myofibrils

The myofibrils are the functional units of muscle contraction. Each myofibril contains sarcomeres, which appear at intervals (Fig. 38-14). The sarcomeres are composed of two contractile proteins, **actin** and **myosin.**

The myofibrils are the most abundant subcellular muscle component, equaling 85% to 90% of the total volume. On cross section, they are irregular polygons with a mean diameter of less than a micrometer. Each myofibril is composed of serially repeating sarcomeres, separated by Z lines, which give the muscle its striped, cross-striated appearance. Each sarcomere has a dark A band and is flanked by two light I bands (Fig. 38-15). The A band is 1.5 to 1.6 μm long and contains the thick myosin filaments. Included in the A band is a lighter zone called the H band, and in the center of the H band is the dark M band, or M line. The I band, which contains actin, is divided at the midpoint of each sarcomere by the Z line. Its length varies with the start of muscle contraction.

Myofibrils are composed of myofilaments. Each myofilament is structured in a closely packed hexagonal arrangement, with two thin filaments for every thick filament. The thick filament, along with C protein and M line protein, is made up of myosin. Myosin has two subunits, heavy and light meromyosin, which resemble twisted golf club shafts. The thin filaments are twisted double strands, made up of actin, troponin, and tropomyosin (see Chapter 26 and Fig. 26-16).

Muscle proteins

Eight proteins have been identified in the muscle fibrils. (Table 38-5 outlines their distribution, localization, and possible functional significance.) The contractile and regulatory functions of actin, myosin, and the troponin-tropomyosin complex (associated with actin) are the most commonly known. They also account for most of the protein found in the myofibril. The structural and regulatory processes of muscle proteins are less well understood. Alpha and beta actin are known to link the filaments. M protein contains the enzyme creatine kinase. Creatine is released when muscle cells are damaged, making serum creatine an important test of pathologic conditions of muscles.

The most abundant proteins, actin and myosin, are also found in other cells, particularly motile cells such as platelets. The complete amino acid sequences of both actin and myosin have been identified. Noteworthy is the presence of the amino acid 3-methylhistidine, which is found only in the thin filament actin. Eighty-five percent to 90% of 3-methylhistidine is found in skeletal muscle. Because it is excreted unchanged (in the urine) after release from muscle and other tissue, 3-methylhistidine has been used to gauge muscle protein degradation. The amino acids lysine and histidine, in addition to leucine, have been used to study protein synthesis by means of stable isotope infusion and muscle biopsy analysis.

Nonprotein constituents of muscle

Substances such as nitrogen, creatine, creatinine, phosphocreatine, purines, uric acid, and amino acids all serve

FIG. 38-15 **Muscle fibers. A,** Lines and bands in striated muscle. **B,** Relationships of bands, actin, myosin, and lines in relaxed and contracted muscle fibers. (From Thompson, McFarland, Hirsch, & Tucker, 1993.)

TABLE 38-5

Contractile Proteins of Skeletal Muscle Fibrils

Name	Percentage of myofibrillar protein	Localization	Function
Myosin	55	A band (thick filament)	Contraction; hydrolyzes ATP and develops tension
Actin	20	I band (thin filament)	Contraction; activates myosin ATPase and interacts with myosin
Troponin	7	Thin filament	Regulatory protein; in presence of Ca^{++}, promotes actin-myosin activation
Tropomyosin	5-7	Thin filament	Regulatory and structural function; links filaments, controls filament length
Alpha (α) actin	10	Z band	Regulatory and structural function; links filaments, controls filament length
Beta (β) actin	2	Z band	Regulatory and structural function; links filaments, controls filament length
M protein	2	M line (center of thick filaments)	Regulatory and structural function; provides enzyme creatine kinase (CK)
C protein	2	A band (thick filaments)	Possible structural role

in the complex process of muscle metabolism. Glycogen and its derivatives are present as energy sources.

Creatine and creatinine metabolism have been used to measure muscle mass. Plasma creatine is taken up by muscle and converted into the high-energy phosphate compound phosphocreatine by the enzyme creatine kinase. Creatinine is formed in muscle from creatine at a constant rate of 2%/day. (Tests for plasma creatine are discussed in Chapter 32.) Creatine excretion is increased in muscle wasting, whereas creatinine excretion is reduced. This change reflects the reduction in total body creatine stores and loss of muscle mass.

Inorganic compounds, anions (phosphate and chloride), and cations (calcium, magnesium, sodium, and potassium) are important in the regulation of protein synthesis, muscle contraction, enzyme systems, and membrane stabilization. Total-body potassium (TBK), measured by the K_{40} method, has been used to measure muscle mass, also called lean body mass. Total-body potassium levels reflect changes in muscle mass seen during growth, malnutrition, and muscle wasting.

Components of Muscle Function

The ultimate function of muscle is to accomplish work. Although variously expressed in such measures as foot-pounds or kilogram-meters, work usually refers to the amount of energy liberated or force exerted over a distance (work = force × distance). Muscles usually contract or tense while doing work. Muscle contraction occurs on the molecular level and leads to the observable phenomenon of muscle movement.

Muscle Contraction at the Molecular Level

Muscle contraction is a four-step process that includes (1) excitation, (2) coupling, (3) contraction, and (4) relaxation. The process involves the electrical properties of all cells and the movement of ions across the plasma membrane (see Chapter 1). The muscle fiber is an excitable tissue. At rest, an electric charge of −90 mV is continually maintained across the sarcolemma. This resting potential, generated by the separation of positive and negative charges on either side of the membrane, creates an electrochemical equilibrium caused by the selective permeability of the sarcolemma to electrolytes in the intracellular and extracellular fluids, particularly potassium and sodium.

Excitation, the first step of muscle contraction, begins with the spread of an action potential from the nerve terminal to the neuromuscular junction. The rapid depolarization of the membrane initiates an electrical impulse in the muscle fiber membrane called the **muscle fiber action potential.** As the action potential advances along the sarcolemmal membrane, it spreads to the transverse tubules. (The velocity of conduction is much slower in muscle fibers than in myelinated nerve fibers, only 3 to 5 m/sec compared with 54 to 90 m/sec in nerve fibers.)

The second stage, **coupling,** follows the depolarization of the transverse tubules. This stage consists of the migration of calcium ions, which are stored in the sarcoplasmic reticulum, to the myofilaments. Calcium affects troponin and tropomyosin, muscle proteins that bind with actin when the muscle is at rest. In the presence of calcium, however, both of these proteins are attracted to calcium ions, leaving the actin free to bind with myosin.

Contraction begins as the calcium ions combine with troponin, a reaction that overcomes the inhibitory function of the troponin-tropomyosin system. The thin filament, actin, then slides toward the thick filament, myosin. The two ends of the myofibril shorten after contraction when the myosin heads attach to the actin molecules, forming a cross-bridge that constitutes an actin-myosin complex. Adenosine triphosphate, located on the actin-myosin complex, is released when the cross-bridges attach. This is the **sliding filament theory** described by A. F. Huxley in the 1950s, but is now called the cross-bridge theory because of the formation of the actin-myosin cross-bridges, the process of contraction (West, 1991). The process is so named because the actin actually slides onto the myosin, causing the sarcomere to shorten. The useful distance of contraction of a skeletal muscle is approximately 25% to 35% of the muscle's length (West, 1991).

The last step, **relaxation,** begins as the sarcoplasmic reticulum absorbs the calcium molecules, removing them from interaction with troponin. Calcium is pumped back into the sarcoplasmic reticulum by means of an active transport process. The cross-bridges detach, and the sarcomere lengthens. (The cross-bridge theory of muscle contraction is discussed in Chapter 26.)

Muscle Metabolism

Skeletal muscle requires a constant supply of ATP and phosphocreatine. These substances are necessary to fuel the complex processes of muscle contraction, driving the cross-bridges of actin and myosin together and transporting calcium from the sarcoplasmic reticulum to the myofibril.

In addition to muscle contraction, other internal processes of the muscular system require ATP. Adenosine triphosphate is required for protein synthesis that replenishes muscle constituents and accommodates growth and repair. The rate of protein synthesis is related to hormone levels (particularly insulin), amino acid substrates, and overall nutritional status. At rest, the rate of ATP formation by oxidation of glucose or acetoacetate is sufficient to maintain internal processes, given normal nutritional status. During activity, the need for ATP increases markedly. The metabolic pathways for muscle activity in Table 38-6 show reactions to the immediate need for increased ATP caused by contraction. Activity lasting longer than 5 seconds expends the available stored ATP and phosphocreatine. Stored glycogen and blood glucose are converted anaerobically to sustain brief activity without increasing the demand for oxygen. Anaerobic glycolysis is much less efficient than aerobic glycolysis, using 6 to 8 times more glycogen to produce the same amount of ATP. With increased activity, such as intense exercise or with ischemia, an increase in lactic acid occurs because of the breakdown of glycogen, thus causing a shift in muscle pH (see Table 38-6). This short-term mechanism "buys time" by allowing ATP formation in spite of inadequate energy stores or oxygen supply. When the anaerobic threshold is reached and more oxygen is required, physiologic changes occur, including an increase in lactic acid and increases in oxygen consumption, heart rate, respiratory rate, and muscle blood flow.

Strenuous exercise requires oxygen, which activates the aerobic glycogen pathway for ATP formation. During maximal exercise, free fatty-acid mobilization and the aerobic glycogen pathways provide ATP over an extended time. These pathways require oxygen both to maintain maximal activity and to return the muscle to the resting state. Maximal exercise increases oxygen uptake by 15 to 20 times over the resting state. When this system becomes exhausted or inadequate to respond to the need for ATP, fatigue and weakness finally force the muscle to reduce activity with a resultant buildup of lactic acid in muscle fibers.

The ability to sustain maximal muscular activity leads to the accumulation of oxygen debt. **Oxygen debt** is the amount of oxygen needed to convert the built-up lactic acid to glucose and replenish ATP and phosphocreatine stores (Seeley et al., 1990; West, 1991). For example, after running at maximal speed for 10 seconds, the average person has consumed 1 L of oxygen. At rest, oxygen consumption for the same period is approximately 40 ml. As the person recovers, the measured oxygen debt is 4 L greater than the amount used during activity.

Measuring oxygen consumption as an indicator of energy expenditure is used to calculate the metabolic cost of activity in normal and diseased muscle. Indirect measures of energy expenditure include oxygen consumption, timed tests of activity, heart rate, and respiratory quotient (ratio of carbon dioxide to expired oxygen consumed). Energy expenditure is measured directly by the production of heat. Heat is released whenever work is accomplished, initially during muscle contraction and then during return to the resting state.

Another factor that changes energy requirements is muscle fiber type. Type II fibers rely on anaerobic glycolytic metabolism and fatigue readily. Type I fibers can

TABLE 38-6		
Energy Sources for Muscular Activity		
Sources	Reactions	
Short-term (anaerobic) sources	Adenosine triphosphate (ATP) $\rightarrow$ Adenosine diphosphate (ADP) + Inorganic phosphate (P_1) + Energy	
	Phosphocreatine + ADP $\rightleftharpoons$ Creatine + ATP	
	Glycogen/glucose + P_1 + ADP $\rightarrow$ Lactate + ATP	
Long-term (aerobic) sources)	Glycogen/glucose + ADP + P_1 + O_2 $\rightarrow$ H_2O + CO_2 + ATP	
	Free fatty acids + ADP + P_1 + O_2 $\rightarrow$ H_2O + CO_2 + ATP	
	Creatine kinase catalyzes the reversible reaction of ATP to ADP: Creatine phosphate + ATP $\underset{kinase}{\overset{Creatine}{\rightleftharpoons}}$ Creatine + ATP	

From Spence, A. P., & Mason, E. E. (1992). *Human anatomy and physiology* (4th ed.). St. Paul, MN: West Publishing Company.

resist fatigue for longer periods because of their capacity for oxidative metabolism.

Muscle Mechanics

Muscle contraction is not a process that can be viewed in isolation. Several factors determine how force is transmitted from the cross-bridges on individual muscle fibers to accomplish whole-muscle contraction. The first factor involves the motor unit. When a motor unit responds to a single nerve stimulus, it develops a phasic contraction, also called "twitch." Because the motor unit contracts in an "all or nothing" manner, the contraction that is generated by the stimulus will be a maximal contraction of the motor unit. The central nervous system smoothly grades the force generated by "recruiting" additional motor units and varying the discharge frequency of each active motor unit. This adding of motor units within the muscle is called **repetitive discharge.**

Recruitment and repetitive discharge of motor units allow the muscle to activate the number of motor units needed to generate the desired force. The total force developed is the sum of the force generated by each motor unit. As the strength, speed, and duration of stimuli increase, the summation of contractions reaches a critical frequency called **tetanus.** When tetanus is reached, no further increase in force can be achieved.

Other variables, such as fiber type, innervation ratio, muscle temperature, and muscle shape, influence the efficiency of muscular contraction. The two muscle fiber types differ in their responses to electrical activity. Tetanus and duration of phasic contractions, which take microseconds to accomplish, are achieved more rapidly in type II than in type I muscle fibers. Low innervation ratios promote control and coordination, whereas high ratios promote strength and endurance. For example, muscles with low innervation ratios, such as the laryn-

geal and ocular muscles, respond more rapidly than muscles with high innervation ratios to achieve fine control over movement. High innervation ratios, for example, in the calf, allow the muscle to sustain movement for prolonged periods or sustain the great forces needed for lifting. Muscle temperature also determines its degree of efficiency. Muscles work best at normal body temperature, 98.6° F (37° C). Muscle efficiency is also altered by the size of the load to be lifted and the shape of the muscle that carries the load. Heavier loads develop tension slowly. In some cases a load is necessary for the muscle to perform optimally. Muscles with a large cross-sectional area, such as the fan-shaped pennate muscles, develop greater contractile forces than smaller-diameter muscles. The initial length of a muscle and the range of shortening that occur when the muscle contracts also determine the force it can generate. The long fusiform muscles have a greater range of shortening and can contract up to 57% of their resting length. A certain amount of elongation is necessary to generate sufficient tension and muscular force. The elongation that occurs during the swing of a golf club or tennis racquet is an example of how stretch improves contractile force.

Types of Muscle Contraction

Two types of functional muscle contraction are isometric and isotonic. During **isometric contraction** (in Greek, *isos* = equal and *metron* = measure), the muscle maintains constant length as tension is increased. Isometric contraction occurs, for example, when the arm or leg is pushed against an immovable object. The muscle contracts, but the limb does not move. Isometric contraction is also called a **static** or **holding contraction.**

During **isotonic contraction** (in Greek, *isos* = equal and *tonus* = tension), the muscle maintains a constant tension as it moves. Isotonic contractions can be **eccentric (lengthening)** or **concentric (shortening)**. Positive work is accomplished during concentric contraction and energy is released to exert force or lift a weight. Typical concentric contractions are stepping up on a stool or flexing the elbow during a pull-up. In contrast, during an eccentric contraction the muscle lengthens and absorbs energy. Negative work is accomplished on the muscle by the load. Examples include stepping down stairs, running downhill, or slowly lowering the forearm into the extended position from the flexed position. Eccentric contraction requires less energy to accomplish and has been said to result in the development of pain and stiffness after unaccustomed exercise.

Movement of Muscle Groups

Muscles do not act alone but in groups, often under automatic control. When a muscle contracts and acts as a "prime mover," or **agonist,** its reciprocal muscle, or **antagonist,** relaxes. This is easily tested by holding the right arm in the horizontal position in front of the body, then bending the elbow while feeling the biceps in the front and the triceps in the back with the other hand. The biceps is firm, and the triceps is soft. As the arm is flexed, the muscles change. When the elbow is completely flexed, the biceps is soft and the triceps firm. Completing this movement causes the agonist and antagonist to change automatically; only the movement is commanded, not the alternate contraction and relaxation of the specific muscle groups.

Most joint movements also involve muscles that act as **synergists,** which are muscles that either act directly on or assist the prime mover or prevent unwanted movements that often occur when a prime mover contracts. For example, flexion may be accompanied by an undesired rotation in a joint (West, 1991). The synergistic muscles would try to oppose the rotation. When a synergistic muscle acts to immobilize a joint or an individual bone, it is referred to as a **fixator.** Fixators act as antagonists by preventing unwanted wrist flexion, for example, when a person makes a fist. Fixator muscle prevents the unwanted wrist flexion (West, 1991).

In addition to the group action of muscles, other associated actions may be unheeded by the casual observer. During walking, as the foot leaves the ground, the paravertebral and gluteal muscles on the opposite sides of the body contract to maintain balance. One notices the loss of the associated muscle's action when paralysis offsets this process and decreases balance. Arm swing is another associated movement that can be reduced with a seemingly mild paralysis. Other associated movements include the involuntary movements of yawning and stretching. These same movements may be preserved when severe paralysis is present.

Muscles have a ligamentous action that prevents com-

pleting movements that would injure tissue. For example, the average person cannot relax the hamstrings sufficiently to touch the toes with the knees straight. This same muscle, if weakened by paralysis, can be damaged if forcibly stretched, for example, when in the supine position, hip flexion was forced while the knees were kept extended, overstretching the paralyzed hamstring.

TESTS OF MUSCULOSKELETAL FUNCTION
Tests of Bone Function
Various diagnostic procedures are used to evaluate bone function, including gait analysis, serum calcium and phosphorus, x-ray films, angiography, and bone scanning. Roentgenograms visualize bone structure because bone absorbs x-ray beams better than soft tissue. Angiography is used to observe bone circulation. Bone scanning is the most frequently used procedure to evaluate bone function and can detect malignancy, trauma, necrosis, infection, metabolic bone disease, and osteoarthritis. The procedure for bone scanning involves the intravenous administration of radioactive isotopes (radionuclides) that have an affinity for bone tissue. The isotopes distribute in bone tissue and emit gamma rays. The spatial distribution of the rays is then visualized by a scanner or camera. Areas of bone that have prolific osteoblastic-osteoclastic activity (tumors, infection, fracture) concentrate greater amounts of isotopes than stable bone so these areas show a localized distribution of rays. Diffuse distribution of gamma rays is seen in metabolic bone disease.

Tests of Joint Function
Procedures used to diagnose joint function include arthrography, arthroscopy, magnetic resonance imaging, and synovial fluid analysis. **Arthrography** (the injection of dye into the joint) is particularly useful to diagnose tears in the fibrocartilage of the knee (meniscus) and the shoulder (rotator cuff). **Arthroscopy** is the direct visualization of a joint through an arthroscope. **Magnetic resonance imaging** (MRI) is a noninvasive procedure that produces images of body tissues through the use of electromagnetic (radio) waves that alter the atoms (hydrogen ions) in the nuclei of cells being examined. When the radio waves are stopped, the nuclear atoms return to their original positions, emitting energy as signals as they move back. The signals are stored in a computer and produce visible images for examination and diagnosis. Magnetic resonance imaging produces excellent contrast of soft tissues for evaluation of musculoskeletal conditions.

Analysis of synovial fluid is an important diagnostic test because the composition of synovial fluid changes dramatically when the joint is injured or diseased. Analysis can disclose inflammatory, septic, and noninflammatory joint diseases. All of these disease conditions cause characteristic changes in the color, clarity, viscosity, and cellular elements of the fluid.

In normal synovial fluid, hyaluronate is joined to proteins. When the fluid is treated with dilute acid, several protein-hyaluronate complexes unite with each other to form a precipitate or clot. The characteristics of the clot, termed a **mucin clot,** provide a crude index of the amount and binding ability of the protein-hyaluronate complexes in the fluid. Normal joint fluid forms a tight, adherent clot, whereas the fluid in an inflamed joint will form a loose clot or a powder precipitate.

The presence of blood in the joint fluid (hemarthrosis) usually indicates joint trauma. Normally, blood in the synovial fluid does not coagulate well because the articular cartilage and synovial membrane release an enzyme that prevents the formation of a firm blood clot. Therefore the formation of a blood clot in the synovial fluid is indicative of a diseased joint.

Normal synovial fluid is sterile, so the presence of bacteria in the fluid is always indicative of disease. Cell fragments and fibrous tissue in the fluid are the result of inflammation or wear and tear on the articular surfaces.

Tests of Muscular Function

When the individual's history and physical examination disclose abnormalities, such as weakness, atrophy, muscle tenderness, cramps, and stiffness, specific tests of muscle function are in order. One of the most useful tests is the serum creatine kinase (CK) concentration. Creatine kinase is found in large quantities in the muscle fibers, and when these are diseased or damaged, CK leaks into the serum. Myoglobin is also detectable in the urine after acute muscle damage caused by crush injury, ischemic disorders, extreme exertion, and some inherited diseases.

Because the muscle membrane tissue is excitable and carries an electrical charge, its capacity to function can be assessed by electromyography. Using sensitive needle electrodes, the **electromyogram** (EMG) records the summation of action potentials of the muscle fibers in each motor unit. The EMG is often compared with the electrocardiogram (ECG), but the activity recorded on the EMG is on a much smaller scale. The amplitude of the ECG is measured in volts, the duration of impulse in seconds, and both are recorded as the heart rate (e.g., 80 volts per 60 seconds). On the EMG, the amplitude is recorded in millivolts and the duration is measured in milliseconds, with a frequency of about 5 to 50 action potentials per second. The motor unit potentials are measured to determine rate of firing, duration, and amplitude. Abnormalities in EMG and nerve conduction

velocities help differentiate muscle diseases (myopathy) from peripheral nerve (neuropathy) and neuromuscular junction disorders. The muscle biopsy (using histologic, histochemical, and electron microscopic studies) is used to further define the presence of myopathic and neuropathic disorders, many of which can be diagnosed only by muscle biopsy.

The forearm ischemic exercise test allows the clinician to determine the integrity of the glycolytic pathways and enzyme systems that function during intensive exercise. To perform this test, a catheter is placed in an antecubital vein and venous blood is collected for up to 20 minutes after intensive graded series of work loads at maximal grip strength. Any defect in the glycolytic pathway are expressed by a lack of lactate production, such as is seen in McArdle disease. Mitochondrial disorders are associated with excessive lactate production at two levels of exercise. The absence of ammonia, usually proportional to the rise in lactate, is seen in myoadenylate deaminase deficiency.

Although manual muscle testing of strength and range of motion is still the most common way to detect changes, myometers are becoming increasingly popular. These hand-held devices measure strength of contraction in several muscle groups, the neck flexors, shoulder abductors, wrist extensors, hip flexors, knee extensors, and foot dorsiflexors.

☐ AGING and the Musculoskeletal System
Aging of Bones

Aging is accompanied by the loss of bone tissue. The haversian systems in compact bone undergo slow erosion, lacunae are enlarged, canals nearest the marrow cavity become widened, and the endosteal cortex converts to spongy bone. The endosteal surface gradually erodes until the rate of loss exceeds the rate of deposition on the subperiosteal surface. Newly forming haversian systems prematurely arrest and show incomplete closure. The end result is a thin and porous cortex. Bone erosion occurs first in the horizontal trabeculae of spongy bone, which considerably decreases the strength of the bone. Consolidation and erosion of the vertical trabeculae follow.

In both types of bone, the bone remodeling cycle takes longer to complete because the bone cells in the basic multicellular units are slower in their ability to resorb and deposit bone tissue. The rate of mineralization also slows down. The number of bone cells decreases because the bone marrow becomes fatty and is unable to provide an adequate supply of precursor cells. (Aging of bone marrow is discussed in Chapter 22.)

As women age, they experience loss of bone density, which becomes accelerated with rapid bone loss during early menopause because of increased osteoclastic bone resorption (Liscum, 1992). By age 70, susceptible women have, on the average, lost 50% of their peripheral cortical bone mass. Bone mass losses to such extent lead to deformity, pain, stiffness, and high risk for fractures. Men experience bone loss also but at later ages and much slower rates than women. Also, initial bone masses in men are approximately 30% higher than in women; therefore, bone loss in men causes less risk of disability than for women. By the age of 60, only 3% of men, but 7% of women, have experienced a fracture of the forearm, spine, or hip, increasing to 8% for men and 25% for women by age 80 (Francis, Scane, Johnson, Sutcliffe, & Sutcliffe, 1992). Men lose 15% to 45% of trabecular bone and 5% to 15% of cortical bone compared with losses of 35% to 50% of trabecular bone and 25% to 30% of cortical bone in women of similar ages (Francis et al., 1992). Men's peak bone mass is related to their race, heredity, hormonal factor (loss of testosterone), physical activity, and calcium intake during childhood. Bone loss in men is related to smoking, alcohol intake, and physical inactivity (Francis et al., 1992).

Bone mass can be gained in healthy young women up to the third decade, which may significantly reduce the risk of osteoporosis in later life (Recker et al., 1992). Bone gain is achieved through physical activity, intake of dietary calcium, and use of oral contraceptives (Recker et al., 1992).

Aging of Joints

With increasing age, cartilage becomes more rigid, fragile, and susceptible to fibrillation. Loss of elasticity and resiliency is attributed to more cross-linking of collagen and elastin, decreasing water content in the cartilage ground substance, and decreasing concentrations of glycosaminoglycans. Decreased range of motion of the joint is related to the changes in ligaments and muscles. Bones in joints develop evidence of osteoporosis with fewer trabeculae and thinner, less dense bones, making them prone to fractures.

Aging of Muscles

As the body ages, muscle bulk and strength decline. Studies of normal men show postpubertal increases in

strength that peak in the third decade, coinciding with an increase in testosterone levels. Strength is maintained into the 50s, with a slow decline in dynamic and isometric strength evident after age 70. A corresponding loss is evident in the number of muscle fibers seen with age, particularly the type II fibers. Other observations include reduced RNA synthesis and loss of mitochondrial volume and reduction in the size of motor units. In one study, the loss of mitochondrial volume seen with aging was not associated with changes in energy production. Changes in RNA synthesis may be responsible for reduced protein synthesis, although the regenerative function of muscle tissue remains normal in aging persons. As much as 30% of skeletal muscles may be lost by age 80 (Spence & Mason, 1992).

Several factors may explain these changes: change in activity level, reduced nerve supply to muscle, cardiovascular disease, and nutritional deficiencies. Reduced activity causes changes in strength and reduced fiber size because of disuse. Although muscle fibers can regenerate into the seventh decade, nerve fibers cannot. Axonal regeneration and nerve terminal sprout are significantly reduced, as is the synthesis of acetylcholine. Signs of neurogenic atrophy are quite common in the aged and may contribute significantly to the reduction in muscle size and strength, and the efficiency of muscle stimulation.

As people age, the maximal oxygen intake decreases. Reduced basal metabolic rate and lean body mass are also seen in the aged population. When the effects of aging are added to poor nutritional status, changes in basal metabolic rate and lean body mass are likely to be significant.

Because mobility is so important to the physiologic and psychologic health of the elderly, it would seem prudent to conduct an exhaustive search for treatable causes of muscle weakness and wasting before ascribing these changes to "old age." Given the normal muscle regenerative capabilities in this population, age should not be a deterrent to developing rehabilitation programs after muscle injury or illnesses that involve loss of muscular strength.

Structure and Function of Bones

1 Bones provide support and protection for the body's tissues and organs and are important sources of minerals and blood cells.

2 Bone formation begins with the production of an inorganic matrix by bone cells. Bone minerals crystallize in and around collagen fibers in the matrix, giving bone its characteristic hardness and strength.

3 Bone tissue is continuously being resorbed and synthesized by basic multicellular units of osteoclasts and osteoblasts.

4 All bones in the body are made up of compact bone tissue and spongy bone tissue. Compact bone is highly organized into haversian systems that consist of concentric layers of crystallized matrix surrounding a central canal that contains blood vessels and nerves. Dispersed throughout the concentric layers of crystallized matrix are small spaces containing osteocytes. Smaller canals, called canaliculi, interconnect the osteocyte-containing spaces. The crystallized matrix in spongy bone is arranged in bars or plates. Spaces containing osteocytes are dispersed between the bars or plates and interconnected by canaliculi.

5 There are 206 bones in the body; these are divided into the axial skeleton and the appendicular skeleton. Bones are classified by shape as long, short, flat, or irregular. Long bones have a broad end (epiphysis), broad neck (metaphysis), and narrow midportion (diaphysis) that contains the medullary cavity.

6 Bone injuries are repaired in stages. Hematoma formation provides the fibrin framework for formation and organization of granulation tissue. The granulation tissue provides a cartilage model for the formation and crystallization of bone matrix. Remodeling restores the original shape and size to the injured bone.

Structure and Function of Joints

1 A joint is the site where two or more bones attach. Joints provide stability and mobility to the skeleton.

2 Joints are classified as synarthroses, amphiarthroses, or diarthroses, depending on the degree of movement they allow. Joints are also classified by the type of connecting tissue holding them together. Fibrous joints are connected by dense fibrous tissue, ligaments, or membranes. Cartilaginous joints are connected by fibrocartilage of hyaline cartilage. Synovial joints are connected by a fibrous joint capsule. Within the capsule is a small fluid-filled space. The fluid in the space nourishes the articular cartilage that covers the ends of the bones meeting in the synovial joint.

3 Articular cartilage is a highly organized system of collagen fibers and proteoglycans. The fibers firmly anchor the cartilage to the bone and the proteoglycans control the loss of fluid from the cartilage.

4 Joints help move bones and muscle.

Structure and Function of Skeletal Muscle

1 Skeletal muscle is the largest organ in the body and is made up of millions of individual fibers.

2 Whole muscles vary in size (2 cm to 60 cm) and shape (fusiform and pennate). They are encased in a three-part connective tissue framework. The fundamental concept of muscle function is the motor unit, defined as all muscle fibers innervated by a single motor nerve.

3 Muscle fibers contain bundles of myofibrils arranged in parallel along the longitudinal axis and include the muscle membrane, myofibrils, sarcotubular system, aqueous sarcoplasm, and mitochondria. There are two types of muscle fibers, type I and type II, determined by motor nerve innervation.

4 Myofibrils and myofilaments contain the major muscle proteins, actin and myosin, which interact to form cross-bridges during muscle contraction. The nonprotein muscle constituents provide an energy source for contraction and regulate protein synthesis, enzyme systems, and membrane stabilization.

5 Muscle contraction includes excitation, coupling, contraction, and relaxation.

6 Muscle strength is graded by the "all or nothing" phenomenon and recruitment. Speed of contraction is affected by several factors: muscle fiber type, temperature, stretch, and weight of the load.

7 There are two types of muscle contraction, isometric and isotonic. Muscle shortening occurs during contraction but can be seen also during pathologic and physiologic contracture.

8 Skeletal muscle requires a constant supply of ATP and phosphocreatine to fuel muscle contraction and for growth and repair. Adenosine triphosphate and phosphocreatine can be generated aerobically or anaerobically.

Tests of Musculoskeletal Function

1 Various diagnostic procedures are used to evaluate bone function including gait analysis, serum calcium and phosphorus, x-ray films, angiography, bone scanning, and magnetic resonance imaging.

2 Procedures used to evaluate joint function include arthrography, arthroscopy, magnetic resonance imaging, and synovial fluid analysis.

3 Tests of muscular function include physical examination, serum creatine kinase, myoglobin, electromyogram, muscle biopsy, myometers, and the forearm ischemic exercise test.

Aging and the Musculoskeletal System

1 Muscle bulk and strength slowly decline although not to a pathologic degree. Age should not be a deterrent to developing an exercise program in the elderly.

KEY TERMS

Actin, 1423
Agonist, 1428
Alpha-glycoprotein, 1408
Amphiarthrosis (slightly movable joint), 1412
Antagonist, 1428
Appendicular skeleton, 1409
Arthrography, 1428
Arthroscopy, 1428
Articular cartilage, 1414
Axial skeleton, 1409
Basement membrane, 1422
Basic multicellular unit, 1410
Bone albumin, 1408
Bone fluid, 1408
Bone matrix, 1406
Bone morphogenic protein (BMP), 1407
Calcification, 1406
Canaliculus, 1408
Chondrocyte, 1414
Collagen fiber, 1407
Compact bone (cortical bone), 1408
Concentric contraction (shortening contraction), 1428
Contraction, 1426
Coupling, 1426
Diaphysis, 1410
Diarthrosis (freely movable joint), 1412
Eccentric contraction (lengthening contraction), 1428
Electromyogram (EMG), 1429
Endomysium, 1420
Endosteum, 1410
Epimysium, 1420
Epiphyseal plate (growth plate), 1410
Epiphysis, 1410
Excitation, 1425
Fascia, 1420
Fascicle, 1420
Fibril, 1407
Fibrous joint, 1412

Fixator muscle, 1428
Flat bone, 1410
Fusiform muscle, 1419
Glycoprotein, 1407
Glycosaminoglycans, 1418
Golgi tendon organ, 1420
Gomphosis, 1412
Ground substance, 1405
Haversian canal, 1408
Haversian system, 1408
Hyaluronate, 1414
Hydroxyapatite (HAP), 1408
Intima, 1414
Irregular bone, 1410
Isometric contraction (static or holding contraction), 1427
Isotonic contraction, 1427
Joint (articulation), 1412
Joint capsule (articular capsule), 1414
Joint cavity (synovial cavity, joint space), 1414
Lacuna, 1407
Lamella, 1408
Laminin, 1408
Link protein, 1418
Long bone, 1409
Magnetic resonance imaging (MRI), 1428
Metaphysis, 1410
Motor unit, 1420
Mucin clot, 1429
Muscle fiber (muscle cell), 1420
Muscle fiber action potential, 1425
Muscle membrane, 1422
Myoblast, 1421
Myofibril, 1421
Myosin, 1423
Osteoblast, 1406
Osteocalcin, 1408
Osteoclast, 1406
Osteocyte, 1406
Osteoid, 1406
Osteonectin, 1408

Oxygen debt, 1426
Pennate muscle, 1419
Perimysium, 1420
Periosteum, 1409
Procallus (granulation tissue), 1412
Protein core, 1418
Proteoglycan, 1407
Relaxation, 1426
Remodeling, 1410
Repetitive discharge, 1427
Sarcolemma, 1422
Sarcomere, 1423
Sarcoplasm, 1423
Sarcoplasmic reticulum, 1423
Sarcotubular system, 1423
Sarcotubule, 1423
Short bone (cuboidal bone), 1410
Sialoprotein (osteopontin), 1408
Skeletal muscle (voluntary, striated, or extrafusal muscle), 1420
Sliding filament theory, 1426
Spindle, 1420
Spongy bone (cancellous bone), 1408
Subintima, 1414
Suture, 1412
Symphysis, 1412
Synarthrosis (immovable joint), 1412
Synchondrosis, 1412
Syndesmosis, 1412
Synergist muscle, 1428
Synovial fluid, 1414
Synovial joint, 1414
Synovial membrane (synovium), 1414
Tendon, 1420
Tetanus, 1427
Tidemark, 1418
Trabecula, 1408
Transverse tubule, 1423
Type A synovial cell, 1414
Type B synovial cell, 1414
Type I fiber, 1422
Type II fiber, 1422
Woven bone (callus), 1412

REFERENCES

Beresford, J. N. (1989). Osteogenic stem cells and the stroma system of bone and marrow. *Clinical Orthopaedics and Related Research, 240*(3), 271-280.

Bonewald, L. F., & Mundy, G. R. (1990). Role of transforming growth factor-beta in bone remodeling. *Clinical Orthopaedics and Related Research, 250*(1), 261-274.

Boskey, A. L. (1990). Bone mineral and matrix: Are they altered in osteoporosis? *Orthopedic Clinics of North America, 21*(1), 19-26.

Bucholz, R. W. (1991). Fracture treatments. In C. A. Rockwood, Jr., & D. P. Green (Eds.), *Fractures in adults* (3rd ed.). Philadelphia: Lippincott.

Einhorn, T. (1991). Mechanisms of fracture healing. *Hospital Practice, 265*(1), 41-45.

Francis, R. M., Scane, F. J., Johnson, C. E., Sutcliffe, D., & Sutcliffe, A. M. (1992). Male osteoporosis. *Journal of Endocrinology, 135*(Suppl.), 9.

Goldring, M. B., & Goldring, S. R. (1990). Skeletal tissue response to cytokines. *Clinical Orthopaedics, 258*(9), 245-263.

Iannotti, J. P. (1990). Growth plate physiology and pathology. *Orthopedic Clinics of North America, 21*(10), 1-10.

Kuettner, K. E., Aydelotte, M. B., & Thonar, E. J. (1991). Articular cartilage matrix and structure: A mini review. *Journal of Rheumatology*, (Suppl. 27), 46-48.

Liscum, B. (1992). Osteoporosis: The silent disease. *Orthopaedic Nursing, 11*(4), 21-25.

Mourad, L. (1991). *Orthopedic disorders*. St. Louis: Mosby–Year Book.

Mundy, G. R. (1991). New concepts in bone metabolism: Clinical implications. *Hospital Practice, 265*(1), 7-12.

Recker, R. R., Davis, K. M., Hinders, S. M., Heaney, R. P., Stegman, M. R., & Kimmel, D. B. (1992). Bone gain in young adult women. *Journal of the American Medical Association, 268*(17), 2403-2407.

Russell, R. G. G. (1992). Hormonal control of bone metabolism. *Journal of Endocrinology, 135*(Suppl.), 8.

Seeley, R. R., Stephens, T. D., & Tate, P. (1990). *Anatomy and physiology*. St. Louis: Mosby–Year Book.

Spence, D B., & Mason, E. E. (1992). *Human anatomy and physiology* (4th ed.). St. Paul, MN: West Publishing.

Thompson, J. M., McFarland, G. K., Hirsch, J. E., Tucker, S. M., & Bowers, A. C. (1989). *Mosby's manual of clinical nursing* (2nd ed.). St. Louis: Mosby–Year Book.

West, J. B. (1991). Excitation and contraction of skeletal muscle. In J. B. West (Ed.), *Best & Taylor's physiological basis of medical practice*. Baltimore: Williams & Wilkins.

SUGGESTED READINGS

Campbell, I. K., Piccoli, D. S., Roberts, M. J., Muirden, K. D., & Hamilton, J. A. (1990). Effects of tumor necrosis factor α and β on resorption of human articular cartilage and production of plasminogen activator by human articular chondrocytes. *Arthritis and Rheumatism, 33*(4), 542-551.

Hulth, A. (1989). Current concepts in fracture healing. *Clinical Orthopaedics and Related Research, 249*(120), 265-282.

Joyce, M. E., Jingushi, S., & Bolander, M. E. (1990). Transforming growth factor-B in the regulation of fracture repair. *Orthopaedic Clinics of North America, 21*(1), 199-209.

Kelm, R. J., & Mann, K. G. (1991). The collagen binding specificity of bone and platelet osteonectin is related to differences in glycosylation. *Journal of Biological Chemistry, 266*(15), 9632-9639.

Larsson, T., Sommarin, Y., Paulsson, M., Antonsson, P., Hedbom, E., Wendel, M., & Heinegard, D. (1991). Cartilage matrix proteins. *Journal of Biological Chemistry, 266*(30), 20428-20432.

Simmons, E. D., Jr., Pritzker, K. P., & Gynpas, M. D. (1991). Age-related changes in the human femoral cortex. *Journal of Orthopaedic Research, 9*(20), 158-167.

Tsukamoto, T., Matsui, T., Nakata, H., Ito, M., Natazuka, T., Fukase, M., & Fujita, T. (1991). Interleukin-1 enhances the response of osteoblasts to platelet-derived growth factor through the α receptor-specific up-regulation. *Journal of Biological Chemistry, 266*(16), 10143-10147.

Wu, L. N. Y., Genge, B. R., & Wuthier, R. E. (1991). Association between proteoglycans and matrix vesicles in the extracellular matrix of growth plate cartilage. *Journal of Biological Chemistry, 266*(2), 1187-1194.

CHAPTER 39

Alterations of Musculoskeletal Function

Leona A. Mourad
Katherine Hoare*
Katharine M. Donohoe*

Chapter Outline

*Contributing authors to first edition.

Musculoskeletal injuries include fractures, dislocation, sprains, and strains. Fracture is the most serious. Alterations in bones, joints, and muscles may be caused by metabolic disorders, infection, inflammatory or noninflammatory disease, or tumors.

MUSCULOSKELETAL INJURIES

Data accumulated by the National Center for Health Statistics show that each year, in the United States, an average of 1 of 10 persons suffers an acute musculoskeletal injury, the most common being fracture, dislocation, sprain, and strain. Bone fracture is the most serious of these injuries.

Skeletal muscles can withstand many penetrating injuries without permanent loss of function. For example, studies of soldiers with severe combat injuries showed that muscle function was preserved after the removal of large portions of muscle tissue. Successful regeneration of skeletal muscle fibers primarily depends on the extent of injury, preservation of vascular supply (and source of nutrition), and the availability of terminal axons for reinnervation.

Skeletal Trauma
Fractures

A **fracture** is a break in the continuity of a bone. A break occurs when force is applied that exceeds the tensile or compressive strength of the bone. The incidence of fractures varies for individual bones according to age and sex. The highest incidence of fractures is in young males (between the ages of 15 and 24) and in the elderly (65 years of age and older). Fractures of healthy bones, particularly the tibia, clavicle, and lower humerus, tend to occur in the young and to be the result of trauma. Fractures of the hands and feet are usually caused by accidents in the workplace. The incidence of fractures of the upper femur, upper humerus, vertebrae, and pelvis is highest in older or elderly adults and is often associated with osteoporosis (see p. 1445). There are more than 200,000 fractures of the hip yearly in the United States alone (Harrison, 1989).

Classification of fractures

Fractures are classified as complete or incomplete and open or closed (Fig. 39-1). In a **complete fracture,** the bone is broken all the way through, whereas in an **incomplete fracture,** the bone is damaged but is still in one piece. Complete or incomplete fractures also can be classified as **open** (formerly referred to as compound) if the skin is broken or as **closed** (formerly called simple) if it is not. A fracture in which a bone breaks into two or more fragments is termed a **comminuted fracture.** Fractures are also classified according to the direction of the fracture line. A **linear fracture** runs parallel to the long axis of the bone. An **oblique fracture** occurs at a 45° angle (oblique angle) to the shaft of the bone. A **spiral fracture** encircles the bone, and a **transverse fracture** occurs straight across the bone.

Incomplete fractures tend to occur in the more flexible, growing bones of children. The three main types of incomplete fractures are greenstick, torus, and bowing fractures. A **greenstick fracture** perforates one cortex and splinters the spongy bone. The name is derived from the damage sustained by a young tree branch (a green stick) when it is bent sharply. The outer surface is disrupted, but the inner surface remains intact. Greenstick fractures typically occur in the proximal metaphysis or diaphysis of the tibia, radius, and ulna. In a **torus fracture,** the cortex buckles but does not break. Torus fractures are common in the metaphyses of persons with osteoporosis. **Bowing fractures** usually occur when longitudinal force is applied to bone. This type of fracture is common in children and usually involves the paired radius-ulna or the fibula-tibia. A complete diaphyseal fracture occurs in one of the bones of the pair, which disperses the stress sufficiently to prevent a complete fracture of the second bone, which bows. Bowing fractures resist correction (reduction) because the force necessary to reduce it must be equal to the force that bowed it. Treatment of bowing fractures is also difficult because the bowed bone interferes with reduction of the fractured bone. (Types of fractures are summarized in Table 39-1.)

Sometimes fractures are further classified by cause as pathologic, stress, or transchondral fractures. A **pathologic fracture** is a break at the site of a preexisting abnormality, usually by force that would not fracture a normal bone. Any disease process that weakens a bone (especially the cortex) predisposes the bone to pathologic fracture. Pathologic fractures are commonly associated with tumors, osteoporosis, infections, and metabolic bone disorders.

Stress fractures occur in normal or abnormal bone that is subjected to repeated stress, such as occurs during athletics. The stress is less than the stress that usually causes a fracture. Two types of stress fractures are recognized: fatigue fracture and insufficiency fracture. A **fatigue fracture** is caused by abnormal stress or torque applied to a bone with normal ability to deform and recover. Fatigue fractures usually occur in individuals (e.g., joggers, dancers, military recruits) who engage in a new or different activity that is both strenuous and repetitive. Because gains in muscle strength occur more rapidly than gains in bone strength, the newly developed

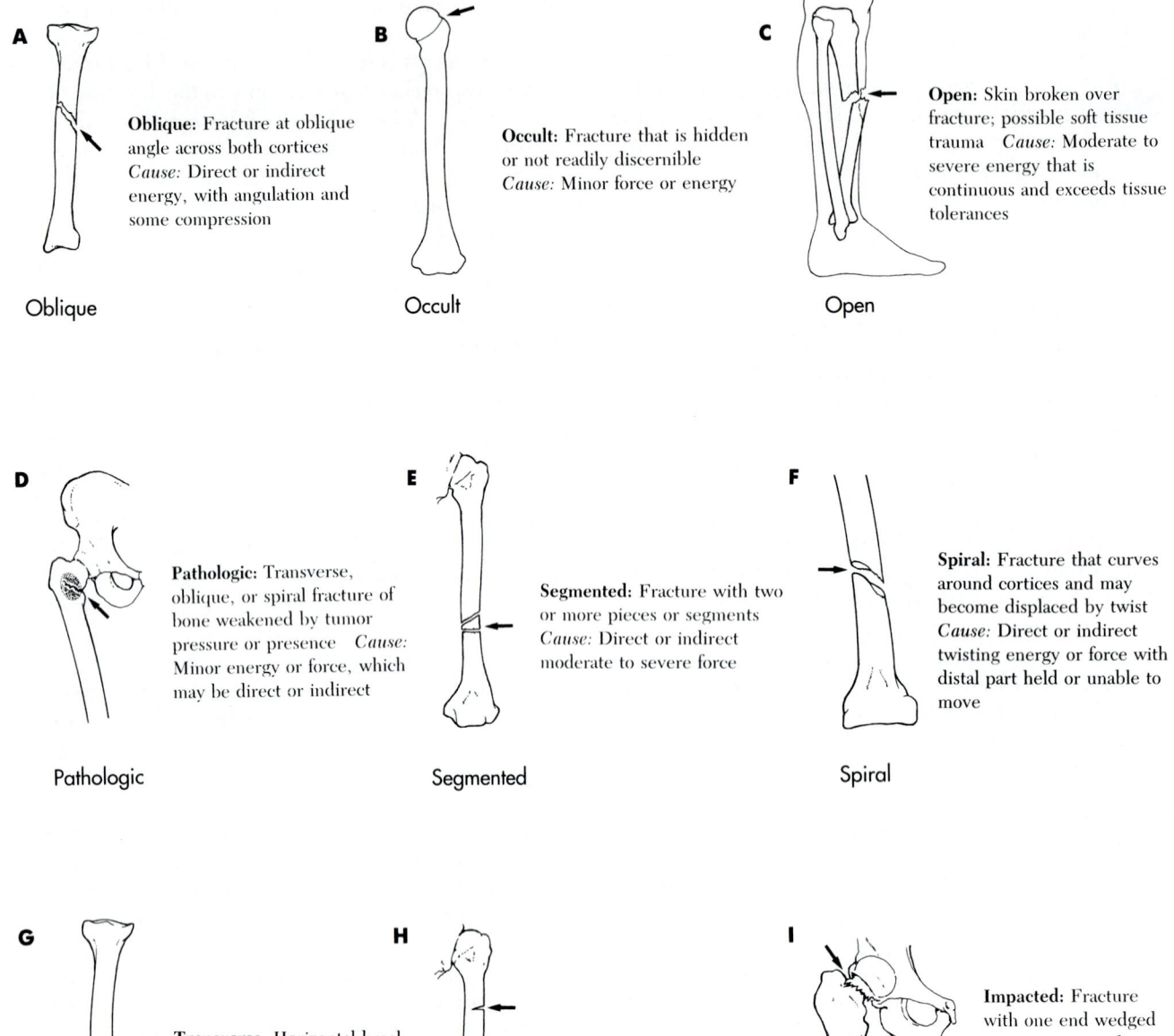

A Oblique

Oblique: Fracture at oblique angle across both cortices *Cause:* Direct or indirect energy, with angulation and some compression

B Occult

Occult: Fracture that is hidden or not readily discernible *Cause:* Minor force or energy

C Open

Open: Skin broken over fracture; possible soft tissue trauma *Cause:* Moderate to severe energy that is continuous and exceeds tissue tolerances

D Pathologic

Pathologic: Transverse, oblique, or spiral fracture of bone weakened by tumor pressure or presence *Cause:* Minor energy or force, which may be direct or indirect

E Segmented

Segmented: Fracture with two or more pieces or segments *Cause:* Direct or indirect moderate to severe force

F Spiral

Spiral: Fracture that curves around cortices and may become displaced by twist *Cause:* Direct or indirect twisting energy or force with distal part held or unable to move

G Transverse

Transverse: Horizontal break through bone *Cause:* Direct or indirect energy toward bone

H Greenstick

Greenstick: Break in only one cortex of bone *Cause:* Minor direct or indirect energy

I Impacted

Impacted: Fracture with one end wedged into opposite end or inside fractured fragment *Cause:* Compressive axial energy or force directly to distal fragment

FIG. 39-1 Examples of types of bone fractures. A, Oblique: Fracture at oblique angle across both cortices. *Cause:* Direct or indirect energy, with angulation and some compression. **B,** Occult: Fracture that is hidden or not readily discernible. *Cause:* Minor force or energy. **C,** Open: Skin broken over fracture; possible soft tissue trauma. *Cause:* Moderate to severe energy that is continuous and exceeds tissue tolerances. **D,** Pathologic: Transverse, oblique, or spiral fracture of bone weakened by tumor pressure or presence. *Cause:* Minor energy or force, which may be direct or indirect. **E,** Segmented: Fracture with two or more pieces or segments. *Cause:* Direct or indirect moderate to severe force. **F,** Spiral: Fracture that curves around cortices and may become displaced by twist. *Cause:* Direct or indirect twisting energy or force with distal part held or unable to move. **G,** Transverse: Horizontal break through bone. *Cause:* Direct or indirect energy toward bone. **H,** Greenstick: Break in only one cortex of bone. *Cause:* Minor direct or indirect energy. **I,** Impacted: Fracture with one end wedged into opposite end or inside fractured fragment. *Cause:* Compressive axial energy or force directly to distal fragment. (From Mourad, 1991.)

TABLE 39-1

Types of Fractures

Type	Definition
Typical complete fractures	
Closed fracture	Noncommunicating wound between bone and skin
Open fracture	Communicating wound between bone and skin
Comminuted fracture	Multiple bone fragments
Linear fracture	Fracture line parallel to long axis of bone
Oblique fracture	Fracture line at 45-degree angle to long axis of bone
Spiral fracture	Fracture line encircling bone (as a spiral staircase)
Transverse fracture	Fracture line perpendicular to long axis of bone
Impacted	Fracture fragments are pushed into each other
Pathologic	Fracture occurs at a point in the bone weakened by disease, for example, with tumors or osteoporosis
Avulsion	A fragment of bone connected to a ligament or tendon breaks off from the main bone
Compression	Fracture is wedged or squeezed together on one side of bone
Displaced	Fracture with one, both, or all fragments out of normal alignment
Extracapsular	Fragment is close to the joint but remains outside the joint capsule
Intracapsular	Fragment is within the joint capsule
Typical incomplete fractures	
Greenstick fracture	Break on one cortex of bone with splintering of inner bone surface, commonly occurs in children and elderly
Torus fracture	Buckling of cortex
Bowing fracture	Bending of the bone
Stress fracture	Microfracture
Transchondral fracture	Separation of cartilaginous joint surface (articular cartilage) from main shaft of bone

muscles place exaggerated stress on the bones that are not ready for it. The imbalance between muscle and bone development causes microfractures to develop in the cortex. If the activity is controlled and increased gradually, new bone formation catches up to increased demands, and microfractures do not occur.

Insufficiency fractures are stress fractures that occur in bones lacking normal ability to deform and recover; normal weight bearing or activity fractures the bone. Rheumatoid arthritis, osteoporosis, Paget disease, osteomalacia, rickets, hyperparathyroidism, and radiation therapy cause bone to lose its normal ability to deform and recover.

A **transchondral fracture** (also known as **osteochondritis dissecans**) consists of fragmentation and separation of a portion of the articular cartilage that covers the end of a bone at a joint. (Joint structures are defined in Chapter 38.) Single or multiple sites may be fractured, and the fragments may consist of cartilage alone or cartilage and bone. Typical sites of transchondral fracture are the head of the femur, the ankle, the knee cap, the elbow, and the wrist. Transchondral fractures are most prevalent in adolescents.

Pathophysiology

When a bone is broken, the periosteum and blood vessels in the cortex, marrow, and surrounding soft tissues are disrupted. Bleeding occurs from the damaged ends of the bone and from the neighboring soft tissue. A clot (hematoma) forms within the medullary canal, between the fractured ends of the bone, and beneath the periosteum (Fig. 39-2). Bone tissue immediately adjacent to the fracture dies. This necrotic tissue (along with any debris in the fracture area) stimulates an intense inflam-

FIG. 39-2 Exuberant callus formation following fracture. (From Rosai, J. [1981]. *Ackerman's surgical pathology* [6th ed]. St. Louis, Mosby–Year Book.)

FIG. 39-3 Bone healing (schematic representation). A, Bleeding at broken ends of the bone with subsequent hematoma formation. B, Organization of hematoma into fibrous network. C, Invasion of osteoblasts, lengthening of collagen strands, and deposition of calcium. D, Callus formation: new bone is built up as osteoclasts destroy dead bone. E, Remodeling is accomplished as excess callus is reabsorbed and trabecular bone is laid down. (From Bucholz, 1991.)

matory response characterized by vasodilation, exudation of plasma and leukocytes, and infiltration by inflammatory leukocytes and mast cells. Within 48 hours after the injury, vascular tissue invades the fracture area from surrounding soft tissue and the marrow cavity, and blood flow to the entire bone is increased. Bone-forming cells in the periosteum, endosteum, and marrow are activated to produce subperiosteal procallus along the outer surface of the shaft and over the broken ends of the bone (Fig. 39-3). Osteoblasts within the procallus synthesize collagen and matrix, which becomes mineralized to form callus (woven bone). As the repair process continues, remodeling occurs, during which unnecessary callus is resorbed and trabeculae are formed along lines of stress (Fig. 39-2). Except for the liver, bone is unique among all body tissues, in that it will form new bone, not scar tissue, when it heals after a fracture.

Clinical Manifestations

The clinical manifestations of a fracture vary according to the type of fracture, site of the fracture, and associated soft tissue injury. In general, the signs and symp-

toms of a fracture include unnatural alignment (deformity), swelling, muscle spasm, tenderness, pain, and impaired sensation. The position of the bone segments is determined by the pull of attached muscles, gravity, and the direction and magnitude of the force that caused the fracture. One or both segments may be rotated inward or outward on the bone's long axis (rotation), misaligned at an angle (angulation), or slide over the other segment (overriding).

The immediate pain of a fracture is severe and usually caused by the trauma. Subsequent pain may be produced by muscle spasm, overriding of the fracture segments, or damage to adjacent soft tissues. Numbness is common and is caused by the pinching or severing of a nerve by the trauma or by bone fragments. Pathologic fractures usually cause angular deformity, painless swelling, or generalized bone pain. Pathologic fractures are not usually associated with trauma or trauma-related pain. Stress fractures are painful, not because of trauma, but because of accelerated remodeling. The pain occurs during activity and is usually relieved by rest. Stress fractures also cause local tenderness and soft tissue swelling. Transchondral fractures may be entirely asymptomatic or painful during movement. Range of motion in the joint is limited, and movement may evoke audible clicking sounds (crepitus).

Evaluation and Treatment

Fracture treatment involves realigning the bone fragments (reduction) close to their normal or anatomic position and holding the fragments in place (immobilization) so that bone union can occur. Several methods are available to reduce a fracture: closed manipulation, traction, and open reduction.

Most fractures can be reduced by closed manipulation: the skin is not opened (closed reduction); the bone is moved or manipulated into place. Closed manipulation is used when the contour of the bone is in fair alignment and can be maintained well with immobilization.

Traction is used to accomplish or maintain reduction. When bone fragments are displaced (not in their anatomic position), weights are used to apply firm, steady traction (pull) and countertraction to the long axis of the bone. Traction stretches and fatigues muscles that pull the bone fragments out of place, allowing the distal fragment to align with the proximal fragment. Traction can be applied to the skin (skin traction) (Fig. 39-4), directly to the involved bone, or distal to the involved bone (skeletal traction). Skin traction is used when only a few pounds of pulling force are needed to realign the fragments or when the traction will be used for brief times only, such as before surgery or, for children with femoral fractures, for 3 to 7 days before applying a cast. A traction bow is applied to the skin, closed with self-adhering straps, with weights attached to the foot area of the traction boot. In skeletal traction, a pin or wire is drilled through the bone below the fracture site, and a traction bow, rope, and weights are attached to the pin or wire to apply tension and to provide the pulling force to overcome the muscle spasm and help realign the fracture fragments.

Open reduction is a surgical procedure that exposes the fracture site; the fragments are brought into alignment under direct visualization. Some form of prosthesis, screw, plate, nail, or wire usually is used to maintain the reduction (internal fixation).

Splints and plaster casts are used to immobilize and hold a reduction in place. Improper reduction or immobilization of a fractured bone may result in nonunion, delayed union, or malunion. **Nonunion** is failure of the bone ends to grow together (Fig. 39-5). The gap between the broken ends of the bone fills with dense fibrous and fibrocartilaginous tissue instead of new bone. Occasionally, the fibrous tissue contains a fluid-filled

FIG. 39-4 Two types of skin traction. **A,** Buck extension traction. **B,** Dunlop traction. (From Mourad, 1991.)

space that resembles a joint and is termed a false joint, or pseudoarthrosis. **Delayed union** is union that does not occur until approximately 8 to 9 months after a fracture. **Malunion** is the healing of a bone in a nonanatomic position.

FIG. 39-5 Nonunion of old fracture of tibia and fibula in 53-year-old white man. Multiple fractures had occurred in 2 years previously and necessitated bone grafting. (From Rosai, J. [1981]. *Ackerman's surgical pathology* [6th ed.]. St. Louis, Mosby–Year Book.)

Dislocation and Subluxation

Dislocation and subluxation are usually caused by trauma. **Dislocation** is the temporary displacement of two bones in which the two bone surfaces lose contact entirely. If the contact between the two bone surfaces is only partially lost, the injury is called a **subluxation.**

Dislocation and subluxation are most common in persons younger than 20 years of age and are generally associated with fractures. Dislocation and subluxation, however, may be due to congenital or acquired disorders that cause (1) muscular imbalance, as occurs with congenital dislocation of the hip or neurologic disorders; (2) incongruities in the articulating surfaces of the bones, as occur with rheumatoid arthritis (see p. 1462); or (3) joint instability.

The joints most often dislocated or subluxated are the joints of the shoulder, elbow, wrist, finger, hip, and knee. The shoulder joint most frequently injured is the glenohumeral joint. The glenohumeral joint is a relatively unstable joint because the articular surface of the glenoid cavity is only one third as large as the surface of the humeral head. Physical trauma to the shoulder can cause anterior, posterior, superior, or inferior dislocation. Anterior dislocation is the most common and

is usually associated with a compression fracture of the humeral head. Posterior dislocations usually occur spontaneously because of a general laxity in the ligaments that normally stabilize the joint. A superior dislocation is usually the result of an extreme forward and upward force on an adducted arm. An inferior displacement is frequently seen in persons with neurologic injuries of the brachial plexus and is believed to be caused by stretching of the supporting muscles or by joint effusion.

Traumatic dislocation of the elbow joint is common in the immature skeleton. In adults, an elbow dislocation is usually associated with a fracture of the ulna or head of the radius. Posterior dislocations occur when the individual falls on an outstretched hand with the arm in extension. Anterior dislocations are usually the result of a direct blow to the flexed elbow.

Traumatic dislocation of the wrist usually involves the distal ulna and carpal bones. Any one of the eight carpal bones can be dislocated after an injury. The most common cause is a fall on the hyperextended hand.

Dislocation in the hand usually involves the metacarpophalangeal and interphalangeal joints. Dislocation of the metacarpophalangeal joint is the result of a fall on the outstretched hand that forces the joint into hyperextension. Dislocation of the interphalangeal joint occurs as a result of injury to the fingers in a hyperextended position.

Considerable trauma is needed to dislocate the hip. Anterior hip dislocation is rather rare and is caused by forced abduction, for example, when an individual lands on the feet from a high fall. Posterior dislocation of the hip can occur in an automobile accident in which the flexed knee strikes the dashboard.

The knee is an unstable joint that depends heavily on the soft tissue structures around it for support. Because the knee is an unstable weight-bearing joint exposed to many different types of motion (flexion, extension, rotation), it is one of the most frequently injured joints. A knee dislocation can be anterior, posterior, lateral, medial, or rotary. It is usually the result of a hyperextension injury that occurs during sports activities.

Pathophysiology

Dislocations and subluxations are often accompanied by fracture because stress is placed on areas of bone not usually subjected to stress. In addition, as the bone separates from the joint, it may bruise or tear adjacent nerves, blood vessels, ligaments, supporting structures, and soft tissue. Dislocation of the shoulder usually damages the shoulder capsule and the axillary nerve. Damage to the axillary nerve causes anesthesia in the sensory distribution of the nerve and paralysis of the deltoid muscle. Elbow dislocations are accompanied by torn periosteum and muscle. Bleeding from the damaged periosteum and muscle puts pressure on adjacent arteries that shuts off circulation to and from the forearm and hand. If the pressure is not promptly relieved, ischemic paralysis develops. Dislocations of the hand often result in permanent disability because of damage to the tendons and intricate mechanisms that allow smooth gliding in the joints. Avascular necrosis of the femoral head is a complication seen in hip dislocations. Knee dislocation usually tears both the collateral and cruciate ligaments.

Clinical Manifestations

The general signs and symptoms of dislocations or subluxations include pain, swelling, limitation of motion, and joint deformity. Pain may be due to effusion of inflammatory exudate into the joint or associated tendon and ligament injury. Joint deformity is usually caused by muscle contractions that exert pull on the dislocated or subluxated joint. Limitation of motion may be a result of effusion into the joint or the displacement of bones.

Tenderness and deformity are prominent in dislocations of the fingers. Unusual muscle pull and pain often result in abnormal posturing of the fingers; for example, the fingers or thumb may be abnormally flexed. A dislocated elbow is often held in a flexed position, and the joint resists active or passive movement. Pain is the key symptom of shoulder injuries. Attempts to lift the arm aggravate the pain. In most shoulder dislocations, the ability to elevate the arms is minimal and the individual supports the injured arm with the opposite hand. Pain and an abnormal gait or limp or inability to bear full weight usually accompany traumatic dislocation of the hip. The pain is constant and severe and is often felt in the inguinal region or thigh. The thigh may assume a position of inward rotation, adduction, or flexion, and appears shortened. In a rare anterior dislocation, the limb is not shortened and the joint is fixed in abduction, outward rotation, and flexion.

Evaluation and Treatment

Evaluation of dislocations and subluxations is based on clinical manifestations and roentgenograms. Treatment consists of reduction and immobilization for 2 to 6 weeks and exercises to maintain normal range of motion in the joint. Depending on the joint, healing is usually complete within months to years.

Support Structures
Sprains and Strains of Tendons and Ligaments

Tendon and ligament injuries can accompany fractures and dislocations. A tendon is fibrous connective tissue that attaches skeletal muscle to bone (see Chapter 38). A **ligament** is a band of fibrous connective tissue that connects bones where they meet at a joint. Tendons and

ligaments support the bones and joints and either facilitate or limit motion. Tendons and ligaments can be torn, ruptured, or completely separated from bone at their points of attachment.

A tear in a tendon is commonly known as a **strain.** Major trauma can tear or rupture a tendon at any site in the body. Most frequently injured are the tendons of the hands and feet, the knee (patellar), the upper arm (biceps and triceps), the thigh (quadriceps), the ankle, and the heel (Achilles). Traumatic rupture of the biceps tendon is often caused by lifting excessive weight with the arms. Rupture of the Achilles tendon occurs when forced dorsiflexion is applied to the foot when it is in plantar flexion (Browner, Jupiter, Levine, & Trafton, 1992). Spontaneous tendon ruptures can occur in individuals receiving local corticosteroid injections and persons with rheumatoid arthritis or systemic lupus erythematosus.

Ligament tears are commonly known as **sprains.** Ligament tears and ruptures can occur at any joint but are most common in the wrist, ankle, elbow, and knee joints. A complete separation of a tendon or ligament from its bony attachment site is known as an **avulsion.** An avulsion is the result of abnormal stress on the ligament or tendon and is commonly seen in young athletes, especially sprinters, hurdlers, and runners.

Pathophysiology

When a tendon or ligament is torn, an inflammatory exudate develops between the torn ends. Later, granulation tissue containing macrophages, fibroblasts, and capillary buds grows inward from the surrounding soft tissue and cartilage to begin the repair process. Within 4 to 5 days after the injury, collagen formation begins. At first, collagen formation is random and disorganized. As the collagen fibers interweave and connect with preexisting tendon fibers, they become organized parallel to the lines of stress. Eventually vascular fibrous tissue fuses the new and surrounding tissues into a single mass. As reorganization takes place, the healing tendon or ligament separates from the surrounding soft tissue. Usually a healing tendon or ligament lacks sufficient strength to withstand strong pull for 4 to 5 weeks after the injury. If strong muscle pull does occur during this time, the tendon or ligament ends may separate again, which causes the tendon or ligament to heal in a lengthened shape with an excessive amount of scar tissue; this renders the tendon or ligament functionless.

Clinical Manifestations

Tendon and ligament injuries are painful and are usually accompanied by soft tissue swelling, changes in tendon or ligament contour, and dislocation/subluxation of bones. The pain is generally sharp and localized, and tenderness persists over the distribution of the tendon

FIG. 39-6 Tendinitis and epicondylitis. **A,** Achilles tendon, site of frequently occurring tendinitis. **B,** Medial or lateral epicondyles of humerus, site of epicondylitis. (From Mourad, 1991.)

or ligament. Painful joint swelling can usually be seen in finger and elbow sprains. Flexion deformities of the fingers and thumb occur in injuries to the extensor tendons. Crepitus may accompany tendon injury in the wrist. Pain in the elbow may be accentuated by flexion, supination, and extension of the elbow or by extension of the wrist. Lifting small objects requires extension of the wrist and therefore aggravates the pain. Tendon injuries in the upper arm cause weakness when the individual tries to flex the forearm. Pain is often the key symptom of shoulder injuries. It may be referred to the deltoid muscle or extend down the arm. The pain is usually aggravated by attempts to lift the arms. Depending on the ligament or tendon involved, tendon and ligament injuries in the knee may produce pronounced mobility, lost lateral movement, instability when walking down stairs, semiflexion, crepitus, or an upward shift of the patella.

Evaluation and Treatment

Evaluation is based on clinical manifestations, stress radiography, arthroscopy, or arthrography. When possible, treatment consists of suturing the tendon or ligament ends in close approximation. If this is not possible because of the extent of damage, tendon or ligament grafting may be necessary.

Tendinitis and Bursitis

Trauma can also cause painful inflammation of tendons (tendinitis) and bursae (bursitis). Other causes of tendinitis include crystal deposits, postural misalignment, and hypermobility in a joint. Achilles tendinitis is inflammation of the Achilles tendon, one that is frequently inflamed.

Epicondylitis is inflammation of a tendon where it attaches to a bone (at its origin). Epicondylar areas of the humerus, radius, or ulna, and around the knee are most frequently inflamed. **Lateral epicondylitis,** commonly called **tennis elbow,** is inflammation of the lateral epicondyle of the humerus, and **medial epicondylitis,** referred to as **golfer's elbow,** is inflammation of the medial humeral epicondyle (Fig. 39-6).

Bursae are small sacs lined with synovial membrane and filled with synovial fluid; they are located between tendons, muscles, and bony prominences. Their primary function is to separate, lubricate, and cushion these structures. Acute bursitis occurs primarily in the middle years and is caused by repeated trauma. Septic bursitis is caused by wound infection or bacterial infection of the skin overlying the bursae. The shoulder is the most common site of bursitis. Bursitis also occurs in the hip, knee, elbow, and the toe with a bunion.

Pathophysiology

Fluid from inflammation accumulates in tendinitis, causing swelling of the tendon and its enclosing sheath.

Inflammatory changes cause thickening of the sheath, which limits movements and causes pain. Microtears cause bleeding, edema, and pain in the involved tendon or tendons. At times, after repeated inflammations, calcium may be deposited in the tendon origin area.

The usual bursitis is an inflammation that is reactive to overuse or excessive pressure. The inflamed bursal sac becomes engorged and the inflammation can spread to adjacent tissues. The inflammation may decrease with rest, heat, and needle puncture. (Inflammation is discussed in Chapter 7.)

Clinical Manifestations

Clinical manifestations are usually localized to one side of the joint. Generally there is local or "point" tenderness (the individual can point to the area of greatest tenderness) and more pain with active motion than with passive motion. With tendinitis, the pain is localized over the involved tendon, and movement in the affected joint is limited. The onset of pain may be gradual or sudden in bursitis, and movement in the joint is limited. Shoulder bursitis impairs arm abduction. Bursitis in the knee produces pain when climbing stairs, and crossing the legs is painful in bursitis of the hip. Lying on the side of the inflamed trochanteric bursa is also very painful. Signs of infectious bursitis include the presence of a puncture site, prior corticosteroid injection, severe inflammation, or an adjacent source of infection (McCune, 1989).

Evaluation and Treatment

Evaluation of tendinitis, epicondylitis, and bursitis is based on clinical manifestations, arthroscopy, arthrography, and possibly magnetic resonance imaging (MRI).

Treatment includes immobilization of the joint with a sling, splint, or cast; systemic analgesics; ice or heat applications; or local injection of an anesthetic and a corticosteroid to reduce inflammation. Physical therapy to prevent loss of function begins after acute inflammation subsides.

Muscle Strains

Mild injury such as **muscle strain** is usually seen after traumatic or sports injuries. Muscle strain is a general term for local muscle damage. It is often the result of sudden, forced motion causing the muscle to become stretched beyond normal capacity. Knife and gunshot wounds also cause traumatic rupture. Strains often involve the tendon as well. Muscles are ruptured more often than tendons in young people; the opposite is true in the older population. Muscle strain may be chronic when the muscle is repeatedly stretched beyond its usual capacity. There is evidence of tissue disruption with subsequent signs of muscle regeneration and connective tissue repair when a biopsy is performed. Hemorrhage into the surrounding tissue and signs of inflammation also may be present. Regardless of the cause of trauma, muscle cells are usually able to regenerate. Regeneration may take up to 6 weeks, and the affected muscle should be protected during this time. (Degrees of acute muscle strain, together with their manifestations and treatment, are summarized in Table 39-2.)

A late complication of localized muscle injury is **myositis ossificans**. This condition is thought to be caused by scar tissue calcification and subsequent ossification. Examples include "rider's bone," in which the adductor muscle of the thigh of equestrians becomes calcified, and "drill bone," in which the same complication is seen

---

TABLE 39-2

Muscle Strain

Type	Manifestations	Treatment
First degree (example: bench press in untrained athlete)	Muscle overstretched, painful	Ice should be applied 5 or 6 times in the first 24-48 hours; complete rest for up to 2 weeks, followed by weight bearing 3 times per week and range of motion daily
Second degree (example: any muscle strain with bruising and pain)	Muscle intact with some tearing pain, mild bruising	Treatment similar to that for first-degree strains, with added mild analgesia; cryokinetics (a treatment system of alternating applications of heat and cold with progressive exercise)
Third degree (example: traumatic injury)	Caused by tearing of fascia, muscle rupture palpable, bleeding present	Surgery to approximate ruptured edges; immobilization and rest for 6 weeks

in the deltoid and pectoral muscles of fencers and infantry soldiers, as well as football players after muscle injury to thigh muscles.

Myoglobinuria

Myoglobinuria, also called rhabdomyolysis, can be a life-threatening complication of severe muscle trauma. Myoglobinuria is named for the principal manifestation of the condition, an excess of myoglobin, an intracellular muscle protein, in the urine. Muscle damage releases the myoglobin. The most severe form is often called crush syndrome. Less severe and more localized forms are called **compartment syndromes,** which can lead to **Volkmann ischemic contracture** in the forearm or leg. Crush syndrome first gained notoriety in the reports of injuries seen after the London air raids in World War II. More recently it has been reported in individuals found unresponsive and immobile for long periods, usu-

ally after a drug overdose. Myoglobinuria also can be seen after viral infections, administration of certain anesthetic agents, strychnine poisoning, tetanus, heat stroke, electrolyte disturbances, and fractures. Excessive muscular activity also has been implicated in reports of myoglobinuria in athletes, such as long-distance runners, ice skaters, skiers, military recruits, and those subjected to fraternity hazing. Status epilepticus, electroconvulsive therapy, and high-voltage electrical shock are also associated with severe and sometimes fatal myoglobinuria.

If the myoglobinuria is caused by fulminant malignant hyperthermia, severe muscle spasm and rhabdomyolysis can lead to renal failure. Other complications include intraoperative rigidity, tachycardia, cardiac arrhythmias, metabolic and respiratory acidosis, and a rapidly rising temperature (elevations of up to 43° C), which can occur at a rate as rapid as 1° every 5 minutes (Millman, 1991). Cerebral edema, cardiogenic and hypovolemic shock, pulmonary edema, and disseminated intravascular clotting can contribute to the death of an individual with malignant hyperthermia.

Pathophysiology

The weight of a limp extremity can generate enough pressure to produce muscle ischemia (Fig. 39-7). This causes edema, rising compartment pressure, and tamponade that leads to muscle infarction and neural injury, and, finally, results in cell loss. Physical interruptions in the sarcolemmal membrane, called holes or delta lesions, suggest that the sarcolemmal membrane

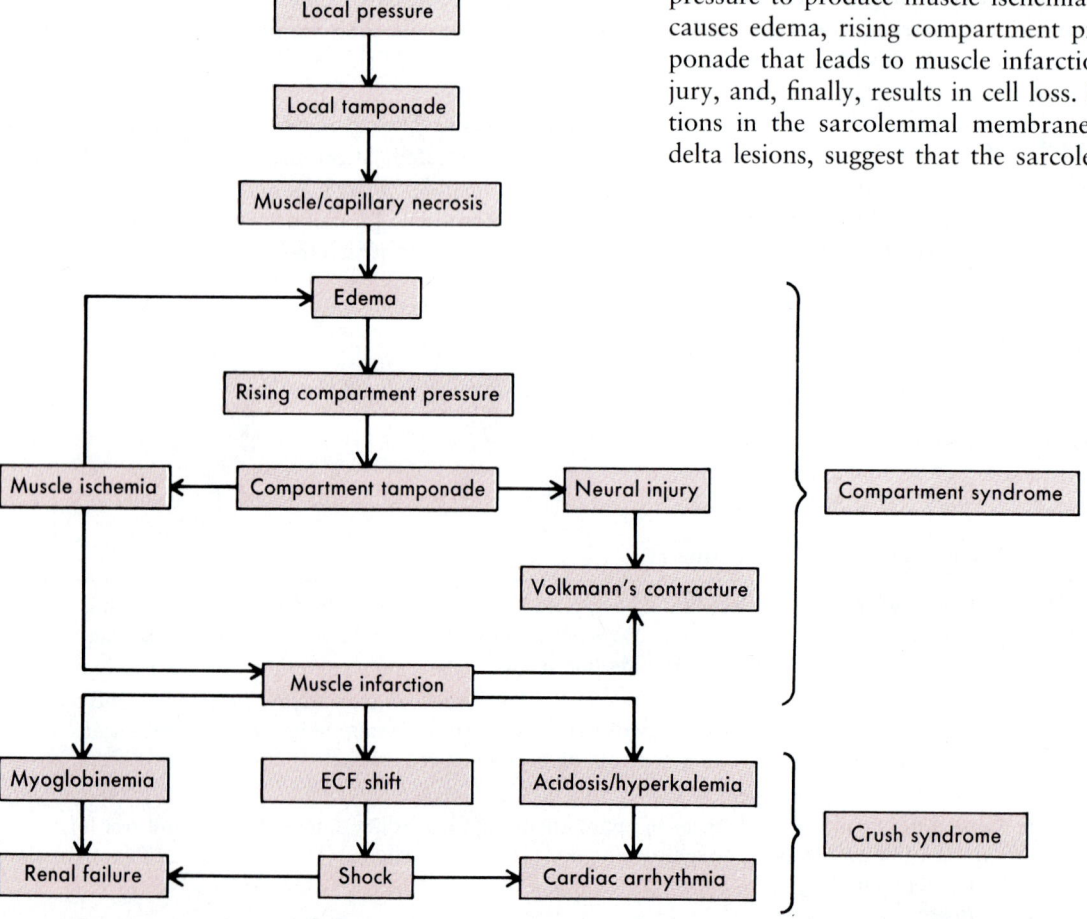

FIG. 39-7 Pathogenesis of compartment syndrome and crush syndrome caused by prolonged muscle compression.

may be the route by which muscle constituents are released. (The sarcolemmal membrane, the plasma membrane of the muscle cell, is described in Chapter 38.)

Clinical Manifestations

When myoglobin is released from the muscle fibers (cells) into the circulation, it can cause a visible, dark reddish brown pigmentation of the urine. The renal threshold for myoglobin is low, approximately 0.5 mg/100 ml urine, so that only 200 g muscle need be damaged to cause visible changes in the urine. Along with the release of myoglobin, creatine kinase and other serum enzymes are released in massive quantities. The creatine kinase level is often 100 times greater than normal (5 to 25 U/ml for women and 5 to 35 U/ml for men). The efflux of proteins and enzymes also includes loss of potassium, phosphate, nucleotides, creatinine, and creatine. Serum hypocalcemia is seen early in the course of myoglobinuria and is followed by late hypercalcemia.

Evaluation and Treatment

Careful and thorough preoperative assessment should alert the anesthesiologist to the possibility of a susceptible individual. A family history of anesthetic problems and previous untoward anesthetic experiences (muscle cramping, unexplained fevers, and dark urine) are criteria that require further clarification before administration of a volatile anesthetic, such as halothane (Millman, 1991).

Priorities in treatment of myoglobinuria include identifying and treating the underlying disorder and preventing life-threatening renal failure. Malignant hyperthermia and myoglobinuria caused by succinylcholine or volatile anesthetic agents can be treated by halting the anesthetic administration and infusing dantrolene sodium (Dantrium). Diluting the pigment using intravenous fluids and administration of mannitol, sodium bicarbonate, and furosemide (Lasix) to "flush" the kidney have been advocated to prevent renal failure. Other secondary problems include electrolyte imbalance, volume depletion, acidosis, hyperuricemia, hyperkalemia, and calcium imbalance. These need specific treatment. Short-term dialysis also may be necessary.

The compartment syndromes may require emergency treatment when blood flow to the affected extremity is compromised because of increased venous pressure, leading to decreased arterial inflow, causing ischemia, and edema. When clinical evaluation is inconclusive, the rising compartment pressure can be directly measured by inserting a wick catheter, needle, or slit catheter into the muscle. Immediate fasciotomy and debridement have been advocated for pressures of more than 30 mm Hg over the individual's normal diastolic pressure (Bourne & Rorabeck, 1989). Most frequently affected are the anterior tibial, deep posterior tibial, volar, hand, and gluteal compartments.

DISORDERS OF BONES

Metabolic Bone Diseases

Metabolic bone disease is characterized by abnormal bone structure that is caused by altered or inadequate biochemical reactions. The altered or inadequate biochemical reactions may be attributable to genetics, diet, or hormones.

Osteoporosis

Osteoporosis is a disease in which the density or mass of bone is reduced. The bone that remains is histologically and biochemically normal, but there is not enough of it to maintain skeletal integrity and mechanical support. The disease can be (1) generalized, involving major portions of the axial skeleton, or (2) regional, involving one segment of the appendicular skeleton. Both spongy and compact bone is lost, but spongy bone loss exceeds compact bone loss.

Healthy young women can gain bone mass during the third decade of life (Recker et al., 1992) through their active physical activity, dietary calcium intake, and the use of oral contraceptives (Recker et al., 1992). Osteoporosis is the most common metabolic disease. Primary osteoporosis has been subdivided into two types, with spinal osteoporosis in the sixth and seventh decades, designated type I, and osteoporotic femoral fractures of extreme old age, designated type II (Harrison, 1989). It is uncertain whether these two subgroups are different manifestations of the same disease or two distinct diseases.

Osteoporosis is the most common medical problem for older women, occurring six to eight times more frequently in women than in men (Liscum, 1992). Because of the decreased bone mass, fractures are major risks for those persons affected with osteoporosis. Wrist fractures in women increase during the sixth decade, and hip fractures increase exponentially from approximately age 70, until in the very elderly, one in three women and one in six men in the United States (approximately 200,000/year) have hip fractures (Harrison, 1989). Vertebral fractures also occur in the latter years of life, mainly in the sixth and seventh decades, with possibly one in three women older than 65 years of age having vertebral fractures (Harrison, 1989). The annual direct and indirect costs of osteoporosis are nearly $6 billion. Approximately 50% of persons with osteoporosis and fractures never walk again (Liscum, 1992). Osteoporosis leads to marked losses of both spongy and trabecular bone, with women losing approximately one half and men approximately one quarter of their spongy bone.

Osteoporosis is most common in whites, probably because members of other races, particularly blacks, have denser bones. Whites are therefore more susceptible than other races to osteoporosis caused by loss of bone density with age.

The cause of generalized osteoporosis is diverse, and in very few cases is the cause certain. Postmenopausal osteoporosis, which occurs in middle-aged and older women, is probably caused by decreased levels of estrogen. Before menopause, higher estrogen levels inhibit bone resorption by decreasing the sensitivity of osteoclasts to circulating parathyroid hormone. Without the inhibitory action of estrogen, parathyroid hormone overstimulates osteoclasts within the basic multicellular units to initiate the remodeling cycle, which begins with resorption. (Remodeling is described in Chapter 38.) The cause of senile (age-related) osteoporosis remains unclear, but it may be that osteoblasts and osteoclasts shrink, regress to a former state, or undergo alterations that diminish their activity. Reduction in physical activity in older persons may also be a major factor in the bone loss, because preservation of bone mass is dependent on skeletal stress through muscle contraction and weight bearing.

Insufficient intake or malabsorption of dietary minerals, particularly calcium, is probably a factor in the development of osteoporosis. Calcium absorption from the intestine decreases with age, and studies of individuals with osteoporosis show that their calcium intake is lower than that of age-matched controls. Deficiencies of protein and vitamins, particularly vitamins C and D, also contribute to bone loss. Excessive intakes of caffeine, alcohol, and nicotine have also been considered risk factors (Harrison, 1989).

A variety of hormonal imbalances also may contribute to osteoporosis. Skeletal homeostasis depends on a very narrow range of plasma calcium and phosphate concentrations, which are maintained by the endocrine system. Therefore, endocrine dysfunction ultimately can cause metabolic bone disease. The hormones most commonly associated with osteoporosis are parathyroid hormone (hyperparathyroidism), cortisol (Cushing syndrome), thyroid hormone (hyperthyroidism), and growth hormone (acromegaly). (Endocrine function is discussed in Unit VI.) Decreased testosterone levels contribute to male osteoporosis (Francis, Scane, Johnson, Sutcliffe, & Sutcliffe, 1992).

Iatrogenic osteoporosis sometimes develops temporarily in individuals receiving large doses of heparin, perhaps because heparin promotes bone resorption by decreasing collagen synthesis or by increasing collagen breakdown. Osteoporosis caused by heparin therapy usually resolves when therapy ceases.

Regional osteoporosis—osteoporosis confined to a region or segment of the appendicular skeleton—usually has a known cause. Classic regional osteoporosis is associated with disuse or immobilization of a limb because of fractures, motor paralysis, or bone or joint in-

flammation. A negative calcium balance develops early and continues throughout the period of immobilization. After 8 weeks of immobilization, significant osteoporosis is present, although it may develop earlier in persons younger than 20 or older than 50 years. The pattern of bone loss may be uniform, spotty, or bandlike. Uniform bone loss usually occurs after long immobilization, for example, in quadriplegics or after an amputation. The bone loss initially appears in the appendicular skeleton or pelvis within 2 to 3 months after the paralysis. A uniform distribution of osteoporosis has also been observed in astronauts and in individuals treated with air suspension therapy as a result of weightlessness.

Pathophysiology

Whatever the cause, osteoporosis develops when the remodeling cycle—the process of bone resorption and bone formation—is disrupted, leading to an imbalance in the coupling process. There are two mechanisms of bone loss occurring in two stages: rapid bone loss and slow bone loss. A complete remodeling cycle, consisting of basic multicellular unit activation (see Chapter 38), bone resorption, and bone formation, takes approximately 4 months in a normal, healthy adult. In an individual with osteoporosis, 2 years may be needed to complete one cycle. In normal bone, the frequency of multicellular unit activation, the rate of resorption, and the rate of new bone formation are relatively constant, so that replacement follows resorption immediately and the amount of bone replaced equals the amount of bone resorbed. In bones affected by osteoporosis, this equilibrium can be disrupted by (1) an increase in the number of basic multicellular units activated, (2) an increase in the frequency of basic multicellular unit activation, (3) an increase in the rate of resorption, (4) a delay in the rate of bone formation, or (5) a deficiency of cells in the multicellular unit. Any one of these changes causes a net decrease in total bone mass. Rapid bone loss occurs during early menopause and is osteoclast-mediated, whereas slow bone loss is osteoblast-mediated, occurring later after early menopause.

If the number of basic multicellular units increases, resorption occurs at more sites, or loci. Loci of resorption become so numerous that new bone is destroyed along with old bone, creating a state of "runaway" resorption. If a normal number of basic multicellular units is activated with abnormal frequency, the result is a net increase in the total amount of bone lost in a given period of time.

Another mechanism causing osteoporosis is an imbalance between the rate of resorption and the rate of new bone formation. Some hormones and drugs are thought to interfere with the relationship between osteoclast activity (bone resorption) and osteoblast (bone formation) activity. Anything that causes resorption to speed up or replacement to slow down causes resorption cavities to persist, weakening the bone.

Osteoporosis also occurs if the basic multicellular units fail to complete the three phases of the remodeling cycle. Failure occurs if there are inadequate numbers of osteoclasts and osteoblasts in bone tissue. Completion of the remodeling cycle requires delivery of a continuous supply of bone cell precursors from the marrow. Any interruption in the bone's vascular system will interfere with the delivery of osteoclast and osteoblast precursors to bone tissue.

Age-related bone loss occurs when bone formation decreases faster than bone resorption, particularly in the fourth decade. Losses are at the rates of 0.3% to 0.5% yearly in both men and women (Liscum, 1992). Men have approximately 30% greater bone mass than women (Scott, 1990), which may be a factor in their later involvement with osteoporosis.

Clinical Manifestations

The specific clinical manifestations of osteoporosis depend on the bones involved. The most common manifestations, however, are pain and bone deformity. Fractures are likely to occur because the trabeculae of spongy bone become thin and sparse, and compact bone becomes porous. As the bones lose volume, they become brittle and weak and may collapse or become misshapen. Vertebral collapse causes kyphosis (hunchback) and diminishes height. Fractures of the long bones (particularly the femur and humerus), the distal radius, ribs, and the vertebrae are most common. Fracture of the neck of the femur—the so-called broken hip—tends to occur in older or elderly women with osteoporosis. Fatal complications of fractures include fat or pulmonary embolism, hemorrhage, and shock. Approximately 20% of persons may die as a result of surgical complications. Male osteoporosis also is noted by hypogonadism in about 20% of persons, low plasma levels of 1,25 dihydroxyvitamin D, and malabsorption of calcium (Francis et al., 1992).

Evaluation and Treatment

Generally, osteoporosis is detected radiographically as increased radiolucency of bone. By the time abnormalities are detected by x-ray examination, approximately 25% to 30% of bone tissue has been lost (Milgrim, 1990). Types of radiologic examinations include single- or dual-photon absorptiometry and computed tomography (CT) scans. Other evaluation procedures include tests for levels of serum calcium, phosphorus, and alkaline phosphatase, and protein electrophoresis. Body calcium levels also can be measured by neuron activation analysis, a procedure involving use of radioactive ^{49}Ca, whose gamma activity can be measured with a whole body counter (Harrison, 1989).

The goals of osteoporosis treatment are to slow down the rate of calcium and bone loss and to stop the disease before it progresses too far. Treatment includes increasing the dietary intake of calcium up to 1500 mg/day and vitamin D supplements to increase the intestinal absorption of calcium. Regular, moderate weight-bearing exercise can slow down the bone loss and, in some cases, reverse demineralization because the mechanical stress of exercise stimulates bone formation. Postmenopausal women are given estrogen and progestins in addition to exercise and dietary supplements of calcium and vitamin D.

An increased risk of endometrial carcinoma is associated with estrogen therapy used to treat postmenopausal women with an intact uterus. With estrogen administered cyclically with progestins, this risk is decreased and the combined estrogen-progestin therapy is given to women, particularly those in the first 10 years after menopause, to aid bone retention. Yet, although controversial, combined estrogen-progestin therapy may be a risk factor for breast cancer (see Chapter 20). A woman taking these hormones needs an annual gynecologic examination because of associated cancer-related side effects, including phlebitis and emboli, and cyclical uterine bleeding. Recent changes to continuous estrogen-progestin administration, however, avoid the cyclical uterine bleeding (Stevenson, 1992).

Other treatments include intramuscular calcitonin given daily, sodium fluoride given orally (experimentally), and etidronate disodium (Didronel) given in a cyclic manner of 400 mg orally daily for 2 weeks every 3 months (Licata, 1991). Males with osteoporosis are treated with testosterone, and one center has reported a 6% increase in spine bone density after this treatment (Francis et al., 1992).

Osteomalacia

Osteomalacia is a metabolic disease characterized by inadequate and delayed mineralization of osteoid in mature compact and spongy bone. In osteomalacia, the remodeling cycle proceeds normally through osteoid formation, but mineral calcification and deposition do not occur. Bone volume remains unchanged, but the replaced bone consists of soft osteoid instead of rigid bone. Rickets is similar to osteomalacia in pathogenesis, but it occurs in the growing bones of children, whereas osteomalacia occurs in adult bone. (Rickets is described in Chapter 40.)

Both osteomalacia and rickets are rare in the United States and western Europe but are significant health problems in Great Britain, Ethiopia, Pakistan, Iran, and India. In the United States, these diseases are prevalent in the elderly, in premature infants of very low birth weight, and in individuals adhering to rigid macrobiotic vegetarian diets.

Many factors contribute to the development of osteomalacia, but the most important is a deficiency of vitamin D. The major risk factors in vitamin D deficiency are diets deficient in vitamin D, decreased endogenous production of vitamin D, intestinal malabsorption of vitamin D, renal tubular diseases, and anticonvulsant therapy. Classic vitamin D deficiency is rare in the United States because of the addition of synthetic vitamin D to dairy products and bread.

Disorders of the small bowel, hepatobiliary system, and pancreas are common causes of vitamin D deficiency in the United States, however. In malabsorptive disease of the small bowel, vitamin D and calcium absorption are decreased, so that vitamin D is lost in feces. Liver disease interferes with the metabolism of vitamin D to its more active form, and diseases of the pancreas and biliary system cause a deficiency of bile salts, which are necessary for normal intestinal absorption of vitamin D.

The mechanism by which anticonvulsant drug therapy results in vitamin D deficiency is incompletely understood, but researchers think that the anticonvulsants phenobarbital and phenytoin interfere with calcium absorption in the intestine and with vitamin D metabolism in the liver.

Pathophysiology

Crystallization of minerals in osteoid requires adequate concentrations of calcium and phosphate. When the concentrations are too low, crystallization (and hence ossification) does not proceed normally.

Vitamin D deficiency disrupts mineralization because vitamin D normally regulates and enhances the absorption of calcium ions from the intestine. A lack of vitamin D causes the plasma calcium concentrations to fall. Low plasma calcium levels stimulate increased synthesis and secretion of parathyroid hormone. Although the increase in circulating parathyroid hormone raises the plasma calcium concentration, it also stimulates increased renal clearance of phosphate. When the concentration of phosphate in the bone decreases below a critical level, mineralization cannot proceed normally.

Abnormalities occur in both spongy and compact bone. Trabeculae in spongy bone become thinner and fewer, whereas haversian systems in compact bone develop large channels and become irregular. Because osteoid continues to be produced but not mineralized, abnormal quantities of osteoid build up, coating the trabeculae and the linings of the haversian canals. Excessive osteoid also can accumulate in areas beneath the periosteum. The excess of osteoid leads to gross deformities of the long bones, spine, pelvis, and skull.

Clinical Manifestations

Osteomalacia causes varying degrees of diffuse skeletal pain and tenderness. Pain is noted, particularly in the hips, and the individual may be hesitant to walk. Muscular weakness is common and may contribute to a waddling gait. Bone fractures and vertebral collapse occur with minimal trauma. Low back pain may be an early complaint, but pain may also involve ribs, feet, other areas of the vertebral column, and other sites.

Evaluation and Treatment

Osteomalacia is evaluated based on radiographic findings of radiolucent bands perpendicular to the surface of the bone and presence of pseudofracture, most commonly in the medial edges of long bone shafts (Marx, 1989). Other tests used to detect osteomalacia are plasma concentrations of calcium and phosphate, and tests of proximal tubular function in the kidney. Ultraviolet radiation therapy and dietary supplements of vitamin D and calcium are used to treat vitamin D deficiency.

Paget Disease

Paget disease (osteitis deformans) is a state of increased metabolic activity in bone. It is characterized by abnormal and excessive bone remodeling, both resorption and formation. Chronic accelerated remodeling eventually enlarges and softens the affected bones.

Paget disease can occur in any bone, but it most often affects the axial skeleton, especially the vertebrae, skull, sacrum, sternum, and pelvis. The femur is often affected in the appendicular skeleton. The disease process may occur in one or more bones without causing significant clinical manifestations.

Paget disease can occur with equal frequency in men and women older than 40 years of age. Because it is often symptomless and can only be diagnosed by invasive procedures, few epidemiologic data are available. Autopsy data from England and Germany indicate that approximately 3% to 4% of the population older than 40 years of age are afflicted with the disease. The disease is most prevalent in Australia, Great Britain, New Zealand, and the United States. Paget disease sometimes affects several members of the same family, leading to some speculation that it is inherited as an autosomal dominant trait.

The cause of Paget disease is unknown, but various researchers have suggested that it is the result of inflammatory processes, viral infection, benign or malignant bone tumors, vitamin D deficiency during childhood, mechanical stress to bone, autoimmune dysfunction, vascular disorders, or hormonal deficiencies. To date, however, little research has been done to support any of these hypotheses. Classic Paget disease arises as a consequence of disorderly bone resorption and formation (Singer & Mills, 1989).

Pathophysiology

Paget disease begins with excessive resorption of spongy bone. The trabeculae diminish, and bone marrow is re-

FIG. 39-8 Paget disease. Extensive Paget disease of clavicle of 60-year-old man. Note distortion and changes in cortex. (From Rosai, J. [1981]. *Ackerman's surgical pathology* [6th ed.]. St. Louis, Mosby–Year Book.)

placed by extremely vascular fibrous tissue (Fig. 39-8).

The resorption phase of Paget disease is followed by the formation of abnormal new bone at an accelerated rate. The collagen fibers are disorganized, and glycoprotein levels in the matrix decrease. Mineralization may extend into the bone marrow. Bone formation is excessive around partially resorbed trabeculae, causing them to thicken and enlarge. Eventually, Paget disease progresses to an inactive phase, in which abnormal remodeling is minimal or absent.

Clinical Manifestations

In the skull, abnormal remodeling is first evident in the frontal or occipital regions; then it encroaches on the outer and inner surfaces of the entire skull. The skull thickens and assumes an asymmetric shape. Thickened segments of the skull may compress areas of the brain, producing altered mentality and dementia. Impingement of new bone on cranial nerves causes sensory abnormalities, impaired motor function, deafness, atrophy of the optic nerve, and obstruction of the lacrimal duct. Headache is commonly noted.

Extensive alterations of the facial bones are rare except in the jaw, where sclerosis and thickening of the maxilla and mandible displace teeth and produce malocclusion. In long bones, resorption begins in the subchondral regions of the epiphysis and extends into the metaphysis and diaphysis. Occasionally, Paget disease affects both ends of a tubular bone. In the femur, Paget disease produces an exaggerated lateral curvature. In the tibia, anterior curvature is also exaggerated. Stress fractures are common in the lower extremities.

Clinical manifestations of Paget disease in the vertebral column depend on the level of involvement and are due to compression of adjacent structures. In the cervical spine, cord compression can lead to spastic quadriplegia. Approximately 1% of persons with Paget disease develop osteogenic sarcoma.

Evaluation and Treatment

Evaluation of Paget disease is made on the basis of radiographic findings of irregular bone trabeculae with thickened and disorganized pattern. Early disease is detected by bone scanning that shows increased uptake of bone radionuclides.

Most individuals require no treatment because the disease is localized and does not cause symptoms. Treatment during active disease is for pain relief, prevention of deformity, or fracture. Etidronate disodium (Didronel), corticosteroids, calcitonin, and cytotoxic drugs are sometimes used to slow excessive resorption.

Infectious Bone Disease: Osteomyelitis

Infectious bone disease is expensive and difficult to treat and often culminates in extensive physical disability. Several factors contribute to the difficulty in treating bone infection:

1. Bone contains multiple microscopic channels that are impermeable to the cells and biochemicals of the body's natural defenses. Once bacteria gain access to these channels, they are able to proliferate unimpeded.
2. The microcirculation of bone is highly vulnerable to damage and destruction by bacterial toxins.

Vessel damage causes local thrombosis (blockage) of the small vessels, which leads to ischemic necrosis (death) of bone.

3. Bone cells have a limited capacity to replace bone destroyed by infections. Initially, osteoclasts are stimulated by infection to resorb bone, which opens up isolated bone channels so that cells of the inflammatory and immune systems can gain access to the infected bone. At the same time, however, resorption weakens the structural integrity of the bone. New bone formation usually lags behind resorption, and the Haversian systems in the new bone are incomplete.

Osteomyelitis is a bone infection caused by bacteria; however, fungi, parasites, and viruses also can cause bone infection (Fig. 39-9). It is further categorized according to the pathogen's mode of entry into bone tissue. **Exogenous osteomyelitis** is an infection that enters from outside the body, for example, through open fractures, penetrating wounds, or surgical procedures. In exogenous osteomyelitis, the infection spreads from soft tissues into adjacent bone. The other type of osteomyelitis, termed **hematogenous osteomyelitis,** is caused by pathogens carried in the blood from sites of infection elsewhere in the body. In hematogenous osteomyelitis, the bone infection spreads from bone outward to adjacent soft tissues. Hematogenous osteomyelitis is commonly found in infants, children, and the elderly. (Osteomyelitis in children is discussed in Chapter 40.) In infants, incidence rates among males and females are approximately equal. In children and older adults, however, males are most commonly affected. Osteomyelitis is a common complication of sickle cell anemia (Milgrim, 1990).

Staphylococcus aureus is the usual cause of hematogenous osteomyelitis. Others include *Streptococcus* B, *Haemophilus influenzae, Salmonella,* and gram-negative bacteria. *Streptococcus* B and *H. influenzae* tend to infect young children; *Salmonella* infection is associated with sickle cell anemia; and gram-negative infections are most common in older adults and individuals with impaired immunity.

Cutaneous, sinus, ear, and dental infections are the primary sources of bacteria in hematogenous bone infections. Soft tissue infections, disorders of the gastrointestinal tract, infections of the genitourinary system, and respiratory infections are also important sources of bacterial contamination.

The vulnerability of specific bone depends on the anatomy of its vascular supply. In children, the long bones of the extremities (tibia, humerus, femur) are particularly susceptible to hematogenous infection. The bacteria pass through the bone's branching blood vessels until they reach the terminal capillaries on the metaphyseal side of the growth plate. In this area, the circulation is sluggish, creating an ideal site for bacterial growth and multiplication. The bacteria lodge in the small vascular channels, where they initiate inflammation.

In adults, hematogenous osteomyelitis is more common in the spine, pelvis, and the small bones. Microorganisms reach the vertebrae through arteries, veins, or lymphatic vessels. The spread of infection from pelvic organs to the vertebrae is well documented. Vaginal, uterine, ovarian, bladder, and intestinal infections can lead to iliac or sacral osteomyelitis.

Exogenous osteomyelitis can be caused by human bites or fist blows to the mouth. Superficial animal or human bites inoculate local soft tissue with bacteria that later spread to underlying bone. Deep bites can introduce microorganisms directly onto bone. The most common infecting organism in human bites is *S. aureus.* In animal bites, the most common infecting organism is

FIG. 39-9 Osteomyelitis. Osteomyelitis of upper femur with massive bone destruction and reactive sclerosis. (Courtesy Dr. H. Rodriguez-Martinez, Mexico City, Mexico. From Rosai, J. [1981]. *Ackerman's surgical pathology* [6th ed.]. St. Louis, Mosby–Year Book.)

Pasteurella multocida, which is part of the normal mouth flora of cats and dogs.

Direct contamination of bones with bacteria can also occur in open fractures or dislocations with an overlying skin wound. Intervertebral disk surgery and operative procedures involving implantation of large foreign objects, such as metallic plates or artificial joints, are associated with exogenous osteomyelitis. Local injections and venous punctures are significant causes of exogenous osteomyelitis. Exogenous osteomyelitis of the arm and hand bones tends to occur in drug abusers. *S. aureus* is the most common pathogen. In general, persons who are chronically ill, have diabetes or alcoholism, or are receiving large doses of steroids or immunosuppressive drugs are particularly susceptible to exogenous osteomyelitis.

Pathophysiology

Regardless of the source of the pathogen, the pathologic features of bone infection are similar to those in any other body tissue (see Chapters 6 and 7). First, the invading pathogen provokes an intense inflammatory response. Inflammation in bone is characterized by vascular engorgement, edema, leukocyte activity, and abscess formation. Once inflammation is initiated, the small terminal vessels thrombose, and exudate seals the bone's canaliculi. Inflammatory exudate extends into the metaphysis and the marrow cavity and through small metaphyseal openings into the cortex. In children, exudate that reaches the outer surface of the cortex forms abscesses that lift the periosteum off underlying bone. Lifting of the periosteum disrupts blood vessels that enter bone through the periosteum, depriving underlying bone of its blood supply, leading to necrosis and death of the area of bone infected, producing **sequestrum,** an area of devitalized bone (Fig. 39-10). Lifting of the periosteum also stimulates an intense osteo-

blastic response. Osteoblasts lay down new bone that can partially or completely surround the infected bone. This layer of new bone surrounding the infected bone is called an **involucrum.** Openings in the involucrum allow the exudate to escape into surrounding soft tissue and ultimately through the skin by way of sinus tracts.

In adults, this complication is rare because the periosteum is firmly attached to the cortex and resists displacement. Instead, infection disrupts and weakens the cortex, which predisposes the bone to pathologic fracture.

Clinical Manifestations

Clinical manifestations of osteomyelitis vary with the age of the individual, the site of involvement, the initiating event, the infecting organism, and whether the infection is acute, subacute, or chronic. Acute osteomyelitis causes abrupt onset of inflammation. If an acute infection is not completely eliminated, the disease may become subacute or chronic. In subacute osteomyelitis, signs and symptoms are usually vague. In the chronic stage, infection is indolent or silent between exacerbations. The microorganisms persist in small abscesses or fragments of necrotic bone and produce occasional flare-ups of acute osteomyelitis. The progression from acute to subacute or chronic osteomyelitis may be due to inadequate or inappropriate therapy or the development of drug-resistant microorganisms.

Acute hematogenous osteomyelitis in the child is usually manifested by a sudden onset of high fever, chills, nausea, and progressive pain at the site of bone involvement. Muscle spasm around the infected bone is common, and the child may refuse to move the affected limb. Tissues overlying the involved bone become edematous and warm because of the vascular changes and edema.

In the adult, hematogenous osteomyelitis has an in-

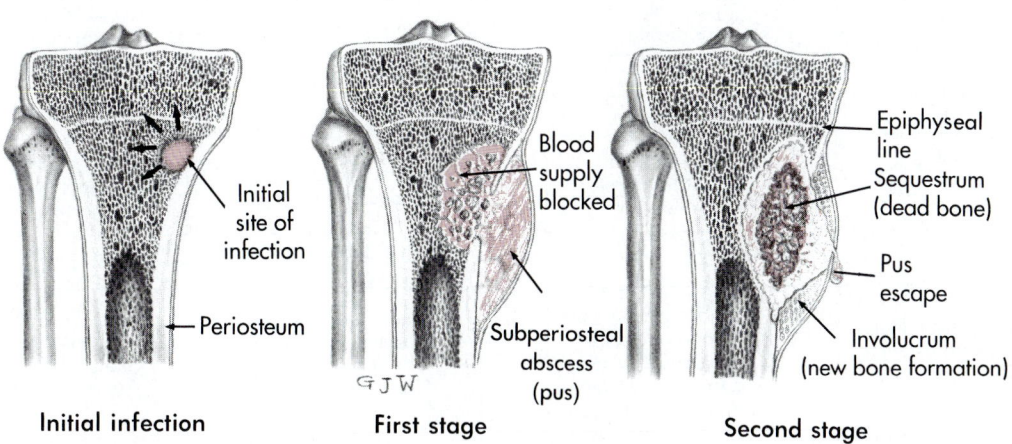

FIG. 39-10 Osteomyelitis showing sequestrum and involucrum. (From Mourad, 1991.)

sidious onset. The symptoms are usually vague and include fever, malaise, anorexia, and weight loss. Recent infection (urinary, respiratory, skin) or instrumentation (catheterization, cystoscopy, myelography, discography) usually precedes onset of symptoms.

The primary symptom of acute osteomyelitis in the spine is back pain. The pain may be intermittent or constant, aggravated by motion, and throbbing at rest. It may radiate in a radicular distribution and is commonly accompanied by spinal tenderness and rigidity. Hip contracture occurs in the presence of soft tissue inflammation as a result of irritation of the psoas muscle.

The signs and symptoms of sacroiliac ("tailbone") osteomyelitis are generally severe and include local pain, tenderness, and a limp. The pain may radiate to the buttock or the abdomen.

Single or multiple abscesses (Brodie abscesses) characterize subacute or chronic osteomyelitis. Brodie abscesses are circumscribed lesions 1 to 4 cm in diameter, usually in the ends of long bones and surrounded by dense ossified bone matrix. The abscesses are thought to develop when the infectious microorganism has become less virulent or the individual's immune system is resisting the infection somewhat successfully.

In exogenous osteomyelitis, signs and symptoms of soft tissue infection predominate. Inflammatory exudate in the soft tissues disrupts muscles and supporting structures and forms abscesses. Low-grade fever, lymphadenopathy, local pain, and swelling usually occur within days of contamination by a puncture wound. Osteomyelitis in the hand causes exquisite tenderness over the course of tendon sheaths. The fingers are usually in a semiflexed position, and extension usually causes severe pain. Palmar swelling or symmetric swelling of the fingers may be present.

Evaluation and Treatment

Evaluation of osteomyelitis is done by radionuclide bone scanning, tomography, and MRI. Tomography is a radiographic technique that produces an image of a slice through the bone rather than the whole bone. Treatment of osteomyelitis includes antibiotics and drainage of the inflammatory exudate. Tubes are placed into holes drilled into the cortex for continuous antibiotic irrigation and drainage. Chronic conditions may require surgical removal of the inflammatory exudate followed by continuous wound irrigation with antibiotic solutions in addition to systemic treatment with antibiotics. **Hyperbaric oxygen therapy** of 100% oxygen, given at 2 atmospheres pressure for 2 hours' duration/day for 30 treatments, is also beneficial for chronic refractory osteomyelitis (Mourad, 1991).

Bone Tumors

Many different types of tumors involve the skeleton. The type is determined by the tissue from which the tumor is derived. Bone tumors may originate from bone cells, cartilage, fibrous tissue, marrow, or vascular tissue. Based on the tissue of origin, bone tumors are classified as osteogenic, chondrogenic, collagenic, and myelogenic. Each of the four types arises from one of the four stem cells that are ultimately derived from the primitive mesoderm (Fig. 39-11). In addition, classifications of bone tumors may include those of histiocytic, notochordal, lipogenic, and neurogenic origins.

The mesoderm contributes the primitive fibroblast

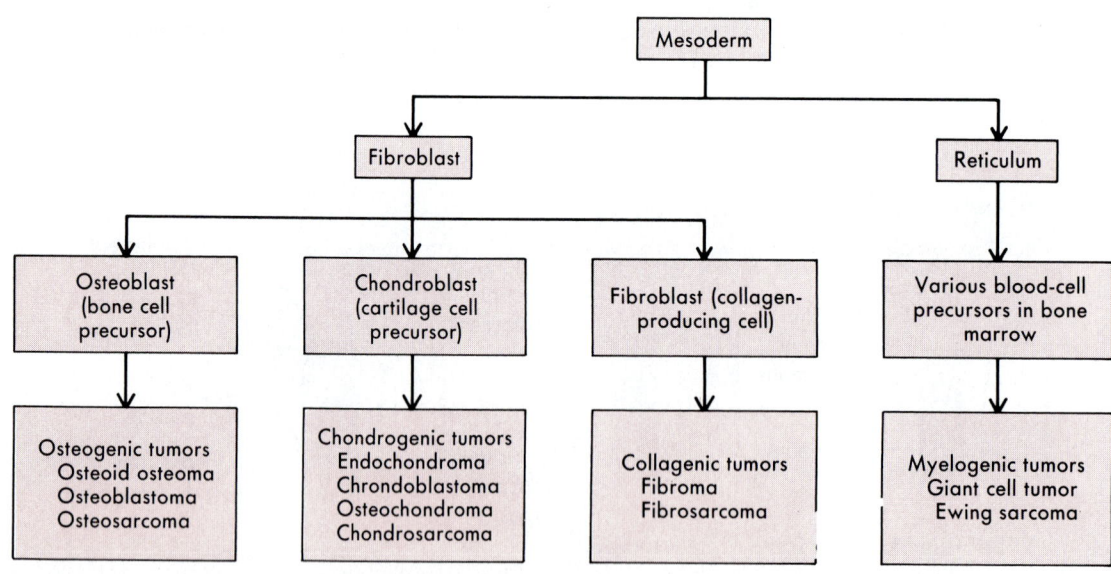

FIG. 39-11 Derivation of bone tumors.

and reticulum cells. The fibroblast is the progenitor of the osteoblast, the chondroblast, and the fibroblast or fibrous connective tissue cell. Each cell synthesizes a specific type of intercellular ground substance, and the tumor derived from the cell is generally characterized by the type of ground substance produced by the cell. For example, osteogenic tumors usually contain cells that have the appearance of osteoblasts and produce an intercellular substance that can be recognized as osteoid. Chondrogenic tumors contain chondroblasts and produce an intercellular substance similar to chondroid (cartilage). Collagenic tumors contain fibrous tissue cells and produce an intercellular substance similar to the type of collagen found in fibrous connective tissue.

Besides being classified according to the tissue of origin, tumors are also classified as benign or malignant. The differences between malignant and nonmalignant bone tumors are nebulous, primarily because the criteria used to differentiate them are vague (see Chapter 10). Generally, malignant bone tumors tend to be larger and more aggressive in their pattern of bone destruction, to invade surrounding tissue, and to initiate independent growth outside the site of origin (i.e., metastasize). Nonmalignant bone tumors, however, are less destructive to the host bone, and tend to be limited to the anatomic confines of the host bone although approximately 2% of benign giant cell tumors metastasize to pulmonary tissues (Kastrup, Buseck, & Lyons, 1992), and have a well-demarcated border. The criteria used to identify tumor cells as malignant are (1) an increased nuclear-cytoplasmic ratio, (2) an irregular nuclear border, (3) excess chromatin, (4) a prominent nucleolus, and (5) an increase in the number of cells undergoing mitosis. These criteria are sometimes confusing and misleading because many young, rapidly growing, normal cells and cells subjected to inflammation and change in their blood supply also exhibit many of these same characteristics. (Tumor characteristics in general are described in Chapter 10.)

Incidence and Cause

The incidence rate of bone tumors varies with age. In children younger than 15 years of age, the rate of bone tumors is relatively low, constituting approximately 3% of all malignancies. Adolescents have the highest incidence of bone tumors, and adults between the ages of 30 and 35 have the lowest incidence. After age 35, the incidence rate slowly increases until, at age 60, it equals the incidence rate in adolescents, primarily related to metastatic tumors.

The cause of bone tumors is highly controversial. Part of the controversy stems from the lack of a common definition for tumor. In general, tumor refers to a new growth (neoplasia) or hyperplasia of cells. The new growth may be an excessive reparative proliferation of

cells that ultimately mature. Thus, some tumors (or masses) may be the result of inflammation or trauma. Other tumors are the result of a spontaneous proliferation of cells that may or may not mature (differentiate), invade surrounding tissue, or metastasize.

Patterns of Bone Destruction

The general pathologic features of bone tumors include bone destruction, erosion or expansion of the cortex, and periosteal response to changes in underlying bone. The least amount of pathologic damage occurs with benign bone tumors, which push against neighboring tissue. Because they usually have a symmetrical, controlled growth pattern, benign bone tumors tend to compress and displace neighboring normal bone tissue, which weakens the bone's structure until it is incapable of withstanding the stress of ordinary use, leading to pathologic fracture, even though the tumor itself may be benign. Other tumors invade and destroy adjacent normal bone tissue. They do this by producing substances that promote resorption by increasing osteoclast activity or by interfering with a bone's blood supply.

Three different patterns of bone destruction by bone tumors have been identified: (1) the geographic pattern, (2) the moth-eaten pattern, and (3) the permeative pattern of bone destruction. The **geographic pattern** of bone destruction is the least aggressive and is generally indicative of a slow-growing or benign tumor. Tumors associated with the geographic pattern have well-defined margins that can be easily separated from the surrounding normal bone. There is a uniform and well-defined lytic area in the bone. The margin may be smooth or irregular, but it is clearly demarcated by a short zone of transition between normal and abnormal bone tissue. A more aggressive pattern of bone destruction is the **moth-eaten pattern.** In this pattern, the tumorous lesion has a less-defined or demarcated margin that cannot be easily separated from normal bone. There are areas of partially destroyed bone adjacent to completely lytic areas (O'Connor & Sim, 1989). The moth-eaten pattern of bone destruction is characteristic of rapidly growing, malignant bone tumors. An aggressive, malignant tumor with rapid growth potential causes the **permeative pattern** of bone destruction. In this pattern, the margins of the tumor are poorly demarcated, and abnormal bone merges imperceptibly with surrounding normal bone tissue.

Tumors that erode the cortex of the bone usually stimulate a periosteal response, that is, new bone formation at the interface between the surface of the bone and the periosteum. Slow erosion of the cortex usually stimulates a uniform periosteal response. Additional layers of bone are added to the exterior surface of the bone so as to buttress the cortex. Eventually, the additional layers expand the bone's contour. Aggressive penetration of the cortex usually elevates the periosteum and stimulates erratic patterns of new bone formation. Examples of erratic patterns include concentric layers of new bone; a sunburst pattern, in which delicate rays of new bone radiate toward the periosteum from a single focus on the underlying surface; and rays of new bone that grow perpendicularly, creating a brush or bristle pattern.

Diagnosis of Bone Tumors

The early recognition of a malignant bone tumor is critical to the survival of the individual and the preservation of the affected limb. Many bone lesions can be diagnosed at an early stage, yet early diagnosis may not occur for several reasons. Frequently, individuals may present with vague symptoms that may be attributed to minor trauma, degenerative changes, or inflammatory conditions. Also, the clinical presentation may be insidious (O'Connor & Sim, 1989). In addition, presence of other conditions may simulate primary bone tumors that may obscure the diagnosis.

Diagnostic studies must be thoroughly done to determine, if possible, the exact type and extent of bone tumor present, which also helps determine the optimal treatment regimen for the individual's specific tumor. Serum alkaline phosphatase levels will be elevated in bone lytic tumors and significantly elevated in osteosarcoma and Ewing sarcoma. Radiologic studies include plain radiologic films, a CT scan, and an MRI, which has become the examination of choice for the local staging of bone tumors, especially the staging of peripheral osteosarcomas (Brylawski, 1991) (Table 39-3). Magnetic resonance imaging is also used to monitor the response of osteosarcomas to radiation or chemotherapy and to detect recurrent disease. A CT scan is used to evaluate involvement of osteosarcoma in flat bones when the tumor is not well defined on a plain film, to assist in differentiating the tumor as a possible osteoid osteoma from a high-grade or blastic type of osteosarcoma, and to locate pulmonary metastases, if present. Such radiologic studies show a hard, firm destructive mass with elevated periosteum of the involved bone. Sunburst striations and "onion skin" of the periosteum are common in osteosarcomas. Radionucleotide bone scans show an increased uptake at the tumor site.

Additional diagnostic studies done for specific bone tumors include a complete blood count and erythrocyte sedimentation rate (to rule out infection, myeloma, or Ewing sarcoma); serum levels of calcium/phosphorus to detect hypercalcemia; serum glucose levels may be elevated in chondrosarcoma; acid phosphatase may show moderate elevations in bone metastases, multiple myeloma, and advanced Paget disease; and serum protein electrophoresis/immunoelectrophoresis to rule out multiple myeloma (Kastrup et al., 1992). Percutaneous or fine needle biopsy is done, usually at the time of surgery, to determine the exact tumor type (Heare, Enneking, & Heare, 1990).

Types of Tumors

An uncommonly large number of lesions are classified as bone tumors. Described here are the bone tumors most representative of the four derivative types (Fig. 39-11): osteogenic, chondrogenic, collagenic, and myelogenic tumors.

Osteogenic tumors: osteosarcoma

Osteogenic tumors (bone-forming tumors) are characterized by the formation of bone or osteoid tissue with a sarcomatous tissue. The tissue can have the appearance of callus or compact or spongy bone. The most common bone-forming tumor is the osteosarcoma.

Osteosarcomas account for 38% of bone tumors. Osteosarcoma occurs 3:2 times as frequently in males as

---

TABLE 39-3

Surgical Staging System for Bone Tumors

Stage	Grade	Site (T)	Metastasis (M)
IA	Low (G_1)	Intracompartmental (T_1)	None (M_0)
IB	Low (G_1)	Extracompartmental (T_2)	None (M_0)
IIA	High (G_2)	Intracompartmental (T_1)	None (M_0)
IIB	High (G_2)	Extracompartmental (T_2)	None (M_0)
IIIA	Low (G_1)	Intracompartmental or extracompartmental (T_1 or T_2)	Regional or distant (M_1)
IIIB	High (G_2)	Intracompartmental or extracompartmental (T_1 or T_2)	Regional or distant (M_1)

From Mourad, L. A. (1991). *Orthopedic disorders*. St. Louis: Mosby–Year Book.

in females, predominantly in adolescents and young adults. Sixty percent of osteosarcomas occur in the under-20 age group. A secondary peak incidence for osteosarcoma occurs in the 50 to 60 age group, primarily in individuals with a history of Paget disease (Fig. 39-12), as a complication of radiation therapy.

Osteosarcoma is a malignant bone-forming tumor. It is large, destructive, and most often found in bone marrow, and it has a moth-eaten pattern of bone destruction. The borders of the tumor are indistinct and merge into adjacent normal bone. Osteosarcomas always contain osteoid and callus, which is produced by anaplastic stromal cells. Anaplastic cells are atypical, abnormal cells not seen in normal developing bone; they are neither normal nor embryonal. The osteosarcoma may also contain chondroid (cartilage) and fibrinoid tissue that may form the bulk of the tumor. The osteoid is deposited as thick masses or "streamers" between the trabeculae of callus, which infiltrate the normal compact bone, destroy it, and replace it with dense callus and masses of osteoid. Demonstrating the presence of osteoid aids in the diagnosis of osteosarcoma. Bone tissue produced by osteosarcomas never matures to compact bone.

Ninety percent of osteosarcomas are located in the metaphyses of long bones, especially the distal femoral metaphysis. Fifty percent of osteosarcomas occur around the knee area. The tumor typically breaks through the cortex, lifts the periosteum, and forms a soft tissue mass that is *not* covered by a smooth shell of new bone. Lifting of the periosteum stimulates bizarre patterns of new bone formation called a periosteal reaction.

Three distinct osteosarcomas occur on the surface of long bones and are now called parosteal, periosteal, and high-grade surface osteosarcoma (Olson & Griffiths, 1990), and dedifferentiated parosteal and central osteosarcoma (Klein, Kenan, & Lewis, 1989).

The most common initial symptoms are pain and swelling. Initially, the pain is slight and intermittent, but within a short time the pain increases in severity and duration. Pain is usually worse at night and gradually requires medication. Systemic symptoms are uncommon. Usually, a coincidental history of trauma is noted. Occasionally, the individual may present with a pathologic fracture.

Surgery is a major treatment of choice, with the location of the tumor, its size, malignancy grade, and evidence of metastasis dictating the type and extent of surgery (Finn & Simon, 1989). Preoperative chemotherapy has greatly increased the number of individuals qualifying for limb salvage surgery.

Amputation was the most common treatment for osteosarcoma; however, in some cases, the tumor and the tissue around it can be removed without amputation. Limb salvaging procedures have been made possible by advances in reconstructive techniques and endoprosthetics. Limb salvage ultimately may be successful in as

B

FIG. 39-12 Osteosarcoma. A, Osteosarcoma of upper end of humerus associated with fracture and Paget disease. B, Point of fracture of humerus shown in A demonstrating extension of hemorrhagic neoplasm up shaft and out into soft tissues. Note porous, thickened cortical bone of Paget disease. (From Rosai, 1981.)

many as 80% of persons. Individuals must have achieved most of their bone growth to be a candidate for limb salvage procedures. Skeletally immature individuals may have a limb salvage operation, referred to as a rotationplasty, in which the major portions of the thigh, including the tumor, together with the contaminated knee are resected while preserving the nerve supply (sciatic) to the leg and foot. The proximal tibia is internally fixed to the stump of the proximal femur after it has been rotated 180°. The foot is positioned at a desired spot or direction, allowing the ankle joint to function as a knee joint with the foot supplying the traditional role of the tibial stump in a below-knee amputation (Krajbich, 1991). Rotationplasty is used for osteosarcomas located in the proximal or distal femur or proximal tibia. A recent study of 16 children and adolescents having rotationplasty yielded results that 11 of the 16 have no evidence of recurrent or residual disease after operation, two individuals have died, and three are alive with pulmonary disease under treatment (Krajbich, 1991).

FIG. 39-13 Gross appearance of peripheral chondrosarcoma of pelvic bone. Huge tumor mass with heavy calcification protrudes into pelvis. (From Rosai, 1989.)

After an amputation, individuals are followed closely with chest roentgenograms and CT. Pulmonary metastases are surgically resected and chemotherapy is now a common therapy given both before and after operation, using combinations of doxorubicin (Adriamycin), cis-diaminedichloroplatinum-II (CDP), and amethopterin (Methotrexate) with citrovorum factor (Brylawski, 1991).

Chondrogenic tumors: chondrosarcoma

Chondrogenic tumors (cartilage-forming tumors) produce cartilage or **chondroid,** a primitive cartilage or cartilagelike substance. The most common chondrogenic tumor is chondrosarcoma.

Chondrosarcoma is a tumor of middle-aged and older adults. Most cases of primary chondrosarcoma are found in persons between 50 and 60 years of age. Secondary chondrosarcoma (a chondrosarcoma derived from an **endochondroma**) occurs most frequently in young adults between 20 and 30 years of age. The tumor is found more frequently in men than in women.

A chondrosarcoma is a large, ill-defined malignant tumor that infiltrates trabeculae in spongy bone. It occurs most often in the metaphysis or diaphysis of long bones, especially the femur, and in the bones of the pelvis (Fig. 39-13). The tumor contains large lobules of hyaline cartilage that are separated by bands of fibrous tissue and anaplastic cells. If located near the end of the bone, the tumor will infiltrate into the joint space. The tumor expands and enlarges the contour of the bone, causes extensive erosion of the cortex, and expands into the soft tissues.

Symptoms associated with the chondrosarcoma have an insidious onset. Local swelling and pain are the usual presenting symptoms. At first the pain is intermittent, then it gradually intensifies and becomes constant. It may waken the person at night.

Diagnostic studies include radiographs, which must be reviewed thoroughly for accurate diagnosis. Biopsy is done at the time of surgery to prevent seeding of tumor cells from earlier biopsy. Sufficient tumor material must be obtained to facilitate an accurate diagnosis.

Surgical excision is generally regarded as the treatment of choice. Many surgically treated individuals demonstrate recurrences, however, so amputation is becoming one treatment of choice. Therefore, tumors located in the limbs have a better prognosis than, for example, pelvic lesions.

Collagenic tumors: fibrosarcoma

Collagenic tumors (collagen-forming tumors) produce fibrous connective tissue. The most typical collagenic tumor is the fibrosarcoma (Fig. 39-14).

Fibrosarcomas represent 4% of the primary malignant bone tumors. The incidence of fibrosarcoma has a broad age distribution. It may occur at any age, but is most common in middle-aged adults between 40 and 50 years of age. The incidence is slightly greater in females. Fibrosarcoma may also be a secondary complication of radiation therapy, Paget disease, and long-standing osteomyelitis.

Fibrosarcoma is a solitary tumor that most frequently affects the metaphyseal region of the femur or tibia. The tumor is composed of a firm fibrous mass of tissue that contains collagen, malignant fibroblasts, and occasional osteoclastlike giant cells. Collagen fibers found within the tumor are quite thin.

The tumor begins in the marrow cavity of the bone and infiltrates the trabeculae. It demonstrates a permeative growth pattern, destroys the cortex, and extends into the soft tissue. Metastasis to the lung is common.

Symptoms associated with the tumor have an insidious onset, which delays diagnosis. Pain and swelling are the usual presenting symptoms and usually indicate that the tumor has broken through the cortex. Local tenderness, a palpable mass, and limitation of motion also may

FIG. 39-14 Fibrosarcoma of tibia. Lesion produced osteolytic defect and was confused roentgenographically with giant cell tumor. (From Rosai, J. [1981]. *Ackerman's surgical pathology* [6th ed.]. St. Louis, Mosby–Year Book.)

be present. A pathologic fracture in the affected bone is frequently the reason for seeking medical help. Diagnostic studies include radiographs and MRI.

Radical surgery and amputation are the treatments of choice for fibrosarcoma. Radiation therapy is generally considered ineffective treatment for this tumor.

Myelogenic tumors

Myelogenic tumors originate from various bone marrow cells. Two types of myelogenic tumors are giant cell tumor and myeloma.

Giant cell tumor. Giant cell tumor is the sixth most common of the primary bone tumors; it accounts for 4% to 5% of the bone tumors (Schwartz & Shives, 1989). Giant cell tumors have a wide age distribution; however, they are rare in persons younger than 10 years and older than 70 years. Most giant cell tumors are found in persons between 20 and 40 years of age. Unlike most other bone tumors, giant cell tumors affect females more frequently than males.

The giant cell tumor is a solitary, circumscribed tumor that causes extensive bone resorption because of its osteoclastic origin. The tumor is rich in osteoclastlike giant cells and anaplastic stromal cells. It also may contain osteoid, callus, and collagen. The giant cell tumor is located in the center of the epiphysis in the femur, tibia, radius, or humerus (Fig. 39-15). The tumor has a slow relentless growth rate and is usually contained within the original contour of the affected bone. It may, however, extend into the articular cartilage. When the tumor extends, it is usually covered by periosteum or periosteal bone growth. The tumor also may extend into local soft tissue, but it has a low rate of metastasis to other organs or tissues, although it has a recurrence rate as high as 80% (Darr, Acker, Pesson, & D'Ambrosia, 1988).

The most common symptoms associated with the giant cell tumor are pain, local swelling, and limitation of movement. Diagnostic studies include radiographs, CT, and MRI. Cryosurgery and resection of the tumor with the use of adjuvant polymethylmethacrylate (PMMA) for bone grafts decrease recurrence and are more successful treatments than curettage and radiation. Depending on the extent of the tumor and its recurrence, amputation may be necessary.

Myeloma. Myeloma is a neoplastic proliferation of immunocytes called plasma cells. The myeloma is the most common of the primary malignant tumors of the skeleton and accounts for 27% of bone tumors. The tumor may be solitary or multifocal (known as a multiple myeloma). Approximately 15% of the detected myelomas are multiple myelomas (see Chapter 24). The myeloma is common in persons older than 40 years of age. Males are affected twice as frequently as females, and blacks have a higher incidence rate than whites.

Myelomas characteristically cause cortical and med-

A

B

FIG. 39-15 **Giant cell tumor. A,** Giant cell tumor of distant end of femur. Lesion was curetted and replaced with bone chips. **B,** Giant cell tumor shown in **A** recurred, necessitating amputation. Gross specimen demonstrates bone chips still in place, with tumor replacing femur. Review of original sections showed benign giant cell tumor, but recuts of curetted material demonstrated malignant stroma. (From Rosai, J. [1981]. *Ackerman's surgical pathology* [6th ed.]. St. Louis, Mosby–Year Book.)

ullary bone lysis and infiltrate the bone marrow. The most common initiating symptom of myeloma is pain, which may be felt in a single bone or the entire skeleton. The usual sites of pain are the lower back, the upper spine, the pelvis, ribs, and sternum. The pain is initially aching, intermittent, and aggravated by weight bearing. As the disease progresses, the pain becomes severe and prolonged. It is common for the individual with myeloma to be treated for a slipped disk or arthritis before the correct diagnosis of myeloma is established. In addition to pain, the individual may also complain of weakness, fatigue, weight loss, and anorexia.

Myeloma has a poor prognosis, and the treatment is generally palliative. Pain is relieved with narcotics and special beds may be used to lessen pain and prevent pathologic fractures. Cord decompression may be necessary in persons with spinal myeloma. Radiotherapy and chemotherapy have very limited success.

DISORDERS OF THE JOINTS

The American Rheumatism Association recognizes 13 groups of joint disease (arthropathies). Most of these disorders can be placed into two major categories: noninflammatory joint disease and inflammatory joint disease.

Noninflammatory Joint Disease

Noninflammatory joint disease is differentiated from inflammatory joint disease by: (1) the absence of synovial membrane inflammation, (2) the lack of systemic signs and symptoms, and (3) normal synovial fluid. **Degenerative joint disease** (osteoarthritis) is the most prevalent noninflammatory joint disease. Its chief pathologic feature is degeneration and loss of articular cartilage in synovial joints (Fig. 39-16). Degenerative joint disease tends to occur in men and women over 40 and becomes more common with increasing age. Although incidence rates are the same in men and women, women are more severely affected.

Medical clinicians are somewhat divided about the use of terms *degenerative joint disease* versus *osteoarthritis*. Some prefer the less accurate term degenerative arthritis (biochemically and metabolically there is no evidence of "degeneration"), and some continue to call the disorder by the descriptive term hypertrophic arthritis to distinguish osteoarthritis from "atrophic arthritis" (an old term for rheumatoid arthritis) (Mankin, 1989). The term *osteoarthritis* has been used in most recent communications and appears to be the more accepted term.

Types of Osteoarthritis

Osteoarthritis (OA) associated with known risk factors, such as joint stress, congenital abnormalities, or joint

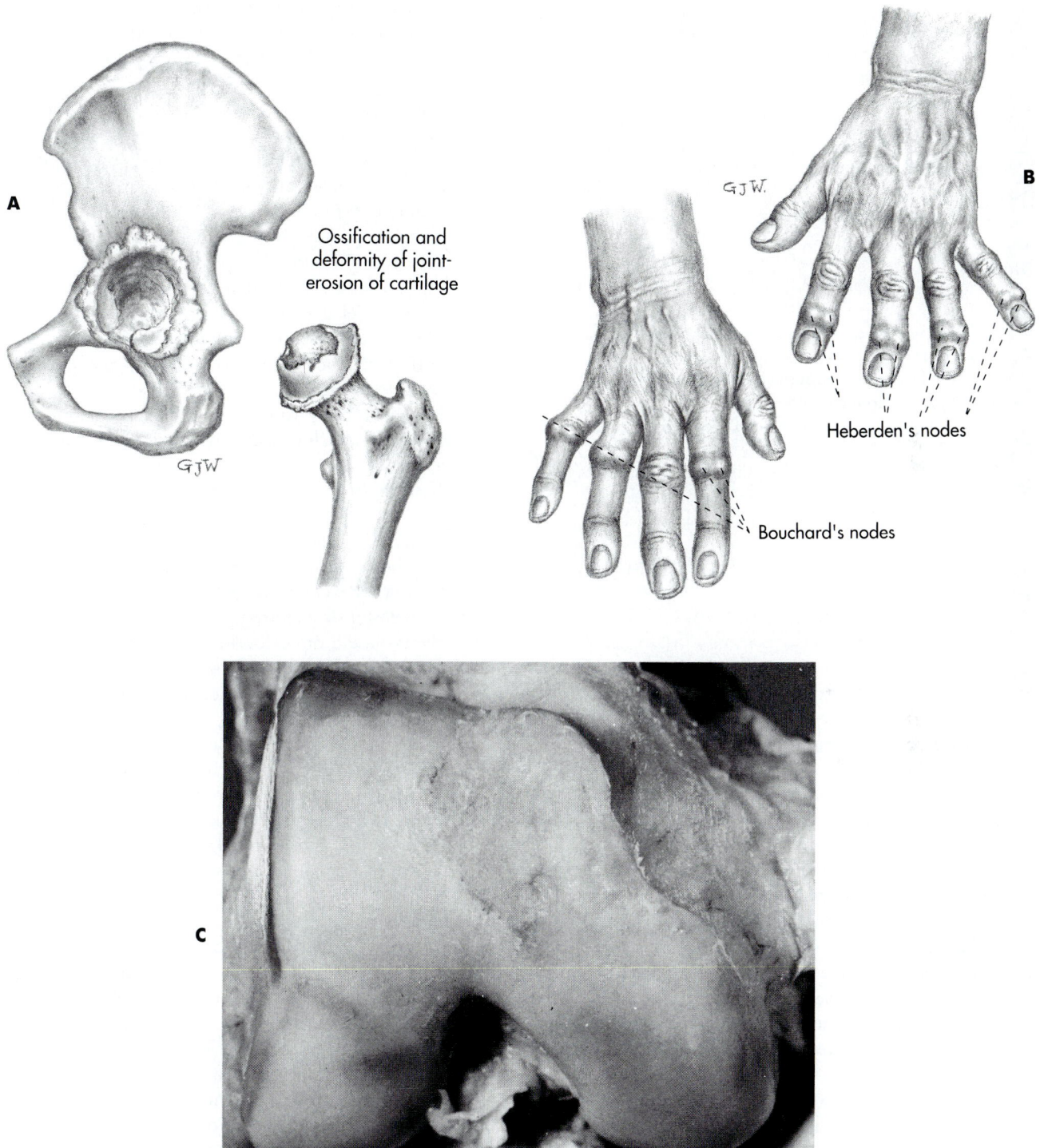

FIG. 39-16 Osteoarthritis. A, Cartilage and degeneration of the hip joint from osteoarthritis. **B,** Heberden's nodes and Bouchard's nodes. **C,** Pronounced degenerative joint disease in 55-year-old man. Note degeneration and destruction of cartilage over wide area. (**A** and **B** from Mourad, 1991; **C** from Rosai, J. [1981]. *Ackerman's surgical pathology* [6th ed.]. St. Louis: Mosby–Year Book.)

CLASSIFICATION OF OSTEOARTHRITIS

Idiopathic

Localized
  Hands (Heberden and Bouchard nodes)
  Feet (hallux valgus, hallux rigidus)
  Knee (patellofemoral, medial, or lateral compartment)
  Hip (eccentric, concentric, diffuse)
  Spine (apophyseal disease, intervertebral joints, spondylosis, Forrestier disease)
  Other single sites
Generalized (general osteoarthritis)

Secondary

Trauma (acute, chronic)
Congenital
  Localized diseases (Perthes disease, CDH, SCE)
  Mechanical factors
  Bone dysplasias (dysplasia epiphysialis multiplex, spondyloepiphyseal dysplasia)
  Metabolic (ochronosis, hemochromatosis, gout, CPPD)
  Endocrine (acromegaly, obesity, diabetes)
  Other bone and joint disease (osteonecrosis, infection, Charcot arthropathy, gout, rheumatoid arthritis)
  Diseases of obscure origin (Kashin-Bek, Mseleni)

From Clinical features of osteoarthritis. (1989). In Kelley, W. N, Harris, E. D., Jr., Ruddy, S., & Sledge, C. B. *Textbook of rheumatology* (3rd ed.). Philadelphia: Saunders.
CDH, Congenital dislocation of the hip; SCE, slipped capital epiphysis; CPPD, calcium pyrophosphate dihydrate.

instability caused by trauma, is referred to as **secondary** (see the box above). Idiopathic, formerly **primary**, OA is not associated with known risk factors. Both idiopathic and secondary OA have the same pathologic characteristics: (1) erosion of the articular cartilage; (2) sclerosis (thickening and hardening) of bone underneath the cartilage; and (3) formation of bone spurs or **osteophytes**, which grossly alter the bony contours and enlarge the joint, possibly even leading to subluxation of the bone from the joint.

Idiopathic OA is the most common type of noninflammatory joint disease, affecting more than 60 million persons in the United States alone. Almost 50% of persons show signs of OA by age 16 (Mankin, 1989), and 70% older than age 65 (Felson, 1990). OA is generally distributed throughout the peripheral and central joints of the body and affects adult men more than women. The joints most characteristically affected are in the hand, wrist, neck (lower cervical spine), lower back (lumbar spine, sacroiliac), hip, knees, ankles, and feet. Although the cause of OA is unknown, aging is the most important associated factor. With aging, the qual-

ity and quantity of the proteoglycans in cartilage decrease, rendering the cartilage more susceptible to breakdown. Evidence also suggests that primary OA may be inherited as an autosomal recessive trait, suggesting that defects in one or more of the genes encoding for the structural components of articular cartilage may cause premature cartilage degeneration (Jimenez, 1991).

Secondary OA can be caused by any condition that damages cartilage directly; subjects the joint surfaces or underlying bone to chronic, excessive, or abnormal forces; or causes instability in the joint. Specific risk factors include the following:

1. Trauma, particularly sprains, strains, joint dislocation, and fractures
2. Long-term mechanical stress associated with athletics, ballet dancing, or repetitive physical tasks
3. The presence of inflammation in joint structures, during which inflammatory cells release enzymes capable of digesting cartilage cells
4. Joint instability caused by damage to supporting structures, such as the joint capsule, ligaments, or tendons
5. Neurologic disorders (e.g., diabetic neuropathy, Charcot neuropathic joint) in which pain and proprioceptive reflexes are diminished or lost, increasing the tendency for abnormal movement, positioning, or weight bearing
6. Congenital or acquired skeletal deformities
7. Hematologic or endocrine disorders, such as hemophilia, which causes chronic bleeding into the joints, or hyperparathyroidism, which causes bone to lose calcium
8. Drugs (e.g., colchicine, indomethacin, steroids) that stimulate the activity of collagen-digesting enzymes in the synovial membrane

All of these factors alter articular cartilage in some way and accelerate the rate of cartilage loss.

Pathophysiology

The primary defect in primary and secondary osteoarthritis is loss of articular cartilage. Early in the disease, the articular cartilage loses its glistening appearance, becoming yellow-gray or brownish-gray. As the disease progresses, surface areas of the articular cartilage flake off, and deeper layers develop longitudinal fissures (fibrillation). The cartilage becomes thin and may be absent over some areas, leaving the underlying bone (subchondral bone) unprotected. Consequently, the unprotected subchondral bone becomes sclerotic (dense and hard). Cysts sometimes develop within the subchondral bone and communicate with the longitudinal fissures in the cartilage. Pressure builds in the cysts until the cystic contents are forced into the synovial cavity, breaking through the articular cartilage on the way. As the articular cartilage erodes, cartilage-coated osteophytes may grow outward from the underlying bone and alter the bone contours and joint anatomy. These spurlike bony projections enlarge until small pieces, called "joint mice," break off into the synovial cavity. If osteophyte fragments irritate the synovial membrane, synovitis and joint effusion result. The joint capsule also becomes thickened and at times adheres to the deformed underlying bone which may figure in the limitation of movement.

Articular cartilage is probably lost through enzymatic breakdown of the cartilage matrix—the proteoglycans, glycosaminoglycans, and collagen. First, the enzymes break down the macromolecules of proteoglycans, glycosaminoglycans, and collagen into large, diffusible fragments. Then the fragments are taken up by the cartilage cells (chondrocytes) and digested by the cell's own lysosomal enzymes. (Processes of cellular uptake and lysosomal digestion are described in Chapter 1.) The loss of proteoglycans from articular cartilage is a hallmark of the osteoarthritic process (Malemud, 1991).

Enzymatic destruction of articular cartilage begins in the matrix, with destruction of proteoglycans and collagen fibers. Enzymes, particularly stromelysin and acid metalloproteinase, affect proteoglycans by interfering with assembly of the proteoglycan subunit or the proteoglycan aggregate (see Chapter 38), and have been found to be elevated at least 150% in OA (Woessner & Gunya-Smith, 1991). Changes in the conformation of proteoglycans disrupts the pumping action that regulates movement of water and synovial fluid into and out of the cartilage. Without the regulatory action of the proteoglycan pump, cartilage imbibes too much fluid and becomes less able to withstand the stresses of weight bearing. Also with aging, the proteoglycan content is decreased, and water content in cartilage can be increased by as much as 8%, affecting the strength of the cartilage. Persons with OA, even those with fairly extensive cartilage destruction, have elevated levels of proteoglycans/fragments in their synovial fluid, perhaps indicative of a more pronounced reparative phase (Heinegard & Saxne, 1991). Other studies indicate that cytokines, such as interleukin-1 (see Chapter 38 for discussion of cytokines) may play a major role in cartilage degradation as a result of release and activation of proteolytic and collagenolytic enzymes (Moskowitz, Boja, & Denko, 1991) associated with an imbalance of cell responses to growth factor activity.

Enzymes that degrade collagen (i.e., collagenases) probably originate in the chondrocytes or in leukocytes. Collagen breakdown destroys the fibrils that give articular cartilage its tensile strength and exposes the chondrocytes to mechanical stress and enzyme attack. Thus a cycle of destruction begins that involves all the components of articular cartilage—proteoglycans, collagen

fibers, and chondrocytes. The serum level of circulating keratan sulfate chains provides a direct measure of the rate of catabolism of the cartilage proteoglycans and is elevated in persons with generalized OA (Thonar et al., 1991).

Clinical Manifestations

Clinical manifestations of idiopathic or secondary osteoarthritis typically appear during the fifth or sixth decade of life, although asymptomatic, articular surface changes are common after the age of 40. Pain in one or more joints is the first symptom of the disease. Examination usually shows general involvement of both peripheral and central joints. Peripheral joints most often involved are in the hands, wrists, knees, and feet. Central joints most often afflicted are in the lower cervical spine, lumbosacral spine, shoulders, and hips.

Joint structures are capable of generating a limited number of signs and symptoms. The primary signs and symptoms of joint disease are pain, stiffness, enlargement or swelling, tenderness, limited range of motion, muscle wasting, instability, partial dislocation, and deformity.

Pain is the predominant symptom of osteoarthritis. It is usually aggravated by weight bearing or use of the joint and relieved by resting the joint. Nocturnal pain is usually not relieved by rest and may be accompanied by paresthesias (numbness, tingling, or prickling). Sometimes pain is referred to another part of the body. For example, osteoarthritis of the lumbosacral spine may mimic sciatica, causing severe pain in the back of the thigh along the course of the sciatic nerve. Osteoarthritis in the lower cervical spine may cause brachial neuralgia (pain in the arm) aggravated by movement of the neck. Osteoarthritic conditions in the hip cause pain that may be referred to the lower thigh and knee area.

The actual mechanisms of joint pain are complex and poorly understood, but several explanations are possible. The pain could be caused by articular distention and stretching of the fibrous joint capsule, which has an abundant nerve supply. Inflammation of the joint capsule also causes fibrous shrinking, so that movement of the joint in any direction causes painful stretching. Pain also can arise from the subchondral or periarticular bone.

The origin of joint stiffness is unknown. Joint stiffness is generally defined as difficulty in initiating joint movement, immobility, or a loss of range of motion. The stiffness usually occurs as joint movement begins, and it dissipates rapidly after a few minutes. Enlargement and bulging of joint contour, commonly described as swelling, may be due to bone enlargement or the proliferation of osteophytes around the margins of the joint. Swelling also occurs if inflammatory exudate or blood enters the joint cavity, thereby increasing the volume of synovial fluid. This condition, termed **joint effusion,** is caused by (1) the presence of osteophyte fragments in the synovial cavity, (2) drainage of cysts from diseased subchondral bone, or (3) acute trauma to joint structures, resulting in hemorrhage and inflammatory exudation into the synovial cavity.

Range of motion is limited to some degree, depending on the extent of cartilage degeneration. Frequently, joint motion is accompanied by sounds of crepitus, creaking, or grating. Hypermobility and subluxation of joints occur in osteoarthritis secondary to a neurologic disorder.

As osteoarthritis of the lower extremity progresses, the person may begin to limp noticeably. Having a limp is distressing because it affects the person's independence and ability to do usual activities of daily living.

Evaluation and Treatment

Evaluation consists of clinical assessment and radiologic studies, CT scan, arthroscopy, and MRI. Treatment is either conservative or surgical. Conservative treatment includes rest of the involved joint until inflammation subsides; range of motion to prevent joint capsule contraction; use of a cane, crutches, or walker to decrease weight bearing; and analgesic and antiinflammatory drug therapy to reduce swelling and pain. Surgery is used to improve joint movement, correct deformity or malalignment, or create a new joint with artificial implants. There are nearly 250,000 total hip replacements yearly in the United States, most of which are related to osteoarthritis ("Robot Succeeds," 1992).

Inflammatory Joint Disease

The second major type of joint disease is **inflammatory joint disease,** commonly termed arthritis. Inflammatory joint disease is characterized by inflammatory damage or destruction in the synovial membrane or articular cartilage, and by systemic signs of inflammation (fever, leukocytosis, malaise, anorexia, hyperfibrinogenemia).

Inflammatory joint disease can be infectious or noninfectious. In infectious inflammatory joint disease, inflammation is caused by invasion of the joint by bacteria, mycoplasmas, viruses, fungi, or protozoa. These agents can invade the joint through a traumatic wound, surgical incision, or contaminated needle, or they can be delivered by the bloodstream from sites of infection elsewhere in the body, typically bones, heart valves, or blood vessels. In noninfectious inflammatory joint disease, which is the most common form, inflammation is caused by immune reactions or the deposition of crystals of monosodium urate in and around the joint. Rheumatoid arthritis and ankylosing spondylitis are noninfectious inflammatory diseases caused by immune reactions; gouty arthritis is a noninfectious inflammatory disease caused by crystal deposition.

Rheumatoid Arthritis

Rheumatoid arthritis (RA) is an autoimmune disease that causes chronic inflammation of connective tissue, primarily in the joints. (Autoimmune disease is described in Chapter 8.) The first joint tissue to be affected is the synovial membrane, which lines the joint cavity (see Chapter 38, Fig. 38-6). Eventually, inflammation may spread to the articular cartilage, fibrous joint capsule, and surrounding ligaments and tendons, causing pain, joint deformity, and loss of function (Fig. 39-17). The joints most commonly afflicted are in the fingers, feet, wrists, elbows, ankles, and knees, but the shoulders, hips, and cervical spine also may be involved, as well as the tissues of the lungs, heart, kidneys, and skin.

Rheumatoid arthritis affects 1% to 2% of adults and, like most autoimmune diseases, develops most often in women, with a female-to-male ratio of 3:1. Besides inflammation of the joints, rheumatoid arthritis can cause fever, malaise, rash, lymph node or spleen enlargement, and Raynaud phenomenon (transient lack of circulation to the fingertips and toes). There is some evidence that RA is declining in incidence and severity (Spector, 1990).

Despite intensive research, the cause of RA remains obscure. It is probably a combination of genetic, environmental, hormonal, and reproductive factors (Spector, 1990). RA probably occurs in a genetically susceptible host because of an aberrant immune response to an unidentified antigen. HLS-DR4 and DR1 have been found to be associated with RA in whites and Asians (Spector, 1990). Infectious microorganisms that may play a role in the cause of RA include bacteria, mycoplasmas, and viruses (especially Epstein-Barr virus). With long-term or intensive exposure to the antigen, normal antibodies (immunoglobulins [Ig]) become autoantibodies—antibodies that attack host tissues (self-antigens). Because they are usually present in individuals with rheumatoid arthritis, the transformed antibodies are termed **rheumatoid factors** (**RFs**). The RFs usually consist of two classes of immunoglobulin-antibodies—antibodies for IgM and IgG—but occasionally involve antibodies for IgA. Their main antigenic targets are portions of the immunoglobulin molecules. Rheumatoid factors bind with their target self-antigens in blood and synovial membrane, forming immune complexes (antigen-antibody complexes). (See Chapter 6 for a discussion about antigen-antibody binding in the immune response.)

Rheumatoid arthritis has a higher incidence in women, with evidence of hormonal involvement (James, 1991). Hormonal changes in RA show that the disease symptoms lessen during pregnancy and exacerbate in the postpartal period. Rheumatoid arthritis is also more severe in winter months (Harris, 1989).

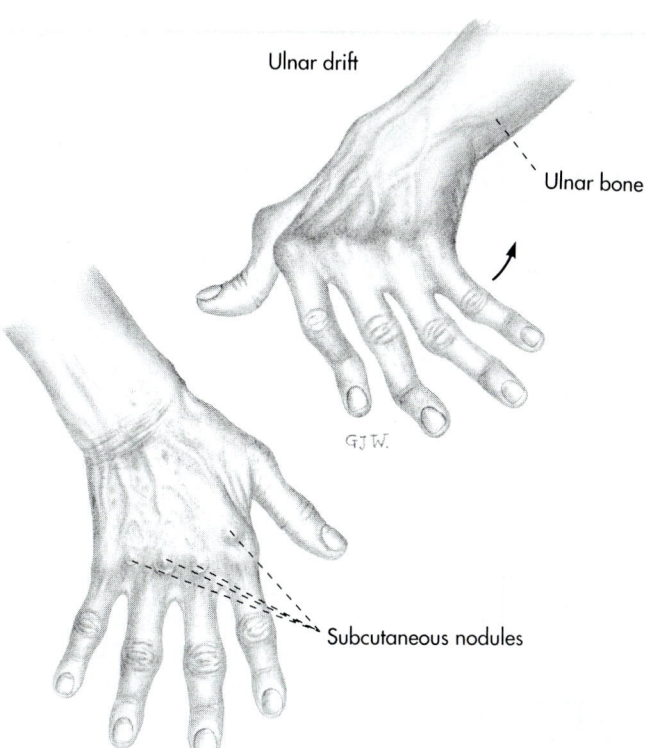

FIG. 39-17 Rheumatoid arthritis of the hand. Note swelling from chronic synovitis of metacarpophalangeal joints, marked ulnar drift, subcutaneous modules, and subluxation of metacarpophalangeal joints with extension of proximal interphalangeal joints and flexion of distal joints. Note also deformed position of thumb. Hand has wasted appearance. (From Mourad, 1991.)

Pathophysiology

Synovial inflammation (synovitis) occurs when immune complexes in blood and synovial tissue trigger the inflammatory response, chiefly by activating the plasma protein complement. (Complement activation by immune complexes is described in Chapter 7.) Complement activation stimulates kinin and prostaglandin release that increases the permeability of blood vessels in the synovial membranes and attracts leukocytes and lymphocytes to the synovial membrane.

Several types of leukocytes are attracted out of the circulation and to the synovial membrane. The phagocytes of inflammation (neutrophils and macrophages) ingest the immune complexes and, in the process of doing so, release powerful enzymes that degrade synovial tissue and articular cartilage. The immune system's B and T lymphocytes are also activated. The B lymphocytes are stimulated to produce more RFs, and the T lymphocytes produce enzymes that amplify and perpetuate the inflammatory response. Unlike the precipitating microorganism, which is killed off and removed from the body, the newly targeted self-antigens (immunoglobulins) are in relatively constant supply and can thus perpetuate in-

flammation and the formation of immune complexes indefinitely (Fig. 39-18).

Inflammatory and immune processes have several damaging effects on the synovial membrane (Fig. 39-19). Along with the swelling caused by leukocyte infiltration, the synovial membrane undergoes hyperplastic thickening as its cells proliferate and enlarge abnormally. As synovial inflammation progresses to involve its blood vessels, small venules become occluded by hypertrophied endothelial cells, fibrin, platelets, and inflammatory cells. These vascular derangements decrease vascular flow to the synovial tissue. Compromised circulation, coupled with increased metabolic needs due to hypertrophy and hyperplasia, causes hypoxia and metabolic acidosis. Acidosis stimulates the release of hydrolytic enzymes from synovial cells into the surrounding tissue, initiating erosion of the articular cartilage and inflammation in the supporting ligaments and tendons.

Inflammation causes hemorrhage, coagulation, and fibrin deposition on the synovial membrane, in the intracellular matrix, and in the synovial fluid. Over denuded areas of the synovial membrane, fibrin develops into granulation tissue called **pannus**. (Granulation tissue is the earliest tissue produced in the process of healing; see Chapter 7.) Researchers disagree about whether pannus is a cause or an effect of articular cartilage involvement in rheumatoid arthritis. Some believe that, as rheumatoid arthritis progresses, pannus extends from the synovial membrane into adjacent articular cartilage and destroys the cartilage. Other researchers think that pannus forms on articular cartilage after the cartilage has been destroyed by inflammation. In any case, pannus formation does not lead to synovial or articular regeneration but rather to formation of scar tissue that immobilizes the joint.

Clinical Manifestations

The onset of rheumatoid arthritis is usually insidious, although 8% to 15% have an acute onset (Harris, 1989). Rheumatoid arthritis begins with general systemic manifestations of inflammation, including fatigue, weakness, anorexia, weight loss, and generalized aching and stiffness. Local manifestations also appear gradually over a period of weeks or months. Typically, the joints become painful, tender, and stiff. Pain early in the disease is caused by pressure from swelling. Later in the disease pain is caused by sclerosis of subchondral bone and new bone formation. Stiffness usually lasts for about an hour after arising in the morning and is thought to be related to synovitis. Initially the joints most commonly involved are the metacarpophalangeal (MCP) joints, proximal interphalangeal (PIP) joints, and wrists.

Joint swelling, which is usually widespread and symmetrical, is caused by increasing amounts of inflamma-

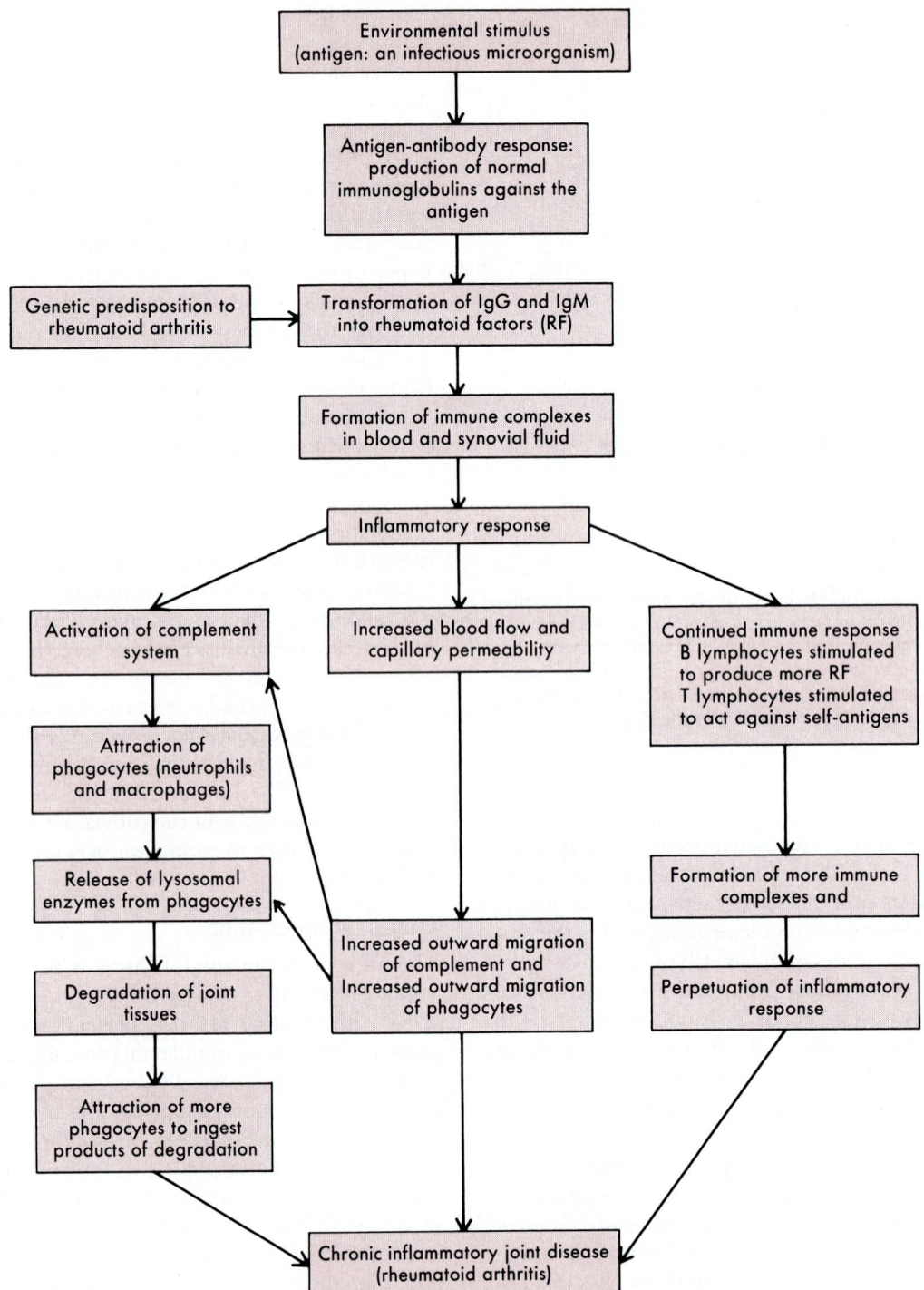

FIG. 39-18 Probable pathogenesis of rheumatoid arthritis.

FIG. 39-19 Advanced rheumatoid arthritis involving femur. There is prominent proliferation of synovium and almost complete destruction of overlying articular cartilage. (From Rosai, J. [1981]. *Ackerman's surgical pathology* [6th ed.]. St. Louis, Mosby–Year Book.)

tory exudate (leukocytes, plasma, and plasma proteins) in the synovial membrane, hyperplasia of inflamed tissues, and formation of new bone. On palpation, the swollen joint feels warm and the synovial membrane feels "boggy." The skin over the joint may have a ruddy, cyanotic hue and may look thin and shiny.

An inflamed joint may lose some of its mobility. Even mild synovitis can lead to loss of range of motion, which becomes evident after inflammation subsides. Extension becomes limited, and is eventually lost if flexion contractures form. Loss of range of motion can progress to permanent deformities of the fingers, toes, and limbs, including ulnar deviation of the hands, boutonniere and swan-neck deformities of the finger joints, plantar subluxation of the metatarsal heads of the foot, and hallux valgus (angulation of the great toe toward the other toes). Flexion contractures of the knees and hips are also common.

Joint deformities cause the physical limitations experienced by persons with rheumatoid arthritis. Loss of joint motion is quickly followed by secondary atrophy of the surrounding muscles. With secondary muscle atrophy the joint becomes unstable, which further aggravates joint pathology.

Two complications of chronic rheumatoid arthritis are caused by excessive amount of inflammatory exudate in the synovial cavity. One of these complications is the formation of cysts in the articular cartilage or subchondral bone. Occasionally, these cysts communicate with the skin surface (usually the sole of the foot) and can drain through passages called fistulas. The second complication is rupture of a cyst or of the synovial joint itself, usually caused by strenuous physical activity that places excessive pressure on the joint. Rupture releases inflammatory exudate into adjacent tissues, thereby spreading inflammation.

Extrasynovial **rheumatoid nodules,** or swellings, are observed in areas of pressure or trauma in 20% of individuals with rheumatoid arthritis. Each nodule is an aggregate of inflammatory cells surrounding a central core of fibrinoid and cellular debris. T lymphocytes are the predominant leukocytes in the nodule. B lymphocytes, plasma cells, and phagocytes are found around the periphery. Nodules are most often found in subcutaneous tissue over the extensor surfaces of elbows and fingers. They may be movable or fixed to tendons or bone.

Rheumatoid nodules also may invade the skin, cardiac valves, pericardium, pleura, lung parenchyma, and spleen. These nodules are identical to those encountered in some individuals with rheumatic fever and are characterized by central tissue necrosis surrounded by proliferating connective tissue. Also noted are large numbers of lymphocytes and occasional plasma cells. The skin nodules appear in approximately 20% of those affected with rheumatoid arthritis, mostly involving the extensor surfaces of the arms and elbows. Less common sites are the scalp, back, hands, feet, buttocks, and knees. Acute glaucoma may result with nodules forming on the sclera. Pulmonary involvement may result in diffuse pleuritis or multiple intraparenchymal nodules. Together, the occurrence of pulmonary nodules and pneumoconiosis (chronic inflammation of the lungs from inhalation of dust) creates the syndrome called **Caplan syndrome.** Diffuse pulmonary fibrosis may occur because of immunologically mediated immune complex deposition.

Rheumatoid nodules within the heart may cause valvular deformities, particularly of the aortic valve leaflets, and pericarditis. Lymphadenopathy of the nodes close to the affected joints may develop. Rheumatoid nodules within the spleen result in splenomegaly. Involvement of blood vessels results in an acute necrotiz-

1988 REVISED ARA CRITERIA FOR CLASSIFICATION OF RHEUMATOID ARTHRITIS

Criteria	Definition
1. Morning stiffness	Morning stiffness in and around the joints lasting at least 1 hour before maximal improvement
2. Arthritis of three or more joint areas	At least three joint areas have simultaneously had soft tissue swelling or fluid (not bony overgrowth alone) observed by a physician. The 14 possible joint areas are (right or left): PIP, MCP, wrist, elbow, knee, ankle, and MTP joints
3 Arthritis of hand joints	At least one joint area swollen as above in wrist, MCP, or PIP joint
4 Symmetric arthritis	Simultaneous involvement of the same joint areas (as in 2) on both sides of the body (bilateral involvement of PIP, MCP, or MTP joints is acceptable without absolute symmetry)
5. Rheumatoid nodules	Subcutaneous nodules, over bony prominences, or extensor surfaces or in juxtaarticular regions, observed by a physician
6. Serum rheumatoid factor	Demonstration of abnormal amounts of serum "rheumatoid factor" by any method that has been positive in fewer than 5% of normal control subjects
7. Radiographic changes	Radiographic changes typical of RA on PA hand and wrist x-ray, which must include erosions or unequivocal bony decalcification localized to or most marked adjacent to the involved joints (osteoarthritis changes alone do not qualify)

For classification purposes, a person is said to have RA if he or she has satisfied at least four of the above seven criteria. Criteria 1 through 4 must be present for at least 6 weeks. Individuals with two clinical diagnoses are not excluded. Designation as classic, definite, or probable rheumatoid arthritis is not to be made. (From Harris, 1989.)

---

ing vasculitis, characteristic of that noted in other immunologic/inflammatory states. Thromboses of such involved vessels may give rise to myocardial infarctions, cerebrovascular occlusions, mesenteric infarction, kidney damage, and vascular insufficiency in the hands and fingers (Raynaud phenomenon). The vascular changes are primarily noted in individuals receiving steroid therapy; thus there is some concern that the therapy may play a role in initiating these lesions. Changes in skeletal muscle are often noted in the form of nonspecific atrophy secondary to joint dysfunction.

Evaluation and Treatment

Evaluation of rheumatoid arthritis is by clinical evaluation, roentgenography of the joint, and serologic tests for rheumatoid factor and circulating immune complexes. The American Rheumatism Association lists 11 diagnostic criteria for rheumatoid arthritis (see box above). The presence of four or more of the criteria is diagnostic of rheumatoid arthritis. Criteria 1 through 4 with joint signs or symptoms must be present for 6 weeks. Designation as classic, definite, or probable rheumatoid arthritis is not to be made (Harris, 1989).

Treatment is conservative or surgical. Conservative treatment includes rest of the inflamed joint and whole-body rest for several hours daily, use of hot and cold packs, physical therapy, antineoplastic medications, diet high in calories and vitamins, corticosteroids, and anti-inflammatory drugs taken orally or injected into the joint. Surgical synovectomy may be done early in the disease to decrease inflammatory effusion and remove pannus. Surgery is used to correct deformity or mechanical deficiency in intermediate or late stages of the disease, and includes arthrodesis, arthroplasty, or total joint replacement. Recently, there is evidence that total fasting induces a substantial reduction in joint pain, swelling, morning stiffness, and other symptoms in individuals with RA (Palmblad, Hafstrom, & Ringertz, 1991).

Ankylosing Spondylitis

Ankylosing spondylitis is a chronic, inflammatory joint disease characterized by stiffening and fusion (ankylosis) of the spine and sacroiliac joints. Like rheumatoid arthritis, ankylosing spondylitis is a systemic, immune inflammatory disease. Although inflammation is the primary pathologic process in both rheumatoid arthritis and ankylosing spondylitis, the two diseases differ in the primary site of inflammation and the end result. In rheumatoid arthritis, the primary site of inflammation is the synovial membrane resulting in the destruction and instability of synovial joints. In ankylosing spondylitis, the primary pathologic site is the **enthesis**—the point at which ligaments, tendons, and the joint capsule are inserted into bone—and the end result is fibrosis, ossification, and fusion of the joint.

The incidence of ankylosing spondylitis is almost equal in men and women (Calin, 1989), but the disease tends to be more severe in men. In women, ankylosing spondylitis may affect the peripheral joints of the appendicular skeleton rather than the axial skeleton, progress less rapidly, and cause less dramatic spinal changes.

The prevalence of ankylosing spondylitis in the United States is approximately 0.5% to 1% among whites, 3% to 4% among blacks, and 18% to 50% among various tribes of American Indians (Khan & van der Linden, 1990). Worldwide, however, the disease appears to be most prevalent in whites. The prevalence of ankylosing spondylitis in males is at least 10 times greater than previously considered, and more prevalent even in females. It is clear that most individuals with ankylosing spondylitis remain undiagnosed (Calin, 1989).

Primary ankylosing spondylitis usually develops in late adolescence and young adulthood, with peak incidence at about age 20. Secondary ankylosing spondylitis affects older age groups and is often associated with other inflammatory diseases (e.g., psoriatic arthropathy, inflammatory bowel disease, or Reiter syndrome).

The cause of ankylosing spondylitis is unknown, but the disease is strongly associated with the presence of histocompatibility antigen HLA-B27 on the chromosomes of affected individuals, suggesting a genetic predisposition to the disease. *Klebsiella* infection or other "triggers" probably perpetuate the inflammatory response (Calin, 1989).

Pathophysiology

Ankylosing spondylitis begins with inflammation of fibrocartilage in cartilaginous joints, primarily in the vertebrae (see Chapter 38, Fig. 38-5). The fibrous tissue of the joint capsule, the cartilage that surrounds intervertebral disks, the entheses, and periosteum are infiltrated by inflammatory cells. As inflammatory cells (chiefly macrophages) and lymphocytes infiltrate and erode bone and fibrocartilage in joint structures, repair begins to occur. Repair is the stage of the disease process that produces disability in individuals with ankylosing spondylitis. Repair of cartilaginous structures begins with the proliferation of fibroblasts. Fibroblasts synthesize and

secrete collagen, which becomes organized into fibrous scar tissue. Eventually, the scar tissue undergoes calcification and ossification. With time, all the cartilaginous structures of the joint are replaced by ossified scar tissue, causing the joint to fuse, or lose flexibility.

Repair of eroded bone begins with osteoblast activation and proliferation. Osteoblasts lay down new bone (callus), which is remodeled and replaced by compact, lamellar bone. Bone repair changes the contour of the bone's surface because the new bone grows outward to form a new enthesis with the end of the eroded ligament. The new enthesis, which forms on top of the old one, is called **syndesmophyte**. As calcification of the spinal ligaments progresses, the vertebral bodies lose their concave anterior contour and appear square. The spine assumes the classic "bamboo spine" appearance of ankylosing spondylitis.

Clinical Manifestations

The most common signs and symptoms of early ankylosing spondylitis are low back pain and stiffness. Typically, the individual with primary disease develops low back pain during the early 20s. The pain is at first insidious but progressively becomes persistent. It is often worse after prolonged rest and is alleviated by physical activity. Early morning stiffness usually accompanies the low back pain, and the individual typically has difficulty sitting up or twisting the spine. Forward flexion, rotation, and lateral flexion of the spine are restricted and painful. Early pain and resultant loss of motion are caused by the underlying inflammation and reflex muscle spasm rather than by soft tissue or bony fusion.

As the disease progresses, the normal convex curve of the lower spine (lumbar lordosis) diminishes, and concavity of the upper spine (kyphosis) increases. The individual becomes increasingly stooped. The thoracic spine becomes rounded, the head and neck are held forward on the shoulders, and the hips are flexed (Fig. 39-20).

Inflammation in the tendon insertions of the many costosternal and costovertebral muscles can cause "pleuritic" chest pain and restricted chest movement. The pain is usually worse on inspiration. Movement in the diaphragm is normal and full. Pressure on the anterior chest wall over the sternum, ribs, and costal cartilages may cause tenderness. Tenderness over the pelvic brim may cause discomfort at night and interfere with sleep because turning onto the iliac crests causes pain. Tenderness over the ischial tuberosities may make sitting on hard seats unbearable. Tenderness in the heels may contribute to a limp or the cautious placement of the feet during walking.

Along with low back pain, many individuals may have peripheral joint involvement, uveitis, fibrotic changes in the lungs, and cardiomegaly, aortic incom-

Ossification of discs, joints, and ligaments of spinal column

Bilateral sacroiliitis

FIG. 39-20 Characteristic posture and sites of ankylosing spondylitis. (From Mourad, 1991.)

petence, amyloidosis, and Achilles tendinitis. Symptoms may include fatigue, weight loss, low-grade fever, hypochromic anemia, and an increased erythrocyte sedimentation rate (Calin, 1989).

Evaluation and Treatment

Diagnosis of ankylosing spondylitis is made from the history and physical examination, roentgenograms, and serum analysis for the presence of the histocompatibility antigen HLA-B27. Erythrocyte sedimentation rate is elevated throughout the disease to 10 to 15 mm/hr in males and 10 to 15 mm/hr in females (normal is 0 to 9 mm/hr in males, 0 to 2 mm/hr in females). Alkaline phosphatase levels are frequently elevated. Treatment of individuals with ankylosing spondylitis consists of physical therapy to maintain skeletal mobility and prevent the natural progression of contractures. Prevention of deformity and maintenance of mobility require a continuous program of physical therapy. Exercises are performed several times a day to maintain chest expansion, full extension of the spine, and complete range of motion in the proximal joints.

Antiinflammatory corticosteroids and analgesic medications are prescribed to suppress some of the pain and stiffness and to facilitate exercise. The medications do not prevent disease progression, but they do provide relief from symptoms. Surgical procedures, such as osteotomy, total hip replacement, and cervical spinal fusion, and radiation therapy are sometimes used to provide relief for individuals with end-stage disease or intolerable deformity. Persons should stop smoking to lessen pulmonary problems.

Gout

Gout is a metabolic disorder that disrupts the body's control of uric acid production or excretion, causing high levels of uric acid in the blood (hyperuricemia) and in other body fluids, including synovial fluid. When the uric acid reaches a certain concentration in fluids, it crystallizes, forming insoluble precipitates that are deposited in connective tissues throughout the body. Crystallization in synovial fluid causes acute, painful inflammation of the joint, a condition known as **gouty arthritis**. With time, crystal deposition in subcutaneous tissues causes the formation of small, white nodules, or **tophi**, that are visible through the skin. Crystal aggregates deposited in the kidneys can form urate renal stones and lead to renal failure.

In classic gouty arthritis, inflammation of the joint is caused by the formation of monosodium urate crystals. Another condition, termed pseudogout, is caused by the formation of calcium pyrophosphate-dihydrate crystals. The effect of either crystal is the same—the onset of an acute inflammatory response (see Chapter 7).

The number of people afflicted by gout is estimated at one-half million, almost all of them men. Approximately 95% of affected individuals have primary gout, in which hyperuricemia is caused by an overproduction of uric acid. The exact biochemical defect in primary gout is unknown, but many researchers suspect inherited enzyme defects. The remaining 5% to 10% of those with gout have secondary gout, in which the hyperuricemia is the result of an acquired chronic disease or a drug that interferes with the normal balance between production and excretion of uric acid.

Both primary and secondary gout are most common in men older than 40 years of age. Primary gout associated with specific enzyme defects has been diagnosed only in men. Secondary gout can afflict both men and women between the ages of 30 and 50, but gout seldom occurs in women until after menopause, probably because estrogen promotes excretion of uric acid.

Familial incidence of primary gout is reported in 18% to 50% of cases. Some studies suggest that gout is autosomal dominant; others that it is X-linked dominant or that it may be a multifactorial inheritance disease (Kelley, Fox, & Palella, 1989). The fact that hyperuricemia is associated with obesity and with alcohol, drug, and purine (a protein) consumption indicates that environmental as well as genetic factors are important in the development of gout. Primary gout is infrequent in blacks.

Secondary gout is caused by drugs or disorders that promote hyperuricemia. Diuretics are the main class of drugs thought to cause secondary gout, particularly chlorothiazide, acetazolamide, ethacrynic acid, and furosemide. These diuretics decrease the renal tubular excretion of urate. Intravenous heparin, cyclosporin, cimetidine, and ranitidine have also led to increased serum urate levels and a goutlike arthritis (Kelley et al., 1989). Other causes of decreased uric acid excretion include chronic renal disease, hypertension, and starvation. Hyperuricemia from overproduction of uric acid can be caused by myeloproliferative disorders of concern, in which metabolic processes are speeded up (e.g., leukemia); hemolytic disorders, in which cellular breakdown is speeded up (e.g., hemolytic anemia); and genetic metabolic disorders in which hyperuricemia is just one of many clinical manifestations (e.g., Lesch-Nyhan syndrome).

Pathophysiology

The pathophysiology of gout is closely linked to (1) purine metabolism (or cellular metabolism of purines) and (2) kidney function. At the cellular level, purines are synthesized to purine nucleotides, which are used in the synthesis of nucleic acids, adenosine triphosphate, cyclic adenosine monophosphate (AMP), and cyclic guanosine monophosphate (GMP). Uric acid is a breakdown product of purine nucleotides. Some individuals with gout have an accelerated rate of purine synthesis accompanied by an overproduction of uric acid. Even with restricted purine consumption, these individuals continue to overproduce uric acid. Other individuals break down purine nucleotides at an accelerated rate that also results in an overproduction of uric acid. Production of uric acid also can be the result of an increased turnover of nucleic acids, which is associated with an increased turnover of cells at other body sites. The increased turnover of nucleic acids leads to increased levels of uric acid with a compensatory increase in purine synthesis.

Kidney function is involved in the pathophysiology of gout because most uric acid is eliminated from the body through the kidneys. Urate (uric acid salt) is normally freely filtered at the glomerulus and undergoes both reabsorption and excretion within the renal tubules. In most individuals with primary gout, urate excretion by the kidneys is sluggish. The sluggish excretion may be the result of a decrease in glomerular filtration of urate or an acceleration in urate reabsorption. In addition, monosodium urate crystals are deposited in renal inter-

stitial tissues causing impaired urine flow. (Kidney function is described in Chapter 32.)

The exact process by which crystals of monosodium urate are deposited in joints and induce gouty arthritis is unknown, but several mechanisms have been proposed: (1) monosodium urate precipitates at the periphery of the body, where lower body temperatures may reduce the solubility of monosodium urate; (2) decreases in albumin or glycosaminoglycan levels decrease urate solubility; (3) changes in ion concentration and decreases of pH enhance urate deposition; and (4) trauma promotes urate crystal precipitation (Kelley et al., 1989). The monosodium urate crystals may form in the synovial fluid or in the synovial membrane, cartilage, or other connective tissues in joints and elsewhere, such as in the heart, earlobes, and kidneys. Mechanical or metabolic changes probably cause release of the crystals from connective tissues into the synovial fluid.

Monosodium urate crystals are capable of both stimulating and perpetuating the inflammatory response (Fig. 39-21). The presence of the crystals triggers the acute inflammatory response, during which neutrophils are attracted out of the circulation and begin to phagocytose (ingest) the crystals. (Processes of acute inflammation and phagocytosis are described in Chapter 7.) Tissue damage begins to occur when the neutrophils release the contents of their digestive vacuoles (lysosomes). Lysosomal contents are released from neutrophils through one of three mechanisms: (1) dissolution of neutrophils that have died of "old age" (neutrophil life span is about 2 days), (2) leakage from neutrophils that have been injured by biochemical reactions with ingested urate crystals, or (3) rupture of neutrophils during attempts to ingest exceptionally large urate crystals.

The neutrophils' lysosomes contain substances that not only damage tissues, but also perpetuate inflammation. Most tissue damage in gouty arthritis is caused by powerful lysosomal enzymes. Other lysosomal substances include the undigested urate crystals and biochemicals that attract more neutrophils to the site and trigger acute inflammation anew.

Clinical Manifestations

Gout is manifested by (1) an increase in serum urate concentration (uricemia), (2) recurrent attacks of monarticular arthritis (inflammation of a single joint), (3) deposits of monosodium urate monohydrate (tophi) in and around the joints, (4) renal disease involving glomerular, tubular, and interstitial tissues and blood vessels, and (5) the formation of renal stones. These manifestations appear in three clinical stages: (1) asymptomatic hyperuricemia, (2) acute gouty arthritis, and (3) chronic tophaceous gouty arthritis.

In asymptomatic hyperuricemia, the serum urate level is elevated but arthritic symptoms, tophi, and renal

```
┌─────────────────────────┐           ┌─────────────────────────┐
│ Overproduction of uric   │           │  Underexcretion of      │
│        acid              │           │     uric acid           │
└─────────────────────────┘           └─────────────────────────┘
              \                               /
               \                             /
                ┌─────────────────────────┐
                │      Hyperuricemia       │
                └─────────────────────────┘
                            │
                ┌─────────────────────────┐
                │ Formation of monosodium  │
                │     urate crystals       │
                └─────────────────────────┘
                            │
                ┌─────────────────────────┐            FIG. 39-21  Pathogenesis of acute gouty arthritis.
                │  Presence of crystals in │
                │     synovial fluid       │
                └─────────────────────────┘
                            │
                ┌─────────────────────────┐
                │ Acute inflammatory response│
                └─────────────────────────┘
                            │
                ┌─────────────────────────┐
                │ Attraction of neutrophils │
                └─────────────────────────┘
                            │
                ┌─────────────────────────┐
                │ Release of lysosomal contents│
                │ following neutrophil death │
                │       or damage          │
                └─────────────────────────┘
```

┌──────────────┐ ┌──────────────┐ ┌──────────────────┐ ┌──────────────────┐
│ Lysosomal   │ │ Urate crystals│ │ Biochemicals that│ │ Biochemicals that│
│   enzymes   │ │   │ │ trigger inflammation│ │ attract more neutrophils│
└──────────────┘ └──────────────┘ └──────────────────┘ └──────────────────┘
       │
┌──────────────┐
│ Tissue damage│
└──────────────┘
       │
┌──────────────┐
│ Debris from │
│ damaged tissues│
└──────────────┘

                ┌─────────────────────────┐
                │ Continued inflammation │
                └─────────────────────────┘

FIG. 39-22 Extensive involvement of knee joint and synovium by gout. In some areas, cartilage of condyles is completely missing and there is involvement of semilunar cartilages as well. Grayish white plaques represent deposits of uric acid crystals. The individual, an 83-year-old woman, had leg amputated because of arterial insufficiency, and finding of gout was unexpected. (From Rosai, J. [1981]. *Ackerman's surgical pathology* (ed. 6). St. Louis, Mosby–Year Book.)

stones are not present. Asymptomatic hyperuricemia may persist throughout life. Attacks of acute gouty arthritis and renal calculi develop with increased serum urate concentrations. Acute gouty arthritis tends to occur with sudden or sustained increases of hyperuricemia, but trauma, drugs, and alcohol also can trigger an acute attack.

Trauma is the most common aggravating factor. The great toe is subject to chronic strain in walking and, subsequently, an acute gout attack may follow long walks. Trauma associated with occupations, such as truck driving, may also precipitate an attack.

Attacks of gouty arthritis occur abruptly, usually in a peripheral joint. The primary symptom is severe pain. Approximately 50% of the initial attacks occur in the metatarsophalangeal joint of the great toe. The other 50% involve the heel, ankle, instep of the foot, knee, wrist, or elbow (Fig. 39-22). The pain is usually noticed at night. Within a few hours the affected joint becomes hot, red, and extremely tender and may be slightly swollen. Lymphangitis and systemic signs of inflammation (leukocytosis, fever, and elevated sedimentation rate) are occasionally present. Untreated, mild attacks usually subside in several hours but may persist for a day or two. Severe attacks may persist for several days or weeks. On recovery, the pain, swelling, and other symptoms resolve completely. The intervals between acute attacks of gouty arthritis are called intercritical periods. Some individuals never have a second attack. Others experience subsequent attacks 5 to 10 years after the first.

Tophaceous gout, the third and chronic stage of disease, can begin as early as 3 years or as late as 40 years after the initial attack of gouty arthritis. Progressive inability to excrete uric acid expands the urate pool until urate crystal deposits (tophi) appear in cartilage, synovial membranes, tendons, and soft tissue. The helix of the ear is the most common site of tophi, which are the characteristic diagnostic lesions of chronic gout. Each tophus consists of a deposit of urate crystals, surrounded by a granuloma made up of mononuclear phagocytes (macrophages) that have developed into epithelial and giant cells. (Granuloma formation is described in and illustrated in Chapter 7.)

Tophaceous deposits produce irregular swellings of the fingers, hands, knees, and feet. Tophi commonly form lumps along the ulnar surface of the forearm, the tibial surface of the leg, the Achilles tendon, and olecranon bursae. Tophi may produce marked limitation of joint movement and eventually cause grotesque deformities of the hands and feet. Although the tophi themselves are painless, they often cause progressive stiffness and persistent aching of the affected joint. Tophi in the upper extremities may cause nerve compressions such as carpal tunnel syndrome. Tophi in the lower extremities may cause tarsal tunnel syndrome. They may also erode and drain through the skin.

Renal stones are 1000 times more prevalent in individuals with primary gout than in the general population. The stones can be the size of a grain of sand or a piece of gravel, or can accumulate in massive deposits called staghorn calculi. They range in color from pale yellow to brown to reddish black, depending on their composition. Some stones consist of pure monosodium urate; others consist of calcium oxalate or calcium phosphate. Renal stones can form in the collecting tubules, pelvis, or ureters, causing obstruction, dilatation, and atrophy of the more proximal tubules and leading eventually to acute renal failure. Stones deposited directly in renal interstitial tissue initiate an inflammatory reaction that leads to chronic renal disease and progressive renal failure.

Treatment

The aims of gout treatment are to (1) terminate the acute gouty attack as promptly as possible, (2) prevent recurring attacks, (3) prevent or reverse complications associated with urate deposits in the joints and kidneys, and (4) prevent formation of kidney stones. Acute gouty arthritis is treated with antiinflammatory drugs. The drugs of choice are colchicine, indomethacin, and phenylbutazone. Hydrocortisone may be injected into the joint to relieve pain. Ice may also relieve some of the inflammation of the joint. Weight bearing on the involved joint is avoided until the acute attack subsides. The individual is put on a low-purine diet and high fluid intake to increase urinary output. Antihyperuricemic drugs are given to reduce serum urate concentrations.

DISORDERS OF SKELETAL MUSCLE

Muscle weakness and fatigue are common symptoms. In many cases, neural, traumatic, and psychogenic causes provide an adequate explanation for the failure to generate force (weakness) or sustain force (fatigue) seen in myopathies. Advances have been made in the understanding of the pathophysiologic mechanisms in some of the metabolic and inflammatory muscle diseases. The cause of many of the myopathies, particularly the muscular dystrophies, remains obscure (see Chapter 40). The complex interaction between muscles and nerves affects muscular function as well. (Discussions of the disorders of neuromuscular transmission are found in Chapter 14; peripheral nerve and anterior horn cell diseases are in Chapter 15.) Only inherited and acquired disorders of skeletal muscles are the focus here.

Secondary Muscular Dysfunction

Muscular symptoms arise from a variety of causes unrelated to the muscle itself. Secondary muscular phenomena (contracture, stress-related muscle tension, and immobility) are common disorders that influence muscular function.

Contractures

Several conditions cause the muscle fibers to shorten without contracting. This shortening, which is called a **contracture,** can be pathologic or physiologic. The physiologic contracture seen in primary muscle disease should be differentiated from the secondary contracture due to spasticity and paralysis. A physiologic muscle contracture occurs in the absence of a muscle action potential in the sarcolemma. Muscle shortening is explained on the basis of failure of the calcium pump in the presence of plentiful adenosine triphosphate (ATP). A physiologic contracture is seen in McArdle disease (muscle myophosphorylase deficiency) and malignant hyperthermia. The contracture is usually temporary if the underlying pathology is reversed.

A pathologic contracture is more commonly viewed as permanent muscle shortening caused by muscle spasm or weakness. Heel cord (Achilles tendon) contractures are examples of pathologic contractures. They are associated with plentiful ATP and occur in spite of a normal action potential. The most common form of contracture is seen in such conditions as muscular dystrophy (see Chapter 40) and central nervous system (CNS) injury. Contractures also may develop secondary to scar tissue contraction in the flexor tissues of a joint, as for example, contracture of burned tissues in the antecubital area of the forearm leading to a flexion contracture.

Stress-Induced Muscle Tension

Although not a uniformly recognized illness, abnormally increased muscle tension has been associated with chronic anxiety as well as a variety of stress-related muscular symptoms, including neck stiffness, back pain, and headache (Riverside Heart Institute, 1992). Abnormalities in the central nervous system, reticular activating system, and autonomic nervous system have been implicated. Although few studies have confirmed these complex interactions, the connection is intuitively plausible. For example, it is known that as an individual progressively relaxes, the amplitude of the knee jerk reflex diminishes. Conversely, individuals with absent reflexes are asked to increase tension by such maneuvers as clenching the teeth or handgrip. The underlying pathophysiology is thought to relate to the fact that as a muscle contracts, the muscle spindle is activated. This gamma-feedback system produces a series of impulses that are transmitted to the brain by the sensitive 1A afferent fibers. Unconscious tension is thought to increase the activity of the reticular-activating system as well. This influences increasing firing of the efferent loop of the gamma fibers, producing further muscle contraction and increasing muscle tension. The connection with the autonomic nervous system that regulates increased blood flow to the muscle during sympathetic activity is thought to be related to increased muscle contraction tension.

In spite of the tentative nature of the pathophysiologic claims, various forms of treatment have been used to reduce the muscle tension associated with stress. Progressive relaxation training, yoga, meditation, and biofeedback are examples of stress-reduction therapies. **Biofeedback** uses an integrated electromyogram (EMG) to make recordings from the skin surface, as opposed to a needle EMG, which records electrical activity from a single muscle. The goal is to teach the individual to control tension that has been functioning maladaptively. It is particularly useful in individuals who have a connection between skeletal muscle tension and pain (Riverside Heart Institute, 1992). **Progressive relaxation training** emphasizes the individual's ability to perceive the difference between tension and relaxation. This technique involves sequential tensing and a relaxing environment. The individual is taught to practice this routine daily, often with the use of audiotaped instructions. By teaching the individual to recognize excessive contraction of skeletal muscle, one hopes to enhance the ability to relax specific muscle groups to relieve tension and, thus, reduce CNS arousal as well as autonomic nervous system (ANS) arousal.

Immobility

The effects of muscular deconditioning associated with lack of physical activity may be apparent in a matter of days. The normal individual on bed rest loses muscle strength from baseline levels at a rate of 3% a day. Bed rest also is associated with cardiovascular, skeletal, and other organ system changes.

The term *disuse atrophy* has been used to describe the pathologic reduction in normal size of muscle fibers after prolonged inactivity from bed rest, trauma (casting), or local nerve damage. Studies of experimental animals show a marked reduction in mitochondrial oxidative metabolism, leaving less energy available for muscle protein synthesis. This would explain the reduction in volume and number of myofibrils that has been demonstrated in studies on the effect of casting a fracture of one leg. These studies show that after 8 weeks, the casted limb demonstrates overall a 50% reduction in the number of muscle fibers, and the individual's maximum oxygen uptake is reduced. Some investigators report that, after knee injury, type I muscle fibers atrophy at a greater rate than type II fibers. Similar studies using the immobilized knee report type I fiber atrophy occurs rapidly after immobilization in a cast.

Measures to prevent atrophy include frequent forceful isometric muscle contractions and passive lengthening exercises. If reuse is not restored within 1 year, regeneration of muscle fibers becomes impaired.

Muscle Membrane Abnormalities

Two defects of the muscle membrane (plasma membrane of the muscle fiber) have been linked to clinical syndromes: the hyperexcitable membrane seen in the myotonic disorders and the intermittently unresponsive membrane seen in the periodic paralyses. Although these are infrequent disorders, research into the pathologic processes has led to an improved understanding of the cell membrane.

Myotonia

Myotonia is both a physical and an electrical phenomenon. It is a delayed relaxation after such voluntary muscle contraction as grip, eye closure, or muscle percussion. The distinctive "dive bomber" noise, audible on needle EMG, is caused by the prolonged depolarization of the muscle membrane. Because the depolarization is not terminated by neuromuscular blocking agents, such as curare, the abnormality has been localized at the muscle membrane, outside the neuromuscular junction and sarcotubular system. (These structures are described in Chapter 38.)

In experimental animals, myotonia can be reproduced by removing extracellular chloride, thus reducing chloride conductance across the plasma membrane. The delicate balance in which sodium diffuses into the intracellular fluid, potassium diffuses out of the intracellular fluid, and chloride is in flux is thus interrupted. Because the normal diffusion processes (described in Chapter 3) stabilize the membrane, the shift in chloride ions is thought to increase membrane excitability. The chloride abnormality may explain the resting membrane hyperexcitability, but it does not explain the delayed relaxation present in myotonia and has not been detected in human myotonia.

Myotonia is seen in several disorders, myotonia congenita, paramyotonia congenita, myotonic muscular dystrophy, and some forms of periodic paralysis. Most are inherited disorders and are mild in symptomatology, with the exception of myotonic muscular dystrophy (see Chapter 40). Myotonia is treated by drugs that reduce muscle fiber excitability, such as procaine, procainamide, phenytoin, and quinine preparations. New treatments include acetazolamide, a carbonic anhydrase inhibitor, and verapamil, a calcium channel blocker.

Periodic Paralysis

During an attack of **periodic paralysis,** the muscle membrane is unresponsive to neural stimuli, and the resting membrane potential is reduced from -90 to -45 mV. Periodic paralysis is triggered by exercise and any process or medication that increases serum potassium. The disorder is often inherited in an autosomal dominant pattern, although it can be seen in hyperthyroidism.

The paralysis, which leaves the individual flaccid and weak, does not affect the respiratory muscles. Many individuals have myotonia present on examination. In most cases the weakness is accompanied by a change in serum potassium, although in some individuals the change may be negligible. Cardiac dysrhythmias have been present during attacks. Although the biochemical defect remains unknown, changes in the muscle membrane and sarcoplasmic reticulum have been described.

Hypokalemic periodic paralysis is triggered by high-carbohydrate meals, prolonged bed rest, or emotional stress. (The effect of potassium on the resting membrane potential is discussed in Chapter 3.) Glucose and insulin infusions and oral potassium loading are used as provocative tests; oral and intravenous potassium can relieve acute attacks. Treatment includes thiazides, diuretics, and a high-salt diet. Acetazolamide and a low-salt diet are useful for long-term therapy.

Metabolic Muscle Diseases

Disorders in muscle metabolism can be caused by endocrine abnormalities, or diseases of energy metabolism, such as glycogen storage disease, enzyme deficiencies, and abnormalities in lipid metabolism and mitochondrial function.

Endocrine Disorders

Often the systemic effects of hormonal imbalance overshadow the individual's muscular symptoms. For example, individuals with thyrotoxicosis may have signs of proximal weakness, paresis of the extraocular muscles (exophthalmic ophthalmoplegia), and, rarely, hypokalemic periodic paralysis. Hypothyroidism is often associated with a decrease in muscle mass and strength, with weak, flabby skeletal muscles and sluggish movements (Seeley, Stephens, & Tate, 1990). Common findings in hypothyroidism, myxedema, and delayed relaxation of the muscle stretch reflexes can be confused with myotonia.

Thyroid hormone is believed to regulate muscle protein synthesis and electrolyte balance. Changes in muscle protein synthesis and electrolyte balance may, therefore, explain the changes in muscle mass and contractility seen in endocrine disorders. The muscular symptoms subside with appropriate treatment of the primary hormonal disorder.

Hyperparathyroidism also causes symptoms of muscular weakness and should be considered when the findings are proximal weakness, wasting and fatigue, brisk reflexes, and defects of neuronal conduction (Allen et al., 1989).

Diseases of Energy Metabolism

The muscle relies on carbohydrates, such as glycogen and lipids (free fatty acids), for energy. When stored glycogen or lipids cannot be used because of a lack of the enzyme necessary to convert energy for contraction, the individual experiences cramps, fatigue, and exercise intolerance. Disorders of muscle metabolism can be self-limiting, such as is seen in McArdle disease and some lipid disorders, or cause widespread irreparable muscle destruction, as in acid maltase deficiency.

McArdle disease

A severe metabolic defect in glycogen metabolism was first described in 1951 by B. McArdle, for whom the illness is named. Since then, three other deficiencies in glycotic enzymes have been described. **McArdle disease** was the first myopathy in which a single enzyme defect was identified. Although it is rare, over 110 cases have been reported from one clinic alone. Individuals with McArdle disease lack muscle phosphorylase, which is responsible for the breakdown of glycogen in muscle. Normally, after the body uses the short-term ATP and phosphocreatine stores, intramuscular lactic acid accumulates as glycogen is used (see Chapter 38). The individual with McArdle disease is not able to break down glycogen or produce lactic acid.

The lactic acid deficiency can be tested by nuclear magnetic resonance or the ischemic exercise test. On the nuclear magnetic resonance scan, lactic acid buildup appears as a change in the ratio of phosphocreatine to ATP and a decrease in muscle pH. The ischemic exercise test normally produces an exponential increase in the serum lactic acid, pyruvate, and ammonia levels after intense muscular work. For the individual with McArdle disease, however, there is no change in muscle pH in response to ischemic exercise.

The altered energy production manifests itself in exercise intolerance, fatigue, and painful muscle cramps. When exercise is carried to an extreme, painful muscle contracture and myoglobinuria develop. Some individuals describe a "second wind" phenomenon, in which exercise tolerance increases if they slow their pace once the initial sensation of fatigue commences. This may be caused by the use of free fatty acids as a secondary source of energy. As the disease progresses, some individuals have pronounced muscle weakness and wasting. Other organs are not involved, because the absence of phosphorylase is limited to muscle.

On muscle biopsy, the muscle does not stain for myophosphorylase, and muscle cells demonstrate subsar-

colemmal glycogen deposition and scattered necrotic fibers. Trials of glucose or fructose administration have been suggested to improve exercise tolerance (Mineo et al., 1990), and a new high-fat, high-protein diet has received some support. Generally, individuals with McArdle disease learn to adapt their daily routine to avoid muscle symptoms.

Acid maltase deficiency

Acid maltase deficiency is an uncommon glycogen storage disease associated with an accumulation of glycogen in the lysosomes of muscle cells and the cells of other tissues. The usual pathways of glycogen degradation are preserved. It appears that the absence of the enzyme acid maltase is responsible for the abnormality in glycogen metabolism, although the exact mechanism is unknown. It is an autosomal recessive disorder, with the gene located on the long arm of chromosome 17. Muscle biopsy shows vacuoles and glycogen deposition similar to the changes in McArdle disease, but this histochemical myophosphorylase reaction is normal.

The two forms of acid maltase deficiency are distinguished by the individual's age at onset. The infantile form is called **Pompe disease** and is recognized shortly after birth by hypotonia, areflexia, and an enlarged heart, tongue, and liver. Hypertrophy of these tissues is thought to be the result of glycogen deposition. The children die of cardiac or respiratory failure within a year of diagnosis. The adult variety becomes evident subacutely. The muscular symptoms resemble those of muscular dystrophy or polymyositis (see p. 1475). A distinguishing feature in adults may be the presence of severe respiratory muscle weakness.

Myoadenylate deaminase deficiency

An enzyme deficiency that produces changes in skeletal muscle and is associated with exercise intolerance is **myoadenylate deaminase deficiency (MDD)**. Because of a lack of the enzyme myoadenylate deaminase, these individuals have a poor capacity for sustained energy production. Myoadenylate deaminase is the catalytic enzyme that forms phosphocreatine and ATP during exercise through a metabolic pathway that binds the purine and phosphate molecules that constitute ATP. Persons with MDD differ from those with McArdle disease in that, during the ischemic exercise test, lactate production is normal and ammonia production is absent. Ammonia is a by-product of the ATP and phosphocreatine synthesis. In muscle biopsies from affected individuals, cells fail to stain for the enzyme myoadenylate deaminase. The enzyme defect has been reported to be quite common, but in practice may be rarely recognized as a cause of exercise intolerance.

Lipid deficiencies

Disorders of lipid metabolism are uncommon but account for severe changes in muscle metabolism. The lipid content of muscle cells consists of the free fatty acids, which are oxidized in the mitochondria. These acids require carnitine and the enzyme carnitine palmityl transferase (CPT) to transport metabolic by-products and energy to the myofibrils. Individuals with CPT deficiency have mild muscular symptoms but can experience bouts of renal failure caused by myoglobinuria. Individuals with a deficiency of carnitine alone have progressive muscle weakness and can experience sudden exacerbations.

Measuring the CPT and carnitine content in muscle aids in the diagnosis. Cells in the muscle biopsy show vacuoles and lipid deposits. Treatments with riboflavin, medium-chain triglyceride, oral carnitine, and prednisone have been suggested.

Inflammatory Muscle Diseases: Myositis
Viral, Bacterial, and Parasitic Myositis

Viral, bacterial, and parasitic infections of varying severity are known to produce inflammatory changes in skeletal muscle, a group of conditions collectively described by the term **myositis.** In the granulomatous diseases, tuberculosis and sarcoidosis, chronic inflammatory changes, and granulomas are found in muscle as well as in other affected tissues. The parasitic infection trichinosis is said to affect up to 4% of the population. In trichinosis, *Trichinella* larvae reside in infected pork and, after ingestion, migrate to the intestinal mucosa and, from there, to the lymphatics. Symptoms include severe pain, rash, and muscle stiffness. Treatment includes administration of corticosteroids, prednisone, and the antiparasitic agent thiabendazole. Toxoplasmosis, a common parasitic infection, is also associated with a generalized polymyositis that responds rapidly to therapy.

In the tropics, more prevalent disorders include bacterial infections with *Staphylococcus aureus* and parasites such as cysticercus, the larva of the tapeworm *Taenia solium.* Viral infections can be associated with an acute myositis. Muscle pain, tenderness, signs of inflammation, and creatine kinase elevation are common manifestations of viral myositis. The self-limiting symptoms of muscle aches and pains during a bout of influenza may actually be a subacute form of viral myopathy.

Polymyositis and Dermatomyositis

Polymyositis (generalized muscle inflammation) and **dermatomyositis** (polymyositis accompanied by skin lesions) are the most common inflammatory muscle diseases requiring chronic care. Prevalence rates are estimated to be up to 6 per 1,000,000 (Robinson, 1991).

Pathophysiology

Polymyositis and dermatomyositis are characterized by inflammation of connective tissue and muscle fibers that presumably causes the extensive necrosis and destruction of muscle fibers. The agent that causes the muscle inflammation has not been identified, but abnormalities in the immune system have been implicated. Experimental studies have not clarified whether the damage is produced by cell-mediated or humoral immune factors. There is growing support for the view that these two diseases should not be considered as a single autoimmune disease. Studies have shown that the inflammatory cells that surround the perimysial and perivascular sites are selectively enriched in B cells and helper T cells in dermatomyositis. (The immune response is discussed in Chapter 6.) Killer and natural killer T cells are rare. This suggests that a humoral immune mechanism may be an important factor.

The deposition of circulating immune complexes in the vascular endothelium makes the presence of cell-mediated response difficult to exclude. There is less vascular involvement in polymyositis, and most of the inflammatory cells, including B cells, T cells, and macrophages, surround the muscle fibers and fascicles. Immune complex deposits have not been located in the muscle fiber in polymyositis, but circulating antigen-antibody complexes were found in most individuals. Again, there is evidence for both cell-mediated and humoral immune responses.

Clinical Manifestations

The constellation of acute symptoms includes many of those seen in any inflammatory process: malaise, fever, muscle swelling, pain and tenderness, lethargy, and listlessness. Both illnesses are usually associated with a symmetric proximal muscle weakness and can be initially confused with other myopathies. They require a thorough evaluation to exclude other disorders. Clinical features common in both polymyositis and dermatomyositis are dysphagia, reduced esophageal motility, vasculitis, Raynaud phenomenon, cardiomyopathy, and interstitial pulmonary fibrosis. Some have other coexisting collagen vascular disorders, such as rheumatoid arthritis, systemic lupus erythematosus, and progressive systemic sclerosis (formerly called scleroderma).

The presence of skin rash, calcinosis, and eyelid edema most often suggests dermatomyositis. The skin rash is a purple (heliotrope) color and involves the eyelids, face, chest, and extensor surfaces of the extremities. Dermatomyositis is slightly more common in children and older adults, with an onset before the age of 15 and after the age of 50. The adult with dermatomyositis occasionally has underlying malignancies. Calcinosis, with calcium deposition in the subcutaneous tissue, can be a severe long-term complication of dermatomyositis.

Evaluation and Treatment

The muscle biopsy is striking in dermatomyositis, with most individuals showing inflammatory cells grouped around blood vessels and atrophy of cells in muscle fascicle. This change, perifascicular atrophy, is absent in polymyositis. Creatine kinase and sedimentation rate are often acutely elevated in both disorders. Electromyogram abnormalities include signs of muscle irritability and myopathic changes, usually large numbers of low-amplitude action potentials of brief duration. The EMG also shows a typical "myopathic" pattern, with short, low-amplitude polyphasic potentials, as well as signs of marked muscle irritability. Muscle biopsy is indispensable to make a definitive diagnosis of polymyositis or dermatomyositis as opposed to other myotonic disease (Fujino, Kobayashi, Goto, & Onitsuka, 1991). Magnetic resonance imaging (MRI) shows inflammation and edema of the muscles (Fujino et al., 1991).

Treatment primarily includes immunosuppressive drugs, although they are not always successful if uniformly applied. Most clinicians choose corticosteroids initially, usually prednisone on a daily or alternating day schedule, tapering the dosage as the symptoms subside. Successful treatment with azathioprine, methotrexate, and cyclophosphamide has also been reported. All immunosuppressives have multiple side effects that require monitoring and frequent follow-up. Individuals with muscle weakness require careful physiotherapy to design a regular exercise program that prevents contractures and maximizes functional ability.

Ocular Myopathies

Several rare muscle disorders cause particular severe ocular findings. One is **oculopharyngeal muscular dystrophy.** The age of onset for this autosomal dominant disorder is usually after age 40, with the symptoms of eyelid drooping (ptosis), ocular muscle weakness, difficulty swallowing (dysphagia), and weight loss. Occasionally, the individual will have mild proximal muscle weakness. Oculopharyngeal dystrophy is a mild, slowly progressive disorder. Findings are initially confined to ocular paresis and ptosis that spares the pupil. Later, the facial muscles may be involved. This disease is rare, but it appears to be clustered in two groups, Spanish-Americans in the southwestern United States and French-Canadians.

Diagnostic studies show only mild elevations in creatine kinase (CK) and a myopathic pattern on EMG.

Muscle biopsy findings are generally similar to those of individuals with other dystrophic disorders, with the exception of intranuclear tubular filaments.

Ptosis and dysphagia are surgically correctable. Surgical elevation of the lids is recommended if visual acuity is impaired, and lid crutches are helpful. The dysphagia seen in this disorder is often associated with a constriction of the cricopharyngeus muscle, which, when released, permits a bolus of food to pass through the pharynx smoothly. Inflammation and edema of the cricopharyngeus muscles and fibrosis of the esophageal inlet mechanism also cause dysphagia in polymyositis (Verma, Bradley, Adesina, Sofferman, & Pendelbury, 1991).

Chronic progressive external ophthalmoplegia (CPEO) is also characterized by ocular weakness. Chronic progressive external ophthalmoplegia is known for the distinctive muscle biopsy finding of "ragged-red" fibers in 100% of cases. Mitochondrial abnormalities of the muscle fiber are an important feature of this disease. Whether a genetic defect causes these mitochondrial changes remains unclear. Individuals with CPEO have associated metabolic, cardiac, and neurologic deficits. Treatment of the lid weakness is the same as for oculopharyngeal muscular dystrophy.

Toxic Myopathies

The most common cause of **toxic myopathy** is alcohol abuse. Two clinical syndromes are prevalent: (1) an acute attack of muscle weakness, pain, and swelling after a binge; or (2) a more chronic, progressive proximal weakness in a drinker of long duration. The incidence of acute alcoholic myopathy has been estimated as up to 20% of individuals admitted with acute alcoholic withdrawal.

The pathologic abnormalities include necrosis of individual muscle fibers; whole segments can be found in the same stage of degeneration. Isolated, damaged fibers can be found next to undamaged fibers. Histochemistry of muscle biopsy specimens reveals patchy loss of oxidative enzymes in type I fibers. Electron microscopy shows a marked accumulation of intracellular fluid and destruction of mitochondria. The mechanism by which alcohol affects the muscle fiber is uncertain, but direct toxic effect and nutritional deficiency have both received experimental support.

Acute alcoholic myopathy can range from benign cramps and pain resolving in a matter of hours, to severe weakness and markedly increased CK associated with myoglobinuria and renal failure. Individuals are prone to repeated attacks following recovery. The only treatment is abstinence from alcohol and improved nutrition. The individual with chronic alcoholic myopathy often has coexisting peripheral neuropathy that complicates the diagnosis.

Chemical agents have also been implicated in the development of myopathy. The drug chloroquine, an antimalarial and amebicidal agent, in high doses has been associated with the development of generalized muscle weakness, particularly of the proximal muscles. Vacuoles and degeneration of muscle fibers, similar to that seen in glycogen storage disease, are present in muscle biopsies. These changes have been attributed to a molecular interaction between the drug and phospholipids in the cell with resultant accumulation on the lysosomes and impairment of the cell's digestive processes. Myopathy has also been caused by emetine (the major constituent of ipecac), vincristine, corticosteroids, and the toxic denatured rapeseed oil.

Rhabdomyolysis and myoglobinuria caused by sedatives and narcotics, particularly street heroin, clofibrate (hypolipidemic agent), and the antifibrinolytic ε-aminocaproate, and by drugs that induce hypokalemia, such as amphotericin B and licorice and azathioprine, have also been reported (Robinson, 1991).

Repeated intramuscular injections have been associated also with changes in muscle fibers. Local necrosis of muscle fiber and elevated CK have been reported after intramuscular injections of cephalothin, lidocaine, diazepam, and digoxin; these effects were not produced with injections of saline. When drugs are injected over long periods, a chronic focal myopathy develops. Proliferation of connective tissue in both the muscle fiber and overlying skin and subcutaneous tissue has been reported. Over time, segments of the muscles, particularly the deltoid and quadriceps, are converted into fibrotic bands. These contractures have functional consequences. Contracture in the deltoid results in the arm becoming fixed in partial abduction. Pathophysiologic mechanisms for these changes include repeated needle trauma and infection, as well as nonphysiologic acidity and alkalinity of the injected material (Robinson, 1991).

Muscle Tumors

Rhabdomyoma

Rhabdomyoma is a benign tumor of muscle, is extremely rare, and generally occurs in the tongue, neck muscles, larynx, uvula, nasal cavity, axilla, vulva, and heart. These tumors are usually treated by surgical excision and do not recur.

Rhabdomyosarcoma

Connective tissue sarcomas constitute 0.7% of all cancers; although they constitute approximately 7% of all cancers in children. (Muscle cancer in children is discussed in Chapter 40.) The malignant tumor of striated muscle is called rhabdomyosarcoma. The incidence of rhabdomyosarcoma ranges from 10% to 20% of all soft tissue cancers. This tumor is highly malignant because of rapid metastasis. The two age peaks in incidence statistics are 2 to 6 years and the early to late teens, although rhabdomyosarcoma also can be seen in adults and the elderly population. These tumors are located in the muscle tissue of the head, neck, and genitourinary tract in 75% of cases. The remainder are in the trunk and extremities.

There are three types of rhabdomyosarcoma differentiated on pathologic section: (1) pleomorphic, (2) embryonal, and (3) alveolar. The pleomorphic, or spindle cell, type is considered to be one of the most highly malignant tumors of the extremities seen in adulthood. Embryonal tumors are most frequently seen in childhood and appear to be shaped like a tadpole or tennis racquet on biopsy. Alveolar-type tumors appear latticelike and look like lung tissue alveoli.

The diagnosis of rhabdomyosarcoma is made by incisional biopsy and examination of the specimen by a pathologist. On electron microscopy, the tissue demonstrates myofilaments and Z-band material; CT scan also helps define the tissue borders. Staging is based on pathologic grade of the tumor and is helpful in determining prognosis and treatment.

Treatment consists of a combination of surgical excision, radiation therapy, and systemic chemotherapy. Those individuals with only regional tumor growth, particularly tumors of the orbit and genitourinary tract, have been reported to have a 5-year survival of 75%, related to earlier diagnosis and vigorous treatments. Childhood rhabdomyosarcoma of any type with only regional involvement can be controlled in 60% of cases. Tumors of the trunk and extremities have a less favorable prognosis. Cure with distant metastasis is unlikely.

Other Tumors

Metastatic deposits of tumors in muscles are rare in spite of the extensive vascular supply of skeletal muscles. It is suggested that local pH or metabolic changes prevent metastatic involvement from other tumors. When adjacent carcinomas do cause muscle damage, it is usually related to the compression of tissue and resultant muscle atrophy.

Musculoskeletal Injuries

1 One of 10 persons in the United States suffers an acute musculoskeletal injury each year.
2 The most serious musculoskeletal injury is a fracture. A bone can be completely or incompletely fractured. A closed fracture leaves the skin intact. An open fracture has an overlying skin wound. The direction of the fracture line can be linear, oblique, spiral, or transverse. Greenstick, torus, and bowing fractures are examples of incomplete fractures that occur in children. Stress fractures occur in normal or abnormal bone that is subjected to repeated stress. Fatigue fractures occur in normal bone subjected to abnormal stress. Normal weight bearing can cause an insufficiency fracture in abnormal bone.
3 Dislocation is complete loss of contact between the surfaces of two bones. Subluxation is partial loss of contact between two bones. As a bone separates from a joint, it may damage adjacent nerves, blood vessels, ligaments, tendons, and muscle.
4 Tendon tears are called sprains and ligament tears are called strains. A complete separation of a tendon or ligament from its attachment is called an avulsion.

Disorders of Bones

1 Metabolic bone diseases are characterized by abnormal bone structure. In osteoporosis, the density or mass of bone is reduced because the bone remodeling cycle is disrupted. Osteomalacia is a metabolic bone disease characterized by inadequate bone mineralization. Excessive and abnormal bone remodeling occurs in Paget disease.
2 Osteomyelitis is a bone infection caused *most frequently* by bacteria. Bacteria can enter bone from outside the body (exogenous osteomyelitis) or from infection sites within the body (hematogenous osteomyelitis).
3 Bone tumors originate from bone cells, cartilage cells, fibrous tissue cells, or vascular marrow cells. Each cell produces a specific type of ground substance that is used to classify the tumor as osteogenic (bone cell), chondrogenic (cartilage cell), collagenic (fibrous tissue cell), or myelogenic (vascular marrow cell). Malignant bone tumors are large, aggressively destroy surrounding bone, invade surrounding tissue, and initiate independent growth outside the site of origin. Benign bone tumors are less destructive, limit their growth to the anatomic confines of the bone, and have a well-demarcated border.

Disorders of Joints

1 Noninflammatory joint disease is differentiated from inflammatory joint disease by the absence of synovial membrane inflammation, the absence of systemic signs and symptoms, and the presence of normal synovial fluid.
2 Degenerative joint disease is a noninflammatory joint disease characterized by the degeneration and loss of articular cartilage, sclerosis of underlying bone, and formation of bone spurs (osteophytes).
3 Rheumatoid arthritis is an inflammatory joint disease characterized by inflammatory destruction of the synovial membrane, articular cartilage, joint capsule, and surrounding ligaments and tendons. Rheumatoid nodules may also invade the skin, lung, and spleen, and involve small and large arteries. Rheumatoid arthritis is a systemic disease that affects the heart, lungs, kidneys, and skin, as well as the joints.
4 Ankylosing spondylitis is a chronic, inflammatory joint disease characterized by stiffening and fusion of the spine and sacroiliac joints.
5 Gout is a metabolic disorder associated with high levels of uric acid in the blood and body fluids. Uric acid crystallizes in the connective tissue of a joint where it initiates inflammatory destruction of the joint.

Disorders of Skeletal Muscle

1 A pathologic contracture is permanent muscle shortening due to muscle spasticity, as seen in CNS injury, or severe muscle weakness.
2 Stress-induced muscle tension is presumably caused by increased activity in the reticular activating system and gamma loop in the muscle fiber. The use of progressive relaxation training and biofeedback has been advocated to reduce muscle tension.
3 Atrophy of muscle fibers and overall diminished size of the muscle are seen after prolonged inactivity. Isometric contractions and passive lengthening exercises decrease atrophy to some degree in immobilized patients.
4 Hyperexcitable membranes cause the physical and electrical phenomenon myotonia. The disorder is treated with drugs that reduce muscle fiber excitability. Periodic paralysis is caused by an unresponsive muscle membrane and is accompanied by changes in serum potassium. The biochemical defect is possibly related to changes in the muscle membrane and sarcoplasmic reticulum.
5 Metabolic muscle diseases are caused by endocrine disorders, glycogen storage disease, enzyme deficiencies, and abnormal lipid function. The muscle de-

pends on a complex system of carbohydrates and fats converted by enzymes to produce energy for the muscle cell. Abnormalities in these pathways can inhibit function or cause damage to the muscle fiber. These illnesses are rare, yet account for significant functional abnormalities.

6 Viral, bacterial, and parasitic infections of muscles produce the characteristic clinical and pathologic changes associated with inflammation. These are usually treatable and self-limiting disorders.

7 Polymyositis (generalized muscle inflammation) and dermatomyositis (polymyositis accompanied with skin rash) are characterized by inflammation of connective tissue and muscle fibers, and muscle fiber necrosis. Cell-mediated and humoral immune factors have been implicated. Treatment with immunosuppressive agents is effective in many cases.

8 Oculopharyngeal muscular dystrophy differs from the more common muscular dystrophies in age of onset and affected musculature. It is a mild illness

in which symptomatic therapy is often successful. Chronic, progressive external ophthalmoplegia is characterized by multisystem deficits and ocular muscle weakness. Mitochondrial abnormality of the muscle fibers has been recognized.

9 The most common toxic myopathy is caused by alcohol abuse. Direct toxic effects of alcohol-producing necrosis of muscle fibers and nutritional deficiency have been suggested. The only treatment is abstinence and improved nutrition. The toxic effects of many drugs on muscle fibers cause local trauma to the muscle fibers caused by direct effects of the needle, secondary infection, and changes caused by nonphysiologic acidity and alkalinity in the fibers.

10 Sarcomas of muscle tissue are rare. Rhabdomyosarcoma has a uniformly poor prognosis because of an aggressive invasion and early, widespread dissemination. The usual treatment includes surgical excision, radiation therapy, and systemic chemotherapy.

KEY TERMS

Acid maltase deficiency, 1474
Ankylosing spondylitis, 1466
Avulsion, 1441
Biofeedback, 1472
Bowing fracture, 1435
Bursae, 1442
Caplan syndrome, 1465
Chemical agents, 1477
Chondrogenic tumor (cartilage-forming tumor), 1456
Chondroid, 1456
Chondrosarcoma, 1456
Chronic progressive external ophthalmoplegia (CPEO), 1476
Closed fracture (simple fracture), 1435
Collagenic tumor (collagen-forming tumor), 1456
Comminuted fracture, 1435
Compartment syndrome, 1444
Complete fracture, 1435
Contracture, 1472
Degenerative joint disease (osteoarthritis), 1458
Delayed union, 1439
Dermatomyositis, 1475
Dislocation, 1440
Endochondroma, 1456

Enthesis, 1467
Epicondylitis, 1442
Exogenous osteomyelitis, 1450
Fatigue fracture, 1435
Fibrosarcoma, 1457
Fracture, 1435
Geographic pattern, 1453
Giant cell tumor, 1457
Gout, 1468
Gouty arthritis, 1468
Greenstick fracture, 1435
Hematogenous osteomyelitis, 1450
Hyperbaric oxygen therapy, 1452
Incomplete fracture, 1435
Inflammatory joint disease (arthritis), 1462
Insufficiency fracture, 1437
Involucrum, 1451
Lateral epicondylitis (tennis elbow), 1442
Ligament, 1441
Linear fracture, 1435
Malunion, 1439
McArdle disease, 1474
Medial epicondylitis (golfer's elbow), 1442
Moth-eaten pattern, 1453

Muscle strain, 1443
Myelogenic tumor, 1457
Myeloma, 1457
Myoadenylate deaminase deficiency (MDD), 1474
Myoglobinuria, 1444
Myositis, 1475
Myositis ossificans, 1443
Myotonia, 1473
Noninflammatory joint disease, 1458
Nonunion, 1439
Oblique fracture, 1435
Oculopharyngeal muscular dystrophy, 1476
Open fracture (compound fracture), 1435
Osteoarthritis (OA), 1458
Osteogenic tumor (bone-forming tumor), 1454
Osteomalacia, 1447
Osteomyelitis, 1450
Osteophyte, 1460
Osteoporosis, 1445
Osteosarcoma, 1454
Paget disease (osteitis deformans), 1448
Pannus, 1463

REFERENCES

Allen, M. A., Boykin, P. C., Drass, J. A., Grasberger, A. A., Hench, K. D., Lincoln, E. C., Loraiux, T. C., Robins, R. A. McC., & Wells, M. (1989). Endocrine and metabolic systems. In J. M. Thompson, G. K. McFarland, J. E. Hirsch, S. M. Tucker, & A. C. Bowers (Eds.), *Mosby's manual of clinical nursing*. St. Louis: Mosby–Year Book.

Bourne, R. B., & Rorabeck, C. H. (1989). Compartment syndromes of the lower leg. *Clinical Orthopaedics, 240*(3), 97-104.

Browner, B. D., Jupiter, J. B., Levine, A. M., & Trafton, P. G. (1992). *Skeletal trauma: Fractures, dislocations, ligamentous injuries* (vol. 1). Philadelphia: Saunders.

Brylawski, R. (1991). Limb salvage surgery over amputation: For most, a superior alternative with patients with malignant bone tumors. *Orthopedic Product News, 9*(3), 1, 9, 14.

Bucholz, R. W. (1991). Healing of the musculoskeletal tissues. In C. A. Rockwood, Jr., & D. P. Green (Eds.), *Rockwood and Green fractures in adults* (3rd ed.). Philadelphia: Lippincott.

Calin, A. (1989). Ankylosing spondylitis. In W. N. Kelley, E. D. Harris, Jr., S. Ruddy, & C. B. Sledge (Eds.), *Textbook of rheumatology* (3rd ed.). Philadelphia: Saunders.

Darr, K. F., Acker, J., Pesson, C., & D'Ambrosia, R. D. (1988). Giant cell tumor of bone. *Orthopedics, 11*(1), 209-221.

Felson, D. T. (1990). Osteoarthritis. *Rheumatic Disease Clinics of North America, 16*(3), 499-512.

Finn, H., & Simon, M. A. (1989). Staging systems for musculoskeletal neoplasms. *Orthopedics, 12*(10), 1365-1371.

Francis, R. M., Scane, F. J., Johnson, C. E., Sutcliffe, D., & Sutcliffe, A. M. (1991). Male osteoporosis. *Journal of Endocrinology, 135*, Suppl., 9.

Fujino, H., Kobayashi, T., Goto, I., & Onitsuka, H. (1991). Magnetic resonance imaging of the muscles in patients with polymyositis and dermatomyositis. *Muscle & Nerve, 14*(7), 716-720.

Harris, E. D., Jr. (1989). The clinical features of rheumatoid arthritis. In W. N. Kelley, E. D. Harris, Jr., S. Ruddy, & C. B. Sledge (Eds.), *Textbook of rheumatology* (3rd ed.). Philadelphia: Saunders.

Harrison, J. E. (1989). Osteoporosis. In C. S. Tam, J. N. M. Heersche, & T. M. Murray (Eds.), *Metabolic bone disease: Cellular and tissue mechanisms*. Boca Raton, FL: CRC.

Heare, C. C., Enneking, W. F., & Heare, M. M. (1990). Staging techniques and biopsy of bone tumors. *Orthopedic Clinics of North America, 21*(1), 277-283.

Heinegard, D., & Saxne, T. (1991). Macromolecular markers in joint disease. *Journal of Rheumatology, 27*(18 [Suppl.]), 27-29.

James, W. H. (1991). Sex ratios and hormones in HLA-related rheumatic disease. *Annals of the Rheumatic Diseases, 50*(6), 401-404.

Jimenez, S. A. (1991). Molecular biological approaches to the study of heritable osteoarthritis. *Journal of Rheumatology, 27*(19 [Suppl.]), 7-9.

Kastrup, J. J., Buseck, M. S., & Lyon, J. C. (1992). Common pitfalls in a bone tumor workup. *Contemporary Orthopaedics, 24*(5), 567-573.

Kelley, W. N., Fox, I. H., & Palella, T. D. (1989). Crystal-associated synovitis. In W. N. Kelley, E. D. Harris, Jr., S. Ruddy, & C. B. Sledge (Eds.), *Textbook of rheumatology* (3rd ed.). Philadelphia: Saunders.

Khan, M. A., & van der Linden, S. M. (1990). Ankylosing spondylitis and other spondyloarthropathies. *Rheumatic Disease Clinics of North America, 16*(3), 551-580.

Klein, M. J., Kenan, S., & Lewis, M. M. (1989). Osteosarcoma: Clinical and pathological considerations. *Orthopedic Clinics of North America, 20*(3), 327-333.

Krajbich, J. I. (1991). Modified Van Nes rotationplasty in the treatment of malignant neoplasms in the lower extremities of children. *Orthopedic Product News, 9*(3), 10, 14.

Licata, A. (1991). Therapies for symptomatic primary osteoporosis. *Geriatrics, 46*(11), 62-63, 66-67.

Liscum, B. (1992). Osteoporosis: The silent disease. *Orthopaedic Nursing, 11*(4), 21-25.

Malemud, C. J. (1991). Changes in proteoglycans in osteoarthritis: Biochemistry ultrastructure and biosynthetic processing. *Journal of Rheumatology, 27*(18, Suppl.), 60-62.

Mankin, H. J. (1989). Clinical features of osteoarthritis. In W. N. Kelley, E. D. Harris, Jr., S. Ruddy, & C. B. Sledge (Eds.), *Textbook of rheumatology* (3rd ed.). Philadelphia: Saunders.

Marx, S. J. (1989). Disorders of vitamin D metabolism—Basic aspects. In C. S. Tam, J. N. M. Heersche, & T. M. Murray (Eds.), *Metabolic bone disease: Cellular and tissue mechanisms*. Boca Raton, FL: CRC.

McCune, W. J. (1989). Monarticular arthritis. In W. N. Kelley, E. D. Harris, Jr., S. Ruddy, & C. B. Sledge (Eds.), *Textbook of rheumatology* (3rd ed.). Philadelphia: Saunders.

Milgrim, J. W. (1990). *Radiologic and histologic pathology of nontumorous diseases of bones and joints* (vols. 1 & 2). Northbrook, IL: Northbrook Publishing.

Millman, M. (1991). Muscle biopsy tests identify patients at risk of malignant hyperthermia. *Hospital Practice, 265*, 8-10.

Mineo, I., Kono, N., Yamada, Y., Hara, N., Kiyokawa, H., Hamaguchi, T., Nakajima, H., Kuyajima, M., & Tauri, S. (1990). Glucose infusion abolishes the excessive ATP degradation in working muscles of a patient with McArdle's disease. *Muscle & Nerve, 13*(7), 618-620.

Moskowitz, R. W., Boja, B., & Denko, C. W. (1991). The role of growth factors in degenerative joint disorders. *Journal of Rheumatology, 27*(18, Suppl.), 147-148.

Mourad, L. (1991). *Orthopedic disorders*. St. Louis: Mosby–Year Book.

O'Connor, M. I., & Sim, F. H. (1989). Early recognition of bone tumors. *Journal of Musculoskeletal Medicine, 6*(4), 124-133.

Olson, P. N., & Griffiths, H. J. (1990). Periosteal osteosarcoma. *Orthopedics, 13*(7), 804.

Palmblad, J., Hafstrom, I., & Ringertz, B. (1991). Antirheumatic effects of fasting. *Rheumatic Disease Clinics of North America, 17*(2), 351-362.

Recker, R. R., Davies, K. M., Hinders, S. M., Heaney, R. P., Stegman, M. R., & Kimmel, D. B. (1992). Bone gain in young adult women. *Journal of the American Medical Association, 268*(17), 2403-2407.

Riverside Heart Institute. (1992). *Healthy lifestyle, healthy heart* (Pamphlet). Columbus, OH: Riverside Heart Institute of Ohio.

Robinson, L. R. (1991). Polymyositis. *Muscle & Nerve, 14*(4), 310-315.

Robot succeeds in hip replacement operation. (1992, November 15). *Columbus Dispatch,* p. 6b.

Rosai, J. (1989). *Ackerman's surgical pathology* (7th ed.). St. Louis: Mosby–Year Book.

Schwartz, H. S., & Shives, T. C. (1989). Surgical management of giant cell tumor of bone. *Complications in Orthopedics, 3*(5), 155-161.

Scott, J. C. (1990). Osteoporosis and hip fracture. *Rheumatic Disease Clinics of North America, 16*(3), 711-722.

Seeley, R. R., Stephens, T. D., & Tate, P. (1992). *Anatomy and physiology,* (2nd ed.). St. Louis: Times Mirror/Mosby College Publishing.

Singer, F. T., & Mills, B. G. (1989). Primary bone cell dysfunction in Paget's disease of bone. In C. S. Tam, J. N. M. Heersche, & T. M. Murray (Eds.), *Metabolic bone disease: Cellular and tissue mechanisms.* Boca Raton, FL: CRC.

Spector, T. D. (1990). Rheumatoid arthritis. *Rheumatic Disease Clinics in North America, 16*(3), 513-538.

Stevenson, F. C. (1992). New treatments for osteoporosis. *Journal of Endocrinology, 135*(Suppl.), 9.

Thonar, E. J-M. A., Manicourt, D. M., Williams, J., Lenz, M. E., Barry, M., Sweet, E., Schnitzer, T. J., Otter, L., Glaut, T., & Kuettner, K. (1991). Circulating keratan sulfate: A marker of cartilage proteoglycan catabolism in osteoarthritis. *Journal of Rheumatology, 27*(18 Suppl.), 24-26.

Verma, A., Bradley, W. G., Adesina, A. M., Sofferman, R., & Pendelbury, W. W. (1991). Inclusion body myositis with cricopharyngeus muscle involvement and severe dysphasia. *Muscle & Nerve, 14*(5), 470-473.

Woessner, J. F., & Gunya-Smith, Z. (1991). Role of metalloproteinases in human osteoarthritis. *Journal of Rheumatology,* (Suppl. 27), 99-101.

SUGGESTED READINGS

Arenas, J., Ricoy, J. R., Encinas, A. R., Pola, P., D'iddio, S., Zeviani, M., Didonato, S., & Corsi, M. (1991). Carnitine in muscle, serum, and urine of unprofessional athletes: Effects of physical exercise, training, and L-carnitine administration. *Muscle & Nerve, 14*(7), 598-604.

Finn, H. A., Nicholas, R. W., & Webb, J. E. (1990). Skeletal reconstruction with allograft segments following bone tumor resection. *Contemporary Orthopaedics, 21*(5), 455-471.

Kaplan, P. E., & Tanner, E. D. (1989). *Musculoskeletal pain and disability.* Norwalk, CT: Appleton & Lange.

Mankin, H. J. (1990). Paget's sarcoma of the femur. *Orthopaedic Consultation, 11*(2), 1-8.

McCully, K., Giger, U., Argov, Z., Valentine, B., Cooper, B., Chance, B., & Bank, W. (1991). Canine X-linked muscular dystrophy studied in in vivo phosphorus magnetic resonance spectroscopy. *Muscle & Nerve, 14*(11), 1091-1098.

Persson, I., Adami, H., Bergkvist, L., Lindgren, A., Petterson, B., Hoover, R., & Schairer, C. (1989). Risk of endometrial cancer after treatment with estrogens alone or in conjunction with progestogens: Results of a prospective study. *British Medical Journal, 298,* 147-151.

Stalberg, E. (1991). Electrodiagnostic assessment and monitoring of motor unit changes in disease. *Muscle & Nerve, 14*(4), 293-303.

Tam, C. S. (1989). The pathogenesis of metabolic bone disease—An overview. In C. S. Tam, J. N. M. Heersche, & T. M. Murray (Eds.), *Metabolic bone disease: Cellular and tissue mechanisms.* Boca Raton, FL: CRC.

Tillman, K. (1990). Recent advances in the surgical treatment of rheumatoid arthritis. *Clinical Orthopaedics, 258*(9), 62-71.

Verity, M. A. (1991). Infantile Pompe's disease, lipid storage, and palmityl carnitine deficiency. *Muscle & Nerve, 14*(5), 435-440.

Weinerman, S. A., & Brockman, R. S. (1990). Medical therapy of osteoporosis. *Orthopedic Clinics of North America, 21*(1), 109-116.

Alterations of Musculoskeletal Function in Children

Frances L. McCullough
Margaret M. Andrews*
Kathleen Hardin Mooney*

Chapter Outline

Musculoskeletal alterations in children are very common. They may be congenital, such as clubfoot; hereditary, such as muscular dystrophy; or acquired, such as Legg-Calvé-Perthes disease. Some of these disorders are acute and the child will recover completely, and others are chronic or, in some cases, terminal. An understanding of the pathophysiology of these alterations will aid in providing the best care possible for these children.

MUSCULOSKELETAL DEVELOPMENT IN CHILDREN

Bone Formation

Bone formation, which begins at about the eighth week of gestation, involves two phases: (1) the delivery of bone cell precursors to sites of bone formation and (2) the aggregation of these cells at **primary centers of ossification,** where they mature and begin to secrete os-

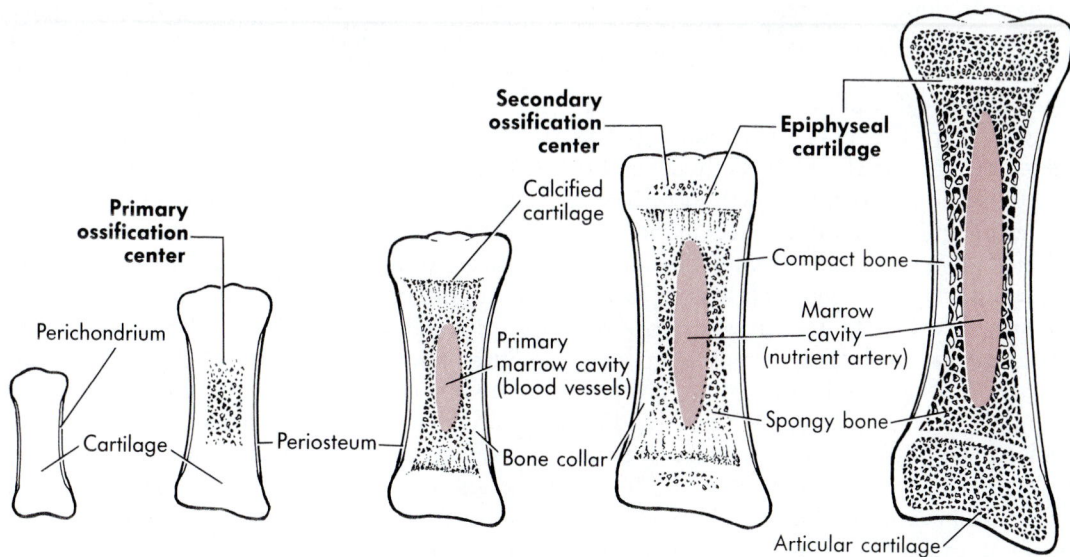

FIG. 40-1 Stages of endochondral bone formation and centers of ossification in long bone.

teoid (see Chapter 38). Some of the bone cell precursors are present in fetal connective tissues, whereas others migrate in blood to sites of bone formation after blood vessels have grown into the tissue.

Cellular aggregation and maturation occur in two types of fetal tissue, depending on which bones are being formed. The cranium, facial bones, clavicles, and parts of the jaw bone arise from a fetal membrane termed the mesenchyme. Bones that develop on or within the mesenchyme grow by the process of **intramembranous formation.** As the mesenchyme becomes vascularized, the immature bone cells aggregate and mature into osteoblasts, which form the centers of ossification. Osteoblasts secrete osteoid, which surrounds them and quickly ossifies, forming the lacunae and canaliculi of compact bone. Spicules of bone radiate from the ossification centers to form the primary trabeculae characteristic of spongy bone. Later, some of the spongy bone is replaced by compact bone.

Endochondral formation is the development of new bone from cartilage. This process, by which the long bones of the appendicular skeleton develop, is more complex than intramembranous formation (Fig. 40-1). First, mesenchymal tissue forms a **cartilage model,** which defines the shape of the bone. The cartilage model is subsequently removed and replaced by bone. Endochondral bone formation begins in the outer layer of the cartilage model, which consists of a layer of dense connective tissue called **perichondrium.** The perichondrium contains cells that develop into osteoblasts, forming a collar of bone, termed the **periosteal collar,** around the cartilage model. Cartilage enclosed within the periosteal collar degenerates, and capillaries from outside the perichondrium invade the degenerating cartilage cells, car-

rying with them osteoblast precursors from the inner layer of the perichondrium and osteoclast precursors from the blood itself.

Endochondral bone formation progresses at the primary center of ossification in the middle of the cartilage model and extends toward either end of the developing bone. At the same time, the periosteal collar thickens and becomes wider toward the epiphyses. By the end of gestation, **secondary centers of ossification,** the epiphyseal centers, begin to lay down bone at both ends of the cartilage model. Here, too, cartilage within the periosteal collar degenerates, and blood vessels grow inward, delivering bone cell precursors. Once the osteoblasts begin to secrete osteoid, ossification spreads from the secondary centers in all directions until all the cartilage within the model is replaced by bone.

Two regions of cartilage remain at the ends of long bones: (1) articular cartilage over the free ends of the bone and (2) the epiphyseal plate, a layer of cartilage between the diaphysis and epiphysis. (These structures are described and illustrated in Chapter 38; see Fig. 38-1.) The epiphyseal plate retains the ability to form and calcify new cartilage and deposit bone until the skeleton matures (at approximately 18 years of age).

Bone Growth

Until adult stature is reached, growth in the length of bone occurs at the epiphyseal plate through endochondral ossification. Cartilage cells in the proximal layer of the epiphyseal plate multiply and enlarge. As rapidly as new cartilage cells form, cartilage cells at the metaphyseal side of the plate are destroyed and replaced by bone.

In the shaft of new bone, where growth is relatively slow, the bone produced by accretion is compact and dense. The compact bone is thickest where it has to withstand the maximal stresses, which generally occur in the middle of the shaft.

More growth always takes place at one end of a long bone than at the other. The more active end is sometimes known as the "growing end" of the bone, and it is the end more likely to sustain a growth disturbance after injury. There are important differences in the rates of growth of individual bones. For example, the growing end of the femur lengthens twice as fast as the growing end of the tibia. The longitudinal growth rate of the extremities is greater at birth than at any other time. Longitudinal growth occurs by division of the cartilage cells on the epiphyseal side of the growth plate and by continued replacement of the calcified cartilage by bone on the metaphyseal side.

Growth in the diameter of bone occurs by deposition of new bone on an existing bone surface. Bone matrix is laid down by osteoblasts on the periosteal surface and subsequently becomes calcified. At the same time, bone resorption occurs on the endosteal surface. Endosteal resorption increases the diameter of the medullary cavity, which contains marrow and spongy bone.

Many factors affect the development, physiology, and rate of growth of the epiphyseal plate. Growth hormone has to be secreted by the pituitary gland at a constant rate to stimulate the growth plate consistently. Other known factors affecting growth include genetic makeup, nutrition, general health, and other hormones, such as thyroid hormone, adrenal and gonadal androgens, and estrogens. These factors influence both the rate of bone growth and the time of appearance of the secondary ossification centers. When the skeleton is mature, the epiphyseal plate is replaced by bone. This process, termed epiphyseal closure, unites the diaphysis and the epiphysis. Epiphyseal closure occurs earlier in females than males because of the accelerating influence of estrogens on cartilage growth and matrix formation.

Throughout life, bone is constantly being destroyed and reformed (see Chapter 38), but the process is at its maximum in children approximately 2½ years of age. By young adulthood, bone turnover, or remodeling, occurs at a relatively slow rate.

Skeletal Development

The axial skeleton changes shape with growth. (The axial skeleton and appendicular skeleton are described and illustrated in Chapter 38; see Fig. 38-3.) In a newborn the entire spine is concave anteriorly; the child's natural posture is "curled up." In the first 3 months of life, with the ability to control the head, the upper (cervical) spine begins to "arch," or become convex anteriorly. The normal arch in the lower (lumbar) spine begins to develop with sitting.

The appendicular skeleton (the extremities) grows faster during childhood than does the axial skeleton. The neonate has a relatively large head and long spine with disproportionately shorter limbs than an adult. By age 1, 50% of the total growth of the spine has occurred (Winter, 1977). Therefore, failure of the spine to grow (e.g., spinal fusion) does not limit eventual height as much as the premature fusion of the growth plates of the lower extremities. In children with congenital curvature of the spine, growth tends to worsen the deformity rather than to increase the length of the spine.

Besides getting longer, growing bones of the extremities undergo changes in rotation and alignment. In the newborn the femur is flexed forward up to 40 degrees, and the tibia is rotated inward. With growth, the femur assumes its normal alignment and tibial rotation disappears, usually at age 8. Bowlegs and knock-knees are normal at certain stages of growth. At birth, the neonate's legs are bowed because of stresses in utero. With growth, the knees gradually turn inward approximately 7 to 8 degrees, which is normal alignment in adults.

Muscle Growth

The composition and size of muscles vary with age. In the fetus, muscle tissue contains a large amount of water and much intercellular matrix. After birth, both are reduced considerably as the muscle fibers (cells) enlarge by accumulating cytoplasm. Little information is available about the numbers of fibers in a given muscle at different ages, but the total mass of muscle in the body can be estimated from the amount of creatinine excreted in the urine because the conversion of creatine to creatinine takes place only in muscle (see Chapter 38). Between birth and maturity, the number of muscle nuclei in the body increases 14 times in boys and 10 times in girls. Muscle fibers reach their maximal size in girls at approximately the age of 10 and in boys by the age of 14. Growth in length occurs at the ends of muscles and the increase in length is accompanied by an increase in number of nuclei in the fibers. Muscle fibers increase in diameter as the fibrils become more numerous. The fibrils themselves do not increase in diameter. Connective tissue components of muscle grow where the tendon and muscle meet.

A potent stimulus to the growth of a muscle is the separation of its attachments as the skeleton grows. The length of a muscle fiber is the direct consequence of the range of movement it is called on to perform. The stimulus for the formation of a tendon is probably the pull of the muscle rudiment on undifferentiated connective tissue. The repair of a tendon from which a segment has been removed does not occur if the muscle is prevented from exercising tension on the damaged tendon. Replacement of muscle by tendon (tendinification) sometimes is the result of limitation of movement. If the normal opponents of a muscle are paralyzed, the muscle fails to grow properly, and it may be that the full development of a muscle is dependent on the progressive rise in the tension exerted on it by its antagonists.

Muscle growth during adolescence is a major factor in weight gain. Sex differences in muscle size and weight are minor in childhood, but become considerable with the onset of puberty.

In the infant, muscle accounts for approximately 25% of total body weight, compared with 40% in the adult. The muscles of the head, trunk, and upper limbs are relatively heavier in the infant because the lower extremities are poorly developed. In the adult, approximately 55% of muscle weight is accounted for by the lower limb muscles. The respiratory and facial muscles are well developed at birth so that the infant can perform the vital functions of breathing and sucking. Other muscle groups, such as the pelvic muscle, take several years to develop fully. Throughout life, the weight of the skeletal muscles can be increased by exercise. Less is known about the development of visceral and cardiac muscle. Visceral muscle fibers increase in both number and size, but the increase in fiber size is most important. Fiber enlargement alone can increase the bulk of visceral muscle by as many as eight times. Cardiac muscle also grows mainly by enlargement of existing fibers.

MUSCULOSKELETAL ALTERATIONS IN CHILDREN

Congenital Defects
Syndactyly

The most common congenital defect of the upper extremity is **syndactyly,** or webbing of the fingers (Fig. 40-2). Simple webbing involves the soft tissue envelope alone and is best released surgically when the child is 3 to 4 years of age. True syndactyly involves fusion of the bones and nails as well as the soft tissues, and may be associated with absence or anomaly of bony or neurovascular units. The primary goal in surgical correction of these defects is to achieve maximal function and appearance. Ideally, corrective surgery is deferred until the child is 6 to 12 months of age and completed before the child enters school. **Vestigial tabs,** such as an extra digit, are best removed during the immediate neonatal period, however. An x-ray examination should be performed before removal to determine whether bone is present, because this may affect the method of removal. Any neonate with a congenital anomaly of the upper extremity is examined for associated systemic anomalies, particularly of the heart and kidneys.

Developmental Dysplasia of the Hip

Developmental dysplasia of the hip (DDH), formerly known as congenital dislocation of the hip, is an abnor-

FIG. 40-2 Syndactyly.

mality in the development of the proximal femur, acetabulum, or both. Although most often present at birth, it may occur at any time in the newborn or infant period.

The incidence of true dislocation of the hip or a dislocatable hip is 1 in 1000 live births. Some degree of instability of the hip is present in approximately 10 per 1000 live births. Girls are affected over males 6:1. The left hip is affected in 60% of cases with the right hip alone affected only 20% of the time. Bilateral DDH occurs 20% of the time.

Although the exact cause of DDH is unknown, it is known to be multifactorial. If there is a family history, there is a higher incidence of DDH; therefore, there is a hereditary component. Other risk factors include first pregnancies and oligohydramnios (deficient volume of amniotic fluid), which are thought to limit fetal movement, and breech presentation that not only limits movement but places the hips in a position of flexion and adduction. Up to 50% of children with DDH have a history of breech presentation. Maternal hormones that reportedly increase joint laxity also have an effect on DDH, although the exact mechanism is unknown. The presence of other anomalies, such as foot deformities and torticollis, increases the risk of DDH. Developmental dysplasia of the hip is more common in Caucasians and those cultures that swaddle infants with the hips in extension and adduction.

Pathophysiology

The hip can be described as subluxed, dislocatable, or dislocated (Fig. 40-3). The subluxed hip maintains contact with the acetabulum but is not well seated within the hip joint. The dislocatable hip is sometimes located but can be dislocated. The dislocated hip has no contact between the femoral head and the acetabulum. Some degree of acetabular dysplasia is present in almost

Normal   Dysplasia   Subluxation   Dislocation

FIG. 40-3 Configuration and relationship of structures in developmental dysplasia of the hip. (From Whaley & Wong, 1991.)

all cases. Typically, the acetabulum is shallow or sloping rather than cup-shaped.

By approximately 10 weeks of gestation, the femur, acetabulum, and hip joint capsule are well developed. Most dislocations occur in the perinatal period, at which time there is maximal joint distention and elasticity. It is hoped that the diagnosis will be made during this period, when the hip can be reduced and returned to its normal anatomic position. If correct alignment is maintained, a stable hip will develop.

If the dislocation is not diagnosed early, secondary changes in both the soft tissues and bony structures will occur. The longer the dislocation has been present, the greater the secondary changes that occur. These secondary changes include stretching of the hip capsule, contracture and shortening of the structures of the hip joint, changes in the blood supply to the hip, flattening of the femoral head, and acetabular dysplasia, sometimes with development of a false acetabulum. It is much more difficult to achieve a normal hip joint at this point, and in some cases it is impossible.

Approximately 2% of dislocations are classified as teratologic. These dislocations occur early in gestation with advanced changes present at birth. Teratologic dislocations are usually associated with other abnormalities, such as arthrogryposis (a syndrome characterized by contractures in multiple joints). It is not usually possible to achieve a normal hip joint in these cases.

Clinical Manifestations

The clinical manifestations vary with the severity of the condition and the age of the child. Signs and symptoms which should be noted include:

1. Asymmetry of gluteal or thigh folds
2. Leg length discrepancy
3. Limitation of hip abduction
4. Positive Ortolani sign
5. Positive Barlow test
6. Positive Trendelenburg sign
7. Abnormal (waddling) gait
8. Pain

The child should also be examined for other anomalies.

Evaluation and Treatment

In the newborn period, clinical examination is the most important diagnostic tool. Real-time ultrasound in which the hip is examined while the ultrasound is performed is extremely valuable in the newborn period. The use of ultrasound allows visualization of the cartilaginous structures of the hip (the femoral head and the outer lip of the acetabulum), which are not seen on plain roentgenogram. Radiographs are used in older infants and children (Boal & Schwentker, 1991).

Treatment depends on the age of the child, severity of dysplasia, and duration of dysplasia. The earlier treatment is begun, the better the result. Nonoperative treatment consists of bracing, traction, casts, or a combination of these. The hip is placed in a position of flexion and abduction and held in this position until the joint capsule tightens and the acetabulum is molded to assume a cup shape. In dislocations discovered in the walking-age child, surgical intervention is usually required (McCullough & Pellino, 1993).

Deformities of the Foot

Foot deformities in children are common and may be the result of intrauterine positioning or true embryonic malformations. **Metatarsus adductus** is the most common foot deformity, occurring in 2 per 1000 live births. It is frequently bilateral and is believed to be the result of intrauterine positioning.

Talipes equinovarus (clubfoot) is another common

FIG. 40-4 Infant with bilateral congenital talipes equinovarus. (From Brashear & Raney, 1978.)

deformity. It occurs in 1 to 2 per 1000 live births and is bilateral 50% of the time. Males are affected more than females (Kyzer, 1991).

Pathophysiology

Arrested or abnormal embryonic development has been implicated in the development of foot deformities. The foot normally goes through a stage of flexion and eversion during early development but gradually assumes a normal position by the seventh month. Arrested development during this early stage tends to result in a rigid deformity. The muscles on the posterior and medial aspect of the leg become unduly short, and the fibrous capsules (joint capsules) of all the deformed joints are thick and contracted on the concave side of the deformity. Soft tissue contractures become progressively resistant to correction, both in utero and after birth, and lead to secondary changes that involve the shape of the actively growing bones and the joints.

Clinical Manifestations

In metatarsus adductus, the forefoot is abducted and in varus, giving the foot its kidney bean shape. The hindfoot is normal. Talipes equinovarus involves both the bony structures and soft tissues of the foot. The forefoot is abducted (turned inward) with the hindfoot in varus and inverted. The entire foot is in equinus (pointing downward) (Fig. 40-4). (Terms that describe foot positions are defined in Table 40-1.) There are deep skin creases on the medial and plantar aspects of the foot. The true clubfoot is rigid and cannot be passively corrected.

Evaluation and Treatment

Metatarsus adductus may resolve without treatment. In many cases, stretching exercises are combined with bracing to bring the foot to a neutral position. Later, reverse-last or straight-last shoes are used for a period of months to maintain the correction. In cases where the foot cannot be passively corrected to neutral, serial cast-

TABLE 40-1

Terms Used to Describe Foot Abnormalities

Term	Definition
Position	
Abduction	Lateral deviation away from the midline of the body
Adduction	Lateral deviation toward the midline of the body
Eversion	Twisting of the foot outward along its long axis
Inversion	Twisting of the foot inward on its long axis
Dorsiflexion	Bending of the foot upward and backward
Plantar flexion	Bending of the foot downward and forward
Abnormality	
Talipes	Congenital abnormality of the foot (clubfoot)
Pes	Acquired deformity of the foot
Varus	Inversion and adduction of the heel and the forefoot
Valgus	Eversion and abduction of the heel and forefoot
Equinus	Plantar flexion of the foot in which the heel is lower than the toes
Calcaneus	Dorsiflexion of the foot in which the heel is lower than the toes
Planus	Flattening of the medial longitudinal arch of the foot (flatfoot)
Cavus	Elevation of the medial longitudinal arch of the foot (high arch)
Equinovarus	Coexistent equinus and varus deformities
Calcaneovarus	Coexistent calcaneus and varus deformities
Equinovalgus	Coexistent equinus and valgus deformities
Calcaneovalgus	Coexistent calcaneus and valgus deformities

Note: The positions listed can all be achieved by voluntary movement of the normal foot; an abnormality exists if the foot is fixed in one or more of the positions while at rest.

ing may be used for several weeks followed by bracing and then shoes.

Treatment of talipes equinovarus should begin in the newborn nursery. Initially, the foot is manipulated and then casted on a weekly basis. This is continued for as long as correction is being achieved (usually 4 to 6 months). Radiographs are taken in a simulated weight-bearing position to assess the alignment of the bones. If the bony architecture is abnormal after casting or a plateau has been reached, surgery may be required. Currently, a single surgical procedure that releases all the tight structures of the foot and allows the foot to come to a normal alignment performed at the age of 6 to 9 months is preferred. After the discontinuation of casting after surgery, reverse-last or straight-last shoes may be used for the next 6 to 12 months to maintain the corrected position. Although a relatively normal appearing and functioning foot can be achieved, it will always be smaller than the nonclubfoot and the muscles of the calf will be less well developed (Ikeda, 1992; Kyzer, 1991; McCullough & Pellino, in press).

Congenital Muscle Disease

Congenital muscle disorders, or myopathies, are rare and are generally mild. The possible congenital myopathies include congenital absence of muscles (failure of muscle cells to differentiate to a given region), congenital hypoplasia (local or generalized), congenital hyperplasia (local or generalized), faulty intrinsic development leading to disfigurement of fibers, and presenile abiotrophy (senescent polymyopathy).

Some persons are born without certain muscles. The muscles may be irrelevant in some instances or very important in others. The most commonly absent muscles are the pectoralis, trapezius, serratus anterior, and quadratus femoris. Congenital muscle absence is associated with other congenital abnormalities.

Many congenital deformities in children are a result of shortened muscles. Some conditions, such as myokymia and neuromyotonia, involve continuous muscle activity. Some true contracture states involve a contracted muscle's inability to relax because of a failure in the metabolic mechanism required for relaxation, such as in McArdle disease (see Chapter 39), in which there is a phosphorylase deficiency and a phosphofructokinase deficiency. Congenital myotonia (Thomsen disease) is a rare hereditary disease having two forms and is characterized by myotonia and muscular hypertrophy. Because no morphologic changes are evident in the muscles, an abnormality in the contracting mechanism must be the cause. Blockage of potassium transfer across the cell membrane or a defect in the formation or use of phosphates also may be the cause of myotonic response (Morrissy, 1990).

Because of new histologic technology in the past 25 years, a group of congenital polymyopathies that show an unusual pattern of central densification of sarcoplasm (cores) has been described. This group of diseases involves a basic morphologic abnormality. Included in this category of congenital myopathies are central core disease, nemaline (rod-body) myopathy, mitochondrial (lipid storage) myopathy, and central myotubular myopathy.

Evidence first suggested that these myopathies are always manifested in infancy as delayed motor development with signs of hypotonia and weakness of the limbs, but now they have been shown to emerge later in life as well—up to middle age. Extremely slow progression characterizes these perhaps misnamed congenital myopathies.

Most diagnoses of congenital muscle disease that are made in childhood involve infants who are "floppy" at birth or show delays in reaching milestones for motor development. The muscle weakness does not fit the genetic pattern or progressive course of the muscular dystrophies (see p. 1497) or equal the distribution and severity seen in anterior horn cell disease. The distribution of weakness is usually greater in the limbs, particularly the quadriceps and elbow flexors, than in the bulbar musculature. Many disorders are not progressive and are associated with spinal deformities and hip dislocations.

Congenital muscle diseases are usually categorized by the striking abnormalities seen on muscle biopsy. Type I fiber predominance and fiber atrophy are also common features on muscle biopsy. Diagnosis is confirmed by histologic stain and phase and electron microscopy.

No specific treatment is yet available. Children require aggressive physiotherapy programs early in the course of the illness to prevent contractures and potentially improve strength. One study reported improvement in strength after a mild isometric exercise program in children with central core disease. In other respects the congenital myopathies require the same treatment programs followed for other individuals with neuromuscular disease. Cardiopulmonary failure is seen in myotubular myopathy and nemaline myopathy. These children should be closely monitored for any treatable complications, and families should be prepared for the difficult decision regarding ventilatory support that may ensue (Brooke, 1977).

A small number of cases are known to have been inherited in an autosomal dominant, autosomal recessive, or X-linked recessive pattern. Therefore genetic counseling, with documentation of a detailed pedigree and calculation of risk factors, is in order for young parents.

Abnormal Density or Modeling of the Skeleton
Osteogenesis Imperfecta

Osteogenesis imperfecta (brittle bone disease) is an inherited disorder of connective tissues that primarily affects bone. The disorder was first described in 1840 as a syndrome in newborns consisting of osteoporosis with fractures and skeletal deformities. Currently, Sillence's (1981) classification is replacing the older classification of tarda and congenita. Sillence's system is based on both models of inheritance and clinical findings. This classification consists of IA, IB, II, III, IVA, and IVB. In the more severe forms, the child is usually stillborn or dies soon after birth, although some survive into childhood. Osteogenesis imperfecta in its more severe forms is evident at birth because fractures and deformity have occurred in utero. The less severe forms may not become evident until the child begins to walk. Some children with this form experience numerous fractures and can be mistaken for battered children until the diagnosis is made.

The incidence of the most common form is about 1 in 40,000 live births. Inheritance is usually autosomal dominant but can be autosomal recessive. At least four syndromes have been identified that have various clinical manifestations and prognoses.

Pathophysiology

The major errors in osteogenesis imperfecta lie in the synthesis of collagen (Sykes, 1987). Very recent genetic studies have shown that the gene responsible for the encoding of collagen is "remarkably feeble," that is, easily mutates (Sykes, 1987). These mutations cause osteogenesis imperfecta. The large range of phenotypes are all mutants of the two collagen structural genes. (Genes are discussed in Chapter 4.) Abnormalities in collagen include: (1) an increase in collagen hydroxylysine residue in bones; (2) a decrease in hydroxylysine-norleucine in skin collagen; and (3) absence of alpha-2-polypeptide production in cultured skin fibroblasts (Zaleske, Doppelt, & Mankin, 1986).

A number of metabolic abnormalities have been reported. Some individuals have increased serum thyroxine levels suggesting hyperthyroidism. This is consistent with the findings of increased sweating, heat intolerance, increased body temperature, a resting tachycardia, and tachypnea. The hyperthyroid findings, however, are not consistent in all individuals with osteogenesis imperfecta. Studies of leukocyte metabolism suggest an uncoupling of oxidative phosphorylation. Reports of alterations of platelet function with defects in adhesion and clot retraction also exist.

Clinical Manifestations

The classic clinical manifestations of osteogenesis imperfecta are bone fractures; osteoporosis; abnormally short, bowed, and deformed limbs; short stature; curvature of the spine; and bluish discoloration of the sclerae (whites of the eyes) (Fig. 40-5). Four syndromes of clinical manifestations, designated type I through IV, have been identified. The most severe, types II and III,

are comparable to osteogenesis imperfecta congenita. These two types are characterized by autosomal recessive inheritance and early onset of manifestations. Both can cause stillbirth or severe neonatal deformity and a short life expectancy. Less severe are types I and IV, which are comparable to osteogenesis imperfecta tarda. Types I and IV are slightly more common than types II and III. Types I and IV are inherited as autosomal dominant traits and vary in age of onset from birth to adulthood. Some children with type IV disease improve at puberty (McCullough & Pellino, in press).

Evaluation and Treatment

Evaluation of osteogenesis imperfecta is based on clinical manifestations and serologic tests. Serum alkaline phosphatase is elevated in all forms of the disease. Osteogenesis imperfecta can be diagnosed prenatally by ultrasound or chorionic villi sampling. Quantitative analysis of cultured skin fibroblast collagen by electrophoresis shows a decreased quantity of collagen in the affected individual.

For osteogenesis imperfecta type II, no therapeutic intervention will be effective. For other types of osteogen-

FIG. 40-5 **Osteogenesis imperfecta.** Severely osteopenic and distorted tibia and fibula of child with osteogenesis imperfecta. Healing fracture shows abundant callus formation. (Courtesy Dr. James W. Debnam, Jr., Chesterfield, MO. From Kissane, 1990.)

esis imperfecta, careful positioning and handling of the neonate may prevent fractures. Beyond the neonatal period, various orthopedic measures are applied, such as prompt splinting of fractures and correction of deformities arising from the progressive bowing or bending of the skeleton. Although no clear benefit has been demonstrated, therapeutic regimens including supplements of calcium or fluoride, vitamin C, or magnesium oxide have been tried. Calcitron has been reported to increase the skeletal mass and decrease the frequency of fracture in some cases. Genetic counseling for affected families should aim at primary prevention (Behrman, Kliegman, Nelson, & Vaughan, 1992).

Rickets

Rickets is a disorder in which growing bone fails to become mineralized (ossified), resulting in "soft" bones and skeletal deformity. Incidence of rickets is greatest in children who receive insufficient dietary vitamin D, a mineral that is necessary for absorption and metabolism of calcium and phosphorus, the main minerals in bone. The pathophysiology of rickets is the same as that of osteomalacia, the "adult form" of rickets (see Chapter 39). The difference between osteomalacia and rickets is that in osteomalacia new bone formed during remodeling fails to ossify, whereas in rickets, new bone formed at the growing ends of bones fails to ossify.

The characteristic bone changes in rickets are identified in the epiphyseal plates (growth plates) before closure. The normal epiphyseal plate is a complex organized structure located at the ends of long bones between the epiphysis and metaphysis. The plate is organized into four distinct layers. The first layer, adjacent to the epiphysis, is composed of a few spherical cartilage cells (chondrocytes) randomly arranged in pairs. Their primary function is to store nutrients. The second layer is composed of flattened chondrocytes arranged longitudinally in parallel columns. The cells in this layer divide and produce cartilaginous matrix (see Chapter 38 for a description of bone formation). The third layer is composed of large spherical cells that participate in ossification of the cartilaginous matrix. The fourth layer is located within the metaphysis. This layer contains bars of collagen fibers that are partially or completely ossified. The bars are sheathed with osteoblasts that produce layers of osteoid.

In rickets, the structure of the growth plate and metaphysis is disorganized. The first and second layers may not be significantly altered, but the third layer is grossly abnormal. There is a disorganized increase in the number of cells that decreases the length and width of the growth plate. In the fourth layer the cartilage bars are disorganized and decreased in size and number. In the metaphysis, there is disorganized formation of lamellae and haversian systems.

Children with rickets are listless and irritable. They have profound hypotonia and muscle weakness and may be unable to walk without support. Abnormal parietal flattening and frontal bossing occur in the skull. The calvaria become soft and the sutures may widen. Cartilaginous attachments of the ribs become prominent, and the long bones of the extremities (tibia, femur, radius, and ulna) may be bowed. Growth is retarded, and fractures are common.

Scoliosis

Scoliosis is a lateral curvature of the spine (Fig. 40-6). It can be classified as nonstructural or structural. **Nonstructural scoliosis** results from a cause other than the spine itself, such as posture, leg length discrepancy, pain, etc. **Structural scoliosis** is curvature of the spine associated with vertebral rotation. Nonstructural scoliosis can become structural if the underlying cause is not found and treated.

Structural scoliosis can be caused by a great variety of conditions. It can result from congenital skeletal abnormalities (15%), neuromuscular diseases (15%), trauma, extraspinal contractures, bone infections that involve the vertebrae, metabolic bone disorders (e.g., rickets, osteoporosis, osteogenesis imperfecta), joint disease, and tumors. Most cases of structural scoliosis, however, have no known cause, although genetic factors are suggested. Structural scoliosis with no known cause, termed **idiopathic scoliosis,** accounts for at least 65% of cases.

Idiopathic scoliosis is classified as infantile, juvenile, or adolescent, depending on the child's age at the time of onset. In infantile scoliosis spinal curvature develops during the first 3 years of life; in juvenile scoliosis, curvature develops between the skeletal age of 4 and the onset of adolescence; and in adolescent scoliosis, it develops after the skeletal age of 12 years in girls and 14 years in boys. Adolescent idiopathic scoliosis is the most common. Scoliosis in its milder forms occurs equally in boys and girls. Girls, however, more often develop more severe curves requiring treatment (Morrissy, 1990; Tachjdian, 1990).

Pathophysiology

It has been hypothesized that in individuals with adolescent scoliosis, there is an abnormality of the central nervous system involving the balance mechanism in the midbrain. Postural and equilibrium dysfunction along with vestibular dysfunction has also been implicated in other studies.

Experimentally, it has also been shown that individuals with adolescent idiopathic scoliosis have an abnormality in the function of the posterior columns of the spinal cord. This results in abnormal proprioception and is not evident clinically except in the presence of

FIG. 40-6 Scoliosis in children. Normal spinal alignment and abnormal spinal curvatures associated with scoliosis. **A,** Normal. **B,** Mild. **C,** Severe. **D,** Rotation and curvature of scoliosis. (From Thompson, McFarland, Hirsch, & Tucker, 1993.)

scoliosis. Presumably this lesion is in the cervical spine as both the upper and lower extremities are affected. It is not known whether these findings are causative or secondary to the scoliosis (Barrack, Whitecloud, Burker, Cook, & Harding, 1984; Barrack, Wyatt et al., 1988; Byrd, 1988).

The earliest pathologic changes, which are actually secondary changes, occur in the soft tissues. The muscles, ligaments, and other soft tissues become shortened on the concave side of the curve long before bone deformities occur. With time, progressive deformities of the vertebral column and ribs develop. In growing children, lateral deviation of the spinal column ceases, and one-sided compression of the vertebral bodies on the concave side of the curve begins. Vertebral deformity occurs as asymmetric forces are applied to the epiphyseal center of the ossification by shortened and tight soft tissues on the concave side of the curve. The degree of compression and twisting varies according to the position of the vertebrae in the curve. The compressive force is greatest on the vertebrae in the apex of the concavity, so that the apical vertebrae become most deformed.

The curves increase most rapidly during periods of rapid skeletal growth. If the curve is less than 40 degrees at skeletal maturity, the risk of progression is quite small. In curves greater than 50 degrees, the spine is biomechanically unstable, and the curve will in all likelihood continue to progress throughout life. The average rate of progression is 1 degree per year. Curves in the thoracic spine greater than 60 degrees result in decreased pulmonary function whereas the most common complication of large curves in the lumbar spine is back pain.

Clinical Manifestations

The clinical manifestations of nonstructural scoliosis are mild spinal curvature with prominence of one hip or rounded shoulders. The curvature disappears with forward flexion of the spine, lying down, or traction of the head. Treatment for nonstructural scoliosis is correction of the underlying disorder. The clinical manifestations of structural scoliosis include asymmetry of hip height, asymmetry of shoulder height, shoulder and scapular (shoulder blade) prominence, rib prominence, and posterior humping of ribs or hips, which are visible when the child bends forward from the waist.

Evaluation and Treatment

Spinal curvature is usually visible or palpable, and muscles on one side of the lower back (the convex side) may be prominent or bulging. Most cases of idiopathic scoliosis are noticed during school screening programs. In girls the deformity may be noticed because clothing does not "hang" properly on the body. Diagnosis is made by x-ray examinations.

Treatment of curves between 25 and 35 degrees in the skeletally immature child is with bracing. In most cases the low-profile brace is used. Occasionally, a Milwaukee brace, which has a metal upperstructure and neck ring, is needed for very high curves. The brace is worn for 23 hours daily until skeletal maturity. Bracing will only prevent progression of the curve; it will not correct the curvature. Currently, there is research being done with night bracing only, but the results are inconclusive at this time. Bracing is not effective in curves greater than 40 degrees or in skeletally mature individuals. Surgical treatment with spinal fusion with instrumentation is recommended for curves greater than 40 to 50 degrees. If surgery, however, is indicated, it is better performed during the adolescent years while there is greater flexibility of the curves and less risk of complications. The surgery can be done at any age, however.

Another treatment is transcutaneous muscle stimulation, in which electrodes are placed on the skin of the back at night, and weak electrical impulses transmitted through the electrodes cause the muscles on the convex side of the curve to contract several times per minute. Theoretically, this treatment strengthens the muscles on the convex side of the curve and pulls the spine into alignment. Initial studies showed this to be a viable alternative to bracing, but as longer follow-up has become available, the results have not been as favorable. Many centers have discontinued the use of electrical stimulation as a treatment modality.

Bone Infection: Osteomyelitis

Osteomyelitis is an inflammation of the bone. Occurring twice as often in males as females, acute osteomyelitis may affect infants and children of any age, but occurs most frequently between 3 and 12 years of age (Behrman et al., 1992).

Bacteria enter the bone through the bloodstream and lodge in the medullary cavity, where a rich phagocytic mechanism frequently prevents most of the bacteria from establishing an infectious state. In some cases, however, the bacteria may lodge at the end of the arterial loops beneath the epiphyseal plate and infection develops because there are no phagocytic cells present to remove the bacteria (Fink & Nelson, 1986; Gillespie, Haywood-Farmer, Fong, & Harding, 1987; Hobbs, 1922; Karlin, 1987; Morrissy & Shore, 1986).

Although bacterial blood infections are common in children, not all infections result in osteomyelitis. Efforts have been made to better understand why some children with blood infections develop osteomyelitis whereas others do not. Investigations into the possible mechanism or mechanisms responsible for osteomyelitis have focused on trauma, an associated factor in the development of osteomyelitis in 30% to 40% of cases in children (Dich, Nelson, & Haltalin, 1975). It has been shown experimentally that osteomyelitis can be induced with a subclinical bacterial infection by making a small crack in the epiphyseal plate. The same bacteria without the injury produce a rare, subclinical form of osteomyelitis that appears to heal spontaneously (Morrissy & Shore, 1986). Thus trauma may be one of the precursors or causative factors that allow the bacteria to settle in the bone or joint.

The organism responsible for osteomyelitis varies and is related to the age of the child (see box on p. 1493). Osteomyelitis in the newborn is caused primarily by *Staphylococcus aureus*. Group B streptococcus and *Escherichia coli* infections are responsible for some cases, especially those of multiple bone involvement and in high-risk infants (Carnsdale, 1992).

Staphylococcus aureus is the responsible organism in 60% to 90% of osteomyelitis in older children. Musculoskeletal infection caused by *Haemophilus influenzae* primarily occurs in children between the ages of 6 months and 4 years. At this age, the child's immunity to the organism, a normal inhabitant of the upper respiratory tract, is lowered because of the loss of passive immunity acquired from the mother at birth. Gram-negative microorganisms account for an increasing number of infections of the vertebrae (Abramovitz, Baston, & Yablon, 1986; Carnsdale, 1992; Ray & Bassett, 1985), whereas *Pseudomonas* infections are associated with heroin addiction (Chandrasekar & Narula, 1986).

Factors that predispose to the development of osteomyelitis include impetigo, furunculosis, infected lesions of varicella (chickenpox), infected burns, cerebral abscesses, immunization with bacillus Calmette-Guérin (BCG) vaccine, prolonged intravenous or central parenteral alimentation, drug addiction, and direct trauma to the area adjacent to the site of osteomyelitis.

Pathophysiology

Osteomyelitis usually begins as a bloody abscess in the metaphysis of the bone. The abscess ruptures under the periosteum and spreads along the bone shaft or into the bone marrow cavity if untreated. Infection rarely spreads down the medullary cavity of the bone but rather first gains entrance to the subperiosteal space in the metaphysis. This is the path of least resistance because the cortex of the bone in this area is porous or mazelike, and the inflammatory response blocks spread within the bone (Morrissy & Shore, 1986). Because of the accumulation of debris caused by the infection, the periosteum may separate and form a shell of new bone around the infected portion of the shaft. Because the periosteum is separated from an adequate blood supply, sections of the bone die with the pieces of dead bone, or **sequestrum** (Fig. 40-7). The periosteum that maintains a blood supply generates new bone and is responsible for the appearance of the periosteal new bone, or **involucrum** (see Fig. 40-7). The presence of the sequestra and involucrum indicates that the disease has progressed to subperiosteal abscess formation.

In cases where the infection in the metaphysis occurs near the joint, the accumulating pus (bacteria, white blood cells, and fluid) creates increasing pressure that may cause a rupture into the joint cavity. If rupture into the joint occurs, the pus causes inflammation and a condition called **secondary suppurative arthritis** (Alderson, Speers, Emslie, & Nade, 1986). Osteomyelitis is most commonly caused by bacteria that reach the metaphysis through the bloodstream but may occur through secondary inoculation of microorganisms caused by trauma or contagious spread of infection from cellulitis in adjacent soft tissue.

Osteomyelitis in infants is frequently associated with septic arthritis because the infant's bone has blood vessels that perforate the growth plate. Because of the unique nature of blood supply to an infant's bones, osteomyelitis and septic arthritis frequently occur together. Normal anatomic variations in infants allow infection to spread directly to the epiphysis, which causes both joint disease and permanent epiphyseal disease.

There are several reasons why children are susceptible to joint involvement. First, capillaries penetrate the epiphyseal plate and provide direct communication between the metaphysis of the bone and the joint cavity during the first month of life. Second, the capsules of the hip joints attach distally to the femur. Because of these two structural differences during infancy, infections originating in the metaphysis of the bone, such as osteomyelitis, can spread rapidly to the joint cavity. The reverse may also occur, i.e., infections of the joint cavity may spread directly to the metaphysis of the bone. Bone growth may be completely arrested in extreme cases.

In the immature infant, there is no epiphyseal plate or an ossific nucleus at the end of the bone, and the cartilage precursor of bone is penetrated by vascular channels. In these infants the infection begins in the vulnerable cartilage precursor of the end-bone itself that results in rapid destruction of the joint and arrested growth of the bone. For this reason, the early detection and treatment of osteomyelitis is crucial if the infant's joint is to be saved from later destruction. As the child matures and the epiphyseal plate forms, a temporary barrier is established against infection because the arterioles end beneath the epiphyseal plate (Morrissy & Shore, 1986; Trueta, 1959).

In children older than 2 years of age, the epiphyseal plate prevents the spread of a metaphyseal abscess into the epiphysis, and the cortex of the metaphysis is thicke   These anatomic differences increase the likelihood that the metaphyseal abscess will extend into the diaphysis and the blood supply of the bone will be disrupted. The periosteum is also more difficult to perforate in older children; this may lead to a larger subperiosteal abscess that could endanger the periosteal blood

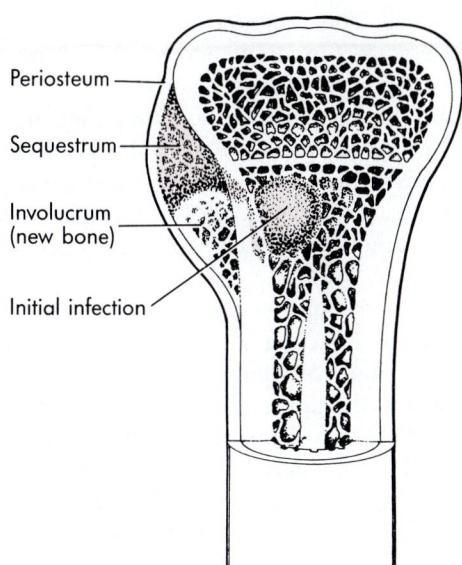

FIG. 40-7 Osteomyelitis in children. Infection starts in the metaphysis of the bone and easily spreads through the adjacent cortex. The inflammatory response decreases the infection's spread down the medullary cavity. In children the periosteum is easily elevated from the bone, allowing formation of a subperiosteal abscess. If allowed to continue, the infection can raise the periosteum from large segments of bone, depriving it of its blood supply and resulting in dead, infected bone called a *sequestrum*. Because the periosteum maintains a normal blood supply, it begins to produce new bone. If extensive, the new bone may surround parts of the dead bone and is called the *involucrum*.

CAUSATIVE MICROORGANISMS OF OSTEOMYELITIS ACCORDING TO AGE

Newborns

Staphylococcus aureus
Group B streptococcus
Gram-negative enteric rods

Infants

Staphylococcus aureus
Haemophilus influenzae

Older children

Staphylococcus aureus
Pseudomonas
Salmonella
Neisseria gonorrhoeae

Adolescents and adults

Pseudomonas
Mycobacterium tuberculosis

supply as well. This process commonly results in extensive sequestrum formation and chronic osteomyelitis (Morrissy & Shore, 1986).

Osteomyelitis is much less common after the epiphyses are closed, except in the vertebral body. Infection may develop in any part of a bone, and abscesses spread slowly. Destruction of the cortex in a localized area may result in a pathologic fracture (Abramovitz et al., 1986; Ray & Bassett, 1985).

Spread of infection to contiguous joints is related to the child's age. Infection may spread to adjacent joints because the epiphyseal plate of the proximal femur is located within the hip joint capsule; the distal femoral plate is partially located within the knee; and the proximal and distal humeral plates are partially located within the shoulder and elbow joints, respectively. There is a common blood supply for the metaphysis and the epiphysis in children younger than 2 years of age that crosses the epiphyseal plate. Infection may be carried through this common circulation into the epiphysis and eventually involves the joint. An unossified epiphysis tends to be the site of initial infection more frequently than an ossified site; this common circulation ceases to exist in older children. After the epiphyses close, infection may extend directly from the metaphysis into the epiphyses and affect the joint. For this reason, osteomyelitis more commonly involves the joints in infants and adults rather than older children. Epiphyseal separation, however, may occur in acute osteomyelitis in infants and children (Carnsdale, 1992; Morrissy & Shore, 1986).

Clinical Manifestations

The clinical manifestations of osteomyelitis are age dependent and are related to the differing vascular patterns found in the skeletal system at various ages. Three distinct groups may be identified: (1) infants younger than 1 year of age, (2) 1 year of age to puberty, and (3) after cessation of bone growth in adolescents and adults.

Infants

Osteomyelitis may be an acute illness characterized by fever and failure to move the affected limb (pseudoparalysis). Infantile osteomyelitis is characterized by permanent arrest in bone growth and involvement of multiple sites within the same bone or in multiple bones.

Children

Osteomyelitis is usually an abrupt illness in children between the ages of 1 year and puberty and is characterized by fever and systemic signs of toxicity. The illness is sometimes subacute, with the child complaining of swelling, redness, tenderness, and slow movement of the affected bone or bones. Osteomyelitis during childhood most frequently affects the long bones but also may be found in the pelvis and small bones of the hands and feet. Clinical manifestations are usually accompanied by elevated white blood cell counts and elevated erythrocyte sedimentation rates. Evidence of infection using x-ray films may not be apparent until 10 to 14 days after the initial appearance of clinical manifestations, and these manifestations may be suppressed in the child receiving antibiotics for management of some other, nonrelated infection.

Adolescents and adults

In addition to the sites previously mentioned, osteomyelitis in adolescents and adults may involve the vertebrae. Back pain, with a duration of several weeks, may be the only clinical complaint.

Evaluation and Treatment

White blood cell counts and erythrocyte sedimentation rates are sometimes elevated, but this is not a consistent finding. Monitoring of erythrocyte sedimentation rates is an indication of response to management. Blood cultures and aspiration of the soft tissue or bone, or both, should be obtained to identify the causative microorganism. Appropriate antibiotics should be prescribed after culture and sensitivity studies have been completed. A tuberculin test is also administered because *Mycobacterium tuberculosis* is sometimes the responsible microorganism. X-ray examinations of the affected area will detect disease processes approximately 10 to 14 days after the appearance of clinical manifestations. Radionuclide imaging and bone scans are also useful.

Treatment includes administration of the appropriate antibiotic, drainage of infected bone, and symptomatic relief of pain and discomfort. Immobilization of the child is sometimes warranted.

Death is rare, but serious sequelae may occur. The course of the disease and prognosis depend on the age of the child, the rapidity with which the diagnosis is established, the initiation of early treatment, and maintenance of the treatment for an adequate time. Dislocation of joints and bone growth arrest are the most serious complications of osteomyelitis (Behrman et al., 1992; Bergdahl, Ekengren, & Eriksson, 1986).

Juvenile Rheumatoid Arthritis

The rheumatic diseases are a group of diverse conditions having in common the inflammation of connective tissues. They include rheumatoid arthritis, systemic lupus erythematosus, dermatomyositis, scleroderma, and polyarthritis. Incidence of these disorders in children is estimated in Table 40-2.

Juvenile rheumatoid arthritis (JRA) is the childhood form of rheumatoid arthritis (see Chapter 39). Like adult-onset rheumatoid arthritis, JRA is a syndrome that is often accompanied by systemic manifestations. Approximately 5% of all cases of rheumatoid arthritis begin in childhood. An estimated quarter of a million children in the United States have JRA.

The basic pathophysiology of JRA is the same as that of adult rheumatoid arthritis. The clinical manifestations of JRA may differ, however, beginning with mode of onset. Unlike adult rheumatoid arthritis, which begins insidiously with systemic signs of inflammation and generalized aches, JRA has three distinct modes of onset: arthritis in fewer than five joints (oligoarthritis), arthritis in more than five joints (polyarthritis), and systemic disease. Onset is less gradual in JRA than in adult rheumatoid arthritis. Juvenile rheumatoid arthritis also differs from the adult form in the following respects (Cassidy, 1982):

1. Systemic disease is most common.
2. The large joints are predominantly affected.
3. Subluxation and ankylosis of the cervical spine are common.
4. Joint pain is not as severe as the adult type.
5. Chronic uveitis is common.
6. Serologic tests often detect antinuclear antibody.
7. Serologic tests seldom detect rheumatoid factor.
8. Rheumatoid nodules are not limited to subcutaneous tissue, but are found in the heart, lungs, eyes, and other organs.

Treatment for children with JRA is supportive but not curative. The aims of treatment are to control inflammation and other clinical manifestations of the disease and to minimize deformity.

Avascular Diseases of the Bone: Osteochondrosis

The avascular diseases of the bone, collectively termed **osteochondroses,** are caused by insufficient blood supply to growing bones. Disturbances of blood supply to primary and secondary centers of ossification (see p. 1483) during periods of rapid bone growth result in a variety of skeletal abnormalities.

The cause of the osteochondroses remains obscure. In the past, infection, nutritional deficiencies, and hormonal imbalances were blamed, but these causes have been largely disproven. Currently, vascular impairment and trauma, coupled with an underlying developmental or genetic predisposition, have been identified as probable causes of osteochondroses. The most common osteochondroses involve the head of the femur, the capital femoral epiphysis (Legg-Calvé-Perthes disease); the epiphyses of the vertebral bodies (Scheuermann disease); the proximal bones of the feet (tarsal navicular bones; Köhler bone disease); the proximal tibial epiphysis (Blount disease); the tibial tuberosity (Osgood-Schlatter disease); and the calcaneus. (These bones are illustrated in Chapter 38.)

The classic clinical course of the osteochondroses consists of three overlapping stages: (1) avascular necrosis, or death of newly formed bone or cartilage associated with diminished blood supply; (2) an acute inflammatory response in tissues adjacent to areas of necrosis; and (3) healing and repair. The first stage of osteochondrosis is characterized by extensive avascular necrosis without any evidence of adjacent tissue inflammation. A secondary defect at the subchondral interface frequently is associated with avascular necrosis of the spongy bone. Because the surface of the articular cartilage receives most of its nutrients from synovial fluid, it is not damaged by avascular necrosis. The deeper layers of the articular cartilage are adversely affected, however, because they depend on vascular support. Later, reabsorption of the spongy bone significantly alters the mechanical strength of the articular cartilage leading to transchondral fractures during joint stress.

In the second or intermediate stage of osteochondro-

TABLE 40-2

Incidence of the Connective Tissue Diseases in Children

Disease	Annual rate/10^5	Sex ratio (F:M)	Race ratio (W:B)	Peak age group at risk (yr)	Childhood onset (%)
Rheumatoid arthritis	40	3:1	Equal	Increases with age (20-50)	5
Systemic lupus erythematosus	6	8:1	1:4	15-45	18
Dermatomyositis	0.8	2:1	1:3	45-65	20
Scleroderma	0.4	3:1	Equal	Increases with age (30-50)	3
Polyarteritis	0.2	1:3	Equal	Midadult	Rare

From Cassidy, 1982.
NOTE: F:M, Female to male; W:B, white to black.

sis, avascular necrosis causes reactive synovitis. Synovitis is often the cause of the first clinical manifestations—pain and muscle spasm. The extent of tissue damage and the outcome of osteochondrosis depend on how long the blood supply was diminished.

Most deformities become evident during the second or intermediate stage of osteochondrosis. Incongruity of the joint surfaces may occur if muscle spasms have resulted in contractures. Necrosis and articular damage are followed by processes of healing: ingrowth of new blood vessels and the appearance of primitive mesenchymal tissues that later differentiate into osteoblasts and contribute to the proliferation of reparative cells and new bone. Cysts in the articular cartilage and endochondral bone affect articular contour and congruity and future function and growth.

In the third or final stage of osteochondrosis, cysts disappear and bone and articular remodeling are completed. Foci of new bone grow outward and ultimately coalesce into remodeled bone tissue.

Osteochondroses have been reported in both primary and secondary ossification centers of all bone. The child is usually bothered by localized discomfort, a deformity, a limp, or an alteration of joint function.

Legg-Calvé-Perthes Disease

Legg-Calvé-Perthes disease, also called coxa plana, is one of the most common of the osteochondroses. This self-limited disease of the hip is presumably produced by recurrent interruption of the blood supply to the femoral head. The ossification center first becomes necrotic and then is gradually replaced by live bone.

Legg-Calvé-Perthes disease is relatively common, usually occurring in children between the ages of 3 and 10 years, with a peak incidence at 6 years. It is more frequent in boys than in girls by a ratio of about 4:1. Incidence is 1 in 750 boys and 1 in 3700 girls. The condition is bilateral in approximately 12% of affected children.

The cause of decreased blood supply to the head of the femur is unknown. Several theories have been proposed, including thyroid deficiency, trauma, and infection. A plausible theory is that acute synovitis (infection

of the synovial membrane) and increased hydrostatic pressure in the hip joint compress blood vessels that supply the femoral head.

Constitutional factors definitely play a role. Birth weight of children with Legg-Calvé-Perthes disease is much lower than that of unaffected children. Skeletal maturation is delayed in children with Legg-Calvé-Perthes disease, and affected children are between 2.5 and 7 cm shorter than unaffected children of the same age. Familial occurrence is common. The disease is rare in blacks and it is frequent in children of Japanese and Central European ancestry.

Pathophysiology

Legg-Calvé-Perthes disease runs its natural course in 2 to 5 years. In the incipient stage, the soft tissues of the hip (synovial membrane and joint capsule) are swollen, edematous, and hyperemic, often with fluid present in the joint (Fig. 40-8). The joint space widens and the joint capsule bulges. The first stage lasts for only a few weeks. In the second, or active avascular necrotic, stage, the entire or anterior half of the epiphysis of the femoral head is dead, and the metaphyseal bone at the junction of the femoral neck and capital epiphyseal plate is softened because of increased blood supply and decalcification. Soon granulation tissue (procallus) and blood vessels invade the dead bone. This stage lasts from several months to 1 year.

The third, or regenerative healing, stage ordinarily lasts 2 to 4 years. The dead femoral head is replaced by procallus and new bone is laid down. Collapse and flattening of the femoral head occur, and the femoral neck becomes short and wide (Fig. 40-8).

In the fourth, or residual, stage, remodeling takes place, and the newly formed bone is organized into a live spongy bone. The restoration of the femoral head to a normal shape is more complete in younger than in older children. A complete return to normal is also more likely if only the anterior epiphysis was involved.

Clinical Manifestations

Injury or trauma precedes the onset of the clinical manifestations in approximately one third of children with

FIG. 40-8 Stages of Legg-Calvé-Perthes disease, a form of osteochondrosis.

Legg-Calvé-Perthes disease. Onset of symptoms is insidious unless trauma aggravates the disease process. The child frequently complains of a limp and pain for several months. The pain usually is referred to the knee, inner thigh, and the groin, following the path of the obturator nerve. In some children, pain may be absent or minimal. If pain is present, it is usually aggravated by activity and relieved by rest.

The typical physical findings include spasm on rotation of the hip in extension, a limitation of internal rotation and abduction, and a hip flexion–abduction deformity. If the child is walking, an abnormal gait termed an **antalgic abductor lurch** is apparent. If the hip pain or limp has been present for a prolonged period, muscles of the hip and thigh atrophy.

Evaluation and Treatment

Diagnosis is confirmed by x-ray examination. The goals of treatment are to preserve normal congruity of the femoral head and acetabulum (hip socket) and maintain spasm-free and pain-free range of motion in the hip joint. In the past, many children were treated successfully with bed rest or the use of braces to keep the affected limb off the ground, but a large percentage were left with distorted femoral heads. Current therapy allows the child to continue weight bearing but with the femur in an abducted position, so that the femoral head is held securely within the acetabulum. This decreases focal areas of increased load and minimizes distortion. Weight bearing in abduction is accomplished by braces that hold the legs in abduction and, occasionally, by short periods of casting in the same position. Surgical procedures can be used that keep the femoral head abducted in relation to the acetabulum.

Factors affecting the outcome of Legg-Calvé-Perthes disease are the age of the child, the extent of necrosis, and the stage of disease at the time treatment is begun. The outcome in 70% to 80% of appropriately treated children with Legg-Calvé-Perthes disease is satisfactory hip joint function.

Osgood-Schlatter Disease

Osgood-Schlatter disease consists of tendinitis of the anterior patellar tendon, within which the patella (kneecap) is embedded, and associated osteochondrosis of the tubercle of the tibia. Osgood-Schlatter disease occurs most frequently in preadolescents and adolescents who participate in sports. The incidence is higher in boys than in girls.

Pathophysiology

The severity of the lesion varies from mild tendinitis to a complete separation of the anterior extension of the tibial epiphysis, which is the part of the epiphysis that contributes to growth of the tibial tubercle. The underlying pathologic alterations also vary. The mildest form of Osgood-Schlatter disease causes ischemic (avascular) necrosis in the region of the bony tibial tubercle, with hypertrophic cartilage formation during the stages of repair. In more severe cases the abnormality involves a true epiphyseal separation of the tibial tubercle, with the characteristics of avascular necrosis described in the section on Legg-Calvé-Perthes disease.

Clinical Manifestations

The child complains of pain and swelling in the region of the patellar tendon and tibial tubercle, which becomes prominent and is tender to direct pressure. The pain is most severe after physical activity that involves vigorous quadriceps contraction or direct local trauma to the tibial tubercle area. Frequently, the child has complaints of sudden onset of acute discomfort referable to the affected region. Sudden onset of pain is caused by a pathologic fracture through an area of ischemic necrosis.

Evaluation and Treatment

Diagnosis is confirmed by x-ray examination. The goal of treatment for Osgood-Schlatter disease is to decrease the stress at the tubercle. Often a period of 4 to 8 weeks of restriction from strenuous physical activity, especially activities requiring deep knee bending, is sufficient. If relief from pain is not achieved, a cast is required to immobilize the knee, a situation that is particularly difficult if the condition is bilateral.

Gradual resumption of activity is permitted after 8 weeks, but return to unrestricted athletic participation requires an additional 8 weeks to allow for revascularization, healing, and ossification of the tibial tubercle.

Muscular Dystrophy

The **muscular dystrophies** are a group of familial disorders that cause degeneration of skeletal muscle fibers. The most prevalent of the muscle diseases in childhood, the muscular dystrophies are characterized by progressive, symmetric weakness, and wasting of skeletal muscle groups, with increasing disability and deformity.

Classification of the muscular dystrophies is based on age of onset, rate of progression, distribution of muscular involvement, and inheritance patterns. The major types that are clinically and genetically distinct are the pseudohypertrophic (Duchenne), facioscapulohumeral, limb girdle, oculopharyngeal, and myotonic muscular dystrophies (Fig. 40-9). Because the clinical findings and genetic inheritance patterns are consistent for each type, some researchers believe that each involves a separate biochemical defect. The precise mechanisms, however, are still unknown. Current research points to defects in muscle fiber (cell) membrane as either a cause or result of an unknown biochemical abnormality. Genetic research has focused on identifying the locus for the ab-

FIG. 40-9 Initial muscle groups involved in three types of muscular dystrophy. **A,** Pseudohypertrophic. **B,** Facioscapulohumeral. **C,** Limb girdle. (From Whaley & Wong, 1991.)

TABLE 40-3

Major Muscular Dystrophy Syndromes

Disease	Mode of inheritance	Age at clinical onset	Usual distribution	Rate of progression	Mental retardation	Distinguished findings
Duchenne dystrophy (DMD)	X-linked recessive	About 3 years	Hips and shoulders, quadriceps femoris, gastrocnemius (pseudohypertrophy)	Rapid	Frequent	Elevated serum enzymes (CPK, LDH, SGOT, aldolase)
Facioscapulohumeral (FSH) dystrophy	Autodomal dominant	In first or second decade	Shoulder girdle, neck, face, pelvic girdle (late)	Moderate	Occasional	Several distinct muscle pathologies
Limb girdle (LG) dystrophy	Poorly defined or recessive	Variable	Pelvic and shoulder girdles	Variable	Variable	Collection of several diseases
Myotonic dystrophy (MyD)	Autosomal dominant	Variable—birth to fifth decade	Distal extensor muscle, eyelids, face, neck, hands, pharynx	Slow, related to age at clinical onset, faster with younger patients	Frequent	Percussion myotonia, cataracts, diabetic GTT despite increased insulin, testicular atrophy, decreased IgC

Modified from Stanbury, 1983.

normal genes. This will permit more accurate carrier detection and, eventually, description of the biochemical aberration (Morrissy, 1990; Tachjdian, 1990). (Table 40-3 summarizes the types of muscular dystrophy.)

Muscle degeneration is characterized by biochemical, morphologic, or neurophysiologic changes that occur alone or in combination. These conditions are not the result of dysfunction of the neuromuscular junctions, peripheral nerves, anterior horn cells, or central nervous system.

The physiology of all types of muscular dystrophy is more or less the same. The genetic abnormality is presumed to cause some abnormality in the intracellular metabolism of the muscle fibers. An abnormality in an enzyme system within the muscle cell or a defect in muscle metabolism may result from inability to absorb or metabolize a substance vital to muscular function. A defect in creatine metabolism and a lowering of levels of intramuscular enzymes in the glycolytic system are involved.

The muscle cells have an increased number of nuclei that form chains and are moved centrally. The muscle cells also show necrosis and phagocytosis. Fragmentation and dissolution of myofilaments occur early. The muscle fibers may be swollen, indistinct, and homogenous, with disturbed striation. Some fibers may be hypertrophic and others atrophic. Muscle fibers are eventually replaced with fat (causing fatty infiltration) and connective tissues (causing fibrosis). The involved muscle fibers are randomly distributed, with no distinct pattern.

Duchenne Muscular Dystrophy

In 1868 the French neurologist G. B. A. Duchenne described a pseudohypertrophic muscular paralysis associated with large amounts of fat and connective tissue. Today, this form of muscular dystrophy, called **Duchenne muscular dystrophy,** is the most common of the muscular dystrophies. Its incidence is approximately 1 in 3500 male births (Scott et al., 1988). Classic Duchenne muscular dystrophy occurs only in boys and has a history of X-linked inheritance in half of the cases.

Pathophysiology

The X-linked inherited type of Duchenne muscular dystrophy is thought to be caused by a deletion of a segment of DNA (Scott et al., 1988) or a single gene defect on the short arm of the X chromosome. A protein encoded by the Duchenne muscular dystrophy gene, called dystrophin, has been identified.

Dystrophin is present in normal muscle cells and absent in Duchenne muscular dystrophy. Other mechanisms causing Duchenne muscular dystrophy are unknown. Areas currently being investigated include: (1) a neurogenic basis, related primarily to abnormal motor neurons; (2) a vascular abnormality in which malformations or physiologic incompetence results in poor small-vessel perfusion, with or without abnormality in biogenic amine metabolism; and (3) an intrinsic abnormality within muscle fibers, possibly related to formation of inappropriate amounts of connective tissue, abnormality in enzyme metabolism, or structural defects (Swaiman & Wright, 1982).

Duchenne muscular dystrophy causes muscle bulk to diminish, and in later stages a predominant pink or yellowish pink replaces the dark red staining of normal muscle. Interstitial connective tissue and fat often replace muscle fibers.

Microscopic changes include a decrease in the number of fibers and necrosis of the fibers with associated phagocytosis. Overall, changes include increase of endomysial connective tissue and fat, loss of striations, and concomitant hyaline, granular, and fatty degeneration of fibers. Disorganization of tendinous insertions is associated with fat accumulation in these areas. Although fibers regenerate in the younger child, they are abnormal in many ways and become nonfunctional with time.

Clinical Manifestations

Duchenne muscular dystrophy is usually identified in children approximately 3 years of age, when the parents notice slow motor development with progressive weakness and muscle wasting. Sitting, standing, and walking are delayed and the child is clumsy, falls frequently, and has difficulty climbing stairs.

Muscular weakness always begins in the pelvic girdle, causing a "waddling" gait. Hypertrophy of the calf muscles is apparent in 80% of cases. The method of rising from the floor by "climbing up the legs" (Gower sign) is characteristic and is caused by weakness of the lumbar and gluteal muscles. The foot assumes a talipes equinovarus position (Fig. 40-4), and the child tends to walk on the toes because of weakness of the anterior tibial and peroneal muscles. Within 3 to 5 years, muscles of the shoulder girdle become involved. The deep tendon reflexes are usually depressed or absent. On rare occasions, a positive Babinski sign and other evidence of upper motor neuron lesions have been reported. Contractures and wasting of the muscles contribute to muscular atrophy and deformity of the skeleton.

Duchenne muscular dystrophy has serious complications. Pulmonary function is compromised greatly because of marked kyphoscoliosis ("humped" upper spine combined with scoliosis), which usually develops after the child is confined to a wheelchair. The incidence of cardiac involvement in Duchenne muscular dystrophy is as high as 95%. Chronic heart failure may occur in 50% of children. A moderate degree of mental retardation causes these children to have a mean IQ of approximately 80. Smooth muscle dysfunction may cause mega-colon, volvulus, cramping pain, and malabsorption in the gastrointestinal tract (McCullough & Pellino, in press).

Evaluation and Treatment

Diagnosis is confirmed by measurement of serum enzymes, electromyography (EMG), and muscle biopsy. The serum enzymes, especially creatine phosphokinase (CPK), are increased to more than 10 times normal, even during infancy and before the onset of weakness. Histologic changes in muscle include degeneration of muscle fibers, with variation in fiber size and central nuclei. Fat and connective tissue replace muscle fibers.

Although intrauterine diagnosis is not yet possible, work is being done in this area (Cole et al., 1988; Evans et al., 1991). Elevated CPK levels at birth are diagnostic indicators of Duchenne muscular dystrophy. Identification of female carriers of the disease cannot be achieved with certainty, but serum CPK is elevated in 60% to 80% of carriers.

There is no effective treatment for Duchenne muscular dystrophy. Maintaining function in unaffected muscle groups for as long as possible is the primary goal. Although activity fosters maintenance of muscle function, strenuous exercise may hasten the breakdown of muscle fibers. Range of motion exercises, bracing, and surgical release of contracture deformities are used to maintain normal function for as long as possible. Genetic counseling is recommended. With X-linked inheritance, male siblings of an affected child have a 50% chance of being affected, and female siblings have a 50% chance of being carriers.

Progressive weakness leads to wheelchair confinement between the ages of 8 and 15 years, after which obesity or excessive thinness, kyphoscoliosis, and other complications of immobility develop. Death, usually resulting from respiratory or cardiac muscle weakness, occurs before age 20. Only 25% of children with Duchenne muscular dystrophy reach the age of 21.

Becker Muscular Dystrophy

Becker muscular dystrophy is often called "benign" Duchenne muscular dystrophy because it shares the X-linked inheritance pattern and similar clinical features. The two diseases are not found in the same pedigree, however, and are thought to involve different biochemical defects. Clinical symptoms often begin between the ages of 5 and 15. Children with Becker muscular dystrophy remain ambulatory into their teens and early 20s; in one study, the age at the time of disability and wheelchair use was 20 to 27 (Brooke, 1977). The incidence is one tenth that of Duchenne muscular dystrophy (Morrissy, 1990; Tachjdian, 1990).

The pattern of muscle weakness for both dystrophies is almost identical, although calf hypertrophy and muscle cramps may precede clinical weakness as in Duchenne muscular dystrophy. Scoliosis and contractures are rare until the child with Becker muscular dystrophy is permanently wheelchair bound. The changes in creatine kinase levels and EMG and ECG readings are the same as those seen in Duchenne muscular dystrophy. Many individuals live well into middle age. Heart failure is infrequent but can be a cause of premature death and disability (Morrissy, 1990; Tachjdian, 1990).

Maintaining ambulation and careful follow-up for evidence of cardiopulmonary complications are essential measures for long-term care. Children with Becker muscular dystrophy rarely show the mental changes seen in Duchenne dystrophy, and with appropriate vocational counseling and support may become exceedingly productive workers. The accurate diagnosis of Becker muscular dystrophy is important. If the affected individual marries and has children, all daughters will be carriers of this X-linked recessive disorder. Of course, genetic counseling should be offered to the mother, female siblings, offspring, and any maternal relatives (Brooke, 1977).

Facioscapulohumeral Muscular Dystrophy

Facioscapulohumeral muscular dystrophy is a mild form of progressive, autosomal dominant muscular dystrophy. Age at onset varies from early childhood to adult life, and the disease affects males and females equally. As the name implies, clinical manifestations begin with weakness and atrophy of facial and shoulder girdle (scapulohumeral) muscles. The illness progresses slowly. Inability to close the eyes completely may be noted from early childhood. The face is expressionless, and pouting of the lips makes whistling impossible. The first symptoms usually include drooping of the shoulders with difficulty in raising the arms above the head. Onset of weakness in the lower limbs often is delayed for 20 to 30 years, and pseudohypertrophy of muscles is rare. Contractures and skeletal deformities develop less frequently and are less prominent than in Duchenne muscular dystrophy.

Treatment includes supportive physiotherapy to prevent contractures and prolong ambulation. Lightweight plastic ankle-foot orthoses (AFO) for footdrop are extremely helpful. Surgery to stabilize the shoulder is sometimes advised (Morrissy, 1990; Tachjdian, 1990).

Some individuals with facioscapulohumeral muscular dystrophy improve with steroid therapy, particularly if the clinical picture includes rapidly progressive weakness. The disease may be arrested for prolonged periods; however, most individuals remain active and have a normal life expectancy. Vocational training and genetic counseling are important to provide them with the information necessary to plan their future.

Scapuloperoneal Muscular Dystrophy

Scapuloperoneal muscular dystrophy is considered a variant of facioscapulohumeral muscular dystrophy, but distal muscles in the lower extremity are involved early instead of the facial and shoulder muscle weakness that is the early sign in facioscapulohumeral dystrophy. Many seek initial treatment for troublesome footdrop and shoulder weakness. Analysis of inheritance patterns shows that the disease can be inherited either as an autosomal dominant trait or as an X-linked recessive trait.

The initial symptoms may resemble those of several other illnesses, including nemaline myopathy (a congenital muscle disease) and early hypertrophic peripheral neuropathy. A careful diagnostic evaluation therefore is in order. Other clinical findings include hypertrophy of the muscle that extends the toes, brought about by a futile attempt to overcome footdrop, and depressed or absent muscle stretch reflexes. Creatinine kinase is elevated two to 20 times normal; EMG readings show myopathy.

Treatment is directed toward treating symptoms and preserving ambulation and functional ability. Footdrop is easily treated with AFOs. Individuals with scapuloperoneal muscular dystrophy remain ambulatory for 40 or more years. Occasionally, walking may be hampered by paraspinal muscle contractures; in this case, a wheelchair may assist the individual to cover long distances. The life span in this disorder is normal (Morrissy, 1990; Tachdjian, 1990). Genetic counseling should be available to all persons (Brooke, 1977).

Limb Girdle Muscular Dystrophy

The diagnosis of **limb girdle muscular dystrophy** is considered when acute causes of proximal weakness are eliminated and the clinical findings and genetic pattern exclude Duchenne and facioscapulohumeral muscular dystrophy. The diagnosis is often determined by exclusion because few consistent clinical features make this type of muscular dystrophy unique. In fact, some researchers think that limb girdle dystrophy actually may be several separate diseases waiting for more sophisticated methods of evaluation to give them precise labels. Most individuals have a negative family history, making sporadic disease or an autosomal recessive pattern of inheritance likely. The prevalence rate for limb girdle muscular dystrophy is set at 20 per million.

The initial symptoms include shoulder and pelvic girdle weakness, which are usually noticed in the early 20s but can be seen as late as the 40s. The muscle weakness is often asymmetric and progresses at a much slower pace than in Duchenne muscular dystrophy. The biceps and deltoid muscles can be extremely atrophic and weak. Individuals can remain ambulatory for extended periods, often up to 20 years after initial diagnosis. When confined to wheelchairs, they show few of the severe effects of other dystrophies, such as contractures and scoliosis. Heart involvement and mental retardation also are rare (Morrissy, 1990; Tachdjian, 1990).

The individual will have mild elevation in creatine kinase levels and a myopathic pattern on EMG. Muscle biopsy is often more characteristic, with fiber splitting and fibers that appear profusely "moth-eaten" and whorled. Treatment includes supportive measures to maintain ambulation and functional ability and frequent follow-up to eliminate secondary complications such as cardiopulmonary disease.

Myotonic Muscular Dystrophy

A multisystemic disorder, **myotonic muscular dystrophy** (MTD) is a common disease with a frequency ranging from 50 to 1200 per million, varying by geographic location. The myotonic muscular dystrophy gene has been identified on chromosome 19, a finding with implications for genetic counseling and for further understanding of biochemical defect.

Pathophysiology

The multisystemic nature of this disorder strongly suggests a defect of widespread involvement, potentially an abnormality of muscle cell membrane. Several studies have advanced this hypothesis. Electron microscopy shows a proliferation of transverse tubules coupled with an abnormal resting membrane potential. Researchers have identified the gene that governs the insulin receptors, and it is also located on chromosome 19. Because many individuals with MTD show severe insulin resistance in skeletal muscle and abnormal insulin-mediated amino acid disposal after a glucose load, insulin studies are an exciting development. Individuals also show reduced protein synthesis; only 40% have normal or stable isotope studies. Because the mechanism of insulin uptake has such important effects on glucose use and protein synthesis in muscle, a defect in the insulin receptor and insulin action would have profound effects on muscle function and in particular may cause muscle wasting (Griggs & Rennie, 1983). Linking both the gene for myotonic muscular dystrophy and the gene for insulin uptake on chromosome 19 further substantiates the relationship between these phenomena.

Clinical Manifestations

The onset of the disease ranges from birth to the fifth decade. The peculiar attitudes of indifference seen in persons with myotonic muscular dystrophy make the onset of the disease and progression of symptoms difficult to qualify. Myotonic muscular dystrophy is typically more severe in the maternally transmitted neonatal and childhood forms than in adult forms.

The early clinical findings are the characteristic facial features and presence of myotonia (tonic muscle spasms). A common observation is that if the diagnosis of MTD is not made at first glance and handshake, the clinician misses it because of the myriad of individual complaints. Many are unrelated to the muscular system and individuals rarely complain of functional difficulties in spite of severe muscle weakness. The prominent temporal and masseter muscle wasting and severe neck flexor weakness give rise to the terms "hatchet facies" and "swan-neck" deformity commonly applied to MTD. Myotonia usually affects the hands more than the eyelids, tongue, or facial muscles. As the disease progresses, weakness in the distal extremities is apparent, and footdrop is common. Weakness of the respiratory muscles and the pharyngeal and esophageal muscles is noted. In fact, abnormalities of all three types of muscles—smooth, skeletal, and cardiac—have been identified in pathologic analysis of sections from biopsies. Other organs are involved; defects in the lens, retina, brain, pancreas, testes, ovaries, skin, bone, gamma globulins, and red blood cells have been reported.

Mental retardation is often associated with neonatal MTD. A mean IQ of 66 was reported in one study (Brooke, 1977). Mental retardation is rarely noted in adolescent, adult-onset, and paternally transmitted disease.

Evaluation and Treatment

Diagnostic tests include the EMG, which shows myopathic findings and audible myotonia, the characteristic "dive bomber" noise heard when the needle is inserted. Creatine phosphokinase level is usually normal. Muscle biopsy shows type I fiber atrophy and type II fiber hypertrophy.

Cardiac abnormalities can be severe and can cause sudden death. Several studies have demonstrated that most individuals have abnormal His bundle conduction and prolonged P-R intervals. In one study, all persons had abnormal His-ventricle intervals in spite of normal P-R intervals. Individuals who complain of syncope should be carefully evaluated for cardiac conduction abnormalities and potential pacemaker insertion.

Other systemic signs include bulbar weakness, with dysarthric nasal speech and swallowing difficulty. Many individuals aspirate and have reduced esophageal motility. If these problems are accompanied by weight loss and aspiration pneumonitis, they can be treated by insertion of a feeding tube. Abnormalities in endocrine function include insulin resistance, testicular atrophy, and infertility.

There is no treatment that alters the severe muscle wasting and weakness, yet treatment is available for many of the common symptoms. Drugs such as phenytoin and quinine can decrease functionally disabling myotonia. Cataract surgery can dramatically improve visual acuity. Hypersomnolence, in which individuals sleep more than 12 hours a day, can be treated with stimulants such as pemoline (Cylert) or methylphenidate (Ritalin). Braces and canes are prescribed when footdrop impedes ambulation.

Genetic counseling should be provided. Analysis of linkage to the ABO blood group has made prenatal prediction of an affected fetus possible in a small number of individuals. Genetic mapping studies have demonstrated that the blood groups ABO and Lutheran are on the same chromosome as myotonic dystrophy. If the patient secretes ABO blood group antigens in body secretions, analysis of the individual's family and spouse would permit prediction of the prenatal diagnosis of myotonic dystrophy (Morrissy, 1990; Tachdjian, 1990).

Musculoskeletal Tumors in Children
Bone Tumors

Bone tumors are uncommon tumors in childhood. They account for less than 5% of childhood malignancies, mostly occurring during adolescence. The two main tumors are osteosarcoma and Ewing sarcoma. Children very rarely develop fibrosarcoma, chondrosarcoma, or non-Hodgkin lymphoma of the bone.

Osteosarcoma

Osteosarcoma, accounting for 60% of childhood bone tumors, is the most common bone tumor during childhood and originates in bone-producing mesenchymal cells. Three fourths of cases occur between the age of 10 and 25 years—most are diagnosed between 15 and 19 years of age. Therefore it is predominantly a tumor that develops during the adolescent growth spurt. The incidence of osteosarcoma before age 15 is the same for males and females.

The cause is unknown, but it has been speculated that osteosarcoma may develop as a result of rapid local growth that increases the likelihood of mutation. Although controversial, there has been some evidence that these tumors occur more commonly in taller individuals, and it has also been well documented in animal studies that osteosarcoma is seen in giant dog breeds, such as Saint Bernards and Great Danes, but not in smaller dogs.

Osteosarcoma can be induced by ionizing radiation, even with relatively low doses. This can be a tragic consequence of therapeutic radiation for other forms of cancer. The latent period after radiation exposure is 5 to 40 years, and it is estimated that 4% of all osteosarcomas occur in previously irradiated bone. Evidence for hereditary links has not been firmly established and no racial tendency is seen, although on rare occasions the tumor has been documented in multiple family members as part of a rare cancer family syndrome. There has also been a link to individuals with retinoblastoma (a hereditary eye tumor). In fact, osteosarcoma is more likely to occur if the individual has bilateral retinoblastoma, confirming a genetic transmission of the eye tumor rather than a spontaneous mutation in the genes. The link between retinoblastoma and subsequent osteosarcoma occurs whether or not radiation has been part of the treatment for retinoblastoma. Osteosarcoma has been associated with a few other medical syndromes. The most well-established association involves older individuals with Paget disease of the bone and is not seen during childhood.

There is no evidence that osteosarcoma can be caused by chemical carcinogens. In addition, there is no convincing evidence that there is a viral link. In the past, there has been some interest in investigating a viral link, because viruses have been shown to cause osteosarcoma in laboratory animals and C-type virus particles have been identified in human osteosarcoma growth in tissue culture. No DNA or RNA virus has been isolated.

Molecular analysis has demonstrated deletion of genetic material on the long arm of chromosome 13 leading to the identification of a tumor-suppressor gene as part of the mechanism for tumor development. The oncogene *src* also has been associated with osteosarcoma.

Pathophysiology

Osteosarcoma occurs mainly in the metaphyses of long bones. Most tumors arise in bones involved with the knee joint at the distal end of the femur or proximal end of the tibia. The ends of long bones are sites of most active epiphyseal growth. As a tumor of mesenchymal cells, osteosarcoma demonstrates production of osteoid cells.

Osteosarcoma is a bulky tumor that extends beyond the bone into a soft tissue mass. It may encircle the bone and destroy the trabeculae of the diseased bone. Osteosarcoma disseminates through the bloodstream, usually to the lung. Up to 25% of children diagnosed with osteosarcoma exhibit lung metastases at diagnosis. Other sites of metastatic spread include other bones and visceral organs.

Clinical Manifestations

The most common presenting complaint is pain. The pain can be intermittent at first, then continue with increasing severity. There may be swelling and warmth and redness caused by the vascularity of the tumor. Symptoms may also include cough, dyspnea, and chest pain if lung metastasis is present. If a lower extremity is involved, a limp may be present and a pathologic fracture may result if the disease is extensive. The child or family member may relate subsequent appearance of the tumor to a traumatic accident; however, osteosarcoma is not the result of trauma, but trauma may call attention to a preexisting tumor.

Initial evaluation includes x-ray examination that shows osteosarcoma's characteristic osteoblastic and osteolytic changes. In addition, a laboratory study of blood serum alkaline phosphate levels may be performed because elevated levels may be caused by osteoid production. Additional imaging studies may include CT or MRI scan of the primary site and bone scan and chest x-ray to evaluate potential metastatic sites.

Evaluation and Treatment

Tissue biopsy confirms the diagnosis, although needle biopsy is often sufficient to establish the diagnosis. Computerized tomography (CT) is necessary to determine the anatomic extent of the tumor. Chest x-ray and chest CT are necessary because of the 10% incidence of lung metastasis present at the time of initial diagnosis. In addition, magnetic resonance imaging (MRI), bone scan with technetium 99, and angiography may be necessary for preoperative planning.

There are five histologic types of osteosarcoma. The histologic type is determined by the predominant cell type. The tumor is then graded according to degree of malignancy; the higher the number, the worse the prognosis (Morrissy, 1990; Tachjdian, 1990).

Surgery and chemotherapy are the primary treatments for osteosarcoma. The tumor is resistant to radiation. Traditionally, surgery includes amputation at the joint above the involved bone; however, more recent limb salvage procedures have gained acceptance, and amputation may be avoided in most children. The primary bone is removed and replaced with an internal prosthesis made of metal, cadaver bone, or bone graft. Better and longer outcomes are achieved with biologic material used in the reconstruction as opposed to metal or other artificial materials. Certain requirements for eligibility for limb salvage surgery include a small tumor with minimal soft tissue involvement and linear bone growth that is nearly complete so that bone asymmetry will not develop as the uninvolved bone grows. The functional performance of the area salvaged must be considered because amputation and a prosthesis are sometimes more appropriate.

Chemotherapy is an important component of treatment because up to 80% of children treated with surgery alone eventually develop metastatic disease. Currently, methotrexate, citrovorum factor rescue, adriamycin, and combinations of bleomycin, cyclophosphamide, and ifosfamide are used. These will change, however, as newer drugs are developed and found to be more effective. The role of preoperative chemotherapy is currently being evaluated. The use of chemotherapy with surgery has increased the 5-year survival rate to 50% or greater.

A number of approaches have been used to treat pulmonary metastases. Because pulmonary metastases are generally solitary, focal lesions, thoracotomy with wedge resection has proven the most effective treatment. Investigators have searched for adjuvant treatment to prevent pulmonary metastases but nothing has proven useful.

Ewing sarcoma

Ewing sarcoma is the second most common and most lethal malignant bone tumor during childhood. This tumor is named after James Ewing, who first identified it as a separate clinical diagnosis in 1921. Ewing sarcoma probably originates from cells within the bone marrow space and does not involve bone-forming cells. The most frequent period of diagnosis is between 5 and 15 years of age and is rare after 30. Like osteosarcoma, Ewing sarcoma is slightly more common in males than females, and the cause is also unknown. Like osteosarcoma, however, there is a link with periods of rapid bone growth. Evidence for hereditary links has not been firmly established; however, Ewing sarcoma is very rare in blacks, in both the United States and Africa, perhaps indicating some genetic resistance.

Pathophysiology

Ewing sarcoma is most commonly located in the midshaft of long bones or in flat bones. The most frequent sites include the pelvis, femur, and humerus. The femur is involved in most cases, with the pelvis being the second most common site. It can occur in any bone.

Arising from bone marrow, Ewing sarcoma can break through the cortex of the bone to form a soft tissue mass. Although the tumor does not form osteoid, it often contains areas of blood vessels and hemorrhage. Ewing sarcoma metastasizes to nearly every organ. Metastasis occurs early and is usually apparent at diagnosis or within 1 year. The most common sites are the lung, other bones, lymph nodes, bone marrow, liver, spleen, and central nervous system.

Clinical Manifestations

Like osteosarcoma, the most common complaint is pain that increases in severity. A soft tissue mass is often present. Additional symptoms may include fever, malaise, and anorexia. Both clinical and x-ray findings may not be diagnostic of Ewing sarcoma.

Evaluation and Treatment

In addition to plain roentgenogram, CT and MRI are needed to help establish the diagnosis and extent of the tumor. Bone scan, chest x-ray, and chest CT are also used to detect metastases. No specific laboratory test is diagnostic; however, the sedimentation rate will be elevated and lactic dehydrogenase (LDH) often is elevated. An elevated LDH is a poor prognostic sign. Biopsy is used to conclusively establish the diagnosis (Morrissy, 1990; Tachjdian, 1990).

Previously, radiation of approximately 1500 rads was the primary treatment modality. The use of multidrug chemotherapy has improved survival rates. Recent treatment protocols call for preoperative chemotherapy followed by radiation or surgical resection, or both, with continuation of chemotherapy for 12 to 18 months afterwards. Amputation is avoided when possible but may be considered in lower limb tumors of children younger than 8 years of age because of the serious discrepancy in bone growth that results if the primary treatment used is radiation—growth is affected in the diseased bone, whereas normal growth continues in the unaffected bone.

Ewing sarcoma has had a dismal prognosis with 5-year survival rates no better than 5% to 10%. Combinations of aggressive radiation, chemotherapy, and surgical resection have, however, improved the survival rate for localized disease to greater than 60%. The major predictor of prognosis appears to be the location of the primary tumor and whether metastases are present at diagnosis. The most favorable sites of involvement are the extremities; the worst prognosis involves tumors of the trunk, particularly the pelvis.

Nonossifying fibroma

The **nonossifying fibroma,** which is believed to be a defect in ossification rather than a true tumor, makes up approximately 50% of benign bone tumors. It is thought to begin as a fibrous, cystlike lesion, called a fibrous cortical defect, in children younger than 2 years of age. Most fibrous cortical defects resolve spontaneously or are obliterated by reparative ossification or remodeling. In some cases, however, the fibrous cortical defect persists and proliferates, becoming a fibroma. Fibromas are found primarily in children and adolescents. Ninety percent of these tumors occur in persons younger than 20 years of age.

The nonossifying fibroma is a sharply demarcated tumor surrounded by a dense border of hardened bone. The tumor itself consists of fibrocytes arranged in whorled bundles, fibroblastic tissue, and osteoclast-like giant cells. As the tumor evolves, the fibrocytes imbibe lipids and assume a foamy appearance; thus they are known as foam cells. The tumor also contains extensive deposits of hemosiderin pigment. The tumor is characteristically located in the metaphyseal region of the bone and may cause a slight bulging of the cortex. The long axis of the tumor parallels the long axis of the bone.

The nonossifying fibroma is usually asymptomatic and is found coincidentally. If the tumor is large enough, it may cause slight swelling or localized pain. An active adolescent may be first seen with a pathologic fracture.

The fibroma is generally not treated until it occupies more than 50% of the diameter of the bone or extends more than 3 to 4 cm into the cortex. When the tumor grows to this size, it is removed by curettage and the area is packed with bone chips (Morrissy, 1990; Tachjdian, 1990).

Muscle Tumors

Most soft tissue tumors in children are benign. Only two malignant soft tissue tumors occur with any frequency, rhabdomyosarcoma in the younger child and synovial cell sarcoma in the teenager. Both of these occur rarely. The annual incidence is 8.0 per million for white children and 7.7 per million for black children. About 230 children are diagnosed with a soft tissue tumor each year in the United States. Soft tissue tumors originate from the primitive mesenchymal cells that normally give rise to muscle, tendons, blood vessels, lymphatic structures, fibrous and connective tissue, and bursa and fascia. Table 40-4 identifies the classification of soft tissue tumors depending on origin. All malignant soft tissue tumors are characterized as highly aggressive tumors that invade surrounding structures and metastasize early.

Rhabdomyosarcoma (RMS) is the most common soft tissue sarcoma of childhood and accounts for more than 50% of soft tissue tumors but less than 3% of all childhood cancers. Rhabdomyosarcoma arises from embryonal rhabdomyoblasts that normally differentiate into mature striated muscle. The annual incidence of RMS is 4.4 per million in white children and 1.3 per million in black children. The five subclassifications of RMS are (1) embryonal (55%), (2) botryoid (7%), (3) alveolar (18%), (4) pleomorphic (2%), and (5) undifferentiated cell types I or II (5% each). The pleomorphic variety of rhabdomyosarcoma occurs in adults, but is uncommon in children.

Rhabdomyosarcoma can develop anywhere striated muscle is located. The primary locations and percentage range of incidence are (1) the head and neck (including the orbit), 61% to 36%; (2) the trunk, 33% to 8%; (3) the extremities, 24% to 14%; and (4) the genitourinary tract, 17% to 10%. Two age ranges (2 to 6 years of age and 15 to 19 years of age) are associated with RMS. More than two thirds of children with RMS are diagnosed by 10 years of age, and RMS is slightly more common in males than females.

The cause of RMS is obscure. It can be induced in laboratory animals with viruses, chemical carcinogens, and heavy metal compounds. Similar links have not been established in humans, however. On rare occasions, familial cases have been reported, sometimes associated with congenital malformations. Rhabdomyosarcoma also has been reported to be a complication of neurofibromatosis and has been associated with breast cancer. Genetic alterations in rhabdomyosarcoma are just beginning to be identified. Some alterations have

TABLE 40-4

Classification of Tumors by Origin

Tissue	Tumor
Muscle	
Striated	Rhabdomyosarcoma
Smooth	Leiomyosarcoma
Adipose	Liposarcoma
Fibrous	Fibrosarcoma
Synovial mesothelium	Synovial sarcoma
Lymphatic structures	Lymphangiosarcoma
Blood vessels	Hemangiopericytoma
Nerve sheath	Neurogenic sarcoma

been described on chromosome 11 (Koufos & Hansen, 1985). Three oncogenes (*src*, H/K *ras*, and c-*myb*) have been associated with this tumor (Israel, 1989).

Pathophysiology

Rhabdomyosarcoma generally appears as a firm, fleshy, grayish-white mass. It sometimes exhibits variations, particularly with the botryoid subclassification that appears as a cystic polypoid mass. Rhabdomyosarcoma has various appearances, depending on the phase of differentiation of the rhabdomyoblast. The cells may be round or spindle shaped, tadpole shaped, or multinucleated giant cells.

The **embryonal subclass of RMS** is the most common. The cells are generally round or spindle shaped because of their primitive stage. These tumors do not show striations and are consistent with the appearance of developing muscle in the 7- to 10-week-old fetus. Embryonal RMS is more common in younger children and is usually found in the head and neck region.

The **botryoides subclass of RMS** is very similar to the embryonal subclass. The gross appearance is often a bizarre polypoid, glistening, edematous "cluster of grapes" that is a mass of stroma and dilated blood vessels, however. Botryoides RMS is most common in young children and favors hollow viscera, including the bladder, vagina, common bile duct, ear, nasopharynx, and uterus.

The **alveolar subclass of RMS** is the most common type of RMS in adolescents. It generally involves an extremity or the perineal and perirectal areas. It appears as a firmer tumor than the embryonal and botryoides types. The tumor is composed of clusters of small, round rhabdomyoblasts and may have multinucleated giant cells. The alveolar subclass represents a higher degree of cellular differentiation than the embryonal or botryoides subtypes. The cell pattern is consistent with the hollow tube stage of normal muscle development seen in the 10- to 12-week-old fetus.

The **pleomorphic subclass of RMS** accounts for only 2% of pediatric RMS and is sometimes seen in adults during the third to fifth decade. It is composed of multinucleated giant cells and racquet-shaped cells. The tumor cells appear as mature striated muscle that has become dedifferentiated.

The **undifferentiated cell types of RMS** are a relatively new subclass. Similar in appearance to Ewing sarcoma (a bone tumor), they are most commonly found in the extremities.

Rhabdomyosarcoma spreads by rapid local infiltration, as well as hematogenous and lymphatic routes. Hematogenous spread is thought to be the more common method of metastatic dissemination. At least 20% of children with RMS have metastatic disease at diagnosis. The preferred sites of metastases include the lungs, the lymph nodes, the bone marrow, the liver, the brain, and the bone.

Clinical Manifestations

The signs and symptoms of RMS depend on the anatomic location of the primary tumor and presence of symptomatic metastases. The tumors are usually painless and early detection of RMS is facilitated by the presence of a palpable or visible mass. Deep-seated tumors cause functional impairment. The clinical manifestations of RMS are outlined in Table 40-5.

Evaluation and Treatment

Diagnostic studies during the pretreatment phase are used to determine the extent of the primary tumor and presence or absence of distant metastases. Specific diagnostic studies depend on the primary site, but a combination of radiographic, nuclear, and CT scanning or MRI technology and blood studies is used. Regional lymph nodes are assessed by lymphangiogram. Liver function, blood studies, and liver scans determine liver involvement, and bone scan determines the presence of bone metastases. Bone marrow aspiration may be used to determine bone marrow involvement. A lumbar puncture is performed to determine central nervous system involvement for tumors adjacent to the central nervous system. A biopsy of the primary tumor is necessary to confirm the diagnosis.

Staging of RMS is based on the classification system of the Intergroup Rhabdomyosarcoma Study, a national cooperative study group. Four stages are proposed based on the resectability of the tumor. Approximately 15% of children have stage I disease (localized disease, completely resected); approximately 28% of children have stage II disease (grossly resected tumor with microscopic residual or regional disease that is totally resected); approximately 36% of children have stage III disease (gross residual disease); and approximately 20% of children have stage IV disease (metastatic disease present).

Rhabdomyosarcoma is treated by a combination of surgery, radiation, and chemotherapy. Complete surgical resection provides the greatest assurance that cure

TABLE 40-5

Clinical Manifestations of Rhabdomyosarcoma

Location	Manifestation
Head and neck	
Orbit	Ptosis
	Exophthalmos
	Proptosis
Paranasal sinuses	Nasal obstruction
	Epistaxis
	Swelling
	Chronic sinusitis
Nasopharynx	Hypernasal speech
	Nasal discharge
	Visible polypoid mass
Oropharyngeal	Dysphagia
	Painful mastication
Middle ear	Chronic serous otitis media
	Discharge from affected ear
	Facial nerve palsy
	Conduction hearing loss
	Visible polypoid mass
Extremities	
All locations	Deep-seated, fixed palpable mass
Retroperitoneal	
All locations	Usually asymptomatic
	May have vague abdominal pain
	Bowel or genitourinary obstruction (late)
	Possible palpable mass
Genitourinary	
Vaginal	Abnormal vaginal bleeding
	Protruding polypoid mass
Prostate	Urinary tract obstruction
Bladder	Urinary retention
	Straining to void
	Hematuria
Paratesticular	Mass in scrotum that may or may not be painful

can be achieved; however, cure occurs in only 16% of children. If surgical resection leads to serious disfigurement or functional disability (e.g., enucleation for orbital tumors or cystectomy for bladder tumors), chemotherapy and radiation serve as the primary treatment and surgery is avoided. If there is a high likelihood of local recurrence, however, as is the case for testicular and prostate tumors, radical orchiectomies and hemiscrotectomy will be used. For all tumors, except stage I disease, local radiation therapy is given. A variety of combination chemotherapies are used with RMS. Agents shown to be effective include vincristine, dactinomycin, doxorubicin, and cyclophosphamide. Other drugs that have been used in combination are ifosfamide, etoposide, carboalatin, and cisplatin. Chemotherapy for stage I or II disease is given for 1 year if there is no disease recurrence. For stage III or IV, treatment continues an additional year combined with radiation therapy. Intrathecal chemotherapy is given to children whose tumor locations favor central nervous system spread.

The primary prognostic factor in RMS is the degree of residual disease that remains after surgical resection. Children with localized disease (stage I and II) have long-term survival rates reported at 70% to 80%. If widespread disease is present, long-term survival rates drop to 20%. Orbital tumors have an overall favorable prognosis, probably because of the lack of lymphatics in the area and early physical signs of disease.

SUMMARY REVIEW

Musculoskeletal Development in Children

1 Skeletal growth and development consist of two concurrent processes in healthy children: (1) the creation of new cells and tissues (growth), and (2) the consolidation of new tissues into a permanent form (maturation).

2 Ossification takes place in two centers in long bones: (1) the primary center or the diaphysis (the long, central portion of the bone), and (2) the secondary center or the epiphysis (the end portions of the bone).

3 Until adult stature is reached, age 17 for females and age 18 for males, growth in length of bones occurs at the epiphyseal plate through endochondral ossification.

4 Fifty percent of the total growth of the spine has occurred by 1 year of age, and most children have achieved 50% of their adult height by 2 years of age.

5 The appendicular skeleton (extremities) grows faster during childhood than does the axial skeleton.

6 Muscle fibers reach their maximal size in females at 10 years of age and at 14 years of age in males.

Musculoskeletal Alterations in Children

1 The most common congenital defect of the upper extremities is syndactyly (webbing of the fingers).

2 Developmental dysplasia of the hip is a serious and disabling condition in children if not diagnosed and treated.

3 Congenital muscle disorders (myopathies) include absence of muscles, hypoplasia, hyperplasia, and faulty intrinsic development.

4 Osteogenesis imperfecta (brittle bone disease) is an inherited disorder of collagen that primarily affects bones and results in serious fractures of many bones.

5 Rickets is a condition caused by deficiencies in vitamin D, calcium, and usually phosphorus, which is characterized by the failure of bones to become mineralized (ossified) and results in skeletal deformity.

6 Scoliosis is a lateral curvature of the spinal column that can be caused by congenital malformations of the spine, poliomyelitis, skeletal dysplasias, spastic paralysis, and unequal leg length, but is most often idiopathic.

7 Osteomyelitis is a local or generalized bacterial infection of bone and bone marrow. Bacteria are usually introduced by direct extension from a nearby infection, through the bloodstream, or by trauma.

8 Juvenile rheumatoid arthritis is an inflammatory joint disorder characterized by pain and swelling.

9 Avascular diseases of the bone are collectively referred to as osteochondroses and are caused by an insufficient blood supply to growing bones.

10 Legg-Calvé-Perthes disease is one of the most common osteochondroses. This disorder is characterized by epiphyseal necrosis or degeneration of the head of the femur followed by regeneration or recalcification.

11 Osgood-Schlatter disease is characterized by inflammation or partial separation of the tibial tubercle caused by chronic irritation, usually as a result of overuse of the quadriceps muscles. The condition is primarily seen in muscular, athletic adolescent males.

12 The muscular dystrophies are a group of genetically transmitted diseases characterized by progressive atrophy of symmetric groups of skeletal muscles without evidence of involvement or degeneration of neural tissue. There is an insidious loss of strength in all forms of the disorder with increasing disability and deformity.

13 The two main types of malignant childhood bone tumors are osteosarcoma and Ewing sarcoma.

14 Osteosarcoma, the most common malignant childhood bone tumor, originates in bone-producing mesenchymal cells and is most often located in the distal end of the femur or proximal end of the tibia.

15 Most childhood osteosarcoma cases are diagnosed between 15 and 19 years of age and occur equally in males and females.

16 Ewing sarcoma originates from cells within the bone marrow space and is most often located in the midshaft of long bones or in flat bones.

17 Ewing sarcoma is more common in males and is most frequently diagnosed between the ages of 5 and 15.

18 Pain is the usual presenting symptom for either osteosarcoma or Ewing sarcoma.

19 The primary treatments for osteosarcoma are surgery and chemotherapy. The primary treatment for Ewing sarcoma is a combination of chemotherapy, radiation, and surgery.

20 The most common type of childhood soft tissue tumor is rhabdomyosarcoma.

21 Rhabdomyosarcoma originates from embryonal rhabdomyoblasts that normally differentiate into mature striated muscle. There are five subtypes.

22 Clinical manifestations of rhabdomyosarcoma depend on the anatomic location; superficial tumors exhibit a painless palpable mass, whereas deep-seated tumors cause functional impairment.

23 Rhabdomyosarcoma is treated with a combination of surgery, radiation, and chemotherapy.

KEY TERMS

Alveolar subclass of RMS, 1505
Antalgic abductor lurch, 1497
Becker muscular dystrophy, 1500
Botryoides subclass of RMS, 1505
Cartilage model, 1483
Developmental dysplasia of the hip (DDH), 1485
Duchenne muscular dystrophy, 1499
Embryonal subclass of RMS, 1505
Endochondral formation of bone, 1483
Ewing sarcoma, 1504
Facioscapulohumeral muscular dystrophy, 1500
Idiopathic scoliosis, 1490
Intramembranous formation of bone, 1483
Involucrum, 1492

Juvenile rheumatoid arthritis (JRA), 1494
Legg-Calvé-Perthes disease, 1496
Limb girdle muscular dystrophy, 1501
Metatarsus adductus, 1486
Muscular dystrophy, 1497
Myotonic muscular dystrophy, 1501
Nonossifying fibroma, 1504
Nonstructural scoliosis, 1490
Osgood-Schlatter disease, 1497
Osteochondrosis, 1495
Osteogenesis imperfecta (brittle bone disease), 1488
Osteomyelitis, 1492
Osteosarcoma, 1502
Perichondrium, 1483
Periosteal collar, 1483

Pleomorphic subclass of RMS, 1506
Primary center of ossification, 1482
Rhabdomyosarcoma (RMS), 1505
Rickets, 1490
Scapuloperoneal muscular dystrophy, 1501
Scoliosis, 1490
Secondary center of ossification, 1483
Secondary suppurative arthritis, 1493
Sequestra (pl., sequestrum), 1492
Structural scoliosis, 1490
Syndactyly, 1485
Talipes equinovarus (clubfoot), 1486
Undifferentiated cell types of RMS, 1506
Vestigial tab, 1485

REFERENCES

Abramovitz, J. N., Baston, R. A., & Yablon, J. S. (1986). Vertebral osteomyelitis: The surgical management of neurologic complications. *Spine, 11*(5), 418-420.

Alderson, M., Speers, D., Emslie, K., & Nade, S. (1986). Acute haematogenous osteomyelitis and septic arthritis: A single disease. An hypothesis based upon the presence of transphyseal blood vessels. *Journal of Bone & Joint Surgery, 68*(2), 268-274.

Barrack, R., Whitecloud, T., Burker, S., Cook, S., & Harding, A. (1984). Proprioception in idiopathic scoliosis. *Spine, 9*(7), 681-685.

Barrack, R., Wyatt, M., Whitecloud, T., Burke, S., Roberts, J., & Brinker, M. (1988). Vibratory hypersensitivity in idiopathic sclerosis. *Journal of Pediatric Orthopaedics, 8*(4), 389-395.

Behrman, R., Kliegman, R., Nelson, W., & Vaughan, V., III (Eds.). (1992). *Nelson textbook of pediatrics.* Philadelphia: Saunders.

Bergdahl, S., Ekengren, K., & Eriksson, M. (1986). Neonatal hematogenous osteomyelitis: Risk factors for long-term sequelae. *Journal of Pediatric Orthopedics, 6*(2), 177-181.

Boal, D. K. B., & Schwentker, E. P. (1991). Assessment of congenital hip dislocation with real-time ultrasound: A pictorial essay. *Clinical Imaging, 15*, 77-90.

Brashear, H. R., & Raney, R. B. (1978). *Shand's handbook of orthopedic surgery* (9th ed.). St. Louis: Mosby–Year Book.

Brooke, M. H. (1977). *A clinician's view of neuromuscular diseases.* Baltimore: Williams & Wilkins.

Byrd, J. (1988). Current theories on the etiology of idiopathic scoliosis. *Clinical Orthopaedics and Related Research, 299*, 114-119.

Carnsdale, P. G. (1992). Osteomyelitis. In A. H. Crenshaw (Ed.), *Campbell's operative orthopaedics* (8th ed., vol. 1). St. Louis: Mosby–Year Book.

Cassidy, J. T. (1982). *Textbook of pediatric rheumatology.* New York: John Wiley & Sons.

Chandrasekar, P. H., & Narula, A. P. (1986). Bone and joint infections in intravenous drug abusers. *Review of Infectious Diseases, 8*(6), 904-911.

Cole, C. G., Coyne, A., Hart, K. A., Sheridan, R., Walker, A., Johnson, L., Hodgson, S., & Bobrow, M. (1988, February 6). Prenatal testing for Duchenne and Becker muscular dystrophy. *Lancet,* 262-265.

Dich, V. Q., Nelson, J. D., & Haltalin, K. C. (1975). Osteomyelitis in infants and children. *American Journal of Diseases of Children, 129,* 1273-1276.

Evans, M. I., Greb, A., Kunkel, L. M., Sacks, A. J., Johnson, M. P., Boehm, C., Hazazian, H. H., & Hoffman, E. P. (1991). In utero fetal muscle biopsy for the diagnosis of Duchenne muscular dystrophy. *American Journal of Obstetrics & Gynecology, 165,* 728-732.

Fink, C. W., & Nelson, J. D. (1986). Septic arthritis and osteomyelitis in children. *Clinics in Rheumatic Diseases, 12*(2), 423-435.

Gillespie, W. J., Haywood-Farmer, M., Fong, R., & Harding, S. M. (1987). Aspects of the microbe: Host relationship in staphylococcal hematogenous osteomyelitis. *Orthopedics, 10*(3), 475-480.

Griggs, R. C., & Rennie, M. J. (1983). Muscle wasting in muscular dystrophy: Decreased protein synthesis or increased degradation? *Annals of Neurology, 13*(2), 125-132.

Hobbs, R. (1922). *Treatment of puerperal infection by drainage.* Westland, MJ, London, xxvii, 16-32.

Ikeda, K. (1992). Conservative treatment of idiopathic clubfoot. *Journal of Pediatric Orthopaedics, 12,* 217-223.

Israel, M. A. (1989). Molecular and cellular biology in pediatric malignancies. In P. A. Pizzo (Ed.), *Principles and practices of pediatric oncology.* Philadelphia: Lippincott.

Karlin, J. M. (1987). Osteomyelitis in children. *Clinics in Podiatric Medicine and Surgery, 4*(1), 37-56.

Kissane, J. M. (Ed.). (1990). *Anderson's pathology* (9th ed.). St. Louis: Mosby–Year Book.

Koufos, A., & Hansen, M. (1985). Loss of heterozygosity in three embryonal tumors suggests a common pathogenetic mechanism. *Nature, 316,* 330-334.

Kyzer, S. P. (1991). Congenital idiopathic clubfoot. *Orthopaedic Nursing, 10*(4), 11-18.

McCullough, F., & Pellino, T. (1993). Congenital and developmental disorders. In A. Maher, T. Pellino, & S. Salmond (Eds.), *Orthopaedic nursing.* Philadelphia: Saunders.

Morrissy, R. (Ed.). (1990). *Lovell and Winter's pediatric orthopaedics* (3rd ed.). Philadelphia: Lippincott.

Morrissy, R. T., & Shore, S. L. (1986). Bone and joint sepsis. *Pediatric Clinics of North America, 33*(6), 1551-1564.

Ray, M. J., & Basset, R. L. (1985). Pyogenic vertebral osteomyelitis. *Orthopedics, 8*(4), 504-506, 510, 512-513.

Scott, M. O., Sylvester, J. E., Heiman-Patterson, T., Shi, Y. J., Fieles, W., Stedman, H., Burghes, A., Ray, P., Warton, R., & Fishbeck, K. H. (1988). Duchenne muscular dystrophy gene expression in normal and diseased human muscle. *Science, 239,* 1418-1420.

Scriver, C. R., Beaudet, A. L., Sly, W. S., & Valle, D. (1989). *The metabolic basis of inherited disease* (6th ed.). New York: McGraw-Hill.

Sillence, D. (1981). Osteogenesis imperfecta: An expanding panorama of variants. *Clinical Orthopaedics and Related Research, 159,* 11-25.

Swaiman, K. F., & Wright, F. S. (1982). *The practice of pediatric neurology.* St. Louis: Mosby–Year Book.

Sykes, B. (1987). Molecular diagnostics: Genetics cracks bone disease. *Nature, 330,* 607-608.

Tachjdian, M. (1990). *Pediatric orthopedics* (2nd ed.). Philadelphia: Saunders.

Thompson, J. M., McFarland, G. K., Hirsch, J. E., & Tucker, S. M. (1993). *Mosby's manual of clinical nursing* (3rd ed.). St. Louis: Mosby–Year Book.

Trueta, J. (1959). The three types of acute hematogenous osteomyelitis. *Journal of Bone and Joint Surgery, 41B,* 671-676.

Whaley, L. F., & Wong, D. L. (1991). *Nursing care of infants and children* (4th ed.). St. Louis: Mosby–Year Book.

Winter, R. B. (1977). Scoliosis and spinal growth. *Orthopaedic Review, 6.*

Zaleske, D. J., Doppelt, S. H., & Mankin, H. J. (1986). Endocrine abnormalities of the immature skeleton. In W. W. Lovell & R. B. Winter (Eds.), *Pediatric orthopaedics* (2nd ed.). Philadelphia: Lippincott.

SUGGESTED READINGS

Arias, F. G., Rodriguez, M., Hernandez, J. G., Gonzalvo, P., & Orense, M. (1987). Osteomyelitis deriving from BCG-vaccination. *Pediatric Radiology, 17*(2), 166-167.

Green, N. E. (1983). Musculoskeletal infections in children. Part II. Primary subacute epiphyseal osteomyelitis. *Instructional Course Lectures, 32,* 37-40.

Green, N. (1990). Adolescent idiopathic scoliosis. In J. Hsu (Ed.), *Spine: State of the art reviews, 4*(1), 211-212.

Gutman, L. T. (1985). Acute, subacute, and chronic osteomyelitis and pyogenic arthritis in children. *Current Problems in Pediatrics, 15*(12), 1-72.

Mason, K. J. (1989). Pediatric orthopaedics: Developmental norms. *Orthopaedic Nursing, 8*(4), 45-50.

Nelson, L. W., & Lydiatt, D. D. (1987). Osteomyelitis of the head and neck. *Nebraska Medical Journal, 72*(5), 154-163.

Riseborough, E. J., & Herndon, J. H. (1975). *Scoliosis and other deformities of the axial skeleton.* Boston: Little, Brown & Co.

Vizkelety, T. L. (1986). Partial destruction of the distal femoral epiphysis as a consequence of osteomyelitis: Regeneration after transplantation of a bone graft. *Journal of Pediatric Orthopedics, 5*(6), 731-733.

Winter, R., & Longstein, J. (1992). Juvenile and adolescent scoliosis. In R. Rothman & F. Simeon (Eds.), *The spine* (3rd ed.). Philadelphia: Saunders.

Wong, S. K., & Wilhelmus, K. R. (1986). Infantile maxillary osteomyelitis with cerebral abscess. *Journal of Pediatric Ophthalmology and Strabismus, 23*(3), 153-154.

UNIT XIV

The Integumentary System

SKIN DISEASES have been known since the early civilizations of the Egyptians, Greeks, Romans, and Arabs. In the time of Hippocrates, superficial ulcers were treated with warm baths, and the temperature of the water was important to prevent chilling and promote bleeding. Ulcers then were cleaned with vinegar, debrided, and covered with wool soaked in a herbal poultice including verdigris (copper acetate), flower of copper (copper oxide), mo-

lybdenum (lead oxide), alum, myrrh, frankincense, gall nuts, vine flowers, and wool grease (Majno, 1975). Both the ancient Romans and Arabs used baths with both hot and cold water for treatment of some skin diseases. The Arabs developed theories of cleanliness in preventing skin diseases, particularly the bites of fleas, lice, and other insects. In the tenth century, Baghdad had more than 27,000 public baths. In second century BC China, "ulcer physi-

THE INTEGUMENTARY SYSTEM

Clay mask, with protruding tongue and skin neoplasm. Pre-Columbian Medicine as told in clay. (Courtesy National Library of Medicine.)

pox and bubonic plague affecting large populations. The major means of treatment were herbal applications, baths, and magical beliefs.

Early medical manuscripts from Britain (fifth to tenth century) indicate that the causes of skin diseases were unknown but often followed pestilence and trauma. Malnutrition, scabies, scurvy, and pellagra commonly occurred during and after wars, with lesions such as ulcers, eczema, impetigo, and erysipelas. Diseases such as psoriasis, scrofula (a tuberculous disease of lymph nodes and bones with draining abscesses), syphilis, and eczema were rampant during this period. Leprosy was associated with eating tainted or rotten meat and fish, and some leper hospitals of the time were noted for their treatment with fresh wholesome food.

cians" were designated to care for swollen ulcers, dripping ulcers, and ulcers caused by piercing instruments or fractures. Such wounds were treated with the five poisons, fortified with the five medicines, and tempered with the five flavors. Celsus, in AD 30, recommended sutures with women's hair to close small wounds and pins to close gaping wounds. He also advocated vinegar washes to avoid inflammation and loose closure for deep draining wounds. Leprosy, syphilis, smallpox, and skin tumors were evident in ancient times with epidemics of small-

Scrofula was known as the "king's evil" because King Edward of Britain (1042 to 1066) believed the condition could be cured by the sovereign's touch. Elizabeth I practiced healing by touch; she knelt in prayer, laying her hands on the sores of her subjects (Huckbody, 1980). Hot herbal baths were often used for treatment. Fennel mint, yarrow, betony, and dill were most effective and are used in more sophisticated forms today. The recognition that pressure caused bedsores was first described by Paget in approximately 1855.

Structure, Function, and Disorders of the Integument

Sue E. Huether
Melva Kravitz

Chapter Outline

The skin is the largest organ of the body. Combined with the accessory structures of hair, nails, and glands, it forms the integumentary system. The skin covers the entire body and accounts for approximately 20% of the body's weight. The primary function of the skin is to protect the body from the environment by serving as a barrier against microorganisms, ultraviolet radiation, loss of body fluids, and the stress of mechanical forces. The skin also regulates body temperature within a very narrow range and is involved in the production of vitamin D. Touch and pressure receptors provide important protective functions and pleasurable sensations.

STRUCTURE AND FUNCTION OF THE SKIN

Layers of the Skin

The skin is formed of two major layers: (1) a superficial or outer layer of **epidermis** and (2) a deeper layer of **dermis** (the true skin) (Fig. 41-1 and Table 41-1). The subcutaneous tissue, or **hypodermis,** is an underlying layer of connective tissue, which contains macrophages, fibroblasts, and fat cells. Each skin layer contains cells that represent progressive stages of skin cell differentiation as the skin grows.

Epidermis

The epidermis grows continually by shedding the superficial layer of **stratum corneum,** which is formed entirely of keratinocytes and melanocytes. These cells are named for the substances they produce. **Keratinocytes** produce **keratin,** a scleroprotein. Keratin is the main constituent of skin, hair, and nail cells. The thickness of the epidermis varies from 0.3 mm on the eyelids to 1.5 mm on the palms of the hands and soles of the feet. New cells (keratinocytes) formed in the **basal layer** (stratum basale) move upward and differentiate, forming the **spinous layer** (stratum spinosum). Together they form the germinative layer (stratum germinativum). The cells enlarge and then become flattened, stacked, and cornified (stratum corneum) as they ascend to the skin surface. Cornification, or keratinization, prevents dehydration of deeper skin layers. The average turnover of the epidermis is about 30 days.

The epidermis has three different types of cells that facilitate its functional characteristics: (1) melanocytes, (2) Langerhans cells, and (3) Merkel cells. The **melanocytes** are usually located near the base of the epidermis. They synthesize and secrete the pigment melanin with

exposure to sunlight in response to melanocyte-stimulating hormone (MSH). Melanin in the epidermis provides a shield against ultraviolet radiation and determines skin color. **Langerhans cells** migrate to the dermis from the bone marrow. The Langerhans cells initiate an immune response and provide defense against environmental antigens. **Merkel cells** are associated with touch receptors, and they function as slowly adapting mechanoreceptors when stimulated by deformation of the epidermis.

Dermis

The dermis varies from 1 to 4 mm in thickness and is composed of three types of fibrous connective tissue: (1) collagen, (2) elastin and reticulin, and (3) a gel-like ground substance. The haphazard arrangement of connective tissue allows the skin to be mobile and stretch and contract with body movement. Hair follicles, sebaceous glands, sweat glands, blood vessels, lymphatic vessels, and nerves are contained in the dermis. The conelike projections of the papillary dermis interface with the epidermis. The papillae provide texture to the surface of the skin by forming what are known as rete pegs.

The cells of the dermis include fibroblasts, mast cells, and macrophages. Fibroblasts secrete the connective tissue matrix. Mast cells release histamine and play a role in hypersensitivity reactions in the skin. Macrophages are phagocytic and participate in immune responses.

Hypodermis (Subcutaneous Layer)

The subcutaneous tissue contains the dermal appendages (nails, hair, sebaceous glands, and the eccrine and apocrine sweat glands), the supplying blood vessels of the dermis, and nerves of the autonomic nervous system. A layer of cushioning fat provides a base for the hypodermis.

Dermal Appendages

The **dermal appendages** include the **nails, hair, sebaceous glands,** and the eccrine and apocrine **sweat glands.** All are variably distributed over the body. The nails are protective keratinized plates that appear at the ends of fingers and toes. The nail is composed of four structural units: (1) the proximal nail fold, (2) the matrix from which the nail grows, (3) the hyponychium (the nail bed), and (4) the nail plate (Fig. 41-2). Nail growth is continuous throughout life at a rate of about 0 mm to 1 mm/day.

Hair follicles and sebaceous glands are integrated units (Fig. 41-1). Hair color, density, grain, and pattern of distribution have considerable variability and depend on age, sex, and race. Hair follicles arise from the matrix (or bulb) located deep in the dermis. They extend from the dermis at an angle and have an erector pili

FIG. 41-1 Structure of the skin. (From Thompson, McFarland, Hirsch, & Tucker, 1993.)

TABLE 41-1

Layers of the Skin

Structure	Characteristics
Epidermis	The most important layer of the skin; normally very thin (0.12 mm) but can thicken and form corns or calluses in areas of constant pressure or friction
Stratum corneum	Dead keratinocytes that provide a tough covering over the body surface
Stratum lucidum	A clear layer of cells containing a substance called eleidin that is transformed into keratin as the cells differentiate into stratum corneum
Stratum granulosum	A layer of cells containing keratohyalin that gives a granular appearance
Stratum spinosum	A layer of cells on top of the basal cells that is polygonal-shaped with spinous processes projecting between adjacent keratinocytes
Stratum germinativum	A basal cell layer closest to the basement membrane; keratinocytes divide and move upward to replace cells normally shed from the surface
Dermis	A 1-4 mm layer of irregular connective tissue composed of collagen and elastic and reticular fibers with a rich blood, lymphatic, and nerve supply; contains sensory receptors and special glands
Papillary layer	An irregular layer of collagen fibers containing capillary loops, sensory receptors, and a horizontal plexus of blood vessels
Reticular layer	A random array or reticulum of collagenous fibers that articulate (connect) with the hypodermis
Hypodermis	Subcutaneous tissue or superficial fascia of varying thickness that connects the overlying dermis to underlying muscle

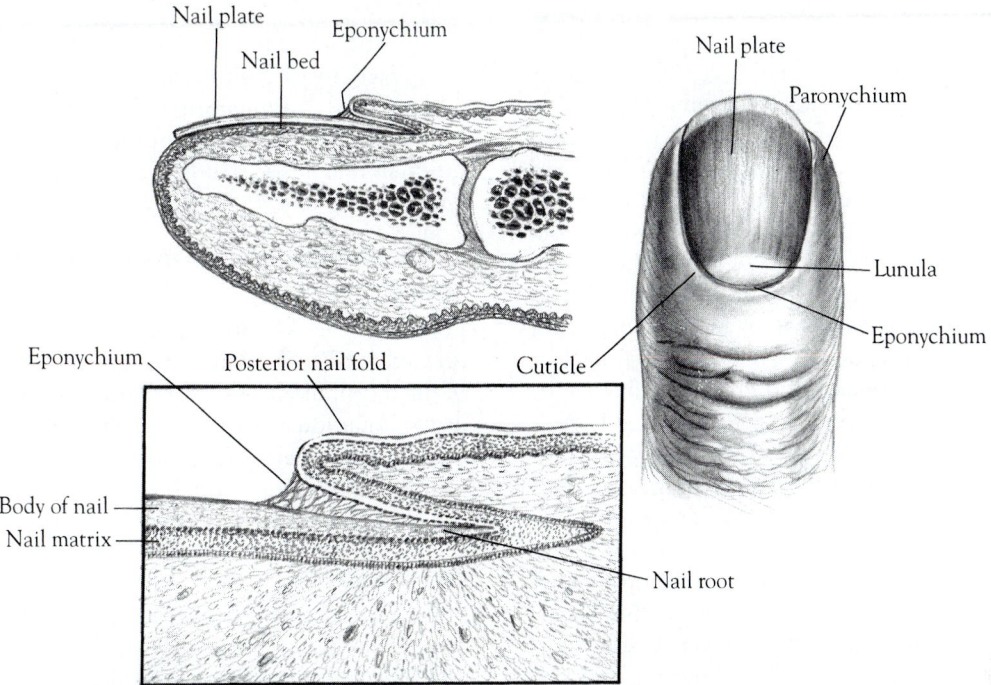

FIG. 41-2 **Structures of the nail.** (From Thompson, McFarland, Hirsch, & Tucker, 1993.)

muscle attached near the mid-dermis that straightens the follicle when contracted, causing the hair to stand up. Hair growth begins in the bulb, with cellular differentiation occurring as the hair progresses up the follicle. Hair is fully hardened, or cornified, by the time it emerges at the skin surface. Hair growth is cyclic with periods of growth and rest that vary over different body surfaces.

The **sebaceous glands** open onto the surface of the skin through a canal. They are found in greatest numbers on the face, chest, and back with modified glands on the eyelids, lips, nipple, glans penis, and prepuce. Sebaceous glands secrete sebum that is composed primarily of lipids, which oils the skin and hair and prevents drying. Growth of sebaceous glands is stimulated by testosterone, and their enlargement is one of the early signs of puberty.

The **eccrine sweat glands** are distributed over the body, with the greatest numbers in the palms of the hands, soles of the feet, and forehead. These secretions are important in thermoregulation and cooling of the body through evaporation. The **apocrine sweat glands** are fewer in number and are located in the axillae, scalp, face, abdomen, and genital area.

Blood Supply and Innervation

The blood supply to the skin is limited to the **papillary capillaries,** or plexus, of the dermis. These capillary loops arise from a subpapillary plexus that is supplied by a deeper horizontal cutaneous arterial plexus. Branches from the deep plexus supply hair follicles and sweat glands. A subpapillary network of veins drains the capillary loops. There are arteriovenous anastomoses at the level of the dermis that facilitate the regulation of body temperature. Heat loss can be regulated by varying blood flow through the skin by opening and closing the arteriovenous anastomoses in conjunction with evaporative heat loss of sweat. The sympathetic nervous system regulates both vasoconstriction and vasodilation. There are only α-adrenergic receptors in the skin. The lymphatic vessels of the skin arise in the papillary dermis and drain into larger subcutaneous trunks, removing cells, proteins, and immunologic mediators.

❑ AGING and Skin Integrity

Many of the age-associated changes in the skin are readily observable and appear over the body surface. Structurally, the skin becomes thinner, dryer, and wrinkled with a change in pigmentation (Kurban & Kurban, 1993). The cellular alterations contributing to the changes include a flattening of the dermoepidermal border with a shortening and decrease in the number of capillary loops. There are fewer melanocytes, with decreased protection against ultraviolet radiation. A significant decrease in the number of Langerhans cells decreases the skin's immune response with aging. The thickness of the dermis also decreases and accounts for the translucent, paper-thin quality of the skin. Loss of the rete pegs gives the skin a smooth, shiny appearance (Gilchrist, 1984).

The decreased vasculature probably contributes to the atrophy of eccrine, apocrine, and sebaceous glands that cause dry skin. Loss of elastin fibers is associated with wrinkling. The collagen fibers become less flexible and decrease the ability of the skin to stretch and regain shape. Decreased cell generation, blood supply, and depressed immune responses also delay wound healing in aging skin. Changes in hair color and distribution also occur. Graying is caused by loss of melanocytes from hair bulbs, and thinning occurs from a gradual decline in the number of hair follicles and growth of finer hair.

The epidermal cells change shape, and the barrier function of the stratum corneum is reduced. There is increased permeability and decreased clearance of substances from the dermis. The accumulation of such substances is related to decreased vascularity and can cause skin irritation. Temperature regulation is compromised in the elderly, and there is increased risk for both heat stroke and hypothermia. Loss of cutaneous vasomotion and subcutaneous fat, decreased vascularity, and decreased eccrine sweat production are contributing factors. The pressure and touch receptors and free nerve endings all decrease in number and reduce sensory perception. In summary, many of the protective functions of the skin are decreased with aging.

Tests of Skin Function

Diagnostic evaluations of skin disorders often can be completed by the gathering of historical information and physical examination and observation of the distribution and characteristics of the presenting lesions. Additional diagnostic studies are summarized in Table 41-2.

Clinical Manifestations of Skin Dysfunction
Lesions

Lesions of the skin are readily observable and easily addressed for distribution and structure. The identification of the morphologic structure and appearance of the skin in combination with a health history are necessary to identify the underlying pathophysiology. Table 41-3 describes and illustrates the basic lesions of the skin. Special skin lesions are described in Table 41-4.

Pressure ulcers

Pressure ulcers, or pressure sores, are the development of ischemic ulcers in normal skin as a result of pressure and shearing forces. The term decubitus ulcer refers to ulcers or pressure sores that develop from being in the recumbent position for a long time. The more general terms of pressure sore or ulcer are used here. Those at greatest risk are individuals who are immobilized, incontinent, or debilitated, particularly the elderly. The

Text continued on p. 1522.

TABLE 41-2

Summary of Skin Diagnostic Procedures

Test	Purpose
Skin biopsy	Differential diagnosis of cellular structure, i.e., benign growths vs. carcinoma, chronic infections, blistering diseases, and vasculitis
Microscopic immunofluorescence	Identification of antibodies, immunoglobulins, and complement components for diseases such as pemphigus, vasculitis, and discoid lupus erythematosus using fluorescent light on slide-mounted biopsies.
Gram stain	Differentiation of gram-positive from gram-negative bacteria according to stain absorption
Culture	Identification of chronic bacterial and fungal infections by incubating skin specimens in culture media
Wood's lamp examination	Examination of skin or hair to identify fungus that fluoresces bright yellow-green under ultraviolet light
Patch and scratch tests	Application of suspected allergens to skin patch or scratch for evaluation of immune system responses to known allergens and evaluation of cell-mediated immune function (*Candida albicans*, skin fungus)
Skin scrapings	Application of potassium hydroxide (KOH) and low heat to skin scrapings on a glass slide to identify fungi
Side lighting	Indirect lighting of the skin using light to the side of the lesions to evaluate patterns of depression and elevation of skin lesions
Diascopy	Use of glass or clear plastic pressed on the skin to differentiate erythema caused by dilated capillaries (blanching) from extravasation of blood (no blanching)

TABLE 41-3

Basic Lesions of the Skin

Type	Characteristics	Example	
Flat lesions			
Macule	A flat circumscribed lesion of any size differentiated from surrounding skin by color	Hyperpigmentation Erythema Telangiectasias Purpura	
Patch	A flat, irregular lesion larger than 1 cm in diameter	Vitiligo	
Elevated lesions			
Papule	Firm elevated lesions 1 cm or less in diameter from infiltration or hyperplasia of the dermis	Verruca (warts) Lichen planus Nevus	
Plaque	Elevated lesions with a large surface area	Psoriasis Eczema	

Continued.

TABLE 41-3

Basic Lesions of the Skin—cont'd

Type	Characteristics	Example	
Nodule	A palpable circumscribed lesion 1-2 cm in diameter located in the epidermis, dermis, or hypodermis; surface features may vary from smooth to ulcerated	Benign or malignant tumors Foreign body inflammation Calcium deposits	
Wheal	A dome or flat-topped elevated lesion with well-defined and often changing borders caused by edema of the dermis	Hives Angioedema	
Vesicle and bulla	A fluid-filled, thin-walled elevated lesion; a bulla is a vesicle greater than 0.5 cm in diameter	Herpes zoster Impetigo Pemphigus Second-degree burn	
Pustule	An elevated lesion containing an exudate of white blood cells that may be sterile or contaminated with bacteria	Acne Pustular psoriasis	

TABLE 41-3

Basic Lesions of the Skin—cont'd

Type	Characteristics	Example	
Scale	Accumulation of the stratum corneum from cellular retention or cellular over-production	Psoriasis	
Crust	Accumulation of dried blood or serum; size may vary	Eczema Impetigo	
Lichenification	Thickening, toughening of the skin with accentuation of skin lines caused by scratching	Chronic dermatitis	
Cyst	An elevated, encapsulated mass of dermis or subcutaneous layers, solid or fluid filled	Sebaceous cyst	

Continued.

TABLE 41-3

Basic Lesions of the Skin—cont'd

Type	Characteristics	Example	
Tumor	A well-demarcated, elevated lesion greater than 2 cm in diameter	Fibroma Lipoma Melanoma Hemangioma	
Scar	Thin or thick elevated fibrous tissue	Healed laceration, burn, or surgical incision	
Depressed lesions			
Atrophy	Thinning of the epidermis or dermis caused by a decrease in cell numbers of connective tissue	Thin facial skin of elderly Striae of pregnancy	
Ulcer	Loss of epidermis and dermis within a distinct border	Pressure sores Basal cell carcinoma	

TABLE 41-3

Basic Lesions of the Skin—cont'd

Type	Characteristics	Example	
Excoriation	Loss of epidermis with exposed dermis	Scratches	
Fissure	Linear crack or break exposing dermis; small, deep, red	Athlete's foot Cheilosis	
Erosion	Depressed, moist, red break in epidermis; follows rupture of vesicle or bulla; larger than fissure	Chicken pox Diaper dermatitis	

TABLE 41-4

Special Skin Lesions

Type	Clinical manifestations
Comedone	A plug of sebaceous and keratin material lodged in the opening of a hair follicle; an open comedone has a dilated orifice (blackhead) and a closed comedone has a narrow opening (whitehead)
Burrow	A narrow, raised, irregular channel caused by a parasite
Petechiae	A circumscribed area of blood less than 0.5 cm in diameter
Purpura	A circumscribed area of blood greater than 0.5 cm in diameter
Telangiectasia	Dilated, superficial blood vessels

highest incidence occurs among individuals with a fractured neck of the femur (Versluysen, 1986).

Individuals with neurologic disorders, such as spinal cord injuries, dementia, or cerebrovascular disease, are particularly at risk, often as a result of loss of sensation rather than immobility. Chronic diseases accompanied by anemia, edema, renal failure, malnutrition, sepsis, and urinary or fecal incontinence increase the risk of pressure sores. The liability for developing a pressure sore is increased when individuals lie for hours on hard x-ray and operating tables or sit in wheelchairs or lie in bed for hours without changing position or relieving pressure. Use of coarse draw-sheets for turning and moving individuals in bed by dragging them about can cause shearing forces that lead to pressure sores.

Pressure sores usually develop over bony prominences. The sacrum, heels, ischia, and greater trochanters are the most common sites. Continuous pressure on tissue between the bony prominence and a resistant outside surface distorts capillaries and occludes the blood supply. If the pressure is relieved within a few hours, a brief period of reactive hyperemia (redness) occurs with no lasting tissue damage. If the pressure continues unrelieved, the endothelial cells lining the capillaries become disrupted with platelet aggregation, forming microthrombi that block blood flow and cause anoxic necrosis of surrounding tissues. Pressure ulcers can be classified by stages:

I. Nonblanchable erythema of intact skin
II. Partial-thickness skin loss involving epidermis or dermis
III. Full-thickness skin loss involving damage or necrosis of subcutaneous tissue that may extend to, but not through, underlying fascia
IV. Full-thickness skin loss with extensive destruction, tissue necrosis, or damage to muscle, bone, or supporting structures ("Clinical guidelines," 1992)

A layer of dead tissue forms that appears as a blister when there is superficial damage, or a reddish blue discoloration when there is deeper tissue damage. Superficial sores are more common on the sacrum as a result of shearing or friction forces (forces parallel to the skin). Deep sores develop closer to the bone as a result of tissue distortion and vascular occlusion from pressure that is perpendicular to the tissue (over the heels, trochanter, and ischia).

The necrotic tissue initiates an inflammatory response, with pain, fever, and leukocytosis. Although bacteria colonize the dead tissue, the infection is usually localized and self-limiting. Proteolytic enzymes from bacteria and macrophages dissolve necrotic tissues and cause a foul-smelling discharge that appears like, but is not, pus.

Pressure sores are often painful in individuals who do not have loss of sensation from spinal cord trauma or neuropathy. The presence of necrotic tissue produces an inflammatory response with hyperemia, fever, and increased white blood cell count. If the ulceration is large, toxicity and pain lead to loss of appetite, debility, and renal insufficiency. Individuals who are immunosuppressed or have diabetes mellitus may develop infection and inflammation of adjacent tissues (cellulitis) or septicemia.

The primary goal for those at risk for pressure ulcers is prevention. Pressure sores are not prevented by topical agents, such as benzoin, vitamin D ointment, zinc oxide, oils, or antibiotics, because they do not relieve the pressure. Turning every 2 hours and use of flotation devices and alternating pressure mattresses are effective preventive techniques.

Superficial ulcers should be covered with flat, nonbulky dressings that cannot wrinkle and cause increased pressure or friction. Spontaneous healing will occur more quickly when the ulcer is kept moist with an occlusive dressing (Monk, Graham-Brown, & Sarkany, 1988). Antibiotics are seldom required. Antiseptics, such as hydrogen peroxide or iodine, are damaging to granulation tissue and should not be used. Successful healing requires continued adequate relief of pressure.

Large, deep pressure ulcers may require surgical debridement of necrotic tissue and opening of deep pockets for drainage. A variety of skin grafting techniques may be used for wound closure. The myocutaneous flap, a single unit of skin with its underlying muscle and vasculature, has been an effective treatment in large avascular areas over bony prominences.

Keloids

Keloids are sharply elevated, irregularly shaped, progressively enlarging scars caused by excessive amounts of collagen in the corneum during connective tissue repair. Seemingly inconsequential trauma may result in a keloidal reaction, particularly in blacks and Orientals. Burns incite this reaction more commonly than other types of injury.

Excessive or poorly aligned tension on a wound, introduction of foreign material into the skin, and certain types of trauma (such as burns) are all provocative factors. Those parts of the body at risk include shoulders, back, chin, ears, and lower legs. Most keloids appear within 1 year of trauma. Individuals 10 to 30 years of age develop lesions much more commonly than do children before puberty or older adults.

The fibrous tissue that accumulates in keloids is associated with increased cellularity and metabolic activity of fibroblasts. **Myofibroblasts,** cells with characteristics of both fibroblasts and smooth muscle cells, have been identified as the principal cell in keloids.

Type III collagen is increased with keloids. The swol-

FIG. 41-3 Keloid formation. Mass of keloids arising from suture marks in a black individual. (From Habif, 1990.)

len appearance of keloids is caused by an abundance of extracellular material. Collagenase activity in keloids has been found to be normal or increased, but the collagen may be protected from degradation by **proteoglycan,** a glycoprotein present in connective tissue that serves as a binding (cementing) material, and by specific inhibitors of proteolytic enzymes. A familial tendency for keloid formation has been found, with both autosomal recessive and autosomal dominant inheritance patterns being reported.

Keloids start as pink or red, firm, well-defined, rubbery plaques that persist for several months after trauma. Later, uncontrolled overgrowth causes extension beyond the site of the original wound and the tumor becomes smoother, irregularly shaped, hyperpigmented, harder, and more symptomatic. The tendency to send out **clawlike prolongations** is typical of keloids (Fig. 41-3).

Preventive measures such as the avoidance of unnecessary, elective surgeries are of paramount importance. When surgery is necessary for cosmetic reasons, early childhood is best. Scalpel surgery with strict aseptic technique and avoidance of wound tension should be imperative. Electrosurgery or chemosurgery should be avoided. Injection of corticosteroids into the lesion often brings excellent results and is the treatment of choice.

Pruritus

Pruritus, or itching, is a symptom associated with many primary skin disorders, such as eczema or lice infestations, or as a manifestation of systemic disease, such as chronic renal failure, cholestatic liver disease, thyroid disorders, iron deficiency, and opiate drugs. It may be localized or generalized and may move from one location to another (Klecz & Schwartz, 1992).

The actual mechanisms causing pruritus are unknown. Multiple stimuli can produce itching, including histamine, heat, and electrical stimulation with a fine probe. In experiments using cowage (a pruritogen or itch-causing substance), itching was most severe when the agent was applied at the junction of the dermis and epidermis (Shelley & Arthur, 1957). It is not known if the cowage stimulates the itching directly or induces histamine release. Antihistamines do not block this type of induced itching. Substance P, a neurotransmitter present throughout the nervous system, induces histamine release and wheal formation with itching when injected into the skin. Antihistamines and local anesthetics block substance P–induced itching. Lymphocytes are also present in many itching skin diseases, and lymphokines may be involved in the pathogenesis of itching (Hagermark, 1992).

Itching also has been linked to pain, because many stimuli that induce pain produce itching at lower intensities. Central nervous system mechanisms can also modulate itching, and itching is less perceptible when the mind is concentrating on other things. How the central nervous system influences the itch sensation is unclear.

Chronic itching is an unpleasant sensation relieved by scratching, often severe enough to cause trauma to the skin, resulting in infection and scarring. Some individuals become so distraught with the constant irritation that they will apply heat with enough intensity and duration to produce burns.

Management of localized itching depends on the cause, and the primary condition must be treated. Symptomatic relief may be obtained from antihistamines, which also have a sedative effect. Minor tranquilizers, such as promethazine, may be effective for some causes of pruritus. Itching related to dry, rough skin (xerosis) can be managed with applications of emollients and increased environmental humidity. Topical steroids are immediately effective with some occurrences of pruritus; however, in some instances, pruritus is resistant to any type of therapy.

DISORDERS OF THE SKIN

Disruptions in skin integrity may be precipitated by trauma, abnormal cellular function, infection and inflammation, and systemic diseases. Many skin disorders are benign and self-limiting, whereas some are severe and life-threatening.

Inflammatory Disorders

The most common inflammatory disorder of the skin is eczema (eczematous inflammation). **Eczema** is an inflammatory response of the skin caused by endogenous and exogenous agents and is often considered synonymous with dermatitis. Endogenous eczemas include atopic dermatitis and seborrheic dermatitis. Exogenous eczemas include irritant dermatitis and allergic contact dermatitis. Eczematous dermatitis is characterized by erythema, vesicles, scales, and itching. Edema, serous discharge, and crusting occur with continued irritation and scratching. In chronic eczema, the skin becomes thickened, leathery, and hyperpigmented from recurrent irritation and scratching. The location of eczema is related to the underlying cause. Eczematous inflammations need to be differentiated from other rashes and dermatoses, particularly psoriasis.

Allergic Contact Dermatitis

Allergic contact dermatitis is a common form of cell-mediated or delayed hypersensitivity. (See Chapter 8 for different types of allergic responses.) A wide variety of allergens (e.g., microorganisms, chemicals, foreign proteins, drugs, metals) can form the sensitizing antigen. Contact with poison ivy is a common example (Fig. 41-4). As the allergen comes in contact with the skin, the allergen is bound to a carrier protein, forming a sensitizing antigen. The Langerhans cells process the antigen and carry it to T cells that then become sensitized to the antigen. Keratinocytes also may activate lymphocytes and endothelial cells in allergic contact dermatitis (Barker, 1992).

Delayed hypersensitivity is characterized by the passing of several hours before an immunologic response is apparent. The T cells play an important role because

FIG. 41-4 Linear eruption caused by contact with poison ivy. Poison ivy dermatitis. Diffuse erythema with linear lesions. (From Habif, T. P. [1985]. *Clinical dermatology: A color guide to diagnosis and treatment.* St. Louis: Mosby–Year Book.)

they differentiate and secrete lymphokines that affect macrophage movement and aggregation, coagulation, and other inflammatory responses (see Chapter 2). Sensitization usually develops with first exposure to the antigen, and symptoms of dermatitis occur with reexposure.

The manifestations of allergic contact dermatitis include erythema and swelling with pruritic (itching) vesicular lesions in the areas of allergen contact. The pattern of distribution provides clues to the source of the antigen (i.e., hands exposed to chemical solutions or boundaries from rings and bracelets). Removal of the irritant is necessary for resolution of the inflammatory response and tissue repair. Topical or systemic steroids may be required for treatment, depending on the severity of the lesion.

Irritant Contact Dermatitis

Irritant contact dermatitis is a nonimmunologically mediated inflammation of the skin. Chemical irritation from acids and prolonged exposure to soaps and detergents are common causes (see box on p. 1525). The skin lesions are similar in appearance to allergic contact dermatitis. Removing the source of irritation and use of topical agents provide effective treatment.

SUBSTANCES KNOWN TO CAUSE CONTACT DERMATITIS

Alkali
  Soaps
  Detergents
  Ammonia preparations
  Lye
  Drainpipe cleaners
  Toilet bowl cleaners
  Oven cleaners

Acids

Metal salts
  Cyanides of calcium, copper, mercury, nickel, silver, zinc
  Chlorides of calcium and zinc

Bromine, chlorine, iodine, fluorine

Insecticides

Dusts of lime, zinc, arsenic

Wood dust from teak, cinchona bark, quinine, pyrethrum

Tobacco dust from cigars

Explosive powders

Hydrocarbons
  Crude petroleum, lubricating oil, cutting oil
  Paraffins, mineral oils
  Asphalt, other tar products

Soot, peat

FIG. 41-5 Stasis dermatitis. The skin is diffusely red, thickened, and bound down by fibrosis. Ulceration occurs with the slightest trauma. (From Habif, 1990.)

Atopic Dermatitis

Atopic dermatitis is a common disease affecting 9% to 12% of the population (Schultz-Larson & Hanifin, 1992). The prevalence is more common in infancy and childhood; however, some individuals are affected throughout life. A family history of asthma, allergic rhinitis, dry skin, and eczema accompanies this disorder.

The dermatitis results from the complex activation of mast cells, T lymphocytes, monocytes, and other inflammatory cells that release histamine, lymphokines, and other inflammatory mediators. The interaction of the allergen with the immune system results in the chronic inflammation (Borish & Joseph, 1992).

During infancy, the eczema is characterized by red, weeping, crusty lesions distributed over the face, neck, and buttocks (see Chapter 42). During adolescence and adulthood, the lesions are usually localized to the hands and feet or flexor surfaces (i.e., antecubital fossa and popliteal space) of the arms and legs. The erythema, scaling, and lichenification (thickened and leatherlike skin) are exacerbated by scratching, because the lesions are manifest by itching. The scratching increases susceptibility to infection from *Staphylococcus aureus* and predisposition to cutaneous dissemination of viruses, particularly herpes simplex and vaccinia. Affected individuals also have a higher incidence of cataracts. Although the cause of atopic dermatitis is unknown, depressed cell-mediated immunity, elevated IgE levels, and increased sensitivity to histamine are related factors.

Management of atopic dermatitis includes avoidance of known irritants, good lubrication, and preservation of skin moisture. During the acute inflammatory stage, application of open wet compresses, using aluminum acetate solution (Burow solution), soothes itching and cools and moistens the skin. Topical steroids in the lowest possible dosages may be used to treat the lesions. Relief of pruritus is difficult, but oral antihistamines are occasionally prescribed. Affected individuals should avoid exposure to herpes simplex and vaccination with live virus.

Stasis Dermatitis

Stasis dermatitis usually occurs on the legs as a result of venous stasis and edema. The disorder is associated with varicosities, phlebitis, and vascular trauma. Initially there is erythema and pruritus with the development of scaling, petechiae, and hyperpigmentation. Progressive lesions become ulcerated, particularly around the ankles and tibia (Fig. 41-5).

Treatment includes elevating the legs as often as possible, not wearing tight clothes around the legs, and not standing for long periods. Acute inflammations are treated with antibiotics. Chronic lesions with ulceration are treated with wet dressings of Burow solution or silver nitrate. Edema is controlled with external compression.

Seborrheic Dermatitis

Seborrheic dermatitis is a common chronic inflammation of the skin involving the scalp, eyebrows, eyelids, ear canals, nasolabial folds, axillae, chest, and back (Fig. 41-6). In infants, the occurrence is known as "cradle cap." The cause is unknown, and the lesions appear from infancy to old age with periods of remission and exacerbation. The lesions appear as scaly, white or yellowish inflammatory plaques with mild pruritus. Mild cases are treated with shampoos containing sulfur, salicylic acid, or tar. Corticosteroid applications are use-

ful for suppression of severe symptoms but should not be used for maintenance therapy.

Papulosquamous Disorders

Psoriasis, pityriasis rosea, and lichen planus are disorders characterized by inflammatory processes associated with papules, scales, plaques, and erythema. Collectively they are described as **papulosquamous disorders.**

Psoriasis

Psoriasis is a chronic relapsing proliferative skin disorder that can occur at any age and affects 1% to 2% of the population. The onset is generally established by 20 years of age. The cause of psoriasis is unknown, but genetic, immunologic, or biochemical alterations have been investigated (Dobson & Abele, 1985; Kragballe & Voorhees, 1985). A family history of psoriasis is often established, but the mode of inheritance is not clear (Fitzpatrick, Eisen, Wolff, Freedberg, & Austen, 1993).

Both the dermis and epidermis are thickened with cellular proliferation and inflammation. The turnover time for shedding the epidermis is decreased from the normal 26 to 30 days to 3 to 4 days. There are increased numbers of germinative cells and an increase in transit time of cells through the dermis. The rapid cellular proliferation does not allow time for cell maturation and keratinization to occur. The cell proliferation contrib-

FIG. 41-6 Seborrheic dermatitis of eyebrow, a common site. (From Stewart, Danto, & Maddin, 1978.)

utes to a thickened epidermis and plaque formation. The loosely cohesive keratin gives the lesion a silvery appearance. There is frequently capillary dilation and increased vascularization to accommodate the increased cell metabolism. The increased vascularity causes erythema. The disease can be classified according to severity as mild, moderate, or severe, depending on the size, distribution, and inflammation of the lesions. The progress of psoriasis is characterized by remissions and exacerbations. Arthritis develops in approximately 5% of individuals with psoriasis.

The typical psoriatic lesion is a well-demarcated, thick, silvery, scaly, erythematous plaque surrounded by normal skin (Fig. 41-7). Initial lesions usually develop insidiously as small erythematous papules that enlarge and coalesce into larger inflammatory lesions. The lesions are commonly located on the face, scalp, elbows, knees, and at sites of trauma. Lesions that develop in skin folds are smooth and have a deep red color. The scales are usually loosely adherent and may cause small bleeding points when removed. Five percent to 7% of

individuals with psoriasis develop psoriatic arthritis. The mechanism of disease is unknown. Genetic and immunologic mechanisms are key factors (Espinoza, Cuellar, & Silveira, 1992).

Guttate psoriasis is the development of few to many small papules appearing suddenly on the trunk and extremities (Fig. 41-8). The lesions may appear a few weeks after a streptococcal respiratory infection and, in younger individuals, reflect a tendency to develop the disease. Guttate psoriasis may resolve spontaneously in weeks or months.

Treatment is related to reducing epidermal cell turnover. Mild lesions are usually treated with emollients, keratolytic agents, and corticosteroids. Moderate lesions may respond to ultraviolet light, tar preparations, or a combination of both, and to methotrexate and etretinate. Vitamin D_3 has recently been used to reduce epidermal proliferation (Kragballe, 1992). Severe disease may require hospitalization with a combination of topical agents and systemic corticosteroids and antimetabolites such as methotrexate. Lesions of the scalp, nails, and genitalia are treated with different lotions and shampoos.

Pityriasis Rosea

Pityriasis rosea is a self-limiting inflammatory disorder that occurs more frequently in young adults, usually during the winter months. The cause is unknown but is thought to be a virus (Ramsey & Hurley, 1985). Pityri-

FIG. 41-7 **Psoriasis.** Typical oval plaque with well-defined borders and silvery scale. (From Habif, 1990.)

FIG. 41-8 **Guttate psoriasis.** Numerous uniformly small lesions may abruptly occur following streptococcal pharyngitis. (From Habif, 1990.)

FIG. 41-9 **Pityriasis rosea.** A ring of tissuelike scale (collarette scale) remains attached within the border of the plaque. (From Habif, 1990.)

FIG. 41-10 **Localized lichen planus.** Early lesions are present on the flexor surface of the wrists, a common site for localized lichen planus. (From Habif, 1990.)

asis rosea begins as a single lesion known as a **herald patch.** The patch is a circular, demarcated salmon-pink lesion approximately 3 to 4 cm in diameter and is usually located on the trunk. Early lesions are macular and papular. Secondary lesions develop within 14 to 21 days and extend over the trunk and upper part of the extremities (Fig. 41-9). Lesions are rarely located on the face. The lesions emerge as small erythematous papules that expand into characteristic oval lesions. There may be few or hundreds of lesions. The pattern of distribution follows the skin lines around the trunk and resembles a drooping pine tree. As scales flake off from the margin of the lesions, a "collarette" pattern is formed. Itching is the most common symptom. Occasionally headache, fatigue, or sore throat precedes the development of the lesions (Ginsburg, 1991).

The diagnosis of pityriasis rosea is made by the clinical appearance of the lesion. It can be confused with secondary syphilis, psoriasis, or seborrheic dermatitis. The disorder is usually self-limiting and resolves in a few months with symptomatic treatment for pruritus. Ultraviolet light or systemic corticosteroids may be used to control itching. Sun exposure facilitates resolution of the lesions.

Lichen Planus

Lichen planus is a benign, inflammatory disorder of the skin and mucous membranes. The cause is unknown, but some individuals develop lichenoid lesions after exposure to drugs or film processing chemicals. The age of onset is usually between 30 and 70 years. The disorder begins with nonscaling, violet-colored pruritic pap-

ules, 2 to 10 mm in size, usually located on the wrists, ankles, lower legs, and genitalia (Fig. 41-10). The papules are flat topped and have a polygonal shape often with a small central depression. New lesions are pale pink and evolve into a dark violet color. Persistent lesions may be thickened and red, forming hypertrophic lichen planus. The lesions often involve the oral mucous membranes, appearing as lacy white rings that must be differentiated from leukoplakia or oral candidiasis. Fine white lines can be seen throughout the oral lesions on magnification. Mucous membrane lesions also can develop on the penis and vulvovaginal area. More commonly, oral lesions do not ulcerate, but localized or extensive painful ulcerations can occur. Chronic ulcerated lesions become malignant in 1% of individuals with the disease. Thinning and splitting of nails is common and part or all of the nail may be shed.

Pruritus is the most distressing symptom. The lesions are self-limiting and may last for months or years, with an average duration of 12 to 18 months. Hyperpigmentation resulting from the inflammation is a common consequence of the lesion. Approximately 20% of individuals have a recurrence. Diagnosis is commonly made by the clinical appearance of the lesion. Antihistamines may be given for itching, and topical or systemic corticosteroids may be used to control inflammation. Mucous membrane lesions are treated with topical steroids or by injection into a single lesion.

FIG. 41-11 Rosacea. A, Pustules and erythema occur on the forehead, cheeks, and nose. **B,** Rosacea and rhinophyma. Chronic rosacea of the nose has caused irreversible hypertrophy (rhinophyma). (From Habif, 1990.)

Acne Vulgaris

Acne vulgaris is an inflammatory disorder of the pilosebaceous follicle (the sebaceous gland contiguous with a hair follicle). It occurs most commonly during adolescence. Details of this disorder are presented in Chapter 42.

Treatment of acne is directed toward the pathogenesis of the lesion, and there is no single effective treatment. Drugs, such as topical vitamin A and benzoyl peroxide, are comedolytic because they produce mild drying and peeling of the skin and facilitate a return of the normal sebum content of follicles. Benzoyl peroxide and an antibiotic (tetracycline, erythromycin, minocycline, or clindamyacin) are also effective for reducing the population of *Propionibacterium acnes*. Overactivity of sebaceous glands can be suppressed with estrogens, and oral contraceptives containing estrogens have been used to treat selected cases of acne in women. 13-Cis-retinoic acid has been used for the successful treatment of nodular cystic acne, but is contraindicated during pregnancy because of deforming effects on the fetus (Strauss, 1985). Prednisone or a single injection of a corticosteroid may be used for painful nodular cystic acne.

Acne Rosacea

Acne rosacea is an inflammation of the skin that develops in middle-aged adults. The disease is chronic with episodes of exacerbation. The most common lesions are erythema, papules, pustules, and telangiectasia. They occur in the middle third of the face, including the forehead, nose, cheeks, and chin (Fig. 41-11). The cause is unknown, but the lesions are associated with chronic flushing and sensitivity to the sun. Hypertrophy of the sebaceous glands may be severe enough to produce an irreversible bulbous appearance of the nose, known as rhinophyma. Disorders of the eye frequently accompany rosacea, particularly conjunctivitis and more rarely, keratitis. Facial application of fluorinated topical steroids may precipitate rosacealike lesions that are difficult to treat.

Hot drinks or alcohol should be taken cautiously because the heat and vasodilation accentuate erythema. Tetracycline is the drug of choice for treatment, and a low maintenance dose may be required after the most severe lesions are controlled. Surgical excision of excessive tissue may be required for rhinophyma.

Lupus Erythematosus

Lupus erythematosus is an inflammatory disease that expresses cutaneous manifestations. Discoid, or cutaneous, lupus erythematosus (DLE) is limited to the skin and can lead to systemic lupus erythematosus. (Systemic lupus erythematosus [SLE], a diffuse, multisystem disease, is discussed in Chapter 8 and on p. 1530.)

Discoid lupus erythematosus

Discoid lupus erythematosus (DLE) usually occurs in adults, but any age can be affected. It is more common in women in their late 30s or early 40s. The lesions may be single or multiple and of various size. Often the lesions are located on light-exposed areas of the skin, and photosensitivity is common. The face is the most common site of lesion involvement, with a characteristic butterfly distribution over the cheeks and bridge of the nose; however, the lesions may occur on any part of the body.

The cause is thought to be an altered immune response to an unknown antigen. Discoid lupus erythematosus may be described as a subset of SLE, with cutaneous manifestations as the only symptom (Callen, 1986) (Fig. 41-12). On skin biopsy with immunofluorescent observation, there are lumpy deposits of immunoglobulins, with IgM as the most common immunoglobulin. There are no deposits in normal skin.

The early lesion is asymmetric, with a 1 to 2 cm raised red plaque with a brownish scale. The scale penetrates the hair follicle and leaves a carpet-tack appearance when removed. The lesions persist for months and then resolve spontaneously or atrophy. Healing progresses from the center of the lesion, with a residual telangiectasia and scarring that is usually hypopigmented. Atrophy of the dermis and epidermis that results in a de-

pressed scar can occur. Scalp lesions may lead to hair loss. Other symptoms of cutaneous lupus erythematosus include alopecia (hair loss), telangiectasias, urticaria, and Raynaud phenomenon. Scarring or atrophic alopecia is a common problem of DLE. Scaling and inflammation lead to destruction of hair follicles, followed by skin that is smooth and white with telangiectasias. Hair loss is random in distribution. Telangiectasias (prominent skin capillaries) are primarily distributed over the palms and fingers in association with erythema. Urticaria of DLE may appear as typical hives but they usually stay localized, are not pruritic, and last for days. They probably result from immune complex deposition rather than an allergic response. Raynaud phenomenon with a history of episodic vasospasm of the arterioles of the fingers and toes with stress or exposure to cold often precedes the onset of DLE by several years. Raynaud phenomenon is characterized by an initial stage of vasospasm that leads to white, numb, and cold digits followed by cyanosis and then a reactive hyperemia as the vasospasm relaxes.

Diagnosis of DLE is made from the presenting symptoms, biopsy of skin lesions, and Wood tests. Individuals with DLE should use sunscreen or limit direct exposure to the sun because this precipitates an exacerbation of lesions. Initial treatment with topical steroids relieves symptoms. Systemic therapy with antimalarial drugs (i.e., chloroquine sulfate) usually leads to clinical improvement within 1 to 3 months, but these medications must be used with caution to prevent serious side effects.

Systemic lupus erythematosus

Systemic lupus erythematosus (SLE) is a chronic inflammatory immune complex disorder that may affect the skin as well as other major body organs. The disease is most common in young women. There is a strong genetic component, with altered cellular immunity resulting in tissue inflammation and injury. The cause is unknown (Arnett, 1992).

The most characteristic clinical manifestations are joint pain, fever, malaise, and diffuse facial erythema, often with a butterfly pattern. Systemic manifestations can include oral ulcers, glomerulonephritis with hypertension and nephrotic syndrome, pleurisy, pericarditis, endocarditis, lymphadenopathy, and splenomegaly. The nervous system may be involved, with polyneuropathy, seizures, and behavioral changes. Anemia and thrombocytopenia are frequently observed in individuals with SLE (Skaer, 1992).

Diagnosis of SLE is based on clinical manifestations and histopathologic findings of low complement levels, the presence of antinuclear antibodies, anti-DNA antibodies, and deposits of immunoglobulin and complement at the dermoepidermal junction.

FIG. 41-12 Chronic cutaneous LE (discoid LE). Lesions that are several months old are hypopigmented and atopic. (From Habif, 1990.)

Avoidance of sun and ultraviolet light is essential to prevent photosensitivity. Treatment of systemic manifestations depends on the degree and extent or organ system involvement. Antimalarials, salicylates, steroids, and immunosuppressive agents may be used. The disease can be controlled but is not curable.

Vesiculobullous Disorders

Vesiculobullous skin disorders represent a group of diseases that have different causes and clinical courses but share a common characteristic of vesicle, or blister, formation. Two such diseases are pemphigus and erythema multiforme.

Pemphigus

Pemphigus is a chronic blister-forming disease of the skin and oral mucous membranes. There are several different types, including **pemphigus vulgaris, pemphigus foliaceus,** and **pemphigus erythematosus.** The blisters form in the epidermis and occur more deeply in pemphigus vulgaris, with separation of the epidermis above the basal layer, and more superficially in pemphigus foliaceus and pemphigus erythematosus, with separation of the upper layer of epidermis. The disease is relatively rare and can occur in all age groups, but is more prevalent between 40 and 50 years of age.

Pemphigus is an autoimmune disease caused by circulating IgG autoantibodies. Serum autoantibodies are formed that react with the intracellular cement or substance that holds the epidermal cells together. The antibody reaction is thought to cause the intraepidermal blister formation and acantholysis (loss of cohesion between epidermal cells) characteristic of pemphigus (Eyre & Stanley, 1989).

Pemphigus vulgaris is the most common form of the disease, with the epidermis separating above the basal layer with blister formation. It usually begins with the formation of a blister in the mouth or on the scalp. Within 6 months to 1 year, flaccid bullous lesions appear that rupture easily, leaving crusty denuded skin. The lesions spread to include the face, back, chest, umbilicus, and groin. Pressure on the blister may cause it to spread to adjacent skin (Nikolsky sign). Secondary infection of the open lesions is a potentially serious complication.

Pemphigus foliaceus and **pemphigus erythematosus** are less severe forms of the disease. Oral lesions are usually absent, and erythema with crusting, scaling, and occasionally bullae develops and is more localized. Blisters that form are in the horizontal plane of the stratum corneum and rupture easily, forming crusts. Both forms of the disease can spread to become more generalized.

The diagnosis of pemphigus is made from the clinical manifestations and histologic examination of the skin.

Immunofluorescence demonstrates the presence of antibodies at the site of blister formation. The clinical course of the disease may range from rapidly fatal to relatively benign. The primary treatment for pemphigus is systemic corticosteroids, usually in high doses during acute episodes or when there is widespread involvement. Immunosuppressive therapy also may be used and decreases the steroid dosage requirement. Newer methods of treatment and a clearer understanding of the pathogenesis have improved the prognosis.

Bullous Pemphigoid

Bullous pemphigoid is a more benign disease with the presence of serum and bound IgG and blistering of the subepidermal skin layer. It occurs more commonly after 60 years of age. The lesions of pemphigoid begin with localized erythema or as pruritic plaques that extend and become edematous. The plaques turn reddish purple by 2 to 3 weeks, with vesicles and bullae emerging on the surface (Fig. 41-13). The bullae do not extend with pressure. The blisters rupture within a week and heal rapidly.

Diagnosis is by skin biopsy and immunofluorescent examination. The presence of subepidermal blistering and eosinophils distinguishes pemphigoid from pemphigus. Treatment usually includes hydroxyzine (Atarax) for itching and prednisone with an immunosuppressive drug to control blistering. Individuals who respond to treatment with sulfapyridine or dapsone do not require prednisone.

FIG. 41-13 Bullous pemphigoid. Generalized eruption with tense blisters arising from an edematous erythematous annular base. (From Habif, 1990.)

Erythema Multiforme

Erythema multiforme is an acute, often recurrent, inflammatory disorder of the skin and mucous membranes, often associated with allergic or toxic reactions to drugs or microorganisms (i.e., *Mycoplasma pneumoniae* and herpes simplex). It can occur at any age, but is more frequent between 20 and 40 years of age. Immune complex formation and deposition of C3, IgM, and fibrinogen around the superficial dermal blood vessels, basement membrane, and keratinocytes are found in most individuals with erythema multiforme. Edema develops in the superficial dermis, leading to the formation of vesicles and bullae. The lesions vary in clinical presentation and may involve the skin or mucous membranes, or both. The characteristic "bull's-eye" or "target" lesions, occur on the skin surface with a central erythematous region surrounded by concentric rings or alternating edema and inflammation. The lesions usually occur suddenly in groups over a period of 2 to 3 weeks. Urticarial plaques, 1 to 2 cm in diameter, can develop without the target lesion. A vesiculobullous form is characterized by mucous membrane lesions and erythematous plaques on the extensor surfaces of the extremities. Single or multiple vesicles or bullae may arise on a part of the plaque accompanied by pruritus and burning. The lesions heal within 3 to 4 weeks.

The most common form in children and young adults is **Stevens-Johnson syndrome** (severe bullous form), in which there are numerous erythematous bullous lesions on both the skin and mucous membranes. The cause is unknown, but an immune mechanism is probably involved (Arnold, Odom, & James, 1990, p. 135). Prodromal symptoms of fever, headache, malaise, sore throat, and cough develop in approximately one third of the cases. The bullous lesions form erosions and crusts when they rupture. The mouth, air passages, esophagus, urethra, and conjunctiva may be involved. Blindness can result from corneal ulcerations. Difficulty eating, breathing, and urinating may develop with severe manifestations. The disease can involve the kidneys and extend from the upper respiratory passages into the lungs. In rare instances, severe forms of the disease can be fatal.

Diagnosis is made by recognition of the target lesion or by skin biopsy if the target lesion is absent. Mild acute forms of the disease last 10 to 14 days. Mild forms of the disease, usually self-limiting, require no treatment. Any ongoing drug therapy should be reevaluated and underlying infections treated. Fluid and electrolyte balance should be monitored in severe forms of the disease, and mucous membranes must be carefully managed with a bland diet, warm saline eyewashes, topical anesthetics, or corticosteroids to maintain comfort and prevent infection. Cutaneous blisters can be treated with wet compresses of Burow solution. Ophthalmic, kidney,

and lung involvement requires special care. Resolution occurs in 8 to 10 days, usually without scarring. Mucosal lesions may take 6 weeks to heal.

Infections

Cutaneous infections are common forms of skin disease. The infections generally remain localized; however, serious complications can develop with systemic involvement. The types of skin infection include bacterial, viral, and fungal. Most infections occur superficially; however, systemic signs and symptoms occasionally develop and rarely are life threatening. The normal flora of the skin consists of aerobes, yeast, and anaerobes. These flora often provide protection against pathogens that cause skin infections, including *Staphylococcus* and *Streptococcus* (Singh, Marples, & Klingman, 1971).

Bacterial Infections

Most bacterial infections of the skin are caused by local invasion of pathogens. Coagulase-positive *S. aureus* and, less frequently, β-hemolytic streptococci are the common causative organisms.

Folliculitis

Folliculitis is a bacterial infection of the hair follicle. *Staphylococcus aureus* is the common causative organism. The infection develops from proliferation of the organism around the opening of the follicle with spread into the follicle. Inflammation is caused by the release of chemotactic factors and enzymes from the bacteria. The lesions appear as pustules with a surrounding area of erythema. They are most prominent on the scalp and extremities and rarely cause systemic symptoms. Prolonged skin moisture, skin trauma, and poor hygiene are associated contributing factors to the development of folliculitis. Cleaning with soap and water and topical application of antibiotics are effective forms of treatment.

Furuncles and carbuncles

Furuncles, or "boils," are an inflammation of the hair follicles. They may develop from a preceding folliculitis with spread through the follicular wall into the surrounding dermis. The invading organism is usually *S. aureus.* The infecting strain may spread to the skin from the anterior nares. Any skin area with hair can be infected, and one or several lesions may be present. The precipitating events are similar to folliculitis. The initial lesion is a deep, firm, red, painful nodule 1 to 5 cm in diameter. Within a few days, the initial erythematous nodules change to a large fluctuant and tender cystic nodule that may be accompanied by cellulitis. No systemic symptoms are present, and the lesion may drain large amounts of pus and necrotic tissue.

Carbuncles are a collection of infected hair follicles. The lesion occurs most frequently on the back of the neck, the upper back, and the lateral thighs. The lesion begins in the subcutaneous tissue and lower dermis as a firm mass that evolves into an erythematous, painful, swollen mass that drains through many openings. Abscesses may develop. Chills, fever, and malaise are systemic symptoms that can occur during the early stages of lesion development.

Furuncles and carbuncles are treated with warm compresses to provide comfort and promote localization and spontaneous drainage. Abscess formation requires incision and drainage, and recurrent infections are treated with systemic antibiotics.

Cellulitis

Cellulitis is an infection of the dermis and subcutaneous tissue usually caused by *Staphylococcus*. Cellulitis can occur as an extension of a skin wound, an ulcer, or from furuncles or carbuncles. The infected area is erythematous, swollen, and painful. The infection responds to systemic antibiotics, and Burow soaks can be used to relieve pain.

Erysipelas

Erysipelas is an acute superficial infection of the skin most often caused by group A streptococci. The face, ears, and lower legs are common sites of involvement, and the site of initial infection may not be identified. Chills, fever, and malaise precede the onset of lesions by 4 hours to 20 days. The initial lesions appear as firm, red spots that then enlarge and coalesce to form a clearly circumscribed, advancing, bright red, hot lesion with a raised border. Vesicles may appear over the lesion and at the border. Itching, burning, and tenderness accompany the development of the lesion. Cold compresses provide symptomatic relief, and systemic antibiotics are required to arrest the infection.

Impetigo

Impetigo is a superficial lesion of the skin caused by coagulase-positive *Staphylococcus* or β-hemolytic streptococci. The disease occurs in adults, but is more common in children (see Chapter 42).

Viral Infections
Herpes simplex virus

There are six types of **herpes simplex virus (HSV)**, HSV-1 (type 1), HSV-2 (type 2), cytomegalovirus (CMV), varicella-zoster virus, Epstein-Barr virus, and human herpes virus 6 (HHV-6) (Wahren & Linde, 1991). A "cold sore" or "fever blister" is a type of HSV-1 infection and is the most common manifestation of the herpes simplex virus (Crumpacker, 1987). Herpes simplex virus-1 usually occurs in nongenital sites

and causes infection of the cornea (herpes keratitis), mouth (gingivostomatitis), and labia (labialis). Individuals receiving cytotoxic therapy for cancer are at risk. Genital infections are more commonly caused by HSV-2. The virus is spread by contact of the virus with the skin, and there is a high risk of infection after sexual contact with infected individuals. After penetrating the skin, HSV is established in the sensory nerve ganglion innervating the primary site. Infection in one area does not protect the other areas from subsequent infection. The primary infection is asymptomatic and can only be determined by a rising antibody titer (Mindel, 1991).

The incubation period ranges from 2 to 14 days, and clinical symptoms last from 1 to 3 weeks. An individual then continues to shed the virus for 2 to 6 weeks. The virus remains dormant within sensory or autonomic nerve ganglia and can lead to recurrence of the disease. A number of factors stimulate recurrence, including sun exposure, fever, or stress, and lesions are usually located at or near the primary site. Because anti-HSV antibodies develop in response to infection, recurrence is also related to the titer or amount of antibodies present.

The lesions of HSV-1 appear as a rash or clusters of inflamed and painful vesicles within the mouth, over the tongue, or on the lips and around the nose (Fig. 41-14). Increased sensitivity, paresthesias, and mild burning may occur before onset of the lesion. The vesicles rupture forming a crust. Lesions may last for 2 to 6 weeks. Occasionally, there is an associated upper respiratory infection. Treatment is symptomatic, and the lesions usually resolve within 2 weeks.

Genital herpes (HSV-2) may also occur in primary or recurrent forms and a large number of infections are sexually transmitted, usually within 3 to 14 days after exposure (see Chapter 21). The lesions begin as small vesicles that progress to ulceration within 3 to 4 days with pain, itching, and weeping. Treatment includes oral or topical administration of acyclovir, an antiviral drug that decreases new lesion formation and promotes healing.

Herpes zoster and varicella

Herpes zoster (shingles) and **varicella** (chickenpox) are caused by the same herpesvirus, varicella-zoster virus (VZV). Varicella occurs as a primary infection followed years later by herpes zoster. Chickenpox usually occurs in children (see Chapter 42).

Herpes zoster, or shingles, has initial symptoms of pain and paresthesia localized to the affected dermatome (the cutaneous area innervated by a single spinal nerve; see Chapter 12), followed by vesicular eruptions that follow along a facial, cervical, or thoracic lumbar dermatome (Fig. 41-15). Some individuals have vesicles scattered outside the area of the dermatome. Lo-

FIG. 41-14 **Herpes simplex labialis.** Typical presentation with tense vesicles appearing on the lips and extending onto the skin. (From Habif, 1990.)

FIG. 41-15 **Herpes zoster.** Diffuse involvement of a dermatome in a 13-year-old boy. (From Habif, 1990.)

cal symptoms are alleviated with compresses, calamine lotion, or baking soda. Antiviral drugs (vidarabine and acyclovir) have provided useful treatment (Gurevich, 1992). Approximately 20% of individuals experience postherpetic neuralgia (Ragozzino, Melton, Kurland, Chu, & Perry, 1982).

Warts

Warts (verrucae) are benign lesions of the skin caused by the human papillomavirus (HPV). There are many different types of HPV, and specific viruses are associated with specific kinds and locations of lesions. The lesions are round and elevated with a rough, grayish surface, and they can occur anywhere on the skin. Warts are transmitted by touch. Common warts (verruca vulgaris) occur most frequently in children and are usually on the fingers, although they may be located on any skin surface or mucous membrane. Warts vary in shape, size (flat, round, or fusiform), and location. Plantar warts are usually located at pressure points on the bottom of the feet (Fig. 41-16).

Condylomata acuminata (venereal warts) are cauliflower-like lesions that occur in moist areas, along the glans of the penis, vulva, and anus (see Chapter 21). Epidermodysplasia verruciformis is a rare condition and is associated with warts all over the body.

Diagnosis of warts is by visualization. Treatment considers age of the individual and size and location of the lesion. Warts can be removed by freezing with liquid nitrogen, electrocautery, vaporization with lasers, application of keratolytics, or application of irritants and corrosives, such as salicylic acid, formaldehyde, interferons, or saturated solution of potassium iodide (Browder, Avaujo, Meyer, & Flowers, 1992). Many warts resolve spontaneously.

Fungal Infections

The fungi causing superficial skin infections are called dermatophytes, and they thrive on keratin (stratum corneum, hair, and nails). Fungal disorders are known as mycoses; when caused by dermatophytes, the mycoses are termed tinea (dermatophytosis or ringworm). **Tinea pedis** is a chronic, superficial fungal infection of the skin of the foot common in adults (Fig. 41-17). In prepubertal children most scaling disorders of the toes and feet are eczema. **Tinea corporis** (ringworm) and **tinea capitis** (a fungal infection of the scalp) are much more common in children than adults. (See Chapter 42 for a discussion of fungal infections in children.)

Tinea infections

Tinea infections are fungal infections of the skin and are classified according to their location on the body. The most common sites are summarized in Table 41-5.

FIG. 41-16 **Verruca plantaris.** Corns (clavi) on the plantar surface are frequently mistaken for warts. (From Habif, 1990.)

FIG. 41-17 **Tinea pedis (toe web infection).** The toe web space contains macerated scale. Inflammation has extended from the web area onto the dorsum of the foot. (From Habif, 1990.)

These infestations are common in children (see Chapter 42). Tinea is diagnosed by culture, microscopic examination of skin scrapings prepared with potassium hydroxide wet mount, or observation of the skin with an ultraviolet light (Wood's lamp). Cultures establish the particular type of fungus and are necessary for hair and nail infections. Fungi have characteristic spores and filaments known as **hyphae** that are more prominent when prepared in potassium hydroxide. The spores fluoresce blue-green when exposed to ultraviolet light. Treatment is related to the type of fungi and includes both topical and systemic antifungal medication.

TABLE 41-5

Common Sites of Tinea Infections

Site	Clinical manifestations
Tinea capitis (scalp)	Scaly, pruritic scalp with bald areas; hair breaks easily
Tinea corporis (skin areas, excluding scalp, face, hands, feet, groin)	Circular, clearly circumscribed, mildly erythematous scaly patches with a slightly elevated ringlike border; some forms are dry and macular, and other forms are moist and vesicular
Tinea cruris (groin, also known as "jock itch")	Small erythematous and scaling vesicular patches with a well-defined border that spreads over the inner and upper surfaces of the thighs; occurs with heat and high humidity
Tinea pedis (foot, also known as "athlete's foot")	Occurs between the toes and may spread to the soles of feet, nails, and skin of toes; slight scaling, macerated painful skin, occasionally with fissures and vesiculation
Tinea manus (hand)	Dry, scaly, erythematous lesions, or moist vesicular lesions that begin with clusters of intensely itching, clear vesicles; often associated with fungal infection of the feet
Tinea unguium or onychomycosis (nails)	A superficial or deep inflammation of the nail that develops yellow-brown accumulations of brittle keratin over all or portions of the nail.

TABLE 41-6

Sites of Candidiasis

	Risk factors	Clinical manifestations	Treatment
Vagina (vulvovaginitis)	Heat, moisture, occlusive clothing Pregnancy Systemic antibiotic therapy Diabetes mellitus Sexual intercourse with infected male	Vaginal itching; white, watery, or creamy discharge Red and swollen vaginal and labial membranes with erosions Lesions may spread to anus and groin	Miconazole cream Clotrimazole tablets or cream Nystatin tablets Ketoconazole cream Loose cotton clothing
Penis (balanitis)	Uncircumcised Sexual intercourse with infected female	Pinpoint red, tender papules and pustules on glans and shaft of penis	Any of creams listed above Topical steroids for severe inflammation
Mouth	Diabetes mellitus Immunosuppressive therapy Inhaled steroids	Red, swollen, painful tongue and oral mucous membranes Localized erosions and plaques appear with chronic infection	Nystatin oral suspension Clotrimazole troches Ketoconazole

Candidiasis

Candidiasis is caused by the yeastlike fungus *Candida albicans* and can normally be found on mucous membranes, on the skin, in the gastrointestinal tract, and in the vagina. *C. albicans* can, under certain circumstances, change from a commensal organism to a pathogen, particularly when the immune system is depressed. Among those factors that predispose to infection are (1) local environment of moisture, warmth, maceration, or occlusion; (2) the systemic administration of antibiotics; (3) pregnancy; (4) diabetes mellitus; (5) Cushing disease; (6) debilitated states; (7) infants younger than 6 months of age, as a result of decreased immune reactivity; (8) immunosuppressed persons; and (9) certain neoplastic diseases of the blood and monocyte/macrophage system. The resident bacteria on the skin, mainly cocci, inhibit proliferation of *C. albicans*. Cell-mediated immunity plays a major role in the defense against monilial infections. *C. albicans* can activate the complement system by the alternative pathway and include small abscesses. Candidiasis affects only the outer layers of mucous membranes and skin and occurs in the mouth, vagina, uncircumcised penis, and large skin folds. Table 41-6 lists the differentiation of different sites of candidiasis.

The initial lesion is a thin-walled pustule that extends under the stratum corneum with an inflammatory base that may burn or itch. The accumulation of inflammatory cells and scale produces a whitish yellow curdlike substance over the infected area. The lesion ceases to spread when reaching dry skin (Levitz, 1992).

Vascular Disorders

Vascular abnormalities are commonly associated with skin diseases, or they may be present as congenital vascular malformations (see Chapter 42), or as vascular responses to local or systemic vasoactive substances. Blood vessels may increase in number, dilate, constrict, or become obliterated by disease processes.

Cutaneous Vasculitis

Vasculitis (angiitis) is an inflammation of the blood vessels. The initiating site of inflammation may be the blood, the vessel wall, or the adjacent tissue. Small vessels are usually affected. Immune complexes, which initiate an uncontrolled inflammatory response, are often the cause of damage, and the lesions are often polymorphic.

Cutaneous vasculitis develops from the deposit of immune complexes in small blood vessels as a toxic response to drugs (phenothiazines, barbiturates, and sulfonamides) or allergens, or as a response to streptococcal or viral infection. The precise mechanism is not known, but the deposit of immune complex activates complement, which is chemotactic for polymorphonuclear leukocytes. The cutaneous form usually resolves in a few weeks and is treated with steroids.

The disorder is also known as allergic vasculitis and occurs primarily in adults. A systemic form (cutaneous systemic vasculitis) can involve other organs, including the kidneys, lungs, and gastrointestinal tract. The extremities are the chief sites, primarily the lower legs and feet. The lesions appear as palpable purpura (from the leakage of blood from damaged vessels) and progress to hemorrhagic bullae with necrosis and ulceration from occlusion of the vessel. Lesions appear in clusters and remain from 1 to 4 weeks. Recurrences are common. Biopsy may disclose the presence of complement or immunoglobulins in the vessel walls.

Identifying and removing the antigen (chemical, drug, or source of infection) is the first step of treatment. Prednisone may be used when symptoms are severe.

Urticaria

Urticarial lesions are most commonly associated with type 1 hypersensitivity reactions to drugs (penicillin, aspirin), certain foods (strawberries, shellfish), systemic diseases (intestinal parasites, lupus erythematosus), or physical agents (heat or cold) (see Chapter 8). The lesions are mediated by histamine release, which causes the endothelial cells of skin blood vessels to contract. The leak of fluid from the vessel appears as wheals, welts, or hives and may be few or many and distributed over the entire body. Most lesions resolve spontaneously within 24 hours, but new lesions may appear. All possible causes should be removed. Antihistamines usually reduce hives and provide relief of itching. Corticosteroids may be required for treatment of severe attacks.

Scleroderma

Scleroderma means sclerosis of the skin, and the cause is unknown. The disease is more prominent in women. Scleroderma may affect the visceral organs or remain localized to the skin. Systemic scleroderma involves the connective tissues of many organs, including the kidney, gastrointestinal tract, and lungs. Only a few organs are involved in some individuals. The cutaneous lesions are most often on the face and hands, the neck, and the upper chest. The entire skin can be involved, however.

The disease is characterized by massive deposits of collagen with fibrosis, accompanied by inflammatory reactions, vascular changes in the capillary network with a decrease in the number of capillary loops, and dilation of the remaining capillaries (Perez & Kohn, 1993). Fibrosis occurs in the papillary and reticular dermis and in the subcutaneous tissue and deep fascia. Autoimmunity and an immune reaction to a toxic substance are both possible initiating mechanisms of the disease,

FIG. 41-18 Scleroderma (acrosclerosis). Fingertips are narrowed and the fingers are shortened as a result of distal bone resorption. (From Habif, 1990.)

and autoantibodies are often recovered from the skin and serum of individuals with scleroderma (Rothfield, 1992).

The skin is hard, hypopigmented, taut, shiny, and tightly connected to the underlying tissue. The tightness of the facial skin projects an immobile masklike appearance, and the mouth may not open completely. The nose may assume a beaklike appearance. The hands are shiny and sometimes red and edematous. The fingers become tapered and flexed, often with depressed scars and loss of fingertips from atrophy. Raynaud phenomenon with episodic arteriolar vasoconstriction of the fingers contributes to ulcer formation. The nails may be shed (Fig. 41-18). Calcium deposits develop in the subcutaneous tissue and erupt through the skin. Progression to body organs may occur, and death is caused by subsequent respiratory failure, renal failure, cardiac dysrhythmias, or esophageal or intestinal obstruction or perforation. There is no specific treatment, and progression of the disease is variable. Fifty percent of individuals die within 5 years from onset of scleroderma.

Suitable clothing and warm environment are essential to protecting the hands. Trauma and smoking should be avoided. Vasodilator drugs or sympathectomy rarely has lasting effects. Symptomatic treatment is required for involved organs (i.e., intestinal resection for obstruction, antibiotics for pneumonitis, and regulation of hypertension) (LeRoy, 1992).

Insect Bites
Ticks

Ticks are significant vectors of transmitted diseases, including Rocky Mountain spotted fever and other rickettsial diseases, tularemia, and Lyme disease. Ticks vary in size from 1 cm to about the size of a comma on this printed page. They embed their heads in the skin to obtain blood. As they gorge themselves on blood, they enlarge to many times their normal size and may release toxins or transmit microorganisms during feeding. In most instances, there is no consequence from a tick bite, with the exception of a papular urticaria at the site of the bite. If mouth parts remain in the skin when the tick is removed, a persistent nodule remains that may require excision; the tick should be removed completely intact. Irritant substances, such as camphor, gasoline, soft wax, or heat from a match, may stimulate the tick to withdraw its head. Applying tick repellant, such as diethyltoluamide (DEET), butopyronoxyl (Indalone), or benzylbenzoate, helps to prevent tick bites.

Lyme disease is a multisystem inflammatory disease caused by *Borrelia burgdorferi* transmitted by tick bites. The highest incidence is among children, and 50% of infected individuals are symptom free. Symptoms of the disease occur in stages. Soon after the bite, there is localized infection (erythema migrans with or without flu-like illness). Approximately 9 months after the onset of the illness, there is disseminated infection (secondary erythema migrans, arthralgias, meningitis, neuritis, and carditis). Late persistent infection can continue for years (arthritis, encephalopathy, and polyneuropathy). The microorganism is difficult to culture.

The diagnosis of Lyme disease is based on the clinical presentation and history of tick bite, if known. Serologic tests may be confirming of the diagnosis. Antibiotics are used for treatment (Cooper & Schoen, 1992; Sigal, 1992).

Mosquitoes and Flies

There are thousands of species of **mosquitoes** throughout the world. Species from the Culicada family are responsible for malaria, yellow fever, dengue fever, filariasis, and St. Louis encephalitis. Mosquitoes can bite through thin, loose clothing and are attracted by warmth and sweat. The edema, pruritus, and papular lesions of the mosquito bite are caused by the disruption of the skin from the insertion of a blood tube by a female mosquito. Irritating salivary secretions also contain anticoagulants. Reactions vary depending on the sensitivity of the victim.

Several species of flies are blood suckers. The black fly (Simuliidae) is usually found in swarms, near moving bodies of water in the late spring and early summer, and is a vicious biter. The initial bite is painless because the fly injects an anesthetic with the bite.

The subsequent lesions are painful and accompanied by significant swelling of surrounding tissues. Systemic reactions, such as fever, headache, and nausea, are common.

Very small flies of the Ceratopogonidae family, also known as "no-see-ums," "midges," "punkies," or sand fleas, are also blood suckers. The bite of the female is particularly miserable and produces immediate pain, erythema, and vesicles. Itching and vesicular reactions may persist for weeks.

The fiercest bloodsucking flies are the Tabanidae, or horseflies, deerflies, gadflies, greenheads, and clegs. These flies vary in size from 1 to 5 cm and produce painful, bleeding bites because of their large mouth parts. The bites produce urticaria that may be accompanied by weakness, dizziness, and wheezing.

Wounds produced by biting insects should be cleansed with soap and water and a local antiseptic should be applied. Local applications of steroid creams or antihistamine will reduce symptoms. Systemic reactions may require more specific medical care.

Benign Tumors

Most benign tumors of the skin are associated with aging. Benign tumors include seborrheic keratosis, keratoacanthoma, actinic keratosis, and moles.

Seborrheic Keratosis

Seborrheic keratosis is a benign proliferation of basal cells that produces elevated lesions that may be smooth or warty in appearance. They are usually seen in older people and occur as multiple lesions on the chest, back, and face. The color varies from tan to waxy yellow, flesh-colored, or dark brown-black. Lesion size varies from a few millimeters to several centimeters, and they are often oval and greasy appearing with a hyperkeratotic scale (Fig. 41-19). Cryotherapy with liquid nitrogen is effective treatment, and the lesions usually slough 2 to 3 weeks after treatment.

Keratoacanthoma

A keratoacanthoma is a benign, self-limiting tumor that arises from hair follicles. It usually occurs on sun-exposed surfaces and develops between 60 and 65 years of age. The most commonly affected sites are the face, back of the hands, forearms, neck, and legs. The lesion develops in stages. The proliferative stage produces a rapid growing dome-shaped nodule with a central crust. In the mature stage, the lesion is filled with whitish-colored keratin (Fig. 41-20). The involution stage usually occurs over a 3- to 4-month period with regression of the lesion. The mature lesion requires differentiation from squamous cell carcinoma. Although the lesions will resolve spontaneously, they can be removed by curettage or excision to improve cosmetic appearance.

FIG. 41-19 Seborrheic keratosis. Typical distal extremity lesion that is broad, flat, and comparatively smooth surfaced. (From Habif, T. P. [1985]. *Clinical dermatology: A color guide to diagnosis and treatment.* St. Louis: Mosby–Year Book.)

FIG. 41-20 Keratoacanthoma. Classic presentation of a fully developed tumor. Round smooth dome-shaped mass with a central keratin-filled crater. (From Habif, 1990.)

Actinic Keratosis

Actinic keratosis is a premalignant lesion found on skin surfaces exposed to the ultraviolet radiation of the sun. The prevalence is highest in individuals with unprotected, light-colored skin. Actinic keratosis is rare in

FIG. 41-21 **Nodular basal cell carcinoma.** Center has ulcerated and is covered with a crust. (From Habif, 1990.)

FIG. 41-22 **Squamous cell carcinoma.** The sun-exposed lower lip is a common site for squamous cell carcinoma. (From Habif, 1990.)

black skin. The lesions appear as pigmented patches of rough, adherent scale. Surrounding areas may have telangiectasias. Freezing with liquid nitrogen provides quick, effective treatment. Excisions also may be performed, providing tissue for cellular analysis. The lesions should continue to be evaluated for progression to squamous cell carcinoma. Protection from the sun with clothing or a sun-blocking agent to prevent lesions from developing elsewhere is advised.

Nevi (Moles)

Nevi are pigmented or nonpigmented lesions that form from melanocytes beginning at ages 3 to 5 years. During the early stages of development, the cells accumulate at the junction of the dermis and epidermis and are macular lesions. Over time the cells move down into the dermis and the nevi become nodular and palpable. Nevi may appear on any part of the skin and they vary in size. They occur singly or in groups and are not disfiguring. Nevi may undergo transition to malignant melanoma (see p. 1542). Nevi irritated by clothing can be excised.

Cancer

Because many cancerous skin lesions are treated and not reported, statistics on the incidence of skin cancer are difficult to obtain. It is estimated that skin cancers are the most prevalent form of cancer and nearly all persons living beyond age 65 will have had at least one skin cancer. The most common types of skin cancer are basal cell carcinoma and squamous cell carcinoma. These carcinomas are 50% greater in men than in women, and incidence increases steadily with age. Malignant melanoma is the most serious skin cancer, affecting 27,000 people per year, and is increasing at a rate of 3.4% per year (American Cancer Society [ACS], 1993). An estimated 8200 people die of skin cancer each year, 6800 from malignant melanoma (ACS, 1993).

Solar radiation causes most skin cancers (Ananthaswamy & Pierceall, 1992). Protection from the sun during the first 10 to 20 years of life significantly reduces the risk of skin cancer (Truhan, 1991). Areas widely exposed to the sun's rays—the face, neck, and hands—are highly vulnerable for such lesions. Outdoor workers (farmers, sailors, fishermen) are high-risk skin cancer populations. For other risk factors, refer to the box on p. 1541.

Basal Cell Carcinoma

Basal cell carcinoma is a surface epithelial tumor of the skin originating from undifferentiated basal or germinative cells. The tumors grow upward and laterally or downward to the dermal epidermal junction (Fig. 41-21). They usually have depressed centers and rolled borders. Early tumors are so small they are not clinically apparent. Generally, these tumors do not invade blood or lymph vessels; thus, they do not metastasize beyond the skin. Basal cell carcinoma can cause severe local destruction, however.

Basal cell carcinoma, as the most common type of skin cancer, is thought to be caused by sunlight exposure (Urbach, 1991). These lesions are seen most frequently in regions with intense sunlight and on those areas most exposed, the face and neck. Dark-skinned persons and those avoiding sunlight are significantly less prone to develop these malignant tumors. In dark-skinned persons, basal cells contain the pigment melanin, a protective factor against sun exposure. Whereas ultraviolet radiation seems to be the primary causative agent, other factors are implicated: arsenic and genetic factors. The use of arsenic in insecticides has recently diminished; however, arsenic is found in drinking water from ground wells. Genetic factors are displayed in the less common nevoid basal cell carcinoma syndrome.

These tumors arise in consequence to a defect that prevents the cells from being shed by the normal keratinization process. The maturing process of epidermal cells is called keratinization; however, the process of keratinization specifically means the synthesis of fibrous protein or keratin. Basal cell tumors lack the normal keratin proteins; however, this may be reversible. Transplantation of basal cell and in vitro cultures shows the property of keratinization can be restored.

The growth rate for these tumors is quite slow. The lesion starts as a nodule (greater than 5 mm across) "pearly" or "ivory" in appearance, slightly elevated above the skin surface with small blood vessels on the surface. As the lesion grows, it often ulcerates, develops crusting, and is firm to the touch. If left untreated, basal cell lesions invade surrounding tissues and, over months or years, can destroy a nose, eyelid, or an ear (for treatment, see the box at right).

Squamous Cell Carcinoma

Squamous cell carcinoma is a tumor of the epidermis characterized by two types: in situ and invasive. Because of the invasive nature of some tumors, squamous cell carcinoma is significantly more malignant if left untreated (Kwa, Campagna, & Moy, 1992).

Both epidemiologic and experimental approaches have demonstrated sunlight as a cause of squamous cell carcinoma. Areas affected are the head and neck (75%), and the hands (15%), with 10% elsewhere on the body. In countries where arsenic is higher in drinking water, these tumors are more predominant. X-rays and gamma rays are also associated with squamous cell carcinoma. Patients who are immunosuppressed also experience a greater occurrence.

The exact mechanism for producing squamous cell carcinoma is unknown. Again, the initiator-promoter model can be applied to conceptually understand the cancer process (see Chapter 11). It is unclear whether ultraviolet light produces its harmful effects because of problems in DNA, synthesis, repair, or replication.

IMPORTANT TRENDS FOR SKIN CANCER

Incidence

Approximately 500,000 cases a year with the majority being the highly curable **basal** or **squamous** cell cancers; not as common is the most serious **malignant melanoma** with an estimated 27,000 cases a year

Mortality

Total estimated deaths in 1993 were 8200; 6800 from malignant melanoma, 2000 from other skin cancers

Risk factors

Excessive exposure to ultraviolet radiation from the sun; fair complexion; occupational exposure to coal tar, pitch, creosote, arsenic compounds, and radium; skin cancer is negligible in blacks because of heavy skin pigmentation

Warning signals

Any unusual skin condition, especially a change in the size or color of a mole or other darkly pigmented growth or spot

Prevention and early detection

Avoidance of sun when ultraviolet light is strongest (e.g., 10:00 A.M. and 3:00 P.M.); use sunscreen preparations, especially those containing ingredients such as PABA (para-aminobenzoic acid); basal and squamous cell skin cancers often form a pale, waxlike, pearly nodule, or a red, scaly, sharply outlined patch; melanomas are usually dark brown or black pigmentation; they start as small molelike growths that increase in size, change color, become ulcerated, and bleed easily from a slight injury

Treatment

There are four methods of treatment: surgery, electrodesiccation (tissue destruction by heat), radiation therapy, or cryosurgery (tissue destruction by freezing); for malignant melanomas, wide and often deep excisions and removal of nearby lymph nodes are required

Survival

For basal cell and squamous cell cancers, cure is virtually assured with early detection and treatment; malignant melanoma, however, metastasizes quickly; this accounts for a lower 5-year survival rate for white patients with this disease

Invasive squamous cell carcinoma can arise from premalignant lesions of the skin. It rarely arises from normal appearing skin or "de novo." The premalignant lesions include sun-damaged skin or dysplasias (actinic dermatitis); leukoplakia, or whitish discolored areas; scars; radiation-induced keratosis; tar and oil keratosis; and chronic ulcers and sinuses. The invasive type grows more rapidly than basal cell carcinomas and can spread to regional lymph nodes. These tumors are firm and increase in both elevation and diameter. The surface may be granular and bleed easily (Fig. 41-22).

In situ squamous cell carcinoma is usually confined to the epidermis (intraepidermal) but may extend into the dermis. Common premalignant skin lesions associated with in situ squamous cell carcinomas are actinic (solar) keratosis and Bowen disease. Actinic keratosis is a white, scaly, keratotic (horny) lesion on the exposed areas of the body. Bowen disease is a dysplasia of the basal layer of the dermis or carcinoma in situ. It often is found on unexposed areas of the body and is demonstrated by flat, reddish, scaly patches. These lesions may enlarge to more than a centimeter in diameter, rarely invading surrounding tissue and almost never metastasizing. Other cellular components in the skin (sweat glands, hair follicles, etc.) can give rise to skin cancer, but these are relatively uncommon.

Malignant Melanoma

Melanoma is a malignant tumor of the skin originating from melanocytes, or cells that synthesize the pigment melanin. Epidemiologists report the incidence of melanoma is doubling every 10 to 20 years (Bellet, Mastrangelo, & Maguire, 1983). Early recognition of cutaneous melanomas can have a major impact on surgically curing this disease.

Causative factors implicated in melanoma induction include genetic predisposition, solar radiation, and steroid hormone activity. There is strong evidence that sunlight is an important promotional factor. Melanomas arise as a result of malignant degeneration of melanocytes located either along the basal layer of the epidermis or in a benign melanocytic nevus. A nevus, or mole, is an aggregation of melanocytes (Fig. 41-23). These clusters of cells may not be apparent until puberty, when the pigmentation process is initiated by steroid hormones. The relationship between nevi and melanoma makes it important for the clinician to understand the various neval forms (Table 41-7). Most nevi never become suspicious; however, suspicious pigmented nevi need removal (Lober, 1992). Indications for biopsy include color change, size change, irregular notched margin, itching, bleeding or oozing, nodularity, scab formation, and ulceration. The clinical varieties of cutaneous melanoma include lentigo malignant melanoma (LMM) (Fig. 41-24), superficial spreading melanoma (SSM) (Fig. 41-25), and primary nodular melanoma (PNM). Clinical characteristics are summarized in the box on p. 1543.

Treatment of melanoma with no evidence of metastatic disease involves surgical excision to the primary lesion site and regional lymph nodes. The extent of surgery is determined by the staging of disease. Lesions of the extremities have the best prognosis, next head and neck lesions, and trunk lesions the poorest. Only 20% to 40% of patients with regional lymph node involvement are alive and cured at 5 years.

Kaposi Sarcoma

Kaposi sarcoma (KS) is a vascular malignancy with different types of presentation. It is associated with immune deficiency states and occurs among kidney transplant recipients taking immunosuppressive drugs. A rapidly progressive form of KS appears with acquired immune deficiency syndrome (AIDS) (see Chapter 21). Kaposi sarcoma is also common among middle-aged, black males in equatorial Africa and those of Mediter-

TABLE 41-7

Classification of Nevi

Type	Common characteristics
Junctional nevus	Flat, well-circumscribed, vary in size up to 2 cm, dark color, hairs may be present; originate in basal layer of epidermis and can eventually reach the cutaneous surface; most likely to develop into a melanoma
Compound nevus	Most common in adolescents and are the majority of pigmented lesions in children; rarely does this lesion develop to melanoma; usually 1 cm in size; hairs may be present; surface is elevated and smooth
Intradermal nevus	Small, less than 1 cm, with regular edges and bristle-like hairs; color ranges from skin tone to light brown; has a slight likelihood of developing into a melanoma

FIG. 41-23 Nevi. **A,** Junctional nevus. Color and shape of this black lesion are uniform. **B,** Dermal nevus. Dome shaped. (From Habif, 1990.)

CLINICAL CHARACTERISTICS OF VARIETIES OF CUTANEOUS MELANOMA

Lentigo malignant melanoma

Frequency	10% to 15% of cutaneous melanomas
Age at diagnosis	50 to 80 years old
Primary location	Head, neck, dorsum of hands
Pigmentation according to thickness	
<1.5 mm (levels I and II)	Tan and brown
>1.5 mm (level III)	Tan, brown, and blue-black
>1.5 mm (levels IV and V)	Nodule formation

Superficial spreading melanomas

Frequency	70% of cutaneous melanomas
Age at diagnosis	20 to 60 years old
Primary location	Legs of females; upper back of both sexes
Pigmentation according to thickness	
<1.5 mm (levels I and II)	Tan and brown
>1.5 mm (levels III)	Tan, brown, and blue-black
>1.5 mm (levels IV and V)	Nodule formation

Nodular melanoma

Frequency	12% of cutaneous melanomas
Age at diagnosis	20 to 60 years old
Primary location	No specific site preference
Pigmentation according to thickness	
>1.5 mm (level III)	Small nodule (any hue)
>1.5 mm (levels IV and V)	Large nodule (any hue)

FIG. 41-24 **Lentigo malignant melanoma.** (From Habif, 1990.)

FIG. 41-25 **Superficial spreading melanoma.** (From Habif, 1990.)

ranean or Jewish descent. Two forms of the disease have been described, classic and epidemic (Safai, 1987). Individuals with AIDS are immunosuppressed, and this allows for opportunistic infection and malignancy. Proliferation of the tumor is dependent on the presence of platelet-derived growth factors (Sturzl et al., 1992).

The human immunodeficiency virus and cytomegalovirus have been proposed as cofactors in the development of KS (Goopman, 1987). The endothelial cell is thought to be the progenitor of KS. The lesions emerge as purplish brown macules and develop into plaques and nodules. They tend to be multifocal rather than spreading by metastasis. The lesions initially appear over the lower extremities in the classic form (Fig. 41-26). The rapidly progressive form associated with AIDS tends to spread symmetrically over the upper body, particularly the face and oral mucosa. The lesions are often pruritic and painful. About 75% of individuals with epidemic KS have involvement of lymph nodes, particularly in the gastrointestinal tract and lungs. Organ involvement is much less common in the classic form. The rapidly progressive form has a poor prognosis and shorter survival rates than the classic form. (See Chapter 21 for further discussion on AIDS.)

Diagnosis is by skin biopsy with a high index of suspicion for those with immune deficiency. Local lesions can be excised. Multiple disseminated lesions may be treated with a combination of α-interferon, radiotherapy, and cytotoxic drugs. Clinical trials for new treatments are in progress. General response to treatment is poor, but a 2-year survival rate is better in individuals with KS alone than in those with KS and an opportunistic infection.

Thermal Injury

It is estimated that about 2 million people are burned in the United States each year (Collins, 1988). Results of an American Burn Association Annual Burn Facility Survey (1991) estimate 60,000 people are hospitalized annually with burn injury. Most significant burns oc-

cur in the home, and the highest percentage of deaths (75%) are from home fires, usually in the kitchen (Hall, 1987).

Burns

Burns may be caused by thermal, chemical, or electrical injury. Thermal injuries result from exposure to direct flames, hot liquids, or radiation. Direct contact, inhalation, and ingestion of acids, alkalies, or blistering agents cause chemical burns. Electrical burns occur with the passage of electrical current through the body to the ground. Associated electrical flames or flashes also can burn the skin.

The physiologic consequences of major **thermal injury** center around the profound, life-threatening hypovolemic shock that occurs in conjunction with cellular and immunologic disruption within a few minutes of the injury. In contrast, the effects of minor and moderate burn injuries are limited to localized skin destruction. Individuals with minor and moderate burn injuries experience discomfort until healing or skin grafting is accomplished, but these burns are not life threatening. With a major burn injury, a systemic pathophysiology ensues that requires therapeutic intervention to sustain life. The American Burn Association (1976) defines severity of burn injury according to depth of injury and extent of injury (Table 41-8). Depth of injury identifies the level

FIG. 41-26 **Kaposi sarcoma.** Purple nodules are most commonly seen on the lower legs. (From Habif, 1990.)

TABLE 41-8

American Burn Association Classification of Burn Injury

Minor burn injury	Moderate, uncomplicated burn injury	Major burn injury
Second-degree burns of less than 15% TBSA in adults or less than 10% TBSA in children	Second-degree burns of 15% to 25% TBSA in adults or 10% to 20% TBSA in children	Second-degree burns of greater than 25% TBSA in adults or 20% TBSA in children
Third-degree burns of less than 2% TBSA not involving special care areas (eyes, ears, face, hands, feet, perineum)	Third-degree burns of less than 10% TBSA not involving special care areas	All third-degree burns of 10% TBSA burn or greater
Excludes electrical injury, inhalation injury, complicated injury (fractures), all poor-risk individuals (extremes of age, intercurrent disease, etc.)	Excludes electrical injury, complicated injury (fractures), inhalation injury, all poor-risk individuals (extremes of age, intercurrent disease, etc.)	All burns involving hands, face, eyes, ears, feet, perineum All inhalation injury, electrical injury, complicated burn injury involving fractures or other major trauma All poor-risk individuals

TBSA: Total body surface area.

of tissue destruction; the extent of injury determines the mortality rate.

Pathophysiology

First-degree burns. The depth of injury is divided into four categories (Table 41-9). First-degree burns are not included in estimates of the extent of total body surface area (TBSA) burn. The skin does not lose its ability to function as a water vapor and bacterial barrier with **first-degree burns.** The most common example of a first-degree burn is a sunburn, which results from indirect

exposure to the heat of the sun. Initially there is local pain and erythema, but no blisters appear for about 24 hours. An extensive first-degree burn may cause systemic responses such as chills, headache, localized edema, and nausea or vomiting. No treatment of extensive first-degree burns is required unless the person is elderly or an infant, in which case severe nausea and vomiting may lead to inadequate fluid intake and dehydration. Therapy consists of intravenous hydration until the nausea and vomiting subside at 24 to 72 hours after burn injury. Comfort measures for previously

TABLE 41-9

Depth of Burn Injury

Characteristic	First degree	Second degree		Third degree
		Superficial partial-thickness	Deep partial-thickness	Full-thickness
Morphology	Destruction of epidermis only	Destruction of epidermis and some dermis	Destruction of epidermis and dermis, leaving only skin appendages	Destruction of epidermis, dermis, and underlying subcutaneous tissue
Skin function	Intact	Absent	Absent	Absent
Tactile and pain sensors	Intact	Intact	Intact but diminished	Absent
Blisters	Present only after first 24 hr	Present within minutes, thin-walled and fluid-filled	May or may not appear as fluid-filled blisters; often is layer of flat, dehydrated "tissue paper" that lifts off in sheets	Blisters rare; usually is a layer of flat, dehydrated "tissue paper" that lifts off easily
Appearance of wound after initial debridement	Skin peels at 24 to 48 hr, normal or slightly red underneath	Red to pale ivory, moist surface	Mottled with areas of waxy white, dry surface	White, cherry red, or black; may contain visible thrombosed veins; dry, hard leathery surface
Healing time	3 to 5 days	21 to 28 days	30 days to many months	Will not heal; may close from edges as secondary healing if wound is small
Scarring	None	May be present, low incidence influenced by genetic predisposition	Highest incidence because of slow healing rate promoting scar tissue development, also influenced by genetic predisposition	Skin graft; scarring minimized by early excision and grafting, influenced by genetic predisposition

healthy children or adults with extensive first-degree burns consist of aspirin for adults or acetaminophen for children, every 4 hours in age-appropriate dosage, and the frequent application of a water-soluble lotion. First-degree burns heal in 3 to 5 days without scarring.

Second-degree burns. Second-degree burns are classified as either superficial or deep partial-thickness injury (Table 41-9). The hallmark of **superficial partial-thickness injury** is the appearance of thin-walled, fluid-filled blisters that develop within just a few minutes after injury. Another dominant characteristic of superficial injury is pain. As blisters break or are removed, nerve endings are exposed to air (Fig. 41-27). Tactile and pain sensors remain intact throughout the healing

process, with each wound care procedure causing extreme pain. Wounds heal in 3 to 4 weeks, provided the individual is adequately nourished and no complications develop (Fig. 41-28). The amount of scarring that develops is a genetically determined trait and is not predictable during the early course of treatment. The tendency to scar is extremely high in black people and people with red hair and extremely low in Asian and American Indian populations, although there is also great variation within these groups.

Deep partial-thickness burns involve the entire dermis, leaving only the epidermal skin appendages located in hair follicles (Table 41-9). The burn tends to be waxy white and is often surrounded by margins of superficial

FIG. 41-27 Second-degree burn (superficial partial thickness). (Courtesy Intermountain Burn Center, University of Utah Health Sciences Center.)

FIG. 41-28 Healing second-degree burn (superficial partial thickness). (Courtesy Intermountain Burn Center, University of Utah Health Sciences Center.)

partial-thickness injury. The injury is initially clinically indistinguishable from a full-thickness injury (Fig. 41-29). By 7 to 10 days after burn injury, hair will appear from hair follicles, indicating that epidermal appendages remain. These wounds take weeks to heal, and current therapy indicates surgical removal of the burn wound (excision) followed by application of the person's own unburned skin from another body area (autograft). Wounds that heal slowly produce more scar tissue and continue to be a potential source of infection until closed. In the presence of extensive wounds or a previous debilitating concomitant disease state such as cardiopulmonary failure, however, deep partial-thickness wounds are not surgically treated but are allowed to heal primarily.

Third-degree burns.   Third-degree, or **full-thickness**, **burns** involve destruction of the entire epidermis, dermis, and some underlying subcutaneous tissue (Table 41-9). On occasion, all underlying subcutaneous tissue is destroyed and muscle or bone may be involved. Some

classification systems designate burns to muscle, tendon, or bone as fourth-degree injury. In burn care facilities, fourth-degree injury is usually a term describing damage from electrical injury. Visible thrombosed veins may be present in some areas of full-thickness injury, with the most common location being the dorsum of the hand. Full-thickness wounds often appear relatively innocuous when their color is white and the delineation between normal and burned skin is not accompanied by a marked color change. Elasticity of the dermis is destroyed, giving the wound a dry, hard, leathery appearance (Fig. 41-30). As marked edema forms, distal circulation may be compromised in areas of circumferential burns. Full-thickness burns are painless because all nerve endings have been destroyed by heat.

FIG. 41-29 **Second-degree burn** (deep partial thickness injury to dorsum of hand). (Courtesy Intermountain Burn Center, University of Utah Health Sciences Center.)

FIG. 41-30 **Third-degree burn** (marked color change). (Courtesy Intermountain Burn Center, University of Utah Health Sciences Center.)

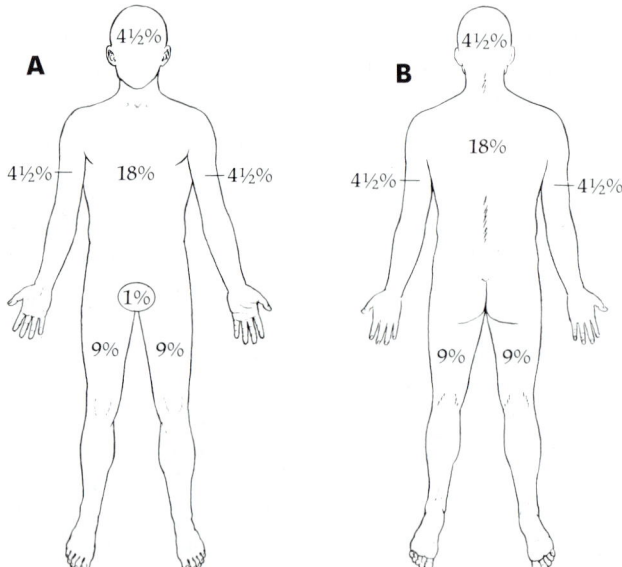

FIG. 41-31 **Estimation of burn injury: rule of nines. A,** Adults (anterior view). **B,** Adults (posterior view). (From Thompson, McFarland, Hirsch, & Tucker, 1993.)

Clinical Manifestations

The extent of the total body surface area (TBSA) burn is estimated using either the "rule of nines" (Fig. 41-31) or the Lund and Browder chart (Fig. 41-32). By convention, burn areas assessed as full-thickness injury are colored in red; areas of superficial or deep partial thickness are colored in blue; and areas of first-degree burn are omitted from the burn diagram and from the TBSA percent burn totals.

Severity of burn injury is a combination of many factors, including age, medical history, extent and depth of injury, and body area involved. Taking these factors into consideration, the American Burn Association has classified burn injury into three categories: (1) minor burn injury; (2) moderate, uncomplicated burn injury; and (3) major burn injury (Table 41-8). In general, people with minor burn injury are expected to be treated as outpatients and those with moderate, uncomplicated burn injury are expected to be treated in a nearby hospital facility, although transfer to a burn care facility may be accomplished at the discretion of health care providers. In both of the previously mentioned categories, treatment is aimed at promoting healing through wound cleansing and nutritional support. Tetanus toxoid is administered prophylactically.

With a major burn injury, a systemic pathophysiology ensues that requires therapeutic intervention to sustain life. The immediate physiologic consequences of major burn injury center around the profound, life-threatening hypovolemic shock that occurs in conjunction with cellular and immunologic disruption within a few minutes of injury. Burn shock is a phenomenon consisting of both a hypovolemic cardiovascular component and a cellular component. Hypovolemic shock results from increased capillary permeability throughout the cardiovascular system, which begins with the onset of burn injury and persists for approximately 24 hours after burn injury, even when adequate resuscitation fluid is given. Researchers have documented the release of many mediators (prostaglandins, thromboxanes, histamine, and serotonin) of the inflammatory response that may play a role in the cardiovascular response to burns (Ferrara, Dyuess, Luterman, & Curreri, 1990). Evidence has also accumulated suggesting that cellular metabolism is disrupted with onset of the burn wound, resulting in altered cell membrane permeability and loss of normal electrolyte homeostasis. This cellular defect may be the pathophysiologic process responsible for the genesis of burn shock. Also, the many circulating factors demonstrated in burn serum may play a role in the generation of cellular abnormalities known to occur. Although it is recognized that the cardiovascular and systemic response is intricately interwoven into the cellular response, they are presented here as separate entities for the purpose of describing their components.

Relative percentages of areas affected by growth
(age in years)

	0	1	5	10	15	Adult
A: half of head	9½	8½	6½	5½	4½	3½
B: half of thigh	2¾	3¼	4	4¼	4½	4¾
C: half of leg	2½	2½	2¾	3	3¼	3½

Second degree _____ and

Third degree _____ =

Total percent burned____

FIG. 41-32 Estimation of burn injury: Lund and Browder chart. Areas designated by letters (*A, B,* and *C*) represent percentages of body surface area that vary according to age. Accompanying table indicates relative percentages of these areas at various stages in life. (From Sabiston, 1977.)

Cardiovascular response to burn injury. Hypovolemic shock develops quickly after major burn injury. The severity of burn shock is directly proportional to the extent of the TBSA burn. Burns involving 25% to 40% TBSA in adults, or 15% to 25% TBSA in children, require cardiovascular support through intravenous fluid, but the treatment is usually tolerated in a fairly predictable manner. Burns involving larger TBSA are potentially lethal injuries that are often accompanied by a stormy clinical course.

The cardiovascular system is normally a closed system with controlled movement of fluid and electrolytes occurring across selected areas, including the capillaries. Within minutes of a major burn injury, however, the capillary bed opens not only in the burn area but also in the entire capillary system. This loss of capillary seal is the mechanism for fluid loss into the interstitium, which leads to the ensuing hypovolemic shock and massive edema. The mechanism of burn shock is not understood, but the sequence is known (Fig. 41-33). As the capillary seal is lost, leakage of intravascular fluid

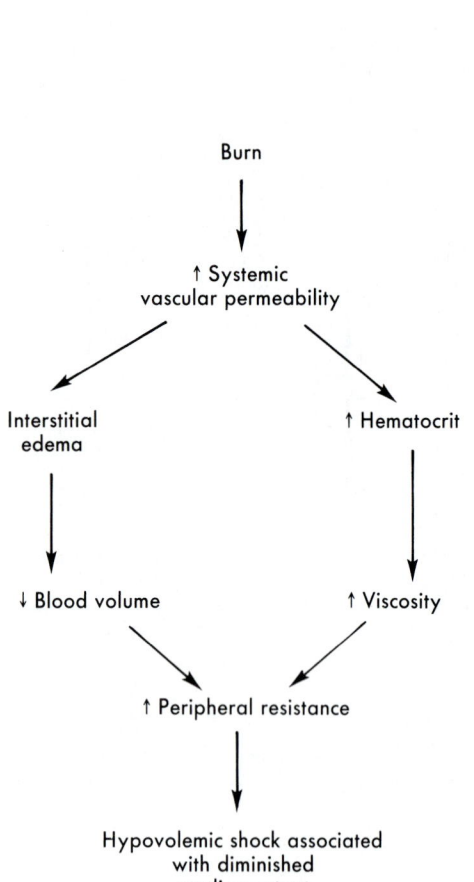

FIG. 41-33 Cardiovascular effects of major burn injury during burn shock. (Courtesy Intermountain Burn Center, University of Utah Health Sciences Center.)

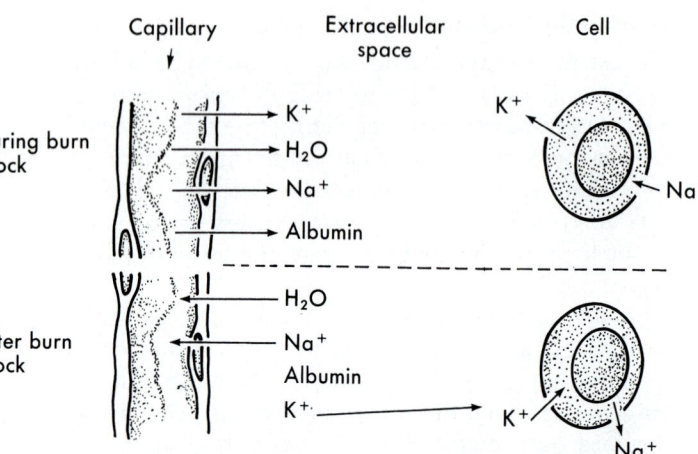

FIG. 41-34 Direction of fluid and electrolyte shifts associated with burn shock. (Courtesy Intermountain Burn Center, University of Utah Health Sciences Center.)

into the interstitial spaces occurs throughout the body with extravasation of water, electrolytes, and proteins (Fig. 41-34). Both red and white blood cells remain in the circulatory system because their relatively larger size does not permit them to leak. Thus an elevated hematocrit and white blood cell count occur. The capillary leak quickly progresses to profound hypovolemic shock that, if not treated, leads to irreversible shock and death within a few hours. Burn shock continues for about 24 hours after burn injury, at which time the capillary seal is restored by an unknown physiologic mechanism.

Burn shock resuscitation involves infusion of intravenous fluid at a rate faster than the rate of the leak of circulating volume fluid for 24 hours after burn injury. Resuscitation for burn shock can be accomplished using one of several available fluid regimens. The most frequently used fluid resuscitation protocol is the Parkland formula (Baxter, 1974). Lactated Ringer solution is the fluid of choice for burn shock because it most closely approximates the fluid being lost from the circulatory system (Table 41-10). Severe electrolyte imbalances occur if fluid resuscitation is accomplished with electrolyte-free intravenous fluid (i.e., D_5W).

The massive edema associated with burn shock is an iatrogenic complication, but failure to administer resuscitation fluid results in irreversible hypovolemic shock and death. The edema occurs over the entire body, not just the burn area (Fig. 41-35). This often leads to mechanical airway obstruction, necessitating tracheal intubation, and increased severity of the interstitial pulmonary edema associated with inhalation injury.

The most reliable criterion for adequate resuscitation of burn shock is urine output. The individual is in hypovolemic shock and will, as a compensatory mechanism, decrease or cease urine output in an effort to pre-

TABLE 41-10

Electrolyte Content of Ringer's Lactate Solution and Extracellular Fluid

Electrolyte	Extracellular fluid* (mEq/L)	Lactated Ringer† (mEq/L)
Sodium	135-145	130
Potassium	3.2-4.5	4
Chloride	95-105	109
Lactate (bicarbonate)	24-28	28

*Normal values may vary slightly between laboratories.
†Plus 80 to 100 ml free water per liter.

FIG. 41-35 Edema of burn shock. (Courtesy Intermountain Burn Center, University of Utah Health Sciences Center.)

MAINTENANCE FLUID REPLACEMENTS FOLLOWING MAJOR BURN INJURY*

1. *Basal fluid* replacements per day
   1500 ml/day/m² body surface area = 24 hour requirements
2. *Evaporative water loss* from burn wound
   a. Adults: (25 + % total body surface area burn) (m² body surface area) = ml/hr
   b. Children: (35 + % total body surface area burn) (m² body surface area) = ml/hr
3. *Total hourly maintenance fluids*
   Basal fluid requirements per day ÷ 24 hours + evaporative water loss per hour = ml/hr maintenance fluids

Example: A 70-kg adult with a 50% total body surface area burn and a body surface area of 2 m requires the following:
   Basal = (1500 ml/day) (2 m² body surface area) = 3000 ml/24 hr or **125 ml/hr**
   Evaporative = (25 + 50% total body surface burn) (2 m² total body surface area) = (75) (2) = **150 ml/hr**
   Total maintenance fluids = **125 ml + 150 ml = 275 ml/hr**

* From end of burn shock until wound closure is achieved.

serve circulating volume. The adult receiving sufficient intravenous fluid will excrete 30 to 50 ml urine/hr: children will excrete 1 ml/kg/hr. If the individual does not have adequate urine output, sufficient fluid is not being administered. The massive amount of intravenous fluid required by burned individuals during the shock phase is often intimidating to the person delivering the fluid. One common concern is that 30 L of intravenous fluid over 24 hours will result in pulmonary edema. It should be remembered that the individual is in hypovolemic shock and that the fluid is leaking out almost as fast as it is infused. Unless the individual is in cardiac failure as a result of a preexisting disease state, the fluid is distributed evenly throughout the body and does not accumulate in the lungs. If the individual is in cardiac failure, there is little chance of survival because without the ability to circulate the administered fluid, hypovolemic shock cannot be resolved. If the fluid is administered, cardiac failure occurs; if the fluid is not administered, irreversible hypovolemic shock occurs. In either case, death is usually inevitable, although cardiac support

drugs such as dopamine may help if the cardiac disease is not too severe.

The end point of burn shock is defined as the time when the individual is able to maintain adequate urine output for 2 hours with the hourly fluid administration rate at the person's maintenance rate (see box above). As burn shock ends, fluid administered remains in the circulating volume and is reflected as increased urine output. The mechanism whereby capillary integrity is restored is unknown but usually occurs about 24 hours after burn injury. After the individual has reached the end point of burn shock, the term used to describe the person's condition is *sealed*. On completion of resuscitation, an infusion of type-specific, fresh frozen plasma or commercially available volume expander solution, equal to 20% of the calculated blood volume, is administered to promote restoration of intravascular volume.

Cardiac dysfunction is also a component of major burn injury. Burn shock is accompanied by a sudden precipitous drop in cardiac output, which does not parallel the gradual reduction of blood volume. Furthermore, infusion of intravenous fluids in amounts sufficient to restore circulating volume does not return cardiac output to preburn levels (Aikawa, Martyn, & Burke, 1978; Dobson & Warner, 1957). The consistent burn shock finding of inappropriately low cardiac output in the presence of vigorous intravenous fluid resuscitation and massive catecholamine release led to the suggestion of a specific myocardial depressant factor (Baxter, Cook, & Shires, 1966; Lefer & Martin, 1970; Rosenthal, Hawley, & Hakin, 1972). Although there is agreement that myocardial dysfunction is present with all major burn injuries, the cause of the depression remains to be described except in the most general terms. It is accepted that there is no simple specific myocardial depressant factor, but rather a cascade of events that is generally termed the cellular response to burn and includes both metabolic and immunologic factors. These factors initiate the cardiovascular sequence of loss of capillary seal and subsequent hypovolemic shock.

Cellular response to burn injury. Major burn injury affects the entire physiologic system; however, survival depends on its ultimate impact at the cellular level. The cellular response to burn injury falls into two categories: (1) metabolic response and (2) immunologic response. The basic syndrome is referred to as the "sick cell syndrome." Welt and colleagues (1967) were among the first to describe this phenomenon as a cell membrane transport defect related to an alteration in the steady state composition characterized by high intracellular concentrations of sodium. Trunkey and colleagues (1973) found a marked decrease in primate muscle extracellular water and an increase in both intracellular sodium and water during hypovolemic shock. In addition, other researchers demonstrated an associated decrease in resting membrane potential, a decrease in amplitude of the action potential, and a prolongation of both the repolarization and depolarization time in association with a decreased intracellular potassium concentration (Cunningham, Shires, & Wagner, 1971; Rosenthal & Tabor, 1945). The cellular dysfunction of burn injury extends beyond the transmembrane potential disruption and the sodium-potassium pump impairment to include a loss of intracellular magnesium and phosphate (Turinsky, Gonnerman, & Loose, 1981) and elevated serum lactic dehydrogenase (LDH) levels (Deets & Glaviano, 1973). This suggests impairments of basic cellular function as the underlying cause of the diminished membrane potentials. The data suggest a decrease in the efficiency of the pump—a change that can be reversed by adequate fluid resuscitation of burn shock over time.

Metabolic reactions to the stress of a major burn injury involve the response of the sympathetic nervous system and other homeostatic regulators. Catecholamines are found in elevated amounts in both the serum and urine of burned individuals. Changes in lipid metabolism are reflected as an elevation in plasma free fatty acids (FFA) and a decrease in plasma cholesterol and phospholipids (Okamoto, Glaviano, & Pindok, 1971).

Burn injury induces an almost immediate hypermetabolic state that persists until wound closure. Wilmore

and colleagues (1974) described the hypermetabolic state of 20 burned individuals as unrelated to ambient temperatures with persistent elevation of core body temperatures. The metabolic rate increased with burn size in a curvilinear relationship with oxygen consumption rarely exceeding 2½ times basal levels. Evaporative water loss and surface cooling are not the primary stimulus for the hypermetabolic state; rather, the hypermetabolism is related to an increase and resetting of the thermal regulatory set point. A core body temperature of 38.5° C is typical. A reflex arc mobilizes neural or hormonal afferent stimuli to the hypothalamus, producing a catecholamine response clinically manifested as hypermetabolism, hyperthermia, and hyperglycemia.

Evidence also exists that the burn wound itself directly mediates the response to injury at both the local and systemic level. The body's priority response to injury is the wound itself, and the general systemic events observed may occur in response to the burn tissue inflammation (Gump, Price, & Kinney, 1970; Wilmore, Aulick, Mason, & Pruitt, 1977; Wilmore et al., 1980). That is, vasodilation, increased capillary permeability, and edema occur to facilitate healing of the local area. The distribution of the peripheral circulation after burn injury transports both heat and glucose preferentially to the wound. The energy cost of these reparative and transport processes is reflected in the increased metabolism and hyperdynamic circulation.

The extensive evaporative water loss that occurs in burn tissue is a heat-consuming process, and the energy need is met, at least in part, by increased visceral heat production. The signal for the response is unknown because individuals whose wounds have been denervated continue to have a posttraumatic hypermetabolic response. Hypothalamic function alterations result in the elevation of human growth hormone (hGH) serum levels in the presence of hyperglycemia, a finding opposite normal states (Wilmore, Orcutt, Mason, & Pruitt, 1975). Furthermore, the hypermetabolic rate is not decreased during rest, sleep, or warmth. Because the increased oxygen consumption cannot be accounted for on the basis of elevated body temperature alone, an elevated metabolic state, not a thermoregulatory drive, is responsible for the increased heat production (Aulick et al., 1979).

Glucose and lactate kinetics are also altered after burn injury. Although tissue hypoxia produces lactic acidosis, its persistence in the presence of adequate tissue perfusion suggests an increased rate of glycogenolysis (Wilmore, Aulick, & Goodwin, 1979). An absolute or relative insulin deficiency in combination with an excess of glucocorticoid, glucagon, or catecholamine is the signal that promotes gluconeogenesis. Evidence of hepatic response to burn injury is characterized by alterations in the clotting factors (Holder & Neely, 1990). A **hyper-**

coagulable state develops as manifested by an elevated plasma fibrinogen concentration in the presence of shortened prothrombin time (PT) and activated partial thromboplastin time (PTT) (McManus, Eurenius, & Pruitt, 1973).

In summary, extensive burn injury initiates the most marked alterations in body metabolism associated with any illness. Much of the work explaining this response has been conducted by Wilmore (Wilmore, 1990; Wilmore & Aulick, 1978), who reported that the persistent tachycardia, hyperpnea, hyperpyrexia, and marked body wasting seen in burn injury reflect heightened metabolic activity and accelerated body catabolism. These systemic alterations occur as a result of the cutaneous inflammatory process and are thought to facilitate wound repair. The neural component of this alteration is in response to a sympathetic reaction that releases catecholamines in large amounts.

The immunologic response to burn injury is immediate, prolonged, and severe. The end result in individuals surviving burn shock is immunosuppression with increased susceptibility to potentially fatal systemic burn wound sepsis. The role of circulating factors has been intensely studied, and the findings clearly show that serum from burned animals induces burn shock in an unburned animal and that burn serum has immunosuppressive qualities in vitro. Leukocyte chemotatic studies in vitro showed a decrease in leukocyte migration with the decrease inversely correlated with burn size (Warden, Mason, & Pruitt, 1974). Placing the burnsuppressed leukocytes into serum obtained from normal donors returned the levels to 107% of normal activity (Warden et al., 1975). Ninnemann (1980) reports the participation of both a serum-borne factor and a specific subset of B lymphocytes in the generation of suppressor cells. Another source of circulating factors appears to be the translocation of microbes and endotoxins across the intestinal wall (Grzygowski, Antos, Sakiel, & Dobke, 1992). Bacterial translocation from the gut may be a mechanism of infection leading to septic shock after burn injury and other major trauma (Deitch & Berg, 1987).

A host of chemicals found in burn plasma in altered concentrations also may play a role in burn shock. These include vasoactive amines (histamine, serotonin), products of complement activation (C3a, C5a), prostaglandins, kinins, endotoxin, and metabolic hormones (catecholamines, glucocorticoids). A decrease in complement components C3a and C5a in the circulation after burn injury suggests a nonspecific activation of the complement system (Heideman, Kaijser, & Gelin, 1978). Activation of the complement system in injured tissue results in an inflammatory response caused by release of histamine and serotonin by C3a and C5a. Because both histamine and serotonin alter capillary per-

meability, some investigators propose this cause for burn shock, because these vasoactive amines initiate the inflammatory response along with kinin polypeptides and other chemical mediators. As a result of these vascular changes, fluid and fibrinogen leave the dilated, permeable vessels. Prostaglandins function in the inflammatory process by regulating metabolism of cells of inflammation (see Chapter 7).

White blood cells are also altered at this time, when their need to inhibit sepsis is vital. Natural resistance to infection in burn wounds is a function of the nonspecific immune system; that is, resistance to microorganisms that infect wounds rests almost solely on the ability of phagocytic cells (namely, granulocytes and macrophages) to leave the bloodstream, migrate to the site of infection, and ingest and kill microorganisms (Benhaim & Hunt, 1992). Normally, opsonin renders bacteria susceptible to phagocytosis, but the burn injury triggers a consumptive opsoninopathy. Burn serum contains an inhibitor of C3 conversion that leads to decreased opsonization and polymorphonuclear (PMN) neutrophil dysfunction (Alexander, McClellan, Ogle, & Ogle, 1976; Bjornson, Altemeier, & Bjornson, 1977).

Individuals with altered immunocompetence prior to burn injury are at additional risk for complications. Included in this group are individuals at the extremes of age and those with cardiac disease, malnutrition, immune deficiency disease, and a history of alcohol or drug abuse (Goff, Purdue, Hunt, & Cochran, 1990; Kelley & Lynch, 1992). Additional risk factors include diabetes mellitus and pulmonary or renal dysfunction.

Evaporative water loss. One of the major purposes of intact skin is to serve as a barrier to evaporative water loss (EWL) from the body. With major burn injury, this ability of the skin to regulate evaporative water loss is totally disrupted. In a classic study done in 1962, Moncrief and Mason (1962) attempted to determine the magnitude of such a loss and determined that daily evaporative water loss was in the range of 20 times normal in the early phase of injury with gradual decreases as wound closure is achieved. Further studies indicated that insensible water loss through burned skin is not from evaporation of water from sweat glands but rather from water vapor formed within the body and lost through the skin (Moncrief, 1974; Roe & Kinney, 1964).

Calculation of the amount of fluid lost by evaporative water loss includes losses from all sources. Normally, the skin is the major source of insensible loss (75%) and the lungs are minor sources (25%), with a total loss of only approximately 600 to 800 ml/day. This changes dramatically with burns because not only does skin loss increase but lung loss also increases by hypermetabolism and hyperventilation, especially in an intubated individual. Total evaporative losses may be up to

FIG. 41-36 Burn scar formation. Scar formation with contractures to the dorsum of the hand after deep partial-thickness burn. (Courtesy Intermountain Burn Center, University of Utah Health Sciences Center.)

1500 ml/day. Replacement of the loss is mandatory to prevent volume deficit.

Evaluation and Treatment

There are three essential elements of survival of major burn injury: (1) meticulous wound management, (2) adequate nutrition, and (3) early surgical excision and grafting. Current therapy for deep-partial and full-thickness burn injury includes surgical removal of the burn tissue (excision) followed by grafting of the person's unburned skin (autograft) to the excised area. New technology currently in development and clinical trial includes use of epidermal sheets of skin grown in a laboratory (Herzog, Meyer, Woodley, & Peterson, 1992) and the use of cultured epithelial autografts (Clugston et al., 1991). Until the grafted epidermis completely cornifies and forms a basement membrane, skin replacements do not function as a semipermeable membrane and are very fragile (Desai et al., 1991; Harriger & Hull, 1992).

Burn recovery is long and stormy, with complications the rule rather than the exception. The goal of burn management is wound closure in a manner that promotes survival. Recovery from a major burn injury is never assured but will usually occur once the burn wound is reduced to less than 20% TBSA. Scar formation with contractures is often a consequence of healing in deep partial-thickness and third-degree burns (Fig. 41-36).

Frostbite

Frostbite is injury to the skin caused by exposure to extreme cold. The most common areas affected are fingers, toes, ears, nose, and cheeks. The mechanism of injury is complex but appears to be related to direct cold injury to cells, indirect injury from ice crystal formation, and impaired circulation with anoxia to the exposed area (Grandberg, 1991). Frozen skin becomes white or yellowish and is waxy. There is numbness and no sensation of pain.

The extent of skin damage can range from mild to severe. There is redness and discomfort with mild frostbite during rewarming followed by a return to normal in a few hours. Cyanosis and mottling develop followed by redness, swelling, and burning pain on rewarming in more severe cases. Within 24 to 48 hours, vesicles and bullae appear that resolve into crusts that eventually slough off, leaving thin, newly formed skin. The most severe cases result in gangrene with loss of the affected part. Frostbite may be classified by depth of injury: superficial includes partial skin freezing (first degree) and full-thickness skin freezing (second degree); deep includes full-thickness skin and subcutaneous freezing (third degree) and deep tissue freezing (fourth degree) (Fisher, Souba, & Ford, 1988).

Immediate treatment of frostbite is to cover affected areas with other body surfaces and warm clothing. The area should not be rubbed or massaged. Local, dry heat should be avoided. Immersion in a warm water bath

(40° C to 44° C) until frozen tissue is thawed is the best treatment. Pain during the thawing period is severe and should be treated with potent analgesics. Gentle cleansing and no pressure on the skin should be maintained during healing. Amputation of necrotic tissue is delayed until a clear line of demarcation is established.

DISORDERS OF THE HAIR

Alopecia

Male-Pattern Alopecia (Androcentric Alopecia)

Alopecia means loss of hair. Localized hair loss in men is not a disease but a genetically predisposed response to androgens. The mechanism of inheritance is unknown. Within the distribution of hair over the scalp, androgen-sensitive hair follicles are on top and androgen-insensitive follicles are on the sides and back. In genetically predisposed men, the androgen-sensitive follicles are transformed into vellus follicles. The normal hair is shed and replaced by fine, light, short hair. Male-pattern baldness begins with frontotemporal recession and progresses to loss of hair over the top of the scalp. Minoxidil is currently being used to stimulate hair growth (Savin & Atton, 1993). Affected men may choose to wear wigs, have hair transplants, or have plastic surgery.

Female-Pattern Alopecia

Some women in their 20s and 30s experience progressive thinning and loss of hair over the central part of the scalp. Contrary to male-pattern baldness, there is no loss of hair along the frontal hairline. Many of these women have elevated levels of serum adrenal androgen dehydroepiandrosterone sulfate (DHEAS) (Rushton, 1993). In rare instances, a male-pattern baldness develops. Laboratory evaluation of serum androgenic hormones shows elevations, and some women have decreased hair loss when treated with daily doses of spironolactone (Kasik et al., 1983).

Alopecia Areata

Alopecia areata is rapid onset of hair loss in multiple areas of the scalp, usually in round patches. The eyebrows, eyelashes, beard, and other areas of body hair are rarely involved. The cause is unknown, but stressful events, cell-mediated immune factors, and genetic susceptibility are linked to hair loss. Metabolic disorders, such as Addison disease, thyroid disease, and lupus erythematosus, are also associated with alopecia areata (Sawaya & Hordinsky, 1992).

The affected areas of skin are smooth or may have short shafts of hair. The hair shaft is poorly developed and breaks at the surface. Regrowth occurs within 1 to 3 months, but there may be recurrent hair loss at the same site. There is usually permanent regrowth of hair. There is total loss of hair (alopecia totalis) in some young people, and the long-term prognosis for total hair regrowth is poor.

Diagnosis is made by observation of the pattern of hair loss. Biopsy may show a lymphocytic infiltrate around the follicle. Intralesional steroids may be used to stimulate hair growth when there are a few small areas of hair loss. Systemic steroids are used for larger areas of alopecia. Topical applications of anthralin are also used to stimulate hair growth. Minoxidil has been tested for use in resistant cases and has been found effective in approximately 18% of cases with severe alopecia areata (Feidler-Weiss, Rumsfield, Cunera, & West, 1987).

Hirsutism

Hirsutism is the growth and distribution of hair on the face, body, and pubic area in a male pattern. There is also frontotemporal hair recession. These areas of hair growth are androgen sensitive. Variations of hair growth in women are great and a male pattern may be normal. Women who develop hirsutism may be secreting hormones associated with ovarian or adrenal disease, and such women should be evaluated for polycystic ovaries, adrenal hyperplasia, or adrenal tumors. If no hormonal pathologic conditions exist, treatment may include cosmetic removal of hair, oral contraceptives, glucocorticoids, or cimetidine (Vigersky, Mehlman, Glass, & Smith, 1980).

DISORDERS OF THE NAIL

Paronychia

Paronychia is an acute or chronic infection of the cuticle. Acute paronychia is manifest by the rapid onset of painful inflammation of the cuticle, usually after minor trauma. An abscess may develop requiring incision and drainage for relief of pain. The most common causative organisms are staphylococci and streptococci. Occasionally *Candida* will be present.

Chronic paronychia develops slowly, with tenderness and swelling around the proximal or lateral nail folds. One or more fingers or toes may be involved. Individuals whose hands are exposed to frequent moisture are at greatest risk. Manipulation of the cuticle can be predisposing because it opens the space between the proximal nail fold and nail plate, leaving a moist, warm medium for the incubation of pathogenic organisms. The skin around the nail becomes more edematous and painful with progressive infection. Pus may be expressed from the proximal nail fold. The nail plate is usually not affected, although it can become discolored with ridges.

Treatment includes keeping the hands dry. Oral antibiotics are not very effective because they do not penetrate the affected tissues. Topical application of thymol is usually effective.

Onychomycosis

Onychomycosis is a fungal or dermatophyte infection of the nail plate. The most common pattern is a nail plate that turns yellow or white and becomes elevated with the accumulation of hyperkeratotic debris within the plate. Fungal infections of the nail are differentiated from psoriasis by the absence of pitting on the nail surface, which is characteristic of psoriasis. Treatment is difficult because topical or systemic antifungal agents do not penetrate the nail plate readily. Surgical excision of the nail may be required.

SUMMARY REVIEW

Structure and Function of the Skin

1 Skin is the largest organ of the body and equals 20% of body weight.
2 The skin has two layers, the dermis and epidermis.
3 The underlying epidermis contains a basal and spinous layer with melanocytes, Langerhans cells, and Merkel cells.
4 The dermis is composed of connective tissue elements, hair follicles, sweat glands, sebaceous glands, blood vessels, nerves, and lymphatic vessels.
5 The papillary capillaries provide the major blood supply to the skin, arising from deeper arterial plexuses.
6 Heat loss and heat conservation are regulated by arteriovenous anastomoses that lead to the papillary capillaries.
7 Older skin is thinner, dryer, and has fewer capillary loops with changes in pigmentation.
8 Loss of melanocytes and hair follicles leads to gray and thinner hair.
9 The skin is more permeable; there is decreased sweating and loss of thermal regulation with decreased protective functions.
10 Pressure ulcers develop from pressure and shearing forces that occlude capillary blood flow with resulting ischemia and necrosis. Areas at greatest risk are pressure points over bony prominences, such as the greater trochanter, sacrum, ischia, and heels. Immobilized individuals with fractures and neurologic deficits are most prone to develop pressure ulcers.
11 Pruritus is itching and is associated with many skin disorders. The exact neurologic mechanism is unknown, but pain receptors with low-intensity stimulation are one theory of irritation. Scratching with skin trauma, potential infection, and scarring are associated with itching.

Disorders of the Skin

1 Contact dermatitis is a form of delayed hypersensitivity that develops with sensitization to allergies, such as metal, chemicals, or poison ivy.
2 Irritant contact dermatitis develops from prolonged exposure to chemicals, such as acids or soaps.
3 Atopic or allergic dermatitis is associated with a family history of allergies, hay fever, elevated IgE levels, and increased histamine sensitivity. Pruritus and scratching predispose the skin to infection, scaling, and thickening.
4 Stasis dermatitis occurs on the legs and results from venous stasis and edema.
5 Seborrheic dermatitis involves scaly, yellowish, inflammatory plaques of the scalp, eyebrows, eyelids, ear canals, chest, axillae, and back. The cause is unknown.
6 Papulosquamous disorders are characterized by papules, scales, plaques, and erythema.
7 Psoriasis is a chronic skin disease with thickening of both the epidermis and dermis, characterized by scaly, erythematous, pruritic plaques.
8 Pityriasis rosea is a self-limiting disease characterized by oval lesions with scales around the edges located along skin lines of the trunk.
9 Lichen planus is a papular, violet-colored inflammatory lesion of unknown origin manifest by severe pruritus.
10 Acne vulgaris is an inflammation of the pilosebaceous follicle.
11 Acne rosacea develops on the middle third of the face with hypertrophy and inflammation of the sebaceous glands.
12 Lupus erythematosus can affect only the skin (discoid) or have a systemic presentation. The inflammatory lesions usually occur in sun-exposed areas with a butterfly distribution over the nose and cheeks.
13 Pemphigus is a chronic, autoimmune, blistering disease that begins in the mouth or on the scalp and spreads to other parts of the body, often with a fatal outcome. There are two forms, pemphigus vulgaris and bullous pemphigus.
14 Erythema multiforme is an acute inflammation of the skin and mucous membranes with lesions that appear targetlike with alternating rings of edema and inflammation, often associated with allergic reactions to drugs. Stevens-Johnson syndrome is a severe form that also involves the mucous membranes.
15 Folliculitis is a bacterial infection of the hair follicle.

16 A furuncle is an infection of the hair follicle that extends to the surrounding tissue.

17 A carbuncle is a collection of infected hair follicles that forms a draining abscess.

18 Cellulitis is a diffuse infection of the dermis and subcutaneous tissue.

19 Erysipelas is a superficial streptococcal infection of the skin commonly affecting the face, ears, and lower legs.

20 Impetigo may have a bullous or an ulcerative form and is caused by *Staphylococcus* or *Streptococcus*.

21 Herpes simplex virus type I (HSV-1) causes cold sores but can infect the cornea, mouth, and labia. HSV-2 causes genital lesions and is usually spread by sexual contact.

22 Herpes zoster and varicella are both caused by the same herpesvirus.

23 Warts are benign, rough, elevated lesions caused by papillomavirus. Condylomata acuminata, or venereal warts, are spread by sexual contact.

24 Tinea infections (fungal infections) can occur anywhere on the body and are classified by location (i.e., tinea pedis, tinea corporis, tinea capitis.)

25 Candidiasis is a yeastlike fungal infection occurring on skin, mucous membranes, and gastrointestinal tract.

26 Cutaneous vasculitis is an inflammation of skin blood vessels with purpura, ischemia, and necrosis resulting from vessel necrosis.

27 Urticarial lesions are associated with hypersensitivity responses and appear as wheals, welts, or hives.

28 Scleroderma is a sclerosis of the skin that may also affect systemic organs and cause renal failure, bowel obstruction, or cardiac dysrhythmias.

29 Ticks cause a local reaction and can cause systemic disease when mouth parts pierce the skin and remain embedded in the tissue.

30 Lyme disease is a multisystem inflammatory disease caused by *Borrelia burgdorferi* transmitted by tick bites.

31 Mosquitoes can transmit infectious diseases, and the saliva from their bite produces the characteristic itching and wheal formation.

32 Bloodsucking flies are represented by many species, including Ceratopogonidae ("no-see-ums"), Tabanidae (horseflies), or Simulidae (blackflies). Their bites are usually painful and produce bleeding, and the itching and local reactions may last for days with systemic symptoms of fever and malaise.

33 Seborrheic keratosis is a proliferation of basal cells that produce elevated, smooth, or warty lesions of varying size. They are most common among the elderly.

34 Keratoacanthoma arises from hair follicles on sun-exposed areas. Three stages of development characterize the lesion, which results in a dome-shaped, crusty lesion filled with keratin that resolves in 3 to 4 months.

35 Actinic keratosis is a pigmented scaly lesion that develops in sun-exposed individuals with fair skin. The lesion may become malignant in the form of a squamous cell carcinoma.

36 Nevi arise from melanocytes and may be pigmented or fleshy pink. They occur singly or in groups and may undergo transition to malignant melanoma.

37 Basal cell carcinoma is the most common skin cancer and occurs most frequently on sun-exposed areas.

38 Squamous cell carcinoma is a tumor of the epidermis and can be localized (in situ) or invasive.

39 Malignant melanoma arises from melanocytes, and if not excised early, metastasis occurs through the lymph nodes.

40 Kaposi sarcoma is a vascular malignancy associated with immune deficiency states.

41 Burns are classified according to depth and extent of injury.

42 First-degree burns involve the superficial skin without loss of protective function.

43 Second-degree burns are superficial (blister formation) or superficial partial thickness with a waxy white appearance and no involvement of dermal appendages.

44 Third-degree burns involve full skin thickness and often underlying tissues. They are painless and can be life threatening from hypovolemic shock and metabolic and immunologic responses.

45 Keloids are sharply elevated scars that extend beyond the border of traumatized skin.

46 Frostbite usually occurs on cheeks and digits, with direct injury to cells and impaired circulation.

Disorders of the Hair

1 Male-pattern alopecia is an inherited form of irreversible baldness with hair loss in the central scalp and recession of the temporofrontal hairline.

2 Female-pattern alopecia is a thinning of the central hair of the scalp beginning in women at 20 to 30 years of age.

3 Alopecia areata is patchy loss of hair usually associated with stress or metabolic diseases; it is usually reversible.

4 Hirsutism is a male pattern of hair growth in women that may be normal or the result of excessive secretion of androgenic hormones.

Disorders of the Nail

1 Paronychia is an inflammation of the cuticle that can be acute or chronic and is usually caused by staphylococci or streptococci.

2 Onychomycosis is a fungal infection of the nail plate.

KEY TERMS

Acne rosacea, 1529
Acne vulgaris, 1529
Allergic contact dermatitis, 1524
Alopecia, 1555
Alopecia areata, 1555
Apocrine sweat gland, 1515
Atopic dermatitis, 1525
Basal cell carcinoma, 1540
Basal layer (stratum basale), 1513
Bullous pemphigoid, 1531
Candidiasis, 1537
Carbuncle, 1533
Cellulitis, 1533
Clawlike prolongations, 1523
Condylomata acuminata, 1535
Cutaneous vasculitis, 1537
Deep partial-thickness burn, 1546
Dermal appendage, 1513
Dermis, 1513
Discoid lupus erythematosus (DLE), 1530
Eccrine sweat gland, 1515
Eczema, 1524
Epidermis, 1513
Erysipelas, 1533
Erythema multiforme, 1532
First-degree burn, 1545
Folliculitis, 1532
Frostbite, 1554
Furuncle, 1532

Hair, 1513
Herald patch, 1528
Herpes simplex virus (HSV), 1533
Herpes zoster, 1533
Hirsutism, 1555
Hypercoagulable, 1552
Hyphae, 1535
Hypodermis, 1513
Impetigo, 1533
Irritant contact dermatitis, 1524
Kaposi sarcoma (KS), 1542
Keloid, 1522
Keratin, 1513
Keratinocyte, 1513
Langerhans cell, 1513
Lichen planus, 1528
Lupus erythematosus, 1529
Lyme disease, 1538
Melanocyte, 1513
Melanoma, 1542
Merkel cell, 1513
Mosquito, 1538
Myofibroblast, 1522
Nail, 1513
Onychomycosis, 1556
Papillary capillary, 1515
Papulosquamous disorder, 1526
Paronychia, 1555
Pemphigus, 1531
Pemphigus erythematosus, 1531

Pemphigus foliaceus, 1531
Pemphigus vulgaris, 1531
Pityriasis rosea, 1527
Proteoglycan, 1523
Psoriasis, 1526
Scleroderma, 1537
Sebaceous gland, 1513, 1515
Seborrheic dermatitis, 1526
Second-degree burn, 1546
Spinous layer (stratum spinosum), 1513
Squamous cell carcinoma, 1541
Stasis dermatitis, 1526
Stevens-Johnson syndrome, 1532
Stratum corneum, 1513
Superficial partial-thickness injury, 1546
Sweat gland, 1513
Systemic lupus erythematosus (SLE), 1530
Thermal injury, 1544
Third-degree burn (full-thickness burn), 1547
Tinea capitis, 1535
Tinea corporis (ringworm), 1535
Tinea infection, 1535
Tinea pedis, 1535
Urticarial lesion, 1537
Varicella, 1533
Warts, 1535

REFERENCES

Aikawa, N., Martyn, J. A. J., & Burke, J. F. (1978). Pulmonary artery catheterization and thermodilution cardiac output determination in the management of critically burned patients. *American Journal of Surgery, 135*, 811-817.

Alexander, J. W., McClellan, M. A., Ogle, C. K., & Ogle, J. D. (1976). Consumptive opsoninopathy: Possible pathogenesis in lethal and opportunistic infections. *Annals of Surgery, 184*, 672-678.

American Burn Association. (1976). American Burn Association committee on specific optimal criteria for hospital resources for care of patients with burn injury. San Antonio: The Association.

American Burn Association. (1991). [American Burn Association annual burn facility survey]. Unpublished raw data.

American Cancer Society (ACS). (1993). Cancer statistics 1993. *CA—A Cancer Journal for Clinicians, 43*(1).

Ananthaswamy, H. N., & Pierceall, W. E. (1992). Molecular alterations in human skin tumors. *Pro Clinical Biologic Research, 376*, 61-84.

Arnett, F. C. (1992). Genetic aspects of human lupus. *Clinical Immunology and Immunopathology, 63*(1), 4-6.

Arnold, H. L., Odom, R. B., & James, W. D. (1990) *Andrew's diseases of the skin* (8th ed., p. 253). Philadelphia: Saunders.

Aulick, L. H., Hander, E. H., Wilmore, D. W., Mason, A. D., Jr., & Pruitt, B. A., Jr. (1979). The relative significance of thermal and metabolic demands on burn hypermetabolism. *Journal of Trauma, 19*, 559-556.

Barker, J. N. (1992). Role of keratinocytes in allergic contact dermatitis. *Contact Dermatitis, 26*(3), 145-148.

Baxter, C. R. (1974). Fluid volume and electrolyte changes of the early postburn period. *Clinical Plastic Surgery, 1*, 693-709.

Baxter, C. R., Cook, W. A., & Shires, G. T. (1966). Serum myocardial depressant factor of burn shock. *Surgical Forum, 17*, 1-4.

Bellet, R. E., Mastrangelo, D. B., & Maguire, H. C. (1983). Primary cutaneous melanoma. In B. S. Kahn, R. R. Love, C. Sherman, R. Chakravorty (Eds.), *Concepts in cancer medicine.* New York: Grune & Stratton.

Benhaim, P., & Hunt, T. K. (1992). Natural resistance to infection: Leukocyte functions. *Journal of Burn Care & Rehabilitation, 13*(Part 2), 287-292.

Bjornson, A. B., Altemeier, W. A., & Bjornson, H. S. (1977). Changes in humoral components of host defense following burn trauma. *Annals of Surgery, 186*, 96.

Borish, L., & Joseph, B. Z. (1992). Inflammation and the allergic response. *Medical Clinics of North America, 76*(4), 765-787.

Browder, J. F., Avaujo, O. E., Meyer, N. A., & Flowers, F. P. (1992). The interferons and their use in condyloma acuminata. *Annual Pharmacotherapeutics, 26*(10), 42-45.

Callen, J. P. (1986). Subsets of lupus erythematosus: Clinical, serologic, and immunologic considerations. In J. P. Callen, M. V. Dahl, L. E. Golitz, J. E. Rasmussen, & S. J. Stegman (Eds.), *Advances in dermatology* (volume I.). Chicago: Year Book Medical.

Clinical guidelines: How to predict and prevent pressure ulcers. (1992). *American Journal of Nursing, 92*(7), 52-60.

Clugston, P. A., Snelling, C. F. T., Macdonald, I. B., Maledy, H. L., Boyle, J. C., Germann, E., Courtemanche, A. D., Wirtz, P., Fitzpatrick, D. J., Dester, D. A., Foley, B., Warren, R. J., & Carr, N. J. (1991). Cultured epithelial autografts: Three years of clinical experience with eighteen patients. *Journal of Burn Care & Rehabilitation, 12,* 533-539.

Collins, J. G. (1988). *Types of injuries and impairments due to injuries—United States* (National Health Survey, Series 10, No. 159; DHHS Publication No. PHS 87-1587). Hyattsville, MD: National Center for Health Statistics.

Cooper, J. D., & Schoen, R. T. (1992). Epidemiology, clinical features, and diagnosis of Lyme disease. *Current Opinions in Rheumatology, 4*(4), 520-528.

Crumpacker, C. S. (1987). Herpes simplex. In T. B. Fitzpatrick, A. Z. Eisen, K. Wolff, I. M. Freedberg, & K. F. Austen (Eds.), *Dermatology in general medicine* (3rd ed.). New York: McGraw-Hill.

Cunningham, J. N., Jr., Shires, G. T., & Wagner, Y. (1971). Changes in intracellular sodium and potassium content of red blood cells in trauma and shock. *American Journal of Surgery, 122,* 650-654.

Deets, D. K., & Glaviano, V. V. (1973). Plasma and cardiac lactic dehydrogenase activity in burn shock. *Proceedings of the Society of Experimental Biological Medicine, 142,* 412-416.

Deitch, E. A., & Berg, R. (1987). Bacterial translocation from the gut: Mechanism of infection. *Journal of Burn Care & Rehabilitation, 8,* 475-482.

Desai, M. H., Mlakar, J. M., McCauley, R. L., Abdullah, K. M., Rutan, R. L., Waymack, J. P., Robson, M. C., & Herndon, D. N. (1992). Lack of long-term durability of cultured keratinocyte burn-wound coverage: A case report. *Journal of Burn Care & Rehabilitation, 12,* 540-545.

Dobson, E. L., & Warner, G. F. (1957). Factors concerned in the early stages of thermal shock. *Circulatory Research, V,* 69-74.

Dobson, R. L., & Abele, D. C. (1985). *The practice of dermatology.* Philadelphia: Harper & Row.

Espinoza, L. R., Cuellar, M. L., & Silveira, L. H. (1992). Psoriatic arthritis. *Current Options Rheumatology, 4*(4), 470-478.

Eyre, R. W., & Stanley, J. R. (1989). Biochemical differentiation of types of pemphigus. *Immunology & Serology, 46,* 317-331.

Feidler-Weiss, V. C., Rumsfield, J., Cunera, B. M., West, D. P., & Wendrow, A. (1987). Evaluation of oral minoxidil in the treatment of alopecia areata. *Archives of Dermatology, 123,* 1488-1490.

Ferrara, J. J., Dyuess, D. L., Luterman, A., & Curreri, P. W. (1990). Transportation of immunosuppressive substances produced at the site of burn injury into the systemic circulation: The role of lymphatics. *Journal of Burn Care & Rehabilitation, 11,* 281-286.

Fisher, R. P., Souba, W. W., & Ford, E. G. (1988). Temperature associated injuries and syndromes. In K. L. Mattox, E. E. Moore, & D. V. Feliciano (Eds.), *Trauma* (p. 662). Norwalk, CT: Appleton & Lange.

Fitzpatrick, T. B., Eisen, A. Z., Wolff, K., Freedberg, I. M., & Austen, K. F. (1993). *Dermatology in general medicine* (3rd ed.). New York: McGraw-Hill.

Gilchrist, B. A. (1984). *Skin and aging processes.* Boca Raton, FL: CRC Press.

Ginsburg, C. M. (1991). Pityriasis rosea. *Pediatric Infectious Disease Journal, 10*(11), 858-859.

Goff, D. R., Purdue, G. F., Hunt, J. L., & Cochran, R. P. (1990). Cardiac disease and the patient with burns. *Journal of Burn Care & Rehabilitation, 11,* 305-307.

Goopman, J. (1987). Neoplasms in the acquired immune deficiency syndrome: The multidisciplinary approach. *Seminars in Oncology, 14*(2) (Suppl. 3), 1-6.

Grandberg, P. O. (1991). Freezing cold injury. *Arctic Medical Research, 50*(Suppl. 6), 76-79.

Grzybowski, J., Antos, M., Sakiel, S., & Dobke, M. K. (1992). Antidietary antigen antibodies in the sera of patients with burns as a potential marker of gut mucosa integrity failure. *Journal of Burn Care & Rehabilitation, 13,* 194-197.

Gump, F. E., Price, J. B. Jr., & Kinney, J. M. (1970). Blood flow and oxygen consumption in patients with severe burns. *Surgical Gynecology and Obstetrics, 130,* 23-28.

Gurevich, I. (1992). Varicella zoster and herpes simplex virus infections. *Heart & Lung, 21*(1), 85-91.

Habif, T. P. (1985). *Clinical dermatology: A color guide to diagnosis and therapy.* St. Louis: Mosby Year—Book.

Hagemark, O. (1992). Peripheral and central mediators of itch. *Skin Pharmacology, 5*(1), 1-8.

Hall, J. (1987, October). *Burn injuries in the U. S., Report of the National Fire Protection Association, Fire Analyses Division.*

Harriger, M. D., & Hull, B. E. (1992). Cornification and basement membrane formation in a bilayered human skin equivalent maintained in an air-liquid interface. *Journal of Burn Care & Rehabilitation, 13,* 187-193.

Heideman, J., Kaijser, B., & Gelin, L. (1978). Complement activation and hematologic, hemodynamic, and respiratory reactions early after soft tissue injury. *Journal of Trauma, 18,* 696-700.

Herzog, S. R., Meyer, A., Woodley, D., & Peterson, H. D. (1988). Wound coverage with cultured autologous keratinocytes: Use after burn wound excision, including biopsy followup. *Journal of Burn Care & Rehabilitation, 28,* 195-198.

Holder, I. A., & Neely, A. N. (1990). Hageman factor—dependent kinin activation in burns and its theoretical relationship to postburn immunosuppression syndrome and infection. *Journal of Burn Care & Rehabilitation, 11,* 496-503.

Huckbody, E. (1980). Dermatology throughout the dark ages. *International Journal of Dermatology, 6,* 344-347.

Kelly, D., & Lynch, J. B. (1992). Burns in alcohol and drug users result in longer treatment times with more complications. *Journal of Burn Care & Rehabilitation, 13,* 218-220.

Klecz, R. J., & Schwartz, R. A. (1992). Pruritus. *American Family Physician, 45*(6), 2681-2686.

Kragballe, K. (1992). Vitamin D analogues in the treatment of psoriasis. *Journal of Cellular Biochemistry, 49*(1), 46-52.

Kragballe, K., & Voorhees, J. J. (1985). Arachidonic acid and leukotrienes in pathogenesis and treatment. In H. H. Roenick & H. I. Maibach (Eds.), *Psoriasis* (pp. 255-264). New York: Marcel Dekker.

Kurban, R. S., & Kurban, A. K. (1993). Common skin disorders of aging. *Geriatrics, 48*(4), 30-42.

Kwa, R. E., Campagna, K., & Moy, R. L. (1992). Biology of cutaneous squamous cell carcinoma. *Journal of the American Academy of Dermatology, 26*(1), 1-26.

Lefer, A. M., & Martin, J. (1970). Origin of myocardial depressant factor in shock. *American Journal of Physiology, 218,* 1423-1427.

LeRoy, E. C. (1992). A brief overview of the pathogenesis of scleroderma (systemic sclerosis). *Annals of Rheumatic Disease, 51*(2), 286-288.

Levitz, S. M. (1992). Overview of host defenses in fungal infections. *Clinics in Infectious Disease, 14*(Suppl. 1), 537-542.

Lober, C. W. (1992). Dysplastic (atypical) nevi: Significance and management. *Southern Medical Journal, 85*(9), 870-877.

Majno, G. (1975). *The healing hand.* Cambridge, MA: Harvard University Press.

McManus, W. F., Eurenius, K., & Pruitt, B. A., Jr. (1973). Disseminated intravascular coagulation in burned patients. *Journal of Trauma, 13,* 416-422.

Mindel, A. (1991). Cutaneous herpes simplex infection. *Scandinavian Journal of Infectious Disease, 80*(Suppl.), 47-52.

Moncrief, J. A. (1974). Burns. In S. I. Schwartz, R. C. Lillehei, G. T. Shires, F. C. Spencer, & E. H. Storer (Eds.), *Principles of surgery* (2nd ed., pp. 253-274). New York: McGraw-Hill.

Moncrief, J. A., & Mason, A. D. (1962). Water vapor loss in the burned patient. *Surgical Forum, 13,* 38-41.

Monk, B. E., Graham-Brown, R. A. C., & Sarkany, I. (1988). *Skin disorders in the elderly.* Oxford: Blackwell Scientific.

Ninnemann, J. L. (1980). Immunosuppression following thermal injury through a B cell activation of suppressor T cells. *Journal of Trauma, 20,* 206-213.

Okamoto, R., Glaviano, V. V., & Pindok, M. (1971). Myocardial lipases and catecholamines in burn shock. *Proceedings of the Society of Experimental Biological Medicine, 137,* 347-353.

Perez, M. I., & Kohn, S. R. (1993). Systemic sclerosis. *Journal of the American Academy of Dermatology, 28*(4), 525-547.

Ragozzino, M. W., Melton, L. J., Kurland, L. T., Chu, C. P., & Perry, H. O. (1982). Population based study of herpes zoster and its sequelae. *Medicine, 5*(61), 310.

Ramsey, D. L., & Hurley, H. J. (1985). Papulosquamous eruptions and exfoliative dermatitis. In S. L. Moschella & H. J. Hurley (Eds.), *Dermatology* (vol. I, p. 522). Philadelphia: Saunders.

Roe, C. F., & Kinney, J. M. (1964). Water and heat exchange in third-degree burns. *Surgery, 56,* 212-220.

Rosenthal, S. M., & Tabor, H. (1945). Electrolyte changes and chemotherapy in experimental burn and traumatic shock and hemorrhage. *Archives of Surgery, 51,* 244-252.

Rosenthal, S. R., Hawley, P. L., & Hakin, A. A. (1972). Purified burn toxic factor and its competition. *Surgery, 71,* 527-536.

Rothfield, N. F. (1992). Autoantibodies in scleroderma. *Rheumatic Disease Clinics of North America, 18*(2), 483-498.

Rushton, D. H. (1993). Management of hair loss in women. *Dermatologic Clinics, 11*(1), 47-53.

Sabiston, D. C., Jr. (Ed.). (1977). *Textbook of surgery: The biological basis of modern surgical practice* (11th ed.). Philadelphia: Saunders.

Safai, B. (1987). Pathophysiology and epidemiology of epidemic Kaposi's sarcoma. *Seminars in Oncology, 14*(2) (Suppl. 3), 7.

Savin, R. C., & Atton, A. V. (1993). Minoxidil: Update on its clinical role. *Dermatologic Clinics, 11*(1), 55-64.

Sawaya, M. E., & Hordinsky, M. K. (1992). Advances in alopecia areata and androgenic alopecia. *Advances in Dermatology, 7,* 211-226.

Schultz-Larsen, F., & Hanifin, J. M. (1992). Secular changes in the occurrence of atopic dermatitis. *Acta Dermato-Venereologica Suppl (Stockholm), 176,* 7-12.

Shelley, W. B., & Arthur. R. P. (1957). The neurohistology and neurophysiology of the itch sensation in man. *Archives of Dermatology, 76,* 296-323.

Sigal, L. H. (1992). Current recommendations for the treatment of Lyme disease. *Drugs, 43*(5), 683-699.

Singh, G., Marples, B. M., & Klingman, A. M. (1971). Staphylococcus infections in humans. *Journal of Investigative Dermatology, 57,* 149.

Skaer, T. L. (1992). Medication induced systemic lupus erythematosus. *Clinical Therapeutics, 14*(4), 496-506.

Stewart, W. D., Danto, J. L., & Maddin, S. (1978). *Dermatology: diagnosis and treatment of cutaneous disorders.* (4th ed.) St. Louis: Mosby–Year Book.

Strauss, J. (1985). Acne. In T. T. Provost & E. R. Farmer (Eds.), *Current therapy in dermatology 1985-1986* (p. 116). St. Louis: Mosby–Year Book.

Sturzl, M., Roth, W. K., Brockmeyer, N. H., Zietz, C., Speiser, B., & Hofschneider, P. H. (1992). Expression of platelet-derived growth factor and its receptor in AIDS-related Kaposi sarcoma in vivo suggests paracrine and autocrine mechanisms of tumor maintenance. *Proceedings of the National Academy of Science, USA. 89,*(15), 7046-7050.

Thompson, J. M., McFarland, G. K., Hirsch, J. E., & Tucker, S. M. (1993). *Mosby's clinical nursing* (3rd ed.). St. Louis: Mosby–Year Book.

Truhan, A. P. (1991). Sun protection in childhood. *Clinical Pediatrics, 30*(12), 676-681.

Trunkey, D. D., Illner, H., Wagner, I. Y., & Shires, G. T. (1973). The effect of hemorrhagic shock on intracellular muscle action potentials in the primates. *Surgery, 74,* 241-250.

Turinsky, J., Gonnerman, W. A., & Loose, L. D. (1981). Impaired mineral metabolism in postburn muscle. *Journal of Trauma, 21,* 417-423.

Urbach, F. (1991). Incidence of nonmelanoma skin cancer. *Dermatology Clinics, 9*(4), 751-755.

Versluysen, M. (1986). How elderly patients with femoral fracture develop pressures sores in hospital. *British Medical Journal, 292,* 1311-1313.

Wahren, B., & Linde, A. (1991). Virological and clinical characteristics of human herpes virus 6. *Scandinavian Journal of Infectious Disease, 80*(Suppl.), 105-109.

Warden, G. D., Mason, A. D., Jr., & Pruitt, B. A., Jr. (1974). Evaluation of leukocyte chemotaxis *in vitro* in thermally injured patients. *Journal of Clinical Investigation, 54,* 1001-1004.

Warden, G. D., Mason, A. D., Jr., & Pruitt, B. A., Jr. (1975). Suppression of leukocyte chemotaxis *in vitro* by chemotherapeutic agents used in the management of thermal injuries. *Annals of Surgery, 181,* 363-369.

Welt, L. G., Smith, E. K. M., Dunn, M. J., Czersinski, A., Proctor, H., Cole, C., Balfer, J. W., & Gitelman, H. J. (1967). Membrane transport defect: The sick cell. *Transactions of the Association of American Physicians, 80,* 217-226.

Wilmore, D. W. (1990). *The metabolic management of the critically ill* (2nd ed.). New York: Plenum.

Wilmore, D. W., Aulick, H. L., Mason, A. D., Jr., & Pruitt, B. A., Jr. (1977). Influence of the burn wound on local and systemic responses to injury. *Annals of Surgery, 186,* 444-458.

Wilmore, D. W., & Aulick, L. H. (1978). Metabolic changes in burned patients. *Surgical Clinics of North America, 58,* 1173-1187.

Wilmore, D. W., Aulick, H. L., & Goodwin, C. W. (1979). Glucose metabolism following severe injury. *Acta Chirurgica Scandinavica, 498,* 43-47.

Wilmore, D. W., Goodwin, C. W., Aulick, L. H., Powanda, M. C., Mason, A. D., Jr., & Pruitt, B. A., Jr. (1980). Effect of injury and infection on visceral metabolism and circulation. *Annals of Surgery, 192,* 491-500.

Wilmore, D. W., Orcutt, T. W., Mason, A. D., & Pruitt, B. A., Jr. (1975). Alterations in hypothalamic function following thermal injury. *Journal of Trauma, 15,* 697-703.

SUGGESTED READINGS

Balfour, H. H., Jr. (1984). Intravenous acyclovir therapy for varicella in immunocompromised children. *Journal of Pediatrics, 104,* 134.

Balin, A. K., & Kligman, A. M. (1989). *Aging and the skin.* New York: Raven Press.

Champion, R. H., Burton, J. C., & Ebling, F. J. G. (1992). *Rook, Wilkinson, Ebling textbook of dermatology* (5th ed.). Boston: Blackwell Scientific.

Friedman, P. S. (1981). Alopecia areata and autoimmunity. *British Journal of Dermatology, 105,* 153.

Krainski, M. M. (1992) Pressure ulcers and the elderly. A review of the literature, 1980-1990. *Ostomy-Wound Management, 35*(5), 22-37.

Kravitz, M. (Guest Editor). (1993). Burn care. *AACN Clinical Issues in Critical Care Nursing, 4*(2), 349-442.

Paget, J. (1873). Clinical lecture on bedsores. *Student Journal and Hospital Gazette, 1,* 144. Reprinted in: J. H. Gibbon & L. W. Freeman. (1946). Primary closure of decubitus ulcers. *American Journal of Surgery, 124,* 1149.

Puhvel, S. M., & Sakamoto, M. A. (1980). Cytotoxin production by comedonal bacteria *(Propionibacterium acnes, Propionibacterium granulosum,* and *Staphylococcus epidermidis). Journal of Investigative Dermatology, 74,* 36.

Seeley, R. R., Stephens, T. D., & Tate, P. (1992). *Anatomy and physiology.* (2nd ed.). St. Louis: Mosby–Year Book.

Thibodeau, G. A., & Patton, K. (1993). *Anatomy and physiology.* (2nd ed.). St. Louis: Mosby–Year Book.

Alterations of the Integument in Children

Noreen Heer Nicol
Sue E. Huether
Margaret M. Andrews*

Chapter Outline

C hildren frequently develop alterations in the skin. The lesions may be minor or severe and localized or generalized. There are often no prodromal symptoms. Skin diseases in children may have different manifestations than in adults, although the causative mechanisms may be similar. Many diseases resolve spontaneously and require no treatment. Diagnosis is commonly made from the history, appearance, and distribution of the lesion or lesions. Common skin diseases of childhood are presented here.

ACNE VULGARIS

Acne vulgaris is the most common skin disease and affects 85% of the population between the ages of 12 and 25. Genetic influences may determine an individual's susceptibility and severity of disease. Severe acne tends to run in families. The incidence of acne is the same in both sexes, although severe disease affects males more frequently.

Distinctive pilosebaceous units, known as "sebaceous

FIG. 42-1 **Acne. A,** Acne vulgaris (open and closed comedones). Comedones (blackheads) are occasionally inflamed. **B,** Pustular acne (erythematous papules and pustules). Many pustules are present and several have become confluent on the chin area. (From Habif, T. P. [1985]. *Clinical dermatology: A color guide to diagnosis and treatment.* St. Louis: Mosby–Year Book.)

follicles," are the sites for development of acne lesions. The follicles are located primarily on the face and upper parts of the chest and back. These follicles have many large sebaceous glands, a small vellus hair, and a dilated follicular canal that is visible as a "pore" on the skin surface. Acne lesions may be divided into inflammatory (pustules, papules, and nodules) and noninflammatory (closed and open comedones) (Fig. 42-1). In **noninflammatory acne,** the comedones are open (blackheads) and closed (whiteheads), with the accumulated material causing distention of the follicle and thinning of follicular canal walls. **Inflammatory acne** develops in closed comedones when the follicular wall ruptures, expelling sebum into the surrounding dermis and initiating inflammation. Pustules form when the inflammation is close to the surface; papules and cystic nodules can develop when the inflammation is deeper, causing mild to severe scarring. Both types of lesions may exist in the same individual.

The exact cause of acne is unknown. The principal factors are abnormal keratinization of the follicular epithelium, excessive sebum production, and proliferation of *Propionibacterium acnes.* An excessive production and accumulation of sebum appear directly related to androgenic hormones and the pathogenesis of acne. Testosterone is converted to dihydrotestosterone in the skin, which increases the size and productivity of the sebaceous glands. Estrogens decrease sebaceous secretion (Forstrom, 1980). Acne begins with sebum accumulation that obstructs the pilosebaceous unit. The mass of accumulated keratinous sebaceous material and bacteria within the pilosebaceous follicle (Fig. 42-1) causes inflammation when it is exposed to the dermis with rupture of a follicle.

The *P. acnes* bacteria produce substances that pro-

mote inflammation, including chemotactic factors and lipolytic and proteolytic enzymes. The hydrolytic action of the enzymes converts triglycerides into free fatty acids that stimulate inflammation and edema with breakdown of the follicle wall. Chemotactic substance also may be released with mediation of inflammation by attraction of polymorphonuclear leukocytes (Arnold, Odom, & James, 1990; Ingham, Eady, Goodwin, Cove, & Cunliffe, 1992). Acne conglobata is a highly inflammatory form of acne with the formation of communicating cysts and abscesses beneath the skin. Remissions tend to occur during the summer, perhaps from more exposure to sunlight.

Treatment of acne should address these causative factors. Topical treatment, including oral antibiotics, benzoyl peroxide, salicylic acid, and tretinoin, should be the first line of therapy because it is the least invasive. Use of systemic therapies, including oral antibiotics, sex hormones, corticosteroids, and isotretinoin, may be limited by side effects. Acne surgery, including comedo extraction, intralesional steroids, and cryosurgery, is useful in selected patients. Severe scarring may be treated with dermabrasion.

DERMATITIS

Atopic Dermatitis

Atopic dermatitis (AD) is the most common cause of eczema in children, with a prevalence of 5% to 10%. The cause of this chronic relapsing form of pruritic eczema is unknown, but 75% to 80% of individuals with atopic dermatitis have a personal or family history of asthma or allergic rhinitis (hayfever). Onset is usually from 2 to 6 months of age, and 85% of cases occur within the

FIG. 42-2 Infantile form of atopic dermatitis. A, Note rash affecting face and trunk. **B,** Note rash affecting trunk and extensor surfaces of arms.

first 5 years of life. There are no specific laboratory features of AD that can be used for diagnostic purposes. An increased serum IgE level and positive immediate skin tests to a variety of common food and inhalant allergens are seen in approximately 80% of patients. Similarly, blood eosinophilia is a common finding in AD. The basis for the elevated serum IgE levels and eosinophilia in AD is thought to relate to various abnormalities of T-cell function (Nicol & Leung, 1992).

There is no single distinguishing feature of AD. Atopic dermatitis has a constellation of clinical features that include severe pruritus, chronic course with frequent exacerbations, and characteristic eczematoid appearance and age-dependent distribution of skin lesions. The skin becomes increasingly dry, sensitive, itchy, and easily irritated because the barrier function is impaired. Microscopic epidermal cracks that let water out and irritants and allergens in lead to further drying and cracking, which results in rubbing and scratching. Rubbing and scratching to relieve the itch are actually responsible for many of the clinical changes that are seen. In children, the rash appears primarily on the face, scalp, trunk, and extensor surfaces of the arms and legs (Fig. 42-2). In older children and adults, the rash tends to be found on the neck, antecubital and popliteal fossae, and hands and feet. Individuals with AD also tend to develop viral, bacterial, and fungal skin infections in the eczematized areas.

Management of patients with AD includes accurate diagnosis and identification and elimination of exacerbating factors, such as irritants, allergens, and reduction of emotional stresses. Hydration of the skin is the key to good therapy but is often difficult to achieve. Antiinflammatory agents, such as topical corticosteroids or tar preparations, are necessary during active flares of eczema. Systemic therapy includes the use of sedating antihistamines and antibiotics. Systemic corticosteroids usually are not warranted in this chronic, non–life-threatening illness.

Diaper Dermatitis

Diaper dermatitis is likely the most common skin disorder of infancy and early childhood. Diaper dermatitis is not a specific disease but rather a variety of inflammatory disorders affecting the lower aspect of the abdomen, genitalia, buttock, and upper portion of the thigh. It is a form of contact dermatitis that is initiated by a combination of factors, including prolonged exposure to and irritation by urine and feces, maceration by wet diapers, and airtight plastic diaper covers. Frequently, diaper dermatitis is secondarily infected with *Candida albicans.*

The lesions vary from mild erythema to erythematous papular lesions. Candidal (monilial) diaper dermatitis is usually very erythematous, with sharp margination and pustulovesicular satellite lesions (Fig. 42-3).

FIG. 42-3 **Diaper dermatitis.** Diaper dermatitis with *Candida albicans* secondary infection characterized with sharp margination and pustulovesicular satellite lesions.

Treatment is frequent diaper changes to keep the area clean and dry or frequently exposing the perineal area to air. Topical antifungal medication is used to treat *Candida albicans*, when present. Short-term use of low-potency topical steroids alternately with antifungals at each diaper change helps to reduce the inflammation. Use of various topicals to provide a barrier from the irritating agents promotes healing.

INFECTIONS OF THE SKIN

Infectious diseases caused by bacteria, viruses, and fungi constitute the major forms of skin disease. Most infections tend to occur superficially; however, systemic signs and symptoms develop occasionally and rarely are life threatening.

Bacterial Infections
Impetigo Contagiosum

Impetigo is a common bacterial skin infection in infants and children. The disease is more common in mid- to late summer, with a higher incidence in hot, humid climates. Impetigo is particularly infectious among those living in crowded conditions with poor sanitary facilities. It affects children in good health, but conditions such as anemia and malnutrition are predisposing factors. There are two types of impetigo: bullous and vesicular. Both start as vesicles with a very thin vesicular roof composed of stratum corneum.

Bullous impetigo

Bullous impetigo is caused by *Staphylococcus aureus*. The staphylococci produce a bacterial toxin called exfoliative toxin (ET), which causes a disruption in cellular adhesion (Leyden, 1991). This form characteristi-

FIG. 42-4 **Impetigo.** Characterized by weeping, crusting lesions.

cally occurs in neonates and is highly contagious. The source of the infection is usually staff in a newborn nursery or a family member with a pustule or who is an asymptomatic carrier. The pathogen is often carried in their anterior nares, perineal region, or fingernails and is transmitted by contact with the individual or contaminated equipment (Ritchie & Thompson, 1992).

The exfoliative toxin stimulates the formation of vesicles, which enlarge or coalesce to form superficial bullae. There may be a few localized lesions or many lesions scattered over the skin. As the bullae rupture, a thin, flat, honey-colored crust appears. The crust is the hallmark of impetigo. A moist, inflamed, serum weeping base is revealed when the crust is removed. The lesions are often located on the face around the nose and mouth, but the hands and other exposed areas are also frequently involved. Regional lymphadenitis is uncommon.

Vesicular impetigo

Vesicular impetigo is a contagious, acute, superficial, vesiculopustular form of impetigo caused by group A *Streptococcus pyogenes* (alone or in combination with *Staphylococcus aureus*). The organisms are disseminated by direct physical contact from other infected individuals or through insect bites. The lesions begin as small vesicles with a honey-colored serum. Yellow to white-brown crusts form as the vesicles rupture and ex-

FIG. 42-5 Staphylococcal scalded-skin syndrome (SSSS). The skin lesions, showing desquamation and wrinkling of the skin margins, appeared 1 day after drainage of a staphylococcal abscess. (From Levine & Norden, 1972.)

tend radially (Fig. 42-4). Untreated lesions may last for weeks and extend to cover a large area. In contrast to bullous impetigo, regional lymphadenitis is common.

The risk of nephritogenic strains of streptococci varies considerably in North America (Weston & Lane, 1991). Aggressive treatment of both patient and patient contacts significantly reduces the chance of acute glomerulonephritis, which is clearly the most significant complication of streptococcal impetigo.

Treatment of choice for both types of impetigo is systemic antibiotics. Antibiotic therapy should be determined by bacterial culture and drug sensitivity. While waiting for these laboratory results, empiric treatment with drugs such as erythromycin or dicloxacillin or topical mupirocin, which give good coverage against staphylococci and streptococci, should be used. Topical antibiotics should be limited to early small localized infections. Removal of crusts and scrubbing the lesions with antibacterial soaps have not been shown to be effective (Weston & Lane, 1991). Good hand-washing techniques and isolation of the infected child's washcloth, towels, drinking glass, and linen are important. The highly contagious nature of this disease should be emphasized.

Staphylococcal Scalded-Skin Syndrome

Staphylococcal scalded-skin syndrome (SSSS) is the most serious staphylococcal skin infection that affects the skin. Staphylococcal scalded-skin syndrome is

caused by infection with group II staphylococci, which produce a toxin, an epidermolysin that causes a separation of the skin just below the granular layer of the epidermis. The toxins are usually produced at body sites other than the skin and arrive at the epidermis through the circulatory system. Staphylococci typically are not found in the skin lesions themselves. The syndrome is more common in children younger than 10 years of age than in adults. Adults have circulating antistaphylococcal antibodies and are better able to metabolize and excrete the toxin. Neonates are at the highest risk because of their lack of immunity, not having prior exposure to the toxin.

The clinical symptoms begin with fever, malaise, rhinorrhea, and irritability followed by generalized erythema with exquisite tenderness of the skin. There may be an associated impetigo, but the infection often begins in the throat or chest. The erythema spreads from the face and trunk to cover the entire body except the palms, soles, and mucous membranes. Within 48 hours, blisters and bullae may form and the pain is severe (Fig. 42-5). Fluid loss from ruptured blisters and water evaporation from denuded areas may cause dehydration. Perioral and nasolabial crusting and fissures develop. In severe cases, the skin of the entire body may slough. When secondary infection can be prevented, healing of the involved skin occurs in 10 to 14 days, usually without scarring.

Before medical intervention, culture, histology, or exfoliative cytology must be done, to differentiate SSSS from toxic epidermal necrolysis (TEN) (see p. 1575). When the infection is confirmed, treatment with oral or intravenous antibiotics is begun. Topical antibiotics are ineffective. The skin should be treated the same as a severe burn, with meticulous aseptic technique. Special care is required when there is involvement of the lips and eyelids.

Fungal Infections

Fungal disorders are known as mycoses and, when caused by dermatophytes (fungi that thrive on keratin), the mycoses are termed tinea (dermatophytosis or ringworm). Tinea pedis (a chronic, superficial fungal infection of the skin of the foot) occurs in children, but is rare. Most scaling disorders of the toes and feet in prepubertal children are eczema (see Chapter 41). Tinea capitis (infection of the scalp) and tinea corporis (infection of the body) are much more common in children than adults. (The different types of tinea are described in Chapter 41.) These dermatophytes invade the stratum corneum and not the remainder of the epidermis or dermis. The inflammatory response is thought, in part, to be secondary to the toxins released by the dermatophyte.

Tinea Capitis

Tinea capitis, a fungal infection of the scalp, is the most common fungal infection of childhood. It rarely affects infants and is seen in children between 2 and 10 years of age. Primary organisms responsible for this disease are *Microsporum canis* or *Trichophyton tonsurans*. *M. canis* is found on cats, dogs, and certain rodents. Hu-

FIG. 42-6 **Tinea capitis.** (From Stewart, Danto, & Maddin, 1978.)

mans appear to be a terminal host for *M. canis,* and children who handle such animals are possible hosts. Human-to-human transmission does not occur. *T. tonsurans* conversely is transmitted human-to-human. Areas of crowding are the most prevalent environments for this organism, which frequently affects inner-city children. The clinical presentations vary, depending on the organism. Frequently, the lesions are circular and manifest by broken hairs 1 to 3 mm above the scalp, leaving a partial alopecia from 1 to 5 cm in diameter (Fig. 42-6). A slight erythema and scaling with raised borders can be observed.

Diagnosis is best confirmed by performing Wood's light examination, potassium hydroxide (KOH) examination, and fungal culture, in that order. *Trichophyton tonsurans* does not fluoresce with Wood's light examination. Oral griseofulvin is the treatment of choice because topical fungicides do not penetrate to the hair bulb.

Tinea Corporis

Tinea corporis is a common superficial dermatophyte infection in children. The organisms most commonly responsible for this disease are *M. canis* and *Trichophyton mentagrophytes*. As in tinea capitis, contact with young kittens and puppies is a common source of the disorder. Tinea corporis has a predilection for the nonhairy parts of the face, trunk, and limbs. Lesions are often erythematous round or oval scaling patches that spread peripherally with clearing in the center, creating the "ring" appearance, which is why this disease is commonly referred to as "ringworm." The lesions are distributed asymmetrically, and multiple lesions, when present, overlap. Potassium hydroxide examination of the scale from the border of the lesions confirms the diagnosis. Most lesions respond well to applications of appropriate topical antifungal medications.

Thrush

Candida albicans infection is a superficial fungal infection that commonly occurs in children. *C. albicans* is part of the normal skin flora in certain individuals and invades susceptible tissue sites if the predisposing factors are not eliminated. *C. albicans* penetrates the epidermal barrier more easily then other organisms because of its keratolytic proteases and other enzymes. *C. albicans* attracts neutrophils to skin sites of invasion and generates inflammation by activation of the complement system within the skin. **Thrush** is the term used to describe the presence of *Candida* in the mucous membranes of the mouth of infants and, less commonly, adults. Thrush is characterized by the formation of white plaques or spots in the mouth that lead to shallow ulcers. The tongue may have a dense, white covering. The underlying mucous membrane is red and tender and may bleed when the plaques are removed. The disease is often accompanied by fever and gastrointestinal irritation. The infection commonly spreads to the groin, buttocks, and other parts of the body. Treatment may be difficult and include oral antifungal washes like nystatin oral suspension. Simultaneous treatment of a *Candida* nipple infection or vaginitis in the mother is helpful in reducing the *C. albicans* surface colonization of the infant. Feeding bottles and nipples should be sterilized to prevent reinfection. The diaper area should be kept clean and dry.

Viral Infections

Viral infections of the skin in children are caused by poxvirus, papovavirus, and herpesvirus. The most common infections are described here.

Molluscum Contagiosum

Molluscum contagiosum is a common, highly contagious viral infection of the skin and, occasionally, conjunctiva that primarily affects children. A poxvirus that induces epidermal cell proliferation causes this disease. The epidermis grows down into the dermis to form saccules containing clusters of virus. The characteristic molluscum body is composed of mature, immature, and incomplete viruses and cellular debris.

The lesions of molluscum are discrete, slightly umbilicated, dome-shaped papules 1 to 5 cm in diameter that appear anywhere on the skin or conjunctiva. The skin distribution in children is mainly on the trunk, face, and extremities (Fig. 42-7). The pubic, genital, and perineal areas are favored in adults (see Chapter 21). There is usually no inflammation surrounding molluscum lesions

FIG. 42-7 Molluscum contagiosum. Waxy pink globules with umbilicated centers. (From Stewart, Danto, & Maddin, 1978.)

unless they are traumatized or secondary infection occurs. Scarring occurs with healing.

The best three diagnostic procedures are (1) staining smears of the expressed molluscum body, (2) examining a biopsy, or (3) inoculating a molluscum suspension into cell cultures to demonstrate the cytotoxic reactions. Most lesions are self-limiting and clear in 6 to 9 months if not manipulated. The papules can be removed by curette or destroyed with liquid nitrogen. If multiple lesions are present, however, these procedures are painful to small children and are not justified. Topical cantharidin can be used to treat these lesions. Measures to prevent spread of infection must be taken. Children must be taught not to manipulate or scratch these lesions. Recurrences are common.

Rubella (German or Three-Day Measles)

Rubella is a common communicable disease of children and young adults caused by an RNA virus that enters the bloodstream through the respiratory route. This disease is mild in most children. The incubation period ranges from 14 to 21 days. Prodromal symptoms are few but may include enlarged cervical and postauricular lymph nodes, low-grade fever, headache, sore throat, runny nose, and cough. A faint-pink to red coalescing maculopapular rash develops on the face with spread to the trunk and extremities 1 to 4 days after the onset of initial symptoms (Fig. 42-8). The rash is thought to be the result of virus dissemination to the skin. The rash subsides after 2 to 3 days, usually without complication.

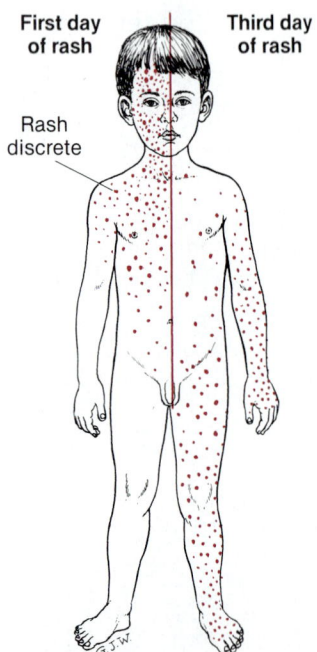

First day of rash

Third day of rash

Rash discrete

FIG. 42-8 Measles. Full-blown maculopapular rash with tendency to coalesce. (From Wehrle & Top, 1981.)

Children are usually not contagious after development of the rash. There is lifelong immunity to rubella, as well as measles, chicken pox, and roseola, after the disease (see Table 42-1 for differential presentations).

Vaccination for rubella is usually combined with vaccines for mumps and measles (rubeola) (MMR). Recommendations now state that MMR vaccine should be given at 15 months of age, so there will not be interference from maternal measles antibody, and again at 11 to 12 years of age (Wallace & Farrington, 1991). Women of childbearing age are immunized if their rubella hemagglutination-inhibition titer is low. Pregnancy should be avoided for 3 months after vaccination because the attenuated virus in the vaccine may remain for this period. Pregnant women who have rubella early in the first trimester may have a fetus that develops congenital defects.

There is no specific treatment. Recovery is spontaneous, although lymph nodes may remain enlarged for weeks. Supportive therapy includes rest, fluids, and use of a vaporizer. In rare cases, a mild encephalitis or peripheral neuritis may follow rubella.

Rubeola (Red Measles)

Rubeola is a highly contagious, acute viral disease of children. Transmitted by direct contact with droplets from infected persons, rubeola is caused by an RNA-containing paramyxovirus with an incubation period of 7 to 12 days, during which there are no symptoms. Prodromal symptoms include high fever up to 40.5° C, malaise, enlarged lymph nodes, runny nose, conjunctivitis, and "barking" cough. Within 3 to 4 days, an erythematous maculopapular rash develops over the head and spreads distally over the trunk, extremities, hands, and feet. Early lesions blanch with pressure, followed by a brownish hue that does not blanch as the rash fades. Characteristic pinpoint white spots surrounded by an erythematous ring develop over the buccal mucosa and are known as Koplik spots. These spots precede the rash by 1 to 2 days. The rash then subsides within 3 to 5 days.

Complications associated with measles may be due to the primary infection or to a secondary bacterial infection. Measles encephalitis occurs in about 1 of 800 cases, and most children recover completely. Only a small minority develop permanent brain damage or die. Bacterial complications include otitis media and pneumonia, usually caused by group A hemolytic streptococcus, *Haemophilus influenzae,* or *Staphylococcus aureus* infection.

Measles is prevented by a single vaccination of live attenuated measles virus as previously discussed. There is no specific treatment for measles, and supportive therapy is the same as for rubella. Antibiotic therapy is initiated if secondary bacterial infections develop.

TABLE 42-1

Differential Presentation of Viral Diseases Producing Rashes

Viral disease	Incubation	Prodromal symptoms	Duration/characteristics	Clinical symptoms
Rubella (German measles)	14-21 days	1-2 days Mild fever Malaise Respiratory symptoms	1-3 days Pink-red maculopapular Face and trunk	Enlarged and tender occipital and periauricular nodes
Rubeola (measles)	7-12 days	2-5 day Fever Cough Respiratory symptoms	3-5 days Purple-red to brown maculopapular Face, trunk, extremities	Koplik spots 1-3 days before rash
Roseola (exanthema subitum)	5-15 days	2-5 days High fever	1-3 days Red macular Neck and trunk	Rash develops when fever subsides
Varicella (chicken pox)	11-20 days	1-2 days Low-grade fever Cough May be asymptomatic	7-14 days Red papules, vesicles, pustules in clusters	Eruption of new lesions for 4-5 days Occasional ulcerative lesion in the mouth

Roseola (Exanthem Subitum)

Roseola is a presumed viral infection of infants between 6 months and 2 years of age and can be seen up to 4 years of age. The exact cause of the disease is unknown (Brunnel, 1987). The incubation period is 5 to 15 days, followed by the sudden onset of fever (38.9° to 40.5° C) that lasts for 3 to 5 days. After the fever, an erythematous macular rash that lasts about 24 hours develops primarily over the trunk and neck. Children usually feel well, eat normally, and have few other symptoms. There is usually no treatment.

Chicken Pox and Herpes Zoster

Chicken pox (varicella) and herpes zoster (shingles) are both produced by the varicella-zoster virus (VZV). Varicella-zoster virus is a complex herpes group DNA virus. The incubation period can be as early as 10 days or as late as 27 days and averages 14 days. Productive infection occurs within keratinocytes such that the vesicular lesions occur in the epidermis and an inflammatory infiltrate is often present. Histologically, VZV lesions form intraepidermal vesicles. Infected keratinocytes degenerate, swell, detach from each other and often contain inclusions surrounded by a clear halo and a circle of darkly staining chromatin. As the vesicle evolves, polymorphonuclear cells enter the vesicle and can lead to a pustular appearance. The vesicle eventually ruptures and is followed by crust formation. On mucous membranes, the vesicles rupture and leave superficial, transient ulcers. Varicella occurs in people not previously exposed to VZV, whereas herpes zoster occurs in partially immune individuals who have had varicella.

Chicken pox

Chicken pox is a disease of early childhood, with 90% of children contracting the disease during the first decade of life. Being a highly contagious virus, chicken pox is spread by close person-to-person contact and by airborne droplets. Introduction of an infected person into a household results in 90% possibility of susceptible persons developing the disease within the incubation period, usually 14 days. Children are contagious for at least 1 day before development of the rash. Transmission of the virus may occur until approximately 5 to 6 days after the onset of the first skin lesions in normal children. In immunocompromised children, the virus is recoverable for a longer period of time, but they must be considered contagious for at least 7 to 10 days. Chicken pox occurs most commonly in the late winter and early spring. Transmission occurs more readily in temperate climates than in tropical climates.

Normal children who develop chicken pox have no prodromal symptoms. The first sign of illness may be itching or the appearance of vesicles, usually on the trunk, scalp, or face. The rash later spreads to the extremities. Characteristically, lesions can be seen in various stages of maturation with macules, papules, and vesicles present in a particular area at the same time (Fig. 42-9). The vesicular lesions are superficial and can be easily ruptured. New lesions will erupt for 4 to 5 days, until there are approximately 100 to 300 in dif-

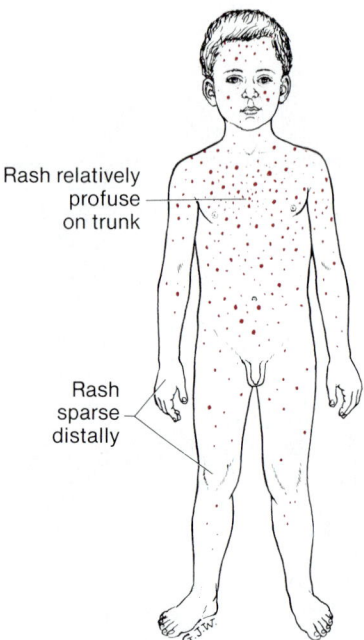

Rash relatively
profuse
on trunk

Rash
sparse
distally

FIG. 42-9 **Chicken pox.** Generalized, polymorphous eruption. (From Wehrle & Top, 1981.)

ferent stages of development. The vesicles become crusted, with only the crust remaining, although there may be an occasional vesicle on the palm later in the disease. Although uncommon, ulcerative lesions are sometimes seen in the mouth and, less commonly, on the conjunctiva and pharynx. Fever usually lasts 2 to 3 days and ranges from 38.5° C to 40° C.

Complications are rare in children but more common in adults. They can include transient hematuria (from rupture of vesicles in the bladder), epistaxis, laryngeal edema, and varicella pneumonia. One case of chicken pox produces almost complete immunity against a second attack. The fetus may be malformed if chicken pox develops in the first trimester of pregnancy (Wheller, 1983). Infants whose mothers have chicken pox at any stage of pregnancy have a higher risk of developing herpes zoster during the first few years of life.

Uncomplicated chicken pox requires no specific therapy. Baths, wet dressings, and oral antihistamines are occasionally helpful to relieve itching and to prevent secondary infection from developing as a result of scratching. Oral antistaphylococcal drugs should be given if secondary bacterial infection is present. Zoster immune globulin may be administered to immunodeficient individuals if given within 72 hours after exposure to chicken pox. Oral acyclovir may be valuable in immunosuppressed or other select groups of children. The use and role of the varicella vaccine in the United States remain unclear.

Herpes zoster

Although herpes zoster (shingles) occurs mainly in adults, approximately 5% of cases are children younger than 15 years of age. The course of the disease in children with an immune defect is more complicated. The eruption of **shingles** consists of groups of vesicles situated on an inflammatory base and following the course of a sensory nerve. Common dermatomal distribution in childhood is thoracic. The base of the lesions frequently appears hemorrhagic, and some of the lesions may become necrotic and ulcerative. In addition to the localized eruption, there are frequently a few scattered lesions resembling chicken pox. Therapy is similar to that for chicken pox unless it is ophthalmic or disseminated zoster, where acyclovir is indicated.

Smallpox

Smallpox (variola) is a highly contagious and deadly but preventable disease. It is caused by poxvirus variolae. Because of worldwide mass immunizations, the world is now virtually free of smallpox.

INSECT BITES AND PARASITES

Insect bites and infestations are common causes of skin disorders in children and adults. Skin damage occurs by various mechanisms, including trauma of bites and stings, allergic reactions, transmission of disease, injection of substances that cause local or systemic reactions, and inflammatory reactions from retained mouth parts.

Scabies

Scabies is a contagious disease caused by the itch mite, *Sarcoptes scabiei* (Fig. 42-10, *A*). It is transmitted by close personal contact (see Chapter 21) and by infected clothing and bedding. Scabies is frequently epidemic in areas of overcrowded housing and poor sanitation. Infestation is initiated by a female mite that tunnels into the stratum corneum, depositing eggs and creating a burrow several millimeters to a centimeter long. Over a 3-week period, the eggs mature into adult mites, which sometimes can be recognized as a tiny dot at the end of an intact burrow.

Symptoms appear 3 to 5 weeks after infestation. The primary lesions are burrows, papules, and vesicular lesions, with severe itching that worsens at night. Itching is thought to be related to sensitization to the larval stages of the parasite. In older children and adults, the lesions occur in the webs of fingers; axillae; creases of the arms and wrists; along the belt line; and around the nipples, genitals, and lower buttocks. Infants and young children have a different pattern of distribution, with involvement of the palms, soles, head, neck, and face (Fig.

A

B

FIG. 42-10 **Scabies. A,** Scabies mite, as seen clinically when removed from its burrow. **B,** A characteristic location, often secondarily infected. (From Stewart, Danto, & Maddin, 1978.)

42-10, *B*). Secondary infections and crusting develop from scratching and eczematous changes.

Norwegian scabies is a relatively rare widespread scabetic infestation with an affinity for the severely mentally retarded, who are unable to effectively scratch. It is highly contagious and is characterized by heavily crusted lesions on the scalp, elbows, knees, palms, soles, and buttocks.

Diagnosis of scabies is made by observation of the tunnels and burrows and scraping of the skin with microscopic examination of the mite or its eggs or feces. Treatment is the application of a scabicide, such as lindane lotion, cream, or shampoo (Kwell), and is curative. In children older than 10 years of age and adolescents, one 6-hour application cures 96% of cases. Care must be given with application instructions, however, because prolonged contact with the skin may result in percutaneous absorption, which will concentrate in the central nervous system. A newer scabicide is permethrin in 5% cream (Elimite), which is applied for 8 to 14 hours and then removed by washing. This product is es-

pecially indicated for infants and young children. One retreatment in 1 to 2 weeks may be necessary. Reassure the family that even with elimination of all viable scabies organisms, itching may persist for 7 to 10 days or longer. All clothing and linens should be washed and dried in hot cycles or dry cleaned.

Pediculosis (Lice Infestation)

There are three known types of human lice: (1) the head louse (*Pediculus capitis*), (2) the body louse (*Pediculus corporis*), and (3) the crab or pubic louse (*Phthirus pubis*). They are parasites and survive by sucking blood. The female louse reproduces every 2 weeks, producing hundreds of nits as newly hatched lice mate with old. The mouth parts are shaped for piercing and sucking and attach to the skin while feeding. When piercing the skin, the louse secretes a toxic saliva and the mechanical trauma and toxin produce a pruritic dermatitis. Head and body lice are acquired by personal contact, combs, or brushes. Crab lice are spread by bodily contact, such as contact with an infected adult (see Chapter 21). Sharing clothing is also a common source of transmission.

Itching is the major symptom of lice. With head lice, the ova attach to hairs above the ears and in the occipital region. The primary lesion of the body louse is a pinpoint red macule, papule, or wheal with a hemorrhagic puncture site. The primary lesion is often not seen, because it is masked by excoriations, wheals, and crusts. The crab louse is found on pubic hairs, but may also involve other body hair such as eyelashes, moustache, beard, and axillae. Young children particularly may become infected with crab lice on their eyebrows or eyelashes.

The live louse, 2 to 3 mm long, is rarely observed, although the ova, or nits, can be observed as oval, yellowish, pinpoint specks fastened to a hair shaft. The ova will fluoresce under an ultraviolet light (Wood lamp) and can be best observed with a microscope. Use of lindane shampoo (Kwell), applied for 5 minutes and rinsed out, is effective for treating head lice. An alternative treatment for head lice, particularly for infants and young children, is permethrin (Nix). Lindane lotion is used for body and crab lice and is left on for 12 hours with retreatment in a week if ova are still visible. All clothes, towels, bedding, combs, and brushes should be washed and dried in hot air, boiled, or clothes ironed. Individuals who have close personal contact should also be treated.

Fleas

Young children are very susceptible to **flea bites,** and the most common are the bites of cat, dog, and human fleas. Bites occur in clusters along the arms and legs or where there are tight-fitting clothes. The bite produces an urticarial wheal with a central hemorrhagic puncture (Fig. 42-11). Treatment includes spraying carpets, crevices, and furniture with malathion or lindane powder. Infected animals should be treated, and clothes and bedding should be washed in hot water.

Bedbugs

Bedbugs live in the crevices and cracks of floors, walls, and furniture, and in bedding or furniture stuffing. They are 3 to 5 mm long and reddish brown. Bedbugs emerge to feed in darkness and attach to the skin to suck blood. Feeding occurs for 5 to 15 minutes, and the bedbug then leaves. It will move long distances to search for food and can travel from house to house.

Two or three bites, commonly referred to as "breakfast, lunch, and dinner," usually appear in a line on exposed areas of the skin. If the host has not been previously sensitized, the only symptom is a red macule that develops into a nodule, lasting up to 14 days. In sensitized children and adults, pruritic wheals, papules, and vesicles may form. Secondary infections require treat-

FIG. 42-11 Flea bites. Flea bite producing an urticarial wheal with central puncture.

ment. Bedbugs are eliminated by spraying with chlordane or lindane and by cleaning or disposing of bedding, mattresses, and furniture.

VASCULAR DISORDERS

Congenital vascular malformations occur in 10% of all infants (Jacobs & Watson, 1976). The lesions are developmental in origin, with islands of angioblastic tissue failing to communicate with normal adjacent blood vessels. The most common disorders are strawberry hemangioma, cavernous hemangioma, nevus flammeus, and salmon patches. They are known collectively as vascular nevi.

Strawberry Hemangioma

The **strawberry hemangioma** is a distinct, raised vascular lesion that may be present at birth but usually emerges 3 to 5 weeks after birth. They proliferate and become bright red and elevated with minute capillary projections that give them a strawberry appearance. There is usually only one lesion and it is located on the head and neck area or trunk (Fig. 42-12). After the ini-

FIG. 42-12 **Strawberry hemangioma.** (From Stewart, Danto, & Maddin, 1978.)

tial growth, the lesion grows at the same rate as the child and then starts to involute at 12 to 16 months of age. Approximately 90% of strawberry hemangiomas involute by 5 to 6 years of age, usually without scarring.

Cavernous Hemangiomas

Cavernous hemangiomas are present at birth and have larger and more mature vessels within the lesion than strawberry hemangiomas. Some lesions, however, are composed of a mixture of strawberry and cavernous hemangiomas. They appear primarily on the head and neck area and have a bluish red color with less distinct borders. Cavernous hemangiomas grow rapidly up to 6 months of age and mature by 1 year of age. A period of involution begins and proceeds for 6 to 12 months with complete involution by 2 to 3 years in 30% of children, and by 9 years of age in 90% of children.

Hemangiomas that require treatment are those located near structures such as the eye, nares, auditory canal, or pharynx, or those that grow rapidly and are susceptible to trauma or secondary infection. No form of treatment is entirely satisfactory. Surgery, liquid nitrogen, or laser ablation can control bleeding or reduce the size of the lesion, however. The best cosmetic results are

obtained when there is spontaneous involution. Ulceration, bleeding, and infection are relatively rare, but cleansing and use of topical antibiotics are effective when they do occur. Open lesions do better when left open to the air, and Telfa dressings are recommended if bandages are required.

Salmon Patches

Salmon patches are macular, pink lesions present at birth and located on the nape of the neck (stork bites), forehead, upper eyelids, or nasolabial fold region. This is one of the most common congenital malformations in the skin. The pink color results from distended dermal capillaries and 95% fade by 1 year of age. They generally do not present a cosmetic problem.

Port-Wine Stain

Port-wine stain (nevus flammeus) is a congenital malformation of the dermal capillaries. The lesions are flat, and their color ranges from pink to dark reddish purple. They are present at birth or within a few days after birth and do not fade with age. Involvement of the face and other body surfaces is common, and the lesions may be large (Fig. 42-13). During adolescence and later adult

FIG. 42-13 **Port-wine hemangioma.** Port-wine hemangioma in an infant (**A**) and adult (**B**). (From Stewart, Danto, & Maddin, 1978.)

years, the port-wine stain may become papular and cavernous. Treatments using cryosurgery or tattooing are not very satisfactory. The pulsed dye laser has been used most recently to successfully lighten the color and flatten the more nodular and cavernous lesions (Goldman et al., 1993). Waterproof cosmetics may be used to cover the lesions.

OTHER SKIN DISORDERS
Miliaria

Miliaria is a dermatosis commonly seen in infants. It is characterized by a vesicular eruption after prolonged exposure to perspiration with subsequent obstruction of

the eccrine ducts. There are two forms of miliaria: **miliaria crystallina** and **miliaria rubra**. In miliaria crystallina, ductal rupture occurs within the stratum corneum and appears as 1- to 2-mm clear vesicles without erythema. They rupture within 24 to 48 hours and leave a white scale. In miliaria rubra, the ductal rupture occurs in the lower epidermis with inflammatory cells attracted to the site of the rupture. Miliaria rubra (prickly heat) is characterized by 2- to 4-mm discrete erythematous papules or papulovesicles (Fig. 42-14). Both forms may become secondarily infected, requiring systemic antibiotics. The key to management is avoidance of excessive heat and humidity, which cause sweating. Light clothing, cool baths, and air conditioning assist in keeping the skin surface dry and cool.

FIG. 42-14 **Miliaria rubra.** Characterized by discrete erythematous papules or papulovesicles.

Erythema Toxicum Neonatorum

Erythema toxicum neonatorum (toxic erythema of the newborn) is a benign, erythematous accumulation of macules, papules, or pustules that appear at birth or 3 to 4 days after birth. The lesions first appear as a blotchy, macular erythematous rash. The macules vary from 1 mm to 1 cm. When papules or pustules develop, they are light yellow or white and 1 to 3 mm in diameter. There may be few or several hundred lesions, and any body surface can be affected, with the exception of the palms and soles, where there are no pilosebaceous follicles. The cause of the lesion is unknown, and it is self-limiting. No treatment is required.

Toxic Epidermal Necrolysis (TEN)

Toxic epidermal necrolysis (TEN) is more common in adults, but is increasing in children. Hypersensitivity re-

actions to drugs (sulfonamides, nonsteroidal antiinflammatory agents, and anticonvulsants) seem to be the cause of most cases of TEN. The onset of skin eruptions is preceded by malaise, anorexia, fever, and mild inflammation of the eyelids, conjunctiva, mouth, or genitalia. Erythema with tenderness is first described in the axillae and groin, extending over the body surface. Blisters and bullae form and the entire epidermis may be shed, leaving open, weeping, painful areas of underlying skin. Toxic epidermal necrolysis must be confirmed by skin biopsy to differentiate from SSSS (see p. 1565) and acute graft versus host disease. Skin biopsy shows full-thickness epidermal necrosis and subepidermal blister formation. Treatment requires intensive burn management, preferably in a burn unit. The offending drug must be discontinued.

Acne Vulgaris

1 Acne is a common disorder that affects susceptible pilosebaceous follicles, primarily of the face, neck, and upper trunk. It is characterized by both noninflammatory and inflammatory lesions.

Dermatitis

1 Atopic dermatitis is associated with elevated IgE levels and a family history of asthma and hay fever. Red, scaly lesions commonly occur on the face, cheeks, and flexor surfaces of the extremities in infants and young children.
2 Diaper dermatitis is a type of contact dermatitis developing from prolonged exposure to urine and feces, which frequently becomes secondarily infected with *Candida albicans*.

Infections of the Skin

1 Impetigo is a contagious bacterial disease occurring in two forms, bullous and vesicular. The toxins from the bacteria produce a weeping lesion with a honey-colored crust.
2 Staphylococcal scalded-skin syndrome (SSSS) is a staphylococcal skin infection that occurs more commonly in young children with low titers of anti-staphylococcal antibody. Painful blisters and bullae form over large areas of the skin, requiring systemic antibiotics for treatment.
3 Thrush is a fungal infection of the mouth caused by *Candida albicans*.
4 Tinea capitis and tinea corporis are fungal infections of the scalp and body caused by dermatophytes.
5 Molluscum contagiosum is a poxvirus of the skin that produces pale papular lesions filled with viral and cellular debris.
6 Rubella (three-day measles) is a communicable disease characterized by fever, sore throat, enlarged cervical and postauricular nodes, and a generalized maculopapular rash that lasts from 1 to 4 days.
7 Rubeola is a contagious disease with symptoms of high fever, enlarged lymph nodes, conjunctivitis, and a red rash that begins on the head, spreads to the trunk and extremities, and lasts from 3 to 5 days. Both bacterial and viral complications may accompany rubeola.
8 Roseola is a benign disease of infants with a sudden onset of fever that lasts 3 to 5 days, followed by a rash that lasts for 24 hours.
9 Chicken pox (varicella) is a highly contagious disease caused by the varicella-zoster virus. Vesicular lesions occur on the skin and mucous membranes. Individuals are contagious from 1 day before the development of the rash until about 5 to 6 days after the rash develops.
10 Herpes zoster (shingles) is a viral eruption of vesicles on the skin along the distribution of a sensory nerve. Children with immune suppression develop more serious complications.
11 Smallpox (variola) is a highly contagious, deadly disease that has been eradicated worldwide by vaccination.

Insect Bites and Parasites

1 Scabies is an itching lesion caused by the itch mite, which burrows into the skin forming papules and vesicles. The mite is very contagious and is transmitted by direct contact.
2 Pediculosis (lice infestation) is caused by blood-sucking parasites that secrete a toxic saliva and damage the skin to produce a pruritic dermatitis. Lice are spread by direct contact and are recognized by the ova or nits that attach to the shaft of body hairs.
3 Flea bites produce a pruritic wheal with a central puncture site and occur as clusters in areas of tight-fitting clothing.
4 Bedbugs are blood-sucking parasites that live in cracks of floors, furniture, or bedding and feed at night. They produce pruritic wheals and nodules.

Vascular Disorders

1 A strawberry hemangioma is a vascular lesion present at birth that proliferates in size and then grows at the same rate as the child. Most lesions resolve spontaneously by 5 years of age.
2 A cavernous hemangioma is present at birth, with larger vessels than a strawberry hemangioma, and is bluish red. They usually involute by 9 years of age and may require surgical removal if located near the eyes, nares, or genitalia.
3 Salmon patches are macular pink lesions with dilated capillaries that usually resolve by 1 year of age.
4 Port-wine stains are congenital malformations of dermal capillaries that do not fade with age.

Other Skin Disorders

1 Miliaria is small pruritic papules or vesicles that result from closure of the sweat duct opening in infants.
2 Erythema toxicum neonatorum is a benign accumulation of macules, papules, and pustules that spontaneously resolves within a few weeks of birth.
3 Toxic epidermal necrolysis (TEN) is similar to SSSS, but the causative agent is usually a drug.

KEY TERMS

REFERENCES

Arnold, H. L., Odom, R. B., & James, W. D. (1990). *Andrew's diseases of the skin* (8th ed., p. 253). Philadelphia: Saunders.

Brunnel, P. A. (1987). Exanthem subitum. In T. B. Fitzpatrick, A. Z. Eisen, K. Wolff, I. M. Freedberg, & K. F. Austen (Eds.), *Dermatology in general medicine: Textbook and atlas* (3rd ed.) (p. 2296). New York: McGraw-Hill.

Forstrom, L. (1980). The influence of sex hormones on acne. *Acta Dermato-Venereologica Supplementum (Stockholm), 89,* 27.

Goldman, M. P., Fitzpatrick, R. E., Ruiz-Esparza, J. (1993). Treatment of port-wine stains (capillary malformation) with the flashlamp-pumped dye laser. *Journal of Pediatrics, 122*(1), 71-77.

Habif, T. P. (1985). *Clinical dermatology: A color guide to diagnosis and therapy.* St. Louis: Mosby–Year Book.

Ingham, E., Eady, E. A., Goodwin, C. E., Cove, J. H., & Cunliffe, W. J. (1992). Pro-inflammatory levels of interleukin-1-alpha like bioactivity are present in the majority of open comedones. *Journal of Investigative Dermatology, 98*(6), 895-901.

Jacobs, A. H., & Watson, R. G. (1976). The incidence of birthmarks in the neonate. *Pediatrics, 58,* 218.

Levine, G., & Norden, C. (1972). *New England Journal of Medicine, 287,* 1339.

Leyden, J. L. (1991). Pathophysiology of certain bacterial diseases. In N. A. Soter & H. P. Baden (Eds.), *Pathophysiology of dermatologic diseases* (2nd ed., pp. 427-440). New York: McGraw-Hill.

Nicol, N. H., & Leung, D. Y. M. (1992). Management of the patient with atopic dermatitis. *The American Journal of Asthma & Allergy for Pediatricians, 5,* 97-105.

Ritchie, S. R., & Thompson, P. J. (1992). Primary bacterial skin infections. *Dermatology Nursing, 4,* 261-267.

Stewart, W. D., Danto, J. L., & Maddin, S. (1978). *Dermatology: diagnosis and treatment of cutaneous disorders* (4th ed.). St. Louis: Mosby–Year Book.

Wallace, C., & Farrington, E. (1991). Vaccines. *Pediatric Nursing, 17,* 372-373.

Wehrle, P. F., & Top, F. H., Sr. (1981). *Communicable and infectious diseases* (9th ed.). St. Louis: Mosby–Year Book.

Weston, W. L., & Lane, A. T. (1991). *Color textbook of pediatric dermatology.* St. Louis: Mosby–Year Book.

Wheller, T. H. (1983). Varicella and herpes zoster: Changing concepts of the natural history, control, and importance of a not-so-benign virus. *New England Journal of Medicine, 309,* 1434.

SUGGESTED READINGS

Ackerman, A. B., Mendonea, A. M. N., & Guo, Y. (1992). *Differential diagnosis in dermatology* (2nd ed.). Philadelphia: Lea & Febiger.

Arndt, K. A. (Ed.). (1989). *Manual of dermatologic therapeutics,* Boston: Little, Brown & Company.

Champion, R. H., Burton, K., & Ebling, F. J. G. (1992). *Rook, Wilkinson, Ebling textbook of dermatology.* Oxford: Blackwell Scientific.

Lever, W. F., & Schaumburg-Lever, G. (1983). *Histopathology of the skin* (6th ed.). Philadelphia: Lippincott.

Nicol, N. H. (1990). Current considerations and management of atopic dermatitis. *Dermatology Nursing, 2,* 129-137.

Sams, W. M., & Lynch, P. J. (Eds.). (1990). *Principles and practice of dermatology.* New York: Churchill Livingstone.

Seidel, H. M., Ball, J. W., Dains, J. E., & Benedict, G. W. (1991). *Mosby's guide to physical examination* (2nd ed.). St. Louis: Mosby–Year Book.

Zaynoun, S. T. (1974). Topical antibodies in pyoderma. *British Journal of Dermatology, 90,* 331-334.

Index

Syndromes and disorders appear in boldface type.

CONVERSION FACTORS TO INTERNATIONAL SYSTEM OF UNITS (SI UNITS)

Component	Normal range in units as customarily reported	Conversion factor	Normal range in SI units, molecular units, international units, or decimal fractions
Biochemical components of blood*			
Acetoacetic acid (S)	0.2-1.0 mg/dl	98	19.6-98.0 μmol/L
Acetone (S)	0.3-2.0 mg/dl	172	51.6-344.0 μmol/L
Albumin (S)	3.2-4.5 g/dl	10	32-45 g/L
Ammonia (P)	20-120 μg/dl	0.588	11.7-70.5 μmol/L
Amylase (S)	60-160 Somogyi units/dl	1.85	111-296 U/L
Base, total (S)	145-160 mEq/L	1	145-160 mmol/L
Bicarbonate (P)	21-28 mEq/L	1	21-28 mmol/L
Bile acids (S)	0.3-3.0 mg/dl	10	3-30 mg/L
		2.547	0.8-7.6 μmol/L
Bilirubin, direct (S)	Up to 0.3 mg/dl	17.1	Up to 5.1 μmol/L
Bilirubin, indirect (S)	0.1-1.0 mg/dl	17.1	1.7-17.1 μmol/L
Blood gases (B)			
P_{CO_2} arterial	35-40 mm Hg	0.133	4.66-5.32 kPa
P_{O_2} arterial	95-100 mm Hg	0.133	12.64-13.30 kPa
Calcium (S)	8.5-10.5 mg/dl	0.25	2.1-2.6 mmol/L
Chloride (S)	95-103 mEq/L	1	95-103 mmol/L
Creatine (S)	0.1-0.4 mg/dl	76.3	7.6-30.5 μmol/L
Creatinine (S)	0.6-1.2 mg/dl	88.4	53-106 μmol/L
Creatinine clearance (P)	107-139 mL/min	0.0167	1.78-2.32 mL/s
Fatty acids (total) (S)	8-20 mg/dl	0.01	0.08-2.00 mg/L
Fibrinogen (P)	200-400 mg/dl	0.01	2.00-4.00 g/L
Gamma globulin (S)	0.5-1.6 g/dl	10	5-16 g/L
Globulins (total) (S)	2.3-3.5 g/dl	10	23-35 g/L
Glucose (fasting) (S)	70-110 mg/dl	0.055	3.85-6.05 mmol/L
Insulin (radioimmunoassay) (P)	4-24 μIU/ml	0.0417	0.17-1.00 μg/L
	0.20-0.84 μg/L	172.2	35-145 pmol/L
Iodine, BEI (S)	3.5-6.5 μg/dl	0.079	0.28-0.51 μmol/L
Iodine, PBI (S)	4.0-8.0 μg/dl	0.079	0.32-0.63 μmol/L
Iron, total (S)	60-150 μg/dl	0.179	11-27 μmol/L
Iron-binding capacity (S)	300-360 μg/dl	0.179	54-64 μmol/L
17-Ketosteroids (P)	25-125 μg/dl	0.01	0.25-1.25 mg/L
Lactic dehydrogenase (S)	80-120 units at 30 °C	0.48	38-62 U/L at 30 °C
	Lactate → pyruvate		
	100-190 U/L at 37 °C	1	100-190 U/L at 37 °C
Lipase (S)	0-1.5 U/ml (Cherry-Crandall)	278	0-417 U/L

From Tilkian, S.M., Conover, M.B., and Tilkian, A.G. (1983). *Clinical implications of laboratory tests* (ed 3). St. Louis, Mosby.
*This is a selected (not a complete) list of biochemical components. The ranges listed may differ from those accepted in some laboratories and are shown to illustrate the conversion factor and the method of expression in SI molecular units. For a more complete listing, see Henry, J.B., (Ed). *Todd-Sanford-Davidsohn clinical diagnosis and management by laboratory methods* (ed. 16). Philadelphia, Saunders.